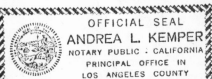

Blakiston's
ILLUSTRATED POCKET
MEDICAL DICTIONARY

Editorial Board

Blakiston's

ILLUSTRATED POCKET
MEDICAL DICTIONARY

Second Edition

Editors
NORMAND L. HOERR, M.D.
ARTHUR OSOL, Ph.D.

With the Cooperation of an Editorial Board

WITH 60 ILLUSTRATIONS, 16 IN COLOR, ON 24 PLATES

The Blakiston Division

McGRAW-HILL BOOK COMPANY, INC.

New York   Toronto   London

CONTENTS

INDEX OF ILLUSTRATIVE PLATES

Illustrative Plates follow page 486

PREFACE

The publication of the second edition of *Blakiston's Illustrated Pocket Medical Dictionary* marks the seventieth anniversary of the medical dictionaries initiated through the extraordinary efforts of Dr. George M. Gould. These dependable and authoritative dictionaries have come to be regarded with the same respect in the medical field as Webster's works are in the general field. It is with considerable pride that the editorial board of *Blakiston's Illustrated Pocket Medical Dictionary* acknowledges its debt to Dr. Gould for the high standards he set for us to follow.

Paramount in considering what to include in the second edition were the needs of the people who use this dictionary and for whom it has proved a valuable tool. To determine which terms are of current importance to nurses, medical assistants and secretaries, dental assistants, pharmacists, medical laboratory technicians, and students, we followed the advice and counsel of many educators and practitioners. Without their help we could not even approach our goal of publishing a concise yet up-to-date and comprehensive dictionary. Their recommendations were based on a study of our larger *Blakiston's New Gould Medical Dictionary,* from which this work is derived.

Reevaluating every entry in the previous edition and reviewing and deciding which of the many new medical terms to include in a dictionary of limited size was exceedingly difficult. Therefore, many decisions had to be arbitrary. The inclusion of a new drug, for example, was based primarily on whether or not it appeared in the latest edition of *New and Nonofficial Drugs;* and decisions on anatomic nomenclature; that is, the new Nomina Anatomica or Basle Nomina Anatomica, were made only after consultation with leading anatomists. In every case final decisions on definitions were based on usage by teachers and other professional workers in the medical and allied fields.

All tables in the Appendix were carefully reviewed and were revised whenever necessary, sometimes to avoid duplication of information available in the vocabulary section. A few tables which contained outdated information were deleted, but whatever valuable information they contained is still available in the vocabulary section. Inclusion of the table of Radioactive and Other Isotopes

Commonly Used in Medicine and Biology indicates the tremendous advances in this important aspect of medical science and extends the usefulness and coverage of the material in the Appendix.

As for any work of this kind, we recommend careful perusal of the Explanatory Notes and the Key to Pronunciation following these pages, which provide detailed information on how to use this dictionary to the greatest advantage. The illustrations, many of them in color, are in a separate section at the end of the book.

With deep regret we record the death of one of our editors, Normand L. Hoerr, which occurred during the preparation of the second edition of *Blakiston's Illustrated Pocket Medical Dictionary*. Dr. Hoerr's contributions to our dictionaries were characterized by scholarly distinction. His editorial colleagues wish to express their deep appreciation for his efforts and guidance, for the privilege of having been associated with him in this undertaking, and for the experience of his warm personal friendship. Dr. Hoerr's editorial responsibilities have been ably discharged by Samuel W. Chase and Carl C Francis, his colleagues on the editorial board and on the faculty of Western Reserve University School of Medicine.

To the many people who have cooperated with the editorial board in the divers ways that publication of a medical dictionary requires, our deep appreciation is expressed.

THE EDITORIAL BOARD

ABBREVIATIONS USED IN DEFINITIONS

Abbreviations with medical significance appear in their proper alphabetic places in the vocabulary section.

adj.	adjective	OT	*In anatomy*, Old Terminology
adv.	adverb		
at. wt.	atomic weight	pl.	plural
ca.	about	q.v.	which see
dim.	diminutive	syn.	synonym
e.g.	for example	v.	verb
i.e.	that is	v.i.	intransitive verb
n.	noun	v.t.	transitive verb
obs.	obsolete		

TRANSLITERATIONS FROM THE GREEK

Greek letters used as symbols with special significance in medicine and allied fields are listed with their meanings in the Table of Signs and Symbols in the Appendix.

Greek Letter		Name	Translit-eration	Greek Letter		Name	Translit-eration
Α	α	alpha	a	Ν	ν	nu	n
Β	β	beta	b	Ξ	ξ	xi	x
Γ	γ	gamma	g	Ο	ο	omicron	o
Δ	δ	delta	d	Π	π	pi	p
Ε	ε	epsilon	e	Ρ	ρ	rho	r, rh
Ζ	ζ	zeta	z	Σ	σ	sigma	s
Η	η	eta	ē	Τ	τ	tau	t
Θ	θ	theta	th	Υ	υ	upsilon	y
Ι	ι	iota	i	Φ	φ	phi	ph
Κ	κ	kappa	k	Χ	χ	chi	ch
Λ	λ	lambda	l	Ψ	ψ	psi	ps
Μ	μ	mu	m	Ω	ω	omega	ō

EXPLANATORY NOTES

Vocabulary Entries

The term to be defined is set in **boldface** type. When a term has more than one meaning, each meaning is numbered (or lettered, if the term is a subentry).

Entries are in alphabetic order, with the noun form usually the main entry. Subentries (phrases containing the main entry word) are also in boldface type and are in alphabetic order.

Derivative forms of a main entry follow main definitions; and their part of speech is identified by a label, as *n., v.,* or *adj.* (See *Abbreviations Used in Definitions,* page ix.)

Syllabification and Pronunciation

Main entries are divided into syllables to show both proper division for spelling and preferred pronunciation. (See *Key to Pronunciation.*) Derivative run-ons are syllabified only when a shift in accent changes the pronunciation.

Trade-marks, proprietary drugs, and proper names are not syllabified or pronounced.

Labels

Definitions or senses with specific meanings in special fields are preceded by labels, such as *In pharmacy, In psychiatry, In bacteriology, In human anatomy.*

Some definitions are followed by a label, such as *obs.* or *O.T.,* indicating usage of the term. (See *Abbreviations Used in Definitions,* page ix.)

Abbreviations

Abbreviations with medical significance appear in their proper alphabetic places in the vocabulary section of the dictionary.

Lexical abbreviations used in definitions are listed and defined on page ix.

Cross References

To locate all information pertinent to a term, the dictionary user is directed to additional or related information by such cross-reference devices as see, see under, or syn., followed by an italicized word or phrase. When the reference is to a compound term or subentry, only the part of the term under which the information is entered is italicized.

Variant Forms

A variant spelling is often shown in boldface type with the preferred form or as a separate entry. When it is a separate entry, the definition refers to the preferred spelling, sometimes after a cross-reference device such as "see" or "same as."

Chemical and Pharmaceutical Terms

Formulas: Definitions for chemical substances usually include the chemical formula of the substance when this is known.

Synonyms: The definition of a medical substance includes the synonyms applied to that substance.

Medicinal Plants: The definitions for a drug representing a structural part of a plant includes its botanical origin, this being distinguished by the use of italicized type. The definition also includes a statement of the active constituents, if any, of the plant.

Biographic Entries

Proper names, biographic entries, and eponyms appear in their proper alphabetic places. When an eponym is fully defined elsewhere under another entry—as a subentry under **disease**, for example—the dictionary user is directed to the proper entry by a cross reference.

KEY TO PRONUNCIATION

A single accent (′) marks the strongest accent, the most heavily stressed syllable in a word. A double accent (″) marks syllables with secondary stress, lighter accent than the primary.

When there is no respelling for pronunciation, the spelling of the entry itself gives the pronunciation. A vowel has its long sound if it is followed immediately by an accent mark. Consonants are pronounced according to the usual rules. For example, c followed by e, i, or y is pronounced as in **cent, de·cide′, cy′press**; otherwise as in **cab, cob, cub, clay, screw**; ch followed by l or r as in **chlo′ro·form, chron′ic**; otherwise as in **chin, rich, church**; g followed by e, i, or y as in **gin′ger, gy′rate, ag′ile, a·gil′i·ty**; otherwise as in **gag, gar′goyle, gun, glue, gray, lig′nite**.

When the ordinary rules do not apply, respellings are given in parentheses immediately after the boldface entries, using the common values of letters, like **aw** in **paw**, **ay** in **pay**, etc., and observing the conventions shown in the following table.

IN THE RESPELLINGS

ah	**calm, fa′ther**	(fah′thur)
ahr	**farm, Dart′mouth**	(dahrt′muth)
ar	**tar′iff, phar″yn·gec′to·my**	(far″in·jeck′to·mee)
err	**mer′ry, dic′tion·ar″y**	(dick′shuh·nerr″ee)
ew	**few, mu″co·hem″or·rhag′ic**	(mew″ko·hem″o·radj′ick)
i	**fas′ci·nate, my″ce·tog′e·nous**	(migh″si·todj′i·nus)
igh	**flight, chei″ma·pho′bi·a**	(kigh″muh·fo′bee·uh)
ye	**dye, ty·phoi′dal**	(tye·foy′dul)
irr	**mir′ror, myr″in·gec′to·my**	(mirr″in·jeck′to·mee)
orr	**hor′rid, cor′o·nar″y**	(korr′o·nerr″ee)
o͞o	**boot** (bo͞ot), **Hoo′ver** (ho͞o′vur)	
o͝o	**foot** (fo͝ot), **pul′ley** (po͝ol′ee)	
oo	**poor, pleu′rae** (ploor′ee)	
uh	**plas′ma·cyte** (plaz′muh·sight), **hap″a·lo·nych′i·a** (hap″uh·lo·nick′ee·uh)	
g	**gag, ex·haus′tion** (eg·zaws′chun)	
ng	**sing′er, con′cha** (kong′kuh)	
s	**sense, oc·cip′i·tal** (ock·sip′i·tul)	
th	**thick, path**	
th	**then** (then), **weath′er** (weth′ur)	
zh	**meas′ure** (mezh′ur), **in·ci′sion** (in·sizh′un)	

Syllables respelled as common words (e.g., *buy, coal, view*) are pronounced like those words: **o″vu·log′e·nous** (o″view·lodj′i·nus)

A

A. 1. *In chemistry*, symbol for argon. 2. *In radiology*, symbol for area of heart shadow. 3. *In physics*, abbreviation for angstrom unit.

a. Accommodation, ampere, anode, anterior, aqua, artery.

a-, an-. A prefix equivalent to *un-* or *in-* and signifying *absence, lack, -less, not.*

āā, āā. Denoting the same quantity of each ingredient in a prescription.

Ab. Chemical symbol for alabamine.

ab-, a-, abs-. A prefix meaning *from* or *away,* or signifying *separation* or *departure.*

a·ba'si·a (a·bay'zhuh, ·zee·uh). Motor incoördination in walking. See *astasia.* **-abasic, abat'ic,** *adj.* **ataxic a.** Awkwardness and uncertainty displayed in locomotion. **choreic a.** Inability to walk due to choreic spasm of muscles in the lower extremities. **paralytic a.** Total inability of the legs to support the body in walking or standing, due to organic paralysis. **paroxysmal trepidant a.** A form of astasia-abasia in which the legs become spastic when the patient attempts to walk. **trembling a.** Incapacity to walk because of exaggerated trembling of the legs.

a·bate'ment. Lessening or moderation of the pain or untoward symptoms of a disease. **-abated,** *adj.;* **abate,** *v.t., v.i.*

ab''at·toir' (ab''uh·twahr'). Slaughterhouse or establishment for the killing and dressing of animals.

ab·ax'i·al. Not situated in the line of the axis.

ab·do'men, ab'do·men. The large, inferior cavity of the trunk, extending from the brim of the pelvis to the diaphragm. It is bounded in front and at the sides by the lower ribs and abdominal muscles, and behind by the vertebral column, the psoas, and the quadratus lumborum muscles. It is artificially divided into nine regions by two lines, the upper parallel with the cartilages of the ninth ribs, the lower with the iliac crests, and by two lines drawn vertically upward from the center of the inguinal ligament. These lines are situated differently by different writers. The regions thus formed are: above, the right hypochondriac, the epigastric, and the left hypochondriac; in the middle, the right lumbar, the umbilical, and the left lumbar; and below, the right inguinal, the hypogastric, and the left inguinal. **-abdom'inal,** *adj.* **acute a.** An acute

pathologic condition within the belly, requiring prompt surgical intervention. **pendulous a.** A relaxed condition of the abdominal wall in which the anterior abdominal wall hangs down over the pubis. **scaphoid a.** A belly characterized by sunken walls, presenting a concavity; seen in starvation and acute meningitis. Also called *navicular a.*

ab·dom'i·no-. A combining form signifying *relating to the abdomen.*

ab·dom''i·no·an·te'ri·or. *In obstetrics,* designating a fetal position in which the belly is forward.

ab·dom''i·no·cen·te'sis. Paracentesis of the abdominal cavity.

ab·dom''i·no·hys''ter·ot'o·my. Hysterotomy through an abdominal incision.

ab·dom''i·no·pos·te'ri·or. *In obstetrics,* designating a fetal position in which the belly is toward the mother's back.

ab·dom''i·nos'co·py. Diagnostic examination of the abdomen externally by the generally practiced physical methods, and internally by endoscopic methods.

ab·dom''i·no·u''ter·ot'o·my. See *abdominohysterotomy.*

ab·dom''i·no·ves'i·cal. Relating to the abdomen and the urinary bladder.

ab·du'cens (ab·dew'senz). The sixth cranial nerve. See Table of Nerves in the Appendix. **-abducent,** *adj.*

ab·du'cent. Abducting.

ab·duct'. Draw away from the median line.

ab·duc'tion. Withdrawal of a part from the axis of the body or of an extremity. *In ophthalmology,* turning of the eyes outward from the central position by the lateral rectus muscles. In refraction, the turning of the eyes outward beyond parallelism under the artificial stimulus of base in prisms and expressed in terms of prism diopters, the measurement being the strongest prism power with which the eyes can maintain single vision at infinity. **total a.** The expression in prism diopters of the capacity for turning the eyes outward from the extreme point of inward or positive convergence to the extreme point of outward or negative convergence beyond parallelism. It is measured from convergence near point. A test of, and an exercise stimulus for, relaxation of the medial recti and convergence.

ab·duc'tor. A muscle which, on contraction, draws a part away from the axis of the body or of an extremity. See

1

Table of Muscles in the Appendix. **a. digiti quinti.** That of the little finger or toe. **a. hallucis.** That of the great toe. **a. pollicis.** One of the two abductor muscles of the thumb known as *abductor pollicis brevis* and *abductor pollicis longus.*

ab·er'rant. Varying or deviating from the normal in form, structure, or course; especially anatomic organs, as aberrant ducts of the testis.

ab"er·ra'tion. 1. A wandering from the correct, the normal, the standard. 2. Slight mental disorder. 3. *In biology,* an abnormal part or individual; a sport. 4. *In optics,* any imperfection in the refraction or the focalization of a lens. **—aber'rant,** *adj.* **chromatic a.** Unequal refraction of different parts of the spectrum producing indistinct images surrounded by a halo of colors. **distantial a.** Indistinct vision due to distance. **lateral a.** Deviation of a ray in any direction from the axis, measured in the focal plane perpendicularly to the axis. **longitudinal a.** Deviation of a ray from the focus, measured along the axis above or below the focal plane. **mental a.** A deviation from normal mental function. **spherical a.** Unequal refraction of monochromatic light in different parts of a spherical lens, producing faulty images which show lack of sharpness or of flatness, or distortion. Also called *monochromatic a.*

a·bey'ance (a·bay'uns). 1. A cessation of activity or function. 2. A state of suspended animation.

ab"i·et'ic ac'id, ab"i·e·tin'ic ac'id. $C_{19}H_{29}COOH$. An acid from the resin of various species of pine.

a·bi'o-. A combining form meaning *without life.*

a"bi·o·gen'e·sis, a"bi·og'e·ny (ay"buy·odj'i·nee). Theory of the production of living from nonliving matter; spontaneous generation. **—abiogenet'ic, abiog'enous,** *adj.;* **abiog'enist,** *n.*

a"bi·ot'ro·phy. Degeneration or loss of vitality in a cell, organ, or part due to defective vital force. Syn., *abionergy.* **—abiotroph'ic,** *adj.*

ab·ir'ri·tant. 1. Tending to diminish irritation; soothing. 2. Relating to diminished sensitiveness. 3. A remedy or agent that allays irritation. **—abirritative,** *adj.;* **abirritate,** *v.t.*

ab"lac·ta'tion. 1. The weaning of an infant. 2. The end of the period of mammary secretion.

ab·la'ti·o (ab·lay'shee-o). Detachment; removal; ablation. **a. placentae.** Premature separation of the placenta. Also called *abruptio placentae.* **a. retinae.** Detachment of a non-pathologic retina.

ab·la'tion. Removal of a part, as a tumor, by amputation, excision, etc. **—ablate',** *v.t.*

a·bleph'a·ry. A congenital defect marked by partial or total absence of the eyelids or palpebral fissure. **—ablepharous,** *adj.;* **ablepharus,** *n.*

ab'lu·ent. 1. Detergent. 2. A cleansing or washing agent, as a soap.

ab·lu'tion. The act of washing or cleansing the body. Syn., *lavation.*

ab·nor'mal. 1. Not normal. 2. Deviating in form, structure, or position; not conforming with the natural or general rule. **—abnormity, abnormal'ity, abnormalism,** *n.*

ab·o'rad. Tending aborally; situated or directed away from the mouth.

ab·o'ral. Opposite to, or remote from, the mouth.

a·bort'. 1. Miscarry; bring forth a nonviable fetus. 2. Prevent complete flare-up of a disease; nip a disease in the bud. 3. Check or fall short of maximal growth and development. 4. An abortion.

a·bor'ti·cide. 1. Killing of an unborn fetus. 2. The agent which destroys the fetus and produces abortion.

a·bor"ti·fa'cient (a·bor"ti·fay'-shunt), **a·bor'tient** (a·bor'shunt). 1. Causing abortion. 2. Drug or agent inducing expulsion of the fetus.

a·bor'tion. 1. Expulsion of the product of conception before the child is viable. When this occurs during the first three months, it is termed *abortion;* from this time to viability, *immature delivery* or *miscarriage;* and from the period of viability to full term, *premature delivery.* 2. A prematurely expelled fetus. **—abortionist,** *n.* **accidental a.** An unexpected premature termination of pregnancy. **artificial a.** Intentional premature termination of pregnancy by medicinal or mechanical means. **criminal a.** Interference with the progress of pregnancy which is not justified by the state of the mother's health; an illegal abortion. **habitual a.** Accidental abortion recurring in successive pregnancies. **incomplete a.** Partial expulsion of the product of conception, with some of the secundines remaining within the uterus. **induced a.** See artificial *a.* **inevitable a.** One which has advanced to a stage where termination of the pregnancy no longer can be prevented. **missed a.** A condition in which the fetus has died but the products of conception are not expelled within two weeks. **partial a.** Premature expulsion of one fetus in the presence of multiple gestation. **psychiatric a.** A therapeutic abortion dictated by the aggravation or inception of mental disease during pregnancy. **spontaneous a.** Unexpected premature expulsion of the product of conception when no ecbolic agent has been employed. **therapeutic a.** Termination of a pregnancy which is a hazard to the life of the mother. **threatened a.** Occurrence of signs and symptoms of impending loss of the embryo. It may be prevented by treatment or may go on to inevitable abortion, *q.v.* **tubal a.** Escape of the product of conception through the abdominal opening of the oviduct into the peritoneal cavity.

a·bor'tive. 1. Prematurely born; undeveloped; immature; rudimentary. 2. Coming to an untimely end. 3. Checking the full development of a disease or cutting short its duration. Syn., *abortifacient, abortient.*

a·bor'tus. Aborted fetus; abortion.

a·bra'chi·us (a-bray'kee-us). 1. Armless. 2. An individual without arms. **–abrachia,** *n.*

ab·ra'sion. 1. A spot denuded of skin, mucous membrane, or superficial epithelium by rubbing or scraping, as a corneal abrasion; an excoriation or attrition. 2. In *dentistry,* the mechanical wearing down of the teeth, as from chewing; a dental abrasion. **–abrade',** *v.t.*

ab·ra'sive. 1. Tending to produce a scraping or abrasion. 2. Agent which scrapes or rubs off the external layers of a part.

ab·ra'sor. A surgeon's rasp; any file or instrument used in dental or surgical abrasion of a surface; a rasp used in pharmacy.

ab"re·ac'tion. In *psychoanalysis,* the mental process by which repressed, emotionally charged material is freed, and forgotten memories are brought to consciousness and relived with appropriate emotional release after insight is obtained; catharsis. Also employed in hypnosis and narcohypnosis, *q.v.* **motor a.** Motor or muscular expression of an unconscious impulse.

ab·rup'ti·o (ab-rup'tee-o). Abruption; a tearing away. **a. placentae.** Premature separation of the placenta. Also called *ablatio placentae.*

ab'scess, ab·sces'sus. Localized collection of pus in any part of the body. According to location, abscesses are named *dorsal, mammary, rectal,* etc. **acute a.** One resulting from an acute inflammation of the part in which it is formed. **alveolar a.** One in a dental alveolus. **amebic a.** A variety found in the liver and lung, containing amebas. It is a complication or sequel of amebic dysentery. **anorectal a.** An abscess of the perirectal celluloadipose tissue near the anus. Also called *ischiorectal a., perirectal a.* **apical a.** One occurring at the end of a root of a tooth. **appendiceal a.** Pus formation about the vermiform proc-

ess secondary to acute suppurative inflammation of the appendix. **caseous a.** One in which the pus has a cheesy appearance, usually tuberculous. **chronic a.** One of slow development, generally about a bone or joint, or in a lymph node; usually tuberculous and containing cheesy material. **cold a.** A slow-growing abscess attended by little or no inflammation. A tuberculous abscess. See chronic *a.* **embolic a.** One formed at the seat of a septic embolus. **hemorrhagic a.** One containing blood. **idiopathic a.** One not attributable to any disease. **ischiorectal a.** See anorectal *a.* **mammary a.** One involving the essential breast tissue. **metastatic a.** One secondary to pyemia and acute or subacute bacterial endocarditis, but not occurring through septicemia. It is usually of embolic origin and generally located in the lungs or liver. **parametritic a.** One occurring between the folds of the broad ligaments of the uterus or in the neighboring cellular tissue. **pelvic a.** One that involves the pelvic fascia. **perinephric a.** One originating in the region immediately surrounding the kidney. **perirectal a.** One situated in the fatty tissue at either side of the anus. **peritonsillar a.** One forming in acute tonsillitis around one or both tonsils; quinsy. **phlegmonous a.** An acute abscess in connective tissue, especially the subcutaneous. **primary a.** One originating at the seat of a pyogenic infection. **psoas a.** A cold abscess arising from diseased lumbar or lower thoracic vertebrae, the pus gravitating through the sheath of the psoas and pointing finally beneath the inguinal ligament. **pyemic a.** One occurring as a complication of pyemia. **retrovesical a.** One situated behind the bladder in the male or between the bladder and the uterus in the female. **secondary a.** An embolic abscess. **septicemic a.** One resulting from septic infection or accompanying septicemia. **stitch a.** One formed about a stitch or suture. **subareolar a.** One beneath the pigmented epithelium of the nipple, sometimes draining through the nipple. **subdiaphragmatic a.** One situated below the diaphragm and above the dome of the liver. **subphrenic a.** One located beneath the diaphragm. **tuberculous a.** See chronic *a.* **tympanitic a.** One containing gas. Also called *abscessus flatuosus, gas a.* **wandering a.** One in which the pus has traveled along the connective-tissue spaces and points at some locality distant from its origin. Syn., *hypostatic a.* Also called *abscessus per decubitum.*

ab·scis'sa (ab-siss'uh). 1. The horizontal of the two coördinates used in plotting the interrelationship of two sets of data. The vertical line is called the ordinate. 2. *In optics,* the point where a ray of light crosses the principal axis.

ab·scis'sion (ab-sish'un, ab-sizh'un). Removal of a part by cutting.

ab'sence. 1. *In psychiatry,* indifference to one's environment. 2. Temporary loss of consciousness, as in epilepsy, melancholia, and individuals with central lesions. 3. Fleeting loss of consciousness occurring in hysterical attacks or at the climax of a completed or very intense sexual gratification (Freud).

ab"sen·tee'ism. The practice of numerous industrial workers of absenting themselves from their jobs due to minor illness or injury, or for personal reasons; the time lost from such practices.

abs. feb. *Absente febre;* in the absence of fever.

ab'so·lute. 1. Simple; pure; free from admixture. 2. Unlimited and unqualified. 3. Complete; entire; real. 4. *In physics,* derived from basic data, not arbitrary.

ab'so·lute al'co·hol. Ethyl alcohol deprived of most of its water.

ab·sorb'. 1. *In physiology,* suck up; take in; imbibe, as fluids or gases, through osmosis and capillarity. 2. Infiltrate into the skin, as ultraviolet rays. 3. Incorporate into the body via the blood and lymph. 4. Stop radiant heat rays.

ab·sor"be·fa'cient (ab-sor"bi·fay'-shunt). 1. Causing or inducing absorption. 2. Any agent which promotes such action.

ab·sorb'ent. 1. Capable of absorbing or sucking up fluids, gases, or light waves. 2. A drug, application, or dressing which promotes absorption of diseased tissues. —**absorp'tive,** *adj.*

ab·sorp'tion. 1. *In physiology,* sucking up, taking in, and assimilation of certain gases, fluids, and suitable matter by the skin, mucous membranes, lacteals, lymphatics, and blood vessels. 2. *In physics,* taking up of a specific gas by a given solid. 3. Extinction of white light or any of its component rays by black or colored objects, or comparable effects on ultraviolet or infrared rays. 4. *In psychology,* inattention to all but a single thought or activity. 5. *In radiology,* loss of energy of an x-ray beam: (a) by the deflection of some photons and (b) by the change of quality or complete disappearance of others through transfer of their energy to the material (thus producing fast corpuscular rays). **cutaneous a.** Absorption through the skin.

ab'sti·nence. Voluntary self-denial of or forbearance from indulgence of appetites, especially for food, alcoholic drink, or sex relations.

ab·strac'tion. 1. Removal or separation of one or more ingredients from a compound, as an abstract from a crude drug. 2. *In psychology,* isolation of a meaning or characteristic from a totality which is unique and inaccessible to comparison; may be performed by thinking, feeling, sensation, or intuition.

a·bu'li·a (ab-yōō'lee-uh, a·bōō'·), **a·bou'li·a** (a·bōō'lee-uh), **ab"u·le'ia** (ab"yoo-lee'yuh). Loss or defect of the ability to make decisions; characteristic of schizophrenia. —**abu'lic,** *adj.*

a·buse'. 1. Wrong use, misuse, or particularly, excessive use. 2. Rape.

a·but'ment, a·but'tal. A tooth used to support or stabilize a prosthetic appliance. —**abut,** *v.i.*

A. C. Air conduction; alternating current; anodal closure.

Ac. Chemical symbol for actinium.

a. c. *Ante cibum;* before meals.

a·ca'cia. Gum arabic, a nearly white, gummy, water-soluble, transparent substance obtained from *Acacia senegal* and other African species. **Acacia mucilage** and **acacia syrup** are used as vehicles and demulcents. The mucilage is also employed intravenously for treating shock following hemorrhage.

a·cal"ci·co'sis. The condition resulting from a diet continuously low in calcium.

a"cal·cu'li·a, ac"al·cu'li·a. An aphasia marked by the inability to work even the simplest mathematical problem.

a·camp'si·a. Inflexibility or rigidity of a joint or limb; an ankylosis.

a·can"thes·the'si·a, **a·can"·thaes·the'si·a** (a·can"thess·thee'zhuh, ·zee·uh). A sensation as of pricking with needles.

a·can'tho-, acanth-. A combining form meaning *thorn, thorny, spine, spiny.*

a·can'thoid. Resembling a spine, spinous.

ac"an·thol'y·sis. Any skin disease in which there is an atrophy of the prickle-cell layer.

ac"an·tho'ma. A neoplasm, or localized excessive growth in any part of the prickle-cell layer of the skin, as cutaneous cancer or papilloma.

a·can"tho·pel'vis. A rachitic pelvis having a sharp, prominent pubic crest. Also called *acanthopelyx, pelvis spinosa.*

ac"an·tho'sis. A thickening of the germinative layer of the epidermis seen in many skin diseases and caused by hyperplasia of the cells. **—acan-thot'ic**, *adj.*

a·cap'ni·a. A condition with a diminished carbon dioxide content of the blood. **—acapnial**, *adj.*

a·cap'su·lar. *In biology*, without a capsule.

a·car'di·a. Congenital absence of the heart. **—acardiac**, *adj., n.*

a·car"di·o·tro'phi·a. Atrophy of the heart.

a·car'i·cide. Agent that destroys acarids.

ac'a·rid. A tick or mite. **—aca'rian, acar'idan, acarid'ian,** *adj., n.*

Ac"a·ri'na. An order of Arachnida comprising the ticks and mites. Many species are important vectors of bacterial, protozoal, rickettsial, and spirochetal diseases. In addition, severe reactions may result from their bites.

ac'a·ro-. A combining form denoting *mites* or *itch.*

ac"a·ro·pho'bi·a. Morbid fear of mites or of certain small animate or inanimate things, as worms or pins.

a·car'pi·a. Sterility, barrenness, unfruitfulness.

Ac'a·rus. A genus of mites. **A. folliculorum.** Synonym for *Demodex folliculorum.* **A. scabiei.** Synonym for *Sarcoptes scabiei.*

ac"a·tap'o·sis. A difficulty in swallowing; dysphagia.

ac"a·thex'i·a. Failure or inability to retain bodily secretions and excretions. **—acathectic**, *adj.*

ac·a·thi'si·a (ack·uh·thigh'zhuh, -thizh'uh). *In psychiatry*, inability to sit down; intense anxiety about sitting.

ACC. Anodal closure contraction.

Acc. Accommodation.

ac·cel'er·a'tion (ack·sel"uh·ray'-shun). 1. Quickening, as of the pulse or the respiration. 2. Change of velocity **(linear acceleration)** or of direction of movement **(centrifugal acceleration)**; important in aviation medicine.

ac·cel'er·a'tor, ac·cel'er·ant. 1. That which hastens. 2. Any agent or part which quickens the speed of a function. 3. A catalyst. **—accelera'tion,** *n.;* **accelerate,** *v.t., v.i.*

ac·ces'so·ry (ack·sess'o·ree). Auxiliary, assisting; applied to a lesser organ or part which supplements a similar organ or part.

ac'ci·dent. 1. *In legal medicine*, an event occurring to an individual without his expectation, and without the possibility of his preventing it at the moment of its occurrence. 2. An intercurrent or complicating symptom or event, not to be looked for in the regular progression of an attack of disease. **cerebral a.** A sudden, unexpected event of an injurious nature that occurs within the cerebrum, as cerebral hemorrhage or apoplexy. **serum a.** A serious allergic reaction which immediately follows the introduction of a foreign serum into a hypersensitive individual. Dyspnea and flushing occur, soon followed by shock and occasionally by fatal termination.

ac·cip'i·ter (ack·sip'i·tur). A facial bandage with tails radiating like the claws of a hawk.

ac·cli"ma·ti·za'tion, ac"cli-ma'tion. Process of adjusting to a strange or foreign climate, soil, water, etc., applied to plants, animals, and people. **—accli'mate, ac'climate, accli'matize,** *v.t., v.i.*

ac·com"mo·da'tion. Adaptation or adjustment of an organ, part, or organism, especially that of the eye. It includes the changes in the ciliary muscle and the lens in bringing light rays from various distances to focus upon the retina. Abbreviated, a., Acc. **—accom'modative,** *adj.* **a. reflex.** Changes which occur when the vision is focused from a distant to a near object; namely, contraction of the pupil, convergence of the eyes, and increased refraction by the lens. **Helmholtz's theory of a.** The increased convexity of the lens is produced by a relaxation of the suspensory ligament, thus removing the influence which tends to flatten the lens and permitting the latter, by its elasticity, to become more convex.

ac·couche'ment (a·kŏŏsh'mahng, uh·kŏŏsh'munt). Childbirth; parturition, *q.v.* **a. forcé.** Rapid delivery by manual dilation of the cervix followed by version or application of forceps and immediate extraction.

ac"cou·cheur' (ack"ŏŏ·shur'). Obstetrician; a professionally trained person attending women in childbirth.

ac"cou·cheuse' (ack"ŏŏ·shuz'). A female obstetrician; a midwife.

ac·cre'tion. 1. Growth characterized by addition to the periphery, as in crystalline and certain organic compounds. 2. Adherence of parts normally separate. 3. A growing together; adhesion. 4. An accumulation of foreign matter, as about a tooth (salivary calculus) or within any cavity. **—accrete',** *adj., v.i.;* **accretive,** *adj.* **-a'ce·ae** (-ay'see·ee). *In botany*, a suffix used in combination with the name of one of the principal genera to form the names of families of plants.

a"ce·nes·the'si·a, a"ce·naes-the'si·a (ay"seh·ness·thee'zhuh, a·sen"ess-). Loss of body sense or well-being; absence of visceral sense, said to occur in melancholia and hypochondriasis. See *cenesthesia.*

a·cen"o·cou'ma·rol. 3-(α-Acetonyl-4-nitrobenzyl)-4-hydroxycoumarin, an intravascular anticoagulant. See *sin-trom*.

a·cen'tric (ay-sen'trick, a·sen'·). 1. Not central; peripheral; eccentric. 2. Not arising centrally, as from a nerve center.

a·ceph'a·lus. Any one of a group of omphalositic monsters characterized by absence of the head. **–acephalous,** *adj.*

a·ceph'a·ly. Absence of the head.

a·cer"a·to'sis (a·kerr"uh·to'sis), **a·ker"a·to'sis** (a·kerr"uh·to'sis). A deficiency or absence of horny tissue, as of the nails.

a·cer'bi·ty. Acidity combined with astringency.

a·cer'vu·lus. Old term for brain sand.

a·ces'o·dyne. A pain-relieving agent; an anodyne. **–acesod'ynous,** *adj.*

acet-. See *aceto-*.

ac"e·tab'u·lec'to·my (ass"i·tab"-yoo·leck'to·mee). Excision of the acetabulum.

ac"e·tab'u·lo·plas"ty. Any plastic operation on the acetabulum, especially an operation aimed at restoring or enlarging the acetabular cavity.

ac"e·tab'u·lum. Cup-shaped depression on the outer aspect of the hipbone for the reception of the head of the femur. **–acetabular,** *adj.*

ac'e·tal (ass'i·tal). 1. $C_6H_{14}O_2$. Ethidene diethylate, a colorless liquid with an ethereal odor, produced by the reaction of alcohol with acetaldehyde. It is moderately soluble in water. Has been used as a soporific in human and veterinary medicine. 2. Generic name for products of the interaction of aldehydes and alcohol.

ac"et·al'de·hyde (ass"it·al'di·hyde, a·seet"al'di·hyde). $CH_3.CHO$. A colorless liquid with a pungent odor resulting from oxidation of ethyl alcohol; taken internally, it causes narcosis and other noxious effects. Also called *acetic aldehyde, ethanal.*

ac"et·an'i·lid (ass"i·tan'i·lid). $C_6H_5NH.OC.CH_3$. Monoacetylaniline, occurring as a white, crystalline powder, soluble in boiling water and alcohol; an analgesic and antipyretic. Syn., *antifebrin.*

ac"et·ar'sone (ass"i·tahr'sohn). 3-Acetylamino - 4 - hydroxyphenylarsonic acid; a white or yellowish powder, slightly soluble in water; used in treatment of amebiasis, also in prophylaxis and treatment in certain cases of syphilis. See *spirocid, stovarsol.*

ac'e·tate. Any salt of acetic acid.

a·cet"a·zol·am'ide. 5-Acetamido-1,3,4-thiadiazole-2-sulfonamide, a carbonic anhydrase inhibitor. See *diamox.*

a·ce'tic ac'id (a·see'tick). An aqueous solution containing 36–37% CH_3COOH. Occasionally used, when diluted,

as an astringent and styptic. **di·luted a. a.** An aqueous solution containing 5.7–6.3% (w/v) CH_3COOH. **glacial a. a.** A colorless liquid containing not less than 99.4% CH_3COOH; formerly used as a caustic for removing warts and corns.

a·ce'tic al'de·hyde. Acetaldehyde.

a·ce'tic an·hy'dride. $(CH_3CO)_2O$. The anhydride of acetic acid; a colorless, mobile liquid having the odor of acetic acid.

a·ce'tic e'ther. Ethyl acetate.

a·ce'tic fer"men·ta'tion. Any process of fermentation resulting in the formation of acetic acid.

ac"e·tim'e·ter (ass"i·tim'i·tur), **ac"e·tom'e·ter.** A device for determining the amount of acetic acid present in vinegar or other solutions. **–acetimet'ric, acetomet'ric,** *adj.;* **acetimetry, acetometry,** *n.*

ac'e·to- (ass'i·to-, a·see'to-), **acet-.** A combining form denoting *connection with,* or *derivation from, acetic acid* or *acetyl.*

ac"e·to·a·ce'tic ac'id (ass"i·to-a·see'tick, a·see"to·a·see'tick). $CH_3.CO.CH_2COOH$. A keto acid eliminated in urine, believed to be a normal product of fat metabolism and found especially when fatty acids are incompletely oxidized, as in diabetes. Syn., *diacetic acid; betaketohydroxybutyric acid.*

ac"e·to·me·naph'thone. Menadiol diacetate or 2-methyl-1,4-naphthohydroquinone diacetate; a white, crystalline powder, almost insoluble in water. Used for its vitamin-K effect.

ac"e·to·mor'phine (ass"i·to-). Heroin.

ac"e·ton·asth'ma (ass"i·ton·az'muh, ·ass'muh). Dyspnea associated with acetonuria, sometimes called uremic asthma. It is marked by restlessness, headache, nausea, vomiting, and transient blindness.

ac'e·tone (ass'i·tone). $CH_3.CO.CH_3$. Dimethylketone, propanone. A colorless, inflammable liquid, miscible with water, alcohol, and ether. Occurs in the blood and urine in minute quantities which may become greatly increased in diabetics. **a. bodies.** Urinary compounds derived from the incomplete oxidation of fats, as butyric, acetoacetic, and β-oxybutyric acids, and acetone. Found in cases of acidosis, as diabetic acidosis. See Table of Normal Values of Blood Constituents in the Appendix. **a.-chloroform.** See *chlorobutanol.*

ac"e·to·ne'mi·a, ac"e·to·nae'mi·a (ass"i·to·nee'mee·uh). The presence of large amounts of acetone bodies in the blood. **–acetonemic,** *adj.*

ac"e·to·nu'ri·a (ass"i·to·new'ree-uh). Abnormal increase in the amount of acetone bodies in the urine, found during fevers, diabetic acidosis, malignancy, and intestinal disorders.

ac″et·o·phe·net′i·din (ass″i·to·fi-net′i·din, a·see″to·). Paraethoxyacet-anilid. A white, crystalline powder; soluble in water. Used as antipyretic and analgesic. Syn., *phenacetin*.

ac′e·tous (ass′i·tus, a·see′tus). Pertaining to, resembling, forming, or containing, vinegar or acetic acid.

a″cet·ri·xo′ic ac′id. 3-Acetylamino-2,4,6-triiodobenzoic acid, the sodium salt of which is used as a roentgenographic contrast medium. See *urokon sodium*.

a·ce′tum. 1. Vinegar; an impure, dilute acetic acid produced by acetous fermentation of fruit juices, as in wine or cider. 2. *In pharmacy*, a solution of the active principles of certain drugs in dilute acetic acid. See *vinegar*. **—ace′tic**, *adj*.

ac′e·tyl (ass′i·til, a·see′til). The univalent radical CH_3CO-. **a. carbinol.** $CH_3CO.CH_2OH$. Hydroxyacetone. A colorless oil possessing a weak, peculiar odor; boils at 145°–150° C. Also called *pyroracemic alcohol, methyl ketol, acetol.*

ac″e·tyl·be″ta·meth·yl·cho′line. A choline compound characterized by sufficient stability in the body and by effectiveness, even if administered orally, to produce increased gastrointestinal tone and motion, and vascular dilation. Its salts are used for treating tachycardia, peripheral vascular diseases, abdominal distention, etc. **a. bromide.** Less hygroscopic than the chloride, this form is preferred for use in tablets. See *mecholyl bromide*. **a. chloride.** The preferred form for administration subcutaneously or by iontophoresis. See *mecholyl chloride.*

ac″e·tyl·cho′line (ass″i·til·ko′leen, a·see″til·). Acetylethanol-trimethylammonium hydroxide. $(CH_3)_3N(OH)CH_2.CH_2.O.CO.CH_3$. Lowers blood pressure, increases peristalsis, and commonly is regarded as the substance released from nerves to activate the muscles (Dale). It is liberated from parasympathetic postganglionic and all preganglionic nerve terminals, and possibly at synapses in the central nervous system. **a. esterase.** See under *esterase.*

a·cet″y·li·za′tion, a·cet″y·la′tion. Chemical introduction of an acetyl radical ($CH_3.CO—$) into an organic compound.

ac″e·tyl·sal″i·cyl′ic ac′id. $C_6H_4.O(CH_3CO).COOH$. A white, crystalline powder, hydrolyzing in moist air to acetic and salicylic acids; soluble in water. Used internally as antirheumatic, analgesic, and antipyretic; locally in acute pharyngitis and tonsillitis. Syn., *aspirin.*

ac″e·tyl·sul·fon′a·mide (ass″i-til·sul·fon′uh·mide). A sulfonamide in which a hydrogen atom of the NH_2 group, attached directly to the benzene ring, is replaced by an acetyl group; a conjugation which occurs in the liver. The resulting acetyl compounds are therapeutically ineffective, and harmful effects may be produced in the renal tubules and urinary tract by their precipitation.

ac″e·tyl·tan′nic ac′id (ass″i·til·tan′ick, a·see″til·). An acetylated tannic acid; a yellowish or grayish powder, slightly soluble in water. In the lower intestine it liberates tannic acid which acts as an astringent. Used in the treatment of diarrhea.

ach″a·la′si·a (ack″uh·lay′zhuh, ·zee·uh). Inability to relax, said of a hollow muscular organ. **a. of the cardia.** Spasmodic constriction of the lower portion of the esophagus with dilatation above; cardiospasm. **sphincteral a.** Failure to relax on the part of one or more sphincter muscles.

ache. 1. A constant or fixed pain, dull to severe in character. 2. Suffer continuous pain.

a·chei′li·a (a·kigh′lee·uh). A condition marked by congenital absence of the lips.

a·chei′rus (a·kigh′rus). An individual without hands. **—acheirous**, *adj.*

a·chieve′ment age. A score, derived from a series of educational tests, expressed in terms of the age at which an average individual attains that score. Also see accomplishment *quotient.*

A·chil′les. According to Homer's Iliad, Achilles was vulnerable only in one heel. His name designates the tendon of the gastrocnemius and soleus muscles (also called *tendo calcaneus* [BNA]) and is applied to certain ailments of the heel. The Achilles jerk or reflex is the ankle clonus reflex. See Achilles tendon *reflex.*

a·chil′lo·bur·si′tis (a·kill′o·bur-sigh′tis). Inflammation of the Achilles bursa.

a·chil′lo·cyn′i·a (a·kill″o·din′ee-uh). Pain in the Achilles tendon or bursa; achillobursitis.

ach″il·lor′rha·phy (ack″il·or′uh-fee). Any suturing operation on the Achilles tendon.

ach″il·lot′o·my (ack″i·lot′o·mee), **a·chil″lo·te·not′o·my** (a·kill″o·ti-not′o·mee). Surgical section of the Achilles tendon.

ACH in′dex. An index of nutrition based on measurements of arm girth, chest depth, and hip width.

a″chlor·hy′dri·a (ay″klor·high′-dree·uh, ack″lor·). The absence of free hydrochloric acid in the stomach, even after the administration of histamine.

a″chlor·op′si·a (ay″klor·op′see·uh, ack″lor·). **a·chlo″ro·blep′si·a.** Green blindness.

ach″lu·o·pho′bi·a (ack″loo·o·fo′bee·uh). Morbid fear of darkness.

a·cho′li·a (ay·ko′lee·uh, a·ko′·). 1. Absence or suppression of biliary secretion. 2. Any condition obstructing the escape of the bile into the small intestine. 3. A mild temperament. **–achol′ic, ach′olous,** *adj.* **pigmentary a.** A deficiency of bile marked by clay-colored feces but no jaundice.

ach″o·lu′ri·a (ack″o·lew′ree·uh). The absence of bile pigments in the urine. **–acholuric,** *adj.*

a·chon″dro·pla′si·a (ay·kon″dro·play′zhuh, a·kon″dro·). **a·chon′dro·plas″ty.** A condition of abnormal osteogenesis resulting in the typical congenital dwarf. The pathologic process begins early in intrauterine life as disordered chondrification and ossification of the ends of the long bones; the membrane bones develop normally. Syn., *chondrodystrophia foetalis.* **–achondroplas′tic,** *adj.*

a·chon′dro·plas″ty. See *achondroplasia.*

a′chor (ay′kor, ack′or). 1. A papular or pustular eruption of the hairy parts. 2. An eczematoid eruption affecting the face and scalp of infants with many scales and scabs, as a milk crust. 3. An acuminate pustule. 4. Barber's itch.

A·cho′ri·on (a·kor′ee·on, ay·kor′ee·on). A former genus of dermatophytes.

a·chre″o·cy·the′mi·a (a·kree″o·sigh·thee′mee·uh). Paleness of the red blood cells due to a deficiency of hemoglobin; anemia.

a·chro′a·cyte (ay·kro′uh·sight, a·kro′·). A colorless cell, or lymphocyte.

a·chro′a·cy·to′sis (ay·kro″uh·sigh·to′sis, a·kro″·). **a·chro″o′cy·to′sis.** An increase in the number of colorless or lymphocytic cells in the blood; lymphocythemia.

a·chroi″o·cy·the′mi·a (a·kroy″o·sigh·thee′mee·uh). 1. Achreocythemia. 2. The general condition associated with this anemia.

a·chro′ma·cyte (ay·kro′muh·sight, a·kro′·). **a·chro′ma·to·cyte″.** A decolorized erythrocyte; a ghost or shadow corpuscle due to loss of hemoglobin. Also called *Ponfick's shadow, Bizzozero's blood platelet, Hayem's corpuscle.*

a″chro·ma′si·a (ay″kro·may′zhuh, ·zee·uh). 1. Loss or absence of normal skin pigmentation, as in albinism, leukoderma, vitiligo. 2. Pallor of cachexia. 3. Failure of cells or tissues to stain normally.

ach′ro·mate (ack′ro·mate). A totally color-blind person.

a″chro·mat′ic (ay″kro·mat′ick). 1. Without color. 2. Containing achromatin. 3. Not decomposing light into its constituent colors. 4. Staining with difficulty, said of cells or tissues.

a·chro·ma·tism. 1. Absence of chromatic aberration. 2. Absence of color.

a·chro′ma·to- (ay·kro′muh·to-, a·kro′muh·to-), **achromat-.** A combining form denoting *achromatic, colorless.*

a·chro″ma·to·phil″. 1. Showing no affinity for stains. 2. A microörganism or histologic element which does not stain readily. **–achromatophil′ic,** *adj.*; **achromatophil′ia,** *n.*

a·chro″ma·top′si·a. Total color blindness.

a·chro″ma·to′sis. Any condition characterized by a deficiency of natural pigment, as albinism, leukoderma, vitiligo.

a·chro″ma·tu′ri·a. A very pale or waterlike urine.

a·chro·mi·a (ay·kro′mee·uh, a·kro′·), **a·chro′ma.** Absence of color; pallor; achromatosis. **–achromic, achromous,** *adj.*

a·chro″mo·der′mi·a, **a·chro″mo·der′ma.** A deficiency or lack of pigment in the skin; leukoderma.

a·chro″mo·trich′i·a (ay·kro″mo·trick′ee·uh, a·kro″·). Absence of pigment from the hair.

achromycin. A trade-mark for tetracycline, 3.

ach″ro·ö·am′y·loid (ack″ro·o·am′i·loyd). Recently deposited amyloid which does not form a blue color with iodine.

a·chyl″a·ne′mi·a, **a·chyl″a·nae′mi·a** (a·kigh″luh·nee′mee·uh). A simple hypochromic anemia associated with gastric achlorhydria. Also called *anemia achylica, achlorhydric anemia.*

a·chyl′i·a (a·kigh′lee·uh). Absence of chyle. **–achylous,** *adj.* **a. gastrica.** Diminution or absence of gastric juice. **a. pancreatica.** An absence of pancreatic juice resulting in fatty stools, intestinal indigestion, and malnutrition.

a·chy′mi·a (a·kigh′mee·uh). Deficient formation of chyme. Also called *achymosis.* **–achymous,** *adj.*

a·cic′u·lar (a·sick′yoo·lur). Needlelike; shaped like a needle.

ac′id. Commonly, a substance containing hydrogen replaceable by metals to form salts, and capable of dissociating in aqueous solution to form hydrogen ions.

ac′id al′co·hol. A solution containing 0.1% hydrochloric acid in 70% ethyl alcohol; used as a decolorizing agent.

ac″id·am″in·u·ri·a (ass″id-am″i-new′ree-uh). Presence of an excess of amino acids in the urine.

ac″i·de′mi·a, ac″i·dae′mi·a (ass″i-dee′mee-uh). A condition of decreased alkalinity of the blood, demonstrated by a lowered pH. See *acidosis.*

ac′id-fast″. Denoting certain bacteria which are not decolorized by mineral acids after staining with aniline dyes, as the bacilli of tuberculosis, leprosy, and smegma.

ac′id in·tox″i·ca′tion. A toxic condition of the body resulting from an excess of acids accumulated from within or introduced from without.

a·cid′i·ty. 1. Quality of being acid; sourness; excess of acid. 2. Acid content of any substance. **a. of the stomach.** Sourness of the stomach due to oversecretion of acid or to fermentation of food. Associated with heartburn, acid eructations, and epigastric pain and distress.

ac″i·do·cy·to′sis (ass″i-do-sigh-to′sis). Morbid increase in the number of circulating eosinophils.

ac″i·do·gen′ic (ass″i-do-jen′ick). Forming acids, especially an acid urine.

a·cid′o·phil″ (a-sid′o-fil″, ass′i-do-fil″). 1. A cell, element, or substance having an affinity for acid stains. 2. One of a group of acid-staining cells, alpha cells, found in the adenohypophysis. 3. Any organism which grows best in acid cultures. Syn., *oxyphil.* **—acidophil′ic, acidoph′ilous,** *adj.*

ac″i·doph′i·lism (ass″i-dof′i-lizum). A condition of overabundance or overactivity of the acidophilic cells of the adenohypophysis.

ac″id·re·sist′ant (ass″i-do-riziss′tunt), **ac″id-re·sist′ant.** Not readily decolorized by acids, applied to certain microörganisms. See *acid-fast.* **—acidoresistance, acid-resistance,** *n.*

ac″i·do′sis (ass″i-do′sis). Reduction of the alkali reserve; acidemia; due to an excess of acid metabolites which are incompletely oxidized or poorly eliminated. When toxic symptoms develop, the condition is called acid intoxication. **—acidot′ic,** *adj.* **carbondioxide a.** The result of CO_2 retention, as in drowning. Also called *gaseous a.* **compensated a.** A condition of reduced blood bicarbonate with the H_2CO_3 to $NaHCO_3$ ratio unchanged because of the blood buffers. In compensated CO_2 acidosis, the blood bicarbonate may be increased, but pH is normal. **diabetic a.** That occurring in diabetes mellitus, due to loss of base in the urine in combination with ketone acids and as a result of polyuria. It may become extremely severe, characterized by air hunger and eventually coma. **uncompensated a.** A condition of reduced blood bicarbonate in which there is a change in the blood pH. In uncompensated CO_2 acidosis, the blood bicarbonate may be normal.

ac′id tide. The temporary increase in the acidity of urine and body fluids which follows the alkaline tide, *q.v.*

ac″i·du′ric (ass″i-dew′rick). Referring to bacteria which can grow in an acid medium but which grow better in an alkaline medium.

ac′i·ni (ass′i-nigh). Plural of acinus.

ac′i·nus (ass′i-nus) (pl: *acini*). A saccular terminal division of a compound gland having a narrow lumen, as contrasted with an alveolus. Several acini combine to form a lobule. **—acinous,** *adj.*

ac·la′sis, a·cla′si·a (a-clay′zhuh, -zee-uh). Morbid continuity of structure, as in chondrodystrophia; especially diaphysial aclasis, marked by imperfect bone formation in cartilage and abnormal cartilaginous growths near the epiphyses, causing multiple exostoses.

a·clas′tic. Not refracting.

a·cleis″to·car′di·a (ay-kly″sto-car′dee-uh, a-kly″sto-). A condition in which the foramen ovale of the heart fails to close.

ac·mas′tic. Designating a disease with a period of progressive symptoms (*epacmastic*), followed by a period of abatement (*paracmastic*).

ac′me (ack′mee). 1. Highest point. 2. Crisis or critical stage of a disease.

ac′ne (ack′nee). A chronic inflammatory condition of the pilosebaceous structures commonly involving the face, back, and chest. The lesions are papular, pustular, or nodular; they affect persons between the age of puberty and 30 years of age, generally are worse in winter, and often are associated with menstrual and gastrointestinal disorders. The primary lesion is the comedo, or blackhead, which later develops into a pink, acuminate papule, pustule, or nodule. Syn., *a. vulgaris.* Also called *adolescent a., a. varis.* **a. agminata.** A facial eruption of small, dusky, reddish papules which develop into pustules and leave scars when healed. Also called *acnitis.* **a. cachecticorum.** An acneform eruption seen in debilitated persons after long wasting diseases, such as tuberculosis. The lesions occur on the trunk and legs, appearing as flat, dull-red papules and pustules varying in size from that of a pinhead to that of a lentil. **a. coagminata.** A pustular acneform eruption often seen after administering any of the halogens or their salts and among industrial workers exposed to hydrochloric acid, tar, tar vapor, oil, wax, or paraffin. The skin is pigmented with many comedos. The pustules form thick clusters and are covered with crusts involving, in addition to the more common sites, the extensor surfaces of the arms and legs, the scalp, the inner thighs, and the genitalia. Syn., *bromine a., chlorine a., iodine a., tar a., a. medicamentosa, a. picealis.* **a. decalvans.** A purulent inflammation of the hair follicles of the scalp causing destruction of the hair with irregular patches of baldness and scarring or atrophy of the skin. Syn., *folliculitis decalvans.* **a. erythematosa.** See *a.* rosacea. **a. hypertrophica.** A stage in the development of acne rosacea in which there is a permanent, intensely red, noninflammatory, nodular thickening of the sides of the nose and the lips. Syn., *rhinophyma.* **a. indurata.** Acne vulgaris in which the lesions are hard and livid due to perifollicular infiltration, and are very resistant to treatment. **a. medicamentosa.** That which results from medication with certain drugs, as the iodides and bromides. See *a.* coagminata. **a. papulosa.** A papular form commonly seen on the foreheads of young adults. **a. punctata.** A superficial papular eruption with pointed lesions marked by slight inflammation about the comedos. **a. pustulosa.** A variety of acne vulgaris with a predominance of small abscesses. **a. rosacea.** A chronic hyperemic skin affection of the nose, forehead, and cheeks, marked by hypertrophy, erythema and flushing, and telangiectasia. Also called *rosacea, telangiectasis faciei, whisky nose.* **a. scrofulosorum.** A variety of acne cachecticorum affecting tuberculous children. **a. vulgaris.** The common type of acne. Also called *a. varis.* **ac'ne·form, ac'ne'i·form.** Resembling acne.

a·co'mi·a. Baldness. A deficiency of hair from any cause. Syn., *alopecia.* **—acomous,** *adj.*

ac'o·nite. A very poisonous drug obtained from the roots of *Aconitum napellus.* It is a cardiac, respiratory, and circulatory depressant and produces sensory paralysis. The principal alkaloid is aconitine. It acts as a diaphoretic, antipyretic, and diuretic. Syn., *monkshood.*

a·con'i·tine (a·kon'i·teen, ·tin), **a·con'i·tin.** $C_{34}H_{47}O_{11}N$. An extremely poisonous alkaloid derived from *Aconitum napellus* and other species.

a·con"u·re'sis. Involuntary passage of urine.

a"cop·ro'sis (ay"kop·ro'sis, ack"o·). Marked deficiency or absence of feces in the bowel. **—acop'rous,** *adj.*

ac"o·re'a. Absence of the pupil.

a·co'ri·a. 1. A form of hunger due to the absence of the feeling of satiety following a meal, to be differentiated from bulimia. 2. Greedy or insatiable appetite because the patient never feels full; a constant desire for food although the appetite may not be large.

a·cos'tate. Without ribs.

acou- (a·koo-), **acouo-.** A combining form denoting *relation to hearing.*

a·cou"es·the'si·a (a·koo"ess·thee'·zhuh, ·zee·uh). The hearing sense, usually suggesting a very acute sense of hearing.

ac"ou·la'li·on (ack"oo·lay'lee·on). An instrument used in teaching speech to deaf-mutes.

a·cou'me·ter (a·koo'mi·tur), **ac"ou·om'e·ter, ac"ou·tom'e·ter.** Instrument for measuring the acuteness of hearing. **—acoumet'ric, acoumomet'ric,** *adj.;* **acou'metry,** *n.* **-a·cou'si·a** (a·koo'zhuh, ·shuh), **-a·cou'sis.** A combining form denoting *hearing.*

a·cous'ma (a·koos'muh, a·kooz'muh). In *psychopathology,* a simple auditory hallucination, as of buzzing or ringing. A borderline condition between illusion and true hallucinosis.

a·cous"mat·ag·no'sis (a·koos"·mat·ag·no'sis, a·kooz"·). Inability to recognize sounds or understand spoken words; mind deafness.

a·cous"ti·co·pho'bi·a (a·koos"ti·ko·). Morbid fear of sounds.

a·cous'tic nerve. The eighth cranial nerve consisting of a cochlear nerve and a vestibular nerve.

a·cous'tics (a·koos'ticks). 1. In *physics,* the science of sound. 2. In *psychology,* that branch dealing with hearing. **—acoustic,** *adj.*

ac·quired'. 1. In *psychology,* gained from experience or learning, as an acquired idea; in contradistinction to innate. 2. In *biology,* developed as a result of environment, or of use or disuse, as an acquired characteristic; in contradistinction to an inherited characteristic.

a·cra'ni·a (ay·kray'nee·uh, a·kray'·). Partial or complete absence of the cranium at birth. **—acranial,** *adj.;* **acranius,** *n.*

a·cra'ti·a (a·kray'shee·uh). Impotence, loss of power.

a·crat"u·re'sis. Inability to micturate due to atony of the bladder.

ac'rid. Pungent; irritating.

ac"ri·fla'vine (ack"ri·flay'veen, ·flav'een). A mixture of 2,8-diamino-10-methylacridinium chloride and 2,8-diaminoacridine. Used chiefly as local antiseptic. Also called *a. base, neutral a.* See *trypaflavin.* **a. hydrochloride.** A mixture of the hydrochlorides of the components of acriflavine; used for the same purposes as acriflavine but more irritant. Also called *acid acriflavine*.

a·crit'i·cal (ay-krit'i·kul, a·krit'·). 1. Without a crisis; not relating to a crisis; applied to diseases which resolve by lysis. 2. Indeterminate, as regards prognosis.

ac'ro-, acr-. A combining form meaning *pertaining to extremes* or *to heights; pertaining to an extremity.*

ac"ro·ag·no'sis. Absence of sense perception in a limb.

ac"ro·an"es·the'si·a, **ac"ro·an"aes·the'si·a** (ack"ro·an"ess·thee'zhuh, ·zee·uh). Anesthesia of the extremities.

ac"ro·as·phyx'i·a. Early symptom of Raynaud's disease characterized by coldness and pallor alternating with heat and redness of the hands and feet.

ac"ro·a·tax'i·a. Incoördination of the muscles of the fingers and toes, as opposed to *proximoatazia*, incoördination of the proximal portions of the extremities.

ac"ro·ceph'a·ly, ac"ro·ce·pha'li·a. Deformity of the head, the top of which is more or less pointed. Syn., *oxycephaly*. **—acrocephal'ic, acrocephalous,** *adj.*

ac"ro·ci·ne'sis (ack"ro·kin·ee'sis). Markedly excessive motion, as in certain cases of hysteria. **—acrocinet'ic,** *adj.*

ac"ro·con·trac'ture. Contracture of the joints of the hands or feet.

ac"ro·cy"a·no'sis. Blueness of the extremities due to vasomotor disturbance. In chronic progressive acrocyanosis there is hypertrophy of the soft tissues of the hands and feet, associated with cyanosis or intense redness.

ac"ro·der"ma·ti'tis. Inflammation of the skin of an extremity.

ac"ro·dyn'i·a, ac"ro·dy'ni·a. See *erythredema polyneuropathy.*

ac"ro·e·de'ma. 1. Swelling of the extremities, sometimes accompanied by acrodynia. Seen particularly in neuropathic individuals. 2. Posttraumatic swelling of a hand or foot, which remains permanent.

ac"ro·es·the'si·a, ac"ro·aes·the'si·a (ack"ro·ess·thee'zhuh, ·zee·uh). 1. Exaggerated sensitiveness or sensibility. 2. Pain in one or more of the extremities.

ac"ro·ger'i·a (ack"ro·jerr'ee·uh, ·jeer'ee·uh). Premature aging of the skin of the hands and feet, marked by looseness and wrinkling.

ac"ro·hy"per·hi·dro'sis (ack"ro·high"pur·hi·dro'sis, ·high"pur·high·dro'sis). Increased perspiration of the hands and feet.

ac"ro·hy'po·ther"my. Abnormal coldness of the extremities.

ac"ro·ker"a·to'sis ver·ru"ci·for'mis. Form of epithelial nevus;

discrete verrucous lesions occurring chiefly on the dorsum of the hands and feet; the palms, wrists, and knees also may be involved.

a·cro'le·in. $CH_2:CH.CHO.$ Acrylic aldehyde. A colorless, mobile liquid with a pungent odor, resulting from the decomposition of glycerin.

ac"ro·mas·ti'tis. Inflammation of the nipple.

ac"ro·me·ga'li·a. See *acromegaly.*

ac"ro·meg'a·ly, ac"ro·me·ga'li·a. Chronic condition resulting from hyperfunction and hyperplasia of the eosinophilic cells of the anterior pituitary. The characteristic features are: increase in size of the viscera (splanchnomegaly), the soft parts, and the bones, especially the short and flat bones (acromegaly), without increase in height, the hands, feet, and face showing most change; metabolic disturbances, chief of which is a change in sugar tolerance; secondary changes in the function of other endocrine organs; and so-called neighborhood symptoms such as bitemporal hemianopsia. *Acromegaloid, forme fruste, transient acromegaly,* and *fugitive acromegaly* are terms which have been used to designate incomplete, arrested, or rapidly changing types of the disease. See *gigantism.* Also called *Marie's syndrome.* **—acromegal'ic,** *adj., n.*

ac"ro·mel·al'gi·a. A peripheral vascular disease. See *erythromelalgia.*

ac"ro·met"a·gen'e·sis. Undue growth of the extremities.

a·cro"mi·o·cla·vic'u·lar. Pertaining to the acromion and the clavicle; applied to the articulation between these two bones and the ligaments joining them. See Table of Joints and Ligaments in the Appendix.

a·cro"mi·o·cor'a·coid. Pertaining to the acromion and the coracoid process. Also called *coracoacromial.*

a·cro'mi·on. The flat, somewhat triangular bony process formed by the lateral extension of the scapular spine, and situated just above the glenoid cavity. It articulates with the clavicle, and serves as a point of attachment for some of the fibers of the deltoid and trapezius muscles. **—acromial,** *adj.*

a·cro"mi·o·tho·rac'ic (a·kro"mee·o·thor·ass'ick). Relating to the shoulder and thorax; designating a branch of the axillary artery.

a·crom'pha·lus. 1. The center of the umbilicus, where the cord attaches. 2. Unusual prominence of the navel, often the first sign of an umbilical hernia. 3. Remains of the umbilical cord attached to the child.

ac"ro·my'o·to'ni·a (ack"ro·my"o·to'nee·uh), **ac"ro·my·ot'o·nus**

(ack″ro·my·ot′o·nus). Tonic muscular spasm of the extremities, usually causing deformity of the hands or feet.

ac″ro·nar·cot′ic. 1. Both acrid and narcotic. 2. An agent which combines a local irritant effect, by acting directly on the peripheral nerves, with a general obtunding effect, by affecting the brain and vital centers in the spinal cord.

ac″ro·neu·rop′a·thy. The simultaneous degeneration of the peripheral nerves in their most distal parts, usually symmetrical. Most common causes: alcohol, arsenic, lead or mercury poisoning, or a deficiency disease such as beriberi. Syn., *polyneuropathy, polyneuritis.*

ac″ro·neu·ro′sis. Any neurosis manifesting itself in the extremities, usually vasomotor in nature or due to deficiency disease.

ac′ro·nyx. Ingrowing of a nail.

ac″ro·pa·ral′y·sis. Paralysis of the extremities.

ac″ro·par″es·the′si·a, ac″ro·par″aes·the′si·a (·par″ess·thee′·zhuh, ·zee·uh). A vasomotor neurosis, seen chiefly in middle-aged women; characterized by tingling or crawling sensations in the hands, hyperesthesia and hyperalgesia of the fingers, coldness, and pallor or cyanosis of the hands.

ac″ro·pa·thol′o·gy. The pathology of the extremities, especially the morbid changes occurring in orthopedic diseases.

a·crop′a·thy. Any disease of the extremities.

ac″ro·pho′bi·a. Morbid dread of being at a great height.

ac″ro·scle·ro′sis. Scleroderma affecting the hands and extending to the upper extremities and the face; seen usually as a sequel of Raynaud's disease.

ac·ro·some. A crescent-shaped body molded to the nucleus; forming the anterior part of the sperm head; the apical body.

ac″ros·te·al′gi·a. Pain in one or more of the bones of an extremity.

ac″ro·ter′ic. Relating to the periphery or most distal parts, as the tips of the toes, fingers, nose, etc. —**acrote′ria,** *n.*

a·crot′ic. Exhibiting any defective beating of the pulse; distinguished by absent or barely perceptible pulse.

ac′ro·tism. Absence or imperceptibility of the pulse.

ac″ro·tro″pho·neu·ro′sis. A trophic disturbance of the extremities caused by a nerve lesion.

a·cryl′ic ac′id. $CH_2{:}CH.COOH$. A liquid acid resulting from oxidation of acrolein.

a·cryl′ics. A group of synthetic thermoplastic substances. They resemble clear glass, but are lighter in weight and permit passage of ultraviolet rays; used in making dental prostheses and temporary artificial eyes. Lucite and plexiglas are commercial forms.

ac′ry·lo-, acryl-. A combining form denoting *relationship to acrylic acid* or *acrylics.*

ac″ry·lo·ni·trile′ (ack″ri·lo·nigh·trill′, ·nigh′tryle). A colorless liquid, $H_2C{:}CH.CN$, used in the manufacture of synthetic rubber. Its toxic action has been said to be due to the formation of hydrocyanic acid. An increase in serum thiocyanates is observed in workers exposed to it. Syn., *vinyl cyanide.*

ACS. Antireticular cytotoxic serum; a specific cytotoxic antiserum produced by the intravenous injection of an antigen prepared from human or heterogenous animal spleen and bone marrow. Minute doses are said to have a stimulating effect, and large doses a depressing effect, on the mesenchymal system. This is the basis for its use in the treatment of such unrelated conditions as wounds, fractures, arthritis, ozena, and even cancer.

act. 1. Any deed, action, or performance. 2. Fulfillment of a purpose or function. **compulsive a.** Any deed or action performed by an individual at the supposed instigation of another's dominant will, but against his own. Also called *imperious a.* **impulsive a.** Any deed or act resulting from a sudden urge rather than the will. **reflex a.** Any action innervated through a reflex arc. **sexual a.** Coitus; cohabitation; sexual intercourse.

ACTH. Adrenocorticotropic hormone from the adenohypophysis; stimulates secretion of steroid substances by the adrenal cortex. Syn., *corticotropin.*

actidione. A trade-mark for an antibiotic produced by *Streptomyces griseus,* highly active against yeasts but relatively innocuous to other microörganisms.

ac′tin. A fiber protein found in muscle.

actin-. See *actino-.*

ac·tin′ic. Pertaining to, or designating, the rays of the spectrum which produce chemical change.

ac·tin′i·um. Ac = 227 *ca.* A radioactive element found in uranium ores, as pitchblende. **a. X.** The disintegration product of radioactinium, *q.v.*

ac′ti·no-, actin-. A combining form meaning *ray, rays,* or *radiated structure.*

Ac″ti·no·ba·cil′lus. A genus of the family Parvobacteriaceae; small, Gram-negative bacteria which attack the soft tissues of cattle and swine, causing a disease resembling actinomycosis. Important species of the group are **A. actinoides, A. actino-**

mycetum-comitans, A. lignie-resi.

ac″ti·no·chem′is·try. Branch of chemistry concerned with the reactions produced by light.

ac″ti·nom′e·ter. 1. An apparatus for determining the intensity of actinic rays. 2. A device which determines the degree of penetration of such rays. **–actinometry,** n.

Ac″ti·no·my′ces (ack″ti·no·migh′-seez). A genus of vegetable parasites belonging to the family Actinomycetaceae. They resemble rosettes of fine filaments, each clubbed at the distal end, surrounding a central group of coccus-like spores. Also called ray fungus. **–actinomyce′tic, actino-myce′tous,** adj. **A. bovis.** The organism which produces actinomycosis in man and lumpy jaw in cattle, the majority of cases being reported in the United States. **A. hominis.** The organism thought by some to be the cause of actinomycosis in man, believed by others to be a contaminant. **A. ma-durae.** Synonym for Nocardia madurae. **A. minutissimus.** Synonym for Nocardia minutissima. **A. necro-phorus.** A species found in lung and liver abscesses and in chronic ulcerative colitis in man; produces necrobacillosis in domestic animals.

Ac″ti·no·my″ce·ta′les (·migh″-see·tay′leez). Any of an order of fungi belonging to the class Schizomycetes, consisting of moldlike, rod-shaped, filamentous, or clubbed forms, many showing considerable branching. The order contains three families: Actinomycetaceae, Mycobacteriaceae, and Streptomycetaceae.

ac″ti·no·my·ce′tin (ack″ti·no-migh·see′tin, ·migh′si·tin). An antibacterial substance obtained from several strains of Actinomyces.

ac″ti·no·my′cin A. Antibacterial agent derived from Actinomyces anti-bioticus.

ac″ti·no·my′cin B. Antibacterial substance derived from Actinomyces antibioticus.

ac″ti·no·my·co′ma (ack″ti·no-migh·ko′muh). A tumor produced by the Actinomyces.

ac″ti·no·my·co′sis (·migh·ko′sis). A parasitic, infectious, inoculable disease affecting cattle, hogs, and sometimes communicated to man; caused by Actinomyces bovis and species of Nocardia. The jaw is most commonly involved, although other organs and systems may be infected. The disease is characterized by the formation of slow-growing granulomatous tumors which usually suppurate, discharging a thick oily pus containing yellowish granules, and by constitutional symptoms of sepsis. Also called lumpy jaw, clyers,

wooden tongue. **–actinomycot′ic,** adj.

ac′ti·non. An = 219. Actinium emanation, an isotope of radon. Half-life 3.9 seconds.

ac″ti·no·neu·ri′tis. Neuritis from exposure to x-rays or radium.

ac″ti·no·phy·to′sis (ack″ti·no·figh-to′sis). A disease, usually caused by Micrococcus aureus, characterized by granulomatous abscesses with granules simulating those of actinomycosis or streptothricosis. Syn., botryomycosis.

ac″ti·nos′co·py. Examination of the body by the x-rays. Syn., skiascopy, radioscopy, fluoroscopy, roentgenoscopy.

ac″ti·no·ther′a·py. Therapeutic use of actinic rays or radiant energy, including sunlight, ultraviolet rays, x-rays, and emanations of radium or other radioactive matter. Syn., radio-therapy. **–actinotherapeu′tic,** adj.

ac′tion. 1. Performance of a function or a movement. 2. Application or wielding of a force—physical, chemical, or mental. 3. In pathology, production of a morbid process. Syn., activity. **an-tagonistic a.** (a) Counteraction; opposition. (b) The effect of an opposing agent or principle. See antagonism. **buffer a.** That exhibited by certain chemical substances which, when added to a fluid, tend to maintain its reaction (pH) within narrow limits. **calori-genic a.** (a) Specific dynamic action, q.v. (b) The total heat liberated by a food or food constituent when metabolized by the body. **cumulative a.** Sudden and marked action of a drug after administration of a number of ineffectual or slightly effective doses. **reflex a.** A response of some peripheral organ to stimulation of the sensory branch of a reflex arc, the action occurring immediately, without the aid of the will or without even entering consciousness. Also called automatic a. **specific dynamic a.** The stimulating effect upon the metabolism produced by the ingestion of food, especially proteins, causing the metabolic rate to rise above basal levels. **trig-ger a.** A sudden stimulus which initiates a physiologic or pathologic process having nothing in common with the action that started it. **vital a.** Physiologic activity or functions which are necessary for maintaining life, as the action of the heart, lungs, and vital centers of the brain and spinal cord.

ac″ti·va′tion. 1. Rendering active; the process of activating. 2. Stimulation of general cellular activity by the use of nonspecific therapy; plasma activation. 3. Stimulation of the egg by the sperm or other agents causing cell division. **–ac′tivate,** v.

ac′ti·va″tor. 1. An agent which is necessary to activate another substance, as a coenzyme to an enzyme; applied to biochemical reactions. An enzyme activator is called *coenzyme* or *kinase.* 2. Internal secretion of the pancreas. 3. Substance which stimulates the development of an embryonic structure. Also called *inductor* or *organizer.* 4. Apparatus which charges water with radium emanations. 5. A catalyst.

ac′tive. 1. Energetic, decisive, as active treatment. 2. Due to an intrinsic as distinguished from a passive force, as active hyperemia. 3. *In optics,* possessing the ability to rotate the plane of a polarized light beam. 4. *In psychoanalysis,* pertaining to masculine qualities.

ac·tiv′i·ty. Capacity for acting; sensibility; vitality; potency; energy. **optical a.** The ability of a substance to rotate the plane of vibration of polarized light. It is characteristic of compounds having an asymmetric atom, usually of carbon.

ac′u-. A combining form meaning *needle.*

a·cu′i·ty. 1.Sharpness;clearness;keenness; distinctness, as of vision. 2. *In optics,* sharpness and clarity of a visual image when a lens is in focus. **auditory a.** The degree of acuteness or clearness of hearing. **minimal visual a.** Smallest image to which the brain responds, threshold illumination being present. **visual a.** Extent of visual perception, dependent upon the clarity of the retinal focus, integrity of the nervous elements, and cerebral interpretation of the stimulus. It is tested usually with Snellen's letters at 20 feet.

a·cu′mi·nate. Sharp-pointed; conical; tapering to a point.

ac′u·pres″sure. An operation to stop hemorrhage by compressing the artery with a needle inserted into the tissues upon either side.

ac′u·punc″ture. Puncture of the tissues with long fine needles; used for centuries for relief of neuralgic pain or the release of fluid.

a′cus. A surgical needle.

ac″u·sec′tion. Cutting with an electrosurgical needle.

ac″u·sec′tor. An electric needle, operating on a high-frequency current, which cuts tissues like a scalpel.

a·cus′ti·cus (a·koos′ti·kus). The auditory or eighth cranial nerve.

a·cute′. 1. Sharp; severe. 2. Having a rapid onset, a short course, and pronounced symptoms; not chronic.

a·cute′ness. 1. The quality of being acute, rapid, or sharp. 2. *In ophthalmology,* acuity; keenness of vision.

a·cu′to-. A combining form meaning *acute* or *acutely.*

a·cy″a·nop′si·a. Inability to see blue colors. Also called *acyanoblepsia, acyoblepsia.*

a·cy′cli·a (ay·sigh′klee·uh, ay·sick′lee·uh). State of arrested circulation of body fluids.

a·cy′clic (ay·sigh′click, ay·sick′lick). 1. Not occurring in cycles; not characterized by a self-limited course; nonintermittent. See *cyclic.* 2. *In chemistry,* denoting organic compounds with an open-chain structure; aliphatic. 3. *In botany,* not whorled.

ac″y·e′sis, ac″i·e′sis (ass″ee·ee′sis, ass″eye·ee′sis). 1. Sterility of the female. 2. Nonpregnancy. 3. Incapacity for natural delivery. **—acyet′ic,** *adj.*

ac′yl (ass′il, ass′eel). An organic radical derived by removal of a hydroxyl group (OH) from an organic acid: thus, R.CO is derived from R.CO.OH.

a·cys′ti·a (ay·sis′tee·uh, a·sis′·). Absence of the urinary bladder.

a. d. *Auris dextra;* right ear.

ad-. A prefix signifying to, *toward, near, addition to,* and *more intense.*

-ad. 1. A suffix used to form *collective numerals.* 2. *In chemistry,* a suffix used to form the names of *elements, atoms,* or *radicals.* 3. *In botany,* a suffix used to form the names of *individual members of groups.*

-ad. *In anatomy* and *zoology,* an adverbial suffix indicating *direction toward.*

A. D. A. American Dental Association, American Dietetic Association.

a·dac′ry·a (ay·dack′ree·uh, a·dack′·). Absence or deficiency of tears.

a·dac·tyl′i·a (ay·dack·til′ee·uh, a·dack·). Congenital absence of fingers or toes, or both. **—adac′tylous,** *adj.;* **adac′tylism, adac′tylus,** *n.;* **adac′tyl,** *adj., n.*

adalin. Trade-mark for a brand of carbromal.

Adam's apple. Common term for the laryngeal prominence. Also called *pomum Adami.*

ad″a·man″ti·no·car″ci·no′ma. An adamantinoma that becomes frankly malignant.

ad″a·man″ti·no′ma, ad″a·man·to′ma. Localized epithelial tumor of low malignancy developing from cells of the enamel organ or dental lamina; occurs usually in the jaws, especially the lower jaw, but may be found rarely in the hypophysis or in the tibia. Syn., *ameloblastoma.*

ad′ams·ite (ad′um·zite, ·sight). A poison gas used in chemical warfare; diphenylaminechloroarsine.

adanon. A trade-mark for amidone hydrochloride.

ad″ap·ta′tion. 1. *In biology,* any change in structure, form, or habits to suit a new environment. 2. *In ophthal-*

mology, normal ability of the eye to adjust to varying intensities of light. See *biophotometer*. 3. Immunization, *q.v.* 4. In *reflex* action, decline in the frequency of impulses when the sensory nerve is stimulated repeatedly. 5. In *dentistry*, proper fitting of a denture or accurate adjustment of bands to teeth; close approximation of filling material to the walls of a tooth cavity. 6. In *psychiatry*, those changes experienced by an individual which lead to adjustment. **dark a.** (a) Adjustment of the iris and retina for night vision. (b) A clinical test for the determination of vitamin-A sufficiency; the eye is exposed to a standard light and its adjustment to darkness is measured.

a·dapt'er, a·dap'tor. 1. A device which permits the fitting of one part of an instrument or apparatus to another, as a glass or rubber tube or metal collar. 2. An apparatus which converts the electric current to the form required in the various types of electrotherapy, or for a particular electric appliance.

ad″ap·tom'e·ter. An instrument for measuring the time taken for retinal adaptation or for regeneration of the rhodopsin (visual purple); used to determine the minimum light threshold and to diagnose night blindness.

ad·ax'i·al. On the side of, or directed toward, the axis.

ADC. Anodal duration contraction.

add. A contraction of *adde* or *additur* in prescription writing, meaning *add*, or *let there be added*.

ad'de. Add; a direction used in prescription writing.

ad de·liq'. *Ad deliquium (animi)*; to the point of fainting.

ad'dict. One who is habituated to some practice, especially the alcohol or drug habit. A **drug addict** is one who uses habitually a narcotic drug for the comfort such indulgence affords, and who has no illness or other legitimate reasons for such practice. **–ad·dict'**, *v.t., v.i.;* **addic'tion**, *n.*

Addison, Thomas [*English physician, diagnostician, and teacher*, 1793-1860]. Described pernicious anemia (called *Addison's anemia*) and studied diseases of the ductless glands, particularly the adrenals. Adrenal cortical hypofunction is also known as *Addison's disease, adrenal insufficiency.*

Ad'di·son·ism. A syndrome sometimes present in pulmonary tuberculosis, consisting of dark pigmentation of the skin, loss of weight and strength; somewhat resembles true Addison's disease.

ad·duc'tion. 1. A movement toward the median line or axis of the body or of a part. 2. In *ophthalmology*, turning of the eyes inward from the central

position, through contraction of the medial rectus muscles. This action may be voluntary, but usually is subconscious, following the stimulus of accommodation. The power of adduction, provoked by fixation of the gaze upon an object placed at the near point, is called **convergence-stimulus adduction. –adduct**, *v.*

ad·duc'tor. Any muscle that produces adduction. See Table of Muscles in the Appendix.

ad″en·al'gi·a. Pain due to an inflamed gland or lymph node.

ad'e·nase. A deamidizing enzyme which converts adenine to hypoxanthine. It is secreted by the liver, pancreas, and spleen.

ad″en·ec'to·my. The excision of a gland or lymph node.

a·de'ni·a. A chronic affection of the lymph nodes characterized by marked hypertrophy but no leukocytosis.

a·den'i·form. Glandlike; like a lymph node.

ad'e·nine (ad'i-neen, ·nin). $C_5H_5N_5$. 6-Aminopurine, one of the two purine bases, the other being guanine, occurring in nucleic acids. With D-ribose it forms adenosine, the phosphoric esters of which are of biochemical importance.

ad″e·ni'tis. Inflammation of a gland or lymph node. **cervical a.** One of a number of various inflammatory conditions, acute and chronic, which affect the lymph nodes of the neck, especially in children. It is often secondary to acute infections of the mouth, throat, and ears; to infestation of the scalp by lice; and is associated with contagious diseases, as German measles, measles, scarlet fever, etc. In chronic tuberculosis, leukemias, and syphilis, it occurs as part of a generalized lymph-node involvement. **primitive syphilitic a.** The enlarged lymphatic nodes associated with a primary lesion, which follow a slow indolent course of six months or more.

ad'e·no-, ad'en-. A combining form denoting *gland, glandular,* or *relation to glands.*

ad″e·no·car″ci·no'ma. See under *carcinoma.*

ad″e·no·cel″lu·li'tis. Inflammation of a gland and the surrounding cellular tissue.

ad″e·no·chon·dro'ma (ad″i-no-kon·dro'muh). A tumor consisting of both glandular and cartilaginous tissue.

ad″e·no·chon″dro·sar·co'ma. A tumor composed of adenomatous, chondromatous, and sarcomatous tissue.

ad″e·no·fi·bro'ma (·figh-bro'muh). Combination of adenoma and fibroma frequently occurring in the uterus.

ad″e·no·fi·bro'sis (·figh-bro'sis). Fibroid degeneration of a gland, particularly the replacement fibrosis following inflammation. See *fibrosis*.

ad″e·nog′e·nous (ad″i·nodj′i·nus), **ad″e·no·gen′ic.** Originating from a gland.

ad″e·no·hy·poph′y·sis (ad″i·no·high·pof′i·sis). Anterior or glandular portion of the pituitary body, as differentiated from the posterior neural portion or neurohypophysis. Syn., *pars anterior hypophyseos.*

ad′e·noid. 1. Glandlike; lymphoid. 2. Designating a structure consisting of reticular connective tissue supporting masses of small lymphocytes, as that found in lymph nodes, spleen, tonsils, and other lymphoid organs. *Rare.* 3. Hypertrophied lymphoid tissue often present in the nasopharynx; occurs especially in children. Also called *pharyngeal tonsil.*

ad″e·noi·dec′to·my. The surgical removal of adenoids.

ad′e·noid·ism. Series of changes in respiration, facial contour, and tooth arrangement resulting from the presence of adenoids.

ad″e·noi·di′tis. Inflammation of adenoids.

ad′e·noids. See *adenoid*.

ad″e·no·lei″o·my″o·fi·bro′ma, ad″e·no·li″o·my″o·fi·bro′ma (ad″i·no·lye″o·my″o·figh·bro′muh). A leiomyofibroma containing gland tissue.

ad″e·no·li·po′ma. A combination of adenoma and lipoma.

ad″e·no·lym·pho′ma. Adenoma of a lymph node. See *lymphadenoma*.

ad″e·no′ma. A tumor which in its growth more or less closely reduplicates glandular acini, tubules, or both. **malignant a.** A well-differentiated adenocarcinoma. **renal a.** Acquired or congenital adenoma of the kidney.

ad″e·no·ma·la′ci·a. Abnormal softening of a gland.

ad″e·no′ma·tome. Cutting forceps or scissors for use in the removal of adenomatous growths; surgical instrument for excising adenoids.

ad″e·nom′a·tous, ad″e·nom′a·toid. Pertaining to an adenoma; characteristic of glandular hyperplasia.

ad″e·no·my·o″ma·to′sis (·migh·o″muh·to′sis). Presence of numerous adenomyomas.

ad″e·no·my″o·sar·co′ma. Malignant tumor composed of muscular and glandular elements.

ad″e·no·myx·o′ma. A growth having the characters of glandular and mucous tissues.

ad″e·no·myx″o·sar·co′ma. A rare type of rapidly growing, malignant, mixed tumor arising from glandular and mucous tissue, the latter undergoing sarcomatous change.

ad″e·nop′a·thy. Any glandular disease, especially the swelling and enlargement of lymph nodes.

ad″e·no·phar″yn·gi′tis. Inflammation of the tonsils and pharynx.

ad″e·no·sar·co′ma. A tumor with the characters of adenoma and sarcoma combined.

ad″e·no·sar″co·rhab″do·my·o′ma (·sahr″ko·rab″do·migh·o′muh). A tumor composed of the elements of sarcoma, adenoma, and rhabdomyoma.

ad′e·nose (ad′i·noce, ·noze). Glandular; abounding in glands; glandlike.

a·den′o·sine (a·den′o·seen, ad′i·no·seen″). A mononucleoside composed of adenine and D-ribose produced by the hydrolysis of adenylic acid.

a·den″o·sine·di·phos′phate (·dye·fos′fate). A compound of one molecule each of adenine and D-ribose and two molecules of phosphoric acid. It is involved in the production of energy for muscular and perhaps other types of cellular work. Syn., *ADP*, *adenosinediphosphoric acid.* See *adenosinetriphosphate.*

adenosinediphosphoric acid. Adenosinediphosphate, *q.v.*

a·den″o·sine·mon″o·phos′·phate. A compound of one molecule each of adenine, D-ribose, and phosphoric acid. It occurs in muscle and other tissues, as well as in yeast; that from the former source is adenosine-5-phosphate, while that from the latter is adenosine-3-phosphate. The acid is involved in the release of energy for muscular and perhaps other types of cellular work. Syn., *adenosinemonophosphoric acid, adenylic acid.*

a·den″o·sine·mon″o·phos·phor′ic ac′id. Adenosinemonophosphate, *q.v.*

a·den″o·sine·tri·phos′pha·tase (·try·fos′fuh·tace, ·taze). An enzymatic substance, possibly myosin; causes hydrolysis of adenosinetriphosphate, and presumably releases sufficient energy for muscular contraction and perhaps also for other types of cellular work. Syn., *adenylpyrophosphatase.*

a·den″o·sine·tri·phos′phate. A compound of one molecule each of adenine and D-ribose with three molecules of phosphoric acid. Hydrolysis of it to similar compounds containing one or two molecules of phosphoric acid is accompanied by release of energy for muscular and perhaps other types of cellular work. Syn., *ATP, adenosinetriphosphoric acid, adenylpyrophosphoric acid.* Also called *adenylpyrophosphate.* See *adenosinetriphosphatase.*

a·den″o·sine·tri″phos·phor′ic ac′id. Adenosinetriphosphate, *q.v.*

ad″e·no′sis. 1. Any glandular disease, especially one involving the lymph nodes. 2. Excessive development of glandular tissue.

ad·e·no·tome. 1. An instrument for incising a gland. 2. An instrument for removing adenoids.

ad″en·ot′o·my. Dissection, incision, or surgical removal of a gland.

ad″en·o·vi′rus. A large group of viruses, members of which can be specifically identified by tissue culture, the causative agents of many respiratory diseases. Also see *APC group.*

ad·e′nyl. $C_5H_4N_5$—. The radical present in adenine.

ad″e·nyl′ic ac′id. Adenosinemonophosphate, *q.v.*

ad″e·nyl·py″ro·phos′pha·tase (ad″i·nil·py″ro·fos′fuh·tace, ·taze). Adenosinetriphosphatase.

ad″e·nyl·py″ro·phos′phate. Adenosinetriphosphate, *q.v.*

ad″e·nyl·py″ro·phos·phor′ic ac′id. Adenosinetriphosphate, *q.v.*

ad′eps. 1. Lard; the purified omental fat of the hog. It contains 38% stearin and margarin, and 62% olein; used in ointments. 2. Animal fat. **a. lanae.** Wool fat; the purified, anhydrous, fatty substance from sheep's wool; anhydrous lanolin. **a. lanae hydrosus.** Hydrous wool fat containing 25–30% water; lanolin.

ad·he′sion. 1. *In physics,* molecular force exerted between two surfaces in contact. 2. Abnormal union of an organ or part to another. 3. *In dentistry,* force which holds an upper denture in place without the aid of vacuum cups. —**adher′ent,** *adj.;* **adher′ence,** *n.;* **adhere′,** *v.t., v.i.* **fibrinous a.** Loose attachment of adjacent serous membranes due to the presence of fibrinous exudate. **fibrous a.** Firm attachment of adjacent serous membranes by bands or masses of fibrous connective tissue; due to organization and cicatrization of exudates, resulting from infection or partial destruction of the surfaces.

ad·he″si·ot′o·my (ad·hee″zee·ot′o·mee). Surgical cutting or division of adhesions.

ad·he′sive. 1. Sticky; tenacious; tending to cling or stick. 2. Resulting in or attended with adhesion. 3. A plaster or emplastrum.

a·di″a·pho·ret′ic. 1. Reducing, checking, or preventing perspiration; anhidrotic. 2. Any such agent or drug. —**adiaphore′sis,** *n.*

a″di·as′to·le (ay″dye·ass′to·lee, ad″eye·). Absence or imperceptibility of diastole.

a·dip′ic. Of, or belonging to, fat.

ad′i·po-, adip·. A combining form denoting *fats, fatty tissue.* See also *lipo-.*

ad′i·po·cele″ (ad′i·po·seel″). A true hernia with hernial sac, containing only fatty tissue. Also called *lipocele.*

ad′i·po·cere″ (ad′i·po·seer″). A waxlike substance which occurs during the decomposition of dead animal tissues (corpses) at suitable temperatures, in the presence of moisture, and in the absence of air, as under earth or water. It consists chiefly of fatty acids and their salts. —**adipocer′atous,** *adj.*

ad″i·po′ma. A fatty tumor; lipoma.

ad″i·po·ne·cro′sis ne″o·na·to′rum. Necrosis of fatty tissue. A self-limiting, localized process, occurring usually in large, well-nourished infants born after difficult labor, characterized by bluish red lesions, becoming manifest 2 to 20 days after birth as deep subcutaneous indurations, and disappearing completely within four months.

ad′i·pose. Fatty, fatlike, fat.

ad″i·po′sis. 1. Corpulence; obesity. 2. Excessive accumulation of fat in the body, local or general; fatty infiltration. Syn., *adiposity.* **a. dolorosa.** A disease marked by deposition of symmetrical masses of fat in various parts accompanied by more or less pain. It affects women oftener and may cause death from pulmonary complications. Also called *Dercum's disease.*

ad″i·po·si′tis. Inflammation in the subcutaneous fatty tissue.

ad″i·pos′i·ty. See *adiposis.*

ad″i·po″so·gen′i·tal. Pertaining to superficial fat of the body and the external genitalia, as adiposogenital dystrophy.

ad″i·po·su′ri·a. Presence of fat in the urine; lipuria.

a·dip′sa (ay·dip′suh, a·dip′suh). 1. Remedies to allay thirst. 2. Foods which do not produce thirst.

a·dip′si·a (ay·dip′see·uh, a·dip′·). **a·dip′sy.** Absence of thirst; avoidance of drinking.

ad′i·tus. *In anatomy,* an entrance. **a. ad antrum.** Outer side of the attic, opening upward, backward, and outward into the mastoid antrum. It gives lodgment to the head of the malleus and the greater part of the incus.

ad·just′ment. 1. Mechanism of a microscope which brings the objective into focus. 2. Chiropractic treatment aimed at reduction of subluxated vertebrae. 3. *In biology,* changes undergone by a plant or animal better to adapt it to the environment. 4. *In psychology,* the establishment of a relationship between the individual and his environment. **absolute a.** Accommodation of each eye, considered alone. Also called *absolute accommodation.* **mental a.** *In psychology,* an adjustment involving an individual's attitudes, traits, or feelings. Also called *intrapsychic a.* **social a.** *In psychiatry,* adaptation of an individual to society and to his social environment.

ad·jus'tor. The central neuron, or neurons, of a reflex arc in the nervous system.

ad'ju·vant. 1. An auxiliary medication; one which is added to enhance the action of a drug. Syn., *synergist.* 2. Assisting the activity of a medicament.

ad lib. *Ad libitum;* at pleasure; the amount desired.

ad·mis'sion rate. Number of admissions to a hospital per thousand of population; often refers to a military population.

ad·mix'ture. 1. That which is added to something to make a mixture; the mixture so made. 2. The act of making a mixture or of mixing.

ad'nate. Congenitally attached or united.

ad nau'se·am (ad naw'shee·um, ·see·um). To the point of producing nausea.

ad·nex'a. Accessory parts or appendages of an organ. Also called *annexa.*
—adnexal, *adj.* **a. uteri.** The uterine tubes and the ovaries.

ad"o·les'cence. The youth period, extending from puberty to maturity.
—adolescent, *adj., n.*

ad·o'ral. Situated near the mouth; toward the mouth.

ADP. Adenosinediphosphate, *q.v.*

ad·re'nal. 1. The adrenal gland, *q.v.* 2. Pertaining to the adrenal gland.

ad·re'nal cor'tex. Cortical substance of the adrenal gland.

ad·re'nal cor'ti·cal hy"po·func'tion. A progressively fatal disease due to a deficiency of the adrenal cortex, usually from tuberculous infection. Characterized by anemia, marked weakness and prostration, low blood pressure, feeble heart action, frequent dizziness, and fainting. There are also gastrointestinal disorders, nervous irritability, psychic changes, and often bronzing of the skin and pigmentation of the mucous membranes. Death occurs in two to three years. Also called *Addison's disease, asthenia pigmentosa, melanoma suprarenale, bronzed skin.*

ad·re'nal·ec'to·mize. Remove the adrenal glands, or an adrenal gland, surgically. **—adrenalectomized,** *adj.;* **adrenalectomy,** *n.*

adrenalin. Trade-mark for epinephrine, *q.v.*

adrenalin chloride. Trade-mark for epinephrine hydrochloride.

ad·re"nal·in·e'mi·a, ad·re"nal·in·ae'mi·a. Presence of epinephrine (adrenalin) in the blood.

ad·re"nal·in·u'ri·a. Presence of epinephrine (adrenalin) in the urine.

ad·re'nal·ism. A condition due to dysfunction of the adrenal gland. See *hyperadrenalism.* Also called *suprarenalism.*

ad·re"na·li'tis, ad"re·ni'tis. Inflammation of the adrenal glands.

ad"ren·er'gic. Designating nerve fibers, mostly postganglionic sympathetic, which produce at their terminals a substance called sympathin, similar to epinephrine (adrenalin).

ad·re'no·chrom, ad·re'no·chrome. $C_9H_9O_3N$. A quinone-type oxidation product of epinephrine. It has the power of controlling capillary bleeding.

ad·re"no·cor"ti·co·tro'phic. See *adrenocorticotropic.*

ad·re"no·cor"ti·co·tro'pic. Affecting the adrenal cortex; denoting a hormone of the adenohypophysis, which stimulates the adrenal cortex.

ad·re"no·lyt'ic. Pertaining to an activity or effect opposed to the action of epinephrine (adrenalin); the opposite of *adrenergic.*

ad"ren·os'te·rone (ad"ren·os'ti·rohn, ad"ri·nos'·). A steroid hormone with androgenic properties; obtained from the adrenal cortex.

ad·re"no·tro'phic. 1. Nourishing the adrenal gland. 2. Incorrectly used for adrenocorticotropic, *q.v.*

ad"re·no·tro'pism. Dominance of the adrenal in endocrine activities.

a·dro'mi·a. Complete failure of impulse conduction in muscle or nerve.

ad·sor'bate. The substance which is adsorbed.

ad·sorb'ent. Any substance which produces adsorption, as activated charcoal, silica gel. See *adsorption.*

ad·sorp'tion. 1. The power possessed by certain substances (*adsorbents*) of taking up fluids, apart from capillary attraction. 2. The process whereby a solid (*adsorbent*) attracts and concentrates upon its surface, in a thin layer, molecules of a gas, liquid, or dissolved substance (*adsorbate*) by adhesion.
—adsorptive, *adj.;* **adsorb',** *v.t., v.i.*

a·dult', ad'ult. 1. Mature; having attained full size and strength; of full legal age. 2. A person of mature age.

a·dul'ter·ant. Any substance that adulterates.

a·dul"ter·a'tion. Admixture or substitution of inferior, impure, inert, or cheaper ingredients for gain, deception, or concealment. **—adul'terate,** *v.t.*

ad·vance', ad·vance'ment. 1. A tenotomy followed by reattachment of the tendon at a more advanced point. 2. *In ophthalmology,* operative correction of strabismus. The muscle tendon opposite to the direction of the squint is removed at its insertion and sutured to the sclera anterior to the original attachment. A modification in which the shortened muscle, rather than its tendon, is attached anterior to the stump, is called **Lancaster's ad-vancement.**

ad″ven·ti·ti·a (ad″ven·tish′ee·uh). The external covering of an organ derived from adjacent connective tissue, as the external coat of a blood vessel or other organ.

ad″ven·ti′tious (ad″ven·tish′us). 1. Accidental, foreign, acquired, as opposed to natural or hereditary. 2. Occurring in unusual or abnormal places. 3. Pertaining to the adventitia.

ae-. For words beginning with ae- not found here, see under e-.

A·ë′des (ay·ee′deez). A genus of mosquitoes, belonging to the family Culicidae, having cosmopolitan distribution. Many species are noxious and troublesome biters. In North America, the species **A. vexans** is found near fresh water; **A. aldrichi, A. dorsalis, A. sollicitans, A. squamiger,** and **A. taeniorhynchus** are found near salt marshes. **A. aegypti** is the principal vector of yellow fever and dengue. It has urban breeding habits.

-ae′mi·a. Same as -emia.

ae′quum (ee′kwum). Amount of food necessary to maintain weight with normal physical activity. It varies with the individual's size and the nature of his activity.

a′er·ate. Charge with air or gas; oxygenate, carbonate, etc.; arterialize. **—aerated,** adj.; **aerator,** n.

a″er·a′tion. 1. Exposure to air. 2. Saturation of a fluid with air or a gas, as carbon dioxide. 3. Conversion of venous to arterial blood.

a·e′ri·al (ay·eer′ee·ul, air′ee·ul). Pertaining to the air, as aerial conduction, hearing through air vibrations.

a′er·i·form (ay′ur·i·form″). Airlike; gaseous.

a′er·o- (ay′ur·o-, air′o-), **aer-.** A combining form denoting air, aerial, or gas, gases.

a″er·o·an·a″er·o′bic (ay″ur·o·an·ay″ur·o′bick, -ob′ick). Applied to organisms which are both aerobic and anaerobic.

A″er·o·bac′ter. A genus of nonpathogenic, Gram-negative, saprophytic bacteria of the Enterobacteriaceae.

a′er·obe. A microörganism which requires air as free oxygen for the maintenance of life. Also called aerobion.

a″er·o′bic (ay″ur·o′bick, -ob′ick), **a″er·o′bi·an.** 1. Requiring air or free oxygen in order to live. 2. Relating to or produced by aerobes.

a″er·o·bi·o′sis (ay″ur·o·buy·o′sis). Life that requires the presence of air, or free oxygen. **—aerobiot′ic,** adj.

a′er·o·cele″ (ay′ur·o·seel″). A tumor caused by the escape of air into an adventitious pouch usually connected with the trachea or larynx, hence its size may vary with respiration. Also called tracheocele, laryngocele, pneumatocele.

a″er·o·col′pos. Distention of the vagina with air or gas.

a″er·o·cys·tos′co·py. Examination of the interior of the urinary bladder with a cystoscope, the bladder being distended with air. **—aerocys′to-scope,** n.

a″er·o·duc′tor. Apparatus to prevent asphyxia of the fetus when the aftercoming head is retained.

a″er·o·dy·nam′ics (ay″ur·o·dye-nam′icks, air″o-). The branch of physics that deals with gases in motion.

a″er·o·em′bo·lism. A condition caused by an abrupt drop from normal to low atmospheric pressure; occurs in aviators in rapid ascents to high altitudes; marked by the formation of nitrogen bubbles in the blood and body tissues. Symptoms include severe pain in the joints and chest, itching of the skin, pulmonary edema, urticaria, paralysis, convulsions, and sometimes coma. Symptoms may be relieved by descent to lower altitude. Syn., aeroemphysema, chokes, decompression sickness. Also see caisson disease.

a″er·o·em″phy·se′ma (-em″fi·see′-muh, -em″figh-). Aeroembolism, q.v.

a′er·o·gen″. Any gas-producing microörganism.

a″er·o·gen·e·sis. Gas formation. **—aerogenic, aerog′enous,** adj.

a′er·o·gram″. An x-ray film of an organ inflated with air.

a″er·o·neu·ro′sis. A form of psychoneurosis found in aviators, characterized by anxiety, restlessness, and various physical manifestations.

a″er·o·ö·ti′tis me′di·a. Traumatic inflammation of the middle ear, occurring during changes of altitude in airplane flights; caused by differences in the pressure of the air in the tympanic cavity and the surrounding atmosphere. It is characterized by pain, congestion, and inflammation, and may be followed by temporary or permanent injury to the hearing. Syn., aviator's ear, otic barotrauma.

a″er·op′a·thy. Any pathologic condition brought about by changes in atmospheric pressure, as caisson disease or aeroembolism.

a″er·o·pha′gi·a, a″er·oph′a·gy. Imbibing and swallowing of air followed by noisy eructations, especially in hysterical patients. Aspiration of air by the rectum is called **rectal aero-phagia.**

a′er·o·phil″. 1. Loving the open air. 2. Aerobic.

a″er·o·pho′bi·a. Morbid fear of drafts or of fresh air.

a′er·o·phore″. 1. Device for inflating the lungs with air in the case of a still-born child or in any case of asphyxia. 2. Apparatus which purifies air for rebreathing, used by firemen and others.

a'er·o·scope". Instrument for the examination of dust in the air and for estimating the purity of the air.

a"er·o·si"nus·i'tis (ay"ur·o·sigh"-nuh·sigh'tis, ·sigh"new·sigh'tis). An acute or chronic inflammation of one or more of the nasal accessory sinuses; caused by a difference in barometric pressure between the gas inside the sinus and that of the surrounding atmosphere.

a'er·o·sol". 1. Atomized particles suspended in the air. 2. Any solution or compressed gas containing an agent for the treatment of the air to remove or destroy insects or microörganisms. 3. In chemistry, a colloid in which gas is the dispersion medium.

aerosol OT dry. Trade-mark for dioctyl sodium sulfosuccinate.

aerosporin. Trade-mark for an antibiotic substance, now called polymyxin B, produced by a soil organism. See polymyxin.

a"er·o·ther"a·peu'tics, a"er·o·ther'a·py. A mode of treating disease by varying the pressure or the composition of the air breathed.

a·er·ot'ro·pism. The inherent tendency of an organism to be attracted to a supply of air, as various bacteria and protozoa collect about an air bubble. —aerotrop'ic, adj.

a"er·o·u·re'thro·scope. A modified endoscope which permits viewing the urethra after it is inflated with air. —aerourethros'copy, n.

Aesculapius. See Asclepius.

aes·thet'ic. Same as esthetic.

aes'ti·val (es'ti·vul, eh·sty'vul). See estival.

aet. Aetatis; of age.

a·fe'brile (ay·fee'bril, ay·feb'ril). Without fever.

af'fect. In psychology, feeling; emotion as it influences a mental state or idea (Freud); the feeling element in emotion; mood.

af·fect"a·bil'i·ty. Capacity for responding to stimulation.

af"fec·ta'tion. Artificiality of manner or behavior.

af·fec'tion. 1. Any pathologic state or condition. 2. In psychology, the emotional factor in consciousness. —affective, adj.

af"fec·tiv'i·ty. 1. Susceptibility to emotional stimuli. 2. In psychology, that part of consciousness comprising affection and affect.

af'fer·ent. Carrying toward; centripetal.

af·fil"i·a'tion. In legal medicine, imputing or fixing the paternity of a child in order to provide for its maintenance.

af·fi'nal, af'fi·nal. 1. Connected through marriage. 2. Having the same origin.

af·fin'i·ty. 1. Inherent attraction and relationship. 2. In biology, the relationship between members of species or more specialized groups, which depends upon their mutual resemblance in structure and form, indicating a similarity of origin. **chemical a.** The force of attraction between atoms which causes them to enter into and maintain certain combinations. **genetic a.** Relationship by direct descent. **morbid a.** The tendency for certain affections to exist simultaneously with, or as sequels of, a particular disease. **vital a.** The selective action or chemotaxis exhibited by the several tissues of an organism for their particular pabulum.

af"fir·ma'tion. During autosuggestion, the stage in which the subject acquires a positive reactive tendency; facilitation of positive reaction tendency.

af'flux, af·flux'ion. Flow of blood or other fluid to a part. Syn., congestion. —af'fluent, adj.; af'fluence, n.

af·fu'sion. Pouring of water upon a part or upon the body, as in fever, to reduce temperature and calm nervous symptoms. The method of treating fevers by pouring cold water over the patient is called **cold affusion.**

aflorone acetate. A trade-mark for fludrocortisone acetate.

aft'er·birth". The placenta and membranes; normally expelled from the uterus following birth of the child.

aft'er·brain". The myelencephalon.

aft'er·care". Care or nursing of convalescents, especially the postoperative treatment of surgical patients. Syn., aftertreatment.

aft'er·cat"a·ract. 1. A portion of lens substance or of lens capsule retained after the extraction of an extracapsular cataract. 2. Any membrane in the area of the pupil following removal or absorption of the lens. Syn., secondary cataract.

aft'er·damp". A poisonous mixture of gases, containing carbon dioxide, found in coal mines after an explosion of inflammable gases.

aft'er·ef·fect". A delayed response to a stimulus or agent, appearing only after the subsidence of the primary response.

aft'er·hear"ing. A sensation of hearing a sound after the stimulus which produces it has ceased; may be a symptom of some neuroses.

aft'er·im"age. A retinal impression continued after the stimulus of the light or image has ceased to act. A **positive afterimage** is a simple prolongation of the sensation; a **negative afterimage** is the appearance of the image in complementary colors. Syn., *accidental image*.

aft'er-pains". Pains from uterine contractions following delivery.

aft'er-sen-sa"tion. A sensation lasting longer than the stimulus producing it.

aft'er-treat"ment. See *aftercare*.

aft'er-vi"sion. Perception of an afterimage.

a-func'tion (ay-funk'shun, a-funk'-shun). Loss or lack of function. **—afunctional,** *adj.*

Ag. *Argentum;* silver.

ag"a-lor-rhe'a, ag"a-lor-rhoe'a. A cessation of the flow of milk.

a-gam'ete. Any protozoan which reproduces asexually.

a-gam'ic, ag'a-mous. *In biology,* asexual; reproducing without sexual union, or asexually.

a'gar (ay'gahr, ag'ahr). 1. A seaweed of the genus *Gelideum,* especially *G. cartilagineum.* 2. Any of various culture mediums containing agar-agar.

a'gar-a'gar. 1. A dried mucilaginous extract obtained from certain species of seaweeds, especially agar; used in bacteriology to solidify culture mediums. Used as laxative because of its marked increase in bulk when moist. 2. See *agar*.

a-gar'ic (a-gar'ick, ag'ur-ick). Touchwood; spunk; tinder; the product of different Basidiomycetes, mostly *Polyporus.* **fly a.** Poisonous mushroom which contains the alkaloid muscarine. Also called *Amanita muscaria.*

A-gar'i-cus. A large genus of fungi. **A. campestris.** The common, nonpoisonous or edible mushroom. **A. muscarius.** Fly agaric, *q.v.*

age. 1. The time elapsed from birth to the present in a living individual. 2. A particular period of life distinguished by development, equilibrium, or involution; especially old age. 3. *In psychology,* a measure of development expressed in terms of the age of an average individual of an equivalent development. 4. Grow old. 5. Ripen artificially, as wine. **achievement a.** Educational accomplishment expressed as equivalent to the age in years of the average child showing similar attainments; determined by tests. Also see accomplishment *quotient.* **a. of consent.** *In legal medicine,* the age at which a minor is considered capable of legally assenting to marriage or to sexual intercourse, varying from 13 years upward according to statute. **anatomic a.** Age as judged by body development. **Binet a.** Mental age as estimated by Binet tests. **bone a.** Age as judged roentgenologically from bone development, when compared with the

normal ossification for that chronologic age. **climacteric a.** The time of the cessation of menstruation. **mental a.** The score obtained on an intelligence test. An adult whose score is the equivalent of that of a normal child of 12 has a mental age of 12. **physiologic a.** Age as judged by the functional development.

ag"e-ne'si-a, a-gen'e-sis. 1. Incomplete and imperfect development. Aplasia. 2. Impotence, barrenness. **—agenet'ic,** *adj.*

a-gen'i-tal-ism. Symptom complex found in persons who lack testes or ovaries.

a'gent. 1. Any force, substance, or person that exerts an action to produce an effect. 2. Any substance, such as a chemical or a medicinal, capable of effecting a reaction or change in an organism.

a"ge-ra'si-a (ay"juh-ray'see-uh, adj"uh-). Vigorous, healthy old age.

a-geu'si-a (ag-yoo'see-uh, a-jew'see-uh), **a-geus'ti-a** (ag-yoos'tee-uh, a-juice'tee-uh). Loss or impairment of the sense of taste. When due to a cortical lesion, it is called **central ageusia;** when due to a disorder of the nerve endings, **peripheral ageusia;** when due to a lesion in the nerve between its origin and distribution, **conduction ageusia.**

ag'ger (ag'ur). *In anatomy,* a projection, eminence, or mound. **a. nasi.** An oblique ridge on the inner surface of the nasal process of the maxilla; the anterior part of the ethmoidal crest.

ag-glu"ti-na'tion. A joining together; an aggregation of suspended particles. **—agglu'tinable, agglu'tinative,** *adj.* **specific a.** Reaction between the suspension of an antigen (bacteria or cells) and its specific antiserum, leading to the clumping of the suspended elements. Used in the diagnosis of certain diseases, as the Widal test for typhoid.

ag-glu'ti-nin. An antibody occurring in a normal or immune serum which, when added to a suspension of its homologous, particulate antigen, causes the antigen elements to adhere to one another, forming clumps. **anti-Rh a.** The anti-Rhesus agglutinin is not found normally in humans, but may occur in Rh-negative mothers, or mothers carrying an Rh-positive fetus, or in an Rh-negative patient treated with multiple transfusions, including Rh-positive blood. **chief a.** An agglutinating antibody in the blood of an individual immunized against a specific disease or microörganism. It is active at higher dilutions than are the group or partial agglutinins. Syn., *major a.* **group a.** One which acts as a specific toward one species and which will agglutinate other related species. Syn., *minor a., partial a.* **major a.** See chief *a.* **minor a.** An agglutinin acting on other organisms related to the one utilized for immunization, but in lower dilution. Also called *group a.*

ag″glu·tin′o·gen (ag″lew-tin′-o·jen, a·glew′tin-o·jen). An antigen which, when injected into the animal body, stimulates the formation of a specific agglutinin. This, in turn, has the capacity to agglutinate the antigen.

ag·glu′ti·noid. 1. An agglutinin which has lost its zymophore group through the action of heat, age, acids, etc., but still possesses its haptophore group. 2. An agglutinin which, as the result of certain chemical or physical treatment, has lost the ability to clump its homologous antigen but retains the capacity to combine with it.

ag·glu″ti·no·phore″. Factor present in an agglutinin, which causes clumping; the zymophore of an agglutinin.

ag″gre·gate. 1. Grouped into a mass; agminate. 2. The mass formed by certain antibodies and their homologous antigens; a clump.

ag″gre·ga′tion. Agmination; a massing together of materials; a congeries or collection of particles, parts, or bodies, usually of a similar nature.

ag·gres′sion. *In psychiatry,* an act or attitude of hostility, commonly arising out of frustration or inferiority.

ag′i·tat″ed de·pres′sion. A type of manic-depressive or involutional psychosis; characterized by marked restlessness, continual activity, despondency, and anxiety.

ag′i·ta″tion. 1. Fatiguing restlessness with violent motion. 2. Mental disturbance. 3. Stirring or shaking a mixture, as in pharmacy.

ag″i·to·graph′i·a (adj″i·to·graf′-ee-uh). A condition characterized by excessive speed in writing, with unconscious omissions of words, syllables, or letters.

ag″i·to·pha′si·a (adj″i·to·fay′zhuh, -xee-uh). A condition marked by excessive rapidity of speech, with sounds or syllables unconsciously slurred, omitted, or distorted.

a·glan′du·lar. Having no glands; without glands, as the brain.

a·glau·cop′si·a, a·glau·kop′si·a (ay·glaw-cop′see-uh, a·glaw-). Green blindness. See color *blindness.*

a″glo·mer′u·lar (ay″glo·merr′yoo-lur, ag″lo-). Without glomeruli, as aglomerular kidney.

a·glos′si·a (ay·glos′ee-uh, a·glos′-). 1. Congenital absence of the tongue. 2. Loss of the ability to speak; mutism.

a·glos′sus (ay·glos′us, a·glos′us). A person without a tongue.

a·glu′cone (a·glue′cone, a·glue′-cone). 1. An older term for the nonsugar portion of a glycoside, now called aglycone. 2. The nonsugar portion of a glucoside, *q.v.*

ag″lu·ti′tion (ag″loo-tish′un). Difficulty in swallowing; inability to swallow; dysphagia.

a·gly·ce′mic (ay·gly·see′mick, a·gly-). Having no sugar in the blood. **—agly·ce′mia,** *n.*

a·gly′cone (ay·gly′cone, a·gly′cone). The nonsugar portion of a glycoside. Also called *genin.*

a·gly″co·su′ric (ay·gly″ko·sue′rick, a·gly″ko-). Free from glycosuria; exhibiting no urinary sugar. **—aglyco·su′ria,** *n.*

ag′mi·nate, ag′mi·nat″ed. Gathered into clumps or clusters; aggregate, as agminated lymph nodules of the intestine.

ag·na′thi·a. Absence or deficient development of the jaws. **—ag′na·thous,** *adj.;* **ag′nathus, ag′nathy,** *n.*

ag·ne′a, ag·noe′a. A condition in which the patient does not recognize things or persons.

ag″no·gen′ic. Of unknown etiology.

ag·no′si·a. Total or partial loss of the perceptive faculty by which persons and things are recognized. It is commonly classified as **auditory agnosia, optic agnosia, tactile agnosia,** etc., according to the sense or senses affected.

ag·nos′ter·ol. $C_{20}H_{47}OH$. A complex terpene alcohol found in wool fat.

-a·gogue. A combining form meaning *inducing, dispelling,* or *guiding.*

ag′o·nal. Struggling; relating to the death struggle or to agony.

ag′o·nist. A contracting muscle engaged in the movement of a part and opposed by an antagonistic muscle. Thus, when flexing the elbow, the biceps is the *agonist* and the triceps is the *antagonist.* Also called *protagonist.*

ag′o·ny. 1. Violent pain; extreme anguish. 2. The death struggle.

ag″o·ra·pho′bi·a. Morbid fear of open places or spaces, as opposed to claustrophobia, *q.v.*

-ag′ra. A combining form denoting *gout,* a gouty *affection,* or a *seizure of pain.*

Agramonte y Simoni, Aristide [Cuban *parasitologist,* 1869–1931]. Member with Reed, Carroll, and Lazear of the U. S. Army Yellow Fever Commission which proved that yellow fever is transmitted to man by mosquitoes (1900–01).

a·gran′u·lo·cyte″ (ay·gran′yoo-lo-sight″, a·gran′-). A nongranular leukocyte. **—agranulocyt′ic,** *adj.*

a·gran″u·lo·cy·to′sis (a·gran″-yoo-lo-sigh-to′sis, ay·gran″yoo-lo-). An acute febrile disease, affecting females oftener than males, frequently caused by coal-tar drugs and some of the sulfonamides. It is characterized by prostration, high fever, ulcerative lesions of the mucous membranes in the mouth, throat, and other areas, and a marked reduction of the granular leukocytes. Syn., *agranulocytic angina, granulocytopenia.*

a·graph'i·a (ay-graf'ee-uh, a·graf'·). Loss of ability to write; a form of aphasia. **amnemonic a.** Inability to write connected sentences, although letters and words can be written. **motor a.** Loss of ability to write because of ataxia. **verbal a.** Inability to write words, although single letters can be written.

ag"ro·ma'ni·a. A morbid desire to live in the open country or in isolation; occasionally occurs in schizophrenia.

ag"ryp·not'ic. Inducing, relating to, or characterized by insomnia.

a'gue (ayg'yŏŏ). 1. Old term for an attack of malaria. 2. A recurrent chill. 3. Neuralgia, as **face ague,** tic douloureux. **a. cake.** The enlarged spleen of chronic malaria. **brass founder's a.** Severe chills which follow the inhalation of fumes of finely divided metal, especially fumes of cadmium, lead, manganese, mercury, magnesium, and zinc (brass). Syn., *metal fume fever, galvo.* **catenating a.** Chills associated with other diseases. **dumb a.** Subacute malaria without definite chills, and only slight periodicity.

a·gy'ri·a (ay-jy'ree-uh, a·jy'·). Congenital absence of cerebral convolutions.

aich"mo·pho'bi·a (ayk"mo-fo'bee-uh, ike"mo·). Morbid dread of sharp or pointed objects, or of being touched by them or by a finger.

ail'ing. Indisposed; in ill health; not well.

ail'ment. A disease; sickness; complaint.

ai·lu"ro·pho'bi·a (ay-lew"ro-fo'-bee-uh, eye"lew-ro·). A morbid fear of cats.

ain'hum (ayn'hum, in'yoom). A tropical disease peculiar to male Negroes, in which a toe is slowly and spontaneously amputated by a fibrous ring. Etiology unknown. Syn., *dactylolysis spontanea.*

air. Atmospheric air is a simple nonchemical mixture of gases 78.03 parts by volume or 75.51 parts by weight of nitrogen, 20.98 parts by volume or 23.15 parts by weight of oxygen, and 0.03 part by volume of carbon dioxide. Air also contains small amounts of ammonia, nitrates, organic matter, and the rare gases argon, neon, krypton, and xenon. By virtue of its oxygen content it is able to sustain respiration.

Syn., *atmosphere.* **alveolar a.** That contained in the air sacs and alveoli. **complemental a.** The amount that can still be inhaled after a normal inspiration. **expired a.** That which is exhaled from the lungs by expiration. **inspired a.** That which is taken in by inspiration. **liquid a.** That which has been liquefied by subjecting it to great pressure; extreme cold is produced by its evaporation. **minimal a.** The small amount left in an excised or collapsed lung. **reserve a.** That which can be expelled after a normal exhalation. Also called *supplemental a.* **residual a.** That remaining in the lungs after the most complete expiration possible. **stationary a.** That remaining in the lungs during normal respiration. **supplemental a.** See under reserve *a.* **tidal a.** That inhaled and exhaled during normal respiration.

air con·di'tion·ing. The modification of the air—by the control of its temperature and humidity, the removal of particulate water, and the sterilization of pathogenic organisms—for better health, bodily comfort, and industrial needs.

air my·e·log'ra·phy. Radiographic examination of the spinal cord after injecting air into the subarachnoid space.

air pi'lots' dis·ease'. Acute emotional shock; aeroneurosis.

air'sick"ness. A form of motion sickness occurring in airplane flights, principally as a result of acceleration; characterized by vertigo, nausea, headache, mental depression and anxiety, pallor, cold sweats, tremor, and vomiting; a feeling of nervous and muscular tenseness is followed by muscular weakness, faintness, and prostration. Airsickness is the same as seasickness and car sickness in etiology and symptoms, but should not be confused with altitude sickness, *q.v.*

air'way". 1. *In anesthesia,* any of several devices used to maintain a clear and unobstructed respiratory passage during general anesthesia. 2. A respiratory passage. **endobronchial a.** One extending down to one of the bronchi. **endotracheal a.** One extending into the trachea. **nasal a.** One through the nose. **oral a.** One through the mouth. **pharyngeal a.** One extending down into the pharynx.

ak-. For words beginning with *ak-* not found here, see under *ac-.*

ak"a·thi'si·a (ack"uth·ee'zhuh, ack"uth-izh'uh). A condition seen in paralysis agitans; because of the severe muscular rigidity, the patient is compelled to change position at frequent intervals or to rise and pace the floor.

ak"i·ne'si·a (ack"i·nee'shuh, ·zhuh).

ak″i·ne′sis. Akinesia. Loss of or impaired motor function; immobility from any cause.

a·kin″es·the′si·a, a·kin″aes·the′si·a (ay·kin″ess·thee′zhuh, a·kin″·), **a·ki·naes′thi·a** (ay·ki·ness′thee·uh, a·ki·). Loss of muscle sense or movement sense.

Al. Chemical symbol for aluminum.

al-. A combining form from *all*.

al-. A combining form from the Arabic definite article *the*.

al-. A form of *ad-* assimilated in Latin before *l*.

-al. *In chemistry,* a suffix indicating the presence of the aldehyde group.

-al. An adjective suffix denoting *belonging to, of* or *pertaining to, having the character of, appropriate to.*

a′la (pl. *alae*). 1. A wing. 2. Any winglike process. —**alar, al′iform, al·ate,** *adj.* **a. of the sacrum.** Flat, triangular surface of bone extending outward from the base of the sacrum.

al″a·bam′ine (al″uh·bam′een, ·in). A rare element found in monazite sand; now called astatine, *q.v.*

al′a·bas″ter. 1. Hydrous calcium sulfate. 2. Calcium carbonate.

a·la′li·a. 1. Impairment or loss of speech due to any organic defect or paralysis. 2. Aphasia due to psychic disorder. —**alal′ic,** *adj.* **mental a.** Speech impairment caused by stammering, especially in children. Also called *relative a.*

al′a·nine (al′uh·neen, ·nin). CH₃·CH(NH₂)COOH. Alpha-aminopropionic acid. It is a constituent of many proteins and is also prepared synthetically. Also called *lactamic acid, lactamine.*

al″a·nyl·gly·cine′ (al″uh·nil·glyseen′, ·glye′seen). A dipeptide formed by the combination of two amino acids, alanine and glycine.

alb-. Same as *albo-.*

al′ba. 1. The white fibrous tissue of the brain; the white matter as opposed to the gray. 2. White.

albamycin. A trade-mark for novobiocin.

Albee, Fred Houdlett [*American surgeon,* 1876–1945]. Noted for his application of mechanical methods to bone operations; for his method of stabilizing tuberculous or fractured spines by the insertion of a tibial graft into the split spinous processes of the vertebrae (spinal fusion); for his bundle-of-reeds technic in which parallel strips of bone are taken from the tibia and used as a bone graft; and for his fracture table, which has had wide use in orthopedic surgery. See also Albee's *saw.*

al′bi·cans (al′bi·kanz) (pl. *albicantia*). 1. White; whitish. 2. One of the corpora albicantia of the ovary.

al″bi·du′ri·a, al″bi·nu′ri·a. 1. Passage of very pale, almost colorless urine, of low specific gravity. 2. Chyluria.

al′bi·nism, al″bi·nis′mus (al″bi·niz′mus), **al·bi′no·ism** (al·buy′no·iz·um, al·bee′no·). Congenital absence of pigment from the skin, hair, choroid coat, and iris. It may be localized, in **partial albinism,** or generalized, in **total albinism.** The latter form is associated with astigmatism, nystagmus, and photophobia. Also called *leukoderma, achromoderma, congenital achroma, achromatosis.*

al·bi′no (al·buy′no, al·bee′no). A person affected with albinism. —**albinot′ic,** *adj.*

al′bo-, alb-. A combining form meaning *white, whitish.*

al″bu·gin′e·a. 1. White or whitish. 2. A layer of white fibrous tissue investing an organ or part. **a. testis.** Tunica albuginea of the testis.

al″bu·gin′e·ous. 1. Whitish. 2. Belonging to a tunica albuginea.

al·bu′men. 1. Egg white, consisting chiefly of albumin. 2. The stored food matter in a vegetable seed. 3. Albumin, *q.v.*

al·bu′min. One of a group of protein substances, the chief constituents of animal tissues. They are soluble in water, coagulable by heat, and composed of carbon, hydrogen, nitrogen, oxygen, and sulfur. —**albuminous,** *adj.* **derived a.** Modified albumin resulting from action of certain reagents upon native albumin. **lactalbumin.** The albumin found in milk. **native a.** Any albumin occurring normally in the tissues. **serum a.** The chief protein of blood plasma and other serous fluids. See Table of Normal Values of Blood Constituents in the Appendix. **urinary a.** Serum albumin, globulin, and other proteins occurring in the urine to produce albuminuria.

al·bu′mi·nate. Any compound of albumin with an acid or base; a product of the hydrolysis of albumin or globulin.

al·bu″mi·nim′e·ter, al·bu″mi·nom′e·ter. An instrument for the quantitative estimation of albumin in a fluid, as in urine.—**albuminimetry, albuminometry,** *n.*

al·bu′mi·noid, al′bu·moid, al·bu′moid. 1. Resembling albumin; applied to certain compounds having many of the characteristics of albumin. 2. Any scleroprotein, a simple protein characterized by being insoluble in neutral solvents, such as collagen, elastin, keratin, etc.

al·bu″mi·nol′y·sin. A lysin which decomposes proteins. Also called *proteolysin.* —**albuminolysis,** *n.*

al·bu″min·u·ret′ic, al·bu″mi·nu′ric. 1. Causing albuminuria. 2. A drug which causes albuminuria.

al·bu″mi·nu′ri·a. The presence in the urine of serum albumin, globulin, and other proteins which may result from disease of the kidneys or from the admixture of blood or pus with the urine; proteinuria. **alimentary a.** That following the ingestion of a heavy protein meal. **cardiac a.** That due to chronic valvular disease. **colliquative a.** A form seen in convalescence from severe fevers. **cyclic a.** The albuminuria of adolescence, in which a small quantity of albumin appears in the urine at stated times of the day. Also called *physiologic a., simple a., functional a.* **dietetic a.** That due to the ingestion of certain forms of food. **emulsion a.** That in which the urine has a milky turbidity which does not clear on heating, filtration, or acidification. **exudative a.** An albuminuria partially due to the filtration of albumin through the membranes of the kidney and also to the presence in the urine of products of inflammation, as in cases of nephritis. **false a.** A mixture of albumin with the urine during its transit through the urinary passages, where it may be derived from blood, pus, or special secretions that contain albumin. **febrile a.** That due to fever, or associated with acute infectious diseases, slight changes occurring in the glomeruli without organic lesion. **functional a.** See *cyclic a.* **hypostatic a.** That which is present when the patient lies flat on his back, but which disappears when he is erect. **nephrogenous a.** That due to renal disease. **neurotic a.** That which is present in epilepsy, exophthalmic goiter, apoplexy, neurasthenia, injuries to the brain, and various psychoses. **orthostatic a.** A form dependent upon an upright posture. **paroxysmal a.** Cyclic albuminuria. **pathologic a.** That which results from a diseased condition, such as that due to degenerative change in the kidney or to an acute febrile disease. **physiologic a.** Albumin in normal urine, without appreciable coexisting renal lesion or diseased condition. **pseudoalbuminuria.** That dependent upon the presence of such fluids as blood, pus, lymph, spermatic fluid, or the contents of an abscess cavity, in the urine. Syn., *adventitious a.* **true a.** That due to the excretion of some albuminous constituents of the blood with the water and salts of the urine. Syn., *intrinsic a.*

al′bu·mose (alb′yōō·moce, alb·yōō′-moze). An albuminous substance, among the first of the decomposition prod-

ucts of proteolysis, not coagulated by heat.

al″bu·mo·su′ri·a. The presence of Bence Jones protein in the urine. Formerly called *Bence Jones albumose.*

Al″ca·lig′e·nes fae·cal′is (al″kuh·lidj′i·neez fi·kal′iss). A species of bacteria found in feces and water, which resembles the typhoid bacillus. Conn has proposed a new genus, *Agrobacterium,* to include this organism.

al′co·hol. 1. A derivative of an aliphatic hydrocarbon which contains a hydroxyl (OH) group. Alcohols are classified on the basis of the number of hydroxyl groups present in the molecule, i.e., monohydric (monatomic), dihydric (diatomic), trihydric (triatomic); or on the basis of the presence of a —CH_2OH (primary alcohol), a =CHOH (secondary alcohol), or a ≡COH (tertiary alcohol) group. 2. Ethyl alcohol, C_2H_5OH (*alcohol*). A liquid containing not less than 92.3% by weight, corresponding to 94.9% by volume, at 15.56° C., of C_2H_5OH. It may be obtained by distillation of fermented grain, starchy substances, or saccharine liquids; it is also prepared by synthesis. The effects of its ingestion are well known, but are generally misinterpreted, since the initial euphoria, increased pulse rate, and sense of warmth give rise to the belief in its value as a stimulant. Larger doses cause increasing exaltation and excitement with muscular incoördination, and, depending on the individual, eventually lead to sleep, stupor, or active delirium. All these manifestations are due to its action as a central nervous system depressant. *In medicine,* it is used internally for its fuel value in the debilitated, and for its cutaneous vasodilative and euphoric effect. On the skin it is antiseptic and astringent. In 70% solution it is used as an antiseptic for instruments. It exists in wine, whisky, brandy, gin, rum, beer, etc. See *alcoholism.* **absolute a.** See *absolute alcohol.* **aromatic a.** One obtained from a hydrocarbon of the aromatic series. **fatty a.** One obtained from a hydrocarbon of the fatty series.

al″co·hol′ic. 1. Pertaining to, containing, or producing alcohol. 2. One addicted to the use of spirituous drinks. **Al″co·hol′ics A·non′y·mous.** A fellowship of persons formerly addicted to alcohol who have banded together to cure others of alcoholism.

al′co·hol·ism. 1. Alcoholic poisoning. 2. Morbid results of excessive or prolonged use of alcoholic liquors. **acute a.** Inebriety; drunkenness. Also called *ebrietas.* **chronic a.** A state produced by repeated and long-continued excesses of alcoholic indulgence, and associated with severe disturbances of the digestive and nervous systems. Syn., *dipsorrhexia, dipsomania, temulence.*

al″co·hol·om′e·ter. A hydrometer or other instrument for determining the amount of alcohol in a liquid. **–alcoholometry,** *n.*

al″co·hol·u′ri·a. Presence of alcohol in voided urine.

alcoometer. Trade name for the apparatus devised by Greenberg and Keator for use in their breath alcohol method of determining the concentration of alcohol in the blood.

al′co·sol (al′ko·sol, ·sole). A colloidal solution in which alcohol is the dispersion medium.

aldarsone. A proprietary arsenical consisting chiefly of sodium 3-amino-4-hydroxyphenylarsonate–N-methanal sulfoxylate, used by insufflation or in the form of a suppository in the treatment of *Trichomonas vaginalis* vaginitis, and by intravenous injection for central nervous system syphilis. See *phenarsone sulfoxylate.*

al′de·hyde. A class of organic compounds intermediate between alcohols and acids. They contain the group —CHO.

al″do·bi·on′ic ac′id (al″do·buy·on″ick). $C_{12}H_{20}O_{12}$. An acid produced by the hydrolysis of gum arabic and other gums, and containing D-glucuronic acid and D-galactose.

al′dol (al′dole, ·dol). 1. $CH_3.CH(OH).$ $CH_2.CHO.$ Beta-hydroxybutyric aldehyde, a condensation product of acetaldehyde. 2. One of a class of condensation products formed from an aldehyde.

al′dol·ase. An enzyme in muscle capable of splitting fructose-1,6-diphosphate into dihydroxyacetone phosphate and phosphoglyceric aldehyde. Syn., *zymohexase.*

al′dose (al′dose, al′doze). Any carbohydrate containing the aldehyde group —CHO.

al·dos′ter·one. An adrenocortical hormone; a potent metabolic regulator of sodium and of potassium.

al·dox′ime (al·docks′im, ·docks′eem). 1. The product derived from an aldehyde when the oxygen of the —CHO group is replaced by —NOH, forming the —CHNOH group. 2. Acetaldoxime, $CH_3.$ CHNOH.

al′e·tris. 1. Star grass; unicorn root; starwort; colic root. 2. The dried rhizome and roots of *Aletris farinosa.* Formerly used in colic, dropsy, and chronic rheumatism.

al′eu·drin (al′yoo·drin, al·yōō′drin). Dichloroisopropyl carbamate, $C_4H_7O_2$ NCl_2, a white crystalline substance, used as a hypnotic and sedative.

a·leu′ro·nat. A vegetable protein

used as a substitute for flour in diabetes.

a·lex′i·a. Word blindness; a form of aphasia in which the patient is unable to recognize or comprehend written or printed words. Also called *optic a., sensory a., visual aphasia.* **motor a.** That in which written or printed words are understood, but cannot be read aloud. **musical a.** Loss of ability to read music.

Al′gae (al′jee). One of the major divisions of primitive plants, living for the most part in water.

al·ge′si·a (al·jee′zee·uh, ·see·uh). 1. Sensitivity to pain. 2. Hyperesthesia. **–algesic,** *adj.*

al″ge·sim′e·ter. Instrument for determining the acuteness of the sense of pain. **–algesimetry,** *n.*

-al′gi·a. A suffix denoting *pain.*

al′gid. 1. Cold or chilly. 2. Denoting a pernicious type of malaria in which the patient is in shock. **–algid′ity,** *n.*

al·gin′ic ac′id. A gelatinous polysaccharide derived from marine algae of the *Fucus* type; the sodium salt produces with water a transparent mucilage, for which reason it is used as a suspending agent in pharmacy.

al′go-, al′gi·o-, alg-. A combining form signifying *pain,* or *of* or *pertaining to pain.*

al″go·gen′ic. Causing neuralgic pain.

al″go·gen′ic. Lowering the body temperature.

al″go·lag′ni·a. A sexual perversion in which the experiencing or infliction of pain heightens sexual gratification, or gives sexual pleasure without intercourse. **–algolagnist,** *n.* **active a.** Sadism. **passive a.** Masochism.

al″go·pho′bi·a. Unreasonable or morbid dread of pain.

al′gor. A sense of chilliness or coldness. **a. mortis.** Chill of death.

al′go·spasm. Painful spasm or cramp. **–algospas′tic,** *adj.*

al′i·ble. Nutritive; absorbable and assimilable, as a food.

al″i·cy′clic (al″i·sigh′click, ·sick′-lick). Having the properties of both aliphatic (open-chain) and cyclic (closed-chain) compounds.

alidase. Trade-mark for hyaluronidase.

a″lien·a′tion (ay″lyen·ay′shun, ay″lee·en·). *In psychiatry,* mental derangement; insanity.

a′lien·ist (ayl′yuh·nist, ay′lee·uh·nist). 1. A psychiatrist; a physician who is expert in the diagnosis and treatment of mental disorders. 2. *In legal medicine,* a medical expert testifying in an insanity hearing. **–alien·ism,** *n.*

al′i·ment. Any food or nutritive substance.

al″i·men′ta·ry. 1. Nourishing, nutritious. 2. Of or relating to food and nutrition. 3. Pertaining to or caused by diet.

al″i·men·ta′tion. Act of nourishing with food; feeding. **rectal a.** The nourishing of a patient by the administration of small quantities of food through the rectum.

al″i·men″to·ther′a·py. The treatment of disease by systematic feeding; dietary treatment.

al″i·phat′ic. 1. Pertaining to a fat. 2. Belonging to the open-chain series of organic compounds.

al″i·sphe′noid. 1. Pertaining to the greater wing of the sphenoid bone. 2. The bone that in adult life forms the main portion of the greater wing of the sphenoid.

a·liz′a·rin. 1,2-Dihydroxyanthraquinone. The reddish coloring matter of *Rubia tinctorum*, dyers' madder; also prepared synthetically. It is a brownish yellow powder or orange-red crystals, insoluble in cold water, soluble in alcohol or ether. Used in dyeing and in the manufacture of dyestuffs; also as pH indicator. **a. blue.** Dihydroxyanthraquinone-quinoline. Dark blue, lustrous crystals used as dye and pH indicator. Syn., *anthracene blue*. **a. carmine.** See *a. red S*. **a. red S.** (C.C.). An acid aniline dye, sodium alizarin sulfonate; an ingredient in some mitochondrial staining methods and used as a stain for bone. Also called *alizarin red, water soluble; alizarin carmine.* **a. yellow.** Sodium p-nitraniline salicylate, used as pH indicator. **a. yellow C.** See *gallacetophenone.* **a. yellow GG.** $O_2N.C_6H_4.$-$N:N.C_6H_3(OH)COONa$, sodium *m*-nitrobenzene-azosalicylate. A yellow powder used as pH indicator. Also called *salicyl yellow.* **a. yellow R.** The p-derivative corresponding to *a. yellow GG*, used as pH indicator.

al″ka·le′mi·a. Decrease of the hydrogen-ion concentration in the blood; increased alkalinity of the blood.

al′ka·li (al′kuh·lye) (pl. *alkalies, alkalis*). 1. Essentially a hydroxide of an alkali metal. 2. A class of compounds which react with acids to form salts, turn red litmus blue, saponify fats, and form soluble carbonates. 3. The term is sometimes applied also to carbonates of alkali metals. **caustic a.** Commonly the hydroxide of potassium or sodium. **fixed a.** Any metallic hydroxide. **volatile a.** Ammonium hydroxide; also ammonium carbonate.

al′ka·li blue. Sodium triphenylrosaniline sulfonate; a dye.

al″ka·lim′e·ter. An instrument for estimating the alkali in a substance. **—alkalimet′ric,** *adj.*; **alkalim′etry,** *n.*

al′ka·line (al′kuh·lyne, ·lin). 1. Containing more hydroxyl than hydrogen ions. 2. Having the qualities of, or pertaining to, an alkali.

al′ka·line-earth met′als. The divalent elements, calcium, strontium, and barium. Some include magnesium in the group.

al′ka·line tide. The temporary decrease in acidity of urine and body fluids after eating, attributed by some to the withdrawal of acid from the blood for gastric digestion.

al″ka·lin′i·ty. Quality of being alkaline.

al′ka·lin·ize, al′ka·lize. Render alkaline. **—alkaliniza′tion, alkaliza′tion,** *n.*

al″ka·li·nu′ri·a. Alkalinity of the urine.

al′ka·lize. See *alkalinize.*

al′ka·loid. A term applied to naturally occurring, basic, organic, nitrogenous compounds, usually of plant origin. Alkaloids are usually colorless, crystalline compounds containing carbon, hydrogen, oxygen, and nitrogen. A few are liquids and, as a rule, contain no oxygen; some are colored. Most are insoluble in water, soluble in organic solvents, and react with acids to form salts which are soluble in water and insoluble in organic solvents. Many alkaloids are medicinally valuable. **—alkaloi′dal,** *adj.* **animal a.** See *ptomaine* and *leucomaine.* **cadaveric a.** See *ptomaine.* **putrefactive a.** See *ptomaine.*

al″ka·lo′sis. A condition in which the bicarbonate content of the blood is relatively high and there is a tendency toward alkalemia. It may be the result of the ingestion of large amounts of sodium bicarbonate, persistent vomiting with the loss of hydrochloric acid, or forced breathing with the reduction of carbon dioxide from blood. (The last is also called *acapnial* or *gaseous alkalosis*.) It is marked by slow pulse, vertigo, and jerky muscular action. **compensated a.** Increased blood bicarbonate without a change of the $H_2CO_3:NaHCO_3$ ratio, and hence no change in pH. **uncompensated a.** Increased blood bicarbonate with a change in the ratio $H_2CO_3:NaHCO_3$, and hence an upward shift of the pH.

al′kane. Any member of the paraffin series of hydrocarbons. See *paraffin.*

al′ka·net. The root of the herb, *Alkanna tinctoria*, yielding a red dye used to give a red color to various pharmaceutical preparations.

al·kan′in. See *alkannin.*

al·kan′nin, al·kan′in. Alkanna-red, a valuable coloring matter obtained from alkanet.

al·kap'ton, al·kap'tone. A yellowish, resinous, nitrogenous substance occasionally found in urine. It is identified as homogentisic acid.

al·kap"to·nu'ri·a. The presence of alkapton (homogentisic acid) in the urine. A hereditary defect of metabolism characterized by the incomplete oxidation of phenylalanine and tyrosine, resulting in the excretion of homogentisic acid in the urine, which may turn dark. In time, ochronosis may develop.

al"ka·ver'vir (al"ka-veer'ver). A mixture of alkaloids from veratrum viride, used as an antihypertensive drug. See *veriloid*.

al'kene. Any member of the series of unsaturated aliphatic hydrocarbons (ethylene series) having one double bond and represented by the general formula, C_nH_{2n}.

al'kine. Any member of the series of unsaturated aliphatic hydrocarbons having a triple bond and represented by the general formula, C_nH_{2n-2}. Acetylene is the first hydrocarbon of the series, hence sometimes called acetylene series.

al'kyl. Any one of the univalent saturated hydrocarbon radicals of the general formula C_nH_{2n+1}; as methyl (CH_3), ethyl (C_2H_5), propyl (C_3H_7), etc.

al"kyl·a·mine' (al"kil-uh-meen', al"kil-am'in). A substance having the constitution of ammonia in which an alkyl replaces hydrogen; one, two, or three hydrogen atoms of the ammonia molecule may be replaced, yielding *primary* or *monalkylamines*, *secondary* or *dialkylamines*, and *tertiary* or *trialkylamines*, respectively.

al"la·ches·the'si·a, al"la·chaes·the'si·a (al"uh-kees-thee'zhuh, -zee-uh), **al"lo·ches·the'si·a, al"lo·chaes·the'si·a.** A tactile sensation experienced remote from the point of stimulation. Syn., *allesthesia*.

al·lan'to-, allant-. A combining form usually meaning *allantoic* or *allantoid* (see under *allantois*).

al·lan"to·cho'ri·on (a-lan"to-kor'ee-on). The allantois and chorion fused together and thus forming a single structure; a chorion supplied by allantoic blood vessels. Syn., *chorion allantoideum*.

al·lan'to·in. A crystallizable substance found in allantoic fluid, fetal urine, amniotic fluid, and some plants. It is produced by the oxidation of uric acid; used as local application to wounds, ulcers, osteomyelitis, etc., to accelerate cell proliferation.

al·lan'to·is (a-lan'toyss, a-lan'to-iss). An extraembryonic membrane arising as an outgrowth of the cloaca in amniotes. It functions as an organ of respiration and excretion in birds and reptiles and plays an important part in the development of the placenta in most mammals, its blood vessels forming the important pathways for the circulation of the blood between fetus and placenta. **—allan·to'ic, allantoid,** *adj.*

al"le·gor"i·za'tion. *In psychiatry* the formation of apparently meaningless new words or sentences, frequently demonstrated in schizophrenia; neologisms.

al·lele', al·lel'. One of a pair, or any one of a series, of genes having the same locus on homologous chromosomes. **—allel'ic,** *adj.*

al·le'lo- (a-lee'lo-, a·lel'o-). A combining form denoting *of one another, reciprocally.*

al·le'lo·morph (a·lee'lo-morf a·lel'o·). One of a pair of sharply contrasted Mendelian characteristics. Also, the genes in identical loci of homologous chromosomes, upon which the characteristics depend. **—allelomor'phic,** *adj.*; **allelomor'phism,** *n.*

al'ler·gen. Any agent capable of producing a state or manifestation of allergy. The commonest allergens are drugs, pollens, fungi, animal hair, and foods. **—allergen'ic,** *adj.*; **aller·genic'ity,** *n.*

al'ler·gist. One skilled in the diagnosis and treatment of allergic diseases.

al"ler·gi·za'tion. Sensitization; the introduction of foreign substances into an organism.

al'ler·gy. 1. Altered reaction capacity to a specific substance which will cause no symptoms of hypersensitivity in the nonsensitive. In the strict sense, this is an antigen-antibody mechanism, although the antibody is not always demonstrable. The allergens (antigens) may be proteins, carbohydrates, lipids and haptens. 2. The branch of medicine that deals with the diagnosis and treatment of allergic diseases. There are four types of allergic diseases: (a) Anaphylaxis, a response induced by previous sensitization; usually refers to the state of hypersensitivity which occurs in experimental animals. (b) Atopic diseases, which depend upon an inherited constitutional capacity; include hay fever, vasomotor rhinitis, asthma, urticaria, infantile type eczema, drug sensitivities, and other rare expressions. (c) Serum sickness. (d) Contact dermatitis. 3. Acquired sensitivities to drugs and biologicals (may be true anaphylaxis). **—aller'gic,** *adj.*

al'li·cin. The antibacterial principle obtained from common garlic.

al"li·ga'tion. *In pharmacy,* the formula for solving problems concerning the mixing of solutions of different percentages; the rule of mixtures. If two substances when mixed retain the specific values of a property, the value for the mixture can be calculated from the equation, $\dfrac{aA + bB}{a + b}$, where a and b are the proportions and A and B equal the respective values for the property.

al'li·ga"tor for'ceps. *In surgery,* a toothed instrument, one jaw of which operates with a double lever.

al·lit"er·a'tion. A form of dysphrasia in which the patient chooses words with the same consonant sounds.

al'lo-, all-. 1. A combining form denoting *differentiation from the normal, extraneousness,* or *reversal.* 2. *In chemistry,* a combining form denoting *an isomer, close relative,* or *variety of a compound;* or denoting the *more stable of two isomers.*

al"lo·che'zi·a (al″o·kee′zee-uh), **al"lo·che'ti·a** (al″o·kee′shee-uh, ·kee′tee·uh). 1. The passage of feces from the body through an abnormal opening. 2. The passing of nonfecal matter from the bowels.

al"lo·cho·les'ter·ol (al″o·ko·les′tur-ole, ·ol). A sterol found in wool fat.

al"lo·er'o·tism, al"lo·e·rot'i·cism. Sexual excitement that is induced by and directed to another, not oneself; opposed to autoerotism, *q.v.*

al'lo·path, al'lop·a·thist. An incorrect designation for a regular medical practitioner.

al·lop·a·thy. System of medical treatment using remedies that produce effects upon the body differing from those produced by disease; the opposite of the homeopathic system. It has been applied erroneously to the so-called regular medical profession. **—allo·path'ic,** *adj.*

al'lo·plas"ty. 1. A plastic operation in which material from outside the human body is utilized, such as ivory, animal bone, gold, silver, plastics, etc. Distinguished from autoplasty and heteroplasty, *q.v.* 2. *In psychoanalysis,* the process whereby the libido of the growing individual directs its energies away from self and toward other individuals and objects. **—alloplas'-tic,** *adj.*

all'-or-none'. See *all-or-nothing.*

all'-or-noth'ing. Occurring either completely or not at all, as the response of a single nerve or muscle unit to a stimulus.

al'lo·some. 1. Originally any chromosome distinguished from ordinary chromosomes (autosomes) by certain peculiarities of form, size, and behavior, but now the term is usually used as synonymous with sex chromosome; an accessory chromosome. Syn.,

heterochromosome. 2. A cytoplasmic inclusion introduced from without. **paired a.** One of a pair of similar allosomes; a diplosome. **unpaired a.** A monosome; an accessory chromosome.

al'lo·therm. An organism whose temperature is directly dependent upon that of its environment.

al'lo·trope. One of the forms in which an element capable of assuming different forms may appear.

al"lo·trop'ic. 1. Pertaining to, or exhibiting, allotropy. 2. *In psychiatry,* denoting a personality which is concerned about others; not egocentric.

al·lot'ro·py (a·lot′ro·pee, al′o·tro″-pee), **al·lot'ro·pism.** 1. Occurrence of an element in two or more distinct forms with differences in physical properties, as carbon, phosphorus, and sulfur. 2. Appearance in an unusual or abnormal form. 3. An attraction or tropism between different cells or structures, as between sperms and ova. 4. Adolf Meyer's term for allopsyche.

al"lox·an' (al″ock·san′, a·lock′sun). Mesoxalyl urea. A crystalline substance produced by oxidation of uric acid. Has been found in the intestinal mucus during diarrhea and is used for production of experimental diabetes through selective necrosis of the islets of Langerhans.

al'loy, al·loy'. The product of the fusion of two or more metals.

al'lyl. The univalent radical —CH_2-CH:CH_2 or C_3H_5—. **a. isopropyl-barbituric acid.** See *alurate.* **a. isothiocyanate.** C_3H_5NCS. Volatile oil of mustard, a colorless or pale yellow liquid. Also called *a. mustard oil, a. isosulfocyanate.* **a. sulfide.** (C_3H_5)$_2$S. A liquid of garliclike odor, possibly present in garlic; formerly used in cholera and tuberculosis. **a. thiourea.** See *thiosinamine.*

N-al"lyl·nor·mor'phine hy"-dro·chlo'ride. Nalorphine hydrochloride.

al'mond (ah′mund, am′und, al′-mund). The seed of the tree *Amygdala communis* var. *dulcis,* which yields the sweet almond, or of *A. communis* var. *amara,* which yields the bitter almond.

al'mond-eyed". Applied to members of the Mongolian race, because of the elliptical form and slanting appearance of their eyelids.

al'mond oil. A fixed oil obtained from kernels of varieties of almonds, used as an emollient. Syn., *sweet almond oil.*

a·lo'chi·a (a·lo′kee·uh). Absence of the lochia.

al'oe (al′o, al′o·ee). The dried juice of the leaves of *Aloe Perryi, A. barbadensis, A. ferox,* and hybrids of this species. Its purgative properties are due to three pentosides (barbaloin, iso-barbaloin, and beta-barbaloin) and to a resin. It is cathartic and tonic. Local application of the leaves is of benefit in the treatment of x-ray burns.

al″o·et′ic. 1. Containing or pertaining to aloe. 2. A medication containing aloe.

al″o·e′tin. 1. Aloe resin. 2. A yellow crystalline principle obtainable from aloes.

a·lo′gi·a. 1. Motor or expressive aphasia, q.v. 2. Stupid or senseless behavior.

al′o·in. A mixture of active principles, chiefly barbaloin and iso-barbaloin, obtained from aloe. It is a yellow, microcrystalline powder with an intensely bitter taste. Used as laxative and purgative. Syn., *barbaloin*.

al″o·pe′ci·a (al″o·pee′shee·uh, ·see·uh). Loss of hair; baldness. The loss may be partial or total; congenital, premature, or senile. Alopecia may complicate various systemic affections. Syn., *calvities*, *baldness*. Also called *defluvium capillorum*. **—alopecic,** *adj*. **a. areata.** Loss of hair in circumscribed patches with little or no inflammation. The scalp and beard areas are usually involved. Syn., a *circumscripta*. Also called *area Celsi*. **a. cachectica.** Baldness due to general malnutrition. **a. cicatrisata.** Circular and irregular patches of alopecia due to atrophy of the skin, causing permanent baldness. Syn., *pseudopelade*. **a. congenitalis.** An unusual form appearing congenitally due to partial or complete absence of hair follicles. **a. prematura.** Baldness which occurs any time after puberty and resembles the senile type. The hair gradually thins and falls out, often beginning at the temples. Also called *presenile a*. **a. prematura symptomatica.** Loss of hair in the course of some diseases, or following prolonged, debilitating fevers, or with changes in endocrine secretion. When baldness follows acute illnesses, it is usually temporary. **a. seborrheica.** Baldness associated with seborrheic dermatitis. Scaliness and varying degrees of inflammation are present. Itching is often associated, and the hair is dry and lusterless. This condition is quite common. Syn., *a. pityrodes*, *pityriasis simplex*. Also called *seborrhea capillitii*. **a. universalis.** Loss of hair from all parts of the body. Also called *a. totalis*.

al′pha. 1. The first letter of the Greek alphabet (A, α). 2. *In chemistry*, it is often combined with the name of a compound to indicate the first of a series, as of isomers or otherwise related substances. 3. In other sciences, it is often employed to differentiate between the members of various groups or series.

al″pha·hy·poph′a·mine (·highpof′uh·meen, ·min). The oxytocin obtained from the neurohypophysis.

al″pha·i′o·dine. Thyroxin, q.v.

al″pha·lo′be·line (·lo′bi·leen, ·lobee′leen). An alkaloid from lobelia used in asphyxia.

al″pha·pro′dine hy″dro·chle′ride. 1,3-Dimethyl-4-phenyl-4-piperidyl propionate hydrochloride, an analgesic. See *nisentil hydrochloride*.

al″pha·to·ceph′er·ol, α-to·ceph′er·ol. 5,7,8-Trimethyltocol, $C_{29}H_{50}O_2$, a light yellow, viscous, oily liquid, obtained from natural sources or prepared synthetically, that is miscible with alcohol. Also called *vitamin E*.

al″ser·ox′y·lon. A fat-soluble alkaloidal fraction from *Rauwolfia serpentina*, used as an antihypertensive and sedative drug. See *rauwiloid*.

al′ter·a″tive (awl′tur·ay″tiv, awl′tur·uh·tiv″). 1. A medicine that alters the processes of nutrition, restoring, in some unknown way, the normal functions of an organ or of the system. Arsenic, iodine, the iodides, mercury, and gold formerly were classed as alteratives, but the term has little if any application now. *Obs*. 2. Changing; alterant; reestablishing healthy nutritive processes. *Obs*.

al′ter·nat″ing. Occurring successively.

al″ter·na′tion. 1. The act of alternating or of performing alternately. 2. *In neurology*, the phenomenon whereby only every other impulse is carried over the eighth cranial (auditory) nerve when the exciting impulse is from 900 to 1800 cycles. Because of the refractory period of nerve impulses, the maximum frequency that can be carried by a nerve is about 900 per second. **—al′ternate,** *adj., n., v*.

al·the′a. Marshmallow root. The peeled root of *Althaea officinalis*. It consists chiefly of starch and gum with some pectin and sugar and contains up to 2% of asparagin. Used in the form of a decoction as a demulcent; also as a pill excipient.

alt. hor. *Alternis horis;* every other hour.

al′ti·tude sick′ness. A symptom complex resulting from anoxia during airplane flights at high altitudes, due to lowered partial pressure of oxygen in the inspired air. **Acute altitude sickness** may occur as the result of a single flight; it is marked by symptoms of acute anoxia, as headache, increased lung ventilation, general bodily distress, mental anxiety, lassitude, sleepiness, fatigue, depression, or euphoria. **Chronic altitude sickness** results from repeated flights at high altitudes; it is characterized by headache, mental and physical fatigue, increased appetite, irritability, nervousness, insomnia, poor mental concentration, lack of volition, disregard for danger in the air, and is accompanied by some nausea, anorexia, indigestion, and vertigo.

aludrine hydrochloride. Trademark for isopropylarterenol hydrochloride.

al′um. 1. Any one of a class of double salts of general formula $M_2′SO_4.M_2′′′(SO_4)_3.24H_2O$　or　$M′M′′′(SO_4)_2.12H_2O$, in which M′ is a monovalent metal or group, and M′′′ is a trivalent metal. 2. The official alum, which may be ammonium alum, $AlNH_4(SO_4)_2.12H_2O$, or potassium alum, $AlK(SO_4)_2.12H_2O$. Both forms are soluble in water, insoluble in alchohol. It is astringent and emetic. **burnt a.** See exsiccated a. **dried a.** See exsiccated a. **exsiccated a.** Official alum (see alum, 2) which has been deprived of most of its water of crystallization. Syn., burnt a., dried a.

al″u·min′i·um. See aluminum.

a·lu′mi·num, al″u·min′i·um. Al = 26.97. Valence, 3. A silver-white, light, ductile metal occurring abundantly in nature. It is soluble in acids and alkalis. It readily forms alloys, as duralumin and magnalium. See thermite. **a. acetate solution.** An astringent and antiseptic used after dilution with from 8 to 10 parts of water as a gargle or a local application. Also called Burow's solution. **a. chloride.** A white or yellow-white, deliquescent, crystalline powder; soluble in water. An astringent and antiseptic. **a. hydroxide gel.** A white, viscous suspension of aluminum hydroxide, used as gastric antacid, especially in the treatment of peptic ulcers. See amphojel, creamalin, fluagel, hydrogel. **a. phosphate gel.** A white, viscous suspension, used like aluminum hydroxide gel, but does not interfere with phosphate absorption. See phosphaljel. **a. subacetate solution.** A clear, colorless, or faintly yellow liquid used, after dilution with about nine parts of water, as an astringent and antiseptic wash, especially as a gargle. **dried a. hydroxide gel.** A white, odorless, tasteless, amorphous powder, used as antacid.

alurate. A trade-mark for allyl isopropylbarbituric acid, a sedative and hypnotic. See aprobarbital. **sodium a.** A soluble sodium salt of alurate.

a·lu′si·a. Hallucination; morbid state of mind.

al′ve·at·ed. Honeycombed; channeled; vaulted.

alveol-. See alveolo-.

al·ve′o·lar. Pertaining to an alveolus.

al·ve′o·late. Pitted like a honeycomb.

al″ve·o·lec′to·my. Surgical removal of part of the alveolar process of the upper or lower jaw.

al·ve′o·li″. Plural of alveolus.

al″ve·o·li′tis. Inflammation of a dental alveolus; especially the inflamed condition following the removal of a tooth. A frequent complication of tooth extraction. See dry socket.

al·ve′o·lo-, alveol-. A combining form denoting alveolus, alveolar.

al·ve″o·lo·den′tal. Pertaining to the teeth and their sockets.

al″ve·o·lot′o·my. Incision into a dental alveolus.

al·ve′o·lus (pl. alveoli). 1. Bony socket of a tooth. 2. An air cell of the lung. 3. A cavity, depression, pit, cell, or recess. 4. A terminal acinus of a racemose gland.

al′ve·us. 1. A trough, tube, or canal; applied to ducts and vessels of the body. 2. A cavity or excavation. 3. See alvus.

al·vi′no·lith, al′vi·no·lith. An intestinal concretion, usually formed from calcareous salts and debris.

al′vus (pl. and gen. alvi). The belly or its contained viscera. —**alvine**, adj.

a·lym″pho·cy·to′sis (ay-lim″fo-sigh·to′sis, a·lim″·). A marked decrease or absence of lymphocytes in the blood.

a·lys′mus. The natural anxiety and restlessness which accompanies any physical disease. Also called alysm.

Am. Chemical symbol for americium.

A. M. A. American Medical Association.

a·mal′gam. 1. An alloy of mercury with any other metal. 2. Any soft alloy. Symbol, āāā.

Am″a·ni′ta. A genus of the Agaricaceae. **A. muscaria.** Fly agaric, q.v. **A. phalloides.** A very poisonous species; the source of amanita toxin and amanita hemolysin.

a·man′i·tine (a·man′i·teen, ·tin). 1. A principle identical with choline, obtained from fly agaric. 2. A poisonous glycoside obtainable from various species of poisonous mushrooms.

am′a·ranth. 1. Any plant of the genus Amaranthus. 2. A dark, red-brown powder used as a color for foods, drugs, and cosmetics, and in dyeing. Also called F.D. and C. Red No. 2.

am′a·roid. Any distinctly bitter vegetable extractive of definite chemical composition other than an alkaloid or a glycoside. Also called bitter principle.

am″a·se′sis. Inability to chew.

a·mas′ti·a, a·ma′zi·a. Congenital absence of the mammae.

am″a·tho·pho′bia. A morbid fear of dust.

am'a·tive·ness. The sexual passion; disposition to love. Syn., *erotism.* —**amative, amatory,** *adj.*

am"au·ro'sis. Partial or total blindness from any cause. **a. fugax.** Temporary blindness resulting from sudden acceleration, as in aerial flight. Syn., *blackout.* **a. partialis fugax.** Partial blindness associated with headache, vertigo, and scotomas. It is usually sudden and transitory. **toxic a.** Blindness which follows the introduction of various poisons and toxic products into the body, as ethyl and methyl alcohol, tobacco, lead, arsenic, quinine, etc., and the metabolites of uremia and diabetes.

am"au·rot'ic. 1. Pertaining to, or affected with, blindness. 2. One suffering from amaurosis. **a. familial idiocy.** (a) A familial disease occurring almost exclusively in Jewish children, and manifesting symptoms in the fourth month of life; characterized by flaccid muscles, convulsions, decerebrate rigidity, and blindness marked by the appearance of a cherry-red spot at the macula lutea; associated with optic atrophy. Also called *Tay-Sachs disease.* (b) A late infantile type in which the symptoms first appear at the age of three or four years. The patient may live about four years. (c) A juvenile type beginning between seven and twelve years; running a longer course; not associated with macular changes; occurring in Gentiles.

am"a·xo·pho'bi·a (am"uk·so·fo'bee·uh, a·mack"so·). Morbid dread of being in, or riding upon, any vehicle.

am'ber. A fossil resin found in alluvial deposits of pine trees in various parts of the world, especially along the shores of the Baltic Sea.

am'ber·gris (am'bur·greece, ·griss). An intestinal concretion of the sperm whale, *Physeter macrocephalus,* found floating on the sea, used in perfumes, particularly as a fixative for floral odors.

am'bi-. A combining form meaning *both.*

am'bi-, amb-. A prefix meaning *about, around.*

am"bi·dex'trous. Able to use both hands equally well. —**ambidexter,** *n.;* **ambidexter'ity, ambidextrism, ambidextral'ity,** *n.*

am"bi·lat'er·al. Relating to or affecting both sides.

am"bi·le'vous. Clumsy in the use of both hands. Syn., *ambisinister.*

am"bi·oc·u·lar'i·ty. Ability to use both eyes equally well.

am"bi·sex'u·al, am"bo·sex'u·al. 1. Denoting feelings and behavior which are neither strictly masculine nor feminine, but common to both sexes. 2. Designating organs, extracts, and substances which evoke activity common to both sexes, as opposed to *bisexual* or *hermaphroditic.* 3. Denoting an individual in whom exist undifferentiated primordia of both sexes. Should both sets develop, hermaphroditism would result. —**ambisexual'ity, ambosexual'ity,** *n.*

am·biv'a·lence, am"bi·va'lence, am·biv'a·len·cy. In *psychiatry,* the coexistence, conscious or unconscious, of the feelings or attitudes of love and hate toward the same person or object. —**ambivalent,** *adj.*

am·biv'a·len·cy. See *ambivalence.*

am'bi·vert. 1. Both introvert and extrovert; or, intermediate between the two. 2. A personality type intermediate between extrovert and introvert. —**ambiver'sion,** *n.*

am'bly-. A combining form meaning *obtuse* or *dulled, faint.*

am"bly·a·cou'si·a (am"bli·a·koo'zhuh, ·zee·uh). Dullness of hearing.

am'bly·ope. A person with amblyopia.

am"bly·o'pi·a. Dimness of vision, especially that not due to refractive errors or organic disease of the eye. It may be congenital or acquired. —**amblyop'ic,** *adj.* **hysterical a.** A unilateral or bilateral disturbance of vision involving great variations in the extent of the visual fields, and, occasionally, inversion of the color fields; seen in hysteria. **toxic a.** A chronic optic neuritis due to poisons, usually alcohol and tobacco.

am"bo·cep'tor. According to the Ehrlich theory, an antibody present in the blood of immunized animals which contains two specialized elements: a cytophile group that unites with a cellular antigen, and a complementophile group that joins with the complement. Syn., *sensitizer.*

am"bo·tox'oid. An immunization agent prepared by reinoculating bacterial toxin with pooled cultures of the bacteria and their bacteriophage, then detoxifying the mixture with formalin and merthiolate. Used especially as a staphylococcus preparation.

Am·bro'si·a (am·bro'zhuh, ·zee·uh). A genus of composite-flowered herbs, including the common ragweeds of North America, **A. artemisifolia** and **A. trifida.**

am·bu·lance. 1. In foreign countries, the staff and equipment of an army medical unit in the field. 2. In the United States, a vehicle for the transportation of the sick or wounded. **air a.** See *a.* plane. **a. company.** Field unit in the U. S. Army Medical Department made up of staff and equipment for the evacuation of the sick and wounded. **a. plane.** An airplane designed for the evacuation of troop casualties. Syn., *air a.* **veterinary a.** One designed to transport sick or injured animals, especially horses.

am'bu·lance chas'er. An unethical lawyer who endeavors to exploit injury cases.

am'bu·la·to''ry, am'bu·lant. Walking or able to walk; designating a patient not confined to bed.

a·me'ba, a·moe'ba (pl. *amebas, amoebae*). A colorless, jellylike, unicellular organism found in sea and fresh waters. It constantly undergoes change in form, progresses by means of pseudopodia, reproduces by simple fission, and obtains nourishment by engulfing tiny neighboring particles. —**amebic, amoebic,** *adj.*

am''e·bi'a·sis. Infection with *Endamoeba histolytica.* **a. cutis.** Ulceration of the skin due to amebas; in association with visceral amebiasis. **intestinal a.** See amebic *colitis.*

a·me'bi·cide, a·moe'bi·cide. 1. Destructive to amebas. 2. An agent fatal to amebas, usually applied to one fatal to *Endamoeba histolytica.* —**amebicid'al,** *adj.*

a·me'boid. Resembling an ameba in form or in movement, as the white blood cells.

a·me'bu·la, a·moe'bu·la. A merozoite having the power of ameboid movement.

a·mel'o·blast (a·mel'o·blast, a·mee'lo·). An enamel cell; one of the columnar cells of the enamel organ which helps in forming dental enamel. Syn., *adamantoblast, ganoblast.*

am''e·lo·gen'e·sis. Histogenesis of the dental enamel.

a·me'lus. An individual with congenital absence of all extremities. —**amel'ia,** *n.*

a·men''o·ma'ni·a, a·moen''o·ma'ni·a. A mild form of mania in which the symptoms are manifested in gaiety, fondness of dress, exaggeration of social condition and the like; a cheerful or joyous delirium; a morbid elevation of the spirits; manic phase of manic-depressive psychosis.

a·men''or·rhe'a, a·men''or·rhoe'a. Absence of menstruation. Syn., *amenia.* —**amenorrheal, a·menorrhoeal,** *adj.* **emotional a.** That which results from sympathetic vasomotor disturbances caused by fright, emotional causes, or hysteria. **pathologic a.** That due to pathologic conditions, such as hysterectomy, oöphorectomy, absence of or damage to endometrium, ovarian failure, debility, or sympathetic vasomotor disturbances. **primary a.** Term applied to those cases in which the menarche has not appeared at the proper time. Also called *radical a., primitive a.* **second-**

ary a. That which occurs after menstruation has been established.

a'ment, am'ent. A person suffering from amentia; an idiot.

a·men'ti·a (a·men'shee·uh, ·shuh). 1. Subnormal mental development; especially, congenital intellectual incapacity. Contrasted with dementia, *q.v.* 2. Proposed by the Viennese school for temporary mental disorder, acute hallucinatory confusion; not generally accepted in U.S.A. **nevoid a.** That associated with a face or scalp nevus, calcification of parts of the brain, glaucoma, epilepsy, and defects of the pyramidal tracts. Also called *Sturge-Weber's disease.*

am'er·i'ci·um (am''ur·ish'ee·um). Chemical element No. 95, symbol Am, produced artificially.

amethone hydrochloride. Trademark for amolanone hydrochloride.

amethopterin. A trade-mark for methotrexate.

a·me'tri·a, a·met'ri·a. Congenital absence of the uterus. —**ametrous,** *adj.*

am''e·tro'pi·a. Imperfect refractive ability due to defects of the media or the structures of the eye, which causes images to fail to focus directly upon the retina. See *myopia, hypermetropia, astigmatism, presbyopia, aphakia.* —**ametrop'ic,** *adj.;* **am'etrope,** *n.*

am''i·an''thi·nop'sy. Violet blindness; inability to distinguish violet rays.

a·mi'cron, a·mi'crone (ay·migh'kron, ·krone, ay·mick'ron, ·rone). A colloid particle, less than 5mμ in diameter.

am'i·dase. A hydrolytic enzyme which splits ammonia from urea; a deamidizing enzyme.

am'ide. 1. Any organic compound containing the monovalent radical, —CO.NH$_2$. 2. A compound formed by the replacement of a hydrogen of ammonia by a metal, such as sodamide, NaNH$_2$. Syn., *ammono base.*

am'i·din. The part of starch that is soluble in water; soluble starch.

am'i·dine (am'i·deen, ·din). Any compound containing the monovalent radical —C(NH$_2$):NH.

a·mi'do- (a·mee'do-, am'i·do-), **amid-.** A prefix denoting a compound containing the —CO.NH$_2$ radical. Also see *amino-.*

am'i·done hy''dro·chlo'ride. 2-Dimethylamino-4,4-diphenylheptanone-5-hydrochloride, an analgesic, more powerful than morphine. See *adanon, dolophine, methadone hydrochloride.*

a·mi''do·py'rine (a·mee''do·pye'reen, am'i·do·). See *aminopyrine.*

a·mim'i·a. 1. Loss of the ability to communicate by gestures or signs. It may be an **amnesic amimia** when the meanings of the signs are not remembered, or an **ataxic amimia** when gestures cannot be made because of muscular defects. 2. *In neurology,* a paralysis of the facial muscles, affecting chiefly the angles of the mouth, apparent when the patient attempts an emotional grimace, as in paralysis agitans.

a·mine′ (a·meen′, am′in), **am′in.** Any member of the group of compounds formed by replacing one or more of the hydrogens of ammonia by one or more organic radicals. **quaternary a.** A compound derived from ammonium hydroxide by replacement of the four hydrogens of the $-NH_4$ group by radicals; tetraalkyl ammonium base.

a·mi·no- (a·mee′no-, am′i·no-). *In chemistry,* a prefix meaning *pertaining to or containing the group* NH_2 *united to a radical other than an acid radical.*

a·mi″no·a·ce′tic ac′id. $H_2N.CH_2.$ COOH. White, crystalline powder, soluble in water; a constituent of many proteins. Syn., *glycocoll, glycine.*

a·mi′no ac′id (a·mee′no, am′i·no). Any one of a large group of organic compounds with the basic formula $NH_2-R-COOH$, R representing any aliphatic radical. These compounds represent the end products of protein hydrolysis. From amino acids, the body resynthesizes its proteins. Ten of them are considered essential to life: arginine, histidine, isoleucine, leucine, lysine, methionine, phenylalanine, threonine, tryptophan, and valine. See Table of Normal Values of Blood Constituents in the Appendix.

a·mi″no·ac′ri·dine (a·mee″no·ack′ri·deen, ·din). An amino derivative of acridine possessing bactericidal power.

a·mi″no·ben′zene·sul·fon′a·mide. See *sulfanilamide.*

a·mi″no·glu′cose. See *glycosamine.*

a·mi″no·lip′id (a·mee″no·lip′id, am′i·no·). A fatty acid ester of an alcohol containing nitrogen in the amino form.

a·mi″no·met′ra·dine. 1-Allyl-3-ethyl-6-aminotetrahydropyrimidinedione, a diuretic. See *mictine.*

aminopterin. Trade-mark for 4-aminopteroylglutamic acid, a substance useful in treating certain types of leukemia.

a·mi″no·pu′rine (a·mee″no·pew′reen, am″i·no·). A purine in which one or more hydrogens are replaced by amino groups, as *adenine, guanine.*

a·mi″no·py′rine (a·mee″no·pye′reen, am″i·no·). Dimethylaminophenyldimethyl pyrazolone; $C_{13}H_{17}N_3O$. An antipyretic and analgesic used in neuralgia, neuritis, migraine, and colds. Syn., *amidopyrine.* See *pyramidon.*

a·mi′no·quin (a·mee′no·kwin, am′i·no·kwin). See *plasmochin.*

a·mi″no·su′ri·a (a·mee″no·sue′ree·uh, am″i·no·), **am″i·nu′ri·a.** The presence of amines in the urine.

a·mi′no·trate phos′phate. Triethanolamine trinitrate diphosphate, a vasodilator. See *metamine, nitretamin.*

am″i·so·met′ra·dine. 1-Methallyl-3-methyl-6-aminotetrahydropyrimidinedione, a diuretic. See *rolicton.*

a″mi·to′sis. Reproduction by direct nuclear cleavage or simple fission. —**amitot′ic,** *adj.*

am·me″ter. A type of galvanometer in which the electric current is measured directly in amperes.

am′mo-, amm-. A combining form meaning *sand.*

am·mo′ni·a. A colorless, pungent gas, NH_3, very soluble in water. **a. water.** See diluted *a.* solution. **aromatic a. spirit.** A flavored, hydroalcoholic solution of ammonia and ammonium carbonate having an aromatic, pungent odor. **diluted a. solution.** A 10% solution of ammonia in water. **strong a. solution.** A 28% solution of ammonia in water. **stronger a. water.** See strong *a.* solution.

am·mo″ni·e′mi·a, am·mo″ni·ae′mi·a. The presence in the blood of ammonia compounds believed to be the result of urea decomposition. The condition is attended by subnormal temperature, digestive disorders, weakened pulse, and coma.

am·mon″i·fi·ca′tion (a·mon″i·fi·kay′shun, a·mo″ni·). Production of ammonia by bacterial action.

am·mo′ni·um. The univalent radical, NH_4. It exists only in combination. **a. acetate solution.** Mindererus spirit, dilute acetic acid neutralized with ammonium carbonate. Used as diaphoretic. **a. bromide.** NH_4Br. Used as sedative and somnifacient. **a. carbonate.** A compound of ammonium acid carbonate and ammonium carbamate in varying proportions. It is a stimulant expectorant and reflex stimulant. **a. chloride.** NH_4Cl. Used as a saline expectorant, a diuretic, and for the acidification of urine. **a. mandelate.** A white deliquescent powder, soluble in water. Used as a urinary antiseptic.

am·mo″ni·u′ri·a. Presence of an excess of ammonia in the urine.

am·mo′no base. An inorganic amide obtained by replacing a hydrogen of ammonia with a metal, as $NaNH_2$, sodium amide.

am″mo·ther′a·py. The use of sand baths in the treatment of disease.

am″ne·mon′ic (am″nee·mon′ick) Relating to impairment of the memory; amnesic.

am·ne'si·a (am-nee'zhuh, -zee-uh). Loss of memory, especially of the ideas represented by words. **—amnesic, amnes'tic,** adj. **anterograde a.** Loss of memory for the period immediately following trauma, shock, or a confused state. **auditory a.** Word deafness. Inability to recognize the spoken word. **lacunar a.** Loss of memory for only certain isolated events, not a complete memory loss. **retro-anterograde a.** A perversion of memory in which recent events are referred to the past, and conversely. **retrograde a.** Loss of memory for events occurring before the onset of the current disease. **tactile a.** Inability to recognize objects by the sense of touch; astereognosis. **visual a.** Word blindness. Inability to recognize the written or printed word, or objects previously seen.

am'ni·a. A plural of amnion.

am'ni·o-. A combining form denoting amnion, amnionic.

am"ni·o·cho'ri·al (am"nee-o-kor'ee-ul). Pertaining to both amnion and chorion.

am"ni·og'ra·phy. Roentgenography of the fetus by injection of a solution of strontium iodide through the abdominal wall and into the amniotic sac; usually used as a diagnostic aid in suspected placenta previa.

am'ni·on (pl. amnia). The innermost of the fetal membranes forming a fluid-filled sac for the protection of the embryo. Its thin, translucent wall is composed of an inner layer of ectoderm and an outer layer of mesoderm continuous with the embryonic somatopleure at the umbilicus. After the second month of development, it obliterates the extraembryonic coelom, forms a sheath about the umbilical cord, and fuses loosely with the chorionic mesoderm. **—amnion'ic, amniot'ic,** adj. **false a.** A temporary cavity in the trophoblastic knob, resembling the early true amnion. Syn., false amniotic cavity, ectoplacental cavity. **true a.** The inner amniotic folds of avian, reptilian, and certain mammalian embryos; the amnion proper.

am'ni·o·tome. An instrument for puncturing the fetal membranes.

am"o·bar'bi·tal. Nonproprietary name for isoamyl-ethylbarbituric acid. See amytal.

am"o·di'a·quin hy"dro·chlo'-ride. 4-(7-Chloro-4-quinolylamino)-α-diethylamino-o-cresol dihydrochloride dihydrate, a synthetic antimalarial drug. See camoquin hydrochloride.

a·moe'ba. See ameba.

a·mok', a·muck'. In or pertaining to a state of murderous frenzy.

a·mol'a·none hy"dro·chlo'ride. 3-(β-Diethylaminoethyl)-3-phenyl-2-benzofuranone hydrochloride, a local anesthetic. See amethone hydrochloride.

a'mor. Love, especially physical attraction and union.

a·mor'phin·ism. State resulting when morphine is withdrawn from an addict.

a·mor'phous, a·mor'phic. 1. Formless, shapeless. 2. In biology, without visible differentiation in structure. 3. In chemistry, not crystalline. **—amorphism, amorphia,** n.

a·mo'ti·o ret'i·nae (a-mo'tee-o ret'i-nee). Detachment of the retina.

am'pere (am'peer, am-peer'). A unit of electric current; the current produced by one volt through a resistance of one ohm.

am·phet'a·mine (am-fet'uh-meen, -min). Racemic 1-phenyl-2-aminopropane, a colorless, volatile, mobile liquid. Inhalation of its vapors causes shrinking of nasal mucosa in head colds, sinusitis, and hay fever. See benzedrine. **a. sulfate.** A white, soluble powder used for its stimulating effect on the central nervous system.

am'phi-, amph-. A prefix signifying both, of both kinds, on both sides, about, around.

am"phi·ar·thro'sis. An articulation of contiguous bony surfaces which are connected by either fibrocartilage, as the vertebrae, or an interosseous ligament, as the distal tibiofibular junction. It permits only slight motion.

am'phi·as"ter. The achromatic figure in mitosis, consisting of two asters connected by a spindle.

Am·phib'i·a. A class of Vertebrata which includes salamanders, newts, frogs, and toads; distinguished by moist, scaleless skin, paired limbs with toes, gills in at least larval stages, lungs in most species, and a three-chambered heart.

am·phib'i·ous. Capable of living both on land and in water.

am"phi·cra'ni·a. Headache affecting both sides of the head, as opposed to hemicrania.

am"phi·di"ar·thro'sis. A mixed articulation such as that of the lower jaw, which partakes of the nature of both amphiarthrosis and diarthrosis.

am·phig'o·ny. Sexual reproduction.

am·phi·tene. The stage of mitosis in which the homologous chromosomes are in the process of conjugation. Syn., synaptene, zygotene.

am'phi·the"a·ter, am'phi·the"-a·tre. A room with seats arranged in tiers; used for students or others to attend surgical operations, lectures, demonstrations, etc.

am'pho-. A combining form meaning *both*.

am"pho·di·plo'pi·a, am·phot"·er·o·di·plo'pi·a. Double vision affecting each of the eyes.

amphojel. Trade-mark for a suspension of aluminum hydroxide used in gastric hyperacidity.

am·phor'ic. Resembling the sound produced by blowing across the mouth of a large, narrow-mouthed jar or bottle.

am·phor'ic breath'ing. See amphoric *respiration*.

am"pho·ter'ic. Having both acid and basic properties.

am"pli·fi·ca'tion. 1. *In microscopy*, the enlargement of the visual area, as *amplification* 200×, or *200 diameters*. 2. *In sound* or *radio*, the magnification of sound. 3. *In electricity*, the increase of electric current in either voltage or amperage, as by a transformer.

am'pli·fi"er. 1. Any device which enlarges, magnifies, or increases the size, strength, or power of an object or force. 2. The concavo-convex lens between the objective and ocular of a microscope. 3. An electron tube in radio or radiotherapy. 4. A transformer.

am'pli·tude. One-half the range of a periodic variation for symmetric vibrations; the maximum displacement from the normal for asymmetric vibrations; largeness; extent; range.

am·poule'. See *ampul*.

am"pro·tro'pine phos'phate. Nonproprietary name for the phosphate of the *dl*-tropic acid ester of 3-diethylamino-2,2-dimethyl-1-propanol. See *syntropan*.

am'pul (am'pul, am'pōol), **am'pule** (am'pewl, am'pōol), **am·poule'** (am-pōol', am'pōol). A container, commonly made of glass and capable of being hermetically sealed, intended to hold sterile preparations usually intended for parenteral use.

am'pule. See *ampul*.

am·pul'la (pl. *ampullae*). The dilated extremity of a canal or duct; as the lacrimal canal, mammary ducts, and semicircular canals. —**ampullar, am"pullary, ampullate,** *adj.* **a. lactifera.** That of a milk duct near its opening on the nipple. **a. of the ductus deferens.** That of the ductus deferens just before its junction with the duct of the seminal vesicle. **a. of the lacrimal duct.** A slight dilatation of the lacrimal duct beyond the punctum. **a. of the uterine tube.** The dilated end of a uterine tube. **a. of the vagina.** The dilated upper end of the vagina, where it joins the cervix of the uterus. **a. of Vater.** The dilatation of the common bile duct and pancreatic duct where they join the duodenum. **membra-**

nous ampullae. Those occurring at one end of the membranous semicircular canals near their junction with the utricle, and containing the end organs of the sense of kinetic equilibrium. **osseous ampullae.** Those parts of the osseous labyrinth of the internal ear which house the membranous ampullae.

am"pu·ta'tion. The removal, generally by surgical means, of a limb, wholly or in part, a projecting part or process, or an organ of the body. Amputation may occur in the course of pathologic processes, such as gangrene or constriction, or as the result of accident. **amniotic a.** Amputation of a fetal limb by a portion of the amnion. **a. appliance.** A prosthesis for an amputated limb. **a. by transfixion.** That performed by thrusting an amputating knife through a limb and cutting the flaps from within out. **a. center.** *In military medicine*, a general hospital in home territory where, prior to discharge, amputees are sent for prosthetic appliances, training in the use of artificial limbs, and rehabilitation. **a. in contiguity.** That performed through a joint (disarticulation, dismemberment). **a. in continuity.** That performed elsewhere than at a joint. **a. neuroma.** A painful bulbous enlargement of the end of a nerve divided at amputation, occurring after the formation of the stump. **a. stump.** The rounded and shaped lower portion of an amputated limb or organ. **central a.** One in which the flaps are joined so that the suture line runs across the end of the stump. **chop a.** One by a circular cut through the soft parts and bone without provision for flaps. **Chopart's a.** An amputation of the foot consisting of a disarticulation of the tarsal bones, leaving only the talus and calcaneus. **cinematic a.** One in which a muscular stump is left so as to allow for movement of an artificial limb. **cineplastic a.** One in which tendons are arranged in the stump to permit their use in moving parts of the prosthetic appliance. Types of cineplastic amputations include the *club*, the *loop*, the *tendon tunnel*, and the *muscle tunnel*. **circular a.** An operation performed with the use of a flap by circular sweeps or incisions around the limb vertical to the long axis of the bone. Syn., *guillotine a.* **coat-sleeve a.** One in which one long skin flap, like a coat sleeve, is left to enclose the stump. **congenital a.** One which takes place in the uterus as the result of some pathologic or accidental process. Syn., *intra-uterine a.* **double-flap a.** One in which there are two opposing skin and muscle flaps. **Gritti-Stokes a.** A supracondylar osteoplastic operation in which the patella, after removal of its articular surface, is retained in the flap and attached to the divided end of the femur, the skin and muscle flap being closed posteriorly. **guillotine a.** See circular *a.* **interpelvioabdominal a.** Amputation of the thigh with a portion of the adjoining half of the pelvis. **interthoracicoscapular a.** Amputation of the upper extremity at the shoulder girdle with disarticulation of the extremity: It includes removal of the scapula and outer portion of the clavicle. **intrauterine a.** See congenital *a.* **Lisfranc's a.** A disarticulation of the metatarsal bones from the tarsus. **major a.** Any amputation through the long bones of the upper or lower extremities; disarticulation at the hip joint or shoulder girdle. **mediotarsal a.** See Chopart's *a.* Also called *midtarsal a.* **osteoplastic a.** One in which there is a portion of bone fitted to the amputated bone end. See Gritti-Stokes *a.* **partial a.** One in which only a portion of a member, part, or organ has been removed. **pathologic a.** One occurring as a result of some pathologic process. **primary a.** One performed immediately after injury, during the period of reaction from shock and before the onset of suppuration. **racket a.** A variety of elliptic or oval amputation with a long cut, like a racket handle, below the elliptic incision. **secondary a.** One performed after suppuration has occurred or for the purpose of improving a temporary circular amputation with flaps left open. **spontaneous a.** (a) Congenital amputation. (b) Amputation not caused by external trauma or injury, as in ainhum, *q.v.* **subperiosteal a.** One in which the divided bone ends are covered by neighboring periosteum. **supracondylar a.** An operation in which the femur is sawed through above the condyles. See Gritti-Stokes *a.* **Syme's a.** Amputation at the ankle joint, the malleoli being sawed through, and a flap made with the skin of the heel. **thigh a.** One through the femur below the hip joint. **traumatic a.** One resulting from direct trauma.

am″pu·tee′. One who has had a major amputation of one or more limbs.

a·muck′. See *amok.*

a·mu′si·a (a-mew′zee-uh, -see-uh). Loss of the ability to produce or comprehend music or musical sounds; an abnormality in regard to music, analogous to aphasia in regard to the faculty of speech. **motor a.** That in which music is understood, but the power of singing or otherwise reproducing music is lost. **sensory a.** Musical deafness, or the loss of the power of comprehension of musical sounds.

am″y·dri′a·sis. Pupillary contraction. See *mydriasis.*

am″y·e′li·a (am″eye-ee′lee-uh, am″ee-). Congenital absence of the spinal cord. **—amyel′ic, amy′elous,** *adj.*

a·my′e·lus. A monster with partial or complete absence of the spinal cord.

a·myg′da·la. See *almond.*

a·myg′da·lin. A glycoside of mandelonitrile, occurring in the bitter almond and other sources.

am′yl, a′myl. The radical $CH_3(CH_2)_3-CH-$, derived from pentane, for which pentyl is a preferred designation. **a. acetate.** $CH_3.COO.C_5H_{11}$, a colorless liquid miscible with alcohol and having a characteristic pearlike odor and taste, used as a flavor, perfume, and solvent. Syn., *banana oil.* **a. alcohol.** Any of the eight isomeric alcohols of the composition $C_5H_{11}OH$, of which the commercial product is also called *fusel oil.* **a. nitrite.** Isoamyl nitrite. A yellowish liquid; used by inhalation to relax arterial spasms and of especial value in angina pectoris. **tertiary a. alcohol.** See *amylene hydrate.*

amyl-. See *amylo-.*

am″y·la′ceous. Containing starch; starchlike.

am′yl·ase (am′i·lace, ·laze). Any amylolytic enzyme which hydrolyzes starch to sugar. See Table of Normal Values of Blood Constituents in the Appendix. **pancreatic a.** Amylopsin. **salivary a.** Ptyalin. **vegetable a.** Diastase.

amylcaine hydrochloride. See *amylsine hydrochloride.*

am′yl·ene hy′drate. Tertiary amyl alcohol, $C_2H_5.(CH_3)_2C.OH$. A narcotic substance; rarely used by itself, but employed as a solvent for and synergist with tribromoethanol, *q.v.*

am′y·lo-, amyl-. A combining form denoting *pertaining to starch.*

am′y·lo-, a·my′lo-, amyl-. A combining form denoting *amyl,* the radical.

am″y·lo·caine′ hy″dro·chlo′ride. The hydrochloride of the benzoyl ester of methylethyldimethylaminomethylcarbinol, a local and spinal anesthetic. See *stovaine.*

am″y·lo·dex′trin. Soluble starch.

am″y·lo·dys·pep′si·a. Inability to digest starchy foods.

a·myl′o·gen. Soluble starch.

am′y·loid. A complex protein deposited in tissues, characterized physically by its hyaline structureless nature, and chemically by special staining reactions. Its exact composition is unknown, and probably variable. It is starchlike only in that it stains brown with iodine.

am·y·loid de"gen·er·a'tion. Formation and deposit of amyloid in tissues and organs; waxy or lardaceous degeneration. See secondary *amyloidosis.*

am"y·loi·do'sis. Widespread deposit of amyloid in various organs of the body or, less commonly, deposit in a particular organ, as amyloidosis of the kidney. **primary a.** A rare disease without known cause; characterized by more or less widespread deposit of amyloid in mesodermal structures, including skeletal muscle, tongue, bone, tendons, cartilage, cardiac muscle, lips, and other sites. This amyloid has less uniform staining reactions than is true in the common secondary forms. **secondary a.** Deposit of amyloid in various organs of the body—especially liver, spleen, and kidney—secondary to chronic diseases, such as chronic ulcerative tuberculosis of the lungs, chronic tuberculosis of the bones, chronic suppurative osteomyelitis, leprosy, tertiary syphilis, and malignant tumors. The material is first found immediately around capillaries and vascular sinuses, then around small arteries and veins, and then later more widely distributed in the organ. Staining reactions are regular and characteristic. Syn., *amyloid degeneration.*

am"y·lol'y·sis. The digestion of starch, or its conversion into maltose. **—amylolyt'ic,** *adj.*

am"y·lop'sin. An enzyme which changes starch into maltose; found in the pancreatic juice.

amylsine hydrochloride. Trade-mark for a local anesthetic, naepaine hydrochloride. Formerly called *Amylcaine hydrochloride.*

am'y·lum. See *starch.*

am"y·lu'ri·a. Presence of starch in the urine.

a·my"o·es·the'si·a, a·my"o·aes·the'si·a (·ess·thee'zhuh, ·zee·uh), **a·my"o·es·the'sis, a·my"o·aes·the'sis.** State of being without muscle sense; lack of the sense of motion, weight, and position.

a·my"o·pla'si·a (a·my"o·play'zhuh, ·zee·uh). Lack of muscle formation and development. **—amyoplas'tic,** *adj.* **a. congenita.** A congenital muscle deficiency attended by joint fixation, malpresentation, and difficult delivery.

a·my"o·sta'si·a (a·my"o·stay'zhuh, ·zee·uh). A tremor of the muscles causing difficulty in standing, often seen in locomotor ataxia. **—amyostat'ic,** *adj.*

a·my"o·tax'i·a, a·my"o·tax'y. Muscular ataxia or incoördination of spinal or cerebellar origin. **—amyotaxic,** *adj.*

a·my"o·tax'y. See *amyotaxia.*

a·my"o·to'ni·a. Lack of muscular tone; myatonia. **a. congenita.** A rare congenital disease of the brain stem and spinal cord of infants; marked by absence of postural tone in the voluntary muscles, absence of reflexes, and with no reaction of degeneration in electrical tests. Mental development is rarely retarded, but the ability to sit up, stand, or walk is badly impaired. Also called *Oppenheim's disease.*

a·my"o·tro'phi·a, am"y·ot'ro·phy. Muscle atrophy. **—amyotroph'ic,** *adj.* **a. spinalis progressiva.** See myelopathic muscular *atrophy.*

amytal. Trade-mark for isoamyl-ethylbarbituric acid or amobarbital, a sedative and hypnotic. **sodium a.** The monosodium salt of amytal. A white, hygroscopic, granular powder, soluble in water or alcohol; used as above.

a·myx'i·a. Absence or deficiency of mucous secretion.

An. 1. Abbreviation for anode. 2. Symbol for actinon.

-an. *In chemistry,* a suffix which indicates *a sugarlike substance, a glycoside, or a gum.*

A. N. A. American Nurses' Association.

an'a. So much of each. Contracted in prescriptions to *āā.*

an'a-. A prefix meaning *back, up, again, through, excessively.*

-a'na (-ay'nuh, -an'uh). A suffix meaning *belonging to, connected with, derived from.* In the naming of subsections or groups of species it is added to the name of a species around which other species naturally cluster.

an"a·bi·ot'ic (an"uh·buy·ot'ick). 1. Apparently lifeless, but capable of being revived. 2. Any agent used to effect such a restoration or revival. **—anabio'sis,** *n.*

a·nab'o·lism. Synthetic or constructive metabolism; the conversion of nutritive material into more complex living matter. **—anabol'ic,** *adj.*

an"a·cid'i·ty. The complete absence of hydrochloric acid in the stomach, demonstrated by lack of response to all secretory stimulants, particularly to histamine; achlorhydria. See *hypoacidity.*

a·nac'li·sis. 1. The act of reclining; decubitus. 2. *In psychiatry,* state of being emotionally dependent upon others. 3. *In psychoanalysis,* state in which the satisfaction of the sex libido is conditioned by some other instinct, such as hunger. **—anaclit'ic,** *adj.*

an·ac'me·sis. The arrest of development in certain bone-marrow cells.

a·nac"ro·a'si·a (a·nack"ro·ay'zhuh, an"uh·kro·). Inability to understand spoken language.

an″a·crot′ic in″ci·su′ra (in″-sigh-sue′ruh). In kymographic tracings, a sharp notch in the upstroke of the central arterial pulse seen in cases of aortic stenosis.

a·nac′ro·tism. The condition in which one or more notches occur on the ascending limb of the pulse curve. **—anacrot′ic,** *adj.*

an″a·cu′si·a (an″uh·cue′zhuh, an″-uh·koo′·), **an″a·cu′sis** (an″uh·cue′-sis, ·koo′sis), **an″a·cou′si·a** (an″-uh·koo′zhuh, ·zee·uh), **an″a·ku′sis.** Complete deafness.

an″a·cu′sis. See *anacusia.*

an″a·did′y·mus. A monster showing inferior duplicity but union above. Syn., *dipygus.* Also called *inferior duplicity.* **—anadidymus,** *adj.*

an″a·dip′si·a. Intense thirst. See *polydipsia.*

a·nae′mi·a. See *anemia.*

an′aer·obe (an′air·ohb, an·air′ohb, an·ay′ur·ohb). A microörganism that will grow in the absence of molecular oxygen. Also called *anaerobion.* **—anaero′bic,** *adj.* **facultative a.** An organism which will grow in the presence or absence of molecular oxygen. **obligatory a.** One which grows only when oxygen is rigorously excluded.

an″aer·o·bi′ase (an″air·o·buy′ace, an·air″o·). A proteolytic enzyme which acts under anaerobic conditions and is present in a number of anaerobes.

an″aer·o·bi·o′sis (an″air·o·buy·o′-sis, an·air″o·). Life sustained in the absence of molecular oxygen. See *anaerobe.* **—anaerobiot′ic,** *adj.*

an″aes·the′si·a (an″ess·thee′zhuh, ·zee·uh). See *anesthesia.*

an″a·gog′ic (an″uh·godj′ick). 1. Relating to the mystical or anagoge. 2. *In psychoanalysis,* pertaining to the efforts of the subconscious to achieve the moral, ideal, or uplifting; also, pertaining to dream material which expresses idealistic and spiritual ideas, as contrasted with that representing the sexual forces of the unconscious.

an″a·kat″a·did′y·mus. A conjoined twin monster exhibiting both inferior and superior duplicity. **—anakatadidymous,** *adj.*

an″a·lep′tic. 1. Restoring consciousness in fainting or coma. 2. Hastening convalescence. 3. A restorative agent or medicine.

an″al·ge′si·a (an″al·jee′zee·uh, ·see·uh), **an·al′gi·a.** Insensibility to pain without loss of consciousness. **a. al′gera.** Severe pain in a part with loss of general sensibility. **continuous caudal a.** A method of relieving the pains of childbirth by bathing the lumbar and sacral nerves with an anesthetic solution, within the epidural space. Can also be used for surgery

below the umbilical plane. **infiltration a.** Paralyzing the nerve endings at the site of operation by subcutaneous injection of an anesthetic. **permeation a.** See surface *a.* **surface a.** Topical application on mucous membranes for local analgesia.

an″al·ge′sic (an″al·jee′zick, ·jee′-sick), **an″al·get′ic, an·al′gic.** 1. Anodyne; relieving pain. 2. Not affected by pain. **—analge′sist,** *n.;* **an′algize,** *v.t.*

an′a·log, an′a·logue. 1. Organ or part having the same function as another but differing in structure and origin, as the wing of an insect and the wing of a bird. 2. One of a group of compounds with similar electronic structure, but with different atoms, as an isologue.

a·nal′o·gy. 1. Resemblance in two or more attributes between two things which differ in other respects. 2. *In biology,* a similarity in function without correspondence in structure and origin. **—analogous,** *adj.*

a·nal′y·sis. 1. The determination of the nature, properties, or composition of a substance. 2. The resolution of a compound body into its constituent parts. 3. *In psychiatry,* psychoanalysis, *q.v.* **chromatographic a.** A method of separating chemical constituents by differential adsorption. **clinical a.** (a) Thorough examination of symptoms, lesions, and history to determine the nature of a disease and its cause. (b) Examination of body fluids and tissues for the diagnosis of diseases. **distributive a.** The method of analyzing a subject's symptoms and complaints according to the concepts of psychobiology, *q.v.,* as distinguished from psychoanalysis. **gasometric a.** Analysis of a solid or liquid substance by conversion to a gas, or the determination of the constituents of gaseous compounds. Also called *eudiometric a.* **gravimetric a.** Quantitative determination, by weight, of the elements of a body. **inorganic a.** Determination of the chemical composition of inorganic matter. **microchemical a.** (a) Chemical analysis with the aid of a microscope. (b) Chemical analysis using small quantities of materials, but employing the conventional reactions. **nephelometric a.** Quantitative determination of a substance by observation of the degree of turbidity produced by it in a suitable dispersion medium. **organic a.** Analysis of organic chemical substances. **proximate a.** Determination of gross constituents, as alkaloids, glycosides, fat, protein, carbohydrate, etc., in drugs. **qualitative a.** Determination of the elements that compose a substance. **quantitative a.** Determination of the amount of an element or compound in a substance. **radiometric a.** Determination of an element that is not itself radioactive by means of an interaction (e.g., precipitation) with a radioactive element. **spectrophotometric a.** Identification and determination of substances through study of the adsorption of energy in the ultraviolet, visible, or infrared spectrum. **ultimate a.** Resolution of a compound into its ultimate elements. **volumetric a.** Quantitative determination of a constituent by titration with standardized volumetric solutions.

an·a·lyst. 1. One experienced in performing analyses. 2. *In psychiatry,* one who analyzes the psyche, usually one who adheres to the formulations of the psychoanalytic school of Freud. See *psychoanalyst.*

an"a·lyt"ic psy·chol'o·gy. The analysis of the psyche according to the concepts of Carl Jung; differs from the psychoanalysis of Freud in that the emphasis in diagnosing and treating a neurosis is not on early complexes but on current maladjustments.

an·a·ly"zer. 1. An analyst. 2. In a polariscope, the Nicol prism which exhibits the properties of light after polarization. 3. An apparatus for recording the excursions of tremor movements.

an"am·ne'sis. 1. Faculty of memory. 2. Information gained from the patient and others regarding the past history of a case. —**anamnes'tic,** *adj.*

An·am'ni·o·ta. A group of vertebrates having no amnion; it includes the fishes and the amphibia.

an·an"a·ba'si·a (an-an"uh-bay'-zhuh, ·zee·uh). Inability to ascend to heights.

an·an"a·phy·lax'is. A condition neutralizing anaphylaxis.

an·an"as·ta'si·a (·ass·tay'zhuh, ·zee·uh). Abulic inability to rise from a sitting posture.

an"a·pau'sis. Hypnotic inducement of calm sleep by allaying excitement.

an"a·pei·rat'ic (an"uh·pye·rat'ick). Denoting a condition which results from overuse, as writer's cramp.

an'a·phase (an'uh·fayz). The stage of mitosis between the metaphase and telophase, in which the daughter chromosomes move apart toward the poles of the spindle, to form the diaster. See *mitosis.*

an·a·phi·a, an·aph'i·a. 1. Defective or absent sense of touch. 2. A state of abnormal sensitiveness to touch. 3. A state in which nothing is learned by palpation. —**anap'tic,** *adj.*

an"a·pho·re'sis. 1. Diminished activity of the sweat glands. 2. The migration of electropositive particles, or ions, into tissues under the influence of an

electric field. —**anaphoret'ic,** *adj.*

an"a·pho'ri·a. An upward tendency of the eyes and of the visual axes. Syn., *anatropia.*

an·aph"ro·dis'i·a (an·af"ro·diz'-ee·uh). Impairment of sexual appetite. —**anaph'rodite,** *n.*

an·aph"ro·dis'i·ac. 1. Relating to or causing anaphrodisia. 2. An agent that allays the sexual desire.

an"a·phy·lac'tic. 1. Relating to the production or state of anaphylaxis, *q.v.* 2. Increasing sensitivity. Syn., *anaphylactoid.*

an"a·phy·lac'tin. The antibody concerned in anaphylaxis. Has been confused with allergen.

an"a·phy·lac'to·gen. A substance which is capable of producing a state of anaphylaxis in a subject previously sensitized to it. —**anaphylactogen'ic,** *adj.*

an"a·phy·lac'toid. Like anaphylaxis.

an"a·phy·lax'is. A state of increased susceptibility, or hypersensitivity, following the parenteral injection of an antigen in an animal. Upon the reintroduction of the antigen after a lapse of time (10 to 12 days) there is manifested a series of characteristic symptoms, including spasms of smooth muscle, capillary dilatation, glandular secretion, altered permeability of the vessels, and varying degrees of shock. The reaction is believed to be due to fixation of a specific antibody in certain tissues, rendering them sensitive to subsequently injected antigen. Also called *active a.* **active a.** Hypersensitization produced by the direct introduction of an antigen. **local a.** A reaction at the site of injections, dependent upon the union in the tissues of the circulating precipitin and its specific antigen; as edema, induration, and necrosis caused by repeated subcutaneous injections of horse serum into rabbits. Also called *Arthus' phenomenon.* **passive a.** Hypersensitivity produced in an animal by parenteral injection of serum from another previously sensitized animal. **reverse passive a.** A type in which the antigen is injected first, then followed by the specific antibody, causing shock.

an"a·pla'si·a (an"uh·play'zhuh, ·zee·uh). 1. Reversion of form of a cell or cells toward the embryonal, together with increased capacity for multiplication. 2. Often used by morphologists to indicate reversion of form only, without reference to capacity for multiplication.

an"a·plas·mo'sis (an"uh·plaz·mo'-sis). A term sometimes used to indicate infection with the sporozoon *Anaplasma;* a disease of cattle.

an"a·plas'tic. 1. Relating to or affected with anaplasia. 2. Pertaining to the replacement of a lost or absent part by surgery.

an'a·plas'ty. An operation for the restoration of lost parts; plastic surgery.

an"a·poph'y·sis. An accessory process of a lumbar or thoracic vertebra, corresponding to the inferior tubercle of the transverse process of a typical thoracic vertebra.

an"a·rith'mi·a. An inability to count.

an·ar'thri·a. Defective articulation in speaking. —**anarthric**, adj. **a. centralis.** Partial aphasia due to a central lesion. **a. literalis.** Stammering.

an"a·sar'ca. An accumulation of serum in the subcutaneous connective tissue and the serous cavities of the body; generalized edema. —**anasarcous**, adj. **a. hystericum.** A transient swelling in a hysterical individual.

a·nas'ta·sis. Recovery; convalescence. —**anastat'ic**, adj.

a·nas"to·mo'ses. Plural of anastomosis.

a·nas"to·mo'sis (pl. anastomoses). 1. The intercommunication of blood vessels by the natural anatomic arrangement which, as a result of an interruption of the chief blood supply, provides an increased growth in other vessels supplying a part. Occasionally, anastomosis of blood vessels is secured by a direct surgical operation upon the vessels themselves. 2. The establishment by surgical means of a communication between two hollow organs or two parts of the same organ, as between the jejunum and stomach, the hepatic duct and small intestine, the ureter and colon. 3. The joining of a nerve to another nerve or to a portion of the same nerve. —**anastomot'ic**, adj.; **anas'tomose**, v.i., v.t. **arteriovenous a.** A modified vessel which connects an artery with a vein without the intervention of capillaries. Such structures are particularly numerous in the palm, the sole, and the skin of terminal phalanges. **crucial a.** An arterial anastomosis in the upper thigh, formed by the inferior gluteal, medial circumflex femoral, lateral circumflex femoral, and first perforating arteries. It is important in the formation of collateral circulation after ligation of the femoral artery. **intersubcardinal a.** A transverse anastomosis between the paired subcardinal veins of the early embryo, ventral to the aorta. **portacaval a.** One joining the portal vein to the vena cava; also known as Eck's fistula. **postcostal a.** A longitudinal anas-

tomosis between successive cervical intersegmental arteries, the first through the seventh, which forms the vertebral artery. **posttransverse a.** A longitudinal anastomosis between intersegmental arteries, dorsal to the transverse processes, forming the deep cervical artery. **precostal a.** A longitudinal anastomosis between cervical and thoracic intersegmental arteries, which forms the thyrocervical trunk and the superior intercostal artery.

a·nas"to·mot'i·ca. A communicating artery or vein.

anat. Anatomic, anatomical, anatomy.

a·nat'o·mist. One who specializes or is skilled in anatomy.

a·nat'o·my. 1. Science or branch of morphology which treats of the structure of organisms and the relation of their parts. 2. Dissection of the various parts of a plant or animal. —**anatom'ic, anatom'ical**, adj. **applied a.** Anatomy as a factor in diagnosis and treatment. **comparative a.** Investigation and comparison of the anatomy of different orders of animals or of plants, one with another. **descriptive a.** Study of the separate and individual portions of the body. **general a.** That which treats of the structure and physiologic properties of the tissues and their arrangement into systems without regard to the disposition of the organs of which they form a part. **gross a.** That which deals with the macroscopic appearance of tissues. **microscopic a.** Histology. Also called minute a. **pathologic a.** Study of the changes in structure caused by disease. Also called morbid a. **physiologic a.** Anatomic study of tissues in respect to their functions. **regional a.** Study of limited parts or regions of the body. **surface a.** Study of superficial landmarks for the location of internal structures. **surgical a.** Application of anatomy to surgery. **topographic a.** Anatomy of a part in its relation to other parts.

an"a·tox'in. A toxin modified by heat and chemical treatment (formaldehyde) so that it is no longer toxic but still retains the capacity for uniting with the antitoxins and stimulating their formation. Syn., toxoid.

an"a·tro'pi·a. A tendency of the eyes to turn upward when at rest; anaphoria.

an"a·ven'in. Venoms which have been altered by physical or chemical agents that eliminate their toxic property but make little or no change in their antigenic qualities.

AnCC. Anodal closure contraction; ACC. Rare.

an'chor·age. 1. The fixation of a floating or displaced viscus, whether by a natural process or by surgical means. **2.** *In dentistry*, the means of retaining a dental filling, particularly its initial portion; also, the means by which a bridge or artificial crown is secured. **3.** *In orthodontics*, a tooth or teeth used for resistance in applying a regulating force.

an″chy·lo- (ang′ki·lo-), **an″cy·lo-** (an′ki·lo-). For words beginning *anchylo-* or *ancylo-* not found here, see under *ankylo-*.

an″co·ne′us, an·co′ne·us. A small triangular muscle at the back of the elbow joint. See Table of Muscles in the Appendix.

An″cy·los′to·ma. A genus of nematodes. **A. duodenale.** A species of hookworm which infests man, the principal and optimum host. Occasionally hogs, dogs, felines, and gorillas are infested.

An″cy·los″to·mat′i·dae (an″ki·los″to·mat′i·dee). A family of hookworms of the superfamily Strongyloidea, characterized by oral cutting organs. The hookworms of man of the genera *Ancylostoma* and *Necator* belong to this family.

an″cy·los″to·mi′a·sis. Infestation of the human intestine with *Ancylostoma duodenale* and the resulting morbid state.

an″dre·o·blas·to′ma. Arrhenoblastoma.

an″dri·at′rics, an·dri′a·try. A branch of medicine dealing with those disorders peculiar to men, especially those of the male genitalia.

an·dri′a·try. See *andriatrics*.

an·dro-, andr-. A combining form signifying *man* or *male, masculine, relating to the male sex*.

an·dro′gen. A hormone which controls the physiologic status of the secondary sex characteristics of males. **—androgen′ic, androg′enous,** *adj.*

an″dro·gen′e·sis. Activation of the egg by the sperm followed by development without the participation of the egg nucleus (Wilson).

an·drog′e·nous. Giving birth to males.

an′dro·gyne (an′dro·jyne, -jin), **an·drog′y·nus** (an·drodj′i·nus), **an·drog′y·na** (an·drodj′i·nuh). A pseudohermaphrodite, *q.v.* **—androg′y·nous,** *adj.*

an·drog′y·nism (an·drodj′i·niz·um). Hermaphroditism.

an·drog′y·ny (an·drodj′i·nee), **an″·dro·gy·ne′i·ty.** Hermaphroditism. **—androg′ynoid,** *adj., n.*

an′droid. Resembling the male.

an″dro·mor′phous. Having the form of a man.

an″dro·pho′bi·a. Morbid fear or dislike of men or of the male sex.

an·dros′ter·one. $C_{19}H_{30}O_2$. 3(a)-Hydroxy-17-ketoandrostane, an androgenic steroid found in the urine of men and women. See also *isoandrosterone*.

a·ne′mi·a. Loss of normal balance between the productive and the destructive blood processes, due to diminution of the normal blood volume (oligemia), as after hemorrhage; or a deficiency in the number of red cells (oligocythemia), hemoglobin (oligochromemia), or both. Microscopically, anemias are classified as normocytic, macrocytic, or microcytic, based upon the mean size of the erythrocytes. Clinically, the condition is marked by varying degrees of pallor, dyspnea, and palpitation. **—anemic,** *adj.* **achlorhydric a.** (a) An anemia associated with an absence of free hydrochloric acid in the gastric juice. (b) A microcytic, hypochromic anemia which responds to iron therapy; characterized by achylia gastrica, glossitis, and epithelial changes. Syn., *achylanemia.* **aplastic a.** That resulting from defects of the bone marrow, as hypoplasia, aplasia, and degenerative changes. It is marked by a deficiency of red cells, hemoglobin and granular cells, and a predominance of lymphocytes. Also called *atrophic a., myelophthisic a., aleukia hemorrhagica.* **deficiency a.** That caused by faulty or inadequate diet or nutrition. Syn., *nutritional a.* **essential a.** See pernicious *a.,* idiopathic *a.* **familial erythroblastic a.** A congenital disease occurring in children of Mediterranean peoples; associated with hypertrophy of the spleen, Mongoloid face and changes in the bones. Also called *thalassanemia, Mediterranean disease, Cooley's disease.* **hemolytic a.** That caused by a hemolytic agent, as cobra venom. **hemorrhagic a.** That following gross hemorrhage. **hyperchromic a.** That in which the hemoglobin deficiency is comparatively less than that of the red cells (where the color index is high). **hypochromic a.** That in which the hemoglobin deficiency is comparatively greater than that of the red cells (where the color index is low). **idiopathic a.** That in which the lesion is in the blood or blood-forming organs. Syn., *primary a., essential a.* **idiopathic hypochromic a.** A severe anemia marked by achylia, very low hemoglobin, and microcytosis. It affects women chiefly, giving them a waxy, apathetic look, brittle nails, and atrophy of lingual papillae. **infantile pseudoleukemic a.** A form of primary anemia peculiar to the young child characterized by anemia and splenomegaly. Probably associated with infantile leishmaniasis and congenital syphilis.

local a. Deficient blood supply to a particular organ or part. **lymphatic a.** Hodgkin's disease. **macrocytic a.** That characterized by abnormally large erythrocytes. Under this type are found *pernicious anemia*, sprue, and *anemia of pregnancy*. **microcytic a.** That in which the erythrocytes are smaller than normal and deficient in hemoglobin. **normochromic a.** (a) A type in which the hemoglobin content of the red blood cell is normal. (b) One with a normal color index and a normal mean corpuscular hemoglobin. **normocytic a.** That in which the erythrocytes are of normal size. **nutritional a.** See deficiency *a*. **pernicious a.** A serious type, formerly fatal, showing a great reduction of the red cells, mostly macrocytic and hyperchromic, many nucleated forms (megaloblasts), and a high color index. Clinically, it is characterized by pallor or a waxy appearance, weakness, languor, dyspnea, persistent achlorhydria, and nervous and digestive disorders. Remission of some or all of the symptoms occurs frequently. The condition is due to a deficiency of a maturation principle derived in part from food (extrinsic factor), and in part from the pyloric and duodenal mucosa (intrinsic factor), and stored in the liver (liver principle). Hence, administration of liver, liver extracts, and stomach preparations causes improvement, usually ushered in by showers of reticulocytes. Also called *Addison's a.*, *Biermer's disease*, *primary a.*, *essential a.*, *idiopathic a.* **physiologic a.** That affecting most infants at about the second month and disappearing usually before the end of the first year. **primary a.** See idiopathic *a.*, pernicious *a.* **secondary a.** That following or resulting from a pathologic condition, as carcinoma and malignancy, poisoning, trauma, or hemorrhagic disease. **sickle-cell a.** That affecting Negroes and dark-skinned individuals, usually hereditary. It is characterized by the crescentic form assumed by the erythrocytes after their removal from the circulation. **splenic a.** That characterized by splenomegaly, marked leukopenia, but no adenopathy. Also called *Gaucher's disease*. **toxic a.** Blood-cell destruction, the result of toxins and poisons. **tunnel a.** Ancylostomiasis.

a·ne″mo·pho′bi·a (a-nee″mo·fo′-bee·uh, an″i·mo-). Morbid dread of drafts or of winds.

an·en″ce·pha′li·a, an″en·ceph′-a·ly. Absence of cerebrum and cerebellum with absence of the flat bones of the skull. **—anenceph′alous, anencephal′ic,** *adj.*

an″en·ceph′a·lus. A monster showing partial or complete anencephalia. **an″en·ceph′a·ly.** See *anencephalia*. **an·ep′i·a, an·e′pi·a.** Inability to speak.

an·ep″i·thym′i·a (an-ep″i-thim′ee-uh, -thigh′mee-uh). Loss or absence of any natural appetite.

an″er·ga′si·a (an″ur-gay′zhuh, -zee-uh). *In psychiatry*, the term coined by Adolf Meyer for a psychosis caused by organic lesions of the nervous system. **an′er·gy.** 1. Lack of energy or activity. 2. Absence of reaction to a specific antigen or allergen. The capacity to resist the effects of potentially harmful agents. **—aner′gic,** *adj.*

an′er·oid. Working without a fluid, as an aneroid barometer.

an·es″the·ki·ne′sis (an-ess″thi·ki·nee′sis, -kigh·nee′-), **an·es″the·ki·ne′si·a** (-ki·nee′shuh, -kigh·nee′-). Sensory and motor paralysis, combined. **an″es·the′si·a, an″aes·the′si·a** (an″ess-thee′zhuh, -zee-uh). Loss of sensation. **a. dolorosa.** Severe pain experienced after complete motor and sensory paralysis; observed in certain diseases of the spinal cord. **angiospastic a.** Loss of sensibility due to spasm of the blood vessels. **balanced a.** That produced by safe doses of two or more agents or methods of anesthesia. **basal a.** An incomplete anesthesia; supplementary anesthetics are usually required. Thus, preliminary narcosis may be induced with an injected drug, requiring but a small amount of inhalation anesthetic to produce surgical anesthesia. Among basal anesthetics are the barbiturates, amytal, sodium amytal, avertin. **block a.** Anesthesia produced by injecting an anesthetic solution into the nerve trunks supplying the operative field (regional block), or infiltrating close to the nerves (infiltration block), or by a wall of anesthetic solution injected about the field (field block). In all these methods the nerve conduction is *blocked*, and painful impulses fail to reach the brain. **bulbar a.** That due to a lesion in the medulla. **carbon-dioxide absorption a.** See closed *a.* **caudal a.** That induced by injection of the anesthetic into the sacral canal. **central a.** That due to disease of the central nervous system. **closed a.** Inhalation anesthesia with complete rebreathing of the anesthetic gases. Soda-lime generally is used to absorb the excess CO_2. **closed circuit a.** That produced by an anesthetizing apparatus in which explosive agents used in anesthesia are prevented from coming in contact with sparks or flame. **combined a.** (a) Anesthesia produced by a combination of anesthetics

—as chloroform, ether, and nitrous oxide—or of methods. (b) That produced by anesthetics plus somnifacient drugs. **conduction a.** See block *a*. **continuous caudal a.** The caudal needle is left in place so that the anesthetic drug can be administered periodically as needed. **continuous spinal a.** The spinal needle is left in place so that the anesthetic drug can be administered periodically as needed. **crossed a.** Anesthesia on one side of the body due to a central lesion on the other side. **cryanesthesia.** See refrigeration *a*. **dental a.** Anesthesia of the teeth for dental operations. **dissociated a.** Loss of pain and temperature sensations, the tactile sense being still present. **electric a.** Transient anesthesia caused by the passage of an electric current through a part. **endotracheal a.** General anesthesia in which the anesthetic is administered by means of a tube which conducts the vapor directly into the trachea. **epidural a.** That induced by the injection of an anesthetic outside the spinal dura mater. **gauntlet a.** anesthesia of the entire hand. Syn., glove *a*. **general a.** Loss of sensation with loss of consciousness. See stages of general *a*. **girdle a.** A zone of anesthesia encircling the body. **glove a.** A loss of sensation in an area corresponding to that covered by a glove; usually a hysterical phenomenon. **hysterical a.** A loss of pain sense in areas of the skin; dictated by suggestion and usually taking on geometric configuration or conforming to zones covered by various articles of apparel. See glove *a*. **ice a.** Refrigeration anesthesia, *q.v.* **infiltration a.** That induced by the injection of the anesthetic solution directly into the tissues that are to be anesthetized. **inhalation a.** That produced by the inhalation of anesthetic gases or vapors. **insufflation a.** That produced by the delivery of anesthetic gases under pressure into the respiratory system. **intravenous a.** The injection of an anesthetic into a vein, as pentothal sodium. **local a.** Anesthesia limited to a local area. See regional *a*. **mixed a.** That produced by two or more anesthetics. **morphine-scopolamine a.** See *twilight sleep.* **olfactory a.** Anosmia. **open a.** Inhalation anesthesia with a minimum amount of rebreathing. **optic a.** Temporary amaurosis. **partial a.** Anesthesia in which some degree of sensibility is still present. **peripheral a.** Loss of sensation due to changes in the peripheral nerves. **pharyngeal a.** Anesthesia of the pharynx occasionally complicating nervous disorders; most common in hysterical patients. **planes of a.** Stages through which the patient passes as anesthesia becomes deeper because of the stepwise depression of the central nervous system. They are as follows: *I. Analgesia or altered consciousness* (higher cortical centers); *II. Delirium or excitement* (basal ganglia and cerebellum); *III. Surgical anesthesia* (spinal cord, motor and sensory); and *IV. Medullary paralysis* (brain stem). **primary a.** The transient anesthesia resulting from a small amount of anesthetic. **rectal a.** That induced by an anesthetic placed within the rectum. **refrigeration a.** A method of rendering a lower limb insensitive by the use of cracked ice applied to the member so as to surround it completely. After two and a half hours of this preparation, amputation may be performed without medication or anesthesia. **regional a.** That limited to a part of the body by blocking nerve conduction from the area. See block *a*. **segmental a.** Loss of sensation of an area supplied by one or a limited group of spinal nerves. **semiopen a.** Inhalation anesthesia with partial rebreathing. **sexual a.** Anaphrodisia. **spinal a.** (a) That due to a lesion of the spinal cord. (b) That produced by the injection of an anesthetic into the spinal subarachnoid space. **stages of general a.** The degree or depth of general anesthesia may be divided into four stages: (1) *Stage of analgesia;* from the beginning of the administration of the anesthetic to the loss of consciousness. (2) *Stage of excitement;* from the loss of consciousness to the onset of muscular relaxation. (3) *Stage of surgical anesthesia;* in this stage, which is divided into four planes, there is sufficient muscular paralysis to permit surgical manipulation. (4) *Stage of paralysis of the muscles of respiration.* **surface a.** See topical *a*. **surgical a.** Stage 3 of general anesthesia where muscles are sufficiently relaxed. See stages of general *a*. **synergistic a.** That combining several anesthetics used simultaneously. **tactile a.** Loss of sense of touch. **thermic a.** Loss of temperature sense. **topical a.** Application of an anesthetic to one of the body surfaces, as with a swab. **traumatic a.** Loss of sensation due to injury of a nerve. **unilateral a.** Hemianesthesia.

an·es″the·sim′e·ter, an″es·the″si·om′e·ter (an″ess·thee″zeeom′i·tur). 1. An instrument that measures the amount of an anesthetic administered in a given time. 2. An instrument that determines the degree of insensibility of a part. Also called *anesthetometer, esthesiometer.*

anesthesin. Brand of ethyl aminobenzoate; used as local anesthetic. See *benzocaine.*

an″es·the″si·ol′o·gy (an″essthee″zee·ol′o·jee). The art and science of administering local and general anesthetics to produce the various types of anesthesia. **—anesthesiologist,** *n.*

an″es·thet′ic, an″aes·thet′ic. 1. Causing anesthesia. 2. Insensible to touch, pain, or other stimulation. 3. A drug which produces local or general loss of sensibility. **general a.** An agent which produces general anesthesia either by injection or by inhalation. **local a.** A drug which, topically applied or injected into the tissues, causes local insensibility to pain.

an·es′the·tize. Subject or place under the influence of an anesthetic; induce anesthesia; render anesthetic. **—anesthetist, anesthetiza′tion, anesthetizer,** *n.*

an·es′trum, an·oes′trum, an·es′trus, an·oes′trus. The interval between the periods of sexual heat of female mammals; diestrum. **—anestrous,** *adj.*

an·es′trus. See *anestrum.*

an′e·thole, an′e·thol. $CH_3O.C_6H_4.$$C_2H_5$, the chief constituent of anise and fennel oils, used as a flavor and carminative.

an″e·to·der′mi·a. Relaxation of the skin; dermatolysis.

a·neu′ri·a. Lack of nervous energy. **—aneuric,** *adj.*

an′eu·rin (an′yoor·in), **a·neu′rin.** Name given to vitamin B_1 by Jansen and Donath who first isolated it in crystalline form. See *thiamine hydrochloride.*

an′eu·rysm, an′eu·rism. A circumscribed axial or lateral communicating dilatation of the wall of an artery forming a blood-containing tumor which pulsates with each systole, produces a bruit, and often is associated with pain, pressure symptoms, and absorption of contiguous parts. Most common in the aorta as a result of syphilis. **—aneurys′mal, aneurysmat′ic,** *adj.* **ampullary a.** A small saccular aneurysm; it is most common in the arteries of the brain. See berry *a.* **anastomotic a.** See cirsoid *a.* **aortic a.** An aneurysm of the aorta. It occurs most frequently in the ascending aorta where it may cause severe pressure symptoms and eventually may rupture. The usual cause is syphilitic aortitis. **arteriovenous a.** Any abnormal communication between arteries and veins, congenital or acquired. Gunshot wounds of the larger vessels of the extremities are the most common cause. A *varicose aneurysm* is produced by the rupture of an aneurysm into a vein. An *aneurysmal varix*

results from the establishment of a communication between an artery and a vein, the latter becoming dilated and pulsating. **berry a.** A saccular aneurysm formed from a congenital defect of the media of a cerebral artery, rupture of which is the most common source of subarachnoid hemorrhage. **cardiac a.** An aneurysm of the heart wall. **circumscribed a.** An aneurysm, either true or false, in which the contents are still within the arterial wall, though there may be rupture of some of its coats. **cirsoid a.** (a) A tortuous lengthening and dilatation of a part of an artery. (b) A dilatation of a group of vessels (arteries, veins, and capillaries), the whole forming a pulsating subcutaneous tumor. Occurs most often on the scalp. **compound a.** One in which one or several of the coats of the artery are ruptured and the others merely dilated. **congenital a.** One due to a developmental defect. **consecutive a.** One following rupture of all the arterial coats, with infiltration of surrounding tissues with blood. **Crisp's a.** Aneurysm of the splenic artery. **diffused a.** See consecutive *a.* **dissecting a.** One in which the blood forces its way between the coats of an artery. Syn., *intramural a.* **ectatic a.** An expansion of a portion of an artery due to yielding of all the coats. **embolic a.** One caused by embolism. **endogenous a.** One formed by disease of the vessel walls. **erosion a.** Aortic aneurysm due to extension from diseased valves breaking down the vessel wall. **exogenous a.** One due to traumatism. **external a.** (a) One remote from the great body cavities. (b) One in which the cavity of the tumor is entirely or chiefly outside the inner coat of the artery. **false a.** One due to a rupture of all the coats of an artery, the effused blood being retained by the surrounding tissues. **fusiform a.** Spindleshaped dilatation of an artery. **hernial a.** One in which the internal coat of the artery, with or without the middle coat, forms the aneurysmal sac which has forced its way through an opening in the outer coat. **intramural a.** See dissecting *a.* **lateral a.** One projecting on one side of a vessel, the rest of the circumference being intact. **medical a.** One which cannot be treated surgically. **miliary a.** A minute saclike dilatation of an arteriole. **mural a.** See cardiac *a.* **mycotic a.** One caused by bacterial infection and inflammation of the wall of a blood vessel. **osteoid a.** Pulsating tumor of a bone. **partial a.** (a) See lateral *a.* (b) Aneurysmal dilatation of a portion of the heart. **peripheral a.** One involving the circumference of an artery. **race-mose a.** See cirsoid *a*. **sacculated a.** A saclike dilatation of an artery communicating with the main arterial trunk by an opening that is relatively small. **spurious a.** See false *a*. **surgical a.** One which can be treated surgically. **syphilitic a.** One occurring in a vessel as a result of syphilitic lesion in its wall. It is most common in the ascending aorta. **traction a.** One due to traction on the aorta by an incompletely atrophied ductus arteriosus. **traumatic a.** One produced by injury, as crushing, or following a gunshot wound, as distinguished from one resulting from disease. **true a.** One in which the sac is formed of one, two, or all of the arterial coats. **varicose a.** See arteriovenous *a*.

an″eu·rys·mec′to·my (an″yoor-iz-meck′to-mee). Excision of an aneurysmal sac.

an″eu·rys′mo·graph. An x-ray film of an aneurysm.

an″eu·rys′mo·plas″ty. Restoration of the artery in aneurysm; reconstructive endoaneurysmorrhaphy.

an″eu·rys·mor′rha·phy (an″yoor-iz-mor′uh-fee). Repair of aneurysm of an artery by means of an obliterative operation of the sac.

an″eu·rys·mot′o·my. Incision of an aneurysm for the purpose of suturing or to promote granulation.

an″eu·tha·na′si·a (an″yoo-thuh-nay′zhuh, ·zee-uh). A painful or difficult death.

an′gei·o- (an′jye·o-). For words beginning *angeio-*, see under *angio-*.

an′gel's wing. Winged scapula; a condition in which the scapula projects posteriorly because of weakness or paralysis of the serratus anterior muscle.

an′gi-. See *angio-*.

an″gi·ec·ta′si·a (an″jee-eck-tay′zhuh, ·shuh), **an″gi·ec′ta·sis.** Abnormal dilatation of a vessel; enlargement of capillaries. —**angiectat′ic,** *adj.*

an″gi·ec′ta·sis. See *angiectasia*.

an″gi·i′tis. Inflammation of a blood or lymph vessel.

an·gi′na, an′gi·na. 1. Any disease marked by attacks of choking or suffocation, particularly an affection of the fauces or throat. 2. Sore throat. 3. Spasmodic, cramplike pain or attack. —**angi′nal, an′ginoid, an′ginose, an′ginous,** *adj.* **agranulocytic a.** Agranulocytosis, *q.v.* **a. abdominis.** Acute attacks of severe, colicky, intraabdominal pain associated with increased pulse rate and tension; attributed to sclerosis of the abdominal blood vessels or abdominal aneurysm. **a. cordis.** See *a.* pectoris. **a. cruris.** Intermittent lameness

with pain and cyanosis caused by arterial obstruction. See intermittent *claudication*. **a. diphtheritica.** Diphtheria of the pharynx or larynx. Also called *a. membranacea, suffocative a.* **a. epiglottidea.** Inflammation of the epiglottis. **a. hypercyanotica.** Severe precordial or substernal pain with cyanosis, occurring in patients with mitral stenosis, due probably to myocardial anoxia. **a. maligna.** (a) Gangrenous or necrotic pharyngitis. See gangrenous *a*. (b) Septic sore throat. **a. necrotica.** See gangrenous *a*. **a. parotidea.** That form due to mumps. Also called *a. externa, a. maxillaris.* **a. pectoris.** Paroxysmal pain of psychosomatic origin, characterized by a sense of oppression and severe constriction about the chest. The pain radiates from the precordium to the left shoulder and down the arm along the ulnar nerve. Associated is a sense of apprehension of impending death. The pain is caused by myocardial ischemia and occurs suddenly because of emotional stress or physical exertion. The condition chiefly affects men over 40, and is rare in women. Syn., *a. cordis, cardiac a.* **a. pectoris vasomotoria.** Angina pectoris in which the breast pain is comparatively mild but is attended by pallor and cyanosis, with marked coldness and numbness of the extremities. Also called *mock a., a. notha, spurious a., false a.* **a. simplex.** Simple sore throat. Also called *a. acuta.* **a. tonsillaris.** Quinsy. Syn., *a. vera.* **a. vera.** Quinsy. **aphthous a.** Throat inflammation associated with the formation of small ulcers. **cardiac a.** See *a.* pectoris. **exudative a.** Croup. Also called *a. canina.* **fibrineus a.** A noninfectious, diphtherialike disease of the throat, characterized by a fibrinous exudate especially over the tonsillar area. Also called *croupous a., pseudomembranous a.* **follicular a.** Follicular tonsillitis. **gangrenous a.** That form characterized by necrotic patches of the fauces, occasionally following scarlet fever or diphtheria. Syn., *a. maligna, a. necrotica.* **herpetic a.** That type marked by the formation of vesicles in the throat, associated with patches of exudation. **hypoleukocytic a.** Agranulocytic angina; agranulocytosis, *q.v.* **Ludwig's a.** An acute streptococcic infection of the floor of the mouth. It begins suddenly with marked constitutional symptoms and swelling under the jaw, rapidly extending into the neck. The floor of the mouth becomes swollen and indurated and the tongue pushed upward. Speech and swallowing are impeded; the disease is frequently fatal. **nerve a.** Neuralgic angina due to spasm of the nutrient arteries of the nerves. **phlegmonous a.** (a) Inflammation of the mucous and submucous tissues of the throat with edema. (b) Acute inflammation of the deep structures of the throat with a tendency to suppuration. **pseudoangina.** A neurosis affecting anemic women, simulating angina pectoris but less severe and never terminating fatally. **pultaceous a.** An affection of the throat with whitish or grayish patches which detach easily and are not true exudates. **serous a.** (a) Edema of the glottis. (b) Catarrhal pharyngitis. **thymic a.** (a) Laryngismus stridulus. (b) Allergic asthma. **Vincent's a.** An ulceromembranous angina and stomatitis of the mucous membranes of the throat and mouth. The organisms constantly associated with this disease are the fusiform bacilli and spirochetes; the causal relation of these organisms to Vincent's angina is not established. *Borrelia vincentii* has been suggested as a causative organism. Syn., *trench mouth*.

an·gi″no·pho′bi·a (an·jye″no·fo′bee·uh, an″ji·no·). Morbid fear of angina pectoris.

an′gi·o- (an′jee·o-), **an′gi-,** A combining form meaning *a vessel* or denoting *a seed, blood vessel,* or pertaining *to* or *covered by* (such) *a vessel.*

an′gi·o·blast″. 1. Special primordium derived from extraembryonic endoderm, which gives rise to the blood cells and blood vessels in the early embryo. 2. That part of the mesenchyme, especially extraembryonic, from which the first blood cells and blood vessels arise. 3. A vasoformative cell of the mesenchyme. **—angioblas′tic,** *adj.*

an″gi·o·blas·to′ma. An angiomatous tumor, consisting of numerous capillary or cavernous spaces, with cell proliferation and with a tendency to extend and infiltrate the surrounding tissue. Syn., *angiosarcoma, endothelioma.*

an″gi·o·car′di·o·gram″. A radiograph of the heart and large vessels.

an″gi·o·car″di·og′ra·phy. Roentgenographic visualization of the thoracic vessels and the heart chambers after intravenous injection of radiopaque material (diodrast). **—angiocardiograph′ic,** *adj.*

an″gi·o·cav″er·no′ma. A cavernous angioma, *q.v.*

an″gi·o·cav′ern·ous. Relating to cavernous angioma.

an″gi·o·chei′lo·scope (an″jee·o·kigh′lo·scope). An instrument which magnifies the capillary circulation of the lips, permitting observation.

an″gi·o·cho·li′tis (an″jee·o·ko·lye′tis). Cholangitis, *q.v.*

an″gi·o·der′ma pig″men·to′sum. Xeroderma pigmentosum, *q.v.*

an″gi·o·der″ma·ti′tis. Inflammation of the vessels of the skin.

an″gi·o·dys·tro′phi·a, an″gi·o·dys′tro·phy. Defective nutrition of the blood vessels.

an″gi·o·en″do·the″li·o′ma. A tumor composed of endothelial cells and blood or lymph vessels. Also called *Ewing's tumor.*

an″gi·o·fi·bro′ma (an″jee·o·fighbro′muh). A fibroma rich in blood vessels or lymphatics.

an″gi·o·gli·o′ma (an″jee·o·glye·o′muh). A glioma which is rich in blood vessels.

an″gi·o·ker″a·to′ma. A rare disease of the skin, usually of the extremities; characterized by telangiectatic warty growths; often preceded by chilblains.

an′gi·o·lith″. A calculus of a blood vessel. **—angiolith′ic,** *adj.*

an″gi·ol′o·gy. The science dealing with blood vessels and lymphatics.

an″gi·o·lu′poid. A cutaneous sarcoid of the type seen in generalized sarcoidosis; usually found on the face; marked by small bluish red nodules with capillary dilatation.

an″gi·ol′y·sis. Obliteration of a blood vessel during embryonal, fetal, or postnatal life; by progressive fibrosis, or by thrombosis followed by organization and cicatrization, as obliteration of the ductus arteriosus.

an″gi·o′ma. A tumor composed of blood or lymphatic vessels; a hemangioma or lymphangioma. Probably derived from embryonal isolation of mesenchymal structures; it is essentially a hamartoma, but many consider it a neoplasm. **—angiom′atous,** *adj.* **a. arteriale racemosum.** A complex meshwork of small blood vessels, near or attached to an artery. **cavernous a.** One in which the vascular spaces are large or cystic, like the cavernous tissue of the penis. Also called *angiocavernoma.* **plexiform a.** One consisting of tortuous capillaries, and sometimes of arteries and veins; usually subcutaneous; produces sessile or wartlike superficial masses. **serpiginous a.** A skin disease in which tiny red vascular dots appear in groups on the skin; called *Hutchinson's disease.* **telangiectatic a.** One in which the component vessels are large, as in angioma of the bone.

an″gi·o·ma·la′ci·a (an″jee·o·malay′shee·uh, -see·uh). Softening of the blood vessels.

an″gi·o·ma·to′sis. A pathologic state of the blood vessels marked by the formation of multiple angiomas. **a. retinae.** An uncommon disease of the retina marked by areas of prolifer-

an″gi·o·meg′a·ly. Enlargement of blood vessels, occurring chiefly in the eyelid.

an″gi·om′e·ter. An instrument for measuring the diameter or tension in a vessel. See *sphygmograph*.

an″gi·o·neu·rec′to·my. 1. Excision of blood vessels and nerves. **2.** The resection of all the elements of the spermatic cord, except the ductus deferens and its artery and vein, for the surgical cure of enlarged prostate.

an″gi·o·neu·ro′ma. A benign tumor composed of vascular tissue and nerve fibers.

an″gi·o·neu″ro·my·o′ma (·new″-ro·migh·o′muh). Glomus tumor, *q.v.*

an″gi·o·neu·ro′sis. A neurosis of the blood vessels; a disturbance of the vasomotor system, either of the nature of a spasm of the blood vessels (*angiospasm*), of a paralysis (*angioparalysis*), or of a paresis (*angioparesis*).—**angioneurot′ic,** *n.*

an″gi·o·no′ma. Ulceration of a vessel.

an″gi·o·pa·ral′y·sis. Paralysis of blood vessels caused by vasomotor defect. —**angioparalyt′ic,** *adj.*, *n.*

an″gi·o·pa·re′sis (an″jee·o·pa·ree′-sis, ·par′i·sis). Partial paralysis of the vasomotor apparatus.

an″gi·op′a·thy. Any disease of the vascular system.

an″gi·o·plas″ty. Plastic surgery upon blood vessels.

an″gi·or′rha·phy. Plastic suture of a blood vessel or vessels.

an″gi·or·rhex′is. Rupture of a blood vessel.

an″gi·o·sar·co′ma. Sarcoma derived from an angioma or a sarcoma rich in blood vessels or lymphatics.

an′gi·o·scope″. An instrument for examining the capillary vessels.

an′gi·o·spasm″. A segmental contracture of a blood vessel. —**angiospas′tic,** *adj.*

an″gi·o·ste·no′sis. Narrowing of the lumen of a vessel.

an″gi·o·tel″ec·ta′si·a (·tel″eck-tay′zhuh, ·zee·uh). A condition in which there is dilatation of groups of capillaries; telangiectasis.

an″gi·o·ti′tis. Inflammation of blood vessels of the ear.

an″gi·ot′o·my. Incision into a blood vessel.

an″gi·ot′o·nin. A polypeptide, the product of the action of the enzyme renin on renin substrate, a pseudoglobulin in the blood plasma. The injection of angiotonin into the blood stream causes an abrupt, fleeting rise of blood pressure. Syn., *hypertensin.*

an′gi·o·tribe″. A clamp with powerful jaws used to crush arteries embedded in tissue.

an′gle. 1. Degree of divergence of two lines or planes that meet each other; the space between two such lines. **2.** A corner. —**angular,** *adj.* **alpha a.** The angle formed by intersection of the optic and visual axes at the nodal point of the eye. In myopia, the alpha angle is smaller than normal and the eye appears to converge; in hyperopia the angle is larger than normal and the eye appears to diverge. **a. of convergence.** The angle between the two visual axes, when the eyes are turned inward. See meter-*a.* **a. of deviation.** (a) *In magnetism*, the angle traversed by the needle when disturbed by some magnetic force. (b) *In optics*, that formed by a refracted ray and the prolongation of the incident ray. **a. of incidence.** The angle between the incident ray and the perpendicular at the point of incidence, at either a reflecting or refracting surface. **a. of inclination of pelvic canal.** *In obstetrics*, that formed by the anterior wall of the pelvis with the conjugate diameter. **a. of inclination of pelvis.** *In obstetrics*, that formed by the pelvis with the general line of the trunk, or that formed by the plane of the inferior strait with the horizon. **a. of iris.** The iridial angle; the angulus iridis [BNA]. That formed by the iris and cornea. Also called filtration *a.* **a. of jaw.** The junction of the inferior border of the mandible with the posterior border of its ramus. **a. of lips.** That formed by the union of the lips at each extremity of the oral opening. **a. of polarization.** *In optics*, the angle of reflection at which light is most completely polarized. **a. of pubes.** That formed by the junction of the pubic bones at the symphysis. **a. of reflection.** *In optics*, that which a reflected ray of light makes with a line drawn perpendicular to the point of incidence. **a. of refraction.** *In optics*, that which exists between a refracted ray of light and a line drawn perpendicular to the point of incidence. **a. of rib.** An angle of the body of a rib, at the attachment of the iliocostalis muscle and the point at which the rib bends ventrally. **a. of sternum.** That between the manubrium and body of the sternum. Also called *a. of Louis, a. of Ludwig.* **angles of the scapula.** The three angles of the triangular scapula. The **inferior angle of the scapula** is that formed by the junction of its axillary and vertebral borders. The **lateral angle of the scapula** is that formed by the junction of its axillary and superior borders; the head of the scapula, bearing the glenoid cavity. The **medial** (or *superior*) **angle of the scapula** is that formed by the junction of its superior and vertebral borders. **carrying a.** Angle between the longitudinal axis of the forearm and that of the arm when the forearm is extended. **cerebellopontine a.** A region bounded laterally by the petrous portion of the temporal bone, medially by the cerebellum and brain stem, below by the floor of the posterior fossa of the skull, and above by the tentorium cerebelli. An angle in which tumors frequently occur. **costal a.** The angle formed by the costal cartilages at the xiphoid process. Also called *infrasternal a., subcostal a.* **costophrenic a.** That formed by the ribs and diaphragm. **facial a.** That formed by a line connecting nasion and gnathion with the Frankfort horizontal plane of the head. This may be measured on the dead skull with a craniostat, or on the living head with the aid of a lateral cephalometric roentgenogram. **filtration a.** The iridial angle, at which point filtration of the aqueous humor supposedly occurs. **meter-a.** *In optics,* the degree of convergence of the eyes when centered on an object one meter distant from each. **nasal a.** The inner canthus of the eye. **sacrovertebral a.** That which the sacrum forms with the last lumbar vertebra. **sternoclavicular a.** That existing between the clavicle and the sternum. **subcostal a.** See costal *a.* **Sylvian a.** The angle formed by the posterior limb of the Sylvian fissure with a line perpendicular to the superior border of the hemisphere. **xiphoid a.** That formed by the sides of the xiphoid notch.

an″go·phra′si·a (ang″go·fray′zhuh, ·zee·uh). A halting, choking, and drawling type of speech occurring in paralytic dementia.

an′gor. Angina; extreme distress. **a. animi.** A sense of imminent dissolution.

an″gos·tu′ra. The bark of *Galipea cusparia.* It is a stimulant bitter tonic.

ang′strom, Ang′ström (ang′strum, awng′strem). An angstrom unit; a unit of length equal to 10^{-8} cm. ($^{1}/_{100}$ millionth of a centimeter); used for measuring wave lengths, as of violet light, x-rays, and radium radiation. Designated by the symbol A., Å., AU., A.U., A.u., Å.u., or a.u.

an″gu·la′tion. 1. The formation of an unnatural angle in a hollow organ following the resection of a portion (as of the intestine or ureter). These angles often become sites of obstruction. 2. Deviation from the normal long axis, as in a fractured bone healed out of line.

an″he·do′ni·a. *In psychology,* a diminution or disappearance of pleasure in life; apathy in the performance of acts which normally give pleasure.

an·hem″a·to·poi·e′sis, an·haem″a·to·poi·e′sis (an-hem″uh-to-poy·ee′sis, an-hee″muh-to-). Defective formation of blood, the result of hypofunction of the bone marrow.

an·he″ma·to′sis. Defective formation of the blood.

an·he″mo·lyt′ic (an-hee″mo-lit′ick, an-hem″o-). Not hemolytic; not destructive of blood corpuscles.

an″hi·dro′sis (an″hi·dro′sis, an″high-). Deficiency or absence of sweat secretion. **—anhidrot′ic,** *adj.*

anhydr-. See *anhydro-.*

an″hy·drae′mi·a (an″high·dree′mee·uh). See *anhydremia.*

an″hy·dra′tion. See *dehydration.*

an″hy·dre′mi·a (an″high·dree′mee·uh). A deficiency of the fluid portion of the blood.

an·hy′dride. A compound resulting from the abstraction of water from a substance. **acid a.** An oxide of a nonmetal; it forms an acid with water. **basic a.** An oxide of a metal; it forms a base with water.

an·hy′drite. Anhydrous calcium sulfate.

an·hy′dro-, anhydr-. A combining form meaning *waterless;* used to denote *deficiency of water* or *an anhydride of a compound.*

an·hy″dro·hy·drox″y·pro·ges′ter·one. 17-Ethinyltestosterone or pregneninolone, a synthetic steroid used like progesterone but active when given orally. See *lutocylol, pranone, progestoral.*

an·hy′drous. *In chemistry,* denoting the absence of water, especially of water of crystallization.

an″hyp·no′sis. Sleeplessness; insomnia.

an″i·an′thi·nop·sy. Inability to recognize violet tints.

an·id′e·us. The lowest form of omphalosite, in which the parasitic fetus is a shapeless mass of flesh covered with skin. Syn., *acardiacus amorphus, holoacardius amorphus.* **—anidian, anidean, ani′dous,** *adj.*

an″i·ler′i·dine. Ethyl-1-(4-aminophenethyl)-4-phenylisonipecotate, an analgesic used in the form of the hydrochloride and phosphate salts. See *leritine.*

an′i·line (an′i·leen, ·lin), **an′i·lin.** $C_6H_5NH_2$. A colorless liquid obtained from coal tar or prepared by reduction of nitrobenzene. **a. oil.** A solvent mixture of aniline, toluidine, xylidine, and other coal distillation products; used in histologic technique.

an'i·line black. See *nigraniline*.

an'i·line blue, W. S. (C.C.). An acid, aniline dye used to stain collagenic fibers and as a general stain. Also called *China blue, soluble blue 3M or 2R, marine blue V, cotton blue, water blue, Berlin blue*.

a·nil'i·ty. Imbecility or childishness. **—an'ile,** *adj.*

an'i·ma. 1. The soul; the vital principle. 2. The active principle of a drug or medicine. 3. *In psychoanalysis,* the image of his feminine ideal, existing in the unconscious of a man.

an'i·mal. 1. Any member of the higher of the two major classes of living things (plants and animals). There is no special test for a strict separation of all plants from all animals. In general, however, animals are distinguished by their mode of nutrition, by a neuromuscular system which permits locomotion, and by a more complex form of development from the egg and a more determinate type of growth. 2. A lower animal as distinguished from the higher. 3. The physical and organic as contrasted with the mental and spiritual. 4. Pertaining to, descended from, or resembling, animals. **control a.** (a) One serving as a check or standard of comparison in experimental studies. (b) A nonimmune animal. See *control*. **decerebrate a.** One in which higher centers of the brain have been removed or disconnected. **experimental a.** One which is the subject of experimentation. **Houssay a.** One in which the pancreas and hypophysis both have been excised. **laboratory a.** See experimental *a*. **spinal a.** One with the cord severed, cutting off connections to the brain. **thalamic a.** One with the brain stem severed just above the thalamus. **an″i·mal'cule.** A minute or microscopic animal; a protozoan.

an'i·mal heat. The heat generated in a living organism by metabolism. Animals fall into two great classes regarding temperature: poikilothermic —those whose temperature varies but seldom exceeds that of the environment, and homothermic—those whose temperature is maintained at a constant level, varying within narrow limits. In man, the normal temperature is 98.6° F. (37° C.) with a normal fluctuation of 1°–3° in 24 hrs.

an'i·mal mag'net·ism. 1. A form of magnetic healing, characterized by a belief that certain men, like certain metals, have remedial powers by virtue of a spiritlike effluvium emanating from their bodies. 2. Mesmer's universal fluid which, he believed, emanates from heavenly bodies and influences the health of man. *Obs.*

an″i·ma'tion. 1. State of being alive, animate. 2. Liveliness; high spirits.

suspended a. A state of interrupted respiration and loss of consciousness; temporary period of apparent death.

an'i·mus. 1. A spirit or feeling of hatred or hostility. 2. *In psychoanalysis,* the image of her male ideal, as it exists in the unconscious of a woman; opposed to *anima*.

an'i″on. An ion carrying one or more negative charges, and migrating to the anode on electrolysis.

an″i·rid'i·a (an″eye·rid'ee·uh, an″-i·rid'ee·uh). Absence or defect of the iris.

an'ise (an'iss). The dried ripe fruit of *Pimpinella anisum*, a mild aromatic carminative. Also called *anise seed, aniseed*. **a. oil.** The volatile oil from anise or star anise; used as carminative and flavor. **star a.** The fruit of *Illicium verum*. It yields a volatile oil. See *a. oil*.

an'i·seed. See *anise*.

an″is·ei·kom'e·ter (an″iss-eye-kom'i·tur). A device for measuring the inequality of size, when the two retinal images differ. Also called *eikonometer*.

an″i·sei·ko'ni·a. A condition in which the image seen by one eye is different from that seen by the other. See iseikonic *lens*. **—aniseikon'ic,** *adj.*

an·i'so-, an'i·so-, anis–. A combining form denoting *unequal, unsymmetrical, dissimilar*.

an·i″so·chro·ma'si·a (a·nigh″so-kro·may'zhuh, an″i·so-). A variation in the color of erythrocytes in which only the peripheral zone of the cell is colored. Occurs as a result of iron deficiency in certain types of anemia.

an·i″so·chro'mi·a. Variation in the intensity of staining of erythrocytes; due to differences in hemoglobin content. **—anisochromic, anisochromat'ic,** *adj.*

an·i″so·co'ri·a. Inequality of the diameter of the pupils.

an·i″so·cy·to'sis (a·nigh″so·sigh·to'sis, an″i·so-). Inequality in the size of the red blood corpuscles.

an·i″so·dac'ty·lous. With unequal digits. **—anisodactylus,** *n.*

an″i·sog'na·thous. Having jaws which do not match, one being considerably wider than the other, especially in the molar region.

an·i″so·me'li·a. An inequality between corresponding limbs. **—anisom'elous,** *adj.*

an·i″so·me·tro'pi·a. A difference in the refraction of the two eyes. **—anisometrop'ic,** *adj.*; **anisomet'rope,** *n.*

an·i″so·ton'ic. Denoting unequal osmotic pressure.

an″i·sot'ro·py. 1. The quality of being doubly refractive or unequally refractive in different directions; or of being unequally responsive to external influences. 2. *In biology,* variation in irritability in different parts or organs. 3. In an ovum, having a predetermined axis or axes. —**anisotrop'ic,** *adj.*

an'kle. The joint between the leg and the foot. It is a ginglymus joint, with four ligaments: anterior, posterior, medial, and lateral. See Table of Joints and Ligaments in the Appendix.

an'ky·lo- (ang'ki·lo-), **an'kyl-.** A combining form denoting *crooked* or *crookedness, bent; adhesion* or *growing together of parts.*

an″ky·lo·bleph'a·ron. The adhesion of the ciliary edges of the eyelids to each other.

an″ky·lo·dac·tyl'i·a. A deformity resulting from the adhesion of fingers or toes to one another.

an″ky·lo·glos'si·a. Tongue-tie.

an'ky·losed (ang'kil·ohzd, ·ohst). Stiff; firmly united; bound down with adhesions; designating a joint immobilized by some pathologic or operative process within or outside the capsule. —**ankylose,** *v.t., v.i.*

an″ky·lo'sis. Stiffness or fixation of a joint. —**an'kylose,** *v.t., v.i.;* **an'kylosed,** *adj.* **bony a.** Complete fixation of a joint due to fusion of the bones. Also called *true a.* **extracapsular a.** That due to rigidity of the parts external to the joint; such as interference resulting from bony block, adhesions of tendons and tendon sheaths, contractures due to muscles, scars, or thickening of skin from scleroderma. Also called *false a., spurious a.* **fibrous a.** That due to fibrosis in the joint capsule or fibrous adhesions between the joint surfaces. **partial a.** That producing limitation of joint motion but not complete fixation.

An″ky·los'to·mum. Old term for a genus of nematode worms. **A. americanum.** See *Necator americanus.* **A. duodenale.** See *Ancylostoma duodenale.*

an'ky·lo·tome (ang'kil·o·tome, ang·kil'o·). 1. A knife for operating on tongue-tie. 2. Any curved knife.

an″ky·lot'o·my. An operation for the relief of tongue-tie.

an'la·ge (ahn'lah·guh) (pl. *anlagen, anlages*). A rudiment; the undifferentiated embryonic cells or tissue from which an organ or part develops. Syn., *primordium, blastema.*

an·nat'to (ah·nah'to, a·nat'o), **an·not'to.** A coloring matter obtained from the pulp surrounding the seeds of the *Bixa orellana.*

an·neal'. Temper; apply a regulated process of heating and subsequent cooling to glass or metal to render it less brittle.

an'ne·lid. 1. Pertaining to the Annelida. 2. One of the Annelida, a phylum of segmented worms.

an'nu·lus (pl. *annuli*). A ring of tissue about an opening. Also see *ring.* —**annular, annulate,** *adj.* **a. fibrosus.** (a) External part of an intervertebral disk. Also called *a. fibrosus fibrocartilaginis intervertebralis* [BNA]. (b) Firm connective tissue containing elastic fibers surrounding the atrioventricular, aortic, and pulmonary openings of the heart. Also called *a. fibrosus atrioventricularis.* (c) Circular fibrous attachment of the tympanic membrane to the tympanic sulcus. Syn., *a. fibrocartilagineus membranae tympani* [BNA]. (d) Fibrous loop holding a tendon in place. **a. inguinalis abdominalis** [BNA]. The deep inguinal ring. **a. inguinalis subcutaneus** [BNA]. The subcutaneous inguinal ring. **a. tendineus communis** [BNA]. Fibrous ring from which arise the four rectus muscles of the eye. It is attached to the dural sheath of the optic nerve and to the upper and medial margins of the optic foramen; it bridges the superior orbital fissure. Also called *ligament of Zinn, tendon of Zinn.* **a. tympanicus** [BNA]. The tympanic ring. **a. umbilicalis** [BNA]. The umbilical ring.

an'o-. A combining form meaning *up, upper, upward.*

a'no-. A combining form signifying *anus* or *anal.*

AnOC. Anodal opening contraction.

an″o·chro·ma'si·a (an″o·kro·may'zhuh, ·zee·uh). 1. Concentration of hemoglobin about the periphery of the red cells with the centers pale; a condition noted in certain types of anemia. 2. Absence of the usual staining reaction in a cell or tissue; achromasia.

a·no″ci·as·so″ci·a'tion, a·no″ci·a'tion. An anesthetic procedure whereby surgical shock, fear, and postoperative neuroses are minimized greatly by excluding most of the painful and harmful stimuli. Syn., *anocithesia.*

an·o'dal clos'ure. The closure of an electric circuit with the anode placed in relation to the muscle or nerve which is to be affected.

an'ode. The positive pole of a galvanic battery or other electric device. Abbreviated, a., An. —**ano'dal,** *adj.*

an″o·don'ti·a. Absence of the teeth. **a. vera.** That due to failure of development of the tooth buds. **senile a.** Absence of the teeth because of their removal, in older persons.

an'o·dyne. 1. A medicine that eases pain. 2. Relieving pain.

a·nom'a·ly. Any deviation from the usual; any organ or part existing in an abnormal form, structure, or location. **—anomalous,** *adj.*

a·no'mi·a. Loss of ability to name objects or to recognize names, usually associated with a hemianopsia. Also called *optic aphasia.*

an"o·nych'i·a (an"o·nick'ee·uh). Absence of the nails.

A·noph'e·les (a·nof'i·leez). A genus of mosquitoes belonging to the family Culicidae. They alone transmit malaria and are important vectors of dengue and filariasis and may transmit yellow fever. **A. albimanus.** A species of mosquito native to tropical America, characterized by white hind feet; a common malarial vector. **A. argyritarsis.** A South American vector of malaria. **A. crucians.** A species carrying the malaria parasite; infrequently molests humans. **A. culicifacies.** A species common to Arabia, India, and Siam. The most important vector of malaria in India. **A. darlingi.** A species from Brazil and British Guiana. A domestic species; it attacks man avidly. **A. gambiae.** A South African and Bazilian species which transmits a very virulent type of malaria. **A. hyrcanus.** A species found from South Europe to China and Japan. Important transmitter of malaria and filariasis. **A. maculipennis.** The type species of this genus, found throughout Europe and many other parts of the world; it is an active vector of malaria. **A. quadrimaculatus.** A species which serves as the chief vector of human malaria in the United States.

an"o·phel'i·cide. An agent which is destructive to anopheles mosquitoes.

an"o·phel'i·fuge. An agent which prevents the bite or attack of anopheles mosquitoes.

A·noph"e·li'ni (a·nof'i·lye'nigh). A tribe of the subfamily Culicinae, or mosquitoes. It includes all the vectors of human malaria.

an"oph·thal'mi·a. Anophthalmos.

an"oph·thal'mos. 1. Congenital absence of the eyes. 2. A person born without eyes.

an·o'pi·a. Absence of sight, especially that due to defect of the eyes.

a'no·plas·ty. Plastic surgery or repair of the anus or anal canal.

An"o·plu'ra. An order of parasitic, sucking insects without wings; lice.

an·op'si·a. 1. Failure to use visual capacity. 2. Upward strabismus.

an·or'chism (an·or'kiz·um, an'or·), **an·or'chi·a** (an·or'kee·uh), **an·or'chid·ism** (an·or'ki·diz·um). Absence of the testes. **—anorchous,** *adj.*

a"no·rec'tal. Pertaining to the anus and the rectum.

an"o·rex'i·a. Absence of appetite. **—anorec'tic, anorec'tous,** *adj.*

a. nervosa. A hysterical aversion t food, which may lead to serious maln trition. **false a.** A condition found i hysteria, in which the patient appa ently eats nothing, but consumes larg quantities of food in secret.

an·or·gas'my (an·or·gaz'mee). condition, usually psychic, in whic there is a failure to reach a clima during coitus.

an"or·thog'ra·phy. Incapacity write correctly; motor agraphia.

a'no·scope. Instrument for examin ing the rectum. **—anos'copy,** *n.*

an·os'mi·a (an·oz'mee·uh, an·oss mee·uh). Absence of the sense of sme In type, it is *afferent* when due to th loss of conductivity of the olfactor nerves; *central,* if due to cerebral di ease; *organic,* if due to disease of th nasal olfactory membrane; *peripheri* if due to disease of the peripheral en of the olfactory nerves. **—anosmi anosmat'ic,** *adj.*

an·o"sog·no'si·a (an·o"sog·no'zhu ·zee·uh). Inability on the part of th patient to recognize that he is hem plegic.

an·o'ti·a (an·o'shuh, ·shee·uh). Co genital absence of the pinnae or e ternal ears. See *anotus.*

an"o·tro'pi·a. The tendency of on eye to latent upward deviation. Syi *anophoria.*

an·o'tus. A person showing congen tal absence of the external ears. **—an otous,** *adj.*

an·o'vu·lar (an·o'view·lur, an·ov yoo·lur), **an·o'vu·la·to"ry** (an·o view·luh·tor"ee, an·ov'yoo·). Not ass ciated with ovulation, applied to me struation. See anovular *menstruatio*

an"ox·e'mi·a. A lack of oxygen the blood from insufficient aeration du to high elevation, low partial pressur of oxygen in anesthesia, cardiac fai. ure, or strangling.

an·ox'i·a. Inadequate supply of oxy gen, or the disturbance of bodily func tions resulting from a deficiency oxygen. **anemic a.** The type due t reduction in the capacity of the bloo to carry oxygen. **anoxic a.** The cor dition arising when the exchange oxygen in the lungs is interfered wit as in pneumonia and in drownin **histotoxic a.** The type due to inter ference with the ability of the cells t utilize oxygen; caused by alcohol, nai cotics, and certain other poison **stagnant a.** The form due to a re duction in the flow of blood. It may b local, as in arterial spasm or embolism or general, as in shock or vasomoto collapse.

an'sa (pl. *ansae*). A loop. **a. hypo glossi.** A loop formed at the side o the neck by the junction of the de scending branch of the hypoglossal nerve with branches of the second and third cervical nerves. **a. lenticularis.** A bundle of efferent fibers from the globus pallidus, passing around the medial border of the internal capsule to join the fasciculus lenticularis. Syn., *a. lentiformis, lenticular loop.*

ansolysen tartrate. Trade-mark for pentolinium tartrate.

ant-. See *anti-.*

antabuse. Trade-mark for tetraethylthiuram disulfide, used in the treatment of alcoholism.

ant·ac'id. A substance which neutralizes acids or relieves acidity.

an·tag'o·nism. Opposition; the mutually opposing or resisting action seen between organisms (antibiosis), muscles, functions, diseases, and drugs; or between drugs and functions; or drugs and diseases. —**antagonis'tic,** *adj.* **bacterial a.** The adverse effect produced by one species of microörganism upon the growth and development of another, as the action of actinomycosis on many Gram-positive organisms.

an·tag'o·nist. 1. A drug that neutralizes the effects of another. 2. *In anatomy,* a muscle that acts in opposition to another. 3. *In dentistry,* a tooth that meets one in the opposing dental arch during occlusion or mastication. **associated a.** One of two muscles or groups of muscles which pull in almost opposite directions. When they contract simultaneously, the affected part moves in a path between their divergent lines of action.

ant·al'ka·line. 1. Neutralizing alkalies. 2. An agent which neutralizes alkalies.

ant"aph·ro·dis'i·ac (ant"af·ro·diz'ee·ack). 1. Lessening the venereal desires. 2. An agent that lessens the venereal impulse; an anaphrodisiac.

an·taz'o·line. 2-(N-Benzylanilinomethyl)-2-imidazoline, an antihistamine used in the form of the hydrochloride and phosphate salts. See *antistine.*

an'te-. A prefix denoting *before, preceding, in front of, prior to, anterior to.*

an"te·au'ral. In front of the ear.

an"te·bra'chi·um (an"tee·bray'kee·um, -brack'ee·um). The forearm. —**antebrachial,** *adj.*

an'te ci'bum. Before meals. Abbreviated, a. c.; used in prescriptions.

an"te·cu'bi·tal. Situated in front of the elbow.

an"te·cur'va·ture. A forward curvature.

an"te·flex'ion. A bending forward. **a. of the uterus.** A condition in which the fundus of the uterus is bent forward on the cervix.

an"te·mor'tem. Before death.

an"te·na'tal. Occurring or existing before birth; prenatal.

an"te·par'tum. Before delivery.

antergan. Trade name for dimethylaminoethyl-benzylaniline, an antihistaminic substance.

an·te'ri·or. Situated before or to the front; designating the forward part, as of an organ. Abbreviated, a. —**anteriad, anteriorly,** *adv.*
In human anatomy, anterior is usually used instead of ventral.

an'ter·o-, anter-. A combining form meaning *anterior, front, from front to.*

an"ter·o·in·fe'ri·or. Situated in front and below.

an"ter·o·lat'er·al. In front and to one side; from the front to one side.

an"ter·o·me'di·an. In front and toward the middle.

an"ter·o·pos·te'ri·or. Extending from before backward; relating to both front and back.

an"ter·o·su·pe'ri·or. Situated in front and above.

an"te·ver'sion. A tipping, tilting, or displacement forward of an organ or part, especially of the uterus. —**antevert'ed,** *adj.;* **antevert',** *v.t., v.i.*

ant·he'lix. See *antihelix.*

an"thel·min'tic, ant"hel·min'tic. 1. Destructive of intestinal worms. 2. A remedy for the destruction or elimination of intestinal worms.

an·the'ma, an'the·ma (pl. *anthemata*). 1. An exanthema. 2. An elementary lesion of the skin.

an'the·mis. English or Roman camomile. The flower heads of *Anthemis nobilis,* variously employed in lay medicine.

anthiomaline. Trade-mark for antimony lithium thiomalate, used for the treatment of filariasis, trypanosomiasis, lymphogranuloma, and schistosomiasis.

an'tho-, anth-. A combining form meaning *flower, floral, flowerlike.*

an"tho·pho'bi·a. A morbid fear of flowers.

an'thra-, anthr-. A combining form denoting *the presence of the anthracene nucleus.*

an"thra·ce'mi·a, an"thra·cae'mi·a. A disease due to the presence in the blood of *Bacillus anthracis;* woolsorter's disease; splenic fever of animals.

an'thra·cene. $C_{14}H_{10}$. A colorless, solid hydrocarbon obtained by distillation from coal tar and other carbon compounds. **a. blue.** See *alizarin* blue.

an'thra·co-, anthrac-. A combining form meaning *coal or carbuncle.*

an"thra·co·sil"i·co'sis. Diffuse fibrosis of the lungs accompanied by black pigmentation, caused by the prolonged inhalation of dusts containing silicon dioxide and carbon; a form of pneumoconiosis. Syn., *coal miner's disease, miner's phthisis, miner's asthma.*

an″thra·co′sis. Black pigmentation of the lungs associated with a mild degree of chronic inflammation; due to the inhalation of carbon dust. A form of pneumoconiosis, *q.v.* **—anthracot′ic,** *adj.*

anthralin. A trade-mark for 1,8-dihydroxyanthranol, a yellow, crystalline powder used externally in ointment form or solution in the treatment of skin diseases. See *cignolin, dithranol.*

an″thra·qui′none′ (an″thruh-kwi-nohn′, -kwin′ohn). A substance produced by oxidizing anthracene. Derivatives of it occur in aloe, cascara, rhubarb, and senna, and are responsible for the cathartic action.

an″thra·ro′bin. 3,4-Dihydroxyanthranol. Yellowish brown crystals used externally in alcoholic solution or as an ointment in skin diseases.

an′thrax. 1. A carbuncle. 2. An acute infectious disease of cattle and sheep, transmissible to man and caused by *Bacillus anthracis.* Syn., *charbon, woolsorter's disease, malignant pustule, malignant a., milzbrand, ragpicker's disease, tanner's disease.* Also called *splenic fever.* **cerebral a.** A complication of intestinal or pulmonary anthrax in which the organisms invade the cerebral vessels. This form is marked by raging and violent delirium. **hemorrhoidal a.** A contagious type of anthrax affecting the rectum of animals and marked by dark bloody evacuations. **malignant a.** Infectious and fatal disease of sheep and cattle marked by ulceration or hard edema at the point of inoculation, followed by symptoms of general sepsis, prostration, and collapse. Transmissible to man. See *anthrax,* 2. **pulmonary a.** The form usually called woolsorter's disease, acquired by inhalation of contaminated dust, resulting in pulmonary gangrene with grave symptoms of systemic infection, coughing, dyspnea, and prostration. **symptomatic a.** An infection of cattle and sheep characterized by subcutaneous, emphysematous swellings and nodules, due to infection by *Clostridium chauvei.* Also called *emphysematous a.*

an′thro·po-, anthrop-. A combining form meaning *human being, man.* **an″thre·po·bi·ol′o·gy** (an″thro-po-buy-ol′o-jee). The biologic study of man and the anthropoid apes.

an″thro·po·gen′e·sis, an″thro·pog′e·ny (an″thro-podj′i-nee). The evolution and development of man, as a race (phylogenesis), and as an individual (ontogenesis). **—anthropogen′ic, anthropogenet′ic,** *adj.*

an′thro·poid. Manlike.

An″thro·poi′de·a. A suborder of Primates, including man, apes, and monkeys.

an″thro·pol′o·gy. The science of man, in all of its ramifications, both physical and cultural. **criminal a.** The study of man in relation to the habitual criminal, utilizing all of the measurements and identification data of anthropology. **cultural a.** The study of man as an intellectual and enlightened being in relation to his own kind and his environment. **physical a.** The study of man in relation to his form, structure, and constitutional characteristics.

an″thro·pom′e·ter. A somatometric caliper used in taking the larger measurements of the human body.

an″thro·pom′e·trist. One skilled in measuring the human body and its parts.

an″thro·pom′e·try. The scientific measurement of the human body, its various parts, and the skeleton. The metric data thus obtained are used extensively in serial and comparative studies and in systems of identification.

an″thro·po·mor′phic. Manlike having a human form.

an″thro·poph′a·gy. 1. Cannibalism. 2. Sexual perversion leading to rape, mutilation, and cannibalism.

an″thro·po·pho′bi·a. Morbid fear of people or society.

ant″hyp·not′ic. 1. Preventing sleep. 2. An agent that tends to induce wakefulness.

an′ti-, ant-. A prefix meaning *against, in return, opposed to, instead, counter.*

an″ti·ac′id. Antacid, *q.v.*

an″ti·ag·glu′ti·nin. A substance having the power of neutralizing the corresponding agglutinin.

an″ti·al·ler′gic. A therapeutic agent that inhibits, arrests, or prevents an allergic reaction. **—antiallergic** *adj.*

an″ti·a·ne′mic. 1. Alleviating or curing anemia. 2. A substance which relieves anemia. See antianemia *factor.*

an″ti·an′ti·bod″y. An antibody to an antibody.

an″ti·ar·thrit′ic. 1. Tending to relieve or cure arthritis. 2. A remedy for arthritis.

an″ti·bac·te′ri·al. Preventing the growth of bacteria or destroying bacteria by physical and chemical agents. **—antibacterial,** *n.*

an″ti·bi·o′sis (an″ti-buy-o′sis). An association between two or more organisms which is harmful to one or them; the opposite of symbiosis.

an″ti·bi·ot′ic (an″ti-buy-ot′ick). 1.

Pertaining to antibiosis. 2. Tending to destroy life; designating the extracts of certain organisms employed against infections caused by other organisms—one commonly used is penicillin. 3. An antibiotic substance.

an″ti·black′out″ suit. A flying suit in which the limbs may be compressed by inflating airtight chambers. This prevents the blackout ensuing from an undue amount of blood leaving the brain and entering the extremities during rapid deceleration in aerial flight.

an′ti·bod′y. One of a class of substances, natural or induced by exposure to an antigen, which have the capacity to react as agglutinins, lysins, precipitins, etc., with the specific or related antigens. In the serum, they are intimately associated with certain globulin fractions. **anaphylactic a.** The antibody concerned in anaphylaxis. Also called *anaphylactin*. **inhibiting a.** A thermostable antibody produced in both allergic and nonallergic individuals as a response to specific immunization, apparently preventing the union of antigen and reagin. Clinical tolerance seems to depend upon the titer of this antibody. **sensitizing a.** An anaphylactic antibody.

an″ti·bra′chi·um (an″ti·bray′kee-um, ·brack′ee-um) [BNA]. The forearm. **—antibrachial,** *adj.*

an″ti·car·cin′o·gen. A substance or agent which opposes the action of carcinogens.

an″ti·car′i·ous (an″ti·kair′ee-us). Inhibiting or preventing dental caries.

an″ti·cat′a·lyst, an″ti·cat′a·lyz·er. Any substance which retards the action of a catalyst by acting directly upon it.

an″ti·ca·thex′is. A condition in which an emotional charge is released from one impulse and shifted to an impulse of an opposite nature. Also called *counterinvestment.*

an″ti·cath′ode, an″ti·kath′ode. The metal plate or target of a Crookes or x-ray tube. It is situated opposite the cathode and is struck by the cathode rays, giving rise to the x-rays.

an″ti·chi·rot′o·nous, an″ti·chei·rot′o·nus (an″ti·kigh·rot′o-nus). Forcible and steady inflexion of the thumb, seen at times in or before attacks of epilepsy.

an″ti·chlor. Sodium thiosulfate.

an″ti·cho″lin·es·ter·ase (an″ti-ko″lin·es′tur·ace, ·aze). A substance which inhibits the enzyme activity of cholinesterase.

an″ti·co·ag′u·lant. 1. Opposed to or preventive of coagulation. 2. A substance preventing coagulation. **—anti-coagulative,** *adj.*

an″ti·com′ple·ment. A substance having the capacity to neutralize, inhibit, or destroy a complement; anti-alexin. **—anticomplemen′tary,** *adj.*

an″ti·con·vul′sant. A therapeutic agent that prevents or arrests convulsions. **—anticonvulsant,** *adj.*

an″ti·con·vul′sive. Of or pertaining to an action or to a therapeutic agent that allays convulsions.

an′ti·cus. Anterior; in front of. *O.T.*

an″ti·di′a·bet′ic. 1. Efficient against diabetes, as the antidiabetic hormone, insulin. 2. A remedy for diabetes.

an″ti·di″ar·rhe′al. Preventing or overcoming diarrhea.

an″ti·di″u·ret′ic. 1. Opposing or decreasing excretion of urine. 2. An agent which decreases excretion of urine. **—antidiure′sis,** *n.*

an″ti·dote. Any agent administered to prevent or counteract the action of a poison. **—antidotal,** *adj.* **a. for arsenic.** A suspension of hydrated ferric and magnesium oxides. **chemical a.** One that changes the chemical nature of the poison so that it becomes an insoluble or harmless compound. **mechanical a.** An agent which prevents absorption of the poison. **physiologic a.** One that counteracts the physiologic effects of a poison.

an″ti·drom′ic. Conducting nerve impulses in a direction opposite to the normal, as when vasodilatation follows peripheral stimulation of an afferent nerve, or dispatching impulses to the spinal cord via the anterior roots by experimental stimulation.

an″ti·dys″en·ter′ic. 1. Serviceable against dysentery. 2. A remedy for or preventive of dysentery.

an″ti·e·met′ic. 1. Relieving or preventing nausea and vomiting. 2. Any agent capable of such action.

an″ti·en′zyme. 1. A substance of enzymatic nature which exerts a specific inhibiting action upon another enzyme. 2. An immune body formed by the injection of an enzyme into an animal; it acts as a defense against the injected enzyme.

an″ti·fe′brile (an″ti·fee′bril, ·feb′-ril). 1. Relieving or reducing fever. 2. An agent that reduces fever.

antifebrin. A proprietary name for acetanilid, *q.v.*

an″ti·fer′ment. 1. An agent that prevents fermentation. 2. Any substance which counteracts an enzyme. Syn., *antienzyme.* **—antiferment′-ative,** *adj.*

an″ti·fi″bri·nol′y·sin. A substance inhibiting the action of fibrinolysin.

an″ti·fi·bro″ma·to·gen′ic (·figh-bro″muh·to·jen′ick). Acting to prevent the formation of fibromas.

an″ti·flash′ gear. Equipment worn by naval gun crews for protection against flash burns.

an″ti·ga·lac′tic. 1. Lessening the secretion of milk. 2. A drug or agent that lessens the flow of milk.

an′ti·gen. 1. Any substance which stimulates the production of antibodies or reacts with them. A **complete antigen** performs both functions. An **incomplete antigen (hapten,** or **partial antigen)** is that part of an antigenic complex responsible for its specificity. Separate from the complex, it reacts with antibodies in vitro, but cannot stimulate their production. 2. A lipoid substance, incapable of eliciting antibodies, employed in syphilis tests; as **beef heart antigen,** that obtained from beef heart by alcoholic extraction. **Acetone-insoluble antigen** is that part of beef heart antigen insoluble in acetone; redissolved in alcohol and reinforced by the addition of cholesterol, it is known as **cholesterinized antigen. a. A.** A group of red blood cell antigens (A₁, A₂, etc.) occurring in types A and AB blood. **a. B.** The red blood cell antigen occurring in types B and AB blood. **artificial a.** (a) A conjugated antigen prepared by compounding an incomplete antigen with a protein, as an azoprotein. (b) An antigen, the specificity of which has been altered through physical or chemical treatment, as through denaturation, nitration, or oxidation. **conjugated a.** An antigen in which an acyl group or a simple compound is attached to the protein. **pollen a.** The antigenic protein or polypeptide extracted from pollen and used for diagnosis and specific pollen desensitization in hay fever.

an″ti·ge·nic′i·ty (an″ti·ji·nis′i·tee). The property of certain substances to produce antibodies.

an″ti·he′lix, ant·he′lix. The curved ridge of the pinna just anterior to the helix and following through most of the course of the helix.

an″ti·he″mo·lyt′ic (an″ti·hee″mo·lit′ick, ·hem″o·lit′ick). 1. Relating to an antihemolysin. 2. Not capable of dissolving blood corpuscles; preventing hemolysis.

an″ti·hem″or·rhag′ic (·hem″o·radj′ick). 1. Checking hemorrhage. 2. Pertaining to vitamin K.

an″ti·hem″or·rhoi′dal. 1. Effective against hemorrhoids. 2. A drug or agent that prevents or relieves hemorrhoids.

an″ti·hi·drot′ic (·hi·drot′ick, ·high-drot′ick) 1. Diminishing the secretion

of sweat. 2. An agent that lessens perspiration.

an″ti·his′ta·mine. A substance capable of preventing or diminishing several of the pharmacological effects o. histamine, by a mechanism other than the production of pharmacologica. responses diametrically opposed t. those produced by histamine.

an″ti·hor′mone. A substance in th. blood of animals which antagonizes th. action of certain pituitary hormones

an″ti·hy·drop′ic, ant″hy·drop′ ic (·high-drop′ick). 1. Relieving drop sical states or conditions. 2. An agen. effective against dropsy.

an″ti·in·fec′tive. 1. A substance that counteracts infection. 2. Counteracting infection.

an″ti·ke″to·gen′e·sis. The diminution of acidosis by the oxidation o sugar and allied substances in the body **—antiketogenic,** adj.; **antike′ togen,** n.

an″ti·li′pase (an″ti·lye′pace, ·lip′ ace). A substance inhibiting or coun. teracting a lipase.

an″ti·lu·et′ic. 1. Efficacious agains the Treponema pallidum. 2. An agen. used to treat syphilis. Syn., antisyphi litic.

an″ti·ma·lar′i·al. Preventing o. suppressing malaria.

an″ti·me·tab′o·lite. A substanc. having a molecular structure similar to but a pharmacologic effect antago. nistic to a metabolite (i.e., a vitamin or hormone). The mechanism of antag. onism is considered to be a competition between antimetabolite and metabolite for a specific protein in an organism

an″ti·me·tro′pi·a. A condition characterized by opposing states of re. fraction in the two eyes, as the exist. ence of myopia in one eye and of hy. peropia in the other.

an″ti·mo′nic (an″·ti·mo′nick, ·mon′ ick). Relating to compounds of penta. valent antimony.

an″ti·mo′ni·ous. See antimonous.

an′ti·mo·nous, **an″ti·mo′ni ous.** Denoting compounds of trivalen. antimony.

an″ti·mo′ny. Sb = 121.76. A metallic crystalline element found native, an. as a constituent of many minerals **a. lithium thiomalate.** See an thiomaline. **a. potassium tartrate** 2KSbOC₄H₄O₆·H₂O, so-called tartar emetic. Occurs in colorless crystals or a. a white powder; soluble in water. Used as a diaphoretic or expectorant, emetic and protozoicide. **a. sodium tartrate.** Used the same as the potas sium compound but more soluble i. water. **a. sodium thioglycollate** White or faintly pink powder, soluble in water, used in the treatment o. granuloma inguinale, kala-azar, an.

filariasis. **a. thioglycollamide.**
$Sb(S.CH_2CONH_2)_3$. White crystals, soluble in water, used in the treatment of granuloma inguinale, kala-azar, and filariasis.

an''ti·mo·nyl. SbO. The univalent radical of antimonous compounds.

an''ti·my·cot'ic (an''ti·migh·cot'ick). Preventing the growth of fungi or the destruction of fungi by physical and chemical agents.

an''ti·nar·cot'ic. Preventing narcosis.

an''ti·neu·ral'gic. Alleviating neuralgia.

an''ti·neu·rit'ic. 1. Efficient in neuritis. 2. A remedy against neuritis.

an''tin·va'sin I. An enzyme found in normal blood plasma of all animals, including man. It acts by destroying the hyaluronidase of bacteria and other sources and, by this action, counteracts invasion and spreading of those organisms and toxins which elaborate hyaluronidase.

an''tin·va'sin II. A protective enzyme observed in normal blood plasma which causes rapid destruction of proinvasin I in pathogenic organisms and venoms. With proinvasin I inactivated, antinvasin I is left intact to destroy hyaluronidase, the enzyme which aids invasion and spreading.

an''ti·o·be'sic. 1. Efficient against corpulence. 2. A remedy for corpulence.

an''ti·o·don·tal'gic. Relieving or preventing toothache.

an''ti·op'so·nin. A substance retarding or destroying the action of an opsonin.

an''ti·ox'i·dant. Any substance which delays the process of oxidation.

an''ti·par''a·sit'ic. 1. Destroying parasites. 2. A substance destructive to parasites.

an''ti·per''i·stal'sis. Reversed peristalsis.

an''ti·phlo·gis'tic. 1. Counteracting fever. 2. An agent subduing or reducing inflammation or fever.

an''ti·phone. An appliance worn in the auditory meatus and intended to protect the wearer from noises.

an''ti·plas'tic. 1. Unfavorable to granulation or to the healing process. 2. Preventing or checking plastic exudation. Not to be confused with aplastic, *q.v.*

an''ti·pneu''mo·coc'cic (·new''-mo·cock'sick). Destructive to the pneumococcus.

an·tip'o·dal. Situated directly opposite.

an''ti·pro·throm'bin. An agent present in the blood which prevents coagulation by neutralizing prothrombin. Substances having similar action

are heparin, hirudin, and dicoumarin, *q.v.*

an''ti·pru·rit'ic. 1. Relieving or preventing itching. 2. A drug or agent that relieves itching.

an''ti·py''o·gen'ic. Preventing or inhibiting suppuration.

an''ti·py·ret'ic (an''ti·pye·ret'ick). 1. Cooling; lowering the temperature. 2. An agent reducing fever. —**antipy·re'sis,** *n.*

an''ti·py'rine (an''ti·pye'rin, an''ti·pye·reen'). 1-Phenyl-2,3-dimethyl-5-pyrazolone. A white, crystalline powder, soluble in water or alcohol; used as antipyretic and analgesic. Locally it is anesthetic and vasoconstrictive. Syn., *phenazone.* **a. salicylate.** A white, odorless, crystalline powder, used as analgesic, antipyretic, and antirheumatic. Syn., *salipyrazolone.* See *salipyrin.*

an''ti·ra'bic, an''ti·rab'ic. Preventing rabies, as the Pasteur treatment.

an''ti·ra·chit'ic (an''ti·ra·kit'ick). 1. Serviceable against rickets. 2. An agent for the prevention or cure of rickets.

an''ti·re·tic'u·lar. Pertaining to a factor operating against the reticuloendothelial system.

an''ti·rheu·mat'ic. 1. Preventing or useful in treating rheumatism. 2. Methods, procedures, or drugs employed in the treatment of rheumatism.

an''ti-Rh se'rum. See *Rh factor.*

an''ti·sca·bet'ic. Effective against the *Sarcoptes scabiei,* which causes scabies.

an''ti·scor·bu'tic. 1. Effective against scurvy. 2. An agent which prevents or cures scurvy; see *vitamin C.*

an''ti·sep'sis. Prevention of sepsis or poisoning by the destruction or exclusion of microörganisms from the body tissues and fluids, or by preventing or checking their growth and multiplication.

an''ti·sep'tic. 1. Checking or preventing decay and putrefaction. 2. Any one of a large group of organic and inorganic compounds which stops or inhibits the growth of bacteria without necessarily killing them, thus checking putrefaction; as alcohol, mercuric chloride, phenol, sodium chloride, phenylmercuric salts, etc.

an''ti·se'rum. 1. The serum of man or animal immunized against bacteria or their products, or other antigenic agents, and therefore containing antibodies specific for these agents. 2. Serums containing natural antibodies such as hemagglutinins. 3. Immune therapeutic agents such as diphtheria and tetanus antitoxins. **Rh antiserums.** Antiserums reacting with one or more of the Rh factors.

an″ti·si·al′ic (·sigh·al′ick). 1. Checking the flow of saliva. 2. An agent that checks the secretion of saliva.

an″ti·so′cial. Denoting a psychopathic state marked by the refusal to accept the obligations and restraints imposed by society. **—antisocialism,** *n.*

an″ti·spas·mod′ic. 1. Tending to relieve spasm. 2. An agent relieving convulsions or spasmodic pains, as the narcotics, diphenylhydantoin, the nitrites, atropine.

an″ti·spas′tic. 1. Antispasmodic. 2. An antispasmodic agent.

an″ti·spi′ro·che′tic (·spy″ro·kee′tick, ·ket′ick). 1. Arresting the growth and development of spirochetes. 2. An agent having this power.

antistine. A trade-mark for antazoline.

an″ti·strep″to·coc′cic (·strep″to·cock′sick). Antagonistic to or preventing the growth of streptococci.

an″ti·strep″to·he″mo·ly′sin (·hee″mo·lye′sin, ·hem·ol′i·sin). An antibody formed in response to the antigen streptohemolysin.

an″ti·strep″to·ly′sin. An antibody which operates against the hemotoxin of hemolytic streptococci.

an″ti·su″dor·if′ic. 1. Checking the excretion of sweat. 2. An agent that checks excretion of sweat. Also called *antisudoral.*

an″ti·syph″i·lit′ic. 1. Effective against syphilis. 2. A remedy used in the treatment of syphilis.

an″ti·throm′bin. A substance present in blood plasma, neutralizing thrombin.

an″ti·throm″bo·plas′tin. A substance which inactivates thromboplastin.

an″ti·tox′i·gen, an″ti·tox·in′o·gen. Any antigen, or toxin, which promotes antitoxin elaboration.

an″ti·tox′in. 1. A substance elaborated in tl body capable of neutralizing a given toxin (bacterial, plant, or animal toxin). 2. One of the class of specific antibodies. **—antitoxic,** *adj.*

an″ti·tra′gus. The projection of the pinna just opposite and posterior to the tragus. **—antitrag′ic,** *adj.*

an″ti·tris′mus. A condition of tonic spasm in which the mouth cannot be closed.

an″ti·ty′phoid. 1. Counteracting or preventing typhoid. 2. An antityphoid serum.

an″ti·ve·ne′re·al. Preventive or curative of venereal disease.

an″ti·ven′in, an″ti·ven′ene (·ven′een, ·vi·neen′). 1. An antitoxin to a venin. 2. An antitoxic serum prepared by immunizing animals against the venom of snakes, insects, or other animals. **bothropic a.** Polyvalent serum for the pit vipers of the genus *Bothrops.* **Crotalus a.** Polyvalent serum for the venom of rattlesnakes.

an″ti·vi′ral. Antagonistic to a virus, weakening or destroying its pathogenicity.

an″ti·vi′rus. A broth culture, filtered of its bacteria and heated to attenuate its toxicity, used in producing local immunity.

an″ti·vi′ta·min. Any substance that prevents the normal metabolic functioning of vitamins, a vitamin-destroying enzyme, or a chemical substance that renders the vitamin unabsorbable or ineffective.

an″ti·viv″i·sec′tion. Opposition to vivisection or animal experimentation. **—antivivisectionist,** *n.*

an″ti·xe″roph·thal′mic. Preventive of xerophthalmia. See *vitamin A.*

an″ti·zy·mot′ic (·zye·mot′ic). 1. Preventing or checking fermentation. 2. An agent preventing the process of fermentation.

ant″lo·pho′bi·a. A morbid fear of floods.

an·trec′to·my. Surgical removal of the walls of an antrum, especially the tympanic antrum.

antrenyl bromide. Trade-mark for oxyphenonium bromide.

an′tro-, antr-. A combining form meaning *cavern, cavity.*

an″tro·at″ti·cot′o·my. *In surgery,* the opening of the tympanic antrum and the attic of the tympanum.

an″tro·na′sal. Pertaining to the maxillary sinus and the nasal cavity.

an″tro·scope″. An instrument for examining the maxillary sinus. **—antros′copy,** *n.*

an·tros′to·my, an·trot′o·my. Opening of an antrum for drainage.

an″tro·tym·pan′ic. Relating to the tympanic antrum and the cavity of the middle ear.

an″trum. 1. A cavity or hollow space, especially in a bone. 2. The maxillary sinus. Also called *a. of Highmore.* **—antral,** *adj.* **a. of the ear.** The mastoid antrum, *q.v.* **a. of the tube.** A saclike dilatation of the uterine tube about an inch from the fimbriated extremity; regarded by some as occurring only in pregnancy. **cardiac a.** A dilatation sometimes found in the esophagus immediately above its passage through the diaphragm. **duodenal a.** The normal dilatation presented by the duodenum near its origin. See duodenal *cap.* **mastoid a.** The pneumatic space between the epitympanic space and the mastoid cavity. Syn., *tympanic a.* **pyloric a.** The cavity of the pylorus (3); the first part of the pyloric region of the stomach, proximal to the pyloric canal.

ANTU. Alpha-naphthylthiourea, a highly specific poison for the common brown, or Norway, rat.

a·nu'cle·ar (ay·new'klee·ur, a·new'·). Lacking cell nuclei; applied to erythrocytes.

an"u·re'sis. See *anuria*.

an·u'ri·a, an'u·ry, an"u·re'sis. Suppression of urine. —**anuret'ic, anu'ric,** *adj.* **traumatic a.** See compression *syndrome.*

a'nus. The termination of the rectum; the outlet of the alimentary canal. —**anal,** *adj.* **artificial a.** A permanent artificial opening made surgically from the exterior into the gut. **fissure of a.** A slight tear in the mucous membrane at the anus, usually due to passage of hardened feces. **fistula of a.** Fistula in ano, a sinus opening from the rectum into the connective tissue about the rectum or discharging externally. **imperforate a.** Absence of the anus, the natural opening being closed by a membranous septum; also called *atresia ani.*

anx·i'e·ty. A state of apprehension and fear, accompanied by restlessness and uncertainty. Also see under *complex, hysteria, neurosis.*

anx·i'e·ty at·tack'. *In psychoanalysis,* a feeling of impending death or physical collapse, acute panic or crisis; occurs in an anxiety neurosis, *q.v.*

A. O. 1. Anodal opening. 2. Opening of the atrioventricular valves.

AOC, AnOC. Anodal opening contraction.

aort-. See *aorto-.*

a·or'ta (ay·or'tuh). The large vessel arising from the left ventricle and distributing, by its branches, arterial blood to every part of the body. It ends by bifurcating into the common iliacs at the fourth lumbar vertebra. The arch extending from the heart to the third thoracic vertebra is divided into an *ascending,* a *transverse,* and a *descending* part. The *thoracic* portion extends to the diaphragm; the *abdominal,* to the bifurcation. See Table of Arteries in the Appendix. —**aortic,** *adj.* **ascending a.** The first part of the aorta. **descending a.** The thoracic and abdominal portions of the aorta.

a"or·tal'gi·a. Severe, constant ache in the upper thorax, neck, and shoulders; due to pressure of an aneurysm against the surrounding tissues, or to periaortitis, usually of syphilitic origin.

a·or"ti·co·re'nal (ay·or"ti·ko·ree'·nul). Near the aorta and kidney, as the aorticorenal ganglion.

a"or·ti'tis (ay"or·tye'tis). Inflammation of the aorta. **acute a.** Inflammation usually observed in the intima, as an infiltration of lymphocytes, plasma cells, large mononuclear cells, and a few polymorphonuclear leukocytes.

rheumatic a. A form of intimal arteriosclerosis with large sausagelike plaques, due presumably to rheumatic fever. **suppurative a.** Suppuration in the wall of the aorta as a result of extension of a neighboring pyogenic infection. **syphilitic a.** Inflammation of the aorta due to syphilis. It affects the proximal part of the aorta but may be more extensive. The principal lesion is destruction of parts of the media as a result of syphilitic inflammation around the medial arterioles. The intima shows stellate lines of depression and often hyaline plaques. It begins probably as deforming or obliterative endarteritis of the vasa vasorum. Also called *syphilitic mesaortitis.*

a·or'to- (ay·or'to-), **aort-.** A combining form meaning *aorta.*

A. O. T. A. American Occupational Therapy Association.

ap-. See *apo-.*

A. P. A. American Physiotherapy Association.

a·pal"les·the'si·a (a·pal"ess·thee'·zhuh, ·zee·uh). Loss of vibration sense. Syn., *pallanesthesia.*

a·pan'dri·a. Morbid dislike of the male sex.

ap"an·thro'pi·a, a·pan'thro·py. 1. Morbid desire for solitude. 2. Morbid aversion to human associations.

a·pas'ti·a. Abstinence from food; seen in mental disorder. —**apastic,** *adj.*

ap'a·thism. Slowness in reacting, as opposed to *erethism.*

ap'a·thy. 1. Want of passion or feeling. 2. Indifference. —**apathet'ic,** *adj.*

APC group. Short for the adenoidal, pharyngeal, conjunctival group of viruses, known to be the causative agents of a number of respiratory infections and of keratoconjunctivitis.

a·pel'lous. 1. Skinless; not cicatrized, applied to wounds. 2. Without a prepuce; circumcised.

a·pe'ri·ent. 1. Laxative; mildly purgative. 2. A mild purgative; a laxative.

a·pe"ri·od'ic (ay·peer"ee·od'ick, a·peer"·). Devoid of periodicity or rhythm. —**aperiodic'ity,** *n.*

a·per"i·stal'sis (ay·perr"i·stal'sis, a·perr"·). Absence of the peristaltic movements of the intestine.

a·per'i·tive (a·perr'i·tiv). 1. Aperient. 2. Deobstruent. 3. Stimulating the appetite.

ap"er·tu'ra (pl. *aperturae*). An opening. **a. aquaeductus cochleae.** The opening of the aqueduct of the cochlea on the petrosa. **a. externa aquaeductus vestibuli.** External opening of the aqueduct of the vestibule. **a. pelvis inferior** [BNA]. Lower opening of the true pelvis (*O.T.,* pelvic outlet). **a. pelvis superior**

[BNA]. Upper opening of the true pelvis (O.T., pelvic inlet).

ap'er·ture. An opening; orifice. **lateral apertures of the fourth ventricle.** Two openings in the lateral recesses of the fourth ventricle through which cerebrospinal fluid passes into the subarachnoid space. Also called *foramens of Luschka*. **medial a. of the fourth ventricle.** One in the center of the roof of the fourth ventricle through which cerebrospinal fluid passes into the subarachnoid space. Also called *foramen of Magendie*. **numerical a.** Capacity of the objective to receive and transmit light rays to the image, expressed by the formula N.A. = sin ½∠a × ir, in which ∠a = angular aperture and ir = index of refraction of the medium in front of the lens. **urogenital a.** External opening of the embryonic urogenital sinus after rupture of the urethral plate.

a'pex. Summit or top of anything; point or extremity of a cone. —**ap'ical**, *adj.* **a. of the lung.** Upper extremity of the lung behind the anterior border of the first rib.

APF. Animal protein factor. A substance, present in animal protein, necessary for normal growth of many animal species. The factor may be vitamin B_{12}.

aph-. See *apo-*.

A. P. H. A. American Public Health Association.

a·pha'gi·a. Loss of the ability to swallow. **a. algera.** Inability or refusal to swallow because of pain.

a·pha'ki·a. The condition of an eye without the lens. —**aphakic, aphakial,** *adj.*

aph"a·lan'gi·a, a·pha"lan·gi·a·sis. Loss or absence of fingers or toes. See *ainhum; ectrodactylia.*

aph"al·ge'si·a (af"al·jee'zee·uh, ·see·uh). A hysterical state wherein pain is induced by contact with a harmless object having symbolic significance.

a·pha'si·a (a·fay'zhuh, ·zee·uh). Loss or impairment of the capacity to use words as symbols of ideas. Aphasia is organic and is caused by a lesion or lesions in the cortex and association paths of the dominant hemisphere. It does not refer to a defect in the mechanics of hearing or speaking but to an impairment of the highest function of the use of language as translating thought. Hysterical speech defects may imitate the symptoms of aphasia. There are many subdivisions according to the degree of loss and specific language function affected. Aphasia may be partial or total (global). The predominant defect may affect the ability to speak, called **motor** or **expressive aphasia.** The lesion responsible is

located in the parolfactory area at the posterior end of the third frontal convolution. The failure may be a lack of comprehension of the spoken word, or **auditory aphasia.** This is a form of **sensory** or **receptive aphasia.** Words are evoked with difficulty, used incorrectly, and do not translate ideas accurately. Sometimes words are uttered fluently but inappropriately, as in jargon or **paraphasia;** this is allied to **amnesic aphasia,** which is a loss of memory for specific words, with hesitant and fragmentary speech. The lesions which cause these types of aphasia lie in the parietal lobe at or near the angular gyrus. Expressive and receptive aphasia are the two most common types, and may occur together in mixed forms. Other varieties are **acaloulia** (loss of ability to do mathematical reckoning); **agraphia** (inability to write); **alexia** or **visual aphasia** (loss of ability to understand the written word); **nominal aphasia** (anomia, dysnomia, loss of ability to name objects); **semantic aphasia** (loss of meaning of words); **syntactic aphasia** (loss of correct grammatical construction). —**aphasiac,** *adj.,* **n. Broca's a.** Motor aphasia, *q.v.* **Wernicke's a.** Cortical sensory aphasia in which both auditory and visual aphasia are present.

a·phelx'i·a. Absent-mindedness; inattention or indifference to external impressions. —**aphelot'ic,** *adj.*

a·phe'mi·a. Motor aphasia; inability to articulate words or sentences, due to a central lesion. See *aphasia.* —**aphem'ic,** *adj.*

aph"e·pho'bi·a. Morbid fear of physical contact with other persons.

a·pho'ni·a (ay·fo'nee·uh, a·fo'nee·uh). 1. Loss of speech due to some peripheral lesion. 2. Hysterical loss of the power of speech. 3. Voicelessness. —**aph'onous, aphon'ic,** *adj.* **a. clericorum.** Clergyman's sore throat. **a. paranoica.** The stubborn silence sometimes encountered in the insane. **paralytic a.** Paralysis of the speech muscles. Syn., *phonetic paralysis.* **spastic a.** Spasm of the vocal muscles initiated by efforts to speak. Syn., *dysphonia spastica.*

a'phose (ay'fohz, a·fohz'). A subjective dark spot or shadow in the field of vision. See *phose.*

a·phra'si·a (a·fray'zhuh, ·zee·uh). Loss of the power to utter connected phrases.

aph"ro·dis'i·a (af"ro·diz'ee·uh). 1. Sexual desire, especially when morbid or immoderate. 2. Sexual union.

aph"ro·dis'i·ac (af"ro·diz'ee·ack). 1. Stimulating the sexual appetite; erotic. 2. An agent stimulating the sexual passion.

aph″ro·dis″i·o·ma′ni·a. Exaggerated sexual interest and excitement. Syn., *erotomania.*

aph′tha (pl. *aphthae*). 1. An ulcer of the oral mucous membranes caused by the herpes simplex virus, characterized by a lesion, usually painful, which has a markedly erythematous border, is covered by a yellowish membrane, and heals without scarring. Syn., *canker sore.* 2. Herpetic stomatitis. **Bednar's a.** One seen in cachectic infants, traumatic in origin.

aph′thous, aph′thoid. Relating to, affected with, or resembling aphthae.

a′pi-. A combining form meaning *bee.*

a″pi·cec′to·my (ay″pi·seck′to·mee, ap″i·). 1. Resection of the tip of a tooth root. 2. Excision of the air cells of the apex of the petrosa.

ap″i·ci′tis. Inflammation of any apex, as of a tooth root or of a lung.

ap″i·col′y·sis. Artificial collapse of the upper portion of a lung by separation of the parietal pleura from the chest wall; used in the treatment of pulmonary tuberculosis with apical cavities.

a″pi·o·ther′a·py. Treatment of disease, especially rheumatism, with bee venom.

a″pi·pho′bi·a (ay″pi·fo′bee·uh, ap″i·). Morbid terror of bees and their sting.

A.P.L. 1. Abbreviation for anterior pituitarylike (see anterior pituitarylike *substance*). 2. Designation of a proprietary preparation of chorionic gonadotrophic hormone used intramuscularly.

a″pla·cen′tal, ap″la·cen′tal. Without a placenta.

a·pla′si·a (a·play′zhuh, ·zee·uh). Defective development or congenital absence of a part. Syn., *agenesia.* **a. axialis extracorticalis congenita.** A heredofamilial disorder appearing in early infancy, manifested by rotary movements of the eyes and head, by spasticity of all limbs, cerebellar ataxia, intention tremor, slurring speech, and dementia; a noninflammatory degeneration of the white matter of the brain and brain stem. Also called *Merzbacher-Pelizaeus disease.* **nuclear a.** A congenital defect in which certain cranial nerve nuclei are absent or imperfectly developed.

a·plas′tic (ay·plas′tick, a·plas′tick). 1. Structureless; formless. 2. Incapable of forming new tissue. 3. Relating to aplasia. 4. Defective in fibrin. 5. Designating an inflammation with little or no production of granulation tissue.

ap·ne′a, ap·noe′a. A transient suspension of respiration because of a decrease of carbon dioxide tension of the blood with the resultant absence of stimulation of the respiratory center. Also called *a. vera.* **a. vagi.** Temporary cessation of breathing due to vagal stimulation. **cardiac a.** The temporary period of suspended breathing in Cheyne-Stokes respiration.

ap·noe′a. See *apnea.*

ap′o-, ap-, aph-. A prefix meaning *away from, from.* It implies derivation or separation.

ap″o·chro·mat′ic. *In optics,* corrected for spherical and chromatic aberration, as an apochromatic lens.

ap″o·clei′sis (ap″o·kly′sis). Aversion to eating.

ap″o·co′de·ine (·ko′dee·een, ·ko′deen). An alkaloid derived from codeine, and having expectorant and emetic qualities.

ap′o·crine (ap′o·kryne, ·krin). Designating a type of secretion in which the secretion-filled free end of a gland cell is pinched off, leaving the nucleus and most of the cytoplasm to recover and repeat the process.

a·poc′y·num (a·poss′i·num). The dried rhizome and roots of *Apocynum cannabinum* or of *Apocynum androsaemifolium.* The physiologic actions are similar to those of digitalis. Syn., *black Indian hemp, Canada hemp.*

ap″o·de″mi·al′gi·a. A morbid dislike of home life, with a desire for wandering; wanderlust.

ap″o·en′zyme (ap″o·en′zime, ·zim). The purely protein part of an enzyme which, with the coenzyme, forms the complete or *holoenzyme.*

ap″o·fer′ri·tin. The protein resulting when iron is removed from ferritin, *q.v.*

a·pog′a·my, ap″o·gam′i·a. The production of a sporophyte from the gametophyte without the formation or union of gametes. Syn., *apomixis, parthenogenesis.* **—apogam′ic, apog′amous,** *adj.*

ap″o·mor′phine (ap″o·mor′feen, ·mor·feen′). A base derived from morphine by the abstraction of a molecule of water.

a·pon″eu·ro′sis, ap″o·neu·ro′sis. An expanded tendon consisting of a fibrous or membranous sheet, serving as a means of attachment for flat muscles at their origin or insertion, or as a fascia to enclose or bind a group of muscles. **—aponeurot′ic,** *adj.* **abdominal a.** The wide, tendinous expanse by which the external oblique, internal oblique, and transversus muscles are inserted. **vertebral a.** A thin aponeurotic lamina extending along the whole length of the back part of the thoracic region, serving to bind down the sacrospinalis muscle and separating it from those muscles that unite the spine to the upper extremity.

a·pon″eu·ro·si′tis (a·pon″yoor·o-sigh'tis, ap''o·new·ro·). Inflammation of an aponeurosis.

a·poph'y·sis. A process, outgrowth, or projection of some part or organ, as of a bone. **—apophys'eal, apophys'ial,** *adj.* **basilar a.** Basilar process of the occipital bone. **true a.** One which has never been an epiphysis.

a·poph''y·si'tis. Inflammation of an apophysis.

ap'o·plex''y. 1. The symptom complex resulting from hemorrhage into or upon the brain, or from embolism or thrombosis of the cerebral vessels, consisting chiefly of hemiplegia, coma, and death. 2. Gross hemorrhage into any organ, as the lungs, spleen, ovary, eye, etc.; designated as apoplexy of the affected organ. *Rare.* **—apoplec'tic, apoplec'tiform,** *adj.* **bulbar a.** That due to hemorrhage into the substance of the medulla oblongata or pons, causing paralysis of one or both sides of the body, inability to swallow, difficulty in protruding the tongue, dyspnea, gastric disorders, and disturbed heart action. **embolic a.** Apoplexy resulting from the plugging of a cerebral vessel by an embolus.

a·pop·nix'is. A choking sensation. Syn., *globus hystericus.*

ap''or·rhip'sis. The throwing off of the clothes or the bedclothes; a symptom seen in some cases of mental disorder.

a·po'si·a (a·po'zhuh, ·zee·uh). Absence of thirst or of the feeling of thirst; adipsia.

ap''o·si'ti·a (ap''o·sish'ee·uh, ·sit'ee·uh). Aversion to or loathing of food. **—aposit'ic,** *adj.*

a·pos'ta·sis. End or crisis of an attack of disease; termination by crisis.

a·poth'e·car''ies' weight. A system of weights and measures used in compounding medicines. The troy pound of 5760 grains is the standard. It is subdivided into 12 ounces. The ounce is subdivided into 8 drachms, the drachm into 3 scruples, and the scruple into 20 grains. For fluid measure the quart of 32 fluidounces is subdivided into 2 pints, the pint into 16 fluidounces, the fluidounce into 8 fluiddrachms, and the fluidrachm into 60 minims. The following symbols and abbreviations are used:

    ℥, *minim.*
    ℈, *scrupulus,* a scruple (20 gr.).
    ℨ, *drachma,* a drachm (60 gr.).
    ℥, *uncia,* an ounce (480 gr.).
    ℔., *libra,* a pound.
    C., *congius,* a gallon.
    O., *octarius,* a pint.
    gr., *granum,* a grain.
    ss., *semissis,* one-half

See Tables of Weights and Measures, Appendix.

a·poth'e·car''y. A druggist or pharmacist; one who prepares and sells drugs, fills prescriptions, etc.

ap''pa·ra'tus. 1. A collection of instruments or devices used for a special purpose. 2. *In anatomy,* used to designate collectively the organs or parts of organs performing a certain function; a mechanism. **juxtaglomerular a.** A cuff of epithelioid cells in the kidney around the afferent arteriole near its entrance into the glomerulus. **lacrimal a.** The mechanism for secreting tears and draining them into the nose, consisting of the lacrimal gland, lake, puncta, canaliculi, sac, and the nasolacrimal duct.

ap·pend'age. Anything appended, usually of minor importance. **—appendic'ulate,** *adj.* **appendages of the eye.** The eyelashes, eyebrows, lacrimal gland, lacrimal sac and ducts, and conjunctiva. **auricular a.** (a) The projecting part of the cardiac atrium. (b) The pinna of the ear. (c) A round or elongated cartilaginous prominence in front of the tragus. **cutaneous appendages.** Nails, hair, sebaceous glands, and sweat glands. **fetal appendages.** Placenta, amnion, chorion, and umbilical cord. **uterine appendages.** Ovaries and oviducts.

ap''pen·dec'to·my, ap·pen''dicec'to·my. Excision of the vermiform process.

ap·pen''di·ci'tis. Inflammation of the vermiform process. **acute a.** That form characterized by sudden onset of abdominal pain, generalized at first, then becoming localized to the right lower quadrant, with nausea, vomiting, and constipation, fever, leukocytosis, localized tenderness, and rigidity. In the absence of operation the attack subsides or goes on to gangrene, perforation, and abscess formation. **chronic a.** That form characterized by recurring attacks of right-sided pain without the signs and symptoms of acute attacks. The appendicular origin of this ailment is doubted by many. **gangrenous a.** Acute appendicitis with formation of pus and necrosis of the appendix. **obliterative a.** That form in which the lumen is narrowed or closed; often found in so-called chronic appendicitis. **perforating a.** This form follows acute gangrenous appendicitis with perforation of the appendix and peritonitis. **suppurative a.** Acute appendicitis with formation of pus.

ap·pen''di·clau'sis. Chronic appendicitis, especially of the obliterative type. See chronic *appendicitis,* obliterative *appendicitis.*

ap·pen''di·cos'to·my. Withdrawal of the appendix and mesoappendix through a McBurney incision, anchoring the former to the abdominal muscle. The tip is then cut off and a catheter passed through the appendiceal lumen into the cecum for subsequent irrigation. Obs.

ap·pen'dix (pl. *appendixes*, *appendices*). An appendage. **—appendic'ular**, *adj*. **appendices epiploicae.** Fatty projections of the serous coat of the large intestine. **appendices epoöphori.** Vestigial remnants of the mesonephric tubules or ducts found in or on the broad ligament of the uterus or near the fimbriae. **a. testis.** A remnant of the cranial part of Müller's duct, attached to the testis. Formerly called *hydatid of Morgagni*. **vermiform a.** The small, blind gut projecting from the cecum.

ap''per·cep'tion. Consciousness of the relation of new events, situations, or sensations to past experience. **—apperceptive**, *adj*.

ap''per·son''i·fi·ca'tion. Unconscious transfer to one's own ego of certain qualities in other persons or objects. Syn., *identification*.

ap'pe·tite. Desire for food, not necessarily prompted by hunger; any natural desire or craving. **a. juice.** The flow of gastric juice initiated by the sight, odor, or thought of food (psychic causes) and by tasting or chewing food, without swallowing it. **perverted a.** A desire for unnatural or indigestible foods, seen occasionally during pregnancy; pica.

ap'pe·ti''zer. A medicine or aperitif taken before a meal to stimulate the appetite.

ap'pli·ca''tor. An instrument used in making local applications.

ap''po·si'tion. The act of fitting together; the state of being fitted together; juxtaposition.

ap·proach'. In surgery, the manner of securing access to a joint, cavity, part, or organ by a suitable incision through the overlying or neighboring structures, as the anterior axillary approach for exposing the shoulder joint.

ap·prox'i·mal, ap·prox'i·mate. Situated close or near; contiguous; next to each other; as approximal fillings.

ap·prox''i·ma'tion. The act or process of bringing together. **—approx'imate**, *v*.

a·prax'i·a (ay·prack'see·uh, a·prack'·). A disorder of the nervous system, caused by lesions in the cortical area; characterized by inability to perform purposeful movements, although no muscular paralysis or sensory disturbance is present. **amnestic a.** Due to inability to remember a command. **ideational a.** That in which there is a lack of ideas for

planning an act, or a distorted sequence of ideas or conception of how to use them; due to diffuse brain disease. **ideomotor a.** That in which simple single acts are correctly performed, but the sequence of associated acts is incorrect and a final, complex act cannot be carried out; due to interruption of the association pathways between ideational and motor kinesthetic areas. **motor a.** Apraxia in which simple movements are clumsy or confused; due to disease of the motor cortex.

apresoline hydrochloride. Trade-mark for hydralazine hydrochloride.

a''pro·bar'bi·tal. Generic name for allyl isopropylbarbituric acid. See *alurate*.

a·proc'ti·a (ay·prock'shee·uh, a·prock'·). Imperforate anus. **—aproctous**, *adj*.

ap''ro·sex'i·a. A mental disturbance consisting in inability to fix attention upon a subject. **a. nasalis.** Inattention and mental dullness often seen in chronic nasal catarrh, especially when associated with adenoids, in children.

ap''ro·so'pi·a. Congenital absence of part or all of the face. **—aprosopous**, *adj*.; **apros'opus**, *n*.

ap''si·thy'ri·a, ap''si·thu're·a. Hysterical aphonia, in which the patient loses the voice, being unable even to whisper.

ap·ty'a·lism (ap·tye'u·liz·um, ay·tye'·), **ap''ty·a'li·a** (ap''tye·ay'lee·uh, ap''ti·). Deficiency or absence of saliva.

a'pus. Lacking feet, or without the entire lower extremities.

a''py·rex'i·a (ay''pye·reck'see·uh, a·pye·). Absence of fever. **—apyrexial, apyret'ic**, *adj*.

AQ. Accomplishment quotient.

aq. *Aqua;* water; water of crystallization.

aq'ua (ack'wuh, ay'kwuh) (pl. *aquae*). Water; medicated water, as aromatic waters, saturated solutions of volatile oils or other volatile substances in water. Abbreviated, a., aq.

aquaphor. A proprietary ointment base with the ability to absorb water or aqueous solutions.

aq'ue·duct. A canal for the passage of fluid; any canal. **a. of the cochlea.** A canal which establishes a communication between the perilymphatic space of the osseous labyrinth and the subarachnoid space, and transmits a vein for the cochlea. **a. of the vestibule.** A canal of the vestibule of the ear running from the vestibule and opening on the back of the petrous portion of the temporal bone and containing the endolymphatic duct and a small vein. **cerebral a.** The elongated, slender cavity of the midbrain which connects the third and fourth ventricles. Also called *a. of Sylvius*.

communicating a. A small canal sometimes found at the junction of the mastoid and petrous portions of the temporal bone; it gives passage to an emissary vein from the transverse sinus.

a'que·ous (ay'kwee·us, ack'wee·us). 1. Watery. 2. The aqueous humor; the transparent fluid of the anterior chamber of the eye.

ar-. 1. *In chemistry*, a combining form denoting *aromatic*. 2. A form of *ad-* assimilated in Latin before *r*.

ar'a·bic ac'id (ar'uh·bick, a·rab'-ick). The acid present in acacia as the calcium salt.

ar'a·bin. Arabic acid. A carbohydrate, obtained from certain gums, soluble in water.

a·rab'i·nose, ar'a·bi·nose''. Pectinose; pectin sugar; gum sugar; a crystalline aldopentose otained by acid hydrolysis of acacia, cherry, and mesquite gums; also from beet pulp.

ar'a·chis oil. Peanut oil.

arachn-. See *arachno-*.

a·rach''ne·pho'bi·a (a·rack''ni-). Morbid fear of spiders.

A·rach'ni·da (a·rack'ni·duh). A large class of the Arthropoda which includes scorpions, spiders, mites, and ticks. They usually lack wings and antennae and, as adults, have four pairs of legs.

a·rach'nid·ism, a·rach'noid·ism. A condition produced by the bite of a poisonous spider; venom poisoning.

a·rach'no- (a·rack'no-), **arachn-.** A combining form meaning *spider*.

a·rach''no·dac'ty·ly. Spider fingers; a condition in which the fingers, and sometimes the toes, are abnormally long. Syn., *dolichostenomelia*.

a·rach'noid (a·rack'noyd). 1. Web-like. 2. The *arachnoidea encephali* [BNA], and *arachnoidea spinalis* [BNA]. The arachnoid membrane; the central of the three meninges covering the brain and spinal cord. It is very fine and delicate in structure, following the pia mater into each sulcus and around each convolution, but separated by the subarachnoid space. The two membranes are often considered as one organ, the piarachnoid. **—arachnoi'dal,** *adj.*

a·rach·noi'de·a [BNA]. The arachnoid membrane. See *arachnoid*.

a·rach''noi·di'tis. Inflammation of the arachnoid membrane.

aralen diphosphate. Trade-mark for the diphosphate of chloroquine.

aramine bitartrate. Trade-mark for metaraminol bitartrate.

a''ra·ro'ba (ahr''uh·ro'buh, ar''uh-ro'buh). Goa powder. An oxidation product of the resin found in the wood of *Andira araroba*, of Brazil. From it is obtained chrysarobin.

ar''bor·i·za'tion. A conformation or arrangement resembling the branching of a tree. **—ar'borize,** *v.t., v.i.*;

arbo'real, arbo'reous, arbo-res'cent, *adj.* **terminal a.** (a) Branched end of a sensory nerve fiber. (b) A motor end plate. (c) Terminal ramifications of the Purkinje system of the heart.

ar'bor vi'tae (ahr'bor vy'tee). 1. Arborescent appearance of the white substance in a median section of the cerebellum. 2. Series of ridges and folds of the mucosa within the uterine cervix.

arc. A part of the circumference of a circle; a more or less curved passageway.

ar·cade'. A series of arches. The term ordinarily is used in reference to blood vessels.

ar·ca'num. A secret medicine.

arch. A structure having a curved outline resembling that of an arc or a bow. **alveolar a.** That formed by the alveolar process of each jaw. **aortic arches.** Six pairs of embryonic vascular arches encircling the pharynx in the visceral arches. In mammals, the left fourth arch becomes a part of the systemic circulatory system and the sixth pair becomes incorporated in the pulmonary circulation. **arches of the foot.** (a) The *metatarsal arch*, a transverse hollow on the inner part of the sole in the line of the tarsometa-tarsal articulations. (b) The *inner longitudinal arch*, consisting of the calcaneus, the talus, the navicular, three cuneiform bones, and the first three toes. (c) The *outer longitudinal arch*, made up of the calcaneus, the cuboid, and the fourth and fifth toes. **a. of the aorta.** The transverse portion of the aorta between its ascending and descending portions. **axillary a.** An occasional muscle slip in the axilla connecting the latissimus dorsi or teres major with the pectoralis major. **branchial arches.** (a) One of the posthyoid gill arches in lower vertebrates. (b) Any one of the visceral arches in the embryos of higher vertebrates. **deep femoral a.** A band of fibers originating apparently in the transversalis fascia, arching across the femoral sheath and attached to the middle of the inguinal ligament and the pectineal line. **deep volar a.** That formed by the anastomosis of the terminal part of the radial artery with the deep volar branch of the ulnar artery. Syn., *deep palmar a.* **dental a.** The parabolic curve formed by the cutting edges and masticating surfaces of the teeth; the alveolar arch. **lumbocostal a.** A ligamentous arch from the twelfth rib to the first lumbar vertebra serving as part of the attachment of the diaphragm. The **lateral lumbo-costal arch** is that lying anterior to the quadratus lumborum; the **medial lumbocostal arch** is that lying anterior to the psoas major. **mandibular a.** The first visceral arch, including the maxillary process. **neural a.** (a) Vertebral arch, q.v. (b) *In comparative anatomy*, the superior loop of the typical vertebra including the neural canal. **pharyngopalatine a.** That formed by the projection of the pharyngopalatinus muscle covered by mucous membrane. Also called *palatopharyngeal a.* Formerly called *posterior pillar of the fauces.* **plantar a.** The arch, in the sole of the foot, made by the lateral plantar artery and the deep plantar branch of the dorsalis pedis artery. **pubic a.** That formed by the conjoined inferior rami of the pubis and ischium. **superciliary a.** The skeletal arch in the anterior region of the frontal bone, underneath the eyebrow. **superficial volar a.** That formed by the ulnar artery in the palm of the hand and completed by a branch of the radial artery. Syn., *superficial palmar a.* **vertebral a.** That formed by the paired pedicles and laminas of a vertebra; the posterior part of a vertebra which together with the anterior part, the body, encloses the vertebral foramen in which the spinal cord is lodged. **zygomatic a.** That formed by the zygomatic process of the temporal bone, the zygoma and the zygomatic process of the maxilla.

arch-. 1. A prefix meaning *first, chief,* or *principal.* 2. A prefix denoting *first in time, original.* 3. A prefix denoting *primitive, original.*

ar·cha'ic. *In psychiatry,* designating elements in the unconscious which are remnants of man's prehistoric past, and which reappear in dreams and other symbolic manifestations.

ar·chen'ter·on (ahr·ken'tur·on). The embryonic alimentary cavity of the gastrula, lined by endoderm. Syn., *archigaster, coelenteron, gastrocoel, primitive* or *primary gut, progaster, primitive stomach.* **—archenter'ic,** *adj.*

ar'che·type (ahr'ki·type). 1. A basic model; prototype. 2. *In comparative anatomy,* an ideal, generalized structural pattern of one of the main kinds of organisms, assumed to be the form of the original ancestor of the group.

ar'chi- (ahr'kee-). 1. A prefix denoting *chief, arch-.* 2. *In anatomy and biology,* a prefix denoting *primitive, original, ancestral.*

ar"chi·neph'ron. The primitive kidney. **—archinephric,** *adj.*

ar"chi·pal'li·um. The olfactory pallium or the olfactory cerebral cortex; the rhinencephalon; the oldest part of the cerebral cortex. **—archipallial,** *adj.*

ar"chi·tec·ton'ic. 1. Pertaining to the structural arrangement or architectural construction of an organ or part. 2. Structure or texture of a tissue or organ. **—architectonics,** *n.*

ar'cho- (ahr'ko-). A combining form formerly used to mean *rectal. Obs.*

ar'ci·form. Arcuate, bow-shaped; especially used to designate certain sets of fibers in the medulla oblongata, and certain veins and arteries of the kidney. See Table of Arteries in the Appendix.

arc·ta'tion. Contraction of an opening or canal; stenosis.

ar'cu·ate, ar'cu·al. Arched; curved; bow-shaped, as the arcuate fibers of the cerebellum and the cerebrum which serve as association fibers.

ar"cu·a'tion. Curvature, especially of a bone. **—ar'cual,** *adj.*

ar'cus. An arch, q.v. **a. juvenilis.** A white ring around the cornea occurring in young individuals and resembling the arcus senilis. **a. senilis.** An opaque ring at the edge of the cornea, seen in the aged. **a. senilis lentis.** An opaque ring in the equator of the crystalline lens; it sometimes occurs in the aged. **a. tendineus.** A thickened band of the parietal pelvic fascia extending from the pubis to the ischial spine and serving as an attachment for part of the fibers of the levator ani muscle.

a're·a. A limited extent of surface; a region; a structural or functional part of the cerebral cortex. **aortic a.** The second right interspace near the sternum, where aortic sounds and murmurs are best heard. **a. acustica.** An area in the lateral angle of the floor of the fourth ventricle overlying the nuclei of the vestibular nerve. **a. cribrosa.** (a) A small perforated space in the internal auditory meatus through which pass filaments of the acoustic nerve. (b) The surface onto which the papillary ducts of a renal pyramid open into a minor calyx. **a. postrema.** One on the floor of the fourth ventricle between the ala cinerea and the taenia of the fourth ventricle, medial to the clava. **associations a.** A term formerly used to designate cortical areas which supposedly had connections only with other parts of the cortex. Now used to designate many areas between the primary projection centers. **auditory projection a.** The cortical receptive center for auditory impulses, located in the transverse temporal gyri. Also called *Brodmann's a. 41, auditosensory a., auditory cortex.* **bare a. of the liver.** Triangular area on the superior surface of the liver devoid of peritoneum, enclosed by the coronary ligament. **Brodmann's areas.** Numbered regions of the cerebral cortex originally differentiated by histologic criteria, now used in discussions of cortical functions; as **areas 1, 2, 3,** the postcentral gyrus, the somesthetic area; **area 4,** the posterior part of the precentral gyrus, the motor area; **area 6,** the anterior part of the precentral gyrus and the adjacent posterior superior part of the frontal cortex, the premotor area; **area 17,** the walls and margins of the calcarine fissure, the visual projection area; **area 41,** the two transverse temporal gyri, the auditory projection area. **calcarine a.** The visual projection area of the occipital cortex in the walls and margins of the calcarine fissure; Brodmann's area 17. **extrapyramidal motor areas.** Those portions of the cortex other than the pyramidal cortex, from which motor responses can be obtained upon stimulation, or motor losses observed after ablation; Brodmann's areas 6, 5, 19, 22. **hypothenar a.** (a) The region of the hypothenar eminence. (b) The medial or ulnar palmar space. **motor a.** The precentral gyrus containing centers for voluntary movement; characterized histologically by the presence of Betz cells. Also called *Brodmann's a. 4, pyramidal a., motor cortex.* **motor speech a.** That located in the triangular and opercular portions of the inferior frontal gyrus; its destruction causes motor aphasia. Also called *Brodmann's a. 44, Broca's a., Broca's center.* **premotor a.** The main cortical extrapyramidal motor area lying immediately in front of the motor area from which it differs histologically by the absence of Betz cells. Also called *Brodmann's a. 6.* **pyramidal a.** The motor area of the cerebral cortex characterized histologically by the presence of giant pyramidal, or Betz, cells; Brodmann's area 4. **sensory a.** The general area of the cerebral cortex in which sensation is perceived. **somesthetic a.** The receptive center for proprioceptive or tactile sensation in the postcentral gyrus. Also called *Brodmann's areas, 1, 2, 3.* **striate a.** The visual projection area of the occipital cortex characterized by the line of Gennari; Brodmann's area 17. **visual projection a.** The cortical receptive center for visual impulses, located in the walls and margins of the calcarine fissure of the occipital lobe, characterized by the line of Gennari. Also called *Brodmann's a. 17, visuosensory a., calcarine a., striate a., visual cortex, visual a.*

a·rec′o·line (a·reck′o·leen, a·ree′ko·). A liquid alkaloid isolated from the seeds of *Areca catechu.* It has anthelmintic properties. *In veterinary medicine,* it is used also as a cathartic.

a″re·flex′i·a (ay″ri·fleck′see·uh, a·ri·). Absence of reflexes.

a·re′o·la. 1. Any minute interstice or space in a tissue. 2. A colored or pigmented ring surrounding some central point or space, as a nipple, pustule. 3. The part of the iris enclosing the pupil. **—areolar,** *adj.* **a. mammae.** The pigmented area surrounding the nipple of the breast. This enlarges during pregnancy, producing the *second areola.* Also called *a. papillaris, mammary a.* **umbilical a.** A pigmented ring which surrounds the umbilicus in some individuals. **vaccinal a.** A red ring surrounding a pustule.

arfonad camphorsulfonate. Trade-mark for trimethaphan camphorsulfonate.

ar·gam″bly·o′pi·a, ar″gi·am″-bly·o′pi·a. Amblyopia due to disuse of the eye.

ar′ge·ma (pl. *argemata*). A white ulcer of the cornea, following phlyctenula.

ar′gent-. See *argento-.*

ar·gen′taf·fin, ar·gen′taf·fine. Referring to the capacity of certain tissue elements to reduce silver in staining solution.

ar·gen′to-, ar′gent-. A combining form denoting *silver, containing silver.*

ar·gen′to·phile, ar·gen′to·phil. See *argyrophile.*

ar·gen′tum. See *silver.*

ar″gil·la′ceous (ahr″ji·lay′shus). Claylike; composed of clay.

ar′gi·nase (ar′ji·nace, ·naze). Enzyme found in the liver, kidney, and spleen of mammals and in the seeds of certain plants. Its action is to split arginine into ornithine and urea.

ar′gi·nine (ahr′ji·neen, ·nin). α-Amino-δ-guanidinovaleric acid. $NH_2C(:NH)NHCH_2CH_2CH_2CH(NH_2)COOH.$ An essential amino acid obtained from both animal and vegetable proteins.

ar′gol. The impure potassium bitartrate deposited during the fermentation of grape juice. See *tartar.*

ar′gon. A = 39.944. An inert gaseous element present in the atmosphere. It may be obtained by fractionation of liquid air.

Argyll Robertson, Douglas Moray Cooper Lamb [*Scottish physician, 1837–1909*]. Remembered for his description of the pupil which reacts to accommodation but not to light, characteristic of certain diseases (1869); called *Argyll Robertson pupil.*

ar·gyr′i·a (ahr·jirr′ee·uh, ahr·jy′ree·uh). A dusky-gray or bluish discoloration of the skin and mucous membranes produced by the prolonged administration or application of silver preparaions, the granules of silver being deposited in much the same sites as those of the natural pigment of the skin. **—argyric,** *adj.*

ar'gy·ro-, argyr-. A combining form meaning *silver.*

ar'gyrol. Proprietary preparation somewhat similar to mild silver protein.

ar'gy·ro·phile, ar·gy'ro·phil (ahr·jy'ro, ahr'ji·ro·). Referring to the capacity of certain fixed tissue elements to retain reduced silver.

arhin"en·ce·pha'li·a, ar·rhin"-en·ce·pha'li·a. A form of partial encephalia in which there is partial or total absence of the rhinencephalon and malformation of the nose.

ari"bo·fla"vi·no'sis (a·rye"bo-flay"vi·no'sis, ·flav"i·no'sis). Deficiency of riboflavin, *q.v.*, a condition formerly confused with pellagra. It is characterized by cheilosis, corneal and other eye changes, and dermatitis seborrheica.

aris"to·gen'ic. Well endowed eugenically. **—aristogenics,** *n.*

aristol. Trade-mark for a brand of thymol iodide.

arith·met'ic mean. The arithmetic average.

arith"mo·ma'ni·a. A morbid impulse to count objects; a preoccupation with numbers.

arlidin hydrochloride. Trademark for nylidrin hydrochloride.

arm. 1. *In anatomy*, the upper extremity from the shoulder to the elbow. **2.** Popularly, the arm and the forearm. **3.** That portion of the stand connecting the body or tube of a microscope with the pillar.

ar"ma·men·tar'i·um (·tair'ee·um). All of the books, journals, medicines, instruments, and laboratory and therapeutic equipment possessed by a physician, surgeon, or medical institution to assist in the practice of his or its profession.

Ar'mor Med'i·cal Re·search' Lab'o·ra·to'ry. An experimental station of the Army Medical Department, for research in the physiologic effects of armor equipment operation on personnel, and having for its object the reduction of operational hazards by the development of armor equipment.

arm'pit". The axilla.

Ar'my Med'i·cal Cen'ter. A centrally situated installation of the Army Medical Department where are located a general hospital, research facilities, training schools for service personnel, laboratories, etc.

Arneth, Joseph [German physician, 1873–]. Classified neutrophil granulocytes according to the number of lobes shown by their nuclei. *Arneth's*

formula gives the percentages found in healthy persons: neutrophils with one lobe, 5%; with two lobes, 35%; with three, 41%; with four, 17%; with five, 2%. Also devised a phagocytic index based on the assumption that those neutrophils with three or more lobes possess the greatest phagocytic power (1904).

ar'ni·ca. The dried flower heads of the *Arnica montana.* Arnica is an irritant, and is popularly used as a tincture for sprains, bruises, and surface wounds.

ar"o·mat'ic. 1. Having a spicy odor. **2.** Characterized by a fragrant, spicy taste and odor, as cinnamon, ginger, or the essential oils. **3.** A qualification applied to any carbon compound originating from benzene, C_6H_6.

ar·rec'tor (pl. *arrectores*). *In anatomy*, an erector muscle. **arrectores pilorum.** Minute, fanlike, involuntary muscles attached to the hair follicles which, by contraction, erect the follicle and cause so-called goose flesh. See Table of Muscles in the Appendix.

ar·rest'. A stopping, checking, or restraining. **cardiac a.** Standstill of the entire heart. **pelvic a.** *In obstetrics*, a condition accompanying labor in which the presenting part of the fetus becomes fixed in its position in the maternal pelvis. **transverse a.** *In obstetrics*, a faulty condition in the mechanism of labor when a flat type of maternal pelvis causes a fixation of the fetal head in the transverse position.

ar"rhe·no·blas·to'ma (ar"i·no-blas·to'muh, a·ree"no·). An infrequent tumor of the ovary, moderate in size, encapsulated, nodular, firm, and nearly always unilateral, occurring most often in earlier life; may be malignant. Three microscopic forms are observed: *testicular tubular adenoma*, a *sarcomatoid* form, and a *mixed tubular and sarcomatoid* form. The latter two forms, especially the sarcomatoid, are usually, if not always, accompanied by virilization, somewhat resembling that in pituitary basophilism.

ar·rhin'i·a, a·rhin'i·a. Congenital absence of the nose. **—arrhinic,** *adj.*

ar·rhyth'mi·a. Absence of rhythm. **—arrhythmic,** *adj.* **phasic sinus a.** Gradual waxing and waning of pulse rate, usually synchronous with the act of breathing. May also be independent of respiration.

ar'row·root". A variety of starch derived from *Maranta arundinacea* of the West Indies and Southern United States.

ar"sa·nil'ic ac'id. $NH_2.C_6H_4.AsO-(OH)_2.$ p-Aminobenzenearsonic acid. The starting compound for the synthesis of many useful medicinal arsenicals.

arsen-. See *arseno-*.

ar'se·nate, ar·se'ni·ate. Any salt of arsenic acid.

ar·se'ni·ate. See *arsenate*.

ar·se'nic, ar·sen'i·cum, ar·se'num. As = 74.91. A brittle, usually steel-gray element of both metallic and nonmetallic properties. It exists in four allotropic modifications. **a. trioxide.** Arsenous oxide, As_2O_3. Syn., *arsenous acid, white a.* **white a.** See *a.* trioxide.

ar·sen'ic ac'id. H_2AsO_4. Orthoarsenic acid; a white, hygroscopic powder used in the manufacture of medicinal and insecticidal arsenates.

ar·sen'i·cal. 1. Pertaining to arsenic. 2. A drug, fungicide, or insecticide the effect of which depends on its arsenic content.

ar·se'ni·ous. Synonym for arsenous, *q.v.*

ar'se·nite. A salt of an arsenous acid.

ar·se·no- (ahr'si·no-, ahr·sen'o-), **ar·sen-.** A combining form designating *a drug combined with arsenic.*

ar"se·no·ther'a·py. Treatment of disease by means of arsenical drugs.

ar·se·nous, ar·se'ni·ous. Containing arsenic in the positive trivalent form.

ar"se·nous ac'id. See *arsenic trioxide*.

ar"se·nox'ide. 3-Amino-4-hydroxyphenyl-arsine oxide. $C_6H_6AsNO_2$. A breakdown product of arsphenamine which accounts for its activity. See *oxophenarsine hydrochloride*.

ar·sine' (ahr·seen', ahr'sin). AsH_3. Hydrogen arsenide, or arsenous hydride. A poisonous gas with a garlicky odor.

ar·sin'ic ac'id. Any acid of the type of $RHAs(:O)OH$ or of $RR'As(:O)OH$, where R is any hydrocarbon radical and R' is the same or a different hydrocarbon radical.

ar·son'ic ac'id. Any acid of the type of $RAs(:O)(OH)_2$, where R is any hydrocarbon radical.

ars·phen'a·mine (ahrs·fen'uh·meen, ahrs"fen·uh·meen'). Diaminodihydroxyarsenobenzene dihydrochloride, a yellow hygroscopic crystalline powder, soluble in water. A specific in syphilis and other protozoan infections. Also called *606*. See *salvarsan*.

ars'thi·nol (ars'thin·ol). The cyclic 3-hydroxypropylene ester of 3-acetamido-4-hydroxydithiobenzenearsonous acid, an intestinal amebicide. See *balarsen*.

artane. Trade-mark for 3-(1-piperidyl)-1-phenyl-1-cyclohexyl-1-propanol hydrochloride, an antispasmodic drug. See *trihexyphenidyl*.

ar'te·fact, ar'ti·fact. 1. *In microscopy* and *histology*, a structure that has been produced by mechanical,

chemical, or other artificial means; structure or tissue that has bee[n] changed from its natural state. 2. [In] *electroencephalography,* a wave n[ot] originating in the brain.

ar·ter'en·ol. Norepinephrine.

arteri-. See *arterio-*.

ar·te'ri·a (pl. *arteriae*). See *artery*.

ar·te"ri·al·i·za'tion. 1. The proc[ess] of making or becoming arteria[l;] the change from venous blood into a[r]terial. 2. Vascularization.

ar·te"ri·arc'ti·a (ar·teer"i·ark[']shee·uh, ·tee·uh). Vasoconstriction stenosis of an artery.

ar·te"ri·ec·ta'sis, ar·te"ri·e[c]·ta'si·a (·eck·tay'zhuh). Dilatation an artery.

ar·te"ri·ec'to·my. Excision of [an] artery or a portion of one.

ar·te'ri·o-, arteri-. A combini[ng] form signifying *artery, arterial.*

ar·te"ri·o·cap'il·lar"y. Blood ve[s]sel between a true artery and a cap[il]lary, usually called arterial capillar[y.]

ar·te"ri·o·gram". 1. A roentge[no]gram of an artery. 2. Arteriograph; tracing of the arterial pulse.

ar·te'ri·o·graph. 1. Instrume[nt] which graphically presents the puls[e.] 2. Tracing of the arterial pulse. 3. A[r]teriogram.

ar·te"ri·og'ra·phy. 1. Graph[ic] presentation of the pulse; sphygmo[g]raphy. 2. Roentgenography of the a[r]teries. —**arteriograph'ic,** *adj.*

ar·te"ri·o'la (pl. *arteriolae*). An a[r]teriole. **a. recta.** One of the straig[ht] arterioles going from the glomeruli [to] the pyramids of the kidney.

ar·te"ri·o'lae (ahr·teer"ee·o'lee[)]. Plural of arteriola.

ar·te'ri·ole. A very small arter[y.] **precapillary arterioles.** T[he] small vessels which terminate in t[he] capillary network.

ar·te"ri·o·lith". A calculus in an a[r]tery.

ar·te"ri·o"lo·ne·cro'sis. Degene[r]ation of the arterioles resulting [in] necrosis, as in nephrosclerosis. —**art[e]riolonecrot'ic,** *adj.*

ar·te"ri·o"lo·scle·ro'sis. Harde[n]ing of the walls of the arterioles. It [is] due mainly to fibrous thickening, h[y]alinization, and infiltration of lip[id] into the intima of an arteriole. T[he] cause is unknown. —**arteriosc[le]rot'ic,** *adj.*

ar·te"ri·o·ma·la'ci·a (ahr·teer"[i]·o·ma·lay'shee·uh, ·see·uh). Soften[ing] of an artery wall.

ar·te"ri·o·ne·cro'sis. Necrosis an artery or arteries.

ar·te'ri·o·plas"ty. Any plastic op[]eration performed on an artery. S[ee] also *aneurysmorrhaphy.* —**arteri[o]plas'tic,** *adj.*

·**te"ri·o·punc"ture.** The surgical
vision or opening of an artery, chiefly
for the abstraction of blood. It usually
performed upon the temporal artery.
·**te"ri·or/rha·phy.** Suture of an
tery, by plication.
·**te"ri·or·rhex'is.** Rupture of an
tery.
·**te"ri·o·scle·ro'sis** (ahr·teer"ee-
sklĭ·ro'sis). Thickening of the intima
of the arteries, the result of prolifera-
on of fibrous connective tissue which
the seat of hyaline degeneration,
oid infiltration, and calcification,
using loss of elasticity and contrac-
ity. The cause is unknown. —**arte-
iosclerot'ic,** adj. **a. obliter-
ns.** Arteriosclerosis associated with
oliferation of the intima to the ex-
nt of obstructing the lumen. **cere-
ral a.** That which affects the vessels
the brain. **decrescent a.** Senile a.
ffuse a. A generalized thickening
the intimal portion of the smaller
ssels and capillaries. It is seen in
ronic nephritis and essential hyper-
nsion. **medial a.** That which af-
cts the middle coat of the small and
edium-sized arteries, showing exten-
ve destruction and atrophy of the
uscular elements and deposition of
lcium. Also called *Mönckeberg's a.*
enile a. That which often occurs in
d age and affects the medium-sized
teries, especially those of the extremi-
es. **syphilitic a.** The arterial scle-
sis due to syphilis. It affects chiefly
e media, but also the adventitia.
·**te"ri·o·spasm".** Spasm of an ar-
ry.
·**te"ri·o·ste·no'sis.** Narrowing of
e caliber of an artery in any part.
·**te"ri·os·to'sis.** Calcification of
a artery.
·**te"ri·ot'o·my.** Cutting or open-
g of an artery for the purpose of
oodletting.
·**te"ri·o·ve'nous.** Both arterial
d venous; involving an artery and a
in, as an arteriovenous aneurysm.
·**te"ri·o·ver'sion.** A method of
resting hemorrhage by turning ves-
ls inside out. —**arteriovert'er,**

"**te·ri'tis.** Inflammation of an
tery. See *endarteritis, periarteritis.*
. deformans. A chronic endarteri-
s with calcareous infiltration. See
darteritis. **a. obliterans.** Inflam-
ation of arteries which leads to ob-
ruction of the lumen. See *endarteri-
s.* **a. syphilitica.** Syphilitic
darteritis. **a. umbilicalis.** Septic
flammation of the umbilical arteries
the newborn.
'**ter·y.** A vessel conveying blood
om the heart. It is composed of three
ats: an outer *adventitia,* consisting
connective tissue and elastic fibers;

an inner *intima* lined with endothelium
and containing collagenous and elastic
fibers; and a middle coat, the *media,*
composed of elastic and muscular
fibers. For arteries listed by name, see
Table of Arteries in the Appendix. Abbreviated, a. —**arte'rial,** adj. **cork-
screw a.** One of the smaller, tortuous, retinal vessels in the macular
region, noted in hypertension. **heli-
cine a.** A spiral vessel which empties
into the cavernous sinuses of erectile
tissue. **hyaloid a.** In the embryo, a
forward continuation of the central
artery of the retina traversing the
vitreous body to ramify on the posterior surface of the lens capsule. **interlobar a.** One lying between the lobes
of an organ. A branch of the renal artery, running in a renal column. **interlobular a.** One lying between the
lobules of an organ. One of the radial
branches of an arciform artery, running
in the renal radial cortex. **intralobular a.** One lying within the lobule
of an organ. **nutrient a.** One which
supplies blood to a bone. **radicular a.** One which supplies the spinal
cord, entering with the anterior and
posterior nerve roots. **venous a.** One
carrying venous blood, as the pulmonary artery. **vitelline a.** One passing to the yolk sac from the primitive
aorta of the embryo. Also called *omphalomesenteric a.*
arthr-. See *arthro-.*
ar·thral'gi·a. Pain in a joint. Syn.,
articular neuralgia. —**arthralgic,**
adj.
ar·three'to·my. Excision of a joint.
**ar"three·de'ma, ar"throe·de'-
ma.** Edema affecting a joint.
ar·thri'tes (ahr·thry'teez). Plural of
arthritis.
ar·thrit'ic. 1. Relating to arthritis or
a joint. 2. An individual affected with
arthritis.
ar·thrit'i·des (ahr·thrit'i·deez).
General term to include the various
types of arthritis.
ar·thri'tis (pl. *arthrites*). Inflammation of a joint. **acute a.** Acute joint
inflammation. **allergic a.** (a) Intermittent hydrarthrosis, usually following ingestion of food allergens. (b)
Serum sickness; usually occurring 7 to
10 days after injection of horse serum;
characterized by fever and urticaria.
There may be pain, redness, swelling,
and stiffness of the joints resembling
rheumatic fever. **a. deformans.** A
general term sometimes used to mean
any chronic, rheumatoid, or degenerative arthritis. **chronic a.** A general
term for any chronic joint disease, but
usually rheumatoid or degenerative arthritis. **chronic infectious a.** See
rheumatoid *a.* **degenerative a.**
(Properly called **degenerative**

joint disease.) A chronic joint disease; characterized by loss of joint cartilage, condensation of bone at the joint surface, and spur formation. Joint crepitus is common, and limitation of motion is due to bony deformity, never to bony ankylosis. Syn., *hypertrophic a., osteoarthritis.* Also called *senescent a.* **fungous a.** Tuberculous disease of the joints; white swelling. **gonorrheal a.** A specific, blood-borne, gonococcal infection in joint tissue. May be very mild and transient, or may be severe, becoming purulent and leading to bony ankylosis. **gouty a.** Arthritis due to gout; characterized by sudden, severe, painful attacks, often coming on in the night; affects one joint, and lasts weeks or months; followed by complete recovery. After repeated attacks in the same joint, degenerative joint disease results. **Heberden's a.** Degenerative joint disease of the terminal joints of the fingers, producing enlargement and flexion deformities. Most common in women, occurring idiopathically and as a result of heredity. May result from trauma. **hemophilic a.** Inflammation due to blood in the joint of a hemophiliac. Repeated episodes lead to thickening of the synovial tissues and finally to degenerative joint disease. **menopausal a.** (a) Degenerative arthritis. (b) An arthralgia without objective or roentgen evidence of disease; occurs in women at the menopause, and is relieved by estrogenic therapy. **mixed a.** A combination of features typical both of rheumatoid arthritis and of degenerative joint disease seen in the same patient or the same joint. **neurotrophic a.** A trophic disease of joints; seen in tabes dorsalis, leprosy, syringomyelia, and other diseases of the nervous system. There is marked enlargement and disorganization of joint structures and hypermotility. It is usually painless. Also called *neuropathic a., Charcot's a.* **rheumatoid a.** A chronic arthritis of unknown etiology; affects multiple joints, producing constitutional effects such as debility, weakness, and loss of weight. The specific lesion is a proliferation of granulation or connective tissue in synovial and periarticular tissues over the joint surfaces and in subchondral spaces. There is pain, limitation of motion, deformity, and sometimes bony ankylosis. Syn., *atrophic a., a. deformans, chronic infectious a., proliferative a.* **scarlatinal a.** A form common in scarlet fever epidemics, usually appearing at the end of 10 days, with redness, pain, and swelling of the wrists, hands, elbows, and knees due to synovial distention. Also called *scarlatinal synovitis.* **syphilitic a.** Painful and swollen joints

due to syphilis, especially during t[?] secondary stage or gumma of the joi[?] **tuberculous a.** Invasion of syn[?] vial tissues or bone with tubercle b[?] cilli; gives rise to tubercle formatio[?] fibrosis, caseation, and causes mark[?] destruction of articular structure[?] healing may occur through ankylos[?]

ar'thro-, arth-. A combining for[?] denoting *relation to the joints.*

ar·throc'a·ce (ahr·throck'uh·see[?] Caries of a joint, as in tuberculo[?] arthritis.

ar'thro·cele. 1. Any swollen joi[?] 2. Hernia of the synovial membra[?] through a joint capsule.

ar''thro·cen·te'sis. Incision into [?] puncture through a joint capsule to r[?] lieve an effusion.

ar''thro·chon·dri'tis (ahr''thr[?] kon·dry'tis). Inflammation of the ca[?] tilaginous parts of a joint.

ar''thro·cla'si·a (ahr''thro·clay[?] zhuh, ·zee·uh), **ar''thro·cla's[?]** (ahr''thro·clay'sis, ahr·throck'luh·si[?] The breaking down of ankylosis in [?] der to produce free movement of [?] joint.

ar·throd'e·sis, ar''thro·de'si- [?] Fusion of a joint by removing t[?] articular surfaces and securing bo[?] union; operative ankylosis.

ar·thro'di·a. A form of joint pe[?] mitting a gliding movement. **—arthr[?] dial,** *adj.*

ar''thro·dyn'i·a. Pain in a joi[?] arthralgia. **—arthrodynic,** *adj.*

ar''thro·dys·pla'si·a (·dis·play[?] zhuh, ·zee·uh). A familial disease [?] which the patellas are rudimentary, t[?] head of the radius dislocated, and t[?] nails generally absent.

ar''thro·em·py·e'sis (·em·pye·e[?] sis, ·em·pee·ee'sis). Suppuration in [?] joint.

ar''thro·en·dos'co·py. Examin[?] tion of the interior of a joint by mea[?] of an endoscope.

ar·throg'ra·phy. 1. Roentgeno[?] raphy of a joint. 2. A treatise or mo[?] graph relating to the joints.

ar''thro·gry·po'sis (ahr''thr[?] grye·po'sis, ·gri·po'sis). 1. Permane[?] flexure of a joint; ankylosis. 2. P[?] sistent idiopathic contracture of [?] joint.

ar'thro·lith''. A calcareous or go[?] deposit or free body within a joint; chalkstone. Syn., *arthrophyte, jo[?] mouse, tophus.* Also called *joint bo[?]* **—arthrolithi'asis,** *n.*

ar·throl'o·gy. The science wh[?] treats of joints.

ar·throm'e·ter. An instrument [?] measuring and recording the extent [?] movement in a joint. Syn., *goniomet[?]* **—arthrometry,** *n.*

ar·throp'a·thy. Any joint disea[?] especially a neurotrophic disorder as[?]

ated with tabes dorsalis and syringo-
yelia, and rarely with general paral-
...is and disseminated sclerosis. —ar-
...hropath'ic, adj. inflamma-
...ory a. Any inflammatory condition
...fecting joints; arthritis. neuro-
...enic a. An osteoarthritis associated
...ith swelling, hypermobility, bone de-
...ruction, and trophic disturbances.
...lso called *Charcot's joint*, *neuro-
...thic a.* osteopulmonary a.
...lubbing of the fingers and toes asso-
...ated with enlargement of the ends of
...e long bones, encountered in chronic
...lmonary disease. psoriatic a. A
...pe of arthritis occurring in associa-
...on with psoriasis. Also called *arthro-
...thic psoriasis*.

...'thro·plas'ty. 1. The making of
...a artificial joint. 2. Reconstruction of
...new and functioning joint from an
...kylosed one; a plastic operation upon
...joint. —arthroplas'tic, adj.

...·throp'o·da. The largest phylum
...the animal kingdom; includes the
...ustacea, insects, myriapods, arach-
...ids, and related forms. The members
...e bilaterally symmetrical, having a
...mited number of segments, a chitin-
...us exoskeleton, and jointed append-
...es. —ar'thropod, adj., n.; ar-
...hrop'odous, adj.

..."thror·rha'gi·a. Hemorrhage
...to a joint.

...'thro·scope. An instrument used
...r the visualization of the interior of
...joint.

...·thros'co·py. The act of examin-
...g the interior of a joint with an
...throscope.

...·thro'sis. 1. Articulation or joint;
...suture. 2. A degenerative process in a
...int.

...·thros'to·my. Incision into a
...int, as for drainage.

...·throt'o·my. Incision into a joint.
..."thro·tro'pi·a. Torsion of a limb.
...'throus. Pertaining to a joint or
...ints; jointed.

...rthus, Nicolas Maurice
..."rench physiologist, 1862–1945]. Known
...r his description of a generalized or
...cal anaphylactic reaction, the result
...the union of antigen and antibody
...ithin the tissues, manifested by local
...ema and inflammation (1903–06);
...lled *Arthus' phenomenon*. Credited
...so with the first mention of the essen-
...al role of calcium in the mechanics of
...ood coagulation (1890).

...·tic'u·late. 1. Divided into joints.
...Distinct, clear. 3. *In dentistry*, posi-
...on artificial teeth.

...·tic'u·la'ti·o (ahr·tick"yoo·lay'-
...ee·o) (pl. *articulationes*). A joint.
...e *articulation*. See Table of Joints
...d Ligaments in the Appendix. **a.
...coxae** [BNA]. Hip joint. **a. genu**

[BNA]. Knee joint. **a. manus** [BNA].
Joint of the hand.

ar·tic"u·la'tion. 1. The enuncia-
tion of speech. 2. A joint; the junction
of two or more bones. The articulations
are divided into: *synarthroses*, or immovable joints, which are subdivided
into (a) schindyleses, or grooved joints,
(b) gomphoses, or sockets, as for the
teeth, and (c) suturae, as the bones of
the skull; *diarthroses*, or movable joints,
which are subdivided into (a) arthro-
dia, or gliding joints, (b) ginglymi, or
hingelike joints, (c) enarthroses, or ball
and socket joints; and *amphiarthroses*,
or those of the mixed type. For articulations listed by name, see Table of Joints
and Ligaments in the Appendix. 3. The
positioning of artificial teeth. 4. Improper term for occlusion (4), *q.v.*
—**artic'ular**, adj. **compound a.**
A diarthrosis in which more than two
bones are involved. **condyloid a.** A
type of diarthrosis in which an ovoid
articular surface, or condyle, is received into an elliptical cavity. Syn.,
ellipsoid a. **false a.** One formed between the end of a dislocated bone and
the contiguous parts, or between the
parts of a broken bone. Syn., *pseudarthrosis.* **hinge a.** Ginglymus; an
articulation in which a convex cylindrical surface is grooved at right angles to
the axis of the cylinder, or trochlea,
and meets a concave cylindrical surface
which is ridged to fit the trochlea in
such a manner as to permit motion
only in one plane. **incongruent a.**
One in which two or more opposing
surfaces may differ in form or present
curves of unequal radii resulting in imperfect fitting. **irregular a.** A type
of diarthrosis in which the surfaces are
small, irregular, flat, or slightly curved.
reciprocal a. A mode of articulation in which the articular surface is
convex on one side and concave on the
other. See condyloid *articulation.*
screw a. A hinge articulation in
which the groove of the trochlea is in
a plane not at right angles with the
axis, and the hinge movement is accompanied by progression at right
angles to the hinge plane. Also called
cochlear articulation or *spiral joint.*
simple a. A diarthrosis in which only
two bones are involved. **spheroid a.**
A type of diarthrosis in which a
rounded head is lodged in a concave
surface. **trochoid a.** A type of diarthrosis in which a pivotlike process rotates within a ring, or a ring rotates
around a pivot, the ring being formed
partly of bone, partly of ligament.
ar·tic"u·la"tor. An instrument used
in dentistry for holding casts of the
jaws or teeth in proper relation during
various steps of artificial denture construction. It may be adjusted so as to

duplicate the mandibular movements of the patient.

ar'ti·fact. See *artefact*.

ar"ti·fi'cial. Imitated by art.

ar"ti·fi'cial res"pi·ra'tion. The artificial promotion of normal breathing in one apparently dead, by the forcing of air into and out of the lungs to aerate the blood. Used in drowning, asphyxia neonatorum, asphyxia from smoke or toxic gases, electric shock, etc. Pulmotors or respirators are used for prolonged application, but numerous hand methods are employed. Chief of these is the *Schafer (prone pressure) method*, in which the patient is placed on his abdomen and his head turned to one side and rested on his arm; intermittent pressure over the lower part of the thorax 15 times per minute causes inspiration and expiration simulating natural breathing. Other methods are: *Buist's method* for asphyxia neonatorum, in which the child is alternately transferred from one hand of the obstetrician to the other, being supine in one and prone in the other; *Drinker's method*, which is the same as the Schafer method, with the addition of a second operator who kneels at the patient's head and raises the arms to assist in inspiration; *Eve's method*, in which the patient is tipped alternately head up and head down on a stretcher, inspiration and expiration occurring as the diaphragm moves up and down from shifting of the abdominal viscera; *Fell-O'Dwyer method*, in which air is forced into the lungs by a bellows through an intubation tube, expiration occurring spontaneously due to elasticity of the chest or being aided by external pressure; *hip-roll prone pressure method*, or *hip-lift prone pressure method*, in which the Schafer method is combined with lifting the hips in expiration; the hips may be rolled to one side which is less effective but less exhausting for the operator; *Holger Nielsen's method*, in which the patient lies prone and the operator extends the patient's arms in inspiration and presses on the scapulae in expiration; *Howard's method*, in which the patient is placed on his back with his head lower than his abdomen and his hands over his head; rhythmic pressure is applied upward and inward against the lower lateral parts of the chest; *Laborde's method*, in which the respiratory center is stimulated by rhythmic traction of the tongue with the fingers or a specially designed forceps; *Marshall Hall's method*, in which the patient is alternately rolled from his side or back to his abdomen to expand or compress the lungs, expiration being augmented by pressure on the chest; *Prochownick's method*, for asphyxia

neonatorum, in which the infant is su pended with the head extended, a intermittent pressure is applied to t chest; the *rocking method*, which synonymous with Eve's method; t *rowing method*, in which the patient supine with the operator at his hea the patient's arms are extended firm above his head and then rapi dropped back toward his chest at rate of 10 to 12 times a minute; *Se terthwaite's method*, in which the p tient is placed on his back and the is alternate pressure and relaxation the abdomen; *Schroeder's method* asphyxia neonatorum, in which the i fant is placed in a bath with its ba supported by the operator, who th effects a forceful expiration by bendi the child's body over the belly, th compressing the thorax; *Schultz method*, in which the newborn child held by the shoulders from behind that the operator has his thumbs the front of the child's shoulders, t index fingers in the axillas, and t other fingers over the back. The chil gradually tipped up until the legs f forward and the body is sharply fle and in an inverted position, so t the abdomen and chest are tightly co pressed, thus producing a forcible piration and allowing fluids to dra out of the nose and mouth; *Silveste method*, in which the patient is plac on his back and his arms raised to t sides of his head and then turned do and pressed against the chest.

ar"y·ep"i·glot'tic, ar"y·ep glot·tid'e·an, ar"y·te"no·ep glot'tic (ar"i·tee"no-, a·rit"i·no 1. Relating to the arytenoid cartila and the epiglottis. 2. Designating t folds of mucous membrane extendi between these structures (aryepiglot folds), each containing an aryepiglot muscle. See Table of Muscles in the A pendix.

ar'yl. An organic radical derived fr an aromatic hydrocarbon by the moval of one hydrogen atom.

a·ryt'e·noid, ar"y·te'noid. 1. I sembling the mouth of a pitcher. 2. P taining to the arytenoid cartilag glands, and muscles. See Table Muscles in the Appendix.

ar"y·te"noi·dec'to·my (ar"i·tee noy·deck'to·mee, a·rit"i·noy·). Remo of an arytenoid cartilage.

As. 1. Chemical symbol for arsenic. Abbreviation for astigmatism; ast matic. **As. H.** Hyperopic astigm tism. **As. M.** Myopic astigmatism.

a.s. *Auris sinistra*; left ear.

as"a·fet'i·da, as"a·foet'i·da. oleo-gum-resin obtained from rhizomes and roots of species of *Feru* It consists of soft masses of yello brown color, bitter taste, and persiste tensive odor. It is a carminative and psychic sedative.

-bes'tos. A soft fibrous silicate mineral of flexible or elastic fibers.

"bes·to'sis. Pneumonoconiosis marked by fibrosis of the lungs from prolonged inhalation of dust laden with asbestos, *q.v.* See *silicatosis.*

"ca·ri·a·sis. An infestation disease caused by the presence of the *caris lumbricoides.* The intestine is most commonly affected, but the infestation may spread to the stomach, liver, and lungs.

-car'i·cide. A medicine that kills caricides.

-car'i·dae (ass·kar'i·dee). A family of nematode worms, to which belong the roundworm and the threadworm.

-car'i·dol, as·car'i·dole. An unsaturated terpene peroxide found in chenopodium oil. It is the active principle of the oil.

'ca·ris. A genus of intestinal nematodes. **—ascarid,** *n.* A. **lumbri·oides.** A species of roundworm causing ascariasis. A. **mystax.** Synonym *Toxocara cati,* the common ascarid of the domestic cat. A. **suum.** A species of roundworm causing ascariasis in the pig.

-ci'tes (a·sigh'teez). An abnormal accumulation of serous fluid in the peritoneal cavity caused by increased venous pressure or a decrease of plasma albumin. The clear, yellowish fluid coagulates on standing but may be turbid, sanguineous, or contain shreds. Physical examination reveals painless abdominal enlargement, dullness over fluid, shifting with position, and fluid wave. The condition is associated most frequently with cardiac failure, cirrhosis of the liver, and renal deficiency. Syn., *abdominal dropsy, hydroperitoneum.* **—ascit'ic,** *adj.* **acute a.** A very sudden and large accumulation of fluid in the abdomen. **a. adiposus.** An accumulation of milky fluid due to contained cells which have undergone fatty degeneration. Seen in chronic peritoneal inflammations as in tuberculosis, carcinoma, etc. **pseudochy·lous a.** Presence in the peritoneal cavity of milky fluid which contains protein but no fat. **sanguineous a.** A bloody form affecting sheep and lambs. Syn., *diarrhemia.*

-cle'pi·as. Pleurisy root; the root of *Asclepias tuberosa.* A popular remedy in the southern states for pleurisy.

clepius (Aesculapius) [Greek *mythological son of Apollo*]. Proficient in the art of healing, he became god of medicine. After his death, he was the object of worship in numerous temples in Greece.

"co·my·ce'tes (ass"ko·migh·see'-teez). One of the four large classes of fungi.

a·scor'bate. A salt of ascorbic acid.

a·scor'bic ac'id. $C_6H_8O_6$. A substance, present in fresh green foods, citrus fruits, and various other uncooked materials, the lack of which in the body eventually leads to scurvy. It is a white or slightly yellowish crystalline powder. Syn., *vitamin C, cevitamic acid, antiscorbutic vitamin.* See Table of Normal Values of Blood Constituents in the Appendix.

as'cus (pl. *asci*). The characteristic spore case of the ascomycetes; usually consisting of a single terminal cell containing eight spores.

-ase (-ace, -aze). Suffix denoting *an enzyme.*

a·se'mi·a. An aphasia in which the patient is unable to understand or use speech, writing, or gestures as a means of communication. Syn., *asemasia, asymbolia.* **—asem'ic,** *adj.*

a·sep'sis. Exclusion of microörganisms producing decay. **—aseptic,** *adj.*

a·sex'u·al (ay·seck'shoo·ul, a·seck'shoo·ul). 1. Not involving the distinction between male and female. 2. Denoting reproduction without sexual union.

ash. The incombustible mineral residue that remains when a substance is incinerated. **bone a.** The white mineral constituents that remain after calcination or incineration of bone.

as"i·a/li·a. Deficiency or failure of the secretion of saliva.

A. S. O. American Society of Orthodontists.

a·so'cial (ay·so'shul, a·so'shul). Withdrawn from interest in others and their activities, and in realities.

a·so'ni·a. Tone deafness.

as·par'a·gin. The amide of asparaginic acid, a constituent of many proteins. Syn., *asparamide.*

as·par"a·gin'ic ac'id. COOH.CH-(NH$_2$).CH$_2$.COOH. Aminosuccinic acid, a hydrolysis product of asparagin and of many proteins. Syn., *aspartic acid.*

as·par·am'ide, as·par'am·ide. Asparagin, *q.v.*

as·par'tic ac'id. Asparaginic acid.

a·spas'tic. Not spastic.

a"spe·cif'ic. Nonspecific; not a specific.

as"per·gil'lic ac'id (ass"pur·jil'-ick). An antibiotic substance produced by *Aspergillus flavus.*

as"per·gil'lin. 1. An antibiotic substance obtained from certain fungi; it is probably identical with flavacidin, flavatin, flavicin, gigantic acid, and parasiticin. 2. A pigment obtained from the spores of *Aspergillus niger.*

as·per"gil·lo'sis (ass·pur"ji·lo'sis, ass"pur·). An infectious disease caused by any species of *Aspergillus.* Infections of lungs, bronchi, external ear, paranasal sinuses, orbit, bones, and meninges have been described.

As"per·gil'lus (ass"pur·jil'us). A genus of fungi important as a contaminant of lesions and as an agent of infection. The species **A. fumigatus** is the most common invader, but **A. flavus, A. nidulans,** and **A. niger** are also found in man.

a·sper'ma·tism (ay·spur"muh·tizum, a·spur'·), **a·sper'mi·a** (ayspur"mee·uh, a·spur'·). 1. Nonemission of semen, whether owing to nonsecretion or to nonejaculation. 2. Defective secretion of semen or lack of formation of spermatozoa. **—aspermat'ic, aspermous,** adj.

as·phyx'i·a. Suffocation; coma the result of deprivation of oxygen causing anoxia in the body and an accumulation of carbon dioxide and fixed acids. Asphyxia should be differentiated from anoxia and apnea. **—asphyxial,** adj. **a. cyanotica.** Traumatic asphyxia, q.v. **a. livida.** Asphyxia neonatorum associated with cyanotic skin, strong pulse, and active reflexes. Syn., blue a. **a. neonatorum.** Asphyxia of the newborn. **a. pallida.** Asphyxia neonatorum attended by a slow, weak pulse, abolished reflexes, and a very pale skin. **intrauterine a.** That due to interference with the fetal blood supply. **local a.** Stagnation of the circulation in a part, as the fingers, hands, toes, or feet. **traumatic a.** Cyanosis of the head and neck from sudden compression of the thorax, upper abdomen, or both. Also called ecchymotic mask, traumatic apnea, pressure stasis.

as·phyx'i·ant. 1. Producing asphyxia. 2. An agent capable of producing asphyxia. **—asphyxiate,** v.t., v.i.

as·pid'i·um. The rhizome and stipes of male fern, Dryopteris Filix-mas; source of the official drug **aspidium oleoresin,** widely used against tapeworms and hookworms.

as"pi·do·sper'ma. Quebracho. The dried bark of Aspidosperma quebrachoblanco; used as respiratory stimulant in asthmatic and cardiac dyspnea.

as"pi·ra'tion. 1. Act of sucking up or sucking in; inspiration; imbibition. 2. Act of using the aspirator. 3. Method of withdrawing fluids and gases from a cavity. **—aspirate,** v.

as'pi·ra"tor. A negative pressure apparatus for withdrawing liquids from cavities.

as'pi·rin. See acetylsalicylic acid.

a·spo"ro·gen'ic (ay·spor"o·jen'ick, a·spor"o·), **as"po·rog'e·nous** (ass"por·odj'i·nus). 1. Producing no spores. 2. Reproduced without spores.

a·spo'rous (ay·spor'us, a·spor'us). Without spores; especially without the

resistant phase, as in the case of ma bacteria.

as·sault'. An unlawful attempt to bodily injury to another. **crim nal a.** In legal medicine, touching attempting to touch any of the sex organs of a female against her w **felonious a.** A malicious att showing criminal intent upon the p son of another.

as·say', as'say. Testing or analy of a metal or drug to determine relative proportion of its constituen

as·sim"i·la'tion. 1. Process transforming food into a state suita for absorption by the circulation a conversion into body tissue; synthe or constructive metabolism; anaboli 2. In psychology, mental reception impressions, and their assignment the consciousness to their proper pla mental assimilation. 3. The abnorn fusion of bones, as the fusion of t transverse processes of the last lu bar vertebra with the lateral mas of the first sacral vertebra, or t atlas with the occipital bone. **—a sim'ilable,** adj.; **assim'ilate,** v. **a. limit.** Amount of starchy or s charine food which a person can ing without the appearance of glycosur **primary a.** Conversion of food i absorbed products. **secondary** Conversion of food elements into bc tissue.

as·so"ci·a'tion. 1. A connecti union, joining, or combination. 2. society or united group of persons. In chemistry, the correlation or agg gation of substances or functions. 4. psychology, a mental linking, as tl of objects, persons, or events with ide thoughts, or sensations. **a. of idea** That established between two simi ideas or two ideas of simultaneous currence. **clang a.** Association words because of their similarity sound; seen in manic patients. **co trolled a.** Directed association relevant ideas, due to a specific stin lus. **free a.** Spontaneous, unrestric association of loosely linked ideas mental images, of very little ratio sequence or continuity; seen in ma or dream states.

as'sue·tude (ass'wi·tewd). 1. Habi ation to disturbing influences. 2. C dition of an organism in which it acquired such tolerance for a drug poison that the effect is lost.

a·sta'si·a (a·stay'zhuh, ·zee·uh). N tor incoördination for standi **a.-abasia.** Apparent inability to w or stand, due to some mental confi not accompanied with organic para sis. It is a symptom of neurosis.

as'ta·tine (ass'tuh·teen, ·tin). At 211. Element number 85, prepared 1940 by bombarding bismuth with alp particles; formerly called alabamine, *q.v.* It is radioactive and forms no stable isotopes.

a·ste″a·to′sis, as″te·a·to′sis. 1. A deficiency or absence of the sebaceous secretion. 2. Any skin disease (as xeroderma) characterized by scantiness or lack of sebaceous secretion, the skin becoming dry, scaly, and often fissured. Syn., *xerosis.* Also called *a. cutis.*

as′ter. The radiating structure surrounding the centrosome of the cell, seen at the beginning of mitosis. —**as·tral,** *adj.*

a·ster″e·og·no′sis. Inability to recognize objects by the sense of touch. Also called *astereocognosy.*

as′ter·o-, aster-. A combining form meaning *star.*

as·the′ni·a. Absence or loss of strength. —**asthen′ic,** *adj.* **a. pigmentosa.** See *adrenal cortical hypofunction.* **a. universalis.** Visceroptosis associated with neurasthenic tendency, vasomotor weakness, and intestinal atony. **grave hypophyseal a.** A serious cachexia of pituitary origin marked by anorexia, emaciation, constipation, amenorrhea, subnormal temperature, hypotonia, and hypoglycemia. **myalgic a.** A state of generalized fatigue associated with muscular pains. **neurocirculatory a.** A psychosomatic disorder characterized by dyspnea, palpitation, vertigo, faintness, fatigue, tremor, precordial pain, tachycardia, and elevated blood pressure. Occurs most frequently in soldiers during the stress and danger of training and combat; may occur physiologically in untrained persons who exercise violently. Also called *effort syndrome, soldier's heart, irritable heart, disordered action of the heart.* Abbreviated, N. C. A.

as·then′ic type. A physical type (Kretschmer) marked by a tall, slender, flat-chested, angular form, and poor muscular development.

as′the·no-, asthen-. A combining form meaning *weak.*

as″the·nom′e·ter. An instrument for detecting and measuring asthenia; especially, a device for measuring muscular asthenopia.

as″the·no′pi·a. Weakness of the ocular muscles or of visual power, due to errors of refraction, heterophoria, overuse, etc. —**asthenop′ic,** *adj.;* **as′thenope,** *n.* **accommodative a.** Subnormal power of the function of accommodation, or the pain or discomfort resulting from accommodative effort. **muscular a.** That due to weakness, incoördination (heterophoria), or strain of the external ocular muscles.

as″the·nox′i·a. Insufficient oxida-

tion of waste products, as ketosis from insufficient oxidation of fatty acids.

asth′ma (az′muh, ass′muh). Paroxysmal dyspnea. Commonly, however, it refers to **allergic asthma,** characterized by dyspnea, cough, wheezing, mucoid sputum, and a sense of constriction of the chest. Pathologic changes consist of bronchiolar spasm, edema of mucosa, hypertrophy of glandular elements, and secretion of mucinlike substance. Is usually due to hypersensitiveness to inhaled or ingested substances, or bacteria. In allergic asthma, the name may include the etiologic factor; as **bacterial asthma, food asthma, horse asthma, pollen asthma.** —**asthmat′ic,** *adj.* **bronchial a.** See allergic a. **cardiac a.** Paroxysmal dyspnea due to cardiac failure occurring, usually at night, in patients with passive congestion of the lungs, secondary to failure of the left side of the heart; accompanied by characteristic rales. **fuller's a.** A pulmonary affection due to the inhalation of lint and dust in the manufacture of wool cloth. **grinder's a.** An interstitial pneumonia due to the inhalation of fine particles set free in grinding steel, etc. See fibroid *phthisis.* **intrinsic bronchitic a.** A form due probably to infection resulting in structural changes. **miner's a.** Dyspnea due to anthracosis. **potter's a.** Pneumoconiosis. **renal a.** Paroxysmal dyspnea occurring as a result of renal failure or uremia. **steam fitter's a.** Asbestosis. **stone a.** Pressure and pain in the chest due to the presence of a calculus in a bronchus. **symptomatic a.** Asthma which is secondary to some other condition. **thymic a.** A rare type due to an enlarged thymus.

asth′ma weed. Lobelia.

a·stig′ma·graph. An instrument for detecting astigmatism of the eye.

a·stig′ma·tism. The faulty vision which results from irregularity in the curvature of one or more refractive surfaces (cornea, anterior and posterior surfaces of the lens) of the eye. When such a condition occurs, rays emanating from a point are not brought into focus at a point on the retina, but appear to spread as a line in various directions depending upon the curvature. The condition may be **congenital** or **acquired.** When the irregularity is in the cornea, it is **corneal astigmatism;** when in the lens, **lenticular astigmatism.** When the greatest refractive power is along the horizontal meridian, it is called **astigmatism against the rule;** when along the vertical meridian, **astigmatism with the rule.**

Astigmatism may complicate myopia or hyperopia, causing **simple hyperopic astigmatism**, where one principal meridian is hyperopic, the other normal, or **compound hyperopic astigmatism** with both meridians hyperopic, one more so than the other. In the same manner, complicating myopia, there may be **simple myopic astigmatism** and **compound myopic astigmatism** (symbol, M + As). When one meridian is myopic and the other hyperopic, **mixed astigmatism** is the result. Also, when the principal meridians are at right angles, the condition is known as **regular astigmatism**, and when different parts of the meridian have different refractive powers, **irregular astigmatism**. —**astigmat′ic, astig′mic,** adj.

a·stom′a·tous (a·stom′uh·tus, a·sto′muh·tus), **as′to·mous, a·sto′mous.** 1. Without a mouth or stoma. 2. In botany, without stomas.

as·trag′a·lec′to·my. Excision of the astragalus, or talus.

as·trag′a·lus. The ankle bone, upon which the tibia rests. O.T. Syn., talus [BNA]. See Table of Bones in the Appendix. —**astragalar,** adj.

as″tra·pho′bi·a, as″tra·po·pho′bi·a. Morbid fear of lightning and thunderstorms.

as·trin′gent. 1. Causing contraction; binding. 2. An agent that produces contraction of organic tissues, or that arrests hemorrhages, diarrhea, etc. —**astringency,** n.

as′tro-, astr-. Combining form signifying pertaining to the stars.

as′tro·blast. A primitive cell which develops into an astrocyte.

as″tro·blas·to·ma. A glioma of the central nervous system, especially of the cerebral hemisphere, composed largely of astroblasts. The cells are loosely arranged, usually mononuclear, with a thick process extending to the neighboring blood vessel.

as′tro·cytes (ass′tro·sights). The many-processed stellate cells of the neuroglia, attached to the blood vessels of the brain and spinal cord by perivascular feet. Also called astroglia, Cajal's cells, macroglia, spider cells. **fibrous a.** Those in the white matter, characterized by long, unbranched processes. **protoplasmic a.** Those in the gray matter, characterized by numerous, freely branching protoplasmic processes.

as″tro·cy·to′ma (·sigh·to′muh). One of the commonest glial tumors of the central nervous system; formed of protoplasmic or fibrillary astrocytes.

as′troid. Star-shaped.

as′tro·sphere. 1. The central mass of the aster, exclusive of the filaments or rays. 2. The entire aster, exclusive of the centriole. Syn., centrosphere, centrosome, attraction sphere.

a·sy′lum. An institution for the support, safekeeping, cure, or education of those incapable of caring for themselves, such as the insane, the blind, etc.

a″sym·met′ric (ay″si·met′rick, ass″i·met′rick). 1. Pertaining to or exhibiting asymmetry. 2. In chemistry, not symmetric; as the 1,2,4-trisubstituted benzene compounds.

a″sym·met′ric at′om. An atom, especially of carbon or nitrogen, which has each of its valence bonds satisfied by a different atom or radical.

a·sym′me·try (ay·sim′i·tree, a·sim′·). 1. In anatomy and biology, lack of similarity or correspondence of the organs and parts on each side of an organism. 2. In chemistry, absence of symmetry in the arrangement of the atoms and radicals within a molecule. —**asymmet′ric, asymmet′rical,** adj.

a″symp·to·mat′ic (ay″simp·to·mat′ick). Without symptoms; exhibiting no symptoms.

a·syn′chro·nism (ay·sing′kro·niz·um, a·sing′·). Absence of synchronism; disturbed coördination.

a·syn′cli·tism (ay·sing′kli·tiz·um, a·sing′·). An oblique presentation of the fetal head at superior strait of pelvis. **anterior a.** Biparietal obliquity; the lateral inclination of the fetal head at the superior pelvic strait, which brings the sagittal suture nearer to the sacral promontory. Also called Naegele's obliquity. **posterior a.** The inclination of the fetal head at the superior strait in anterior presentations; the posterior part of the parietal bone or ear is the presenting part. Also called Litzmann's obliquity.

a″syn·ech′i·a (ay″si·neck′ee·uh, ·nee′kee·uh). Absence of continuity in structure.

as″y·ner′gi·a. See asynergy.

a·syn′er·gy, as″y·ner′gi·a. Faulty coördination of groups of organs or muscles normally acting in unison; particularly, the abnormal state of muscle antagonism in cerebellar disease. —**asyner′gic,** adj. **progressive locomotor a.** See tabes dorsalis.

a·sys′to·le. See asystolia.

a″sys·to′li·a (ay″sis·to′lee·uh, a·sis·), **a·sys′to·le** (ay·sis′to·lee, a·sis′·). Faulty or imperfect contraction of the cardiac ventricles, especially of the right ventricle, as seen in the last stages of mitral disease. —**asystol′ic,** adj. **cardiataxic a.** Temporary asystolia due to rapid heart rate. **cardioplegic a.** That resulting from weakness or injury of the heart muscle.

A.T.10. A preparation of dihydrotachysterol used in the treatment of parathyroid tetany.

At. Chemical symbol for astatine.

atabrine dihydrochloride. Trade-mark for a brand of quinacrine hydrochloride. Also called *atabrine*.

a·tac'tic. Irregular; incoördinate. Pertaining to muscular incoördination, especially in aphasia; ataxic.

at"a·rac'tic. An ataraxic.

at"a·rac'tic. Of or pertaining to ataraxia or an ataraxic.

atarax hydrochloride. Trademark for hydroxyzine hydrochloride.

at"a·rax'i·a (at"a-rak'see-uh). A state of tranquility or calmness.

at"a·rax'ic. A drug capable of promoting peace of mind; a tranquilizer.

at"a·rax'ic. Pertaining to a tranquilizing drug.

at'a·vism. The reappearance of remote ancestral characteristics in an individual. Syn., *reversion.* —**atav'ic, atavis'tic,** adj.

a·tax"a·pha'si·a (a-tack"suh-fay'-zhuh, -zee-uh). Inability to arrange words into sentences.

a·tax'i·a. Incoördination of muscular action. —**ataxic,** adj. **bulbar a.** That due to a lesion in the pons or medulla oblongata. **cerebellar a.** That due to disease of the cerebellum or the brain. **diphtheritic a.** A sequel of diphtheria preceding diphtheritic paralysis, in which the chief phenomena of locomotor ataxia are present. **Friedreich's a.** A progressive, familial disease occurring in childhood and characterized by ataxia, absent deep reflexes, positive Babinski sign, speech disturbance, nystagmus, and clubfoot. The specific lesions are degenerations of lateral and posterior columns of the cord and to some extent in the cerebellum and medulla. **locomotor a.** Tabes dorsalis, *q.v.* **moral a.** The inconstancy of ideas and will, attended with convulsions and pain, observed in hysterical subjects. **motor a.** Inability to coördinate the muscles in walking. **spinal a.** That due to disease of the spinal cord. **static a.** Lack of muscular coördination in standing still, or in fixed positions of the limbs. **thermal a.** Large and irregular fluctuations of the body temperature. **vasomotor a.** Instability of the circulatory mechanism, due to lack of coördination between the sympathetic and the parasympathetic nervous systems in relation to the vasomotor phenomena.

a·tax'i·a·graph". A device for recording the degree of ataxia.

a·tax"i·o·pho'bi·a. A morbid fear of disorder.

at"e·lec'ta·sis. 1. Imperfect expansion of the lungs at birth. 2. A collapsed or airless state of the lungs caused by occlusion of a bronchus, with subsequent absorption of the air, or by external compression, as from a pleural effusion or a tumor. Syn., *lung collapse.* —**atelectat'ic,** adj.

a·te"li·o'sis (a-tee"lee-o'sis, a-tel"ee-), **a·te"lei·o'sis** (a-tee"lye-o'sis). Infantilism or dwarfism; a generalized type of underdevelopment characterized by a childish face, thin voice, slender limbs, and normal intelligence. All parts are proportionately smaller, giving the impression of an adult in miniature, as differentiated from cretinoid or achondroplastic dwarfs, where disproportion is the rule. —**ateliot'ic, ateleiot'ic, ate'lio,** adj.

at'el·o-, atel-. Combining form signifying *imperfect* or *incomplete development.*

a·the'li·a. Absence of the nipples.

ath"er·o'ma. 1. A sebaceous cyst; steatoma. 2. The fatty degeneration and infiltration by lipids of the walls of the arteries in arteriosclerosis. —**atherom'atous,** adj.

ath"er·o"ma·to'sis. Generalized atheromatous condition of the arteries.

ath"er·o"scle·ro'sis. A form of simple intimal arteriosclerosis with atheromatous deposits within and beneath the intima.

ath"e·to'sis. A condition chiefly affecting children, characterized by recurrent, slow, and continual change of position of the fingers, toes, hands, feet, and other parts of the body, usually the result of a central brain lesion. Also called *posthemiplegic chorea.* —**ath'etoid, athetosic, athetot'ic,** adj.

ath·lete's foot. See *dermatophytosis.*

a·thy'mic (ay-thy'mick). Without feeling, as an athymic psychopath.

at·lan'to-. A combining form signifying *relation to the atlas.*

at·lan"to·ax'i·al. Pertaining to the atlas and the axis or epistropheus; applied to the joints between these two vertebrae and the ligaments which join them. Syn., *atlantoepistrophic.*

at·lan"to·ep"i·stroph'ic. Pertaining to the atlas and the epistropheus or axis; applied to the joints between these two vertebrae and the ligaments joining them. Syn., *atlantoaxial.* See Table of Joints and Ligaments in the Appendix.

at·lan"to·oc·cip'i·tal (-ock-sip'i-tul). Pertaining to the atlas and the occipital bone; applied to the joints between these two bones and the ligaments joining them. See Table of Joints and Ligaments in the Appendix.

t'las. The first cervical vertebra. It articulates with the occipital bone of the skull and with the axis. See Table of Bones in the Appendix.

atmo-, atm-. A combining form denoting *steam* or *vapor.*

at·mol'y·sis. A method of separating mixed gases or vapors by means of diffusion through a porous substance.

at·mom'e·ter. An instrument which measures the amount of water evaporated from a given surface in a given time, to determine the humidity of the atmosphere.

at'mos·phere. 1. Layer of air surrounding the earth to a height of approximately 200 miles. 2. Climatic conditions of a locality. 3. *In physics,* one atmosphere is equivalent to the pressure of a column of mercury 760 mm. high, at sea level and 0° C. 4. *In chemistry,* gaseous medium surrounding a body. **—atmospher'ic,** *adj.*

at'om. The smallest particle of an element capable of existing individually or in combination with one or more atoms of the same or another element. It consists of a dense inner core or nucleus, made up of neutrons and protons, with electrons vibrating in a relatively empty surrounding space. **—atom'ic,** *adj.*

at"om·i·za'tion. Mechanical process of breaking up a liquid into a fine spray. **—at'omizer,** *n.*

at'om smash'er. Any device able to bring about artificial atomic disintegration.

a·to'ni·a, at'o·ny. Abnormally low degree of tonus; absence of tonus. **—aton'ic,** *adj.;* **atonic'ity,** *n.* **a. of bladder.** Inability to expel the urine, due to deficient muscular power or disturbance of innervation.

at'o·ny. See *atonia.*

at'o·pen. An antigen or allergen, usually inhaled or ingested, which produces an atopic disease.

atophan. Trade-mark identifying the original cinchophen.

a·top'ic (ay·top'ick, a·top'ick). 1. Pertaining to atopy or to an atopen. 2. Old term for ectopic.

a·top"og·no'si·a, a·top"og·no'sis. Lack of ability to locate a sensation accurately.

at'o·py. A peculiar form of allergy, which is believed to occur only in humans. Marked by a familial tendency to certain hypersensitivities, as hay fever, asthma, atopic dermatitis; an immediate vascularization and exudation of the sensitive tissue when exposed to the stimulant; and the presence of certain antibodies, called atopic reagins.

a·tox'ic (ay·tock'sick, a·tock'sick). Not venomous; not poisonous.

ATP. Adenosinetriphosphate, *q.v.*

a·tre'mi·a. Hysterical inability to walk, stand, or sit without general discomfort and paresthesia of the head and back, all movements being readily executed without tremor in the recumbent posture. Also called *Neftel's disease.*

a·tre'si·a (a·tree'zhuh, ·zee·uh). Imperforation or closure of a normal opening or canal, as of the anus, vagina, auditory meatus, or pupil. **—atresic, atret'ic,** *adj.*

a·tre'to-. A combining form meaning *imperforation; absence or closure of a passage.*

a'tri·a. Plural of atrium.

at"ri·cho'sis (at"ri·ko'sis), **a·trich'i·a** (a·trick'ee·uh). A condition characterized by absence of hair. **a. congenitalis.** The congenital absence of hair.

a'tri·o-. A combining form denoting *atrium* or *atrial.*

a"tri·o·ven·tric'u·lar. Relating to the atria and the ventricles of the heart.

a'tri·um (pl. *atria*). 1. A cavity, entrance, or passage. 2. Either of the two chambers of the heart that receives blood from veins first. 3. The end of the alveolar duct. **—atrial,** *adj.* **a. of infection.** The point of entrance of bacteria, as in infectious disease. **primitive a.** The unpaired chamber of the embryonic heart. See *sinus venosus.*

At'ro·pa. A genus of the Solanaceae; source of belladonna, *q.v.,* and atropine, *q.v.*

at"ro·pho·der'ma. Atrophy of the skin.

at"ro·pho·der"ma·to'sis. A class of skin diseases characterized by atrophy.

at'ro·phy. A reduction in size of an organ or cell which had previously reached a larger size; hypoplastic organs may exhibit atrophy. It may be physiologic or pathologic, the latter type being accompanied by some degree of degeneration. **—atrophied, atroph'ic,** *adj.* **acute yellow a.** Acute diffuse necrosis of the liver; icterus gravis. **brown a.** A form in which the atrophic organ is of a deeper brown than normal because of an increase of pigment (hemosiderin and hemofuscin); observed in the heart, skeletal muscles, and liver. **cardiac a.** Atrophy of the heart observed especially in chronic, wasting diseases. **chronic spinal muscular a.** See progressive muscular *dystrophy.* **compression a.** See pressure *a.* **concentric a.** That which proceeds from without inward, as atrophy of bone beginning at the periosteal portion. **correlated a.** Atrophy secondary to the removal or destruction of other parts of the body, as atrophy of bone and muscle following amputation of an extremity. **cyanotic a.** Atrophy of the liver accompanying prolonged passive hyperemia, largely degenerative. **degenerative a.** A form in which cellular degeneration is conspicuous. **disuse a.** That form resulting from inactivity, usually affecting glandular or muscular structures. Also called *inactivity a.* **eccentric a.** That which proceeds from within outward, as atrophy of bone beginning next to the marrow cavity. **gray a.** Degeneration in the optic disk with assumption of a gray color. **halisteretic a.** Atrophy of bone, or osteoporosis, due to a withdrawal of calcium from the bone. **inanition a.** That due to inadequate nutrition. **Leber's optic a.** A rare hereditary form of axial neuritis of the optic nerve. **linear a.** Atrophy of the papillary layer of skin, resulting in striae atrophicae. **muscular a.** That in which muscle becomes atrophic, especially skeletal muscle; may be hereditary or acquired, idiopathic, myelopathic, myopathic, neuropathic, primary, secondary, simple, or progressive; often a part of a disease, such as progressive muscular atrophy, myasthenia gravis, and various forms of myotonia. **myelopathic muscular a.** A progressive muscular wasting due to degeneration of the cells of the anterior horns of the spinal cord. Beginning usually in the small muscles of the hands, but in some cases (scapulohumeral type) in those of the upper arm and shoulder; the atrophy progresses slowly to the muscles of the lower extremities. Also called *progressive spinal muscular a., Duchenne-Aran muscular a.* **myotonic a.** A hereditary, progressive weakening and atrophy of muscles; usually begins in early life. Syn., *dystrophia myotonica.* **neurotrophic a.** A form particularly observed in muscle as the result of interruption of motor nerve supply; due partly to inactivity and partly to absence of nutritional influences. **numerical a.** Reduction in the number of cells of an organ; necrobiotic atrophy. **olivopontocerebellar a.** A heredodegenerative disease occurring in the later decades of life; causes ataxia, hypotonia, and dysarthria. **olivorubrocerebellar a.** A heredodegenerative disease involving the postural centers of the brain stem, particularly the superior cerebellar peduncle; causes ataxia, coarse tremor, and hypotonia. **optic a.** Atrophy of the optic nerve. **pathologic a.** That due to disease or other abnormality. **physiologic a.** That which affects

certain organs at different times of life, as involution of the thymus at puberty, atrophy of the mammary glands and ovaries after the menopause. **pressure a.** That following prolonged pressure on a part, chiefly the result of local inanition. **progressive muscular a.** A chronic disease characterized by progressive wasting of individual muscles, or physiologic groups of muscles, and by an associated and proportional amount of paralysis; due to a degeneration and atrophy of the motor cells in the anterior gray horns of the cord, with consecutive degeneration of the anterior nerve roots and muscles. Syn., *chronic anterior poliomyelitis, wasting palsy.* **progressive nervous a.** Atrophy of spinal nerve roots due to pressure from fibrosis of the spinal arachnoid. **progressive neuropathic (peroneal) muscular a.** A form of muscular atrophy due to degeneration of the cells of the posterior columns of the spinal cord and of the peripheral motor nerves. It begins in the muscles supplied by the peroneal nerves, progressing slowly to involve the muscles of the hands and arms. Also called *peroneal muscular a., Charcot-Marie-Tooth disease, progressive neural muscular a.* **progressive unilateral facial a.** Slowly progressive atrophy of skin, subcutaneous tissue, bone, and, less often, of the muscles of one side of the face. **red a.** See cyanotic *a.* **senile a.** That which occurs in old age. **serous a.** Atrophy of fat associated with accumulation of serous fluid. **sympathetic a.** Rarely observed in one member of paired organs secondary to atrophy of its fellow. **syphilitic spinal muscular a.** Progressive spinal muscular atrophy due to destruction of the anterior horn cells of the spinal cord by syphilis. **toxic a.** Atrophy which appears in the course of prolonged wasting and infectious diseases, due probably to malnutrition rather than toxins. **trophoneurotic a.** See neurotrophic *a.*

at·ro·pine (at'ro-peen, -pin). A white, crystalline alkaloid obtained from *Atropa belladonna* and other solanaceous plants. It causes paralysis of all responses to parasympathetic stimulation.

at·ro·pin·ize. 1. Bring under the influence of, or treat with, atropine. 2. Administer belladonna or atropine until physiologic effects become manifest. **—atropiniza'tion,** *n.*

A. T. S. Antitetanic serum; American Temperance Society.

at'tar. A general name for any of the volatile oils.

at·ten'u·at·ed. Weakened; used for a microörganism with decreased capacity to produce disease because of growth in an unfavorable environment.

at·ten″u·a′tion. A thinning, weakening, or diluting; especially a reduction of the virulence of a virus or pathogenic microörganism, as by successive culture, repeated inoculation, or exposure to light, heat, air, or a weakening agent. —**atten′uant,** *adj., n.;* **atten′uate,** *v.t., v.i.;* **atten′uated,** *adj.*

at′tic. Part of the tympanic cavity situated above the atrium. It contains the incus and the head of the malleus. Syn., *epitympanic recess.*

at′ti·tude. Posture; the position of the body and limbs. **a. of fetus.** Relation of the fetal members to one another *in utero.* **crucifixion a.** In hysteroepilepsy, a rigid state of the body, the arms stretched out at right angles. **discobolus a.** A position of the body assumed as a result of stimulation of one labyrinth. The trunk, head, and arms are turned toward the side stimulated in order to counteract the false sensation of falling in the opposite direction. **frozen a.** A peculiar stiffness of the gait characteristic of disease of the spinal cord, especially of amyotrophic lateral sclerosis. **passionate a.** Assumption of a dramatic or theatrical expression, a position assumed by some hysterical patients.

at·ton′i·ty. A state of stupor with complete or partial immobility; occurs most frequently in the catatonic form of schizophrenia, but also in some forms of melancholia.

at·trac′tion. The force exerted by one mass upon another, drawing them together. Syn., *gravitation, affinity, cohesion.* **capillary a.** The force which draws fluids into and along the lumen of a capillary tube. **chemical a.** The force which unites the atoms of one element to those of others, forming compounds. See *affinity.* **electric a.** The tendency of bodies to draw together when carrying opposite charges of electricity. Also called *magnetic a.*

at·tri′tion (a·trish′un). An abrasion, rubbing, or chafing of the skin or any surface; thus the wearing away of tooth enamel by mastication, brushing, or clasp friction is called attrition of enamel.

at. wt. Atomic weight.

a·typ′i·cal. Not typical; irregular. **primary a. pneumonia.** See under *pneumonia.*

A.U. Angstrom unit.

Au. Chemical symbol for gold.

au′di·o-, au′di·to-. A combining form denoting *pertaining to hearing.*

au″di·o·gen′ic. Caused or induced by sound.

au″di·o·gram″. A graphic record showing the variations of auditory acuity of an individual, as indicated by the audiometer.

au″di·ol′o·gy. Science of hearing.

au″di·om′e·ter. An instrument for measuring the acuity and range of hearing. There are two main types: the pure tone audiometer and the speech or phonograph audiometer. Either may be used for an individual test or in screening large groups of people. —**audiomet′ric,** *adj.;* **audiometry, audiometrist,** *n.*

au″di·o·vis′u·al. Pertaining to, or using, both sound and visual impressions, as the sound movies.

au·di′tion. Hearing; ability to hear.

au″di·to·psy′chic. Pertaining to the auditory association area of the temporal cortex, Brodmann's area 42.

au′di·to″ry. Pertaining to the act or the organs of hearing.

aug′ment, aug″men·ta′tion. 1. Exacerbation; aggravation of symptoms or signs. 2. Reproduction by growths greater than normal. —**augment′,** *v.*

aug·men′tor. An agent which increases or accelerates the action of auxetics, *q.v.,* though it is unable to initiate cell division when used alone. **a. nerves.** Those which increase the force as well as the rate of cardiac contractions. See *accelerator.*

aug·na′thus. An individual with an accessory lower jaw.

au′ra. 1. A premonitory sensation preceding a convulsion, usually experienced by epileptics. 2. *In electricity,* the current of air which attends the receipt of a static electric discharge. **auditory a.** An acoustic sensation which sometimes ushers in an epileptic seizure. **a. asthmatica.** Oppression of the chest, flatulence, or other subjective phenomena which usher in an asthmatic attack. **a. hysterica.** Sensations similar to those experienced in epilepsy, which introduce a hysterical attack. **cephalic a.** A diffuse head sensation often described as heaviness, fullness, or pressure. **epigastric a.** A midline sensation over the gastric area which may ascend to the throat. **olfactory a.** A sudden disagreeable sensation of smell. **somatosensory a.** A sensation of tingling, numbness, or of invisible movement in a part of the body. **vertiginous a.** Dizziness announcing an epileptic seizure. **visual a.** Flashing of bright light, whirling or colored light, or sudden darkness in the visual fields.

au′ral. Relating to the air or to an aura.

au′ral. Relating to the ear or to the hearing.

au′ra·mine″ O (aw′ruh·meen″) (C.C.). A basic aniline dye of the diphenyl methane series used in fluorescence microscopy. Also called *canary yellow, pyoktanin yellow, pyoktaninum aureum.*

aureomycin hydrochloride. Trade-mark for chlortetracycline hydrochloride.

au′ri-. A combining form denoting *the ear.*

au′ri-. A combining form denoting *gold,* and more precisely, *in chemistry, the presence of gold in the trivalent or auric state.*

au′ric. 1. Pertaining to or containing gold. 2. *In chemistry,* referring to compounds of trivalent gold. See *aurous.*

au′ric ac′id. H_3AuO_3. Gold trihydroxide; insoluble in water but soluble in alkalis to form aurates.

au′ri·cle. 1. The pinna of the ear; the ear flap or external ear; auricula. 2. An appendage to an atrium of the heart; auricular appendix. 3. Any earshaped structure or appendage. 4. Old term for *atrium.* 1. **–auric′ular,** *adj.* **cervical a.** Accessory auricle; a projection of the skin, sometimes containing cartilage, found over the sternocleidomastoid muscle; a developmental anomaly of the region around the second visceral groove.

au′ris. The ear. **–auriform,** *adj.* **a. dextra.** Right ear. Abbreviated, a.d. **a. externa.** The outer ear; auricle, pinna. **a. interna.** The internal ear, labyrinth. **a. media.** The middle ear, tympanic cavity. **a. sinistra.** Left ear. Abbreviated, a.s.

au′ro-. A combining form denoting *gold,* and more precisely, *in chemistry, the presence of gold in the univalent or aurous state.*

au″ro·ther′a·py. The administration of gold salts. Has been employed for the treatment of arthritis and various skin diseases.

au″ro·thi″o·glu′cose. The active component of solganol-B oleosum, containing approximately 50% of gold, used in the treatment of rheumatoid arthritis and lupus erythematosus.

au′rous. 1. Pertaining to gold and its compounds. 2. *In chemistry,* referring to compounds of monovalent gold.

au′rum. See *gold.*

aus″cul·ta′tion. The detection and study of sounds arising from various organs, chiefly the heart and lungs, to aid in the determination of their physical condition. **–auscul′tatory,** *adj.;* **auscult′,** *aus′cultate,* *v.* **a. tube.** *In otology,* an instrument for listening to the forced passage of air into the middle ear of a patient. **immediate a.** The direct application of the examiner's ear to the patient's skin. **mediate a.** Listening with the aid of a stethoscope.

aut-. See *auto-.*

au′ta·coid. A chemical messenger released into the blood by the cells of one organ to stimulate or inhibit activity in a remote organ (Schäfer). Thus hormones, for the most part, stimulate and chalones inhibit.

au·te·me′si·a (aw·ti·mee′shuh, ·see·uh). Idiopathic vomiting; vomiting at will by certain psychiatric patients.

au′tism. A tendency to morbid concentration on oneself; an interest in daydreaming and phantasy. **–autis′tic,** *adj.*

au′to-, aut-. A combining form meaning *pertaining to, by, or for oneself or the same individual.*

au″to·ag·glu″ti·na′tion. 1. Agglutination which occurs without the addition of a specific antiserum. 2. Agglutination of the blood corpuscles of an individual by his own serum.

au″to·ag·glu′ti·nin. An agglutinin contained in the serum of an individual which causes an agglutination of his red cells.

au″to·a·nal′y·sis. Analysis by a patient of his own mental disorder; employed as a psychotherapeutic method.

au″to·an″ti·bod″y. Antibodies produced by a host to tissues of his own body that ordinarily are not accessible to the blood stream, such as the lens of the eye.

au″to·ca·thar′sis. Psychotherapy by having the patient describe his difficulties, thus gaining insight into his mental complexes and conflicts.

au·toch′tho·nous (aw·tock′thon·us). 1. Formed in the place where found, as a clot. 2. Native; aboriginal.

au′to·clave. 1. An apparatus for sterilizing objects by steam heat at high pressure. 2. Sterilize in an autoclave.

au″to·cy″to·tox′in. A cell toxin produced against the cells of one's own body, due to retained degenerated and dead cells acting as an antigen.

au″to·di·ges′tion. Digestion of the stomach walls by gastric juice, in disease of the stomach; autolysis, *q.v.*

au″to·ech″o·la′li·a (aw″to·eck″·o·lay′lee·uh). Stereotypy in which the patient continually repeats some word or phrase of his own.

au″to·ech″o·prax′i·a (·eck″o·prack′see·uh). Stereotypy in which the patient continually repeats some action he has previously experienced.

au″to·er′o·tism, au″to·e·rot′i·cism. 1. A combination of sexual emotion and self-admiration. 2. Self-gratification of sexual instinct. See *masturbation.* **–autoerot′ic,** *adj.*

au″to·fel·la′ti·o (·feh·lay′shee·o). Fellatio practiced upon oneself.

au·tog′e·nous (aw·todj′i·nus), **au″to·ge·net′ic, au″to·gen′ic.** 1. Self-generated; endogenous. 2. Arising within the organism, applied to toxins, pathologic states, vaccines, and the like.

au′to·graft″. Any tissue removed from one part of a person's body and applied to another part.

au″to·he·mol′y·sis, au″to·hae·mol′y·sis (aw″to·hee·mol′i·sis, ·hem·ol′i·sis). Hemolysis of an individual's red blood cells by his own serum.

au″to·he″mo·ther′a·py, au″to·hae″mo·ther′a·py (aw″to·hee″mo·therr′uh·pee, aw″to·hem″o·). Treatment of disease with the patient's own blood, withdrawn through a venepuncture and injected directly into his body, usually intramuscularly.

au″to·hy·drol′y·sis (aw″to·high·drol′i·sis). Spontaneous hydrolysis.

au″to·hyp·no′tism, au″to·hyp·no′sis. Self-induced hypnosis. —**au·tohypnot′ic,** *adj., n.*

au″to·im·mun″i·za′tion. Immunization obtained by natural processes within the body.

au″to·in·fec′tion. Infection by an organism existing within the body or transferred from one part of the body to another.

au″to·in·fu′sion. Forcing of the blood toward the heart by applying firm bandages to the extremities distoproximally, compression of the abdominal area, etc., to raise blood pressure and get blood to the vital centers.

au″to·in·tox″i·ca′tion. Poisoning by faulty metabolic products elaborated within the body; generally synonymous with toxemia of morbid states. Formerly considered to occur in constipation.

au″to·i″so·lys′in (aw″to·eye″so·lye′sin, ·eye·sol′i·sin). An antibody which dissolves the corpuscles of the individual from which it was obtained; also the red cells of others of the same species.

au·tol′o·gous. Derived from, or a part of, an organism. Contrasted with homologous (same species) and heterologous (different species).

au·tol′y·sate. That which results from or is produced by autolysis.

au″to·ly′sin, au·tol′y·sin. A substance which produces autolysis, *q.v.*

au·tol′y·sis. 1. Self-digestion of tissues within the living body. 2. The chemical splitting-up of the tissue of an organ by the action of an enzyme peculiar to it. 3. The hemolytic action of the blood serum or plasma of an animal upon its own corpuscles. —**au·tolyt′ic,** *adj.;* **au′tolyze,** *v.*

automat-. See *automato-.*

au″to·mat′ic. Performed without the influence of the will; spontaneous.

au·tom′a·tin. 1. A theoretical substance present in the heart which normally initiates the contraction. 2. An extract of bovine heart muscle used therapeutically in various circulatory disorders.

au·tom′a·tism. 1. Performance of acts without apparent volition, as in somnambulism and in hysterical and epileptic states. 2. *In biology,* spontaneous activity of cells and tissues, as the spontaneous beating of a heart freed from its nervous connections.

au·tom′a·to-, automat′. A combining form meaning *self-moving* or *self-acting;* used to denote *automatic.*

au·tom′a·ton. One who acts in an involuntary or mechanical manner.

au″to·nom′ic, au·ton′o·mous. Independent in origin, action, or function; self-governing.

au″to·phil′i·a. Morbid self-esteem.

au″to·pho′bi·a. A morbid dread of one's self or of solitude.

au′to·plas″ty. Repair of a defect by grafting tissue taken from another area of the patient's body. —**autoplas′tic,** *adj.;* autoplast, *n.*

au′top·sy. A post-mortem examination of the body.

au″to·psy·cho′sis. A mental derangement in which the patient's ideas about himself are distorted. —**autopsy′chic,** *adj.*

au″to·re·in·fu′sion. Intravenous infusion in a patient of his own blood.

au′to·some. Any ordinary chromosome as distinguished from an allosome, *q.v.* —**autosomal,** *adj.*

au″to·sug·ges′tion. 1. The acceptance of a thought or idea, predominantly from within one's own mind, which induces some mental or physical action or change. 2. Self-suggestion. The persistence in consciousness of impressions gained while in a hypnotic state. 3. The highly suggestible state of mind existing after accidents, where a very slight injury may be the cause of hysterical pain, paralysis, and other disorders. Also called *traumatic suggestion.* —**autosuggestibil′ity,** *n.*

au″to·syn·noi′a. A state of introversion in which the subject is so concentrated in his thoughts or hallucinations that he loses all interest in the outside world.

au″to·trans·form′er. A step-down transformer used extensively in varying the voltage to the primary windings of a high-voltage x-ray transformer.

au″to·trans·fu′sion. 1. Forcing of blood into vital regions after severe hemorrhage or to prevent shock, by elevation of, and application of Esmarch bandages to, three of the extremities. See *autoinfusion*. 2. Intravenous injection of blood or serum lost during an operation or hemorrhage, especially when it occurs in the abdominal cavity. See *autoreinfusion*.

au″to-trans″plan·ta′tion. The operation of transplanting to a part of the body tissue taken from another area in the same body.

auxano-. A combining form denoting *growth*.

aux·e′sis. 1. Increase in size or bulk; growth. 2. Growth in size by cell expansion without cell division; hypertrophy. *Obs.*

aux·et′ic. 1. Stimulating the increase of cells. 2. A hypothetical substance which excites cell reproduction; an agent which causes proliferation of human cells, especially leukocytes.

aux′in. A plant hormone which governs cell extension or growth.

aux′o-. 1. A combining form signifying *increase*. 2. In biochemistry, a combining form denoting *accelerating* or *stimulating*. 3. In biology, a combining form denoting *concerned with*, or *due to*, *growth*.

aux′o·chrome. 1. That which increases color. 2. A chemical group which, added to a chromophore group, will produce a dye. 3. Increase or development of color. **—auxoch′romous,** *adj.*

aux′o·drome. A standard schedule of development.

aux·om′e·ter, aux·i·om′e·ter. A device for measuring the magnifying power of lenses.

A. V., AV. Atrioventricular; auriculoventricular.

Av. Avoirdupois weight.

a·vas″cu·lar·i·za′tion (ay-vas″-cue·lur·i·zay′shun, a·vas″·). Act of rendering a part bloodless, as by compression or bandaging. **—avas′cular,** *adj.;* **avas′cularize,** *v.t.*, *v.i.*

av′er·age. 1. The medial sum; the figure arrived at by adding together several quantities and dividing by the number of quantities; arithmetic average. 2. Usual; typical of a group; ordinary.

avertin. Trade-mark for tribromoethanol or tribromoethyl alcohol. **a. with amylene hydrate.** A solution containing tribromoethanol and amylene hydrate, used for basal anesthesia by rectal administration and for the control of certain convulsive conditions. See *bromethol*.

a′vi·an. Pertaining to birds.

a″vi·a′tion med′i·cine. That branch of medicine concerned with the pathologic conditions and physiologic and emotional disturbances resulting from airplane flights.

av′i·din. A biotin-inactivating protein in raw egg white.

a·vid′i·ty. 1. Obsolete term for chemical affinity. 2. In immunology, that characteristic of antitoxic serum which determines the rate of neutralization; it is distinct from the antitoxin content.

a·vir′u·lent (ay-virr′yoo·lunt, a-virr′·). Without virulence.

a″vi·tam′ic ac′id (ay″vi·tam′ic). Ascorbic acid.

a·vi″ta·min·o′sis (ay·vy″tuh·mi·no′sis, a·vy″·). Any disease resulting from a deficiency of one or more vitamins.

Avogadro, Amadeo [*Italian physicist,* 1776–1856]. Stated the physical law that equal volumes of all gases at the same temperature and pressure contain equal numbers of molecules (1811). See also Avogadro's *number*.

av″oir·du·pois′ (av″ur·duh·poyz′). The English system of weights and measures. See Tables of Weights and Measures in the Appendix.

avosyl. Trade-mark for mephenesin, *q.v.*

a·vul′sion. A forcible tearing or wrenching away of a part, as a polyp or a limb. **a. of the bulb.** Forcible separation of the eyeball by tearing the muscles, the vessels, and the optic nerve. **nerve a.** Surgical tearing away of a nerve from its origin by traction, as a phrenic avulsion, for paralyzing one side of the diaphragm to obtain rest for a tuberculous lung.

ax-. See *azo-*.

a″xe·roph′thol. Vitamin A.

ax·il′la. The armpit. **—ax′illary,** *adj.*

ax′is. 1. An imaginary line passing through the center of a body; also the line about which a rotating body turns. 2. The second cervical vertebra; the epistropheus [BNA]. See Table of Bones in the Appendix. 3. The spinal column. 4. The cerebrospinal nervous system. 5. The odontoid process of the epistropheus. 6. A very short artery which breaks up into several branches. **—axial,** *adj.* **cardiac a.** A line passing through the center of the base and apex of the heart. **craniofacial a.** Axis through the bones forming the base of the skull. **optic a.** (a) An imaginary line on which the refracting surfaces of the eye are more or less centered; it passes from the midpoint (approximately) of the cornea (anterior pole) to the midpoint of the optic fundus (posterior pole); the principal axis of the eye. (b) An imaginary line passing from the center of the eyepiece of a microscope through the body, objective, stage, and substage to the mirror. **pelvic a.** An imaginary line passing through all the median anteroposterior diameters of the pelvic canal at their centers. **principal a.** *In op-*

tics, a line which passes through the centers of curvature of the surfaces of a lens. *In ophthalmology*, same as optic axis, *q.v.* Also called *optical center nodal point*. **visual a.** Line of vision; a line extending from the object of vision, through the center of the pupil, to the macula lutea.

ax'is cyl'in·der. The conducting or essential part of a nerve fiber.

ax'o-, ax-. A combining form meaning *axis* or denoting *the axis cylinder*.

ax"o·fu'gal, ax·of'u·gal. Pertaining to nerve impulses transmitted from the cell body to the periphery. Also called *axifugal, centrifugal.*

ax'on, ax'one. The efferent process of a nerve cell. Also called *neuraxon, neurite, axis cylinder process.* **—axonal,** *adj.*

ax·op'e·tal. Pertaining to nerve impulses transmitted along an axon toward the cell body. Also called *axipetal, centripetal.*

ax'o·plasm". Undifferentiated cytoplasm, neuroplasm, of the axon in which neurofibrils are embedded.

Ayerza, Abel [*Argentinian physician*, 1861–1918]. Remembered for his description of the syndrome of chronic cyanosis, dyspnea, and sclerosis of the pulmonary artery (1901), called *Ayerza's syndrome*. This is now classified as syphilis of the pulmonary artery, dilatation of the pulmonary artery due to mitral stenosis, hypertension of lesser circulation due to disease of the lungs, or arteriosclerosis of the lesser circulation.

ax"a·cy'clo·nol hy"dro·chlo'ride. *a,a*-Diphenyl-4-piperidinemethanol hydrochloride, an agent counteracting hallucinations. See *frenquel.*

axap'e·tine phos'phate. 6-Allyl-6,7-dihydro-5H-dibenz[o,e]-azepine phosphate, an adrenergic blocking agent. See *ilidar phosphate.*

az'i-. A prefix denoting *the presence of the group* N_3.

ax'ide (az'ide, -id). A compound containing the monovalent —N_3 group.

az'o- (az'o-, ay'zo-), **ax-.** A combining form indicating *the presence of nitrogen or of the group* —$N:N$— *within a compound.* **—azo,** *adj.*

azochloramid. Trade-mark for the germicide N,N'-dichloroazodicarbonamidine, or chloroazodin.

az'o dyes (az'o, ay'zo). A group of synthetic organic dyes derivable from azobenzene, containing the chromophore —$N:N$—.

az"o·lit'min. A dark-red coloring matter obtained from litmus and used as an indicator, especially in routine bacteriologic work with milk.

a·zo"o·sper'mi·a, a·zo"o·sper'ma·tism. Absence of spermatozoa in the semen.

az"o·pro'te·in. One of a group of synthetic antigens formed by coupling proteins with diazo compounds.

az"o·te'mi·a. The presence of excessive amounts of nitrogenous compounds in the blood; uremia.

a·zot'ic ac'id. Nitric acid.

a·xo"ti·fi·ca'tion. Fixation of atmospheric nitrogen.

az"o·tom'e·ter. A device for gasometrically measuring the nitrogen content of compounds in solution.

az"o·tor·rhe'a, az"o·tor·rhoe'a. Excess of nitrogenous matter in the urine or feces.

az"o·tu'ri·a. An increase of the nitrogenous substances in the urine. **—azoturic,** *adj.*

azulfidine. Trade-mark for salicylazosulfapyridine.

az'ure (azh'ur, ay'zhur). A basic thiazine dye; used in blood and connective-tissue stains. **a. A** (C.C.). Asymmetrical dimethyl thionine; used in 0.1–1.5% aqueous solution as a nuclear stain for sections of fixed tissue, or in combination with other dyes. **a. B** (C.C.). The trimethyl derivative of thionine. **a. C.** A basic dye, monomethyl thionine. **a. I.** Trade name for a mixture of azure A and azure B. Syn., *methylene a.* **a. II.** A mixture of equal parts of azure I and methylene blue. **methylene a.** See *a. I.*

az'u·rin. Theobromine sodium acetate; used as a diuretic. See *theobromine.*

a·zu"ro·phile" (a·zhuo'ro·file", -fil"), **a·zu'ro·phil".** Staining promptly with an azure dye. **—azurophil'ic,** *adj.*

ax'y·gos, a·xy'gos. 1. Unpaired; without a fellow. 2. An unpaired anatomic structure. **—azygous,** *adj.*

a·xy'mi·a, a·xym'i·a. The absence of an enzyme or ferment.

a·xym'ic, a·xy'mic. 1. Not rising from a fermentation; unfermented. 2. Not containing enzymes.

B

B. 1. Chemical symbol for boron. 2. Abbreviation for *Bacillus;* formerly abbreviation for *Bacterium.*

Ba. The chemical symbol for barium.

Babcock, Stephen Moulton [*American agricultural chemist*, 1843-1931]. Remembered for his invention of a test for determining the percentage content of butterfat in milk by means of centrifuging a mixture of equal quantities of the specimen and sulfuric acid (1890).

Babcock, William Wayne [*American surgeon*, 1872-]. Known for his originality in devising a number of surgical procedures, as proctosigmoidectomy by the combined method; a plastic operation for the relief of extrophy of the bladder; a method of extirpating varicose veins by means of a pliable, acorn-shaped probe which is inserted into the greater saphenous vein, tied in place, and withdrawn with the vein. See also *Jackson-Babcock operation* under *Chevalier Jackson.* The author of *Principles and Practice of Surgery.*

Babinski, Joseph François Félix [*French neurologist*, 1857-1932]. Noted for his description of a reflex (extension of the great toe with fanning of the other toes on exciting the sole) connected with a lesion in the pyramidal tract and found in organic, but not in hysterical, hemiplegia; called *Babinski's sign.* He also described a sign in true sciatica, a diminution of the Achilles reflex, and a syndrome in which lightning pains, absent patellar reflex, Argyll Robertson pupil, and arterial disease indicate tabes. In association with Nageotte, he described a syndrome, now called tegmental medullary syndrome, marked by contralateral hemiplegia and hemianesthesia with hemiasynergia and hemiataxia, due to multiple lesions of the pyramidal tracts and cerebral peduncle; known as the *Babinski-Nageotte syndrome.* See also adiposogenital *dystrophy,* called *Babinski-Froehlich's disease.*

ba′by. An infant; a newborn child; a child up to the time he talks. **b. farm.** Institution for rearing infants. **blue b.** A newborn child suffering from cyanosis, transitory or permanent. The former is due to a passing obstruction, irregular respiration, or may follow crying or exercise; the latter occurs when venous blood is shunted to the arterial side because of a cardiac anomaly, as an open foramen ovale. See *cyanosis.*

bac′ci·form (back′si·form) Berry-shaped.

bac′il·lar″y (bas′i·lerr″ee), **ba·cil′lar.** 1. Relating to bacilli or to a bacillus. 2. Consisting of or containing rods.

bac″il·le′mi·a, bac″il·lae′mi·a (bas″i·lee′mee·uh). Presence of bacilli in the blood.

ba·cil′li (ba·sil′eye). Plural of bacillus.

ba·cil′li·form. Having the shape or appearance of a bacillus; rod-shaped.

ba·cil′lo- (ba·sil′o-, bas′i·lo-), **ba·cil′li-** (ba·sil′ee-, bas′i·lee-). A combining form meaning *bacillus.*

ba·cil″lo·my′cin. An antibiotic substance isolated from cultures of *Bacillus subtilis;* it is active against a variety of fungi but has little effect against bacteria.

ba·cil″lo·pho′bi·a. Morbid fear of bacilli.

bac″il·lu′ri·a (bas″i·lew′ree·uh). The presence of bacilli in the urine.

Ba·cil′lus (pl. *Bacilli*). A genus of rod-shaped, nonflexuous forms of the family Bacillaceae, described by Cohn in 1872 with *Bacillus subtilis* as the type. They may occur as slender, short, straight, or slightly bent rods. **B. aerogenes capsulatus.** Synonym for *Clostridium welchii.* **B. aertrycke.** See *Salmonella typhimurium.* **B. agni.** The lamb dysentery bacillus, which has also been designated as *Clostridium welchii B.* **B. anthracis.** A species pathogenic to man, although in nature it is primarily a pathogen of cattle and horses. The *B. anthracis* is one of the largest of the pathogenic bacteria and is nonmotile. **B. botulinus.** Synonym for *Clostridium botulinum.* **B. enteritidis.** See *Salmonella enteritidis.* **B. faecalis alcaligenes.** See *Alcaligenes faecalis.* **B. fusiformis.** Synonym for *Fusobacterium plauti-vincenti.* **B. influenzae.** See *Hemophilus influenzae.* **B. lacunatus.** Synonym for *Morazella lacunata.* **B. leprae.** See *Mycobacterium leprae.* **B. mallei.** See *Malleomyces mallei.* **B. oedematiens.** Synonym for *Clostridium novyi.* **B. oedematis maligni.** Synonym for *Clostridium novyi.* **B. ovitoxicus.** Synonym for *Clostridium welchii.* **B. paratyphosus A.** Synonym for *Salmonella paratyphi A.* **B. paratyphosus B.** Synonym for *Salmonella paratyphi B.* **B. pertussis.** Synonym for *Hemophilus pertussis.* **B. pestis.** See *Pasteurella pestis.* **B. proteus.** See *Pro-*

teus vulgaris. **B. subtilis.** The type species of the genus Bacillus, which infects human beings only rarely. Its medical importance lies in the fact that the antibiotic substance, subtilin, is prepared from this species. **B. tetani.** Clostridium tetani. **B. vaginalis.** A common organism found in the vagina, contributing to the acidity of the vaginal secretions. It is thought to be identical with the Lactobacillus acidophilus.

ba·cil'lus (pl. bacilli). A term used loosely to include any member of the class Schizomycetes. **abortus b.** Brucella abortus. **anthrax b.** Bacillus anthracis. **Bordet-Gengou b.** Hemophilus pertussis. **colon b.** Escherichia coli. **comma b.** Vibrio comma. **diphtheria b.** Corynebacterium diphtheriae. **diphtheroid bacilli.** Bacilli similar to the diphtheria bacillus but which do not produce toxin. **Döderlein's b.** Bacillus vaginalis. **Ducrey's b.** Hemophilus ducreyi. **Duval's b.** Shigella sonnei. **Flexner's b.** Shigella paradysenteriae. **Friedländer's b.** Klebsiella pneumoniae. **fusiform b.** A common designation for bacteria of spindle-shaped or cigar-shaped morphology, belonging to the genus Fusobacterium. **gas gangrene b.** Clostridium perfringens Type A. **glanders b.** Malleomyces mallei. **Hansen's b.** Mycobacterium leprae. **hay b.** Bacillus subtilis. **Hiss and Russell's Y b.** Shigella paradysenteriae. **hog cholera b.** See Salmonella choleraesuis. **Klebs-Loeffler b.** Corynebacterium diphtheriae. **Koch-Weeks b.** An attenuated (or pleomorphic) form of Hemophilus influenzae. **Morax-Axenfeld b.** Morazella lacunata. **Morgan's b.** Proteus morganii. **Pfeiffer's b.** Hemophilus influenzae. **pneumobacillus.** Klebsiella pneumoniae. **pseudodysentery b.** Shigella paradysenteriae. **Schmitz's b.** Shigella ambigua. **Shiga b.** Shigella dysenteriae. **streptobacilli.** Those bacilli which remain attached end to end producing a chainlike group. **tubercle b.** Mycobacterium tuberculosis. Abbreviated, t. b. **typhoid b.** Synonym for Eberthella typhosa.

ba·ci·tra'cin. An antibiotic obtained from Bacillus subtilis isolated from a wound (in the patient Margaret Tracy, after whom the antibiotic was named).

back. 1. The dorsum; the posterior aspect. 2. The posterior part of the trunk from the neck to the pelvis. **b. rest.** Any device used to support the back in an upright or semireclining position. **hollow b.** One with excessive lumbar lordosis. **poker b.** A back stiffened by ankylosing spondylitis. **trench b.** Dorsolumbar pain and rigidity experienced by troops engaged in trench warfare.

back'ache". Pain in the lower lumbar or lumbosacral regions of the back. Also called lumbago, lumbosacral pain.

back'bone". The vertebral column.

back'ward·ness. 1. Retarded growth or mental development; due to any cause, as general illness or sense-deprivation, except mental deficiency. 2. Educational retardation due to extrinsic causes. **—backward,** adj.

bac"te·re'mi·a. The presence of bacteria in the blood.

bac·te'ri·a. Plural of bacterium.

Bac·te"ri·a'ce·ae (back-teer"ee-ay'see-ee, back"teer-ee-). A family of Eubacteriales containing one genus: Bacterium.

bac·te'ri·cide (back-teer'i-side, ·terr'i-side). 1. Destructive to bacteria. 2. An agent that destroys bacteria. **—bactericid'al,** adj.

bac"te·ri·ci'din, bac·te"ri·o·ci'din. An antibody that in the presence of complement kills bacteria.

bac'te·rid. An eruption of the skin due to absorption of bacteria or their toxins by the blood.

bac"te·rin·ert'ness. The failure to support bacterial growth because of the absence of the necessary nutrients; to be distinguished from bacteriostasis, q.v. **—bacterinert',** adj.

bac"te·ri·o·ci'din. See bactericidin.

bac·te"ri·o·gen'ic, bac·te"ri·og'e·nous (back-teer"ee-odj'i-nus). Caused by bacteria; of bacterial origin.

bac"te"ri·o·he"mo·ly'sin, bac·te"ri·o·hae"mo·ly'sin (·hee"mo-lye'sin, ·hem-ol'i-sin). A very unstable substance which liberates hemoglobin from the red blood cells, and is formed in the body by bacterial action, as streptolysins, staphylolysins, tetanolysins, etc. A single bacterial strain may produce multiple hemolysins.

bac·te"ri·ol'o·gist. One versed in bacteriology. One whose profession is the study and practice of bacteriology.

bac·te"ri·ol'o·gy. The science and study of bacteria. **—bacteriolog'ic,** adj.

bac·te"ri·o·ly'sin (back-teer"ee-o-lye'sin, back"teer-ee-ol'i-sin). A specific antibody which, in coöperation with other substances (complements), is capable of causing the dissolution of the homologous bacterium.

bac·te"ri·ol'y·sis. The intracellular or extracellular dissolution of bacteria. When mediated by a specific antibody and complement, it is called immune bacteriolysis. **—bacteriolyt'ic,** adj.

bac·te'ri·o·phage (back-teer"ee-o-faydj, ·o·fahzh"). An ultramicroscopic agent which produces a transmissible dissolution of certain bacterial cells. The agent is considered by some to be living, and by others as enzymatic. —**bacteriophag'ic**, *adj.*; **bacterioph'agy**, *n.*

bac·te″ri·o·pho'bi·a. A morbid dread of bacteria or other m'croörganisms.

bac·te″ri·o·pro'te·in. Any one of a number of protein substances contained in bacteria; often the cause of fever, inflammation, and suppuration.

bac·te″ri·op'so·nin. An opsonin which acts upon bacteria, as distinguished from one affecting erythrocytes. —**bacteriopson'ic**, *adj.*

bac·te″ri·os'ta·sis (back-teer″eeos'tuh·sis, ·o·stay'sis). Arrest or hindrance of the growth of bacteria; to be distinguished from *bacterinertness*, *q.v.* —**bacteriostat'ic**, *adj.*

bac·te'ri·o·stat″. Any agent which arrests or hinders the growth of bacteria.

bac·te″ri·o·ther'a·py. The treatment of disease by the introduction of bacteria or their products into the system. —**bacteriotherapeu'tic**, *adj.*

bac·te″ri·o·tox'in. 1. A toxin destructive to bacteria. 2. A toxin produced by bacteria. —**bacteriotoxic**, *adj.*

bac·te″ri·o·trop'ic. Denoting substances which render bacteria susceptible to phagocytosis.

bac·te″ri·ot'ro·pin. An immune, thermostable opsonin; an antibody aiding the phagocytic action of certain cells, as leukocytes.

Bac·te'ri·um. A genus of the Bacteriaceae. Abbreviated, **Bact. Bact. ambiguum.** Synonym for *Shigella ambigua.* **Bact. cholerae-suis.** Synonym for *Salmonella choleraesuis.* **Bact. coli.** Synonym for *Escherichia coli.* **Bact. dispar.** Synonym for *Shigella madampensis.* **Bact. dysenteriae.** Synonym for *Shigella dysenteriae.* **Bact. flexneri.** Synonym for *Shigella paradysenteriae.* **Bact. friedländeri.** Synonym for *Klebsiella pneumoniae.* **Bact. fusiformis.** Synonym for *Fusobacterium plauti-vincenti.* **Bact. monocytogenes.** Synonym for *Listeria monocytogenes.* **Bact. paradysenteriae.** Synonym for *Shigella paradysenteriae.* **Bact. paratyphosum A.** Synonym for *Salmonella paratyphi A.* **Bact. paratyphosum B.** Synonym for *Salmonella paratyphi B.* **Bact. pneumoniae.** Synonym for *Klebsiella pneumoniae.* **Bact. shigae.** Synonym for *Shigella dysenteriae.* **Bact. sonnei.** Synonym for *Shigella sonnei.* **Bact. suipestifer.** Synonym for *Salmonella choleraesuis.* **Bact. tularense.** Synonym for

Pasteurella tularensis. **Bact. typhimurium.** Synonym for *Salmonella typhimurium.* **Bact. typhosum.** Synonym for *Eberthella typhosa.*

bac·te'ri·um (pl. *bacteria*). 1. Formerly the schizomycetes. 2. Any of a very large group of unicellular, vegetable microörganisms existing morphologically as oval or spherical cells (cocci), rods (bacilli), spirals (spirilla), or a smaller group of comma-shaped organisms (vibrios). The first two forms occur singly or are grouped in pairs (diplococci), or chains (streptococci). Some cocci are grouped in clusters (staphylococci). Bacteria are aerobic, requiring free oxygen, or anaerobic, living without oxygen. Some can flourish under both conditions, being facultative aerobes or anaerobes. The cells are either motile or nonmotile and exist as parasites on living hosts, or saprophytes on dead hosts, some being facultative parasites while others are true parasites. A relatively small group is pathogenic, causing disease, while most are nonpathogenic. The organisms react differently to Gram's stain, being Gram-positive when they retain the stain, and Gram-negative when they decolorize. A few are acid-fast, retaining stain even when subjected to acid-alcohol. Some bacteria cause fermentation (zymogenic), others produce pigment (chromogenic), while another group produces gas (aerogenic). —**bacterial**, *adj.*

bac·te″ri·u'ri·a. The presence of bacteria in the urine.

bac'ter·oid. 1. Resembling bacteria. 2. A bacterium modified in form or structure.

bag. 1. Sac or pouch. 2. The scrotum. 3. A cow's udder. **b. of waters.** The amniotic sac and fluid which serve during pregnancy to protect the fetus and during labor to dilate the cervix. See *amnion.* **caked b.** In cows, an inflammation of the udder. **colostomy b.** One of rubber worn as a belt, especially constructed to receive the intestinal excreta from a colostomy opening. **ice b.** One of rubber to hold cracked ice; used to reduce localized inflammation. **Politzer b.** A rubber bag used to inflate the middle ear. One end is tightly fixed into one external naris while the other is held closed during the act of swallowing water or saying the letter *k.*

ba″gas·so'sis, ba″gas·sco'sis. A disease of the lungs occurring in workmen who handle bagasse, the dry residue of sugar cane after the juice has been expressed. It is characterized by abrupt onset, dyspnea, cough, fever; there is fine mottling in the roentgenogram, and small fibrils of sugar cane are present in the lungs. Also called *bagasse disease*.

Bag'dad boil. See *oriental sore*.

Ba·hi'a ul'cer (buh-high'uh, bah-ee'ah). See *leishmaniasis americana*.

bak'er. *In medicine*, a heating chamber for applying dry heat to a part; used especially in joint diseases. **–bake,** *v*.

bak'ing so'da. Sodium bicarbonate.

BAL. CH₂SH.CHSH.CH₂OH. British anti-lewisite. 2,3-Dimercaptopropanol or dimercaprol, an antidote to poisoning by arsenic, mercury and other metals.

bal'ance. 1. A device for weighing. 2. The normal, harmonious interaction between related parts and organs of the body; equilibrium. **acid-base b.** Physiologic processes whereby acids and alkalies are maintained in a state of equilibrium by buffers, respiration, and elimination, thus keeping the pH of the blood constant; as distinguished from an excess of acid (acidosis) or an excess of alkali (alkalosis). **allergic b.** A state of equilibrium between the patient and his environment, in which the amount of a specific noxious allergen does not exceed the patient's threshold of allergic tolerance. **calcium b.** Physiologic tendency of the body to equalize the outgo and intake of calcium. **energy b.** The relation of the amount of utilizable energy taken into the body to that which is employed for internal work, external work, and the growth and repair of tissues. **fluid b.** Physiologic tendency of the body to maintain the optimum water content by a special water-regulating mechanism. **heat b.** The relation of the amount of heat produced in the body to that which is lost. **hemogenic-hemolytic b.** Physiologic processes by which the normal red-cell production equals the red-cell destruction, thus maintaining the count and the hemoglobin at the optimum level. **nitrogen b.** The difference between the nitrogen intake (as protein) of an individual and his total nitrogen excretion. If the nitrogen intake equals the nitrogen excretion, a subject is in nitrogen equilibrium. If the nitrogen intake exceeds the nitrogen excretion, the nitrogen balance is positive. If the nitrogen excretion is greater than the nitrogen intake, the nitrogen balance is negative. Syn., *nitrogen equilibrium.* **torsion b.** Instrument which measures small torques by their torsional effect upon elastic fibers or wires. **water b.** See *fluid b.*

bal'a·nism. The application of a pessary or suppository. *Obs.*

bal''a·ni'tis. Inflammation of the glans penis, or glans clitoridis.

bal'a·no-, balan-. A combining form

meaning *relating to the glans penis* or *glans clitoridis.*

bal'a·no·plas''ty. Plastic surgery of the glans penis.

bal''a·no·pos·thi'tis. Inflammation of the glans penis and of the prepuce.

bal''a·nor·rha'gi·a (bal''uh-no-ray'juh, ·radj'uh). Hemorrhage from the glans penis.

Bal''an·tid'i·um. A genus of ciliated, parasitic protozoans. **B. coli.** A common parasite of the hog; occasionally infects man, causing severe dysentery.

bal'a·nus. The glans of the penis or of the clitoris.

balarsen. Trade-mark for arsthinol.

bald'ness. Loss or absence of hair. Syn., *acomia, alopecia, calvities.* **–bald,** *adj.*

Bal'kan frame. An overhead quadrilateral supported by uprights fastened to the bedposts; used to suspend immobilized fractured limbs and to apply continuous traction by weights and pulleys.

ball. An object having a round or spherical shape. **hair b.** Bezoar, *q.v.*

bal'lism (bal'iz-um), **bal·lis'mus** (ba-liz'mus). 1. Chorea characterized by jerky, swinging movements of arms and legs. 2. Paralysis agitans. *Obs.*

bal·lis''to·car'di·o·graph. An instrument which records the movements of the body caused by the impact and recoil of the blood after ejection from the ventricles; used in estimating the cardiac output. The record made by this instrument is called a **ballisto-cardiogram.**

bal·lis''to·pho'bi·a. Morbid fear of projectiles or missiles.

bal·loon'ing. Surgical distention of any body cavity by air or other means for examination or therapeutic purposes.

bal·lotte·ment' (bal·awt·mahn', balot'munt). Diagnostic rebound of an organ after palpation.

balm (bahm). A popular synonym of balsam, *q.v.*

bal''ne·o·ther'a·py. Therapeutic use of baths.

bal'sam (bawl'sum). The resinous, aromatic, liquid, or semisolid substance obtained from certain trees by natural exudation or by artificial extraction and usually consisting chiefly of resins and volatile oils containing esters of cinnamic and benzoic acids. **Canada b.** A turpentine gathered from the natural blisters of the bark of *Abies balsamea;* used as a mounting medium by microscopists. Syn., *Canada turpentine.* **friar's b.** Compound benzoin tincture. Also called *Turlington's b.* **Peruvian b.** That obtained from *Myroxylon Pereirae.* A stimulating and antiseptic dressing for indolent ulcers, local tuberculosis, wounds, etc. An expectorant in asthma and chronic bronchitis. Also called *b. of Peru*, *Indian b.* **tolu b.** Is obtained from *Myroxylon balsamum*. It is a feeble stimulant and expectorant.

ba·nan'a oil. Amyl acetate.

band. 1. That which binds. 2. *In zoology*, a stripe. 3. *In anatomy*, a ligament or long slender muscle. Also a disk, *q.v.*, of a striated muscle fiber as seen in longitudinal section. 4. *In dentistry*, a strip of thin metal, formed into a hoop, for encircling a natural tooth or its root. **amniotic b.** A fibrous band connecting amnion and fetus. **iliotibial b.** A thickened portion of the fascia lata extending from the lateral condyle of the tibia to the iliac crest. **moderator b.** A muscle band in the right ventricle of the heart, between the anterior papillary muscle and the ventricular septum, which is supposed to prevent overdistention of the right ventricle.

band'age. A strip of gauze, muslin, flannel, or other material; usually in the form of a roll of various widths and lengths, but may be triangular or tailed. The chief functions of a bandage are: to hold dressings in place, to apply pressure, to immobilize a part, to support a dependent or injured part, to obliterate tissue cavities, and to check hemorrhage. **adhesive b.** One composed of adhesive plaster or moleskin for immobilization or support of a part. **capeline b.** One resembling a cap or hood, suitable for the head, shoulder, or amputation stump. **circular b.** One in which the bandage is wound about the limb or part. **cohesive b.** One of a number of bandages, under various trade names, which has the property of sticking to itself, but not to other substances. **compression b.** One in which a high degree of compression is exerted on the tissues in order to shrink a part, as an amputation stump. **cravat b.** A triangular bandage folded to form a band and wound about a part. **demigauntlet b.** A bandage covering the wrist and hand but not the fingers. **double-headed roller b.** A strip of material rolled from both ends to meet in the middle. **elastic b.** One of rubber or woven elastic material. Used to exert continuous pressure on swollen extremities or joints, fractured ribs, the chest, or varicose veins. **Esmarch's b.** A live rubber compression bandage with tourniquet, used to render a limb bloodless. **figure-of-eight b.** One in which the successive turns cross like the figure eight. **four-tailed b.** A strip of cloth with the ends split, used to cover prominent parts, as the elbow, chin, nose, or knee.

gauntlet b. One which covers the hands and fingers, like a glove. **hammock b.** One which retains scalp dressings. The dressings are covered by a broad strip of gauze brought down over the ears and anchored by a circular bandage around the head. The ends of the broad strip are then turned up over the circular bandage and secured by a few more turns. **immovable b.** A bandage for immobilizing any part. **impregnated b.** A wide-meshed bandage impregnated with such substances as plaster of Paris, sodium silicate, starch, or dextrin; put up in rolls and used for stiffening, immobilizing, and making molds of various parts of the body. **jelly b.** One used in treating varicose veins and ulcers. See Unna's paste *boot*. **many-tailed b.** An irregular bandage having four or more cut or torn ends which are tied together to hold a dressing. **oblique b.** A bandage which covers the part by oblique turns. **plaster b.** An impregnated bandage, *q.v.* **pressure b.** One used to stop hemorrhage or support varicose veins. **quadrangular b.** A towel or large handkerchief, folded variously and used as a bandage. **recurrent b.** One in which each turn comes back to the point of starting; used in bandaging the head or an amputation stump. **reversed b.** An oblique bandage applied to a limb; for each turn, the roll is given a half twist to make a snug fit over the expanded part of the limb. **roller b.** A long strip of material from one-half to six inches in width, rolled on its short axis. **rubber b.** An elastic bandage, *q.v.* **scultetus b.** One used in compound fractures, usually of the lower extremity, composed of short pieces which overlap each other, thereby permitting their removal without movement of the limb. Also called *Scultet's b.* **silica b.** An impregnated bandage, *q.v.* **spica b.** One with successive turns and crosses, as in a modified figure-of-eight bandage; so called because it resembles the folded edges of the husk of an ear of corn. **spiral b.** An oblique bandage, *q.v.* **spiral reverse b.** One in which the oblique turns are reversed and folded back at each turn, to adapt the bandage to the part. **suspensory b.** One for supporting the scrotum. **T b.** A bandage with three arms which form a letter T; especially used about the waist and the perineum to hold a dressing. **triangular b.** A square of muslin cut diagonally to make two triangles. Useful as slings, and for inclusive dressings of a part, as a whole hand. **Velpeau's b.** One which completely fixes the arm against the side, with the forearm flexed at an angle of 45°, the palm resting upon the mid-clavicular region opposite. By successive turns about the body, the bandage envelops the shoulder, arm, forearm, and hand.

Bandl, Ludwig [German obstetrician, 1842–92]. Described a thickened line, observed during labor, at the lower limit of the upper contractile segment of the uterus. Called *Bandl's contraction ring, Lusk's contraction ring.*

bank. A reserve stock of body fluids and parts usually maintained at a hospital or Red Cross Center under suitable storage facilities. The stocks kept now are: whole blood, plasma, blood vessels, bone, arteries, nerves, cartilage, and corneas (for corneal grafts).

banthine bromide. Trade-marked name for β-diethylaminoethylxanthene-9-carboxylate methobromide, an anticholinergic drug. See *methantheline* bromide.

bar. 1. A band or stripe. 2. A fetal or visceral arch. 3. A unit of atmospheric pressure representing one megadyne per square centimeter. 4. *In prosthetic dentistry,* a piece of metal connecting two parts of a bridge or partial denture. 5. *In orthodontics,* a wire extending from an anchorage in one part of the mouth to another tooth or teeth in the same jaw. The opposite end may be free, that is, not inserted in a second anchorage. **b. of bladder.** The transverse ridge joining the openings of the ureters on the inner surface of the urinary bladder; it forms the posterior boundary of the trigone. **episternal b.** See episternal *cartilage.* **median b.** Contracture of the vesical neck, or constriction of the prostatic urethra, caused by prostatic hyperplasia (*glandular bar*) or by overgrowth of connective tissue across the posterior lip of the vesical orifice or of the vesical trigone (*fibrous bar*). A "muscular" bar due to congenital hypertrophy of muscle at the vesical neck, and a "prefibrotic" bar due to inflammatory changes associated with urethritis and prostatitis, have also been described.

bar″ag·no′sis (bar″ag·no′sis). Loss of the perception of weight; loss of barognosis.

bar·ba. 1. The beard. 2. A hair of the beard. 3. The heavy beard which appears after puberty as a secondary male sex character [BNA].

bar·bal′o·in. A pentoside chiefly responsible for the purgative action of aloe. See *aloin.*

bar′ber″ry. See berberis.

bar′bi·tal (bahr′bi·tol). Diethylmalonylurea. A white, crystalline powder, soluble in alcohol and water; used as hypnotic with prolonged action. Also called *barbitone, diethylbarbituric acid.* Also see *veronal.* **b. sodium.** The sodium salt of barbital, a white

powder soluble in water. Also called *soluble b., sodium diethylbarbiturate.*

bar′bi·tone. British name for barbital.

bar·bit′u·rate, bar″bi·tu′rate. A general term denoting a derivative of barbituric acid, $C_4H_4O_3N_2$. Barbiturates are used in medicine as hypnotic and sedative drugs.

bar″bi·tu′ric ac′id. $C_4H_4O_3N_2$. Malonyl urea, the parent compound of the barbiturates.

bar′bi·tu·rism. An acute intoxication following an overdose of drugs of the barbiturate group; often the result of attempted suicide. It is characterized by delirium, followed by coma and sometimes death. There are pathologic changes in the tissues; tremor, ataxia, and mental confusion are present, and cutaneous eruptions are sometimes observed.

bar·bo·tage′ (bahr·bo·tahzh′, ·tazh′). Method of spinal anesthesia; part of the anesthetic solution is injected into the subarachnoid space; spinal fluid is then aspirated into the syringe and reinjected. This may be repeated several times before the entire contents of the syringe is finally injected.

bar″es·the′si·a (bar″ess·thee′zhuh, ·zee·uh). Perception of weight or pressure; pressure sense.

bar″i·to′sis. Chronic inflammation of the lungs due to the inhalation of barium. A form of pneumoconiosis.

ba′ri·um, bar′i·um. Ba = 137.36. A metal belonging to the alkaline earths. All of its soluble salts are poisonous. **b. chloride.** $BaCl_2.2H_2O$. A violent stimulant of all smooth muscles; occasionally used to increase the force of cardiac contraction in atrioventricular dissociation (Adams-Stokes disease). **b. sulfate.** $BaSO_4$; a white, odorless, tasteless powder, insoluble in water; employed as an opaque roentgenographic contrast medium. **b. sulfide.** BaS; soluble in water; used in depilatories and in luminous paint.

bar′ley. Any cereal grass of the genus *Hordeum,* family Gramineae. Used as a food, and also in the preparation of malt. **b. water.** A decoction prepared from 2 ounces of pearl barley boiled in 1½ pints of water; used as demulcent and food in children's diarrheas. **pearl b.** Husked barley grains, rounded and polished.

bar′o-. A combining form implying *heaviness.*

bar″og·no′sis. The ability to estimate weight; the perception of weight.

bar′o·graph. A self-registering barometer.

bar″o·ma·crom′e·ter. An apparatus to measure the weight and length of newborn infants.

ba·rom′e·ter. An instrument which

measures atmospheric pressures. —**baromet'ric**, *adj.*; **barometry**, *n.* **aneroid b.** A barometer in which changes in pressure are indicated by the collapsing or bulging of a thin, corrugated cover of a partially evacuated metallic box.

bar'o·pho'bi·a. A morbid fear of gravity.

bar'o·scope. Any instrument which indicates variations in atmospheric pressure.

bar'ri·er. An obstacle, barricade, or impediment. **blood-brain b.** The theoretical concept of a barrier between blood vessels and brain tissue to explain the phenomenon that certain dyes when injected into the blood system fail to stain brain tissue but will stain other organs. The actual mechanism and location of the barrier is not known. Also called *hematoencephalic b.* **hematoencephalic b.** See bloodbrain *barrier.* **placental b.** The tissues intervening between the maternal and the fetal blood of the placenta, which prevent or hinder certain substances or bacteria from passing from mother to fetus.

Barton, Clara [*American philanthropist and nurse*, 1821–1912]. Famed for her organization of nursing and medical aid during the American Civil War. First president of the American Red Cross Society (1881–1904).

Bar"to·nel'la. A genus of microorganisms which multiply in fixed tissue cells and parasitize erythrocytes. They occur without an intermediate host in man; in arthropod vectors, are found only as **B. bacilliformis**, the causative agent of Oroya fever.

bar'y-. A combining form signifying *heavy.*

bar"y·la'li·a. An indistinct, thick speech; occurs in organic lesions; common in advanced general paresis.

bar"y·pho'ni·a. A heavy or deep quality of voice.

ba·ry'ta (ba·rye'tuh, bar'ĭ·tuh), **ba·ry'tes** (ba·rye'teez, bar'ĭ·teez). BaO. Barium oxide. **b. water.** An aqueous solution of barium hydroxide.

ba'sal met"a·bol'ic rate. The amount of energy expended per unit of time under basal conditions, usually expressed as large calories per square meter of body surface (or Kg. of body weight) per hour.

bas"cu·la'tion. Replacing a retroverted uterus by pressing upward on the fundus and downward on the cervix.

bas'cule move'ment. The recoil of the heart in its systolic motion.

base. 1. The lowest part of a body or the foundation upon which anything rests. 2. The principal ingredient of a substance or compound. 3. *In chemistry,* commonly a compound which yields

hydroxyl ions (OH⁻) in aqueous solution and which reacts with an acid to produce a salt and water. 4. *In dentistry,* the support for the teeth in an artificial denture; a base plate. —**ba'sal, ba'sic, bas'ilar**, *adj.*

Basedow, Karl Adolph von [*German physician,* 1799–1854]. Famed for his early description of exophthalmic goiter (1840), called *Basedow's disease, Flajani's disease, Graves's disease, Parry's disease.* Described his syndrome of the disease: tachycardia, heat flashes, and sweating crises; called *Basedow's syndrome.*

basergin. Trade-mark for ergonovine, $C_{19}H_{23}O_2N_3$, an alkaloid from ergot.

ba'si- (bay'see-, bas'ee-). A combining form meaning *basis, base, forming a base; walking.*

ba"si·chro'ma·tin. That portion of the nuclear reticulum stained by basic aniline dyes.

ba·sic'i·ty (bay·sis'ĭ·tee). 1. The quality of being basic. 2. The number of replaceable hydrogens of an acid.

ba"si·cra'ni·al. Relating to the base of the skull.

Ba·sid"i·o·my·ce'tes (ba·sid"ee·o·migh·see'teez). A large class of fungi comprising genera which produce spores upon basidia. It includes the smuts, rusts, mushrooms, puffballs, and their allies.

ba"si·fa'cial. Pertaining to the lower portion of the face.

ba·sil'ic. Important; prominent; said of a drug or of a structure, as the basilic vein. See Table of Veins in the Appendix.

ba·sil'i·con oint'ment. Rosin cerate.

ba·sil'ic vein. Large vein of the arm on the medial side of the biceps muscle.

ba"si·oc·cip'i·tal (bay"see·ock·sip'ĭ·tul, bas"ee·). Referring to the basilar process of the occipital bone.

ba'si·o·tribe" (bay'see·o·, bas'ee·o·). Instrument used for basiotripsy, *q.v.*

ba'si·o·trip'sy. The operation of crushing or perforating the fetal head to facilitate delivery. *Obs.*

ba"si·pho'bi·a. A morbid fear of walking.

ba'sis. A base, foundation, or fundamental part; the part opposite the apex. —**bas'ilar**, *adj.* **b. cranii externa** [BNA]. External aspect of the base of the skull. **b. cranii interna** [BNA]. Internal aspect of the base of the skull. **b. linguae.** The root of the tongue. **b. pedunculi** [BNA]. The base of the cerebral peduncle containing descending tracts. Also called *crus cerebri, pes pedunculi.*

bas'ket. 1. The fibrillar network in which the Purkinje cell body rests, formed by large arborizations from the axis cylinder process of certain neurons.

See *basket cells* under *cell*. 2. A condensation of intracellular neurofibrils seen in senile dementia. **fiber baskets.** The delicate fibrils extending from the outer limiting membrane of the retina to surround neighboring rods and cones.

Basle an"a·tom'i·cal no'men·cla"ture. A list of anatomic terms (in Latin) adopted by the German Anatomical Society in Basle, Switzerland, in 1895. Abbreviated, BNA (Basle Nomina Anatomica).

ba'so·phil, ba'so·phile. 1. Showing an affinity for basic dyes. 2. A substance, cell, or tissue element showing an affinity for basic dyes. See *basophilia*, basophil *leukocyte*.

ba'so·phile. See *basophil*.

ba"so·phil'i·a. 1. Increased number of basophils in the circulating blood. 2. Stippling of the red cells with basic staining granules, representing a degenerative condition as seen in severe anemia, leukemia, malaria, lead poisoning, and other toxic states. Syn., *granular degeneration, basophilic degeneration, stippling*. Also called *punctate b*.

ba"so·phil'ic, ba·soph'i·lous (bay-sof'i·lus). Susceptible to staining by basic rather than by acid dyes.

ba·soph'i·lism. Basophilia. **pituitary b.** A condition ascribed to an excess of basophil cells (adenoma) of the adenohypophysis; characterized by painful, plethoric obesity of the face and trunk, weakness, osteoporosis, amenorrhea or impotence, arterial hypertension, polycythemia, hyperglycemia, adrenal cortical hypertrophy, and gonadal atrophy. Also called *Cushing's disease*.

ba"so·pho'bi·a (bay"so·fo'bee·uh, bas"o·). A morbid fear of walking or standing erect, without muscular impairment. —**basophobic,** *adj.;* **basophobiac,** *n*.

bas'si·net'. An infant's crib or bed; a wicker basket with a hood at one end, used as a cradle.

bas'so·rin. A tasteless, odorless, vegetable gum, insoluble in cold water, found in gum tragacanth.

bath. 1. A bathing place or room. 2. Any yielding medium such as air, vapor, sand, or water, in which the body is wholly or partially immersed for therapeutic purposes. It may be designed to cleanse, to soothe, to stimulate, to irritate, to heat, or to cool. **air b.** The therapeutic exposure of the naked body to air. **alcohol b.** The sponging of the body with dilute alcohol for its soothing and cooling effect. **astringent b.** One in which the body or a part is immersed in a solution of alum, tannic acid, or other astringent. **bed b.** One given to a patient in his own bed.

bland b. Immersion in a bath containing bran or starch for relief of irritation, itching, or urticaria. **bran b.** See bland *b*. **brine b.** Immersion of the body in a strong solution of salt water. **cabinet b.** An air bath given by placing the patient in a cabinet which is heated by means of numerous electric light bulbs. **cold b.** One given in water of 50°–60° F. **continuous b.** One in which a patient is restrained in a tub and immersed in water from 90°–98° F. for hours at a time. It is used for its sedative effect on agitated or maniacal patients. Also called *continuous tub*. **contrast b.** The alternate immersion of the hands or feet in hot and cold water. **cool b.** One in water 60°–75° F. **effervescent b.** Immersion of the patient in water in which carbon dioxide is released. This may be natural or introduced. **electric cabinet b.** See cabinet *b*. **foot b.** One restricted to the feet. **full b.** One in which the entire body except the head is immersed. **graduated b.** One in which the temperature is gradually lowered. **hafussi b.** A form of Nauheim bath in which only the hands and feet of the patient are immersed. **half b.** One restricted to the lower half of the body. Also called *hip b*. **hot air b.** Exposing the whole body to hot air circulating in a bath cabinet. **hot b.** One in which the water has a temperature of 98°–108° F. **hydroelectric b.** Applying faradic, galvanic, or sinusoidal currents to a patient through water. **medicated b.** One to which a medicinal substance has been added. **mustard b.** One in which powdered mustard has been included. **Nauheim b.** An effervescent bath popularized at Nauheim, using naturally hot, carbonated water. **needle b.** Shower bath which throws very fine jets of water under forceful pressure. **oxygen b.** An effervescent bath employing oxygen instead of carbon dioxide. **paraffin b.** Apparatus for the infiltration of pieces of tissues with molten paraffin before imbedding them for sectioning. **radioactive b.** One which is given in water having radioactive properties. **Russian b.** Hot vapor bath followed by a rubdown and a cold plunge. **sand b.** Covering the body with warm, dry sand. **Scotch b.** Usually called *Scotch douche*. One given to a patient in the erect position by playing a forceful stream of alternately hot and cold water on the patient's body. **sea b.** A bath in sea water, usually heated. Also called *salt water b*. **sedative b.** A prolonged, warm, full bath. **sheet b.** A cooling bath given by sprinkling tepid water on a sheet which is spread over the patient. **shower b.** One given by spraying the patient with water from an overhead fixture. **sitz b.** One given in a specially built tub so that only the patient's lower back, hips, and upper thighs are immersed. **sponge b.** One in which the body is sponged one part at a time without being immersed. **starch b.** A bland bath using starch. **stimulating b.** One containing tonic, astringent, or aromatic substances which increase the cutaneous effect and stimulate the body circulation. **sun b.** The exposure of part or all the body to the sun for the actinic effect. **sweat b.** Given by any one of several methods to apply heat to the body and produce sweating. **tannic acid b.** The immersion of all or part of the body in a solution of tannic acid for its astringent effect; formerly used in the treatment of extensive burns. **tepid b.** One employing water at about 80°–92° F. **tub b.** Any bath in which the body is immersed in a tub. **Turkish b.** One in which the bather is placed in steam rooms of successively higher temperature, then is rubbed and massaged and finally stimulated by a cold shower. **vapor b.** One in which the bather is exposed to vapors. **warm b.** One in which the water has a temperature of 85°–95° F. **water b.** In chemistry, an apparatus for drying solids containing moisture or for evaporating fluids without subjecting them to a heat that will cause disintegration or dissipation of the contained substance. **whirlpool b.** One in which an arm, or leg, or the greater part of the body is immersed in hot water which is agitated by a whirling or churning current of equally hot water mixed with air.

bath″o·pho′bi·a. Morbid fear of depths.

bath″y·car′di·a. A condition in which the heart is in a lower position than usual; the condition is an anatomic one, and is not the result of disease.

bat″o·pho′bi·a. 1. Dread of high objects, as fear of passing near a high building or of going through a deep valley. 2. Morbid fear of being at great heights.

bat′ter·y. 1. A device which converts chemical to electric energy. 2. A series of two or more pieces of apparatus connected so as to augment their effects, as a battery of boilers, prisms, or galvanic cells.

Bau′ru ul′cer. See *leishmaniasis americana*.

bay′ber″ry. The wax myrtle *Myrica cerifera* or *M. pennsylvanica*.

BCG. Bacillus Calmette-Guérin, or the vaccine prepared from this organism, recommended for immunization against tuberculosis. It has been suggested that the vaccine might also give some protection against leprosy.

b.d. *Bis die;* twice a day; used in prescriptions.

bdel′li·um (del′ee·um). A resinous gum exuding from various species of *Commiphora*. It resembles myrrh.

Be. Chemical symbol for beryllium.

bead′ed. 1. Beadlike. 2. *In bacteriology,* the term is applied to the nonuniform appearance of certain organisms such as the diphtheria bacillus when stained.

bead′ing of ribs. See *rachitic rosary.* Also called *rachitic beads.*

bear′ing down. The feeling of weight or pressure in the pelvis in certain diseases. **b.-d. pains.** Expulsive pains in labor.

beat. An impulse or throb, as of the heart and blood vessels. **anomalous b.** An abnormally distributed excitation wave in the ventricles. **apex b.** The striking of the chest wall by the heart apex during each systole. It can be felt, and sometimes seen, in the fifth left intercostal space. Syn., *point of maximum impulse.* **dropped b.** Condition noted in extrasystoles, when an occasional ventricular beat is lost. **ectopic b.** A beat or rhythmic series of beats initiated by ectopic impulses. **forced b.** An extrasystole initiated by artificial stimulation. **idioventricular b.** One following a long diastole, originating in the atrioventricular node or below it. **premature b.** An extrasystole. **retrograde b.** Excitation of the atrium by the ventricle; the P wave following the R of the ECG.

Beaumont, William [*American Army surgeon,* 1785–1853]. Internationally famous for his observations and experiments on human digestion (1822–33). By means of his access to the gastric fistula suffered by Alexis St. Martin, he was the first to study the process of digestion in life, and his work on this subject was the most important in existence, up to the time of Pavlov.

be·bee′rine (bi·bee′reen, ·rin). An alkaloid, from the root of *Cissampelos pareira* or from *Ocotea rodioei* (*Nectandra*). Also called *chondrodendrine.*

bed. The couch or support on which the body may rest in sleep or in sickness. **air b.** One with an inflatable rubber mattress. **fracture b.** One especially devised for patients with broken bones. **hydrostatic b.** One with a rubber mattress partially filled with water to prevent bedsores. **metabolic b.** One especially arranged to save fluid and solid waste of the patient. **surgical b.** One equipped with a double windlass which raises and lowers, independently, the foot and the head of the bed. **vasoscillator b.**

One which may be tipped to provide postural vascular exercise. Also called *Sanders b.* **water b.** Hydrostatic bed, *q.v.*

bed'bug''. A blood-sucking insect belonging to the genus *Cimex* which lives and lays its eggs in the crevices of bedsteads, upholstered furniture, and walls. It is apparently not a vector of pathogenic organisms, although it has been suspected. *Cimex lectularius* is the most common species in the temperate zone; *C. hemipterus* is the most common in the tropics.

bed'fast''. Bedridden, *q.v.*

bed net. A mosquito bar or netting suspended over the bed, its edges being tucked in about the mattress to prevent the entrance of insects.

bed'pan''. A shallow, suitably shaped receptacle for receiving solid and fluid waste from patients confined to bed.

bed'rid''den. Designating an individual permanently confined to bed. Syn., *bedfast.*

bed'sore''. An ulceration caused by pressure against the bed, generally occurring in those confined to bed for long periods; decubitus ulcer.

bees'wax. Yellow wax, *q.v.*

Bekhterev, Vladimir Mikhailovich [*Russian neurologist,* 1857–1927]. Widely known for his many contributions in the fields of neurology, especially in cerebral localization and experimental psychology. Described an kylosing spondylitis (1892), called *Bekhterev's disease, Strümpell-Marie disease, atrophic spinal arthritis, rheumatoid spinal arthritis.*

bel. A unit frequently used to measure the intensity of sound, commonly the intensity above the normal threshold of hearing. See *decibel.*

bel, bael (bell, bay'el). The dried, half-ripe fruit of *Ægle marmelos,* of India. Has been used as a remedy for chronic diarrhea and dysentery.

Bell, Charles [*Scottish physician,* 1774–1842]. Internationally known for his studies in anatomy, physiology, and neurology. His *System of Dissections* (1798–1803) was published while he was studying medicine. His experimental work on the motor functions of ventral spinal nerve roots is the earliest of its kind (1811). He demonstrated the sensory and motor functions of the fifth cranial nerve and the cause of facial palsy (1821); neuropathy of the facial nerve is also called *Bell's palsy.*

bel''la·don'na. Deadly nightshade. A perennial plant, *Atropa belladonna,* the leaves and root of which are used in various forms for antispasmodic, cardiac, and respiratory stimulant, secretion inhibiting, and anodyne effects. See *atropine.*

bel''la·don'nine (bel''uh·don'een ·in). $C_{17}H_{21}O_2N$. An alkaloid found in solanaceous plants as belladonna, hyoscyamus.

bel'ly. The abdominal cavity or abdomen, *q.v.* See words beginning *celi-* **b. button.** Navel or umbilicus. **b. of a muscle.** The most prominent fleshy, central portion of a muscle.

bel'ly·ache''. Pain in the abdomen colic.

ben·ac'ty·zine hy''dro·chlo'-ride. Benzilic acid diethylaminoethyl ester hydrochloride, a psychotherapeutic agent. See *suavitil.*

benadryl hydrochloride. Trademark for diphenhydramine hydrochloride.

Benedict's reagents. See under *reagent.*

Benedict's solution. See under *solution.*

Benedict's test. See under *test.*

benemid. Trade-mark for probenecid.

be·nign', be·nig'nant. Not endangering health or life; not malignant, innocent; applied to certain tumors.

ben'ne oil. Sesame oil.

benodaine hydrochloride. Trademark for piperoxan hydrochloride.

benoquin. Trade-mark for monobenzone.

ben·ox'i·nate hy''dro·chlo'ride. β-Diethylaminoethyl 4-amino-3-n-butoxybenzoate hydrochloride, a local anesthetic. See *dorsacaine hydrochloride.*

ben'ton·ite. A native, colloidal, hydrated aluminum silicate used as a suspending agent.

benz·al'de·hyde. $C_6H_5.CHO$. A colorless liquid, used as a flavoring agent

ben''zal·ko'ni·um chlo'ride. A mixture of alkyl dimethyl-benzylammonium chlorides. In solution of proper concentration it is an effective surface disinfectant. See *zephiran chloride.*

benz·an'thra·cenes. A group of hydrocarbons in which a benzene and anthracene ring have a double bond in common.

benz'a·thine pen'i·cil'lin G. N,N'-Dibenzylethylenediamine dipenicillin G, a long-acting penicillin which can be taken orally. See *bicillin, neolin permapen.*

benz·az'o·line hy''dro·chlo'-ride. Tolazoline hydrochloride.

benzedrex. Trade-mark for propyl hexedrine.

benzedrine. A trade-mark for amphetamine.

ben'zene, ben·zene'. A liquid hydrocarbon, C_6H_6, obtained chiefly as by-product in the manufacture of coke It is used extensively as a solvent **b. hexachloride.** $C_6H_6Cl_6$. Commonly, the gamma isomer of 1,2,3,4,5,6 hexachlorocyclohexane, a potent insecticide. See *gammexane*, *lindane*.

ben·zes'trol. A synthetic estrogenic substance, 2,4-di(p-hydroxyphenyl)-3-ethyl-hexane.

benz''e·tho'ni·um chlo'ride. Benzyldimethyl{2-[2-(p-1,1,3,3-tetramethylbutylphenoxy) ethoxy] ethyl} ammonium chloride, a detergent and antiseptic. See *phemerol chloride*.

ben'zi·dine (ben'zi·deen, ·din). Diaminodiphenyl, a colorless crystalline compound; used in identification of occult blood. See under *test*.

ben'zin, ben'zine (ben'zin, ben'zeen, ben·zeen'). A mixture of hydrocarbons obtained in the fractional distillation of petroleum. Also called *petroleum* b.

ben'zo-, benz-. A combining form denoting *relation to benzene*, *presence of the benzene ring*, or *azo colors used for direct dyeing of cotton*.

ben'zo·ate. Any salt of benzoic acid, as sodium benzoate.

ben'zo·caine (ben'zo·cane, ·kay·in). Ethyl aminobenzoate. See *anesthesin*.

ben·zo'ic ac'id. C_6H_5COOH. White scales or needles, soluble in water. A mild antiseptic.

ben·zo'ic al'de·hyde. See *benzaldehyde*.

ben'zo·in (ben'zo·in, ·zoyn). A balsamic resin obtained from *Styrax benzoin*, *S. tonkinensis*, and other species of *Styrax*. Used as a stimulating expectorant, as an inhalant in respiratory-tract inflammations, and as an external antiseptic and protective. Syn., *gum benjamin*. Also called *gum* b. —**benzo'inated**, *adj.* **compound b. tinc·ture.** Prepared from benzoin 10, aloe 2, storax 8, tolu balsam 4, alcohol to make 100. Also called *friar's* or *Turlington's balsam*.

ben'zol, ben'zole. See *benzene*.

ben''zo·naph'thol. Betanaphthyl benzoate, *q.v.*

ben''zo·py'rene. $C_{20}H_{12}$. A carcinogenic substance obtained from tar.

ben''zo·sul'fa·mide. Saccharin.

ben'zo·yl (ben'zo·il, ·eel). The monovalent radical C_6H_5CO-, derived from benzoic acid. **b.·gly·co·coll.** Hippuric acid. **b.·gly·col'ic acid.** Mandelic acid. **b. green.** Malachite green.

benz''py·rin'i·um bro'mide. 1-Benzyl-3-(dimethylcarbamyloxy)-pyridinium bromide, a cholinergic agent. See *stigmonene bromide*.

benz·tro'pine meth''ane·sul'fon·ate. 3-Diphenylmethoxytropane methanesulfonate, a parasympatholytic agent. See *cogentin methanesulfonate*.

ben'zyl (ben'zil, ·zeel). The univalent radical, $C_6H_5CH_2-$. **b. alcohol.** $C_6H_5CH_2OH$. Phenyl methyl alcohol, a colorless liquid, soluble in water; employed as a local anesthetic. Syn.,

phenylcarbinol. **b. benzoate.** $C_6H_5·CO_2.CH_2.C_6H_5$. Colorless crystals or oily liquid; insoluble in water. Used as a remedy for scabies.

ben·xyl'i·dene. The divalent radical, $C_6H_5CH=$ or $C_6H_5CH<$.

ber'ber·ine (bur'bur·een, ·in). $C_{20}H_{19}NO_5$. An alkaloid found in *Berberis* and many other plants.

ber'ber·is. Barberry; the dried rhizome and roots of various shrubs of the genus *Mahonia*. Used as a bitter tonic.

Berger, Hans [*German neurologist*, 1873–1941]. Remembered for his descriptions of the alpha rhythm and the waves recorded in encephalography.

Bergey, David Hendricks [*American bacteriologist*, 1860–1937]. Celebrated for his systematic arrangement or key for the identification of the class Schizomycetes in his *Manual of Determinative Bacteriology* (1923).

ber'i·ber'i. A disease due to deficiency of thiamine; seen endemically in those living mainly on a polished rice diet, and sporadically in other countries when the diet is similarly limited. Various manifestations occur, depending upon the severity and duration of the vitamin lack. Multiple neuritis, general weakness, paralysis, progressive edema, mental deterioration, and finally heart failure make up the classic picture.

Berkefeld filter. See under *filter*.

berke'li·um. Chemical element No. 97, symbol Bk, produced artificially in minute amounts.

Ber·lin' blue. See *aniline blue*.

Bernard, Claude [*French physiologist*, 1813–78]. One of the greatest figures in the history of physiology, he introduced experimental methods (1855). Demonstrated nerve paralysis by the use of curare, showing the independent excitability of muscle. Discovered the vasoconstrictor and dilator nerves. Demonstrated the glycogenic function of the liver and the digestive action of pancreatic juice (1848). He is said to have coined the term internal secretions (1855). The syndrome following section or paralysis of the cervical sympathetic trunk is known as the *Bernard-Horner syndrome*, *Horner's syndrome*. See Johann Friedrich Horner.

Ber''ti·el'la. A genus of tapeworm parasites. **B. mucronata.** A species parasitic to man, found in the intestine.

Bertillon, Alphonse [*French criminologist*, 1853–1914]. Inventor of the system of identification which bears his name (1886). It consists of selected measurements of various parts of the body. The *Bertillon system* has been largely superseded by the use of fingerprints.

Bertin, column of. See renal *column.*

be·ryl″li·o′sis. Pneumonoconiosis due to inhalation of beryllium oxide dust. **acute b.** Acute pneumonitis in beryllium workers. **chronic b.** Chronic pulmonary granulomatosis in beryllium workers.

be·ryl′li·um. Be = 9.02. A divalent metallic element. Formerly called *glucinum.*

bes″ti·al′i·ty. 1. Behavior resembling that of an animal. 2. *In psychiatry*, sexual relations between human beings and animals.

be′ta (bee′tuh, bay′tuh). The second letter of the Greek alphabet, β; used in chemical nomenclature to indicate the second of two isomeric compounds.

be″ta·eu·caine hy″dro·chlo′ride. Eucaine hydrochloride, *q.v.*

be″ta·hy·poph′a·mine (-high·pof′-a-meen, ·min). The pressor principle of neurohypophysis.

be′ta·ine. 1. Any one of a group of compounds characterized by the radical (CH₃)₃N<. 2. Trimethylglycocoll.

be″ta·ke′to·hy·drox″y·bu·tyr′ic ac′id. Acetoacetic acid.

be″ta·naph′thol. C₁₀H₇OH. White crystalline leaflets or powder; an effective intestinal antiseptic and also useful, in the form of an ointment or alcoholic solution, as a parasiticide. Also called *naphthol, β-naphthol.*

be″ta·naph′thyl. The radical C₁₀H₇—. **b. benzoate.** C₆H₅COO·-C₁₀H₇. White, crystalline powder used as intestinal antiseptic and as parasiticide. Also called *benzonaphthol, beta-naphthol benzoate.*

be″ta·ox″y·bu·tyr′ic ac′id. CH₃·CHOH.CH₂.COOH. Beta-hydroxybutyric acid, an acid formed when fatty acids are incompletely oxidized.

be′ta par′ti·cle. One of the radiations emitted by certain radioactive materials, identical with the electrons found in the outer structure of all atoms. It has a unit negative charge equal and opposite to the positive charge of the proton and is nearly weightless, having less than ¹⁄₁₈₀₀ the mass of a proton.

be′ta·tron (bay′tuh·tron, bee′tuh·tron). An instrument with which electrons are accelerated to millions of electron volts by magnetic induction.

be′ta·zole hy″dro·chlo′ride. 3-(β-Aminoethyl)pyrazole dihydrochloride, a diagnostic agent for gastric anacidity. See *histalog.*

be·thane′chol chlo′ride. β-Methylcholine carbamate chloride, a parasympathomimetic agent not destroyed by cholinesterase. See *urecholine chloride.*

be·tween′brain. The diencephalon.

be′zoar (bee′zor, bee′zo·ar). A concretion found in the stomach or intestine of some animals (especially ruminants), most commonly composed of ingested hair. Also found in some psychopathic patients. Also called *hair ball.*

bhang. See *cannabis.*

B.H.C. Abbreviation for the insecticide benzene hexachloride (hexachlorocyclohexane).

Bi. Chemical symbol for bismuth.

bi- (buy-). 1. A prefix meaning *two, twice, double.* 2. *In anatomy*, a prefix denoting *connection with* or *relation to each of two symmetrically paired parts.* 3. *In chemistry*, a prefix denoting *the presence of two atoms* or *equivalents of* the constituent to the name of which it is attached or *the presence of this* constituent *in double the usual proportion* or *in double the proportion of the other component.*

bi′ased sam′ple. A sample which is not representative of its field.

bi″a·stig′ma·tism. Condition of the eye in which both corneal and lenticular astigmatism exist.

bib″li·o·klep″to·ma′ni·a. Morbid desire to steal books.

bib″li·o·ma′ni·a. An abnormal or intense desire to collect rare or curious books.

bib″li·o·pho′bi·a. A morbid fear or hatred of books.

bi·bo′rate. See *borate.*

bi·cap′i·tate. Having two heads; bicephalous; dicephalous.

bi·car′bon·ate. Any carbonic acid salt in which only one of the hydrogen atoms has been replaced by a metal. The radical —HCO₃. **blood b.** The amount of bicarbonate present in the blood indicating the alkali reserve. Also called *plasma b.*

bi′ceps. A muscle having two heads as the biceps brachii, the biceps femoris. See Table of Muscles in the Appendix. **—bicip′ital,** *adj.*

bi·chlo′ride. 1. Any salt containing two equivalents of chlorine. 2. A careless designation of mercury bichloride.

bicillin. A trade-mark for benzathine penicillin G.

bi·cor′nate, bi·cor′nu·ate, bi″cor·nute′ (buy′kor·newt′, buy·kor′-newt), **bi·cor′nous.** Having two horns, as a bicornate uterus.

bi·cus′pid. Having two cusps, as bicuspid teeth.

b. i. d. *Bis in die*; twice daily.

bi·dac′ty·ly. Congenital absence of all fingers or toes except the first and fifth; lobster-claw deformity.

Bie′brich scar′let (bee′brick). An acid disazo dye used in aqueous solution as a plasma stain. Also called *croceine scarlet, double scarlet BSF, Ponceau B, scarlet B* or *EC.*

Bielschowsky, Max [*German neuropathologist, 1869–1940*]. Known for his discoveries relating to tumors of the glial and reticuloendothelial systems. Devised silver staining methods for the nervous system. Described late infantile amaurotic familial idiocy.

bi′fid. Divided into two parts; cleft, as bifid uvula.

bi·fo′cal. Having two foci; applied to a system of lenses or spectacles called **bifocals**. The latter are used in the correction of presbyopia, where there is a refractive error for distant vision. The distance lens is above. Three types of bifocals are commonly used, the greater refractive power being obtained by: (a) cementing a wafer onto the front or back of the lens (**cement bifocals**); (b) fusing an insert of denser glass, as flint glass, into a crown-glass lens (**fused bifocals**); or (c) grinding the two different curvatures on one glass (**one-piece bifocals**).

bi′fur·ca′tion. Division into two branches. —**bi′furcate**, *adj.*, *v.t.*, *v.i.*

Bigelow, Jacob [*American physician and botanist, 1787–1879*]. One of the great botanists of America and celebrated as the author of a discourse on self-limited disease (1835). Said to have rescued medicine from the slavery of the drugging system.

bi·gem′i·nal. Occurring in pairs; double; twin.

bi′labe. A surgical instrument for removing foreign bodies from the bladder through the urethra.

bi·lat′er·al. Relating to two sides; pertaining to or affecting both sides of the body. —**bilateralism**, *n.*

bile. A very bitter, alkaline, greenish yellow to golden-brown fluid, secreted by the liver and poured into the duodenum. It contains bile salts, cholesterol, lecithin, fat, various pigments, and mucin. Functionally, it aids in the emulsification, digestion, and absorption of fats, in the alkalinization of the intestines, and in the prevention of putrefaction.

bile ac′id. Any one of the naturally occurring acids of bile formed by the conjugation of glycine or taurine with a cholic acid, *q.v.*, forming glycocholic and taurocholic acids, respectively. **unconjugated b. a.** The residual cholic acid remaining when glycine or taurine is removed from a bile acid.

Bil·har′zi·a. Old term for *Schistosoma*.

bil″har·xi′a·sis. See *schistosomiasis*, 1.

bil′i- (bil′i-, buy″li-). A combining form signifying a *relationship to bile or the biliary system*.

bil′i·ar″y. Pertaining to or conveying bile, as a biliary duct.

bil″i·cy′a·nin. A blue pigment obtained by the interaction of bilirubin and zinc chloride.

bil″i·fla′vin. A yellow coloring matter derivable from biliverdin.

bil″i·ful′vin. Bilirubin.

bil″i·fus′cin (bil″i-fuss′in, buy″li-). A dark brown powder obtained from bile pigment.

bil″i·hu′min. An insoluble residue left after treating gallstones with various solvents.

bil″i·neu′rine (bil″i-new′reen, -rin). Choline.

bil′ious. 1. Pertaining to bile. 2. Popular term designating disorders arising from an excess of bile.

bil′ious·ness. Popular term for a condition marked by general malaise, headache, anorexia, indigestion, coated tongue, constipation, and lassitude; attributed to disorders of biliary secretions, but probably due to a digestive disorder.

bil″i·pha′in. Bilirubin.

bil″i·pra′sin. A bile pigment formed in the oxidation of bilirubin to biliverdin. Syn., *choleprasin*.

bil″i·pur′pu·rin. Cholehematin, *q.v.*

bil″i·ru′bin (bil″i-roo′bin, buy″li-). Orange-red crystals or powder. The principal pigment of bile. See Table of Normal Values of Blood Constituents in the Appendix.

bil″i·ru″bi·ne′mi·a, bil′i·ru″bi·nae′mi·a (bil″i-roo″bi-nee′-mee-uh, buy″li-). The presence of bilirubin in the blood; jaundice, icterus.

bil″i·ru″bi·nu′ri·a. Presence of bilirubin in the urine.

bil″i·u′ri·a. The presence of bile salts in the urine.

bil″i·ver′din. Dark green, amorphous powder. A bile pigment.

bil″i·xan′thine (bil″i-zan′theen, buy″li-), **bil″i·xan′thin.** See *choletelin*.

Billings, John Shaw [*American Army medical officer and librarian, 1838–1913*]. Well-known medical bibliographer and authority on public health and vital statistics. Compilation of the *Index-Catalogue of the Library of the Surgeon General* was begun under his direction (1880). With Robert Fletcher, founded the monthly *Index Medicus* (1879). Author of *History of Surgery* (1895). Responsible for the plans of the Johns Hopkins Hospital.

bill of health. An authenticated document issued by quarantine or other public health officials to a ship's master after inspection, to indicate the state of health of the ship's company and of the port.

bi·lo′bate (buy·lo′bait). Having, or divided into, two lobes.

bi·loc′u·lar, bi·loc′u·late. Having two cells, compartments, or chambers.

bi·man'u·al. Pertaining to both hands; done by both hands.

bi'na·ry. 1. *In chemistry*, compounded of two elements. 2. *In anatomy*, separating into two branches or parts.

bi·na'sal (buy·nay'zul). Referring to both nasal visual fields, as binasal hemianopsia.

bin·au'ral. Pertaining to or having two ears. Also called *binauricular*, *binotic*.

bind. 1. To bandage; join together with a band. 2. *In chemistry*, unite with, as in the combination of two substances having affinity.

bind'er. A wide bandage or girdle worn to support the abdomen or breasts after childbirth or operations, as an obstetric or abdominal binder.

Binet, Alfred [*French psychologist*, *1857–1911*]. Devised an intelligence test, with Théodore Simon, in which the intellectual capacity of the subject is estimated by comparison with that of normal children and adolescents of various ages; the mental age divided by the chronologic age gives the intelligence quotient (I.Q.). Called *Binet's test*, *Binet-Simon test*. *Binet's formula* states that children under nine whose mental development is retarded by two years probably are mentally deficient, and that children of nine or more who are retarded by three years are definitely deficient.

bin·oc'u·lar. Pertaining to both eyes. *In optics*, instrument with two eyepieces for use with both eyes at once. See *horopter*.

bin·ox'ide. See *dioxide*.

bi'o-, bi-. A combining form denoting *relation to*, or *connection with*, *life*, *vital phenomena*, or *living organisms*.

bi'o-as·say". Estimation of the concentration of a given drug by comparing it with a standard preparation, and by noting the amounts of each necessary to produce a definite effect on a test animal under the same conditions. Syn., *biological assay*.

bi"o·chem'is·try. The chemistry of the living tissues or of life; physiological chemistry. **—biochemical,** *adj*.

bi"o·chem·or'phic. Noting the relationship between chemical structure and biologic activity; relating to biochemorphology.

bi"o·chem"or·phol·o·gy.   The science dealing with the chemical structure of foods and drugs and their reactions on living organisms.

bi"o·cli'ma·tol'o·gy. The study of the effect of climate on life. Also called *bioclimatics*.

bi"o·cy'tin. A complex of biotin occurring in yeast and possibly in other natural products.

bi"o·e·lec"tric'i·ty. Electric phenomena occurring in living tissues; effects of electric currents upon living tissues.

bi"o·en"er·get'ics. The science of the transformation of energy in biologic functions.

bi'o·fla'vo·noids. A classification for flavone compounds or derivatives having biological activity in various animal species.

bi"o·gen'e·sis. 1. The doctrine that living things are produced only from living things—the reverse of abiogenesis. 2. Also a general term to include both ontogeny and phylogeny. **—biogenet'ic, biog'enous,** *adj*.

bi·og'e·ny (buy·odj'i·nee). Biogenesis.

bi"o·ki·net'ics (buy"o·ki·net'icks, ·kigh·net'icks). The kinetics of life; the science of the movements of developing organisms. See *karyokinesis*.

bi"o·ki·net'ic   tem'per·a·ture lim'its. The lowest and highest temperatures beyond which no form of life can be sustained: −273° C. to approximately 150° C.

Biol. Biology.

bi"o·log'i·cal as·say'. A method of determining the potency of a substance by comparing its effects on living material quantitatively with those of a standard substance. Syn., *bio-assay*.

bi"o·log'i·cals. Medicinal preparations of a complex biologic nature, their action depending on numerous phases of immunity. They include serums, vaccines, antitoxins, and antigens. **lyophilized b.** Any biologic substance, such as blood plasma, antitoxins, toxins, serums, etc., which has been prepared in dry form by rapid freezing and dehydration, while in the frozen state, under high vacuum.

bi·ol'o·gist. One learned in biology.

bi·ol'o·gy. The science of life. It includes botany, zoology, and all their branches. **—biolog'ic, biolog'ical,** *adj*.

bi"o·lu"mi·nes'cence. Luminescence caused by living organisms; phosphorescence.

bi"o·math"e·mat'ics. Mathematics applied to biologic phenomena.

bi"o·me·chan'ics. The science dealing with the mechanics of the living organism, especially of the levers and arches of the skeleton, and the forces applied to them by the muscles and by gravity.

bi·om'e·try. 1. The statistical study of biologic problems; biometrics. 2. Calculation of the expectancy of life, for life insurance purposes.

bi"o·pho·tom'e·ter. An instrument designed to measure the rate and degree of dark adaptation.

bi"o·phys'ics. The study of life processes by physical apparatus and methods; the physics of life processes.

bi'op·sy. 1. Observation of the living subject, as opposed to necropsy. 2. The excision, during life, of tissue to establish a diagnosis by means of a microscopic examination of the excised piece. **muscle b.** The most specific means of diagnosis for trichinosis.

bi'os I. See *inositol*.

bi'os IIb. See *biotin*.

bi'ose. 1. A disaccharide. 2. A sugar containing two carbon atoms.

bi"o·sta·tis'tics. The branch of biometry which deals with the laws and data of demography, natality, morbidity, and mortality; vital statistics.

bi·os'ter·ol. Old term for vitamin A.

bi"o·syn'the·sis. The formation of a substance occurring in the presence of or due to the metabolism of living cells or tissues.

bi'o·tin (buy'o·tin, buy·ot'in). A member of the vitamin-B complex, widely distributed in plant and animal tissues; essential for growth of certain bacteria and yeasts. Syn., *vitamin H, coenzyme R.*

bi'o·type. 1. A group of individuals all of which have the same genotype. 2. Constitutional (body) type. **–biotyp'ic,** *adj.*

bip'a·ra. A woman who has borne two children at different labors.

bi"pa·ri'e·tal. Relating to both parietal bones; as the biparietal diameter, the distance from one parietal eminence to the other.

bi'ped. 1. Having two feet. 2. An animal with two feet. **–bipedal,** *adj.*

bi·pen'nate. See *bipenniform.*

bi·pen'ni·form (buy·pen'i·form), **bi·pen'nate** (buy·pen'ate). Having the appearance of a feather with barbs on both sides, as certain muscles.

bipp. Dressing for wounds, composed of bismuth subnitrate 1 part, iodoform 2 parts, petrolatum 1 part. Also called *B.I.P.,* bismuth iodoform paste.

bi"re·frac'tive. Doubly refractive; anisotropic.

bi"re·frin'gence. Double refraction, *q.v.,* in biologic objects three types occur: crystalline, form, and strain birefringences. **stream b.** That occurring when solutions containing asymmetric particles are set into motion and the particles tend to orient as a result of the flow. When the flow stops, the solution becomes isotropic. The tobacco mosaic virus is such a particle.

birth. 1. The delivery of offspring. 2. That which is born. See *labor.* **cross b.** Transverse presentation, *q.v.* **multiple b.** The occurrence of two or more offspring at a birth. **partial b.** In labor, the incomplete expulsion of offspring, as in a macerated fetus. **plu-**

ral **b.** See multiple *b.* **premature b.** See premature *labor.* **stillbirth.** The birth of dead offspring.

birth cer·tif'i·cate. A legal form on which the date and place of birth, name and sex of child, names of parents, and other pertinent information are recorded.

birth con·trol'. The prevention or regulation of conception by whatever means; contraception.

birth in'ju·ry. Any injury suffered by a child during parturition, such as fracture of a bone, subluxation of a joint, injury to peripheral nerves, or intracranial hemorrhage.

birth'mark". A nevus, either vascular, nonvascular, or pigmented.

birth rate. The proportion of births in a given year to the total population, known as the **crude birth rate. Specific birth rates** are figured for the female population, for the females of certain age or race groups, or for other variables.

birth reg"is·tra'tion a're·a. That territory from which the United States Bureau of the Census collects birth records. Since 1933, this has been the entire United States.

bis-. 1. A prefix meaning *twice, both.* 2. *In chemistry,* a prefix denoting *the doubling of a complex expression.*

bi·sex'u·al (buy·seck'shoo·ul). Having male and female sex organs; hermaphroditic.

bis"hy·drox"y·cou'ma·rin (·koo'muh·rin). A white, crystalline compound, 3,3'-methylene-bis-(4-hydroxycoumarin), occurring in spoiled sweet clover and hay, and prepared synthetically. It is an anticoagulant of use in thromboses. Syn., *dicoumarin, dicoumarol, melitoxin.* See *dicumarol.*

Bis'marck brown Y (C.C.). An aniline dye of the azo series; used as a biological stain. Also called *Vesuvin; phenylene brown; Manchester brown; excelsior brown; leather brown; basic brown G, GX,* or *GXP; aniline brown.*

bis'muth (biz'muth). Bi = 209.00. A white, crystalline metal with a reddish tint. Its insoluble salts are employed chiefly for their protective action on mucous membranes; the salts are also feebly antiseptic. Various compounds of bismuth are employed for the treatment of syphilis. **b. and emetine iodide.** A reddish orange salt, practically insoluble in water; used in the treatment of amebic dysentery. **b. and potassium tartrate.** A basic bismuth potassium bismuthotartrate, soluble in water. Employed in the treatment of syphilis. **b. and sodium tartrate.** A water-soluble salt used like bismuth and potassium tartrate. **b. carbonate.** The official British Pharmacopoeia name for bismuth subcarbonate. **b. oxychloride.** A white, water-insoluble salt approximating the composition BiOCl; may be used internally for the same purposes as bismuth subnitrate; also used as an antisyphilitic. **b. salicylate.** The name occasionally applied to bismuth subsalicylate, but used properly only for a mixture of salicylic acid and bismuth subsalicylate. **b. subcarbonate.** A white salt, insoluble in water; used as a protective in gastrointestinal diseases as well as for local application. **b. subgallate.** A bright yellow powder, practically insoluble in water. Employed externally as a dusting powder; sometimes used internally in treating enteritis. **b. subnitrate.** A basic salt of varying composition, practically insoluble in water. It is used like bismuth subcarbonate. **b. subsalicylate.** A basic salt of varying composition; practically insoluble in water. It is used in the treatment of enteritis, and as an antisyphilitic. **precipitated b.** A finely subdivided form of metallic bismuth, used as an injection in the treatment of syphilis.

bis'muth·yl (biz'muth-il, ·eel). The univalent radical BiO—.

bis'tou·ry (biss'too-ree). A long, narrow knife, either straight, curved, sharp-pointed, or probe-pointed, used for cutting from within outward. Its use in surgery is confined to the incision of abscesses, the opening of sinuses or fistulas, or, occasionally, the cutting of the constriction in strangulated hernia.

bi·sul'fide (buy-sul'fide, ·fid). A binary compound containing two atoms of sulfur. Syn., *disulfide.*

bi·sul'fite. Any compound containing the radical —HSO₃. An acid sulfite.

bit. *In dentistry,* a rotary drill.

bi·tar'trate. Any compound containing the radical —HC₄H₄O₆. An acid tartrate.

bite. 1. The forcible closure of the lower against the upper teeth; the measure of force exerted by such closure as recorded in pounds by the gnathodynamometer. 2. A skin puncture produced by the teeth or mouth parts of an insect, snake, or other animal. 3. *In dental prosthetics,* a plastic impression of the relationship of the upper and lower teeth in occlusion; known as *the bite.* 4. Seize or grasp with the teeth. 5. Corrode or eat into by chemical action. **check b.** A plastic impression of the teeth, serving as a guide for alignment in the articulator; used in orthodontics and dental prosthetics. It consists of bites taken in hard wax or soft modeling compound, which record centric and eccentric occlusion. **closed b.** One in which the lower incisors and canines are posterior

to the upper, almost touching the gum line when the jaws are closed; extreme overbite. **edge-to-edge b.** The meeting of the cutting edges of the upper and lower anterior teeth. Also called *end-to-end b.* **jumping the b.** A forcible shifting forward of a retruded lower jaw to obtain a normal occlusion. **mush b.** A record of the relation of upper and lower jaws obtained in a mass of wax into which the patient bites. **open b.** A condition in which the upper and lower incisors do not occlude. **opening the b.** Elevation of the occlusal plane of some or all of the posterior teeth by orthodontic manipulations or prosthetic restorations.

bite'wing. A type of dental x-ray film having a central fin or wing upon which the teeth can close to hold the film in place.

bi·thi'o·nol. 2,2'-Thiobis(4,6-dichlorophenol), a bacteriostatic agent used in some soaps.

Bi·thyn'i·a. A genus of snails whose species serve as intermediate hosts of the trematodes of man. The species **B. tentaculata** of Eastern Europe is the host of the cat liver fluke, *Opisthorchis felineus.* **B. fuchsiana** and **B. longicornis** of China are hosts of *Clonorchis sinensis.*

bit'ters. 1. Medicines characterized by a bitter taste. 2. An alcoholic drink, an appetizer. **angostura b.** See *angostura.* **aromatic b.** Medicines that unite the properties of aromatics with those of simple bitters. **astringent b.** Medicines that add styptic and astringent properties to that of bitterness. **simple b.** Medicines that stimulate the gastrointestinal tract without influencing the general system.

bi·tu'men (bi-tew'mun, buy·). Any one of a group of native, solid, or semisolid hydrocarbons. **sulfonated b.** An unofficial synonym for ichthammol.

bi''u·ret' (buy''yoo·ret', buy'yoo·ret). NH(CO—NH₂)₂. A compound obtained by heating urea.

bi''u·ret' re·ac'tion. A blue or blue-violet color given by biuret on the addition of copper sulfate and strong alkali.

bi·va'lent (buy-vay'lunt, biv'uh-lunt). 1. Denoting the ability to combine with or displace two atoms of hydrogen or their equivalent; having a valence of two. Syn., *divalent.* 2. *In biology:* see bivalent *chromosome.* 3. *In psychiatry:* see *ambivalence.* —**biva·lence,** *n.*

bi'valve''. 1. Having two valves or shells, as a speculum. 2. A mollusk with double shells, as a clam or oyster.

Bk. Symbol for berkelium.

black'damp''. Carbon dioxide gas which collects in mines and deep shafts; chokedamp.

Black Death. The plague which ravaged Europe and Asia in the fourteenth century. See *plague*.

black haw. *Viburnum prunifolium*.

black'head''. An enlarged, chronically disordered, sebaceous gland; comedo, *q.v.*

black'out''. *In aviation*, temporary loss of vision and even consciousness; due to cessation of the blood flow to the cranial cavity; caused by linear or centrifugal accelerations of considerable magnitudes. Syn., *amaurosis fugax, stagnant anoxia*.

black'wa''ter fe'ver. A severe, usually fatal, form of malaria associated with bloody urine. See *hemoglobinuria*.

Blackwell, Elizabeth [*American physician*, 1821-1910]. The first woman to receive a medical degree in America (1849).

blad'der. 1. A membranous sac serving for the reception of fluids or gases. 2. The hollow organ which serves as a reservoir for the urine. **cord b.** Dysfunction of the bladder due to a lesion in the spinal cord, such as tabes dorsalis. **encysted b.** A urinary bladder with communicating cysts. **hypertonic b.** A condition of increased muscular activity of the bladder which appears after recovery from the shock following section of the voluntary innervation to the bladder. **irritable b.** Condition characterized by a constant desire to urinate. **multilocular b.** A sacculated bladder having many pouches. **nervous b.** A condition in which there is a frequent desire to urinate, with inability to perform the act perfectly. Syn., *irritable b.* **neurogenic b.** A bladder in a state of dysfunction due to lesions of the central or peripheral nervous system. **sacculated b.** Condition due to overextension; pouches in which urine may be held are formed by the forcing out of the mucous coat between the muscular bundles. **spastic b.** A condition appearing after the return of reflex activity following partial section of the cord in which the bladder is overactive, exhibits a reduced capacity, and urine is ejected involuntarily because the detrusor mechanism is stimulated at lower pressures than normal.

blad'der train'ing. Establishing the control of urination as a habit during infancy or early childhood.

blade. 1. The cutting portion of a surgical knife or of surgical scissors. 2. One of the two arms or limbs of forceps.

Blalock, Alfred [*American surgeon*, 1899-]. Known for his operation for the relief of congenital obstruction at the origin of the pulmonary artery by the creation of an artificial ductus arteriosus. A surgical anastomosis is made of an artery arising from the aortic arch (innominate or subclavian) to the side of one of the pulmonary arteries, thus permitting a larger quantity of blood to reach the lungs. Called *Blalock-Taussig operation*.

blast. The compression or suction wave which is set up by the detonation of high explosives.

-blast. Combining form denoting *a sprout, shoot, or germ*; specifically, *in biology*, denoting *a formative cell, a germ layer, or a formative constituent of living matter*.

blas·te'ma (pl. *blastemata*). 1. The formative cellular matrix from which an organ or part is derived. 2. A small bud of competent cells from which begins the regeneration of an organ or appendage. 3. Budding or sprouting part of a plant. 4. The formative lymph or fluid from which cells or organs are formed. *Obs.* **—blastemal, blastemat'ic, blastem'ic,** *adj.*

blas·te'ma·ta. Plural of blastema, *q.v.*

blast in'ju·ry. Trauma resulting from short-range exposure to the detonation of high explosives. **atmospheric b.** i. The pressure on the body causes capillary hemorrhages of the lungs with hemoptysis; dyspnea and cyanosis are constant, lobar pneumonia may develop, and shock is often pronounced. The eardrums may be ruptured. **immersion b. i.** Trauma caused by underwater explosion of a depth charge in close proximity. The abdominal viscera are most often injured, the injuries being serious due to the greater force exerted on the body in water. Symptoms and prognosis vary.

blas'to-, blast-. A combining form denoting *connection with, or relation to, a bud, budding, a germ,* and especially *the early stages of the embryo.*

blas'to·coele, blas'to·coel (blas'to-seel), **blas'to·cele.** The central cavity of the blastula or blastocyst.

blas'to·cyst. 1. A blastula. 2. The modified mammalian blastula consisting of trophoblast, inner cell mass, and blastocoele. 3. Rarely, the egg nucleus or germinal vesicle. See *blastula*.

blas'to·derm. *In embryology:* 1. The cellular disk of cleavage cells derived from the blastodisk of meroblastic ova. 2. The primitive germ layer or epithelium of a blastula or blastocyst from which the primary germ layers are derived. 3. By extension, the germinal membrane after the formation of the several germ layers. **—blastoder'mal, blastoder'mic,** *adj.* **embryonic b.** That part of a blastoderm forming the embryo proper. Syn., *embryonic disk, embryonic shield.* **extra-**

embryonic b. That part of a blastoderm forming the extraembryonic membranes.

blas'to·disk, blas'to·disc. 1. The uncleaved cytoplasmic disk capping the embryonic pole of meroblastic ova. 2. The embryonic or germinal disk of mammals.

blas·to'ma. 1. A term employed to indicate that a particular tumor originates from embryonal cells, as fibroblastoma, chondroblastoma. 2. A true tumor. **—blastom'atous,** adj.

blas'to·mere. A cleavage or segmentation cell; any one of the cells into which the fertilized ovum divides.

Blas"to·my'ces (blas"to·my'seez) (pl. Blastomycetes). A genus of yeastlike organisms. **B. brasiliensis.** Synonym for Paracoccidioides brasiliensis. **B. dermatitidis.** A fungus; the causative agent of North American blastomycosis, a cutaneous or systemic, suppurative, granulomatous disease. The organism is spheroid and buds in tissues; it produces aerial hyphae in culture.

Blas"to·my·ce'tes (blas"to·migh·see'teez). Plural of Blastomyces.

blas"to·my·co'sis. Originally this term represented a more or less definite clinical syndrome, but it has come to mean all diseases produced by budding, yeastlike organisms. Diseases vary in different countries and have different causative agents, but are similar in that they are granulomatous and may involve not only the skin but the viscera and bony structures as well.

blas'to·pore. External opening of the archenteron in a gastrula. The avian and mammalian primitive streaks have been regarded by some as closed blastopores; hence the primitive pit, or the opening into the notochordal canal, may be considered a remnant of a blastopore. Also called archistome, gastropore, primitive mouth.

blas'tu·la. A spherical mass consisting of a central cavity surrounded by a single layer of cells produced by the cleavage of the ovum; frequently modified by the presence of yolk. Syn., blastodermic vesicle, germ or germinal vesicle, blastosphere, blastocyst. Also called vesicular morula. **—blastular,** adj.; **blastula'tion,** n.

Bla·tel'la. A genus of cockroaches whose species are important as transmitters of human pathogens. **B. germanica.** A species which serves as an obligatory intermediate host of Hymenolepis diminuta. Syn., Croton bug.

Blat'ta. A genus of cockroaches of the Blattidae. The species **B. orientalis,** the oriental cockroach, has been incriminated as an intermediate host of Hymenolepis diminuta.

bleach'ing pow'der. Chlorinated lime.

bleb. A skin blister or vesicle filled with serum or blood; bulla, q.v.

bleed'er. One who is subject to frequent hemorrhages, as a hemophiliac.

bleed'ing. The escape of blood from the vessels; venesection, q.v.

bleed'ing time. The time required for bleeding to cease from a deep cut in the skin, normally from one to three minutes. Bleeding time is determined in clinical laboratories to aid in diagnosis or to ascertain the state of the blood prior to operation. Also see clotting time; prothrombin time.

blen'no-, blenn-. A combining form denoting presence of, or relation to, mucus.

blen"noph·thal'mi·a. Catarrhal conjunctivitis.

blen"nor·rha'gi·a. 1. An excessive mucous discharge. 2. Gonorrhea.

bleph'a·ral. Relating to the eyelids.

bleph"a·rec'to·my. Excision of a part or the whole of an eyelid.

bleph"ar·e·de'ma, bleph"a·ro·e·de'ma. Swelling or edema of the eyelids.

bleph'a·rism. Rapid involuntary winking; spasmodic nictitation.

bleph"a·ri'tis. Inflammation of the eyelids. **b. angularis.** That involving the medial commissure with blocking of punctum. **b. ciliaris.** Inflammation of the hair follicles and sebaceous glands along the margins of the lids. **b. gangraenosa.** Carbuncle of the lids. **b. marginalis.** See b. ciliaris. **b. parasitica.** Marginal blepharitis caused by lice and/or mites. **b. simplex.** Mild inflammation of the borders of the eyelids with the formation of moist yellow crusts on the ciliary margins which glue the eyelids together. **b. squamosa.** Marginal blepharitis with the formation of branny scales. **b. ulcerosa.** Marginal blepharitis with ulcer formation.

bleph'a·ro-, blephar-. A combining form denoting relating to the eyelid.

bleph"a·ro·ath"er·o'ma. Sebaceous cyst of the eyelid.

bleph"a·ro·blen"nor·rhe'a. Conjunctivitis with a purulent discharge.

bleph"a·ro·chal'a·sis (blef"uh·ro·kal'uh·sis). A redundance of the skin of the eyelids which causes the skin to fold over and hang down. In some persons it hides the tarsal margin when the lids are open.

bleph"a·ro·chrom"hi·dro'sis. Colored sweat of the eyelids, usually of a bluish tint.

bleph"a·ro·con·junc"ti·vi'tis. Inflammation of both the eyelids and the conjunctiva.

bleph″a·ro·di·as′ta·sis (blef″uh-ro-dye-ass′tuh-sis). Excessive separation of the eyelids; inability to close the eyelids completely.

bleph′a·ron (pl. *blephara*). The eyelid; palpebra.

bleph″a·ron′cus (blef″uh-rong′-kus). A tumor or swelling of the eyelid. —**blepharonco′sis**, *n.*

bleph″a·ro·pa·chyn′sis (blef″uh-ro-pa-kin′sis). Morbid thickening of the eyelid.

bleph″a·roph′ry·plas″ty. Plastic surgery of the eyebrow and eyelid. —**blepharophryplas′tic**, *adj.*

bleph′a·ro·plast″. 1. A basal body from which a cilium or flagellum grows. 2. A centriole which forms such basal bodies.

bleph″a·ro·plas″ty. An operation for the restoration of any part of the eyelid. —**blepharoplas′tic**, *adj.*

bleph″a·ro·ple′gi·a. Paralysis of an eyelid.

bleph″a·rop·to′sis. Drooping of the upper eyelid.

bleph″a·ro·py′or·rhe′a. A flow of pus from the eyelid.

bleph″a·ror′rha·phy. Repair by suturing of a cut or lacerated eyelid.

bleph′a·ro·spasm″. Spasm of the orbicularis oculi muscle; excessive winking.

bleph″a·ro·sphinc″ter·ec′to·my. An operation to lessen the pressure of the upper lid upon the cornea.

bleph′a·ro·stat″. An instrument for holding the eyelids apart while performing operations upon the eyes or lids.

bleph″a·ro·ste·no′sis. Pathologic narrowing of the space between the eyelids, or palpebral space.

bleph″a·ro·sym′phy·sis. The adhesion or growing together of the eyelids; blepharosynechia.

bleph″a·ro·syn·ech′i·a (blef″uh-ro-si-neck′ee-uh, -sin″i-kigh′uh). Adhesion or growing together of the eyelids.

bleph″a·rot′o·my. Incision into the eyelid.

blep″so·path′i·a, blep·sop′a·thy. Eyestrain.

blight. A fungus disease of plants.

blind. Without sight; deprived of sight.

blind gut. The cecum.

blind′ness. Loss or absence of vision; inability to see. Also called *caecitas*, *typhlosis*. **amnesic color b.** A form of aphasia in which colors are seen normally, but the names cannot be recalled. **color b.** Inability to perceive one or more, rarely all, colors; achromatopsia. **cortical b.** That resulting from a lesion of the cortical visual center. **day b.** Hemeralopia. **elec-**

tric-light b. A condition similar to snow blindness, due to exposure of the eyes to intense and prolonged electric illumination. **green b.** A variety of color blindness in which green is not distinguished; aglaucopsia. **night b.** See *night blindness*. **psychic b.** Loss of conscious visual sensation from destruction of the cerebral visual center while pupillary reactions remain intact. **red b.** Defective vision for red. Also called *green-sightedness*. See *protanopia*. **snow b.** Photophobia and conjunctivitis due to exposure of the eyes to the ultraviolet rays. **violet b.** Amianthinopsy.

blind spot. That spot on the retina not affected by light; the place where the optic nerve enters.

blink′ing. Involuntary winking.

blis′ter. 1. A vesicle resulting from the exudation of serous fluid between the epidermis and true skin. 2. The agent by which the blister is produced. **blood b.** One that contains blood. **fever b.** Herpes simplex of the lips. **flying b.** One that remains long enough to produce redness of the skin but not vesication. **pus b.** One containing purulent matter, usually from infection of the serum in a blister. **water b.** One with watery contents.

blis′ter·ing. Forming a vesicle upon the skin. Syn., *epispastic*.

bloat. 1. Puffiness; edema; turgidity from any cause, as from anasarca. 2. *In veterinary medicine*, an abnormal accumulation of gas in the stomach or intestines, resulting in distention of the abdomen. Also called *wind colic*, *hoven*.

block. 1. Obstruct the path of sensory impressions by the injection of an anesthetic agent in the nerve trunks in the area of surgical operation connecting with the sensorium. 2. Any blockage of a passage or opening. 3. *In dentistry*, a set of two or more artificial teeth (block teeth) carved as one piece on a porcelain base to which the corresponding section of the gum (gum block) has been added. 4. *In dentistry*, a mass of gold foil for filling teeth, made by folding a tape of foil upon itself several times to secure a block of the thickness desired. **air b.** An air leak from the lung alveoli into the pulmonary connective tissue and mediastinum, which obstructs the normal inflow and outflow of air and pulmonary blood. **arborization b.** Impaired intraventricular conduction, due supposedly to subendocardial fibrosis, with characteristic electrocardiographic findings. **bite b.** (a) *In dentistry*, a device for registering the proper interrelation of upper and lower jaws, with or without the presence of teeth. (b) Hard rubber device used in bronchoscopy. **bundle**

branch b. See *bundle branch block.*
field b. Regional anesthesia by surrounding an operative field with an anesthetic wall. **heart b.** See *heart block.* **nerve b.** See regional *anesthesia.* **sinoatrial b.** Due to failure, at times, of the stimulus arising in the sinoatrial node to cause contraction of the atrium. The pause resulting is usually shorter than two normal cycles. Also called *sinus arrest.* **spinal b.** Obstruction to the flow of spinal fluid when the spinal canal is blocked. **subarachnoid b.** A condition in which some obstructing mass prevents the normal flow of cerebrospinal fluid. Evidenced by failure of a rise of pressure in the lumbar manometer during jugular compression. **ventricular b.** Block of the interventricular foramens, the cerebral aqueduct, or the lateral and medial apertures of the fourth ventricle; interfering with the flow of spinal fluid from the brain ventricles and causing internal hydrocephalus.

block′ing. 1. Obstructing a sensory nerve pathway by injection of an anesthetic agent, as a novocain block. 2. *In psychoanalysis,* a sudden obstruction of the flow of speech; an interruption of free association when a painful complex is revived. 3. *In psychiatry,* the process of sudden interruption of thought in schizophrenia, resulting in an abrupt change of subject, stopping or slowing down of speech. 4. Fastening a histologic specimen on a microtome block, in preparation for cutting.

blood. The fluid tissue which circulates through the heart, arteries, capillaries, and veins, supplies oxygen and food to the other tissues of the body, and removes from them carbon dioxide and waste products of metabolism. It is made up of plasma and cellular elements. The latter consist of red cells, white cells, and blood platelets. One cu. mm. of normal blood contains about 6,000 white and 5,000,000 red cells. The bright red color of arterial blood is due to the oxyhemoglobin of the red cells, the darker red of venous blood to reduced hemoglobin or methemoglobin. The total amount of blood is equal to about $\frac{1}{13}$ of the body weight. On removal from the body and under abnormal conditions in the body, blood coagulates, forming a red clot from which a yellowish fluid, the serum, can be expressed. Healthy blood contains about 78% water and 22% solids. For normal values of blood constituents, see Table in the Appendix. Also see blood *island,* hematogenous *pigment,* Rh *factor, serum, typing.* **b. cell.** A cellular element of the blood. The red cells are biconcave disks, circular in mammals (except the camel), and elliptical in other vertebrates. In man they

are about 7.7μ in diameter and 1.9μ thick. The white cells have a diameter of 5–16μ. Some exhibit movements similar to those of the ameba. See *leukocyte.* **b. corpuscle.** A blood cell. **b. count.** See *blood count.* **b. groups.** In the human, there are four classifications of blood, depending on agglutinogens in the red cells and agglutinins in the serum which lead to hemolysis or agglutination when incompatible bloods are mixed, as in transfusion. These groups are variously classified as below:

O, A, B, AB—Adopted by the Permanent Commission on Biology Standards.
IV, II, III, I—Moss's grouping.
I, II, III, IV—Jansky's grouping.

b. platelets. Spheroidal or ovoid, light-gray bodies found in blood, averaging in diameter about 2.5μ, and numbering about 300,000 per cubic millimeter; an important factor in blood coagulation. **b. vessel.** An artery, vein, or capillary. **cord b.** Blood obtained from the umbilical cord. **defibrinated b.** That from which the fibrin is removed by agitation. **Do b. group.** A blood group in dogs; analogous to Rh in humans, it may cause jaundice in the young because of incompatibility with the mother. **laked b.** That in which the red blood cells are hemolyzed. **occult b.** Small amounts of blood, as in gastric contents, which are not visible. Their presence is determined by chemical tests. **Rh b. types.** Tests with Rh₀, anti-Rh′, and anti-Rh″ yield eight standard types, whose names and approximate frequencies among white persons in New York City are as follows: type Rh₁Rh₂, 13%; Rh₁, 54.5%; Rh₂, 15%; Rh₀, 2.5%; Rh′Rh″, 1 in about 10,000; Rh′, 1.2%; Rh″, 0.3%, and Rh−, 13.5%. There are striking differences in the distribution among different races. In Negroes, type Rh₀ exceeds 40% and in Mongolian races Rh− is virtually absent.

blood bank. A reserve stock of whole blood or plasma, obtained from suitable donors, stored under refrigeration for use in emergencies when erythrocytes, serum proteins, or antibodies are needed. See *bank.*

blood count. The determination of the number of red and white cells per cubic millimeter of blood. This is done with a hemocytometer, *q.v.* The **differential blood count** is that made to estimate the percentage of each different type of leukocyte per cubic millimeter of blood. The **absolute blood count** determines the total number of each different type of leukocyte; this is obtained by multiplying the total leukocyte count per cubic millimeter by the percentage of each type, as shown by the differential count.

blood do'nor cen'ter. A central establishment where facilities are provided for the collection, processing, storage, and distribution of blood and plasma. During World War II, such a center was operated by the Red Cross in most large cities.

blood'less. Without blood; blanched; exsanguinated.

blood'let"ting. Venesection, q.v.

blood poi'son·ing. Septicemia, q.v.

blood pres'sure. The pressure exerted by the blood within the arteries, depending upon the force of the heart beat, elasticity of the vessel walls, resistance of the capillary bed, and volume and viscosity of the blood. The systolic pressure depends upon the ventricular systole, and the diastolic upon the diastole. The difference between the systolic and the diastolic is the pulse pressure. **negative b. p.** Pressure which is less than that of the atmosphere. It exists in the large veins near the heart, owing to the aspirating action of the thorax.

blood sub'sti·tute. Some substance, or combination of substances, used in place of blood, such as plasma, albumin, acacia, gelatin, or mineral salts.

blood typ'ing. The method used to determine to which blood group an individual belongs. This consists of matching the unknown blood cells with known serum, one serum containing *a* agglutinin for type A cells, and the other serum containing *β* agglutinin for type B cells. If a corresponding agglutinogen is present on the unknown cells, the red cells will show clumping which can be observed under a microscope.

Blumer's shelf. Carcinomatous metastases in the rectouterine pouch felt as a firm ridge on digital rectal examination; occurs especially in carcinoma of the stomach.

blutene chloride. Trade-mark for tolonium chloride.

B. M. A. British Medical Association.

B. M. R. Basal metabolic rate.

BNA. Basle Nomina Anatomica. See *Basle anatomical nomenclature.*

board of health. An official board in a municipality, state, or province, responsible for maintaining public health through sanitation and preventive medicine.

bod'y. 1. The animal frame with its organs. 2. A cadaver or corpse. 3. The largest and primarily central part of an organ, as the body of the uterus. 4. A mass of matter. 5. A small organ, as the carotid body. Also see *corpus.*

amyloid bodies. Corpora amylacea, q.v. under *corpus.* **anococcygeal b.** A fibromuscular mass between the anal canal and the coccyx, forming in part a point of attachment for the external sphincter and the levator ani muscles. Also called *anococcygeal ligament.* **aortic bodies.** Irregular epithelioid masses associated with the aortic arch; probably chemoreceptive in function, stimulated by changes in the carbon dioxide content of the blood. Also called *glomus aorticum.* **basal bodies.** Minute granules at the bases of cilia or flagella, derived from the centriole and producing the cilia or flagella. Also called *blepharoplast.* **carotid bodies.** Epithelioid masses similar in structure and function to the aortic bodies; situated at or near the carotid bifurcation. Formerly called *glomus caroticum.* **cavernous bodies.** The corpora cavernosa, q.v. under *corpus.* **chromaffin bodies.** Small bodies on either side of the abdominal aorta, which give a brown coloration with chromic acid or its salts. Also called *paraganglions.* Formerly called *Zuckerkandl's bodies.* **chromatin bodies.** Chromosomes. **ciliary b.** The ciliary muscle and processes. **coccygeal b.** A small, vascular nodule at the tip of the coccyx. Formerly called *glomus coccygeum.* **Donovan bodies.** Short rod- or oval-shaped capsulated organisms occurring in the cytoplasm of large mononuclear cells from ulcers of granuloma inguinale; best demonstrated by Wright's or Giemsa stain. **epithelial b.** A parathyroid gland. **foreign b.** A substance present in any organ or tissue where it is not normally found. **geniculate bodies.** Four oval, flattened bodies on the posterior inferior aspect of the thalamus. The **medial geniculate bodies** receive auditory impulses by way of the brachia of the inferior colliculi and relay them to the temporal cortex via the auditory radiations. The **lateral geniculate bodies** receive optic impulses by way of the optic tracts and relay them to the occipital cortex via the geniculocalcarine tracts. **immune b.** Old term for immune hemolysin. See *antibody.* **inferior quadrigeminal b.** Inferior colliculus. **ketone b.** A group name for any of the compounds, *β*-hydroxybutyric acid, acetoacetic acid, or acetone, which simultaneously increase in blood and urine in diabetic acidosis, starvation, pregnancy, and after ether anesthesia. **Leishman-Donovan bodies.** Small, parasite-like bodies on the liver and spleen of those suffering from kala-azar. **Malpighian b.** (a) A renal corpuscle. (b) A lymph nodule of the spleen. Also called *Malpighian corpuscle*.

mammillary bodies. Two small, spherical masses of gray matter in the interpeduncular space at the base of the brain. They receive olfactory impulses from the hippocampus by means of the fornix and relay them to the anterior nucleus of the thalamus via the mammillothalamic tract and to the tegmentum of the pons and medulla oblongata via the mammillotegmental bundle. Also called *corpora mammillaria*.

Negri bodies. Inclusion bodies in the Purkinje cells and cells of the hippocampus of animals with rabies. **Nissl bodies.** Chromop'1 substance of nerve cells. **perineal b.** The dense connective tissue between the vulva and the anus or between the scrotum and the anus. **pituitary b.** Pituitary gland. **polar bodies.** The minute, abortive cells extruded by the oöcyte in the process of maturation. Also called *polocytes*. **primitive perineal b.** The primary perineum; the projecting wedge formed by the cloacal septum, which separates the anus and the orifice of the urogenital sinus after the rupture of the cloacal membrane. **psammoma bodies.** Sandlike, laminated, calcareous deposits seen typically in the psammoma, a type of meningeal fibroblastoma. Similar deposits are found in chronic inflammation, in benign and malignant tumors, and, as brain sand, in the pineal body. Also called *corpora arenacea*. **purine bodies.** Compounds that contain the purine ring; compounds derived from purine by the substitution of their hydrogen atoms. **restiform b.** A large bundle of nerve fibers running from the medulla oblongata to the cerebellum. It contains the dorsal spinocerebellar tract from the nucleus dorsalis of the spinal cord, olivocerebellar fibers from the inferior olivary nuclei, dorsal external arcuate fibers from the lateral cuneate nucleus, and ventral external arcuate fibers from the arcuate and lateral reticular nuclei. **ring bodies.** Peculiar ring-shaped bodies found in the erythrocytes in pernicious anemia, leukemia, and lead poisoning. **threshold b.** Any substance in the blood plasma which, above a certain concentration, is excreted by the kidneys. The critical concentration is called the excretion threshold. **ultimobranchial bodies.** Those considered by some to be rudimentary fifth visceral pouches; by others, to be lateral thyroid primordia and fourth pouch derivatives. Syn., *postbranchial bodies*. Also called *lateral thyroids*. **vertebral b.** A short column of bone forming the anterior, weight-bearing segment of a vertebra. **vitreous b.** The vitreous; the transparent, colorless, gelatinous body filling the space between the retina and the lens of the eye.

bod'y ar'mor. Clothing reinforced with armor; used by aviators as a protection against antiaircraft fire.

bod'y snatch'ing. Unauthorized removal of a corpse from the grave.

boil. A furuncle; a localized inflammation of the skin and subcutaneous connective tissue, attended by suppuration; usually at the site of a hair follicle. It has but one opening for drainage in contrast to a carbuncle, *q.v.*, which is larger and has several openings. See *furuncle*. Also see *sore*. **blind b.** One not attended by the formation of a core; nonsuppurating.

bol'do. The dried leaves of the boldutree, *Peumus boldus*, formerly used as an aromatic stimulant and diuretic.

bole. A translucent, soft variety of clay formerly much used in medicine.

bo·lom'e·ter. A device for measuring minute differences in radiant heat. Syn., *thermic balance*.

bo'lus. 1. A large pill. 2. The rounded mass of food prepared by the mouth for swallowing, called an **alimentary bolus.** 3. Bole, *q.v.*

bonamine. A trade-mark for meclizine hydrochloride.

bond. The linkage between atoms believed by some to consist of a pair of electrons vibrating or rotating between two kernels.

bone. 1. Osseous tissue; a supportive, rigid connective tissue consisting of an abundant calcified matrix enclosing many much-branched cells, the osteocytes. The body of each osteocyte occupies an ovoid space, the lacuna; its branches lie in minute, branching tubules, the canaliculi. Many varieties of osseous tissue are differentiated according to method of formation, relation to other tissues, and architecture. See also *endosteum, ossein, ossification, osteogenesis, osteoid, periosteum*. 2. An element or individual member of the skeleton, as the femur, the parietal bone. For Bones listed by name, see Table of Bones in the Appendix. —**bony,** *adj.* **alveolar b.** The alveolar processes of the maxilla and the mandible. Within the alveolar bone, a distinction should be made between the "alveolar bone proper" and the "alveolar supporting bone" due to their biologic and functional differences. The alveolar bone proper may be defined as that thin bony plate surrounding the root to which fibers of the periodontal membrane are attached. *In radiography*, this bony plate is called "lamina dura" as it appears more radiopaque than the surrounding spongy bone. The alveolar supporting bone consists of the compact alveolar plates and of the spongy bone of the alveolar processes.

other than the alveolar bone proper.
ankle b. The talus, *q.v.* **bundle-b.**
Bone traversed by coarse collagenous
fibers (Sharpey's penetrating fibers), as
where tendons or ligaments are affixed.
cancellous b. A form in which the
matrix is arranged in a network of
rods, plates, or tubes (the trabeculae),
between which are spaces filled with
marrow. Syn., *spongy b.*, *substantia
spongiosa.* **cartilage b.** (a) Bone
(1) preceded during development by a
mass of hyaline cartilage which it
largely replaces. (b) A bone (2) which
has been preceded by a cartilaginous
primordium. **compact b.** Bone (1) in
which marrow spaces are replaced by
cylindrical, concentrically laminated
Haversian systems, each with an axial
vascular channel, the Haversian canal.
Syn., *substantia compacta.* **endochondral b. formation.** The replacement of a cartilaginous primordium by cartilage bone. **flat b.** A bone
(2) more or less in the form of a plate,
as the parietal bone. **incisive b.** The
premaxilla or intermaxillary bone
which bears the upper incisor teeth.
Fused with the maxilla in man; a separate bone in most mammals. **intra-
cartilaginous b. formation.**
See endochondral *b.* formation. **intramembranous b. formation.** The
formation of bone by or within a connective tissue without involvement of a
cartilage stage. **lamellar b.** Bone
(1) which exhibits microscopic lamina-
tions (lamellas) of its matrix. **long b.**
One in which the length markedly exceeds the width. **membrane b.** Bone
(1) formed by or within a connective
tissue, as by a periosteum. **periosteal b.** Membrane bone formed by
the periosteum. Syn., *subperiosteal b.*
primary b. The first bone formed in
a given location. **rider's b.** An ossification of the lower tendon of the adductor longus or magnus; due to pressure. **secondary b.** Bone which replaces primary bone. **sesamoid b.** A
small bone developed in a tendon subjected to much pressure. **short b.** One
having the three dimensions nearly
equal. **spongy b.** See cancellous *b.*
tabular b. A flat bone; composed of
an outer and an inner table of compact
bone with cancellous bone or diploë between them. **Wormian b.** Any of the
small supernumerary bones in the sutures of the skull.
bone on'lay. A strip of transplanted
bone laid across a fracture and held in
position by wires, pins, screws, or other
device.
bone′set″. An herb used in making a
therapeutic tea. See *Eupatorium.*
bone′set″ter. One who specializes in
setting bones, especially an uneducated

empiric, and often a pretender to hereditary skill in the business.
bone wax. A material used for packing bone, especially during skull operations, for the arrest of bone bleeding.
Bonjean's ergotin. See under *ergotin.*
Bo·öph′i·lus. A genus of ticks.
B. annulatus. The cattle tick which
carries the organism responsible for
Texas fever.
boot, Unna's paste. Used in treating varicose ulcers and veins by relieving venous hydrostatic pressure; a
paste of zinc oxide, gelatin, and glycerin is applied to the leg and a bandage
is placed over the paste. Commonly
three layers of paste and three layers
of bandages are applied alternately.
bo·rac′ic ac′id. Boric acid.
bo′rate. Any salt of boric acid.
bo′rax. Sodium borate, *q.v.*
bor″bo·ryg′mus. The rumbling
noise caused by flatus in the intestines.
Bor″deaux′ mix′ture (boar″do′).
A fungicide containing copper sulfate
1.5, lime 1.0, water to make 100.
Bor″deaux′ red. An acid monoazo
dye, used as a plasma stain. Also called
*acid Bordeaux; archelline 2B; azo-Bor-
deaux; cerasin R; fast red B, BN, or P.*
bo′ric ac′id. H_3BO_3. Colorless crystals, or a white crystalline powder,
soluble in water. Used as a mild antiseptic, but may be toxic. Syn., *boracic
acid, orthoboric acid.*
bor′ne·ol. $C_{10}H_{17}OH$. A substance
which occurs in fissures in trees of the
genus *Dryobalanops,* growing in Borneo
and Sumatra. Used in the preparation
of perfumes and incense. Syn., *Borneo
camphor.* Also called *Sumatra camphor.*
bor′nyl. The monovalent $-C_{10}H_{17}$
radical derived from borneol by removing the hydroxyl group.
bo′ro-, bor-. A combining form for
boron.
bo″ro·glyc′er·ide (bo″ro·gliss′ur-
ide, ·id). See *boroglycerin.*
bo″ro·glyc′er·in (bo″ro·gliss′ur-
in). A product formed by heating together boric acid and glycerin.
bo′ron. B = 10.82. A nonmetallic element; it is the characteristic element
of boric acid, the borates, metaborates,
and perborates.
Bor·re′li·a, Bor·rel′i·a. A genus
of spirochetes parasitic in man and
other warm-blooded animals; consists
of many species, which are the causative agents of relapsing fever. **B. duttonii.** The causative agent of tick-
borne relapsing fever. **B. recurrentis.** The causative agent of louse-
borne relapsing fever. **B. vincentii.**
May be the causative agent of Vincent's
angina.
boss. A rounded or knoblike protuber-

ance, as on the side of a bone or tumor; may result from disease of the spine (kyphosis). **—bos'celated,** *adj.;* **bossela'tion,** *n.*

bot. The larva of the botfly, especially the species infesting the horse and related animals.

bot'a·ny. That branch of biology dealing with plants. **—botan'ic,** *adj.*

both'ri·o-, both'ri-. A combining form signifying bothrium.

Both''ri·o·ceph'a·lus. Synonym for *Diphyllobothrium.*

both'ri·um. A grooved sucker, such as is seen on the head of the tapeworm *Dibothriocephalus latus.* Syn., *bothrion.* Also called *bothridium.*

bot''o·gen'in, bo''to·gen'in. A steroidal sapogenin obtained from the Mexican yam *Dioscorea mexicana;* of interest as a possible source for the synthesis of cortisone.

bots. *In veterinary medicine,* infestation with botflies, which pass through one period of development in the bodies of animals, as larvae. They infest the cavities of the facial bones, the stomach and intestine, and the subcutaneous connective tissue, causing severe damage to the affected animals. Also called *bot larvae infestation.*

bot'tle. A vessel, usually of glass, with a narrow neck. **nursing b.** A feeding bottle; a narrow- or wide-mouthed flask with a rubber nipple attached; used for feeding infants.

bot'u·lism. Food poisoning due to the production of toxins by *Clostridium botulinum* in improperly canned foods; characterized by the abrupt onset of violent symptoms; often fatal. **—bot·uli'nus, botuliform,** *adj.*

bou'gie' (boo''zhee', boo'zhee). 1. A slender cylindrical instrument of rubber, waxed silk, or other material, for introduction into body passages, as the urethra, anus, or other canal. It may be plain or tipped, angled, or straight, being intended for use in exploration, in dilatation of strictures, as a guide for the passage of other instruments, or for the induction of labor. 2. A suppository, *q.v.* **armed b.** One having a caustic attached to the tip. **b. à boule.** A bulbous or bulb-tipped instrument. **cylindrical b.** One which is circular in cross section. **dilatable b.** One which can be increased in diameter for dilating a stricture. Also called *dilating b.* **elastic b.** One made of some elastic material. **filiform b.** One of very slender caliber and variously tipped. **fusiform b.** One with a spindle-shaped shaft. **medicated b.** (a) One charged with some medicated substance. (b) A rectal or other suppository for the application of a medicinal substance into a cavity. **olive-tipped b.** A bulbous bougie

with an olive- or acorn-shaped tip. **soluble b.** One containing substances which dissolve at body temperature. **wax b.** One made of linen or gauze impregnated with melted wax. **whip b.** A variety of filiform bougie.

bouil''lon' (boo-yon'). Broth, *q.v.*

bo'vine. 1. Cattlelike. 2. Relating to, or derived from, a cow or ox.

bow'el. The intestine, *q.v.*

bow'el com·plaint'. Diarrhea, *q.v.*

bow'el train'ing. The establishing of regular habits of defecation during early childhood.

bow'leg''. An arching outward of the lower limbs, usually rachitic. Syn., *genu varum.*

Boyle, Robert [*English physicist,* 1627–91]. Discovered *Boyle's law:* at any given temperature the volume of a given mass of gas varies in inverse proportion to the pressure exerted upon it. Studied the elasticity and compressibility of air. His demonstration that air is necessary for life (1669) was an important contribution to the knowledge of respiration.

B.P. Blood pressure.

B.P., B. Ph. British Pharmacopoeia.

B. P. C. British Pharmaceutical Codex.

BR. *In anatomy,* indicating a term adopted in the British Revision of the BNA terminology.

Br. Chemical symbol for bromine.

brace. Apparatus which gives support to any movable part of the body; for permanent use, in contradistinction to a splint; may assist in locomotion, and is frequently attached to clothing, as to shoes; sometimes jointed to permit flexion.

bra'chi·a (bray'kee-uh, brack'ee-uh). Plural of brachium, *q.v.*

bra''chi·al'gi·a (bray''kee-al'juh, brack''ee-). Severe pain in the arm or in the brachial plexus.

bra''chi·a'lis (bray''kee·ah'liss, brack''ee-). A muscle lying under the biceps brachii and covering the front of the elbow joint. See Table of Muscles in the Appendix.

bra'chi·o- (bray'kee-o-, brack'ee-o-), **brachi-.** A combining form denoting *the arm* or *connection with the arm.*

bra''chi·o·ceph·al'ic. 1. [NA] The artery arising from the right side of the aortic arch and dividing into the right subclavian and right common carotid arteries. 2. [BNA] The innominate artery.

bra''chi·ot'o·my. Surgical or obstetric cutting or removal of an arm.

bra'chi·um (bray'kee-um, brack'ee-um) (pl. *brachia*). 1. The arm, especially the upper arm. 2. Any armlike structure. **—brachial,** *adj.*

brach'y- (brack'i-). A combining form meaning *short.*

brach″·y·ce·pha·li·a, brach″·ceph′a·lism, brach″·y·ceph′·a·ly. Shortness of the head, the cephalic index being 81.0 to 85.4. **—brachycephal′ic, brachyceph′alous,** adj.

brach″·y·chei′li·a (brack″i·kigh·lee-uh), **brach″·y·chi′li·a** (brack″i·kigh′lee·uh, ·kill′ee·uh), **bra·chych′il·y** (bra·kick′i·lee). Abnormal shortness of the lip. Syn., microcheilia.

brach″·y·chei′rous, brach″·y·chi′rous (brack″i·kigh′rus). Having short hands. **—brachychiria, brachychirism, n.**

brach″·y·dac·tyl′i·a, brach″·y·dac′ty·ly. Abnormal shortness of the fingers or toes. **—brachydac′tylous, brachydactyl′ic,** adj.

brach″·y·glos′sal. Having a short tongue. **—brachyglossia, n.**

brach″·yg·nath′ous (brack″ig·nath′us). Having an abnormally short lower jaw. **—brachygna′thia, brachygnathus, n.**

brach″·y·ker′kic. Denoting a forearm disproportionately shorter than the upper arm.

brach″·y·mor′phy. Short stature. **—brachymorphic,** adj.

brach″·y·pel′vic. Denoting an oval type of pelvis with a transverse diameter measuring about 13 cm.

brach″·y·pha·lan′gi·a. A condition in which the phalanges are abnormally short. **—brachyphalangous,** adj.

brach″·y·pro·sop′ic (brack″i·pro·sop′ick, ·so′pick). Having a short face.

brach″·y·rhin′i·a. Abnormal shortness of the nose.

brach″·y·skel′ic. Characterized by extreme shortness of the legs.

brach″·y·sta′sis. A process in which a muscle does not relax to its former length following a contraction and maintains its original degree of tension in its new state. Also called brachy-static contraction.

Bradford, Edward Hickling [American orthopedic surgeon, 1848–1926]. Known for his invention of orthopedic appliances and especially for his canvas-covered, gas-pipe frame made in various sizes. It was devised originally for handling children with tuberculous disease of the spine, but was later extended to the care of joint disease and for immobilization after operations. Where young children are involved, restraint is imposed by webbing straps and a pelvic band.

brad′y-. A combining form meaning slow.

brad″y·ar′thri·a. Slow speech; due to organic disturbance of the speech apparatus.

brad″y·car′di·a. Slowness of the heart; manifested in a pulse rate usu-ally less than 60 per minute. **—bradycardic,** adj.

brad″y·crot′ic. Characterized by a slow pulse.

brad″y·di·as′to·le (brad″i·dye·ass′to·lee), **brad″y·di′as·to′li·a** (brad″i·dye″ass·to′lee·uh). Prolongation of the diastolic interval; associated with myocardial lesions.

brad″y·glos′si·a. Slow speech; due to difficulty in tongue movement.

brad″y·ki·ne′si·a (brad″i·ki·nee′shuh, brad″i·kigh·nee′·), **brad″y·ki·ne′sis** (·ki·nee′sis, ·kigh·nee′sis). Slow or retarded movement, as in melancholia or catatonia. **—bradykinet′ic,** adj.

brad″y·la′li·a. Slowness of utterance.

brad″y·lex′i·a. Abnormal slowness in reading.

brad″y·pha′si·a (brad″i·fay′zhuh, ·zee·uh). Slow speech.

brad″y·phre′ni·a. Sluggish mental activity, such as that following encephalitis lethargica.

brad″y·pra′gi·a. Abnormally slow action; usually applied to physical activity.

brad″y·prax′i·a. Slow or retarded physical movement.

brain. That part of the central nervous system contained in the cranial cavity, consisting of the cerebrum, cerebellum, pons, and medulla oblongata. Syn., encephalon.

brain sand. Psammoma bodies in the pineal body; corpora arenacea.

brain stem. See under stem.

bran′chi·al. (brang′kee·ul). 1. Pertaining to the branchiae or gills. 2. By extension, pertaining to the embryonic visceral arches. See arch, cyst, cleft.

bran′chi·o- (brang′kee·o-), **bran′chi-** (brang′ki-). A combining form denoting connection with or relation to branchiae or gills.

bran″chi·og′e·nous (brang″kee·odj′i·nus), **bran″chi·o·gen′ic.** Produced or developed from a branchial or visceral cleft.

bran′chi·o·mere″. A segment of the visceral mesoderm which develops into a branchial or visceral arch.

bran″chi·om′er·ism. Serial arrangement of the visceral arches or branchiomeres.

bran′dy. The product of the distillation of fermented grape juice or other fermented fruit juice.

brass. An alloy of copper with zinc.

brass chills. See metal fume fever.

brass found′er's a′gue (ayg′yoo). See metal fume fever; brass founder's ague.

brass poi′son·ing. Synonym for brass founder's ague. See metal fume fever; brass founder's ague.

brawn′y. Fleshy; muscular.

bra·ye'ra (bra·yair'uh, bray·yair'uh). The dried panicles of the pistillate flowers of *Hagenia abyssinica*, the kusso tree. Used as an anthelmintic against tapeworms.

break'bone" fe'ver. Dengue, *q.v.*

breast. 1. The front of the chest. 2. One of the mammary glands. **caked b.** Colloquial term for puerperal mastitis, *q.v.* **chicken b.** A chest with a prominent sternum due to rickets or obstructed infantile respiration. Also called *pigeon b.* **funnel b.** A thoracic wall anomaly characterized by a depression or groove involving the sternum and neighboring cartilages.

breast'bone". Sternum.

breath. The air inhaled and exhaled during respiration. **saturnine b.** The peculiar sweet breath characteristic of lead poisoning.

breath'ing. See *respiration*.

breath'ing ma·chine'. Respirator, *q.v.*

breech. The buttocks or nates. **b. presentation.** See under *presentation*.

breg'ma (pl. *bregmata*). The junction of the coronal and sagittal sutures; in infants, the anterior fontanel. —**breg·mat'ic,** *adj.*

brei (bry). Tissue that has been mashed or ground to a pulp; a preparation useful in studying tissue metabolism.

bribe. *In psychoanalysis,* a compromise in which the ego accepts the symptoms of a neurosis and, in turn, placates the superego by suffering.

bridge. 1. *In anatomy,* any ridge or spanlike structure. 2. *In dentistry,* a partial denture supported by one or more natural teeth. See *bridgework*. 3. *In electricity,* an apparatus for measuring the resistance of a conductor. **arterial b.** A segment of vein, fresh or preserved by the rapid freeze technique, used to bridge a gap in an injured artery. The anastomosis between artery and vein is carried out by a nonsuture technique over two funnel-shaped vitallium tubes or one long vitallium tube through which the vein is threaded. Also called *Blakemore's operation*. **b. of the nose.** That formed by the union of the two nasal bones. **intercellular bridges.** Protoplasmic bridges which connect adjacent cells.

bridge'work". *In dentistry:* 1. An appliance made of artificial crowns of teeth to replace missing natural teeth. Such crowns are connected to natural teeth or roots for anchorage by means of a bridge. A *fixed bridge* is one which is permanently fastened to its abutments; a *removable bridge* one which, though held firmly in place, may be removed by the wearer; a *removable fixed*

bridge one which may be removed, without mutilation of any of its parts, by the dentist, but not by the patient. 2. The technic of making bridges.

Bright, Richard [*English physician and clinician,* 1789–1858]. Known universally for his description of chronic nephritis, which received the name *Bright's disease* (1827).

bril'liant cres'yl blue (kress'il, kree'sil) (C.C.). A basic dye, having highly metachromatic properties; chiefly used for staining blood to demonstrate the platelets and reticulated corpuscles. Also called *brilliant blue C, cresyl blue 2RN* or *BBS.*

bril'liant green (C.C.). Tetraethyl-diamino-triphenylcarbohydride sulfate, $C_{27}H_{34}N_2O_4S$. A surgical antiseptic used in 1:1000 aqueous solution. Also called *ethyl green, malachite green G.*

bril'liant vi'tal red. See *vital red.*

Brit'ish an"ti·lew'is·ite. BAL, *q.v.*

broach. *In dentistry,* a delicate, tapered, flexible steel instrument having a spring temper; used for removing the dental pulp and for opening, enlarging, and treating the root canals. Various forms are: the **barbed broach, hooked broach, smooth broach,** and **spiral broach,** all of which are operated by a removable handle. The **root canal broach** is used for root canal surgery, and the **watchmaker's broach,** a four- or five-sided, very gradually tapering, sharp-angled instrument, is used as a reamer to enlarge the root canals.

brom-. See *bromo-.*

bro'mate. A salt of bromic acid containing the monovalent radical —BrO_3.

bro"ma·tom'e·try. The estimation of the amount of food required for an individual.

bro"ma·to·ther'a·py. Dietotherapy.

bro"ma·to·tox'in. A basic poison generated in food by the growth of microörganisms.

bro"ma·to·tox'ism. Poisoning with infected food.

brom"di·eth"yl·ac"e·tyl·u·re'a (brohm"dye·eth"il·ass"i·til·yoo·ree'uh). Carbromal, *q.v.*

bro'me·lin, bro·mel'in. A protein-digesting enzyme from the pineapple.

bro'me·thol. British Pharmacopoeia title for solution of tribromoethanol. See *avertin.*

bro'me·tone. Tribromtertiarybutyl alcohol. $Br_3C.C(OH)(CH_3)_2$. A white, crystalline powder with sedative action similar to that of the bromides.

brom"hi·dro'sis (brohm"hi·dro'sis, brom"hi-), **bro"mi·dro'sis** (bro"mi·dro'sis, brom"i-). Excretion of sweat with an unpleasant odor. Various odors may occur, usually disagreeable, and are characteristic in some races. Syn., *osmidrosis, fetid perspiration*.

brom·hy'dric ac'id. Hydrobromic acid.

bro'mid. See *bromide*.

bro'mide, bro'mid. Any binary salt in which monovalent bromine is the anion; as sodium bromide, NaBr.

bro'mine (bro'meen, ·min). Br = 79.916. A reddish brown liquid which gives off a heavy, suffocating vapor. It is a very active escharotic and disinfectant. **—bromated, brominated,** *adj*.

bro'mine poi'son·ing. A diseased state caused by the prolonged administration of bromides; characterized by headache, sleepiness, apathy, cold extremities, fetid breath, and a typical acneform eruption. There may be loss of strength and sexual drive, associated with atrophy of the testes or mammae.

bro'mi·pin. A liquid composed of bromine and sesame oil, containing 10% of bromine. It is used as a sedative in epilepsy. A similar compound containing 33% of bromine is used as an x-ray contrast medium.

brom"i·so·val'um. (α-Bromoisovaleryl)urea, a sedative and hypnotic. See *bromural*.

bro'mo-, brom-. 1. A combining form denoting *a bad smell*. 2. *In chemistry*, a combining form denoting the *presence of bromine*.

bro"mo·ben"xyl·cy'a·nide. C₆H₅·CHBrCN. A lacrimator used in chemical warfare.

bro"mo·cre'sol green. Tetrabromo-metacresolsulfonphthalein, an indicator used for determination of hydrogen-ion concentration.

bro"mo·cre'sol pur'ple. Dibromorthocresolsulfonphthalein, an indicator used for determination of hydrogen-ion concentration.

bro"mo·der'ma. A skin eruption due to ingestion of bromides.

bro'mo·form. CHBr₃. Tribromomethane. A heavy, colorless, mobile liquid of sweetish taste; slightly soluble in water.

bro"mo·hy"per·hi·dro'sis (·hidro'sis, ·high·dro'sis), **bro"mo·hy"per·i·dro'sis.** The excessive secretion of malodorous sweat.

bro"mo·ma'ni·a. Psychosis from the excessive use of bromides.

bro"mo·men"or·rhe'a, bro"mo·men"or·rhoe'a. Disordered menstruation marked by offensiveness of the flow.

bro"mo·phe'nol blue. Tetrabromophenolsulfonphthalein, an indicator used for determination of hydrogen-ion concentration.

bro"mo·thy'mol blue. Dibromothymolsulfonphthalein, an indicator used for determination of hydrogen-ion concentration.

bromsulphalein. Trade-mark for a brand of sulfobromophthalein sodium; a compound used for quantitative evaluation of liver function.

brom"te·trag'nost (brohm"ti-trag'nohst, ·nost). Sulfobromophthalein sodium, a diagnostic agent.

bromural. Trade-mark for bromisovalum.

bron'chi (brong'kigh). Plural of bronchus.

bron"chi·ec'ta·sis (brong"kee-eck'tuh·sis). Dilatation of bronchi due to an inflammatory or degenerative process; usually associated with chronic suppuration. **—bronchiectat'ic,** *adj*.

bron'chi·o- (brong'kee·o-), **bron'-chi-** (brong'ki-). A combining form signifying *bronchial*.

bron"chi·o·gen'ic. Bronchogenic, *q.v.*

bron'chi·ole (brong'kee·ole). One of the small (1 mm. or less in diameter) subdivisions of the bronchi. **—bron-chi'olar,** *adj*. **respiratory b.** The last bronchiolar subdivision; one which has pulmonary alveoli in its wall. **terminal b.** The next to the last bronchiolar subdivision; the last bronchiole without pulmonary alveoli in its wall.

bron"chi·o·lec'ta·sis. Dilatation of bronchioles. See *bronchiectasis*.

bron"chi·o·li'tis. Inflammation of the bronchioles; capillary bronchitis. **acute obliterating b.** Pulmonary cirrhosis affecting the smaller bronchioles, causing occlusion of the lumens by induration of the walls. **b. fibrosa obliterans.** Bronchiolitis resulting in occlusion of the bronchioles by the growth of connective tissue from the terminal bronchi. **vesicular b.** Bronchopneumonia.

bron·chi'tis (bron·kigh'tis, brong·kigh'tis). Inflammation occurring in the mucous membrane of the bronchi. **—bronchit'ic,** *adj*. **acute b.** That due to extension of an acute nasopharyngitis, to the inhalation of irritant vapors, or to certain infectious agents. It is characterized by fever, cough, substernal pain, and by dry rales in the early, and moist rales in the later, stages. **asthmatic b.** A form characterized by hyaline thickening of the mucosa, degeneration of epithelium, and hypertrophy of muscle, with eosinophilia. **b. convulsiva.** Whooping cough. **capillary b.** An acute bronchitis of the finer bronchioles; bronchiolitis. Bronchopneumonia is a common complication. **catarrhal b.** A form attended with profuse, mucopurulent discharges. **chronic b.** A form of bronchitis usually occurring in middle or advanced life; characterized by cough and by dry and moist rales. It may be due to repeated attacks of acute bronchitis, to gout, rheumatism, or tuberculosis, or it may be secondary to cardiac and renal disease. **croupous b.** A rare variety of bronchitis attended with expectoration of casts of the bronchi, containing Charcot-Leyden crystals and eosinophil cells, after a paroxysm of dyspnea and violent coughing. **dry b.** That unattended by expectoration. **fibrinous b.** See croupous b. **fusospirochetal b.** A type of chronic bronchitis caused by a spirochete; it is amenable to treatment by neoarsphenamine. **mechanical b.** A form caused by the inhalation of dust, etc. **putrid b.** A variety of chronic bronchitis characterized by the discharge of a copious, half-liquid, extremely offensive sputum. **secondary b.** One which develops as a complication of some preceding disease.

bron·cho- (brong'ko-), **bronch-.** A combining form signifying *relating to a bronchus* or *to the bronchi.*

bron'cho·cele". A swelling or dilatation of a bronchiole.

bron"cho·con·stric'tor. Any substance having the property of decreasing the caliber of the pulmonary air passages.

bron"cho·dil"a·ta'tion (brong"ko·dil"uh·tay'shun, ‑dye"luh·tay'shun). The widening of the caliber of the pulmonary air passages by the use of drugs or surgical instruments.

bron"cho·di·la'tor (‑dye·lay'tor, ‑di·lay'tor). 1. Any drug which has the property of increasing the caliber of the pulmonary air passages. 2. An instrument used for this purpose.

bron"cho·e·de'ma. Swelling of the bronchi, and thus diminishing their lumens, hindering the passage of air through them, and causing dyspnea.

bron"cho·e·soph"a·gos'co·py. Visual examination of the interior of the larger tracheobronchial tubes and the esophagus with the aid of an instrument.

bron"cho·gen'ic, bron"chi·o·gen'ic. 1. Arising in a bronchus or in the bronchi. 2. *In embryology,* capable of forming the bronchi.

bron'cho·gram. Radiograph of the bronchial tree made after the injection of a radiopaque substance.

bron·chog'ra·phy (brong·cog'ruh·fee). Roentgenographic visualization of the bronchial tree after the introduction of an opaque contrast material, usually iodized oil.

bron'cho·lith (brong'ko·lith). A calculus or concretion in a pulmonary air passage. **—broncholithi'asis,** *n.*

bron·chop'a·thy. Any abnormality in a bronchus.

bron·choph'o·ny (brong·kof'o·nee). An abnormal increase in the intensity of the voice sounds; heard by auscultation over the chest wall when the density of the lung tissue has been increased by disease. Also see *pectoriloquy.*

bron'cho·plas"ty. *In surgery,* repair of a bronchial defect.

bron"cho·pleu'ral (brong"ko·ploor'ul). Pertaining to a bronchus and the pleural cavity, as bronchopleural fistula.

bron"cho·pneu·mo'ni·a. Inflammation of the lungs which has spread from infected bronchi; includes all forms of pneumonitis which are not suppurative or with lobar distribution. Common in the very young or very old, and may be due to a variety of causative organisms.

bron"cho·pul'mo·na·ry. Relating to both the bronchi and the lungs.

bron·chor'rha·phy (brong·kor'uh·fee). The suturing of a bronchus.

bron"chor·rhe'a, bron"chor·rhoe'a (brong"ko·ree'uh). Excessive discharge from the bronchial mucous membranes. **—bronchorrheal,** *adj.*

bron'cho·scope. Instrument for the visual examination of the interior of the bronchi; also used for treatment and/or operation. **—bronchoscop'ic,** *adj.;* **bronchos'copy,** *n.*

bron'cho·spasm. Temporary narrowing of the bronchioles due to violent, involuntary contraction of the muscles.

bron"cho·spi"ro·che·to'sis (brong"ko·spy"ro·kee·to'sis). Chronic bronchitis, usually complicated by bronchiectasis; caused by infection with symbiotic anaerobic spirochetes and fusiform bacilli.

bron"cho·spi·rog'ra·phy (‑spy·rog'ruh·fee). The graphic recording of the functional capacity of the lungs.

bron"cho·spi·rom'e·ter (‑spy·rom'i·tur). A spirometer connected with a special type of catheter designed for intrabronchial use.

bron"cho·spi·rom'e·try. The determination of various aspects of the functional capacity of a single lung.

bron"cho·ste·no'sis. Narrowing of the lumen of one or more bronchi.

bron·chos'to·my. Fistulization of a bronchus through the chest wall.

bron"cho·ve·sic'u·lar. Pertaining to an intermediate stage in the transition from normal vesicular to completely bronchial breath sounds; characterized by elevation of pitch and prolongation of the expiratory phase.

bron'chus (brong'kus) (pl. *bronchi*). One of the primary branches of the trachea or such of its branches within the lung as contain cartilage in their walls. **—bronchial,** *adj.* **eparterial b.** The first branch of the right primary bronchus, situated above the right pulmonary artery. **extrapulmonary b.** One which is not surrounded by lung substance. Also called *primary b.* **hyparterial b.** Any one of the first collateral branches of the stem bronchi except the eparterial bronchus. **stem b.** The continuation of the main, or primary, bronchus which extends lengthwise in each lung, giving off anterior and posterior branches to the lobes.

bron″to·pho′bi·a. Morbid fear of thunder.

broth. A liquid nutritive medium for the culture of microörganisms, prepared from finely chopped lean meat or dehydrated meat extract. Syn., *bouillon.*

brow. 1. The forehead; the upper anterior portion of the head. 2. The superciliary ridge; the eyebrow.

Brown-Séquard, Charles Edouard [*British physiologist in France,* ca. 1817–94]. Widely known for his experimental work on internal secretions (1856), on the adrenal glands and testicular extracts (1889–90), on the functions of the sympathetic nerves (1852–54), and for his excellent exposition of the pathways of conduction in the spinal cord (1863). Described a lesion of one lateral half of the spinal cord, causing paralysis of motion on one side and of sensation on the opposite (1851); called *Brown-Séquard paralysis, syndrome.* He has been regarded as a successor of Claude Bernard and as one of the founders of modern endocrinology.

brown mixture. Compound opium and glycyrrhiza mixture. See under *opium.*

Bru·cel′la. A genus of small, Gram-negative, nonmotile, short bacilli or coccobacilli which are not acid-fast and do not form endospores; the cause of brucellosis (undulant fever in man and contagious abortion in cattle). There are three species recognized: **Br. abortus,** the bovine strain; **Br. melitensis,** the goat strain; **Br. suis,** the porcine strain. These three species are the causative agents of infectious abortion and undulant fever. **—brucellar,** *adj.*

bru·cel′ler·gin. A suspension of *Brucella* nucleoproteins used in the intradermal test for the diagnosis of brucellosis.

bru·cel′lin. A preparation from the combined cultures of the three species of *Brucella,* used in the diagnosis, prophylaxis, and treatment of brucellosis.

bru″cel·lo′sis. A remittent febrile disease caused by infection with bacteria of the genus *Brucella.* In humans, brucellosis may occur in acute or chronic form and leads to weakness, loss of weight, and anemia. The disease is rarely transmitted from person to person, but spreads readily from animal to animal and from animal to man. Cattle, goats and hogs are the chief sources of infection. Syn., *Malta fever, Mediterranean fever, undulant fever, brucelliasis.*

bru′cine (brew′seen, ·sin). A poisonous alkaloid found in various species of *Strychnos.*

bruise. Contusion, *q.v.*

bruisse·ment′ (brwees·mong′). A purring sound heard on auscultation.

bruit (broo·ee′). Old term for an adventitious sound heard on auscultation. See *heart sound; heart murmur.*

brux′ism. The unconscious habit of gnashing or grinding the teeth, often limited to the sleeping period but sometimes occurring during mental or physical concentration or strain.

brux″o·ma′ni·a. Grinding or pounding of the teeth as a manifestation of neurosis, usually occurring during sleep.

bry·o′ni·a (brigh·o′nee·uh). The root of *Bryonia alba* or *B. dioica.* It is an irritant emetic, drastic cathartic, and vesicant.

bry·on′i·din (brigh·on′i·din). A glycoside from *Bryonia alba.*

bry′o·nin. A glycoside from *Bryonia alba.*

B.T.U., B.t.u. British thermal unit. See under *unit.*

bu′bo (bew′bo, boo′bo). Inflammation, swelling, and hypertrophy of one or more lymph nodes, often going on to suppuration, and usually located in the groin and axilla. It occurs commonly with chancroid, gonorrhea, and venereal lymphogranuloma. Syn., *sympathetic abscess.* Also called *inguinal adenitis.* **—bubon′ic,** *adj.* **serpiginous b.** An ulcerated bubo which changes its seat or in which the ulceration extends in one direction while healing in another. **syphilitic b.** That which appears in syphilis a few days after the primary lesion. **venereal b.** That due to venereal disease.

bu″bon·ad″e·ni′tis. Inflammation of an inguinal lymph node.

bu″bon·al′gi·a. Pain in the inguinal region.

bu·bon′ic plague. See under *plague.*

bu·car′di·a (bew·kahr′dee·uh, boo·kahr′·). Bovine heart; extreme hypertrophy of the heart.

buc′ca (pl. *buccae*). The cheek; the hollow of the cheek, or its inner surface. **—buccal,** *adj.*

buc′ci·na″tor (buck′si·nay″tor).

The muscular foundation of the cheek. See Table of Muscles in the Appendix.

buc'co-. A combining form denoting *of or pertaining to the cheeks.*

buc″co·gin'gi·val (buck″o·jin'ji-vul, ·jin·jy'vul). Pertaining to the cheek and the gums.

buc″co·la'bi·al. Pertaining to the cheek and the lip.

buc″co·lin'gual. Relating to the cheek and the tongue. **—buccolingually,** *adv.*

buc″co·me'si·al (buck″o·mee'zhul, ·mee'see·ul). Pertaining to the buccal and the mesial walls of a tooth or cavity.

buc″co·na'sal (buck″o·nay'zul). Pertaining to the oral and nasal cavities.

buc″co·na″so·pha·ryn'ge·al (·nay″zo·fa·rin'jul, ·far″in·jee'ul). Pertaining to the mouth and upper part of the pharynx.

buc″co·pha·ryn'ge·al. Relating to the mouth and to the pharynx.

buc'cu·la. The fleshy fold beneath the chin which forms what is called a double chin. *Obs.*

bu'chu (bew'cue, boo'koo). The leaves of several species of *Barosma,* yielding a volatile oil. Formerly used as a diuretic in cystitis.

Bucky's diaphragm. See under *diaphragm.*

bud. 1. *In embryology,* a protuberance or outgrowth which is the primordium of an appendage or an organ. 2. *In anatomy,* an organ or structure shaped like the bud of a plant. **limb b.** A lateral swelling of the embryonic trunk; the anlage of an appendage. **lung b.** One of the primary outgrowths of the embryonic trachae whose growth and subsequent division produce a primary bronchus and all its branches. **taste b.** End organ of the sense of taste; one of the oval, flask-shaped bodies embedded, most commonly, in the epithelium of the tongue. Also called *calyculus gustatorii.*

bud'ding. *In biology,* a form of asexual reproduction occurring in the lower animals and plants, in which the parent organism develops projections which become separated and develop into independent organisms.

Buerger, Leo [*American physician,* 1879–1943]. Known for his observations on thromboangiitis obliterans, a term he originated. His observations furnished the first clear report of the clinical course and the pathology of the disease, which is known as *Buerger's disease* (1908). Devised passive exercises as routine treatment of the condition.

buff'er. A substance which, when present in or added to a solution, re-sists any change of hydrogen-ion concentration when either acid or alkali is added.

buff'er. To treat with a buffer.

buff'y coat. The white blood cells which separate and form a layer on top of the erythrocytes when whole blood is centrifuged.

bug. An insect of the order Heteroptera. **assassin b.** Any one of the Triatomidae. Syn., *conenose.* Also called *flying bedbug, kissing b., Mexican* or *Texas bedbug.* **bedbug.** Any bug of the genus *Cimex.* **Croton b.** The cockroach. See *Blatella germanica.* **red b.** Harvest mite; a mite of the genus *Trombicula, q.v.*

bug'ger·y. *In legal medicine,* sodomy, *q.v.*

bulb. 1. An oval or circular expansion of a cylinder or tube. 2. Old term for the medulla oblongata. **—bulb'ar,** *adj.* **arterial b.** The anterior part of the embryonic heart from the division of which the aortic and pulmonary stems have their origin. Syn., *bulb of the heart* (bulbus cordis). **brachial b.** The expansion of the spinal cord at the place of distribution of the nerves forming the brachial plexus. **b. of the eye.** The eyeball. **b. of the heart.** The anterior division of the embryonic heart within the pericardial cavity. Its proximal part is incorporated into the right ventricle; its distal part forms the aortic and pulmonary valve region of the heart. **b. of the penis.** The expanded proximal portion of the corpus cavernosum urethrae. Syn., *b. of the urethra.* **duodenal b.** *In radiology,* the first part of the duodenum, immediately beyond the pylorus. Also called *duodenal cap.* **hair b.** The swelling at the deep end of the root of a hair. **inferior b. of the internal jugular vein.** An enlargement of the jugular vein immediately above its union with the subclavian vein. **nerve b.** An eminence of protoplasm within the sarcolemma of a muscle fiber, representing the termination of a motor nerve fiber. **olfactory b.** The bulb of the olfactory nerve; one is situated on each side of the longitudinal fissure upon the undersurface of each anterior lobe of the cerebrum. **vestibular b.** One of the paired masses of erectile tissue located on either side of the vestibule of the vagina, homologous to the bulb and adjacent corpus cavernosum urethrae in the male.

bul'bo-. A combining form denoting *a bulb or bulbar.*

bul″bo·cap'nine (bul″bo·cap'neen, ·nin). An alkaloid in the tubers of *Bulbocapnus cavus.*

bul″bo·cav″er·no'sus. A muscle encircling the bulb and adjacent, proximal parts of the penis in the male and encircling the orifice of the vagina and covering the lateral parts of the vestibular bulbs in the female. See Table of Muscles in the Appendix.

ul″bo·u·re′thral. Relating to the bulb of the urethra, as the bulbourethral glands.

ulb′ous. Having or containing bulbs; bulb-shaped; swollen; terminating in a bulb.

u·lim′i·a (bew·lim′ee·uh, boo·), **bou·lim′i·a** (boo·lim′ee·uh). Excessive, insatiable appetite, seen in psychotic states; a symptom of diabetes mellitus and of certain cerebral lesions. Syn., *adephagia, cynorexia.* —**bulim′ic,** *adj.*

ul′la (bool′uh, bul′uh) (pl. *bullae*). A large bleb or blister. —**bullous,** *adj.* **b. ethmoidalis.** A rounded projection into the middle meatus of the nose, due to an enlarged ethmoid cell.

ul′late (bool′ate, bul′ate). 1. Blistered; marked by bullae. 2. Inflated, bladderlike, vesiculate. —**bulla′tion,** *n.*

uMed. The Bureau of Medicine and Surgery, U. S. Navy.

UN (bee·you·en). Abbreviation for blood urea nitrogen.

un′dle. In *biology,* a fascicular grouping of elementary tissues, as nerve fibers or muscle fibers. Old term for *nerve fiber tract.* **atrioventricular b.** That part of the conduction system of the heart arising from the atrioventricular node and dividing into two branches, which run down either side of the interventricular septum and ramify among the muscle bundles of the ventricle. Syn., *b. of His.* **b. of His.** See atrioventricular b. **b. of Kent.** A bridge of muscular tissue joining the atria and ventricles at the right margin of the septum. It is considered an anomalous or aberrant atrioventricular bundle which, in some cases, may conduct impulses.

un′dle branch block. Interruption of excitation through either division of the atrioventricular bundle.

un′ion. A swelling of a bursa of the foot, especially of the metatarsophalangeal joint of the great toe; associated with a thickening of the adjacent skin and a forcing of the great toe laterally, into adduction.

un″ion·ec′to·my. Excision of a bunion; plastic repair of the first metatarsophalangeal joint.

unsen, Robert Wilhelm [*German chemist and physicist,* 1811–99]. Celebrated for his invention of the gas burner which is provided with holes near the base, permitting admixture of air so that the gas is completely oxidized, giving a hot blue flame.

bur, burr. 1. *In botany,* a rough, prickly shell or case. 2. The lobe of the ear. 3. *In dentistry,* a cutting instrument with a rounded, pointed, cylindrical, or ovoid head having numerous blades; used in the dental engine for excavating carious dentine and for other purposes. 4. *In surgery,* an instrument similar in form to a dental bur, but larger, designed for surgical operations upon the bones.

bur′bot liv′er oil. The oil extracted from the liver of the burbot, *Lota maculosa;* used like cod liver oil.

Bur′gun·dy pitch. See under *pitch.*

burn. 1. The tissue reaction or injury resulting from the application of heat, caustics, or electricity. Burns are classified as simple hyperemic (*first degree*); vesicant (*second degree*); destructive of skin and underlying tissues (*third degree*). 2. Feel the sensation of heat. 3. Char or destroy by fire. 4. *In chemistry,* to oxygenize. **brush b.** Mechanical injury produced by friction. **chemical b.** That produced by caustics (acid or alkaline), irritant gases, etc. **electric b.** One caused by high-frequency currents. **flash b.** One produced by ignition of high explosives such as cordite, especially in naval warfare. Also called *powder b.* **radiation b.** One resulting from exposure to radiant energy as x-ray, radium, sunlight, or other form. These may be severe, and x-ray and radium burns heal very slowly. **sunburn.** Injury to the skin of varying degrees of intensity, produced by actinic rays of the sun or sun lamps. See *sunburn.* **thermal b.** One caused by contact with fire, hot objects, or hot liquids. **x-ray b.** See radiation b.

bur′sa (pl. *bursae*). A small sac interposed between parts that move upon one another. **Achilles b.** The bursa lying between the Achilles tendon and the calcaneus. Also called *b. tendinis calcanei.* **cystic b.** A subhyoid bursa which has become cystic. **gluteal b.** One or more lying under the gluteus maximus. **gluteofascial b.** One lying between the greater trochanter and the gluteus maximus. Also called *gluteotrochanteric b.* **iliac b.** One lying between the tendon of the iliacus muscle and the lesser trochanter. **iliopsoas b.** One separating the tendon of the iliopsoas muscle from the hipbone and the capsule of the hip joint. **ischial b.** One over the ischial tuberosity. **olecranon b.** One over the olecranon process. **omental b.** The lesser peritoneal sac; formed in the embryo by a lateral outgrowth of the mesentery, dorsal to the stomach, and after rotation of the gut forming a cavity back of the stomach and into the great omentum. **patel-**

lar b. One of several bursae about the patella which may communicate with the knee joint. See prepatellar *b.* **pharyngeal b.** A small pit caudal to the pharyngeal tonsil, resulting from the ingrowth of the epithelium along the course of the degenerating tip of the notochord. Also called *Luschka's b.* **popliteal b.** A bursa situated in the popliteal space between the tendon of the semimembranosus and the tendon of the inner head of the gastrocnemius, where they rub against each other. **prepatellar b.** A bursa situated over the patella and the upper part of the patellar ligament. **sacral b.** One found in the aged, over the sacrococcygeal articulation or over the spine of the fourth or fifth sacral vertebra. **subacromial b.** See subdeltoid *b.* **subdeltoid b.** One lying beneath the deltoid muscle and extending beneath the acromion and coracoacromial ligament; it separates these structures from the capsule of the shoulder joint. It is frequently inflamed. Syn., *subacromial b.* [BNA]. **subhyoid b.** One lying between the thyrohyoid membrane and hyoid bone and the conjoint insertion of the omohyoid, sternohyoid, and stylohyoid muscles. **subscapular b.** One between the tendon of the subscapularis muscle and the capsule of the shoulder joint; it communicates with the joint cavity. **synovial b.** One found between tendons and bony surfaces.

bur·sec'to·my. The surgical removal of a bursa.

bur·si'tis. Inflammation of a bursa. **Achilles b.** Inflammation of the bursa beneath the tendo calcaneus. **popliteal b.** Inflammation of the popliteal bursa. Syn., *Baker's cyst.* **prepatellar b.** Inflammation of bursa in front of the patella. Syn., *housemaid's knee.* **radiohumeral b.** Inflammation of the olecranon bursa. See *tennis arm.* **subdeltoid b.** Inflammation of the subdeltoid bursa.

bur'so·lith. A calculus formed within a bursa.

bu·sul'fan. 1,4-Di(methanesulfonyloxy)butane, a neoplastic suppressant. See *myleran.*

but-. *In chemistry,* a combining form denoting the presence of a grouping containing four carbon atoms.

bu"ta·bar'bi·tal. Nonproprietary name for 5-ethyl-5-*sec.*-butyl barbituric acid. See *butisol.*

bu'ta·caine" sul'fate (bew"tuh-cane", bew"tuh·kay'een). γ-Di-*n*-butylaminopropyl-*p*-aminobenzoate sulfate, a water-soluble local anesthetic. See *butyn.*

bu"ta·di'ene. 1,3-Butadiene. $CH_2:$ $CH.CH:CH_2$. A gaseous hydrocarbon derived from petroleum and which is used in the manufacture of synthetic rubber.

but"al·lyl·o·nal. Nonproprietary name for 5-*sec.*-butyl-5-β-bromallyl barbituric acid. See *pernoston.*

bu·tam'ben. Nonproprietary name for butyl aminobenzoate. See *butesin.*

bu"ta·no'ic ac'id. Butyric acid, *q.v.*

butazolidin. Trade-mark for phenylbutazone.

butesin. Trade-mark for a brand of butyl aminobenzoate. See *butamben.*

bu"te·thal. Nonproprietary name for 5-*n*-butyl-5-ethylbarbituric acid. See *neonal.*

bu·teth'a·mine. Nonproprietary name for 2-isobutylaminoethyl-*p*-aminobenzoate. See *monocaine.*

butisol. Trade-mark for butabarbital.

butoben. A trade-mark for butyl parahydroxybenzoate.

bu"to·pyr"o·nox'yl. Butyl mesityl oxide, a yellowish liquid, insoluble in water; used as an insect repellent and toxicant. See *indalone.*

but'ter. 1. The fatty part of milk, obtained by rupturing the fat globules by churning or mechanical agitation. 2. Various vegetable fats having the consistency of butter. 3. Certain chemical products having the appearance or consistency of butter. **antimony b.** Antimonic chloride. **cacao b.** See *theobroma* oil. **tin b.** Stannic chloride. **zinc b.** Zinc chloride.

but'ter yel'low. *p*-Dimethylaminoazobenzene. A yellow dye used to color fats and in the preparation of Töpfer's reagent for the determination of free HCl in gastric juice.

but'tock. One of the two fleshy parts of the body posterior to the hip joints, formed by the masses of the glutea muscles.

but'ton·hole". *In surgery,* a small straight opening into an organ or part **mitral b.** An advanced case of mitral stenosis, usually of rheumatic origin.

bu'tyl. The monovalent hydrocarbon radical, C_4H_9—. It occurs as **normal-b.**, $CH_3.CH_2.CH_2.CH_2$—; **iso-b.**, abbreviated i-butyl, $(CH_3)_2CH.CH_2$— **secondary-b.**, $CH_3.CH_2.(CH_3)CH$— and **tertiary-b.**, $(CH_3)_3C$—. **b. aminobenzoate.** A white, crystalline powder, almost insoluble in water; used as a local anesthetic. See *butesin.* **b.-chloral hydrate.** Trichlorobutylidene glycol. White, lustrous scales, soluble in water; an analgesic and hypnotic. Syn., *croton chloral hydrate.* **b.-ethylbarbituric acid.** Also called *b.-ethylmalonyl urea.* See *neonal.* **b. parahydroxybenzoate.** White, crystalline powder, soluble in water, used as preservative of medicinals, foods, etc. See *butoben.*

butyn. A trade-mark for butacaine sulfate.

bu″tyr·a′ceous (bew″ti·ray′shus). Resembling butter; containing or yielding butterlike substances.

bu·tyr′ic ac′id. $CH_3.CH_2.CH_2.COOH$. Butanoic acid; occurs in butter as a glyceride.

bu′tyr·in. $(C_3H_7COO)_3C_3H_5$. Glyceryl tributyrate, a constituent of butterfat. Also called *tributyrin*.

bu′tyr·in·ase′. An enzyme found in blood serum which hydrolyzes butyrin.

bu′tyr·oid. Buttery; having the consistency of butter.

bux′ine (buck′seen, ·sin). An alkaloid from the leaves of *Buxus sempervirens.*

bys″si·no′sis. Irritation of the pulmonary air passages; caused by the inhalation of cotton dust. Formerly thought to be a form of pneumoconiosis.

Bywaters, Eric George Lapthorne [*English physician*, 1910–]. With Desmond Beall, described crush syndrome with impairment of renal function (1941).

C

C. 1. Chemical symbol for carbon. 2. Abbreviation for Celsius, centigrade, closure, congius, contraction, cylinder, cylindrical lens.

c. 1. *Cum;* with. 2. *Centum;* one hundred.

C′. Symbol for complement.

Ca. 1. Chemical symbol for calcium. 2. Abbreviation for cathode.

ca′ble. The flexible arm of the dental engine.

Cabot, Hugh [*American urologic surgeon*, 1872–1945]. Known for his many contributions to the knowledge of urology.

Cabot, Richard Clarke [*American physician and clinician*, 1868–1939]. Widely known for his teachings of differential diagnosis by means of the case-history system and for his interest in the problems of social service.

ca·ca′o (ka·kay′o, ka·kah′o). Seeds from *Theobroma cacao* from which cacao butter, chocolate, and cocoa are prepared. See *Theobroma.* **c. butter.** Theobroma oil, obtained from the roasted seeds of *T. cacao;* used in the preparation of suppositories, in ointments, and as an emollient.

ca·chet′ (ka·shay′, cash′ay). Two rounded or oblong, concave pieces of wafer (rice paper) enclosing an ill-tasting medication when the opposing edges are pressed together.

ca·chex′i·a (ka·keck′see·uh). Weakness and emaciation caused by some serious disease such as syphilis, tuberculosis, or carcinoma. **—cachec′tic,** *adj.* **c. exophthalmica.** That associated with exophthalmic goiter. **c. hypophysiopriva.** The symptoms of hypopituitary cachexia observed when the pituitary has been removed. **c. strumipriva.** That following ablation of the thyroid. Also called *c. thyropriva.* **cancerous.** That associated with malignant disease.

malarial c. Anemia, weakness, mental depression, and emaciation associated with chronic malaria. Also called *paludal c.* **urinary c.** That associated with chronic suppurative infections of the urinary tract.

cach″in·na′tion (kack″i·nay′shun). Immoderate laughter, as in hysteria.

ca′chou′ (kah″shoo′, ka·shoo′). An aromatic pill or tablet for deodorizing the breath.

cac′o-, cac-. A combining form signifying *bad, diseased, deformed,* or *vitiated.*

cac″o·de·mo′ni·a, cac″o·demon″o·ma′ni·a. A psychosis in which the patient believes he is possessed by or of an evil spirit.

cac′o·dyl. $(CH_3)_2As-As(CH_3)_2$. Tetramethyldiarsenic. A colorless, heavy liquid with an extremely offensive odor.

cac′o·dyl·ate. A salt of cacodylic acid. The sodium, calcium, and iron salts are used in medicine.

cac″o·dyl′ic ac′id. Dimethylarsinic acid, $AsO(CH_3)_2OH$.

cac″o·geu′si·a (kack″og·yoo′see·uh, kack″o·jew′see·uh). The sensation of bad taste; frequently a symptom in idiopathic epilepsy.

ca·coph′o·ny, cac″o·phe′ni·a. An abnormally harsh or discordant sound. **—cacophon′ic,** *adj.*

ca·dav′er. A dead body, especially that of a human being; a corpse. **—cadaver′ic,** *adj.*

ca·dav′er·ous. Resembling a cadaver; of a deathly pallor.

cad′mi·um. Cd = 112.41. A bluish white metal used as a constituent of easily fusible alloys. Its salts have physiologic actions similar to those of zinc.

ca·du′ce·us (ka·dew′see·us). The symbol or insigne of medicine consisting of the staff of Asclepius about which a single serpent is coiled. The Medical Corps of the United States Army has modified the symbol to consist of a staff with two formal wings at the top, and two serpents entwined about the remainder. The latter is not regarded as a medical, but as an administrative emblem, implying neutral, noncombatant status.

cae-. For words beginning with *cae-* not found here, see under *ce-*.

Caes"al·pin'i·a (sez"al·pin'ee·uh, ses"al·). A genus of tropical trees of the Leguminosae.

caf·fe'ic ac'id. (OH)$_2$.C$_6$H$_3$.CH:CH.-COOH. Dihydroxycinnamic acid, obtained from coffee.

caf'fe·ine (kaf'ee·in, kaf'een). An alkaloid, chemically 1,3,7-trimethylxanthine, found in the leaves and beans of the coffee tree, also in tea and in guarana. It is a cerebrospinal, circulatory, and renal stimulant. Syn., *guaranine, methyltheobromine, theine, trimethylxanthine.* Also called *psoraline.* **c. and sodium benzoate.** A white powder containing 47-50% of caffeine, soluble in water. A form of caffeine especially suited for subcutaneous injection. **c. with sodium salicylate.** A white powder, soluble in water, and containing 48-52% of caffeine. **citrated c.** A mixture of equal parts of caffeine and citric acid, the latter increasing the solubility of caffeine in water. **caf'fe·in·ism.** Chronic poisoning due to the excessive use of coffee or other caffeine-containing preparations.

cai"no·pho'bi·a (kigh"no·fo'bee·uh, kay"no·). Neophobia; morbid fear of newness.

caj'e·put, caj'u·put (kadj'uh-putt). An East Indian tree, *Melaleuca leucadendron,* which yields a volatile oil resembling turpentine oil.

caj'e·put·ol", caj'u·put·ol". Cineol; eucalyptol, *q.v.*

caj'u·put. See *cajeput.*

caked. Compressed, tense, or hardened, due to engorgement or induration.

Cal. Large or great calorie.

cal. Small calorie.

cal'a·mine (kal'uh·myne, ·min). Native zinc carbonate. Official calamine, also called prepared calamine, is zinc oxide with a small amount of ferric oxide. Used as a local application in the treatment of skin diseases.

cal'a·mus. Sweetflag. The rhizome of *Acorus calamus,* an ingredient of many popular bitters.

cal·ca'ne·o-. A combining form signifying *pertaining to the calcaneus.*

cal·ca"ne·o·dyn'i·a, cal"ca·no·dyn'i·a. Pain in the heel, or calcaneus, when walking or standing. Syn., *achillodynia.*

cal·ca'ne·um. BR term for calcaneus, the heel bone.

cal·ca'ne·us. 1. The heel bone. See Table of Bones in the Appendix. 2. Clubfoot in which the heel alone touches the ground; talipes calcaneus. **—calcaneal, calcanean,** *adj.*

cal·car'e·ous (kal·kair'ee·us). 1. Pertaining to or of the nature of limestone. 2. Having a chalky appearance or consistence. 3. Containing calcium.

cal·car"i·u'ri·a. The presence of calcium salts in the urine.

cal·ce'mi·a, cal·cae'mi·a (kal·see'mee·uh). The occurrence of an excessive amount of calcium in the blood. Syn., *hypercalcemia.*

cal"ci·co'sis. A form of pneumoconiosis due to the inhalation of marble dust.

cal·cif'er·ol. Vitamin D$_2$, obtained by irradiation of ergosterol. One mg. represents 40,000 units of vitamin-D activity.

cal"ci·fi·ca'tion. The deposit of calcareous matter within the tissues of the body. **pathologic c.** Abnormal deposition of calcium salts, of two forms: (a) *dystrophic,* deposition in degenerated or necrotic tissues; (b) *metastatic,* deposition of calcium salts, mobilized from a natural site, in tissues not demonstrably injured; commonly associated with destructive lesions of bone.

cal'ci·fy. To deposit mineral salts, as in the process of calcification. **—calcified,** *adj.*

cal·cig'er·ous (kal·sidj'ur·us). Containing lime or a lime salt.

cal'ci·grade. Walking on the heels. *Obs.*

cal·cim'e·ter. An apparatus for determining the amount of calcium in the blood.

cal"ci·na'tion. The process of driving off organic matter and volatile chemical constituents from inorganic compounds by heat. **—calcine,** *v.t.*

cal"ci·no'sis. The deposition of calcium salts in the skin and subcutaneous tissues; presumed to be a disorder of hyperparathyroidism. **circumscribed c.** Calcified nodules limited to the skin and subcutaneous tissues of the upper extremities, particularly the hands; frequently seen in scleroderma. **diffuse c.** Widespread calcified nodules which tend to ulcerate and heal slowly, and involve subcutaneous tissues, muscles, tendons, and nerve sheaths; seen especially in children. Also called *universal c.*

cal"ci·pe'ni·a. Calcium deficiency.

cal'ci·um. Ca = 40.08. A brilliant, silver-white metal, characterized by strong affinity for oxygen. **c. acetylsalicylate.** A white powder, readily soluble in water; used as an antirheumatic and analgesic. **c. bromide.** $CaBr_2$. A nerve sedative. **c. carbonate.** Any of the forms of $CaCO_3$, such as chalk, marble, or whiting. See precipitated *calcium* carbonate. **c. chloride.** $CaCl_2$. It occurs as white, deliquescent fragments or granules, soluble in water; used internally in the treatment of hemorrhage, tuberculosis, hay fever, and other allergies, etc. **c. creosotate.** A mixture of the calcium compounds of creosote, representing about 50% of creosote; used as an expectorant. **c. gluconate.** $[CH_2OH(CHOH)_4.COO]_2Ca.-H_2O$. A white, crystalline or granular powder, soluble in water. It is less irritating than other calcium salts and can be given in large doses orally or intravenously. **c. glycerophosphate.** $CaC_3H_5(OH)_2PO_4$. A white, crystalline powder, soluble in cold water; has been recommended as a nerve tonic. **c. hydrate.** See c. hydroxide. **c. hydroxide.** $Ca(OH)_2$. Slaked lime. It is the active ingredient of lime water. Syn., c. *hydrate.* **c. hypochlorite.** $Ca(ClO)_2$. White cubes decomposing readily. It is antiseptic and is used as a disinfectant and strong bleaching agent. **c. iodobehenate.** Contains principally $(C_{22}H_{42}O_2I)_2Ca$. It is a white or yellowish powder, insoluble in water. In the body, it slowly liberates iodide ions, for which effect it is used. Syn., *calioben.* See *sajodin.* **c. lactate.** $Ca(C_3H_5O_3)_2.5H_2O$. A white powder, soluble in water; used when calcium therapy is indicated. **c. mandelate.** $(C_6H_5.CHOH.COO)_2Ca$. A white powder, slightly soluble in cold water. It is used for the effect of mandelic acid as urinary antiseptic. **c. oxide.** CaO. Lime; quicklime; burnt lime. It is not used medicinally. **c. sulfate.** This substance occurs in several forms: (a) $CaSO_4.2H_2O$. Found naturally as the minerals alabaster, gypsum, mineral white, satin spar, and selenite. (b) $CaSO_4.\frac{1}{2}H_2O$. Plaster of Paris, made by heating gypsum to 120° to 130° C. (c) $CaSO_4$, completely dehydrated calcium sulfate prepared by heating gypsum or plaster of Paris above 200° C. **dibasic c. phosphate.** $CaHPO_4.2H_2O$. A white powder, almost insoluble in water; used in rickets and other bone diseases. **monobasic c. phosphate.** $CaH_4(PO_4)_2.H_2O$. It occurs in granules or as a powder, partially soluble in water, used in certain baking powders and is the calcium superphosphate used as a fertilizer. **precipitated c. carbonate.** $CaCO_3$. A white powder practically insoluble in water. It is antacid. Externally, it is used as a desiccant. **tribasic c. phosphate.** $Ca_3(PO_4)_2$. A white powder, almost insoluble

in water; used as an antacid. Also called precipitated c. phosphate.

cal"co·glob'u·lin. A combination of calcium with protein such as is found in calcospherites, probably representing an early stage in the process of laying down calcium in teeth and bone.

cal"co·sphae'rite. See *calcosphe-rite.*

cal"co·sphe'rite, cal"co·sphae'-rite. One of the granules found in tissues like bone or shell, or formed into loose proteid combinations by calcium salts obtained from the blood.

cal'cu·li (kăl'cūe-lye). Plural of calculus.

cal"cu·lo'sis. The presence of a calculus, or abnormal concretion.

cal'cu·lus (pl. *calculi*). A solid concrement composed chiefly of mineral substances and salts found principally in ducts, passages, hollow organs, and cysts. Organic materials such as cells, mucus, etc., may form a centrum or nidus and may be dispersed as a matrix for the mineral deposits, as salts of calcium, of uric acid, of bile acids, etc. **—calculous,** *adj.* **arthritic c.** A deposit near a joint of salts of uric acid, as in gout. **biliary c.** One containing mineral material and originating in the biliary passages. If composed of cholesterol or pigment, or both, without mineral constituents, it is a concrement rather than a calculus. **bronchial c.** A concretion of mucus or exudate, infiltrated with mineral salts, situated in the bronchial tree. **cystic c.** One found in either the urinary bladder or the gallbladder. **dental c.** Calcareous deposits on the teeth. Syn., *tartar.* **mammary c.** A calcified mass of secretion or exudate in the ducts of the mammary gland. **mulberry c.** A urinary calculus with a finely nodular outer surface resembling a mulberry and usually composed largely of calcium oxalate. **prostatic c.** Calcified nodules in prostatic acini, probably derived from corpora amylacea. **renal c.** A concretion in the kidney. **salivary c.** One situated in the duct of a salivary gland, or a deposit upon the surfaces of the teeth. **serumal c., serumnal c.** Formerly believed to be a calcareous deposit formed about the teeth by exudation from diseased gums. Also called *sanguinary c.* **staghorn c.** A large, irregularly branched calculus in the renal pelvis. **tonsillar c.** A calcified mass of detritus in the tonsillar crypts. **urinary c.** One situated in any part of the urinary system. **vesical c.** A stone in the urinary bladder.

cal"e·fa'cient (kal"1·fay'shunt). 1. Warming, producing a sensation of

heat. 2. A medicine, externally applied, that causes a sensation of warmth.

ca·len'du·la. 1. A plant of the genus *Calendula*, of the Compositae; marigold. 2. The dried ligulate floret of plants of this genus, especially *C. officinalis*.

calf. The thick, fleshy part of the back of the leg, formed by the gastrocnemius and soleus muscles.

cal"i·bra'tion. The measurement of the caliber of a tube, or the determination or rectification of the graduations on a tube, pipet, or balance weights. —**cal'ibrator,** *n.;* **cal'ibrate,** *v.t.*

cal'i·ces (kal'i·seez, kay'li·seez). Plural of calyx.

cal"i·for'ni·um. Chemical element No. 98, symbol Cf, produced artificially in minute amounts.

cal·i'o·ben. Calcium iodobehenate.

cal'i·pers (kal'i·purz). An instrument for measuring the thickness or the outside or inside diameters of objects.

cal"i·sa'ya. Cinchona bark, especially that of *Cinchona calisaya*. See *cinchona*.

cal"is·then'ics. The practice of light gymnastics by various rhythmical movements of the body; intended to develop the muscles and graceful carriage.

cal"li·pe'di·a. The desire to give birth to a beautiful child.

cal"lo·ma'ni·a. A mania characterized by delusions of beauty.

cal·los'i·tas. A hard, thickened patch of skin with hypertrophy of the horny layer caused by irritation, friction, or pressure. Syn., *keratoma, tyloma, tylosis, callus,* 1.

cal·los'i·ty. A circumscribed area of thickened skin due to friction or pressure.

cal'lus. 1. A callosity; an area of hardened and thickened skin, seen usually in the palm or the sole; a hypertrophic reaction of the epidermis to pressure and friction. 2. New growth of incompletely organized bony tissue surrounding the bone ends in fracture; a part of the reparative process. **fibrous c.** The connective tissue that precedes the formation of cartilage and bone in the reparative process of a fracture. **permanent c.** The thickening of the bony tissues in bone fractures, indicating complete repair. —**callous,** *adj.*

cal'o·mel. HgCl, mercurous chloride. A white powder; formerly used popularly as a purgative, also as an alterant and antisyphilitic.

cal'or (kal'or, kay'lor). 1. Heat; one of the four classic signs of inflammation: calor, rubor, tumor, dolor. 2. Body heat or moderate fever heat. 3. Localized heat associated with inflammation.

calori-. A combining form signifying heat.

ca·lor'ic. 1. Pertaining to a calorie or to heat. 2. Heat.

cal'o·rie, cal'o·ry. A heat unit; the amount of heat required to raise the temperature of 1 kg. of water from 0° to 1° C. This is also known as a **large calorie** or **kilocalorie**, and is the unit used in the study of metabolism. Abbreviated, Cal. The **small calorie** is the amount of heat required to raise the temperature of 1 Gm. of water 1° C., and is one one-thousandth of the large calorie. Abbreviated, cal.

cal"o·rif'ic. Heat-producing.

cal"o·rim'e·ter. Instrument for measuring the heat production of an individual or system. **respiration c.** Apparatus which determines the heat production of an individual by measuring the gaseous exchange of the lungs.

cal"o·rim'e·try. The determination of the heat change in any individual or system by use of the calorimeter. —**calorimet'ric,** *adj.*

ca·lum'ba. Colombo, the dried root of *Jateorrhiza palmata*, native to East Africa and Madagascar. It is a simple bitter.

cal·va'ri·a (pl. *calvariae*). The upper part of the skull; the skullcap; also called *calvarium*. —**calvarial,** *adj.*

cal·vi'ti·es (kal·vish'ee·eez). Baldness. Loss of hair, especially of the upper part of the head. Syn., *alopecia*.

cal'y·ces (kal'i·seez, kay'li·seez). Plural of calyx.

ca'lyx, ca'lix (kay'licks, kal'icks) (pl. *calyxes, calyces, calices*). 1. A cup. 2. *In anatomy*, one of the cuplike divisions of the pelvis of the kidney into which the pyramids project. —**calycine, calyc'inal, calyc'iform, calicine,** *adj.* **major c.** A primary subdivision of the renal pelvis; derived from the embryonic pole tubules, usually two or three in number. **minor c.** One of the 4 to 13 cuplike divisions of the major calyces; derived from tubules of the second, third, and fourth orders, each receiving one or more of the renal papillae.

cam'bi·um. A layer of tissue formed between the wood and the bark of exogenous plants. **c. layer.** The cellular layer of the periosteum.

cam'er·a. 1. Chamber or compartment. 2. Apparatus used for photography. **c. lucida.** An optical device used to project onto paper the image of an object so that an accurate drawing can be made. There are two main types: (a) that equipped with a Wollaston prism which projects an image in reduced, enlarged, or natural size; (b) that equipped with an Abbe prism, mirror, and microscope, used where a magnified image is desired.

cam'i·sole. A kind of straitjacket; a canvas shirt with very long sleeves; used to restrain violent psychotics.

camequin hydrochloride. Trademark for amodiaquin hydrochloride.

cam'phene. $C_{10}H_{16}$. Terpene hydrocarbon occurring in several volatile oils.

cam'pho-, camph-. A combining form denoting *camphor.*

cam'phor. $C_{10}H_{16}O$. A ketone obtained from the volatile oil of *Cinnamomum camphora*, a tree indigenous to eastern Asia, or produced synthetically. It is a mild irritant and antiseptic and is used as a carminative and stimulant. —**camphorated, camphor'ic**, *adj.*

cam'phor·at"ed oil. Camphor liniment.

cam·phor'ic ac'id. $C_{10}H_{16}O_4$. A dibasic acid obtained by the oxidation of camphor.

cam'phor lin'i·ment. A solution of camphor in cottonseed oil. Syn., *camphorated oil.*

cam'phor oil. A volatile oil obtained from the camphor tree *Cinnamomum camphora*, usually used as a solvent and, occasionally, as a rubefacient.

cam·pim'e·ter. Instrument for measuring the field of vision. See *perimeter.* —**campimetry**, *n.*

amp"to·cor'mi·a. A special form of hysteria, seen most often in soldiers; characterized by extreme forward flexion of the spine, the eyes usually being focused on the ground. The person affected apparently walks with great difficulty and frequently has associated tremors. Also called *bent back.*

amp"to·dac'ty·ly. A condition in which one or more fingers are constantly flexed at one or both phalangeal joints.

an'a·dine (kan'uh·deen, ·din). *l*-Tetrahydroberberine, an alkaloid from *Hydrastis canadensis.*

a·nal'. Any tubular channel; duct. **adductor c.** A triangular, aponeurotic tunnel bounded by the sartorius, vastus medialis, and adductor muscles; it extends from the femoral triangle to the hiatus adductorius and gives passage to the femoral artery and vein, the saphenous nerve, and the nerve to the vastus medialis. Also called *Hunter's c., subsartorial c.* **alimentary c.** The whole digestive tube from the mouth to the anus; the gastrointestinal tract. **alveolar canals** [BNA]. Those in the maxilla or mandible giving passage to vessels and nerves to the teeth. A **superior alveolar canal** is one located in the maxilla. An **inferior alveolar canal** is one located in

the mandible. Syn., *dental canals.* **anal c.** The terminal portion of the large intestine extending from the rectum to the anus. **birth c.** See *parturient c.* **carotid c.** One in the petrous portion of the temporal bone; it gives passage to the internal carotid artery. **central c. of the spinal cord.** The small canal that extends through the center of the spinal cord from the conus medullaris to the lower part of the fourth ventricle. It represents the embryonic neural canal. **facial c.** A canal in the temporal bone for the passage of the facial nerve. **hair c.** A canal in the epidermis through which the hair shaft erupts. **Haversian canals.** The canals penetrating the compact substance of bone in a longitudinal direction and anastomosing with one another by transverse or oblique branches. They contain blood vessels and connective tissue. **incisive c.** The bifurcated bony passage from the floor of the nasal cavity to the incisive fossa. On each side, the branches open by a median and a lateral incisive foramen transmitting respectively the nasopalatine nerve and a branch of the greater palatine artery. **infraorbital c.** A canal running obliquely through the bony floor of the orbit; it gives passage to the infraorbital artery and nerve. **inguinal c.** A canal about one and one-half inches long, running obliquely downward and medially from the abdominal to the subcutaneous inguinal ring; the channel through which an inguinal hernia descends; it gives passage to the ilioinguinal nerve and to the spermatic cord in the male and to the round ligament of the uterus in the female. **intestinal c.** The portion of the gastrointestinal tract extending from the pylorus to the anus. **lacrimal c.** (a) The nasolacrimal canal. (b) See lacrimal *duct.* **medullary c.** The cavity of a long bone, containing the marrow. **membranous semicircular canals.** That portion of the membranous labyrinth of the ear consisting of three loop-shaped tubes lying at right angles to one another and communicating with the utricle. The **superior** (*frontal*) **semicircular canal** and the **posterior** (*sagittal*) **semicircular canal** lie in vertical planes making a right angle which opens laterally. The **lateral** or **horizontal canal** lies in the horizontal plane. Syn., *semicircular ducts.* **nasolacrimal c.** The bony canal that lodges the nasolacrimal duct. **osseous semicircular canals.** That part of the osseous labyrinth of the ear which houses the membranous semicircular canals: three loop-shaped canals in the petrous portion of the temporal bone, the **superior semi-circular canal**, the **posterior semicircular canal**, and the **lateral** or **horizontal semicircular canal**. They lie at right angles to one another and communicate with the osseous vestibule. **parturient c.** The channel through which the fetus passes in parturition; the cavities of the uterus and vagina, considered as a single canal. Also called *birth c.* **pelvic c.** The cavity of the true pelvis from inlet to outlet. **portal c.** An interlobular artery, vein, bile duct, nerve and lymph vessel, and the interlobular connective tissue in which they lie, between the corners of the anatomic lobules of the liver. **pterygopalatine c.** The connection between the pterygopalatine fossa and the palate; it gives passage to the palatine nerves and vessels. Its inferior openings are the greater and lesser palatine foramens. **pudendal c.** A passage within the inferior fascia of the obturator internus muscle for the transmission of the pudendal nerve and internal pudendal vessels. **semicircular canals.** (a) The osseous semicircular *canals.* (b) The membranous semicircular *canals.* **uterine c.** Cavity of the uterus, including the body and cervix. **uterocervical c.** Cavity of the cervix of the uterus. **vertebral c.** That formed by the foramens of the vertebrae; it contains the spinal cord and its meninges. Also called *spinal c., neural c.*

can″a·lic′u·li (kan″uh-lick′yoo-lye). Plural of canaliculus.

can″a·lic′u·lus (pl. *canaliculi*). 1. A small canal, *q.v.;* especially that leading from the punctum to the lacrimal sac of the eye. 2. Any one of the minute canals branching from the lacunas of bone. —**canalicular,** *adj.;* **canaliculiza′tion,** *n.*

ca·nal″i·za′tion (ka·nal″i·zay′shun, kan″ul·i·zay′shun). 1. The formation of new channels in tissues, as the formation of new blood vessels in a clot or thrombus. 2. A system of wound drainage without tubes.

can·cel′lous. Characterized by reticulated or latticed structure, as the spongy tissue of bones or, in botany, certain leaves consisting largely of veins. Syn., *cancellate, cancellated.* —**cancella′tion,** *n.*

can′cer. Any malignant neoplasm, including carcinoma and sarcoma; formerly a synonym of carcinoma. **c. en cuirasse.** Widely infiltrating carcinoma of the skin of the thorax, usually arising in mammary carcinoma; also applied to widespread carcinoma of the pleura. **c. occultus.** Carcinoma identified first by the appearance of

metastasis. **claypipe c.** Carcinoma of the lip and tongue, presumably due to the stem of the clay pipe. See smoker's c. **contact c.** One occurring on a surface, as the lip, which has been in contact with a cancer of the opposing surface. Rare and not proved to be due to direct implantation. **osteolytic c.** Metastasis of cancer to bone with destruction of bone. **osteoplastic c.** Metastasis of cancer to bone which stimulates new production of bone in the immediate neighborhood. **primary c.** An original malignant tumor as contrasted with a metastatic or secondary, cancer. **smoker's c.** Squamous-cell carcinoma of the lip, usually the lower lip, observed in habitual smokers.

can″cer·ol′o·gist. A cancer specialist.

can″cer·ol′o·gy. Study and science of cancer.

can″cer·o·pho′bi·a, can″cer·pho′bi·a. Morbid fear of acquiring cancer.

can′croid. 1. Cancerlike. 2. An epithelioma. 3. A variety of skin cancer of low or moderate malignancy.

Can′di·da. A genus of yeastlike pathogenic microörganisms. **C. albicans.** A species of considerable importance which produces thrush and other types of moniliasis. Also called *Monilia albicans.*

ca·nel′la. The bark of *Canella winterana,* native to the West Indies. It is called white cinnamon and is an aromatic tonic and bitter stomachic.

ca′nine. 1. Relating to, resembling dogs. 2. Pertaining to the sharp tearing teeth of mammals, located between the incisors and the premolars. 3. A canine tooth; also called *cuspid.*

ca·ni′ti·es (ka·nish′ee·eez). Poliosis; hoariness; grayness or whiteness of the hair. **c. unguium.** White spots, streaks, or bands of the nails.

can′ker. 1. An ulceration, especially one of the mouth and lips; also a festering or gangrenous ulcer, as noma gangrenous stomatitis. 2. Aphthous stomatitis; thrush. 3. *In veterinary medicine,* a disease of the horn-forming membrane of horse's hoofs, leading to destruction of the cells and loss of the horn-secreting function.

can″na·bid′i·ol. A constituent of cannabis which, on isomerization to tetrahydrocannabinol, exhibits to a great degree the activity of cannabis.

can′na·bin, can′na·bine (kan′uh-bean, -bin). A resinous substance from Indian hemp; it is hypnotic but is no longer used medicinally.

can·nab′in·ol. A substance resulting from the spontaneous dehydrogenation of tetrahydrocannabinol in cannabis.

an·nab'i·non, can·nab'i·none.
An amorphous bitter resinoid from cannabis.

an'na·bis. Hemp. The flowering tops of the pistillate plants of *Cannabis sativa*, of which there are two varieties, Indian and American, the former being the more potent. The active constituents appear to be tetrahydrocannabinols. Cannabis is antispasmodic and narcotic. *Guaca, gunjah, bang, bhang, cunjah, churrus, hashish,* and *marihuana* are among the various names by which the drug is known.

an'na·bol. A constituent of cannabis; it is believed to be an isomer of cannabidiol.

an"ni·bal·is'tic. Pertaining to the eating of human flesh, an impulse sometimes observed in psychotics.

Cannon, Walter Bradford [*American physiologist,* 1871–1945]. Renowned as one of the great physiologists of his time. Was the first to suggest the connection between the endocrine glands and the emotions (1915). Credited with originating the word *sympathin* (1931). With Binger and Fitz, showed that exophthalmic goiter could be produced artificially (1915).

an'nu·la. An artificial tube often fitted with a trocar for insertion into a tube or cavity of the body, as an artery or the trachea. Clinically, numerous cannulas of various sizes and shapes have been devised for specific uses. —**cannular, cannulate,** *adj.* **perfusion c.** A double cannula, one tube of which is used for the inflow of a fluid, the other for its escape; used in irrigating a cavity.

an·thar'i·des (kan·thar'i·deez). The dried insects, *Cantharis vesicatoria,* containing cantharidin. Locally applied, cantharides is rubefacient and vesicant; internally, it is irritant, causing pain and vomiting. —**cantharidal, cantharidic,** *adj.*

an·thar'i·dic ac'id (kan·thar'i·dick, kan"thuh·rid'ick). $C_{10}H_{14}O_5$. A cyclohexanedicarboxylic acid derivative; the hydrated form of cantharidin.

an·thar'i·din. $C_{10}H_{12}O_4$. The active principle contained in cantharides and other insects. It is the anhydride of cantharidic acid.

an'tha·ris. Singular of cantharides, *q.v.*

an·thec'to·my. Excision of a canthus.

an·thi'tis. Inflammation of a canthus.

an'tho-, canth-. A combining form denoting *canthal.*

an·thol'y·sis. Canthotomy with section of the lateral palpebral ligament.

an·tho·plas"ty. Increasing the length of the palpebral fissure by slit-

ting the outer canthus. Also, any plastic restoration of a canthal defect.

can·thor'rha·phy. In *plastic surgery,* shortening of the palpebral fissure by suture of the canthus.

can·thot'o·my. Surgical division of a canthus.

can'thus. Either of the two angles formed by the junction of the eyelids, designated outer or lateral, and inner or medial; palpebral angle. —**canthal,** *adj.*

cap. 1. A covering or an organ like a cover; a tegmen. 2. In *dentistry,* a substance or a structure designed to cover an exposed pulp. **cradle c.** An area of seborrhea often seen on the scalp of an infant or small child. See *crusta lactea.* **duodenal c.** The first part of the duodenum, immediately beyond the pylorus. From radiographic appearance, it is called bishop's cap. Syn., *duodenal bulb.* **knee c.** Patella. **skull c.** (a) Cranium. (b) Sinciput.

cap. 1. *Capiat;* let him take. 2. *Capsula;* a capsule.

ca·pac'i·tance (ka·pas'i·tunss). The quantity of electricity which a condenser or other structure can hold per volt of electric pressure applied.

ca·pac'i·tor (ka·pas'i·tur). An instrument for holding or storing charges of electricity; condenser.

ca·pac'i·ty. 1. The power of receiving, containing, holding, or absorbing. 2. Cubic volume. 3. Mental ability to acquire and hold knowledge, accomplish, or understand. 4. Physical ability to perform muscular work; maximum output. —**capacitate,** *v.t.* **cranial c.** Volume of the cranial cavity. **electric c.** (a) The amount of electricity a condenser can hold. (b) The amount of electricity that can be delivered under specific conditions, as by a battery or generator. (c) Maximum output of a generator. (d) Capacitance. **respiratory c.** (a) Vital capacity, *q.v.* (b) The ability of the blood to combine with oxygen from the lungs, and with the carbon dioxide from the tissues. **testamentary c.** In *legal medicine,* the mental ability requisite to make a valid will. **thermal c.** The amount of heat necessary to raise the temperature of a body from 15° to 16° C. **vital c.** The volume of air that can be expelled by the most forcible expiration after the deepest inspiration.

cap"il·lar'i·ty. Capillary attraction; elevation or depression of liquids in capillary tubes.

cap"il·la·ros'co·py, cap"il·lar"i·os'co·py. Microscopic examination of the cutaneous capillaries for diagnosis.

cap·il·lar"y (kap'i·lerr"ee). 1. Hairlike; relating to a hair, to a hairlike filament, or to a tube with a minute bore. 2. A minute blood vessel, one of a network connecting the smallest arteries and veins. **arterial c.** The first part of a capillary network; the continuation of an arteriole; precapillary. **c. fragility.** Weakness of the capillaries, as in purpura. **venous c.** The terminal part of a capillary network, opening into a venule; postcapillary.

ca·pil'lus. A hair; specifically, a hair of the head.

cap'i·tate. 1. In biology, having a head or a headlike termination; headshaped. 2. See Table of Bones, Appendix.

cap"i·ta'tum. The large bone of the wrist; the os magnum.

cap"i·tel'lum. 1. A small head or rounded process of bone. 2. The rounded process at the lower end of the humerus, articulating with the radius.

ca·pit'u·lum. 1. A small head or small, bony eminence. 2. Head of a rib articulating with the centrum. 3. Upper extremity or head of the fibula. —**capitular,** adj.

ca'pri-. A combining form meaning goat.

cap'ric ac'id. $CH_3(CH_2)_8COOH$. A solid fatty acid occurring as a glyceride in butter and other animal fats.

ca·pro'ic ac'id. $CH_3(CH_2)_4COOH$. A liquid fatty acid occurring as a glyceride in butter and other animal fats.

caprokol. Trade-mark for a brand of hexylresorcinol, q.v.

ca·pryl'ic ac'id. $CH_3(CH_2)_6COOH$. A solid fatty acid occurring in butter, coconut oil, and other fats and oils.

cap·sa'i·cin. The vanillylamide of isodecenoic acid, the most important constituent of capsicum.

cap'si·cum. The dried fruit of Capsicum frutescens (bush red-pepper) or of several other varieties (tabasco or Louisiana long or short peppers). Its characteristic pungent constituent is capsaicin; used internally as tonic and carminative, externally to produce counterirritation. Also called Cayenne pepper, red pepper.

cap'sule. 1. A membranous sac enclosing a part. 2. An envelope surrounding certain organisms. 3. A soluble shell for administering medicines. 4. In physiology, an instrument used for the optical recording of pressure changes or vibrations, as pressure pulses or heart sounds. It consists of a cylindrical chamber closed on one end by a thin membrane to which is glued a small mirror. Pressure changes cause movement of the membrane and deflections of a beam of light which is reflected to a photokymograph. —**capsular,** adj. **articular c.** Joint capsule. **c. of the eyeball.** The

fascial envelope of the eyeball. **c. of the kidney.** The fat-containing connective tissue encircling the kidney. **c. of the lens.** A transparent, structureless membrane enclosing the lens of the eye. **c. of the liver.** The connective tissue and capsule derived from a part of the transverse septum of the embryo. Also called Glisson's c. **cartilage c.** The lining of the cavities containing the cartilage cells. **external c.** A layer of white nerve fibers forming part of the external boundary of the lenticular nucleus. **Glisson's c.** The stroma of the liver. **glomerular c.** The sac surrounding the glomerulus of the kidney; the first part of the uriniferous tubule. Also called Bowman's c. **internal c.** A layer of nerve fibers on the outer side of the thalamus and caudate nucleus, which it separates from the lenticular nucleus; it is continuous with the cerebral peduncles and the corona radiata and consists of fibers to and from the cerebral cortex. **joint c.** The fibrous sheet enclosing a joint. **periotic c.** The structure surrounding the internal ear. **renal c.** The connective-tissue capsule of the kidney. Also called the fibrous c. of the kidney. **segment c.** A capsule used for the optical recording of pressure changes or vibrations, the cylindrical chamber being flattened on one side with a mirror pivoting on the chord of the circular membrane-covered surface. Also called Frank's segment c. **Tenon's c.** The fascia of the bulb of the eye.

cap"su·lec'to·my. Surgical excision of a capsule.

cap"su·li'tis. Inflammation of a capsule, as that of the lens, liver (perihepatitis), or the labyrinth (otosclerosis).

cap'su·lo-, capsul-. A combining form meaning capsule.

cap"su·lo·plas'ty. Operation for plastic repair of a joint capsule.

cap"su·lor'rha·phy. Suture of a capsule; especially suture of a joint capsule to repair a rent or to prevent dislocation.

cap"su·lo·tome". 1. See cystotome. 2. Instrument used in capsulotomy of the crystalline lens.

cap"su·lot'o·my. The operation of incising the capsule of the crystalline lens in cataract operations, or a joint capsule. **renal c.** Incision of the kidney capsule.

cap·ta'tion. The first or opening stage of hypnotism.

ca'put (kay'put, kap'ut). The head; also the chief part or beginning of an organ. **c. galeatum.** A child's head which emerges at birth covered with the caul. **c. Medusae.** The peculiar plexus of veins surrounding the umbilicus in periportal cirrhosis of the liver. It represents collateral paths for the return of the venous blood from the abdominal viscera. **c. succeda'neum.** A tumor composed of a serosanguineous infiltration of the connective tissue situated upon the presenting part of the fetus.

ca·ram'i·phen hy''dro·chlo'ride. Nonproprietary title for the hydrochloride of β-diethylaminoethyl-1-phenylcyclopentane-1-carboxylate, a drug possessing atropine-like action. See *panparnit.*

car'ba·chol (kahr'buh·coal, ·kol). Carbamylcholine chloride, or carbaminoylcholine chloride. A potent parasympathomimetic, effective orally. See *carcholin, doryl.*

car'ba·mate, car·bam'ate. A salt of carbamic acid; it contains the monovalent radical, NH₂COO—. See *ethyl carbamate.*

car·bam'ic ac'id. NH₂COOH. The mono-amide of carbonic acid existing only in the form of salts and esters, the latter known as urethanes.

car·bam'ide, car'ba·mide. Urea, *q.v.*

car·bam'i·dine (kahr·bam'i·deen, din). Guanidine.

car·bam''i·no·yl·cho'line chlo'ride. Carbachol.

car''ba·myl·cho'line chlo'ride. Carbachol.

car'bar·sone. A white powder containing from 28.1 to 28.8% of pentavalent arsenic, only slightly soluble in water; used in the treatment of intestinal amebiasis and *Trichomonas vaginalis* vaginitis.

car'ba·sus. Gauze; thin muslin used in surgery. *O.T.* **c. absorbens.** Absorbent gauze. **c. absorbens adhaesivus.** Adhesive absorbent gauze.

car·be''ta·pen'tane cit'rate. 2-(Diethylaminoethoxy)ethyl-1-phenylcyclopentyl-1-carboxylate citrate, an antitussive. See *toclase.*

car'bi·nol. 1. Methyl alcohol. 2. The monovalent radical, —CH₂OH, characteristic of primary alcohols. 3. A generic term for the primary alcohols.

carbitol. 1. Trade-mark for diethylene glycol monoethyl ether; used principally as a solvent. 2. Trade-mark for various ethers of diethylene glycol, the specific ether being indicated by a qualifying adjective.

car'bo. See *charcoal; carbon.*

car'bo-, carb-. A combining form signifying carbon.

car''bo·cy'clic (kahr''bo·sigh'click, sick'lick). In chemistry, pertaining to compounds of the closed-chain type in which all the ring atoms are carbon. See *heterocyclic.*

car''bo·hy'drase. An enzyme capable of converting the higher carbohydrates into simple sugars.

car''bo·hy'drate. An organic substance belonging to the class of compounds represented by the sugars, dextrins, starches, and celluloses; it contains carbon, hydrogen, and oxygen.

car''bo·hy''dra·tu'ri·a. Presence of an abnormally large proportion of carbohydrates in the urine; glycosuria.

car'bo·late. 1. Phenate. 2. Impregnate with phenol.

car·bol'ic ac'id. Phenol.

car''bol·xy'lene (kahr''bol·zy'leen). A mixture of phenol, one part, and xylene, three parts; used for clearing sections for microscopy.

car·be·my'cin. An antibiotic from *Streptomyces halstedii,* that possesses strong inhibitory activity against certain Gram-positive bacteria. See *magnamycin.*

car'bon. C = 12.010. A nonmetallic element widely distributed in nature. Its three allotropic forms are exemplified by the diamond, graphite, and charcoal. **c. bisulfide.** See *c. disulfide.* **c. black.** Finely divided carbon obtained by the incomplete combustion of natural gas, animal tissues, oils, wood, or other organic substances. **c. dioxide.** CO₂. An odorless, colorless gas which neither burns nor supports combustion. Also called *carbonic acid gas.* See *carbonic acid.* Also see Table of Normal Values of Blood Constituents, Appendix. **c. disulfide.** CS₂. A colorless or slightly yellow, highly inflammable liquid. A solvent of wide application. **c. monoxide.** CO. A colorless, odorless, poisonous gas resulting from the combustion of carbonaceous compounds in an insufficient supply of oxygen. It combines firmly with hemoglobin, preventing subsequent union with oxygen. See *carboxyhemoglobin.* **c. tetrachloride.** CCl₄. Tetrachloromethane. A colorless, noninflammable liquid, useful as an anthelmintic, especially against the hookworm. It is also used as a fire extinguisher, a solvent, and an insecticide. See *carbon tetrachloride poisoning.*

car'bon·ate. The divalent radical =CO₃; any salt containing this radical, as salts of carbonic acid. **acid c.** See *bicarbonate.*

car'bon·a''ted. Containing or charged with carbon dioxide.

car·bon'ic ac'id. H₂CO₃. When carbon dioxide dissolves in water, a portion of it forms this feebly ionizing acid. Its salts are carbonates. See *carbon dioxide.*

car·bon'ic an·hy'drase. An enzyme found in erythrocytes and in tissues which catalyzes the reaction $H_2O + CO_2 \rightleftharpoons H_2CO_3$. In the transport of CO_2 in the body, the reaction proceeds to the right in the tissues and to the left in the lungs, and in each instance is catalyzed by carbonic anhydrase.

car″bon·i·za′tion. 1. Decomposition of organic compounds by heat in the absence of air, driving off the volatile matter and leaving the carbon. 2. Charring. —**car′bonize,** v.t.

car″bon·om′e·ter. Apparatus for measuring the amount of carbon dioxide in a room or in exhaled breath. —**carbonom′etry,** n.

car″bon·u′ri·a. Presence of carbon compounds in the urine, particularly carbon dioxide.

car·bon·yl. The divalent radical =CO. **c. chloride.** $COCl_2$. Phosgene.

carbowax. The trade-mark for certain polyethylene glycols, of the general formula $HOCH_2(CH_2OCH_2)_xCH_2$-OH, having a molecular weight above 1000.

carboxide. Trade-mark for a mixture of ethylene oxide and carbon dioxide, used as a fumigant.

car·box″y·hae″mo·glo′bin. See carboxyhemoglobin.

car·box″y·he″mo·glo′bin (kahr-bock″see-hee″mo·glo′bin, ·hem″o·glo′bin). The compound of carbon monoxide and hemoglobin formed when CO is present in the blood. The carbon monoxide displaces the oxygen and checks the respiratory function of the red corpuscles.

car·box′yl. The group —COOH characteristic of organic acids. The hydrogen of this can be replaced by metals, forming salts.

car·box′yl·ase. An enzyme causing the splitting off of carbon dioxide from an aliphatic acid. Specifically, the enzyme involved in the conversion of pyruvic acid to acetaldehyde and carbon dioxide.

carboxymethocel. Trade-mark for the sodium salt of carboxymethylcellulose, q.v.

car·box″y·meth″yl·cel′lu·lose. A substance obtained from cellulose; it is available as the sodium salt, a white, granular, odorless, and tasteless powder. Used as a suspending agent and colloid laxative. See carboxymethocel.

car·box″y·pep′ti·dase. A pancreatic enzyme which catalyzes the splitting of a terminal amino acid from a polypeptide.

car·box″y·pol″y·pep′ti·dase. A proteolytic enzyme in pancreatic secretion, active in splitting amide linkages of certain amino-acid compounds.

car·bro′mal. Bromdiethylacetylurea, a white, crystalline powder. Used as a nerve sedative. See adalin.

car′bun·cle. A hard, circumscribed, deep-seated, painful, suppurative inflammation of the subcutaneous tissue. It is larger than a boil, having a flat surface discharging pus from multiple points. There is usually fever with generalized constitutional reaction. Eventually, the entire mass sloughs away healing as a scarred excavation. —**car·bun′cular,** adj.

car·bun″cu·lo′sis. Condition characterized by the formation of carbuncles in rapid succession or simultaneously.

carcholin. Trade-mark for carbacho supplied in powder form for preparing solutions and ointments for use in the treatment of glaucoma simplex.

car″ci·no-, carcin-. 1. In zoology, a combining form denoting a crab. 2. In medicine, a combining form denoting cancer.

car′ci·no·gen. Any cancer-producing substance or agent. —**carcinogen′ic,** adj.; **carcinogenic′ity,** n.

car″ci·no·gen′e·sis. Origin or production of cancer. —**carcinogenet′ic,** adj.

car′ci·noid. A tumor derived from argentaffin (enterochromaffin) cells; i is usually benign, and commonly occurs in the appendix and ileum. Also called argentaffinoma.

car″ci·no′ma. A malignant neoplasm of epithelial origin. The two principal varieties are **epidermoid carcinoma** and **cylindrical-cell carcinoma,** both of which may show various degrees of differentiation and may be graded accordingly. The chief forms of epidermoid carcinoma are **squamous-cell carcinoma, basal-cell carcinoma,** and in **termediate-cell carcinoma,** al derived from surface or lining epithelium. The principal form of cylindrical cell carcinoma is the **adenocarcinoma,** derived from glandular epithelium. Completely undifferentiated carcinoma, or **carcinoma simplex** is usually a cylindrical-cell carcinoma but may also be a form of epidermoid carcinoma. Metastasis is chiefly through lymphatics, either by embolism of cells or by permeation growth of the tumor through the vessels. Metastasis sometimes occurs through blood vessels spread may also occur by direct extension or by surface implantation. —**carcinom′atous,** adj. **adenocarcinoma.** One originating in glandular or ductal epithelium and tending to produce acinic structures. Differentiation of the adenocarcinomas depend on the degree of resemblance which the acinic structures bear to the gland; the completely undifferentiated form is the carcinoma simplex, and the most highly differentiated tumor is often named *malignant adenoma.* **basal-cell c.** A variety of epidermoid carcinoma probably derived from basal cells of the epidermis and reproducing the basal type of cell in its growth. Found in skin of exposed parts, especially in elderly people. Grows slowly and is not highly malignant. Metastasizes late if at all; may extend laterally and ulcerate. *Rodent ulcer* is a form of basal-cell carcinoma. **c. in situ.** Carcinoma growing within a mucosa and not clearly invasive. Also called *intraepithelial c.* **c. simplex.** Carcinoma in which differentiation is absent or poor. Usually a cylindrical-cell carcinoma but may be derived from epidermis or other lining epithelium. As a rule, highly malignant. **chimney sweep's c.** Squamous-cell carcinoma of the scrotum. Occurs usually in chimney sweeps and is probably due to tar in soot, but may occur in persons working in other occupations. Also called *soot cancer.* **chorionic c.** A type derived from trophoblast or the chorionic villi or multipotential cells of the testis, the ovary, or other parts of the body. Also called *choriocarcinoma.* **colloid c.** A misnomer for carcinomas of glandular or undifferentiated forms in which the cells produce mucin either in acinic spaces or within the cells. **epidermoid c.** A type derived by metaplasia from surfaces covered by stratified squamous epithelium or from other epithelial surfaces. Tends to reproduce basal, intermediate, and squamous cells, but may be undifferentiated. The squamous cells may be concentrated in balls with concentric laminas, the so-called cancer pearls. The most highly differentiated form is often called *acanthoma.* Another variety is the *basal-cell carcinoma.* Formerly called *epithelioma.* **glandular c.** Adenocarcinoma. **intermediate-cell c.** One derived from surface epithelium, but composed almost entirely of intermediate cells with intercellular bridges, the prickle cells. **medullary c.** A form of cylindrical-cell carcinoma which is soft in consistency because it is made up principally of carcinoma cells with little supporting connective tissue. Usually grows rapidly and metastasizes early and widely. **papillary c.** A type derived from a papilloma, and papillary in structure; villous carcinoma. **papilliferous c.** An adenocarcinoma which shows in the acinic structures an ingrowth of the lining cells to produce papillae. **scirrhous c.** Cylindrical-cell carcinoma which is hard, because the connective-tissue component is large in amount and collagenous, while the epithelial component is small in amount. Usually grows

slowly and metastasizes late; the metastases usually have the same proportionate amount of the components. Syn., *scirrhus.* **squamous-cell c.** A form of epidermoid carcinoma. **tar c.** Carcinoma, usually epidermoid, produced experimentally by application of tar, its distillation products, or other agents of the same order. **thymic c.** A thymoma made up of cells resembling epithelium which may be so arranged as to resemble squamous-cell carcinoma but with little keratinization. **transitional-cell c.** Derived from and made up of transitional epithelial cells. Prevalent in the urinary tract, especially the urinary bladder.

car″ci·nom′a·toid (kahr″si·nom′-uh·toyd, ·no′muh·toyd). 1. Resembling a carcinoma. 2. *In experimental oncology,* epithelial proliferation in induced papillomas without invasion of adjacent tissue.

car″ci·no″ma·to′sis. A condition of widespread dissemination of cancer throughout the body.

car″ci·no·sar·co′ma. A mixed tumor having the characteristics of carcinoma and sarcoma. Not to be confused with collision tumor, in which a sarcoma invades a carcinoma or vice versa.

car′da·mom oil. A volatile oil obtained from the seeds of an East Indian herb *Elettaria cardamomum,* used as a flavoring and, sometimes, as a carminative.

car′da·mom seed (kahr′duh·mum, ·mom). The dried, ripe seed of *Eletaria Cardamomum,* found chiefly in Ceylon. It is an aromatic, carminative stomachic.

car′di·a. The esophageal orifice of the stomach.

car′di·ac. 1. Relating to the heart. 2. Pertaining to the cardia. 3. A person with a heart lesion. 4. A tonic acting especially on the heart.

car′di·ac fail′ure. The syndrome resulting from failure of the heart as a pump. The etiology is varied, the symptoms depending on whether the left or right ventricle preponderantly fails. Dyspnea is most marked in left ventricular failure; and engorgement of organs with venous blood, edema, and ascites, most marked in right ventricular failure.

car′di·ac in″suf·fi′cien·cy. See *cardiac failure.*

car′di·ac out′put″. Blood volume in liters ejected per minute by the left ventricle.

car″di·al′gi·a. Pain in the region of the heart; heartburn.

car″di·am′e·ter. An apparatus for determining the position of the cardiac orifice of the stomach.

car″di·asth′ma (kahr″dee-az′muh, ·ass′muh). Asthmalike dyspnea from left ventricular failure. See *cardiac asthma.*

cardiazol. Trade-mark for pentylenetetrazol. See *metrazol.*

car″di·ec′ta·sis. Dilatation of the heart.

car″di·ec′to·my. Excision of the cardiac end of the stomach.

car′di·nal flow′er. A common name for several species of *Lobelia,* chiefly *Lobelia cardinalis.*

car′di·o-, cardi-. A combining form denoting *of,* or pertaining to, *the heart; cardiac.*

car″di·o·ac·cel′er·a″tor. 1. An agent which quickens the action of the heart. 2. Speeding up cardiac action.

car″di·o·ac′tive. Affecting the heart.

car″di·o·an″gi·ol′o·gy (kahr″dee-o-an″jee-ol′o-jee). Branch of medicine dealing with the heart and blood vessels.

car′di·o·cele. Hernia of the heart.

car″di·o·cen·te′sis, car″di·cen·te′sis. Puncture of one of the chambers of the heart to relieve engorgement.

car″di·o·cir·rho′sis. Cirrhosis of the liver due to chronic congestive heart failure.

car″di·o·cla′sis, car″di·o·cla′si·a (kahr″dee-o-clay′zhuh, ·zee-uh). Rupture of the heart.

car″di·o·di·la′tor (kahr″dee-o-dye-lay′tur, ·di-lay′tur). Instrument for dilating the esophageal opening of the stomach.

car″di·o·di·o′sis (kahr″dee-o-dee-o′sis, ·dye-o′sis). Dilatation of the cardiac end of the stomach by means of an instrument passed through the esophagus.

car″di·o·dy·nam′ics (kahr″dee-o-dye-nam′icks, ·di-nam′icks). Kinetic mechanisms by means of which the heartbeat insures the circulation of the blood from the heart to the periphery and back to the heart. —**cardiody-namic,** *adj.*

car″di·o·dyn′i·a. Pain in or about the heart.

car″di·o·gram″. A record of the heart's pulsation taken through the chest wall; the tracing made by the cardiograph.

car″di·o·graph″. An instrument for registering graphically the cardiac cycle. —**cardiograph′ic,** *adj.*

car″di·og′ra·phy. 1. Analysis of cardiac action by instrumental means, especially by tracings which record its movements. 2. A description of the heart.

car″di·o·he·pat′ic. Pertaining to the heart and the liver, as the cardiohepatic angle.

car″di·o·in·hib′i·to″ry. Diminishing, restraining, or suppressing the heart rate, as the cardioinhibitory fibers which pass to the heart through the vagus nerves.

car″di·o·ki·net′ic (kahr″dee-o-ki-net′ick, ·kigh-net′ick). 1. Exciting the heart action. 2. An agent which excites heart action.

car″di·o·ky·mog′ra·phy (·kigh-mog′ruh·fee). A roentgenographic method for recording changes in the size of the heart by kymographic means. See *kymography, radiokymography.*

car″di·o·lip′in. A class of phospholipids isolated from beef heart and consisting of a phosphorylated polysaccharide esterified with fatty acids. Essential for the reactivity of beef heart antigens in the serologic test for syphilis, and may be the pure antigen.

car″di·ol′o·gist. A specialist in the diagnosis and treatment of disorders of the heart.

car″di·ol′o·gy. The study of the heart.

car″di·ol′y·sis. 1. Resection of the precordial ribs and sternum to free the heart and its adherent pericardium from the anterior chest wall, to which they are bound by adhesions, as in adhesive mediastinopericarditis. 2. Cardiac degeneration or destruction.

car″di·o·men′to·pex″y. The operation of bringing vascular omentum through the diaphragm and attaching it to the heart for improving cardiac vascularization. Also called *O'Shaughnessy's operation.*

car″di·om′e·ter. An apparatus which envelops the ventricles of a mammalian heart, recording their changes in volume during a cardiac cycle.

car″di·o·my′o·pex″y. The operation of suturing living muscular tissue, generally from the pectoral region, to the abraded surface of the heart, to provide improved vascularization of the heart. Also called *Beck's operation.*

car″di·o·my·ot′o·my (kahr″dee-o-migh-ot′o-mee). An operation to relieve stenosis of the cardia; consists of freeing the esophagus from the diaphragm and pulling it into the abdominal cavity, where the constricting muscle is divided anteriorly and posteriorly without dividing the mucous coat.

car″di·o·neph′ric. Pertaining to the heart and the kidneys.

car″di·o·neu′ral. Pertaining to the nervous control of the heart's mechanism.

car″di·o·pal′u·dism. Disturbance of the heart due to malaria, characterized by gallop rhythm, dilatation of the right heart, and reduplication of the diastolic sound.

ar'di·o·path. A sufferer from heart disease; a cardiac. —**cardiopath'ic**, *adj.*

ar″di·op'a·thy, car″di·o·path'i·a. Any disease of the heart. The various types are: arteriosclerotic, hypertensive, inflammatory, nephropathic, thyrotoxic, toxic, and valvular.

ar″di·o·per″i·car'di·o·pex″y. The surgical establishment of adhesive pericarditis, to improve a deficient coronary circulation resulting from coronary disease.

ar″di·o·per″i·car·di'tis. Associated carditis and pericarditis; inflammation of the heart and pericardium.

ar″di·o·pho'bi·a. Morbid fear of heart disease.

ar'di·o·phone. An instrument which makes the heart sounds audible; useful when presenting cases to a large group.

ar'di·o·plas″ty. Plastic surgery of the cardiac portion of the stomach, as for cardiospasm.

ar″di·o·pneu·mat'ic (kahr″dee-o·new·mat'ick). Pertaining to the heart and respiration, as the cardiopneumatic movements of the air in the lungs, caused by the pulsations of the heart and great vessels.

ar″di·o·pneu'mo·graph. An instrument designed for graphically recording cardiopneumatic movements. —**cardiopneumog'raphy,** *n.*

ar″di·op·to'sis (kahr″dee-op·to'sis, kahr″dee-o·to'sis), **car″di·op·to'si·a** (kahr″dee-op·to'shuh, kahr″dee-o·). Downward displacement of the heart from excessive mobility; prolapse of the heart.

ar″di·o·pul'mo·nar·y. Relating to the heart and lungs. Also called *cardiopulmonic.*

ar″di·o·punc'ture. 1. Cardiocentesis. 2. Any surgical or vivisectional puncture of the heart.

ar″di·o·py'lor·ic (kahr″dee-o·pye-lor'ick, ·pi·lor'ick). Referring to both the cardiac and the pyloric portions of the stomach.

ar″di·o·re'nal. Relating to the heart and kidney.

ar″di·o·re·spir'a·to″ry (kahr″dee·o·ri·spy'ruh·tor″ee, ·res'pi·ruh·tor″ee). Of or pertaining to the heart and respiration.

ar″di·o·roent'gen·o·gram″ (·rent'ghin·o·gram″). Roentgenogram of the heart.

ar″di·o·roent'gen·og'ra·phy. Roentgenographic examination of the heart.

ar″di·or·rhex'is. Rupture of the heart. *Rare.*

car'di·o·scope″. A lag-screen belt electrocardiograph; the electrocardiogram can be visualized immediately for a few seconds' time on a rotating fluorescent belt.

car'di·o·spasm″. Contraction of the cardia, a condition usually associated with spasm of the cardiac end of the stomach and dilatation and hypertrophy of the esophagus above the contracted region.

car″di·o·ste·no'sis. Constriction of the heart, especially of the conus arteriosus; the development of such a constriction.

car″di·o·ta·ohom'e·ter (kahr″dee-o·ta·kom'i·tur). Instrument that counts the total number of heartbeats over long periods of time.

car″di·o·ther'a·py. Treatment of heart disease.

car″di·ot'o·my. Dissection or incision of the heart or the cardiac end of the stomach.

car″di·o·ton'ic. 1. Increasing the tonus of the cardiac muscle; generally applied to the effect of digitalis and related drugs. 2. Any drug which produces such action.

car″di·o·tox'ic. Poisonous to the heart.

car″di·o·vas'cu·lar. Pertaining to the heart and the blood vessels.

car″di·o·vas'cu·lar·re'nal. Pertaining to the heart, blood vessels, and kidney.

car·di'tis. Inflammation of the heart. —**cardit'ic,** *adj.* **internal c.** Endocarditis.

cardrase. Trade-mark for ethoxzolamide.

Car'i·ca. A genus of the Caricaceae. **C. papaya.** The papaw tree of tropical America; contains in its leaves and fruit papain (papayotin) and other enzymes, the alkaloid carpaine, and also the glycoside carposide. The dried latex and leaves are used as a digestant.

ca'ri·es (kair'ee·eez, kair'eez). A molecular death of bone or teeth, corresponding to ulceration in the soft tissues. —**car'ious,** *adj.* **c. of the spine.** Tuberculous osteitis of the bodies of the vertebrae and intervertebral fibrocartilage, producing curvature of the spine. Also called *Pott's disease, tuberculosis of vertebra.* **c. sicca.** A form of tuberculosis caries characterized by absence of suppuration, obliteration of the cavity of the joint, and sclerosis and concentric atrophy of the articular extremity of the bone. **dental c.** A localized progressive disease of the calcified tissue of a tooth beginning with decalcification and followed by disintegration of the organic substance, leaving the so-called cavity of decay.

car·in'a·mide. 4'-Carboxyphenyl-methanesulfonanilide. A substance having the power of retarding excretion of penicillin by the kidneys, presumably by action on an enzyme system.

car·min'a·tive (kahr·min'uh·tiv, kahr'min·). Having the power to relieve flatulence and colic.

car·mine (kahr'min, ·myne) (C.C.). A bright red coloring matter prepared from cochineal, the active staining principle being carminic acid.

car"na·u'ba (kahr"nuh-ōō'buh). The root of *Copernicia cerifera*, a wax-producing palm tree of tropical America; used in Brazil as an alterative.

car"ni·fi·ca'tion. Alteration of tissue so that it resembles skeletal muscle in color and consistency. It sometimes affects the lungs.

car'no·sine (kahr'no·seen, ·sin). Alanyl histidine, a dipeptide said to occur in muscle tissue.

car'o·tene, car'o·tin, car'rot·ene, car'rot·in. A red, orange, or yellow hydrocarbon ($C_{40}H_{56}$) belonging to the group of carotenoids. It is synthesized by many plants and is the precursor of vitamin A. See Table of Normal Values of Blood Constituents in Appendix.

car"o·te·ne'mi·a. Presence of carotene in the circulating blood. When excessive (*hypercarotenemia*), it may cause a yellowish pigmentation of the skin called pseudojaundice.

ca·rot'e·noid, ca·rot'i·noid (ka-rot'i-noyd, kar'o·ti·noyd). 1. A group of plant pigments occurring in carrots, tomatoes, and other vegetables, and in fruits and flowers. Chemically, they are unsaturated hydrocarbons. 2. Like carotene; colored like carotene.

car"o·te·no'sis. Pigmentation of the skin due to carotene in the tissues.

ca·rot'ic. Pertaining to stupor.

ca·rot'id. 1. The carotid artery, the principal large artery on each side of the neck. 2. Of or relating to the carotid artery. See Table of Arteries in the Appendix.

car'o·tin. See carotene.

ca·rot'i·noid. See carotenoid.

car'pa·ine (kahr'pay-een, kahr'puh·). An alkaloid from the leaves of *Carica papaya*.

car'pal. Pertaining to the wrist or carpus.

car·pec'to·my. Excision of a carpal bone.

car·phol'o·gy, car"pho·lo'gi·a. Aimless picking and plucking at bedclothes, seen in delirious states, fevers, and exhaustion. Syn., *floccillation*.

car'po-, carp-. A combining form meaning *carpus* or *wrist*.

car"po·met"a·car'pal. Pertaining to the carpal and the metacarpal bones; applied to the joints between

them and to the ligaments joining them. See Table of Joints and Ligaments in the Appendix.

car"po·pe'dal (kahr"po·pee'dul, ·ped'ul). Affecting the wrists and feet or the fingers and toes.

car"po·pha·lan'ge·al. Pertaining to the wrist and the phalanges.

car'po·side. A crystalline glycoside from *Carica papaya*.

car'pus. The wrist, consisting of eight wrist bones. See Table of Bones in the Appendix. **—carpal,** *adj*.

Carrel, Alexis [*French surgeon 1873–1944*]. Introduced the extravital cultivation of tissues. Demonstrated that arteries can be transplanted after being stored for some time. Successfully transplanted a kidney from one animal to another. Developed a method of suturing blood vessels end-to-end; correct apposition is maintained by three traction sutures, the arteries assuming a triangular shape. Called *Carrel method* or *suture*. With Dakin, developed a method of treating wounds by irrigation with a solution of chlorinated soda and sodium bicarbonate, called *Carrel-Dakin treatment*. With Lindbergh, devised a perfusion apparatus with which organs can be kept alive outside the body; called *Carrel-Lindbergh pump*. Nobel laureate (1912).

car'ri·er. 1. A normal person or one convalescing from an infectious disease who shows no signs or symptoms of the disease but who harbors and eliminates the microörganism, and so spreads the disease. 2. A quantity of a naturally occurring element added to a minute amount of pure isotope to facilitate the chemical handling of the isotope. **chronic c.** One who eliminates the infectious element for an indefinite period. **temporary c.** A convalescent who eliminates the infectious element for only a short time after recovery. Also called *transitory c.*

car'ri·er-free". Of, or pertaining to, a pure isotope.

car'ron oil. A liniment consisting of equal parts of linseed oil and lime water, used in the treatment of burns.

car'rot·ene. See carotene.

car'rot·in. See carotene.

car sick'ness. A form of motion sickness occurring as a result of movement of a train or automobile. See *airsickness*. Also called *motion sickness*.

Car'tha·mus. A genus of Eurasian herbs of the Carduaceae. **C. tinc·torius.** Safflower; American or bastard saffron. The dried flowers are used in making an infusion used popularly as a diaphoretic.

car'ti·lage (kahr'ti·lidj). Gristle; a white, semiopaque, nonvascular connective tissue composed of a matrix containing nucleated cells which lie in cavities or lacunas of the matrix. When boiled, cartilage yields a substance called chondrin. **—cartilag'inous,** *adj.* **alar cartilages.** The **major alar c.** is the lower lateral cartilage of the nose, and the **minor alar c.,** one of the lesser alar cartilages of the nose. **articular c.** That lining the articular surfaces of bones. **arytenoid c.** One of two cartilages of the larynx regulating, by means of the attached muscles, the tension of the vocal folds. **auricular c.** The cartilage of the pinna of the ear. **bronchial c.** Plates of cartilage, in some instances very minute, that are found in the bronchi. **costal c.** That occupying the interval between the true ribs and the sternum or adjacent cartilages. **cricoid c.** The ring-shaped cartilage of the larynx. **cuneiform cartilages.** Two small, rod-shaped cartilages of the larynx, located in the aryepiglottic folds anterior to the arytenoid cartilages. Formerly called *Wrisberg's cartilages.* **elastic c.** A type in which a network of elastic fibers pervades the matrix. **epiglottal c.** The cartilage of the epiglottis. **episternal c.** One of a pair of small embryonic cartilages articulating with the clavicle and forming part of the manubrium. **floating c.** A detached segment of cartilage in a joint cavity. **hyaline c.** That in which the matrix is clear and homogeneous. **interarticular cartilages.** Flat fibrocartilages situated between the articulating surfaces of some of the joints. Also called *interarticular fibrocartilages, articular disks.* **intermediary c.** (a) Cartilage bone in process of transformation into true bone. (b) That interposed between the epiphysis and diaphysis of a bone. **intervertebral cartilages.** See *intervertebral disks* under *disk.* **laryngeal cartilages.** The cartilages supporting the larynx. **Meckel's c.** The cartilage bar of the mandibular arch. **palpebral c.** Incorrect term for the connective tissue forming the framework of the eyelids; the tarsal plate. It is not composed of cartilage. **paranasal c.** One of the paired extensions of the nasal septal cartilage lying laterally to the nasal cavity and forming the primordium of the right or left ethmoidal labyrinth. **Reichert's c.** The cartilage of the hyoid arch. **semilunar cartilages.** Two interarticular cartilages of the knee. **septal c. of the nose.** Cartilage of the nasal septum. **tubal c.** A rolled triangular cartilage running from the osseous part of the auditory tube to the pharynx. **xiphoid c.** The lower cartilaginous tip of

the sternum. **yellow c.** Elastic cartilage.

ca'rum. Caraway; the dried ripe fruit of *Carum Carvi.* Its odor and taste are due to a volatile oil; used chiefly as a flavor.

car'un·cle, ca·run'cle. A small, fleshy, red mass or nodule. **—carun'cular, carun'culate, carun'culated,** *adj.* **lacrimal c.** A small, reddish mass at the inner canthus. **urethral c.** A small, benign, spherical or elliptical, strawberry-colored mass, sessile or pedunculated, situated on the posterior wall of the external urinary meatus of women; observed most frequently at the menopause, and a cause of pain and bleeding.

car'vone. $C_{10}H_{14}O$. A terpene ketone found in various volatile oils.

car'y·o-, car'y-. A combining form signifying *nut* or *kernel.* Also see *karyo-.*

car″y·o·phyl'lin (kar″ee·o·fill'in, kar″ee·off'i·lin). The nonnitrogenous crystalline principle of cloves.

car″y·o·phyl'lus (kar″ee·o·fill'us, -off'i·lus). See *clove.*

cas'ca bark. Sassy bark; the bark of *Erythrophleum guineense,* an African tree. See *erythrophleine.*

cas·car'a (kas·kair'uh, kas·kar'uh). Cascara sagrada. **c. amarga.** Honduras bark. The bark of *Sweetia panamensis,* native to Mexico, which has been used as a bitter tonic. **c. sagrada.** The bark of *Rhamnus Purshiana,* the chief constituents of which are anthraquinone derivatives. It is useful in chronic constipation. Also called *chittem bark, sacred bark.*

cas″ca·ril'la. The bark of *Croton eluteria,* native to the Bahama Islands; an aromatic bitter.

cas″ca·ril'lin. $C_{12}H_{18}O_4$. The bitter principle of cascarilla; white crystals, slightly soluble in water.

cas'ca·rin. A glycosidal cathartic fraction isolated from the bark of *Rhamnus Purshiana* (cascara sagrada).

case. 1. A single instance or example of a disease. 2. A covering; a boxlike structure.

ca'se·ate. 1. A lactate. 2. Caseinate, a casein compound. 3. Undergo caseous degeneration.

ca″se·a'tion. 1. The precipitation of casein during the coagulation of milk. 2. A form of necrosis which changes tissue into a soft, cheeselike substance, characteristic of tubercular infection.

ca'se·ic ac'id (kay'see·ick, ka·see'ick). Lactic acid.

ca'se·i·form. Like cheese or casein.

ca'se·in. A protein obtained from milk by the action of rennin or acids. **vegetable c.** A protein of plant origin resembling the casein of milk, as conglutin.

ca″se·in·o·gen. A compound protein of milk, yielding casein when acted upon by digestive enzymes; the precursor of casein.

ca·se·o-, ca·se-. A combining form denoting *casein.*

ca·se·ous. Resembling, or having the nature or consistency of, cheese. See *caseation,* 2.

Cas″i·mi·ro′a (kas″i·mi·ro′uh, kas″i·mirr′o·uh). A genus of plants belonging to the Rutaceae.

cas·sa′va (ka·sah′vuh). 1. Any of several plants of the genus *Manihot.* 2. The starch obtained from rhizomes of *Manihot esculenta* and *Manihot aipi;* nutrient. Tapioca is prepared from it by heating while moist.

cas″sette′ (kah″set′, ka·zet′). A holder for a roentgenographic film or plate.

Cas′si·a (cash′ee·uh, kas′ee·uh). A genus of the Leguminosae, several species of which afford senna.

cas′sia (cash′uh, cash′ee·uh). An old name, still used commercially, for the coarser varieties of cinnamon. **c. bark.** Chinese cinnamon. **c. buds.** The dried flowers of Chinese cinnamon; used chiefly as spice. **c. oil.** Cinnamon oil. **purging c.** *Cassia fistula.* Dried fruit of a tree growing in tropical regions. The pulp is a mild laxative.

cast. 1. A mass of fibrous material or exudate that has taken the form of some cavity in which it has been molded. From their source, casts may be classified as bronchial, intestinal, nasal, esophageal, renal, tracheal, urethral, vaginal, etc. Of these, the renal casts, by reason of their significance in diseases of the kidney, are the most important. Classed according to their constitution, casts are blood, epithelial, fatty, fibrinous, granular, hyaline, mucous, waxy, etc. 2. An accurate reproduction in form of an object, structure, or part in some plastic substance which has taken form in an impression or mold. 3. A lay term for strabismus. **plaster of Paris c.** A mixture of gypsum and water which becomes hard upon drying; when incorporated into gauze as a binder it may be used to immobilize fractured bones, arthritic joints, the spine, etc. Syn., *plaster c.* **waxy c.** A tubal renal cast composed of translucent, usually amyloid, material.

cas′tor. Castoreum.

cas′tor bean. The seed of the plant *Ricinus communis,* from which castor oil is expressed.

cas·to′re·um. Dried preputial follicles and their secretion, obtained from the beaver, *Castor fiber.*

cas′tor oil. The fixed oil obtained from the castor bean, containing glycerides of ricinoleic acid and possessing cathartic properties.

cas′tor xy′lene. A mixture of castor oil and xylene, used to clear or clarify collodion or celloidin and objects imbedded in them.

cas·tra′tion. Orchiectomy; the excision of one or both testes or ovaries. **—cas′trated,** *adj.;* **cas′trate,** *n., v.t.* **female c.** Removal of the ovaries; oöphorectomy; spaying.

cas′u·al·ty. 1. An accident causing injury or death. 2. *In military medicine,* a member of the armed forces who is wounded, disabled, or killed.

cas″u·is′tics (kazh″oo·iss′ticks, kaz″yoo·). Study of individual cases as a means of arriving at the general history of a disease.

cat′a-, cat-, cath-. A prefix denoting *downward, in accordance with, against, back, completely.*

ca·tab′o·lin, ca·tab′o·lite. Any product of catabolism.

ca·tab′o·lism. Destructive phase of metabolism concerned with the breaking down by the body of complex compounds, often with the liberation of energy; the opposite of anabolism. **—catabol′ic,** *adj.*

cat″a·crot′ic. Designating the descending limb of the arterial pulse wave or any irregularities in it.

cat′a·lase (cat′uh·lace, ·laze). 1. An enzyme, found in tissues, capable of decomposing peroxides. 2. Any one of a group of oxidizing enzymes.

cat′a·lep′sy. A morbid state of consciousness, usually trancelike, in which there is a loss of voluntary motion and a peculiar plastic rigidity of the muscles, by reason of which they retain for an indefinite time any position in which they are placed. The condition is associated with hysteria and schizophrenia, and is a stage of hypnotic sleep. In **local catalepsy,** a single organ or group of muscles is affected. Also called *catalepsis.* **—catalep′tiform, catalep′toid,** *adj.;* **catalep′tic,** *adj., n.;* **catalep′tize,** *v*

Ca·tal′pa. A genus of American and Asiatic trees of the Bignoniaceae. The seeds of **C. bignonioides** and **C. speciosa,** of North America, have been used in asthma.

ca·tal′y·sis. An increase in the rate at which a chemical reaction proceeds to equilibrium. **—catalyza′tion,** *n.*

cat′a·lyst. A substance which increases the velocity of a chemical reaction. Syn., *catalyzer.* See *enzyme.* **—catalyt′ic,** *adj.*

cat″a·me′ni·a. Menstruation. **—catamenial,** *adj.*

cat″am·ne′sis. The medical history of a patient after an illness or a behavior disorder. **—catamnes′tic,** *adj.*

at″a·pha′si·a (cat″uh·fay′zhuh, zee·uh). A speech disorder in which the patient keeps repeating the same word or series of words.

at″a·pho·re′sis (cat″uh·fo·ree′sis, ·for′i·sis). The migration of charged colloidal particles through the medium in which they are dispersed, when placed under the influence of an applied electric potential. Preferably called *electrophoresis.* —**cataphoret′ic,** *adj.*

at″a·pla′si·a (cat″uh·play′zhuh, ·shuh). 1. Stage of decline in life. 2. Degenerative changes affecting cells and tissues, especially reversion to an earlier or embryonic type of cell or tissue. 3. Application of a plaster or coating. *Obs.*

at′a·plasm. A poultice, *q.v.,* of various substances; usually applied when hot. **kaolin c.** A mixture of kaolin, glycerin, and boric acid, with small amounts of thymol, methyl salicylate, and peppermint oil.

at′a·plex″y. 1. A sudden and overwhelming emotion, fright, or shock causing muscular rigidity in some animals. 2. In man, the sudden loss of muscle tone provoked by exaggerated emotion, often associated with a tendency to narcolepsy. 3. Prostration by the sudden onset of disease. 4. Hypnotic sleep. —**cataplec′tic,** *adj.*

at′a·ract. Partial or complete opacity of the crystalline lens or its capsule. —**catarac′tous,** *adj.* **black c.** A nuclear cataract with a dark opacity. **capsular c.** Cataract due to opacity of the capsule. **immature c.** One in which only a part of the lens substance is cataractous. **irradiation c.** One caused by the use of radium and roentgen rays in large doses or by exposure to intense radiation and high temperatures for long periods of time in the glass-blowing and iron-puddling industries. Also called *glassblower's c., puddler's c.* **lamellar c.** One due to opacity of certain layers between the cortex and nucleus, the remaining layers being transparent. **mature c.** One in which the whole lens substance is cataractous. **polar c.** Either anterior or posterior; a form in which the opacity is confined to one pole of the lens. **senile c.** The cataract of old persons, the most frequent form, and that understood when not specified as congenital, juvenile, traumatic, soft, etc. **soft c.** A form occurring especially in the young; the lens matter is of soft consistence and milky in appearance.

a·tarrh′. Old term once widely used for inflammation of mucous membranes, particularly those of the air passages of the nose and throat, with an exudation containing mucin and epithelial cells. —**catarrhal,** *adj.*

cat″a·stal′sis. The downward moving wave of contraction occurring in the stomach during digestion. There is no preceding wave of relaxation.

cat″a·thy′mi·a. The existence of a complex in the unconscious mind which is heavily charged with affect or feeling so as to produce a pronounced effect in consciousness.

cat″a·to′ni·a. A phase or form of schizophrenia in which the patient seems to lack the will to talk or move and stands or sits in one position, assumes fixed postures, and resists attempts to activate motion or speech. A benign stupor which frequently may be punctuated by violent outbursts, hallucinosis, and panic. —**caton′ic,** *adj., n.*

cat″a·tro′pi·a. Turning of both eyes downward.

cat′e·chol (cat′i·coal, ·kol). See *pyrocatechol.*

cat′e·chu (cat′i·choo, ·koo). Extract prepared from the wood of *Acacia catechu,* a native tree of the East Indies. It contains catechutannic acid and is a powerful astringent.

cat′gut″. A suture and ligature material made from the submucosa of sheep's intestine, cleansed, treated, and twisted. Put up aseptically in glass tubes, in sizes from 00000 to 8. Varieties are: *plain* (untreated), *chromicized* (treated with chromic trioxide), and *iodized* (immersed in a solution of iodine and potassium iodide).

ca·thar′sis. 1. Purgation. 2. *In psychoanalysis,* mental and emotional purge by abreaction.

ca·thar′tic. 1. Purgative. 2. A medicine used to produce evacuations of the bowels; a purgative.

ca·thar′tic ac′id. An active principle from several species of *Cassia.*

ca·thep′sin. Any one of several proteolytic enzymes present in tissue, catalyzing hydrolysis of proteins to proteoses and peptones.

ca·ther′e·sis, ca·thaer′e·sis (katherr′i·sis, kath″i·ree′sis). 1. Prostration or weakness induced by medication. 2. A feebly caustic action.

cath″e·ret′ic. 1. Reducing; weakening; prostrating. 2. Caustic. 3. A reducing or caustic agent.

cath′e·ter. A hollow tube of metal, glass, hard or soft rubber, rubberized silk, etc., for introduction into a cavity through a narrow canal, for the purpose of discharging the fluid contents of a cavity or for establishing the patency of a canal. Specifically, one intended to be passed into the bladder through the urethra for the relief of urinary retention. **c. fever.** The rise in temperature ascribed to the passage of a catheter, associated especially with cystitis. **c. gauge.** A metal sheet having circular holes punched in it which fit exactly certain sized catheters or sounds. See following illustration:

The upper number indicates the size of American catheters: the lower, the French.

c. life. A term employed to indicate constant employment of catheterization on the part of persons who are unable to void urine naturally or who can evacuate only a portion of the bladder contents because of high residual urine. **c. specimen.** Urine obtained under aseptic technic, to insure its being uncontaminated when examined for diagnostic purposes. **elbow c.** One of metal or stiff, rubberized material with one or two 45° bends at or near the proximal end. **Eustachian c.** A small catheter having a bend at one end; used for introduction into the auditory tube to relieve obstruction. **female c.** A short catheter, usually of glass, for catheterizing women. **indwelling c.** A catheter which is allowed to remain in the bladder after passing through the urethra, for establishing constant drainage; used to clear up infected bladders and, especially, in preparation for surgical operations upon the genitourinary tract. **rat-tail c.** A sharp, narrow-ended catheter shaped somewhat like a rat's tail and used in urethral strictures. **self-retaining c.** One which has a bulbous or mushroomlike end, usually made of rubber, which offers enough resistance in withdrawal

to allow of its retention in the bladder under ordinary care. **sigmoid c.** One shaped like an S, for passage into the female bladder. **two-way c.** A double-current uterine catheter. Also called *Bozeman's catheter.*

cath'e·ter·ism. The habitual use of a catheter

cath'e·ter·ize. 1. Insert a catheter. 2. Withdraw urine by means of a catheter. **—catheteriza'tion,** *n.*

cath'ode. The negative electrode or pole of an electric circuit. Abbreviated, ca. **—cathodal,** *adj.*

ca·thod'ic. 1. Relating to a cathode. 2. Proceeding downward; efferent or centrifugal (applied to a nerve current or nerve impulse).

cathomycin. A trademark for novobiocin.

cat'i"on. A positive ion moving toward, or being evolved at, the cathode in electrolytic cells or discharge tubes. **—cation'ic,** *adj.*

cat's'purr". A peculiar purring sound heard on auscultation; due to stenosis of the mitral valve.

can'da. A tail. **—caudal, caudate,** *adj.;* **cauda'tion,** *n. c.* **equina.** A term applied collectively to the roots of the sacral and coccygeal nerves, from their resemblance to a horse's tail.

cau'dad. Toward the tail or cauda; in man, downward; opposed to *cephalad.*

cau'do-, caud-. A combining form denoting *caudal, connected with* or *related to the caudal vertebrae.*

caul. 1. A portion or all of the fetal membranes covering the head and carried out in advance of it in labor. 2. The great omentum.

cau'li·flow"er ear. Thickening and irregularity of the external ear following repeated blows; seen in pugilists.

cau'lo-, caul-. A combining form meaning *stem.*

can"lo·phyl'lum. The dried rhizome and roots of *Caulophyllum thalictroides;* contains the alkaloid caulophylline, several glycosides, and two crystallizable saponins. It produces intermittent contractions of the gravid uterus and is also said to possess diuretic and anthelmintic properties. Syn., *blue cohosh, papoose root.* Also called *squaw root.*

cau·sal'gi·a. The burning pain that is sometimes present in injuries of the nerves, particularly those sensory nerves supplying the palms and soles. The disturbance may be associated with many vasomotor, trophic, and dermal changes in the affected parts. **cause.** The sources, conditions, and origins of a result. The preceding factors that unite to produce a given condition. **antecedent c.** See predisposing c. **determining c.** One that precipitates the action of another or other causes. **essential c.** One that secures the effect independently of the action of other causes. **exciting c.** The immediately preceding and conditioning factor. **immediate c.** See proximate c. **predisposing c.** That which favors the development of a condition. **proximate c.** That one of several causes which is direct and effective. **secondary c.** An ultimate cause. **ultimate c.** One that eventually comes into play aided by a proximate cause.

caus'tic. 1. Very irritant; burning; capable of destroying tissue. 2. A substance that destroys tissue. 3. *In optics,* a curve to which the rays of light reflected or refracted by another curve are tangent; it is called a *catacaustic* or a *catacaustic curve* when caused by reflection; and a *diacaustic* or a *diacaustic curve* when caused by refraction. **c. alkali.** The hydroxide of an alkali element. **c. potash.** Potassium hydroxide. **c. soda.** Sodium hydroxide. **lunar c.** Toughened silver nitrate. See *silver* nitrate.

cau'ter·ant. A caustic or escharotic substance.

cau''ter·i·za'tion. The application of a cautery or a caustic; the effect of such an application. See *cautery.* —**cau'terize,** *v.*

cau'ter·y. 1. Destruction of tissue by the application of a cauterizing agent. 2. A device to produce tissue coagulation by chemical or mechanical means. —**cauteriza'tion,** *n.* **actual c.** The white-hot or red-hot iron. **chemical c.** A caustic substance used to destroy tissue. **cold c.** Cauterization by extreme cold, as carbon dioxide snow. **galvanocautery.** Cauterization by means of a wire loop or needle heated by a direct galvanic current. Also called *electrocautery.* **linear streak c.** A type used in an everted cervix uteri, in which the cautery strokes radiate like spokes of a wheel.

cav'ern. A cavity in the lung due to necrosis of the parenchyma; also the cavity of a dilated bronchus.

cav'ern·ous. Having hollow spaces.

cav''i·ta'tion. 1. The formation of a cavity or cavities, as in tuberculosis of the lung. 2. The process of amnion formation in man and certain mammals.

cav'i·ty. 1. A hole or hollow space. 2. *In dentistry,* the lesion produced by dental caries, *q.v.* **abdominal c.** The space within the body between the diaphragm and the pelvic floor, containing the abdominal viscera. **body c.** The coelom; the peritoneal cavity; any serous cavity, *q.v.* **c. preparation.** *In dentistry:* (a) The removal of carious tooth substance and the proper shaping of a cavity to receive and retain a filling material. (b) The cavity so prepared. **cranial c.** The hollow of the cranium. **glenoid c.** The depression in the scapula for the reception of the head of the humerus. **nasal c.** The cavity of the nose. The two **primary nasal cavities** are derived from the nasal pits; and the **secondary nasal cavities,** in turn from them and from a part of the primary oral cavity, by the formation of the maxillary part of the palate. **oral c.** That of the mouth. The **primary oral cavity** is that derived from the stomodeum before it contributes to the buccal cavity; and the **secondary oral cavity,** the definitive oral cavity after the formation of the palate. **pelvic c.** (a) The cavity within the bony pelvis, including both false and true pelves. (b) *In obstetrics,* the cavity of the true pelvis from inlet to outlet, containing the pelvic viscera. **pericardial c.** A potential space within the pericardium between the serous layer of the pericardium and the epicardium of the heart and roots of the great vessels. **peritoneal c.** A potential space between the visceral and parietal layers of the peritoneum. **pleural c.** The potential space included between the parietal and visceral layers of the pleura. Like the peritoneal and pericardial cavities, it is not an actual space unless opened. **pulp c.** The space within the dentine of the crown and neck of a tooth; it is continuous with the root canal and contains pulp. **serous c.** A potential space between two layers of serous membrane, as the pericardial, peritoneal, or pleural cavity. **thoracic c.** The space within the walls of the thorax, between the base of the neck and the diaphragm, containing the thoracic viscera. **tympanic c.** The cavity of the middle ear; an irregular, air-containing, mucous membrane-lined space in the temporal bone. The chain of auditory ossicles extends from its lateral wall, the tympanic membrane, to its medial wall, the osseous labyrinth. It communicates anteriorly with the nasopharynx through the auditory tube and posterosuperiorly with the mastoid air cells through the tympanic antrum.

Cb. Symbol for columbium.

C.C. Commission Certified; indicating that a sample of the stain so marked has been submitted to the Biological Stain Commission and has been found by them to be true to type, up to specification in respect to dye content, and satisfactory in the procedures listed on the label. Only one batch of dye may be sold under each certification number.

cc. Cubic centimeter.

Cd. Symbol for cadmium.

Ce. Symbol for cerium.

ce″bo·ce·pha′li·a (see″bo·si·fay′-lee·uh), **ce″bo·ceph′a·ly.** A condition, related to incipient cyclopia, in which there is absence or marked defect of the nose, with, however, two orbital cavities and two eyes, the region between the eyes being narrow and flat.

ce·cec′to·my (see·keck′to·mee). Excision of the cecum.

ce′co·cele (see′ko·seel). A hernia of the cecum.

ce″co·co·los′to·my. The formation of an anastomosis between the cecum and some part of the colon.

ce″co·il″e·os′to·my. The formation of an anastomosis between the cecum and the ileum.

ce′co·pex″y. Fixation of the cecum by a surgical operation.

ce″co·pli·ca′tion. Operation for the relief of dilated cecum, consisting in taking tucks or folds in the wall.

ce″cop·to′sis. Downward displacement of the cecum.

ce·cos′to·my. In surgery, the establishment of a permanent artificial opening into the cecum.

ce·cot′o·my. Incision into the cecum.

ce′cum, cae′cum (see′kum). The large blind pouch or cul-de-sac in which the large intestine begins. —**cecal,** adj.

ce′dar. A tree of the genus Cedrus.

cedilanid. Trade-mark for crystalline lanatoside C from Digitalis lanata. See digoxin.

ceepryn. A proprietary surgical antiseptic and detergent, cetylpyridinium chloride, $C_5H_5N(C_{16}H_{33})$ Cl. See cepacol.

cel′an·dine (sel′an·dyne). See chelidonium.

Ce·las′trus. A genus of trees and shrubs of the Celastraceae.

-cele (-seel). A suffix denoting a tumor, hernia, pathologic swelling, or cavity.

-cele. See -coele.

ce′li·ac (see′lee·ack). Abdominal; pertaining to the belly.

ce″li·a·del′phus. Conjoined twins united at the abdomen. Syn., omphalopagus, gastrodidymus.

ce″li·ec·ta′si·a, coe″li·ec·ta′si·a (see″lee·eck·tay′zhuh, ·shuh). Abnormal distention of the abdominal cavity.

ce′li·o-. See coelio-.

ce″li·o·hys″ter·ec′to·my, coe″li·o·hys″ter·ec′to·my. Removal of the uterus through an abdominal incision; abdominal hysterectomy.

ce″li·o·par″a·cen·te′sis, coe″li·o·par″a·cen·te′sis. Tapping, or paracentesis of the abdomen.

ce″li·os′co·py, coe″li·os·co·py. Method of examining the peritoneal cavity by filling it with sterile filtered air through a hollow needle, plunging a trocar through the distended abdominal wall, and passing through the trocar a cystoscope by means of which the adjacent peritoneal surface may be inspected.

ce″li·ot′o·my. In surgery, the opening of the abdominal cavity.

cell. 1. A mass of protoplasm containing a nucleus. The protoplasm of the nucleus is the karyoplasm; that of the remainder of the cell (cytosome) is the cytoplasm. The cell body, or perikaryon, is the mass of cytoplasm, exclusive of processes, immediately surrounding the nucleus. 2. One of the units consisting of electrodes and an electrolyte in a voltaic battery. 3. A compartment; particularly, a hollow space in a bone. —**cell′ular,** adj. **adventitial c.** A branched cell found in the perilymphatic and perivascular tissues; generally regarded as belonging to the reticuloendothelial system. **alpha cells.** Certain granular cells that are found in the pancreatic islets or in the adenohypophysis. **ameboid c.** One capable of changing its form and moving about like an ameba. **argentaffin c.** A type of cell found in the intestinal and gastric glands which reduces silver salts in staining; enterochromaffin cell. **Aschoff c.** The characteristic cell of the Aschoff nodule in rheumatic fever; a large, elongated cell with one or more vesicular nuclei having a central mass of chromatin from which fibrils radiate toward the nuclear membrane. **basal c.** One of the cells of the deepest layer of a stratified epithelium. **basket cells.** (a) Deep, stellate cells of the molecular layer of the cerebellar cortex. The terminal arborizations of their axons envelop Purkinje cells to form the baskets. (b) The myoepithelial cells of salivary, lacrimal, and sweat glands. (c) Degenerating leukocytes in blood smears. **beta cells.** (a) Cells in the pancreatic islets in which the cytoplasm contains alcohol-soluble granules. (b) Cells, containing basophilic granules, that are found in the adenohypophysis. **bipolar nerve c.** One having two prolongations of the cytoplasm, as in the vestibular ganglion of the eighth nerve. **cells of Paneth.** Coarsely granu

r cells found in the crypts of Lieber-
ühn in the small intestine. **centro-
cinar cells.** Those of the inter-
lated ducts of the pancreas which,
certain planes of section, appear
rrounded by the zymogenic cells of
e pancreatic acini. **chief c.** (a)
ne of the columnar, granular cells of
e fundic glands of the stomach; the
urce of pepsin. Also called *zymogenic
central c., adelomorphous c., peptic*
(b) A chromophobe cell of the pitui-
ry gland. **chromaffin cells.** See
romaffin. Formerly called *pheo-
rome cells.* **chromophil cells.** The
pha and beta cells of the pituitary gland.
romophobe cells. The faintly
aining cells of the anterior lobe of the
tuitary gland. Also called *chief cells,
incipal cells, reserve cells.* **colum-
ar c.** An epithelial cell in which the
ight is markedly greater than the
dth. **cuboidal c.** An epithelial cell
which height and width are nearly
ual. **decidual c.** One of the large,
unded, modified, connective-tissue
lls characteristic of the deciduae in
egnancy and responsible for their
pertrophy. **demilune cells.**
rous cells forming a cap at the end
a mucous tubule in mixed glands.
so called *cells of Giannuzzi, serous
escent.* **Dorothy Reed c.** One of
e extremely large cells observed in
ained tissue specimens in Hodgkin's
sease. See Reed-Sternberg *c.* **dust
lls.** Macrophages in the pulmonary
veoli. **endothelial c.** One of the
in, flat cells forming the lining (en-
thelium) of the heart and blood and
mph vessels. **enterochromaffin c.**
ne of the chromaffin cells scattered
roughout the epithelium of the glands
the small intestine and stomach;
gentaffin cell. **ependymal c.** (a)
cell of the ependymal zone in the
veloping neural tube. (b) A type of
uroglia cell lining the central canal
the spinal cord and brain. **eth-
oid cells.** The paranasal sinuses
hich lie in the ethmoid bone. Also
lled *ethmoid sinuses.* **fat c.** A con-
ctive-tissue cell in which fat is
ored. **follicular cells.** The epi-
ielial cells of the ovarian follicle ex-
usive of the ovum. **foreign-body
iant c.** A multinucleated giant cell
ith centrally placed nuclei; found in
reign-body reactions and in certain
anulomatous lesions. **ganglion c.**
nerve cell in a ganglion. Formerly
y neuron of the central nervous
stem. **germ c.** A spermatozoon or an
vum, or a formative stage of either.
ormerly called *gonoblast.* **giant c.**
large, multinucleated cell, as the
egakaryocytes of bone marrow, the
teoclasts, and Langhans' giant cells
tubercles. **goblet c.** One of the

unicellular mucous glands found in the
epithelium of certain mucous membranes, notably those of the respiratory
passages and the intestine. **hair c.** An
epithelial cell with delicate, hairlike
processes, as that of the organ of Corti,
which responds to the stimuli of sound
waves. **interstitial c.** (a) A cell
which lies between the germ cells of a
gonad. (b) A cell with short, branched
processes in an enteric plexus, possibly
of microglial nature. **Kupffer cells.**
Fixed macrophages lining the hepatic
sinusoids. **Langhans' giant c.** A
multinucleated giant cell with peripheral, radially arranged nuclei found
in certain granulomatous lesions, as
tuberculosis, leprosy, tularemia. **L.E. c.**
Lupus erythematosus cell. A mature
polymorphonuclear neutrophil with a
vacuole containing lysed nuclear material which has been phagocytized;
found in bone marrow and peripheral
blood preparations from patients with
systemic lupus erythematosus. **Leydig c.** One of the interstitial cells of
the testis, thought to be the source of
male sex hormone. **lutein cells.**
Cells of the corpus luteum. **Follicular (granulosa) lutein cells** are
derived from the follicular cells of the
ovarian follicle; **paralutein (theca
lutein) cells** are modified connective-tissue cells from the theca folliculi.
lymphoid c. A mononuclear cell resembling a lymphocyte. **lymphoid
stem cells.** Lymphoblasts; hemo-
cytoblasts. **mast c.** One found in connective tissue; characterized by large,
basophil, metachromatic granules.
microglia c. A small glia cell which
becomes phagocytic under pathologic
conditions and acts to remove debris.
motor c. An efferent neuron; specifically, one of the large multipolar neurocytes of the ventral horn of the spinal
cord. **myoepithelial c.** One of the
smooth muscle cells of ectodermal origin in sweat, mammary, lacrimal, and
salivary glands. **parietal c.** One of
those found in the periphery of the
fundic glands of the stomach, farther
from the lumen than chief cells.
Their function is the secretion of
hydrochloric acid. Also called *acid c.,
delomorphous c., oxyntic c.* **plasma
cells.** Derivatives of lymphocytes,
common in serous membranes and in
chronically inflamed regions; these
cells have an eccentric nucleus, basophil, usually clear cytoplasm, and a
lightly staining zone about the cyto-
centrum. **prickle c.** A cell possessing
delicate rod-shaped processes by which
it is connected with neighboring cells.
Purkinje cells. (a) Cells of the
cerebellar cortex with large, flask-
shaped bodies forming a single cell
layer between the molecular and granu-

lar layers. Their dendrites branch in the molecular layer in a plane at right angles to the long axis of the folia, and their axons run through the granular layer into the white substance to end in the central cerebellar nuclei. (b) See *Purkinje fibers* under *fiber*. **pus c.** A degenerate or necrotic leukocyte; the characteristic cell of suppurative inflammation. **pyramidal c.** A nerve cell of the cerebral cortex, usually somewhat triangular on longitudinal section, with one large apical dendrite and several smaller dendrites at the base. The axon is given off from the base of the cell or from one of the basal dendrites. **red blood c.** Erythrocyte, *q.v.* **Reed-Sternberg c.** The characteristic cell of Hodgkin's disease; a giant cell with homogeneous cytoplasm and one or more large oval vesicular nuclei; the nuclei in the multinuclear forms are overriding. **reticular c.** (a) A cell of the cytoreticulum of reticular tissue. (b) a reticulocyte or reticulated red blood cell of the bone marrow or peripheral blood. **Schwann cells.** See *neurilemma*. **septal cells.** Macrophages in the interalveolar septa of the lung. **Sertoli cells.** The sustentacular cells of seminiferous tubules. **sickle c.** A crescent-shaped erythrocyte found in a form of anemia occurring almost exclusively in Negroes. **sperm c.** Spermatozoon, *q.v.* **spindle c.** (a) A fibroblast or smooth muscle cell which is spindle-shaped. (b) A fusiform or spindle-shaped cell, typical of a variety of sarcoma. **squamous c.** A thin, flat epithelial cell. **stellate c.** Any cell with numerous processes making it appear star-shaped, as a Kupffer cell or astrocyte. Also called *star c.* **target c.** An abnormal erythrocyte which, when stained, shows a central and peripheral zone of hemoglobin separated by an intermediate unstained area and thus resembles a bull's eye target. Found after splenectomy and in several types of anemia, etc. Also called *Mexican hat c.* **unipolar c.** A nerve cell with one process only, as a cell of the dorsal root ganglions. **white blood c.** Leukocyte, *q.v.* **zymogenic c.** A cell which forms an enzyme, as that in a pancreatic acinus.

cel'lo-. *In chemistry*, a combining form denoting *cellulose*.

cel''lo·bi'ose. A disaccharide, $C_{12}H_{22}O_{11}$, formed by the partial hydrolysis of cellulose. On hydrolysis it yields two glucose molecules.

cel'lu·lin. Cellulose, *q.v.*

cel''lu·li'tis. A diffuse inflammation of connective tissue. **ischiorectal c.** Inflammation of the connective tissue of the ischiorectal fossa. **pelvic c.** In-

flammation of the connective tissue of the pelvis. Also see *parametritis*.

cel'lu·lose. $(C_6H_{10}O_5)$ n. The principal carbohydrate constituent of the cell membranes of all plants. Absorbent cotton is one of the purest forms of cellulose. **absorbable c.** Cellulosic acid. **oxidized cellulose.** Cellulosic acid.

cel''lu·lo'sic ac'id. Cellulose, in the form of cotton or gauze, which has been oxidized to introduce carboxyl groups, thereby making the material absorbable in tissues to which it is applied. Syn., *absorbable cellulose, oxidized cellulose.*

ce'lom. See *coelom*.

ce''lo·so'ma. Congenital body cleft with eventration; associated with various anomalies of the extremities, of the genitourinary apparatus, of the intestinal tract, and even of the whole trunk. Syn., *gastroschisis, abdominal fissure.*

Cel'si·us. A centigrade thermometer or scale. Abbreviated, C., Cels.

ce·ment'. 1. Any plastic material capable of becoming hard and of binding together the objects that are contiguous to it. 2. Filling material for the teeth. 3. The crusta petrosa of the teeth. See *cementum.* **c. substance.** The substance holding together the endothelial cells of the intima of blood vessels. **intercellular c.** The substance holding epithelial cells together.

ce·men'ti·cle. A calcified body found free in the connective tissue of the periodontal membrane, or fused with the cementum of a tooth.

ce·men'to·blast. An osteoblast that takes part in the development of the cementum.

ce·men''to·gen'e·sis. Formation of the cementum.

ce''men·to'sis (see''men·to'sis, sem''en-). A thickening of the cementum on the root of a tooth; sometimes associated with excess stresses, or may result from bacterial or other irritations.

ce·men'tum. The layer of bone deposited on the root of a tooth.

ce''nes·the'si·a, ce''naes·the-si·a, coe''nes·the'si·a, coe''naes·the'si·a (see''ness·thee'zhuh, sen''ess-). The general sense of bodily existence, the irreducible level of consciousness. **—cenesthet'ic,** *adj.*

ce''nes·thop'a·thy, coe''nes-thop'a·thy, ce''naes·thop's-thy, coe''naes·thop'a·thy (see''-ness·thop'uth·ee, sen''ess-). The general feeling of discomfort or fatigue in illness.

cen'sor·ship. *In psychoanalysis,* the restrictions imposed upon a pure instinctual impulse by counterforces that the unconscious and conscious levels of the mind before it discharges itself upon the environment.

cen'tau·ry. 1. A popular name for various plants of the genus *Centaurium.* 2. The dried flowering plant of *Centaurium umbellatum;* has been used as a stomachic.

cen'ter. 1. The middle point of any surface or of a body. 2. A nucleus or collection of nuclei in the brain or spinal cord regulating a particular function. See also *area, nucleus.* **autonomic c.** Any center of the brain or spinal cord regulating visceral functions by way of the parasympathetic and thoracolumbar outflows. **cardioaccelerator c.** (a) See spinal cardioaccelerator c. (b) Any one of the three postulated higher centers. The precise locations of these centers are not known; they are thought to be in the floor of the fourth ventricle, in the posterior hypothalamic region, and in the motor and premotor areas of the cerebral cortex. **cardioinhibitory c.** The dorsal motor nucleus of the vagus from which arise inhibitory fibers to the heart. **c. of curvature.** *In ophthalmology,* the center of the sphere of which a lens curvature is the segment. **c. of ossification.** The region at which bone first appears in cartilage or membrane. **c. of rotation.** *In ophthalmology,* the point around which the eyeball rotates under the action of the extrinsic muscles. **chondrification c.** The region at which cartilage is first formed. **defecation centers.** Those controlling the defecation reflex. The **medullary defecation center** is located in the floor of the fourth ventricle; the subsidiary **spinal defecation center,** in the second, third, and fourth sacral segments of the spinal cord. **germinal c.** The actively proliferating region of a lymphatic nodule. Also called *germ c.* **heat-regulating centers.** Centers in the hypothalamus for the control of heat production and heat elimination and for regulating the relation of these. **higher c.** A center usually located in the cerebrum; associated on the sensory side with consciousness, on the motor side with regulation of primary efferent nuclei. **hypothalamic centers.** Superior centers for the autonomic nervous system. Those for the sympathetic system are located in the posterior group of hypothalamic nuclei; those for the parasympathetic system, in the anterior and middle nuclei. **lower c.** A center of the brain stem or spinal cord, one concerned with a reflex pathway or one receiving impulses from a higher center. **micturition centers.** Those governing the micturition reflex. Higher centers are located in the mesencephalon and in

the medulla oblongata; the **spinal micturition center** is located in the second, third, and fourth sacral segments of the spinal cord. **receptive centers.** *In physiology* and *in psychophysics,* nerve centers which receive influences that may excite sensations or some kind of activity not associated with consciousness. **reflex c.** Any nerve cell or group of nerve cells in the central nervous system which transforms an afferent impulse into an efferent one. **respiratory c.** A region at the calamus scriptorius, probably including the nucleus of the tractus solitarius and the dorsal sensory nucleus of the vagus, which regulates respiratory movements. **spinal cardioaccelerator c.** That in the lateral column of the upper five thoracic segments of the spinal cord from which arise the preganglionic fibers of the accelerator nerves to the heart. **taste c.** The gustatory nervous center, located in the anterior end of the nucleus of the solitary fasciculus. **trophic centers.** Centers regulating the nutrition of nerves, or, through them, of organs. **vasoconstrictor c.** That located in the floor of the fourth ventricle at the apex of the ala cinerea, regulating constriction of the blood vessels. **vasodilator c.** That located in the floor of the fourth ventricle just lateral to the obex, regulating dilation of the blood vessels. **vasomotor centers.** The vasoconstrictor and vasodilator centers.

cen·te'sis. Puncture; perforation.

cen'ti·bar. A unit of atmospheric pressure; it is one one-hundredth of a bar.

cen'ti·grade. Having 100 divisions or degrees. Abbreviated, C.

cen'ti·gram, cen'ti·gramme. The hundredth part of a gram, equal to 0.1543 grain. Abbreviated, cg.

cen'ti·li''ter, cen'ti·li''tre (sen'-ti·lee''tur). The hundredth part of a liter, equal to 0.6102 cubic inch. Abbreviated, cl.

cen'ti·me''ter, cen'ti·me''tre. The hundredth part of a meter, equal to 0.3937 (or about ⅜) inch. Abbreviated, cm. **cubic c.** The one one-thousandth part of a liter. Abbreviated, cc. See also *milliliter.*

cen''ti·nor'mal. Having one one-hundredth of the normal strength, said of a solution containing one one-hundredth of a gram equivalent of the solute in 1 liter of solution.

centr-. See *centro-.*

cen'trad. Toward the center, or toward the median line.

cen'tra·phose (sen'truh·foze). A subjective sensation of darkness originating in the optic centers.

cen·trif′u·gal. Proceeding from the center to the periphery.

cen′tri·fuge. 1. An apparatus for separating substances of different densities by centrifugal force. 2. Submit to the action of a centrifuge. See *ultracentrifuge.* —**centrifuga′tion, centrifugaliza′ton,** *n.*

cen′tri·ole. A minute body, rod, or granule, usually found in the centrosome and frequently considered to be the active, self-perpetuating, division center of the cell. See *blepharoplast, diplosome.*

cen·trip′e·tal. Traveling toward the center from the periphery.

cen′tro-, centr-. A combining form denoting *center* or *centrosome.*

cen′tro·phose (sen′tro-foze). A subjective sensation of light originating in the optic centers.

cen′tro·some. The centrosphere together with the centriole or centrioles. Also called *central body.*

cen′tro·sphere″. A hyaline body of differentiated cytoplasm found at the center of the astral rays in mitosis and miosis. Also called *astrosphere.*

cen′trum. The center or middle part; the body of a vertebra, exclusive of the bases of the neural arches. **c. ovale.** Medullary center; the central white matter seen on making a section of the brain at the level of the upper surface of the corpus callosum. **c. semiovale.** See *c. ovale.* **c. tendineum.** Central tendon of the diaphragm.

cepacol. A proprietary antiseptic mouth wash containing cetylpyridinium chloride. See *ceepryn.*

ceph′al-. See *cephalo-.*

ceph′al·ad. Toward the head.

ceph″a·lal′gi·a, ceph″a·lal′gy. Headache. —**cephalalgic,** *adj.*

Ceph″a·lan′thus. A genus of the Rubiaceae. **C. occidentalis** is the common buttonbush of North America; its bitter bark has been used as laxative and tonic.

ceph″al·he″ma·to′ma (·hee″muh-to′muh, ·hem″uh-). 1. A collection of blood beneath the pericranium, forming a tumorlike swelling. 2. Caput succedaneum, *q.v.*

ceph″al·hy′dro·cele. Effusion of cerebrospinal fluid beneath the scalp in fractures of the skull.

ce·phal′ic. Pertaining to the head.

ceph′a·lin. 1. A phospholipid found in brain and spinal tissues of mammals. 2. A crystalline acid principle from the bark of *Cephalanthus, q.v.*

ceph″a·lo-, ceph′al-. A combining form denoting *the head.*

ceph″a·lo·cau′dal. In anatomy, relating to the long axis of the body, head to tail.

ceph′a·lo·cele″ (sef′uh-lo-seel″, si-

fal′o-). Hernia of the brain; protrusion of a mass of the cranial contents.

ceph″a·lo·graph″. An instrument for diagrammatically recording the size and form of the head.

ceph″a·lo·men″in·gi′tis. Inflammation of the meninges of the brain.

ceph″a·lom′e·ter. In *craniometry,* an instrument for measuring the head.

ceph″a·lop′a·gus. Conjoined twins united by their heads. Syn., *craniopagus, q.v.* —**cephalopagous,** *adj.*

ceph″a·lo·ple′gi·a. Paralysis of the muscles about the head and face.

ceph′a·lo·tome. An instrument for performing cephalotomy on the fetus.

ceph″a·lot′o·my. The opening or division of the head of the fetus to facilitate delivery.

ceph″a·lo·tribe. An instrument for crushing the fetal head.

-ceph′a·lous. A combining form meaning *having a head of a* (specified) *type,* as in *microcephalous.*

-ceph′a·lus. A combining form meaning *a* (specified) *type of cephalic abnormality; a type of head.*

-ceph′a·ly. A combining form meaning *a* (specified) *condition of the head,* as in *hydrocephaly.*

ce′ra. Wax; obtained from plants or made by insects; consists of esters of monohydric, high molecular-weight alcohols plus various mixtures of fatty acids, hydrocarbons, and other materials, depending on the source. —**cera′ceous,** *adj.* **c. alba.** White wax; prepared by bleaching yellow wax. **c. flava.** Yellow wax; the purified wax from the honeycomb of the bee. Its chief constituent is myricyl palmitate. The color is due to carotene.

cer′a·sin. 1. A resin from the bark of cherry, peach, and plum trees. 2. Kerasin. A cerebroside associated with phrenosin in brain tissue.

ce′rate. In *pharmacy,* an unctuous preparation consisting of wax mixed with oils, fatty substances, or resins. —**cerated,** *adj.*

cer′a·to-, cerat-. See *kerato-.*

Cer″a·toph′yl·lus. A genus of fleas. **C. fasciatus.** The common rat flea of the United States and Europe; a vector of typhus fever and a host of *Hymenolepis diminuta.*

cer·ca′ri·a. Any trematode worm in its second stage of larval life. —**cerca′rial,** *adj.;* **cerca′rian,** *adj., n.*

cer″e·bel′lum. The inferior part of the brain lying below the cerebrum and above the pons and medulla, consisting of two lateral lobes and a middle lobe. —**cerebellar,** *adj.*

cer′e·bral (ser′e-bral, se·re′bral). Of or pertaining to the cerebrum.

cer″e·bra′tion. Mental activity.

cer'e·bric ac'id (serr'i·brick, si·reb'rick), **cer''e·brin'ic ac'id.** A fatty acid from brain tissue.

cer'e·brin. $C_{17}H_{33}O_3N$. A nitrogenous glycoside obtained from brain and similar tissue.

cer'e·brin'ic ac'id. See *cerebric acid.*

cer'e·bro-, cerebr-. A combining form denoting *the cerebrum* or *the brain.*

cer'e·bron. See *phrenosin.*

cer''e·bron'ic ac'id. An acid obtained by hydrolysis of white brain substance.

cer'e·brose. $C_6H_{12}O_6$. Galactose.

cer''e·bro·side. One of a class of nitrogenous, fatty substances occurring in brain tissue, containing galactose.

cer''e·bro·spi'nal. Pertaining to the brain and spinal cord.

cer''e·bro·to'ni·a. *In constitutional medicine,* the motivational drive in personality associated with the inhibitory and attentional functions of the cerebrum. The third component of temperament.

cer'e·brum. The chief portion of the brain, occupying the whole upper part of the cranium, and consisting of the right and left hemispheres; the endbrain; telencephalon.

cer'e·sin, cer'e·sine (seer'i·sin, ·seen). A naturally occurring solid mixture of hydrocarbons somewhat resembling white beeswax. Syn., *ozocerite, earth wax, mineral wax.*

cer'e·sine. See *ceresin.*

ce'ri·um. Ce = 140.13. One of the rarer metals. It forms two series of salts, cerous and ceric. **c. oxalate.** A mixture of the oxalates of cerium, lanthanum, praseodymium, and other associated elements; occurs as a white or slightly pink powder and is insoluble in water; useful in treating vomiting of pregnancy.

ce'ro- (seer'o-, serr'o-), **cer-.** A combining form denoting *presence of,* or *resemblance to, wax.*

ce·ro'sis. Morbid condition of a membrane in which it seems to consist of waxlike scales.

cer'ti·fi'a·ble. A term applied to certain infectious diseases which should be reported to the health authorities. See *notifiable.*

ce·ru'men. Wax of the ear. —**ceru·minous,** *adj.*

ce·ru''mi·no'sis. An excessive secretion of cerumen.

cer''vi·cec'to·my. Excision of the cervix of the uterus.

cer''vi·ci'tis. Inflammation of the cervix of the uterus.

cer'vi·co-, cervic-. A combining form denoting *relation to the neck or cervix of an organ.*

cer''vi·co·vag'i·nal (sur''vi·ko·vadj'i·nul, ·va·jy'nul). Relating to the cervix of the uterus and to the vagina.

cer''vi·co·vag''i·ni'tis (·vadj''i·nigh'tis). Inflammation involving the cervix of the uterus and the vagina.

cer''vi·co·ves'i·cal. Pertaining to the urinary bladder and the cervix uteri.

cer'vix. A constricted portion or neck. —**cervical,** *adj.* **c. of the uterus.** The cylindrical lower portion of the uterus between the isthmus and internal os and the external os. **c. vesicae.** Neck of the urinary bladder. **conoid c.** Malformation of the cervix of the uterus marked by a conical shape and elongation, with constriction of the external os.

ce'ryl. $C_{27}H_{55}$. An organic radical found in combination in beeswax.

Ce·sar'e·an sec'tion (si·zair'ee·un). Delivery of the fetus through an abdominal incision. **low cervical C. s.** Delivery by the supravesical extraperitoneal route in contradistinction to the median abdominal route. **post-mortem C. s.** Delivery of the fetus by section after the mother's death. **radical C. s.** Section followed by hysterectomy.

ce'si·um (see'zee·um). Cs = 132.91. A member of the alkali group of elements. The physiologic actions of cesium are similar to those of potassium.

Ces·to'da. Cestoidea.

Ces·toid'e·a. A class of endoparasitic, usually segmented flatworms belonging to the phylum Platyhelminthes. Syn., *Cestoda.*

ces'tode, ces'toid. 1. Resembling a tapeworm. 2. A parasitic worm; one of the Cestoidea.

ces''to·di'a·sis. Infestation with tapeworms.

ce·ta'ce·um (see·tay'shee·um, ·see·um). Spermaceti; a waxy substance obtained from the head of the sperm whale, *Physeter macrocephalus.* It is employed as a base for ointments and cerates.

cetavlon. Trade-mark for cetyltrimethylammonium bromide or cetrimide, *q.v.*

ce'tin. $C_{32}H_{64}O_2$. Cetyl palmitate, cetyl cetylate. The chief constituent of commercial, purified spermaceti. —**cetic, cetin'ic,** *adj.*

Ce·tra'ri·a. 1. A genus of lichens. 2. Iceland moss—a lichen, **C. islandica,** found in Iceland and other northern countries. It contains a form of starch, lichenin, that gelatinizes when boiled with water. It has been used as a demulcent and nutrient in the form of a jelly or decoction.

cet'ri·mide. $C_{16}H_{33}N(CH_3)_3Br$. Cetyltrimethylammonium bromide, a synthetic detergent having antiseptic power; useful for skin cleansing and washing of wounds. See *cetavlon*, *CTAB*.

cet'yl (set'il, see'til). The radical $C_{16}H_{33}$, compounds containing which are found in beeswax and spermaceti.

cet'yl al'co·hol. $C_{16}H_{33}OH$. A waxy solid, insoluble in water; used as ingredient of many washable ointment bases. Also called *palmityl alcohol*.

cet''yl·pyr''i·din'i·um chlo'ride. $C_5H_5N(C_{16}H_{33})Cl$. A quaternary ammonium compound, soluble in water; used as a germicide and fungicide. See *ceepryn*.

cev''a·dil'la. Sabadilla, *q.v.*

cev'a·din. See *cevadine*.

cev·a·dine (sev'uh-deen, -din), **cev'-a·din.** A crystalline alkaloid of sabadilla.

ce'vine (see'veen, sev'een). An alkaloid found in sabadilla seed and veratrum. Syn., *sabadinine*.

ce''vi·tam'ic ac'id (see''vigh-tam'-ick, see''vi·). Ascorbic acid, *q.v.*

Cf. Chemical symbol of californium.

cg. Centigram.

C. G. S. Centimeter-gram-second—denoting that system of scientific measurements which takes the centimeter, the gram, and the second as the units, respectively, of distance, mass (or weight), and time.

cha'fing. Irritation of the skin, usually due to rubbing.

Cha'gres fe'ver (chah'gres, shag'-rus). A malignant form of malaria, endemic on the Isthmus of Panama.

chain of e·vac''u·a'tion. A term used in the U. S. Army to denote the various medical installations through which a sick or wounded soldier passes in evacuation from the front line to the rear, such as the aid station, the surgical hospital, the evacuation hospital, the general hospital, etc.

chain saw. A surgeon's saw, the teeth of which are linked together like a chain.

cha·la'zi·on (ka·lay'zee-on, kay·lay'·). A tumor of the eyelid from retained secretion of the Meibomian glands; a Meibomian cyst or infection.

chal'co- (kal'co-). A combining form denoting *copper, brass*.

chal·co'sis (kal·ko'sis). A deposit of copper particles in the tissues, especially in the cornea and the lens of the eye. **ocular c.** A characteristic inflammation, due to the effects of copper in the eye; seen in brass and copper workers.

chal''i·co'sis (kal''i·ko'sis). A type of pneumoconiosis caused by inhalation of lime dust. Syn., *flint disease*.

chalk. $CaCO_3$. An impure, native form of calcium carbonate. **c. gout.** Circumscribed calcinosis. **prepared c.**

A native form of calcium carbonate freed from most of its impurities by elutriation. Used as an antacid and in diarrhea.

chal'one. An internal secretion that depresses activity.

cha·lyb'e·ate (ka·lib'ee·ate). 1. Containing iron; having the color or taste of iron. 2. A medicine containing iron.

cham'aer·rhine (kam'uh·ryne). See *platyrrhine*.

cham'ber. 1. A cavity or space. 2. An apparatus in which material to be investigated may be enclosed. **air c.** A vessel or tank in which air pressure can be increased or decreased at will. **aqueous c. of the eye.** That between the posterior surface of the cornea and the anterior surface of the lens, containing aqueous humor. It is divided by the iris into the anterior and posterior chambers. **c. of the heart.** An atrium or a ventricle of the heart. **cloud c.** Apparatus for studying ionizing rays. When nuclear particles, such as alpha particles, are shot into a chamber containing supersaturated water vapor, the particle produces gas ions, each of which condenses a droplet of water, thus marking the path of the particle. **counting c.** An apparatus with a ruled chamber of fixed depth used for counting cells in a fluid; especially, that in which diluted blood is placed for counting the erythrocytes, leukocytes, and platelets. **ionization c.** An instrument for collecting and measuring ions produced in a definite volume of air by a beam of roentgen rays or rays emitted from radioactive substances. **moist c.** A type of large culture plate made of heavy glass and having a loosely fitting cover; used in bacteriologic work. **monitor ionization c.** An ionization chamber, usually with large volume of air, employed for checking the constancy of performance of a roentgen-ray tube. **posterior c.** The space between iris and lens. **pulp c.** The coronal portion of the central cavity in a tooth. **resonance c.** One attached to a tuning fork for acoustic investigation. **respiratory c.** A respiratory cavity. **thimble c.** A small, thimble-sized, enclosed ionization chamber. An **air-wall thimble chamber** is one with walls of material having approximately the same effective atomic number as atmospheric air. **vitreous c.** The portion of the globe of the eye posterior to the crystalline lens.

chan're (shang'kur). The lesion formed at the site of primary inoculation; usually an ulcer. Generally refers to the initial lesion of syphilis, although the term may be used for the primary focus of such diseases as sporotrichosis and tularemia. **c. re-dux.** A syphilitic lesion which is a recurrent ulcer at the site of a previous syphilitic chancre. **hard c.** The primary lesion of syphilis. Also called *Hunterian c., true c.* **soft c.** Chancroid, *q.v.*

chan′croid (shan′kroyd). A lesion produced by an infection with *Hemophilus ducreyi*, involving the genitalia, usually of venereal origin. The lesions are, as a rule, multiple and painful, and cause local lymph-node involvement with the formation of buboes. See *chancre.* Syn., *soft chancre, ulcus molle.* —**chancroi′dal**, *adj.*

chapped. Cracked or roughened by cold, as chapped hands. —**chap**, *n., v.*

char′ac·ter. *In biology,* any structural or functional property of an organism. **acquired c.** A modification of the organism, caused by an environmental factor. **dominant c.** The member of a pair of contrasted traits which manifests itself in the heterozygote. **recessive c.** The member of a pair of contrasted traits which fails to manifest itself in the heterozygote.

char′coal″. The residue, largely amorphous carbon, obtained by incomplete combustion (destructive distillation) of animal or vegetable matter. **activated c.** Charcoal which has been treated, as with steam and carbon dioxide or with other substances, to increase its adsorptive power. **animal c.** Charcoal derived from roasting animal bones and other tissue. Also called *bone black.* **wood c.** Charcoal prepared by incomplete combustion of wood.

charge. A quantity of electricity.

char′la·tan (shahr′luh·tun). One who claims to have more knowledge or skill than he really has; a quack.

char′la·tan·ism, char′la·tan·ry. Unwarranted pretension to skill or knowledge; quackery.

char′ley horse. A rupture or strain of muscle or tendon fibers generally resulting from athletic efforts.

char′ta (kahr′tuh). *In pharmacy,* a medicated paper.

char′tu·la (kahr′tew·luh). A small paper, especially one containing a single dose of a medicinal powder.

chaulmestrol. A brand of ethyl chaulmoograte used in the treatment of leprosy.

chaul·moo′gra oil. A yellow oil from the seeds of *Taraktogenos Kurzii, Hydnocarpus Wightiana* or *Hydnocarpus anthelmintica,* trees of Burma and India. It contains chaulmoogric, gynocardic, and hydnocarpic acids; used in the treatment of leprosy.

chaul·moo′grate. An ester of chaulmoogric acid.

chaul·moo′gric ac′id. 13-(2-Cyclopenten-1-yl) tridecanoic acid. An unsaturated crystalline acid obtained from chaulmoogra oil.

cheek. The side of the face; composed of skin, mucous membrane, and the fat, connective tissue and muscles intervening. Syn., *bucca, gena.*

chei·lal′gi·a (kigh·lal′juh, ·jee·uh). Neuralgia of the lips.

chei·lec′to·my (kigh·leck′to·mee). Excision of a portion of the lip.

chei′lec·tro′pi·on (kigh″leck·tro′pee·on). Eversion of the lip.

chei·li′tis (kigh·ligh′tis). Inflammation of the lips. **c. actinica.** A form in which the lips are irritated by sunlight; usually seen in persons whose skin is sensitive to light. **c. exfoliativa.** Persistent peeling of the lips. **c. glandularis.** A chronic disorder of the lips; characterized by swelling due to hypertrophy of the labial glands and their ducts, with secondary inflammatory symptoms. Also called *c. glandularis apostematosa.* **c. venenata.** A contact dermatitis of the lips, often caused by lipstick or cosmetics.

chei′lo- (kigh′lo-), **cheil-** (kyle-), **chi′lo-** (kigh′lo-), **chil-** (kyle-). A combining form denoting *relation to the lips.*

chei·log″na·tho·pal″a·tos′chisis (kigh·log″nath·o·pal″uh·tos′ki·sis, kigh″lo·nath″o·). Unilateral or bilateral cleft of the lip, alveolar process, and palate.

chei′lo·plas″ty (kigh′lo·plas″tee). Any plastic operation upon the lip.

chei·los′chi·sis (kigh·los′ki·sis). Harelip.

chei·lo′sis (kigh·lo′sis). A disorder of the lips; due to avitaminosis. There is pallor of the mucosa at the angles of the lips in the early stages, followed by maceration and piling up of tissue. Later, fissures appear which may become deep and extend into the cheek. Also called *riboflavin deficiency.*

chei·los″to·mat′o·plas″ty (kigh·los″to·mat′o·plas″tee, kigh″lo·sto′·mat·o·plas″tee). Plastic repair of the lips and mouth.

chei′ro- (kigh′ro-), **cheir-.** See *chiro-.*

che′late (kee′late). Of, pertaining to, or designating chelation or its characteristic ring structure. —**che-late,** *v.*

che′lat·ing a′gent. Any compound, usually organic, with two or more points of attachment at which an atom of a metal may be joined, forming a characteristic heterocyclic ring.

che·la′tion. The action between a chelating agent and a metal ion, which forms a heterocyclic ring.

chel′i·do·nine (kel′i·do·neen, kel″-

i-do'-). A crystalline alkaloid of celandine, related to papaverine.

chel"i·do'ni·um (kel"i·do'nee·um). The leaves and stems of *C. majus*, with properties due to a number of alkaloids and acids. Syn., *celandine*.

chem/i·cal. 1. Of or pertaining to chemistry. 2. A substance of known or definite composition.

Chem'i·cal Corps. A department of the U. S. Army; responsible for the use and manufacture of toxic gases, incendiary materials, and chemicals used in warfare, and for defense apparatus used against such materials.

chem'i·cal war'fare". The use in war of toxic gases, incendiary mixtures, and other chemicals, for defensive or offensive purposes. See war *gas*.

chem'i·cal war'fare a'gent. Any agent, as a war gas, used in chemical warfare.

chem'i·co-. A combining form signifying *relation to*, or *connection with*, *chemistry*.

chem"i·co·cau'ter·y. Cauterization by means of chemical agents.

chem"i·lu"mi·nes'cence. Light produced by means of a chemical reaction and entirely independent of any heat involved. The so-called cold light.

chem'ist. One skilled in chemistry.

chem'is·try. The science of the structure of matter and the composition of substances, their transformation, analysis, synthesis, and manufacture. **analytical c.** That concerned with the detection (qualitative analysis) and determination (quantitative analysis) of substances. **applied c.** Chemistry applied to some useful end, as in industry. **biological c.** The chemistry of life, or that which deals with the composition of animal and vegetable matter, the changes occurring in living organisms, the transformation of food into living tissues, and the elimination of waste products. **colloid c.** Study of the properties developed by substances in the colloidal state of subdivision. **food c.** That dealing with the composition and examination of foods. **forensic c.** The application of chemical knowledge in the solution of legal problems, especially in the detection of crime. **histological c.** Chemistry of the tissues of plants and animals. **immunochemistry.** Chemistry of the changes associated with the phenomena of immunity. **inorganic c.** That branch which treats of substances other than carbon compounds. **nuclear c.** That dealing with changes occurring in the nucleus of an atom. **organic c.** Chemistry of carbon compounds. **pathological c.** Chemistry of abnormal tissues and the changes caused by disease. **pharmaceutical c.**

Chemistry applied to the preparation, the testing, and the composition of drugs. **physical c.** That dealing with the generalizations or laws and the theories of chemistry. **physiological c.** Study of the composition and chemical changes in plants and animals. **toxicological c.** A branch of forensic chemistry dealing with the detection and estimation of poisons.

chem'o-, chem-. A combining form denoting *relation to chemical action* or *to chemicals*.

chem'o·cep"tor, chem'o·re·cep"tor. One of the side chains or receptors in a living cell, having the power of fixing chemical substances in the same way that bacterial toxins are fixed.

chem"o·pro"phy·lax'is. Prevention of disease by the administration of chemical drugs, as sulfanilamide.

chem'o·re·cep"tor. Chemoceptor, *q.v.*

che·mo'sis (ki·mo'sis). Swelling of the conjunctiva. —**chemot'ic,** *adj.*

chem'o·stat. A device used for keeping a bacterial population growing at a reduced rate over an indefinite period by controlling the inflow of nutrients and the outflow of the bacterial suspension; used in experimental bacteriology.

chem"o·sur'ger·y. Removal of malignant and other tissue after it has been fixed chemically in situ so that it may be used for microscopic sections. The technic is used chiefly for the systematic microscopic control of the excision of external cancer.

chem"o·tax'is, chem'o·tax"y. Response of organisms to chemical stimuli; attraction toward a substance is positive while repulsion is negative chemotaxis; chemotropism. —**chemotac'tic,** *adj.*

chem"o·ther'a·py. Prevention or treatment of infective diseases by chemicals which act as antiseptics within the body, without producing serious toxic effects on the patient.

che·mot'ro·pism. 1. Attraction of cells by chemical substances. 2. *In immunology*, the positive attraction of phagocytes to microörganisms, cellular debris, and areas of inflammation. Syn., *chemotaxis*.

Che"no·po'di·um (kee"no·po'dee·um, ken"o·). A genus of herbs of the family Chenopodiaceae.

che"no·po'di·um oil. A volatile oil, obtained from the flower and fruit of a variety of the herb *Chenopodium*, containing ascaridol, used as an anthelmintic. Syn., *wormseed oil*.

cher"o·pho'bi·a (kerr"o·fo'bee·uh, keer"o·). A morbid fear of gaiety or happiness.

cher'ry. Any of a number of species of the genus *Prunus*, trees having typical globose drupes. **wild c.** The stem bark of *Prunus serotina*. It is frequently used as a flavoring agent, especially for cough syrups. Also called *wild black c. bark*.

chest. The thorax, *q.v.*

chi·as'ma (kigh·az'muh) (pl. *chiasmata*). 1. The optic commissure. Also called *chiasm*. 2. A crossing. Also called *chiasm*. 3. *In genetics,* the crossing of two chromatids at the prophase of the first maturation division of the germ cells, as a result of crossing over.

chick'en·pox". An acute, contagious disease of childhood, characterized by a superficial eruption of macular transparent vesicles which appear in successive crops on different parts of the body. Varicella, *q.v.*

chig'ger. A larval mite of the genus *Trombicula;* the bite of the common chigger causes severe inflammatory lesions in warm-blooded animals, including man.

chig'oe, chig'o. See *Tunga* penetrans.

chil'blain". Congestion and swelling of the skin, due to cold, and attended with severe itching or burning; vesicles and bullae may form, and these may lead to ulceration. Syn., *erythema pernio, pernio.*

child. One who has not reached the age of puberty.

child'bed". Condition of a woman being in labor; parturition. **c. fever.** Puerperal fever.

child'birth". Parturition. **natural c.** A method of preparing an expectant mother, emotionally through an understanding of the birth process and physically by a regimen of special exercises and breathing techniques, for labor without fear and thus reducing or eliminating the need for anesthetics.

chill. A sensation of cold accompanied by shivering; frequently the initial symptom of acute infections, as pneumonia; a prominent symptom of various forms of malarial fever. The subjective sensation of chilliness results from constriction of the blood vessels of the skin and is accompanied by a rise of body temperature.

chi'lo- (kigh'lo-), **chil-** (kighl-). See *cheilo-*.

chi·me'ra, chi·mae'ra (kigh-meer'uh, ki-meer'uh). 1. A plant composed of two genetically distinct types of tissue resulting from somatic mutation, segregation, or from artificial fusion, as in graft hybrids; mosaic. 2. A compound embryo produced by grafting approximately equal halves of two embryos, usually of different species.

chin. The mentum; the lower part of the face, at or near the symphysis of the lower jaw. **c. reflex.** See jaw-jerk *reflex.*

chinacrin hydrochloride. Trade name for quinacrine hydrochloride.

chin'i·o·fon (kin'ee·o·fon, chin'ee·). A mixture of 7-iodo-8-hydroxyquinoline-5-sulfonic acid, its sodium salt, and sodium bicarbonate, employed as an amebicide and as a surgical dusting powder.

chin'o- (kin'o-, kee'no-), **chin-** (kin-). A combining form denoting *presence of* or *relation to quinine.*

chinosol. Trade name for 8-hydroxyquinoline sulfate (oxyquinoline sulfate), an active bactericide.

chi"o·na·blep'si·a, chi"o·na·blep'sy (kigh"o·nuh·). Loss of sensibility of the retina resulting from the exposure of the eyes to reflection of the sunlight upon snow; snowblindness.

chi'ro- (kigh'ro-), **chir-, chei'ro-** (kigh'ro-), **cheir-.** A combining form denoting *pertaining to the hand.*

chi·rol'o·gy (kigh·rol'o·jee). 1. Method of communicating with deaf-mutes by means of the hands. *Obs.* 2. Study of the hand.

chi"ro·meg'a·ly (kigh"ro·meg'uh·lee). Enlargement of one or both hands, but not of acromegalic nature. Also called *pseudoacromegaly.*

chi'ro·plas"ty (kigh'ro·plas"tee). Plastic operation on the hand.

chi·rop'o·dist (kigh·rop'o·dist, ki·rop'·). One who treats minor ailments of the feet. Syn., *podiatrist.*

chi·rop'o·dy (kigh·rop'o·dee, ki·rop'·). The medical specialty dealing with diseases of the feet.

chi"ro·prac'tic (kigh"ro·prack'tick). A system of therapeutics based upon the theory that disease is caused by abnormal function of the nervous system; attempts to restore normal function are made through manipulation and treatment of the structures of the body, especially those of the spinal column. **—chi'roprac'tor,** *n.*

chi'tin (kigh'tin). $C_{15}H_{26}N_2O_{10}$. The substance forming the skeleton of many invertebrates. **—chitinous,** *adj.*

chlo·as'ma (klo·az'muh). Deposit of pigment in the skin, occurring in patches of various sizes and shapes, and of a yellow, brown, or black color; often associated with some endocrine derangement. Syn., *discolorations, melanoderma, melasma.* **c. hepaticum.** Liver spots, a term used by the laity for any pigmentation of the face or chest. **c. uterinum.** Located chiefly on the forehead, temples, cheeks, nipples, and median line of abdomen. They may be marked during pregnancy, menstruation, functional derangements of the uterus, or ovarian disorders and tumors.

chlor-. See *chloro-*.

chlo'ral. 1. Trichloroacetaldehyde, CCl₃.CHO. A colorless, caustic liquid of pungent odor. 2. Chloral hydrate. **camphorated c.** A liquid prepared from equal parts of chloral hydrate and camphor; used as a counterirritant and anodyne. Syn., *chloral camphor*. **c. hydrate.** CCl₃.CH(OH)₂. White crystals, soluble in water; used as rapid somnifacient and anticonvulsant.

chlor·am'bu·cil. 4-{p-[Bis(2-chloroethyl)amino]phenyl}butyric acid, an antineoplastic agent. See *leukeran*.

chlo'ra·mine"-T. Sodium para-toluenesulfonchloramide. A white or faintly yellow powder, unstable in air. A surgical disinfectant in 0.5–4.0% solution. Syn., *chlorazene*.

chlor"am·phen'i·col. D(-)-Threo-1-p-nitrophenyl-2-dichloroacetamido-1,3-propanediol, an antibiotic produced by *Streptomyces venezuelae* Burkholder, also synthetically. See *chloromycetin*.

chlo'rate. A salt of chloric acid; the radical ClO₃⁻.

chlo'ra·zene. Chloramine-T.

chlo'ra·zol black E (C.C.). An acid poly-azo dye; used as a vital dye and as a nuclear stain. Also called *Erie black G X 00, Pontamine black E*.

chlor·bu'ta·nol. Chlorobutanol.

chlor·bu'tol. Chlorobutanol.

chlorcosane. Trade name of chlorinated paraffin.

chlor·cre'sol. See *chlorocresol*.

chlor·cy'cli·zine. Nonproprietary title for N-methyl-N'-(4-chlorobenzhydryl)piperazine dihydrochloride, an antihistaminic drug. See *di-paralene, perazil*.

chlor'dan, chlor'dane. 1,2,4,5,6,-7,8,8-Octachloro-2,3,3a,4,7,7a-hexahydro-4,7-methanoindene, an insecticide.

chlo·rel'lin. A substance produced by certain algae, notably species of *Chlorella*, which inhibits the growth of various Gram-positive and Gram-negative bacteria.

chloresium. Trade-mark for certain medicinal products containing chlorophyll.

chlor·eth'yl. See *ethyl chloride*.

chloretone. A trade-mark for chlorobutanol.

chlor·hy'dri·a. Excess of hydrochloric acid in the stomach.

chlo'ric ac'id. HClO₃. An acid known only in solution and in the form of its salts (chlorates).

chlo'ride. A salt of hydrochloric acid; a binary compound containing Cl⁻. **lime c.** Chlorinated lime.

chlo'ride shift. The exchange of chloride ion for bicarbonate ion between intracellular and extracellular

fluid without a corresponding movement of cations.

chlo"ri·du'ri·a. Excess of chlorides in the urine.

chlo"rin·a'tion. Act or process of treating with chlorine, as for disinfecting sewage or drinking water.

chlo'rine (klo'reen, ·rin). Cl = 35.457. A greenish yellow gas of suffocating odor; very irritant. A powerful germicide in the presence of moisture. **—chlorinated,** *adj.*

chlor"i·son'da·mine chlo'ride. 4,5,6,7-Tetrachloro-2-(2-dimethylaminoethyl)isoindoline dimethylchloride, a hypotensive drug. See *ecolid chloride*.

chlo'rite. A salt containing the radical ClO₂⁻, derived from chlorous acid.

chlor·mer'o·drin. [3-(Chloromercuri)-2-methoxypropyl]urea, a diuretic. See *neohydrin*.

chlo·ro-, chlor-. 1. A combining form meaning *pale green*. 2. In chemistry, a combining form meaning *having chlorine as a substitute for hydrogen*.

chlo"ro·ac"e·to·phe'none (klor"-o·ass"i·to·fee'nohn). C₈H₇OCl. A white solid used as a lacrimator in chemical warfare. See *war gas*.

chlo"ro·az'o·din. See *azochloramid*.

chlo"ro·bu'ta·nol. Trichloro-*tert*-butyl alcohol. White crystals; soluble in water. Hypnotic, sedative, anticonvulsant, local anesthetic and antiseptic. Syn., *chlorbutol, acetone-chloroform*.

chlo"ro·cre'sol. Parachlorometacresol. Colorless, slightly soluble crystals used for the sterilization and preservation of injections.

chlo"ro·form. Trichloromethane, CHCl₃. A heavy, colorless liquid having a characteristic ethereal odor. It is used as an organic solvent and, medicinally, as an anesthetic, anodyne, and antispasmodic. **acetone-c.** Chlorobutanol.

chlo"ro·form·ism. 1. Habitual use of chloroform for its narcotic effect. 2. Symptoms produced by this use of the drug.

chlor"o·gua'nide hy"dro·chlo'ride. The nonproprietary title for N¹-(p-chlorophenyl)-N⁵-isopropylbiguanide hydrochloride, an antimalarial drug. See *paludrine hydrochloride*.

chlo·ro'ma. Multiple tumors of marrow of bones, and of soft tissues near bones, lymph nodes, and viscera. Grossly, the nodules are green; microscopically, they resemble focal lesions of leukemia. Chloroma is usually accompanied by the blood picture of leukemia.

chloromycetin. Trade-mark for the antibiotic chloramphenicol.

chlo"ro·per'cha. Solution of gutta-percha in chloroform; used in dentistry.

chlo'ro·phe'nol. Monochlorophenol. $C_6H_4Cl.OH$. The *ortho* variety is a colorless liquid; the *meta* and *para* isomers are crystalline. Antiseptic and caustic. *Trichlorophenol* occurs as white crystals; it is used as a 5–10% antiseptic ointment.

chlo'ro·phen'o·thane. United States Pharmacopeia name for the medicinal grade of DDT, *q.v.* Syn., *dicophane.*

chlo'ro·phy'lase. An enzyme which splits or hydrolyzes chlorophyll.

chlo'ro·phyll. The green coloring matter responsible for photosynthesis in plants. It consists of chlorophyll-α and chlorophyll-β. It is used in the treatment of various infections. See *pheophytin.* **crystalline c.** Consists chiefly of ethyl chlorophyllide, a product of the extraction of green leaves with ethyl alcohol.

chlo'ro·pic'rin. Trichloronitromethane. A liquid used as an insecticide and as a lacrimator and emetic chemical warfare agent. Syn., *chlorpicrin.* Also called *nitrochloroform.*

chlo'ro·plast, chlo'ro·plas'tid. In plant cells, the cytoplasmic structures which bear the chlorophyll.

chlo·rop'si·a, chlo·ro'pi·a. Defect of vision in which all objects appear green. It occurs occasionally in digitalis poisoning.

chlo'ro·quine (klor'o·kwine, ·kween). 7-Chloro-4-(4-diethylamino-1-methylbutylamino)-quinoline; a synthetic antimalarial. Introduced as *SN 7618.* See *aralen diphosphate.*

chlo·ror'a·phin. An antibiotic substance obtained from *Chromobacterium.*

chlo·ro'sis. Greensickness; a form of anemia; most common in young women; characterized by a marked reduction of hemoglobin in the blood, with but a slight diminution in number of red cells. —**chlorot'ic,** *adj.*

chlorothen. Trade-mark for the antihistaminic substance N,N-dimethyl-N'-(2-pyridyl)-N'-(5-chloro-2-thenyl)-ethylenediamine hydrochloride.

chlo"ro·thi'a·zide. 6-Chloro-7-sulfamyl-1,2,4-benzothiadiazine-1, 1-dioxide, an orally effective diuretic. See *diuril.*

chlor"o·thy'mol. Monochlorothymol. A white, crystalline powder used as a germicide and fungicide. Syn., *chlorthymol.*

chlo"ro·vi"nyl·di"chlo·ro·ar'·sine. $CHCl:CH.AsCl_2$. Lewisite; a potent lacrimator, lung irritant, and vesicant, developed for use as a chemical warfare agent. See *war gas.*

chlo"ro·xy'le·nol (klor"o·zy'li·nole, ·nol). 2-Chloro-5-hydroxy-1,3-dimethylbenzene. Creamy-white, crystalline powder used as an antiseptic.

chlor"phen·ir'a·mine ma·le'ate (klor"fen·eer'a·meen). 2-[p-Chloro-α-(2-dimethylaminoethyl)benzyl]pyridine maleate, an antihistaminic drug. See *chlor-trimeton maleate.*

chlor·phe'nol. See *chlorophenol.*

chlor·pic'rin. See *chloropicrin.*

chlor·pro'ma·zine hy"dro·chlo'ride. 2-Chloro-10-(3-dimethylaminopropyl)phenothiazine hydrochloride, an antinauseant and tranquilizer. See *thorazine hydrochloride.*

chlor"quin·al'dol. 5,7-Dichloro-8-hydroxyquinaldine, a topical antibacterial agent. See *sterosan.*

chlor"tet·ra·cy'cline hy"dro·chlo'ride. A broad-spectrum antibiotic of the tetracycline group biosynthesized by *Streptomyces aureofaciens,* active against many Gram-negative and Gram-positive bacteria as well as rickettsiae and certain viruses. See *aureomycin hydrochloride.*

chlor·thy'mol. See *chlorothymol.*

chlor-trimeton maleate. A trade-mark for chlorpheniramine maleate.

cho·a'na (ko·ay'nuh, ko·ah'nuh). 1. A funnel-like opening. 2. Either of the posterior nasal orifices. Also called *internal naris.* —**choanal,** *adj.*

choke. Suffocate; prevent access of air to the lungs by compression or obstruction of the trachea or larynx.

choke'damp". A name given by miners to carbon dioxide gas; blackdamp.

choked disk. See *papillitis.*

chok'ing. Partial or complete suffocation from mechanical obstruction by a foreign body or external pressure, or from laryngeal spasm caused by an irritating gas or liquid.

chol-. See *cholo-.*

chol'a·gogue, chol'a·gog (kol'uh·gog, ko"luh·). 1. Stimulating the flow or the secretion of bile. 2. Any agent that promotes the flow of bile.

cho·lal'ic ac'id (ko·lal'ick, ko·lay'·lick). See *cholic acid,* 1.

cholan-DH. Trade-mark for dehydrocholic acid.

cho'lane (ko'lane, kol'ane). $C_{24}H_{42}$. A hydrocarbon, parent substance of sterols, hormones, bile acids, and digitalis aglycones.

chol"an·gi·ec'ta·sis. A dilatation of extrahepatic or intrahepatic biliary passages.

chol"an·gi·og'ra·phy (kol"an·jee·og'ruh·fee, ko"lan·). Roentgenography of the bile ducts.

chol·an"gi·o·li'tis (ko·lan"jee·o·lye'tis). Inflammation of the bile canaliculi within the liver.

chol"an·gi·os'to·my (kol"an·jee·os'to·mee, ko"lan·). *In surgery,* the drainage of any of the bile ducts by means of abdominal incision and penetration into the hepatic, cystic, or common duct.

chol″an·gi·ot′o·my (kol″an·jee-ot′o·mee, ko″lan·). Incision into any of the bile ducts, usually for removal of a calculus.

chol″an·gi′tis (kol″an·jy′tis, ko″lan·). Inflammation of the biliary ducts, especially the intrahepatic ducts in the portal canals. Syn., *angiocholitis*.

cho′late (ko′late). Any salt of cholic acid.

chol″e·bil″i·ru′bin (kol″i·bil″i·roo′bin, ko″li·). 1. Bilirubin after passage through the hepatic cells. 2. The form of bilirubin present in bile and blood in hepatic or obstructive jaundice, giving a positive direct van den Bergh reaction. Also see *hemobilirubin*.

chol″e·cal·cif′er·ol (kol″e·kal·sif′er·ol). Vitamin D₃, prepared from cholesterol.

chol′e·cy′a·nin (kol″i·sigh′uh·nin, ko″li·). Bilicyanin.

chol′e·cyst (kol′i·sist, ko′li·), **chol″e·cys′tis**. The gallbladder. **—chole·cys′tic**, *adj.*

chol″e·cyst′a·gogue (kol″i·sist′uh·gog, ko″li·). An agent or agency which causes or promotes the evacuation of the gallbladder, by inducing contraction of its musculature, or by relaxation of the sphincter of Oddi.

chol″e·cyst·al′gi·a (kol″i·sist·al′juh, ko″li·). Biliary colic.

chol″e·cyst·ec′to·my. Excision of the gallbladder.

chol″e·cyst·en″ter·or′rha·phy. *In surgery*, suturing the gallbladder to the small intestine.

chol″e·cyst·en″ter·os′to·my. *In surgery*, the establishment of a communication between the gallbladder and the small intestine.

chol″e·cys·ti′tis. Inflammation of the gallbladder.

chol″e·cys″to·co·los′to·my. Formation, by operation, of an anastomosis between the gallbladder and some portion of the upper colon.

chol″e·cys″to·du″o·de′nal (kol″i·sis″to·dew″o·dee′nul, ·dew·odd′i·nul). Pertaining to the gallbladder and duodenum.

chol″e·cys″to·du″o·de·nos′·to·my. *In surgery*, the establishment of a communication between the gallbladder and the duodenum.

chol″e·cys″to·e·lec″tro·co·ag″u·lec′to·my. Electrosurgical obliteration of the gallbladder.

chol″e·cys′to·gram. A roentgenray picture of the gallbladder.

chol″e·cys·tog′ra·phy. Roentgenography of the gallbladder after it has been prepared by ingestion or injection of radiopaque substances, which are excreted into it.

chol″e·cys″to·il·e·os′to·my. *In surgery*, establishment of a communication between the gallbladder and the ileum.

chol″e·cys″to·jej″u·nos′to·my. *In surgery*, the establishment of a communication between the gallbladder and the jejunum.

chol″e·cys″to·ki·net′ic (kol″i·sis″to·ki·net′ick, ko″li·). Possessing the property of causing or promoting gallbladder contraction.

chol″e·cys″to·ki′nin (kol″i·sis″to·kigh′nin, ·kin′in). A hormone produced by the upper intestinal mucosa. It causes the gallbladder to contract.

chol″e·cys″to·li·thi′a·sis. Presence of one or more gallstones in the gallbladder.

chol″e·cys·tor′rha·phy. Suture of the gallbladder, especially to the abdominal wall.

chol″e·cys·tos′to·my. *In surgery*, establishment of an opening into the gallbladder, usually for drainage of its contents.

chol″e·cys·tot′o·my. Incision into the gallbladder to remove gallstones, etc.

cho·led′o·chal (ko·led′o·kul). Pertaining to the common bile duct.

cho·led″o·chec′to·my (ko·led″o·keck′to·mee). Excision of a part of the common bile duct.

cho·led″o·chi′tis (ko·led″o·kigh′tis). Inflammation of the common bile duct.

cho·led″o·cho·du″o·de·nos′·to·my. *In surgery*, the establishment of a passage between the common bile duct and the duodenum.

cho·led″o·cho·en″ter·os′to·my. *In surgery*, establishment of a passage between the common bile duct and the small intestine.

cho·led″o·cho·lith·i′a·sis. The presence of a calculus in the common bile duct.

cho·led″o·cho·li·thot′o·my. Surgical removal of a calculus by incision of the bile ducts. **transduodenal c.** Removal of a biliary calculus in the common bile duct through an opening made into the duodenum.

cho·led″o·cho·lith′o·trip′sy (ko·led″o·ko·lith′o·trip″see, ·li·thot′·rip·see). Crushing of a gallstone in the common bile duct without opening the duct. *Obs.*

cho·led″o·chos′to·my (ko·led″o·kos′to·mee). *In surgery*, draining of the common bile duct through the abdominal wall.

cho·led″o·chot′o·my (ko·led″o·kot′o·mee). An incision into the common bile duct. **transduodenal c.** Incision for the removal of gallstones from the ampulla of Vater.

cho·led′o·chus (ko·led′o·kus). Receiving or holding bile, as ductus choledochus.

chol″e·he′ma·tin (kol″i·hee′muh·tin, ·hem′uh·tin). Bilipurpurin; pigment found in the bile and biliary concretions of ruminants. It is identical with the pigment phylloerythrin, a pigment obtained from chlorophyll.

cho·le′ic (ko·lee′ick, kol′ee·ick), **cho′lic** (ko′lick, kol′ick). Pertaining to the bile.

cho·le′ic ac′id. Any one of the several stable molecular compounds formed by desoxycholic acid with other substances, especially fatty acids.

chol′e·lith (kol′i·lith, ko′li·lith). A biliary calculus or gallstone.

chol″e·li·thi′a·sis. The presence of, or a condition associated with, calculi in the gallbladder or in a bile duct.

chol″e·li·thot′o·my. Incision for the removal of gallstones.

cho·le′mi·a (ko·lee′mee·uh). Presence of bile in the blood. —**cholemic,** *adj.* **congenital familial c.** A condition characterized by microcytic erythrocytes. Usually seen in childhood in successive generations of the same family. Occurs in both sexes. Also called *acholuric familial jaundice, Chauffard-Minkowski syndrome.*

chol″e·poi·e′sis (kol″i·poy·ee′sis, ko″li·). The process of formation of bile by the liver.

chol″e·poi·et′ic. 1. Possessing the property of stimulating the processes or a process concerned in the formation of bile. 2. An agent which stimulates the formation of bile.

chol″e·pra′sin (kol″i·pray′zin, ·pray′sin). Biliprasin; a bile pigment.

chol″e·pyr′rhin. Bilirubin, *q.v.*

chol′er·a. An acute, specific, infectious disease caused by *Vibrio comma;* characterized by profuse, effortless diarrhea, rice-water stools, vomiting, collapse, muscular cramps, and suppression of urine. Case fatality varies from 10 to over 50 per cent. The source is exclusively human. Food or water may be the vehicle. Epidemics are common in the tropical Orient, especially in India. A vaccine prepared from the causative organism killed by heat probably gives protection for several months. Also called *Asiatic c., c. indica.* —**cholera′ic,** *adj.* **c. infantum.** Old term applied indiscriminately to diarrheal conditions in infants and young children. **c. morbus.** Old term applied to any inflammatory enteritis with pain and purging. **c. sicca.** Fatal cholera without diarrhea. At autopsy, the bowel is often found filled with rice-water material.

chol·er·e′sis (kol·er·e′sis). An increased secretion of bile by the liver.

chol·er·et′ic. A therapeutic agent that produces or stimulates choleresis.

chol·er·et′ic. Of or pertaining to choleresis or to a choleretic.

chol′er·ic. Easily angered; irritable.

chol″er·o·pho′bi·a. Morbid fear of cholera.

chol″er·rha′gi·a (kol″uh·ray′juh, ·radj′ee·uh). A flow of bile.

cho·les·tane (kol′es·tane, ko′les·tane). A saturated hydrocarbon, $C_{27}H_{48}$, from which all sterols may be considered to be derived.

cho·les′ta·nol (ko·les′tuh·nole, ·nol). A sterol, found in the feces of human beings, and probably resulting from the action of bacteria on cholesterol.

cho·les″te·a·to′ma (ko·les″tee·uh·to′muh, kol″es·). Pearly tumor; a tumor derived from embryonal inclusions of ectoderm, lined by stratified squamous epithelium, and containing squames and a mixture of lipids including cholesterol and, occasionally, dermal structures such as sebaceous glands; occurs in the middle ear, and rarely about the base of the brain and in the spinal cord. —**cholesteatom′atous,** *adj.*

chol′es·tene (kol′es·teen, ko′les·teen). The unsaturated hydrocarbon $C_{27}H_{46}$. It is the parent hydrocarbon of cholesterol.

cho·les″ter·e′mi·a (ko·les″tur·ee′mee·uh). An excess of cholesterol in the blood.

cho·les″ter·i·nu′ri·a. The presence of cholesterol in the urine.

cho·les′ter·ol. $C_{27}H_{45}OH$. A solid monohydric alcohol, a constituent of all animal fats and oils; insoluble in water. It is important in metabolism and derivatives may be activated to form a vitamin D. See Table of Normal Values of Blood Constituents in Appendix.

cho·les′ter·yl. $C_{27}H_{45}$. The radical of cholesterol.

cho·let′e·lin (ko·let′i·lin). $C_{16}H_{18}$-N_2O_6. An amorphous, soluble, yellow pigment and oxidation product derived from biliverdin. It is readily soluble in alkalis, alcohol, and chloroform.

chol″e·ver′din (kol″i·vur′din, ko″li·). See *biliverdin.*

cho′lic (ko′lick, kol′ick). Choleic, *q.v.*

cho′lic ac′id. 1. $C_{24}H_{40}O_5$. The 3,7,12-trihydroxycholanic acid, one of the unconjugated bile acids. Syn., *cholalic acid.* 2. Any one of the several unconjugated bile acids which are hydroxy derivatives of cholanic acid.

cho′line (ko′leen, kol′een). $C_5H_{15}NO_3$. A nitrogenous base widely distributed in nature as a component of lecithin and other phospholipids. See also *acetylcholine.*

cho″lin·er′gic (ko″lin·ur′jick, kol″in·). Applied to parasympathetic or preganglionic sympathetic nerves which liberate acetylcholine at the nerve terminals.

cho″lin·es′ter·ase (ko″li-nes′tur-ace, -aze). An enzyme found in blood and in various other tissues, which catalyzes the hydrolysis of acetylcholine to acetic acid and choline.

chol′o- (kol′o-, ko′lo-), **chol-**. A combining form denoting *bile* or *gall*.

chol′o·gogue. A substance which stimulates the flow of bile.

cholografin. Trade-mark for iodipamide.

chol′o·lith. A gallstone. **—chololith′ic**, *adj.*

chol″or·rhe′a. Profuse secretion of bile.

cho·lu′ri·a (ko-lew′ree-uh). The presence of bile in the urine.

Chon″do·den′dron. A genus of South American climbing plants of the Menispermaceae. **C. tomentosum** is the source of pareira.

chon′dral (kon′dral). Cartilaginous; relating to cartilage.

chon·drec′to·my (kon-dreck′to-mee). *In surgery*, the excision of cartilage.

chon′dri·fy (kon′dri-figh). Convert into cartilage; become cartilaginous. **—chondrifica′tion**, *n.*

chon′dri·gen (kon′dri-jen). The protein of cartilage which is converted by boiling into chondrin; similar to collagen.

chon′drin (kon′drin). A protein material obtained by boiling cartilage; primarily gelatin obtained from the collagen component of the cartilage.

chon′dri·o- (kon′dree-o-). *In biology*, a combining form denoting *grit, grain, cartilage, chondriosome,* or *chondriosomal.*

chon′dro- (kon′dro-), **chondr-**. A combining form denoting *grain, cartilage, composed of cartilage,* or *connection with cartilage.*

chon′dro·blast. A cartilage-forming cell.

chon″dro·blas·to′ma. Chondroma.

chon·droc′la·sis (kon-drock′luh-sis, kon″dro-clay′sis). 1. Crushing of a cartilage. 2. Resorption of cartilage.

chon′dro·clast (kon′dro-klast). A cell concerned in the resorption of cartilage.

chon″dro·cos′tal. Relating to the ribs and their cartilages.

chon″dro·cra′ni·um. The embryonic cartilaginous cranium.

chon′dro·cyte. A cartilage cell.

chon″dro·der″ma·ti′tis. Inflammation of a cartilage and overlying skin. **c. nodularis helicis**. Painful nodules of the ear; usually seen in men on the rim of the ear. Frostbite has often preceded their occurrence.

chon″dro·dys·tro′phi·a. A defect

in the formation of bone from cartilage, congenital in origin. **c. hyperplastica**. Enlarged cartilage with possible formation of massive, nodular, irregularly ossified projections at the ends of poorly developed bones. Also called *multiple cartilaginous exostoses.*

chon″dro·dys′tro·phy. 1. See *chondrodystrophia*. 2. See *lipochondrodystrophy*.

chon′dro·gen. See *chondrigen*.

chon″dro·gen′e·sis. Formation of cartilage. **—chondrogenic**, *adj.*

chon′droid (kon′droyd). Resembling cartilage.

chon·dro′i·tin (kon-dro′i·tin). A complex nitrogenous substance which, in the form of chondroitinsulfuric acid, occurs combined with protein as chondromucoid, a constituent of cartilage.

chon·dro″i·tin·sul·fu′ric ac′id. A compound which on hydrolysis yields sulfuric acid, acetic acid, galactosamine, and glycuronic acid. It is the prosthetic group of the glycoprotein, chondromucoid. Syn., *chondroitic acid.*

chon·dro′ma (kon·dro′muh). A tumor which in its growth simulates the structure of cartilage (either hyaline cartilage or fibrocartilage); may grow from bone, cartilage, or other tissue; is generally benign, but tends to recur after removal.

chon″dro·ma·la′ci·a (kon″dro-muh·lay′shuh, -see-uh). Softening of a cartilage.

chon″dro·mu′coid. A mucoid found in cartilage; a glycoprotein in which chondroitinsulfuric acid is the prosthetic group.

chon″dro·myx·o′ma. A chondroma with myxomatous elements, or one which has undergone mucoid degeneration.

chon″dro·myx″o·sar·co′ma. A sarcoma which contains immature cartilage and mucoid tissue. One form occurs as a highly malignant, primary, osteogenic, periosteal sarcoma in young persons; located usually about the knee, lower end of the femur, or upper part of the tibia. May occur in later life secondary to otherwise benign skeletal lesions such as chondroma, exostosis, osteoarthritis, and dyschondroplasia.

chon″dro·os″te·o·dys′tro·phy. A disease encountered in children; characterized by irregular metaphyses with increased thickening of the epiphyseal cartilage; resembles achondroplasia, *q.v.*, but apparently is not congenital. Club hand and coxa vara are frequent. Also called *Morquio's disease.*

chon″dro·os″te·o′ma. See multiple osteocartilaginous *exostoses.*

chon′dro·plas″ty. Plastic operation on cartilage.

chon"dro·ster'nal. Pertaining to the costal cartilages and the sternum.

chon'dro·tome. An instrument for cutting cartilage.

chon·drot'o·my (kon·drot'o·mee). *In surgery,* the division of a cartilage.

Chon'drus (kon'drus). Irish moss; a small genus of red algae of the Gigartinaceae.

chor'da (kor'duh). 1. A cord, tendon, or nerve filament. 2. The notochord; chorda dorsalis. —**chordal, chordate,** *adj.* **c. gubernaculum.** That part of the genital ligament which develops in the inguinal crest and adjacent body wall. It forms a part of the gubernaculum testis in the male, and a part of the round ligament of the uterus in the female. **c. tendinea.** Any one of the tendons of the papillary muscles of the ventricles of the heart, attached to the atrioventricular valves. **c. tympani.** A nerve which originates from the facial, traverses the tympanic cavity, and joins the lingual branch of the mandibular nerve. See Table of Nerves in the Appendix.

Chor·da'ta (kor·day'tuh, ·dah'tuh). A phylum of the animal kingdom whose members are characterized by having at some point in their development a notochord, a tubular central nervous system lying dorsal to the notochord, and lateral clefts in the walls of the pharynx.

chor'date. 1. Possessing a notochord; belonging or pertaining to the phylum, Chordata. 2. A member of the phylum, Chordata.

chor·dee' (kor·dee'). A painful curved erection of the penis with concavity downward; caused by gonorrheal inflammation of the corpus cavernosum urethrae (corpus spongiosum).

chor·di'tis. 1. Inflammation of a spermatic cord. 2. Inflammation of a vocal fold. Also called **c. vocalis. c. nodosa.** Singer's node, a small inflammatory nodule on a vocal fold, which occurs in singers and public speakers.

chor·dot'o·my. *In surgery,* the division of an anterolateral column of the spinal cord.

cho·re'a (ko·ree'uh). A nervous disorder, characterized by irregular and involuntary action of the muscles of the extremities and the face; seen in many conditions as part of a syndrome following an infection. It is also a disease entity, and as such is identical with *Sydenham's chorea, St. Vitus' dance, choromania, dancing chorea,* or *chorea minor.* —**choreal, choreic, choreat'ic,** *adj.* **c. gravidarum.** Intractable chorea occurring during pregnancy, toward its close sometimes aggravated and attended with fever. **c. insaniens.** Maniacal chorea; a severe form usually seen in pregnant

women. It is associated with mania and generally ends fatally. **chronic progressive hereditary c.** A disease characterized by jerky, irregular movements of the entire body, beginning in middle life and associated with progressive dementia. Heredity is the chief etiologic factor. Also called *hereditary c., Huntington's c., Huntington's disease.* **chronic progressive nonhereditary c.** A form of chorea in which the symptoms become progressively more severe; however, the disease shows no hereditary traits. It may or may not be accompanied by mental deterioration. **congenital c.** Chorea due to birth palsy. **essential c.** That occurring independently and not as a symptom of some other disease. **general c.** A form of chorea in which all or almost all of the voluntary muscles are subject to irregular contractions. **hereditary c.** See chronic progressive hereditary c. **Huntington's c.** See chronic progressive hereditary c. **posthemiplegic c.** A form of involuntary movement seen in patients after an attack of hemiplegia. Also called *postparalytic c., athetosis.*

cho·re'i·form. Resembling chorea.

cho"re·o·ath'e·toid (kor"ee·o·ath'i·toyd). Referring to both chorea and athetosis, as in the involuntary movements seen in both chorea and athetosis.

cho"re·o·ath"e·to'sis. A condition characterized by both choreiform and athetoid movements.

cho"ri·o·ad"e·no'ma (kor"ee·o·ad"i·no'muh). A tumor associated with a history of hydatidiform mole and characterized by invasion of the uterine wall and formation of metastases. Also called *chorioadenoma destruens.*

cho"ri·o·al'lan·to'ic. Pertaining to the chorion and allantois, or to the chorioallantois. See *placenta.*

cho"ri·o·al·lan'to·is (kor"ee·o·a·lan'to·iss, ·a·lan'toyss). The membrane formed by the union of chorion and allantois in birds and certain mammals and vascularized by the allantoic blood vessels. That of chicks is used for the culture of viruses in the preparation of vaccines.

cho"ri·o·cap"il·la'ris. Network of capillaries over the inner portion of the choroid coat of the eye.

cho"ri·o·ep"i·the"li·o'ma. See chorionic *carcinoma.*

cho"ri·o·gen'e·sis. The development of the chorion.

cho'ri·oid-. For words beginning with *chorioid-* see under *choroido-.*

cho"ri·o·men"in·gi'tis. A nonpurulent meningitis, characterized by involvement of arachnoid membrane and choroid plexus. **lymphocytic c.**

A rare form of acute viral meningitis, occurring in the absence of any evident focal or general cause of infection; characterized clinically by the rapid onset of symptoms of meningeal irritation, pleocytosis in the cerebrospinal fluid, and a short, benign course with recovery. Syn., *acute aseptic meningitis.* Also called *acute benign lymphocytic meningitis, acute lymphocytic c., benign lymphocytic c., epidemic serous meningitis.*

cho'ri·on (kor'ee·on). The outermost of the fetal membranes, consisting of an outer trophoblastic epithelium lined internally by extraembryonic mesoderm. Its villous portion, vascularized by allantoic blood vessels, forms the fetal part of the placenta. Also called *serosa.* —**chorial, chorion'ic,** *adj.* **c. laeve.** The smooth membranous part of the chorion devoid of villi. Also called *c. avillosum.*

cho'roid (kor'oyd). 1. Vascular tunic of the eye, continuous with the iris in front, and lying between the sclera and the retina; the choroid membrane. 2. Pertaining to the choroid. —**choroi'dal,** *adj.*

cho'roid·i'tis. Inflammation of the choroid coat of the eye. It may be *anterior,* the foci of exudation being at the periphery of the choroid; *central,* the exudate being in the region of the macula lutea; *diffuse* or *disseminated,* characterized by numerous round or irregular spots scattered over the fundus; *exudative* or *nonsuppurative,* when there are isolated foci of inflammation scattered over the choroid; *metastatic,* when due to embolism; or *suppurative,* when proceeding to suppuration. **c. gut·tata.** Familial degeneration of the macula combined with characteristically grouped hyaline bodies. Also called *Tay's c.*

cho·roi'do- (ko·roy'do-), **choroid-.** A combining form signifying *choroid.*

cho·roi'do·cy·cli'tis (ko·roy'do·sick·ligh'tis, ·sigh·kligh'tis). Inflammation of the choroid and ciliary body.

cho·roi''do·i·ri'tis (ko·roy''do·eye·rye'tis, ·i·rye'tis). Inflammation of the choroid and the iris. See *uveitis.*

cho·roi''do·ret'i·ni'tis. Choroiditis associated with retinitis, *q.v.*

chro·maf'fin (kro·maf'in, kro'muh·fin). Staining deeply with chromium salts.

chro·mal'um. Chrome alum, *q.v.*

-chro·ma'si·a. Combining form meaning *condition of pigmentation* or *of staining.*

chromat-. See *chromato-.*

chro'mate. Any salt of chromic acid.

chro''ma·te·lop'si·a, chro''ma·te·lop'sis. Color blindness. Syn., *chromatopseudopsis.*

chro·mat'ic. Relating to or possessing color.

chro'ma·tin. The protoplasmic substance in the nuclei of cells which is readily stainable, as contrasted with the achromatic constituents which include the nuclear membrane, linin network, and nuclear sap. *Basichromatin* stains with basic dyes; *oxychromatin* with acid dyes.

chro'ma·to-, chromat-. A combining form denoting *color, chromatin, pigment,* or *pigmentation.* Also see *chromo-.*

chro''ma·to·dys·o'pi·a. Color blindness.

chro''ma·tog'ra·phy. A technic for resolving a mixture into its components by spatial separation resulting from selective adsorption when a solution of the mixture is passed through a column of an adsorbing substance or along a strip of paper. —**chromatograph'ic,** *adj.*

chro''ma·tol'y·sis. Disintegration and disappearance of the Nissl granules from nerve cells. —**chromatolyt'ic,** *adj.*

chro''ma·top'a·thy, chro''ma·to·path'i·a. Any pigmentary skin disease.

chro''ma·to·phore'' (kro'muh·to·for'', kro·mat'o·for''). 1. *In botany,* a colored plastid. 2. *In zoology,* a cell containing pigment granules.

chro''ma·top·tom'e·try. Testing of the sensibility of the eye with respect to color perception.

chro''ma·to'sis. 1. Pigmentation. 2. A pathologic process or pigmentary disease consisting in a deposit of coloring matter in a locality where it is usually not present, or in excessive quantity in regions where pigment normally exists.

chrome. A name occasionally given to the element chromium or to one of its ores or compounds. **c. alum.** CrK(SO₄)₂.12H₂O. Chromium potassium sulfate. **c. alum, ammonium.** CrNH₄(SO₄)₂.12H₂O. Chromium ammonium sulfate.

chrom''es·the'si·a, chrom''aes·the'si·a (krohm''ess·thee'zhuh, ·zee·uh). The association of colors with words, letters, and sounds.

chro'mi·um. Cr = 52.01. A hard, bright, silvery metal; largely used as a protective plating for other metals and in the manufacture of alloys. It forms *chromous* and *chromic* salts, wherein its valence is two and three respectively. **c. trioxide.** CrO₃. Dark, purplish red crystals, deliquescent, soluble in water. It is astringent and caustic. Syn., *chromic acid.* Also called *chromic anhydride.*

chro'mo-, chrom-. A combining

form denoting *color, pigment, pigmentation,* or *chromium.*

hro'mo·gen. Any substance which, under suitable conditions, is capable of producing color. See *chromophore.*

hro'mo·mere. One of the beadlike chromatin granules, arranged in a linear series in a chromosome.

hro'mo·phil. 1. Any easily stained cell. 2. Readily stainable. **—chro·moph'i·lous,** *adj.*

hro''mo·pho'bi·a. 1. Abnormal fear of colors. 2. Excessive dislike of certain colors. 3. *In histology,* staining little or not at all, said of intracellular granules or of certain cells, as the chromophobic cells of the hypophysis. **—chro'mophobe, chromopho'bic,** *adj.*

hro'mo·phore. The chemical group which is responsible for the color of a compound.

hro'mo·phose (kro'mo·foze). A subjective sensation of color.

hro''mo·pro'te·in. A conjugated protein containing a prosthetic group which imparts a color to the compound, as hemoglobins, flavoproteins, and cytochromes.

hro'mo·some (kro'mo·sohm). Any one of the separate, deeply staining bodies, commonly rod-, J-, or V-shaped, which arise from the nuclear network during mitosis. They carry the genes, and there is generally a constant number for each species. **—chromoso'mal,** *adj.* **bivalent c.** A pair of chromosomes, one maternal and the other paternal, temporarily united in the process of synapsis. **X c.** A sex-determining factor in both ovum and sperm. Spermatozoa containing the X chromosome give rise to female offspring. **Y c.** A sex-determining factor in the sperm giving rise to male offspring.

hro'nax·ie, chro'nax·y. The duration of time that a current of twice the rheobasic (galvanic threshold) intensity must flow in order to excite the tissue being tested. Chronaxie is related to irritability and is used in testing for irritability changes in nerve and muscle.

hron'ic. Long-continued; of long duration; opposed to *acute.* **—chron·ic'ity,** *n.*

hron'o-, chron-. A combining form denoting *time.*

hron'o·graph. Instrument for recording small intervals of time in physiologic and psychophysical experiments.

hro·nom'e·try. The measuring of time.

hrys'a·lis. A stage in which the pupas of certain insects are enclosed in a cocoon.

hrys''a·ro'bin. A mixture of principles obtained from Goa powder, a substance deposited in the wood of *Andira Araroba,* a Brazilian tree. It is a brown to orange-yellow powder, useful in psoriasis.

chrys'o-, chrys-. A combining form signifying *gold, golden yellow,* or *yellow.*

chrys·oi'din Y. 2,4-Diaminoazobenzene hydrochloride. A brown dye used in some procedures as a substitute for Bismarck brown.

chrys''o·phan'ic ac'id. $C_{15}H_{10}O_4$. 1,8-Dihydroxy-3-methylanthraquinone, a constituent of rhubarb, aloes, cascara, and other species of *Rhamnus.* It is more properly called *chrysophanol.*

chrys''o·phan'ol. 1,8-Dihydroxy-3-methylanthraquinone; a constituent of rhubarb, aloes, cascara, and other species of *Rhamnus,* and of chrysarobin. Syn., *chrysophanic acid.*

chrys''o·ther'a·py. Treatment by the use of a gold compound.

chthon''o·pha'gi·a (thon''o·fay'juh, ·jee·uh), **chtho·noph'a·gy** (tho·nof'uh·jee). Dirt eating; geophagy.

chur'rus. See *cannabis.*

chyle (kyle). A milk-white emulsion of fat globules in lymph formed in the small intestine during digestion. **—chy'lous,** *adj.*

chy·le'mi·a. Presence of chyle in the blood.

chy'lo- (kigh'lo-), **chyl-.** A combining form denoting *connection with,* or *relation to, chyle.*

chy'lo·cele. Accumulation of fatty lymph in the tunica vaginalis of the testis; seen especially as a result of rupture of lymphatics in elephantiasis.

chy''lor·rhe'a. 1. An excessive flow of chyle. 2. A diarrhea characterized by a milky color of the feces.

chy''lo·tho'rax. An accumulation of chyle or a milky fluid in the pleural cavity, the turbid appearance being due to fat droplets.

chy·lu'ri·a (kigh·lew'ree·uh). The presence of chyle or lymph in the urine, usually due to a fistulous communication between the urinary and lymphatic tracts or to lymphatic obstruction.

chyme (kime). Viscid, fluid contents of the stomach consisting of food which has undergone gastric digestion, and has not yet passed into the duodenum. **—chy'mous,** *adj.*

chy'mo·sin (kigh'mo·sin). Rennin; the rennet enzyme.

chy''mo·sin'o·gen. The precursor of chymosin or rennin.

chy''mo·tryp'sin (kigh''mo·trip'sin). A proteolytic enzyme found in the intestine and formed from the chymotrypsinogen of the pancreatic juice by the action of trypsin.

chy''mo·tryp·sin'o·gen. An enzyme occurring in the pancreas and giving rise to chymotrypsin.

C. I. Color index.

cic'a·trix, ci·ca'trix. A scar. The connective tissue which replaces a localized loss of substance. It is usually white and glistening when old, red or purple when newly developed. —**cica·tri'cial** (sick″uh·trish′ul), *adj.*; **cicatriza'tion,** *n.*; **cic'atrize,** *v.*

-cid'al. A suffix signifying *killing* or *having power to kill.*

-cide. A suffix signifying *a killing; destroyer* or *killer.*

cignolin. A proprietary name for anthralin.

cili-. See *cilio-.*

cil″i·ar·ot'o·my (sil″ee·ur·ot′o·mee, sigh″lee·). Surgical section of the ciliary zone for glaucoma.

cil'i·o-, cili-. 1. *In zoology,* a combining form denoting *having* or *like cilia.* 2. *In anatomy,* a combining form signifying *ciliary.* 3. *In surgery,* a combining form denoting *the ciliary margin* or *nerves.*

cil'i·um (pl. **cilia**). 1. One of the eyelashes. 2. One of the threadlike cytoplasmic processes of cells which beat rhythmically, thereby causing the locomotion of certain aquatic organisms or propelling fluids over surfaces covered by ciliated cells. —**ciliary, ciliated,** *adj.*

cil·lo'sis. A spasmodic trembling of the eyelid. —**cillot'ic,** *adj.*

Ci'mex. A genus of insects of the family Cimicidae; bedbug. It can be infected (a) with *Pasteurella tularensis* and can transmit the infection to mice, (b) with other bacteria, and (c) with *Trypanosoma cruzi.* **C. hemipterus.** An important bloodsucking species parasitic to man; the Oriental bedbug. **C. lectularius.** The common bedbug; parasitic to man.

cin·cham'i·dine (sin·kam′i·deen, ·din). An alkaloid found in various cinchona species. Also called *hydrocinchonidine, dihydrocinchonidine.*

cin·cho'na (sin·ko′nuh). The dried bark of the stem or the root of *Cinchona succirubra* or its hybrids, known as red cinchona, or of *Cinchona ledgeriana, Cinchona calisaya,* or hybrids of these with other species of *Cinchona,* known as calisaya bark or as yellow cinchona. Cinchona contains quinine, quinidine, cinchonine, cinchonidine, and other alkaloids. Cinchona has the action and uses of quinine. Also called *Peruvian bark, Jesuit's bark.* —**cinchon'ic,** *adj.*; **cinchoniza'tion,** *n.*; **cin'chonize,** *v.*

cin″chon·am'ine (sin″kon·am′een, sin·kon′uh·meen). An alkaloid of cuprea bark.

cin·chon'i·dine (sin·kon′i·deen, ·din). An alkaloid derived from cinchona.

cin'cho·nine (sin′ko·neen, ·nin). An alkaloid derived from cinchona.

cin'cho·nism (sin′ko·niz·um). The systemic effect of cinchona or its alkaloids when given in full doses. The symptoms produced are a ringing in the ears, deafness, headache, giddiness, dimness of sight, and a weakening of the heart's action.

cin'cho·phen (sin′ko·fen). Phenylcinchoninic acid; a white powder, almost insoluble in cold water. It increases the elimination of uric acid and is used in treating rheumatism.

cin″cho·tan'nic ac'id (sin″ko·tan′ick). The characteristic tannic acid of cinchona bark. Syn., *cinchotannin, quinotannic acid.*

cin″cho·tan'nin. The characteristic tannin of cinchona; it exists as a glycoside. Syn., *cinchotannic acid, quinotannic acid.*

cine-. For words beginning with *cine-* not found here, see under *kine-.*

ci·ne're·a. Gray matter of the brain or spinal cord.

cin'gu·lum. 1. A girdle or zone; the waist. 2. Herpes zoster or shingles. 3. A bundle of association fibers running in the cingulate gyrus of the brain from the anterior perforated substance to the hippocampal gyrus. 4. The lingual lobe of incisor teeth, notably of the superior laterals, and of cuspids; a bandlike ridge rising crownwise from the cervix and often accentuated to a blunt point or a rudimentary cusp.

cin″na·mal'de·hyde. Cinnamic aldehyde, the chief constituent of cinnamon oil.

cin·nam'ic ac'id (si·nam′ick, sin′uh·mick), **cin″na·myl'ic ac'id.** $C_6H_5CH:CHCOOH$. An acid occurring in Peruvian and tolu balsams, in storax, and in some benzoin resins.

cin·nam'ic al'de·hyde. $C_6H_5CH:CH.CHO$. The chief constituent of cinnamon oil. Syn., *cinnamaldehyde.*

cin'na·mon. The dried bark of several species of *Cinnamomum,* native to Ceylon and China, the latter variety being known in commerce under the name of *cassia.* It is used as a carminative. —**cinnam'ic,** *adj.*

cin'na·mon oil. A volatile oil distilled from leaves and twigs of species of cinnamon trees, used as a carminative, fungicide, and flavor. Syn., *cassia oil.*

cin″na·myl'ic ac'id. See *cinnamic acid.*

cir'ci·nate (sur′si·nayt). Having a circular outline or a ring formation.

cir'cle. 1. A ring; a line, every point on which is equidistant from a point called the center. 2. A ringlike anastomosis of arteries or veins. **c. of diffusion.** The imperfect image formed by incomplete focalization, the position of the true focus not having been reached by some of the rays of light, or else having been passed. **c. of Willis.** The arterial anastomosis at the base of the brain, formed in front by the anterior communicating artery joining together the anterior cerebral arteries; laterally, by the internal carotids and the posterior communicating arteries joining them with the posterior cerebral arteries; behind, by the posterior cerebral arteries branching from the basilar.

cir'cuit. 1. The course of an electric current. 2. The path of a circulating fluid in a system of tubes. 3. The path of nerve impulses in reflex arcs. **Geiger-Müller counting c.** An amplifier and accessories which make visible or audible, or in other ways record, the pulses from a Geiger-Müller tube.

cir'cu·lar. 1. Ring-shaped. 2. Pertaining to a circle. 3. Marked by alternations of despondency and excitation, as circular insanity.

cir'cu·la'tion. Passage in a circle, as the circulation of the blood. —**cir'culatory,** *adj.* **collateral c.** That established for an organ or a part through anastomotic communicating channels, when the original direct blood supply is obstructed or abolished. **coronary c.** The circulation of the blood through the muscular walls of the heart. **fetal c.** That of the fetus, including the circulation through the placenta and the umbilical cord. **intervillous c.** The circulation of maternal blood in the intervillous spaces of the placenta. **placental c.** (a) The umbilical circulation. (b) The intervillous circulation. **portal c.** The passage of the blood from the gastrointestinal tract and spleen through the liver. **pulmonary c.** The circulation of blood through the lungs by means of the pulmonary artery and veins, for the purpose of oxygenation and purification. Also called *lesser c.* **systemic c.** The general circulation, as distinct from the pulmonary circulation. Also called *greater c.*

cir'cu·la'tion time. The rate of blood flow; the time required for blood to flow from arm to lung or arm to tongue, etc.

cir'cu·la·to'ry fail'ure. Failure of the circulatory system to deliver sufficient blood to the tissues for their metabolic needs; due either to cardiac failure, *q.v.*, or to peripheral circulatory failure. **peripheral c. f.** A syndrome due to insufficient venous return to the heart to permit normal output, because of some disturbance in the vasomotor mechanism. The fundamental cause of the condition is not clear. The symptoms of pallor, cyanosis,

cold and clammy skin, lowered blood pressure and temperature, restlessness, and syncope give a typical clinical picture and are seen following surgical or accidental trauma, hemorrhage, burns, and, in a less degree, emotional factors. Also see under *shock.*

cir'cu·lin. An antibiotic substance produced by *Bacillus circulans.*

cir'cum-. A prefix meaning *around, about, on all sides.*

cir"cum·a'nal. Periproctal; surrounding the anus.

cir"cum·ar·tic'u·lar. Around a joint.

cir"cum·ci'sion (sur″kum·sizh′un). The removal of the foreskin; excision of a portion of the prepuce.

cir"cum·cor'ne·al. Around or about the cornea.

cir"cum·duc'tion. The movement of a limb in such a manner that its distal part describes a circle, the proximal end being fixed.

cir"cum·flex. Winding around; designating a number of arteries, veins, and nerves which have a winding course.

cir"cum·stan'ti·al'i·ty. *In psychiatry,* indulging in many irrelevant and unnecessary details when answering a simple question; usually observed in mania.

cir'cus move'ment. An excitation wave that re-enters excitable tissues and continues to circulate; believed to be the mechanism responsible for the continuance of atrial and ventricular contraction.

cir·rho'sis (si·ro′sis). 1. A chronic, progressive disease of the liver, essentially inflammatory; characterized by proliferation of connective tissue, degeneration and death of parenchymal cells, regeneration of parenchymal cells, and distortion of architectural pattern. Liver may be enlarged or much reduced in size. 2. Incorrectly used to mean interstitial inflammation of other organs, as pulmonary cirrhosis, interstitial pneumonia. —**cirrhot'ic,** *adj.* **cardiac c.** Progressive fibrosis of central lobular structures as well as of portal spaces, the result of prolonged passive hyperemia often of cardiac origin. Also called *congestive c.* **hypertrophic c.** Enlargement with intralobular fibrosis, accompanied by icterus, but without ascites. Also called *Charcot's c., Hanot's c.* **juvenile c.** Usually of Laennec's type, due to congenital syphilis, congenital atresia or malformation of bile ducts (obstructive biliary); perhaps due to erythroblastosis foetalis or to unknown cause. **Laennec's c.** A type formerly thought to be due to excessive use of alcohol; now known to be due to the associated nutritional disturbances. The liver is slightly nodular, with fibrosis especially in the portal canals; characterized by degeneration and regeneration of the hepatic parenchymal cells, often accompanied by ascites, esophageal varices, and ultimately icterus. Syn., *alcoholic c., atrophic c., diffuse nodular c.* **syphilitic c.** (a) Syphilitic nodular cirrhosis (hepar lobatum) in which gummas or their scars lead to irregularly disposed retractions of outer surface. (b) Packet liver, in which the cross section shows interlaced thin bands of connective tissue with relatively normal lobular structures within the network. **toxic c.** Extensive cicatrization of the liver following various forms of acute, diffuse necrosis of the organ. Also called *postnecrotic c.*

cir′soid (sur′soyd). Resembling a varix or dilated vein.

cis-. A prefix denoting *on this side, on the same side, since, following.*

cis′tern. 1. A reservoir. 2. A large, subarachnoid space of the brain. **basal c.** The subarachnoid space at the base of the brain, divided by the optic chiasma into the cistern of the chiasma and the interpeduncular cistern. **cerebellomedullary c.** The cisterna magna, *q.v.* **c. of the great cerebral vein.** That containing the great cerebral vein, formed by the arachnoid stretching over the transverse cerebral fissure from the splenium of the corpus callosum to the superior surface of the cerebellum. Formerly called *superior c. c. of the lateral cerebral fossa.* The subarachnoid space of the lateral fossa of the cerebrum, formed by the arachnoid stretching over the lateral cerebral fissure. **pontine c.** That ventral to the pons.

cis·ter′na. 1. Cistern, *q.v.* 2. The cisterna chyli, the saclike beginning of the thoracic duct opposite the twelfth thoracic vertebra. **c. magna.** A large cistern formed by the arachnoid stretching across from the inferior surface of the cerebellum to the dorsal surface of the medulla oblongata. Syn., *cerebellomedullary cistern.*

cit′ral. An aldehyde found in the oils of lemon, lemon grass, orange, and others. Syn., *geranial.*

cit′rate. Any salt of citric acid.

cit′ric ac′id. $H_2C_6H_5O_7 \cdot H_2O$. A tribasic acid occurring in the juice of many fruits and in various animal tissues. Translucent crystals or a white, crystalline powder soluble in water.

cit′rin. A crystalline substance, said to be a mixture of hesperidin, quercitrin, and eriodictyol glycoside, isolated from lemon juice. It combats the increased permeability of capillary walls. Syn., *vitamin P.*

cit′rine oint′ment (sit′reen, ·rin). Ointment of mercuric nitrate.

cit′ron. The tree, *Citrus medica,* or its fruit. The fruit rind is used in conserves.

cit″ron·el′lal. $C_{10}H_{18}O$. An aldehyde occurring in many essential oils, including citronella oil.

cit″ron·el′la oil. A volatile oil obtained from the citronella grass, containing geraniol and citronellal, used as an insect repellant.

ci·trul′lin. A resinoid from *Citrullus colocynthis.* It is a cathartic used in veterinary practice.

Cit′rus. A genus of trees of the Rutaceae. From this genus come the orange, lemon, citron, and lime.

cit·to′sis. Pica; a longing for strange or improper food.

Cl. 1. Chemical symbol for chlorine. 2. Abbreviation for *Clostridium.*

cl. Centiliter.

clamp. An instrument for holding and compressing vessels or hollow organs to prevent hemorrhage or the escape of contents during the progress of an operation, as a **pedicle clamp** for grasping and holding a pedicle during removal of an organ or a tumor, or a **stomach clamp** for securing an entire segment of the stomach. Also see *clip, forceps.*

clang as·so″ci·a′tion. A symptom observed in the manic phase of manic-depressive psychosis in which resonant sounds bring to mind certain words or ideas.

cla·rif′i·cant. An agent used to make a turbid liquid clear.

clar″i·fi·ca′tion. The operation of removing the turbidity of a liquid or a naturally transparent substance. It may be accomplished by allowing the suspended matter to subside; by the addition of a clarificant or substance that precipitates suspended matters; or by moderate heating. —**clar′ify·ing,** *adj.;* **clar′ify,** *v.*

clas·mat′o·cyte (klaz·mat′o·sight, klass·mat′·). Old term for macrophage, *q.v.,* of the connective tissue.

clas′tic. Breaking up into fragments; causing division.

clau″di·ca′tion. Lameness. **intermittent c.** Cramplike pains and weakness in the legs, particularly the calves; induced by walking and relieved by rest; associated with excessive smoking, vascular spasm, and arteriosclerosis. Syn., *angina cruris, dysbasia intermittens angiosclerotica.* **venous c.** Lameness due to venous stasis. Also called *angiosclerotic paroxysmal myasthenia.*

claus″tro·pho′bi·a. Morbid fear of being in a room or a confined space.

cla′va. An enlargement of the funiculus gracilis; the nucleus gracilis —**claval,** *adj.*

clav′a·cin. An antibiotic substance produced in cultures of several differ ent fungi; it is identical with *clavatin*, *claviformin*, and *patulin*.

clav′a·tin. Clavacin.

Clav′i·ceps. A genus of fungi. **C. purpurea.** The fungus producing the ergot of rye.

clav′i·cle (klav′ĭ·kul). A bone of the shoulder girdle articulating medially with the sternum and laterally with the acromion of the scapula; the collarbone. See Table of Bones in the Appendix. —**clavic′ular,** *adj.*

cla·vic″u·lec′to·my. Surgical removal of the clavicle. The operation is indicated in cases of thyroid cancer, osteomyelitis of the clavicle, and limitation of arm motion where the shoulder joint has become fused.

clav′i·for′min. Clavacin.

cla′vus. 1. A cone-shaped, circumscribed hyperplasia of the horny layer of the epidermis, in which there is an ingrowth as well as an outgrowth of horny substance forming epidermal thickenings, chiefly about the toes; caused by friction or pressure. 2. *In psychiatry,* a severe pain in the head described as the sensation of a nail being driven into the head. **hard c.** A dense and callous hypertrophy at points of pressure on the toes. **soft c.** That type which develops on opposing surfaces of the toes. It is soft as a result of heat and moisture.

claw′foot″. A foot having an abnormally high longitudinal arch, a depression of the metatarsal arch, and dorsal contractures of the toes. It exists in two forms: that in which the outstanding deformity is an exaggeration of the longitudinal arch, and that in which the exaggeration of the longitudinal arch is associated with contraction of the plantar fascia and limitation of dorsiflexion at the ankle. Also called *hollow foot, contracted foot, pes cavus, nondeforming clubfoot.*

claw′hand″. An acquired deformity of the hand. In the extreme type, due to a paralysis of the ulnar and median nerves, it is characterized by extension of the thumb, hyperextension and abduction of the proximal phalanges of the fingers, and flexion of the other phalanges. Lesser degrees of the deformity result from paralysis of the ulnar or median nerve separately.

clear′ance. 1. The complete removal of a substance from the blood by the kidneys. 2. A test of renal function. See under *test.*

clear′ing sta′tion. A divisional medical unit operating in war, set up with or without shelter, for emergency treatment, including medical record. It is charged with rapid disposal of army casualties either by return to duty or by evacuation.

cleav′age. 1. The linear clefts in the skin indicating the general direction of the fibers. They govern to a certain extent the arrangement of the lesions in skin diseases. The **lines of cleavage** run, for the most part, obliquely to the axis of the trunk, sloping from the spine downward and forward; in the limbs, they are mostly transverse to the longitudinal axis. 2. Cell division, especially of the zygote and blastomeres. Syn., *segmentation.* 3. An early stage of the process of development between fertilization and the blastula, when the embryo consists of a mass of dividing cells, the blastomeres.

cleft. 1. A fissure. 2. Divided. **branchial c.** (a) One of the slitlike openings between the gills, as in fish. (b) See visceral *c.* **c. cheek.** Transverse facial cleft. Syn., *macrostomia.* **c. foot.** Division of the foot due to absence of one or more digits and the corresponding metatarsal(s). **c. hand.** Division of the hand due to absence of one or more digits and the corresponding metacarpal(s). **c. lip.** See *harelip.* **c. palate.** A congenital defect, due to failure of fusion of embryonic facial processes resulting in a fissure through the palate. This may be *complete,* extending through both hard and soft palates into the nose, or any degree of *incomplete,* or *partial,* cleft. Often associated with harelip, *q.v.* **facial c.** An embryonic fissure between facial processes; the facial anomaly produced by failure of these processes to fuse. A **median facial cleft** (median harelip, median fissure) is one between the mandibular or the median nasal processes which may involve both mandible and maxilla or only one; an **oblique facial cleft,** one between the maxillary and frontonasal processes; a **transverse facial cleft,** a fissure at the angle of the mouth causing macrostomia. **visceral c.** An embryonic fissure between the visceral arches, produced by rupture of the closing plate between a visceral pouch and its corresponding external visceral groove.

clei′do- (kly′do-), **cleid-.** A combining form denoting *the clavicle,* or *pertaining to the clavicle.*

clei″do·mas′toid. Pertaining to the clavicle and to the mastoid process.

clei″do·ster′nal. Pertaining to the clavicle and the sternum.

clei·dot′o·my. *In obstetrics,* section of the clavicles when the shoulders of the fetus are too broad to pass; an operation performed when the head is delivered, and the child dead.

clei″thro·pho′bi·a (kly″thro·fo′bee-uh). Morbid fear of being locked in.

cli″ma·co·pho′bi·a. A morbid fear of staircases.

cli·mac'ter·ic (klye·mack'tur·ick, kly"mack·terr'ick). A period of life at which the system was believed to undergo marked changes. These periods were thought to occur every seven years. The word is now generally applied to the menopause. **male c.** The male menopause; due to impaired testicular function.

cli'mate. The sum of those conditions in any region or country that relate to the air, the temperature, moisture, sunshine, and winds, especially in so far as they concern the health or comfort of mankind. —**climat'ic,** adj.

cli'ma·to-. A combining form denoting climate.

cli"ma·tol'o·gy. In medicine, the study of climate in relation to health and disease.

cli'max. 1. The height of a disease; period of greatest intensity. **2.** The sexual orgasm.

clin-. See clino-.

clin'ic. 1. Medical instruction given at the bedside, or in the presence of the patient whose symptoms are studied and whose treatment is considered. **2.** A place where such instruction is given. **3.** A gathering of instructors, students, and patients for the study and treatment of disease. **4.** A place where medical care is given to ambulant patients who live at home.

clin'i·cal. 1. Relating to bedside treatment or to a clinic. **2.** Pertaining to the symptoms and course of a disease as observed by the physician, in opposition to the anatomic changes found by the pathologist.

cli·ni'cian. 1. A physician whose opinions, teachings, and treatment are based upon experience at the bedside. **2.** A clinical instructor. **3.** One who practices medicine.

clin'i·co-. In medicine, a combining form denoting clinical.

clin"i·co·pa·thol'o·gy. The study of disease in the living patient; applied particularly to the study of the blood, urine, feces, and other secretions and excretions and to parts of the body, such as tumors, removed for examination.

cli'no-, clin-. A combining form denoting inclination or declination.

cli'noid. Resembling a bed; applied to sundry bony structures of the body, as the clinoid processes.

clip. In surgery, a device or appliance that grips skin or other tissue to secure apposition or to control hemorrhage. Also see clamp, forceps. **dura c.** A thin wire suture applied by a special forceps to check hemorrhage in brain operations. Also called brain c. **skin c.** A band of malleable metal with pointed ends; held in a magazine and applied by a special forceps to the

apposed edges of a skin wound; a more rapid method of closure than the use of sutures. Also called Michel c., wound c.

clit"o·ri·dec'to·my. Excision of the clitoris.

clit'o·ris (klit'o·ris, kly'to·ris). In the female the homolog of the penis, attached to the ischiopubic rami by two crura, which meet in front of the pubic symphysis to form the body, or corpus. It possesses erectility. —**clitorid'ean,** adj.

clit'o·rism (klit'o·riz·um, kly'to·). **1.** Enlargement or hypertrophy of the clitoris. **2.** A condition of painful and persistent erection of the clitoris; analogous to priapism in the male.

clit"o·ri'tis (klit"o·rye'tis, kly"to·). Inflammation of the clitoris.

cli'vus. 1. A slope. **2.** The slanting surface of the body of the sphenoid bone between the sella turcica and basilar part of the occipital bone.

clo. In aviation medicine, an arbitrary unit of thermal insulation, used in expressing the thermal insulation value of clothing. A suit of clothing has a thermal insulation value of one clo when it will maintain in comfort a resting-sitting human adult male whose metabolic rate is approximately 50 kilogram calories per square meter of body surface per hour, when the environmental temperature is 70° F. In terms of absolute thermal insulation units, one clo is 0.18° C. per square meter kilogram calorie per hour.

clo·a'ca. 1. In the early embryo, the endodermal chamber common to hindgut and allantois; later, to hindgut and urogenital duct or sinus. **2.** In certain vertebrates, an endodermal chamber common to hindgut, bladder, and urogenital ducts. —**cloacal,** adj. **urogenital c.** An abnormal common opening of the urethra and vagina due to a defective urethrovaginal septum. **vesicorectovaginal c.** A common aperture of the bladder, rectum, and vagina; due to deformity or trauma.

clo"nor·chi'a·sis (klo"nor·kigh'uh·sis, klon"or·kee·ay'sis), **clo"nor·chi·o'sis** (klo"nor·kee·o'sis, klon"or·). Condition due to the presence of Clonorchis sinensis in the bile ducts, causing marked dilatation and proliferation of the biliary epithelium and atrophy of the liver cells; characterized by edema, diarrhea, and hepatomegaly in moderate cases, and cirrhosis, anasarca, and cachexia in severe cases.

Clo·nor'chis (klo·nor'kis, klon·or'kis). A genus of flukes indigenous in the Orient. **C. sinensis.** The most common of the liver flukes, having as definitive hosts man or other mammalia.

clo'nus (klo'nus, klon'us). A series of

movements characterized by alternate contractions and relaxations; a clonic spasm. Involuntary, reflex, irregular contractions of muscles when put suddenly upon the stretch. According to the part affected, the phenomenon is spoken of as ankle clonus, wrist clonus, etc. —**clon'ic**, *adj.*; **clonic'ity**, *n.*

toe o. Contraction of the great toe on sudden extension of the first phalanx.

clopane hydrochloride. Trademark for cyclopentamine hydrochloride.

orarsen. Trade-mark for dichlorophenarsine hydrochloride.

Clos·trid'i·um (klos·trid'ee·um, klo·trid'·). A genus of anaerobic sporebearing bacteria of ovoid, spindle, or club shape; widely distributed in nature. —**clostridial**, *adj.* **Cl. botulinum.** A species which produces a very powerful toxin in canned food. The disease is a toxemia; the organism is not invasive but produces its toxin outside the body. **Cl. novyi.** This species is important in gas gangrene; also produces a strong soluble toxin. **Cl. perfringens Type A.** The gas gangrene bacillus. **Cl. septicum.** A species found in gas gangrene but not so frequently as some of the other anaerobic bacilli. It is also responsible for some cases of blackleg in cattle. **Cl. tetani.** The species which causes tetanus. It is characterized by spherical terminal spores and the production of tetanus toxin, a potent exotoxin. **Cl. welchii.** A species of plump, nonmotile, Gram-positive rods of varying length, occurring in chains and singly. This organism produces a variety of toxins and is the most important cause of gas gangrene. It has also been found to be the cause of dysentery of sheep.

closure. 1. The act of completing or closing an electric circuit. 2. The closing of a wound by suture. Abbreviated, C.

clot. 1. A semisolid coagulum of blood or lymph. 2. Coagulate. **chicken-fat c.** That formed after death, consisting of a light yellow, serumal, nonfibrinous clot in its upper portion, and an accumulation of red cells in its dependent portion. **c. retraction time.** The time required after clotting for the clot to retract to a firm mass at 38° C.

clotting time. The time required for a small amount of blood, obtained by skin puncture and removed to a glass slide or capillary tube, to clot. Also see *bleeding time*, prothrombin time.

clove. The dried flower bud of the tree *Eugenia caryophyllata*.

clove oil. A volatile oil, distilled from the dried flower buds of the clove tree, containing eugenol; used as a

local anesthetic, especially for toothache, and as a carminative.

club'foot". A congenital malformation, either single or bilateral, in which the forefoot is inverted and rotated, accompanied by shortening of the Achilles tendon and contracture of the plantar fascia. Also see *talipes*.

club'hand". A rare congenital malformation usually characterized by complete or partial absence of one of the bones of the forearm, the hand being in an abnormal position; talipomanus.

clump'ing. Agglutination. —**clump**, *v.*

clu'ne·al. Pertaining to the buttock.

clu·pan"o·don'ic ac'id. An unsaturated fatty acid occurring in certain fish oils.

clu·pe·ine (kloo'pee·een, ·in). $C_{30}H_{57}N_{17}O_8 + 4H_2O$. A protamine from the herring. Syn., *salmine*.

cly'sis. Administration of an enema; cleansing by means of an enema.

Cm. Symbol for curium.

cm. Centimeter.

C.N.S. Central nervous system.

Co. Symbol for cobalt.

Co60 (see"oh·six'tee). Symbol for cobalt-60.

co"a·cer'vate (ko"a·sur'vayt, ko·ass'ur·vayt). The product formed when two hydrophilic colloids of opposite charge are mixed and form a stable particle which may form a separate phase. —**coacerva'tion**, *n.*

co·ag'u·lant. 1. Causing the formation of a clot or coagulum. 2. A coagulating agent. —**coagulable**, *adj.*

co·ag'u·lase (ko·ag'yoo·lace, ·laze). A clotting enzyme.

co·ag'u·late. 1. Curdle; clot. 2. Cause to change from a fluid state to a compact, jellylike mass; solidify.

co·ag"u·la'tion. 1. The formation of a coagulum or clot, as in blood or in milk. 2. A clot. —**coag'ulated, co·ag'ulative**, *adj.*

co·ag'u·lum (pl. *coagula*). A clot; a curd; a coagulated mass.

co"a·les'cence. The union of two or more parts or things previously separate. —**coalescent**, *adj.*

coal tar. A by-product in the destructive distillation of coal; a black, viscid fluid. It is employed locally in the treatment of certain skin diseases.

co"ap·ta'tion. The proper union or adjustment of the ends of a fractured bone or the lips of a wound.

co"arc·ta'tion. A compression of the walls of a vessel or canal, narrowing or closing the lumen; reduction of the normal or previous volume, as of the aorta; shriveling and consequent detachment, as of the retina. A stricture.

coat. A cover or membrane covering a part or substance.

coat'ing. A covering or layer of a substance, as of a wound or the tongue. **c. of pills.** A covering of various substances to conceal the taste in swallowing. **c. of tongue.** A condition of the tongue indicative of abnormality of the digestive tract. **enteric c.** A coating for pills or tablets or capsules, intended as a protection against solutions found in the stomach, but dissolving in the intestines.

co·bal'a·min. 1. The generic name for the vitamin-B_{12} group, specific members of which are identified by prefixes, as cyanocobalamin. 2. That portion of the molecule of crystalline vitamin B_{12} occurring in all vitamin-B_{12} analogs.

co'balt (ko'bawlt). Co = 58.94. A hard, gray, ductile metal used in alloys.

co'balt-60 (ko'bawlt-six'tee). A radioactive isotope of cobalt, which emits beta and gamma rays, used in the treatment of cancer. Symbol, Co^{60}.

co''bra·ly'sin (ko''bruh·lye'sin, ko-bral'i·sin).** The hemolytic toxin of cobra venom.

co'ca. The leaves of *Erythroxylon coca*, *E. truxillense*, or *E. novogranatense*, containing cocaine and other alkaloids.

co·caine' (ko·kayn', ko'kayn). $C_{17}H_{21}NO_4$; methylbenzoylecgonine; an alkaloid obtained from the leaves of *Erythroxylon Coca* and other species of *Erythroxylon*. **—cocainist,** *n.*; **cocainize,** *v.* **c. bug.** Itching, crawling, and sticking skin sensations experienced in cocaine poisoning. **c. hydrochloride.** The hydrochloride of the alkaloid cocaine; occurs as colorless crystals, or as a white, crystalline powder; soluble in water. A paralyzant to the peripheral ends of the sensory nerves.

co·cain'ism (ko·kayn'iz·um, ko'kayn-iz·um). The cocaine habit.

co''car·box'yl·ase. Thiamine pyrophosphate; the coenzyme of carboxylase, an enzyme catalyzing the decarboxylation of pyruvic acid in animal tissues and in yeast.

co''car·cin'o·gen. A noncarcinogenic agent which augments the carcinogenic process.

cocc-. See cocco-.

Coc·cid'i·a (cock·sid'ee·uh). An order or group of cell parasites of the class Sporozoa, found in vertebrates and invertebrates, usually common in lower animals but rare in man.

Coc·cid'i·oi'des (cock·sid''ee·oy'deez, ·oi'·deez). A genus of parasitic fungi. **C. immitis.** The causative agent of coccidioidomycosis, an infectious, systemic, suppurative, and granulomatous disease. The organism is spheroid, nonbudding, and endosporu lating in the tissues; it produce branching, septate, aerial hyphae i culture.

coc·cid''i·oi''do·my·co'sis (cock sid''ee·oy''do·migh·ko'sis). A diseas caused by inhalation of spores of Coc cidioides immitis, causing pulmonar symptoms and later cutaneous nodule Syn., San Joaquin Valley fever.

coc'co-, cocc-. A combining for meaning *a grain, seed, or berry*.

coc'cu·lus. The dried fruit of *Ana mirta cocculus*; fishberry; a convulsan poison which has been used external against pediculi. See picrotoxin.

coc'cus (pl. *cocci*). 1. A bacteriu whose greatest diameter is not mor than twice its shortest. 2. Latin nam for cochineal. **—coccal, coccoid** *adj.*

coc''cy·gec'to·my (cock''si·jeck'to mee). Surgical excision of the coccy

coc·cyg'e·us (cock·sidj'ee·us). On of the pelvic muscles. See Table Muscles in the Appendix. **—coccys eal,** *adj.*

coc'cyx (cock'sicks). The last bone the spinal column, formed by the unic of 4 rudimentary vertebrae. See Tab of Bones in the Appendix. **—coccys eal,** *adj.*

coch''i·neal' (kotch''i·neel', kotch i·neel). The dried female insects, *Co cus cacti*, from which the coloring ma ter carmine may be prepared.

coch'le·a (cock'lee·uh). A cavity the internal ear resembling a sna shell; it contains the essential organ of hearing. It describes two and on half turns about a central pillar call the modiolus or columella, forming th spiral canal, which is about one an one-half inches in length. Also see *co* **—cochlear,** *adj.*

co''cil·la'na (ko''si·lay'nuh, ·lan'uh The bark of the tree *Guarea Rusbyi* nauseating expectorant.

cock'roach''. See *Blatella, Blatta.*

co'co·nut oil. A fixed oil obtaine from coconuts, used chiefly in th manufacture of soap.

coc''to·sta'bile (cock''to·stay'b ·stab'il), **coc''to·sta'ble.** Able withstand the temperature of boili water without change.

cod. The common cod, *Gadus morrhu* which furnishes cod liver oil.

co''de·car·box'yl·ase. Pyridox phosphate; the prosthetic compone of the enzyme carboxylase which ca alyzes decarboxylation of L-ami acids, as well as of certain transan nating enzymes, in which latter ca it is commonly referred to as *cotran aminase.*

co''de·hy'drase. See *coenzyme I a II.*

o″de·hy′dro·gen·ase. See co-enzyme I and II.

o·de′ia. See codeine.

o′de·ine (ko′dee·een, ko′dēn). A white, crystalline alkaloid of opium, resembling morphine in action, but weaker. Syn., codeia, methylmorphine. **c. phosphate.** Soluble in water; most soluble codeine salt. **c. sulfate.** The sulfate of the alkaloid.

od liv′er oil. The partially desteacinated fixed oil obtained from fresh livers of Gadus morrhua and other species of the family Gadidae. Contains vitamins A and D.

o″ef·fi′cient. Multiplier; figure indicating the degree of physical or chemical alteration characteristic of a given substance under stated conditions. **c. of correlation.** A measure of the degree of association between two characteristics in a series of observations. Its value ranges from −1, representing perfect negative correlation, to +1, representing perfect positive correlation. **c. of fecundity.** The number of conceptions per 1000 women-years of exposure to risk of conception, both taken after two years of married life. **c. of solubility of a gas.** The amount of a gas which is dissolved at a given temperature in 1 cc. of a liquid, when the pressure of gas on the liquid is 760 mm. Hg. **c. of variation.** The standard deviation of a series of observations expressed as a per cent of the mean of the series.

coele, -cele (-seel). A combining form denoting a chamber, ventricle, or a normal cavity of the body.

oe′li·o- (see′lee·o-), **coe′li-** (see′lee-), **ce′li·o-, ce′li-.** A combining form denoting abdomen or belly.

oe′lom, ce′lom (see′lum). The embryonic body cavity formed in the lateral mesoderm, which subsequently becomes divided into pericardial, pleural, and peritoneal cavities in developing mammals. **—coelom′ic,** adj. **extraembryonic c.** The cavity in the extraembryonic mesoderm; between chorionic mesoderm on one hand and the mesoderm of the amnion and yolk sac on the other. It is continuous with the embryonic coelom in the region of the umbilicus, and is obliterated by the growth of the amnion.

o·en′zyme. A substance associated with and activating an enzyme; prosthetic group of an enzyme. **c. I.** A nucleotide composed of two molecules each of D-ribose and phosphoric acid, and one molecule each of adenine and nicotinic acid amide. Occurs chiefly in yeast. Syn., codehydrase I, codehydrogenase I, cozymase, diphosphopyridine nucleotide. **c. II.** A nucleotide composed of one molecule each of adenine and nicotinic acid amide, two mole-cules of a pentose, and three molecules of phosphoric acid. Syn., codehydrase II, codehydrogenase II, triphosphopyridine nucleotide. **c. R.** Biotin.

co·fer′ment. Coenzyme, q.v.

cof′fee. The dried and roasted ripe seeds of various species of Coffea.

cogentin methanesulfonate. Trade-mark for benztropine methanesulfonate.

co·hab″i·ta′tion. 1. The living together of a man and woman, with or without legal marriage. 2. The sexual act, without legal marriage.

co·her′ence. Reasonable connectedness of thought shown in speech or writing.

co·he′sion. The attractive force between the same kind of molecules, that is, the force which holds the molecules of a substance together. **—cohesive,** adj.

coil. A spiral or helix. **induction c.** Turns of wire used to transform a current of low potential into a current of high potential by electric induction. **primary c.** The inner coil of an induction apparatus. **resistance c.** A coil of wire of known electric resistance, used for estimating resistance. **secondary c.** The outer coil of fine insulated wire in an induction apparatus.

co·i′tion (ko·ish′un). Coitus.

co″i·to·pho′bi·a. Morbid dread of coitus.

co′i·tus. The act of sexual connection; copulation.

col-. See colo-.

co′la nut. See kola.

co·la′tion. In pharmacy, the operation of straining.

col″a·to′ri·um (kol″uh·tor′ee·um, ko″luh·). In pharmacy, a sieve, colander, or strainer.

col′a·ture (kol′uh·choor, ko′luh·). 1. In pharmacy, a liquid that has been subjected to colation. 2. Colation.

col′chi·cine (kol′chi·seen, kol′ki·). An alkaloid of colchicum; employed in the treatment of gout.

col′chi·cum (kol′chi·kum, kol′ki·kum). Meadow saffron. The corm and seed of Colchicum autumnale, the properties of which are due to colchicine.

cold. 1. The comparative lack of heat. Cold in the form of baths or ice packs is used therapeutically to lower fever, stop convulsions, or allay irritation and inflammation. 2. See common cold.

cold′-blood′ed. Poikilothermic; without ability to regulate the body temperature; said of fishes, reptiles, and amphibians, whose temperatures correspond to that of the environment.

cold cream. A type of cosmetic cream of varying composition; sometimes, the official rose water ointment.

co·lec'to·my. Excision of all or a portion of the colon.

co'le·o- (ko''lee-o-, kol'ee-o-), **cole-** (ko''lee-, kol'ee-). A combining form denoting a sheath.

co''le·o·cys·ti'tis. Inflammation of vagina and urinary bladder.

Co''le·op'ter·a (ko''lee-op'tur-uh, kol''ee-). An order of insects which includes species of carnivorous and herbivorous beetles.

co''le·op·to'sis. Prolapse of the vaginal wall.

co''le·ot'o·my. A cutting operation upon the vagina; colpotomy.

col'ic. 1. Pertaining to the colon. 2. Paroxysmal abdominal pain due to smooth-muscle spasm. A symptom of many different conditions; inflammatory, as that associated with appendicitis; obstructive, as that due to calculi in biliary or urethral passages; toxic, as in lead poisoning; overdistention from overeating or air swallowing; or due to emotional factors such as that associated with nervous indigestion.

col'i·form (kol'i·form, ko''li·form). 1. Sievelike; ethmoid; cribriform. 2. A group of nonsporeforming, Gram-negative, lactose-fermenting, aerobic bacilli; the demonstration of such organisms in water is accepted as presumptive evidence of fecal contamination. The coliform or colon-aerogenes group of bacteria includes members of the *Escherichia* and *Aerobacter* genera.

co'li group (ko'lye). Colon-aerogenes group. See *coliform*.

co·li'tis. Inflammation of the colon. **acute c.** That seen with acute infections or irritations; characterized by diarrhea. Also called *simple c.* **amebic c.** An infectious disease due to infection of the colon with *Endamoeba histolytica.* **balantidial c.** That due to infection by *Balantidium coli;* characterized by diarrhea and dysentery. Also called *balantidiasis.* **mucous c.** A chronic affection of the mucous membrane of the colon; characterized by colicky pain, constipation, or diarrhea, and the passage of mucous or membranous threads or masses. Also called *chronic exudative enteritis, croupous c., desquamative c., diphtheritic c., follicular c., intestinal c., membranous c., mucomembranous c., plastic c.* **spastic c.** That associated with an increased tonus of the colon. **ulcerative c.** An idiopathic, nonspecific, inflammatory disease of the colon; of unknown cause; characterized by friability and ulceration of the mucosa.

col'la·gen. The albuminoid substance of the white fibers of connective tissues, cartilage, and bone. It is converted into gelatin by boiling. **—collagen'ic, collag'enous,** adj.

col·lapse'. 1. Extreme depression, exhaustion, or prostration; from failure of circulation, as in shock, hemorrhage, or vasomotor disturbance. 2. An abnormal sagging of an organ or falling together of its walls. **lung c.** Decreased volume of any portion of a lung, with decrease or absence of its air content, due to any cause. See *atelectasis.* **massive c.** The airless state of an entire lung, usually due to bronchial occlusion by accumulated secretions; often follows a surgical operation. Also called *massive atelectasis.*

col'lar·bone'. The clavicle.

col·lat'er·al. 1. Accessory or secondary; not direct or immediate. 2. One of the first branches of an axis cylinder of a nerve cell passing at a right angle.

col·lic'u·lus. A small eminence. **inferior c.** One of the posterior pair of rounded eminences arising from the dorsal portion of the mesencephalon. It contains centers for reflexes in response to sound. Also called *inferior quadrigeminal body.* **superior c.** One of the anterior pair of rounded eminences arising from the dorsal portion of the mesencephalon. It contains centers for reflexes in response to visual stimuli. Also called *superior quadrigeminal body.*

col'li·ma''tor. 1. The diaphragm of a spectroscope, the purpose of which is to provide a beam of parallel rays of light by means of a small slit at the focus of its lens. 2. A fixed telescope for adjusting the optical axis of an instrument, as a photomicrographic camera.

col·lo'di·on. A dressing for wounds made by dissolving pyroxylin in ether and alcohol. See *pyroxylin.* **flexible c.** Collodion with the addition of castor oil and camphor.

col'loid. A state of subdivision of matter in which the individual particles are of submicroscopic size and consist either of single large molecules, as of proteins, or aggregates of smaller molecules. The dimension of a colloid particle, arbitrarily fixed, is between 1 and 100 millimicrons ($m\mu$). **—colloi'dal,** adj. **hydrophilic c.** One capable of combining with, or attracting to it, water to form a stable dispersion. **hydrophobic c.** One incapable of combining with, or attracting to it, water. **irreversible c.** One which, on being precipitated or otherwise separated from its dispersion medium, cannot be restored to its original state merely by adding the dispersion medium. **lyophilic c.** One capable of combining with, or attracting to it, the dispersion medium. **lyophobic c.** One incapable of combining with, or attracting to it, the dispersion medium. **protective c.** A lyophilic colloid which, when added to a lyophobic colloid, confers upon the latter the stability of the former. **reversible c.** One which, on being precipitated or otherwise separated from its dispersion medium, can be restored to its original state merely by adding the dispersion medium.

col·loid'o·pha"gy. Invasion and ingestion of colloid by macrophages, as in the thyroid gland.

col'lum. Neck, q.v.

col·lyr'i·um (pl. *collyriums, collyria*). A preparation for local application to the eye, usually a wash or lotion.

co'lo- (ko'lo-, kol'o-), **col-.** A combining form denoting *the colon.*

col"o·bo'ma. Any congenital, pathologic, or operative defect of the eye; occurs most commonly in the iris, ciliary body, or choroid, usually as a cleft placed inferiorly. May be a congenital fissure of the eyelid, usually the upper. **atypical c.** One located other than inferiorly in any part of the eye. **bridge c.** A form affecting the iris, in which the cleft is separated from the pupil by a bridging strand of iris or by persistent pupillary membrane. **c. of the choroid.** Congenital cleft of the choroid coat (and retina) of the eye. **c. of the iris.** Congenital cleft of the iris. **c. of the lens.** A congenital notch or groove in the lens. **c. of the optic nerve.** One caused by partial closure or nonclosure of the fetal fissure of the optic stalk. **c. of the retina.** One caused by partial closure or nonclosure of the fetal fissure of the optic cup. **c. palpebrae.** Congenital cleft of an eyelid.

col'o·cynth. The dried pulp of the unripe but full-grown fruit of *Citrullus Colocynthis*, a powerful purgative.

co·logne' wa'ter. Perfumed spirit.

co'lon. The part of the large intestine beginning at the cecum and terminating at the end of the sigmoid flexure. In the various parts of its course it is known as **ascending c., transverse c., descending c.,** and **sigmoid c.** The last is sometimes divided into the **iliac c.** and the **pelvic c. —col'ic, colon'ic,** adj. **redundant c.** One with congenitally increased length, causing looping or reduplication; commonly associated with constipation.

col'o·ny. *In bacteriology,* a group or mass of microörganisms in a culture, derived from a single cell. **rough c.** An irregular, flattened, and wrinkled colony of bacteria. R-type. **smooth c.** Round, convex, and shining colonies. S-type.

col'o·ny coun'ter. A device for counting bacterial colonies; usually consists of an illuminated transparent plate, divided into spaces of known

area, over which a Petri dish containing the colonies is placed.

col'o·pex"y (kol'o·peck"see, ko'lo-). Suturing of the sigmoid flexure to the abdominal wall.

col'or. 1. A visual sensation due to radiated or reflected light. 2. Tint or hue; that quality of an object perceptible to sight alone. 3. A pigment. **complementary colors.** Two colors which, when combined, produce white. **primary colors.** (a) *In painting,* those whose various combinations make all other colors; red, yellow, and blue; or, more loosely, a classification of distinct color sensations to which other shades or tints may be referred, as green, light or dark. (b) *In psychology,* red, yellow-green, and blue.

col"or·im'e·ter (kul"o·rim'i·tur). An instrument for determining color intensity, as for measuring the proportion of hemoglobin in blood. Also see *photoelectric colorimeter.* **—colorimet'ric,** adj.; **colorimetry,** n.

co"lo·sig"moid·os'to·my. Formation of an anastomosis between the sigmoid and some other part of the colon.

co·los'to·my. The formation of an artificial anus in the anterior abdominal wall or loin. The opening into the colon may be anywhere depending on the location of the diseased condition, as cecostomy, sigmoidostomy, etc.

col"os·tra'tion. Diarrhea of infants caused by colostrum.

co·los'trum. The first milk from the mother's breasts after the birth of the child. It is laxative, and assists in the expulsion of the meconium. Contains greater quantities of lactalbumin and lactoprotein than later milk.

co·lot'o·my. Incision of the colon; may be abdominal, lateral, lumbar, or iliac, according to the region of entrance.

colp-. See colpo-.

col·pal'gi·a (kol·pal'juh, ·jee·uh). Vaginal pain or neuralgia.

col·pec'to·my. Excision of the vagina.

col·pi'tis. Inflammation of the vagina.

col'po-, colp-. A combining form meaning *the womb,* denoting *connection with* or *relation to the vagina.*

col'po·cele. Hernia or tumor in the vagina.

col"po·per"i·ne·o·plas"ty. Plastic surgery of the perineum and vagina.

col"po·per"i·ne·or'rha·phy. Suture of a cut or lacerated vagina and perineum.

col'po·pex"y. Fixation of the vagina by suturing it to a surrounding structure.

col'po·plas"ty. Plastic repair of the vagina.

col'po·scope. An instrument for the

visual examination of the vagina; a vaginal speculum. **—colposcop'ic**, *adj.*; **colpos'copy**, *n.*

col·pot'o·my. Surgical incision of the vagina.

colts'foot". A European herb, *Tussilago farfara*; its leaves are used as a demulcent and bitter.

co·lum'bi·um. See *niobium*.

col'umn. A supporting pillar; a pillar-shaped structure. **—colum'nar**, *adj.* **columns of the gray matter.** Divisions of the longitudinal column of gray matter in the spinal cord; usually classified as the **anterior column**, the **lateral column**, and the **posterior column**. Also called *cornua of the gray matter.* **rectal c.** One of the vertical folds of the mucous membrane of the upper part of the anal canal. Also called *anal c., c. of Morgagni.* **renal c.** That part of the cortical substance of the kidney between the sides of any two pyramids. Also called *c. of Bertin.* **vertebral c.** The flexible, supporting column of the body made up of vertebrae separated by intervertebral disks and bound together by ligaments. Syn., *spinal c.* Also called *backbone.*

col'umn·ing, col"um·ni·za'-tion. The placing of vaginal tampons to support a prolapsed uterus.

co'ma. 1. Unconsciousness from which the patient cannot be aroused. It may be due to ingested poison such as opiates or alcohol; to a poison developed in the body, as in uremia or overwhelming toxemias; to profound disturbances of the acid-base balance, as in diabetic acidosis; or to brain injury, trauma, apoplexy, or tumor. 2. *In ophthalmology,* spherical aberration in oblique incidence. **c. vigil.** A comatose condition in which the patient lies with eyes open but is unconscious. **hypochloremic c.** That due to reduced blood chloride.

com'a·tose (kom'uh·toce, ko'muh·). In a condition of coma.

com'e·do, co·me'do (pl. *comedos, comedones*). A collection of sebaceous material and dead cells retained in the hair follicle and excretory duct of the sebaceous gland, the surface covered with a dark crust due to hyperkeratosis at the follicular orifice. It is the primary lesion of acne vulgaris; usually found over the face, chest, and back, and more commonly during adolescence. Syn., *blackhead.*

com"e·do'nes (kom"i·do'neez). Plural of comedo, formerly used.

com'mi·nute. 1. *In chemistry,* pulverize; divide into fine particles. 2. *In surgery,* fracture a bone so that it is shattered in several pieces. **—comminute, comminuted**, *adj.*; **com·minu'tion**, *n.*

com'mis·sure. 1. Strands of nerve fibers uniting like structures in the two sides of the brain or spinal cord. 2. The point of union of the lips, eyelids, labia majora, or mitral leaflets. **—commis'sural**, *adj.*

com"mis·sur·ot'o·my. The surgical section of any commissure.

com·mit'ment. *In legal medicine,* an act consigning a patient to an institution.

com'mon cold. An acute upper respiratory infection, due to a filtrable virus, which leads to invasion of the respiratory tract by pathogenic organisms such as pneumococcus, streptococcus, staphylococcus, and influenza bacillus. The disease is mild, of short duration, endemic. It has a high morbidity and is highly contagious. Attacks produce only temporary immunity. The onset is marked by a chilly sensation followed by sneezing, watering of the eyes, nasal discharge, cough and is often accompanied by mild pyrexia. Syn., *coryza, rhinitis.* Also called *upper respiratory infection.*

com·mo'ti·o (kuh·mo'shee·o). A concussion, commotion, or shock. **c. cerebri.** Concussion of the brain. **c. retinae.** Concussion or paralysis of the retina from a blow on or near the eye. It is characterized by sudden blindness, but there is little or no ophthalmoscopic evidence of any lesion. The sight is usually regained, and its loss is supposedly due to disturbance of the retinal elements.

com·mu'ni·ca·ble. Transmissible from one person to another.

com·mu'ni·cans (ko·mew'ni·kanz). Communicating; connecting.

com·pan'ion·ate mar'riage. Form of marriage for sexual companionship without legal obligation, economic responsibility, or desire for children.

com'pa·ny aid man. A medical department soldier attached to a company of combat troops, whose principal duties are to administer emergency treatment to casualties, to examine and tag the dead, and to instruct the walking wounded as to location of the nearest aid station.

com·par'a·scope. An apparatus attached to two microscopes for the simultaneous comparison of two different specimens.

com·pat"i·bil'i·ty. Congruity; the power of a medicine or a substance in a medicine to mix with another without deleterious chemical change or loss of therapeutic power. **—compat'ible**, *adj.*

compazine. Trade-mark for prochlorperazine.

com"pen·sa'tion. 1. The act of making good a deficiency; the state of counterbalancing a functional or structural defect. 2. *In psychopathology*, a psychic phenomenon in which strong feelings of guilt or inferiority prompt excessive defensive reactions. **—compensating, compen'satory,** *adj.*

com·pen'sa·to"ry pause. *In cardiology*, any pause which, immediately following a premature beat, compensates by its length for the prematurity of the beat.

com'pe·tence. *In embryology*, the ability to react to a developmental stimulus; a state of reactivity or unstable equilibrium necessary for induction to occur. See *potency, determination*.

com·plaint'. Lay term for disease or ailment.

com'ple·ment. A group of substances with enzymatic properties, formed in the blood, plasma, or serum of animals, having the capacity, in coöperation with antibody and cellular elements, to destroy a variety of pathogenic organisms and other foreign substances. The common functions of complement are bacteriolysis, bactericidal action, hemolysis, and acceleration of opsonic actions. Complement (C') may be fractionated into four components, indicated by C'1, C'2, C'3, and C'4. Syn., *addiment, alexin, cytase.* **c. fixation.** See *fixation* of complement.

com'plex. 1. *In psychoanalysis*, a group of ideas with strong emotional tone, which have been transferred by the conscious mind into the unconscious, and from there influence the personality. 2. A combination of symptoms or related factors, as a symptom complex or syndrome; complexus. **anxiety c.** A symptom of a neurosis, marked by fear and apprehension, especially with regard to beginning any task, or to impending accident, castration, infection, and the like. **Eisenmenger's c.** An anomaly of the heart consisting of a defect in the interventricular septum, dextroposition of the aorta, and hypertrophy of the right ventricle. There is no pulmonary stenosis as in the tetralogy of Fallot. **Electra c.** The female analog of the Oedipus complex. *q.v.* **Oedipus c.** A carry-over into adult life of a son's childhood sexual desire for his mother, usually accompanied by hostility toward, or envy of, the position of his father. According to Freud, every male child experiences this Oedipus situation.

com·plex'ion. Color and appearance of the skin of the face.

com"pli·ca'tion. *In medicine*, an accidental condition or second disease occurring in the course of a primary disease. **—com'plicated,** *adj.*

compocillin-V hydrabamine. Trade-mark for hydrabamine phenoxymethyl penicillin.

com·po'nent. Constituent part. **nerve c.** The group of fibers in a nerve having similar functions, as the sensory and motor components of a mixed nerve.

com"po·si'tion. 1. The constitution of a mixture. 2. The kind and number of atoms which are contained in the molecule of a compound.

com'pos men'tis. Of sound mind.

com'pound. A substance composed of two or more elements chemically combined in definite proportion. Abbreviated, comp. **—compound'ing,** *n.;* **compound',** *v.t.*

com'pound E (Kendall's). Cortisone, *q.v.*

com'pound F (Kendall's). Hydrocortisone.

com'pound G-11. Hexachlorophene, *q.v.*

com'press. A folded cloth or pad of other soft material, wet or dry, applied firmly to a part for the relief of inflammation or the prevention of hemorrhage. **cold c.** One moistened with cold or ice water. **cribriform c.** A compress with holes for drainage or a hole for observation of the skin beneath. Also called *fenestration c.* **graduated c.** A compress with folds of varying size, thick in the center and thinner toward the periphery. **hot c.** One moistened with warm or hot water. **pressure c.** One which is held in place with a bandage in order to produce pressure on the wound and prevent oozing.

com·pres'sion. 1. The state of being compressed. 2. The act of pressing or squeezing together. **cerebral c.** Compression of the brain by any spacetaking, intracranial lesion such as tumors, hemorrhage, etc. **c. fracture.** See under *fracture*.

com·pres'sor. 1. An instrument for compressing an artery or other part. 2. A muscle having a compressing function, as the sphincter urethrae (compressor urethrae). See Table of Muscles in the Appendix.

com·pul'sion. An act which is against the conscious will of the individual at the time it is performed.

con-. 1. A prefix meaning *with, together*. 2. *In chemistry*, a prefix denoting *a substance found with a substance*.

co·na'tion. The exertive power of the mind, including will and desire; a special act or exercise of the exertive power.

con'cave. Possessing a curved, depressed surface; opposed to *convex*. **—concav'ity,** *n.*

con·ceive'. Become pregnant.

con'cen·trate. 1. To increase the

strength of a substance as by condensation. 2. To intensify an effort.

con'cen·trate. That which is produced by concentration, 1.

con"cen·tra'tion. 1. The act or result of increasing the intensity or strength of a substance. 2. A measure for the composition of a solution.

con·cen'tric. Having a common center.

con·cep'tion. 1. The fecundation of the ovum by the spermatozoon, occurring in humans usually about the twelfth to fifteenth day after the first day of menstrual flow. 2. The abstract mental idea of anything; the power or act of mentally conceiving. —**conceptive,** *adj.*

con'cha (kong'kuh) (pl. *conchae*). 1. A shell; a shell-like organ, as the hollow part of the external ear. 2. Any one of the three nasal conchae; a medial projection of thin bone from the lateral wall of the nasal cavity, covered by mucous membrane and designated by position as superior, middle, or inferior. Also called *turbinate bone.* See Table of Bones in the Appendix. —**conchal,** *adj.*

con'chi·nine (kong'ki·neen, ·nin). See *quinidine.*

con·com'i·tant. Accompanying.

con·cres'cence. 1. A growing together of the roots of two teeth. 2. A process by which the formative embryonic cells of the germ ring converge and fuse at the blastopore to form the axial part of the embryo during gastrulation. Syn., *convergence.*

con·cre'tion. 1. A calculus. 2. Union of parts normally separate, as the fingers. 3. *In dentistry,* a deposit.

con·cus'sion. Shock; the state of being shaken; a severe shaking or jarring of a part; also, the morbid state resulting from such a jarring. **air c.** Aerial compression generated at the moment of detonation of a high explosive. See *blast.* **c. of the brain.** A condition produced by a fall or blow on the head, and marked by unconsciousness, feeble pulse, cold skin, pallor, at times the involuntary discharge of feces and urine; this is followed by partial stupor, vomiting, headache, and eventual recovery. In severe cases, inflammation of the brain or a condition of feeblemindedness may follow. **c. of the labyrinth.** Deafness and tinnitus from a blow or an explosion. **c. of the spinal cord.** A condition caused by severe shock of the spinal column, with or without appreciable lesion of the cord, leading to functional disturbances.

con"den·sa'tion. 1. Making more compact or dense. 2. The changing of a gaseous substance to a liquid, or a

liquid to a solid. 3. *In chemistry,* the union of two or more molecules by the linking of carbon atoms and the formation of more complex carbon chains. 4. The pathologic hardening, with or without contraction, of a soft organ or tissue. 5. *In dentistry,* the compression of gold pellets in building a gold-foil filling. 6. *In psychopathology,* a psychic mechanism whereby one idea becomes the symbolic expression of many incompatible, repressed ideas; the meaning of this symbol may not be clear to the conscious mind or to others.

con·dens'er. 1. A lens or combination of lenses used in microscopy for gathering and concentrating rays of light. 2. An apparatus for condensing gases. 3. An apparatus for the accumulation of electricity. **dark-field c.** An apparatus attached to a microscope which reflects light through a microscopic field so that it illuminates the object only, the surrounding field remaining unilluminated.

con·di'tion·ing. 1. *In psychology,* the process of attaching a new stimulus to an old response or a new response to an old stimulus. 2. The development of better physiologic condition through physical exercise.

con'dom. A sheath worn over the penis during copulation for preventing conception or infection.

con·duc'tion. The passage or transfer of electrons, heat, or sound waves through suitable media, or of nerve and muscle impulses through those tissues. —**conductiv'ity,** *n.* **air c.** (a) Transmission of sound stimuli to the eardrum through the external auditory canal. (b) A test for hearing, using a watch or tuning fork at various distances from the ear. Abbreviated, A. C. **antidromic c.** A conduction in the reverse direction from the normal. **bone c.** Transmission of sound vibrations to the internal ear via the bones of the skull. **decremental c.** A conduction in which the intensity of the impulse decreases progressively. **reflex c.** The passage of a nerve impulse from the afferent to the efferent components of the reflex arc.

con·duc'tor. 1. A body or substance that transmits energy by direct molecular transfer; applied to carriers of heat, electric currents, and sound. 2. An instrument serving as a guide for the surgeon's knife.

con"du·ran'go. The dried bark of a South American vine, used as a bitter and astringent stomachic.

con'dyle (kon'dyle, ·dil). Any rounded eminence such as occurs in the joints of many of the bones, especially the femur, humerus, and mandible. —**condylar,** *adj.*

con"dy·lec'to·my. Excision of a condyle.

con'dy·lo-, condyl-. A combining form denoting a *knuckle, joint,* or *knob.*

con"dy·lo'ma. A wartlike growth or tumor, usually near the anus or pudendum. **—condylom'atous,** *adj.* **c. acumina'tum.** The pointed condyloma or wart of the genital organs of nonsyphilitic origin. Syn., *verruca acuminata.* **c. la'tum.** A moist, syphilitic papule occurring where two surfaces of skin come in opposition, often warty and vegetative, very communicable, and usually teeming with *Treponema pallidum.* Syn., *moist papule.* **syphilitic c.** See *c.* latum.

con"dy·lot'o·my. Extraarticular osteotomy; division through the condyles of a bone.

cone. 1. A solid body having a circle for its base and terminating in a point. 2. The mechanical element of the tooth crown. 3. One of the light-receptive, flask-shaped cells which, with the associated rods, forms an outer layer, the neuroepithelial layer, of the retina. Also called *retinal c.* 4. Conus, *q.v.* **—con'ical, co'noid,** *adj.* **ether c.** An apparatus used in the administration of ether.

con·fab"u·la'tion. The fabrication of ready answers and fluent recitals of fictitious occurrences; found in certain mental disorders such as Korsakoff's psychosis and senile dementia.

con·fec'tion. *In pharmacy,* a soft mass of sugar and water, or of honey; used as an excipient. Syn., *electuary.* Also called *conserve.*

con·fig"u·ra'tion. The structure of a chemical compound, especially the relative positions in space of atoms in a molecule. Also see *isomerism.*

con·fine'ment. Lying-in; giving birth to a child; accouchement.

con'flict. *In psychiatry,* the clash of pure instinct with various psychic forces in its attempt to discharge its energies without modification, or between opposing forces within the psyche, as wishes.

con·flu·ens si'nu·um (kon'floo-enz sin'yoo-um) [BNA]. Confluence of the sinuses; the dilated junction of the superior sagittal, the straight, the occipital, and the transverse sinuses of the dura mater. Formerly called *torcular Herophili.*

con·flu·ent. 1. Running together; the opposite of *discrete.* 2. *In anatomy,* coalesced or blended; applied to two or more bones originally separate, but subsequently formed into one.

con"fron·ta'tion. A method for measuring visual fields in which the patient sits on the same level three feet from the examiner and fixes with one eye on the examiner's corresponding eye. The examiner then raises his hands until he just sees them. Any movement at this point should be perceived readily by the patient.

con·fu'sion. 1. State of mental bewilderment. 2. A mixing or confounding.

con"ge·la'tion. 1. Freezing; frost bite; intense cold or its effect on the animal economy or any organ or part. 2. Coagulation.

con·gen'i·tal. Existing at birth.

con·ges'tion. An abnormal collection of blood in a part or organ; hyperemia, *q.v.* **—congested, congestive,** *adj.* **passive c.** Stasis in various parts of the body, caused by myocardial insufficiency. **pleuropulmonary c.** Congestion of the lungs marked by symptoms similar to those of pleurisy. Also called *pulmonary c., Potain's type of c.*

con'gi·us. A term frequently employed in the apothecaries' measure meaning a gallon. Abbreviated, C., cong.

con·glo'bate. Forming a rounded mass.

con·glom'er·ate. 1. Massed together; aggregated. 2. A mass of units without order. **—conglomera'tion,** *n.*

con·glu'tin. A simple protein of the globulin type; found in lupines, almonds, beans, and seeds of various leguminous plants.

con·glu'ti·nant. Adhesive; promoting union, as of the edges of a wound. **Con'go red** (C.C.). An acid aniline dye of the azo group; used as a diagnostic agent, histologic stain, and indicator. Also called *Congo; cotton red A, B,* or *C; direct red C, R,* or *Y.*

con'gress. 1. An assemblage for deliberative purpose. 2. A coming together. **sexual c.** Coitus, or carnal intercourse.

con·hy'drine (kon·high'dreen, -drin). A crystalline alkaloid, $C_8H_{17}ON$; obtained from conium.

co·nic'e·ine (ko·niss'ee-een, kon-i-see'in). A liquid alkaloid, $C_8H_{15}N$, in conium.

co·nid'i·o-, co·nid'i-. A combining form denoting *conidium.*

co·nid'i·o·phore". The mycelial thread of a fungus which bears conidia.

co·nid'i·o·spore". A conidium.

co·nid'i·um (pl. *conidia*). An asexual spore cut from the end of a fungus filament. **—conidial,** *adj.*

co'ni·ism. Poisoning by conium. It begins with paralysis of the legs and extends to the arms and respiratory muscles, leading to unconsciousness and death.

co·ni·o-, coni-. A combining form signifying *dust.*

co"ni·om'e·ter. See *konimeter.*

co"ni·o'sis. A disease or morbid condition due to inhalation of dust.

co'ni·um. Poison hemlock, *Conium maculatum,* the fruit and leaves of which were formerly official. Conium alkaloids produce motor paralysis without loss of sensation or consciousness. It has been used in the treatment of spasmodic disorders.

con"ju·ga'ta ve'ra. The true conjugate. The distance from the middle of the sacral promontory to the upper margin of the symphysis pubis.

con'ju·gate. 1. Yoked or coupled. 2. The anteroposterior diameter of the inlet of the pelvis, the plane of the inlet being regarded as an ellipse. **obstetric c.** The minimum diameter of the pelvic inlet; usually a little shorter than conjugata vera. **true c.** Conjugata vera, *q.v.*

con"ju·ga'tion. The process in lower organisms, analogous to fertilization, involving the fusion of gametes or the temporary union of individuals with exchange of nuclear material.

con"junc·ti'va. The mucous membrane covering the anterior portion of the globe of the eye, reflected upon the lids and extending to their free edges. Its parts are called palpebral and bulbar or ocular. **—conjunctival,** *adj.* **bulbar c.** That covering the anterior third of the eyeball, from the retrotarsal fold to the margin of the cornea. Also called *ocular c.* **palpebral c.** The conjunctiva of the eyelid.

con·junc"ti·vi'tis. Inflammation of the conjunctiva. **acute contagious c.** Pinkeye. **allergic c.** Characterized by mild irritation and more or less abundant mucus; accompanies other symptoms of hay fever, but frequently occurs without rhinitis. **catarrhal c.** The most common form, usually mild, resulting from cold or irritation. Also called *acute catarrhal c.* **follicular c.** A form characterized by numerous round, pinkish bodies found in the retrotarsal fold. **gonorrheal c.** A severe form of purulent conjunctivitis caused by infection with gonococci. **hypertrophic c.** Chronic catarrhal conjunctivitis attended with enlargement of the conjunctival papillae. **klieg c.** A condition caused by ultraviolet rays from klieg lights used in motion picture studios. Also called *klieg eyes.* **phlyctenular c.** A form characterized by the presence on the ocular conjunctiva of small vesicles surrounded by a reddened zone. **subacute c.** Redness and thickening of the conjunctiva, largely confined to the conjunctiva of the lids and fornixes, a scanty secretion of mucus, with some pus corpuscles, due to the presence of an infection. **vernal c.** A form recurring each

spring or summer and disappearing with frost. Syn., *c. catarrhalis aestiva.*

con"junc·tiv'o·plas"ty. Plastic surgery of the conjunctiva.

co'no-, con-. A combining form denoting *cone.*

co·quin'a·mine (kon·kwin'uh-meen, ·min). An alkaloid of cuprea bark.

con"san·guin'i·ty. The relationship arising from common parentage; blood relationship. **—consanguineous,** *adj.*

con'scious·ness. State of being aware of one's own existence, of one's own mental states, and of the impressions made upon one's senses; ability to take cognizance of sensations. **—conscious,** *adj.* **double c.** That morbid condition in which there are two separate and alternating states of mental consciousness, in either one of which the events that have occurred in the other state are not remembered by the patient.

con·sent', 1. *In legal medicine,* willing participation in unnatural or illegal intercourse. 2. Agreement.

con·serv'a·tive. Aiming at the preservation and restoration of injured parts; as conservative surgery or dentistry.

con·sol"i·da'tion. Process of becoming firm or solid, as a lung in pneumonia.

con'stant. 1. Fixed, not changing. 2. *In physics,* a property which remains numerically the same, and which may serve as a unit of measurement. 3. *In mathematics,* a quantity, having a definite and fixed value in a certain stage of investigation; an **absolute constant** retains the same value under all circumstances.

con"stel·la'tion. *In psychiatry,* a group of allied thoughts held together by a common emotional experience around a nuclear idea.

con"sti·pa'tion. A condition in which the bowels are evacuated at long intervals or with difficulty. **atonic c.** That due to decreased tonus of the colon. **spastic c.** That due to increased tonus of the colon.

con"sti·tu'tion. 1. Genotype, *q.v.* 2. *In medicine,* the total individuality of the person, including his inherited qualities and the cumulative effects of his reactions to all the environmental factors which influenced his physical and emotional development. **allergic c.** The inherited tendency to develop allergy.

con·stric'tor. Any muscle that contracts or tightens any part of the body. See Table of Muscles in the Appendix.

con·sult'ant. A consulting physician; one summoned by the physician in attendance to give counsel in a case.

on″sul·ta′tion. A deliberation between two or more physicians concerning the diagnosis and the proper method of treatment in a case.

con·sump′tion. An old term, formerly used to designate progressive tuberculosis. **—consumptive,** *adj.* **galloping c.** Popular term for a rapidly fatal form of pulmonary tuberculosis. Also called *florid phthisis.*

con′tact. 1. Direct or indirect exposure to a source of infection usually to a person affected with a contagious disease. 2. A person who has been exposed to a contagious disease. **—con·tac′tile, contac′tual,** *adj.*

con·ta′gion. The transmission of a disease directly or indirectly from one individual to another. **—contagious,** *adj.*

con·tam″i·na′tion. 1. Soiling with bacteria. 2. In *psychology,* the fusion of words (Freud). **—contam′inating,** *adj., n.;* **contam′inant,** *n.;* **contam′inate,** *v.t.*

conteben. Trade-mark for p-acetylaminobenzaldehyde-thiosemicarbazone, a tuberculostatic agent. See *tibione.*

con·tig′u·ous. In contact, or adjacent.

con′ti·nence. Self-restraint, especially in regard to sexual intercourse. **—continent,** *adj.*

con·tin′gen·cy ta′ble. A two-way frequency table showing the frequency of occurrence of classifications of one variable for specified classification of the other variable; a cross-classification table.

con·tor′tion. A twisting or writhing, as of the body.

con′tour. 1. The line that bounds, defines, or terminates a figure. 2. In *operative dentistry,* to effect the restoration of lost parts of teeth by building them up with gold, etc.

con′tra-. A prefix meaning *against, contrary,* or *in opposition.*

con″tra·cep′tion. Prevention of conception.

con″tra·cep′tive. An agent which prevents conception, such as medicated jelly in the vagina, the condom or thin rubber sheath for the penis, the cervical pessary or soft rubber diaphragm to cover the cervix of the uterus.

con·trac′tile (kon-track′tile, ·til). Having the power or tendency to contract.

con″trac·til′i·ty. The property of shortening upon the application of a stimulus.

con·trac′tion. Shortening, especially of the fibers of muscle tissue. Abbreviated, C. **aerobic c.** A phase of muscular contraction in which oxygen is utilized. **anaerobic c.** A phase of muscular contraction utilizing no oxygen. **Braxton Hicks c.** A pain-

less, intermittent uterine contraction occurring throughout pregnancy; valuable but not conclusive in diagnosing pregnancy. **clonic c.** Alternate muscular contraction and relaxation. **front tap c.** Contraction of the gastrocnemius muscle when the muscles of the front of the leg are tapped. **hourglass c.** A contraction of an organ, as the stomach or uterus, at the middle. **tetanic c.** In *obstetrics,* a state of continued contraction of the uterine muscle; occurs in prolonged labors, usually in the second stage. Results from a pathologic retraction ring. Abbreviated, Te. **vermicular c.** Peristaltic contraction.

con′tract prac′tice. Partial or complete medical service furnished to an individual, or a group of individuals, by a physician, or a group of physicians, for compensation that has been mutually agreed upon.

con·trac′ture. 1. Shortening, as of muscle or scar tissue, producing distortion or deformity. 2. Retarded relaxation of muscle, as when it is injected with veratrin. **Dupuytren's c.** A painless, chronic contracture of the hand, marked by thickening of the digital processes and of the palmar fascia, and flexion of the fingers, especially of the third and fourth, upon the palm. The disease is of uncertain etiology, and affects chiefly adult males. **hypertonic c.** That due to continuous discharge of nervous impulses; disappears during sleep or anesthesia. Seen in spastic paralysis. **ischemic c.** Shortening of muscle due to interference with the blood supply. Also called *Volkmann's c.* **myostatic c.** Assumption of shortened length after fixation in cast or tendon section with innervation intact. **myotatic c.** That occurring in a degenerating muscle when tapped or suddenly stretched; may also occur when a fatigued muscle is struck.

con″tra·in″di·ca′tion, con″tra·in′di·cant. A symptom, indication, or condition in which a remedy or a method of treatment is inadvisable.

con″tra·lat′er·al. Opposite; acting in unison with a similar part on the opposite side of the body.

con″tre·coup′ (kawn″ truh-kōō′). Counterstroke; injury of a part opposite to that struck, due to transmission of the shock, especially when the force is exerted against an organ or part containing fluid, as the skull, stomach, intestine, or urinary bladder.

con·trol′. A standard by which to check observations, and insure the validity of their results. May refer to a **control animal** (one used experimentally) or to a **control experiment.**

con·trol' ex·per'i·ment. One used to check or verify other experiments, using conditions identical except for one factor.

con·tu'sion. A bruise; an injury in which the skin is not broken. **—con·tuse',** v.

co'nus (pl. *coni*). 1. A cone. 2. A crescentic patch of atrophic choroid tissue near the optic papilla in myopia.

con"va·les'cence. 1. The restoration of health after disease. 2. The time spent in recovery. **—convalescent,** *adj.,* n.

con·val"la·mar'in (kon·val"uh-mair'in, kon"vuh·lam'ur·in). 1. A glycoside obtained from *Convallaria majalis.* 2. A mixture of the glycosides of convallaria used as an uncertain cardiac stimulant.

con"val·la'ri·a. The dried rhizome and roots of *Convallaria majalis,* the lily of the valley. Its properties are due to glycosides which give an unreliable digitalislike action.

con·vec'tion. A transmission or carrying, as of heat.

con·ver'gence. 1. Inclination or direction toward a common point, center, or focus, as of the axes of vision upon the near point. 2. Concrescence, *q.v.* **—convergent,** *adj.*

con·ver'sion. 1. *In psychiatry,* a mental defense mechanism whereby unconscious emotional conflict is transformed into physical disability. The affected part always has symbolic meaning pertinent to the nature of the conflict in contrast to the physiologic responses to strong emotion, which are without symbolic meaning. See conversion *hysteria.* 2. *In obstetrics,* an alteration in the presentation of the fetus to facilitate delivery.

con'vex. Rounded, as a swelling of round or spherical form on the external surface; gibbous; opposed to concave. **—convex'ity,** n.

con·vex'o-con'cave. Having one convex and one concave surface.

con·vex'o-con'vex. Having two convex surfaces; biconvex, as a lens.

con·vo·lu"ted. Folded in curves or contorted windings; coiled, as tubules.

con"vo·lu'tion. A fold, twist, or coil of any organ, especially any one of the prominent convex parts of the brain, separated from each other by depressions or sulci. See *gyrus.*

con·vol'vu·lin. $C_{31}H_{50}O_{16}$. A glycosidal resin, one of the chief constituents of the roots of jalap.

con·vul'sant. A medicine that causes convulsions.

con·vul'sion. An involuntary general paroxysm of muscular contraction, that is either tonic (without relaxation) or clonic (having alternate contractions of opposite groups of muscles). **—convul-**sive, *adj.,* **convulsionary, convulsivant,** n. **epileptiform c.** One characterized by total loss of consciousness. **hysterical c.** One due to hysteria; consciousness is only apparently lost. **infantile c.** One due to a number of causes, such as rickets, exhaustion, cerebral birth injury; sometimes called screaming fits. **local c.** One affecting one muscle, member, or part of a member. **mimetic c.** A facial convulsion. **oscillating c.** One in which the separate fiber bundles of a muscle are affected successively and not simultaneously. Also called *oscillatory* c. **puerperal c.** See *eclampsia.* **tetanic c.** General tonic convulsions without loss of consciousness. **toxic c.** One due to the action of some toxic agent upon the nervous system. **uremic c.** One that occurs in kidney disease due to retention in the blood of matter that should be eliminated by the kidney.

co·ör"di·na'tion. 1. The harmonious activity and proper sequence of those parts that coöperate in the performance of any function. 2. *In neurology,* the combination of nervous impulses in motor centers to insure coöperation of the appropriate muscles in a reaction.

co·pai'ba (ko·pay'buh, ko·py'buh). Balsam of copaiba. The oleoresin of *Copaifera* species (Leguminosae); native to South America. Has been used as stimulant, diuretic, diaphoretic, and expectorant.

co'pe·pod. A small fresh-water or salt-water crustacean. Some copepods are intermediary hosts to worms parasitic in man.

cop"i·o'pi·a (kop"ee·o'pee·uh, ko"pee·). Eyestrain; weariness of the eyes; asthenopia, *q.v.*

cop'per. Cu = 63.54. A reddish brown, malleable metal, various salts of which are used in medicine. They are employed as emetics, and, externally, as caustics. **c. sulfate.** $CuSO_4.5H_2O$, occurring as blue crystals or powder, soluble in water, valuable as an emetic, tonic, and astringent.

cop'per·as (cop'ur·us). Ferrous sulfate.

cop·rem'e·sis. Vomiting of fecal matter.

cop'ro-, copr-. A combining form meaning *feces* or *dung.*

cop'ro·lith. A hard mass of fecal matter in the intestine.

cop·roph'a·gy. Eating of feces; a symptom occasionally seen in severe psychoses. **—coprophagous,** *adj.*

cop"ro·phil'i·a. An abnormal interest in fecal matter, seen in certain mental patients.

cop·roph'i·lous. Growing upon fecal matter; said of certain bacteria.

cop″ro·pho′bi·a. A morbid fear of fecal matter.

cop·ros′ter·ol. $C_{27}H_{47}OH$. A derivative of cholesterol, found in the lower intestine.

cop″ro·xo′ic. Living in feces, as protozoans found in fecal matter outside the body but not in the intestine.

Cop′tis. A genus of herbs of the Ranunculaceae, the crowfoot family.

cop″u·la′tion. The sexual union of male and female.

cor. The heart, *q.v.* **c. triloculare biventriculare.** A serious defect of the upper part of the interatrial septum. The person may live to adulthood.

cor′a·co-. A combining form denoting *pertaining to the coracoid process.*

cor″a·co·a·cro′mi·al. Relating to the coracoid and the acromion processes.

cor″a·co·bra″chi·a′lis (kor″uh-ko-bray″kee-ay′liss, ·brack″ee-ay′liss). A muscle of the upper and medial part of the arm, arising from the coracoid process of the scapula. See Table of Muscles in the Appendix.

cor″a·co·cla·vic′u·lar. Relating to the coracoid process and the clavicle.

cor″a·co·hu′mer·al. Relating to the coracoid process and the humerus.

cor′a·coid. 1. Having the shape of a crow's beak. 2. The coracoid process.

cor′a·mine. A trade-mark for nikethamide, the product supplied as a 25% solution.

cord. 1. Any stringlike body. 2. The long, cylindrical structure bearing the umbilical arteries and vein and connecting the placenta and the fetus. Also called *umbilical c.* 3. A column of cells. **hepatic cords.** The anastomosing columns of liver cells separated by the hepatic sinusoids. Also called *liver cords.* **medullary cords.** (a) The primary invaginations of the germinal epithelium of the embryonic gonad that differentiate into rete testis and seminiferous tubules or into rete ovarii. Also called *primary cords, testis cords.* (b) The cords of dense, lymphatic tissue separated by sinuses in the medulla of a lymph node. **red pulp cords.** The anastomosing, cordlike columns of reticular connective tissue separating the venous sinuses of the spleen; the splenic red pulp. Also called *Billroth's cords.* **spermatic c.** That extending from the testis to the abdominal inguinal ring and consisting of the ductus deferens, the vessels and nerves of the testis and of the epididymis, and the accompanying connective tissue. **spinal c.** That part of the central nervous system contained within the vertebral canal and extending from the medulla oblongata at the level of the foramen magnum to the filum terminale at the level of the first or second lumbar vertebra. **tendinous c.** Chorda tendinea, *q.v.* **true vocal c.** Vocal fold, *q.v.*

cor·dec′to·my. Excision of a cord, as removal of a vocal fold. Also called *chordotomy.*

cor′di·form. Cordate; shaped like a heart.

cor·di′tis. Inflammation of the spermatic cord; funiculitis.

cor′do·pex′y. The operation of suturing a vocal fold to a new support to relieve the stenosis resulting from bilateral abductor paralysis.

cor·dot′o·my. Chordotomy; section of the anterior lateral white columns of the spinal cord for relief of intractable pain. Syn., *tractotomy.*

cor″e·cli′sis. Pathologic closure or obliteration of the pupil.

cor·ec′ta·sis. Dilatation of the pupil.

cor″ec·to′pi·a. Anomalous position of the pupil; displacement of the pupil.

cor″e·di·as′ta·sis (·dye·ass′tuh·sis). Dilatation of the pupil.

co″re·duc′tase (ko″ri·duck′tace, ·taze). See *coenzyme I.*

cor″e·mor′pho·sis. The operation for establishing an artificial pupil.

cor″en·cli′sis. The formation of a new pupil by displacement, the iris being drawn aside and in part excised.

cor′e·om′e·ter. An instrument for measuring the pupil of the eye. —**core·ometry,** *n.*

cor′e·plas″ty. Any operation for forming an artificial pupil.

cor″e·to·me″di·al′y·sis (kor″i·to-mee″dye·al′i·sis). Iridectomy, *q.v.*

co″ri·an′der. Coriander seed. The dried ripe fruit of *Coriandrum sativum,* (Umbelliferae). An aromatic, carminative, and stimulant.

co′ri·um. The deep layer of the skin. Syn., *cutis vera, derma.*

corn. A lay term for clavus, *q.v.*

cor′ne·a. The transparent anterior portion of the eyeball, its area occupying about one-sixth the circumference of the globe. It is continuous with the sclera, and is nourished by lymph from the looped blood vessels at its peripheral border. —**corneal,** *adj.* **transplantation of c.** Operation of engrafting a section of transparent cornea into the space of an excised central portion of an opaque human cornea.

cor′ne·o-. A combining form denoting *cornea* or *corneal.*

cor″ne·o·bleph′a·ron. Adhesion of the palpebral conjunctiva to the cornea.

cor′ne·ous. Horny or hornlike.

cor′ne·um. The stratum corneum or horny layer of the skin.

cor″ni·fi·ca′tion. The degenerative

process by which the cells of a stratified squamous epithelium are converted into dead, horny squames as in the epidermis and such epidermal derivatives as hair, nails, feathers. Syn., *keratinization, hornification.* —**cor'nified,** *adj.*

corn oil. A fixed oil obtained from the kernels of maize, used as a food and as a solvent for injectable medicaments, especially hormones. Syn., *maize oil.*

cor'nu (pl. *cornua*). A horn; a horn-shaped process or excrescence. —**cornual,** *adj.* **cornua of the hyoid bone.** Segments of the hyoid bone. The **greater cornu** projects backward from the lateral border of the body; the **lesser cornu** projects upward from the angle of junction of the body and the greater cornu. **cornua of the lateral ventricle.** Prolongations of the lateral ventricle of the cerebral hemisphere. The **anterior cornu** is that extending into the frontal lobe; the **inferior cornu,** that extending into the temporal lobe; and the **posterior cornu,** that extending into the occipital lobe. **cornua of the thyroid cartilage.** Processes of the thyroid cartilage; prolongations of its posterior border upward as the **superior cornu of the thyroid cartilage,** and downward as the **inferior cornu of the thyroid cartilage. c. cutaneum.** A corneous excrescence, varying in size and shape, occurring most frequently on the face and scalp and occasionally on the glans penis and scrotum. Considered a precancerous lesion. Syn., *cutaneous horn.* **dorsal c.** The posterior column of gray matter of the spinal cord. **lateral c.** The lateral column of gray matter of the spinal cord. **ventral c.** The anterior column of gray matter of the spinal cord.

cor'nus. The bark of the root of *Cornus florida,* the flowering dogwood. It is a simple bitter.

co·ro'na. 1. A crown. 2. The corona radiata. —**coronal,** *adj.* **c. capitis.** The crown of the head; the top of the head. **c. dentis.** The crown of a tooth. **c. radiata.** (a) A radiating mass of white nerve fibers ascending from the internal capsule to the cerebral cortex. (b) A zone of follicular cells circumjacent to the zona pellucida of the ovum, which persists for some time after ovulation.

cor'o·nar"y (korr'o·nerr"ee). A term applied to vessels, nerves, or attachments that encircle a part or an organ.

cor'o·ner. An officer who inquires by authority of the law into the causes of sudden or violent deaths.

cor'o·noid. Shaped like the beak of a crow, as the coronoid process of the ulna or of the mandible.

cor'po·ra. Plural of corpus, *q.v.*
cor'po·rin. Progesterone, *q.v.*
corpse. A cadaver.
cor'pu·lent. Excessively fat; obese. —**corpulence, corpulency,** *n.*
cor'pus (pl. *corpora*). Body, *q.v.* —**corpo'real,** *adj.* **corpora amylacea.** Microscopic, concentrically laminated, hyaline bodies occurring in the acini of the prostate, in the meninges, in diseased lungs, occasionally in other sites, and staining like amyloid with metachromatic aniline dyes. Syn., *amyloid bodies.* **corpora cavernosa.** Cylindrical bodies of erectile tissue; the basic structures of the penis and clitoris. The two **corpora cavernosa clitoridis** form the crura and body of the clitoris; they are analogous to the two **corpora cavernosa penis** which form the crura of the penis, and, together with the **corpus cavernosum urethrae** which surrounds the male urethra, form the body of the penis. **corpora quadrigemina.** The inferior and superior colliculi collectively. **c. adiposum orbitae.** The fat body of the orbital cavity; fatty connective tissue filling the space between the eyeball, optic nerve, ocular muscles, and lacrimal glands, and supporting the orbital vessels and nerves. **c. albicans.** A white, fibrous scar in an ovary; it is produced by the degeneration of a corpus luteum. **c. callosum.** The great transverse commissure connecting the cerebral hemispheres; a broad, arched band of white matter at the bottom of the longitudinal fissure of the cerebrum. **c. delicti.** The body of facts necessary to establish that a crime has been committed. **c. hemorrhagicum.** A collapsed Graafian follicle containing blood; an early phase of a corpus luteum. **c. luteum.** The yellow endocrine body formed in the ovary in the site of a ruptured Graafian follicle. The large **corpus luteum of pregnancy** is called a **true corpus luteum;** the smaller **corpus luteum of menstruation** is called a **false corpus luteum.**

cor'pus·cle (kor'pus·ul, kor'pus"ul). 1. A small rounded body. 2. An encapsulated sensory nerve end-organ. 3. Old term for cell, especially a blood cell. —**corpus'cular,** *adj.* **blood corpuscles.** See *erythrocyte, leukocyte.* **colostrum c.** One of the phagocytic cells of the mammary glands, found in the colostrum, containing fat globules. These corpuscles are present for the first two weeks after parturition and may again appear when the milk is diminishing. After the third day, the globules are freed by the bursting of cells, to form the true milk. Also called *colostrum body.* **lamellar c.** See Pacinian *c.* **Meissner's c.** An ovoid corpuscle connected with one or more myelinated nerve fibers which lose their sheaths as they enter the capsule, make several spiral turns, and break up into a complex network of branches. Found, especially, in the papillae of the volar surfaces of the fingers and toes. **milk c.** (a) The detached, fat-drop filled, distal portion of a glandular cell of the mammary gland, constricted off from the rest of the cell body in apocrine secretion. It breaks down, freeing milk globules. (b) See milk *globule.* **Pacinian c.** A large, ellipsoidal corpuscle made up of many concentric lamellas of connective tissue around a core containing the termination of a nerve fiber. Found in the deeper layers of the skin, under mucous membranes, in association with tendons, intermuscular septums, periosteum, and serous membranes. Also called *lamellar c., c. of Vater-Pacini.* **red c.** See *erythrocyte.* **renal c.** The glomerulus together with its glomerular capsule in the cortex of the kidney. Once called *Malpighian c., Malpighian body.* **splenic c.** A lymph nodule of the spleen. Once called *Malpighian c., Malpighian body.* **stellate c.** A type of sensory nerve ending in the skin. Also called *Langerhans' c.* **tactile c.** Any encapsulated nerve end-organ or end-bulb having to do with the sense of touch. Also called *touch c.* **thymic c.** A characteristic, rounded, acidophil body in the medulla of the thymus; composed of hyalinized cells concentrically arranged about a core which is occasionally calcified. Also called *Hassall's body, Hassall's c.*

cor·pus'cu·lum (pl. *corpuscula*). A little body; a corpuscle.

cor·rec'tion. Rectification of any abnormality, as a refractive or muscular defect, or of any undesirable quality, as in a medicine.

cor·rec'tive. 1. Modifying favorably. 2. A substance used to modify or make more pleasant the action of the principal ingredients of a prescription.

cor"re·la'tion. 1. *In biometry,* the degree of association between two characteristics in a series of observations, usually expressed as the coefficient of correlation. 2. *In neurology,* the combination of nervous impulses in sensory centers resulting in adaptive reactions.

cor"re·spond'ence. The adaptation of things to each other. **abnormal retinal c.** A condition found in concomitant strabismus, in which the retinal image formed at the macula of the fixing eye is associated with the image formed at the extramacular area of the retina of the squinting eye. Also called *binocular false projection, retinal incongruity.*

cor·ro'sion. Process of eating away or the resulting state.

cor·ro'sive. 1. Eating away. 2. A substance that destroys organic tissue either by direct chemical means or by causing inflammation and suppuration. **cor·ro'sive sub'li·mate.** See *mercury* bichloride.

cor'set. *In surgery,* a removable appliance embracing the trunk from pelvis to chest; used for correction of deformities, for support of injured bones and muscles of spine or thorax, or in control of ventral hernia, etc. Also called *surgical c.*

cortate. Trade-mark for desoxycorticosterone acetate.

cortef. A trade-mark for hydrocortisone.

cor'tex (pl. *cortices*). 1. The bark of an exogenous plant. 2. The surface layer of an organ. 3. The external gray layer of the brain; cerebral cortex. 4. The peripheral portion of an organ, situated just beneath the capsule. —**cortical,** *adj.* **fetal c. of the adrenals.** See *androgenic zone.*

cor'ti·ces. Plural of cortex, *q.v.*

cor'ti·co-. A combining form denoting *cortex* or *cortical.*

cor"ti·co·ster'oid (kor"ti·ko·ster'-oid). Any steroid that has certain properties characteristic of the hormones secreted by the adrenal cortex.

cor"ti·cos'te·rone. An adrenal cortical hormone, steroid in nature, which has an influence on carbohydrate metabolism, electrolyte metabolism, muscular efficiency, and protects against stress.

cor"ti·co·tro'phin. World Health Organization designation for corticotropin.

cor"ti·co·tro'pin (kor"ti·ko·tro'-pin). A hormone secreted by the anterior pituitary that controls the activity of the adrenal cortex. Also called *corticotropic hormone, pituitary adrenocorticotropic hormone, ACTH.*

cor'tin. An extract of adrenal cortex; contains several hormones; is life-sustaining in bilaterally adrenalectomized individuals.

cortinoral. Trade-mark for a lipid fraction of adrenal cortex extract offered in capsule form.

cor'ti·sone. 17-Hydroxy-11-dehydrocorticosterone, an adrenal cortex hormone, also prepared by partial synthesis from desoxycholic acid; has been found to exert a beneficial influence on rheumatoid arthritis, rheumatic fever, and many other collagen diseases, as well as in asthma, hay fever, and states caused by hypersensitivity. Also called *Kendall's Compound E.*

cortone. Trade-mark for 17-hydroxy-11-dehydrocorticosterone, *q.v.*

cortril. A trade-mark for hydrocortisone.

cor″us·ca′tion. The subjective sensation of light flashes.

co·ryd′a·line. An alkaloid from *Corydalis tuberosa.*

co·ryd′a·lis. The tuber of *Dicentra canadensis*, squirrel corn, or of *D. cucullaria*, Dutchman's-breeches, containing several alkaloids. Corydalis has been used as a tonic and alterative.

cor″y·loph′il·line (kor″i·lof′i-leen, ·lin). An antibiotic identical with *Escherichia coli* factor, mycoin, notatin, penatin, and penicillin-B.

Co·ry″ne·bac·te′ri·um. A genus of slender, aerobic, nonmotile, nonspore-forming, Gram-positive bacteria of which **C. diphtheriae** is the type species; varying from slightly curved to club-shaped and branching forms; showing irregular staining. This genus includes a large group of diphtheroid bacilli, such as **C. acnes**, and **C. pyogenes**, mainly saprophytic and morphologically similar to *C. diphtheriae;* found in normal tissues and secretions as well as in pathologic conditions; probably not causative. **C. diphtheriae.** The causative organism of diphtheria; the varieties *gravis* and *mitis* have been described; produces both an exotoxin and an endotoxin.

co·ry′za. See *common cold.*

cos·met′ic. 1. Beautifying. 2. A preparation applied to the skin or its appendages to alter its appearance, to protect it, to beautify, or to promote attractiveness.

cos′ta (pl. *costae*). A rib. **—costal,** *adj.* **costae fluctuantes.** Floating ribs. **costae spuriae.** False ribs. **costae verae.** True ribs.

cos·tal′gi·a. Intercostal neuralgia; pain in the ribs.

cos·tec′to·my. Excision of a rib or a part of one.

cos′to-. A combining form denoting a rib or costa.

cos″to·car′ti·lage. A costal cartilage or unossified sternal rib.

cos″to·chon′dral (kos″to·kon′-drul). Pertaining to the ribs and their cartilages.

cos″to·phren′ic. Pertaining to the ribs and the diaphragm.

cos′to·tome. Heavy curved shears or forceps with a hooked limb against which the knife blade acts; used for rib resection.

cos·tot′o·my. Division of a rib.

cos″to·trans″ver·sec′to·my (·trans″vur·seck′to-mee, ·tranz″vur·). Excision of part of a rib and a transverse vertebral process.

cos″to·ver′te·bral. Pertaining to a rib and the vertebral column; applied to the joints between them.

cot. A small bed.

cot. The finger of a glove, or other covering to protect a finger.

co·tar′nine (ko-tahr′neen, ·nin). $C_{12}H_{15}NO_4$. An oxidation product of narcotine. **c. chloride.** Small yellow crystals, soluble in water and alcohol; has been used in uterine hemorrhage and hemoptysis. See *stypticin.*

co′to. Coto bark; the bark of a tree native to Bolivia, *Aniba coto.* It contains a bitter principle, cotoin, irritant to the skin and mucous membranes.

co″trans·am′in·ase. Pyridoxal phosphate; the component of certain transaminating enzymes, as well as of the enzyme carboxylase which catalyzes decarboxylation of L-amino-acids, in which latter case it is commonly referred to as *codecarboxylase.*

cot′ton. The hairs of the seed of cultivated varieties and some species of *Gossypium.* **absorbent c.** Cotton prepared so as to absorb moisture readily. **c. wool.** Raw cotton. **styptic c.** Cotton saturated with a styptic substance.

cot′ton-oil. Cottonseed oil.

cot′ton-seed oil. A fixed oil obtained from the seeds of the cotton plant, used as a nutrient, emollient, cathartic, vehicle for injectable medicinals, and in the manufacture of soap.

cot″y·le′don. 1. Any one of the groups of villi separated by smooth chorion characteristic of the ruminant semiplacenta. 2. Any one of the rounded lobules bounded by placental septums into which the uterine surface of a discoidal placenta is divided. 3. Any plant of the genus *Cotyledon.* 4. The primary or seed leaf in the embryo of a flowering plant.

cough. A sudden, violent expulsion of air after deep inspiration and closure of the glottis. **dry c.** That unattended by expectoration. **moist c.** One with free expectoration. **pleuritic c.** The dry, short, frequent cough of pleurisy, pneumonia, and phthisis, which accompanies the pain and friction sounds of pleurisy and disappears with effusion or when bronchitis supervenes. **productive c.** One in which mucus or exudate is raised by coughing. **reflex c.** One produced by irritation of a remote organ. **whooping c.** See *whooping cough.* **winter c.** A short troublesome cough of old people due to chronic bronchitis and recurring every winter.

cou·lomb′ (kōō-lom′, kōō′lom). A unit of electric quantity; the amount of electricity conveyed per second by a current of one ampere.

coumadin sodium. Trade-mark for warfarin sodium.

cou'ma·rin (koo'muh·rin). The lactone of orthohydroxycinnamic acid; found widely distributed in the vegetable kingdom, especially in tonka bean, and also prepared synthetically. It is used solely for its odorous quality.

cou·min'gine (koo·min'jeen, ·jin). An alkaloid having a digitalislike action; obtained from *Erythrophleum couminga.*

count. The number obtained by reckoning the units of a series or collection, as blood count, the number of blood cells per unit volume of blood. **Addis c.** The number of cells found in 10 cc. of a 12-hr. specimen of urine indicates the total precipitation. **direct platelet c.** Using the red cell pipet, platelet diluting fluid is drawn to the 1 mark, blood from a fresh puncture wound is quickly drawn to the 0.5 mark, and diluting fluid then drawn to the 101 mark. The pipet is shaken for two minutes and the platelets counted on the counting chamber by the method used for red blood cells. Normal ranges are 250,000 to 350,000 per cubic millimeter. **parasite c.** The number of parasites infecting a certain volume of blood. This has been used in trypanosomiasis and malaria. It is considered to be unreliable in the latter since there may be no organisms in the peripheral blood at certain times in the course of the disease. Originally used to estimate the susceptibility of a community. See parasite *index.*

coun"ter·ac'tion. Action of a drug or agent opposed to that of some other drug or agent.

coun"ter·ex·ten"sion. Traction made in a direction opposite to that in which traction is made by another force.

coun"ter·ir'ri·tant. An agent which produces an inflammation of the skin for the relief of a more deep-seated inflammation. **—counterirrita'tion,** *n.*

coun'ter·o"pen·ing. A second incision into an abscess or cavity, made opposite to the first, for purposes of drainage.

coun'ter·pres"sure. Manipulation to counterbalance pressure by exercising force in the opposite direction.

coun'ter·trac"tion. In *surgery,* a traction which offsets another, as in reducing fractures. See *counterextension.*

cov'er glass. In *microscopy,* the thin slip of glass covering the object mounted on the slide.

cow'pox". Vaccinia, *q.v.*

cox'a (pl. *coxae*). The hip or hip joint. See Table of Bones in the Appendix. **c. plana.** Osteochondritis deformans

juvenilis. **c. valga.** A condition, the reverse of coxa vara, in which the angle between the neck and the shaft of the femur is increased above 140 degrees. **malum coxae senile.** Hypertrophic arthritis of the hip.

cox·al'gi·a, cox'al"gy. Literally, pain in the hip joint, but generally used synonymously with hip disease. **—cox·algic,** *adj.*

cox·i'tis. Inflammation of the hip joint. **senile c.** A rheumatoid disease of the hip joint occurring in old people; marked by pain, stiffness, and wasting, with no tendency to suppuration.

C.P. Chemically pure.

Cr. Chemical symbol for chromium.

cracked'-pot sound. A peculiar sound, elicited by percussion over a pulmonary cavity communicating with a bronchus.

cra'dle. A frame of wicker, wood, or wire, used to prevent the bedclothes from coming in contact with a fractured or injured part.

cramp. 1. Painful, involuntary contraction of a muscle, such as occurs in swimmers. 2. Any cramplike pain, as of the gut. 3. Paralysis of certain muscles; may be intermittent, as in tetany, or occupational, resulting from their excessive use. 4. In *gynecology,* a colloquial term for dysmenorrhea. **heat cramps.** Pain in the muscles, with nausea and vomiting; occurring during hard work in a hot environment; due to loss of salt through perspiration. Also called *miner's c., stoker's c.* **writer's c.** An occupational neurosis occurring in those who write constantly with a pen or pencil; characterized by painful spasm of the muscles of the forearm, hand, and fingers; now seen infrequently.

cra'ni·ad. Cephalad.

cra'ni·al. Pertaining to the cranium.

cra'ni·ec'to·my. Surgical removal of strips or pieces of the cranial bones.

cra'ni·o-. A combining form denoting *the cranium, the fetal head, cranial.*

cra'ni·oc'la·sis, cra'ni·o·clas"ty. Operation of breaking the fetal head by means of the cranioclast.

cra'ni·o·clast. Heavy forceps for crushing the fetal head.

cra"ni·o·clei"do·dys·os·to'sis (kray"nee·o·kly"do·dis·os·to'sis). Congenital defect of the clavicles associated with imperfect ossification of the bones of the cranium.

cra"ni·o·did'y·mus. Craniopagus.

cra"ni·om'e·ter. A caliper used for measuring the dimensions of the skull.

cra"ni·om'e·try. The science and technic of measuring the skull in order to establish exact, comparable, metric records for use in the comparative study of physical types, variation, and individual peculiarities in the skulls of man and the other primates. —**cra·niomet'ric**, *adj.*

cra"ni·op'a·gus. Conjoined twins united by their heads.

cra"ni·op'a·thy. Any disease of the head.

cra"ni·o·plas"ty. Surgical correction of cranial deficiencies.

cra"ni·o·sa'cral. Of or relating to the cranium and the sacrum, as craniosacral outflow.

cra"ni·os'chi·sis (kray"nee-os'ki-sis). Congenital fissure of the cranium.

cra"ni·o·ste·no'sis. Premature closing of the cranial sutures, resulting in a small cranium.

cra"ni·o·ta'bes (kray"nee-o·tay'-beez). An atrophy of the cranial bones occurring in infancy, with the formation of small, shallow, conical pits in the bone substance. It results from rickets, syphilis, or marasmus. —**cra·niotabet'ic**, *adj.*

cra"ni·ot'o·my. 1. Operation of reducing the size of the fetal head by cutting or breaking when delivery is otherwise impossible. 2. Excision of a part of the skull.

cra'ni·um. The part of the skull that contains the brain, its membranes and vessels. See *skull.* See Table of Bones in the Appendix.

cra"ter·i·za'tion (*of bone*). The removal of a piece of bone, leaving a crater, as in operations for osteomyelitis.

cream. The part of milk rich in butterfat.

creamalin. Trade-mark for an aluminum hydroxide gel.

cream of tar'tar. Potassium bitartrate, $KHC_4H_4O_6$; it is diuretic and aperient.

cre'a·tine (kree'uh-teen, -tin). Methylguanidinoacetic acid, present in animal tissues, particularly muscle. See Table of Normal Values of Blood Constituents in the Appendix. **c. phosphate.** Phosphocreatine. **dehydrated c.** Creatinine.

cre"a·tine·phos·phor'ic acid (kree"uh-teen-, -tin-). See *phosphocreatine.*

cre·at'i·nine (kree-at'i-neen, -nin). A normal constituent of blood and urine, and a waste product of creatine, excreted in the urine at a constant rate. See Table of Normal Values of Blood Constituents in the Appendix.

cre·mas'ter (kree-mass'tur). The muscle that draws up the testis. See Table of Muscles in the Appendix. —**cremaster'ic**, *adj.*

cre·ma'tion. Destruction of a dead body by burning, as distinguished from interment. —**cre'mate**, *v.*

cre'ma·to"ry. 1. Establishment for burning the bodies of the dead. 2. Incinerator.

cre'nate, cre'nat·ed (kree'nay-tid). 1. Notched or scalloped. 2. *In botany,* denoting leaves that are serrated.

cre·na'tion (kree-nay'shun). A notched or cogwheel-like appearance of shrunken red blood corpuscles. Seen when they are exposed to the air or to hypertonic saline solutions.

cre'o·sol. 4-Hydroxy-3-methoxy-methylbenzene, one of the principal phenols contained in creosote.

cre'o·sote. A mixture of phenols obtained by the distillation of wood tar. Creosote is antiseptic, astringent, styptic, anesthetic, and escharotic. Used in pulmonary tuberculosis. **beechwood c.** That obtained from beechwood. **c. carbonate.** A mixture of the carbonates of various constituents of creosote.

crep"i·ta'ti·o (krep"i·tay'shee-o), **crep"i·ta'tion, crep'i·tus.** 1. The grating of fractured bones. 2. The crackling of the joints. 3. The noise produced by pressure upon tissues containing an abnormal amount of air or gas, as in cellular emphysema. 4. The sound heard at the end of inspiration in the first stage of croupous pneumonia. It closely resembles the sound produced by rubbing the hair between the fingers held close to the ear. —**crep'itant**, *adj.*

cre'sol. $CH_3.C_6H_4.OH$. A mixture of isomeric cresols obtained from coal tar. A liquid of phenol-like odor; soluble in water. It is used chiefly as a surgical disinfectant, usually in the form of **saponated cresol solution.** Syn., *cresylic acid.*

cre·sot'ic ac'id (kree-sot'ick, -so'-tick), **cres"o·tin'ic ac'id.** Hydroxytoluic acid, methylhydroxybenzoic acid, of which 10 isomers are possible.

crest. A ridge or linear prominence, especially of bone. Also see *crista.* **alveolar c.** The rim of a socket for the root of a tooth in the alveolar process. Syn., *limbus alveolaris.* **iliac c.** The thickened and expanded upper border of the ilium. **neural c.** A band of ectodermal cells on either side of the neural tube which is the primordium of the cranial and spinal ganglions. Syn., *ganglionic c.*

cres'yl·ate. Any compound of cresol with a metallic radical.

cres'yl blue. See *brilliant cresyl blue.*

cres'yl·ic ac'id. Cresol.

cres'yl vi'o·let (kress'il, kree'sil) (C.C.). A basic dye of the oxazine group, having strongly metachromatic properties; used for staining nervous tissue and fresh tumor tissue. Also called *cresylecht violet, cresyl fast violet.*

cre'ta. Chalk. Native calcium carbonate. —**creta'ceous**, *adj.*

cre'tin·ism. A condition originating in fetal life or early infancy, due to severe thyroid deficiency; characterized by stunting of physical and mental development. Typically, the large tongue protrudes, the subcutaneous tissue is thickened, the skin is dry, the abdomen protrudes, the mentality is of idiot grade, and the stature is dwarfish. Commonest in regions where endemic goiter is severe; elsewhere it occurs sporadically. —**cretinous,** *adj.;* **cretinoid,** *adj., n.;* **cretin,** *n.* **acquired c.** Myxedema. Also called *adult c.*

crib'ri·form. Perforated like a sieve.

crick. Any painful spasmodic affection, as of the back or neck.

cri'coid. 1. Ring-shaped. 2. The signet-ring-shaped cartilage of the larynx.

cri"co·thy'roid. 1. Pertaining to the cricoid and thyroid cartilages. 2. The muscle, attached to the cricoid and thyroid cartilages, which tenses the vocal folds.

crin'o·gen'ic. Stimulating the production of secretions.

cri'sis. 1. A turning point, as that of a disease or fever; especially, the sudden favorable termination of the acute symptoms of an infectious disease. 2. Paroxysmal disturbance of function accompanied with pain. —**crit'ical,** *adj.* **anxiety c.** Anxiety attack, *q.v.* **cardiac c.** A paroxysm of cardiac distress or disordered action. **Dietl's c.** Severe nephralgia, chills, nausea, vomiting, and collapse resulting from angulation of the ureter. **gastric crises.** Attacks of intense, paroxysmal pain in the abdomen, often attended with vomiting. They occur in tabes dorsalis. **hemoclastic c.** A condition occurring during anaphylactic shock; characterized by temporary leukopenia, relative lymphocytosis, red cell destruction, altered blood coagulability, and fall in blood pressure. Seen in those who have poor liver function. **oculogyric crises.** Recurrent attacks of tonic conjugate deviation of the eyes, usually upward, lasting from a few seconds to an hour or more; a sequel of lethargic encephalitis. **spastic vasoconstrictive c.** One characterized by increased distress on lying down, pain, tympanites, and a marked and sudden increase of arterial hypertension. **tabetic c.** Paroxysmal pain occurring in the course of tabes dorsalis. **vesical c.** Paroxysmal attack of bladder pain, with difficulty in urination, seen in tabes dorsalis.

cris'ta. Crest, *q.v.* —**cristate,** *adj.* **c. galli.** The superior triangular process of the ethmoid bone, so called because it is shaped like a cock's comb.

cross match'ing. A test to establish blood compatibility before trans-fusion, by mixing the blood serum of the recipient with the blood cells of the donor, and vice versa. If agglutination or hemolysis does not occur in either test, the bloods are considered compatible. See also *blood groups.*

cross sec'tion. A section or slice made at a right angle to an axis, most commonly the longer axis.

crot'a·line (krot'uh·leen, kro'tuh·). 1. A protein found in the venom of rattlesnakes. 2. A preparation of venom from the rattlesnakes, *Crotalus horridus* and *C. adamanteus,* which has been used for immunization against snake bites.

crotch'et. A hook used in extracting the fetus after craniotomy.

cro·tam'i·ton. N-Ethyl-o-crotonotoluide, a scabicide. See *eurax.*

Cro'ton. A genus of plants of the Euphorbiaceae. **C. eluteria.** Yields cascarilla. **C. tiglium.** Yields croton oil.

cro'ton oil. A fixed oil obtained from seeds of the tree *Croton tiglium,* which acts as a drastic purgative and as a skin irritant. See croton tiglium *poisoning.*

cro"ton·al'de·hyde. CH₃CH:CH-CHO. A colorless, pungent liquid; used as a component of tear gas and as an intermediate in chemical syntheses.

cro'ton chlo'ral hy'drate. See *butyl-chloral hydrate.*

croup (kroōp). A condition of the larynx seen in children; characterized by a harsh, brassy cough and crowing, difficult respiration. It may be due to edema, inflammation with or without exudate or membrane formation, or spasm. **catarrhal c.** Usually occurs at night, during the course of an upper respiratory infection.

croup ket'tle. A small boiler with an attached inhaling tube. Water or medicament is placed in the receptacle, heated, and the steam inhaled or allowed to escape to humidify the air in the room.

crown. Corona; the top part of anything; any structure like a crown. **c. of a tooth.** That part covered with enamel. **jacket c.** An artificial restoration of the crown of a tooth; consists of a covering of metal, porcelain, or acrylic. **pivot c.** *In dentistry,* a tooth crown of porcelain or other material, attached to the root by means of a pin or post.

cru'cial. Resembling or pertaining to a cross, as a crucial incision.

cru'ci·ble. Vessel of clay or other suitable material used in melting substances which require a high degree of heat.

cru'ci·form. Crucial; shaped like a cross.

crus (pl. *crura*). A term applied to

certain parts of the body, from their resemblance to legs or roots. —**cru'ral**, adj.

crust. A covering; especially, a dried exudate on the skin.

crus'ta. A thin layer; crust, q.v.

c. lactea. Seborrhea of the scalp in infants.

crutch. A staff used as a support in walking, having a concave, padded crosspiece to fit the axilla, and a grip for the hand. **Canadian c.** A hand crutch. Also called *Toronto c.* **hand c.** A crutchlike support in which the weight of the body is partially borne by the hand and arm instead of by the axilla. The device is used in training the individual to use an artificial leg or legs after the usual crutch stage of training is ended. **perineal c.** A support or brace attached to an operating table to hold a patient in certain positions.

cry. The utterance of an inarticulate vocal sound, or the sound so uttered; the sound of the voice in lamentation. **cry-.** See *cryo-*.

cry·an″es·the'si·a (cry-an″ess-thee'zhuh, -zee-uh). Loss of sensation or perception of cold.

cry″es·the'si·a (cry″ess-thee'zhuh, -zee-uh). 1. Temperature sense for cold. 2. Sensitiveness to cold.

cry'o-, cry-. A combining form meaning *cold* or *freezing.*

cry'o·cau'ter·y. The destruction of tissues by application of extreme cold which causes an obliterative thrombosis; used especially in removing moles.

cry'o·glob'u·lin. Globulin which precipitates in the cold; it is found in cases of leukemia or myeloma.

cry·om'e·ter (crye-om'i·tur). Thermometer for measuring low temperatures.

cry'o·scope. Device for determining the freezing point of a liquid.

cry'o·stat. Any device for maintaining very low temperatures: specifically, a refrigerator that operates by compressing, regeneratively cooling, and then expanding helium gas until part of the gas becomes liquid; can cool contents to −450° F.

cry″o·ther'a·py. The therapeutic application of cold.

crypt. 1. A small sac or follicle. 2. A glandular cavity. **crypts of Lieberkühn.** Simple tubular intestinal glands. Also called *Lieberkühn's glands.* **tonsillar c.** A deep epithelium-lined invagination in the palatine or lingual tonsils, surrounded by lymphatic tissue.

cryp·ten'a·mine. A mixture of alkaloids from veratrum viride, used as a hypotensive. See *unitensen.*

cryp'to-, crypt-. A combining form meaning *hidden, covered, secret.*

cryp'to·gam. In botany, one of the Cryptogamia, a division of the vegetable kingdom comprising all plants without flowers or seeds, as the algae, fungi, mosses, and ferns. —**cryptog'amous,** adj.

cryp″to·gen'ic. Of unknown or obscure cause; the opposite of *phanerogenic.*

cryp'to·lith. A concretion or calculus formed within a crypt, as in the tonsil.

cryp″toph·thal'mos. 1. Congenital union of the eyelids, usually over imperfect eyes. 2. A person who has congenital union of the eyelids.

cryp'to·pine (krip'to-peen, -pin). One of the minor alkaloids of opium; colorless and odorless.

crypt·or'chism (kript-or'kiz·um). A developmental defect in which the testes fail to descend, and remain within the abdomen or inguinal canal. —**cryptorchid, cryptorchis,** n.

cryp″to·xan'thin (krip″to-zan'thin). A carotenoid pigment found in yellow corn and certain other natural sources, and which acts like vitamin A in the body.

crys'tal. In chemistry, a substance that assumes a definite geometric form. **Charcot-Leyden crystals.** Colorless, pointed, often needle-like crystals occurring in the sputum in bronchial asthma and in the feces in amebic dysentery and other ulcerative diseases of the colon. Also called *asthma crystals.* **hematoidin crystals.** Yellowish or brown, needle-like or rhombic crystals which may occur in the feces after hemorrhages in the gastrointestinal tract. Formerly called *Virchow's crystals.*

crys'tal·line (kris'tuh·lin, -lyne). Like a crystal.

crys″tal·li·za'tion. The process by which the molecules of a substance arrange themselves in geometric forms when passing from a gaseous or a liquid state to a solid state.

crys″tal·log'ra·phy. The science of crystals, their formation, structure, and classification.

crys'tal·loid. Having a crystal-like nature, as distinguished from colloid.

crys″tal·lo·mag'net·ism. The property common to certain crystals of orienting themselves in a magnetic field.

crys″tal·lo·pho'bi·a. A morbid fear of glass.

crys'tal·lose. Sodium saccharinate.

crys″tal·lu'ri·a. The presence of crystals in the urine; often a normal condition but of importance when the crystals are of the sulfa drugs since the crystals may form in the kidney tubules and cause blocking.

crys'tal vi'o·let (C.C.). A basic dye of the triphenylmethane group, hexamethyl pararosaniline. A constituent of all the bluer shades of methyl violet and gentian violet. Also called *hexamethyl violet, methyl violet 10B, gentian violet.*

CTAB. Trade-mark for cetyltrimethylammonium bromide or cetrimide, *q.v.*

Cten″o·ce·phal′i·des (ten″o-si-fal′i-deez, tee″no-). A genus of fleas which are cosmopolitan in distribution. The species **Ct. canis,** the dog flea, and **Ct. felis,** the cat flea, while they infest primarily dogs and cats, may attack man and other mammals. Members of this genus also serve as intermediate hosts of the *Dipylidium caninum.*

Cu. Chemical symbol for copper.

cu′beb. The dried, unripe, nearly full-grown fruit of *Piper cubeba,* cultivated in Java and the West Indies and containing a volatile oil. It has been used as a diuretic, urinary antiseptic, and expectorant.

cu′bo-. A combining form denoting *a cube* or *cubital.*

cu′boid. Resembling a cube.

cu·boi′de·o-. See *cubo-.*

Cu′cu·mis. A genus of plants of the Cucurbitaceae. **C. melo.** Muskmelon; a species indigenous to the old-world tropics and widely cultivated. **C. sativus.** Cucumber; the juice of the fruit has been used in skin diseases and as a cosmetic.

Cu·cur′bi·ta. A genus of plants of the Cucurbitaceae. Several species, such as **C. pepo,** the pumpkin, yield seeds that have been used as anthelmintics.

cud′bear. A powder prepared from species of *Roccella, Lecanora,* or other lichens; it is used as a red coloring agent.

cui·rass′ (kwee·rass′, kwee′rass). A close-fitting or immovable bandage for the front of the chest.

cul-de-sac (kul′-di-sack′, kōōl′-). 1. A closed or blind pouch or sac. 2. The rectouterine pouch; the prolongation of the peritoneal cavity between the anterior surface of the rectum and the posterior surface of the uterus. Also called *pouch of Douglas.*

cul′do·scope. An instrument for the visual examination of the uterus, tubes, and ovaries. **—culdos′copy,** *n.*

Cu′lex. A genus of mosquitoes which are vectors of disease. **C. fatigans.** The most important intermediate host of *Wuchereria bancrofti.* **C. pipiens.** This species is known as the common house mosquito and is found in temperate regions; of medical importance as a vector of filariasis. **C. quinquefasciatus.** A mosquito which is the most common vector of *Wuchereria bancrofti.* Also called *C. fatigans.*

cu′li·cide. Any agent which destroys mosquitoes.

Cu″li·ci′nae (cue″li·sigh′nee). A subfamily of the Culicidae; contains all species of mosquitoes of medical significance, which are important as vectors of filariasis, malaria, hemoglobinuric fever, dengue, and yellow fever.

Cu″li·coi′des (cue″li·koy′deez). A genus of flies, several species of which serve as intermediate hosts of filarial parasites. **C. austeni** and **C. grahami** are species which transmit the nonperiodic filarial worm, *Acanthocheilonema perstans;* **C. furens** has been found to transmit *Mansonella ozzardi.*

cult. Any spurious or unorthodox system of healing, usually based on the belief that all disease is due to a single underlying cause and can be cured by some simple treatment.

cul″ti·va′tion. Successive transferring of organisms to different mediums favorable to growth. See *culture.*

cul′ture. 1. Growth of microörganisms on artificial mediums. 2. Act of cultivating microörganisms on artificial mediums. 3. A group of microörganisms grown in an artificial medium. **c. medium.** A substance used for cultivating bacteria. Culture mediums are either liquid or solid, bouillon and milk being the important liquid mediums, and gelatin, agar, blood serum, and potato the principal solid mediums. **hanging-drop c.** A culture in which the microörganism is inoculated into a drop of fluid on a cover glass and the latter is inverted over a glass slide having a central concavity. **plate c.** A culture of bacteria on a medium spread upon a flat plate or in a Petri dish. **pure c.** A culture of a single microörganism. **slant c.** One made on the slanting surface of a medium, to get a greater surface for growth. **stab c.** One in which the medium is inoculated by means of a needle bearing the microörganisms, which is inserted deeply into the medium. **thrust c.** Stab culture. **tissue c.** The growing of tissue cells in artificial mediums.

cu′mene. C₆H₁₂. Cumol; isopropyl benzene. A hydrocarbon occurring in pine tar, petroleum, and some volatile oils.

cu′mu·la″tive. Increasing; adding to.

cu′mu·lus. A heap or mound. **c. oöphorus.** The mass of follicular cells surrounding the ovum and protruding into the liquid-filled cavity of a Graafian follicle. Syn., *discus proligerus.*

cu′ne·ate. Wedge-shaped, as cuneate fasciculus, a fiber tract in the posterior funiculus of the spinal cord.

cu·ne′i·form, **cu′ne·i·form.** Wedge-shaped; cuneate.

cu′ne·o-. A combining form meaning *a wedge* and denoting *cuneiform.*

cun″ni·lin′gus. An abnormal sexual practice consisting of the licking of the vulva. **—cunnilinguist,** *n.*

cu′o·rin. $C_{71}H_{125}O_{21}NP_2$. A phospholipin which has been isolated from heart muscle.

cup. 1. A drinking vessel. 2. To bleed. **feeding c.** A cup used in the forcible feeding of the insane. **suction c.** A cupping glass.

cu′po·la. The dome of the diaphragm.

cup′ping. 1. A method of bloodletting by means of the application of cupping glasses to the surface of the body. 2. Formation of a cuplike depression. **c. glass.** A small bell-shaped glass capable of holding three to four ounces, in which the air is rarefied by heat or by exhaustion; the glass is applied to the skin, either with or without scarification of the latter. **dry c.** A form of counterirritation in which the blood is drawn to the surface by means of a cup. This is used mainly in inflammatory affections of the lung. **wet c.** The abstraction of blood after scarification.

cu′pre·a bark. The bark of certain species of *Remijia.* It was at one time used as a substitute for cinchona bark.

cu′pre·ine (cu′pree·een, ·in). An alkaloid, $C_{19}H_{22}O_2N_2.2H_2O$, derived from cuprea bark.

cu′pric. Containing copper as a bivalent element. See *copper.*

cu′prous. Containing copper as a univalent element. See *copper.*

cu′prum. See *copper.*

cu·ra′re (cu·rah′ree). A drug of uncertain and variable composition prepared from several species of *Strychnos* and *Chondodendron* plants. Curare from *Chondodendron tomentosum,* currently of chief medical interest, owes its characteristic action to the base *d*-tubocurarine, which paralyzes the skeletal muscles by a selective blocking of the neuromuscular junction. **—cu′rarize,** *v.*

cu·ra′ri·form. Pertaining to or designating a drug that acts like curare.

cu·ra′rine (cu·rah′reen, cure′uh·). An alkaloid isolated from a curare by Boehm (1898); now called *d-tubocurarine.*

cu″ra·ri·za′tion. The subjection to the full influence of curare. Voice and power of motion are generally abolished, but not sensibility to pain.

cu·ra·tive. Having a healing tendency.

cur′cu·ma. Turmeric. The rhizome of *Curcuma longa,* of India, a plant of the Zingiberaceae, with properties similar to ginger. Used as a coloring matter, and indicator.

cur′cu·min. The crystalline coloring matter of curcuma. Used as an indicator and dye.

curd. The coagulum that separates from milk on the addition of rennin or acids.

cure. 1. Heal or make well. 2. The successful treatment of an illness or a wound. 3. Special treatment for a disease or an invalid.

cu·ret′. 1. An instrument, shaped like a spoon or scoop, for scraping away exuberant or dead tissue. 2. Scrape with a curet. **suction c.** A small hollow tube with a cutting window to which suction may be applied; used for obtaining endometrial biopsy.

cu·ret′tage (cue·ret′idj, cure″i·tahzh′). *In surgery,* scraping of the interior of a cavity with a curet, or by the finger.

Curie, Marie Sklodowska [*Polish-French chemist,* 1867–1934]. Internationally renowned for her discovery of radium (with her husband, Pierre Curie) and for her continued investigation of the nature of radium and radioactive substances. Received Nobel award jointly with Pierre Curie and A. H. Becquerel (1903) and the undivided award (1911).

cu′rie (cure′ee, koor′ee). 1. Formerly, the amount of radon in equilibrium with one gram of radium. 2. That quantity of any radioactive species (radioisotope) undergoing exactly 3.70×10^{10} disintegrations per second.

cu′rie·gram (cure′ee·gram, koor′ee·gram). A photographic print made by radium rays, similar to a roentgenogram.

cu′rine (cure′een, ·in). An alkaloid obtained from a kind of curare.

cu′ri·um. Chemical element No. 96, symbol Cm, produced artificially.

cur′rent. The rate at which electricity (electrons) flows through a circuit. **action c.** The electric current accompanying activity of any reacting tissue. **alternating c.** A current which changes its direction a number of times per second. Abbreviated, A. C. **convection c.** A current of a liquid or gas heated to a temperature above that of the surrounding medium; it rises due to its lesser density, resulting in the circulation of the entire fluid or gas until it acquires the same temperature. **D′Arsonval c.** A high-frequency oscillating current used in electrotherapy; it is of low voltage and high amperage. **direct c.** A current which flows continuously in one direction, in contradistinction to an alternating current. **eye c.** The normal electric current that passes from the retina to the optic nerve under the stimulus of light. **faradic c.** A current produced by an induction coil. **galvanic c.** A direct current from a galvanic battery. **high-frequency** c. A rapidly alternating electric current. See D'Arsonval c., Oudin c., Tesla c. **induction** c. Current produced in a coil of insulated wire by a changing magnetic field of force surrounding the coil. **interrupted** c. A current that is alternately opened and closed. **Oudin** c. A high-frequency current from only one pole or terminal, used in electrotherapy. **primary** c. A current which, on opening and closing, produces an induced current in an adjacent coil. **secondary** c. Momentary current produced in a coil of insulated wire, introduced within the field of another coil, when the circuit is made or broken in the latter. **Tesla** c. A high-frequency oscillating current used in electrotherapy; it is of medium voltage.

cur'va·ture. A bending or curving. See *curve*. **angular** c. The deformity resulting from tuberculosis of the vertebrae. Also called *Pott's c.* **compensatory** c. In spinal curvature, a secondary curve, occurring as the result of the efforts of the trunk to maintain its upright position. **c. of the spine.** Bending of the vertebral column. See *kyphosis; lordosis; scoliosis*.

curve. 1. A bending or flexure; a curvature, *q.v.* 2. *In biometry*, a line, usually curved, which in a graphic representation indicates the relationship between an independent and a dependent variable. **temperature** c. A graphic curve showing variations in temperature for a given period.

cus'co bark. The bark of *Cinchona pelletierana* (Rubiaceae), yielding several minor alkaloids of the quinoline group.

cush'ion. *In anatomy*, an aggregate of adipose and fibrous tissue relieving pressure upon tissues lying beneath.

cusp. 1. A pointed or rounded eminence on or near the masticating surface of a tooth. 2. One of the leaflets of a valve in the heart or in a vessel. **—cus'pate, cus'pated,** *adj.*

cus'pid. A canine tooth, *q.v.* **—cuspidal, cuspidate, cuspidated,** *adj.*

cu·ta'ne·ous. Pertaining to the skin.

cu'ti-. A combining form meaning *skin*.

cu'ti·cle. 1. A horny or chitinous, sometimes calcified, layer formed by and covering an epithelium. 2. Popular term for epidermis. **—cutic'ular,** *adj.;* **cuticulariza'tion,** *n.* **hair** c. The outermost layer of cells of a hair shaft.

cu·tic'u·la. Cuticle, *q.v.*

cu''ti·fi·ca'tion. Formation of skin.

cu'tin. A waxlike substance found over most of the aerial parts of vascular plants. It serves to protect the underlying cells from too rapid loss of moisture.

cu'tis. The skin. **c. vera.** The corium, or derma.

cu·ti'tis. Dermatitis, *q.v.*

cu''ti·za'tion. Transformation of an exposed mucous membrane into true skin at the mucocutaneous margins.

Cy. Symbol for cyclonium, *q.v.*

cy''an·am'ide (sigh''uh·nam'ide, sigh·an'uh·mide). 1. HN:C:NH. Colorless deliquescent crystals. 2. Calcium cyanamide.

cy'a·nate. The monovalent radical, —C≡N:O.

cy''an·he''mo·glo'bin (sigh''an·hee''mo·glo'bin, ·hem''o·glo'bin). A compound of hydrocyanic acid with hemoglobin formed in cases of poisoning with this acid. It gives the blood a bright red color.

cy·an'ic ac'id (sigh·an'ick). HCNO. A poisonous liquid.

cy'a·nide. The monovalent radical —CN; any compound containing this radical, as potassium cyanide, KCN.

cy'a·no-, cyan-. 1. A combining form meaning *dark blue.* 2. *In chemistry*, a combining form denoting *the presence of the cyanogen group.*

cy·an''o·co·bal'a·min. Crystalline vitamin B_{12}. Also see *cobalamin.*

cy·an'o·gen (sigh·an'o·jen). 1. NC·CN. A colorless toxic gas having the odor of bitter almonds. 2. The radical —CN. See *cyanide.*

cy''a·no·met''he·mo·glo'bin (sigh''uh·no·met''hee·mo·glo'bin, ·hem·o·glo'bin). A relatively nontoxic compound formed by the combination of cyanide and methemoglobin.

cy·an'o·phose (sigh·an'o·foze, sigh'·uh·no·foze''). A blue phose.

cy'a·nosed (sigh'uh·nosed). Affected with cyanosis.

cy''a·no'sis. A bluish tinge in the color of mucous membranes and skin, due to the presence of excessive amounts of reduced hemoglobin in capillaries, less frequently to the presence of methemoglobin. Certain drugs, such as the sulfonamides, may cause cyanosis. **—cyanot'ic,** *adj.* **congenital** c. Cyanosis due to a congenital lesion of the heart or of the great vessels. **delayed** c. See tardive c. **tardive** c. That due to arteriovenous shunt which is terminal or transient, resulting in venous blood entering the systemic circulation in patent ductus arteriosus, or localized defects of aortic, interatrial, and interventricular septums. Syn., *delayed* c.

cy·as'ma (sigh·az'muh) (pl. *cyasmata*). The peculiar pigmentation sometimes seen upon pregnant women.

cy''ber·net'ics. The science of communication and communication-control theory, as applied to mechanical devices and to animals. Also see *servomechanism*.

cycl-. See *cyclo-*.

cyclaine hydrochloride. Trademark for hexylcaine hydrochloride.

cy'cla·mate. The anion cyclohexylsulfamate, calcium and sodium salts of which are used as sweetening agents. See *sucaryl*.

cyclamycin. Trade-mark for triacetyloleandomycin.

cy'cle. A regular series of changes which involve a return to the original state or condition, and repetition; a succession of events or symptoms. **cardiac c.** The complete series of events occurring in the heart during systole and diastole of all of its chambers up to the return to the beginning point. **Cori c.** A series of enzymatic reactions which purport to show the mode of conversion of lactic acid (formed during muscular activity from glycogen) to glucose in the liver, and its subsequent anabolism to glycogen in muscle. **c. of generation.** Haeckel's term for the successive changes through which an individual passes from its birth to the period when it is capable of reproducing its kind. **estrous c.** The periodically recurring series of changes in uterus, ovaries, and accessory sexual structures associated with estrus and diestrus in lower mammals. **Krebs c.** A series of enzymatic reactions originally described by H. A. Krebs as occurring in pigeon breast muscle and now believed to occur, in a modified form, in most living cells of aerobic organisms. It aims to define a cycle of reactions whereby the pyruvate (or a two-carbon derivative thereof), formed during the anaerobic phase of carbohydrate oxidation, is converted to carbon dioxide and water. As intermediates of the Krebs cycle are also formed in the oxidation of fatty acids and amino acids, it is thought to be the final common path for the burning of all foodstuffs to carbon dioxide and water. Syn., *citric acid c.*, *tricarboxylic acid c.* **life c.** Life history, including metamorphoses, hosts, habitats, and modes of reproduction. **menstrual c.** The periodically recurring series of changes in the uterus, ovaries, and accessory sexual structures associated with menstruation and the intermenstrual periods in primates. **Meyerhof c.** A series of enzymatic reactions which have been shown to occur in a variety of animal, plant, and microbial tissues, whereby glucose (or glycogen or starch) is converted to pyruvic acid. This conversion may occur anaerobically, and then lactic acid or ethanol and carbon dioxide are the end products; aerobically the pyruvate is further oxidized by the

Krebs cycle or other mechanisms. The entire series of reactions is reversible. At present the Meyerhof cycle is believed to be the main pathway of the catabolism and of the anabolism of carbohydrate. Also called *Emden-Meyerhof scheme*, *Emden-Meyerhof-Parnas scheme.*

cy'clic (sigh'klick, sick'lick). 1. Having cycles or periods of exacerbation or change; intermittent. 2. Having a self-limited course, as certain diseases.

cy·cli'tis (sigh-kly'tis, sick-lye'tis). Inflammation of the ciliary body, manifested by a zone of congestion in the sclerotic coat surrounding the cornea. It may be serous, plastic, or suppurative.

cy'cli·zine. 1-Diphenylmethyl-4-methylpiperazine, the hydrochloride and lactate salts of which are used as antinauseants. See *marezine*.

cy'clo- (sigh'klo-, sick'lo-), **cycl-.** A combining form meaning *circular*, *a cycle*, or *pertaining to the ciliary body.*

cy"clo·bar'bi·tal. Cyclohexenylethylbarbituric acid, a rapidly eliminated sedative used in insomnia. See *phanodorn.*

cy"clo·di·al'y·sis (·dye·al'i·sis). Detaching the ciliary body from the sclera in order to effect reduction of intraocular tension in certain cases of glaucoma, especially in aphakia.

cy"clo·di'a·ther·my. Destruction, by diathermy, of the ciliary body.

cyclogyl hydrochloride. Trademark for cyclopentolate hydrochloride.

cy"clo·hex"yl·sul'fam·ate. A salt containing the anion C_6H_{11}· NHSO₃-.

cy'cloid. *In psychiatry*, pertaining to a type of personality characterized by alternating periods of well-being and mild depression.

cy·clo'ni·um. Cy. A name proposed for a synthetic form of element 61. See also *florentium, illinium, promethium.*

cyclopal. A trade-mark for the sedative and hypnotic substance cyclopentenylallylbarbituric acid.

cy"clo·pen'ta·mine   hy"dro·chlo'ride. N,α-Dimethylcyclopentaneethylamine hydrochloride, a sympathomimetic agent. See *clopane hydrochloride.*

cy"clo·pen·te'no·phen·an'threne. $C_{17}H_{34}$. A hydrocarbon representing the fusion of three benzene rings and one cyclopentane ring which is considered the basic structure of sterols and steroids.

cy"clo·pen·ten'yl·al·lyl·bar"bi·tu'ric ac'id. See *cyclopal.*

cy"clo·pen'to·late   hy"dro·chlo'ride. β-Dimethylaminoethyl(1-hydroxycyclopentyl)phenylacetate hydrochloride, a cycloplegic and mydriatic agent. See *cyclogyl hydrochloride.*

cy"clo·phor'ase. An enzyme catalyzing oxidation of members of the Krebs cycle.

cy"clo·pho'ri·a. An insufficiency of the oblique muscles of the eye, giving the eyes a tendency to roll outward or inward, so that the naturally vertical meridians would diverge at either the upper or lower extremities.

cy·clo'pi·a (sigh·klo'pee·uh). A large group of terata; characterized externally by fusion of the orbits and various degrees of fusion of the eyes; internally by severe defects of the facial skeleton and brain. A proboscis may or may not be present. Syn., *synopsia, synophthalmia.*

cy"clo·ple'gi·a. Paralysis of ciliary muscle of the eye. **—cycloplegic,** adj.

cy"clo·pro'pane. A saturated cyclic hydrocarbon gas, C_3H_6, used as an inhalation anesthetic.

Cy'clops. A genus of minute crustaceans having a large, median eye; widely distributed throughout fresh and salt waters but found most commonly in still water. Species of *Cyclops* have been found to be intermediate hosts of *Dracunculus medinensis, Diphyllobothrium latum, Drepanidotaenia lanceolata,* and *Gnathostoma spinigerum.*

cy'clops. A monster with a congenital fusion of the two eyes into one.

cy"clo·ser'ine. A broad-spectrum antibiotic produced by *Streptomyces orchidaceus,* effective in treating tuberculosis and genitourinary infections. See *seromycin.*

cy"clo·thy'mi·a (sigh"klo·thigh'-mee·uh, ·thim'ee·uh). *In psychiatry,* a disposition marked by alternations of mood between elation and depression; may precede a manic-depressive psychosis. Also called *cyclothymosis.* **—cyclothymic,** adj. n.; **cyclothymiac,** n.; **cyclothyme,** n.

cy'clo·tome. A knife used in cyclotomy.

cy·clot'o·my (sigh·clot'o·mee, si·clot'·). An operation for the relief of glaucoma, consisting of an incision through the ciliary body.

cy'clo·tron. A device for imparting high speeds to protons or deuterons by a combination of a constant powerful magnet and an alternating high-frequency charge.

cy'cri·mine hy"dro·chlo'ride. 1-Phenyl-1-cyclopentyl-3-piperidino-1-propanol hydrochloride, a drug effective as a muscle relaxant in Parkinsonism. See *pagitane hydrochloride.*

cy·do'ni·um (sigh·do'nee·um). Quince seed. The seeds of *Cydonia oblonga;* employed mainly for the mucilage contained in the covering.

cy"e·si·og·no'sis. Diagnosis of pregnancy.

cy·e"si·ol'o·gy (sigh·ee"see·ol'o·jee).

The science of gestation in its medical aspects.

cy·e'sis (sigh·ee'sis). Pregnancy.

Cyl. Cylinder; cylindrical lens.

cy·lin'dro-, cylindr-. A combining form denoting *cylindrical.*

cyl'in·droid. A long, pale, ribbonlike structure found in normal and pathologic urines. The diameter is usually smaller than that of a true renal cast. The ends may be tapered. The clinical significance of cylindroids is uncertain, although they may result from inflammation of the urinary tract.

cyl"in·dru'ri·a. The presence of cylindroids in the urine.

cym'bi·form. *In biology,* boat-shaped.

cym'bo-. A combining form denoting *boat-shaped.*

cy'mene. $C_{10}H_{14}$. 1-Methyl-4-isopropylbenzene, a hydrocarbon that occurs in various other volatile oils. Syn., *cymol.* **—cymic,** adj.

cy'me·nyl. Cymyl; the radical $C_{10}H_{13}$ derived from cymene.

cy'mol. Cymene.

cy'myl. Cymenyl.

cy·nan'thro·py (si·nan'thro·pee, sigh·nan'·), **cyn"an·thro'pi·a.** A mania in which the patient believes himself to be a dog and imitates one.

cyn'o- (sin'o-, sign'no-), **cyn-.** A combining form denoting *dog.*

cyn"o·pho'bi·a (sin"o·fo'bee·uh, sigh"no·). 1. Morbid fear of dogs. 2. A psychosis reproducing the symptoms of rabies.

cyn"u·ren'ic ac'id. A crystalline acid found in dog's urine. It is a decomposition product of proteins.

cyn'u·rin. A base derived from cynurenic acid.

cy·ot'ro·phy (sigh·ot'ro·fee). Nutrition of the fetus.

cy·prid"o·pho'bi·a (si·prid"o·fo'bee·uh, sigh"prid·o·). A morbid fear of acquiring a venereal disease.

cyp"ri·pe'di·um. Lady-slipper. The dried rhizome and roots of *Cypripedium calceolus (pubescens).* Has been used as an antispasmodic and tonic.

cyr'to- (sur'to-). A combining form meaning *curved* or *convex.*

cyr·tom'e·ter. An instrument for measuring or delineating the curves of parts of the body. Used to demonstrate the dilation and deformation of the chest in certain diseases, or to measure the shape and size of the head. **—cyr·tometry,** n.

cyr·to'sis. A curvature or deformity of the spinal column; kyphosis.

cyst. A sac with a distinct wall, containing fluid or other material. May be a normal or a pathologic structure. **adventitious c.** One enclosing a foreign body or substance. **blue dome c.** A bluish cyst occurring in disorders of the mammary gland. **bone c.** A tumor distending and thinning bone, filled with serum or bloody fluid. **branchial c.** One due to anomalous development of the embryonal visceral pouches or grooves. Also called *branchiogenic c., cervical c.* **cervical c.** A closed, epithelial sac in the neck arising by retention of a visceral groove, of a visceral pouch, or of the cervical sinus. Also called *branchial c., branchiogenic c.* **chocolate c.** (a) Any cyst filled with degenerated blood. (b) The lesion characteristic of endometriosis. **colloid c.** One containing a hyaline material resembling the colloid of the thyroid gland. **corpus luteum c.** Cystic distention of a corpus luteum. Also called *luteal c.* **c. of broad ligament.** One developing within the broad ligament; derived from embryonal tubules in the ligament or from cysts of adherent ovary. **dentigerous c.** One originating in the enamel organ of a developing tooth. Syn., *follicular c.* **dermoid c.** A congenital cyst containing sebaceous material, hairs, and other dermal appendages; the wall is lined by skin and contains derivatives of all three embryonal layers. **echinococcus c.** (a) A cyst formed by growth of the larval form of *Echinococcus granulosus*, usually in the liver. (b) The cysticercus stage of the life cycle of *Echinococcus granulosus.* **epidermoid c.** A cyst lined by stratified squamous epithelium without associated cutaneous glands. **extravasation c.** A cyst formed by encapsulation of extravasated fluid, usually blood, as a hematoma. **follicular c.** (a) A cyst due to retention of secretion in a follicular space, as in the ovary. (b) A dentigerous cyst, *q.v.* **hemorrhagic c.** See extravasation c. **inclusion c.** A cyst due to embryonal or traumatic implantation of epithelium into another structure, as an epidermoid cyst. **involutional c.** Cystic dilatation of glands or ducts during the course of involution of a gland, as in the mammary gland in abnormal involution. **mucous c.** A retention cyst of a gland, containing a secretion rich in mucin. Also called *mucinous c.* **multilocular c.** One with several more or less separate compartments. **Nabothian c.** Cystic distention of the mucous (Nabothian) glands of the uterine cervix. **pilonidal c.** Cystic distention of a congenital tract, opening on the skin of the sacrococcygeal region; lined by stratified squamous epithelium, often contains hairs and the products of bacterial contamination; it may extend as deeply as the spinal dura. **retention c.** A cyst due

to obstruction of outflow of secretion from a gland. **sanguineous c.** One containing blood-stained fluid. **sebaceous c.** A retention cyst of a sebaceous gland. **sublingual c.** See ranula. **thyroglossal c.** Cystic distention of the remnants of the thyroglossal duct, filled with secretion of lining epithelial cells. **tubo-ovarian c.** A fusiform dilatation of the oviduct due to communication with an ovarian cyst. **unilocular c.** One with but a single cavity. **urinary c.** A retention cyst in the kidney.

cyst-. See *cysto-.*

cyst″ad·e·no′ma. An adenoma containing cysts. **c. adamantinum.** Cystic adamantinoma. **c. papilliferum.** An adenoma containing cysts with papillae on the inner aspect of the cyst walls. **pseudomucinous c.** The most frequent tumor of the ovary, lobulated, multilocular, lined with nonciliated columnar epithelium and filled with pseudomucin in fluid or semisolid form. This tumor may attain great size, may become carcinomatous and may rupture, leading to pseudomyxoma peritonei. **serous c.** Cystic tumor of the ovary; often intraligamentous, not infrequently bilateral, usually small, grossly monolocular. Contains a watery fluid, is lined by low cuboidal, ciliated epithelium with centrally placed nuclei. Usually papilliferous and disposed to become a cystadenocarcinoma with involvement of peritoneum.

cyst″ec·ta′si·a (sis″teck·tay′zhuh·shuh), **cys·tec′ta·sy.** Dilatation of the urinary bladder.

cys·tec′to·my. 1. Excision of the gall bladder, or part of the urinary bladder. 2. Removal of a cyst.

cys·te·ine (sis′tee·in, sis·tee′in). α-Amino-β-thiolactic acid; obtained by reduction of cystine and important as a constituent of many proteins.

cyst′ic. 1. Pertaining to or resembling a cyst. 2. Pertaining to the urinary bladder or to the gallbladder.

cys″ti·cer′coid. A larval tapeworm, differs from the cysticercus, *q.v.*, in that it has a slightly developed bladder and a solid posterior.

cys″ti·cer·co′sis. Infestation by cysticerci; characterized by muscular pain, general muscular weakness, fatigue, loss of weight, and nervousness; or, in severe cases, where the infestation is general and the brain is invaded, general paralysis, epileptic attacks, and convulsions.

cys″ti·cer′cus (pl. *cysticerci*). The larval tapeworm; develops in man after ingestion of the ova of *Taenia solium* or *T. saginata*. The ova infestive to man develop only into the larval forms, complete development failing to take place.

cys'tine (sis'teen, ·tin). Di-(α-amino-β-thiopropionic) acid. An amino acid component of many proteins, especially keratin. It may be reduced to cysteine.

cys"ti·nu'ri·a. The presence of cystine in the urine.

cys·ti'tis. Inflammation of the urinary bladder.

cys'to-, cyst-. A combining form denoting likeness to or connection with a bladder or cyst.

cys'to·cele. Prolapse of the bladder into the vagina.

cys'to·gram. Radiograph of the urinary bladder made after the injection of a contrast medium, either of a greater or lesser density than the surrounding soft tissues.

cys·tog'ra·phy. Radiography of the urinary bladder after the injection of a radiopaque medium. —**cystograph'ic,** adj.

cys·to'ma. A cystic mass, especially in or near the ovary; may be either neoplastic, inflammatory, or due to retention. **parovarian c.** Dilation and sometimes proliferation of the tubules of the epoöphoron, a remnant of the mesonephros, situated at the junction of the uterine tube and the ovary. **tubo-ovarian c.** A cyst formation which may occur when an ovarian cyst communicates with a fused uterine tube.

cys'to·pex"y. Surgical fixation of the urinary bladder, or a portion of it, in new location.

cys'to·plas"ty. Plastic operation upon the urinary bladder.

cys"to·py"e·li'tis. Inflammation of the urinary bladder and the pelvis of the kidney.

cys"to·py"e·lo·ne·phri'tis. Cystopyelitis plus involvement of the kidney.

cys'to·scope. An instrument used in diagnosis and treatment of lesions of the bladder, ureter, and kidney. It consists of an outer sheath bearing the lighting system, a well-fitted obturator, space for the visual system, and room for the passage of operative devices to be used under visual control.

cys·tos'co·py. The procedure of using the cystoscope.

cys'to·tome. 1. A knife used in cystotomy. 2. A knife used in rupturing the capsule of the lens in cataract operations.

cys·tot'o·my. Incision of the bladder.

cys"to·u·re'thro·gram. A radiograph of the urinary bladder and urethra, made following injection of an opaque contrast medium.

cys"to·u·re'thro·scope. An instru-

ment for inspecting the urinary bladder and posterior urethra.

-cyte (-sight). A suffix denoting a cell.

cyt'i·sine (sit'i·seen, ·sin). A poisonous alkaloid from *Laburnum anagyroides,* goldenchain laburnum, from baptisia and other plants. It stimulates, then paralyzes, autonomic ganglions. Syn., *baptitoxine, sophorine, ulexine.*

cy'to-, cyt-. A combining form denoting connection with, relation to, or derivation from a cell, cells, or cytoplasm.

cy"to·chem'is·try. That science dealing with the chemical constitution of cells and cell constituents.

cy'to·chrome. 1. A nerve cell which has only a small amount of cytoplasm and no Nissl bodies. 2. A mixture of three hemochromogen-like compounds (**cytochromes A, B,** and **C**) occurring in animal tissues and yeast and capable of being oxidized and reduced by accepting and transferring hydrogen.

cy'to·chrome ox'i·dase (ock'si·dace, ·daze). A widely distributed enzyme which causes the oxidation of phenols, amines, etc., through the medium of cytochrome C. It reoxidizes reduced cytochrome C, which is then ready to accept more hydrogen.

cy"to·di"ag·no'sis. The determination of the nature of a pathogenic liquid by the study of the cells it contains.

cy"to·gen'e·sis. The genesis and differentiation of the cell. —**cytogen'ic, cytogenet'ic,** adj.

cy·tol'o·gy (sigh·tol'o·jee). The subdivision of biology which deals with cells. —**cytolog'ic,** adj.; **cytologist,** n.

cy"to·ly'sin. An antibody produced by injection of foreign cells, which causes dissolution of cells. May be specific or nonspecific.

cy·tol'y·sis. The disintegration or dissolution of cells. —**cytolyt'ic,** adj.

cytomel. Trade-mark for sodium liothyronine.

cy·tom'e·ter (sigh·tom'i·tur). A device for counting cells, especially blood corpuscles. Also see *hemocytometer.*

cy"to·mor'pho·sis (sigh"to·mor'fo·sis, ·mor·fo'sis). All the structural alterations which cells or successive generations of cells undergo from the earliest undifferentiated stage to their final destruction.

cy"to·path·o·gen'ic. Pertaining to the destruction of cells, as in tissue culture, by a transmissible agent, such as a virus; also, pertaining to or denoting the agent itself.

cy"to·pa·thol'o·gy. The branch of pathology concerned with alterations within cells.

cy"to·pe'ni·a. A cell count less than

normal. See *leukopenia, anemia, thrombocytopenia.*

cy'to·plasm (sigh'to·plaz·um). 1. Protoplasm. 2. The protoplasm of a cell other than that of the nucleus, as opposed to *karyoplasm.*

cy·tos'co·py (sigh·tos'ko·pee). Cytodiagnosis, *q.v.* **—cytoscop'ic,** *adj.*

cy'to·sine (sigh'to·seen, ·sin). 2-Oxy-6-amino-pyrimidine. A pyrimidine base found in nucleic acid.

cy'to·tox'in. A serum, natural or immune, capable of injuring certain cells without lysis (a toxic action). **—cytotoxic,** *adj.*

cy''to·troph'o·blast (·trof'o·blast, ·tro'fo·blast). The inner, cellular layer of the trophoblast, covering the chorion and the chorionic villi during the first half of pregnancy. Also called *Langhans' layer.*

cy·tot'ro·pism (sigh·tot'ro·piz·um). The tendency of cells to move toward or away from a stimulus. **—cytotrop'ic,** *adj.*

cy'to·zyme. A substance in various tissues, capable of activating thrombin, the fibrin ferment. Also see *thrombokinase.*

D

D. Deuterium.

D-. *In chemistry,* a prefix, printed as a small capital letter, used to indicate the structural configuration of a particular asymmetric carbon atom, with reference to the standard substance D-glyceraldehyde, so designated because its asymmetric carbon atom has the configuration represented by

HC.OH, rather than by HO.CH which

is the configuration of the asymmetric carbon atom in L-glyceraldehyde. Also see *d-, dl-,* isomerism. L-, l-.

d. Abbreviation for da (*give*), density, detur (*let it be given*), dentur (*let them be given*), dexter, diopter, dose, duration.

d-. 1. *In chemistry,* an abbreviation used as a prefix, meaning *dextrorotatory.* See also *dl-, l-.* 2. *In chemistry,* formerly the same as D-.

dac'ry-. See *dacryo-.*

dac''ry·ad''e·no·scir'rhus (dack''ree·ad''l·no·skirr'us). An indurated tumor of the lacrimal gland.

dac''ry·ag''o·ga·tre'si·a (dack''ree·ag''o·ga·tree'zhuh, ·shuh). Obstruction of a tear duct.

dac'ry·a·gogue (dack'ree·uh·gog), **dac'ry·a·gog.** 1. Inducing tears. 2. An agent causing a flow of tears. Syn., *lacrimator.*

dac'ry·o-, dac'ry-. Combining form meaning *a tear,* or denoting *relation to tears* or *to the lacrimal apparatus.*

dac''ry·o·ad''e·nal'gi·a. Pain in a lacrimal gland.

dac''ry·o·ad''e·nec'to·my. Excision of the lacrimal gland.

dac''ry·o·ad''e·ni'tis. Inflammation of a lacrimal gland.

dac''ry·o·blen''nor·rhe'a. Chronic inflammation of and discharge of mucus from the lacrimal sac.

dac''ry·o·cys·tec'to·my. Excision of any part of the lacrimal sac.

dac''ry·o·cys·ti'tis. Inflammation of the lacrimal sac. **blennorrheal d.** Purulent inflammation of the lacrimal sac. **phlegmonous d.** Inflammation of the tissues composing the lacrimal sac and of the surrounding soft parts.

dac''ry·o·cys'to·cele. Protrusion of a lacrimal sac. Also called *dacryocele.*

dac''ry·o·cys''top·to'sis. Prolapse or downward displacement of a lacrimal sac.

dac''ry·o·cys''to·rhi·nos'to·my (dack''ree·o·sis''to·rye·nos'to·mee). An operation to restore drainage into the nose from the lacrimal sac when the nasolacrimal duct is obliterated.

dac''ry·o·cys·tos'to·my. Incision into the lacrimal sac, particularly to promote drainage.

dac''ry·o·cys'to·tome. Instrument for dividing strictures of the lacrimal passages.

dac''ry·o·cys·tot'o·my. Incision of the lacrimal sac.

dac''ry·o·lith'', dac'ry·o·lite''. A calcareous concretion in the lacrimal passages.

dac''ry·o·li·thi'a·sis. The formation and presence of dacryoliths.

dac''ry·o'ma. 1. A lacrimal tumor. 2. Obstruction of the lacrimal puncta causing epiphora.

dac'ry·on. The point where the frontomaxillary, the lacrimomaxillary, and the frontolacrimal sutures meet.

dac'ry·ops. 1. Watery eye. 2. A cyst of the duct of a lacrimal gland. *Ray.*

dac''ry·or·rhe'a. An excessive flow of tears.

dac''ry·o·so''le·ni'tis. Inflammation of a lacrimal duct.

dac″ry·o·ste·no′sis. Stenosis or stricture of a lacrimal duct.

dactil. Trade-mark for piperidolate hydrochloride.

dac′tyl. In zoology, a digit; a finger or a toe. —**dac′ty·lar, dac′ty·late,** adj.

dac″ty·li′tis. Inflammation of a finger or a toe.

dac′ty·lo-, dactyl-. A combining form meaning finger, toe, or digit.

dac″ty·lo·gram″, dac·tyl′o·gram″. A fingerprint, generally used for purposes of identification.

dac″ty·lo·meg′a·ly. A condition in which one or more of the fingers or toes is abnormally large.

dac″ty·lo·sym′phy·sis. Syndactyly, q.v.

dac′ty·lus. 1. A finger or toe. 2. A toe, in opposition to digitus, a finger.

Dakin, Henry Drysdale [English chemist in the United States, 1880-　　]. With Carrel, developed a method of treating open wounds by irrigation with a solution of chlorinated soda and sodium bicarbonate; called Carrel-Dakin solution. See also diluted sodium hypochlorite solution, called modified Dakin's solution.

Dalton, John [English chemist and physicist, 1766-1844]. Developed the atomic theory. Discovered Dalton's laws: (1) The pressure of a mixture of gases equals the sum of the partial pressures of the constituent gases. (2) So long as no chemical change occurs, each gas in a mixture of gases is absorbed by a given volume of solvent in proportion not to the total pressure of the mixture but to the partial pressure of that gas.

Dal′ton·ism (dawl′tun·iz·um, dal′tun-). Color blindness.

dam. In dentistry or surgery, a thin sheet of rubber used to keep fluids away from a part; also, a piece of dam used as a drain, q.v.

da″mal·u′ric·ac′id (day″mul·yoor′ick, dam″ul-). $C_7H_{12}O_2$. An acid found in human urine.

dam′ar. See dammar.

dam′i·an′a (dam″ee·an′uh, ·ay′-nuh). The dried leaves of Turnera diffusa. Formerly used as a stimulant and laxative, and by the laity as an aphrodisiac.

dam′mar, dam′ar. A resinous exudate from Shorea wiesneri (Dipterocarpaceae) and other related genera. A solution of dammar is a mounting medium used in microscopy.

D and C. Short for dilatation of the cervix and curettage of the uterus.

dan′der. Scales of the hairy skin of any animal; dandruff. May act as an allergen, dog, cat, and horse dander being the most common.

dan′druff. Scales formed upon the scalp in seborrhea; dander.

Dandy, Walter Edward [American surgeon, 1886–1946]. Introduced ventriculography as an aid in the diagnosis of cerebral disease. Devised numerous neurologic procedures, including operations for ruptured intervertebral disk.

danilone. A trade-mark for phenindione.

daraprim. Trade-mark for pyrimethamine.

darbid. Trade-mark for isopropamide iodide.

dar′tos. The contractile, musculofibrous layer in and beneath the skin of the scrotum. —**darto′ic,** adj.

darvon. Trade-mark for dextro propoxyphene hydrochloride.

Darwin, Charles Robert [English naturalist, 1809–82]. One of the great thinkers of all time; author of On the Origin of Species (1859) and The Descent of Man (1871). The word Darwinism denotes adherence to his theory of evolution by natural selection. He described the tuberculum auriculae, called Darwin's tubercle, which he considered evidence of the simian connections of the human species. See under tubercle.

da·tu′rine (dat-yoor′een, dat′yoo-reen). An alkaloid from Datura stramonium, identical with hyoscyamine.

Davy, Humphry [English chemist and physicist, 1778–1829]. Widely known for his contributions to science, especially to industrial hygiene by the invention of a coal miner's safety lamp (1815) which revolutionized mining methods and saved many lives. Discovered the anesthetic properties of nitrous oxide and suggested its use in surgery as early as 1800.

DBE. aa-Di-(p-ethoxyphenyl)-β-phenyl bromoethylene; a synthetic estrogen.

D. C. Doctor of Chiropractic, direct current, Dental Corps.

D. D. S. Doctor of Dental Surgery.

DDT. 1,1,1-Trichloro-2,2-bis(p-chlorophenyl) ethane, an insecticide the medicinal grade of which is called chlorophenothane.

de-. A prefix denoting down, away from; separation, off, away; intensification, completely, quite; or the reversing or undoing of an action, depriving or ridding of, or freeing from.

de·ac″ti·va′tion. 1. Process of becoming inactive or of making inactive. 2. Loss of radioactivity.

dead. Without life; destitute of life.

dead′ly night′shade. Belladonna.

de·af″fer·en·ta′tion. The process of interrupting afferent (sensory) nerve fibers.

deaf-mute. One who is unable to

utter articulate speech because of deafness before the establishment of speech.

deaf'ness. Loss, lack, or impairment of the sense of hearing. It may be due to disease of the external auditory canal, the middle ear, the internal ear, the auditory nerve, or the brain. **—deaf,** adj. **bass d.** Deafness to certain bass notes, while higher notes are heard. **boilermakers' d.** Deafness resulting from working among loud noises; characterized by inability to hear ordinary conversation in conditions of quiet, but an increase in hearing power in the midst of noise; paracusia Willisii. **cerebral d.** That due to a brain lesion. **clang d.** A defect of hearing in which sounds are heard, but their more delicate qualities are not perceived. **conduction d.** That due to disease or defect of the external ear or middle ear, or of both. **cortical d.** That due to disease of the cortical hearing centers. **mind d.** Inability to comprehend sounds heard, due to injury of the auditory center; auditory aphasia. Also called psychic d. **psychogenic d.** Any deafness that has 50% or more of a psychic factor. Persons so affected do not know they can hear better than they manifest. Must be distinguished from malingering deafness. **speech d.** A variety of mind deafness in which the faculty of repeating and writing after dictation is retained. **tone d.** Sensory amusia; a form of mind deafness. **word d.** Inability to understand words, although they are heard; a form of mind deafness.

de·am'i·dase (dee-am'i-dace, -daze). An enzyme that catalyzes oxidative deamination of purines and pyrimidines.

de·am'i·nase (dee-am'i-nace, -naze). An enzyme which catalyzes the splitting off of an amino group from an organic compound.

de·am'i·nize. Remove the —NH₂ group from an organic compound, particularly from an amino acid, with the formation of the corresponding —OH compound or further decomposition products. **—deamida'tion, deamina'tion, deaminiza'tion,** n.

de·an"es·the'si·ant (dee-an"ess-thee'zhunt, -zee-unt). Any means of arousing a patient from a state of anesthesia.

death. The cessation of life, beyond the possibility of resuscitation. Syn., abiosis. **local d.** Death of one part of the body. **molecular d.** Death of individual cells; ulceration. **muscular d.** A state in which the muscles no longer react to stimuli. **serum d.** Sudden death occurring in a sensitized person during the intravenous injection of serum. **somatic d.** Death of

the whole organism. **thymic d.** Sudden death assumed to be due to enlargement of the thymus gland.

death cer·tif'i·cate. A form, usually required by law, for recording the event of death, its time, place, cause, the name and age of decedent, and other pertinent data. **standard d. c.** The form recommended by the United States Bureau of the Census and in common usage in the United States.

death rate. The proportion of deaths in a given year to the total population, known as the **crude death rate. Specific death rates** are figured on the basis of the number of deaths reported in a given group; specific for age, race, sex, or cause, or for a combination of these variables.

death rat'tle. A gurgling sound heard in dying persons, due to the passage of the air through fluid in the trachea.

death reg"is·tra'tion a're·a. That territory from which the United States Bureau of the Census collects death records. Since 1933, this has been the entire United States.

death strug'gle. The semiconvulsive twitches often occurring before death.

de·bil'i·tant. 1. An agent allaying excitement. 2. Weakening.

de·bil'i·ty. Weakness; asthenia, q.v. **nervous d.** Neurasthenia, q.v.

de"bride'ment (day"breed"-mahn', di-breed'mint). In surgery, removal from a wound of foreign material and devitalized tissue.

dec'a-, dec-. A prefix denoting ten times.

dec'a·gram. A metric measure of weight equal to 10 grams.

de·cal"ci·fi·ca'tion (dee-kal"si-fi-kay'shun). Withdrawal or removal by acid of the mineral salts of bone or other calcified substance. **—decal'cify,** v.

dec'a·li"ter (deck'uh-lee"tur). A metric measure of volume equal to 10 liters.

dec'a·me"ter. A metric measure of length equal to 10 meters.

dec"a·me·tho'ni·um. A compound containing a methonium ion with ten CH₂ groups, that possesses powerful skeletal muscle relaxant activity. Also see methonium. See syncurine.

de·can"cel·la'tion (dee-can"suh-lay'shun). The removal of cancellous bone either for use as bone chips in grafting operations or for correcting deformity.

dec'ane. C₁₀H₂₂. A hydrocarbon of the paraffin series.

dec'a·nor·mal. Having 10 times the strength of the normal; said of solutions.

de·cant'. Gently pour off a liquor or

solution without disturbing the sediment. —**decanta'tion,** n.

de·cap″i·ta'tion (dee·cap″i·tay″-shun). Beheading; removal of the head of a person, a fetus, or a bone; decollation. —**decap'itate,** v.

de·cap″i·ta″tor (dee·cap'i·tay″tur). Instrument used in performing decapitation in embryotomy.

Decapryn. Trade-mark for the antihistaminic substance 2-[α-(β-dimethylaminoethoxy)-α-methylbenzyl]pyridine, commercially available as the succinate salt.

de·cap″su·la'tion (dee·cap″suh·lay'shun, ·cap″sue·lay'shun). Removal of a capsule or enveloping membrane, as the capsule of a kidney.

de·car″bon·i·za'tion (dee·kahr″-bun·i·zay'shun, ·eye·zay'shun). Removal of carbon, as from the blood. —**decar'bonize,** v.

de″car·box'yl·ase. See carboxylase.

de″car·box″yl·a'tion, de″car·box″yl·i·za'tion. The splitting off of one or more molecules of carbon dioxide from organic acids, especially amino acids. —**decarboxylate,** v.

dec″a·vi'ta·min. A U.S. Pharmacopeia preparation containing the recommended daily requirement of vitamins supplied in a single capsule or tablet.

de·cay'. 1. In bacteriology, the progressive chemical decomposition of organic matter in the presence of atmospheric oxygen; due generally to aerobic bacteria. 2. Decline in health or strength. 3. Senility. 4. Lay term for dental caries, q.v. **radioactive d.** The alteration of an element because of its radioactive disintegration; the sum total of the processes by which unstable nuclear configurations are spontaneously converted into stable ones. The term as distinguished from radioactivity usually implies the statistical laws which govern these processes.

de'cem-. A combining form meaning ten.

de·cen'tered (dee·sen'turd). Out of common center; said of a lens in which the visual axis and the axis of the lens do not coincide. —**decentra'tion,** n.

de·cer″e·bra'tion (dee·serr″i·bray'-shun). Removal of the brain in physiologic experiments. —**decer'ebrated,** adj.; **decer'ebrate,** adj., v.t.; **decer'ebrize,** v.t.

Deceresol OT. Trade-mark for dioctyl sodium sulfosuccinate, used as a wetting agent.

de·chlo″ri·da'tion (dee·klor″i·day'shun). Reduction of the quantity of chlorides in the body by the removal of salt from the diet.

de·chlo″ru·ra'tion (dee·klor″oo-

ray'shun). Reduction of the amount of chlorides excreted in the urine.

decholin. Trade-mark for dehydrocholic acid.

deci- (dess'i-). A combining form meaning tenth; used in the metric system to indicate a measure one-tenth as large as the unit.

dec'i·bel. A tenth of a bel, q.v.

de·cid'u·a. The mucous membrane (endometrium) of the uterus, especially that part subject to special modification in preparation for and during pregnancy and which is cast off at parturition and menstruation. Also called membrana d., tunica d. —**decidual,** adj. **d. basalis.** That part of the endometrium between the chorionic vesicle and the myometrium that forms the maternal part of the placenta. Also called d. serotina. **d. capsularis.** That part of the endometrium between the chorionic vesicle and the uterine lumen; the outer investing envelope of the fetus. Also called d. reflexa. **d. marginalis.** That part of the endometrium at the junction of the decidua basalis, decidua parietalis, and decidua capsularis. **d. menstrualis.** The outer layer of the uterine mucosa which is shed during menstruation. **d. parietalis.** The endometrium exclusive of the region occupied by the embryo. Also called d. vera.

de·cid″u·a'tion. Act or process of dropping off or shedding.

de·cid″u·i'tis. An acute inflammation of the decidua, frequently the result of attempts to induce abortion.

de·cid″u·o'ma. 1. Decidual tissue produced in the uterus by mechanical or other methods in the absence of an embryo, so named by its discoverer, Leo Loeb (1908). 2. An intrauterine tumor containing decidual relics, and believed to arise from some hyperplasia of a retained portion of the decidua. —**deciduomal,** adj.

de·cid'u·ous. Falling off or shed at maturity.

dec'i·gram (dess'i·gram). One-tenth of a gram.

dec'i·li″ter (dess'i·lee″tur). One-tenth of a liter.

dec'i·me″ter (dess'i·mee″tur). One-tenth of a meter.

dec″i·nor'mal (dess″i·nor'mul). Having one-tenth the strength of the normal.

de·cip'a·ra. A woman who has been in labor ten times.

de·coc'tion. In pharmacology, a liquid preparation obtained by boiling medicinal vegetable substances in water.

de″col·la'tion. Decapitation, q.v.

de′col·la″tor (dee″kuh·lay″tur, dee-kol'ay·tur). Instrument used for fetal decapitation.

de·col'or·ant (dee-kul'ur·unt). 1. Capable of removing color. 2. An agent for the altering or removal of color. —**decoloriza'tion**, *n.*; **decolor·ize,** *v.*

de·com"pen·sa'tion (dee-kom"pen·say'shun). Failure of compensation, as of the circulation or of the heart.

de"com·po·si'tion. 1. The separation of the component principles of a body. 2. Putrefaction. —**decompose',** *v.t., v.i.* **double d.** The mutual reaction of two substances upon each other with formation of new substances; metathesis.

de"com·pres'sion. The removal of compression or pressure; particularly, various technics for reducing intracranial pressure in divers and caisson workers to prevent caisson disease. **explosive d.** *In aviation medicine,* a reduction of barometric pressure which is so rapid as to cause expansion of the involved gases in an explosive manner. **intestinal d.** Release of pressure by means of suction through a tube inserted into the intestine, usually by way of the nose. **intracranial d.** Removal of part of the cranium to release intracranial pressure; subtemporal, suboccipital, and orbital routes are employed.

de"com·pres'sion sick'ness. See *aeroembolism.*

de·con·ges'tant. A therapeutic agent that reduces congestion. —**decongestant,** *adj.*

de"con·ges'tive. Relieving congestion.

de"con·tam"i·na'tion. The destruction or inactivation of poison gas, or removal of a radioactive contaminant. —**decontam'inate,** *v.*

de·cor"ti·ca'tion. 1. Stripping of the bark or husk of a plant. 2. Removal of the cortex or external covering from any organ or structure, as the removal of portions of the cortical substance of the brain from the summits of the gyri; decapsulation. **pulmonary d.** Pleurectomy.

de"cu·ba'tion. The period in the recovery from an infectious disease beginning with the disappearance of the symptoms and lasting until the final exit of the microörganisms from the body. *Obs.*

de·cu'bi·tus. 1. The recumbent or horizontal posture. 2. Decubitus ulcer; a bedsore. —**decubital,** *adj.* **acute d.** A form of bedsore due to cerebral lesions.

decurvon. Trade name for a pectin insulin.

de·cus'sate, dec"us·sate. Intersect; cross.

de"cus·sa'tion (dee"kuh·say'shun, deck"uh·). A chiasma or X-shaped crossing, especially of symmetrical parts, as of nerve fibers that unite structures in the two sides of the brain or spinal cord. **d. of the optic nerve.** The optic chiasma. **pyramidal d.** The oblique crossing in the medulla oblongata of the corticospinal tracts (pyramidal tracts, O.T.) from the opposite sides of the anterior median fissure.

de"den·ti'tion (dee"den·tish'un). Loss of teeth, especially in old age as a result of atrophy of the alveoli.

de"dif·fer·en"ti·a'tion. Loss of differentiation; a process of giving up specific characters and returning to a more generalized morphologic state.

deep sen"si·bil'i·ty. Perception of pressure, tension, and pain in the muscles, joints, tendons, and deep layers of the skin, as contrasted with sensations derived from the superficial layers of the skin.

deer fly. *Chrysops discalis,* the vector of tularemia. Most common in western U.S.A.

def"e·ca'tion. Evacuation of the bowels.

de·fect', de'fect. A lack or failure; absence of any part or organ; absence or failure of a normal function.

de"fem·i·na'tion. The loss or diminution of female characteristics.

de·fense' mech'a·nism. A psychic device for guarding oneself against blame, guilt, anxiety, and unpleasant or disagreeable memories or experiences, or for concealing unacceptable desires, feelings, and beliefs; an unconscious attempt at self-justification and the maintenance of self-esteem. Rationalization is a common defense mechanism. Syn., *defense reaction.*

de·fense' re·ac'tion. Defense mechanism, *q.v.*

def'er·ent. 1. Carrying away or down; efferent. 2. Pertaining to the ductus deferens.

def"er·en'tial. Pertaining to the ductus deferens.

def"er·en"ti·o·ves'i·cal (def"ur·en"shee·o·). Pertaining to both the ductus deferens and the urinary bladder.

def"er·en·ti'tis. Inflammation of the ductus deferens.

de"fer·ves'cence. Disappearance of fever.

de·fi"bri·na'tion (dee·figh"bri·nay'shun). Removal of fibrin from blood or lymph.

de·fi'cien·cy. Absence, lack, or inadequacy of a substance or of a quality.

def"i·ni'tion. *In optics,* the power of a magnifying lens to show clear outlines of the object examined; free from aberration or distortion.

de·flec'tion. A turning, or state of being turned, aside.

def"lo·ra'tion. Loss of the physical sexual characteristics which in woman indicate virginity, usually regarded as typified by the rupture of the hymen at the first intercourse. The surgical removal or piercing of the hymen is not considered as defloration.

de"flo·res'cence. Disappearance of the eruption of an exanthematous disease.

de·form'i·ty. 1. The state of being misshapen. 2. Marked deviation from the normal in size or shape of the body or of a part. **_deforming,_** adj. **deforma'tion,** n. **gunstock d.** One following fracture of either condyle of the humerus in which the long axis of the fully extended forearm deviates outwardly from the arm. **silver-fork d.** Displacement of the wrist, seen in Colles' fracture.

de·fuse' (dee-fewz'). In psychoanalysis, separate two primal instincts.

de·gan'gli·on·ate (dee-gang'glee-un-ate). Remove a ganglion or ganglions.

de·gas'sing. The freeing of an area from toxic gas. **—degas',** v.

de·gen'er·a·cy. A state marked by the deterioration of the mind and body. **criminal d.** That characterized by a tendency to commit criminal acts, especially sexual crimes.

de·gen'er·ate. 1. Undergo the retrogressive changes of degeneration. 2. Deteriorate in mental or psychic characters. 3. An individual so deteriorated.

de"gen·er·a'tion. 1. A retrogressive, pathologic process in cells in which the cytoplasm undergoes deterioration and the nucleus is preserved. 2. A retrogressive process including even the death of nerves, axons, or tracts of the central nervous system. 3. Deterioration of mentality. **—degen'erative,** adj. **albuminous d.** Cloudy swelling, q.v. **ascending d.** Degeneration of the myelin sheath and axons of sensory tracts progressing cranially from the point of cord injury. **atheromatous d.** A retrogressive change, with the deposition of lipids in the degenerated tissue; observed especially in the hyalinized connective tissue of arteriosclerosis. **calcareous d.** Not a true degeneration, but rather a deposit of calcareous material in degenerate or necrotic tissue. **colloid d.** Abnormal production of colloid, as in the thyroid gland. **cystic d.** Any form of degeneration with cyst formation. **descending d.** Deterioration of myelin sheath and axons of descending tracts progressing caudally from the point of cord injury. **fatty d.** A deteriorative process in which the cytoplasm of the cell contains microscopically visible, small droplets of fat, accompanied by other lipids. The fat is derived partly from lipids and proteins of the cell and partly from transported fat. **fibrofatty d. of placenta.** Fatty necrosis of placenta, usually the result of infarction. **granular d.** Cloudy swelling, q.v. **hepatolenticular d.** An affection marked by muscular tremors, weakness, loss of weight, cirrhosis of the liver, mental deterioration, and the presence of the Kayser-Fleischer ring. Also called _Wilson's disease._ **hyaline d.** A form in which there is produced a clear, structureless or homogeneous, translucent change in tissues or cells. **hydropic d.** Cellular degeneration with imbibition of so much water into the cytoplasm that microscopically visible droplets of water are formed. **lardaceous d.** Amyloid degeneration. Also see _amyloidosis._ **mucoid d.** A retrogressive change in mesodermal tissues in which mucoid is produced. **mucous d.** Degeneration of epithelial cells or structures associated with abnormal production of mucus. **myelin d.** A deterioration or necrosis of myelin sheaths of nerves. **pigmentary d.** A retrogressive change, especially in nerve cells, with abnormal deposit of pigmentary substances. **primary d.** Degeneration of nerves at the point of injury or disease. **progressive lenticular d.** A rare familial disease in young people consisting of hobnail cirrhosis and degeneration of the lenticular nucleus. There is considerable emotional disturbance; bilateral athetoid movements of the hands, arms, legs, and face; spasticity and contracture of the limbs; no actual weakness of muscles or loss of sensation; dysarthria; and dysphagia. **secondary d.** Ascending or descending degeneration of nerves or tracts. Also called _Wallerian d._ **subacute combined d. of spinal cord.** Combined degeneration of posterior and lateral columns of the spinal cord, with relatively little gliosis, such as occurs in pernicious anemia. Incorrectly named posterolateral sclerosis. **traumatic d.** The degeneration of the ends of nerves at the point of section, extending to the nearest node of Ranvier, after which fatty degeneration occurs. **Wallerian d.** Usually applied to degenerations as described under ascending and descending degenerations; due to interruption of nerve fibers.

de·gen"i·tal'i·ty (dee-jen·#i·tal'i-tee). In psychoanalysis, a condition wherein genital instincts are expressed through activities of a nongenital character.

de·glu·ti·tion (dee″gloo-tish′un, deg″loo-). The act of swallowing. **—deglu′titive, deglu′titory,** adj.

deg″ra·da′tion. The conversion of one organic compound to another containing a smaller number of carbon atoms.

de·grease′ (dee-grees′, -greez′). Remove fat, as from bones in the preparation of skeletons.

de·gree′. 1. A position in a graded series. 2. One of the units or intervals of a thermometric or other scale. 3. The unit for measuring arcs or angles. One degree is ¹⁄₃₆₀ of a circle. 4. A rank or title conferred by a college or university in recognition of attainment. 5. In law, the relative amount of guilt. 6. One remove in the direct line of descent; a remove in the chain of relationship, as a cousin of fourth degree.

de·gree′ of free′dom. 1. In mechanics, any of the ways in which a point, body, or system may change or move. 2. In physical chemistry, a system's capacity for variation due to the variability of one of its factors. 3. In biometry, the number of independent values in a statistical table.

de″gus·ta′tion. Act of tasting.

de·his′cence. 1. The act of splitting open. 2. A defect in the boundary of a bony canal or cavity.

de″hy·dra′tion (dee″high-dray′shun). The removal of water, as from the body or a tissue. **—dehy′drate,** v.

de·hy′dro-, dehydr-. In chemistry, a combining form signifying dehydrated or dehydrogenated.

de·hy″dro·an·dros′ter·one. Old term for dehydroisoandrosterone, q.v.

de·hy″dro·a·scor′bic ac′id. The relatively inactive acid resulting from elimination of two hydrogen atoms from ascorbic acid when the latter is oxidized by air or other agents.

7-de·hy″dro·cho·les′ter·ol (-ko-less′tur-ole, -ol). A provitamin of animal origin in the skin of man, in milk, and elsewhere, which upon irradiation with ultraviolet rays becomes vitamin D_3.

de·hy″dro·cho′lic ac′id (dee-high″dro-ko′lick, -kol′ick). 3,7,12-Triketocholanic acid. An acid resulting from oxidation of cholic acid; used for its hydrocholeretic and choleretic effects. See cholan-DH, cholic acid, 1; decholin, procholon.

de·hy″dro·cor″ti·cos′te·rone. 11-Dehydrocorticosterone. A steroid of the adrenal cortex possessing biologic activity similar to that of corticosterone.

de·hy′dro·gen·ase. An enzyme

which catalyzes the oxidation of [a] specific substrate by removal of hydrogen. Some dehydrogenases (aerobic) can transfer hydrogen directly t[o] gaseous oxygen, whereas other dehy[-] drogenases (anaerobic) require a hy[-] drogen acceptor. Also called dehydrase.

de·hy′dro·gen·ize, de·hy′dro[-] gen·ate. Remove hydrogen from [a] **—dehydrogeniza′tion, dehy[-] drogena′tion,** n.

de·hy″dro·i″so·an·dros′te·rone. $C_{19}H_{28}O_2$; Δ⁵-androstene-3(β)-ol-17-one. A 17-ketosteroid, having androgenic activity, found in urine.

de·hy″dro·stil·bes′trol. See di[-] enestrol.

dé″jà″vu′ (day″zhah″view′). A feel[-] ing of familiarity; a dream state in which experiences seem to have oc[-] curred before. A symptom found in tu[-] mors or other lesions of the temporal lobe of the brain. Syn., dreamy state; epilepsy.

de·jec′tion. 1. Depression, lowness o[f] spirits. 2. Discharge of fecal matter[;] defecation. 3. Feces; excrement.

de″lac·ta′tion. 1. Weaning. 2. Ces[-] sation of lactation.

de·lam″i·na′tion (dee-lam″i-nay′[-] shun). Separation or splitting int[o] layers, as in the dividing of cells t[o] form new layers.

De Lee, Joseph Bolivar [Ameri[-] can obstetrician, 1869–1942]. Known fo[r] his contributions in the field of opera[-] tive obstetrics and modern maternity care and for his textbook, Principle[s] and Practice of Obstetrics.

de·lim″i·ta′tion. The fixing of lim[-] its or boundaries.

de·lin′quen·cy. 1. An offense or vio[-] lation, especially that committed by [a] minor, as truancy, vandalism, lyin[g,] stealing, overt sex practices. 2. Th[e] tendency to commit delinquencies; th[e] committing of such offenses.

del″i·ques′cence. Process of lique[-] faction by absorption of water from th[e] atmosphere, or the resultant stat[e.] **—deliquescent,** adj.; **deliquesce,** v.

de·lir″i·fa′cient (di-lirr″i-fay′[-] shunt, -shee-unt). Producing delirium. Also called deliriant.

de·lir′i·um. A condition of menta[l] excitement, confusion, and cloude[d] sensorium, usually with hallucination[s,] illusions, and delusions; precipitated b[y] toxic factors in diseases or drugs. **—de[-] lirious,** adj. **abstinence d.** Tha[t] occurring upon withdrawal of alcoho[l] or of a drug from one addicted to i[t.] **acute d.** That form marked by con[-] vulsions and usually death. **alco[-] holic d.** See d. tremens. **co[l-] lapse d.** Delirium produced b[y] physical collapse. **d. grandiosu[m]**

That in which the individual has greatly exaggerated ideas of his own importance or possessions; megalomania. **d. nervosum.** That following severe surgical operations or injuries, or that associated with organic brain disease. **d. tremens.** A delirious state marked by distressing delusions, illusions, hallucinations, constant tremor, fumbling movements of the hands, insomnia, and great exhaustion. Usually associated with alcoholic poisoning, but may appear in acute inflammatory brain diseases, arteriosclerosis, or senile encephalopathy, or in schizophrenia or manic-depressive psychoses. Syn., *alcoholic d.* **emotional d.** That in which the state of mind is such that the individual will accept a false idea without qualifications. **exhaustion d.** That brought about by fatigue and extreme lowering of psychologic tension. Syn., *asthenic d.* **oneiric d.** Dream delirium; one occurring at night, made up of parts of dreams which vary uninterruptedly and may continue after the patient wakes. **quiet d.** A mental condition marked by delirious, scarcely audible mumbling. Syn., *d. mite.* **traumatic d.** Acute delirium resulting from head or brain injury.

e·liv·er·y. 1. Liberation; release. 2. Parturition; expulsion or extraction of a fetus and its membranes. 3. Removal of a part, as a lens in cataract extraction, or of a tumor. **—deliver,** *v.* **post-mortem d.** Extraction of the fetus after the death of the mother. **premature d.** Expulsion of the fetus after the twenty-eighth week and before term.

e"lo·mor'phous (dee"lo·mor'fus, del"o·). Having a conspicuous form, as a delomorphous cell, the acid-secreting parietal cell of the fundic glands.

e·louse' (dee-louse', ·louze'). Free from lice; destroy lice. **—delous'ing,** n.

el·phin'i·um. A genus of plants of the Ranunculaceae; the larkspurs.

elta cortef. A trade-mark for prednisolone.

eltasone. A trade-mark for prednisone.

el'toid. 1. Shaped like a Δ (capital delta), as the deltoid ligament of the ankle joint. 2. The large, thick, delta-shaped muscle covering the shoulder joint. See Table of Muscles in the Appendix.

eltra. A trade-mark for prednisone.

e·lu'sion. A belief maintained in the face of incontrovertible evidence to the contrary.

elvinal sodium. Trade-mark for sodium ethyl (1-methyl-1-butenyl) barbiturate, a rapidly acting sedative and hypnotic.

de"mar·ca'tion. Separation, establishing of limits. **line of d.** A line forming at the edge of a gangrenous area and marking the limit of the process.

de·ment'ed. Deprived of reason. **—dement',** n., v.

de·men'ti·a. Deterioration or loss of the intellectual faculties, the reasoning power, the memory, and the will; characterized by confusion, disorientation, apathy, and stupor of varying degrees. **alcoholic d.** A dementia more prolonged but less intense than delirium tremens, occurring in late stages of chronic alcoholism. **apoplectic d.** Dementia due to cerebral hemorrhage or to softening of brain tissue from other causes. **circular d.** That characterized by alternating phases of excitement and depression. **d. agitata.** Old term for a form distinguished by great excitement, motor activity, and continuous hallucinations; seen in patients with schizophrenia. **d. paralytica.** A meningoencephalitic type of psychosis in syphilis of the central nervous system. There are three recognised types: **dementia paralytica without psychosis, juvenile dementia paralytica,** and the **tabetic form of dementia paralytica.** Formerly called *general paralysis of the insane, q.v.* **d. precox.** The name given by Kraepelin to a form of insanity occurring during adolescence or early adulthood; was formerly thought to be a single psychotic disease, but is now known to be a group of heterogeneous psychoses. Four types are recognized—simple, hebephrenic, paranoid, and catatonic. Now more properly called schizophrenia, *q.v.* **epileptic d.** Mental deterioration in an epileptic person. **senile d.** The progressive cerebral manifestation of deterioration associated with old age. A less intense mental involvement than senile psychosis, *q.v.* **traumatic d.** That due directly or indirectly to an injury, usually of the head.

demerol hydrochloride. Trade-mark for a brand of meperidine hydrochloride.

dem'i-. A prefix signifying *half.*

dem"i·fac'et (dem"ee·fass'it). One-half of an articulation surface adapted to articulate with two bones.

de·min"er·al·i·za'tion (dee·min"·ur·ul·i·zay'shun, ·eye·zay'shun). Loss of mineral salts from the body, as from the bones. **coefficient of d.** The quantity of mineral matter as compared with the total solids in the urine.

de'mo-, dem-. A combining form denoting *populace.*

Dem'o·dex (dem'o·decks, dee'mo·). A

genus of parasitic arachnids. **D. folliculorum.** Species of mites which are parasites of the sebaceous glands and hair follicles.

de·mog'ra·phy (dee·mog'ruh·fee). The science of peoples collectively considered; social science, including that of vital statistics. **dynamic d.** A study of the activities of human communities, their rise, progress, and fall.

de'mon·o-, de'mon-. A combining form signifying *demon.*

de"mon·ol'a·try. Worship of a demon or spirit.

de"mon·o·ma'ni·a. A form of madness in which a person imagines himself possessed of a devil. **—demonomaniac,** n.

de"mon·o·pho'bi·a. Morbid fear of devils and demons.

de·mor"phin·i·za'tion (dee·mor'fin·i·zay'shun, ·eye·zay'shun). Treatment of morphinism by gradual withdrawal of the drug.

de·mul'cent. 1. Soothing; allaying irritation of surfaces, especially mucous membranes. 2. A soothing substance, particularly a slippery, mucilaginous liquid.

de·my'e·lin·ate. Remove or destroy the myelin sheath of nerves or nerve tracts.

de·nar'co·tized (dee·nahr'ko·tized). 1. Deprived of narcotizing qualities. 2. Deprived of narcotine, said of opium.

de·na"tur·a'tion. See *denaturization.*

de·na'tured. Changed, made different from normal.

de·na'tured al'co·hol. Alcohol into which some other substance has been introduced, rendering it unfit for drinking but still useful for other purposes.

de·na"tur·i·za'tion (dee·nay"chur·i·zay'shun, ·eye·zay'shun). Alteration in the characteristics of an organic substance, especially a protein, by physical or chemical action.

den'drite. A process of a neuron which carries the nerve impulse to the cell body. It is usually branched, like a tree. **—dendrit'ic,** adj.

den'dron. See *dendrite.*

de·ner'va·ted (dee·nur'vay·tid). Having the nerve supply interfered with, or the nerve removed.

de"ner·va'tion. 1. Sectioning or removal of a nerve to interrupt the nerve supply to a part. 2. *In veterinary medicine,* the cutting off of the nerve supply to the lower leg and foot to relieve certain types of lameness in the horse.

den'gue (deng'ghee, deng'gay). An acute, infectious, endemic, and epidemic disease; caused by a filtrable virus transmitted by mosquitoes, especially by the *Aëdes aegypti.* Dengue is characterized by a febrile paroxysm, severe pains in the bones and muscles,

and swelling, reddening, and pain ⌐ the joints. At times there is a cutaneo⌐ eruption. The period of incubation ⌐ from three to five days, and the inv⌐ sion is sudden. The high fever (106° F⌐ lasts for three or four days and su⌐ sides for an interval, which is followe⌐ by a second paroxysm. Convalescen⌐ is slow and complications are rar⌐ The disease is widespread throughou⌐ the tropics and the subtropics. Syr⌐ *breakbone fever.* Also called *danc⌐ fever.*

den"i·da'tion (den"i·day'shu⌐ dee"nigh·). Disintegration and eje⌐ tion of the superficial part of t⌐ uterine mucosa.

de·ni'tri·fy (dee·nigh'tri·figh). R⌐ move nitrogen.

dens (denz) (pl. *dentes*). 1. A tooth. ⌐ The toothlike process on the body ⌐ the axis, going through the front pa⌐ of the ring of the atlas. **d. acutu⌐** An incisor tooth. **d. adultus.** A too⌐ of second dentition. **d. adversu⌐** An incisor tooth. **d. angularis.** ⌐ canine or cuspid tooth. **d. bicusp⌐ datus.** A bicuspid tooth. **d. ca⌐ ninus.** A canine or cuspid toot⌐ **d. cariosus.** A carious toot⌐ **d. columellaris.** A molar toot⌐ **d. cuspidatus.** A cuspid toot⌐ **d. exsertus.** A tooth which projec⌐ or is in front of the dental arch; a⌐ plied more particularly to the cuspi⌐ **d. incisor.** An incisor tooth. **d. la⌐ teus.** A milk, temporary, or deciduo⌐ tooth. **d. molaris.** A molar toot⌐ **d. primoris.** An incisor tooth; ⌐ called because it occupies the front ⌐ anterior part of the dental arc⌐ **d. sapientia.** A wisdom tooth; ⌐ name given to the third molar tooth ⌐ each half of each jaw. **d. serotinu⌐** A wisdom tooth. **d. tomici.** An i⌐ cisor tooth.

den·sim'e·ter. An appliance f⌐ ascertaining the specific gravity of ⌐ liquid. Syn., *hydrometer.* **—dens⌐ met'ric,** adj.

den"si·tom'e·ter. See *densimeter.*

den'si·ty. Closeness of any space di⌐ tribution; for example, **electro⌐ density** signifies the number of ele⌐ trons per unit volume. Abbreviated, **absolute d.** (a) The ratio of t⌐ mass of a substance to its volume. S⌐ specific *gravity.* (b) The light-absor⌐ ing power of the silver image in ph⌐ tographic materials.

dent-. See *denti-.*

den·tag'ra (den·tag'ruh, den'ta⌐ ruh). 1. Toothache. 2. A tooth forcep⌐

den'tal. Pertaining to the teeth.

den'tal en'gine. *In dentistry,* t⌐ apparatus used to operate rotatin⌐ cutting, or polishing devices such ⌐ burs, abrasive disks or wheels, a⌐

brushes. These interchangeable parts are held in a handpiece which is connected by a flexible arm to a controlled driving mechanism, usually an electric motor.

den'tal floss. A soft thread, usually flat and waxed; used to clean interdental spaces and tooth surfaces.

den·tal'gi·a. Toothache.

den'tate. *In botany,* having teeth or toothlike projections; having a toothed or serrated edge. **—denta'tion,** *n.*

den'tes (den'teez). Plural of dens, *q.v.*

den'ti-, dent-. A combining form meaning *tooth* or *dental.*

den'ti·a pre'cox. The presence of erupted teeth at birth.

den'ti·cle. 1. A small tooth or projecting point. 2. The deposit of calcareous material within the pulp of the tooth; associated with degenerative or retrogressive changes of the pulp; pulpstone.

den·tic'u·late. Having minute dentations; furnished with small teeth or notches.

den"ti·fi·ca'tion. Formation of teeth; dentition.

den'ti·form. Odontoid; tooth-shaped.

den'ti·frice (den'ti·friss). A substance or preparation used to aid the mechanical cleaning of the teeth.

den·tig'er·ous (den·tidj'ur·us). Bearing or containing teeth.

den'ti·lave. A mouthwash or toothwash.

den'tin (den'tin, ·teen), **den'tine.** The calcified tissue which forms the major part of a tooth. Dentin is related to bone but differs from it in the absence of included cells. It is covered by the enamel over the crown of the tooth, by the cementum over the roots, and itself surrounds the pulp chamber and root canals which contain the dental pulp. Syn., *substantia eburnea, ivory, ebur.* **—dentinal,** *adj.* **cir·cumpulpar d.** The major part of the dentin which lies next the pulp. **interglobular d.** A small region of poorly calcified dentin found along the course of the incremental lines. **mantle d.** The thin superficial layer of dentin. **secondary d.** The dentin of repair; that which is deposited on the walls of the pulp chamber by the dental pulp in response to loss of tooth substance.

den"ti·nal'gi·a. Pain in the dentin.

den"ti·no·gen'e·sis. The formation of dentin. Also called *dentinification.* **d. imperfecta.** A hereditary hypoplasia of the dentin in which the teeth are brown, subject to rapid wear, and easily fractured. Also called *hereditary opalescent dentin.*

den'ti·noid. A calcified structure having some but not all of the characteristics of dentin.

den"ti·no'ma. A tumor of the dentin.

den"ti·nos'te·oid. A hard, calcified structure having some of the histologic appearance of both dentin and bone.

den'tist. One who practices dentistry.

den'tis·try. That department of medicine concerned with the prevention, diagnosis, and treatment of diseases of the teeth and adjacent tissues, and the restoration of missing dental and oral structures. **aesthetic d.** The preservation, repair, and restoration of the teeth and adjacent tissues, performed so that the work has a natural and pleasing appearance. **operative d.** The branch of dentistry concerned with actual operations upon the natural teeth or the soft tissues of the oral cavity, as distinguished from those operations performed in the dental laboratory. **prosthetic d.** That branch of dentistry which deals with the replacement of missing teeth or oral tissues by artificial means.

den·ti'tion. 1. The process of teething; the eruption of the teeth through the alveolar ridge. 2. The character and arrangement of the teeth of an individual or species. **primary d.** (a) The eruption of the deciduous teeth. (b) The deciduous teeth. See under *tooth.* Syn., *deciduous d.* **secondary d.** (a) The eruption of the adult teeth. (b) The permanent teeth. See under *tooth.* Syn., *permanent d.*

den'to-. Combining form meaning *dental, pertaining to dentistry.*

den"to·al·ve·o'lar. Pertaining to the alveolus of a tooth.

den"to·al"ve·o·li'tis. See *periodontosis.*

den"to·fa'cial (den"to·fay'shul). Pertaining to both the teeth and the face.

den·tog'ra·phy. A description of teeth.

den'toid. Toothlike.

den"to·le'gal. Pertaining to dental jurisprudence.

den·ton'o·my. Classification of the teeth.

den'ture. The natural or artificial teeth of an individual considered as a unit. **artificial d.** A complete artificial replacement of either the upper or the lower teeth. **continuous gum d.** An appliance with the artificial gum portion of fused porcelain. **full d.** A replacement of the complete dental equipment of both jaws. **partial artificial d.** A replacement of less than the full number of teeth in either arch; a removable appliance is used, which is attached to the adjoining natural teeth.

de·nu·cle·a"ted (dee·new'klee·ay"tid). Deprived of a nucleus.

de·nude'. Deprive of covering, strip,

lay bare; said of the root of a tooth. —**denuda'tion,** n.

de·ob'stru·ent. Any agent or drug which removes an obstruction or obstructive material, as in the alimentary canal.

de"o'dor·ant. 1. Removing or concealing offensive odors. 2. A substance that removes or conceals offensive odors. —**deodorizer,** n.; **deodorize,** v.t.

de"or·al'i·ty. In psychoanalysis, the shifting of instinctual activity away from gratification through oral expression.

de·or"sum·duc'tion. A turning downward of a part.

de·or"sum·ver'gence. A downward inclination, as of the eyes.

de·os"si·fi·ca'tion. The absorption of bony material; the deprivation of the bony character of any part.

de·ox'y-, des·ox'y. A combining form denoting loss of oxygen from a compound, frequently by replacement of a hydroxyl group by a hydrogen atom.

de·ox"y·cho'lic ac'id (dee-ock*"*si-ko'lick, ·kol'ick). Desoxycholic acid.

de·ox"y·cor'tone ac'e·tate. British Pharmacopoeia title for desoxycorticosterone acetate.

de·ox"y·gen·a'tion. The process of removing oxygen from a compound.

de·ox"y·ri"bo·nu'cle·ase, des·ox"y·ri"bo·nu'cle·ase. An enzyme capable of hydrolyzing deoxyribonucleic acid; abbreviated, DNase. Also called streptodornase.

de·ox"y·ri"bo·nu·cle'ic ac'id, des·ox"y·ri"bo·nu·cle'ic ac'id. A nucleic acid present in the nucleus of cells, thought to be the carrier of genetic determinants. Abbreviated, DNA.

de·per"son·al·i·za'tion (dee-pur*"*-sun·ul·i·zay'shun, ·eye·zay'shun). Loss of the sense of one's own reality or identity; a feeling of being someone else.

de·pig"men·ta'tion (dee-pig*"*men-tay'shun). 1. The removal of natural pigments from the skin. 2. The removal of pigments from microscopic preparations by the action of weak preparations of bleaching or oxidizing solutions.

dep'i·late. Remove the hair. —**depil'atory,** adj., n.; **depila'tion,** n.

dep'i·lous. Hairless.

de·ple'tion. 1. The act of diminishing the quantity of fluid in the body or in a part, especially by bleeding. 2. The condition of the system produced by the excessive loss of blood or other

fluids; reduction of strength; exhaustion. —**deplete',** v.t.

de"plu·ma'tion. Loss of the eyelashes. Rare.

de·po"lar·i·za'tion (dee-po*"*lux-i·zay'shun, ·eye·zay'shun). The neutralization of polarity; the breaking down of polarized semipermeable membranes, as in nerve or muscle cells in the conduction of impulses.

de"po·lym'er·ase (dee*"*po·lim'ur·ace, dee·pol'i·mur·ace). One of a group of enzymes which depolymerize high molecular weight plant and animal nucleic acids, forming mononucleotides without the liberation of phosphoric acid.

de·pos'it. A sediment; a collection of morbid particles in a body. **dental d.** Hard or soft material adherent to the surface of a tooth.

de·pres'sant. 1. Lowering functional activity. 2. A medicine that diminishes functional activity.

de·pres'sion. 1. A hollow or fossa. 2. Inward displacement of a part, as of the skull. 3. Lowering of vital function under the action of some depressing agent. 4. In psychopathology, an emotional state of dejection usually associated with manic-depressive psychosis, q.v. Mild depression with anxiety and hypochondria is frequently seen in youth of either sex (**adolescent depression**) and often occurs when ever the adult sex problem becomes acute, as after engagement or marriage. Depression may also occur as a result of an external situation, being relieved when the external situation is removed (**reactive depression**). See melancholia. —**depressed, depressive,** adj.

de·pres'sor. 1. A muscle, instrument, or apparatus that depresses. 2. A nerve stimulation of which lowers arterial blood pressure by reflex vasodilatation and by slowing the heart, as the depressor nerve. **tongue d.** A spatula for pushing down the tongue during the examination of the mouth and throat.

depth. Measurement of distance from top to bottom or from front to back; deepness. **focal d.** The power of a lens to give clear images of objects at different distances from it. Also called field d.

de·pu"li·za'tion (dee-pew*"*li·zay'shun, ·lye·zay'shun). The destruction or removal of fleas, as from infested animals or premises.

der"a·del'phus. A monocephalic dual monster, with the body fused above the umbilicus, and with four lower extremities and three or four upper. Syn., cephalothoracopagus.

de·range'ment. Disorder of intellect; insanity. **internal d. of the**

knee. A condition of abnormal joint mobility with painful symptoms usually due to injury to the medial semilunar cartilage.

e're·ism. *In psychiatry,* a mental state in which the subject is lost in phantasy, showing no interest in external experiences or reality; autism. **—dereis'tic,** *adj.*

er'ic. External; pertaining to the skin.

er″i·va'tion. The deflection of blood from one part of the body to another, as by counterirritation; formerly thought to relieve inflammatory congestion. *Obs.*

e·riv'a·tive. 1. Producing derivation. 2. An agent that produces derivation. 3. A substance derived from another substance.

erm-. See *dermato-.*

ierm. Suffix signifying *skin, integument,* or *covering.*

er'ma, derm. The layer of the skin between the epidermis and subcutaneous tissue; the connective tissue of the true skin. Syn., *corium, cutis vera, ermis.* **—dermal, dermic,** *adj.*

er'ma-. See *dermato-.*

ier'ma. A combining form denoting *a type of skin, a type of skin disease, or a genus characterized by a type of skin.*

er″ma·cen'tor. A genus of ticks some species of which are vectors of disease. **D. andersoni.** The wood tick; medically, it is the most important North American species, transmitting Rocky Mountain spotted fever and tularemia as well as producing tick paralysis. **D. variabilis.** A species widely distributed in North America which has as its principal host the dog, although man and other mammals may be attacked.

er″ma·cen·trox′e·nus rick·tt′si. Synonym for *Rickettsia rickettsii.*

er·man′a·plas′ty. Skin grafting.

er″ma·nys′sus. A genus of itch mites. **D. gallinae.** A species which is a serious pest of poultry and sometimes attacks man.

er″ma·tag′ra (dur″muh·tag′ruh, ay′gruh). 1. Pellagra, *q.v.* 2. Dermatalgia.

er″ma·tal′gi·a. Pain, burning, and other sensations of the skin, unaccompanied by any structural change; probably caused by some nervous disease or reflex influence.

er″ma·ta·neu′ri·a. Derangement of the nerve supply of the skin, causing anesthesia or paresthesia.

er″mat·he′mi·a (dur″mat·hee′·ee-uh, dur″muh·tee′mee-uh). A congestion of the skin. Also called *deraemia, dermohemia.*

der·mat′ic. 1. Relating to the skin. 2. A remedy for diseases of the skin.

der″ma·ti′tis. An inflammation of the skin. **atopic d.** That due to sensitization to substances by ingestion or inhalation. There is usually a familial history of some type of allergy. **berlock d.** A brownish pigmentation seen on skin exposed to sun after the use of cologne. **blastomycetic d.** A skin disease caused by one of the several yeastlike fungi. **caterpillar d.** A form due to the highly irritating hairs of the larvae of certain lepidoptera; characterized first by erythematous macules and then by wheals. **contact d.** That due to sensitization to a substance coming in contact with the skin. **d. actinica.** That due to the action of actinic rays, from sunlight or artificial ultraviolet light. **d. calorica.** That due to burns and scalds. **d. dysmenorrheica.** An eruption seen during the menstrual period in women having dysmenorrhea. Wheals, vesicles, or erythematous areas are seen over the body. Many eruptions are exaggerated during the menses. Also called *catamenial d.* **d. escharotica.** A severe ulcerative type due to exposure to escharotic agents. **d. exfoliativa.** An acute or chronic inflammation of the skin, in which the epidermis is shed more or less freely in large or small scales. See *pityriasis rubra.* **d. factitia.** An eruption induced by the patient; varies from simple erythema to gangrene. Usually produced by some irritant in neurotic or hysterical subjects. Also called *feigned eruptions, d. autofactitia, hysterical dermatoneuroses.* **d. gangrenosa.** Sphaceloderma; gangrenous inflammation of the skin. **d. gangrenosa infantum.** A form of ecthyma marked by brown discolorations of the skin, usually surrounded by a halo; the center of these efflorescences rapidly becomes necrotic. Due to *Pseudomonas aeruginosa.* **d. herpetiformis.** An inflammatory, recurring skin disease of a herpetic character, the various lesions showing a tendency to group. It is protean, appearing as erythema, vesicles, blebs, and pustules; associated with intense itching and burning. **d. hiemalis.** A recurrent inflammation of the skin, associated with cold weather and allied to the erythemas. **d. hypostatica.** One occurring in an area of poor blood supply, usually the lower legs. **d. medicamentosa.** Eruptions due to the action of certain drugs. **d. nodularis necrotica.** A necrosis of the epidermis and superficial layers of the corium; due primarily to changes and consequent obstruction in the blood vessels between the cutis and subcutis. **d. papillaris capillitii.** A chronic skin disease affecting the nape of the neck and adjacent parts; characterized by minute red papules, which occasionally suppurate and are usually traversed by a hair. They unite to form hard white or reddish keloids. **d. repens.** An infectious dermatitis of the extremities, more frequently of the hands, consisting of a flaccid bulla which spreads peripherally, undermining the corneous layer of the epidermis and separating it from the subjacent epithelial layers. **d. rhus.** Contact dermatitis due to poison ivy or poison oak. **d. seborrheica.** An acute inflammatory form, occurring usually on oily skin in areas having large sebaceous glands; may be due to a fungus. Characterized by dry, moist, or greasy scales and by crusted yellowish patches, remissions, exacerbations, and itching. Syn., *eczema seborrheicum, seborrhea sicca.* **d. traumatica.** That resulting from traumatism. **d. vegetans.** Elevated, vegetating lesions covered with crusts; very prone to bleeding and believed to be due to some infection. **d. venenata.** That produced by the local action of irritant substances, usually plants. A type of contact dermatitis. **infectious eczematoid d.** A low-grade skin infection; produces oozing, erythematous patches. **roentgen d.** That due to prolonged exposure to roentgen rays, or radium. Also called *radium d., x-ray d.*

der/ma·to-, dermat-. A combining form meaning *skin* or *hide.*

Der/ma·to·bi·a. A genus of botflies whose larvae are obligatory sarcobionts, producing cutaneous myiasis in many animals. **D. hominis.** A species found in tropical America, causing dermal myiasis in man. The eggs are deposited by the adult female, or by another insect parasitized by the egg, on the skin of the host. Upon emergence, the larva burrows into the skin, producing a swelling very much like an ordinary boil.

der/ma·to·cel/lu·li/tis. Acute inflammation of the skin and subcutaneous tissue.

der/ma·to·cha·la/sis. Diffuse relaxation of the skin, with associated folding and excess of elastic and collagenous fibers.

der/ma·to·co/ni·o/sis, der/ma·to·ko/ni·o/sis. Any skin disease due to dust.

der/ma·to·cyst/. A cyst of the skin.

der/ma·to·fi·bro/ma len·tic/u·la/re (dur/muh·to·figh·bro/muh len·tick/yoo·lah/ree). A skin disease producing hard, nodular lesions; few in number and often permanent. Syn., *fibroma durum.*

der/ma·to·fi/bro·sar·co/ma. fibrosarcoma of the skin.

der/ma·to·glyph/ics. Study [of?] skin-pattern lines and whorls of t[he] hands and feet; used for identificat[ion] purposes. These patterns are individ[u]ally characteristic and do not chan[ge] during a person's lifetime.

der/ma·tog/ra·phy. 1. A descr[ip]tion of the skin. 2. Dermograph[y] *q.v.*

der/ma·tol/o·gist. A skin sp[e]cialist: a physician who makes a spec[ial] study of diseases of the skin.

der/ma·tol/o·gy. Science of t[he] skin, its structure, functions, diseas[es] and their treatment. —**derma[to]tolog/ic, dermatolog/ical,** a[dj.]

der/ma·tol/y·sis. 1. Abnormal la[xi]tion of the skin, usually congenit[al] producing folds. 2. Fibromas of the sk[in] with masses of pendulous skin. A[lso] called *chalazodermia, cutis pendu[la]fibroma pendulum, lax skin.*

der/ma·tome. 1. An instrument f[or] cutting skin, as in grafting. 2. T[he] lateral part of an embryonic som[ite] cutis plate. —**dermatom/ic,** *adj.*

der/ma·to·my·co/sis (·migh·k[o]·sis). Any skin disease caused by a ve[ge]table parasite; a fungus infection [of] the skin.

der/ma·to·my·o/ma (·migh·[o]·muh). Myoma located in the skin.

der/ma·to·my/o·si/tis. Degene[ra]tive changes of skin and muscles ca[us]ing weakness and pain; the condit[ion] may be extensive or minimal. T[he] cutaneous reaction may be severe w[ith] edema and erythema or complet[ely] absent.

der/ma·to·neu·rol/o·gy. Study [of] the nerves of the skin.

der/ma·to·neu·ro/sis. A skin d[is]ease of nervous origin. **hysterical** [d.] A self-produced eruption in a hyste[ri]cal person.

der/ma·to·pa·thol/o·gy. Path[ol]ogy of the skin.

der/ma·to·path/o·pho/bi·[a]. Morbid fear of having a skin diseas[e.]

der/ma·top/a·thy. Any skin d[is]ease. —**dermatopath/ic,** *adj.*

Der/ma·toph/i·lus pen/e·tra[ns] (pen/i·tranz). Synonym for *Tu[nga penetrans.*

der/ma·to·phyte/. A group [of] fungi which invade the superficial sk[in] The dermatophytes are now divi[ded] into three genera—*Microsporum, E[pi]dermophyton,* and *Trichophyton* (E[m]mons' classification based on dif[fer]ences in morphologic features). F[or]merly, the dermatophytes were cla[ssi]fied according to the type of lesion fr[om] which they were isolated, without [re]gard to the form or structure of [the] organisms.

der/ma·toph/y·tid. A rash asso[ciated]

...ted with a skin disease caused by a vegetable parasite.

er″ma·to·phy·to′sis (·figh·to′sis). A skin eruption characterized by the formation of small vesicles on the hands and feet, especially between the toes, with cracking and scaling. There is sometimes secondary infection. The cause may be any one of the dermatophytes. Syn., *ringworm, athlete's foot.*

er″ma·to·plas″ty. A plastic operation on the skin whereby skin losses or defects are replaced by skin flaps or grafts.

er″ma·tor·rha′gi·a. Hemorrhage from the skin.

er″ma·tos′co·py. Examination of the skin; particularly, microscopical examination of the superficial capillaries of the skin.

er″ma·to′sis. Any disease of the skin. **d. papulosa nigra.** An eruption commonly seen in Negroes, usually on the face, consisting of many tiny tumors of the skin; probably nevoid in origin. **occupational d.** One that results from chemicals or irritations resulting from the nature of an occupation. **postvaccinal d.** A dermatosis following vaccination, marked by lesions similar to those of urticaria pigmentosa except that desquamation is present and dermographia is absent. **precancerous d.** A skin condition that sometimes develops into a malignant skin lesion. **progressive pigmentary d.** A reddish, purpuric, papular eruption; it is seen principally on the legs and is progressive in character. Also called *Schamberg's disease.*

er″ma·to·stom″a·ti′tis (·stom″-h·tye′tis, ·sto″muh·tye′tis). A rare, severe form of erythema multiforme with involvement of the conjunctiva and oral mucosa.

er″ma·to·ther′a·py. Treatment of cutaneous affections.

er″ma·to·thla′si·a (dur″muh·to·thlay′zhuh, ·zee·uh). A morbid state marked by an uncontrollable impulse to pinch or rub the skin.

er″ma·tot′o·my. Anatomy or dissection of the skin.

er′mis. Derma, *q.v.*

er″mo-, derm-, der′ma-. See *ermato-.*

er″mo·blast. That part of the mesoderm which develops into the corium.

er″mo·ep″i·der′mal. Pertaining to both the superficial and the deeper layers of the skin; said of skin grafts.

er″mo·graph′i·a (dur″mo·graf′e·uh, ·gray′fee·uh), **der·mog′ra·phy.** A condition in which the skin is peculiarly susceptible to irritation; characterized by elevations or wheals caused by tracing the fingernail or a blunt instrument over the skin. May or may not be accompanied by urticaria.

Also called *dermographism, autographism, urticaria factitia.* —**dermograph′ic,** *adj.*

der′moid. 1. Resembling skin. 2. A dermoid cyst.

der″moid·ec′to·my. Excision of a dermoid cyst.

der″mo·la′bi·al. Having relation to the skin and the lips.

der″mo·phle·bi′tis. Inflammation of the cutaneous veins.

der″mo·skel′e·ton. The exoskeleton, 2.

der″mo·ste·no′sis. A tightening of the skin, due to swelling or to disease.

der″mos·to′sis. Ossification occurring in the true skin.

der″mo·syn″o·vi′tis (·sin″o·vy′tis, ·sigh″no·vy′tis). Inflammation of a subcutaneous bursa together with the adjacent skin.

der″mo·syph″i·lop′a·thy. A syphilitic skin disease.

der′o-, der-. A combining form denoting the neck.

des-. A prefix denoting the *reversing* or *undoing* of an action, *depriving* or *ridding of,* or *freeing from;* used before vowels, especially in chemistry. Also see *de-.*

Descemet's membrane. See under *membrane.*

des″ce·me·ti′tis. A pseudoinflammation of Descemet's membrane; keratitis punctata, *q.v.*

des″ce·met′o·cele. Hernia of Descemet's membrane.

de·scend′ens (di·send′enz). Downward. **d. hypoglossi.** A branch of the hypoglossal nerve which forms, with the descending cervical nerve, the ansa hypoglossi. The fibers come from the first and second cervical nerves and not from the hypoglossal nucleus. See Table of Nerves in the Appendix.

de·scen′sus (di·sen′sus). A descent, fall, prolapse.

de·scent′. Derivation from an ancestor, especially in regard to evolutionary origin.

de·sen″si·ti·za′tion (dee·sen″si·ti·zay′shun, ·tigh·zay′shun). 1. A condition of insusceptibility to infection; established in experimental animals by the injection of an antigen which produces sensitization or an anaphylactic reaction. After recovery, a second injection of the antigen is made, bringing about no reaction, thus producing desensitization. 2. *In psychiatry,* the alleviation or removal of a mental complex. —**desen′sitize,** *v.t.*

de·ser′pi·dine. 11-Desmethoxyreserpine, an alkaloid from *Rauwolfia canescens,* used, like reserpine, as a sedative and antihypertensive drug.

de·sex″u·al′i·ty (dee·seck″shoo·al′i·tee). A state in which a sexual impulse is deprived of that quality by being diverted into other activities, as in sublimation.

de·sex"u·al·i·za'tion (dee-seck"-shoo·ul·i·zay'shun, ·eye·zay'shun). Depriving an individual of his sexual powers.

des'ic·cant. 1. Causing desiccation; drying. 2. A drying medicine or application.

des"ic·ca'tion. Process of drying up.

des'ic·ca"tor. A vessel containing a strongly hygroscopic substance, such as calcium chloride or sulfuric acid, used to absorb moisture from any substance placed therein or to maintain it in a moisture-free state.

des'mo- (dez'mo-, des'mo-), **desm-** Combining form meaning *bond, ligament,* or *fastening.*

des'mo·cyte. Any kind of supporting tissue cell.

des'moid. Like a ligament; fibrous.

des'mo·lase. An enzyme which breaks or forms a carbon chain of an organic substrate.

des'mone. A general term for growth-promoting substances, theoretically present in all cells.

des·mot'o·my. Incision of a ligament.

des·ox'y-. Same as *deoxy-.*

des·ox"y·cho'lic ac'id (dess·ock"-si·ko'lick, ·kol'ick), **de·ox"y·cho'lic ac'id.** 3,12-Dihydrocholanic acid. One of the unconjugated bile acids; in bile it is largely conjugated, with glycine or taurine, to form glyco-desoxycholate and taurodesoxycholate salts.

des·ox"y·cor"ti·cos'te·rone. A potent steroid hormone of the adrenal cortex. **d. acetate.** The acetate ester of desoxycorticosterone and the form in which the hormone is used clinically. Syn., *deoxycortone acetate, deoxycostone acetate.* See *cortate, doca, percorten.*

des·ox"y·e·phed'rine (·eh·fed·rin, ·ef'i·dreen). Phenylisopropylmethylamine, $C_6H_5.CH_2.CH(CH_3).NH(CH_3)$. A substance related to both amphetamine and ephedrine, employed in the form of its salts as a cerebral stimulant and a vasoconstrictor. Syn., *methamphetamine, methylamphetamine.*

des·ox"y·ri"bo·nu'cle·ase. Deoxyribonuclease.

des·ox"y·ri"bo·nu·cle'ic ac'id. Deoxyribonucleic acid.

des·ox"y·ri'bose. A pentose found in all cells, and particularly in nucleic acid.

des"qua·ma'tion. Shedding; a peeling and casting off, as of the superficial epithelium of mucous membranes, renal tubules, or the skin. The horny layer of the epidermis is constantly shed as a normal physiologic process. In disease, an exaggerated process pro-

duces various-sized flakes and scale Desquamation from newborn infan (desquamatio neonatorum) takes pla during the first week of life. —de quam'ative, *adj.;* des'quamate *v.i.*

des·sert'spoon". A spoon of mediu size, equal to approximately 2 flu drachms or 8 cc.

de·stru'do. *In psychopathology,* th basic energy that is associated with th destructive or death instinct.

det. *Detur;* let it be given.

de·ter'gent. 1. Purifying; cleansin 2. A drug, compound, or solution use for cleansing wounds, ulcers, etc.

de·ter'mi·nant. *In biology,* a hyp thetical unit of the germ plasm whic according to Weismann's theory heredity, determines the final fate the cell or the part which receives during development.

de·ter"mi·na'tion. 1. Tendency the blood to collect in a part. 2. Fixatio of the embryologic fate of a tissue a part of an embryo by an evocator other agent. **sex d.** Determination the sex of an embryo at fertilization b the complement of sex chromosomes.

de·tox'i·cate (dee·tock'si·kayt). lessen or remove the poisonous proper of a substance. —**detoxica'tion,** *ad n.;* **detoxica'tion,** *n.*

de·tox'i·fy (dee·tock'si·figh). Detox cate. —**detoxifica'tion,** *n.*

de·tri'tion (di·trish'un). Wearin away by abrasion.

de·tri'tus. 1. Waste matter from di integration. 2. *In dentistry,* waste ma terial adherent to a tooth, or disinte grated tooth substance.

de"trun·ca'tion. Decapitation, e pecially of the fetus.

de·tru'sion. An ejection or expulsion thrusting down or out.

de"tu·mes'cence. 1. Subsidence any swelling. 2. Subsidence of th erectile sexual organs.

deu"ter·a·no'pi·a (dew"tur·uh·no pee·uh). Inadequate green vision; rec sightedness.

deu·te'ri·um (dew·teer'ee·um Heavy hydrogen. The isotope of hydr gen of atomic weight approximate. 2.0, symbol H^2, H^b, or **D. d. oxide** Water of composition D_2O. Syn., *heav water.*

deu'ter·o- (dew'tur·o-), **deuter** (dew'tur-). A combining form mean ing *second* or *secondary.*

deu'ter·on. The nucleus of a heav hydrogen atom.

deu'ter·o·plasm. 1. The passive o lifeless components of cytoplasm, espe cially reserve foodstuffs such as yol 2. The store of nutrient material in th ovum. Syn., *food yolk.* Also calle *deutoplasm.*

deu"ter·o·tox'in. One of the second group into which Ehrlich classifies toxins, according to the avidity with which they combine with antitoxins, deuterotoxin having less affinity than has prototoxin and more than tritotoxin.

deu'ton. Deuteron.

de·vel'op·ment. In biology, the series of events occurring in an organism during the change from the fertilized egg to the adult stage. **arrested d.** Failure of an organism to carry out its normal evolution, stopping at an initial or intermediate stage of the process. **postnatal d.** That portion of development occurring after birth. **prenatal d.** That portion of development occurring before birth.

de"vi·a'tion. 1. Turning from a regular course, standard, or position; deflection. 2. In optics, the inability of the two eyes to fix upon an object at the same time; squint; strabismus. When the healthy eye is fixed upon the object, the squinting eye is unable to fix and consequently deviates; this is known as **primary deviation.** When the squint-eye is the one fixed, there is a corresponding deviation of the healthy eye, known as **secondary deviation. axis d.** In electrocardiography, a term indicating that the mean electric axis is beyond the normal limits (0°–90°), but without other electrocardiographic abnormalities. Due to variations in the position of the heart. **conjugate d.** The forced and persistent turning of the eyes and head toward one side; observed with some lesions of the cerebrum. **mean d.** The arithmetic average of the differences between each observation in a series and the mean of the series, disregarding the sign of the differences.

de"vi·om'e·ter. A variety of strabismometer.

de·vi'tal·ize (dee-vy'tul·ize). Destroy vitality. **—devitaliza'tion,** n.

dev"o·lu'tion. 1. The reverse of evolution; involution. 2. Catabolism. Degeneration.

Dex'edrine. A trade-mark for the dextrorotatory isomer of amphetamine.

dex'ter. Right; upon the right side. Abbreviated, d.

dex'trad. Toward the right side.

dex'tral. Pertaining to the right side; right-handed.

dex·tral'i·ty. Condition in which the right side of the body is more efficient than the left; right-handedness.

dex'tran. A generic term for a high molecular weight polysaccharide which yields dextrose on hydrolysis. A dextran synthesized from sucrose by Leuconostoc mesenteroides is used as a plasma substitute.

dex·trau'ral. Pertaining to the right ear.

dex'trin. ($C_6H_{10}O_5$) $n.xH_2O$. A white or yellow, amorphous powder, dextrorotatory, produced by incomplete hydrolysis of starch. Used as an emulsifying, protective, and thickening agent. **animal d.** Glycogen.

dex"tri·nu'ri·a. Presence of dextrin in the urine.

dex'tro-. A combining form meaning toward, of, or pertaining to the right.

dex"tro·car'di·a. Transposition of the heart to the right side of the thorax. Also called dexiocardia. **—dextrocardial,** adj.

dex"tro·car'di·o·gram". That component of the normal electrocardiogram for which the right ventricle is responsible.

dex"tro·cer'e·bral. Located in the right cerebral hemisphere.

dex·troc'u·lar. Right-eyed; using the right eye in preference to the left. **—dextrocular'ity,** n.

dex"tro·duc'tion. Movement of the visual axis toward the right.

dex"tro·glu'cose. Dextrose, q.v.

dex"tro·gy'rate. Dextrorotatory, q.v.

dex"tro·man'u·al. Right-handed. **—dextromanual'ity,** n.

dex"tro·pe'dal, dex·trop'e·dal. Right-footed.

dex"tro·pho'bi·a. Morbid fear of objects on the right side of the body.

dex"tro·pho'ri·a. A tending of the visual lines to the right.

dex'tro pro·pox'y·phene hy"dro·chlo'ride. α-d-4-Dimethylamino-1,2-diphenyl-3-methyl-2-butanol propionate hydrochloride, an analgesic. See darvon.

dex"tro·ro·ta'to·ry. Turning the rays of light to the right. Abbreviated, d-. Also see (+) in Table of Signs and Symbols in the Appendix.

dex'trose (decks'troce, ·troze). $C_6H_{12}O_6.H_2O$. A dextrorotatory monosaccharide occurring as a white powder; soluble in water. It is an essential constituent of blood, being not only a source of energy but also a necessity for the complete combustion of fats. See glucose. Syn., dextroglucose, grape sugar, starch sugar. Also called d-glucose.

dex"tro·sin'is·tral (decks"tro·sin'·is·trul, ·sin·iss'trul). Extending from right to left.

dex"tro·su'ri·a. Presence of dextrose in the urine.

dex"tro·tar·tar'ic ac'id (decks"·stro·tahr·tar'ick, ·tahr·tahr'ick). Tartaric acid.

dex"tro·tor'sion. A twisting to the right.

dex″tro·ver′sion (decks″tro-vur′-zhun, ·vur′shun). Version to the right side.

DFP. [(CH₃)₂CH]₂FPO₃. Diisopropyl fluorophosphate. An oily liquid, soluble in water but hydrolyzing rapidly; miscible with oils. A powerful inhibitor of cholinesterase; used in the treatment of glaucoma.

dho′bie itch (do′bee). See *tinea cruris.*

di- (dye-, *even when unstressed*). See *dis-.*

di′a-, di-. A prefix denoting *through, between, apart, asunder,* or *across.*

di′a·be′tes (dye″uh-bee′teez, ·bee′tiss). A disease characterized by the habitual discharge of an excessive quantity of urine and by excessive thirst; used without qualification, the word means diabetes mellitus. **biliary d.** Hypertrophic cirrhosis of the liver with icterus. **bronze d.** Diabetes mellitus associated with hemochromatosis. **d. decipiens.** Diabetic glycosuria, without any of the cardinal symptoms. **d. insipidus.** A disease due to a disorder of the hypothalamus, either congenital or following injury or infection; characterized by the passage of a large quantity of urine of low specific gravity, associated with intense thirst and dehydration; usually relieved by extracts of the neurohypophysis. Formerly called *neuropituitary syndrome.* **d. mellitus.** An inheritable, constitutional disease of unknown cause, characterized by the failure of the body tissues to oxidize carbohydrate at a normal rate. The metabolic disturbance, which has as its most important factor a deficiency of insulin, manifests itself in an excess of sugar in the blood (hyperglycemia), presence of sugar in the urine (glycosuria), and, in more advanced stages, acidosis (ketosis), and coma, with symptoms of intense thirst and hunger, weakness, and loss of weight. The disease may be further attended in later life by degenerative changes such as arteriosclerosis, cataract, neuritis. **experimental d.** Diabetes mellitus produced in animals by various methods, such as puncture of the diabetic center, pancreatectomy, injection of extracts of the anterior pituitary or of alloxan. **meta d.** A permanent diabetes produced by stresses sufficient in intensity and duration to cause permanent damage to the pancreatic beta cells. Overstimulation of other endocrine glands can produce forms of it, such as *metadrenocortical d., metathyroid d.,* and *metahypophysial d.* **pancreatic d.** A variety of diabetes mellitus dependent upon disease of the pancreas. **renal d.** See renal *glycosuria.*

di′a·bet′ic. 1. Pertaining to diabet 2. A person suffering from diabetes.

di″a·be″to·gen′ic (dye″uh-bee″jen′ick, dye″uh·bet″o·). Causing d betes.

di″a·be·tog′e·nous (dye″uh-todj′i·nus). Produced by diabetes.

di″a·be″to·pho′bi·a. Morbid fe of becoming a diabetic.

di·ab′o·lep″sy. Diabolical seizure possession; delusion of supernatu possession. **—diabolep′tic,** n.

di″a·ce·te′mi·a. Presence of diace acid in the blood.

di″a·ce′tic ac′id (dye″uh-see′ti ·set′ick). Acetoacetic acid.

di·ac′e·tu′ri·a (dye·ass″i·tew′r uh), **di·ac′e·to·nu′ri·a** (dye·ass i·to·new′ree·uh). Presence of diace acid in the urine.

di·ac″e·tyl·mor′phine (dye·ass i·til·mor′feen, ·mor·feen′). Heroin.

di·ac′la·sis (dye·ack′luh·sis, dye″clay′sis), **di″a·cla′si·a** (dye″ clay′zhuh, ·zee·uh). 1. Refraction. 2. fracture produced intentionally. **—** **aclas′tic,** *adj.*

di′a·clast. Instrument for breaki the fetal head.

di·ac″o·la′tion. A method of dr extraction involving percolation a suitable solvent through long narr columns packed with the drug.

di″a·crit′ic, di″a·crit′i·cal. agnostic, distinctive.

di″ac·tin′ic. Capable of transmitti actinic rays.

di′ad. 1. An element or radical havi a valence of two. 2. A bivalent chrom some resulting from synapse, 2.

di′a·derm. A two-layered blastode composed of ectoderm and endoder O.T.

di·ad″o·cho·ki·ne′si·a (dye·ad o·ko·ki·nee′shuh, ·kigh·nee′·), **di·ad o·cho·ki·ne′sis** (dye·ad″o·ko· nee′sis, ·kigh·nee′sis), **di·ad″o·k ki·ne′si·a, di·ad″o·ko·ki·ne′s** The normal power of performing alt nating movements in rapid successio

di″ag·no′sis. 1. The art or the act determining the nature of a disease. The decision reached. **—diagnos** *v.* **anatomic d.** 1. A diagnosis bas upon the recognition of definite a tomic alterations underlying speci phenomena. 2. A post-mortem diagr sis. **clinical d.** One made from re ognition of the symptoms alone. **d ductive d.** A diagnosis made by physician after a consideration of the manifestations of the disease, a after forming a conception of the d order in terms of physiology, hence the anatomic localization of the lesi and, finally, by inference, of the path logic process and its etiology. **d.** **exclusion.** The recognition of a d ease by excluding all other known conditions. **differential d.** The distinguishing between diseases of similar character, as by comparing their symptoms. **laboratory d.** One arrived at from the results of tests on and examination of various tissues and excretions. **microscopical d.** That made by means of microscopical examination of tissues or specimens. **pathologic d.** One based on the study of the structural lesions present. **physical d.** The determination of disease by inspection, palpation, percussion, or auscultation. **topographic d.** One determined by the location of a lesion.

di″ag·nos′tic. Pertaining to or serving as evidence in diagnosis.

di″ag·nos·ti′cian. One skilled in making diagnoses.

dial. Trade-mark for 5,5-diallylbarbituric acid, a sedative and hypnotic.

di·al′y·sate (dye·al′ĭ·sayt). See *dialyzate*.

di·al′y·sis (dye·al′ĭ·sis). Separation of substances from one another in solution by taking advantage of their differing diffusibility through porous membranes. **—dialyt′ic, di′alyza·ble,** *adj.;* **di′alyze,** *v.*

di·al′y·zate, di·al′y·sate. The portion of a liquid which passes through the membrane in dialysis, and contains the crystalloids in solution.

di′a·ly″zer. Apparatus for effecting dialysis; also the porous septum or diaphragm of such an apparatus.

di·am′e·ter. A straight line joining opposite points of a body or figure and passing through its center. **anteroposterior d. of the pelvic inlet.** That which joins the sacrovertebral angle and pubic symphysis. See internal conjugate *d.,* external conjugate *d.* **anteroposterior d. of the pelvic outlet.** That between the lower margin of the symphysis pubis and the tip of the sacrum or the tip of the coccyx. Syn., *sacropubic d., coccygeopubic d.* **anterotransverse d.** That joining the tips of the greater wings of the sphenoid. Syn., *temporal d.* **biparietal d.** That joining the parietal eminences. **bispinous d.** That joining the spines of the ischia. **bitemporal d.** That joining the extremities of the coronal suture. **craniometric d.** A line connecting two corresponding points on opposite surfaces of the cranium. **diagonal conjugate d.** That connecting the sacrovertebral angle and the subpubic ligament. **external conjugate d.** That connecting the depression above the spine of the first sacral vertebra and the middle of the upper border of the symphysis pubis. Also called *Baudeloque's d.* **fetal cranial diameters.** Those includ-

ing the biparietal, bitemporal, occipitofrontal, occipitomental, and suboccipitobregmatic diameters. **intercristal d.** The widest distance between the iliac crests. **internal conjugate d.** That connecting the sacrovertebral angle and the most prominent portion of the posterior aspect of the symphysis pubis. Also called *true conjugate d., conjugata vera, anatomic conjugate d.* **interspinous d.** That connecting the anterior superior iliac spines. **oblique d. of the pelvic inlet.** That joining the iliopectineal eminence to the sacroiliac articulation on the opposite side. **occipitofrontal d.** That joining the root of the nose and the most prominent point of the occiput. **occipitomental d.** That joining the occipital protuberance and the chin. **pelvic d.** Any one of the diameters of the pelvis. **sacropubic d.** See anteroposterior *d.* of the pelvic outlet. **transverse d. of the pelvic inlet.** That connecting the two most widely separated points of the pelvic inlet. **transverse d. of the pelvic outlet.** That between the two ischial tuberosities. Also called *biischial d., biischiatic d., bituberal d., intertuberal d.*

di·am′i·dine (dye·am′ĭ·deen, ·din). Any compound consisting of two amidine groups, $NH:C(NH_2)-$, linked together by a hydrocarbon chain.

di″a·mine′ (dye″uh·meen′, dye′uh·meen, dye·am′in). An amine formed by replacing hydrogen in two molecules of ammonia by a hydrocarbon radical. See *amine.* **d. oxidase.** See *histaminase.*

di″a·mi·nu′ri·a. Presence of diamine compounds in the urine.

di″a·mor′phine hy″dro·chlo′ride (dye″uh·mor′feen, ·fin). British Pharmacopoeia title for the hydrochloride of heroin.

diamox. Trade-mark for acetazolamide.

di·am′tha·zole di·hy″dro·chlo′ride. 6-(β-Diethylaminoethoxy)-2-dimethylaminobenzothiazole dihydrochloride, a water-soluble agent used topically in treating superficial fungous infections.

diaparene chloride. Trade-mark for methylbenzethonium chloride.

di″a·pa′son (dye″uh·pay′zun, ·sun). A tuning fork; used in the diagnosis of diseases of the ear, especially in determining the presence and extent of deafness.

di″a·pe·de′sis. Passage of blood cells, especially erythrocytes, through the unruptured vessel into the tissues. **—diapedet′ic,** *adj.*

di′a·phane. 1. The transparent investing membrane of an organ or cell. 2. A small electric lamp used in transillumination. 3. A commercial mounting medium for histologic sections.

di·aph″a·nom′e·ter. Instrument for measuring the transparency of fluids.

di·aph′a·no·scope (dye·af′uh·no·scope, dye″uh·fan′o·). Device for lighting an interior body cavity so as to render it visible from the exterior. **—diaphanos′copy,** n.

di·aph″e·met′ric (dye·af″i·met′rick, dye″uh·fi·). Pertaining to measurements of tactile sensibility.

di·aph′o·rase. The enzyme which catalyzes the oxidation of reduced coenzyme I.

di″a·pho·re′sis. Perspiration, especially perceptible perspiration.

di″a·pho·ret′ic. 1. Causing an increase of perspiration. 2. A medicine that induces diaphoresis.

di′a·phragm (dye′uh·fram). 1. *In anatomy,* a musculotendinous partition; especially that partition muscular at the circumference and tendinous at the center, which separates the thorax and abdomen and is the chief muscle of respiration and expulsion. See Table of Muscles in the Appendix. 2. A thin septum such as is used in dialysis. 3. *In microscopy,* an apparatus placed between the mirror and object to regulate the amount of light that is to pass through the object. **Bucky's d.** *In roentgenography,* a moving grid of alternate thin strips of lead and wood which permits only radiation traveling in the direction of the x-ray beam to strike the photographic film; thus producing pictures with sharper contrast. **central stop d.** *In microscopy,* a diaphragm having a circular slit just within its margin, the center remaining opaque. **condensing d.** A diaphragm containing lenses for converging the light rays. **contraceptive d.** A rubber device fitted over the cervix of the uterus. **d. opening.** The opening in the disk or apparatus of a microscope through which the rays of light pass. **iris d.** A device for changing or regulating the amount of light directed upon an object under the microscope. **pelvic d.** That formed by the levator ani and the coccygeus muscles; the concave floor of the pelvis, separating it from the perineum. **urogenital d.** That stretching across the pubic arch, formed by the deep transverse perineal and the sphincter urethrae muscles. Also called *trigonum urogenitale, triangular ligament.*

di″a·phrag′ma. Diaphragm, *q.v.*

di″a·phrag·mat′o·cele (dye″uh·frag·mat′o·seel). Hernia through the diaphragm.

di″a·phrag·mi′tis. Inflammation of the diaphragm. *Rare.*

di″aph·y·sec′to·my (dye″af·i·seck′-to·mee, ·zeck′to·mee). Excision of a portion of the shaft of a long bone.

di·aph′y·sis. The shaft of a long bone. **—diaphys′eal,** *adj.*

di·ap′la·sis. Reduction of a dislocation or of a fracture.

di″a·poph′y·sis. The superior or articular part of a transverse process of a vertebra. **—diapophys′ial,** *adj.*

di″ar·rhe′a. A common symptom of gastrointestinal disease; characterized by increased frequency and more or less fluid consistency of the stools; may be due to various causes from acute infections to psychogenic factors. Also see *dysentery.* **acute d.** Characterized by the sudden onset of frequent liquid stools, usually with constitutional symptoms of weakness and pain, and often with fever and vomiting; may be of infectious origin (as bacillary dysentery) or noninfectious origin (as arsenic poisoning). **choleraic d.** Old term for a severe, acute type with serous stools, vomiting, and collapse; so called because of its resemblance to cholera. **chronic d.** That characterized by frequent stools over an extended period of time, occurring as a manifestation of an intestinal lesion or of a constitutional disease. **epidemic d. of the newborn.** A form, seen in newborns in hospital nurseries, which occurs as an epidemic and is of unknown origin. **fermentative d.** That associated with fermentation of the intestinal contents. **green d.** A form of infantile diarrhea, characterized by the passage of green stools. **infantile d.** An acute form seen in infants, most frequently during the summer; due primarily to damage of the intestinal mucosa by infection. Many organisms have been thought to be causative. Seen most frequently in artificially fed infants, and associated with poor hygiene. The cholera infantum of older writers. **inflammatory d.** A general term for diarrhea caused by poisons or infections which induce local inflammation of the intestinal mucosa. **nervous d.** That due to disturbances of the autonomic nervous system. **pancreatic d.** A persistent form, due to absence of pancreatic digestive enzymes; characterized by the passage of large, greasy stools having a high fat and nitrogen content. **parenteral d.** That due to infections outside of the intestinal tract. **putrefactive d.** That associated with putrefaction of the intestinal contents. **simple d.** A form in which the evacuations consist of fecal matter only. **summer d.** An acute form seen during the intense heat of summer; usually caused by bacterial contamination of poorly refrigerated food.

di″ar·rhoe′a (dye″uh-ree′uh). See *diarrhea*.

di·ar′thric. Relating to two joints.

di″ar·thro′sis. A freely movable articulation. See *articulation*. —**diar·throdial,** *adj.*

di″ar·tic′u·lar. Diarthric.

di·as·chi·sis (dye-ass′ki-sis). An inhibition of function in a region of the nervous system, due to a localized injury in another region with which it is connected by fiber tracts.

di′a·scope. Device consisting of a thin piece of glass, used to press against the skin so that superficial lesions may be observed. —**dias′copy,** *n.*

diasone. Trade-mark for disodium formaldehyde sulfoxylate diaminodiphenylsulfone.

di″a·stal′sis. The downward moving wave of contraction, occurring in the small intestine during digestion.

di′a·stase. An enzyme from malt which converts starch to maltose by hydrolysis; vegetable amylase. Also called *vegetable d.* **animal d.** Any of the amylolytic enzymes of animals, such as ptyalin, amylopsin, etc. **pancreatic d.** Amylopsin. **salivary d.** Ptyalin.

di·as′ta·sis. 1. Any simple separation of parts normally joined together, as the separation of an epiphysis from the body of a bone without true fracture, or the dislocation of an amphiarthrotic joint. 2. The final phase of diastole in which ventricular filling is reduced to the minimum. **d. recti abdominis.** Separation in the median line of the two rectus abdominis muscles, usually from repeated childbirth.

di″a·ste′ma. 1. A cleft or fissure, especially if congenital. 2. *In dentistry,* an abnormal space between the teeth.

di″a·stem″a·to·my·e′li·a (dye″-uh-stem″uh-to-migh-ee′lee-uh, dye″uh-stee″muh-to·). Congenital division of the spinal cord, usually associated with spina bifida. Syn., *diplomyelia*.

di·as′to·le (dye-ass′to-lee). The rhythmic period of relaxation and dilatation of a chamber of the heart during which it fills with blood; used alone the word means ventricular diastole. —**diastol′ic,** *adj.* **atrial d.** The dilatation of the cardiac atria. **ventricular d.** That of the cardiac ventricles.

di″a·tax′i·a. Bilateral ataxia, as opposed to *hemiataxia.*

di″a·ther″mo·co·ag″u·la′tion. Coagulation secured by the use of a high-frequency electrosurgical knife.

di″a·ther·mom′e·ter. *In physics,* an instrument for measuring the heat-conducting capacity of substances.

di′a·ther″my (dye″uh·thur″mee, dye″uh·thur′mee), **di″a·ther′mi·a.**

1. The therapeutic use of an oscillating electric current of high frequency to produce local heat in the body tissues below the surface. 2. The electric current so used. 3. The machine producing it. —**diather′mic, diather′manous, diather′mal,** *adj.;* **diather′mize,** *v.* **conventional d.** The use of a current of moderately high frequency, 500–3000 kilocycles per second, at wave lengths of 600–100 meters. **medical d.** That form in which the tissues are heated to a point less than destructive temperature. **short-wave d.** That form making use of a current of extremely high frequency, 10,000–100,000 kilocycles per second, at wave lengths of 30 to 3 meters.

di·ath′e·sis. Constitution; hereditary influence. A state or condition of the body or a combination of attributes in one individual causing a susceptibility to disease. —**diathet′ic,** *adj.* **exudative d.** A condition formerly recognized in children, associated with an irritable skin and chafing, intertrigo, seborrhea, eczema, and hypersusceptibility to external irritants of the skin and mucous membranes. There are also frequent respiratory infections with resulting lymphoid hyperplasia. **hemorrhagic d.** An abnormal bleeding tendency as in hemophilia, purpura, scurvy, or vitamin-K deficiency. **uratic d.** A condition in which there is a tendency to the deposition of urates in the joints and elsewhere; gout.

di′a·tom (dye′uh·tom, ·tome). Any of the Diatomaceae, a small family of microscopic, unicellular algae having a cell wall of silica, the skeleton persisting after death of the organism.

di″a·to·ma′ceous earth. A sedimentary rock composed of empty shells of diatoms and other unicellular plants; used as an absorbent.

di″a·tom′ic. 1. Consisting of two atoms. 2. Divalent.

di″a·tri·zo′ate so′di·um. Sodium 3,5-diacetamido-2,4,6-triiodobenzoate, a roentgenographic contrast medium. See *hypaque sodium.*

di·az′o- (dye-az′o-, dye-ay′zo-), **diaz-.** *In chemistry,* a combining form indicating the presence in a compound of a group involving two nitrogen atoms, usually arranged in the form of $R-N=N-$, where R is an aryl group. —**diazo,** *adj.*

di·ba′sic (dye-bay′sick). Of a salt, containing two atoms of a monobasic element or radical; of an acid, having two replaceable hydrogen atoms.

dibenamine. Trade-mark for N,N-dibenzyl-beta-chloroethylamine, used in the form of the hydrochloride experimentally as a sympatholytic and adrenolytic agent.

di″ben·zan′thra·cene. A hydrocarbon; said to be the first pure chemical found experimentally to produce cancer in an animal.

dibenzyline. Trade-mark for phenoxybenzamine.

di·both″ri·o·ceph″a·li′a·sis. Old term for diphyllobothriasis, *q.v.*

Di·both″ri·o·ceph′a·lus. Synonym for *Diphyllobothrium.*

di·bu′caine hy″dro·chlo′ride. 2-Butoxy-N-(2-diethylaminoethyl)-cinchoninamide hydrochloride, a local anesthetic similar in action to cocaine hydrochloride when applied to mucous surfaces and to procaine or cocaine hydrochloride when injected. See *nupercaine hydrochloride.*

dibuline sulfate. Trade-mark for dibuline sulfate.

di·bu′to·line sul′fate. Bis[dibutyl-carbamate of ethyl (2-hydroxyethyl)-dimethylammonium] sulfate, a parasympatholytic agent. See *dibuline sulfate.*

di·car″box·yl′ic ac′id. An organic compound with two —COOH groups.

di·ceph′a·lism, di·ceph′a·ly. The condition of having two heads.

di·ceph′a·lus. A monster with two heads. —**dicephalous,** *adj.*

di·ceph′a·ly. See *dicephalism.*

di·chei′lus, di·chi′lus (dye-kigh′-lus). Double lip; due to a fold of mucous membrane giving the appearance of duplicity.

di″chlor·a·mine′-T (dye″klor-uh-meen′, ·klor′uh-meen). Paratoluenesulfondichloramide, a pale yellow powder with the odor of chlorine, used as a surgical antiseptic in 2–10% oil solution. Syn., *dichloramine.* See *chloramine-T.*

di·chlo″ro·a·ce′tic ac′id. CHCl₂.COOH. A colorless liquid at ordinary temperatures, soluble in water. Used as an escharotic.

di·chlo″ro·di·eth″yl·sul′fide (·dye·eth″il·sul′fide, ·fid). (C₂H₄Cl)₂S. Mustard gas. A fluid vesicant used in chemical warfare.

di·chlo″ro·di·flu″o·ro·meth′·ane (dye·klor′o-dye·floo″o·ro-meth′-ane). CCl₂F₂. A noninflammable gas used as a refrigerant. See *freon.*

di·chlo″ro·phen·ar′sine hy″·dro·chlo′ride (dye·klor″o-fen·ahr′-seen, ·fen·ahr′sin). 3-Amino-4-hydroxyphenyl-dichlorarsine hydrochloride. A white powder used as an antisyphilitic.

di·chlo″ro·phe′nol-in″do·phe′nol so′di·um. Sodium 2,6-dichlorophenol-indophenol. Dark-green powder, soluble in water and alcohol; used in analytical determination of ascorbic acid.

di·chlo″ro·phen·ox″y·a·ce′tic ac′id. 2,4-Dichlorophenoxyacetic acid; substance regulating plant growth; also found to be an effective herbicide. Also called *2,4-D.*

di·chot′o·mize (dye·cot′o·mize). Divide a distribution, variable, or series into two parts according to a specified classification, as persons with or without a known disease or characteristic.

di·chro′ic. Having or showing two colors; applied to doubly refracting crystals which show different colors when viewed from different directions; or to solutions that show different colors in varying degrees of concentration. —**di′chroism,** *n.*

di″chro·mat′ic. 1. *In biology,* exhibiting two colors, regardless of sex or age. 2. *In psychology,* pertaining to that form of color blindness in which only two of the fundamental colors can be seen.

di·chro″ma·top′si·a. A form of color blindness in which only two primary colors can be distinguished.

di·chro′mic. 1. Marked by two colors. 2. Containing two atoms of chromium.

di′chro·mism, di·chro′mism. Dichroism; the state of being dichroic, *q.v.*

di·chro′mo·phil. Characterizing a tissue or cell which stains with both an acid and a basic dye.

di″chro·moph′i·lism. Capacity for double staining. —**dichro′mophil, dichro′mophile,** *adj.*

Dick, George Frederick [*American physician,* 1881–   ]. Known as one of the originators of the test for individual susceptibility to scarlet fever; see *Dick test* (1924). Prepared immunizing antitoxin against the disease with his wife, Gladys Rowena Henry Dick (1924).

Dick, Gladys Rowena Henry [*American physician,* 1881–   ]. Co-originator of a test for individual susceptibility to scarlet fever; see *Dick test* (1924). Prepared immunizing antitoxin for the disease with her husband, George Frederick Dick (1924).

dicodid. Trade-mark for dihydrocodeinone.

di′co·phane. A name sometimes applied to the medicinal grade of DDT. Syn., *Chlorophenothane.*

di·cou′ma·rin (dye·koo′muh·rin). A white, crystalline compound, 3,3′-methylene-bis-(4-hydroxycoumarin), occurring naturally and prepared synthetically. It is an anticoagulant of use in thromboses. Syn., *bishydroxycoumarin, melitoxin.* See *dicumarol.*

di·cou′ma·rol. British Pharmacopoeia title for bishydroxycoumarin.

Di″cro·coe′li·um (dye″kro·see′lee-um, ·dick″ro·). A genus of trematodes. **D. dendriticum.** A species of flukes which has as its definitive host sheep and other herbivorous animals, with some cases of human infestation reported.

di·crot'ic notch. A notch in the descending limb of the pulse of a peripheral artery, as recorded in a pulse tracing.

di'cro·tism. A condition of the pulse in which with every wave there is given to the finger of the examiner the sensation of two beats; occurs in fever and after inhalation of amyl nitrite. —**di·crot'ic,** *adj.*

dicumarol. A collective trade-mark for bishydroxycoumarin.

di·dac'tic (dye-dack'tick, di-dack'-tick). *In medicine*, teaching by lectures and textbooks, as opposed to instruction by the clinical method.

di·dac'tyl·ism (dye-dack'til-iz-um). The congenital condition in which there are but two digits on a hand or foot.

di·del'phic. Having a double uterus.

did·y·mi'tis. Orchitis, *q.v.*

did'y·mous. Growing in pairs; arranged in a pair, or in pairs.

did'y·mus. 1. A twin. 2. A double monstrosity. 3. A testis.

die. An exact reproduction in metal of any object or cast. Used in dentistry for the swaging of prosthetic appliances; referred to as the **male die,** and is usually made of zinc or babbitt metal. The **counter-die** is the product of casting a lower fusing metal, lead, or an alloy to fit in opposition to the die. This is known as the **female die.** Prosthetic appliances are constructed by swaging a metal plate between the die and the counter-die.

die. Cease to live; expire.

di·el'drin. An insecticide containing not less than 85% of the chemical 1,2,3,4,10,10-hexachloro-6,7-epoxy-1,4,-4a,5,6,7,8,8a-octahydro-1,4,5,8-dimethanonaphthalene.

di"e·lec·trol'y·sis. Electrolysis of a compound, the current passing through a diseased portion of the body and carrying one of the elements of the compound with it.

di"en·ceph'a·lon. That part of the brain between the telencephalon and the mesencephalon. It includes the thalami and most of the third ventricle. Syn., *betweenbrain.* —**diencephal'ic,** *adj.*

di"en·es'trol (di"en-es'trol). 3,4-Bis-(*p*-hydroxyphenyl)-2,4-hexadiene or dehydrostilbestrol, an estrogenic substance.

Di·en"ta·moe'ba (dye-en"tuh-mee'-buh). A genus of parasitic protozoa having two nuclei.

di·es'trum, di·oes'trum (dye-ess'-trum), **di·es'trus, di·oes'trus** (dye-ess'trus). The period of quiescence or sexual rest of a polyestrous animal;

the longest stage of the estrual cycle in which there is a gradual build-up of the uterine mucosa or endometrium in preparation for the reception of a fertilized ovum. —**diestrous,** *adj.*

di·es'trus. Diestrum, *q.v.*

di'et. 1. Food and drink regularly consumed. 2. Food prescribed as to kind and amount, for therapeutic or other purposes. 3. Take food according to a regimen. 4. Cause to take food according to a regimen. For special diets, see Table of Diets in the Appendix. —**dietet'ic,** *adj.*; **dietist,** *n.* **acid-ash d.** One used to lower the pH of the urine. **alkaline-ash d.** One used to raise the pH of the urine. **bland d.** One free of stimulating or irritating ingredients. **Coleman d.** A high-caloric, largely liquid diet introduced by Coleman for the treatment of typhoid fever. **diabetic d.** One used in the treatment of diabetes, usually containing weighed or measured amounts of carbohydrate, protein, and fat. **elimination d.** A severely restricted diet designed to demonstrate to what foods, if any, a patient reacts allergically. **gout d.** A low-purine, more or less low-protein diet used in gout. **high-caloric d.** One containing a large number (3,000–5,000) of calories. **high-protein d.** One containing a large amount of protein, used especially in anemia, hypoproteinemia, and obesity. **high-vitamin d.** One rich in vitamins, used in vitamin-deficiency diseases, anemia, hyperthyroidism, tuberculosis, etc. It is often combined with a high-caloric diet. **Karell d.** A restricted-fluid, low-salt regimen at one time much used in cases with edema, especially when due to myocardial failure. **ketogenic d.** One in which fat is high in relation to carbohydrate, so that ketosis is produced; it was formerly used in the treatment of epilepsy and urinary-tract infections. **Lenhartz d.** A low-caloric regimen for the treatment of gastrointestinal ulcer; it consists chiefly of milk and eggs. **low-caloric d.** One containing a small number (600–1500) of calories. **low-salt d.** One low in its content of sodium salt; once widely used in the treatment of hypertension, its chief use has been in cases of edema. **Meulengracht d.** One especially recommended for patients with bleeding peptic ulcer; it includes liberal amounts of food. **Minot-Murphy d.** A diet high in protein, purines, and iron, the chief constituent of which is liver; used in the treatment of pernicious anemia. **obesity d.** A low-caloric diet, used to reduce weight; also called *reducing diet.* **Rowe diets.** A regimen of elimination diets. **salt-free d.** A term used erroneously to describe diets low in sodium chloride. A diet without added salt will contain approximately 3–5 Gm. of NaCl; when salt is not used in cooking, 2–3 Gm.; using only foods containing a minimum of salt may bring the total down to 0.5–1.0 Gm. **S.H.G. d.** Sauerbruch, Herrmannsdorfer, Gerson diet; used in the treatment of tuberculosis; characterized chiefly by the exclusion of sodium chlor'de from the diet. **Sippy d.** One used in the treatment of gastric and duodenal ulcer; it combines alkalies with neutralizing foods. **soft d.** One consisting of easily consumed, easily digested foods.

di·e·tar′y. 1. A rule of diet. 2. A treatise describing such rule or rules. 3. A fixed allowance of food.

di′e·tet′ics. The science of the systematic regulation of the diet for hygienic or therapeutic purposes.

di·eth″yl·bar″bi·tu′ric ac′id. Barbital, *q.v.*

di·eth″yl·stil·bes′trol. α,β-Diethyl-4,4′-stilbenediol; occurs as a white, crystalline powder; insoluble in water. A synthetic estrogen used as a substitute for the natural hormones of this type. Syn., *stilbestrol, stilboestrol.*

di″e·ti′cian. Dietitian, *q.v.*

di″e·ti′tian, di″e·ti′cian. One who is proficient in dietetics.

di″e·to·ther′a·py. That branch of dietetics which has to do with the use of food for therapeutic purposes.

dif″fer·en′tial. Pertaining to or creating a difference.

dif″fer·en″ti·a′tion. 1. The act or process of distinguishing or making different. 2. An increase in complexity and organization of cells and tissues during development.

dif·frac′tion. The separation of light into component parts by means of prisms, parallel bars in a grating, or layers of atoms in a crystal. **x-ray d.** When x-rays are passed through crystals they are diffracted in a manner similar to light rays passed through a ruled diffraction grating.

dif·fuse′ (di·fews′). Scattered; not limited to one tissue or spot; opposed to *localized.*

dif·fus″i·bil′i·ty (di·few″zi·bil′i·tee). Capacity for being diffused. **—diffus′ible,** *adj.*

dif·fu′sion. 1. A spreading-out. 2. Dialysis.

di·fla′vine (dye·flay′veen, ·flav′een). 2,7-Diaminoacridine hydrochloride; an antiseptic related to proflavine.

di·gal′lic ac′id. Tannic acid.

di·gas′tric. 1. Having two bellies; said of a muscle having a fleshy part at each end and a tendinous portion in the middle. 2. The digastric muscle. See

Table of Muscles in the Appendix. 3. Relating to the digastric muscle.

Di″ge·ne′a. A subclass of the Trematoda, which in their life cycle exhibit alternation of generations and alternation of hosts. It includes all the species of flatworms parasitic in man, such as the liver flukes.

di·gen′e·sis. Alternation of generations.

di″ge·net′ic. 1. Relating to alternation of generations. 2. Referring to the Digenea.

di·gest′ant (di·jest′unt, dye·jest′unt). 1. Concerning or promoting digestion. 2. An agent that promotes digestion.

di·gest′er (di·jest′ur, dye·jest′ur). An apparatus used to subject substances to high temperature and pressure in order to decompose, soften, or cook them; autoclave.

di·ges′tion (di·jes′chun, dye·jes′chun). 1. The act or process of converting food into assimilable form. 2. The softening of substances by moisture and heat. 3. The disintegration of materials by strong chemical agents. **—digest′ible,** *adj.;* **digestibil′ity,** *n.;* **digest′,** *v.t., v.i.* **artificial d.** Digestion carried on outside of the body. **gastric d.** Digestion by the action of the gastric juice. **intestinal d.** Digestion by the action of the intestinal juices, including the action of the bile and the pancreatic fluid. **pancreatic d.** Digestion by the action of the pancreatic juice. **peptic d.** See gastric *d.* **primary d.** Gastrointestinal digestion. **salivary d.** Digestion by the saliva. **secondary d.** The assimilation by body cells of appropriate pabulum.

dig′i- (didj′i-). A combining form signifying digitalis.

dig″i·lan′id (dij″i·lan′id). A mixture of the cardioactive glycosides lanatoside A, lanatoside B, and lanatoside C.

dig′it (didj′it). A finger or toe. Also see *digitus.* **—digital,** *adj.*

dig″i·ta′le·in (didj″i·tay′lee·in, ·tal′ee·in). A term used to designate a mixture of active and inactive glycosides of digitalis.

dig″i·ta′lin (didj″i·tal′in, didj′i·tuh·lin). The original *Digitalinum verum* of Schmiedeberg and Kiliani; a mixture of amorphous alcohol-soluble glycosides from the seeds of *Digitalis purpurea.* **crystallized d.** Digitoxin. Also called *Nativelle d.* **French d.** A yellowish, odorless, bitter powder; said to consist of digitalin, digitonin, and digitoxin. Also called *chloroformic d., Homolle's amorphous d., insoluble d.* **German d.** A white or yellowish powder said to consist of a mixture of

glycosides, chiefly digitonin. **soluble d.** See German d.

dig″i·tal′is (didj″i·tal′is, ·tah′lis).
Common foxglove. The dried leaf of
Digitalis purpurea. Its activity is due
to a number of glycosides, notably digitoxin. Digitalis is a powerful cardiac
stimulant. It also acts indirectly as a
diuretic. **powdered d.** The leaf reduced to powder and standardized to
contain 1 U.S.P. Digitalis Unit in each
0.1 Gm.

dig″i·tal·i·za′tion (didj″i·tul·i-
zay′shun, ·eye·zay′shun). Administration of digitalis in sufficient amount by
any of several types of dosage sched-
ules to build up the concentration of
digitalis glycosides in the body of a
patient. In this way therapeutic effects
are attained and thereafter only a
maintenance dose is required.

dig″i·ta·lose (didj″i·tay′loce, didj/i-
tuh·loce). A sugar obtained in the hydrolysis of certain digitalis glycosides.

dig″i·ta′tion. A fingerlike process,
or a succession of such processes, especially that of a muscle attachment.

dig′i·ti·form″. Finger-shaped.

dig″i·to·gen′in (didj″i·to·jen′in,
·todj/uh·nin). The aglycone of digitonin.

dig″i·to′nin. A glycoside from digitalis.

dig″i·tox″i·gen′in. The aglycone
from digitoxin.

dig″i·tox′in. The principal active
glycoside of digitalis; it occurs in crystals practically insoluble in water.

dig″i·tox′ose. The sugar resulting
when certain digitalis glycosides, notably digitoxin, gitoxin, and gitalin,
are hydrolyzed.

dig′i·tus (didj/i·tus). A finger or toe;
digit. **d. annularis.** The ring finger.
d. minimus. Old term for the little
finger. **d. quintus.** The little finger
or toe.

di·glos′si·a (dye·glos′ee·uh). A form
of schistoglossia in which the lateral
lingual swellings fail to fuse, producing a bifid tongue.

di·gox′in (dye·gock′sin, didj·ock′sin).
A cardioactive, crystalline product de-
rived from one of the glycosides of
Digitalis lanata.

di·hy′drate. A compound containing
two molecules of water.

di·hy′dric. Containing two hydroxyl
groups in the molecule.

di·hy″dro·co·de′i·none. A synthetic alkaloid related to codeine;
used as a cough sedative. See *dicodid.*

di·hy″dro·co·en′zyme I. Coenzyme I to which two hydrogen atoms
are added, important in many hydrogen transfer reactions.

di″hy·dro·co·en′zyme II. Coenzyme II to which two hydrogen atoms

are added, important in many hydrogen transfer reactions.

**di·hy″dro·di·eth″yl·stil·bes′-
trol.** See *hexestrol.*

di·hy″dro·er″go·cor′nine. The
hydrogenated derivative of the ergot
alkaloid ergocornine; possesses adrenergic-blocking action.

di·hy″dro·er·got′a·mine. A derivative of ergotamine, *q.v.,* employed
in the treatment of migraine.

di·hy′drol. An associated form of
water having the composition $(H_2O)_2$.

**di·hy″dro·mor′phi·none hy″-
dro·chlo′ride.** An alkaloid prepared
by hydrogenation of morphine; a white
powder soluble in water. A respiratory sedative and analgesic more
powerful than morphine. See *dilaudid
hydrochloride.*

di·hy″dro·strep″to·my′cin. A
derivative of streptomycin having the
actions of, and used clinically like,
streptomycin, but exhibiting less neuro-
toxicity.

di·hy″dro·ta·chys′te·rol (dye-
high″dro·ta·kiss′tuh·rol, ·tack″i·steer′-
ol). A synthetic steroid derived from
ergosterol; useful in treating hypopara-
thyroidism. See *A.T. 10, hytakerol.*

di″hy·dro·the′e·lin (dye″high·dro-
thee′uh·lin, ·thee′lin). Estradiol.

di″hy·drox″y·a·ce′tic ac′id
(dye″high·drock″see·a·see′tick, ·a·set′-
ick). Glyoxylic acid.

di″hy·drox″y·ac′e·tone (dye″-
high·drock″see·ass′i·tone). $C_3H_6O_3$. A
simple 3-carbon keto-sugar.

**di″hy·drox″y·a·lu′mi·num
a·mi″no·ac′e·tate.** A basic aluminum salt of aminoacetic acid containing small amounts of aluminum hydroxide and aminoacetic acid, used as
a gastric antacid and for controlling
hyperacidity in peptic ulcer.

di″hy·drox″y·an′thra·nol. $C_{14}H_7$-
(OH)₃. Anthrarobin, *q.v.* See also *anthralin.*

di″hy·drox″y·es′trin. Estradiol.

di″hy·drox″y·pro′pane. Propylene glycol.

di″i·o·do·form. $I_2C:Cl_2$. Ethylene
tetraiodide. Light yellow crystals occasionally used as an antiseptic similar to
iodoform.

di″i·o″do·hy′drox·y·quin. Diio-
dohydroxyquinoline, an antiprotozoan
agent. See *diodoquin.*

di″i·o″do·ty′ro·sine (dye″eye·o″-
do·tye′ro·seen, ·sin). A substance found
in skeletons of marine organisms. It is
one of the constituent amino acids of
thyroglobulin and has been used in
hyperthyroidism.

**di·i″so·pro′pyl flu″o·ro·phos′-
phate.** See *DFP.*

dik″ty·o′ma. See *neuroepithelioma.*

di·lac″er·a′tion (dye·lass″uh·ray′-

shun, di·lass"uh·). 1. Act of tearing apart; being torn in pieces. *Obs.* 2. *In dentistry*, a partial alteration of the position of the formative organ during development, resulting in teeth with sharp angulation of the root and crown.

dilantin sodium. A trade-mark for diphenylhydantoin sodium, an anticonvulsant in the treatment of epilepsy. See *diphenylhydantoin sodium.*

dil"a·ta'tion (dil"uh·tay'shun, dye"luh·). 1. The state of being stretched. 2. Enlargement, as of a hollow part or organ. **congenital d. of the colon.** Megacolon due to a congenital defect in innervation. Also called *Hirschsprung's disease.* **digital d.** Dilatation of a body cavity or orifice by means of one or more fingers. **d. of heart.** An increase in the size of one or more of the cavities of the heart, arising from a relaxation or weakening of the heart muscle. It is associated with evidences of failure of circulation, resulting in congestion of the lungs and other viscera. **d. of stomach.** Increase in size of the stomach from relaxation of the walls or expansion with gas or fluid. **hydrostatic d.** Dilatation of a cavity or part by an introduced elastic bag which is subsequently distended with water.

di·la'tion (dye·lay'shun, di·lay'shun). The act of stretching or dilating, as contrasted with dilatation, which is the state of being stretched. The two words are often used synonymously.

di·la·tor (dye'lay·tur, dye·lay'tur). 1. An instrument for stretching or enlarging a cavity or opening. 2. A dilating muscle. **d. naris.** A dilating muscle of the nostril. See Table of Muscles in the Appendix. **d. pupillae.** The set of radiating involuntary muscle fibers in the iris, dilating the pupil. Also called *d. iridis.* See Table of Muscles in the Appendix.

dilaudid hydrochloride. Trademark for dihydromorphinone hydrochloride.

dil'u·ent. 1. Diluting. 2. Agent that dilutes the strength of a solution or mixture. 3. Medication which dilutes any one of the body fluids.

di·lute' (di·lute', dye·lute'). Make weaker and thinner by the addition of liquid, especially water; or thin and dissolve.

di·lu'ted al'co·hol. Contains 41–42% by weight, or 48.4–49.5% by volume at 15.56° C., of C_2H_5OH.

di·lu'tion. 1. Process of adding a neutral fluid to some other fluid or substance, in order to diminish the qualities of the latter. 2. A diluted substance; the result of a diluting process.

di"men·hy'dri·nate. Nonproprietary title for the drug supplied under the trade-marked name *dramamine.*

di"mer·cap'rol. BAL, *q.v.*

di"mer·cap"to·pro'pan·ol. BAL, *q.v.*

di"meth·i'so·quin **hy"dro·chlo'ride.** 3-Butyl-1-(2-dimethylaminoethoxy)isoquinoline hydrochloride, a local anesthetic. See *quotane hydrochloride.*

di·meth'yl. A combining form denoting the presence of *two methyl groups.*

dimethylane. Trade-mark for promoxolane.

di·meth"yl·ar·sin'ic ac'id. $(CH_3)_2AsO.OH$. A deliquescent, crystalline solid; soluble in water. Usually employed in the form of sodium cacodylate. Syn., *cacodylic acid.*

di·meth"yl·xan'thine (dye·meth"il·zan'theen, ·thin). 1. Theobromine (3,7-dimethylxanthine). 2. Theophylline (1,3-dimethylxanthine).

di·me'tri·a. Condition in which the uterus is a double organ. Also called *uterus duplex.*

di·mor'phism. Property of existing in two distinct structural forms. —**dimorphous,** *adj.*

dimp'ling. An abnormal skin depression from retraction occurring in subcutaneous carcinomas.

di·ni'tro·phen"yl·hy'dra·zine (dye·nigh"tro·fen"il·high'druh·zeen, dye·nigh"tro·fee"nil·). $C_6H_3(NO_2)_2NH·NH_2$. Red, crystalline powder. Used in identification and analysis of aldehydes and ketones.

di'nus. Vertigo or dizziness.

Di·oc"to·phy'ma. A genus of large nematodes of the superfamily Dioctophymoidea.

di·oc'tyl so'di·um sul"fo·suc'ci·nate (sul"fo·suck'sin·ate). $C_{20}H_{37}O_7SNa$. A white, waxlike solid, soluble in water; employed as a wetting agent in the formulation of lotions, creams, ointments, and shampoos. See *aerosol OT dry, deceresol OT.*

di'o·done. A product consisting of the diethanolamine salt of 3,5-diiodo-4-pyridone-N-acetic acid. See *diodrast, iodopyracet injection.*

diodoquin. Trade-mark for an antiprotozoan agent, chemically 5,7-diiodo-8-hydroxyquinoline.

diodrast. Trade-mark for the diethanolamine salt of 3,5-diiodo-4-pyridone-N-acetic acid, used as a contrast agent for intravenous urography. See *diodone, iodopyracet injection.*

di·oes'trum (dye·ess'trum). See *diestrum.*

di·oes'trus (dye·ess'trus). See *diestrum.*

di'o·nin. Ethylmorphine hydrochloride. A white or faintly yellow, microcrystalline powder, soluble in water. An analgesic and hypnotic, somewhat more powerful than codeine.

di″op·sim′e·ter. An instrument for determining the visual field.

di·op′ter (dye-op′tur). Unit of measurement of the refractive power of an optic lens. It is the refractive power of a lens having a focal distance of one meter. Abbreviated, d. **—diopter′ic, dioptral,** adj. **prism d.** A unit of prismatic refractive power; the refractive power of a prism that deflects a ray of light 1 cm. on a tangent plane situated at a distance of 1 meter.

di″op·tom′e·ter. Instrument for determining ocular refraction. Syn., optometer. **—dioptometry,** n.

di·op′tric. 1. Pertaining to transmitted and refracted light. 2. A diopter.

di·op′trics. The branch of optics treating of the refraction of light by transparent media, especially by the media of the eye.

di″or·tho′sis. Surgical correction of a deformity, or repair of an injury done to a limb; diaplasis. **—diorthot′ic,** adj.

di″os·co′re·a. Wild yam root. The dried rhizome of Dioscorea villosa.

di′ose (dye′oce, ·oze). A monosaccharide containing only two carbon atoms; it is the simplest form of sugar.

diothane hydrochloride. Trademark for piperidinopropanediol-diphenylurethane hydrochloride, a local anesthetic for mucous membranes. See diperodon hydrochloride.

di·o′tic (dye-o′tick, ·ot′ick). Binaural; pertaining to both ears.

di·ox′ane, di·ox′an. 1,4-Diethylene dioxide, $(CH_2CH_2)_2O_2$, a colorless liquid employed as a solvent, and a dehydrating agent in the process of paraffin-embedding in histologic technic.

di·ox′ide. A molecule containing two atoms of oxygen and one of a base.

di·ox″y·an′thra·nol. Dihydroxyanthranol, q.v.

di·ox″y·ben′zene. See hydroquinone.

dip. 1. Submerge an animal either partially or completely. 2. Preparation for the destruction of skin parasites in animals. 3. A sudden drop, or downward inclination, as in the audiometric curve. **4000-cycle d.** A marked dip in the audiometric curve at the 4000-cycle area. Loss of acuity in this area, the most vulnerable in the human hearing, may be due to congenital lesion or to acoustic trauma.

di·paralene. Trade-mark for chlorcyclizine, an antihistaminic.

diparcol. Trade-mark for 10-(β-diethylaminoethyl)-phenothiazine hydrochloride, a drug possessing atropine-like actions.

dipaxin. Trade-mark for diphenadione.

di·pep′ti·dase. The enzyme which splits dipeptides to amino acids.

di·pep′tide. A chemical combination of two molecules of amino acids obtained by condensation of the acids or by hydrolysis of proteins.

di·per′o·don hy″dro·chlo′ride. Nonproprietary name for the substance available under the trade-mark diothane hydrochloride.

di·phem′a·nil meth″yl·sul′-fate. 4-Diphenylmethylene-1,1-dimethylpiperidinium methylsulfate, a parasympatholytic agent. See prantal methylsulfate.

di″phen·a·di′one. 2-Diphenylacetyl-1,3-indandione, an intravascular anticoagulant. See dipaxin.

di·phen′an. $C_6H_5CH_2\cdot C_6H_4O\cdot CONH_2$. Para-benzylphenylcarbamate, a white powder, almost insoluble in water; employed in the treatment of oxyuriasis.

di″phen·hy′dra·mine hy″dro·chlo′ride (dye″fen·high′druh·meen). 2-(Benzhydryloxy)-N,N-dimethylethylamine hydrochloride, an antihistaminic drug. See benadryl hydrochloride.

di·phen″yl·a·mine (dye-fen″il-uh-meen′, ·am′een). $(C_6H_5)_2NH$. Used as a reagent for nitrates, chlorates, and other oxidizing substances.

di·phen″yl·a·mine″chlo·ro·ar′sine (dye-fen″il-uh-meen″klo-ro-ahr′seen, dye-fee″nil·). $(C_6H_4)_2NH.AsCl$. Adamsite, a sternutator used in chemical warfare. See war gas.

di·phen″yl·chlo″ro·ar′sine. $(C_6H_5)_2AsCl$. A solid used as a sternutator in World War I.

di·phen″yl·hy·dan′to·in so′di·um (dye-fen″il-high-dan′to-in, ·high-dan′toyn). A white powder, soluble in water. An anticonvulsant particularly useful in grand mal seizures and automatisms. See dilantin sodium. Syn., phenytoin sodium.

di·pho′ni·a. The production of two distinct tones during speech; double voice.

di·phos′gene. $ClCOOCCl_3$, a gas similar in its effects to phosgene, q.v.

di·phos″pho·pyr′i·dine nu′cle·o·tide (dye-fos″fo-pirr′i-deen, ·din). Coenzyme I; cozymase; a nucleotide made up of adenine, nicotinamide, ribose, and phosphoric acid. It is a coenzyme for numerous dehydrogenase reactions.

diph·the′ri·a. An acute, communicable disease caused by the Corynebacterium diphtheriae (Klebs-Loeffler bacillus); characterized by the formation of a false, adherent membrane on mucous membranes, usually of the pharynx, larynx, and trachea, and rarely of the conjunctiva and vagina. Locally, the disease produces pain, swelling, and obstruction; systemically, the toxin causes fever, prostration, cardiac damage, in some cases paralysis, and often death. **—diphtherit′ic, diph·**

ther'ic, *adj.* **d. antitoxin.** Blood serum from a horse or other animal immunized against diphtheria toxin. **d. toxin.** A toxalbumin produced by *Corynebacterium diphtheriae;* capable of causing in susceptible animals the same phenomena induced by inoculation with the living bacilli. **d. toxin-antitoxin.** A mixture of toxin and antitoxin used to produce active immunity against diphtheria; now superseded by toxoid. **d. toxoid.** A detoxified diphtheria toxin used to produce active immunity against diphtheria. It has the advantage over toxin-antitoxin of not producing sensitivity to serum. **surgical d.** Formation of a diphtheritic membrane on the surface of a wound.

diph·the'ri·a·phor. A diphtheria carrier.

diph'the·roid. 1. Resembling diphtheria or the diphtheria bacteria. 2. Any bacterium resembling the diphtheria bacteria, though not producing diphtheria toxin. 3. Any pseudomembranous formation not due to *Corynebacterium diphtheriae.*

diph''the·ro·tox'in. Diphtheria toxin, *q.v.*

diph·thon'gi·a. Production of a double tone of the voice; due to incomplete unilateral paralysis of the recurrent laryngeal nerve, or to some lesion of the vocal folds which causes each to produce its own sound.

diph''y·gen'ic. In zoology, characterized by or having two types of development.

di·phyl''lo·both·ri'a·sis. Infestation with *Diphyllobothrium latum.*

Di·phyl''lo·both'ri·um. A genus of tapeworms, formerly called *Dibothriocephalus.* **D. erinacei.** A species of which only the larval stage is found in man, the adult worm being found only in dogs and cats. **D. latum.** The fish tapeworm, a large tapeworm found in the intestine. The head has two suckers or bothridia. The adult worm ranges from 3 to 10 meters in length, and may have over 4000 proglottids. The definitive hosts are man, dog, and cat. The first intermediate hosts are fresh-water copepods, and the secondary intermediate hosts are various fresh-water fishes. Infestation in man may cause disorders of the nervous and digestive systems, malnutrition, and anemia.

di·phy'o·dont. Having two sets of teeth, as the milk teeth and the permanent teeth.

dip''la·cu'sis. Hearing of the same sound differently by the two ears. **d. binauralis.** Perception of a single tone as having a higher fundamental pitch in one ear than in the other. **d. uniauralis.** Hearing of

two tones by one ear when only one tone is produced.

di''plas·mat'ic (dye''plaz·mat'ick). Containing matter other than protoplasm; said of cells.

di·ple'gi·a. Paralysis of similar parts on the two sides of the body. —**diple'gic,** *adj.* **spastic d.** Spastic paralysis of the legs; due to organic changes in the infantile brain, such as diffuse degeneration or atrophic lobar sclerosis, malformations or developmental defects, and microscopic cellular alterations. This disorder is sometimes associated with convulsions and mental deficiency.

dip'lo-, dipl-. A combining form signifying *two, twice, twofold, double, twin,* etc.

dip''lo·al·bu''mi·nu'ri·a. The coexistence or alternation of physiologic and pathologic albuminuria in the same subject.

dip''lo·blas'tic. Having two germ layers, ectoderm and endoderm.

dip''lo·car'di·ac. Having a double heart, or one in which the two sides are more or less separate, as in birds and mammals.

dip''lo·coc'cin (dip''lo·cock'sin). An antibiotic substance obtained from cultures of certain streptococci.

Dip''lo·coc'cus. A genus of bacteria of the family Lactobacteriaceae of the tribe Streptococceae. **D. gonorrhoeae.** Synonym for *Neisseria gonorrhoeae.* **D. pneumoniae.** A species that is oval or spherical, typically paired, encapsulated, nonmotile, and usually Gram-positive. It has been subdivided into types, of which 31 are recognized at present, but at least 55 have been described. It is one of the causes of pneumonia, especially lobar, but may also cause other infectious diseases, as meningitis, otitis media, pericarditis, and arthritis. Formerly called *Pneumococcus.*

dip''lo·coc'cus. A micrococcus that occurs in groups of two, such as the pneumococcus.

dip''lo·co'ri·a. Double pupil.

dip''lo·ë (dip'lo·ee). The cancellous bone between the outer and inner tables of the skull. —**diplo'ic, diploet'ic,** *adj.*

dip'loid. Having double the haploid or gametic number of chromosomes.

dip''lo·mel''li·tu'ri·a. Coexistence or alternation of diabetic and nondiabetic glycosuria in the same subject.

dip''lo·my·e'li·a (dip''lo·migh·ee'lee·uh). An anomaly occurring in certain types of spina bifida, consisting of doubling of the spinal cord. Syn., *diastematomyelia.*

dip''lo·neu'ral (dip''lo·new'rul). Pertaining to a muscle supplied by two nerves from different sources.

di·plop′a·gus (di-plop′uh-gus). A double monster consisting of conjoined twins equally developed or having one or more vital organs in common.

di·plo′pi·a (di-plo′pee-uh). Double vision, one object being seen as two. **—diplop′ic,** adj. **binocular d.** The most common type; due to a derangement of muscular balance of the two eyes; the images of an object are thrown upon nonidentical points of the retina. **crossed d.** The result of divergent strabismus; the image of the right eye appears upon the left side, and that of the left eye upon the right side. Also called heteronymous d. **homonymous d.** The reverse of crossed diplopia; found in convergent strabismus. Also called direct d. **introspective d.** Formation of images on noncorresponding retinal points, giving a perception of depth and perspective. Also called physiologic d. **monocular d.** Diplopia with a single eye; usually due to hysteria, to double pupil, or to beginning cataract.

dip″lo·pi·om′e·ter. Instrument for measuring the degree of diplopia.

dip′lo·scope. Instrument for the investigation of binocular vision.

dip′lo·some. The pair of centrioles commonly found in certain cells.

di′pole″. 1. A particle or object bearing opposite charges. 2. A pair of electric charges, positive and negative, situated near each other in a conducting medium. Syn., doublet.

di′pole mo′ment. The measure of the electric asymmetry of a molecule. It is equal to the product of the ionic charges and their spatial separation.

dip′ping. 1. Palpating the liver by quick depression of the abdomen. 2. In veterinary medicine, the act of submerging an animal for the application of the dip.

dip″ro·so′pi·a (dip″ro·so′pee-uh, dye″pro-), **di·pros′o·py** (dye-pros′-o-pee). In teratology, duplication of the face or of its parts.

di·pro′so·pus (dye-pro′so-pus, dye″-pro·so′pus). A monster characterized by a duplicity of the face. Such monsters occur with all degrees of duplicity, as **diprosopus dirhinus** (a monster with a double nose) and **diprosopus tetrotus** (one with four ears), and grade into dicephaly.

dip″so·ma′ni·a. The recurrent periodic compulsion to excessive drinking of alcoholic beverages. **—dipsoma′niac,** n.

dip″so·pho′bi·a. A morbid fear of drinking.

dip″so·ther′a·py. Treatment of certain diseases by reducing the amount of fluid allowed the patient.

Dip′ter·a. An order of two-winged insects; includes mosquitoes, flies, botflies, midges.

dip′ter·ous. In biology, having two wings or winglike processes.

di·py′gus, dip′y·gus. A monster with more or less duplication of the pelvis and lower parts of the back. Syn., dilecanus.

Di″py·lid′i·um (dye″pye-lid′ee-um). A genus of tapeworms. **D. caninum.** A species of which the dog and cat are definitive hosts, and man is an occasional host; these worms vary from 20–40 cm. in length. Fleas are the host of the larval stage.

di·rec′tor. Anything that guides or directs. **grooved d.** An instrument grooved to guide the knife in surgical operations.

di·rhi′nus, di·rhy′nus, dir·rhi′-nus. A partial or complete doubling of the nose; a mild degree of diprosopia.

dirt eat′ing. See chthonophagia; geophagy.

dis-, di-. A prefix signifying two, twice, or double.

dis-. A prefix meaning separation, the opposite of, reversal.

di·sac′cha·rid. See disaccharide.

di·sac′cha·ride (dye-sack′uh-ride, -rid), **di·sac′cha·rid** (dye-sack′uh-rid). A carbohydrate formed by the condensation of two monosaccharide molecules.

dis·ag″gre·ga′tion. 1. A state of perpetual distraction which prevents an individual from entertaining any idea other than the one which dominates or occupies his mind, as in obsessive, ruminative states. 2. In hysteria, an inability to coördinate various new sensations and to connect them with visual impressions.

dis″ar·tic″u·la′tion. Separation at a joint; amputation at a joint.

dis·az′o-, dis·a′zo-. In chemistry, a combining form indicating the presence in a compound of two azo (—N=N—) groups. **—disazo,** adj.

disc. See disk.

dis·charge′. 1. An emission, unloading, evacuation, or secretion. 2. That which is emitted. 3. To emit, to unload. 4. In electricity, a setting free or escape of stored-up energy; the equalization of differences of potential between the poles of a condenser or other source of electricity by connecting or nearly connecting them with a conductor.

dis·charg′ing. Unloading; flowing out, as pus.

dis·cis′sion. (di-sish′un, -sizh′un). 1. State of being torn apart. 2. In eye surgery, an operation for soft cataract in which the capsule is lacerated a number of times to allow the lens substance to be absorbed.

disc·i′tis (disk·eye′tis). Inflammation of a disk, especially of an intervertebral or interarticular disk.

dis'co-, disc-. A combining form denoting *connection with,* or *resemblance to, a disk.*

dis'coid. 1. Shaped like a disk. 2. *In dentistry,* an excavator having a blade in the form of a disk.

dis·col″or·a′tion. Change in or loss of the natural color of a part.

dis″co·pla·cen′ta. A discoid placenta.

dis·crete′. Not running together; separate; opposed to *confluent.*

dis·crim″i·na′tion. The act of distinguishing or differentiating. **one-point d.** The act of distinguishing by localization a point of pressure on the surface of the skin. **tonal d.** The act of distinguishing tone values. This function is located in the cochlea. **two-point d.** The act of differentiating or identifying two points of pressure on the surface of the skin. The normal ability for this is proportional to the distance between the points.

dis'cus. A disk. **d. articularis.** Interarticular fibrocartilage. **d. proligerus.** The cumulus oöphorus, *q.v.*

dis·cu′tient. 1. Dispersing; scattering. 2. A remedy which causes dispersion or disappearance, as of a swelling.

dis·ease′. An illness or sickness. A disturbance in function or structure of any organ or part of the body. **acute d.** One marked by rapid onset and short course. **Adams-Stokes d.** Cerebral syncope with bradycardia. **Addison's d.** A condition brought about by hypofunction or dysfunction of the suprarenal glands; adrenal insufficiency. It is characterized by extreme emaciation, anemia, and deep bronzing of the skin, ending in death. The name also was applied formerly to pernicious anemia. **Australian X d.** An epidemic virus encephalitis, prevalent in children; first appeared in Australia in 1917; it resembles poliomyelitis, and can be transmitted to some animals. **Ayerza's d.** A syndrome of chronic cyanosis, dyspnea, and sclerosis of the pulmonary artery. **Bang's d.** Infectious abortion of cattle. **Banti's d.** Splenomegaly of undetermined origin; characterized by anemia, leukopenia, hemorrhage, and cirrhosis of the liver. **Barlow's d.** Infantile scurvy. **Basedow's d.** Exophthalmic goiter. **Bekhterev's d.** Chronic arthritis of unknown etiology, with progressive deformity, stiffness, and bony fusion of vertebrae. **Bell's d.** Neuropathy of the facial nerve. **Bernhardt's d.** Abnormal sensations, especially of numbness, with hyperesthesia and pain on exertion, in the region supplied by the lateral cutaneous nerve of the thigh. **Bowen's d.**

A disease involving the skin and sometimes the mucous membranes; may be a precancerous dyskeratotic process or a superficial epithelioma with lateral intraepithelial spread. Marked by reddish papules covered with a thickened horny layer. **Bright's d.** Chronic nephritis. **Brill's d.** A recrudescent attack of epidemic, louse-borne typhus fever; the Weil-Felix test is unreliable. **Buerger's d.** Thromboangiitis obliterans, a chronic arteritis and phlebitis of the extremities, with thrombotic occlusion leading to gangrene; generally affects portions of the toes and feet. **caisson d.** A condition caused by a too rapid return from high to normal (sea level) atmospheric pressure; affects tunnel and caisson workers, divers, and others who work under high atmospheric pressure; due to the formation of nitrogen bubbles in the blood and body tissues. Symptoms vary with the location of the bubbles and include pain in the abdomen, joints, and extremities, vertigo, various sensory or motor disturbances, itching of the skin, asphyxia, collapse, and unconsciousness. Prompt treatment usually assures recovery. Syn., *aeremia, bends, compressed-air illness, diver's neurosis.* Also see *aeroembolism.* **celiac d.** A chronic disturbance of nutrition, seen most frequently in children of two or three years; characterized by a distended abdomen, diarrhea, and large, frothy, foul-smelling stools. In adults this condition is known as nontropical sprue. **Charcot-Marie-Tooth d.** Progressive, familial, neuropathic muscular atrophy, characterized by weakness and atrophy of the peroneal muscles. This is accompanied by diminution of proprioceptive and cutaneous sensation and loss of deep reflexes. Talipes cavus frequently is present. **Christian-Weber d.** Nodular, nonsuppurative panniculitis. **chronic d.** One which is slow in its course and of long duration. **collagen d.** Any one of a group characterized by widespread alterations of connective tissue, as rheumatic fever, polyarteritis, or dermatomyositis. **communicable d.** One which is readily transmitted from person to person by direct contact or through the agency of a vector. **complicating d.** A secondary or independent disease superimposed upon one already existing. Syn., *intercurrent d.* **congenital d.** One acquired in utero, and therefore present at birth. **constitutional d.** (a) An inherent disease, owing to the individual's inherited genotypic characteristics. (b) A general disease involving the entire body, as contrasted to local disease confined to one part. **contagious d.**

Any infectious disease in which the pathogenic organism is transmitted directly or indirectly from one individual to another. **Cooley's d.** Familial erythroblastic anemia. **Cushing's d.** Pituitary basophilism resulting from basophilic adenomas. The condition occurs generally in young women and is associated with amenorrhea, male hirsutism, and a peculiar obesity of the face, neck, and trunk only, with a greatly altered physiognomy. The disease is rare and should not be confounded with many of the variable syndromes of adrenal insufficiency. **deficiency d.** One resulting from the lack of a necessary dietary constituent, as minerals, vitamins, or fatty acids. **degenerative d.** A general wearing-out process, in which no specific deficiency is recognized; common in old age. **degenerative joint d.** Preferred name for degenerative arthritis, *q.v.* **demyelinating d.** One of a large group of diseases of the nervous system which possess, as a common pathologic feature, foci in which the myelin sheaths of the nerve fibers are destroyed. **Dercum's d.** Adiposis dolorosa. **diffused d.** One which involves several tracts of the spinal cord. **Duchenne-Aran d.** Progressive myelopathic muscular atrophy. **Durand-Nicolas-Favre d.** Lymphogranuloma of venereal origin. **Eddowes' d.** A familial syndrome of fragile bones and dark scleras. **endemic d.** One which occurs continuously or repeatedly at the same season in a certain locality. **epidemic d.** One attacking a large number of people in one locality at the same time. **Erb-Charcot d.** Syphilitic spastic spinal paralysis. **familial d.** One occurring in several members of the same family. Often restricted to mean several members of the same generation, in contrast to hereditary disease, *q.v.* **foot-and-mouth d.** An acute febrile disease due to a filtrable virus; causes a vesicular eruption of the mucous membranes of the nose and mouth and the skin of the feet. It is contagious to ruminants and pigs and is often transmitted to other domestic animals as well as to man. Syn., *epidemic stomatitis, epizootic stomatitis.* **fourth d.** A syndrome occurring in childhood, characterized by an acute, reddish exanthem extending over the entire body, with the exception of the face, and followed by desquamation. It resembles scarlatina, but runs a mild course. The etiology is unknown. **Fox-Fordyce d.** A chronic, itching, papular eruption, seen about the areola, the pubic area, the axillas; probably due to a disorder of the apocrine sweat glands. Most common in women. **functional d.** One in which no definite cause or no demonstrable pathologic lesion can be discovered. **Gaucher's d.** A rare familial disease occurring in infancy or childhood. Characterized by anemia and marked enlargement of the spleen and liver. **glass-blower's d.** Enlargement of the parotid gland; seen in glass blowers. **glycogen d.** See *glycogenosis.* **Graves's d.** Exophthalmic goiter. **Hanot's d.** Hypertrophic cirrhosis of the liver. **Hansen's d.** A chronic disease, occurring almost exclusively in tropic and subtropic countries, caused by the microörganism *Mycobacterium leprae;* commonly called *leprosy.* See also indeterminate *leprosy,* lepromatous *leprosy,* tuberculoid *leprosy.* **Heberden's d.** The condition associated with bony enlargement about the terminal phalangeal joints. **hemorrhagic d.** Disease in which pathologic hemorrhage occurs, due to a disturbance in blood coagulation or to increased permeability of the walls of the blood vessels. **hemorrhagic d. of the newborn.** A disease occurring in the first two weeks of life, usually between the second and fifth day; marked by spontaneous bleeding in any body tissues. Due to hypoprothrombinemia, resulting from a vitamin-K deficiency in the mother. **hereditary d.** One transmitted from the parent to his offspring through the genes. May be dominant, recessive, or sex-linked. **Hirschsprung's d.** Congenital hypertrophic dilatation of the colon. **Hodgkin's d.** A disease of the lymph nodes of unknown origin, characterized by their painless, progressive enlargement, progressive anemia, enlargement of the spleen, periodic fever, itching, and weight loss; occurs most frequently in young adult males, terminating fatally. Syn., *lymphogranulomatosis.* **Holla d.** Epidemic hemolytic jaundice. **Huntington's d.** Chronic progressive hereditary chorea, *q.v.* **idiopathic d.** One in which no causative factor is recognized. **infectious d.** One due to invasion of the body by pathogenic organisms. **Legg-Calvé-Perthes d.** Osteochondritis deformans juvenilis. **malignant d.** (a) Cancer, *q.v.* (b) Any disease in a particularly violent form, threatening to produce death in a short time. **Marie's d.** Rheumatic spondylitis involving the spine only, or invading the shoulders and hips (Strümpell-Marie type). **occupational d.** One arising from the particular toxic substances, characteristic hazards, or frequently repeated mechanical operations of a particular industry or trade. **organic d.** One associated with recognizable structural changes in the organs or tissues of the body. **Osgood-Schlatter d.** Osteochondritis in the tibial tuberosity. **Paget's d.** (a) Osteitis deformans, a rare disease of unknown etiology in which there is loss of calcium from the long bones and sometimes of the bones of the skull with replacement later of the calcium. This is accompanied by deformity and sometimes by fractures. Affects principally middle-aged males. (b) The eczematous area about the nipple observed in subjects who shortly develop mammary cancer formerly was called *Paget's disease of the nipple*. **pandemic d.** One epidemic over a large area, as an entire country or several countries. **parasitic d.** One due to invasion of the body by animal or vegetable parasites. **Parkinson's d.** Paralysis agitans, *q.v.* **Parry's d.** Exophthalmic goiter. **Pel-Ebstein's d.** Pseudoleukemia; multiple lymphadenoma. **periodic d.** One occurring at regular intervals or at the same season of the year. **Pick's d.** (a) Polyserositis, *q.v.* (b) Lobar atrophy. **Pott's d.** Tuberculosis of the spine. **ragpicker's d.** Anthrax. Also called *ragsorter's d.* **Raynaud's d.** A trophoneurosis characterized by three grades of intensity: (a) Local ischemia, observed most frequently in the extremities, and producing the condition known as dead fingers or dead toes. (b) Local asphyxia, which usually follows local ischemia, but may develop independently; the fingers, toes, and ears are the parts usually affected. (c) Local or symmetrical gangrene; small areas of necrosis appear on the pads of the fingers and of the toes, also at the edges of the ears and tip of the nose. Occasionally symmetrical patches are seen on the limbs or trunk and, in severe cases, terminate in extensive gangrene. **rickettsia d.** Any disease caused by rickettsia. The most important groups are the typhus fever group, caused by *Rickettsia prowazekii*; the Rocky Mountain spotted fever group, caused by *R. rickettsii*; the scrub typhus group, caused by *R. tsutsugamushi*; and the Q fever group, caused by *Coxiella burneti*. **sacroiliac d.** An inflammation of the sacroiliac joint, characterized by pain and tenderness over the joint, and thought to produce sciatica. **Schüller-Christian d.** A disease of childhood, insidious in onset and progressive; characterized by exophthalmos, diabetes insipidus, and softened areas in the bones, particularly those of skull, thigh, shoulder, and pelvic girdle. Pathologically the changes are due to lipoidosis of the xanthoma type. Syn., *lipoid granulomatosis*. **septic d.** One due to the presence and multipli-

cation of pyogenic or putrefactive organisms in the body. **sexual diseases.** Diseases of the sexual organs. **sporadic d.** One occurring only occasionally and in single cases. **Still's d.** A type of chronic, infectious polyarthritis occurring in children. In the later stages, splenomegaly and glandular enlargement appear. **subacute d.** One which is more prolonged and less active than an acute disease. **Tay-Sachs d.** Infantile form of amaurotic familial idiocy, *q.v.* **vagrant's d.** A discoloration of the skin occurring especially in elderly persons who are uncleanly and infested with pediculi over a long period. **venereal diseases.** Gonorrhea, syphilis, chancroid, granuloma inguinale, and venereal lymphogranuloma. Abbreviated, V.D.

dis″en·gage′ment. Emergence from a confined state; especially the emergence of the head of the fetus from the vaginal canal during parturition.

dis″in·fect′ant. An agent which destroys or inhibits the microörganisms causing disease. **complete d.** One that destroys the spores as well as the vegetating cells. **incomplete d.** One that destroys the vegetating cells but not the spores.

dis″in·fec′tion. The destruction or removal of pathogenic organisms, especially by means of chemical substances. —**disinfect′**, *v.t.* **concurrent d.** Prompt disinfection and disposal of infective material continuously throughout the course of a disease. **steam d.** The destruction of pathogenic bacteria by application of live steam under pressure. Moist heat is regarded as a more effective germicide than dry heat. **terminal d.** Disinfection and disposal of infectious material after the termination of a disease.

dis·in″fes·ta′tion. Extermination of insects or animal parasites; delousing.

dis·in′te·grate. Break up or decompose.

disipal. Trade-mark for orphenadrine hydrochloride.

dis·joint′. Disarticulate; separate, as bones from their natural relations.

disk, disc. A circular, platelike organ or structure. **anisotropic d.** The doubly refractive, dark, broad disk of a myofibril of a striated muscle fiber. Also called *A d., Q d.* **articular d.** One of fibrocartilage, dividing the joint cavity of certain joints. **choked d.** Papillitis, *q.v.* **embryonic d.** In mammals, the central, round, or oval area of the bilaminar blastoderm in which the primitive streak arises and from which the embryo proper develops. Also called *area germinativa, area embryonalis, embryonic blasto-*

derm. **herniated d.** Ruptured disk. **intervertebral disks.** The disks of fibrocartilage between the adjacent surfaces of the bodies of the vertebra. **isotropic d.** The singly refractive, light, broad disk of a myofibril of a striated muscle fiber. **optic d.** The circular area in the retina that represents the convergence of fibers from the ganglion cells of the retina to form the optic nerve. Syn., *optic papilla.* **ruptured d.** An intervertebral disk in which the nucleus pulposus has protruded through the surrounding fibrocartilage. **Z d.** The thin membrane which bisects the isotropic disk in a relaxed muscle fiber and forms the boundary of a sarcomere. Syn., *Z band, Z line, intermediate d.* Also called *Krause's membrane, Dobie's line, telophragma.* See also Z, 2.

dis″lo·ca′tion. The displacement of one or more bones of a joint or of any organ from the original position. See *diastasis, displacement, subluxation.* Syn., *luxation.* —**dis′located**, *adj.;* **dis′lo·cate**, *v.t.* **complete d.** One in which there is complete separation of the joint surfaces. **compound d.** One in which there is a communication with the joint from outside, through an external wound. **congenital d.** One existing since birth. **d. of lens.** A displacement of the crystalline lens of the eye. **diverging d.** A dislocation of the radius and ulna at the wrist, involving rupture of the annular ligament. **double d.** One in which there are two similar joint dislocations, on opposite sides of the body. **fracture-d.** One in which there is a fracture accompanying the dislocation. **habitual d.** One in which there are frequently relapsing dislocations of a particular joint, as the shoulder. Also called *recurrent d., relapsing d.* **incomplete d.** A partial dislocation; subluxation. **intrauterine d.** One which occurs during fetal life. **paralytic d.** One resulting from flaccid paralysis of the muscles and muscular atrophy. **pathologic d.** One resulting from joint disease with destruction of tissue, or from paralysis. **traumatic d.** A dislocation as a result of violence. **unreduced d.** One in which the dislocated bone has not been replaced in normal position. Syn., *old d.*

is·mem′ber. Amputate an extremity or a major portion thereof. —**dismemberment,** *n.*

dis″oc·clude′. Grind or level a tooth surface so that it will fail to touch the corresponding tooth in the other jaw during mastication.

dis·or′der. A disturbance or derangement of physical, emotional, or mental health or function. See also *disease, reaction, syndrome.*

dis·or″gan·i·za′tion. Act of deranging or the state of abnormal structure.

dis·o″ri·en·ta′tion. Loss of normal relationship to one's surroundings; particularly the inability to comprehend time, place, and people, such as occurs in organic brain disease.

dis′pa·rate. Not alike; unequal or unmated.

dis·par′i·ty. Difference; inequality.

dis·pen′sa·ry. 1. A place where medicine or medical aid is given free or at low cost. 2. In a place of business, a medical office provided by the owner to serve sick or injured employees.

dis·pen′sa·to″ry. A book containing a systematic discussion of medicinal agents, including origin, preparation, description, use, and mode of action.

dis·pense′. Prepare and distribute medicines for the sick.

dis·pens′ing. Preparation and distribution of medicines to those who are to use them.

di·sper″my, di·sper′my. Entrance of two spermatozoa into the ovum.

dis·per′sion. 1. Act of scattering. 2. Any scattering of light, as that passed through ground glass.

dis·pers′oid. A colloid or finely divided substance.

dis·place′ment. 1. Removal from the normal position; dislocation, luxation. 2. *In pharmacy,* a process occurring in percolation. 3. *In chemistry,* a change in which one element is removed by another element. 4. *In psychopathology,* a device whereby the emotional tension arising out of a repressed feeling, as of guilt or inadequacy, is discharged through an unrelated, trivial act or conscious expression; such as a compulsive ritual or a senseless fear. The original intolerable situation or experience is thereby barred from entering the consciousness. **fish-hook d.** A term referring to a vertical type of stomach, not an actual displacement; an orthotonic stomach. **toe d.** Overlapping toes. **uterine d.** Any change in position of the uterus from the accepted normal. See *anteversion, prolapse, retroversion.*

dis″po·si′tion. A tendency to acquire a certain disease; a peculiar predisposing factor, partly or wholly dependent upon heritable factors.

dis·rup′tive. Bursting; rending.

dis·sect′. Cut tissues apart carefully and slowly, in order to allow study of the relations of a part.

dis·sec′tion. The cutting of tissues of the body for purposes of study.

dis·sec′tor. 1. One who makes a dissection. 2. Handbook or manual of anatomy and instructions for use in dissection.

dis·sem″i·na′tion. The scattering or dispersion of disease or disease germs. —**dissem′inated,** *adj.*

dis·sim″u·la′tion. Act of feigning, disguising, or malingering.

dis·so″ci·a′tion. 1. Separation; especially of a chemical compound into ions. 2. *In cardiology,* completely independent action of atria and ventricles; heart block, *q.v.* 3. *In psychology,* the segregation from consciousness of certain components of mental processes, which then function independently; the separation of ideas from their natural and appropriate affects or feelings. 4. *In bacteriology,* a change in colony form, often occurring in a new environment, and associated with modified growth or virulence. —**disso′ciant,** *adj., n.* **atrioventricular d. with interference.** That condition in which there is a unidirectional block which prevents impulses from passing from the atrioventricular node back to the atria. This block is exhibited by a series of ventricular beats, representing responses to the atrioventricular node, and a premature ventricular beat, representing a response to the sinus node.

dis·so″ci·a′tion con′stant. The constant pertaining to a reversible reaction in which a compound breaks up into two or more products. See K_a, K_b.

dis″so·lu′tion. 1. Separation of a body or compound into its parts. 2. Death; decomposition.

dis·solve′. Make a solution of. —**dis·sol′vent,** *adj., n.*

dis′tad. Toward the periphery; in a distal direction.

dis′tal. 1. Extreme; at the greatest distance from a central point; peripheral. 2. *In dentistry,* referring to a position which lies away from the sagittal plane along the curve of a dental arch. See *mesial.* —**distad, distally,** *adv.*

dis′tance. The measure of space between two objects. **focal d.** The distance between the center of a lens and its focus. **hearing d.** The distance at which a certain sound can be heard. **infinite d.** *In optics,* a distance of 20 feet or more, so established because the rays from an object at that distance to the lens of the eye are practically parallel.

dis·tem′per. The common name applied to certain infectious diseases of animals.

dis·ten′tion. A state of dilatation.

dis·tich′i·a (dis·tick′ee·uh), **dis″tichi′a·sis** (dis″ti·kigh′uh·sis). The presence of a row of cilia at the inner lid border, which turn in and rub on the cornea. This row of cilia is additional to the two or three rows arising at the outer lid border.

dis′til·land. The substance being distilled.

dis′til·late. The condensate obtained by distillation.

dis″til·la′tion. Process of vaporization and subsequent condensation; it is used principally to separate liquids from nonvolatile substances. —**distill′,** *v.t., v.i.* **destructive d.** Decomposition of complex organic substances by heat and distillation of the products. **fractional d.** Separation of a liquid into its components by means of gradually increasing temperature, the different products being vaporized in the order of their respective boiling points. **molecular d.** That under high vacuum, the condensing surface being close to the distilland.

dis′to-, dist-. A combining form signifying *posterior, distant from the center.*

Dis′to·ma, Dis′to·mum. Old generic name for a genus of trematode worms. **D. haematobium.** Synonym for *Schistosoma haematobium.* **D. hepaticum.** Synonym for *Fasciola hepatica.*

Di·sto′ma·ta. A suborder of the Trematoda or flukes.

di·sto′mi·a (dye·sto′mee·uh). Congenital duplication of the mouth.

dis″to·mi′a·sis. Infestation with flukes.

dis·tor′tion. 1. A twisted or bent shape; deformity or malformation, acquired or congenital. 2. A writhing or twisting motion, as of the face. 3. *In optics,* a form of aberration in which objects viewed through certain lenses appear changed in shape but not broken in continuity. 4. *In psychoanalysis,* the adaptive alteration of an idea to conform with the subject's wishes or prejudices.

dis″tri·bu′tion. *In anatomy,* the branching of a nerve or artery, and the arrangement of its branches within those parts that it supplies.

dis″tri·chi′a·sis (dis″tri·kigh′uh·sis). Two hairs growing from a single follicle.

dis′trix. Splitting of the distal ends of the hair.

di·sul′fide (dye·sul′fide, ·fid). Bisulfide.

di′thi·zone. Diphenyl-thiocarbazone. A reagent used as a sensitive test for heavy metals, particularly lead.

di′thra·nol. British Pharmacopoeia name for 1,8-dihydroxyanthranol, used locally in the treatment of skin diseases. See *anthralin, cignolin.*

di·thy″mol·di·i′o·dide. Thymol iodide.

di·u′re·ide. 1. A derivative of urea in

which a hydrogen of both NH₂ groups is replaced by an acyl radical. 2. An acyl derivative of urea containing residues of two urea molecules.

di″u·re′sis. Increased excretion of urine.

di″u·ret′ic. 1. Increasing the volume of urine. 2. Agent that increases the volume of urine. **acidifying d.** Substance that produces diuresis because of its acid-forming properties in the body. **cardiac d.** Substance, such as digitalis, which produces diuresis by increasing the efficiency of the heart in patients with cardiac edema. **mercurial d.** An organic mercurial compound, which acts primarily by reducing tubular reabsorption of water. **osmotic d.** A substance producing diuresis because of the osmotic effect of the unabsorbed fraction in the renal tubules with resulting loss of water. **saline d.** A salt which produces diuresis because of its osmotic effect in the tubules.

di′uril. Trade-mark for chlorothiazide.

di·ur′nule. A medicinal product that contains the full quantity of a drug to be administered in 24 hours.

di″va·ga′tion. Rambling speech and thought.

di·va′lent (dye-vay′lunt, dye′vay-lunt). 1. Bivalent. 2. Having the ability to exist in two valence states.

di·ver′gence (dye-vur′junss, di-vur′junss). *In ophthalmology*, the abduction of both eyes simultaneously, or of one eye when the other is fixed. **—divergent,** *adj.*

di′ver's ear. An inflammation of the middle ear and auditory tube; caused by sudden changes in atmospheric pressure that may occur during an underwater diver's ascent or descent. Seen in caisson disease, *q.v.* Similar to aerootitis media.

di″ver·tic′u·la. Plural of diverticulum, *q.v.*

di″ver·tic″u·lec′to·my. Surgical removal of a diverticulum.

di″ver·tic″u·li′tis. Inflammation of a diverticulum.

di″ver·tic″u·lo′sis. Presence of many diverticula of the intestine.

di″ver·tic′u·lum (pl. *diverticula*). A pouch or sac springing from a hollow organ or structure; may be congenital or acquired. **congenital d.** One present at birth; the most common varieties are the esophageal diverticulum, intestinal diverticulum, and the diverticulum ilei. **esophageal d.** A saclike protrusion of a part of the wall of the esophagus or of the pharynx just above the esophageal opening. See pulsion d., traction d. **Eustachian d.** A small abnormal pouching of the lower portion of the auditory tube.

false d. One involving the large intestine, having only mucosal and serosal coats and lacking the muscular coat present in true diverticula. **gastric d.** A pouching of the stomach generally seen near the pylorus in connection with duodenal or gastric ulcer. **giant d.** A congenital enteric cyst or duplication of a portion of the ileum, jejunum, duodenum, and occasionally the stomach; the cyst has a common wall with the gastrointestinal tract. **hepatic d.** The primordium of the liver, gallbladder, and their ducts. Also called *hepatic gutter*. **intestinal d.** A sacculation of the intestinal wall. **pulsion d.** A thin-walled sac in the posterior wall of the hypopharynx opposite the cricoid cartilage just above the esophageal opening. **synovial d.** Abnormal pouches found in large joints such as the knee. **traction d.** A circumscribed sacculation of the esophagus due to the pull of adhesions. **ureteral d.** A chronic localized bulging of the ureter, usually the result of obstruction; generally associated with hydronephrosis. **vesical d.** One occurring in the urinary bladder, usually in males over 60 and generally secondary to urinary obstruction.

di·vi′nyl e′ther (dye-vy′nil). (CH₂:-CH)₂O. A highly volatile, unsaturated ether used as an inhalation anesthetic for short operations. Syn., *divinyl oxide, vinyl ether.* See vinethene.

di·vi′nyl ox′ide. See *divinyl ether.*

di·vi′sion. Act or process of dividing into parts. **equational d.** A nuclear division in which daughter chromosomes separate from each other, as in ordinary somatic cell division; applied especially to the second miotic division in contrast with the reduction division in which maternal and paternal homologous chromosomes disjoin.

di·vul′sion (dye-vul′shun). A tearing apart. **—divulse′,** *v.t.*

di·vul′sor (dye-vul′sur, di-vul′sur). Instrument for the forcible dilation of a part or of stricture in any organ.

diz′zi·ness. An unpleasant sensation of disturbed relations to surrounding objects in space; giddiness, *q.v.* **—dizzy,** *adj.*

dl-. *In chemistry*, an abbreviation used as a prefix, meaning a *racemic mixture containing equal amounts of both dextrorotatory and levorotatory forms* of an organic compound. See also d-, l-.

D.M.D. Doctor of Dental Medicine. Equivalent to the more common *D.D.S.*

DNA Abbreviation for deoxyribonucleic acid.

DNase Abbreviation for deoxyribonuclease.

doca. Trade-mark for desoxycorticosterone acetate.

doc'tor. 1. One licensed, usually after special study, and qualifying by examination, to practice medicine, dentistry, or veterinary medicine. 2. Recipient of an academic title signifying competence in a special branch of learning. 3. Treat medically. *Colloq.*

do'dec·a-, dodec-. A prefix denoting *twelve.*

do·lan'tin. Meperidine hydrochloride.

dol'i·cho- (dol'i·ko-), **dol'ich-** (dol'ick-). A combining form meaning *long, narrow.*

dol″i·cho·ceph'a·ly. The condition in which the length-breadth index of the head is 75.9 or less, indicating that the head is much longer than it is broad. **—dolichocephal'ic, dolichocephalous,** *adj.*

dol″i·cho·mor'phic. Marked by a long or narrow form or build.

dol″i·cho·pel'ic, dol″i·cho·pel'vic. Designating a pelvis the pelvic index of which is 95.0 or more.

dolophine. A trade-mark for amidone hydrochloride, *q.v.*

do'lor (pl. *dolores*). Pain. **dolores praesagientes.** Fleeting, false pains occurring a few days before the onset of labor.

do″lo·rim'e·ter. A device for measuring sensitivity to pain and the degree of pain experienced in any nerve irritation caused by disease.

dol″or·o·gen'ic (dol″or·o-, do″lor·o·). Possessing the quality of pain; causing or arousing pain.

do″ma·to·pho'bi·a. Morbid fear of being in a house; a variety of claustrophobia.

dom'i·nant. 1. *In biology,* a characteristic of one of the parents of a hybrid which is present in the offspring, the contrasting recessive characteristic of the other parent being absent. 2. Pertaining to such a characteristic. See *Mendel's law,* under Gregor Johann *Mendel.* **—dominance,** *n.*

do'nee'. The patient who receives transfused blood or other tissue.

do'nor. A person who gives blood for transfusion to another, or skin for grafting. **universal d.** One whose blood is of group O; one whose blood corpuscles are not agglutinated by the blood of anyone.

do'pa. 3,4-Dihydroxyphenylalanine; an amino acid intermediate in the formation of melanin from tyrosine.

do'pa ox'i·dase, do'pase. An enzyme of the skin that catalyzes the oxidation of dihydroxyphenylalanine (dopa) to melanin. This enzyme plays an important role in skin pigmentation.

dope. 1. Any drug administered to stimulate or to stupefy, temporarily, or taken habitually. *Slang.* 2. Administer such drug. *Slang.* **d. fiend.** One addicted to the use of a drug. *Slang.*

do″ra·pho'bi·a. Morbid fear of touching the skin or fur of animals.

doriden. Trade-mark for glutethimide.

dorsacaine hydrochloride. Trade-mark for benoxinate hydrochloride.

dor'sal. *In human anatomy,* pertaining to the back or to the posterior part of an organ. See also *posterior.* **—dorsally, dorsad,** *adv.*

dor·sal'gi·a. Pain in the back.

dor·sa'lis pe'dis (pee'diss, ped'iss). The main artery of the dorsum of the foot. See Table of Arteries, Appendix.

dor'si-. A combining form meaning *of* or *on the back.*

dor″si·flex'ion (dor″si·flek'shun). Bending the foot upward. See *plantar flexion.*

dor'so-. A combining form denoting *the back, dorsal,* or *dorsally.*

dor″so·an·te'ri·or. Applied to a fetus having its back toward the ventral aspect of the mother.

dor″so·ceph'al·ad. Toward the dorsal aspect of the head.

dor″so·lat'er·al. Relating to the back and the sides.

dor″so·me'di·an. Situated in or relating to the middle region of the back.

dor″so·pos·te'ri·or. Applied to the position of a fetus having its back toward the dorsal aspect of the mother.

dor″so·ra'di·al. Relating to or situated upon the dorsal aspect and radial border of the hand, finger, or arm.

dor″so·ul'nar. Relating to or situated upon the dorsal aspect and ulnar border of the arm, hand, or finger.

dor″so·ven'tral. Pertaining to the dorsal and ventral regions; extending in a direction from the dorsal surface toward the ventral. Syn., *posteroanterior.*

dor'sum (pl. *dorsa*). 1. The back. 2. Any part corresponding to the back, as the dorsum of the foot or hand. **d. linguae.** The upper surface of the tongue.

doryl. Trade-mark for carbachol suitable for oral or subcutaneous administration.

do'sage. The proper amount of a medicine or other agent for a given case or condition. **electric d.** The regulation of the strength of an electric current for therapeutic purposes.

dose. 1. The measured portion of medicine to be taken at one time. Abbreviated, d. 2. *In radiology,* the measure expressed in number of roentgens, of property of the x-rays at a particular place, whether in air, tissue, or other material, or even in a vacuum; exposure. **air d.** The number of roentgens in the air at the center of the field

mployed in treatment with roentgen
rays. **average d.** One which may be
expected ordinarily to produce the
therapeutic effect for which the ingredient or preparation is most commonly
employed. **daily d.** The total amount
to be administered in 24 hours.
depth d. The number of roentgens
within the body at a specified depth
below the surface field of roentgen irradiation. **exit d.** The skin dose of
roentgen rays or gamma rays of radioactive substances in the exit field of
the body. **field d.** The total number
of roentgens which affect the skin
during treatment with roentgen rays.
lethal d. A dose sufficient to kill.
maximum d. The largest dose consistent with safety. **minimum d.**
The smallest quantity of a medicine
that will produce physiologic effects.
minimum lethal d. (a) The
amount of a drug which is fatal to 50%
of the experimental animals of a group
studied under controlled conditions.
(b) Formerly the quantity of a toxin
which will kill a guinea pig of 250 Gm.
weight in from 4 to 5 days. **skin d.**
The number of roentgens on the surface of the skin at the center of the
field of treatment. **tissue d.** The
number of roentgens of radioactive
substances at specified points in the
tissues of the body.

dosim'e·try. 1. Accurate determination of medicinal doses. 2. A system of
therapeutics consisting in the use of
only a few drugs, mainly alkaloids, in
the form of granules administered according to certain fixed rules. 3. Measurement of exposures or doses of x-rays.
dosimet'ric, adj.

douche (dōōsh). 1. A stream of water
or air directed against the body or into
a body cavity. In physiotherapy,
douches are commonly used on the body
surface for their stimulating effect.
They may be hot, cold, or alternating.
In gynecology, lavage of the vagina;
used for cleansing or for the application of heat or medication to the part.

Do'ver's pow'der. A diaphoretic
and sedative powder containing 10 per
cent each of ipecac and opium.

DPN. Abbreviation for diphosphopyridine nucleotide.

drachm (dram), **dram.** The eighth
part of the apothecary's ounce. (Symbol, 3.) Also, less commonly, the sixteenth part of the avoirdupois ounce.
(Abbreviated, dr.) **fluidrachm.** The
eighth part of a fluidounce. Symbol, f3.

Dra·cun'cu·lus. A genus of thread-
worms belonging to the superfamily
Dracunculoidea. **D. medinensis.** A
species of filarial worms of which certain species of Cyclops are the intermediate hosts and man is a definitive
host. Human infestation is caused by

drinking raw water containing infested
Cyclops.

draft, draught. 1. A current of air.
2. A quantity of liquid, usually medicine, taken at one swallow.

dra·gee' (drah-zhay'). A sugar-coated
pill.

drain. 1. A material, such as gauze,
rubber tubing, rubber tissue, or twisted
suture material, which affords a channel of exit for the discharge from a
wound or cavity. 2. In surgery, procure
the discharge or evacuation of fluid
from a cavity by operation, tapping,
or otherwise. **capillary d.** One of
horsehair or silkworm gut used to keep
a wound open for a short period. **ciga-
rette d.** A drain of gauze surrounded
by rubber tissue, rubber dam, or split
rubber tubing. Also called Penrose d.
lamp chimney d. A tubular drain
of large caliber glass or metal, anchored over selected areas within the
abdomen and adapted to gastric, co-
lonic, and bladder surgery. **Miku-
licz d.** A large gauze tampon formed
by placing continuous or cut strips upon
a square which lines the interior of the
wound, the strip ends remaining outside. **sump d.** An aspirating tubular
drain of rubber, plastic, glass, etc.,
sometimes with lateral openings and
fishtail ends.

drain'age. The method of draining.
See drain. **basal d.** Removal of cerebrospinal fluid from the cisterna
magna. **continuous d.** Constant
emptying of a viscus by a retained
catheter or tube. Used especially of the
bladder. **negative pres-
sure d.** A closed system for draining
an empyema cavity. **postural d.**
Removal of bronchial secretions or of
the contents of a lung abscess by placing the patient's head downward.

dram. Synonym of drachm, q.v.

dramamine. Trade-mark for β-di-
methylaminoethyl benzohydryl ether 8-
chlorotheophyllinate, useful in motion
sickness. See dimenhydrinate.

dram'a·tism. Stilted and lofty
speech or behavior, observed in the insane.

drape. Arrange sterile linen about a
part preparatory to operation or examination.

drap"e·to·ma'ni·a. A morbid desire
to wander from home; dromomania.

draw. 1. Cause to soften and discharge, said of a poultice. 2. In dentistry, pull; remove a tooth from its
socket.

draw'-sheet". A narrow sheet, covering a rubber sheet, across the bed
under the patient's buttocks; can easily
be withdrawn and replaced if soiled.

dread. Extreme fear or apprehension.

dream. 1. An involuntary series of
images, emotions, and thoughts presented to the mind during sleep. Ac-

cording to Freud, a dream is a vehicle which conveys impulses from the unconscious to the conscious levels of mind. 2. Experience such images and emotions during sleep. —**dream′y**, *adj.* **day d.** Idle reverie. **waking d.** An illusion or hallucination. **wet d.** Seminal emission during sleep, generally accompanying an erotic dream.

dress′er. An attendant in British hospitals, usually a medical student, whose special duty is to dress and bandage wounds.

dress′ing. 1. Application of various materials for protecting a wound and favoring its healing. 2. Material so applied.

drib′ble. 1. Drool. 2. Void in drops, as urine from a distended or paralyzed bladder.

Drinker, Philip [*American industrial hygienist*, 1894–]. Invented the iron lung or *Drinker respirator;* see under *respirator.* Invented a negative-pressure cabinet for maintaining respiration in the newborn. See also *Drinker's method* under *artificial respiration;* Drinker-Collins *resuscitation.*

drip. 1. Fall in drops. 2. The continuous slow, intravenous introduction of fluid containing nutrients or drugs.

driv′el·ing. 1. An involuntary flow of the saliva, as in old age, infancy, idiocy, and mental stupor. 2. Talking, as in senile weakness of the mind, idiocy, and mental stupor.

drom′o·graph, dro′mo·graph. Instrument for registering the velocity of the blood current.

drom″o·ma′ni·a (drom″o·may′nee-uh, dro′mo·). An insane desire to wander; vagabondage.

drom″o·pho′bi·a (drom″o·fo′bee-uh, dro′mo·). Morbid fear of walking or roaming about.

drop. 1. A minute mass of liquid which in falling or in hanging from a surface forms a spheroid. 2. The falling of a part, as from paralysis. **ear drops.** Liquid medication instilled by drops into the external auditory meatus. **foot d.** See toe d. **toe d.** Inability to dorsiflex the foot; generally due to paralysis of the dorsiflexor muscles of the foot and toes, or to severance of a tendon. **wrist d.** Inability to extend the hand; due to paralysis of the extensor muscles of the hand and fingers, or to severance of a tendon.

drop′let. A minute particle of moisture expelled by talking, sneezing, or coughing, which may carry infectious microörganisms from one individual to another.

drop′per. A bottle, tube, or pipet, fitted for the emission of a liquid drop by drop.

drop′sy. An infiltration of the tissues with diluted lymph, or the collection

of such lymph in the body caviti… anasarca. —**dropsical**, *adj.* **ca**… **diac d.** Edema due to congesti… heart failure. **famine d.** Nutritio… edema; war edema. A form of ede… occurring in individuals suffering fro… protein deprivation, either as the r… sult of disease, or from inadequate i… take. **general d.** (a) Dropsy of o… or more of the large serous sacs of t… body combined with anasarca. (b) S… perficial dropsy when it affects th… trunk and arms as well as the leg… **mechanical d.** That due to m… chanical obstruction of the veins o… lymphatics. **renal d.** Anasarca due … disease of the kidneys.

Dro·soph′i·la. A genus of Dipte… containing the common fruit flie… **D. melanogaster.** The best know… species because of its extensive use … genetic analysis.

drug. A substance used as a medicin…

drug′gist. A dealer in medicines.

drum. The tympanic membrane; ea… drum.

drunk′en·ness. Intoxication; us… ally produced by drinking alcoho… liquor. **ether d.** That produced … drinking ether.

drupe. A fruit which has a thin ep… carp, a fleshy mesocarp, and a sto… endocarp which encloses a seed, as t… plum or peach.

Dry·op′ter·is (dry·op′tur·iss). … large genus of medium-sized ferns … the Polypodiaceae; woodfern.

D. Sc., D. S. Doctor of Science.

du″al·is′tic the′o·ry. The theo… that the lymphoblast of lymphatic t… sue and the myeloblast of myeloid t… sue are stem cells having entirely di… ferent potencies in hemopoiesis.

duck heart. Enlargement of the le… ventricle as a result of aortic insu… ciency, giving the heart a duck-shap… configuration in its fluoroscopic a… radiographic appearance. Also call… *wooden-shoe heart.*

duct. 1. A tube or channel, especia… one for conveying the secretions o… gland. 2. A small enclosed channel co… ducting any fluid, as the cochlear du… *q.v.* **accessory pancreatic d.** T… proximal part of the dorsal pancreat… duct that usually persists. Also call… **d. of Santorini. allantoic d.** T… proximal part of the allantois openi… into the cloaca. Also called *allantoe… teric d.* **alveolar d.** One of the a… passages in the lung branching from … respiratory bronchiole and leading … alveolar sacs. **Bartholin's d.** (… The duct of a major vestibular gla… at the vaginal introitus. (b) The du… of the major sublingual gland. O… **bile d.** A general term for the cyst… hepatic, or common duct or any of t… small ducts of the liver connecting w…

he hepatic duct. Also called *biliary d.* **branchial d.** The tubular second or fourth visceral grooves opening into the cervical vesicle of the embryo. **cervical d.** The temporary, external duct of the cervical vesicle formed as the cervical sinus is closed over by the opercular fold of the hyoid arch. **cloacal d.** The caudal part of the cloaca before the urorectal septum completely divides rectum and urogenital sinus. Also called *reichel's d.* **cochlear d.** The ductus cochlearis; the endolymph-filled, triangular (in cross-section) canal between the scala tympani and scala vestibuli; it contains the organ of Corti. Syn., *membranous cochlea, membranous cochlear canal.* Formerly called *scala media.* **common bile d.** The duct formed by the union of the cystic and the hepatic ducts. Syn., *ductus choledochus.* **common pharyngobranchial d.** The medial part of the fourth visceral pouch forming a common duct for the ultimobranchial body (fifth pouch) and the lateral part of the fourth pouch. **cystic d.** The duct of the gallbladder. **d. of Cuvier.** One of the two common cardinal veins. **d. of the testis.** That made up of the epididymal duct, the ductus deferens, and the ejaculatory duct. **ejaculatory d.** The terminal part of the ductus deferens imbedded in the prostate gland and opening into the urethra on the colliculus seminalis. **endolymphatic d.** (a) The duct which unites the endolymphatic sac with the utriculosaccular duct. (b) *In embryology,* a dorsomedian diverticulum of the otocyst, the anlage of the endolymphatic sac. **epididymal d.** The highly convoluted part of the duct of the testis which forms the main mass of the epididymis. Syn., *d. of the epididymis, ductus epididymidis.* **excretory d.** A duct, lined by nonsecretory epithelium, which is solely conductive. **hepatic d.** The common duct formed by the union of the left hepatic duct which drains the left and caudate lobes of the liver and the right hepatic duct which drains the right and quadrate lobes of the liver. Also called *common hepatic d.* **hepatocystic d.** A bile duct connected directly with the gallbladder. **hepatopancreatic d.** The terminal part of the embryonic common bile duct which also drains the ventral pancreas. **intercalated d.** The narrow portion of the intralobular ducts of the pancreas, or the parotid or submaxillary glands. **lacrimal d.** One of the 7 to 14 ducts extending obliquely from the gland to the fornix conjunctivae, carrying the tears to the conjunctival surface of the eyeball. (b) See *nasolacrimal d.* **lactiferous d.** One of the excretory ducts of the mammary gland, opening on the nipple.

Also called *milk d.* **Luschka's d.** One of the aberrant bile ducts found in the wall of the gallbladder. It may connect with a bile duct, but never with the lumen of the gallbladder. **mesonephric d.** The duct of the mesonephros or embryonic kidney. It becomes the excretory duct of the testis and gives rise to the ureteric bud in both sexes. Syn., *Wolffian d.* **milk d.** See *lactiferous d.* **Müllerian d.** The paramesonephric duct, *q.v.* Also called *Müller's d.* **nasofrontal d.** That between the frontal sinus and the middle meatus of the nose. Also called *frontonasal d.* **nasolacrimal d.** The membranous duct lodged within the nasolacrimal canal; it gives passage to the tears from the lacrimal sac to the inferior meatus. **pancreatic d.** The main duct of the pancreas formed from the dorsal and ventral pancreatic ducts of the embryo. Also called *d. of Wirsung.* **papillary d.** Any one of the largest collecting tubules of the kidney, opening into the minor calyces of the renal pelvis. **paramesonephric d.** An embryonic genital duct. In the female, the anlage of the oviducts, uterus, and vagina; in the male, it degenerates, leaving the appendix testis. Syn., *Müllerian d.* **paraurethral d.** That of a paraurethral gland. Formerly called *Skene's duct.* **parotid d.** That of the parotid gland. It passes horizontally across the lateral surface of the masseter muscle, pierces the buccinator muscle, and opens into the oral vestibule opposite the second upper molar tooth. Also called *Stensen's d., d. of Steno.* **perilymphatic d.** Aqueduct of the cochlea; a minute canal uniting the scala tympani with the subarachnoid space. **pharyngobranchial d.** The narrow medial part of a visceral pouch. **prostatic d.** Any of the ducts conveying the secretion of the prostate into the urethra. **right lymphatic d.** The common lymph trunk receiving the right jugular, subclavian, and bronchomediastinal trunks, and emptying into the right subclavian vein at its junction with the right internal jugular vein. **salivary d.** That of a salivary gland. **semicircular ducts.** The membranous semicircular canals. **seminal d.** The duct of the testis, especially the ductus deferens and the ejaculatory duct. Syn., *spermatic d.* **spermatic d.** The seminal duct. **Stensen's d.** See *parotid d.* **sublingual ducts.** Those of the sublingual gland opening into the oral cavity. Some unite to form the **major sublingual duct.** Others, the **minor sublingual ducts,** open on the sublingual plica. **submaxillary d.** That of the submaxillary gland receiving the major sublingual duct and emptying into the oral cavity at the side of the frenulum of the tongue. Also called *Wharton's d*. **thoracic d.** The common lymph trunk beginning in the cisterna chyli, passing upward, and emptying into the left subclavian vein at its junction with the left internal jugular vein. **thymopharyngeal d.** The third pharyngobranchial duct which may elongate and persist between thymus and pharynx. **thyrocervical d.** The fourth branchial duct. **thyroglossal d.** A slender temporary duct connecting the thyroid anlage with the surface of the tongue. **thyropharyngeal d.** The fourth pharyngobranchial duct. **urogenital d.** (a) The male urethra from the orifices of the ejaculatory ducts to the fossa navicularis. (b) In certain vertebrates, the mesonephric duct. **utriculosaccular d.** A membranous tube uniting the utricle and the saccule; from it arises the endolymphatic duct. **vitelline d.** The constricted part of the yolk sac opening into the midgut in the region of the future ileum. Syn., *omphalomesenteric d.* Formerly called *umbilical duct*. **Wolffian d.** The mesonephric duct.

duct'ule. A small duct. **aberrant ductules.** Blindly ending epithelial tubules associated with the epididymis; the ductuli aberrantes superiores and inferiores. **efferent d.** Any one of eight to fifteen coiled ducts which connect the rete testis with the duct of the epididymis and form the head of the epididymis; derived from paragenital mesonephric tubules. Syn., *lobule of the epididymis, vascular cone, efferent duct.*

duc'tu·li (duck'tew·lye). Plural of *ductulus*.

duc'tu·lus (pl. *ductuli*). A small duct. Also see *ductule*.

duc'tus (pl. *ducti*). Duct, *q.v.* **d. arteriosus.** The distal half of the left sixth aortic arch forming a fetal blood shunt between the pulmonary artery and the aorta. Also called *Botallo's duct, duct of Botal*. **d. choledochus.** The common bile duct, *q.v.* **d. cochlearis.** The cochlear duct, *q.v.* **d. deferens.** That portion of the excretory duct system of the testis which runs from the epididymal duct to the ejaculatory duct. Syn., *vas deferens*. Also called *deferent duct*. **d. endolymphaticus.** Endolymphatic duct, *q.v.* **d. epididymidis.** Epididymal duct, *q.v.* **d. reuniens.** A membranous tube in the inner ear uniting the saccule with the cochlear duct; it contains endolymph. Also called *Hensen's canal*. **d. venosus.** A venous channel of the embryonic liver shunting blood from the left umbilical vein to the enlarging right sinus venosus of the heart. Also called *duct Arantius*.

du·ip'a·ra. A woman who has been in labor twice.

dul'cin. *p*-Phenetolcarbamide-4-et oxy-phenylurea; occurs as whi needles, soluble in water. It is abo 250 times as sweet as cane sugar a has been suggested as a substitute saccharin. Syn., *sucrol, valzin*.

dul'ci·tol. $C_6H_{14}O_6$. Sugar from M *lampyrum nemorosum* and oth plants.

dul'cose. Dulcitol.

dull. 1. Slow of perception. 2. Not res nant on percussion; may be normal over the heart or pathologic as over area of pulmonary consolidation. Not bright in appearance. 4. Not shan blunt. —**dull'ness,** *n.*

dumb. Unable to utter articul speech. —**dumb'ness,** *n.*

Dunant, Jean Henri [*Swiss ph anthropist*, 1828–1910]. Aroused pub opinion with his account (1863) of t battlefield of Solferino (1859). Orga ized the first Geneva Convention (186 which founded the International R Cross Society.

du'o-. A combining form meaning tv

du"o·de·nec'ta·sis. Chronic dilat tion of the duodenum.

du"o·de·nec'to·my. Excision part of the duodenum.

du"o·de·ni'tis. Inflammation of t duodenum.

du"o·de'no- (dew"o·dee'no-, de od'i·no-), **duoden-.** A combini form meaning *related to* or *connect with the* duodenum.

du"o·de"no·chol"an·gi't (·kol"an·jy'tis, ·ko"lan·jy'tis). Inflan mation of the duodenum and the co mon bile duct about the ampulla.

du"o·de"no·chol"e·cys·tos't my (·kol"i·sis·tos'to·mee, ·ko"l The formation of an anastomosis b tween the duodenum and gallbladde

du"o·de"no·cho·led'o·chot' my (·ko·led"o·cot'o·mee, ·ko"led·o A modification of choledochotomy incising the duodenum in order to a proach the common duct.

du"o·de"no·cys·tos'to·m Duodenocholecystostomy, *q.v.*

du"o·de"no·en"ter·os'to·m Surgical formation of a passage b tween the duodenum and another p of the intestine.

du"o·de'no·gram (dew"o·dee' gram, dew·od'i·no·). A roentgenogr of the duodenum.

du"o·de"no·il"e·os'to·my. T surgical formation of a passage b tween the duodenum and the ileum

du"o·de"no·je"ju·nos'to·m (dew"o·dee"no·jee"jew·nos'to·m dew·od"i·no·). Surgical anastomosis

...e duodenum to the jejunum for duo-
...nal obstruction.

...**"o·de'no·plas"ty.** A reparative
...eration upon some portion of the
...odenum. See *pyloroplasty.*

...**"o·de·nos'co·py.** Inspection and
...sual examination of the duodenum by
...strumental means.

...**"o·de·nos'to·my.** The formation,
...mporarily, of a duodenal fistula by
...rgical procedure.

...**"o·de·not'o·my.** Surgical in-
...sion of the duodenum.

...**"o·de'num, du·od'e·num.** The
...rst part of the small intestine, be-
...nning at the pylorus. It is from eight
... ten inches long and is the most fixed
...rt of the small intestine; consists of
...perior, descending, and inferior por-
...ons, and contains the openings of the
...ncreatic duct and the common bile
...cts. —**duodenal,** *adj.* **giant d.**
...n enormously enlarged duodenum,
...milar to that seen in congenital
...egacolon. **inversed d.** A congenital
...normality associated with acute
...gulation and dilatation. **mobile d.**
... movable condition of the duodenum.
...otal. A trade-mark for guaiacol
...rbonate.

...**'pli·ca"ture.** A fold, as a mem-
...ane folding upon itself.

...**"pli·ca'tus cru"ci·a'ta.** Ex-
...rimentally produced double monsters
...tained by grafting on inversion of
...e two-celled stage in amphibia.

...**·plic'i·tas** (dew·pliss'i·tus). A
...onstrosity with duplication of either
...e cephalic or pelvic end, or both.
...**·plic'i·ty** (dew·pliss'i·tee). *In tera-
...logy,* the condition of being double;
...plexity.

...**ponol C.** Trade-mark for a U.S.P.
...ade of sodium lauryl sulfate.

...**'ra.** The dura mater, *q.v.*

...**racillin.** Trade-mark for a com-
...und of penicillin G and procaine sus-
...nded in sesame oil.

...**ralumin.** A noncorroding alloy of
...uminum and copper, used in surgical
...lints and appliances.

...**'ra ma'ter.** The fibrous mem-
...ane forming the outermost covering
... the brain and spinal cord. Syn.,
...ra. —**dural,** *adj.*

...**'ra·plas"ty.** Repair of defects in
...e dura mater.

...**st count.** The number of particles
... dust in a given atmosphere, usually
...pressed as the number of particles
...ss than 10μ in diameter per cu. ft. of
...r when counted by the light field
...thod. Used chiefly in evaluation of
...lcosis hazards in industry.

...**V. M.** Doctor of Veterinary Medi-
...e.

...**V. M. S.** Doctor of Veterinary
...dicine and Surgery.

...**V. S.** 1. Doctor of Veterinary

Science. 2. Doctor of Veterinary Surgery.

dwarf. 1. A diminutive human being.
2. Prevent normal growth. 3. Become
small. 4. Of smaller than normal size.
—**dwarfism,** *n.* **achondroplastic d.** See *achondroplasia.* **asexual d.** One with deficient sexual development. **cretin d.** One due to thyroid deficiency; a cretin. **diabetic d.**
One with retarded growth due to diabetes. **micromelic d.** One with very
small limbs. **normal d.** One abnormal only in size. Also called *hypoplastic d.* **ovarian d.** One due to
absence of the ovaries. The person is
not a true dwarf but is undersized and
seldom over 54 inches in height; the external genitalia are undeveloped; premature aging is said to be common.
pituitary d. One due to deficiency
of pituitary growth hormone. **rachitic d.** One due to severe rickets.
sexual d. One with normal sexual
development. **true d.** One with general underdevelopment, characterized
by delayed ossification of the epiphyses.
dwt. Abbreviation for pennyweight.
Dy. Chemical symbol for dysprosium.
dy'ad. 1. A pair or a couple. 2. One of
the groups of two chromosomes formed
by the division of a tetrad in miosis.
3. *In chemistry,* a divalent element or
radical.

dyclone. Trade-mark for dyclonine
hydrochloride.

dy·clo'nine hy"dro·chlo'ride.
4′ - Butoxy - 3 - piperidinopropiophenone
hydrochloride, a topical anesthetic.
See *dyclone.*

dy·nam'ic (dye·nam'ick, di·nam'ick).
Pertaining to energy; sthenic; characterized by energy or great force.

dy·nam'ics. The science which treats
of matter in motion. **vital d.** The
science of the inherent power of an organism.

dy'na·mo. A machine for converting
mechanical energy into electric energy
by means of coils of insulated wire revolving through magnetic fields of
force.

dy'na·mo-. A combining form denoting *power.*

dy"na·mo·gen'e·sis. The generation of power, force, or energy.

dy·nam'o·graph (dye·nam'o·graf,
di·nam'·). An instrument designed to
measure and record graphically muscular strength. —**dynamog'raphy,** *n.*

dy"na·mom'e·ter. An instrument
for the measurement of muscular
strength, particularly of the hand, such
as a spring balance.

dy·nam'o·neure (dye·nam'o·newr,
di·nam'·). A spinal motor neuron.

dys-. 1. A prefix meaning *hard* or *ill;*
used to signify *ill, bad, hard,* or *difficult.* 2. *In biology,* a prefix denoting

unlike. 3. *In medicine,* a prefix denoting *difficult* or *painful; faulty* or *impaired;* or *abnormal* or *morbid.*

dys·ad″ap·ta′tion. Inability of the iris and retina to accommodate themselves to variable intensities of light.

dys·an″ti·graph′i·a (·graf′ee·uh, ·gray′fee·uh). Inability to do copy writing or to print.

dys·a′phi·a, dys·aph′i·a. Disordered sense of touch.

dys″ar·te″ri·ot′o·ny. Abnormal blood pressure.

dys·ar·thri·a. Impairment of articulation; stammering. **—dysar′thric,** *adj.*

dys″ar·thro′sis. 1. Deformity, dislocation, or disease of a joint. 2. A false joint. 3. Dysarthria.

dys·ba′si·a (dis·bay′zhuh, ·shuh). Difficulty in walking.

dys·bu′li·a. Impairment of will power.

dys·chi′ri·a (dis·kigh′ree·uh). Inability to tell which side of the body has been touched.

dys·chi′zi·a (dis·kigh′zhuh, ·zee·uh), **dys·che′zi·a** (dis·kee·zhuh, ·zee·uh). Painful or difficult defecation.

dys·chon″dro·pla′si·a (dis·kon″dro·play′zhuh, ·shuh). A disease of unknown etiology, attacking the long bones and the metacarpal and phalangeal skeleton of the hand. It is characterized by cartilaginous tissue developing regularly but ossifying very slowly. Also called *skeletal enchondromatosis.*

dys′chro·a (dis′kro·uh, dis·kro′uh), **dys·chroi′a.** Discoloration of the skin; a bad complexion.

dys″chro·ma·top′si·a. Partial color blindness; difficulty in distinguishing colors. **—dyschro′matope,** *n.*

dys·chro′mi·a. Discoloration, especially of the skin.

dys′chro·nous. Not agreeing as to time. **—dyschrona′tion,** *n.*

dys″di·ad″o·cho·ki·ne′si·a, dys″di·ad″o·ko·ki·ne′si·a (dis″dye·ad″o·ko·ki·nee′shuh, ·kigh·nee′·). Impairment of the power to perform alternating movements in rapid succession, such as pronation and supination; a sign of cerebellar disease.

dys″e·coi′a. Deafness.

dys″e·me′si·a (dis″i·mee′zhuh, ·zee·uh), **dys·em′e·sis.** Painful vomiting; retching.

dys″en·do·crin·ism (dis″en·dock′rin·iz·um, dis·en′do·krin·iz·um). Any abnormality in the function of the endocrine glands. **—dysen′docrine,** *adj.*

dys″en·ter′y. An inflammation of the colon; characterized by pain, rectal tenesmus, intense diarrhea with the frequent passage of small amounts mucus and blood, and symptoms toxemia. **—dysenter′ic,** *adj.* **am**bic d. See amebic **colitis.** bacillary d. An infectious disease which primarily involves the colon, caused a species of the genus *Shigella.*

dys″er·ga′si·a (dis″ur·gay′zhu ·shuh). *In psychobiology,* a mental disturbance due to toxic factors which a capable of producing delirium, such uremia or alcohol.

dys″es·the′si·a, dys″aes·the si·a (dis″ess·thee′zhuh, ·zee·uh). Impairment of the senses, especially the sense of touch. 2. Painfulness any sensation not normally painful.

dys·func′tion. Any abnormality impairment of function, as of an orga

dys″ga·lac′ti·a (dis″ga·lack′tee·u ·shee·uh). Loss or impairment of m secretion.

dys·gen′ic. Detrimental to the b reditary constitution of the race; contrast to *eugenic.*

dys″ger·mi·no′ma. A firm, elasti usually well-encapsulated, solid tum of the ovary, not disposed to metast size. Occurs usually before 30 years age, and microscopically resembles t embryonal carcinoma (seminoma) the testis with lymphoid stroma.

dys·geu′si·a (dis·gew′see·uh, d jew′·). Morbidity or perversion of t sense of taste.

dys·glan′du·lar. Pertaining to a abnormality in the function of glane particularly the glands of intern secretion.

dys·gram′ma·tism. Inability make the proper use of words; a sym tom of certain cerebral diseases; pa ticularly diseases of the temporal lol

dys·graph′i·a (dis·graf′ee·uh, ·gra fee·uh). Impairment of the power writing as a result of a brain lesion.

dys″hi·dro′sis, dys″i·dro′sis. Any disturbance in sweat producti or excretion. 2. Pompholyx, *q.v.* **—d** hidros′iform, *adj.*

dys″ki·ne′si·a (dis″ki·nee′sh dis″kigh·nee′·). Impairment of power of voluntary motion.

dys·la′li·a, dys·lal′i·a. Impa ment of the power of speaking, due a defect of the organs of speech.

dys·lex′i·a. Impairment of the abil to read.

dys·lo′gi·a. Difficulty in the expr sion of ideas by speech.

dys″ma·se′sis, dys″ma·se′si (dis″ma·see′zee·uh). Difficulty of ma tication.

dys″men·or·rhe′a, dys″men·o rhoe′a. Difficult or painful menstru tion. **congestive d.** A form of pa ful menstruation due to an inter congestion of the pelvic viscera. Sy plethoric d., vascular d. d. inte

menstrualis. Pain between the menses. **functional d.** (a) That without anatomic or pathologic explanation. (b) That contributed to or caused by pelvic congestion from unsatisfied sexual stimulation. **inflammatory d.** That due to inflammation. **mechanical d.** That due to mechanical obstruction to the free escape of the menstrual fluid. Syn., *obstructive d.* **membranous d.** That characterized by discharge of casts or shreds of uterine mucosa. **ovarian d.** That form due to disease of the ovaries. **psychogenic d.** Menstrual pain of mental or psychic origin. **secondary d.** That type associated with organic pelvic disease. Syn., *acquired d.* **spasmodic d.** That due to sudden and severe uterine contraction. **tubal d.** That form associated with disease of the oviduct. **uterine d.** That type caused by uterine disease. **vaginal d.** The type associated with disease of the vagina.

dys·me·tri·a, dys·met·ri·a. Inability to control accurately the range of movement in muscular acts, as observed in cerebellar lesions.

dys·mim·i·a. Impairment of the power to use signs and gestures as a means of expression; inability to imitate; caused by a disturbance in the emotional innervation of the facial muscles.

dys·mne·si·a (dis-mnee′zhuh, dis-nee′-). An impaired or defective memory.

dys·mor′pho·pho·bi·a. Morbid fear of deformity.

dys·no′mi·a. Nominal aphasia.

dys″o·don·ti′a·sis (dis″o·don·ty′-uh·sis, -tee′uh·sis). Difficult or painful dentition.

dys·o′pi·a. Painful or defective vision.

dys″o·rex′i·a. A disordered or unnatural appetite.

dys·os′mi·a (dis-oz′mee-uh). Impairment of the sense of smell.

dys″os·to′sis. Defective formation of bone. **d. cleidocranialis.** A congenital complex consisting in incomplete ossification of the skull, malformation of the palatine arch, and more or less aplasia of the clavicles.

dys·par″a·thy′roid·ism. Any functional disorder of the parathyroid gland.

dys″pa·reu′ni·a (dis″puh·roo′nee-uh). Painful or difficult intercourse. **psychologic d.** That form of dyspareunia having an emotional basis with no anatomic or pathologic explanation.

dys·pep′si·a. Disturbed digestion. **acid d.** That attended with hyperacidity of the gastric juice. **an·acidic d.** That accompanied by lack of the normal acidity of the gastric

juice. **bilious d.** Intestinal dyspepsia due to impaired secretion of bile. **flatulent d.** That marked by almost constant eructation of gas. Also called *gaseous d.* **gastric d.** That confined to the stomach. **gastrointestinal d.** That in which both the stomach and the intestine are concerned. **inflammatory d.** That due to some form of gastritis. **intestinal d.** That due to imperfect digestive action of the intestinal juices or a lack of tone in the muscular coat of the bowel. **muscular d.** That due to atony of the muscular coat of the stomach or intestine. **nervous d.** That characterized by gastric pains, precipitated by emotional states.

dys·pep′tic. 1. Relating to or affected with dyspepsia. 2. A person suffering from dyspepsia.

dys″per·i·stal′sis. Violent or abnormal peristalsis.

dys·pha′gi·a. Difficulty in swallowing, or inability to swallow. **d. constricta.** That due to stenosis of the pharynx or esophagus. **d. lusoria.** That caused by compression of the esophagus and trachea between the aorta and ductus arteriosus in the case of right-sided aortic arch, or between the two sides of the arch when it is double, or due to pressure on the esophagus by an anomalous right subclavian artery. **d. spastica.** That due to hysterical spasm of the esophagus or pharynx.

dys·pha′si·a (dis-fay′zhuh, -zee-uh). Difficulty in speaking or in understanding language; caused by a central lesion.

dys·phe′mi·a. Stammering.

dys·pho′ni·a. An impairment of the voice.

dys·pho′ri·a. Impatience and restlessness; mental anxiety; fidgets. —**dys·phor′ic,** adj.

dys·pho′ti·a. Nearsightedness.

dys·phra′si·a (dis-fray′zhuh, -zee-uh). Imperfect speech due to impairment of mental power.

dys″pi·tu′i·ta·rism. A condition due to abnormal functioning of the pituitary body.

dys·pla′si·a (dis-play′zhuh, -shuh. Abnormal development or growth. **hereditary ectodermal d.** A hereditary disease involving the ectodermal structures, skin, sweat glands, teeth, etc., where development is markedly retarded. **macular d.** An irregularly circular or oval defect of the macula, occurring in young children and causing a reduction in visual acuity. **neuroectodermal d.** A congenital derangement of cerebral tissues associated with skin tumors, as neurofibromatosis.

dysp·ne′a. Difficult or labored breathing. **—dyspneal, dyspneic,** *adj.* **cardiac d.** That due to cardiac failure. **renal d.** That due to acidosis in uremia.

dys·pra'gi·a. Dyspraxia, *q.v.*

dys·prax'i·a. Disordered or painful functioning of a part.

dys·pro'si·um (dis·pro'shee·um, ·see·um). Dy = 162.46. A rare earth metal.

dys·rhyth'mi·a (dis·rith'mee·uh, dis·rith'·). Disordered rhythm. **cere·bral d.** Any abnormal rhythm in brain waves, as revealed by the electroencephalogram. The waves may be too fast, too slow, or may alternate between the two types. Dysrhythmia is frequently associated with an epileptiform condition.

dys·sper'ma·tism, dys·sper'·mi·a. 1. Difficulty of depositing the sperm within the vagina. 2. Occurrence of pain or discomfort in discharge of seminal fluid.

dys·sta'si·a (dis·stay'see·uh, ·zee·uh). Difficulty in standing. **—dys·stat'ic,** *adj.*

dys·tax'i·a. Ataxia or partial ataxia. **d. agitans.** Tremor due to irritation of the spinal cord. Also called *pseudoparalysis agitans.*

dys"tha·na'si·a (dis"thuh·nay'zhuh, ·zee·uh). A slow and painful death.

dys·the'si·a (dis·thee'zhuh, ·zee·uh). Impatience; fretfulness; ill temper in the sick. **—dysthet'ic,** *adj.*

dys·thy'mi·a (dis·thigh'mee·uh, ·thim'ee·uh). 1. Melancholy or mental perversion. 2. A state due to malfunction of the thymus during childhood.

dys·tith'i·a. Difficulty of nursing or inability to nurse at the breast

dys·to'ci·a. Difficult labor. **—dys·tocic,** *adj.* **fetal d.** Difficult labor due to abnormalities of position or size and shape of the fetus. **mater·nal d.** Difficult labor due to deformities within the mother.

dys·to'ni·a. Disorder or lack of tonicity. **—dyston'ic,** *adj.*

dys·to'pi·a. Displacement of any organ. **—dystop'ic,** *adj.*

dys·tre'phi·a. Dystrophy. **d. myo·tonica.** Muscular dystrophy.

dys'tro·phy. 1. Defective nutrition. 2. Defective or abnormal development; degeneration. **—dystroph'ic,** *adj.* **adiposogenital d.** A syndrome characterized by adiposity, retarded development of gonads, and, occasionally, diabetes insipidus, due to impaired function of the pituitary gland and hypothalamus. **muscular d.** A progressive, familial disorder marked by atrophy of the muscles and by stiffness, observed when initiating voluntary action after rest. Syn. *dystrophia myotonica.* **progressive muscu·lar d.** A primary wasting disease of muscles characterized by progressive muscular weakness; apparently due to peripheral rather than central nervous degeneration. **pseudohyper·trophic muscular d.** A progressive, familial disorder beginning in childhood; characterized by early hypertrophy and later atrophy of the muscles with lordosis, weakness, inability to rise from the ground, a waddling gait, and progressive helplessness.

dys·u'ri·a. Difficult or painful urination.

E

E. 1. Abbreviation for eye, emmetropia, electromotive force. 2. An einstein, 6.06×10^{23} quanta.

e. Symbol for an electron, as $H = H^+ + e$.

e-. A prefix denoting *without, out, out of, from.*

Eagle, Harry [*American pathologist, 1905– *]. Known for his flocculation test for syphilis, employing inactivated serum with antigen made of lecithin from beef heart, fortified with cholesterol and corn germ sterol, and for a complement-fixation test for syphilis. See Eagle *test.*

Eales, Henry [*English physician, 1852–1913*]. Known for his description of a condition characterized by repeated retinal and vitreous hemorrhages, called *Eales's disease.*

ear. The organ of hearing, consisting of the external ear, the middle ear, and the internal ear or labyrinth. The **external ear** is made up of an expanded portion, the pinna, and the external auditory canal. The **middle ear** consists of the tympanic cavity, with the auditory ossicles, the auditory tube, and the mastoid cells. The **in·ternal ear** consists of the osseous and membranous labyrinths, which are separated from each other by a space containing the perilymph. The osseous labyrinth consists of three parts: the vestibule, the semicircular canals, and the cochlea. **congenital deform·**

ity of e. See Darwin's *tubercle.*
flat e. A large, prominent ear, characterized by effacement of the ridges and grooves.

ear′drum″. The tympanic membrane.

ear′plug″. A device, usually made of rubber, plastic, or cotton kneaded with glycerin or petrolatum; to protect the ear, as from loud noises.

earth. The soil. **diatomaceous e.** Purified siliceous earth. **fuller's e.** A clay related to kaolin, and used similarly as an adsorbent and protective. **infusorial e.** Purified siliceous earth. **purified siliceous e.** A form of silica (SiO_2) consisting of the whole or broken shells of diatoms.

ear′wax″. Cerumen.

E″ber·thel′la (ee″bur-thel′uh, ·tell′uh). Formerly considered to be a genus of the tribe Salmonelleae, family Enterobacteriaceae. Organisms of this genus are now classified as belonging to the genus *Salmonella, q.v.* **E. typhosa.** See *Salmonella typhosa.*

Ebner, Victor von [*Austrian histologist, 1842–1925*]. Remembered for his description of the serous glands opening into the trenches of the vallate papillae of the tongue, called *serous lingual glands, Ebner's glands.*

e′bur. A tissue similar to ivory in appearance or structure. **e. dentis.** Dentin, *q.v.*

e″bur·na′tion. An increase in the density of tooth or bone following some pathologic change. **—eburnated,** *adj.*

ec-. A prefix meaning *out of.*

Ec·bal′li·um. A genus of the Cucurbitaceae. See *elaterium.*

ec·bol′ic. 1. Producing abortion or accelerating labor. 2. Any agent which initiates or accelerates parturition.

ec′bol·ine (eck′bo-leen, ·lin). An alkaloid of ergot.

ec·cen′tric. Situated away from the center or median line.

ec·cen′tro-os″te·o·chon″dro·dys·pla′si·a (eck-sen′tro-os″tee-o·kon″dro·dis·play′zhuh, ·shuh). A type of imperfect ossification due to eccentric centers of ossification in which the bones of the extremities fail to develop normally and become rarefied and deformed. Also called *Morquio's disease.*

ec·ceph″a·lo′sis (eck·sef″uh·lo′sis). Removal of the brain of the fetus to facilitate delivery. Syn., *cephalotomy, excerebration.*

ec″chon·dro′ma (eck″on·dro′muh). A nodular outgrowth from cartilage at the junction of cartilage and bone; usually a hyperplasia (ecchondrosis) but may be neoplastic.

ec″chon·dro′sis (eck″on·dro′sis). A benign cartilaginous outgrowth.

ec″chy·mo′sis (eck″i·mo′sis). An

extravasation of blood into the subcutaneous tissues. It is marked by a purple discoloration of the skin, the color gradually changing to brown, green, and yellow. **—ecchymot′ic,** *adj.*

ec″cy·e′sis (eck″sigh·ee′sis). Extrauterine gestation.

ec·dem′ic. Applied to diseases brought into a region from without; not endemic or epidemic.

ec′dy·sis. Sloughing or casting off of the outer epidermis; desquamation.

ECG, EKG. Electrocardiogram.

ec′go·nine (eck′go·neen, ·nin). An alkaloid, $C_9H_{15}NO_3.H_2O$, produced by acid hydrolysis of cocaine.

e·chid′nin (eh·kid′nin). 1. Snake poison; the poison or venom of the viper and other similar snakes. 2. A nitrogenous and venomous principle found in the poisonous secretion of various snakes.

Ech″id·noph′a·ga (eck″id·nof′uh·guh). A genus of fleas. **E. gallinacea.** The species known as the sticktight or tropical hen flea, which attacks poultry in many parts of the world; may also become a human pest.

e·chid′no·tox′in (eh·kid″no·tock′sin). A principle of snake venom which produces a general reaction in the human body and has a powerful effect on the nervous system.

ech″i·na′ce·a (eck″i·nay′shuh, ·see·uh). Cone flower. The dried rhizome and roots of *Echinacea pallida* and *E. angustifolia;* formerly used to treat ulcers, septicemia, etc.

e·chin′e·none (eh·kin′i·nohn, eh·kigh′ni·). A precursor of vitamin A found in sea urchins.

e·chi′no- (eh·kigh′no-, eck′i·no-), **echin-.** A combining form usually denoting *spiny, bearing spines,* or *relation* or *resemblance to the sea urchins.*

e·chi″no·coc·ci′a·sis (·cock·sigh″uh·sis). Infestation with cysticercus of the dog tapeworm.

e·chi″no·coc·co′sis. Infestation of man with the *Echinococcus granulosus* in its larval or hydatid stage. Most important site of infestation is the liver, and secondly, the lungs.

E·chi″no·coc′cus. A genus of tapeworms. **E. granulosus.** That species whose ova, when ingested by man or other intermediate hosts, develop into echinococcus cysts.

E·chi″no·rhyn′chus (·ring′kus, ·rin′kus). Formerly a genus of acanthocephalan worms. **E. moniliformis.** Synonym for *Moniliformis moniliformis.*

ech″i·no′sis (eck″i·no′sis). Crenation, *q.v.*

E·chi″no·sto′ma (eh·kigh″no·sto′muh, eck″i·no·). A genus of flukes parasitic in man, but of little pathologic importance.

ech'o. A reverberated sound. **am-phoric e.** A vocal resonance in which the voice, when transmitted, sounds as if it were spoken into a narrow-necked bottle.

ech"o·a·cou'si·a (eck"o·a·kōō'zhuh, ·zee-uh). The subjective sensation of hearing echoes following sounds heard normally.

ech"o·graph'i·a (·graf'ee-uh, ·gray'-fee-uh). A form of aphasia in which questions submitted to the patient are copied without ability to comprehend the inquiry; also, in writing, the last word or letter is repeated.

ech"o·la'li·a. The meaningless repetition of words spoken by others; commonly seen in the catatonic form of schizophrenia. Syn., *echophrasia.* —**ech·olal'ic,** *adj.*

ech·op'a·thy (eck-op'uth-ee). *In psychiatry,* a morbid condition marked by the automatic and purposeless repetition of a word or sound heard or of an act seen. Also see *echolalia, echopraxia.*

ech·oph'o·ny. An echo of a vocal sound heard in auscultation of the chest.

ech"o·prax'i·a. Automatic imitation by the patient of the examiner's movements or mannerisms; seen in the catatonic form of schizophrenia. Syn., *echokinesis, echomatism, echomimia, echomotism.*

ECHO vi'rus (ek'oh). Short for enteric cytopathogenic *human* orphan virus, a heterogenous group of enteric viruses thought to be the causative agents of many varied disorders and diseases, such as acute gastroenteritis, benign aseptic meningitis, and acute febrile diarrhea in children.

ech'u·gin (eck'yoo-jin). A glycoside from *Adenium boehmianum,* Apocynaceae. It is probably related to the digitalislike group of glycosides.

Eck, Nikolai Vladimirovich [*Russian physiologist,* b. 1847]. Reported experimental study of diseases of the liver and liver metabolism by means of an artificial communication made between the portal vein and inferior vena cava. Called *Eck's fistula.*

ec·la'bi·um. Eversion of the lip.

ec·lamp'si·a. A convulsive or epileptiform seizure, usually of peripheral origin. —**eclamptic,** *adj.* **e. nu-tans.** A condition characterized by paroxysms, in which the head and upper part of the body are bowed forward several times in succession; the attacks are accompanied by disordered consciousness. Syn., *nodding spasm, salaam convulsion.* **puerperal e.** A convulsion occurring toward the end of pregnancy, or during or after labor, associated with uremia or other toxic

states; the end state of preeclampsia. **uremic e.** Convulsive seizures associated with suppression of urine.

ec·lamp'sism. The preeclamptic toxemia of pregnancy which may lead to convulsions and coma; includes the preconvulsive prodromata, from true toxemia, nephritis, and vascular disease.

ecolid chloride. Trade-mark for chlorisondamine chloride.

e·col'o·gy. The study of the environmental relations of organisms.

e"co·ma'ni·a, eo"i·o·ma'ni·a (eck"ee·o·may'nee-uh). A psychosis marked by a domineering and haughty attitude toward members in the family, but an attitude of humility toward those in authority; domestic perversity.

ECS. Electroconvulsive shock. See electroshock *therapy.*

ec'sta·sy. A trancelike state with mental exaltation. —**ecstat'ic,** *adj.*

ECT. Electroconvulsive therapy. See electroshock *therapy.*

ec'tad. Outward.

ec'tal. External; superficial.

ec·ta'si·a (eck·tay'zhuh, ·zee-uh), **ec'ta·sis.** Dilatation of a tubular vessel. —**ectat'ic,** *adj.* **hypostatic e.** Dilatation of a blood vessel, due to gravitational settling of the blood. **papillary e.** Circumscribed dilatation of the capillaries, resulting in an elevated red spot on the skin. **se-nile e.** Varices or dilated tufts of capillaries in the skin. Usually seen in older people as red or purplish areas on the trunk.

ec·thy'ma. An inflammatory skin disease attended with an eruption of large, flat pustules that ulcerate and become crusted. They vary in size from a half to two centimeters in diameter, and are surrounded by a distinct inflammatory areola. The lesions as a rule appear on the legs and thighs, and occur in crops which persist for an indefinite period.

ec'to-, ect-. A combining form signifying *without, upon the outer side.*

ec"to·car'di·a. An abnormal position of the heart. It may be outside the thoracic cavity (ectopia cordis) or misplaced within the thorax.

ec"to·cho·roi'de·a (eck"to·ko·roy'-dee-uh). The outer layer of the choroid.

ec'to·derm. The outermost of the three primary germ layers of the embryo from which the epidermis and neural tube develop. —**ectoder'mal,** *adj.* **amniotic e.** The internal epithelium of the amnion continuous with the epidermis of the embryo at the umbilicus. **basal e.** That part of the trophoblast covering the eroded uterine surface of the placental sinuses, continuous with the tips of the chorionic villi; it partly disappears in late pregnancy. **neural e.** That part of the ectoderm destined to form the neural tube and neural crest. Syn., *neuroblast.* **primitive e.** The undifferentiated external layer of a gastrula or of the bilaminar blastodisk. Syn., *ectoblast.* Also called *primary e.*

ec″to·der·mo′sis e″ro·siv′a plu″ri·or″i·fi·ci·a′lis. A form of erythema multiforme, usually limited to the extremities but may be accompanied by inflammation of the orifices of the body.

ec″to·en′zyme. An extracellular enzyme; one excreted into the surrounding medium or tissue.

ec·tog′e·nous (eck·todj′i·nus). Capable of growth outside of the body of its host; applied to bacteria and other parasites.

ec′to·mere. A blastomere destined to take part in forming the ectoderm.

ec″to·mes′o·derm. Mesoderm derived from the primary ectoderm of a bilaminar blastodisk or gastrula, in contrast to *endomesoderm.*

ec″to·mor″phy. A component of physique denoting linearity, fragility, and delicacy of structure in association with the presence quantitatively of ectodermally derived tissues. The third component of the somatotype.

-ec′to·my. A combining form denoting *surgical removal.*

ec″to·par′a·site. A parasite that lives on the exterior of its host. **—ec″to·par·a·sit′ic,** *adj.*

ec″to·phyte. An external parasitic plant growth; a vegetable parasite on the skin. **—ec·to·phyt′ic,** *adj.*

ec·to′pi·a. An abnormality of position of an organ or a part of the body; usually congenital. **—ec·top′ic,** *adj.* **e. testis.** A rare, congenital anomaly in which the testis descends into an abnormal location, generally in the perineum or near the pubic bone. **vis·ceral e.** A congenital hernia into the umbilical cord.

ec″to·pla·cen′ta. The growing, functional part of the trophoblast that develops into the placenta, especially in rodents. Syn., *trophoderm.* **—ecto·placental,** *adj.*

ec′to·plasm. The outer, denser layer of cytoplasm of a cell or unicellular organism. **—ectoplas′mic,** *adj.*

ec″to·pot′o·my. Laparotomy for the removal of the contents of an extra-uterine gestation sac.

ec′to·thrix. A type division of the genus *Trichophyton, q.v.*

Ec″to·trich″o·phy′ton (eck″to·trick″o·fy′ton). A name sometimes given to the ectothrix type of the genus of fungi, *Trichophyton, q.v.*

ec″to·xo′on. An external animal parasite; ectoparasite.

ec″tro-. A combining form denoting *congenital absence.*

ec″tro·dac·tyl′i·a, ec″tro·dac′·tyl·ism, ec″tro·dac′ty·ly. Congenital absence of any of the fingers or toes or parts of them.

ec·trog′e·ny (eck·trodj′i·nee). Loss or congenital absence of any part or organ. **—ectrogen′ic,** *adj.*

ec·tro′pi·on. Eversion of a part, especially of an eyelid. **—ectropioni·za′tion,** *n.;* **ectropionize,** *v.*

ec″tro·syn·dac′ty·ly. A developmental defect in which some of the digits are missing while others are fused.

ec·trot′ic. Tending to cut short; preventing the development of disease; abortive; abortifacient.

ec″tyl·u·re′a. 2-Ethyl-*cis*-crotonylurea, a central nervous system depressant. See *nostyn.*

ec′ze·ma (eck′si·muh, eck′zi·muh). Tetter; salt rheum. An acute or chronic, noncontagious, itching, inflammatory disease of the skin; usually characterized by irregular and varying combinations of edematous, vesicular, papular, pustular, scaling, thickened, or exudative lesions. The skin is reddened, the redness shading off into the surrounding unaffected parts. The cause is unknown. Eruptions of similar appearance due to such known causes as ingested drugs or local irritants are properly referred to as *dermatitis medicamentosa, contact dermatitis,* or *dermatitis venenata,* etc. **—eczem′atous, eczem′atoid,** *adj.* **e. erythematosum.** The mildest form of eczema in which the skin is reddened and slightly swollen. **e. hypertrophicum.** A form characterized by permanent hypertrophy of the papillae of the skin, giving rise to general or limited warty outgrowths. **e. nummularis.** A patchy variety, localized chiefly on the surfaces of the upper limbs and the trunk. The patches are small, poorly defined, erythematous, vesicular, and often exudative. **e. papulosum.** A variety showing minute papules of deep-red color and firm consistency; accompanied by intense itching. **e. vesiculosum.** An eczema characterized by the presence of vesicles. **hyperkeratotic e.** That type in which the stratum corneum is thickened. **lichenoid e.** That marked by acuminate papules on reddened and infiltrated bases, and accompanied by intense itching. **weeping e.** Moist eczema; one marked by fluid exudation on the surface.

ec·zem″a·ti·za′tion (eg·zem″uh·ti·zay′shun, eck″si·mat·i·zay′shun). A condition of the skin marked by persistent eczemalike lesions, due to continued injury from physical or chemical irritation.

ed·a·tham'il cal'ci·um-di·so'-di·um. Calcium disodium ethylenediaminetetraacetate, used in treatment of lead poisoning. See *versenate*.

e·de'ma. Dropsy; excessive accumulation of fluid in the tissue spaces; due to disturbance in the mechanisms of fluid exchange. There may be decrease of osmotic pressure of the plasma from reduction in protein concentration, increased hydrostatic pressure in the capillaries due to cardiac failure, increased permeability of the capillary walls from injury or inflammation, or there may be obstruction of the lymph channels. —**edem'atous,** *adj.* **angioneurotic e.** That marked by acute, transitory, localized swellings, usually about the face; the lesions resemble those of urticaria, but are larger and of less distribution. Some cases are hereditary, others appear to be due to food allergy. Syn., *giant urticaria, giant e.* Also called *Quincke's disease.* **cardiac e.** That occurring in cardiac failure, due to increased venous pressure; most marked in dependent parts where hydrostatic pressure is the greatest. **cerebral e.** Edema of the brain; due to toxic causes or nutritional or vitamin deficiencies. It is usually associated with delirium, convulsions, or coma. **nephrotic e.** A type found in patients with chronic lipoid nephrosis or the nephrotic stage of glomerulonephritis, resulting from the loss of protein through proteinuria. **nutritional e.** That occurring in starvation or in a poorly nourished state; due to an abnormally low plasma protein concentration of the blood. **pitting e.** Edema of sufficient degree that the surface can be indented by pressure. Such indentation is temporary, lasting only several minutes after pressure is released. **pulmonary e.** An effusion of fluid into the air vesicles and interstitial tissue of the lungs.

e·den'tate. 1. Without teeth. 2. Referring to the order of mammals Edentata.

e·den'tu·lous. Without teeth.

e·de'o-, e'de-. A combining form meaning *relating to the external genitals.* Most words from this stem are now obsolete.

e·des'tin, e'des·tin. A globulin type of simple protein; obtained from the seeds of hemp.

ed'i·ble. Fit to eat.

ed'i·pism. Self-inflicted injury to the eyes. *Rare.*

ed"ro·pho'ni·um chlo'ride. Dimethylethyl(3-hydroxyphenyl)ammonium chloride, an antagonist to curariform drugs. See *tensilon chloride.*

EDTAA. Abbreviation for ethylenediaminetetraacetic acid.

EEG. Electroencephalography, electroencephalogram, electroencephalograph.

ef·fec'tor. A motor or secretory nerve ending in an organ, gland, or muscle, which is consequently called an effector organ; opposed to *receptor.*

ef'fer·ent. Carrying away, as efferent nerves, conveying impulses away from the central nervous system; or as efferent lymphatics, conveying lymph from the lymph nodes. Opposed to *afferent.*

ef"fer·ves'cence. 1. The escape of a gas from a liquid; a bubbling. 2. In infectious diseases, that period following the prodrome; the onset or invasion of the disease.

ef"fer·ves'cent. Capable of producing effervescence.

ef"fleu·rage' (ef"loo-rahzh'). The stroking movement used in massage. It may be superficial, for producing reflex action, or deep, for actual emptying of the veins and lymphatic vessels.

ef"flo·res'cence. 1. The spontaneous conversion of a crystalline substance into powder by a loss of its water of crystallization. 2. The eruption of an exanthematous disease.

ef'flu·ent. 1. An outflow. 2. A fluid discharged from a basin or chamber for the treatment of sewage.

ef·flu'vi·um (pl. *effluvia*). That which emanates from an animal, especially an unwholesome or foul-smelling exhalation.

ef·fuse' (ef-yōōss', ef-yōōz'). Said of a type of growth produced by bacteria on solid mediums. The growth does not project above the surface, in contrast with the raised type of growth.

ef·fu'sion. 1. A pouring-out of fluid, either serous, purulent, or bloody, into serous or other spaces. 2. The effused fluid.

Egas Moniz, Antonio Caetano de Abreu Freire [Portuguese neurologist, 1874–   ]. Described frontal or prefrontal lobotomy in the treatment of certain mental disorders. Nobel laureate, 1949.

e·ges'ta (i-jes'tuh). The discharges of the intestines or other excretory organs.

egg. Ovum, *q.v.*

egg'-white in'ju·ry. A syndrome developed in experimental rats fed on raw white of egg; characterized by dermatitis, and emaciation resulting in death; caused by the presence of avidin in the white of egg which renders unavailable the biotin of the diet.

e'go. 1. *In psychology,* the self, regarded as a succession of mental states, or as the consciousness of the existence of the self as distinct from other selves. 2. *In psychoanalytic theory,* that part of the personality in conscious contact with reality.

e·go·cen'tric. Self-centered. **—egocentric'ity, egocentrism,** n.

e"go·ma'ni·a. Abnormal self-esteem.

e·goph'o·ny. A modification of bronchophony, in which the voice has a bleating character, like that of a goat. It is heard over a compressed lung, as above the level of fluid in hydrothorax.

Ehrlich, Paul [German bacteriologist and pathologist, 1854–1915]. A pioneer in the fields of bacteriology, immunology, and chemotherapy. Developed the differential blood-count technic. Introduced methylene blue as a tissue stain (1881), and developed various staining technics. See Ehrlich's acid hematoxylin, under stain. Advanced his side-chain theory of immunity (1885); see under theory. Was the first to recognize aplastic anemia. His research on chemotherapy for experimental trypanosomiasis (1907) led to his discovery, with Hata, of arsphenamine, also called salvarsan, Ehrlich's 606, for the treatment of syphilis and yaws (1909); this marked the beginning of a new era in the treatment of bacterial diseases. Shared Nobel prize in physiology and medicine with Metchnikoff (1908).

i'do·gen (eye'do·jen). A chemical substance having the power of modifying the form of an embryonic organ after induction has occurred; a second-grade inductor involved in regional differentiation about the neural axis.

Eijkman, Christiaan [Dutch pathologist, 1858–1930]. Produced beriberi in fowls (1893), discovering that a diet of overmilled rice causes the disease. The first experimental demonstration of the dietetic origin of a deficiency disease. Discovered vitamin B_1. Nobel laureate (1929).

Ei·me'ri·a (eye·meer'ee·uh). A genus of protozoans living in the body fluids or tissues of vertebrates and invertebrates, and having a life cycle characterized by alternation of generations. Only one species, **E. gubleri,** is perhaps a parasite of man.

Einstein, Albert [American theoretical physicist, 1879–1955]. Famous for his theory of relativity, his formula for Brownian movement, and for his contributions to the quantum theory. Did much to prepare the theoretical ground for the development of atomic research. Nobel laureate (1921).

ein'stein. A unit of energy (6.06×10^{23} quanta) analogous to the faraday (6.06×10^{23} electrons); the amount of radiation absorbed by a system to activate one gram molecule of matter. Abbreviated, E.

e·jac"u·la'tion. The ejection of the semen.

e·jec'ta. Materials cast out; excretions or excrementitious matter; dejecta.

e·jec'tion. 1. The act of casting out, as of excretions or of excrementitious matter. 2. That which is cast out. **systolic e.** The discharge of blood by the ventricles into the pulmonary artery and aorta after a previous short phase of isometric contraction.

e·jec'tor. One that casts out, expels, or draws off. **saliva e.** A suction tube for removing saliva from the mouth during dental operations.

e'ka. In chemistry, a combining form meaning first, used as a prefix to a recognized chemical element to designate provisionally a predicted but as yet undiscovered element which should adjoin the former in the same group of the periodic system.

e"ka-i'o·dine (ee"kuh-eye'o·deen, ay"kuh-). The provisional name of the element of atomic no. 85, adjoining iodine in the halogen group of the periodic table. Now called astatine.

EKG. Abbreviation for electrocardiogram, from the German elektrokardiogram.

e·lab"o·ra'tion. In physiology, any anabolic process, such as the making of crude food into higher tissue products, or the formation of secretory products in gland cells.

el'a·cin. The product of degeneration of elastin.

e·la'i·din. A white, crystalline, fatty substance, produced by the action of nitric acid upon olein and isomeric with the latter.

E·lap'i·dae. A family of venomous snakes possessing short, erect, immovable front fangs; includes cobras, tiger snakes, death adders, kraits, etc. **—elapine,** adj.

e·las'tic. Capable of returning to the original form after being stretched or compressed.

e·las'ti·ca. 1. Elastic. 2. The tunica elastica of a blood vessel. **lamina e.** The elastic layer of the mucous membrane of the pharynx and respiratory tract.

e·las'tin. The albuminoid base of elastic tissue.

e·las'ti·nase (i·lass'ti·nace, ·naze). An enzyme that digests or hydrolyzes the protein elastin.

e·las'to·mer. A generic term for all substances having the properties of natural or synthetic rubber. **—elastomer'ic,** adj.

e·las·to'sis se·ni'lis. Degeneration of the elastic fibers of the skin and subcutaneous tissue in old age.

e·lat'er·in. Neutral principle from juice of the fruit of Ecballium elaterium; a hydragogue cathartic.

el"a·te'ri·um. The dried sediment from the juice of the squirting cucumber, Ecballium elaterium. It is a powerful hydragogue cathartic.

el'bow. The junction of the arm and forearm; the bend of the arm. **ten·nis e.** Inflammation of the olecranon bursa, or of a bursa over the head of the radius.

el'der. Sambucus, q.v.

el'drin. See *rutin*.

el"e·cam·pane', el"e·cam'pane. Inula, q.v.

e·lec'tric al"ter·na'tion. Alternation in amplitude of the QRS waves of the electrocardiogram; a sign of cardiac fatigue. Of grave importance if the heart rate is slow.

e·lec"tric'i·ty. One of the basic quantities in nature, consisting of the fundamental particles, electron and proton, q.v. Electricity in rest and in motion can be produced by friction, by magnetism, and by chemical methods. **—elec'tric, elec'trical,** adj. **fa·radic e.** That produced by induction. **galvanic e.** Primary direct current generated by chemical action in a battery.

e·lec"tro-. A combining form denoting *connection with electricity.*

e·lec"tro·cap"il·lar'i·ty. The effect of an electric current upon the interface between two liquids in a capillary; due to changes in the surface tension.

e·lec"tro·car'di·o·gram'. A graphic record, made by an electrocardiograph, of the electric potential differences due to cardiac action, taken from the body surfaces. A typical normal record shows P, Q, R, S, T, and U waves: the P wave is due to excitation of the atria; Q, R, and S, to excitation of the ventricles; T, to repolarization of ventricles; U is a diastolic wave of unknown origin. Electrocardiograms furnish important aid in the diagnosis and management of patients with heart disease. Abbreviated, ECG, EKG. Also see *lead, wave.*

e·lec"tro·car'di·o·graph'. An instrument for making a permanent record of small voltages, due to the beating heart, that exist between different parts of the body.

e·lec"tro·car"di·og'ra·phy. The specialty of recording and interpreting electrocardiograms. See also axis *deviation, interval, preponderance,* ventricular *hypertrophy,* ventricular *strain.*

e·lec"tro·ca·tal'y·sis. Catalysis or chemical changes produced by the action of electricity.

e·lec"tro·cau'ter·y. Galvanocautery. See under *cautery.*

e·lec"tro·chem'is·try. The science treating of the chemical changes produced by electricity.

e·lec"tro·co·ag"u·la'tion. The destruction or hardening of tissues by coagulation induced by the passage of high-frequency currents; surgical diathermy.

e·lec"tro·con·vul'sive shock. Electroshock therapy. Abbreviated ECS.

e·lec"tro·con·vul'sive ther'·a·py. Electroshock therapy. Abbreviated, ECT.

e·lec"tro·cor'ti·co·gram'. A recording of the electric activity of the brain by means of electrodes placed directly on the cerebral cortex.

e·lec"tro·cu'tion. Causation of death by electricity.

e·lec"tro·cys'to·scope. A cystoscope combined with an electric light. **—electrocystos'copy,** n.

e·lec'trode. 1. A surface of contact between a metallic and a nonmetallic conductor. 2. One of the terminals of metal, salts, or electrolytes through which electricity is applied to, or taken from, the body or an electric device or instrument. **active e.** A small one used for its exciting effect in a sharply localized area for stimulating muscles or nerves. **antimony e.** One made of antimony for determining hydrogen-ion concentration. **brush e.** One consisting of a wire brush, used to apply faradic current over a large area of skin. **calomel e.** One used as a standard, as in determining hydrogen-ion concentration. **dispersing e.** A large electrode used in treatment or testing which has little or no localizing effect. **glass e.** An electrode used in determining hydrogen-ion concentration. **hydrogen e.** An electrode used in determining hydrogen-ion concentration. **indifferent e.** Dispersing electrode. **positive e.** The anode.

e·lec"tro·des"ic·ca'tion. The diathermic destruction of small growths of the bladder, skin, cervix, etc., by means of a single terminal electrode with a small sparking distance.

e·lec"tro·di·al'y·sis (i·leck"tro·dye·al'i·sis). A method for rapidly removing electrolytes from colloids by dialysis of the colloidal sol while an electric current is being passed through it.

e·lec"tro·di'a·phane. An apparatus for illumination of body cavities; a diaphanoscope. **—electrodiaph'·any,** n.

e·lec"tro·en·ceph'a·lo·gram'. A graphic record of the minute changes in electric potential associated with the activity of the cerebral cortex, as detected by electrodes applied to the surface of the scalp. Also see under *rhythm, wave.* Abbreviated, EEG.

e·lec"tro·en·ceph'a·lo·graph'. An instrument for recording the electric activity of the brain. Abbreviated, EEG. **—electroencephalograph'·ic,** adj.

e·lec″tro·en·ceph″a·log′ra·phy. A method of recording graphically the electric activity of the brain, particularly the cerebral cortex, by means of electrodes attached to the scalp. Electroencephalography is used in the diagnosis of epilepsy, trauma, tumors, and degenerations of the brain. Abbreviated, EEG.

e·lec″tro·gas′tro·gram. A record of electrical potential patterns of the stomach; used in studies of gastric ulcer, gastric carcinoma, and atrophic gastritis.

e·lec″tro·he″mo·sta′sis. Arrest of hemorrhage by means of a high-frequency clamp, which causes desiccation of the tissue.

e·lec″tro·ky·mog′ra·phy. A method of continuously recording pulsations of the heart or large vessels by means of roentgen rays projected through a slit onto a fluoroscopic screen; the varying light intensity is recorded by a string galvanometer attached to a multiplier phototube.

e·lec″trol′y·sis. The decomposition of a chemical compound by a direct electric current. —**e·lec′trolyze,** v.

e·lec′tro·lyte. A substance which in solution is capable of conducting an electric current, and is decomposed by it. —**electrolyt′ic,** adj. **amphoteric e.** One that can act as either an acid or a base.

e·lec′tro·ly″zer. An instrument for removing urethral strictures by electricity.

e·lec″tro·mag′net. A core of soft iron surrounded by a coil of wire. A current passing through the wire will make the iron temporarily magnetic.

e·lec″tro·mas·sage′. The transmission of electricity through a kneading instrument; electric treatment combined with massage.

e·lec″tro·my′o·gram. 1. A record of the response of a muscle to an electric stimulation. 2. A record of eye movements during reading, obtained by measuring the potential difference between an electrode placed at the center of the forehead and one placed at the temple.

e·lec″tro·my·og′ra·phy (i·leck″tro·migh·og′ruh·fee). Production and study of the electromyogram. —**electromyograph′ic,** adj.

e·lec′tron. The smallest particle of negative electricity. The mass of an electron at rest is 9.035×10^{-28} grams, or $\frac{1}{1845}$ that of a hydrogen atom. Its unit electric charge is 4.77×10^{-10} electrostatic units. Symbol, e. —**electron′ic,** adj. **photoelectron.** An electron set into swift motion by the impact of a photon, and to which the primary photon transmits all of its energy. **recoil e.** An electron removed

from its place in an atom and set into motion by impact of a photon; as a result of the collision the photon gives up only part of its energy to the electron and proceeds along a new path. Also called *Compton electron*. **secondary e.** Any photoelectron or recoil electron produced when roentgen rays strike an atom.

e·lec″tro·neg′a·tive. Pertaining to or charged with negative electricity.

e·lec′tron volt. A unit of energy equal to the energy acquired by an electron when it falls through a potential difference of one volt.

e·lec″tro·os·mo′sis. The movement, produced by application of an electric potential, of the liquid component of a dispersion of colloidal particles when migration of the latter is prevented by a barrier. See also *electrophoresis.*

e·lec″tro·pho·re′sis. The migration of charged colloidal particles through the medium in which they are dispersed, when placed under the influence of an applied electric potential. Also called, though less preferably, *cataphoresis*. The process of ion transfer, *q.v.,* is sometimes erroneously called electrophoresis.

e·lec″tro·pos′i·tive. Pertaining to or charged with positive electricity.

e·lec″tro·py·rex′i·a (i·leck″tro·pye·reck′see·uh). The production of high body temperatures by means of an electric current.

e·lec″tro·scis′sion. (i·leck″tro·sizh′un). Cutting of tissues by an electrocautery knife.

e·lec″tro·scope. An instrument for detecting the presence of static electricity and its relative amount.

e·lec″tro·sec′tion. Tissue division by a knifelike electrode operated by a high-frequency machine.

e·lec″tro·shock′. Shock produced by electricity. See electroshock *therapy.*

e·lec″tro·ther″a·peu′tics (i·leck″tro·therr″uh·pew′ticks). Electrotherapy.

e·lec″tro·ther′a·py. The use of electricity for therapeutic purposes.

e·lec″trot′o·nus (i·leck″trot′o·nus, i·leck″tro·to′nus). The change of condition in a nerve or a muscle during the passage of a current of electricity. —**electroton′ic,** adj.

e·lec″tro·va′lence. The number of planetary electrons that an atom tends to lose or accept by transfer in chemical reaction.

el′e·ment. 1. Any one of the ultimate parts of which anything is composed, as the cellular elements of a tissue. 2. *In chemistry,* any one of the 102 ultimate chemical entities of which matter now is believed to be composed. Each element is composed wholly of atoms of the same atomic number (having the same charge on their nuclei), although their atomic weights may differ due to differences in nuclear weight. See *isotope*. For elements listed by name, see Table of Elements in the Appendix.

electronegative e. An element having a tendency to attract additional electrons.

el'e·mi (el'i-mee). A resinous exudation derived from *Canarium commune* and other plants of the Burseraceae. Its action is similar to that of the turpentines.

el"e·om'e·ter. An apparatus for ascertaining the specific gravity of oil.

el"e·op'tene. The permanent liquid portion of volatile oils, as distinguished from stearoptene. Syn., *oleoptene*.

el"e·phan·ti'a·sis. A chronic enlargement of the subcutaneous and cutaneous tissues as a result of lymphatic obstruction. In the form commonest in the tropics, the recurrent lymphangitis is caused by *Wuchereria bancrofti*. The legs and scrotum are most commonly affected. **—elephan'tiac, elephantias'ic,** *adj.* **e. con·genita cystica.** A state of malformation marked by skeletal defects, general anasarca, and formation of cysts in the subcutaneous tissue. **e. dura.** A variety of elephantiasis marked by density and sclerosis of the subcutaneous connective tissues. Also called *e. scirrhosa*. **e. filariensis.** That due to infection with *Wuchereria bancrofti*.

el'e·va"tor. An instrument for elevating or lifting a part, or for extracting the roots of teeth.

e·lim"i·na'tion. The process of expelling or casting out; especially, the expelling of the waste products of the body.

e·lin"gua'tion (e·lin"gway'shun, e·ling"·). Surgical removal of the tongue.

e·lix'ir. A sweetened, aromatic, spirituous preparation, containing soluble medicaments, usually in small amount. **aromatic e.** A tasteful vehicle prepared from compound orange spirit, syrup, and alcohol. It contains 22–24% of alcohol. **compound digestive e.** Compound pepsin elixir. **isoalcoholic e.** An elixir of the particular alcohol concentration which is most suitable for the intended medicament. It is prepared by combining in suitable proportions a high-alcoholic elixir and a low-alcoholic elixir. Also called *iso-elixir*. **red aromatic e.** Aromatic elixir colored with cudbear tincture. **simple e.** Aromatic elixir.

elkosin. Trade-mark for sulfisomidine.

el·lip'sin. The protein constituents of the cell responsible for maintaining its form and structure.

elm. See *Ulmus*.

e·lon"ga'tion. 1. The process of lengthening. 2. A lengthened condition, as of the cervix of the uterus through hypertrophy.

clorine chloride. A trade-mark for tricyclamol chloride.

el'u·ant. The solvent used in elution in chromatography. Also called *eluent*.

el'u·ate. The extract obtained from elution in chromatography; it consists of the eluant and the formerly adsorbed substance.

e·lu'tion. The process for the extraction of the adsorbed substance from the solid adsorbing medium in chromatography.

e·lu"tri·a'tion. A process whereby the coarser particles of an insoluble powder are separated from the finer by mixing the substance with a liquid and decanting the upper layer after the heavier particles have settled.

el'y·tro-, elytr-. A combining form meaning *connection with*, or *relation to, the vagina*, as in *elytritis*, inflammation of the vagina.

e·ma"ci·a'tion. The process of losing flesh so as to become extremely lean, or the resultant state; a wasted condition; cachexia.

e·mac"u·la'tion. The removal of freckles or other skin lesions, especially skin tumors.

em"a·na'tion. 1. That which flows or is emitted from a substance; effluvium. 2. Gaseous, radioactive products formed by the loss of alpha particles from radium (radon), thorium X (thoron), and actinium X (actinon).

e·man'si·o (e·man'see·o, ·shee·o). A failing. **e. mensium.** Delay in the first appearance of the menses.

e·mas"cu·la'tion. Castration; removal of the testes, or of the testes and penis.

Em"ba·do·mo'nas (em"buh·do·mo'nus, ·dom'o·nus). A genus of protozoan flagellates. **E. intestinalis.** A species found in the intestine of man.

em·balm'ing. The treatment of a cadaver with antiseptic and preservative substances for burial or for dissection.

em·bed'. *In histology*, surround a specimen with a substance, as paraffin or celloidin, to give support during the process of cutting it into sections for microscopic examination. **—embedding,** *n.*

Em·be'li·a. A genus of shrubs of the Myrsinaceae. **E. ribes.** An Asiatic species; the berries contain embelin, an anthelmintic principle.

em·bel'ic ac'id. Embelin.

em'be·lin. 2,5-Dihydroxy-3-laurylpara-benzoquinone, the taeniacidal principle of *Embelia ribes*. Syn., *embelic acid*.

m″bo·lec′to·my. Surgical removal of an embolus.

m″bo·le′mi·a. Presence of emboli in the blood.

m·bol′ic. 1. Relating to an embolus or an embolism. 2. Pushing or growing in.

m′bo·lism. The occlusion of an artery by an embolus, causing various syndromes depending on the size of the vessel occluded, the part supplied, and the character of the embolus. Also see *embolus.* **air e.** Large amounts of air in the blood stream, such as may gain entrance through wounds of the great veins in the neck, and, reaching the heart, cause cardiac arrest; small amounts are resorbed and cause no symptoms. **cerebral e.** The blocking of a cerebral vessel by any type of embolus that gives rise to a syndrome resembling cerebral hemorrhage. **coronary artery e.** The blocking of a coronary artery by an embolus is rare, and clinically gives rise to a syndrome similar to that seen in coronary thrombosis or spasm. **fat e.** A crushing injury of adipose tissue or of bone liberates fat into the blood stream and results in multiple, widely disseminated embolism of parenchymatous organs which is often fatal. Fat embolism may also occur following the injection of oily solutions. Also called *oil e.* **pulmonary artery e.** Obstruction of the pulmonary artery, or its large branches, by large blood-clot thrombi, originating in peripheral veins or the right side of the heart; occurs not infrequently postoperatively or in cardiac disease, and results in sudden death.

m″bo·lo·la′li·a, em″bo·la′li·a. The insertion of meaningless words into speech, occurring in some aphasic and schizophrenic states.

m′bo·lus (pl. *emboli*). A bit of matter foreign to the blood stream—it may be blood clot, air, cancer or other tissue cells, fat, cardiac vegetations, clumps of bacteria, or a foreign body, such as a needle or bullet—which either gains entrance to the circulation from the individual's body or is carried by the blood stream until it lodges in an artery and obstructs it, causing embolism. **embol′iform, emboloid,** *adj.* **·iding e.** An embolus at the bifurcation of an artery, blocking both branches. Also called *saddle e.,* *straddling e.*

n·bra′sure (em·bray′zhur, ·shur). In *dentistry,* the space between the sloping proximal surfaces of the teeth. The opening may be toward the cheek (*buccal*), toward the lips (*labial*), or toward the tongue (*lingual*).

n″bro·ca′tion. 1. The application, especially by rubbing, of a liquid to a

part of the body. 2. The liquid so applied; liniment.

em″bry·ec′to·my. The surgical removal of an extrauterine embryo.

em′bry·o. 1. A young organism in the early stage of development. 2. The product of conception up to the third month of pregnancy. **embryon′al, embryon′ic,** *adj.* **presomite e.** An embryo from the time of fertilization until the appearance of the first somite, about 21 days. **somite e.** An embryo during the period when somites are formed, approximately the twenty-first to the thirty-first days of development.

em′bry·o-, embry-. A combining form signifying *fetus, embryo, embryonic.*

em″bry·ol′o·gy. The science dealing with the embryo and its development. **—embryolog′ic, embryolog′ical,** *adj.;* **embryol′ogist,** *n.*

e·mer′gen·cy the′o·ry. The concept that the major function of adrenal medulla is to liberate epinephrine in states of emergency so as to increase heart rate, raise blood pressure, reduce blood flow to viscera, and mobilize blood glucose, thereby creating optimal conditions for function of skeletal muscles.

em′e·sis. Vomiting.

em″e·ta·mine′ (em′i·tuh·meen′, i·met′uh·meen). An alkaloid found in ipecac.

e·met″a·tro′phi·a. Atrophy or wasting away, due to persistent vomiting.

e·met′ic. 1. Having the power to induce vomiting. 2. An agent causing emesis.

em′e·tine (em′i·teen, ·tin). An alkaloid derived from ipecac root; it is emetic, diaphoretic, and expectorant. It is also a specific for amebiasis.

em′e·to-, emet-. 1. A combining form denoting *vomiting.* 2. A combining form denoting an *emetic.*

em″e·to·ca·thar′sis. Vomiting and purgation at the same time, or produced by a common agent.

em″e·to·mor′phine (em″i·to·mor′feen, ·fin). Apomorphine.

emf. Electromotive force. **E, e.m.f., E.M.F.** are also used.

-e′mi·a, -ae′mi·a. A suffix used in the naming of diseases to denote *a condition of the blood.*

e·mic′tion. Urination.

e·mic′to·ry. 1. Diuretic. 2. A diuretic agent.

em″i·gra′tion. The outward passage of wandering cells or leukocytes through the walls of a small blood vessel.

em′i·nence. A projecting, prominent

part of an organ, especially a bone. **articular e.** [BR]. The articular tubercle of the zygomatic process of the temporal bone, forming the anterior boundary of the mandibular fossa. **frontal e.** One of two rounded elevations of the frontal bone above the superciliary ridges. **hypothenar e.** An elevation on the ulnar side of the palm corresponding to the muscles of the little finger. **intercondyloid e.** The spinous process lying between the two articular facets on the superior articular surface of the tibia. **parietal e.** The rounded part of the parietal bone. This is sometimes bossselated, due to rickets. **thenar e.** A rounded elevation on the radial side of the palm corresponding to the muscles of the thumb.

em·is·sar″y (em′i·serr″ee). A venous channel through the skull, communicating the venous sinuses with the diploic veins and veins of the scalp.

e·mis·sion. 1. An ejaculation, or sending forth. 2. A seminal discharge, voluntary or involuntary.

em·men·a·gogue (eh·men′uh·gog, eh·mee′nuh·). 1. Stimulating the menstrual flow. 2. An agent that stimulates the menstrual flow. —**emmenagog′ic,** adj.

em·men′i·a (eh·men′ee·uh, ·mee′nee·uh). The menses.

em″me·tro′pi·a. Normal or perfect vision. The condition in which parallel rays are focused exactly on the retina without effort of accommodation. Abbreviated, E. —**emmetrop′ic,** adj.; **em′metrope,** n.

em′o·din. An anthraquinone derivative; product of hydrolysis or oxidation of glycosidal compounds found in aloe, senna, rhubarb, cascara, and other plants. It is an irritant cathartic.

e·mol′li·ent. 1. Softening; relaxing; soothing. 2. A substance used externally to soften the skin; or, internally, to soothe an irritated or inflamed surface.

e·mo′tion. 1. A mental feeling or sentiment. 2. Strong feeling, usually of an agitated nature, accompanied frequently by physical and psychic reactions, as changes in heart action and vasomotor disturbances. —**emotional,** adj.

em·pasm′ (em·paz′um, em′paz·um), **em·pas′ma** (em·paz′muh). A perfumed powder for dusting the person.

em′pa·thy. In psychology, the emotional appreciation of another's feelings.

em′phly·sis. Any vesicular or exanthematous eruption terminating in scales.

em·phrac′tic. 1. Obstructive; closing the pores of the skin. 2. Any agent that obstructs the function of an organ,

especially the excretory function of the skin.

em·phrax′is. An obstruction, infarction, or congestion.

em″phy·se′ma (em″fi·see′muh, em″figh·). A condition where there is overdistention of the air spaces in the lungs, or there is abnormal presence of air or gas in the body tissues. —**emphysem′atous,** adj. **acute pulmonary e.** Distended lungs and alveoli with little or no rupture of alveolar walls. **chronic pulmonary e.** Coalescence of groups of air sacs or permanent dilatation of alveoli with atrophy of alveolar walls and blood vessels, resulting in decreased elasticity of the involved lung. **interstitial e.** Air in tissue spaces between alveoli or lobules, or under the pleura; usually due to trauma. **subcutaneous e.** The accumulation of air or gas in the connective tissue spaces under the skin, due to trauma or to infection with a gas-producing organism.

em·pir′ic. 1. Based on practical observation and not on scientific reasoning or education. 2. One who in practicing medicine relies solely on experience and not on scientific training and reasoning; a quack, or charlatan —**empirical,** adj.

empirin. Trade-mark for a brand of acetylsalicylic acid.

em″pros·thot′o·nos. Tonic muscular spasm in which the body and head are forcibly flexed forward.

em″py·e′ma (em″pye·ee′muh, em″·pee·ee′muh). A term used to indicate the presence of pus in a cavity, hollow organ, or space; such as the pleura, cavity, the gallbladder, the maxillary sinus, or the pericardial cavity. —**empyemic, empyem′atous,** adj.

em″py·e′sis. A pustular eruption, as smallpox; any disease characterized by phlegmonous pimples gradually filling with purulent fluid.

e·mul′si·fi″er. An agent used to assist in the production of an emulsion.

e·mul′si·fy″. Make into an emulsion —**emulsifica′tion,** n.

e·mul′sin. An enzyme found in bitter almonds and other seeds. It induces hydrolysis of amygdalin into benzaldehyde, hydrocyanic acid, and glucose Sometimes called glucosidase.

e·mul′sion. A product consisting of minute globules of one liquid dispersed throughout a second liquid. The portion which exists as globules is known as the internal, dispersed, or discontinuous phase; the other liquid is the external or continuous phase or the dispersion medium.

e·mul′soid. A colloid system whose internal phase is liquid; a lyophilic colloid.

e·munc'to·ry. Excretory.

en-. A prefix signifying *in*, *into*.

-en. A suffix meaning *to make*, *to render*.

-en. An adjectival suffix meaning *made of*.

en·am'el. The hard, calcified substance that covers the crown of a tooth. **mottled e.** Imperfectly calcified or hypoplastic dental enamel that is the result of excessive ingestion of fluorides; chronic dental fluorosis, *q.v.*

en″an·the'ma, en·an'them. An eruption on a mucous membrane, or within the body; in distinction from *exanthema*. —**enanthem'atous**, *adj.*

en·an″ti·o·la'li·a. Talking contrariwise; a disturbance in mental and speech function which prompts ideas and words opposite to those presented as a stimulus.

en″ar·thro'sis. A ball-and-socket joint, like that of the hip. —**enarthrodial**, *adj.*

en·can'this. A neoplasm in the inner canthus of the eye.

en·cap″su·la'tion. The process of surrounding a part with a capsule.

en·ceph″a·li'tis. Inflammation of the brain; may be a specific disease, or a sequela or complication of another disease. —**encephalit'ic**, *adj.* **e. periaxialis diffusa.** A disease, primarily of children, due to extensive inflammation and early demyelination of the white matter in the cerebral hemispheres; characterized by marked loss of hearing, speech, and sight. Also called *Schilder's disease.* **lethargic e.** An epidemic form, frequently occurring with influenza and characterized by drowsiness, apathy, muscular weakness, and paralysis of various cranial nerves. Also called *sleeping sickness*, *von Economo's disease*. **postinfectious e.** That occurring as a sequela of any one of a variety of infectious diseases, such as influenza, measles, and chickenpox. Also called *acute disseminated e.*, *encephalomyelitis.* **postvaccinal e.** An acute form following vaccination against smallpox or rabies. **suppurative e.** A type caused by pyogenic organisms and characterized by abscess formation. **toxic e.** An acute cerebral disturbance of unknown etiology, occurring chiefly in children, characterized clinically by delirium or coma and convulsions, cerebral palsies, and symptoms of meningeal irritation.

en·ceph'a·lo-, encephal-. A combining form meaning *the encephalon* or *brain*.

en·ceph'a·lo·cele″. Hernia of the brain through a congenital or traumatic opening in the cranium.

en·ceph'a·lo·gram″. A roentgenogram of the brain made in encephalography.

en·ceph″a·log'ra·phy. Roentgenography of the brain following removal of cerebrospinal fluid, by lumbar or cisternal puncture, and its replacement by air or oxygen.

en·ceph″a·lo·ma·la'ci·a (en·sef″-uh·lo·ma·lay'shuh, ·see·uh). A softening of the brain caused by a deficient blood supply; the symptoms vary according to the part affected, and consist of partial or complete loss of function. Depending upon the appearance, the softening is distinguished as red, yellow, or white.

en·ceph″a·lo·me·nin'go·cele. Hernia of the membranes and brain substance through an opening in the cranium.

en·ceph″a·lo·my'e·li'tis. Inflammation of the brain and spinal cord. **acute disseminated e.** An acute disorder of the brain and cord with variable symptoms, due to various causes, as vaccination or acute exanthema.

en·ceph″a·lo·my″e·lo·ra·dic″-u·li'tis. Any acute inflammatory disease of the entire nervous system, particularly affecting the nerves to the extremities, the spinal roots, the cord and the bulbar nuclei; symptoms include paresthesia and weakness in the distal parts of the extremities, absence of tendon reflexes, and facial diplegia. Essential in diagnosis is an albumino-cytologic dissociation in the spinal fluid.

en·ceph'a·lon. The brain. —**encephal'ic**, *adj.*

en·ceph″a·lo·spi'nal. Pertaining to the brain and to the spinal cord.

en·ceph'a·lo·tome. 1. An instrument for dissecting the brain. 2. A surgical instrument for incising the brain. 3. A surgical instrument for destroying the brain of a fetus to facilitate delivery.

en·ceph″a·lot'o·my. 1. Surgical incision of the brain. 2. Operative destruction of the fetal brain to facilitate delivery. 3. Dissection of the brain.

en″chon·dro'ma (en″kon·dro'muh). A true chondroma, composed of irregularly arranged cells and hyaline or fibrocartilage. May occur in organs where cartilage is not normally found; when in bones, usually seen in the diaphysis near the epiphysis. —**enchondrom'atous**, *adj.*

en″chon·dro'sis (en″kon·dro'sis). The occurrence of multiple enchondromas in a single bone. Also called *enchondromatosis.*

en·clit'ic. Presenting obliquely; not synclitic; designating the inclination of the pelvic planes to those of the fetal head.

en″co·pre′sis. Psychic incontinence of feces in children.

en·cyst′ed. Enclosed in a cyst or capsule.

en·cyst′ment. The state of being enclosed in a cyst, or sac, or the process of forming a cyst. —**encysted,** adj.

En″da·moe′ba (en″duh·mee′buh). A genus of protozoan parasites which includes species parasitic in humans. **E. coli.** A nonpathogenic species inhabiting the intestinal tract. **E. histolytica.** The etiologic agent of amebic, or tropical, dysentery.

en″dar·te·ri′tis. Inflammation of the inner coat of an artery. **obliterating e.** A form in which the production of new intimal connective tissue obliterates the lumen of a vessel.

end·au′ral. Pertaining to the inner surface or part of the external auditory canal, as endaural approach for mastoidectomy.

end′brain. The telencephalon.

en·dem′ic. Peculiar to a certain region; said of a disease which occurs more or less constantly in any locality.

en·der′mic. Acting through the skin by absorption, as medication applied to the skin.

en″der·mo′sis. 1. A method of administering medicines through the skin, by rubbing. 2. Any herpetic affection of a mucosa.

en′do-, end-. A combining form signifying within.

en″do·an″eu·rys·mor′rha·phy (en″do·an″yoor·iz·mor′uh·fee). The operation for aneurysm consisting of opening the sac and folding and suturing the walls of the aneurysm, thus leaving a lumen of approximately normal size.

en″do·bron′chi·al (en″do·brong′kee·ul, ·bron′kee·ul). Within a bronchus.

en″do·car·di′tis. Inflammation of the endocardium or lining membrane of the heart and its valves. The condition may be acute, subacute, or chronic. **Acute endocarditis** is either warty or ulcerative, the most frequent causes being rheumatism and the infectious diseases. The disease usually affects the valves of the left side of the heart and gives rise to a murmur, fever, dyspnea, and rapid pulse. **Chronic** or **sclerotic endocarditis** is a terminal process following the acute or recurrent rheumatic forms, or is a primary endocarditis due to gout, rheumatism, alcoholism, syphilis, and to other obscure causes, and usually is associated with general arteriosclerosis. Both the acute and the chronic forms give rise to insufficiency or obstruction of the valvular orifice, or to

both combined. —**endocardit′ic** adj. **subacute bacterial e.** A form which runs a somewhat prolonged course, usually due to alpha streptococcus (S. viridans). Syn., e. lenta.

en″do·car′di·um. The membrane lining the interior of the heart, consisting of endothelium and the subjacent connective tissue. —**endocar′di·al,** adj.

en″do·cer″vi·ci′tis. Inflammation of the lining membrane of the cervix uteri.

en″do·cho·led′o·chal. Within the common bile duct.

en″do·cra′ni·um. The inner lining of the skull; the dura mater. —**endocranial,** adj.

en′do·crine (en′do·kryne, ·krin). 1. Secreting internally. 2. Any one of the ductless glands, such as the adrenals, the thyroid, the pituitary, whose secretions pass directly into the blood stream. See under gland.

en″do·cri·nol′o·gy (en″do·kri·nol′o·jee, ·cry·nol′o·jee). The study of the internal secretions and the endocrine glands.

En″do·der·moph′y·ton. Formerly a genus of the dermatophytes, now included in the genus Trichophyton.

en″do·en′zyme. An intracellular enzyme; one retained in the originating cell.

en·dog′e·nous (en·dodj′i·nus). 1. Produced within; due to internal causes; applied to the formation of cells or of spores within the parent cell. 2. Relating to the metabolism of the nitrogenous elements of tissues. 3. In psychology, arising from within the body and directly affecting the nervous system, as a hereditary or constitutional disorder.

en·dog′e·ny (en·dodj′i·nee). In biology, growth from within; endogenous formation.

En″do·li′max. A genus of protozoans of the family Amoebidae, parasitic in man, but nonpathogenic. **E. nana** A species of nonpathogenic amoeba containing a characteristic single small nucleus in which the chromatin is clustered in a single, coarse, irregular shaped karyosome; widely distributed in both temperate and tropical countries. Man is the common host, though these amoebae are also found in the intestine of various species of monkeys. Formerly called Entamoeba nana and Endolimax intestinalis.

en′do·lymph. The fluid of the membranous labyrinth of the ear. —**endolymphat′ic, endolym′phic,** adj.

en″do·ly′sin, en·dol′y·sin. An intracellular, leukocytic, bactericidal substance.

en″do·me″tri·o′sis. The presence of endometrial tissue in abnormal loca ions, as in the perimetrium or in the wall of the urinary bladder.

en″do·me·tri′tis. Inflammation of the endometrium. Formerly a common clinical diagnosis; now, for the most part, a laboratory term.

en″do·me′tri·um. The mucous membrane lining the uterus. —**endometrial,** *adj.*

en′do·mor″phy. A component of physique denoting the presence quantitatively of endodermally derived tissues, expressed in terms of soft roundness and the tendency to laying on of fat. The first component of the somatotype.

en″do·my′ces (en″do-migh′seez). An invalid name for a genus of fungi.

en″do·my″o·car·di′tis. Inflammation of both endocardium and myocardium.

en″do·mys′i·um (en″do-miss′ee-um, miz′ee-um). The connective tissue between the fibers of a muscle bundle, or fasciculus. —**endomysial,** *adj.*

en″do·na′sal. Within the nasal cavity, as endonasal approach in sinus drainage.

en″do·neu′ri·um. The delicate connective tissue holding together the fibers of a nerve bundle, or fasciculus. —**endoneurial,** *adj.*

en″do·par′a·site. A parasite living within its host. —**endoparasit′ic,** *adj.*

en′do·plasm. The inner cytoplasm of a protozoan or of certain cells.

end organ. The expanded termination of a nerve fiber in muscle, skin, mucous membrane, or other structure.

en′do·scope. An instrument, equipped with an electric light or a system of lenses, used for the visual examination of the interior of a body cavity or viscus through its natural outlet. —**en·doscop′ic,** *adj.;* **endos′copy,** *n.*

en″dos·mo′sis (en″dos-mo′sis, en″doz-), **en′dos·mose** (en′dos-moce, en′doz-). The passage of a liquid inward through a porous septum. —**en·osmo′sic, endosmot′ic,** *adj.*

en′do·sperm. *In biology,* the protein of a seed.

en′do·spore. 1. A spore formed within the parent cell. 2. The inner coat of a spore.

en·dos″te·o′ma, en″dos·to′ma. A tumor within a bone.

en·dos′te·um. The membranous layer of connective tissue lining the medullary cavity of a bone. —**endosteal,** *adj.*

en″do·the″li·o·an″gi·i′tis. A systemic infection similar to, and possibly the same as, lupus erythematosus, *q.v.,* and marked by fever, arthritis, and meningitis.

en″do·the″li·o′ma. A group of

tumors made up of large cells morphologically like endothelium and supposedly derived from cells lining blood vessels, lymphatics, and various serous spaces. The different forms vary as to malignant character, and may affect solid organs, such as lymph nodes, skin, etc., because of growth from vascular or tissue spaces.

en″do·the′li·um. 1. The simple squamous epithelium lining the heart, blood vessels, and lymph vessels; vascular endothelium. 2. The mesodermally derived, simple, squamous epithelium lining any closed cavity in the body. *Obs.* —**endothelial,** *adj.*

en″do·ther′mic. 1. *In chemistry,* relating to the absorption of heat. 2. Pertaining to endothermy.

en′do·thrix. A type division of the genus *Trichophyton, q.v.*

en″do·tox′in. A toxin produced within a microörganism which does not diffuse out of the bacterial cell until the cell is disintegrated.

end pleas′ure. *In psychoanalysis,* the pleasure accompanying sexual discharge or detumescence, brought about by a relief of the tension built up during the forepleasure, *q.v.*

-ene. *In chemistry,* a suffix used in the naming of certain hydrocarbons; specifically, indicates the presence of one double bond.

en′e·ma. A rectal injection for therapeutic, diagnostic, or nutritive purposes. **high e.** An injection into the colon. **retention e.** Liquid injected into the rectum, the expulsion of which is delayed voluntarily in order to liquefy the rectal contents or to provide medication.

en″er·get′ics (en″ur-jet′icks). The branch of physics dealing with energy and the laws and conditions governing its manifestations.

en′er·gy. The capacity for doing work. **kinetic e.** That part of the total energy of a body in motion which is due to its motion. **nuclear e.** Energy involved in the intertransformations of mass and energy in nuclear reactions. **potential e.** The power possessed by a body at rest, by virtue of its position, as the potential energy of a suspended weight. Also called *latent e.* **radiant e.** Energy transmitted through electromagnetic or thermal radiation.

en″er·va′tion. Weakness, lassitude, neurasthenia; reduction of strength.

en·gage′ment. *In obstetrics,* the entrance of the presenting part of the fetus into the superior pelvic strait.

en·gorge′ment. Hyperemia; an excessive amount of blood in a part, usually with local edema. —**engorged′,** *adj.*

en′ni·a·tine. A multiple antibiotic

from *Fusarium orthoceras* var. *enniatinum*; it is active against several species of mycobacteria.

e'no·lase. The enzyme that converts 2-phosphoglyceric acid to phosphopyruvic acid.

en″oph·thal'mos. Recession of the eyeball into the orbit.

en″os·to'sis. A bony ingrowth within the medullary canal of a bone.

en'si·form. Shaped like a sword, as the ensiform cartilage.

en'stro·phe (en'stro-fee). Inversion, as of the margin of an eyelid.

en″ta·cous'tic (en″tuh-kōōs'tick). Subjective auditory sensations having their origin within the ear or in its vicinity.

en'tad. Inward.

En″ta·moe'ba (en″tuh-mee'buh). Synonym for *Endamoeba*.

en·ta'si·a (en-tay'zhuh, -zee-uh), **en'ta·sis.** A generic term for spasmodic muscular action; tonic spasm. **—entat'ic**, *adj*.

en·tel'e·chy (en-tel'i-kee). 1. The complete realization or expression of some principle. 2. A vital influence which guides living organisms in the right direction.

en'ter·al. Intestinal.

en″ter·ec'to·my. Excision of a part of the intestine.

en·ter'ic. Of or pertaining to the intestines.

en″ter·i'tis. Any intestinal inflammation, acute or chronic. **acute fibrinous e.** An acute inflammatory process associated with desquamation and fibrin deposition on the mucosa; not a clinical entity but a pathologic classification. **acute follicular e.** An acute inflammation characterized by hyperplasia of the lymph nodules in the intestine; occurs commonly in children suffering from summer diarrhea. **chronic catarrhal e.** A form due to passive hyperemia in which the mucosa is thickened and covered by mucus, and, in cases of long standing, is associated with atrophy.

en'ter·o-, **enter-.** A combining form denoting the *intestine*.

En″ter·o·bac·te″ri·a'ce·ae (en″tur-o-back-teer″ee-ay'see-ee). A family of bacteria including many animal and some plant parasites, causing blight and soft rot; the five tribes are the Eschericheae, Erwineae, Serrateae, Proteae, and Salmonelleae.

en″ter·o·bi'a·sis. Infestation of the small intestine, colon, and rectum with the *Enterobius vermicularis*; characterized by mild catarrhal inflammation of the intestinal mucosa, occasionally by secondary bacterial invasion, and, if the infection is very severe, obstruction of the intestine.

En″ter·o'bi·us. A genus of nematode parasites of man. **E. vermicularis.** The human pinworm or seatworm; the etiologic agent of enterobiasis.

en″ter·o·cele″. A hernia containing a loop of intestine.

en″ter·o·cen·te'sis. Surgical puncture of the intestine.

en″ter·oc'ly·sis. Injection of a fluid preparation into the rectum for nutrient, medicinal, or cleansing purposes.

en″ter·o·coc'cus. Any streptococcus found in the human intestine.

en″ter·o·coele″ (en'tur·o·seel″). A coelom formed by evagination of the wall of the primitive gut. **—enterocoe'lic**, *adj*.

en″ter·o·co·li'tis. Inflammation of small intestine and colon.

en″ter·o·co·los'to·my. Operation for the formation of a communication between the small intestine and colon; enterocolic anastomosis.

en″ter·o·crin'in (en″tur·o·krin'in, en″tur·ock'rin·in). A hormone produced by the intestinal mucosa which stimulates the glands of the small intestine.

en″ter·o·cyst″. An intestinal cyst.

en″ter·o·cys'to·cele. Hernia involving urinary bladder and intestine.

en″ter·o·en″ter·os'to·my. The surgical formation of a passage between two parts of the intestine.

en″ter·o·gas'tro·cele. A hernia containing the stomach and intestine or portions of them; ventral hernia.

en″ter·o·gas'trone. A hormone from the upper intestinal mucosa. It inhibits gastric motility and secretion.

en″ter·og'e·nous (en″tur·odj'i·nus). Originating in the intestine.

en″ter·o·ki'nase (en″tur·o·kigh'nace, -kin'ace). An enzyme present in the intestinal juice which converts inactive trypsinogen into active trypsin.

En″ter·o·mo'nas (en″tur·o·mo'nas -om'o·nas). A genus of intestinal flagellates of the family Cercomonadidae; contains only one species parasitic in man, **E. hominis.**

en″ter·o·my·co'sis (-migh·ko'sis). Intestinal mycosis.

en″ter·o·my'ia·sis (en″tur·o·migh'yuh·sis, -migh·eye'uh·sis). Disease due to the presence of the larvae of flies in the intestine.

en″ter·o·sta'sis (en″tur·o·stay'sis -os'tuh·sis). Intestinal stasis; delay in the passage of the intestinal contents.

en″ter·o·ste·no'sis. Stricture or narrowing of the intestinal canal.

en″ter·os'to·my. The formation of an artificial opening into the intestine through the abdominal wall.

en″ter·o·tox'in. A toxin produced by the *Micrococcus pyogenes* var. *aureus* (*Staphylococcus aureus*) which gives rise to typical symptoms of food poisoning.

en″ter·o·zo′on. An animal parasite of the intestine.

en′the·sis. The employment of metallic or other inorganic material to replace lost tissue.

en·ti′ris. The uvea of the iris, forming its inner and pigmentary layer.

en·to-, ent-. A combining form signifying *within, inner.*

en″to·cho·roi′de·a (en″to·ko·roy′-dee·uh). The inner lining of the choroid membrane of the eye, made up mainly of capillaries.

en′to·cone. The posterior lingual cusp of a maxillary molar tooth.

en″to·co′nid. The posterior lingual cusp of a mandibular molar tooth.

en′to·derm. The innermost of the three primary germ layers, which forms the lining of the gut, from pharynx to rectum, and its derivatives. Syn., *endoderm.* **primitive e.** The internal layer of the gastrula; the group of cells that segregate from the inner cell mass on the ventral surface of the primitive ectoderm and from which are derived the yolk-sac and embryonic gut. Syn., *entoblast, hypoblast.* Also called *primary e.* **yolk-sac e.** The epithelial lining of the yolk sac, continuous with that of the gut.

en″to·mol′o·gist. A specialist in that department of zoology which deals with insects.

en″to·mol′o·gy. The study of insects.

ent″oph·thal′mi·a. Inflammation of the internal parts of the eyeball.

ent″os·to′sis, ent·os″te·o′sis. A benign growth of bone extending from the compacta near the endosteum into a medullary cavity; enostosis.

ent·o′tic (ent·o′tick, -ot′ick). Pertaining to the internal ear.

en″to·zo′on. An animal parasite living within another animal. **—entozo′al,** *adj.*

en·tro′pi·on. Inversion of the eyelid, so that the lashes rub against the globe of the eye. **—entropioniz′e,** *v.t.* **cic·atricial e.** That due to scar tissue on the inner side of the lid; affects the upper lid most commonly. **spastic e.** That caused by excessive contraction of the ciliary portion of the orbicularis muscle; occurring almost always in the lower lid.

en′tro·py. That portion of the energy of a system, per degree of absolute temperature, which cannot be converted to work.

e·nu′cle·ate. Remove an organ or a tumor in its entirety, as an eye from its socket. **—enuclea′tion, enucleator,** *n.*

en″u·re′sis. Incontinence of urine. **nocturnal e.** That occurring at night during sleep.

en·vi′ron·ment. Those external conditions which surround, act upon, and influence an organism or its parts.

en′zyme (en′zime, -zim). A catalytic substance formed by living cells and having a specific action in promoting a chemical change. Syn., *ferment.* **—enzymat′ic, enzy′mic,** *adj.* **autolytic e.** That producing autolysis or digestion of the cell in which it exists, usually at the death of the cell. **bacterial e.** That existing in, or produced by, bacteria. **deaminating e.** One splitting off $-NH_2$ groups; usually followed by a secondary oxidative reaction, as guanase, adenase. **decarboxylating e.** That splitting CO_2 from organic acids, as carboxylase. **digestive e.** An enzyme concerned with digestion in the alimentary tract. **extracellular e.** An enzyme which retains its activity when removed from the cell in which it is formed, or which normally exerts its activity at a site removed from the place of formation. Also called *unorganized ferment, lyoenzyme.* **glycolytic e.** One capable of decomposing sugars, either by hydrolysis or by oxidation. **intracellular e.** An enzyme which exerts its activity within the cell in which it is formed and which loses its activity when removed from the cell. Also called *organized ferment.* **phosphorylating enzymes.** Enzymes which catalyze the phosphorylation or dephosphorylation of compounds. **proteolytic e.** Protease; an enzyme involved in the breaking down of protein, as pepsin, rennin, etc. **respiratory e.** An enzyme concerned with the mechanism by which molecular oxygen produces oxidations in the living cell. Indophenol oxidase, cytochrome oxidase.

e′on·ism. The adoption of feminine habits, manners, and costume by a male. Also see *sexo-esthetic inversion, transvestitism.*

e′o·sin. Tetrabromofluorescein. A bacteriologic stain and diagnostic reagent. Commercially several rose-colored fluorescein dyes of the xanthine series are called eosins. **alcohol-soluble e.** The potassium or sodium salt of the ethyl ester of tetrabromofluorescein. A moderately coarse, red powder; used as histologic stain. Also called *ethyl e.* **soluble e.** The sodium salt of tetrabromofluorescein.

e″o·sin′o·phil. 1. Having an affinity for eosin or any acid stain. **2.** One of the eosinophil leukocytes of the blood or connective tissues. **—eosinophil′ic, eosinophil′ious,** *adj.*

e″o·sin″o·phil′i·a. An increase above the normal number of eosinophils in the circulating blood or in the tissues.

e·pac′tal. 1. Intercalated, supernumerary. **2.** An epactal bone, as the interparietal or Inca bone, or a sutural or Wormian bone.

ep″ar·te′ri·al. Situated upon or above an artery; applied especially to the first branch of the right primary bronchus.

ep·en′dy·ma. The lining membrane of the cerebral ventricles and the central canal of the spinal cord. **—ependymal,** adj.

ep·en″dy·mo′ma. A glioma which originates in or near the ependyma and grows into a ventricle; the cells are of moderate size and polygonal, with blepharoplasts in their cytoplasm.

E·phe′dra, Eph′e·dra. A genus of shrubs of the Gnetaceae, from some species of which is obtained the alkaloid ephedrine. Under the name *ma·huang*, species of *Ephedra* have been used in China for many years.

e·phed′rine (eh·fed′rin, ef′i·dreen). $C_2H_5CHOH.CH(CH_3).NH.CH_3$. An alkaloid from *Ephedra equisetina*, *E. sinica*, and other species, or produced synthetically. Soluble in water and alcohol; slowly soluble in liquid petrolatum. Used in hay fever and asthma, urticaria, surgical shock and as a topical application to mucous membranes in congestions such as colds, etc. **e. hydrochloride.** White crystals or powder soluble in water. **e. sulfate.** White crystals or powder soluble in water. Locally, solutions of 0.5–3.0% are used.

e·phem′er·al. Temporary; applied to fevers that are of short duration.

eph″i·dro′sis. Excessive perspiration; hyperhidrosis.

ephynal. Trade-mark for a synthetic a-tocopherol, a substance having potent vitamin-E activity.

epi-, ep-. 1. A prefix meaning *upon, beside, among, above, anterior, over, on the outside.* 2. *In chemistry*, a prefix denoting relation of some kind to a (specified) compound.

ep″i·a·gnath′us (ep″ee·a·nath′us, ep″ee·ag′nuth·us). An individual with a deficient upper jaw.

ep″i·bleph′a·ron. A congenital fold of skin on the lower eyelid, causing lashes to turn inward. *Rare.*

ep″i·can′thus. A congenital anomaly in which a fold of skin covers the inner canthus and caruncle. Epicanthus is a racial characteristic of the Mongolian race, and is not uncommon in infants of other races in whom the nasal bone is underdeveloped.

ep″i·car′di·um. The visceral layer of the pericardium. **—epicardial,** adj.

ep″i·cho′ri·on (ep″i·ko′ree·on). The decidua capsularis.

ep″i·con′dyle. An eminence upon a bone above its condyle. **—epicon-**

dylar, **epicondyl′ian, epicon·dyl′ic,** adj.

ep″i·con″dy·li′tis. Inflammation of the epicondyle of the humerus; often applied to synovitis of the radiohumeral articulation.

ep″i·cri′sis. The disease phenomena succeeding crisis.

ep″i·crit′ic. Pertaining to sensory nerve fibers which enable one to appreciate very fine distinctions of temperature and touch. These fibers are found in the skin and oral mucosa.

ep″i·dem′ic. Unusual prevalence of a disease; ordinarily affecting large numbers or spreading over a wide area. An arbitrary standard of normal incidence is used to determine the presence of an epidemic. The number of cases occurring for the equivalent chronological period during the previous five years is used to determine the median. **—epidemic′ity** (ep″i·di·miss′i·tee), n.

ep″i·de″mi·ol′o·gist (ep″i·dee″mee·ol′o·jist, ep″i·dem″ee·). One who has made a special study of epidemiology.

ep″i·de″mi·ol′o·gy. The study of occurrence and distribution of disease; usually restricted to epidemic and endemic, but sometimes broadened to include all types of disease. **—epidemiolog′ic,** adj.

ep″i·der″ma·to·plas′ty (ep″i·dur″muh·to·plas′tee, ep″i·dur′muh·to·plas″tee). Skin grafting by transplanting small pieces to denuded areas.

ep″i·der′mis, ep′i·derm. The protective, epithelial outer layer of the skin apposed to the dermis or corium. **—epider′mal, epider′mic, epidermat′ic,** adj.

ep″i·der″mi·za′tion. 1. The formation of epidermis. 2. Skin grafting.

ep″i·der′mo-. A combining form denoting *epidermis.*

ep″i·der″mo·dys·pla·si·a ver·ru″ci·for′mis (ep″i·dur″mo·dis·play′zhuh verr·oo″si·for′miss). A congenital defect in which verrucous lesions occur on the hands, feet, face, or neck.

ep″i·der′moid. 1. Resembling epidermis. 2. A neoplasm occurring as a cyst in the epidermis; containing keratin, hair, or any other parts arising from epidermis.

ep″i·der·mol′y·sis bul·lo′sa. A skin disease in which bullae and vesicles, containing serum or serum and blood, are formed at a point of trauma; may be congenital or hereditary. *Rare.*

ep″i·der″mo·my·co′sis (·migh·ko′sis). Any dermatitis caused by a fungus.

ep″i·der·moph′y·tid. A secondary allergic skin eruption thought to occur when the fungus *Epidermophyton floccosum*, or its products, is carried through the blood stream to sensitized areas of the skin.

Ep″i·der·moph′y·ton (ep″i·dur-mof′i·ton, ep″i·dur″mo·figh′ton). A genus of fungi of the dermatophyte group; contains but one recognized species. **E. floccosum**. The single species of this genus, found in infections of the skin and nails.

ep″i·der″mo·phy·to′sis (ep″i·dur″mo·figh·to′sis). Infection by the *Epidermophyton floccosum*. It has commonly been used to include any fungus infection of the feet producing scaliness and vesicles with pruritus.

ep″i·der·mo′sis. A collective name for anomalous growths of the skin of epithelial origin and type.

ep″i·did″y·mec′to·my. Surgical removal of an epididymis.

ep″i·did′y·mis (pl. *epididymides*). That portion of the seminal duct lying posterior to the testis and connected to it by the efferent ductules of the testis. **—epididymal**, *adj*.

ep″i·did″y·mi′tis. Inflammation of the epididymis.

ep″i·did′y·mo-. A combining form signifying *epididymis*.

ep″i·fol·lic″u·li′tis. Inflammation of the hair follicles of the scalp.

ep″i·gas′tri·um. The upper and middle part of the abdominal surface between the two hypochondriac regions; the epigastric region. **—epigas′tric**, *adj*.

ep″i·gen′e·sis. The theory that the fertilized egg gives rise to the organism by the progressive production of new parts, previously nonexistent as such in the egg's original structure. Distinguished from preformation. **—epigenet′ic**, *adj*.

ep″i·glot′tis. An elastic cartilage covered by mucous membrane forming that superior part of the larynx which guards the glottis during swallowing. **—epiglottic**, *adj*.

ep″i·la′tion. Removal of the hair by the roots by the use of forceps, chemical means, or roentgentherapy. **—ep′ilate**, *v*.

ep″i·lep″sy, ep″i·lep′si·a. A disorder of the central nervous system; characterized by recurring explosive nerve cell discharges and manifested by transient episodes of unconsciousness or psychic dysfunction, with or without convulsive movements. The discharge or seizure is associated with a pronounced change in the electric activity of the brain cells, and the normal synchrony is disturbed by a dysrhythmia. **—epilep′tic**, *adj*. **cerebellar e.** A condition marked by short seizures, during which the patient falls suddenly with extremities rigidly

extended and trunk and neck stiff; a symptom of cerebellar disease. **continuous e.** A generalized convulsion associated with fever, delirium, paralysis, and loss of consciousness; recovery is followed by a long period of focal muscular twitching and weakness. Attributed to a brain infection. Also called *epilepsia partialis continua, Kozhevnikov's (Kojewnikoff's) e.* **di-encephalic autonomic e.** A condition characterized by a paroxysmal discharge into the autonomic nervous system, with sudden excitement, dilated pupils, excessive sweating, lacrimation, salivation, tachycardia, tremor, apnea, and generalized muscular twitching. Usually caused by an irritating lesion of the floor of the third ventricle. **grand mal e.** A complete epileptic seizure; characterized by sudden loss of consciousness, tonic convulsion, cyanosis, and dilated pupils, followed by a clonic spasm of all voluntary muscles, with the eyes rotated upward, the head extended, a frothing at the mouth, and, frequently, incontinence of urine. After the convulsion subsides, the patient is confused and then falls into a deep sleep. The electric rhythm or brain wave during a grand mal attack is one of increased rate and high voltage. Also called *epilepsia gravis.* **hysterical e.** A functional disorder in which the seizures occur in the presence of others; they are violent, marked by disorganized muscular movements, do not cause injury, and are abruptly terminated without the confusion and lethargy which usually occur in true epilepsy. **idiopathic e.** A convulsive disorder not caused by a known or specific brain disease. **Jacksonian e.** Spasmodic contractions in certain groups of muscles or paroxysmal paresthesias in certain skin areas; due to local disease of the cortex. May be limited to one side of the body with retention of consciousness, or progress and become generalized with loss of consciousness. Syn., *focal e., cortical e.* **petit mal e.** A form characterized by very short lapses of consciousness and by a sudden momentary pause in conversation or movement, the duration of which is rarely more than 30 seconds. Petit mal attacks are frequent in children, and may occur as often as 200 times a day, but rarely cause the patient to fall or to show muscular spasm. The brain wave disturbance is a very slow rate of three or four waves per second. Also called *epilepsia mitis, epilepsia vertiginosa.* See *pyknolepsy.* **psychomotor e.** That in which transient mental disturbances replace the typical convulsions.

ep″i·lep′toid. 1. Resembling epilepsy. 2. A person subject to nervous attacks of the general nature of epilepsy.

ep″i·mere. 1. The somite or dorsal part of the mesoderm. 2. The dorsal part of a myotome.

ep″i·mys′i·um (ep″i·miz′ee·um, ·miss′ee·um). The sheath of connective tissue surrounding a muscle.

ep″i·neph′rine (ep″i·nef′reen, ·rin). l-3,4-Dihydroxyphenyl-2-methylaminoethanol. White or light-brown powder obtained from suprarenal glands or synthesized. It is a sympathomimetic drug; sometimes used as a vasoconstrictor and cardiac stimulant in acute circulatory failure; as a local vasoconstrictor in hemorrhage and local congestion; to relax the bronchi in asthmatic paroxysms. Its action is fleeting. See *adrenalin, suprarenalin, suprarenin.* **slow e.** An epinephrine suspension in a vegetable oil which retards and prolongs its action.

ep″i·neu′ral. Attached to a neural arch.

ep″i·neu′ri·um. The connective-tissue sheath of a nerve trunk. —**epineurial**, *adj.*

ep″i·ot′ic (ep″ee·ot′ick, ·o′tick). Situated above or on the cartilage of the ear.

ep″i·pas′tic. 1. Having the qualities of a dusting powder. 2. A powder for use on the surface of the body, as talc.

ep″i·phe·nom′e·non. An unusual or peculiar event or process in the course of a disease, not necessarily due to the same cause, for example, epituberculosis in lungs, the site of focal atelectasis or nontuberculous pneumonia.

e·piph′o·ra. A persistent overflow of tears, due to excessive secretion or to impeded outflow.

ep″i·phy·lax′is (ep″i·figh·lack′sis, ·fi·lack′sis). The reinforcing or increase of the defensive agencies of the body.

ep″i·phys″i·ol′y·sis, ep″i·phys″e·ol′y·sis (ep″i·fizz″ee·ol′i·sis). The separation of an epiphysis from the shaft of a bone.

e·piph′y·sis. A portion of bone attached for a time to another bone by cartilage, but subsequently becoming consolidated with the principal bone. —**epiphys′eal**, *adj.* **slipping e.** Displacement of the upper femoral epiphysis; of uncertain etiology. It occurs in children.

e·piph′y·sis ce·re′bri. The pineal body.

e·piph″y·si′tis. Inflammation of an epiphysis.

ep′i·phyte. 1. A vegetable parasite growing on the exterior of the body. 2. A plant growing upon another plant, but deriving the moisture required for its development from the air.

e·pip′lo·on. The omentum; specifically, the great omentum. —**epiplo′ic**, *adj.*

ep″i·plo·pex″y. The operation of suturing the great omentum to the anterior abdominal wall, for the purpose of establishing a collateral venous circulation in cirrhosis of the liver. *Obs.*

ep″i·scle′ra (ep″i·skleer′uh). The loose connective tissue lying between the conjunctiva and the sclera.

e·pi′si·o- (eh·pis′ee·o-, eh·piz′ee·o-). A combining form indicating *relation to* the vulva.

e·pi″si·ot′o·my (eh·pee″see·ot′o·mee, eh·pis″ee·). Medial or lateral incision of the vulva during childbirth, to avoid undue laceration.

ep′i·sode. An event having a distinct effect on a person's life, or on the course of a disease.

ep″i·spa′di·as (ep″i·spay′dee·us, ·spad′ee·us). A condition in which the urethra opens on the dorsum of the penis. —**epispadial**, *adj.;* **epispadiac** *adj., n.*

ep″i·spas′tic. 1. Causing blisters. 2. A blistering agent.

ep″i·sta′sis. 1. A scum or film of substance floating on the surface of urine. 2. A checking or stoppage of a hemorrhage or other discharge.

ep″i·stat′ic. *In genetics,* dominating or suppressing, as a gene which suppresses the effect of another mutant gene that affects the same part of the organism. —**epis′tasy**, *n.*

ep″i·stax′is. Bleeding from the nose.

ep″i·stro′phe·us [BNA]. Axis; the second cervical vertebra. See Table of Bones in the Appendix.

ep″i·tha·lax′i·a. Shedding of epithelial cells, especially in the lining of the intestine.

ep″i·the″li·o·cho′ri·al (ep″ith·ee″lee·o·kor′ee·ul). Pertaining to the uterine epithelium and the chorionic ectoderm, as epitheliochorial placenta.

ep″i·the′li·oid. Resembling epithelium.

ep″i·the″li·o′ma. Any benign tumor derived from epithelium and composed largely of epithelial cells; formerly applied to epidermoid carcinoma. —**epitheliomatous**, *adj.*

ep″i·the·li′tis. Inflammation and overgrowth of epithelium of a mucous membrane, due to an x-ray burn.

ep″i·the′li·um (pl. *epithelia*). A tissue composed of contiguous cells with a minimum of intercellular substance. It forms the epidermis and lines hollow organs and all passages of the respiratory, digestive, and genitourinary systems. Special types include **endothelium**, lining blood and lymph vessels; and **mesothelium**, lining body cavities. Epithelium is divided, according to the shape and arrangement of the cells, into columnar, cuboidal, and squamous; simple, pseudostratified, and stratified epithelium; according to function, into protective, sensory, and glandular or secreting. **—epithelial,** adj. **ciliated e.** A form in which the cells bear vibratile filaments or cilia on their free extremities. **columnar e.** Distinguished by elongated, prismatic, or columnar cells. **cuboidal e.** Distinguished by prismatic cells in which height and width are approximately equal. **germinal e.** A region of the dorsal coelomic epithelium, lying between the dorsal mesentery and the mesonephros. It becomes the covering epithelium of the gonad when it arises from the genital ridge. Some believe that it gives rise to the germ cells. Also called *germ e.* **pseudostratified e.** One in which all cells are seated on the basement membrane, but not all reach the free surface. **respiratory e.** The pseudostratified, ciliated epithelium lining most of the respiratory tract. **sensory e.** Epithelium in which sensory cells combined with ordinary epithelial cells form the peripheral terminations of the nerves in the organs of sense. **simple e.** That consisting of only one layer of cells. **squamous e.** The form in which the cells have been reduced to thin plates. **stratified e.** A form in which the cells are arranged in distinct layers. **transitional e.** The epithelium of the urinary tract. The cells of this form vary in shape between squamous, when the epithelium is stretched, and columnar, when not stretched.

ep″i·the″li·za′tion. The growth of epithelium over a raw surface.

ep′i·them. Any local application, as a compress, fomentation, lotion, or poultice.

ep″i·to′nos, ep″i·to′nus. Anything exhibiting abnormal tension or tone, or stretched from one point to another. **—epiton′ic,** adj.

ep″i·trich′i·um (ep″i·trick′ee·um). 1. The superficial layer of fetal epidermis, the remnant of which forms the cellular component of the vernix caseosa. Syn., *periderm.* 2. The superficial layers of squamous cells overlying a hair shaft in its canal before it breaks through the epidermis. **—epitrichial,** adj.

ep″i·troch′le·ar (ep″i·trock′lee·ur). Applied to a lymph node which lies above the trochlea of the elbow joint.

ep″i·tu·ber″cu·lo′sis. A pulmonary lesion occurring in tuberculin-positive children; characterized by a massive or lobar density in the x-ray films, paucity of clinical symptoms, and eventual complete resolution. Originally interpreted as nonspecific pneumonia modified by association with tuberculous infection, but no longer accepted as a single pathologic entity.

ep″i·tym′pa·num. The attic of the middle ear, or tympanic cavity. **—epitympan′ic,** adj.

ep″o·nych′i·um (ep″o·nick′ee·um). 1. A horny condition of the epidermis from the second to the eighth month of fetal life, indicating the position of the future nail. 2. The horny layer (stratum corneum) of the nail fold attached to the nail plate at its margin.

ep′o·nym. A name formed or derived from that of a person known or assumed to be the first, or one of the first, to discover or describe a disease, symptom complex, theory, etc. Eponyms often honor persons who are proponents of systems and procedures, methods, surgical operations, etc., even though these are not original with the person so honored. **—eponym′ic, epon′ymous,** adj.

ep″o·öph′o·ron. A vestigial structure in the female; derived from paragenital mesonephric tubules, a part of the mesonephric duct, and perhaps the rete ovarii.

eprolin-S. A trade-mark for α-tocopherol.

Ep′som salt. Magnesium sulfate.

ep·u′lis (pl. *epulides*). Any solitary tumorlike lesion developing from the periosteum of the maxilla or mandible, appearing clinically as a circumscribed swelling beneath the gum. It may be a true giant-cell tumor, a fibroma, or a reparative hyperplasia. **—ep′uloid,** adj.

equanil. A trade-mark for meprobamate.

e·qua′tion. A means of expressing equality between two parts.

e·qua′tor, ae·qua′tor. Any imaginary circle which divides a body into two equal and symmetrical parts in the manner of the equator of a sphere. **—equato′rial,** adj. **e. of the eye.** A line encircling the eyeball midway between its anterior and posterior poles; aequator bulbi oculi. **e. of the lens.** The periphery of the crystalline lens between the two layers of the ciliary process; aequator lentis.

e′qui-. A prefix meaning *equally.*

e″qui·ax′i·al. Having equal axes.

e″qui·len′in, e·quil′e·nin. An estrogenic steroid hormone, chemically 3-hydroxy-17-keto-1,3,5,6,8-estrapentaene, occurring in the urine of pregnant mares.

e″qui·li·bra′tion (ee″kwi·li·bray′shun). Maintenance of equilibrium.

e″qui·lib′ri·um. 1. A state of balance; a condition in which opposing forces equalize one another so that no movement occurs. 2. A well-balanced condition of mind or feeling. **membrane e.** A state of ionic balance created on opposite sides of a membrane which is impermeable to an ion. Also called *Donnan e.* **nitrogen e.** A state of balance between the intake of nitrogen as proteins and its excretion, in urine, feces, sweat, etc. See *nitrogen balance.* **nutritive e.** A condition of balance between the intake of a nutritive material and the excretion of the products of its metabolism.

e'qui·lin (ee'kwi·lin, eck'wi·lin). An estrogenic steroid hormone, chemically 3-hydroxy-17-keto-1,3,5,7-estratraene, occurring in the urine of pregnant mares.

e"qui·mo·lec'u·lar. 1. Containing or representing quantities of substances in the proportion of their molecular weights. 2. Containing or representing an equal number of molecules.

Eq"ui·se'tum (eck"wi·see'tum, ee"-kwi·). A genus of cryptogamous plants, some of which have been shown to have a diuretic effect.

e·quiv'a·lent. 1. Having an equal value. 2. That which is equal in value, size, weight, or in any other respect, to something else. 3. *In chemistry,* the weight of a substance which is chemically equal to 8 parts by weight of oxygen; the weight is commonly expressed in grams. The weight of a substance which combines with or replaces one gram atomic weight of hydrogen. Syn., *equivalent weight.* **combustion e.** The amount of heat obtained by burning one gram of fat or carbohydrate. **mechanical e. of heat.** The mechanical energy required to raise the temperature of one gram of water one degree centigrade; it is 4.185 × 10⁷ ergs per calorie (15°); Joule's equivalent. **thermometric e.** A change of 180 Fahrenheit degrees is equivalent to a change of 100 centigrade degrees and a change of 80 Réaumur degrees. See Tables of Thermometric Equivalents in the Appendix. **toxic e.** The quantity of poison capable of killing, by intravenous injection, one kilogram of animal.

Er. Chemical symbol for erbium.

e·ra'sion (e·ray'zhun). 1. Surgical removal of tissue by scraping. 2. Excision of a joint; arthrectomy.

Er"a·ty'rus. A genus of bugs of the Triatomidae. **E. cuspidatus.** A species found in South America which has been incriminated in the transmission of American trypanosomiasis.

er'bi·um. Er = 167.2. A rare earth metal.

e·rec'tile. Capable of being dilated or erected.

e·rec'tion. The enlarged state of erectile tissue when engorged with blood, as in the penis or clitoris. **—erect',** *adj., v.*

e·rec'tor. 1. A muscle that produces erection of a part. 2. A prism attached to the eyepiece of a microscope for correcting the inversion of the image.

e·rec"tor spi'nae [NA]. A large, compound deep muscle of the back, arising from the posterior aspect of the sacrum and inserted above on the vertebral spines and transverse processes and on the ribs. Syn., *sacrospinalis.*

e·rep'sin. An enzyme mixture produced by the intestinal mucosa, consisting of various peptidases which split peptones and proteoses into simpler products; it has no effect on native proteins.

er'e·thism. 1. An abnormal increase of nervous irritability. 2. Quick response to stimulus. **—erethis'mic, erethis'tic, erethit'ic,** *adj.*

erg. A unit of work; representing the work done in moving a body against the force of one dyne through a distance of one centimeter.

er·ga'si·a (ur·gay'zhuh, ·shuh). 1. *In psychobiology,* the sum total of the functions and reactions of an individual; the actions or responses which spring from the whole organism or personality. 2. A tendency toward work.

er·ga"si·o·ma'ni·a (ur·gay"see·o·may'nee·uh, ur·gass"ee·o·). An exaggerated desire for work of any kind; seen in the manic state of manic-depressive psychoses. *Rare.*

er'go-, erg-. A combining form denoting *work.*

er"go·ba'sine (ur"go·bay'seen, ·sin). Ergonovine.

er"go·ba'si·nine (ur"go·bay'si·neen, ·nin). Ergometrinine.

er"go·cor'nine. An alkaloid from ergot.

er"go·cris'tine (ur"go·kris'teen, ·tin). A levorotatory alkaloid from ergot.

er"go·cris'ti·nine. The dextrorotatory isomer of ergocristine; it is nearly devoid of therapeutic activity.

er'go·graph. An instrument which, by means of a weight or spring against which a muscle can be contracted, records the extent of movement of that muscle or the amount of work it is capable of doing.

er·gom'e·ter. An instrument which permits calculation of the work performed (weight multiplied by shortening) by a muscle or muscles over a period of time. One form of this instrument is the **ergometer bicycle**, a stationary bicycle on which the subject pedals against a measurable load.

er"go·met'rine (ur"go·met'reen, ·rin). Ergonovine.

er″go·met′ri·nine (ur″go·met′ri-neen, ·nin). The dextrorotatory, relatively inactive isomer of ergonovine. Syn., *ergobasinine*.

er″go·no′vine (ur″go·no′veen, ·vin). An alkaloid obtained from ergot, also known as ergotocin, ergometrine, ergostetrine, and ergobasine. It is more prompt but less persistent in its action than other ergot alkaloids. **e. maleate.** $C_{19}H_{23}N_3O_2 . C_4H_4O_4$. See *ergotrate*.

er′go·phore group. A chemical group which determines the specificity of the antibody.

er′go·sine (ur′go·seen, ·sin). An alkaloid, $C_{30}H_{37}O_5N_5$, of ergot, having physiologic activity similar to that of ergotoxine.

er·go′si·nine. The dextrorotatory isomer of ergosine; it is nearly devoid of therapeutic activity.

er·gos′ter·ol. An inert alcohol derived from yeast and other fungi. It is provitamin D_2; on ultraviolet radiation, it is activated to vitamin D_2, and is then known as irradiated ergosterol or viosterol.

er″go·stet′rine (ur″go·stet′reen, ·rin). Ergonovine.

er′got. The dried sclerotium of *Claviceps purpurea*, a fungus developed on rye plants. It contains at least five optically isomeric pairs of alkaloids. Ergot causes powerful uterine contractions, and is useful in menorrhagia and metrorrhagia and in preventing and checking post-partum hemorrhage. Through its vasoconstrictor action, it is useful in cerebral or spinal congestion, and in conditions where there is local passive congestion.

er·got′a·mine (ur·got′uh-meen, ur″-guh·tam′een). An alkaloid from ergot, having activity qualitatively identical with that of ergotoxine but two-thirds as strong. **e. tartrate.** Used as uterine contractor and in migraine. See *gynergen*.

er″go·tam′in·ine. The dextrorotatory isomer of ergotamine; nearly devoid of therapeutic activity.

er″go·thi″o·ne′ine. See *thioneine*.

er′got·in. Ergot extract. **Bonjean's e.** An aqueous ergot extract.

er·got′i·nine (ur·got′i·neen, ·nin). An alkaloid from ergot. It is practically inert physiologically.

er′got·ism. The constitutional effects following the prolonged use of ergot, or of grain containing the fungus *Claviceps purpurea*. There are two types: a spasmodic form with contractions and cramps of the muscles, and a form characterized by dry gangrene.

er″go·to′cin. Ergonovine.

er″go·tox′ine (ur″go·tock′seen, ·sin). An alkaloid from ergot. **e. eth-**

anesulfonate. A useful salt of ergotoxine.

ergotrate. Trade-mark for ergonovine maleate.

E·rig′er·on (i·ridj′ur·on). A genus of the Compositae. Several species have been used in urinary diseases, diarrhea, and dysentery. Syn., *fleabane*.

E″ri·o·dic′ty·on (eer″ee·o·dick′tee-on, err″ee·o·). A genus of shrubs of the Hydrophyllaceae. **E. californicum.** California yerba santa; mountain balm. The leaves of this California shrub have been used as an expectorant and in fluid preparations to mask the taste of bitter drugs.

E·ro′di·um. A genus of herbs of the Geraniaceae. **E. cicutarium.** Alfilaria; has been used as a substitute for hydrastis.

e·rog′e·nous (i·rodj′i·nus), **er″o·gen′ic.** Producing or stimulating the sexual appetite.

e·ro′si·o in″ter·dig″i·ta′lis blas″to·my·ce′ti·ca (eh·ro′see·o in″tur·didj″i·tah′lis blas″to·migh·see′ti-kuh, ·set′i·kuh). A form of moniliasis which involves the webs of the fingers and particularly the third or fourth interdigital web. This disease is seen in laundresses and in others whose hands are exposed to the macerating effects of water and strong alkalies.

e·ro′sion. Superficial destruction of a surface area by inflammation or trauma. —**erosive,** *adj.*; **erode′,** *v.* **dental e.** A process, probably chemical, which results in the loss of calcified tissues at the neck of a tooth. **e. of cervix uteri.** Destruction of the stratified squamous epithelium of the vaginal cervix, the eroded area being covered by columnar cells.

e·rot′ic. 1. Pertaining to the libido or sexual passion. 2. Moved by or arousing sexual desire. 3. A lustful or amorous person; one activated by sexual desire.

er′o·tism, e·rot′i·cism. 1. Sexual excitement or desire. 2. *In psychoanalysis,* any manifestation of the sexual instinct or love life.

er″o·to·gen′ic (err″o·to·jen′ick, i·ro″to·). Causing, or originating from, erotic feelings.

er″o·to·ma′ni·a. Morbid exaggeration of the affections, usually toward the opposite sex. Also called *eromania, eroticomania.* —**erotomaniac,** *n.*

e·ru′cic ac′id. $CH_3(CH_2)_7CH:CH-(CH_2)_{11}COOH$. An unsaturated acid found in the glycerides of rape seed oil and mustard oil.

e″ruc·ta′tion (ee″ruck·tay′shun, err″uck·). Belching.

e·ru′ga·to″ry. Tending to remove wrinkles.

e·rup′tion. 1. Lesions on the skin, especially applied to those of the exanthematous diseases. 2. The **appear-**

ance of a tooth through the gums. **drug e.** Dermatitis medicamentosa, *q.v.* **miliary e.** An eruption of little vesicles occurring in the course of febrile diseases.

e·rup'tive. Attended by or producing an eruption, as an eruptive fever.

E·ryn'gi·um. A genus of plants of the Umbelliferae. **E. aquaticum.** Button snakeroot eryngo; a species indigenous to the western prairies and southern barrens of the United States. The root is reputedly diaphoretic, expectorant, and emetic.

er″y·sip′e·las (err″i·sip′i·lus, irr″i·). An acute, infectious disease due to *Streptococcus pyogenes*; characterized by a spreading inflammation of the skin and subcutaneous tissues, rarely of the mucous membranes. Sulfa drugs are very effective in treatment. —**erysipel′atous**, *adj.* **e. diffusum.** That in which the affected area is not sharply defined, the redness merging gradually with the color of the surrounding skin. **e. glabrum.** That in which the skin is tightly stretched and has a smooth, shining appearance. **e. medicamentosum.** A rash resembling erysipelas, but marked by rapid development, the absence of well-defined areas, and tenderness on pressure; produced by ingested drugs. **facial e.** Erysipelas of the face; the most common form. After an initial chill, the temperature rises very high and there are severe symptoms of toxemia; there may be vomiting and delirium, and the disease may spread rapidly over a great part of the body. The affected area is swollen, itches, has a deep-red color and an elevated margin, and tends to heal centrally while spreading peripherally. **wandering e.** A form in which the erysipelatous process successively disappears from one part of the body to appear subsequently in another part.

er″y·sip′e·loid. An infection caused by *Erysipelothrix rhusiopathiae;* occurs on the hands of those who handle infected meat or fish. Characterized by circumscribed, multiple lesions of a red color; extreme hyperemia is present in some cases.

Er″y·si·pel′o·thrix (err″i·si·pel′o·thricks, err″i·sip′i·lo·). A genus of filamentous, branching bacteria of the family Corynebacteriaceae.

e·rys′i·phake. An instrument shaped like a small spoon, with blunt edges and a long handle, connected with an apparatus for producing a vacuum; used in an operation for cataract known as phakoerisis. Also spelled *erisophake.*

er″y·the′ma. Hyperemia of the skin occurring in patches of variable size and shape. —**erythem′atous** (err″ith·em′uh·tus, ·eem′uh·tus), *adj.* **epi-**demic arthritic e. An acute, infectious disease; characterized by abrupt onset with chills, fever, back and joint pains; after a few days a rubelliform or morbilliform eruption appears. Syn., *Haverhill fever.* **e. circinatum.** A form of erythema multiforme showing lesions with depressed centers and erythematous borders. **e. diffusum.** A form resembling scarlatina, with ill-defined outline, the red color of the affected skin merging gradually with that of the surrounding parts. **e. elevatum diutinum.** A clinical variety of granuloma annulare, characterized by firm, painless nodules which, discrete at first, later coalesce to form flat, raised plaques or nodular tumors. **e. gyratum persistens.** An eruption characterized by persistent erythematous patches in annular, marginate, or gyrate forms. Syn., *erythema figuratum perstans.* **e. induratum.** A chronic recurrent disorder; characterized by deep-seated nodosities and subsequent ulcerations; usually involves the skin of the legs of younger women, often tuberculous. Also called *Bazin's disease.* **e. marginatum.** A type of erythema multiforme in which an elevated, well-defined band remains as a sequela of an erythematous patch. **e. multiforme.** An acute, inflammatory skin disease; characterized by reddish macules, papules, or tubercles; the lesions, varying in appearance, occur usually on neck, face, legs, and dorsal surfaces of hands, forearms, and feet; initial symptoms are often gastric distress and rheumatic pains. The term *Stevens-Johnson syndrome* is applied when lesions of mucous membrane are also present. **e. nodosum.** An eruption, usually on the anterior surfaces of the legs below the knees, of pink to blue, tender nodules appearing in crops; more frequently seen in women, often associated with joint pains. **e. perstans.** Persisting, recurring erythema; a group including erythema figuratum perstans, erythema annulare centrifugum, erythema simplex gyratum, erythema chronicum migrans. **e. simplex.** A hyperemia showing various shades of redness, either diffuse or circumscribed. The symptomatic erythemas may be precursors of systemic disturbances or febrile disorders. Also called *e. hyperemicum.* **e. venenatum.** Redness of the skin produced by external irritants. **e. vesiculosum.** A type of erythema multiforme characterized by vesicles. **tertiary circinate e.** Skin lesions of pink to red color occurring as circular or oval patches with normal or pigmented centers, or in segments of circles which may form gyrate figures by coalescence; occurring several years after syphilitic infection. Also called *neurosyphilid, circinate syphilitic erythema.*

er″y·the′moid, er″y·the′ma·toid. Resembling erythema.

er″y·thras′ma (err″i·thraz′muh). A skin disease seen in the axillas or the inguinal or pubic regions. It forms reddish or brownish, sharply defined, slightly raised, desquamating patches which cause little or no inconvenience. It is due to the fungus *Nocardia minutissima.*

·ryth″re·de′ma pol″y·neu·rop′a·thy (eh·rith″ri·dee′muh pol″i·new·rop′uth·ee). An afebrile disease of unknown etiology, seen in young children of 9–12 months; characterized by typical skin lesions on the hands and feet and by vasomotor and emotional disturbances. The extremities are dusky pink, swollen, and itch intolerably; there is profuse sweating, photophobia, anorexia, insomnia, and irritability. The disease usually runs a course of several months, with spontaneous recovery. Also called *pink disease, acrodynia, Selter's disease, Feer's disease.*

er″y·thre′mi·a. Erythrocytosis.

Er″y·thri′na. A genus of tropical and subtropical trees and shrubs, various species of which have long been used in folk medicine. The seeds of some species contain one or more alkaloids having curarelike action; of these beta-erythroidine and its derivative dihydro-β-erythroidine are potentially of clinical importance.

·ryth·ri′tyl tet″ra·ni′trate. A vasodilator which gives its maximum effect in about 20 minutes and lasts for five or six hours. It is available in tablet form. Syn., *erythrol tetranitrate.*

·ryth′ro-, er′yth·ro-. A combining form signifying *red.*

·ryth′ro·blast. In general use it indicates any nucleated hemoglobiniferous cell. Red blood cells of the embryo are primitive erythroblasts, those in the fetal liver and normal bone marrow are definitive erythroblasts. According to their size and nuclear pattern erythroblasts may be subdivided into microblasts, normoblasts, macronormoblasts, and megaloblasts. In specific usage, erythroblasts may indicate a cell stage in erythropoiesis. —**erythroblas′tic,** *adj.* **basophilic e.** The youngest erythroblast, characterized by basophilic cytoplasm and large vesicular nucleus. **polychromatic e.** An erythroblast containing various amounts of acidophil hemoglobin inversely proportional to the basophilic cytoplasm.

·ryth″ro·blas·to′ma. A tumor of bone marrow which is composed of cells that resemble large erythroblasts.

e·ryth″ro·blas·to′sis foe·tal′is (fee·tah′lis). A hemolytic anemia of the newborn, characterized by icterus and an increased number of nucleated red blood cells. Occurs when a mother is Rh negative and develops antibodies against the fetus, which is Rh positive.

erythrocin. A trade-mark for erythromycin.

e·ryth″ro·cy″a·no′sis. Irregular reddish blue markings on the skin, usually reticular in arrangement; due to a circulatory disturbance of the skin.

e·ryth′ro·cyte. A red blood cell. —**erythrocyt′ic,** *adj.* **crenated e.** One with indented edges, due to withdrawal of fluid from the inside of the cell.

e·ryth″ro·cy″to-. A combining form signifying *erythrocyte.*

e·ryth″ro·cy″tol′y·sis. The plasmolysis of red corpuscles; the escape of soluble substances and the reduction of the volume of the corpuscle; hemolysis.

e·ryth″ro·cy″to·poi·e′sis. The formation or development of red blood corpuscles.

e·ryth″ro·cy″tor·rhex′is. Breaking up or fragmentation of the red blood corpuscles. Syn., *erythrorrhexis.*

e·ryth″ro·cy·to′sis (·sigh·to′sis). 1. Excessive formation of red corpuscles, especially in response to a known stimulus. 2. An increase in the number of red blood cells in the fetus and newborn.

e·ryth″ro·der′ma. A dermatosis characterized by an abnormal redness of the skin; erythema; erythrodermia. **e. desquamativa.** A generalized redness and scaly eruption seen in children. The nails, scalp, and intestinal tract are usually involved. May be fatal. Differentiated from dermatitis exfoliativa. Also called *Leiner's disease.* **e. ichthyosiforme congenitum.** A type of congenital dermatosis in which there is a thickening and reddening of the skin, and a tendency to resemble lichen. **e. maculosa perstans.** A plaquelike variety of psoriasis in which the areas involved are about one-half inch in diameter and without marked desquamation. **exfoliative e.** A dermatosis having a scarlatiniform eruption lasting from six to eight weeks, with free desquamation. See *pityriasis rubra.*

e·ryth″ro·dex′trin. A dextrin formed by the partial hydrolysis of starch with acid or amylase. It yields a red color with iodine.

er′y·throid. Reddish; of a red color.

e·ryth·roi′dine (eh·rith′roy·deen, ·din). An alkaloid obtained from species of *Erythrina.* It occurs in α- and β-varieties. β-Erythroidine and its derivative dihydro-β-erythroidine may be useful because of their curare-like action.

er′y·throl. A crystalline alcohol, tetrahydroxybutane, $C_4H_6(OH)_4$, from certain algae and lichens. Also called *erythritol.*

e·ryth″ro·leu·ke′mi·a (eh·rith″ro·lew·kee′mee·uh, err″ith·ro·). An acute disease characterized by the presence in the blood of both immature leukocytes and immature erythrocytes.

e·ryth″ro·leu·ko′sis (eh·rith″ro·lew·ko′sis, err″ith·ro·). A condition characterized by an increase in the number of immature erythrocytes and leukocytes in the blood.

e·ryth″ro·me·lal′gi·a. A cutaneous vasodilatation of the feet or, more rarely, of the hands; characterized by redness, mottling, changes in skin temperature, and neuralgic pains. It is thought to be an angioneurosis of the sympathetic system, of unknown etiology.

e·ryth″ro·me′li·a. A condition of the extensor surfaces of the arms and legs; characterized by painless progressive redness of the skin; distinct from erythromelalgia.

e·ryth″ro·my′cin. Antibiotic isolated from cultures of *Streptomyces erythreus,* administered orally, and effective against many Gram-positive and some Gram-negative pathogens. See *erythrocin, ilotycin.*

e·ryth″ro·ne″o·cy·to′sis (·nee″o·sigh·to′sis). The presence of regenerative forms of red corpuscles in the circulating blood.

Er′y·thro′ni·um. A genus of plants of the Liliaceae. **E. america′num.** A species indigenous to the United States; the dried plant is emetic in large doses.

er″y·thro·pe′ni·a. Deficiency in the number of red blood corpuscles.

e·ryth″ro·phle′ine (eh·rith″ro·flee′een, err″ith·ro·). An alkaloid from casca bark having a digitalislike action.

e·ryth″ro·phle′um. Casca bark.

e·ryth″ro·phose (eh·rith′ro·fohz, err′ith·ro·). A red phose.

e·ryth″ro·pla′si·a of Quey·rat′ (eh·rith″ro·play′zhuh uv kay·rah′, err″ith·ro·). A condition characterized by a circumscribed, erythematous, velvety lesion affecting mucocutaneous junctions or mucosa of the mouth, tongue, vulva, glans penis, or prepuce. Considered precancerous to squamous-cell carcinoma.

er″y·throp′si·a, er″y·throp′i·a. An abnormality of vision in which all objects appear red; red vision.

er″y·throp′sin. Visual purple. See *rhodopsin.*

e·ryth′ro·sin (eh·rith·ro·sin, err″·ith·ro′sin), **e·ryth′ro·sine** (eh·rith′-

ro·seen, err″ith·ro′sin). A red dye, an iodine derivative of fluorescein. **e., yellowish.** Di-iodofluorescein; valuable counterstain after Delafield hematoxylin or methylene blue. Also called e. R or G, *pyrosin J, dianthin G, iodoeosin G.*

e·ryth′ro·sin B (C.C.). Tetraiodofluorescein; used as a counterstain. Also called *bluish e., pyrosin B, eosin J, iodoeosin B, dianthin B.*

e·ryth′ro·sin BB (C.C.). See *phloxine.*

er″y·throx′y·lon. Coca, *q.v.*

es·cape′. *In medicine,* leakage or outflow, as of nervous impulses. **vagal e.** One or more spontaneous beats of the heart, occurring in spite of the fact that the function of the sinus node that normally initiates heart beats has been arrested by stimulation of the vagus nerve.

es·cape′ mech′a·nism. A mode of adjustment to difficult and/or unpleasant situations by utilizing a means easier or pleasanter than that required for a permanent solution of the difficulty; an evasion of responsibility.

es′char (ess′kahr). A dry slough, especially that produced by heat or a corrosive or caustic substance.

es″cha·rot′ic (ess″kuh·rot′ick). 1. Caustic; producing a slough. 2. A substance that produces an eschar; a caustic or corrosive. —**escharo′sis,** *n.*

Esch″er·ich′i·a (esh″ur·ick′ee·uh). A genus of nonsporeforming, Gram-negative bacteria, widely distributed in nature. **E. coli.** A normal inhabitant of the intestine of man and all vertebrates. It occasionally causes peritonitis and infections of the urinary tract.

es·cor′cin. Escorcinol, prepared from esculetin. One drop of a 10–20% aqueous solution is used in observation of corneal defects and lesions of the conjunctival epithelium; it imparts a red color to the lesions.

es″cu·le′tin, es·cu′le·tin. 6,7-Dihydroxycoumarin. A cleavage product of esculin.

es·cu·lin. A glycoside from the bark of the horse chestnut, *Aesculus hippocastanum.* Being fluorescent, it absorbs ultraviolet rays and has been used as a protective against the sun.

es·cutch′eon. The pattern of the pubic hair growth which differs in men and women.

-ese. *In biochemistry,* a suffix denoting an enzyme which exerts a synthetic action.

e·ser′i·dine (eh·serr′i·deen, ·din). An alkaloid found in Calabar beans. Syn. *geneserine.*

es′er·ine (ess′ur·een, ·in). Physostigmine.

Esmarch, Johann Friedrich August von [*German military sur-*

geon, 1823–1908]. Celebrated in surgical annals for his introduction of the first-aid packet for use on the battlefield (1869). Devised the widely used rubber bandage and tourniquet, a pure rubber elastic bandage about three inches in width, of great value in operations upon limbs where a bloodless field is desired. His name is associated also with a chloroform inhaler which consists of a drop bottle and a wire frame over which is stretched a double layer of gauze; adapted to the open method of ether inhalation. A resourceful surgeon, he devised a number of operations, including an amputation at the hip joint, which bore his name but are now obsolete.

e·soph″a·gec′to·my. Surgical resection of part of the esophagus.

e·soph′a·go-, e·soph′a·go- (e-sof′-uh-go-), e·soph′a·g-, oe·soph′a·g-. A combining form denoting *relation to the esophagus.*

e·soph′a·go·scope″ (i-sof′uh-go-scope″, ee″so·fag′o-). An electrically illuminated instrument for direct visualization of the interior of the esophagus. —esophagos′copy, *n.*

e·soph″a·go·ste·no′sis. Constriction of the esophagus.

e·soph′a·gus, oe·soph′a·gus. The gullet; the musculomembranous canal, about nine inches in length, extending from the pharynx to the stomach. —esophag′eal, *adj.*

es″o·pho′ri·a. Form of heterophoria in which the visual lines tend inward.

es″o·tro′pi·a. Convergent concomitant strabismus; one eye fixes upon an object and the other deviates inward.

ESR. Erythrocyte sedimentation rate.

es′sence. 1. That which gives to anything its character or peculiar quality. 2. A solution of an essential oil in alcohol.

es·sen′tial. 1. Pertaining to the essence of a substance. 2. Of diseases, idiopathic; occurring without a known cause.

es′ter. A compound formed from an alcohol and an acid by elimination of water, as ethyl acetate, $CH_3CO.OC_2H_5$.

es′ter·ase (ess′tur·ace, ·aze). Any enzyme which catalyzes the hydrolysis of an ester into an alcohol and an acid. acetylcholine e. An enzyme found in the blood which rapidly hydrolyzes any excess of acetylcholine to acetic acid and choline.

es·the′si·a (ess·thee′zhuh, ·zee·uh). Capacity for perception, feeling, or sensation. Opposed to *anesthesia.*

s·the′si·o-, aes·the′si·o- (ess-thee′zee-o-, ·see-o-). A combining form meaning *pertaining to the perceptive faculties.*

es·the″si·om′e·ter. An instrument for measuring tactile sensibility.

es·thet′ic, aes·thet′ic. Of or pertaining to the senses, sensation, or feelings; especially, pertaining to an appreciation of beauty.

es″thi·om′e·ne (ess″thee-om′i-nee). A term applied to the chronic ulcerative lesion of the vulva in venereal lymphogranuloma.

estinyl. Trade-mark for ethinyl estradiol.

es′ti·val, aes′ti·val (es′ti·vul, es-tye′vul). Of, or belonging to, the summer.

es·tra·di′ol (es″truh·dye′ol). 3,17-Dihydroxy-1,3,5-estratriene. An estrogenic hormone secreted in the ovarian follicular fluid and placenta. It is also found in pregnancy urines. Syn., *dihydrotheelin.* ethinyl e., ethynyl e. $C_{20}H_{24}O_2$. An orally active, synthetic estrogen. See *estinyl, lynoral.*

es′trin. Old term for estrogen.

es′tri·ol (es′tree-ole, ·ol). A crystalline estrogenic hormone, 3,16,17-trihydroxy-1,3,5-estratriene, from human pregnancy urine. Formerly called *theelol.*

es′tro·gen. Any substance possessing the biologic activity of estrus-producing hormones, either occurring naturally or prepared synthetically. —es·trogen′ic, *adj.*

es′trone. 3-Hydroxy-17-keto-1,3,5-estratriene. An estrogenic hormone present in the ovary, adrenal glands, placenta, and urine. Syn., *theelin.*

es′trus, oes′trus (es′trus). 1. Sexual desire in the lower animals; the mating period of animals, especially of the female; heat; rut. 2. The whole sequence of changes in the uterine mucosa of animals, corresponding to the various phases of ovarian activity. —estrous, estrual, *adj.*

etamon chloride. Trade-mark for tetraethylammonium chloride, $(C_2H_5)_4$·NCl, available in solution for parenteral use. See *tetraethylammonium.*

eth′ane. A saturated, gaseous hydrocarbon, $CH_3.CH_3$; found in natural and illuminating gas. Syn., *methylmethane.*

eth″ane·di·sul′fon·ate. A salt containing the anion $(CH_2SO_3)_2^=$.

eth′a·nol. Ethyl alcohol.

eth″chlor·vy′nol. Ethyl β-chlorovinyl ethynyl carbinol, a hypnotic agent. See *placidyl.*

e′ther, ae′ther. 1. An all-pervading and permeating medium, formerly believed to exist and to transmit light and similar energy. 2. A compound formed hypothetically from H_2O by the substitution of two hydrocarbon radicals for the H. 3. Ethyl ether $(C_2H_5)_2O$; a thin, colorless, volatile, and highly inflammable liquid. Its chief use is as an anesthetic. Also called *ethyl oxide, sulfuric ether, diethyl ether, diethyl*

oxide, although the United States Pharmacopeia recognizes as *ethyl oxide* a less pure form of the substance for use as a solvent. —**ethe'real**, *adj.* **anesthetic e.** Ethyl ether. See under *ether*, 3. **compound e. spirit.** A solution containing 32.5% ethyl oxide, and 2.5% of ethereal oil, by volume, in alcohol. Used as an anodyne and antispasmodic. Also called *Hoffmann's anodyne.* **e. spirit.** A solution containing 32.5% by volume of ethyl oxide in alcohol; used like compound ether spirit. Also called *Hoffmann's drops.* **ethyl e.** See under *ether*, 3. **isopropenyl vinyl e.** See propethylene *e.* **nitrous e.** Ethyl nitrite. **propenyl ethyl e.** $CH_3CH:CH.O.C_2H_5$. An inhalation anesthetic which produces irritation of the upper respiratory tract. **propethylene e.** Isopropenyl vinyl ether. $H_2C:C(CH_3).O.CH:CH_2$. An inhalation anesthetic less volatile and more potent than ether. **vinyl e.** $CH_2:CH.O.CH:CH_2$. An inhalation anesthetic used for short operations. Syn., *divinyl ether.* See *vinethene.*

eth'ics. A system of moral principles. **medical e.** The principles of ethical conduct and practices for members of the medical profession.

eth"in·am'ate. 1-Ethynylcyclohexyl carbamate, a hypnotic agent. See *valmid.*

17-eth·i·nyl"tes·tos'ter·one, 17-eth·y·nyl"tes·tos'ter·one. Anhydrohydroxyprogesterone.

eth'mo-. A combining form signifying *ethmoid.*

eth"mo·fron'tal. Relating to the ethmoid and frontal bones.

eth'moid. 1. A bone of the base of the skull perforated for the olfactory nerves and forming the upper bony nose. 2. Relating to the ethmoid bone. See Table of Bones in the Appendix. —**ethmoi'dal**, *adj.*

eth"moid·ec'to·my. Surgical removal of the ethmoid sinuses or part of the ethmoid bone.

eth"moid·i'tis. Inflammation of the ethmoid bone or of the ethmoid sinuses.

eth"mo·tur'bi·nal. Relating to the turbinal portions of the ethmoid bone, forming what are known as the superior and middle turbinates.

eth'nic. Pertaining to races and to their traits and customs.

eth·nog'ra·phy. A description of the races of mankind.

eth"o·pro'pa·zine hy"dro·chlo'ride. 10-(2-Diethylaminopropyl)phenothiazine hydrochloride, a parasympatholytic agent. See *parsidol hydrochloride.*

eth"o·to'in. 5-Ethyl-5-phenylhydantoin, an anticonvulsant. See *peganone.*

eth·ox'y-. A combining form denoting the univalent radical C_2H_5O.

eth"ox·ol'a·mide. 6-Ethoxy-2-benzothiazolesulfonamide, a diuretic. See *cardrase.*

eth'yl. The monovalent radical, C_2H_5—. **e. acetate.** $CH_3CO.OC_2H_5$. A colorless, pleasantly odorous liquid used chiefly as a solvent and in artificial fruit essences. Syn., *acetic ether.* **e. alcohol.** See *alcohol*, 2. **e. aminobenzoate.** $H_2N.C_6H_4.CO.OC_2H_5$. A white, crystalline powder used as a local anesthetic. Syn., *benzocaine.* See *anesthesin.* **e. carbamate.** $H_2N.CO.OC_2H_5$. Colorless crystals, easily soluble in water. A somnifacient, also used in treating myeloid and lymphatic leukemia, it has brought about disappearance of nodules of anaplastic undifferentiated cancer. Syn., *urethan.* **e. cellulose.** A product useful for increasing the viscosity of aqueous or oily liquids and as a dispersing agent. **e. chaulmoograte.** The ethyl esters of the mixed acids of chaulmoogra oil; used in leprosy. **e. chloride.** $CH_3.CH_2Cl$. A colorless liquid. Acts as a local anesthetic of short duration through the superficial freezing produced by rapid vaporization from the skin. **e. chlorophyllide.** The chief constituent of crystalline chlorophyll, *q.v.* **e. green.** See *brilliant green.* **e. nitrite.** $C_2H_5O.NO$. A pale yellow liquid of pleasant ethereal odor. Syn., *nitrous ether.* **e. nitrite spirit.** An alcoholic solution of 3.5–4.5% of ethyl nitrite. A popular diaphoretic in mild fevers. Also called *spirit of nitrous ether, sweet spirit of niter.* **e. parahydroxybenzoate.** A preservative

eth'yl·ene. Ethene; olefiant gas, C_2H_4. A colorless gas of slightly sweet odor and taste; used as an inhalation anesthetic. The ripening of certain fruits is hastened by its application. **e. glycol.** $HOCH_2CH_2OH$. A colorless, viscid hygroscopic liquid of sweet taste. It has been used in the manufacture of some pharmaceutical products intended only for external use. It is markedly toxic. Also called *glycol, ethylene alcohol.* **e. oxide.** $(CH_2)_2O$. A colorless gas used as a fumigant. See *carboxide.* **e. series.** A group of hydrocarbons of the general formula, C_nH_{2n}, having one double bond. Also called *ethene, alkene series.*

eth"yl·ene·di"a·mine' (eth"i·leen dye"uh·meen', ·dye'uh·meen). $H_2N.CH_2.CH_2.NH_2$. A colorless, strongly alkaline liquid of ammoniacal odor. It is used to increase the solubility of certain medicinal substances. **e. dihydrochloride.** A urine acidifier.

eth"yl·ene·di"a·mine·tet"ra·ace'tic ac'id. A synthetically produced amino acid of which the water soluble salts are powerful chelating and sequestering agents, and the di sodium salt prevents the coagulation of blood. Abbreviated, EDTAA.

eth″yl·e·phed′rine (eth″il·eh·fed′rin, ·ef′i·dreen). *l*-N-Ethylephedrine hydrochloride, a white, odorless, crystalline compound having pharmacologic action and toxicity similar to *l*-ephedrine hydrochloride. See *nethamine*.

eth″yl·hy″dro·cu′pre·ine (·high″dro·cue′pree·een, ·in). A synthetic derivative of cupreine; it is also related to quinine and possesses the latter's antimalarial and anesthetic action. See *optochin*. **e. hydrochloride.** A 1 or 2% solution is instilled into the conjunctival sac in pneumococcic infections of the eye. See *optochin*.

eth″yl·mor′phine hy″dro·chlo′ride (eth″il·mor′feen, ·fin). A sedative used especially in diseases of the bronchi. Syn., *dionin*.

N-eth″yl·pi·per′i·dine. C₆H₁₀NC₂H₅. A compound used in a chemical assay for penicillin-G.

eth″yl·stib′a·mine (eth″il·stib′uh·meen, ·min). A nonproprietary title for the trade-marked product neostibosan.

e″ti·o·la′tion. Pallor caused by the exclusion of light.

e″ti·ol′o·gy. The science or study of the causes of disease, both direct and predisposing, and the mode of their operation; not synonymous with cause or pathogenesis of disease. **—etiolog′ic,** *adj.*

e″ti·o·path′o·gen′e·sis. The cause and course of development of a disease or lesion.

Eu. Chemical symbol for europium.

Eu″bac·te′ri·a′les (yoo″back·teer″ee·ay′leez). An order of Schizomycetes, including forms least differentiated and least specialized; the true bacteria. According to Bergey, suborder I, the Eubacteriineae, is composed of the following 13 families: Nitrobacteriaceae, Pseudomonadaceae, Azotobacteriaceae, Rhizobiaceae, Micrococcaceae, Neisseriaceae, Lactobacteriaceae, Corynebacteriaceae, Achromobacteriaceae, Enterobacteriaceae, Parvobacteriaceae, Bacteriaceae, and Bacillaceae. Suborder II, the Caulobacteriineae, is composed of five families: Nevskiaceae, Gallionellaceae, Caulobacteriaceae, Siderocapsaceae, and Pasteuriaceae. Suborder III, the Rhodobacteriineae, is composed of three families: Thiorhodaceae, Athiorhodaceae, and Chlorobacteriaceae.

eu·caine′ hy″dro·chlo′ride (yoo·cane′, yoo·kay′in). The hydrochloride of benzoyl vinyl-diacetone alkamine, a local anesthetic introduced as a substitute for cocaine but rarely used today. Also called *betaeucaine hydrochloride*.

eu″ca·lyp′tene (yoo″kuh·lip′teen). C₁₀H₁₆. A terpene derived from eucalyptol. **e. hydrochloride.** Eucalypteol, *q.v.*

eu″ca·lyp′te·ol. C₁₀H₁₆.2HCl. Eucalyptene hydrochloride. Yellowish crystals; camphorlike odor. Formerly used like eucalyptol. Syn., *terpilene dihydrochloride*.

eu″ca·lyp′tol. Cineol. A substance obtained from the volatile oil of Eucalyptus. A mild local irritant; used in bronchitis, coryza, etc.

eu″ca·lyp′tus. The leaf of *Eucalyptus globulus*, formerly used medicinally. **e. gum.** The dried gummy exudate from *E. camaldulensis* containing 46% kinotannic acid; used as an astringent. **e. oil.** A volatile oil from the leaves of *E. globulus*; contains eucalyptol. Used as a stimulant antiseptic.

eu·cat′ro·pine hy″dro·chlo′ride (yoo·cat′ro·peen, ·pin). A white powder freely soluble in water; used as a mydriatic of brief duration. See *euphthalmine*.

eu″chlor·hy′dri·a (yoo″klor·high′dree·uh, ·hid′ree·uh). Presence of a normal amount of hydrochloric acid in the gastric juice.

eu·chro′ma·tin. 1. The deeply staining substance of the chromosomes, rich in nucleic acid, which is genetically active (contains the genes). 2. The substance of the euchromosomes, more usually called autosomes, in contrast to the substance of heterochromosomes. See *heterochromatin*. **—euchromat′ic,** *adj.*

eu·chro″ma·top′si·a. Capacity for correct recognition of colors.

eu′co·dal. A synthetic, narcotic alkaloid, dihydro-hydroxycodeinone hydrochloride. Used for pain, spasmodic cough, and as a miotic.

eucupin. Trade-mark for isoamylhydrocupreine, a local anesthetic.

eu″es·the′si·a (yoo″ess·thee′zhuh, ·zee·uh). The sense of well-being; vigor and normal condition of the senses.

euflavine. Trade-mark for acriflavine.

eugallol. Trade-mark for a brand of pyrogallol monoacetate.

Eu·ge′ni·a. A genus of trees and shrubs of the Myrtaceae, mostly tropical. **E. caryophyllata.** A species which yields cloves.

eu·gen′ics. The applied science concerned with improving the genetic constitution of a stock or race, usually limited now to man. **Positive eugenics** includes all those measures under social control which aim to increase the families of the better types; **negative eugenics,** those measures which aim to decrease the worse types. **—eugenic,** *adj.*

eu′ge·nol. 4-Allyl-2-methoxyphenol.

A colorless or pale yellow liquid obtained from clove oil and other sources. Used as a local anesthetic and antiseptic.

eu·glob'u·lin. True globulin; a globulin fraction insoluble in distilled water but soluble in dilute salt solutions. Also see *pseudoglobulin*.

eu·gnath'ic (yoo·nath'ick, ·nay'·thick). Pertaining to jaws that are well developed and in proper relation to each other.

eu·gon'ic. Growing luxuriantly; used to describe bacterial cultures.

eu"ki·ne'si·a (yoo"ki·nee'shuh, ·zhuh). Normal power of movement.

eumydrin. Trade-mark for a brand of atropine methylnitrate.

eu'nuch (yoo'nuck). A male whose testes have been removed. **—eunuch·ism,** *n.*

eu'nuch·oid·ism (yoo'nuck·oyd·iz·um). A condition in which the testes are present but physiologically inactive. **—eunuchoid,** *adj.*

eu·on'y·mus. The dried bark of *E. atropurpureus;* used as a cathartic. Syn., *wahoo bark.*

eu'pa·ral. A mixture of resins used as a mounting medium for histologic sections. The colorless form lacks (the green form contains) a copper salt for intensification of hematoxylin stain.

Eu"pa·to'ri·um. A genus of composite-flowered plants. The leaves and flowering tops of *E. perfoliatum,* thoroughwort or boneset, are used principally by the laity, as a bitter tonic, diaphoretic, and feeble emetic.

eu·pav'er·in. A synthetic alkaloid, related to papaverine. It is antispasmodic for smooth muscle.

eu·pho'ni·a. A normal, good, and clear condition of the voice.

Eu·phor'bi·a. A genus of plants of the Euphorbiaceae. **E. corollata** and **E. ipecacuanhae,** the American species, were formerly employed in medicine because of their emetic and cathartic properties. **E. pilulifera** of South America and Australia is used in asthma and bronchitis. **E. resinifera** of Africa produces euphorbium.

Eu·phor"bi·a·ce·ae. A plant family of herbs, shrubs, or trees.

eu·phor'bi·um. The dried resinous latex from *Euphorbia resinifera.* It is strongly purgative and vesicant; now mainly employed in veterinary medicine.

eu·pho'ri·a. *In psychology,* the exaggerated sense of well-being. **—eu·phor'ic,** *adj.*

euphthalmine. Trade-mark for eucatropine hydrochloride; a mydriatic.

eu'ploid. *In biology,* having an exact multiple of the basic haploid number of chromosomes. **—euploidy,** *n.*

eu·prax'i·a. Normal and perfect performance of coördinated movements.

eu·qui'nine (yoo·kwye'nyne, yoo'·kwi·neen). Quinine ethylcarbonate, *q.v.*

eurax. Trade-mark for crotamiton.

euresol. Trade-mark for resorcinol monacetate, used in certain skin diseases.

eu"ro·don'ti·a. Dental caries.

eu·ro'pi·um. Eu = 152.0. A rare earth metal found in cerium minerals.

eu"ry·ce·phal'ic. Designating a head that is unusually broad. Sometimes used to designate a brachycephalic head with a cephalic index of 81 to 85.4. Also called *eurycephalous.*

eu"ry·gnath'ism (yoo"i·nath'iz·um, yoo·rig'nuh·thiz·um). A condition in which the jaws are unusually broad. **—eurygnath'ic, eurygnathous,** *adj.*

Eu·sta'chi·an (yoo·stay'kee·un, ·stay'shun). Pertaining to the auditory tube.

eu·sys·to·le (yoo·sis'to·lee). A normal contraction of the heart.

eu·tec'tic. *In physical chemistry,* the specific mixture of two or more substances which has the lowest melting point of any mixture of the substances. **e. mixture.** Through common usage, any mixture which has a lower melting point than the individual constituents; more usually a mixture which softens or melts at room temperature.

eu"tha·na'si·a (yoo"thuh·nay'shuh, ·zee·uh). 1. An easy or calm death. 2. The painless killing of people who are suffering from an incurable or painful disease.

eu·then'ics. The science which deals with the improvement of the human race by means of the betterment of living conditions. Also see *eugenics.* **—euthenist,** *n.*

eu·to'ci·a (yoo·to'shee·uh, ·see·uh). Natural or easy childbirth; normal labor.

e·vac'u·ant. 1. Emptying. 2. A medicine which empties an organ, especially the bowels; a purgative.

e·vac"u·a'tion. 1. The voiding of any matter either by the natural passages of the body or by an artificial opening; specifically, defecation. 2. *In military medicine,* the withdrawal of sick and wounded troops, as in **air evacuation.**

e·vac'u·a"tor. An instrument for the removal of fluid or particles from the bladder or intestine.

e·vag"i·na'tion (i·vadj"i·nay'·shun). Outpouching.

ev"a·nes'cent. Unstable; tending to vanish quickly.

e"ven·tra'tion. Protrusion of the abdominal viscera through the abdominal wall, as in ventral hernia, to be distinguished from evisceration, *q.v.* **e. of**

the diaphragm. A condition where there is defective muscular action of the diaphragm, as when the left leaf is abnormally high, not moving through the normal excursion.

e·ver'sion. A turning outward. **—evert', v.t. e. of the eyelid.** (a) A method of folding the lid upon itself for the purpose of exposing the conjunctival surface or sulcus. (b) Ectropion, q.v.

evi·dence. In legal medicine, the means by which the existence or non-existence of the truth or falsehood of an alleged fact is ascertained or made evident; proof, as of insanity. **circumstantial e.** Evidence which is beyond actual demonstration, but upon which conclusions are based. **expert e.** That given before a jury by an expert in any science, art, profession, or trade.

evipal, Trade-mark for hexobarbital, a rapidly acting narcotic.

evipal sodium. Trade-mark for hexobarbital sodium.

ev''i·ra'tion (ev''i·ray'shun, ee''vi·). 1. Castration; emasculation. 2. A psychic process in which there is a deep and permanent assumption of feminine qualities, with corresponding loss of manly qualities. In contrast to defemination.

e·vis''cer·a'tion. 1. Removal of the abdominal or thoracic viscera. 2. Protrusion of the viscera through an abdominal incision following an operation; burst belly. 3. Removal of the contents of an organ, such as the eye. **obstetric e.** Removal of the abdominal or thoracic viscera of a fetus to permit delivery.

ev''o·lu'tion. The view that present-day species of plants and animals have originated by descent with modification from preëxisting species. The development has been through a series of progressive changes, leading from the simpler and more generalized to the complex and more specialized forms, although there has been some retrogression and degeneration, as in parasitic forms.

e·vul'sion. Forcible tearing or plucking away of a part. See avulsion.

Ewing, James [American pathologist, 1866–1943]. Widely acclaimed for his evaluation of different varieties of tumors in a masterly work on neoplastic disease (1919). Described a form of bone sarcoma involving the shaft of the long bones, characterized by cells of endothelial type, and seen most frequently before the twentieth year; called Ewing's tumor, angioendothelioma, endothelial myeloma.

ex-. A prefix denoting beyond, from, off, out of, thoroughly, or without.

ex·ac''er·ba'tion (eg-zass''ur·bay'-shun, eck-sass''ur·). Increase in the manifestations of a disease.

ex''al·ta'tion. A mental state characterized by self-satisfaction, ecstatic joy, abnormal cheerfulness, optimism, or delusions of grandeur.

ex·am''i·na'tion. Investigation for the purpose of diagnosis. Qualified as: bimanual, digital, oral, physical, etc.

ex''an·the·ma, ex·an'them (pl. exanthemas, exanthems). 1. An eruption upon the skin. 2. Any eruptive fever such as measles or scarlet fever. **—exanthem'atous, exanthemat'ic,** adj.

ex''ca·va'tion. 1. A hollow or cavity, especially one with sharply defined edges. 2. Act or process of making hollow. **dental e.** (a) The cavity prepared in a tooth, prior to filling or the insertion of an inlay. (b) The preparation of such a cavity. **e. of the optic disk.** A cupping of the optic disk, which is more pronounced than the normal physiologic cupping, seen in glaucoma and certain other ophthalmic diseases. **rectouterine e.** [BNA]. The rectouterine pouch, q.v.; cul-de-sac.

ex''ca·va'tor. 1. An instrument like a gouge or scoop used to scrape away tissue. 2. A dental instrument for removing decayed matter from a tooth cavity.

ex·cer''e·bra'tion. Removal of the fetal brain in the process of embryotomy.

ex·cip'i·ent. Any substance combined with an active drug to give the latter an agreeable or convenient form.

ex·ci'sion (eck·sizh'un). The cutting out of a part; removal of a foreign body or growth from a part, organ, or tissue.

ex·cit''a·bil'i·ty (eck·sight''uh·bil'-i·tee). Readiness of response to a stimulus; irritability. **—excit'able,** adj.

ex''ci·ta'tion (eck''sigh·tay'shun). The act of stimulating or irritating an organ or tissue. **—excit'ing,** adj.; **excite',** v.t.

ex·clu'sion. 1. The process of extruding or shutting out. 2. A surgical operation by which part of an organ is disconnected from the rest, but not excised.

ex·co''ri·a'tion. Abrasion of a portion of the skin. **—exco'riate,** v.

ex'cre·ment. An excreted substance; the feces. **—exorementi'tious,** adj.

ex·cres'cence. Abnormal outgrowth upon the body.

ex·cre'ta. Waste material cast out or separated from an organism.

ex·cre·tin. That fraction of secretin which stimulates pancreatic secretion. Also see incretin.

ex·cre'tion. 1. The discharge of waste products. 2. The matter so discharged. **—ex'cretory,** adj., n.; **excrete',** v.t.

ex″cre·to·lic ac′id. A fatty acid occurring in feces.

ex·cur′sion. 1. A wandering from the usual course. 2. The extent of movement, as of the eyes from a central position, or of the chest during respiration.

ex·cy″clo·pho′ri·a. A latent outward tilting of the upper pole of the eye. See cyclophoria.

ex·cy″clo·tro′pi·a. A defect of vision in which the vertical median superior pole of the eye is turned outward.

ex″cys·ta′tion. The escape from a cyst by the bursting of the surrounding envelope; a stage in the life of an intestinal parasite which occurs after the parasite has been swallowed by the host.

ex·en″ter·a′tion. 1. Evisceration or surgical removal, as of the orbital contents. 2. Destruction of the cells of a sinus by removing the bony partitions and forming a single, large cavity, as of the petrosa.

ex′er·cise. Functional activity of the muscles; such activity when its purpose is the preservation or restoration of the health, or the development of physical prowess or athletic skill. **active e.** That done with the cooperation of, or voluntarily by, the patient. **passive e.** The moving of parts of the body by another without help or hindrance by the patient. **postural e.** That designed to improve posture for the correction of minor deformities. **underwater e.** That done under water so that buoyancy makes movement easy enough for weakened muscles to control.

ex″fe·ta′tion. Ectopic or extrauterine fetation.

ex·fo″li·a′tion. 1. The separation of bone or other tissue in thin layers; a superficial sequestrum. 2. A peeling and shedding of the horny layer of the skin. A normal process that may be exaggerated after an inflammation or as part of a skin disease. —**exfo′liative,** adj.

ex″ha·la′tion. 1. The giving off or sending forth in the form of vapor; expiration. 2. That which is given forth as vapor; emanation.

ex·haus′tion. 1. Loss of vital and nervous power from fatigue or protracted disease. 2. The pharmaceutical process of dissolving out one or more of the constituents of a crude drug by percolation or maceration. **e. from cold.** The condition seen when the body is no longer able to compensate for exposure to cold; marked by fatigue, drowsiness, and coma. **heat e.** Heat prostration.

ex″hi·bi′tion·ism. A sexual perversion in which pleasure is obtained by exposing the genitals to one of the opposite sex. —**exhibitionist,** n.

ex·hil′a·rant. 1. Exhilarating. 2. An agent to enliven and cheer the mind. —**exhilara′tion,** n.

ex″hu·ma′tion. Removal from the ground after burial; disinterment. —**exhume′,** v.

ex′o-, ex-. A prefix signifying outside, outer layer, out of.

ex′o·crine (eck′so·kryne, ·krin, ·kreen). Ecrine; applied to glands which deliver their secretion or excretion to an epithelial surface, either directly or by means of ducts.

ex″o·don′ti·a, ex″o·don′tics. The art and science of the extraction of teeth.

ex·og′a·my. Union of gametes of different ancestry; outbreeding; crossfertilization.

ex·og′e·nous (eck·sodj′i·nus), **ex″o·gen′ic, ex″o·ge·net′ic.** 1. Due to an external cause; not arising within the organism. 2. In physiology, pertaining to those factors in the metabolism of nitrogenous substances obtained from food.

ex″o·pho′ri·a. A type of heterophoria in which the visual lines tend outward.

ex″oph·thal′mos, ex″oph·thal′mus. Abnormal protrusion of the eyeball from the orbit. —**exophthal′mic,** adj.

ex″o·skel′e·ton. 1. The skeleton of invertebrates. 2. Bone in skin of vertebrates.

ex″os·mo′sis (eck″sos·mo′sis, eck″soz·), **ex′os·mose** (eck′sos·mohss, eck′soz·). Passage of a liquid outward through a porous membrane. —**exosmot′ic,** adj.

ex″os·to′sis. A bony outgrowth from the surface of a bone. —**exos′tosed, exostot′ic,** adj. **multiple osteocartilaginous exostoses.** An obscure, hereditary, and familial bone disease characterized by sessile tumors on the shaft or central tumors expanding the shaft of long bones. Occurs chiefly in males. Also called dyschondroplasia, chondro-osteoma.

ex″o·ther′mic, ex″o·ther′mal. 1. Relating to the giving out of energy, especially heat energy. 2. A substance formed with liberation of heat.

ex″o·tox′in. A toxin which is excreted by a living microörganism and can afterwards be obtained in bacteria-free filtrates without death or disintegration of the organisms. —**exotoxic,** adj.

ex″o·tro′pi·a. Divergent concomitant strabismus; occurring when one eye fixes upon an object and the other deviates outward.

ex·pan′sive. 1. Comprehensive; wide-extending. 2. *In psychiatry,* characterized by megalomania, euphoria, talkativeness, overgenerosity, grandiosity. **—expansiveness,** *n.*

x"pec·ta'tion of life. 1. *In biometry,* the average number of years lived by a group of individuals after reaching a given age, as determined by the mortality experience of a specific time and geographic area; mean afterlifetime. 2. Commonly, the probable number of years of survival for an individual of a given age.

x·pec'to·rant. 1. Promoting expectoration. 2. A remedy that promotes or modifies expectoration.

x·pec"to·ra'tion. 1. Ejection of material from the mouth. 2. The fluid or semifluid matter from the lungs and air passages expelled by coughing and spitting; sputum.

x·pel'. Drive or force out, as the fetus, by means of muscular contractions.

x·per'i·ment. A trial or test; a procedure undertaken to discover some unknown principle or effect, to test a hypothesis, or to illustrate a known principle or fact. **—experimen'tal,** *adj.;* **experimenta'tion,** *n.*

x'pert. A person specifically qualified in a certain subject, as a science or an art.

x"pi·ra'tion. Act of breathing forth or expelling air from the lungs. **—expi'ratory,** *adj.*

x"plan·ta'tion. Removal of living tissue from its habitat for cultivation in artificial mediums; tissue culture. **—explant',** *v.*

x"plo·ra'tion. The act of exploring for diagnostic purposes, through investigation of a part hidden from sight, by means of operation, by touch, by artificial light, or by instruments. **—explor'atory,** *adj.*

x·plor'er. An instrument, such as a probe, used in exploration. **—explore,** *v.*

x·po'sure. 1. Act of exposing or laying open. 2. State of being open to some action or influence that may affect detrimentally, as cold or wet. 3. *In radiology,* dose, *q.v.* **e. of person.** *In legal medicine,* the exhibiting of the genitalia in public, before a person of the opposite sex. Also called *indecent exposure.* See *exhibitionism.*

x·pres'sion. 1. Act of pressing out. The product of the act of pressing out. **e. of fetus.** Pressure exerted upon the uterus through the abdominal walls to aid in the expulsion of the fetus.

x·pul'sion. 1. Act of forcing out. 2. Summary dismissal from membership. **expulsive,** *adj.*

x·san'gui·nate. 1. Drain of blood. Bloodless. **—exsanguine,** *adj.;*

exsanguina'tion, exsanguin'ity, *n.*

ex·sic'cant. 1. Drying or absorbing moisture. 2. A dusting powder.

ex"sic·ca'tion. Act of drying; especially, depriving a crystalline body of its water of crystallization. **—exsic'cative,** *adj.*

ex·stro·phy. Eversion; the turning inside out of a part. **e. of bladder.** A congenital malformation in which the lower part of the abdominal wall, the anterior wall of the bladder, and usually the symphysis pubis are wanting, and the posterior wall of the bladder is pressed through the opening.

ext. *Extractum;* extract.

ex·ten'sion. 1. A straightening out, especially the muscular movement by which a flexed limb is made straight. 2. Traction upon a fractured or dislocated limb. **Counterextension** is traction made on a part in a direction opposite to that in which traction is made by another force.

ex·ten'sor. A muscle which extends or stretches a limb or part, as opposed to a *flexor.* See Table of Muscles in the Appendix.

ex·te"ri·or·i·za'tion. 1. *In psychiatry,* the act of objectivating one's interests; the turning of one's interests outward. 2. *In surgery,* the operation of marsupialization, *q.v.*

ex·ter'nal. 1. Exterior, acting from without. 2. *In anatomy,* on or near the outside of the body; away from the center or middle line of the body. 3. Not essential, superficial. **—externad,** *adv.*

ex·ter'nal·ize. 1. *In psychology,* transform an idea or impression which is in the percipient's mind into a phantasm apparently outside him. 2. Refer to some outside source, as the voices heard by the subject of hallucinations.

ex"ter·o·cep"tor (eck"stur·o·sep"-tur, eck"stur·o·sep'tur). An end organ, in or near the skin or a mucous membrane, which receives stimuli from the external world.

ex·tinc'tion. 1. The act of putting out or extinguishing; destruction. 2. *In psychology,* the disappearance of a conditioned reflex when excited repeatedly without reinforcement.

ex"tir·pa'tion. Complete removal of a part or surgical destruction of a part.

ex·tor'sion. 1. Outward rotation of a part. 2. *In ophthalmology,* a turning outward of the vertical meridians.

ex'tra-. A prefix denoting *outside of, beyond the scope of.*

ex"tra·cap'su·lar. Outside a capsule; outside the capsular ligament of a joint.

ex"tra·cel'lu·lar. External to the cells of an organism.

ex″tra·cra′ni·al. Outside of the cranial cavity.

ex′tract. A pharmaceutical preparation obtained by dissolving the active constituents of a drug with a suitable menstruum, evaporating the solvent, and adjusting to prescribed standards, generally so that one part of the extract represents four to six parts of the drug. Abbreviated, ext. **—extract′,** v. **fluid e.** See *fluidextract*. **liver e.** A water-soluble, thermostable preparation of a fraction of mammalian livers used in the therapy of pernicious anemia. **powdered e.** A powder form of an extract, more suitable for encapsulation. **protein e.** A protein substance dissolved out of materials such as foods or inhaled matter. Used in testing and treating allergic patients.

ex·trac′tion. 1. The act of drawing out. 2. The process of making an extract. **e. of cataract.** The surgical removal of a cataractous lens. **e. of tooth.** The surgical removal of a tooth from its alveolus.

ex·trac′tor. 1. An instrument or forceps for extracting bullets, sequestra, or foreign bodies. 2. *In dentistry*, an instrument for extracting the root of a tooth.

ex″tra·du′ral. Situated outside of or upon the dura.

ex″tra·mu′ral. Outside the wall of an organ.

ex″tra·sys′to·le (eck″struh·sis′to-lee). A heartbeat occurring before its normal time in the rhythm of the heart and followed by a compensatory pause, due to abnormal or re-entry stimuli in various parts of the heart—atria, ventricles, atrioventricular bundle, and even the nodes themselves—and named from the origin of the stimuli, as ventricular extrasystole. Also called *premature beat, premature contraction.* **interpolated e.** One of ventricular origin, occurring early in diastole and not disturbing the normal rhythm.

ex″tra·tu′bal. Outside of a tube, as the uterine tube.

ex″tra·u′ter·ine (·yōō′tur·in, ·yne). Outside of the uterus.

ex·trav′a·sa′tion. 1. Passing of a body fluid out of its proper place, as blood into surrounding tissues after rupture of a vessel, or urine after rupture of the bladder or urethra. 2. Material so discharged.

ex″tra·vas′cu·lar. Outside of a vessel.

ex·trem′i·ty. The distal, or terminal, end of any part. **lower e.** The hip, thigh, leg, ankle, and foot. **upper e.** The shoulder girdle, arm, forearm, wrist, and hand.

ex·trin′sic. Originating outside of part.

ex′tro·phy. 1. Malformation of a organ. 2. Incorrect spelling of exstrophy, q.v.

ex′tro·vert, ex′tra·vert. 1. O whose interests center in the outsi world rather than in subjective acti ity. 2. Turn one's interests to extern things rather than to oneself. **—extr vert′, extravert′,** v.

ex·tru′sion (ecks·trōō′zhun). 1. forcing out; expulsion. 2. *In dentistr* thrust out, as a tooth that extends b yond the occlusal plane. **—extrude** n., v.

ex′u·date. The material that h passed through the walls of vesse into adjacent tissues or spaces in i flammation. **fibrinous e.** One which fibrin is the main solid constit ent. **purulent e.** An exudate co taining a large proportion of pu **sanguineous e.** One containing vi ible blood. Also called *hemorrhagic*

ex″u·da′tion. The passage of vario constituents of the blood through t walls of vessels into adjacent tissues spaces in inflammation. **—exu′d tive,** adj.; **ex′udate,** v.

eye. The organ of vision. It occupi the anterior part of the orbit, and nearly spherical. It is composed three concentric coats: the sclero and cornea; the choroid, ciliary bod and iris; and the retina. **dom nant e.** The eye which is unco sciously and preferentially chosen guide decision and action.

eye′ball. The globe of the eye.

eye′brow″. The supercilium; the ar above the eye; the hair covering t arch.

eye′cup″. 1. The optic vesicle. 2. small cup which fits over the eye; us for bathing the conjunctiva.

eye ground. The fundus of the ey the internal aspect of the eye as se through an ophthalmoscope.

eye′lash″. One of the stiff hairs gro ing on the margin of the eyelid; a ciliu

eye′lid″. One of the two protecti coverings of the eyeball; a curtain movable skin lined with conjuncti having the tarsus, glands, and cilia the distal part, muscle in the proxim part. **fused eyelids.** (a) The no mal fusion between the epithelia of t fetal eyelid folds, occurring about t ninth week and persisting until t seventh or eighth month. (b) A co genital anomaly caused by the failu of the two fetal eyelids to separate

eye′wash″. A medicated solution the eye; a collyrium.

F. 1. Abbreviation for Fahrenheit, field of vision, formula. 2. Chemical symbol for fluorine.

F₁. The first filial generation. The offspring of a given mating.

F_1. The first filial generation. The offspring of a given mating.

F_2. The second filial generation. The grandchildren of a given mating.

Fa. Chemical symbol for francium.

fa·bel'la. A sesamoid fibrocartilage or small bone occasionally developed in a head of the gastrocnemius muscle.

F.A.C.D. Fellow of the American College of Dentists.

face. The anterior part of the head including forehead and jaws, but not the ears. See Table of Bones in the Appendix. —**fa'cial**, *adj.* **adenoid f.** One showing the characteristic openmouthed and stupid appearance associated with adenoid growths which interfere with nasal breathing. **bird f.** One characterized by a receding chin and beaklike appearance of the nose; the result of mandibular hypoplasia (micrognathia). **mask f.** A condition present in paralysis agitans; the facial muscles are fixed and do not react to motions. Also called *Parkinsonian mask*. **masklike f.** A face often seen in alcoholic multiple neuritis; expressionless and immobile between the eyes and lips, while the eyebrows, forehead, and lips may be moving freely.

fac'et (fass'it). A small plane surface, especially on a bone or a hard body; may be produced by wear, as a worn spot on the surface of a tooth.

fa'ci·es (fay'see·eez, ·shee·eez). 1. The appearance of the face. 2. A surface. **f. hippocratica.** An appearance of the face indicative of the rapid approach of dissolution: the nose is pinched, the temples hollow, the eyes sunken, the ears leaden and cold, the lips relaxed, the skin livid.

fa·cil'i·ta'tion. 1. Increased ease in carrying out an action or function. 2. The furtherance of neural activities by conditioning or by previous or simultaneous stimulation.

fa'ci·o-. A combining form denoting the face.

F.A.C.P. Fellow of the American College of Physicians.

F.A.C.S. Fellow of the American College of Surgeons.

fac'tor. 1. A circumstance, fact, or influence which tends to produce a result; a constituent. 2. *In biology*, a gene. 3. An essential or desirable element in diet. **accessory food factors.** Substances, present in foods, which are necessary to life, or for proper growth and development. See *vitamin*. **antianemia f.** A specific substance in the liver; effective in the treatment of pernicious anemia. Syn., *erythrocyte-maturing f.* **CH f.** A substance in liver extract that intervenes in the metabolic process to correct deficiencies of methionine or choline. It protects against lathyrism. **erythrocyte aggregation f.** A serum or plasma factor first discovered in cases of lupus erythematosus and demonstrable by cold conglutination tests. **external f.** An external component of the environment of an organism, as heat or gravity. **extrinsic f.** A substance in food, identified as vitamin B_{12}, which, with the intrinsic factor, makes an antianemic principle. **internal f.** An internal component of the environment of an organism. **intrinsic f.** A substance, produced by the stomach, which combines with the extrinsic factor in food to yield an antianemic principle; lack of the intrinsic factor is believed to be a cause of pernicious anemia. **Jarrell f.** A dominant hereditary blood factor; in persons lacking it, the presence of the antibody may be related to the development of cancer in some cases. **maturation f. of liver.** A substance believed to be stored in the liver which is necessary for the production of mature erythrocytes. Pernicious anemia is believed to be caused by the absence of this factor. **milk f.** A filtrable, noncellular agent in the milk and tissues of certain strains of inbred mice; transmitted from the mother to the offspring by nursing. It seems to be an essential factor in the genesis of mammary cancer in these strains. **Rh f.** See *Rh factor*. **semilethal f.** A gene which causes the death of the individual soon after development is completed or before reproductive age.

fac'ul·ta"tive. Voluntary; optional; having the power to do or not to do a thing.

fae'ces (fee'seez). See *feces*.

fa'gar·ine (fay'gur·een, fag'ur·). The name applied to the three alkaloids of *Fagara coco*, a tree of Argentina; they are differentiated by the prefixes α, β, and γ.

Fahr. Fahrenheit scale or thermometer. Also abbreviated F.

Fahrenheit, Gabriel Daniel [*German physicist*, 1686–1736]. The inventor of the thermometer and scale bearing his name, in which the interval between the freezing point of water

(32°) and its boiling point (212°) is divided into 180 degrees.

fail'ure. See *cardiac failure, circulatory failure, metabolic failure.*

faint. 1. Weak; wanting strength. 2. A state of syncope or swooning. 3. Swoon; suffer syncope. **—faint'ing,** *n.*

faith cure. The system or practice of treating disease by religious faith and prayer.

fal'ci·form (fal'si·form). Having the shape of a sickle.

false. Not genuine; not real; imitating.

falx. A sickle-shaped structure. **—fal'cial,** *adj.* **f. cerebelli.** A sicklelike process of dura mater between the lobes of the cerebellum. **f. cerebri.** The process of the dura mater separating the hemispheres of the cerebrum.

fa'mes (fay'meez). Hunger.

fa·mil'ial. Of, pertaining to, or occurring among, the members of a family, as a familial disease.

fam'i·ly. 1. A group of closely related persons; parents and children; those descended from a common ancestor. 2. *In biology,* a classification group higher than a genus; the principal division of an order.

fa·nat'i·cism. Perversion and excess of the religious sentiment; unreasoning zeal in regard to any subject. Sometimes a manifestation of mental disease.

fang. 1. A sharp or pointed tooth; especially, the tooth of a wild beast or serpent. 2. The root of a tooth. *Obs.*

fan"go·ther'a·py. Treatment with imported mud; used in arthritis or gout.

fan'ta·sy. 1. Imagination; the ability to form mental pictures of scenes, occurrences, or objects not actually present; fanciful, whimsical image making. 2. An image. Also see *phantasy.*

far'ad. The unit of electric capacitance, corresponding to one coulomb per volt. **—fa·rad'ic,** *adj.*

far'a·day. The quantity of electricity which will liberate one gram equivalent of an element in electrolysis. It equals 96,489 coulombs.

far'a·dism. 1. Induced rapidly alternating currents. 2. Faradization.

far"a·di·za'tion. Faradism; the therapeutic application of induced rapidly alternating currents to a diseased part. **—far'adize,** *v.*

far'a·do-. A combining form signifying *faradic.*

far"i·na'ceous. Having the nature of or yielding flour; starchy; containing starch.

far'-point". The most distant point at which an eye can see distinctly when accommodation is completely relaxed.

far'-sight". Hypermetropia. **—far'sight'edness,** *n.*

fas'ci·a (fash'ee·uh) (pl. *fasciae*). 1.

The areolar tissue layers under the skin (superficial fascia), or between muscles and forming the sheaths of muscles, or investing other deep, connective structures, as nerves and blood vessels (deep fascia). 2. A bandage. *Obs.* **—fascial,** *adj.* **Buck's f.** The deep fascia of the penis. Also called *f. penis.* **Camper's f.** The superficial, loose, fat-containing layer of the superficial fascia of the lower abdomen. **Colles' f.** The deep layer of the superficial perineal fascia. **cremasteric f.** A thin covering of the spermatic cord, enclosing the fibers of the cremaster muscle. **cribriform f.** The sievelike covering of the fossa ovalis of the thigh. **deep cervical f.** That which invests the muscles of the neck and encloses the vessels and nerves. It consists of three fascial planes, one surrounding the trapezius and sternocleidomastoid muscles, a second surrounding the cervical viscera, and a third, the prevertebral fascia. **external spermatic f.** The outer covering of the spermatic cord and testis, continuous with the aponeurosis of the external oblique muscle at the subcutaneous inguinal ring. **f. lata.** The dense fascia surrounding the muscles of the thigh. **f. lunata.** The deep fascia of the ischiorectal fossa. **intercolumnar f.** (a) fascia attached to the crura of the external inguinal ring. (b) That portion of the diaphragmatic pelvic fascia located between the two pubococcygeus muscles. **internal spermatic f.** The inner covering of the spermatic cord and testis, continuous with the transversalis fascia at the abdominal inguinal ring. **ischiorectal f.** That covering the perineal aspect of the levator ani muscle and filling the ischiorectal fossa. **lumbodorsal f.** Variously described as the sheath of the sacrospinalis muscle alone, or the sheaths of the sacrospinalis and the quadratus lumborum muscles. **palpebral f.** Fascia of the eyelids; orbital septum. **pectoral f.** Deep fascia over the pectoralis major muscle on the anterior aspect of the thorax. Also called *pectoralis f.* **prevertebral f.** The third layer of the deep cervical fascia; a band of connective tissue covering the front of the cervical vertebrae and the prevertebral muscles. It is attached to the esophagus and pharynx by loose connective tissue. **Scarpa's f.** The deep, membranous layer of the superficial fascia of the lower abdomen. **Sibson's f.** A domelike expansion of fascia strengthening the pleura over the apex of the lung, extending from the first rib to the transverse process of the seventh cervical vertebra. **transversalis f.** That

ing between the transversus abdominis muscle and the peritoneum. **Waldeyer's f.** That portion of the pelvic fascia surrounding the distal end of each ureter.

fas·cic″u·la″ted (fa-sick″yoo-lay″-tid). United into bundles or fascicles.

fas·cic″u·la′tion (fa-sick″yoo-lay″-shun). 1. An incoördinate contraction of skeletal muscle in which groups of muscle fibers innervated by the same neuron contract together. 2. The formation of fasciculi.

fas·cic′u·lus (fa-sick′yoo-lus). 1. In histology, a bundle of nerve, muscle, or tendon fibers separated by connective tissue; as that of muscle fibers, by perimysium. 2. In neurology, a bundle or tract of nerve fibers presumably having common connections and functions. Also see tract. —**fascicular,** adj. **dorsal longitudinal f.** A bundle of long association fibers in the cerebrum, connecting the frontal lobe with the occipital and temporal lobes. **f. cuneatus.** The lateral part of the dorsal funiculus. Also called Burdach's column. **f. gracilis.** The medial part of the dorsal funiculus of the spinal cord carrying proprioceptive impulses from the lower regions of the trunk and legs. Also called Goll's column. **f. interfascicularis.** Comma tract, q.v. **f. proprius.** That which immediately surrounds the gray columns of the spinal cord, containing short ascending and descending correlation fibers. Syn., ground bundle. **f. retroflexus.** A bundle of nerve fibers connecting the habenular nucleus with the interpeduncular nucleus. It is concerned with olfactory impulses. Syn., habenulopeduncular tract. Also called Meynert's bundle. **inferior longitudinal f.** A bundle of long association fibers coursing horizontally in the lateral wall of the inferior and posterior horns of the lateral ventricle, extending from the occipital to the temporal lobe. **medial longitudinal f.** One of two heavily medullated bundles close to the midline, just ventral to the central gray matter and extending from the upper spinal cord to the rostral end of the midbrain. **occipitofrontal f.** A bundle of long association fibers extending from the cortex of the frontal lobe to the cortex of the occipital lobe. **occipitothalamic f.** A bundle of nerve fibers connecting the thalamus with the occipital lobe. **subcallosal f.** A tract of long association fibers lying under the corpus callosum and connecting the frontal, parietal, and occipital lobes. **uncinate f.** A bundle of medullated fibers extending between the uncus and the basal portions of the frontal lobe and connecting the orbital gyri of the

frontal lobe with the rostral part of the temporal lobe. Also called unciform f.

fas″ci·ec′to·my (fash″ee-eck′to-mee, fass″ee·). Surgical excision of fascia; specifically, excision of strips from the lateral part of the fascia lata (iliotibial tract) for use in plastic surgery.

fas·ci′num. Belief that certain persons possess the so-called evil eye; a frequent delusion expressed by patients with the paranoid form of schizophrenia.

fas′ci·o- (fash′ee·o-, fass′ee·o-). In anatomy, a combining form for fascia.

fas″ci·od′e·sis (fash″ee-od′i-sis, fass″ee·). The operation of suturing a tendon to a fascia.

Fas·ci′o·la (fa-sigh′o-luh, fa-see′·). A genus of trematodes. **F. hepatica.** A species which is a natural parasite of sheep and cattle and, occasionally, man.

fas″ci·o·li′a·sis. Infestation with the Fasciola hepatica; normally occurs in sheep and other herbivorous animals, but man has served as an accidental host. The liver is usually the site of infestation. Also called liver rot.

Fas″ci·o·loi′des (fass″ee-o-loy′deez, fash″ee·o·). A genus of digenetic trematodes. **F. magna.** A species of flukes occurring in the liver, rarely the lungs, of cattle and other herbivores in North America and northern Europe.

Fas″ci·o·lop·si′a·sis (fash″ee-o-lop-sigh′uh-sis, fass″ee-o·). Intestinal infestation of man and the hog by the Fasciolopsis buski; characterized by toxic diarrhea with visceral complications in severe cases.

Fas″ci·o·lop′sis. A genus of flukes parasitic in both man and the hog. **F. buski.** Largest intestinal fluke of man; endemic only in the Orient; the causative organism of fasciolopsiasis.

fas′ci·o·plas″ty. Plastic surgery upon fascia.

fas″ci·or·rha·phy. Suture of cut or lacerated fascia.

fas″ci·ot′o·my (fash″ee-ot′o-mee, fass″ee·). Incision of a fascia.

fas·ci′tis (fass-eye′tis, fash-eye′tis). Inflammation of a fascia.

fast. 1. Resistant to the action of a drug or chemical, especially to the action of a stain. 2. Refrain from eating. **-fast.** A combining form meaning securely attached, narrowly confined, as in bedfast; resistant to a (specified) dye, chemical agent, or microörganism, as in acid-fast.

fas·tig′i·um (fas-tidj′ee-um). 1. The acme of a disease. 2. The angle between the superior lamina and the inferior medullary velum in the roof of the fourth ventricle.

fat. Any of a class of naturally occurring mixtures consisting of glyceryl esters of certain acids (in animal fat chiefly oleic, palmitic, and stearic). **—fat'ty,** *adj.* **depot f.** Fat occurring in certain regions like the abdominal wall or the buttocks, which are called fat depots.

fa'ther. 1. Male parent. 2. Beget.

fat'i·ga·ble. Susceptible to fatigue; easily tired. **—fatigableness, fatigabil'ity,** *n.*

fa·tigue'. 1. Exhaustion of strength; weariness from exertion. 2. Condition of cells or organs in which, through overactivity, the power or capacity to respond to stimulation is diminished or lost. 3. Induce a condition of fatigue in. 4. Become weary. 5. Suffer fatigue. **battle f.** A euphemism for a neurotic or psychotic reaction developed in combat. Formerly called *shellshock.* **flying f.** (a) That occurring in flyers. (b) A euphemism for a neurosis occurring in flyers. **operational f.** A euphemism for a neurosis developed during combat flying.

fat'-sol'u·ble. Soluble in fats or fat solvents; specifically, used with a letter to designate certain vitamins, as fat-soluble A.

fau'ces (faw'seez). The space surrounded by the soft palate, palatine arches, and base of the tongue. **—fau'cial,** *adj.*

fau'na. The entire animal life peculiar to any geographic area or geologic period.

fa·ve'o·late. Honeycombed; alveolate.

fa·ve'o·lus. A pit or cell like that of the honeycomb. See *foveola.*

fa'vi·des (fay'vi·deez). Allergic skin reactions to favus.

fa'vism (fay'viz·um, fah'viz·um). An acute hemolytic anemia, common in Sicily and Sardinia; caused by sensitivity to the broad bean, *Vicia faba.* May result from ingestion of the seeds or from inhalation of the pollen. Also called *fabism, fabismus.*

fa'vus (fay'vus, fah'vus). A parasitic skin disease due to the presence of the vegetable parasite, *Trichophyton schoenleini, T. violaceum,* or *Microsporum gypseum.* It is characterized by the presence of round, sulfur-yellow, cup-shaped crusts **(favus cups)** having a peculiar mousy odor. This crust formation, scutulum, is found on microscopic examination to contain the elements of the fungus. The disease affects the scalp most frequently, but may occur elsewhere. Syn., *tinea favosa.*

F.D.I. *Fédération Dentaire Internationale;* International Dental Federation.

Fe. Chemical symbol for iron.

fear. An emotion marked by dread, apprehension, or alarm. An irrational

and persistent fear is called a phobia q.v.

fear re·ac'tion. A euphemism for neurosis, particularly one developed combat, in which anxiety is manifeste by the conscious fear of a particula object or event.

fea'ture. Any single part or lineament of a structure, as of the face.

feb'ri·fa'cient (feb"ri·fay'shunt Producing fever.

fe'brile (fee'bril, feb'ril). Pertaining to or characterized by fever.

feb"ri·pho'bi·a. A morbid fear fever; pyrexeophobia.

fe·ca·lith (fee'kuh·lith, feck'uh·). concretion or calcified mass of fec material; coprolith.

fe'cal·oid (fee'kuh·loyd, feck'uh. Resembling feces.

fe'ces, fae'ces (fee'seez). The excr tions of the bowels. The excretio from the intestine of unabsorbed foo indigestible matter, and intestin secretions. **—fe'cal,** *adj.*

fec'u·la. 1. The starchy part of a see 2. The sediment subsiding from an in fusion.

fec'u·lent. 1. Having sediment. Excrementitious.

fe"cun·da'tion (fee"kun·day'shu feck"un·). The act of fertilizin **—fe'cundate,** *v.t.* **artificial** Artificial insemination, q.v.

fe·cun'di·ty. The innate potent reproductive capacity of the individu organism, as denoted by its ability form and separate from the bo mature germ cells. **—fe'cund,** *adj.*

fee"ble·mind'ed·ness. Mental d ficiency, q.v.

feed'ing. The taking or giving food. **artificial f.** (a) The introduc tion of food into the body by means artificial devices. (b) The nourishi of an infant by any means other tha breast milk. **extrabuccal f.** The i troduction of food into the system channels other than the mouth; fee ing by nutritive enema, by intravasc lar injection, or through gast fistulas. **forced f.** The administr tion of food against the will of t patient. **sham f.** That in which t food is swallowed and then diverted the exterior by fistula or other mean

feel'ing. 1. The sense of touch. 2. sensation, as a sensation of touc bodily consciousness, temperatu pain. 3. An emotion or emotional sta 4. *In psychology,* any conscious pro ess; consciousness, including sensatic thought, and emotion. 5. Of great se sibility; easily moved. **—feel,** *v.*

fee split'ting. A division of the co sultant's fee between consultant a referring physician.

fel·la'ti·o (feh·lay'shee·o). An act sexual perversion in which the penis introduced into the mouth of another; friction by the lips or tongue produces the orgasm. Syn., *irrumation*.

fel'on. A deep infection in the distal closed space on the palmar surface of a finger; it may progress to osteomyelitis of the distal phalanx.

e'male. 1. Pertaining to the sex which produces the ovum. Symbol, ◯, ♀. (That of the male is ◻, ♂.) 2. Denoting that part of a double-limbed instrument that receives the complementary part.

em'i·nism. The presence in a male of various mental and physical approximations to the characters of the female sex. **—feminiza'tion,** *n.*

em″o·ro·tib'i·al. Relating to the femur and the tibia.

e'mur (pl. *femora*). 1. Thigh bone. See Table of Bones in the Appendix. 2. Old term for the thigh. **—fem'oral,** *adj.* **pilastered f.** A femur with exaggerated backward concavity and prominent linea aspera.

e·nes'tra (pl. *fenestrae*). 1. *In anatomy*, a name given to two apertures of the medial tympanic wall of the ear; the **fenestra cochleae** or round window and the **fenestra vestibuli** (or **fenestra ovalis**) or oval window. 2. An opening in a bandage or plaster splint for examination, drainage, etc. 3. The open space in the blade of a forceps. **—fenestral,** *adj.*

en″es·tra'tion. 1. The presence of fenestrae or openings in a structure. 2. An operation to create a permanently mobile window in the lateral semicircular canal; used in cases of deafness caused by stapedial impediment to sound waves. Sometimes referred to as *Lempert operation.* **—fenes'trated,** *adj.*

n'nel. The dried, ripe fruit of cultivated varieties of *Foeniculum vulgare.* **en'nel oil.** A volatile oil distilled from the seeds of the herb *Foeniculum vulgare*, which contains anethole, used as a carminative and as a flavoring.

eosol. A trade-mark for certain preparations of ferrous sulfate.

er″-de-lance' (fair″-duh-lahns′, -lans′). A large, venomous snake of Central America; the *Bothrops atrox.*

er'ment. A catalytic agent produced by, and associated with, a living organism (*organized ferment*), as distinguished from an enzyme which may be separated from the living organism (*unorganized ferment*). This distinction is no longer commonly made, having been replaced by intracellular and extracellular enzymes. See under *enzyme.*

er″men·ta'tion. The decomposition of complex molecules under the influence of ferments or enzymes.

acetic f. The fermentation whereby weak alcoholic solutions are converted into vinegar. **alcoholic f.** That resulting in the conversion of carbohydrates into alcohol. **butyric f.** That resulting in the conversion of sugars, starches, milk, etc., into butyric acid. **caseous f.** That resulting in the conversion of milk into cheese. **lactic f.** That resulting in the souring of milk.

fer'ra·ted. Combined with iron; containing iron.

fer'ri-. A combining form indicating *ferric* compounds, *containing iron as a trivalent element.*

fer'ric. 1. Pertaining to or of the nature of iron. 2. Containing iron as a trivalent element.

fer'ri·cy·a·nide. A salt containing the trivalent [Fe(CN)$_6$] anion.

fer'ri·heme. Heme in which the ferrous iron normally present is in the ferric, or oxidized, state and which may form hematin in alkaline solution or hemin in hydrochloric acid solution.

fer″ri·he″mo·glo'bin. Methemoglobin.

fer'ri·tin. A protein, containing a variable amount of iron, occurring in various tissues of humans and animals. See *apoferritin.*

fer'ro-. A combining form generally used to indicate a *ferrous* compound; sometimes to designate a *substance containing metallic iron.*

fer″ro·cy·a·nide. A salt containing the divalent [Fe(CN)$_6$] anion.

fer'ro·heme. See *heme.*

fer″ro·he″mo·glo'bin. Hemoglobin in which the iron is normally in the ferrous state.

fer″ro·ther'a·py. Treatment of disease by the use of iron compounds.

fer'rous. Containing iron in divalent form.

fer·ru'gi·nous. 1. Chalybeate. 2. Having the color of iron rust.

fer'rum. See *iron.*

fer'tile. Prolific; fruitful. **—fertil'ity,** *n.*

fer·til'i·ty clin'ic. A clinic to diagnose the causes of sterility in human beings and to assist reproductive ability; often called *sterility clinic.*

fer″ti·li·za'tion. The act of making fruitful; impregnation; union of male and female gametes. **cross-f.** *In biology*, the fertilization of the ovules of one species by the seed germs of another.

Fer'u·la (ferr′yoo·luh, ferr′oo·luh). A genus of the family Umbelliferae whose species yield asafetida and sumbul.

fes'ter. 1. Superimpose a suppuration on a lesion such as an ulcer. 2. Suppurate.

fes″ti·na'tion. An involuntary increase or hastening in gait, seen in paralysis agitans.

fes·toon'. The papilliform interproximal gingiva which fills each buccal and lingual embrasure between the necks of adjacent teeth.

fe'tal·ism. The presence or persistence of certain prenatal conditions in the body after birth.

fe·ta'tion. 1. The formation of a fetus. 2. Pregnancy, q.v.

fe'ti·cide. The killing of the fetus in the uterus.

fet'id (fet'id, fee'tid). Having a foul odor.

fe'tish, fe'tich (fee'tish, fet'ish). 1. Any material object thought to have magical power or to bring supernatural aid. 2. In psychiatry, a personalized inanimate object, love object, or any maneuver or body part which, through association, arouses erotic feelings. —**fetishism, fetishist,** n.

fet'lock. That region of the leg of the horse extending from the lower extremity of the metacarpal or metatarsal bone to the pastern joint.

fe·tom'e·try (fee-tom'i-tree). The measurement of the fetus, especially of its cranial diameters.

fe'tor, foe'tor (fee'tur, -tor).Stench. **f. ex ore.** Bad breath.

fe'tus, foe'tus (fee'tus). The unborn offspring of viviparous mammals in the later stages of development; especially, in man, from the ninth week until birth. —**fetal,** adj. **calcified f.** See lithopedion. **f. compressus.** See f. papyraceus. **f. cylindricus.** A malformed, abortive fetus with but little indication of head and extremities, being roughly cylindrical in form. **f. papyraceus.** A dead twin fetus which has been compressed by the growth of its living twin. **parasitic f.** A more or less completely formed fetus which is attached to its twin host.

fe'ver. 1. Elevation of the body temperature above the normal; in human beings, above 37° C. or 98.6° F. 2. A disease whose distinctive feature is elevation of body temperature. Syn., pyrexia. —**feverish,** adj. **algid pernicious f.** A severe attack of malaria; characterized by collapse, extremely cold skin, and a tendency to fatal syncope. **artificial f.** One purposefully produced for therapeutic benefit, as by the induction of malaria, by the injection of foreign protein, or by means of a fever cabinet. **brain f.** Cerebrospinal meningitis. **bullous f.** That which accompanies pemphigus. **camp f.** Typhus, q.v. **catarrhal f.** Old term for the common cold. **cat-scratch f.** A disease characterized by a history of domestic cat scratches followed by a systemic infection, with

malaise, fever, lymphadenopathy, an occasionally, exanthemas. **cerebr spinal f.** Cerebrospinal meningiti **childbed f.** See puerperal f. **Cold rado tick f.** An acute, febrile infec tion occurring in western U.S.A.; asse ciated with the bite of the tick Derm centor andersoni. The disease is rare. fatal, and no rickettsia has been di covered to be associated with it. **co tinued f.** One which does not va more than 1° or 2° F. during 24 hour **double quartan f.** A form malaria with a three-day cycle; pa oxysms occurring on two successiv days are followed by a one-day interva **drug f.** That resulting from the a ministration of a drug, often by sen sitization, as by the sulfonamides. **en teric f.** Typhoid. **epidemic ca tarrhal f.** Influenza. **eruptive** Any fever with a skin rash. **essen tial f.** One of unknown caus **harvest f.** A form of spirochetos affecting field workers. **hectic f.** On recurring daily, with the highest tem perature in the evening; accompanie by chills and sweats. It occurs fre quently in tuberculosis. **hemoglo binuric f.** A severe form of malari associated with hematuria; occu mainly in endemic areas of malignan tertian malaria. **herpetic f.** On with chills, sore throat, and herpet eruption on the face. **intermi tent f.** Malaria, q.v. **jungle ye low f.** A form of yellow fever endem in parts of Brazil; occurs in or ne forested areas where the Aëdes aegyp has not been found. **Malta f.** Bruce losis, q.v. **Mediterranean f.** Bru cellosis, q.v. **metal fume f.** A febri reaction following the inhalation finely divided particles of metall oxides. Also called brass chills, bras founder's ague, metal ague, zinc chill spelter shakes. **miliary f.** An acut infectious disease; characterized b fever, profuse sweating, and a papula rash later forming pustules. Syn sweating sickness. **milk f.** A mi nomer for a fever during the pue perium, once thought to be due to great accumulation of milk in th breasts, but now generally believed be due to actual puerperal infectio **papular f.** A disease characterize by fever, papular eruption, and rhe matic pains. **paratyphoid f.** Par typhoid, q.v. **parenteric f.** One r sembling typhoid or paratyphoid, b due to a different organism. **Pe Ebstein f.** A type of remittent fev occurring in Hodgkin's disease which characterized by periods of temper ture elevation up to 104° F. for 7 to days followed by normal temperatur for 2 or 3 weeks. **pretibial f.** febrile disease of unknown origi

Characterized by an erythematous rash in the pretibial region, frontal, postorbital, and lumbar aching, nausea, vomiting, leukopenia, and enlargement of the spleen. **protein f.** Artificial fever produced by the intravenous or intramuscular injection of a foreign protein. **puerperal f.** Infection of the endometrium and septicemia following delivery. Also called *childbed f., puerperal sepsis.* **Q f.** An acute infection transmitted by *Rickettsia burnetii* (Australian type) or *R. diaporica* (American type); characterized by pneumonitis, fever, nausea, and vomiting. The disease is of short duration, without mortality. Also called *quadrilateral f., Queensland f.* **quartan f.** Malaria, with paroxysms every 72 hours. **quinine f.** A disease marked by fever and skin eruption; occurs in persons exposed to quinine during its preparation. **rabbit f.** Tularemia, *q.v.* **ragweed f.** See *hay fever.* **rat bite f.** A form which includes two distinct diseases contracted from the bite of infected rats or other animals. One caused by *Streptobacillus moniliformis* is identical with epidemic arthritic erythema, *q.v.* The other, due to a spirochete, *Spirillum minus,* is characterized by an indurated ulcer at the site of inoculation, remittent fever, and a purplish maculopapular rash. Also called *sodoku.* **recurrent f.** See relapsing *f.* **relapsing f.** Any one of a group of specific infectious diseases caused by spirochetes, *Borrelia recurrentis* and *Borrelia duttonii* being the most common, and transmitted to man by lice or ticks. Both varieties are widespread and resemble each other in having an acute onset with chills, fever, pain in the back and legs, enlargement of the spleen, delirium, and sometimes convulsions; a rapid disappearance of symptoms by crisis is followed after an interval of a week or more by another paroxysm. This cycle may be repeated from two to six times. Also called *famine fever, remittent fever, spirillum fever, tick fever, louse fever.* **remittent f.** A paroxysmal fever with exacerbations and remissions, but without intermissions. **rheumatic f.** A febrile disease characterized by painful migratory arthritis and a predilection to heart damage, leading to chronic valvular disease. Permanent joint damage never occurs. The cause is not definitely known, but it is related to streptococcal infection of the throat, to climate, and to hereditary susceptibility. It is essentially a disease of childhood. Girls are more frequently affected than boys, and multiple attacks are the rule. **Rocky Mountain spotted f.** A form of fever with a characteristic rash occurring throughout the Western Hemisphere; formerly thought to be limited to the Rocky Mountain area. The causative organism is *Rickettsia rickettsii,* and it is transmitted to man by several varieties of ticks, principally *Dermacentor andersoni* and *D. variabilis* in the United States. **rose f.** See *hay fever.* **scarlet f.** An acute, contagious, febrile disease, having a period of incubation varying from several hours to a week, setting in with vomiting or chill, which is followed by high fever, rapid pulse, sore throat, cervical adenitis, and the appearance of a punctiform, scarlet-red eruption from one to five days thereafter. The tongue, at first heavily coated and red at the tip and edges, soon shows prominence of the papillae, which are red and swollen (strawberry tongue). The eruption, at the appearance of which all the symptoms become intensified, gradually fades after five or six days, and is followed by a scaly desquamation. A peculiarity of scarlet fever is its tendency to involve the kidneys. The causal agent is a hemolytic streptococcus. See *Dick test.* Also called *scarlatina.* **seven-day f.** A disease similar to dengue, lasting about one week; due to the spirochete *Leptospira hebdomadis.* **tertian f.** A form of malaria due to *Plasmodium vivax,* which completes its life cycle in 48 hours. Chills recur every two days. **Texas f.** An infectious disease of cattle; due to the parasite *Babesia bigemina,* which is transmitted by the cattle tick *Boöphilus annulatus,* and invades the red blood corpuscles. Characterized by high fever, hemoglobinuria, and enlargement of the spleen. **therapeutic f.** See artificial *f.* **thermic f.** Sunstroke, *q.v.* **threshing f.** A form of pneumonoconiosis affecting threshers; characterized by headache, fever, and irritation of the respiratory tract. **traumatic f.** That following a wound or an injury. Syn., *symptomatic f.* **trench f.** An acute infection lasting several days; caused by *Rickettsia quintana* and transmitted by the body louse. Syn., *Volhynia f.* **typhomalarial f.** Malaria with typhoidlike symptoms. **typhus f.** See *typhus.* **undulant f.** Brucellosis, *q.v.* **vaccinal f.** That following vaccination. **yellow f.** An acute infectious disease of tropical and subtropical regions of America; caused by a filtrable virus disseminated by the *Aëdes aegypti* (*Stegomyia fasciata calopus*). After a period of incubation varying from a few hours to several days, the disease begins with a chill and pain in the head, back, and limbs. The temperature rises rapidly to from 103° to 105° F., vomiting occurs, the bowels are constipated, the urine scanty and albuminous. A remission follows, after which, in severe cases, the temperature rises to its original height, jaundice develops, and the vomited material becomes dark from the presence of blood (black vomit). Hemorrhages may occur from the intestinal mucous membrane. The disease is often fatal, death occurring from exhaustion or from uremia.

F.F.T. Flicker fusion test; flicker fusion threshold.

fi'at (pl. *fiant*). Let there be made; used in the writing of prescriptions. Abbreviated, *ft*.

fi'ber, fi'bre. A filamentary or threadlike structure. —**fibrous,** *adj.* **accelerating fibers.** Sympathetic nerve fibers which convey impulses that hasten the rapidity and increase the force of the heartbeat. Also called *augmentor fibers.* **adrenergic fibers.** Nerve fibers which liberate an adrenalin-like substance at their terminations; include most of the postganglionic fibers of the sympathetic nervous system. **argyrophil fibers.** The delicate, branching connective-tissue fibers forming the reticular framework of lymphatic tissue, myeloid tissue, the red pulp of the spleen, the finest stroma of many glands, and most basement membranes. They differ from collagenous fibers chemically and in their response to silver impregnation, in which they are blackened. Syn., *lattice fibers, precollagenous fibers.* Also called *reticular fibers.* **association fibers.** White nerve fibers situated just beneath the cortical substance and connecting the adjacent cerebral gyri. **axial f.** (a) The axis cylinder of a nerve fiber. (b) The central spiral filament, probably contractile, of the flagellum of the spermatozoon. **cholinergic fibers.** Nerve fibers which liberate an acetylcholine-like substance at their terminations; include most of the motor nerves of the body except postganglionic sympathetics. **collagenous fibers.** The flexible, fibrillar, nonelastic, connective-tissue fibers which are the commonest type. They make up the main mass of such structures as the corium, fasciae, tendons, ligaments, aponeuroses, periostea, and capsules of organs, and form also the fibrillar, intercellular substance of bone and cartilage. Syn., *white fibers.* **commissural fibers.** Fibers joining an area of the cortex of one cerebral hemisphere to a similar area of the other. **dentinal fibers.** The processes of odontoblasts in the dentinal tubules. Syn., *Tomes's fibers.* **elastic fibers.** The nonfibrillar, branching, highly elastic fibers of fibroelastic connective tissue. They form also the fenestrated membranes of large arteries. Syn., *yellow fibers.* **f. cell.** Any cell elongated to a fiberlike appearance; for example, muscle cells are commonly referred to as muscle fibers. **lens fibers.** The highly modified epithelial cells which form the main mass of the lens of the eye. **muscle f.** The ultimate element of which muscular tissue is made up. Voluntary muscles consist of transversely striated fibers, involuntary muscles of spindle-shaped fibers or cells. **nerve f.** The long process of a neuron, usually the axon. **perforating fibers.** Collagenous fibers of a tendon, ligament, or periosteum buried in the matrix of subperiosteal bone. Also the similar fibers in the cementum of a tooth. Syn., *Sharpey's fibers.* Also called *penetrating fibers.* **Purkinje fibers.** The modified cardiac muscle fibers of the conduction system of the heart. **secretory fibers.** Centrifugal nerve fibers exciting secretion. **smooth muscle fibers.** The straight, or slightly bent, elongated, spindle-shaped, nucleated cells, bearing more or less distinct longitudinal striations, which make up involuntary, or unstriped, muscles. Also called *involuntary fibers, nonstriated fibers, unstriated fibers, unstriped fibers.* See muscular tissue. **Tomes's fibers.** Dentinal fibers, *q.v.* **vasoconstrictor fibers.** Nerve fibers which, upon stimulation, produce constriction of blood vessels. **vasodilator fibers.** Nerve fibers whose function is to dilate blood vessels. **white fibers.** See *collagenous fibers* under *fiber.* **yellow fibers.** See *elastic fibers* under *fiber.* **zonular fibers.** The fibers of the ciliary zonule of Zinn.

fi·bre'mi·a, fi·brae'mi·a (figh-bree'mee-uh). The presence of fibrin in the blood.

fi'bril. A component filament of a fiber as of a muscle or of a nerve. Also called *fibrilla.* —**fibrillar, fibrillary,** *adj.* **fi·bril'la** (pl. *fibrillae*) (figh-bril'uh) See *fibril.*

fi"bril·la'tion. 1. The formation of fibrils. 2. A local quivering of muscular fibers. —**fi'brillated,** *adj.* **atrial f.** A cardiac arrhythmia due to a disturbed spread of excitation through atrial musculature; generally believed to be due to waves of excitation circulating irregularly and continuously at rapid rates around a variable "ring" of muscle in the atria from where excitation of the rest of the atria and ventricles occurs, giving rise to an irregular, usually rapid, rate of ventricular excitation. Also called *auricular f.* **auricular f.** A term often used clinically for atrial f., q.v. **ventricular f.** A cardiac arrhythmia characterized by an absolutely irregular spread of idioventricular excitation whose origin and spread are completely disordered, analogous to atrial fibrillation. It produces only limited, ineffectual, and irregular ventricular contractions and, being almost always irreversible in man, usually is fatal.

fi'brin. The fibrous protein, formed by the interaction of thrombin and fibrinogen, in the network of which blood corpuscles are enmeshed in the clotting of shed blood. **f. film.** A pliable, elastic, translucent film of fibrin, prepared from human blood plasma. **f. foam.** A spongy material made from human fibrin which, when treated with human thrombin, is a useful hemostatic agent.

fi'bri-no-, fi'brin-. A combining form meaning *relating to* fibrin.

fi-brin'o-gen (figh-brin'o-jen). A protein of the globulin class, obtained from blood plasma and serous transudations; one of the chief elements forming fibrin. See Table of Normal Values of Blood Constituents in the Appendix. —**fibrinogen'ic, fibrin-og'enous** (figh″bri-nodj′i-nus), *adj.*

fi-brin″o-gen″o-pe′ni-a (figh-brin″o-jen″o-pee′nee-uh). Decrease in the fibrinogen of the blood plasma; usually due to liver disease but may be congenital. Formerly called *fibrino-penia.*

fi″brin-o-glob′u-lin. A protein present in blood serum and derived from fibrinogen.

fi′bri-noid. The fibrinlike material of the placenta; produced by necrosis of the mucosa and trophoblast and by fibrin from maternal blood. It occurs as an incomplete layer in the chorion and decidua and as patches on the chorionic villi. Also called *stria.* **canalized f.** The layered fibrinoid material having a striated or canalized appearance, found especially on the chorionic plate during the last half of pregnancy.

fi″bri-no-ly′sin, fi″bri-nol′y-sin. An enzyme formed by the action of pathogenic streptococci; present in plasma, and capable of causing solution of fibrin clots.

fi″brin-ol′y-sis. The slow digestion and solution of fibrin which occurs when a blood clot is allowed to stand aseptically in the serum in which it was formed.

fi′bro-, fibr-. A combining form signifying *pertaining to fibers, relation to fibrous tissue or structure.*

fi″bro-ad′e-no′ma. Adenofibroma.

fi″bro-ad′i-pose. Both fibrous and fatty.

fi″bro-an″gi-o′ma. A benign tumor composed of blood or lymph vessels, with abundant connective tissue.

fi′bro-blast. A stellate or spindle-shaped cell (rod-shaped, if seen on edge) with a large, oval, flattened nucleus and a thin layer of cytoplasm; found in fibrous tissue. Syn., *fibrocyte.* Also called *connective-tissue cell.*

fi″bro-bron-chi′tis. Bronchitis with expectoration of fibrinous casts.

fi″bro-cal-car′e-ous (figh″bro-kal-kair′ee-us). Both fibrous and calcareous, as a deposit of calcific material in tissues (occurring in fibromas or in a seat of fibrosis).

fi″bro-car″ci-no′ma. A carcinoma with fibrous elements.

fi″bro-car′ti-lage. Dense, white, fibrous connective tissue in which the cells have formed small masses of cartilage between the fibers, and have impregnated the fibers with chondrin. —**fibrocartilag′inous** (figh″bro-kahr″ti-ladj′i-nus), *adj.*

fi″bro-cel′lu-lar. Both fibrous and cellular.

fi″bro-chon-dro′ma (figh″bro-kon-dro′muh). A chondroma with a considerable amount of fibrous tissue.

fi″bro-cys-to′ma. A fibrous tumor accompanied by cystic degeneration.

fi″bro-cyte. Fibroblast, *q.v.*

fi″bro-e-las′tic. Applied to connective tissue in which interlacing collagenous fibers are interspersed by more or less strongly developed networks of elastic fibers.

fi′broid. Composed of fibrous tissue; said of a tissue or structure which has become the seat of extensive fibrosis.

fi″broid-ec′to-my. Removal of a uterine fibroid.

fi″bro-li-po′ma. A lipoma with a considerable amount of fibrous tissue. —**fibrolipom′atous,** *adj.*

fi-bro′ma (figh-bro′muh). A benign tumor composed principally of whorls of white fibrous connective tissue. —**fibrom′atous,** *adj.* **f. durum.** A hard fibroma, firm because of large quantities of collagenous material in comparison with the number of cells. **f. lipomatodes.** See *xanthoma.* **f. molle.** A soft fibroma, soft because cellular components are rich as compared with collagen; a fibroma may be soft because of edema. **f. molluscum.** Cutaneous neurofibroma. Syn., *molluscum fibrosum.* **papillary f.** A superficial fibroma with papillary projections.

fi-bro″ma-to′sis (figh-bro″muh-to′sis). The simultaneous occurrence of many fibromas.

fi″bro-mus′cu-lar. Made up of connective tissue and muscle.

fi″bro-my-o′ma (·migh-o′muh). A myoma in which connective tissue is so intermingled with the muscle as to constitute a fibromatous component.

fi″bro-my″o-mec′to-my. Excision of a fibromyoma.

fi"bro·myx"o·li·po'ma. A mixed, fatty tumor with fibrous and myxomatous tissues.

fi"bro·myx·o'ma. Fibroma with mucoid degeneration; rarely, a combination of fibroma and myxoma.

fi"bro·myx"o·sar·co'ma. A fibrosarcoma with mucoid degeneration; rarely, a combination of fibrosarcoma and myxosarcoma.

fi"bro·neu·ro'ma. See *neurofibroma*.

fi"bro·pla'si·a (figh"bro·play'zhuh, ·shuh). The growth of fibrous tissue, as in the second phase of wound healing. **—fibroplas'tic,** *adj.* **retrolental f.** A blinding disease of the eye affecting premature infants with low birth weight. The name is derived from the fact that in the ultimate stage the contracture of organized fibrous tissue, occupying the area back of the lens, detaches the retina.

fi"bro·pu'ru·lent. Consisting of pus containing flakes of fibrin.

fi"bro·sar·co'ma. Spindle-cell sarcoma, mature in type, with production of collagenous fibrils. **f. mucocellulare carcinomatodes.** A secondary carcinoma of the ovary which is most frequently primary in the gastrointestinal tract, especially the stomach, composed of groups of small spheroidal or ovoid cells. Also called *Krukenberg tumor*.

fi·bro'sis (figh·bro'sis). The growth of white fibrous connective tissue in an organ or part in excess of that naturally present. **—fibrot'ic,** *adj.*

fi"bro·si'tis. Inflammatory hyperplasia of fibrous connective tissue. **—fibrosit'ic,** *adj.*

fi'brous. Containing fibers; similar to fibers.

fib'u·la. The slender bone at the outer part of the leg, articulating above with the tibia and below with the talus and tibia. See Table of Bones in the Appendix. **—fibular,** *adj.*

fi'cin. A proteolytic enzyme from fig-tree sap. It is an active vermicide for *Ascaris* and *Trichuris*.

F.I.C.S. Fellow of the International College of Surgeons.

field. 1. An open space or area. 2. A concept of development in which the whole and the parts of a structure or organism are dynamically interrelated, reacting to each other and to the environment. 3. A region of the embryo that is the anlage of some organ or part. **auditory f.** The area within which a given sound is audible to the ear. **f. of fixation.** *In optics,* the region bounded by the utmost limits of distinct or central vision, which the eye has under its direct control throughout its excursions when the head is not moved. **f. of microscope.** The area within which objects can be seen through a microscope at one time. **f. of vision.** The space visible to the patient when the eye is fixed steadily on an object in the direct line of vision. Abbreviated, F.

fig'ure. The visible form of anything; the outline of an organ or part. **chromatic f.** The chromosomes or the pattern formed by the chromosomes in miosis or mitosis. **nuclear figures.** The peculiar arrangement of the chromosomes during karyokinesis.

fi·la'ceous (fi·lay'shus, figh·lay'shus). Consisting of threads or threadlike fibers or parts.

fil'a·ment. A small, threadlike structure. **—filamen'tous,** *adj.* **axial f.** The central contractile fibril of a cilium or flagellum which arises from a centriole or blepharoplast. **terminal f.** The end piece or naked axial filament of the tail of a spermatozoon.

fil"a·men·ta'tion. Thread formation; a peculiar reaction observed when bacteria are grown in an immune serum. Long threads of bacteria occur. The reaction is shown by the typhoid and proteus bacilli. Also called *Pfaundler's reaction, thread reaction.*

fi'lar. Filamentous.

fi·la'ri·a (pl. *filariae*). A long filiform nematode which is a member of the superfamily Filarioidea. The adults may live in the circulatory or lymphatic systems, the connective tissues, or serous cavities of a vertebrate host. The larval forms, or microfilariae, are commonly found in the circulating blood or lymph spaces from which they are ingested by some form of blood-sucking arthropod. After a series of metamorphoses in the body of the arthropod, the larvae migrate to the proboscis as infestive forms. **—filarial,** *adj.*

fil"a·ri'a·sis. A diseased state due to the presence of filariae in the body.

fi·lar'i·cide. A drug which destroys filariae. **—filarici'dal,** *adj.*

fil'i·form. Threadlike.

fill'ing. 1. The material used in closing cavities in carious teeth. 2. The process of inserting, condensing, shaping, and finishing a filling substance. **contour f.** *In dentistry,* a filling in which the material is so built out as to restore the lost portion of the crown of the tooth. **root canal f.** The closure and filling of the prepared root canal from the apex to the coronal portion of the tooth with an impervious material to prevent subsequent infection. **temporary f.** A substance, as cement or gutta percha, used in teeth as a filling which is to be replaced later by a permanent restoration.

film. 1. A pellicle or thin skin. 2. An opacity, as of the cornea. 3. *In micros-*

copy, a thin spread of blood, usually on a glass slide or cover slip.

fil′ter. 1. An apparatus which separates one or more components of a mixture from the others. 2. *In roentgen therapy,* a thin layer of any one of several materials used to absorb a greater percentage of the soft rays than of the hard rays of a roentgen beam, thus hardening the beam. Aluminum filters are used for superficial and medium therapy; copper or Thoraeus filters, *q.v.,* for deep therapy; and lead or tin filters, for supervoltage therapy. **Berkefeld f.** An apparatus for sterilizing any liquid or solution by separating bacteria and spores by means of diatomaceous earth. **pollen f.** A means of removing pollen from the air; may either make the atmosphere pollen-free, as by means of a forced draft through various sized filters, or filter the respired air, as with a gauze mask worn over mouth and nose, or an adjustable device worn in the nostrils. **Thoraeus f.** A combination filter consisting of tin, copper, and aluminum, used in x-ray therapy. **ultraviolet f.** One which passes ultraviolet radiation but which is relatively opaque to longer wave lengths.

fil′ter. To separate one or more components of a mixture; to pass through a filter.

fil′tra·ble. Capable of passing through a filter.

fil′trate. The liquid that has passed through a filter.

fil·tra′tion. The operation of straining through a filter.

fi′lum (pl. *fila*). Any threadlike or filamentous structure. **f. terminale.** The atrophic slender inferior end of the spinal cord, the caudal part of which is mostly pia mater.

fim′bri·a (pl. *fimbriae*). 1. A fringe. 2. One of the irregular processes which form the fringelike margin of the infundibulum of a uterine tube. 3. A flattened band of white fibers along the medial margin of the hippocampus, continuous with the crus of the fornix. Formerly called *f. cornu Ammonis.* —**fimbrial,** *adj.*

fim′bri·ate, fim′bri·a″ted. Fringed with slender processes which are larger than filaments; said of bacterial cultures and of the ostium of the uterine tube.

fin′ger. A digit of the hand. **baseball f.** Luxation of a distal phalanx with rupture of the distal portion of the extensor tendon, resulting in a drop of the phalanx; caused by a baseball injury. **clubbed f.** A finger, the terminal phalanx of which is short and broad, with an overhanging nail; seen in some cases of pulmonary and cardiac disease. Also called *Hippocratic f., chronic hypertrophic pulmonary osteoarthropathy, drumstick f.* **hammer f.** A congenital flexion deformity, usually of middle phalanx of middle finger. **lock f.** A peculiar affection of the fingers in which they suddenly become fixed in a flexed position, due to the presence of a small fibrous growth in the sheath of a flexor tendon. **seal f.** An infection occurring in Norway believed to be contracted from seals, characterized by the glistening appearance of the swollen and painful finger. It is similar clinically to erysipeloid. **springfinger.** Condition in which there is an obstruction to flexion and extension of one or more fingers; due to injuries or inflammation of the tendinous sheaths. **trigger f.** A condition in which flexion or extension of a finger is at first obstructed, but finally accomplished with a jerk or sweep. It is due to chronic tenosynovitis. **webbed fingers.** Union of adjacent fingers by interdigital tissue; fingers fused at the lateral aspects. Syn., *syndactyly.*

fin′ger cot. A covering of rubber or other material to protect the finger or to prevent infection. Also called *finger stall.*

fin′ger·print″. An ink impression of the cutaneous ridges of a finger tip. May be a direct pressure print or a rolled print, the latter recording the entire flexor and lateral aspects of the phalanx. See *dermatoglyphics.* —**fingerprinting,** *n.*

fin′ger stall″. A rubber cap for a finger.

fire′damp″. An explosive mixture of methane and air.

first aid. Emergency treatment given before regular medical care can be obtained in cases of accident, injury, or illness. —**first′-aid′,** *adj.;* **first′aid/er,** *n.*

first′-aid′ kit. A pouch, bag, or box containing sterilized dressings, adhesive plaster, iodine, bandages, and simple instruments; for use in giving first aid in an emergency.

first′-aid′ pack′et. A hermetically sealed, waterproof case containing emergency first-aid material, which is issued to each soldier of the U. S. Army, and is not to be opened until needed.

first in·ten′tion. See *healing* by first intention.

fis′sion. 1. Any splitting or cleaving. 2. *In biology,* asexual reproduction by the division of the body into two or more parts, each of which grows into a complete organism. It is the common method of reproduction among the bacteria and protozoa. **atomic f.** The splitting of the nucleus of an atom by neutron bombardment into two main fragments. For example, the uranium isotope 235 can be split in two, barium and krypton resulting, with the release of a vast amount of energy. Also called *nuclear f.* **binary f.** The division of first the nucleus and then the cytoplasm into two equal parts; common in the Protozoa. **multiple f.** A series of divisions of the nucleus followed by a division of the body into as many parts as there are nuclei. **nuclear f.** Fission or splitting of the nucleus, the center of an atom. Also called *atomic f.* **uranium f.** See atomic *f.*

fis'sure. A groove or cleft; applied to the clefts or grooves in various organs, as the skull, the brain, the liver, the spinal cord; also to cracks in the skin or linear ulcers in mucous membranes. Also see *sulcus.* —**fissured, fissural,** *adj.*; **fissura'tion,** *n.* **anal f.** A linear ulcer at the mucocutaneous junction of the anus, causing intense suffering on defecation. **anterior median f.** A groove extending the entire length of the spinal cord in the midline anteriorly, and incompletely dividing it into two symmetrical parts. **central f.** See central *sulcus.* **choroid f.** (a) The ventral fissure in the optic cup and the optic stalk of the embryo. (b) The line of invagination of the tela choroidea of the lateral ventricles of the brain. Syn., *fetal f.* **decidual f.** Fissured spaces developing in the decidua basalis, parallel with the uterine wall, in the later months of pregnancy. **fetal f.** See choroid *f.* **inferior orbital f.** That of the orbit which gives passage to the infraorbital blood vessels and ascending branches from the sphenopalatine ganglion. **lateral cerebral f.** A deep fissure of the brain, beginning on the outer side of the anterior perforated space, and extending outward to the lateral surface of the hemisphere. It has two branches, a short vertical and a long horizontal, the latter separating the temporal from the frontal and parietal lobes. Also called *Sylvian f.* **longitudinal f. of the cerebrum.** The deep fissure that divides the cerebrum into two hemispheres. **longitudinal f. of the liver.** A fissure on the lower border of the liver, through which passes the round ligament. **palpebral f.** The space between the eyelids extending from the outer to the inner canthus. **precentral f.** A fissure in front of the central sulcus and parallel to it. **Rolandic f.** Old term for central sulcus, *q.v.* **superior orbital f.** The elongated opening between the small and the great wings of the sphenoid. **Sylvian f.** Lateral cerebral fissure, *q.v.* **transverse f. of the**

liver. A fissure crossing transversely the lower surface of the right lobe of the liver. It transmits the portal vein, hepatic artery and nerves, and hepatic ducts.

fis'tu·la. A narrow tube or canal formed by incomplete closure, as of an abscess, wound, disease process, or (congenitally) a part. Usually transmits some fluid, either pus or the secretions or contents of some organ, viscus, or body cavity. Fistulas opening from a viscus to the exterior of the body are named according to the viscus involved, as biliary, gastric, cecal, vesical. When the communication is between two organs, the names are combined, as esophagotracheal, gastrocolic, vesicovaginal, anorectal. —**fistular, fistulate, fistulous,** *adj.* **abdominal f.** One opening through the abdominal wall and communicating with an abdominal viscus or space. **alveolar f.** One communicating with a diseased alveolar process. **blind f.** One having an opening at one end only; may be an internal or external opening or, more properly, a sinus. **bone f.** One leading to an osteomyelitic process or to the site of an ostitis. **bronchial f.** (a) An abnormal tract communicating between the pleural cavity and a bronchus and generally closing when the empyema is healed. (b) An abnormal tract leading from a bronchus to a cutaneous opening, the result of gangrene or abscess of the lung. **cervical f.** An open communication between the pharynx and the surface of the neck arising by retention of a visceral groove and pouch with perforation of their closing plate. **esophageal f.** An abnormal tract of congenital origin, communicating between the esophagus and some portion of the skin through an external opening, or between esophagus and some viscus or organ through an internal opening. A similar fistula may result from trauma or disease. **fecal f.** An opening from the intestine through the abdominal wall to the skin, with discharge of intestinal contents; usually applied to openings from the ileum and colon. **internal f.** A fistula in which the openings are within the body without communication through the skin. **labial f.** A minute fistulous tract or congenital pit near the vermilion border of the lower lip. **lateral f. of the neck.** A congenital fistula opening lateral to the midline, anywhere from the mandible to the sternum, and connecting with the pharynx, a cyst, a cell rest, or a duct; due to faulty closure of visceral pouches or the thymopharyngeal duct, or to other developmental defects. **pilonidal f.** Pilonidal *cyst.* **rectovaginal f.** An opening between the vagina and the rectum. **rectovesical f.** A congenital or acquired opening between the rectum and the urinary bladder. **sacrococcygeal f.** One communicating with a dermoid cyst in the coccygeal region. **salivary f.** One communicating with a salivary gland or its duct, usually the parotid, with discharge of saliva through an external opening in the skin. **thyroglossal f.** A developmental abnormality, due to incomplete obliteration of the thyroglossal duct, resulting in a midline cervical fistula. **urinary f.** An abnormal tract from any portion of the urinary system; discharges urine through an opening on the skin or into some organ, viscus, or cavity.

fix·a′tion. 1. The act of fixing or making firm. 2. The operation of rendering fixed a displaced or floating organ by means of sutures. 3. *In microscopy*, fixing, *q.v.* 4. *In psychiatry*, the arrest of development of an emotion or desire at an immature level. **external skeletal f.** *In dentistry and surgery*, a method of immobilizing bony fragments of fractures by the use of metal pin or screw devices applied externally; adapted especially to edentulous mouths. **f. of complement.** The entering of complement into combination with an antigen-antibody aggregate so that it is not available for subsequent reaction in the indicator systems of hemolysis or bacteriolysis. The basis of the Wassermann test and other serologic tests. **intramedullary f.** A method of holding a fractured bone in proper alignment by means of a metal pin in the marrow cavity. See Küntscher *nail*.

fix′a·tive. Any substance used to fix tissues in the structural condition and shape found in life, or that used for fastening a microscopical section to a slide.

fix′ing. The preparation of tissue for microscopical study by means of some agent that hardens it and preserves the form and arrangement of the cells.

fix′ing flu′id. A solution, or mixture of solutions, used to prepare tissues for microscopical study. Formalin, Zenker's fluid, and Regaud's fluid are the most widely used. Also see *fixing*. **Bouin's f.f.** A mixture of saturated aqueous picric acid, Formalin, and acetic acid, generally, the most useful of all the picric acid fixatives. **Müller's f.f.** A mixture of potassium bichromate, sodium sulfate, and distilled water, used to harden nerve tissue after preliminary fixation and, with addition of Formalin, to make other fixing fluids, such as Regaud's. **Regaud's f.f.** A mixture of 3%

aqueous potassium bichromate and Formalin, used for many purposes. **Zenker's f.f.** A mixture of potassium bichromate, mercuric chloride, distilled water, and glacial acetic acid, used in numerous fixing technics. When the acetic acid is replaced by an equal volume of Formalin, it is called **Helly's fixing fluid**; when replaced by twice its volume of Formalin, it is called **Bensley's Formalin-Zenker.**

Fl. Symbol for florentium.

fl. Fluid.

flac′cid (flack′sid). Soft; flabby; relaxed. —**flaccid′ity,** *n.*

flag′el·late (fladj′uh·late). A protozoan furnished with slender, whiplike processes.

flag″el·la′tion (fladj″uh·lay′shun). 1. Flogging or beating. 2. Beating or whipping as a means of producing sexual gratification. 3. Massage by strokes or blows.

fla·gel′lum. A whiplike process consisting of an axial filament enclosed in a thin cytoplasmic sheath; the organ of locomotion of sperm cells, and of certain bacteria and protozoa.

flank. The fleshy or muscular part of an animal or a man between the ribs and the hip; the thigh of an animal; the outer side of the thigh, hip, and buttock of a human.

flap. A partially detached portion of skin or other tissue, either accidentally formed, or created by the surgeon to be used as a graft to fill a defect or to improve contour. Flaps which are composed of special tissue, such as mucous membrane, conjunctiva, dura, wall of intestinal tract, omentum, muscle, etc., are named after the tissue contained, as muscle flap, etc. They may also be named according to the special purpose for which they are used, as a rhinoplastic flap, for repair of the nose. **amputation f.** A simple, broad-based flap which needs no advancement, and is shaped to provide proper contour of the part to be covered. **osteoplastic f.** A flap of skin and underlying bone, commonly of scalp and skull, raised for the purpose of exploring the underlying structures. **pedicle f.** A type which obtains its blood supply through a narrow base, or pedicle; used when length is required to fill a remote defect, or on a movable part which can be approximated to the donor site. The pedicle flap has many forms for specific purposes and therefore many named varieties. For instance, a pedicle flap which has the ends reversed to gain more distance is called a **jump, caterpillar,** or **waltzing flap.** Long pedicle flaps are usually tubed or rolled on themselves, so the free edges are sutured together: such a **tubed flap** attached at both ends is a **bipedicled flap;** attached also in the center, it is a **bridge flap.** A flap raised and applied to a movable part, such as one from the abdominal wall applied to the hand, may be a **pocket** or **tunnel flap.** A pedicle flap may include a large artery in its base; it is then called an **artery flap.** It may be lined with skin or mucous membrane, for repair of cheek or nose, or contain other tissue, as bone, cartilage, etc.; it is then called a **compound flap. sliding f.** A simple flap which is rotated on a broad base to fill an adjacent defect. **z f.** A means of lengthening a linear contracted scar by transposing two triangular flaps of skin, the sutured incision having a z shape.

flare. An abnormal vasomotor reaction manifested by a prolonged, widespreading flush of the skin after a pointed instrument has been drawn heavily across it.

flare'-up. An increase in the intensity of a disease or reaction.

flask. A glass or metal vessel having a narrow neck. **Erlenmeyer f.** A conical flask with a flat bottom. **Fenwall f.** Flask having a heavy rubber cap with a central outlet fitted with a stainless steel secondary stopper; used for sterilizing fluids by steam. **Florence f.** A round-bottomed flask used in distillation.

flat. 1. Lying on one plane. 2. A percussion note that is low-pitched and without resonance. —**flat'ness,** n.

flat'foot". Pes planus; a depression of the plantar arch of varying degree. It may be congenital, or acquired as a result of loss of muscle tone often caused by ill-fitting shoes, incorrect walking habits, and/or standing long hours at certain occupations. The acquired form is usually associated with eversion.

flat'sedge". A genus of plants of the family Cyperaceae.

flat'u·lence. The presence of gas in the stomach and intestinal canal. —**flatulent,** adj.

fla'tus. Gas, especially gas or air in the gastrointestinal canal.

flat'worm". Any worm of the phylum Platyhelminthes.

fla·ve'do. Yellowness of the skin.

fla'vi·cid. The dye 3,7-dimethyl-8-amino-2-dimethylamino-10-methylacridinium chloride. Used as a local germicide.

flav'i·cin (flav'i·sin, flay'vi·sin). An antibiotic substance from certain fungi. It is identical with aspergillin, flavacidin, flavatin, gigantic acid, and parasiticin.

fla'vin, flav'in. 1. One of a group of

yellow pigments, derived from isoalloxazine, isolated from various plant and animal sources. 2. Quercetin, q.v.

fla'vine (flay'veen, flav'een). 1. Flavin, q.v. 2. Acriflavine, q.v.

fla'vo-. 1. In botany, a combining form designating a yellow tint. 2. In chemistry, a combining form designating a series of complex yellow salts of cobalt.

Fla"vo·bac·te'ri·um. A genus of the Achromobacteriaceae whose species become orange-yellow in cultures.

fla'vone. 1. $C_{15}H_{10}O_2$. 2-Phenylbenzopyrone. 2. One of the yellow vegetable dye derivatives of flavone, 1.

flav'o·nol (flav'o·nol, ·nawl). 1. $C_{15}H_{10}O_3$. 3-Hydroxyflavone. 2. One of a group of vegetable dyes, including the anthocyanins, derived from flavonol, 1. Also spelled flavanol.

fla'vo·none. $C_{15}H_{12}O_2$. 2,3-Dihydroflavone, derivatives of which include hesperetin and citrin.

fla"vo·pro'te·in. One of a group of conjugated proteins of the chromoprotein type which constitute the yellow enzymes.

flaxedil. Trade-mark for gallamine triethiodide.

flax'seed". Linseed, q.v.

flax'seed oil. Linseed oil.

flea. Any blood-sucking, laterally compressed, wingless insect of the order Siphonaptera. Fleas are of medical importance as hosts and transmitters of disease and their bites produce a form of dermatitis. **cat f.** See Ctenocephalides felis. **dog f.** See Ctenocephalides canis. **human f.** See Pulex irritans. **rat f.** See Xenopsylla cheopis.

Fleming, Alexander [Scottish bacteriologist, 1881–1955]. Discovered that cultures of Penicillium inhibited the growth of certain bacteria (1928); hence the development of penicillin. Known also for his work in immunology and chemotherapy. Nobel laureate with E. B. Chain and H. Florey (1945).

flesh. The soft tissues of the body, especially the muscles. —**flesh'y,** adj. **goose f.** A rough condition of the skin, due to erection of the hairs; caused by cold or fear. Syn., cutis anserina. **proud f.** See exuberant granulation.

flex. Bend.

flex"i·bil'i·tas ce're·a (fleck"si·bil'i·tass seer'ee·uh). The tendency of a cataleptic or catatonic patient to maintain with seemingly indifferent passivity any posture in which he is placed.

flex'i·ble. Capable of being bent, without breaking; pliable. —**flexibil'ity,** n.

flex'ile (fleck'sill). Easily bent.

flex·im'e·ter. An instrument for measuring the amount of flexion possible in a joint.

flexin. Trade-mark for zoxazolamine.

flex'ion (fleck'shun). The act of bending; the condition of being bent.

Flexner, Simon [*American pathologist and bacteriologist*, 1863–1946]. Made many contributions to our knowledge of the transmission of infectious diseases. With William Henry Welch, made experimental studies of the action of diphtheria toxin (1891–92). Isolated *Shigella paradysenteriae*, called *Flexner's bacillus* (1900). This bacillus, at first incorrectly identified with *Shigella dysenteriae*, was found in tropical dysentery. It produces acid, indole, and endotoxin. With Noguchi, Flexner studied the effects of snake venom. Developed *Flexner's serum* for cerebrospinal meningitis (1907). With Paul A. Lewis, transmitted poliomyelitis to monkeys by means of cultures of a filtrable virus (1909). An experimentally transmissible carcinoma of the rat is called *Flexner-Jobling tumor.*

flex'or (fleck'sur, ·sor). A muscle that bends or flexes a limb or a part, as opposed to an *extensor*. See Table of Muscles in the Appendix.

flex'u·ous (fleck'shoo-us, flecks'yoo-us). Curving in an undulant manner.

flex'ure (fleck'shur). A bend or fold. **duodenojejunal f.** The abrupt bend at the junction of the duodenum and jejunum. **hepatic f.** An abrupt bend in the ascending colon to the right of the gallbladder. **perineal f.** The second curve of the rectum; its concavity is directed posteriorly. **sacral f.** The curve of the rectum in front of the sacrum; its concavity is directed anteriorly. **sigmoid f.** An S-shaped bend in the colon between the descending portion and the rectum. **splenic f.** An abrupt turn of the colon beneath the lower end of the spleen, connecting the transverse with the descending colon.

flick'er. A sensation of fluctuating vision; caused by a light of such slow intermittence that the visual impressions produced do not fuse.

flight of i·de'as. A condition in acute mania in which disconnected ideas and fancies flow rapidly through the mind. Also called *idea chase.*

float'ing. Abnormal movability or situation of a structure, due to natural lack, abnormal stretching, or destruction of its attachments. **f. kidney.** One which is displaced from its bed, becoming more freely movable, sometimes causing symptoms of disease, as by kinking the ureter.

floc"cu·la'tion (flock"yoo·lay'-shun). The coagulation or coalescence of finely divided or colloidal particles into larger particles which precipitate.

floc'cu·lent. 1. Flaky, downy, or woolly, said of a liquid containing irregularly shaped particles. 2. *In bacteriology*, a fluid culture characterized by small adherent masses of bacteria of various shapes.

floor. The basal limit of any hollow organ or open space. **f. of the pelvis.** The united mass of tissue forming the inferior boundary of the pelvis, consisting mainly of the levator ani muscles.

flo'ra. The entire plant life of any geographic area or geologic period.

flor·an'ty·rone. γ-Oxo-γ-(8-fluoranthene)butyric acid, a hydrocholeretic agent. See *zanchol.*

flo·ren'ti·um. Fl. The name given by Rolla and Fernandez to element 61, which has been called *illinium* by Hopkins, and for synthetic forms of which the names *cyclonium* and *promethium* have been proposed.

flo'res (flor'eez). 1. The flowers or blossoms of a plant. 2. A flocculent or pulverulent form assumed by certain substances after sublimation.

flor'id. Bright red in color.

flo·ta'tion. *In colloid chemistry*, the process of separating the valuable constituents (minerals) of ores from the valueless portion by agitation with water, a small proportion of an oil, and a foaming agent, causing the mineral to rise with the foam.

flow. 1. The free discharge of a liquid, as the blood. 2. The menses. 3. Menstruate profusely. **intermenstrual f.** Metrorrhagia, polymenorrhea, *q.v.* **streamline f.** A flow in which particles in the axial stream move more rapidly than those in the periphery, as the corpuscles in the capillaries.

flow'ers. 1. The blossoms of a plant. See *flores.* 1. 2. A sublimated drug, usually sulfur. See *flores,* 2. 3. The menses. *Obs.*

flow'me"ter. A physical device for measuring the rate of flow of a gas or liquid, as blood in the blood vessels; a stromuhr.

fluagel. Trade-mark for aluminum hydroxide gel.

fluc"tu·a'tion. 1. The wavelike motion produced when a body containing fluid is tapped between the fingers or hands. 2. A slight deviation from the average of the sort which gives rise to the continuous variability of a normal frequency curve.

flu"dro·cor'ti·sone ac'e·tate. 9α-Fluoro-17-hydroxycorticosterone-21-acetate, a derivative of hydrocortisone acetate used as an anti-inflammatory agent.

flu'id. 1. A substance whose molecules move freely upon one another. 2. Any liquid secretion of the body. 3. Liquid or gaseous. Abbreviated, fl. **allantoic f.** The fluid contents of the allantois. **amniotic f.** The transparent, almost colorless, albuminous fluid contained within the amniotic sac surrounding the fetus. **cerebrospinal f.** The fluid within the cerebral ventricles and between the arachnoid membrane and pia mater of the brain and spinal cord. **serous f.** Normal lymphatic fluid. **subarachnoid f.** See cerebrospinal *f.* **synovial f.** The clear fluid, resembling white of egg, found in various joints, bursae, and sheaths of tendons. An example of tissue fluid in general, being produced by dialysis from the plasma.

flu'id·ex'tract. A hydroalcoholic solution of vegetable principles so made that each cc. contains the therapeutic constituents of 1 Gm. of the standardized drug which it represents. Syn., *fluid extract.* See *extract, diacolation.*

flu'id·ounce'. A liquid measure; 8 fluidrachms. Equivalent to approximately 29.57 cc. Symbol, f℥.

flu'i·drachm", flu'i·dram" (floo'i-dram", floo"i·dram'). A liquid measure equal to one-eighth fluidounce, roughly equivalent to one teaspoonful. 60 minims = 1 fluidrachm. Symbol, f℈.

fluke. A trematode worm of the order Digenea. **blood f.** *Schistosoma haematobium, S. mansoni, S. japonicum.* **intestinal f.** *Fasciolopsis buski, Heterophyes heterophyes, Metagonimus yokogawai.* **liver f.** *Clonorchis sinensis, Fasciola hepatica, Opisthorchis felineus.* **lung f.** *Paragonimus westermani.*

flu'o-. *In chemistry,* a combining form indicating *the presence of fluorine.*

flu"o·res'ce·in, flu"o·res'cin. C₂₀H₁₂O₅ + H₂O. Resorcinolphthalein, a condensation product of resorcinol and phthalic anhydride. The water-soluble sodium salt is used diagnostically. **f. sodium.** C₂₀H₁₀O₅Na₂, freely soluble in water. A 2% solution is employed in diagnosing corneal lesions and in the detection of minute foreign bodies in that tissue; it is suggested as a means of determining apparent death by injection of the salt; if circulation remains, the mucosae will be stained yellow within a few minutes. Syn., *soluble fluorescein, uranin.*

flu"o·res'cence. A property possessed by certain substances of radiating, when illuminated, a light of a different, usually greater, wave length. —**fluorescent,** *adj.*

flu"o·res'cin. See *fluorescein.*

flu"o·ri·da'tion. The addition of fluorides to the water supply of a community as an aid in control of dental caries.

flu'o·ride. A salt of hydrofluoric acid.

flu"o·ri·na'tion. The addition of fluorine in one of several compounds to the water supply of a community as an aid in control of dental caries.

flu'o·rine (floo'o·reen, ·rin). F = 19.00. A gaseous element belonging to the halogen group. Its salts, the fluorides, may prevent dental caries but in excessive amounts in drinking water may cause mottling of tooth enamel.

flu'o·rite. Native calcium fluoride, CaF₂; used as a source of fluorine compounds, as a flux, and in manufacture of certain lenses.

flu"or·og'ra·phy. A combination of fluoroscopy and photography whereby a photograph of small size is made of the fluoroscopic image. Used to reduce the cost of making large numbers of chest examinations for tuberculosis surveys. Also called *miniature fluorography.* —**fluorograph'ic,** *adj.*

flu"o·ro·pho·tom'e·try. The quantitative study of fluorescent substances in solution. —**fluorophotomet'ric,** *adj.*

flu'o·ro·scope. The instrument used for examining the form and motion of the internal structures of the body by means of roentgen rays. It consists of a fluorescent screen composed of crystals of cadmium tungstate. —**fluoros'copy,** *n.* **biplane f.** One having two fluorescent screens and two x-ray tubes at right angles to each other for examination of foreign bodies, fractures, and other lesions in two planes.

flu"o·ro'sis. Poisoning by absorption of toxic amounts of fluorine. **chronic dental f.** Hypoplasia and discoloration of the teeth; resulting from the continued use, during the formative period of the tooth, of water containing toxic amounts of fluorine. Syn., *mottled enamel.*

flu"ox·y·mes'ter'one. 9α-Fluoro-11β-hydroxy-17β-methyltestosterone, a potent anabolic and androgenic agent. See *halotestin.*

flush. 1. Blush, become suffused, as the cheeks; due to vasodilation of small arteries and arterioles especially when these vessels are hypotonic. Occurs in emotional states, hyperthyroidism, local inflammation, pyrexia, and in states of chronic malnutrition of the skin. 2. Cleanse a wound or cavity by a rapid flow of water. —**flush,** *n.*

flut'ter. Quick, irregular motion; agitation. **atrial f.** A cardiac irregularity closely resembling atrial fibrillation, consisting of regular but abnormal atrial contractions said to be caused by a wave of excitation and contraction constantly circulating, about 300 times per minute, around a fixed ring of muscle in the atria. The ventricles respond at a fraction of the atrial rate (usually about 150 per minute). Electrocardiograms indicate two types of atrial flutter: impure, in which the events are not accurately repeated from cycle to cycle; pure, in which the events are constant from cycle to cycle. **flux.** 1. An excessive flow of any of the excretions of the body, especially the feces. 2. *In chemistry,* material added to minerals or metals to promote fusion. **fly.** Any insect of the order Diptera. Many insects not belonging to the Diptera are popularly called flies, such as dragonflies, caddis flies, May flies, butterflies, sawflies, gallflies, etc. Some insects belonging to the Diptera are not popularly known as flies, notably the mosquitoes. **black f.** See *Simulium.* **botfly.** See *Oestridae.* **flesh f.** See *Sarcophagidae.* **gadfly.** See *Tabanidae.* **horsefly.** See *Tabanidae.* **sand f.** See *Phlebotomus.* **stable f.** See *Stomoxys.* **tsetse f.** See *Glossina.* **foam.** *In physicochemistry,* a heterogeneous mixture of a gaseous phase, or finely divided gas bubbles, suspended in a liquid. **fibrin f.** See *fibrin* foam.

fo'cal length. The distance from the second principal point of a lens to a point on the axis where rays from an infinitely distant source converge to a common point or focus.

fo'cus (pl. *foci*). 1. The principal seat of a disease. 2. The point (called **principal focus** or **real focus**) at which rays of light converge that pass through a convex lens or are reflected from a concave mirror. —**focal,** *adj.* **conjugate foci.** Two interchangeable points at corresponding distances from a lens; the focal point of the image and the point of the object. **virtual f.** The point at which divergent rays would meet if prolonged in a backward direction. Also called *negative f.*

fog'ging. 1. In repression treatment of esophoria, the reduction of vision to about 20/80 by combining prisms (varying with the muscular imbalance), bases in, with a convex sphere; the patient reads with these glasses for a half hour at night before retiring. 2. A method of refracting the eye by using a convex lens sufficiently strong to cause the eye to become artificially myopic and fog the vision. Astigmatism is then corrected by means of minus cylinders, after which the fog is removed by gradually reducing the convex lens. Generally used in adults or when cycloplegia might precipitate glaucoma.

foil. A thin sheet of metal, especially gold or tin.

fold. A plication or doubling of various parts of the body. **amniotic f.** One of the folds of the blastoderm that unite over the embryo to form amnion and chorion in Sauropsida and many mammals. Also called *amnionic f.* **aryepiglottic f.** A fold of mucous membrane that extends from each arytenoid cartilage to the epiglottis. **body f.** One of the various folds formed by the rapid growth of the embryonic area. **circular folds.** The shelflike folds of the mucous membrane of the small intestine. Also called *valvulae conniventes, valves of Kerckring, plicae circulares.* **fimbriated f.** A fold of mucous membrane having a fringed, free edge, on either side of the frenulum of the tongue. **glossoepiglottic f.** A fold separating the glossoepiglottic fossa into the two vallecolae. **gluteal f.** Crease between buttock and thigh. **head f.** A ventral fold formed by rapid growth of the head of the embryo over the embryonic disk, resulting in the formation of the foregut accompanied by anteroposterior reversal of the anterior part of the embryonic disk. **lateral umbilical f.** A fold of peritoneum covering the obliterated umbilical artery. **median umbilical f.** A fold of peritoneum covering the urachus. **neural f.** One of the paired, longitudinal folds of the neural plate which unite in the midline to form the neural tube. **palpebral f.** That formed by the reflection of the conjunctiva from the eyelids onto the eye. There are two folds, the superior and the inferior. **salpingopharyngeal f.** A vertical fold of mucous membrane which covers the salpingopharyngeal muscle from the torus tubarius to the oropharynx. **semilunar f.** A conjunctival fold in the inner canthus of the eye, the rudiment of the nictitating membrane of birds. **sublingual f.** A fold of mucous membrane caused by the projection of the sublingual gland. **tail f.** A fold formed by rapid growth of the caudal end of the embryo over the embryonic disk, resulting in the formation of hindgut and ventral body wall in this region. **transverse rectal folds.** Large, semilunar folds projecting into the lumen of the upper part of the rectum. Also called *Houston's valves.* **urethral f.** One of a pair of folds flanking the urethral groove on the caudal surface of the genital tubercle or phallus. **ventricular f.** A fold of mucous membrane on either side of the larynx, inclosing the superior thyroarytenoid ligament. Also called *false vocal fold, plica ventricularis.* **vocal f.** One of the two membranous bands extending from the thyroid cartilage to the arytenoid cartilage; their tension controls the pitch of the voice. Also called *true vocal fold, plica vocalis.*

fo''li·a'ceous. Leaflike.

fo'lic ac'id. Pteroylglutamic acid; a substance occurring in green leaves, liver, and yeast, also produced by synthesis. It is essential for the growth of *Lactobacillus casei* and possesses hematopoietic activity for animals. Also called *liver L. casei factor, vitamin B₄*. See *folvite*.

fo″lie′ (fo″lee′). 1. A mental disorder or psychosis. 2. Old term for insanity. **f. à deux.** A type of communicated psychosis involving two persons, one of whom has an essential psychosis. His control of and influence over the other person is so potent that the latter will simulate or accept the elements of the psychosis without question. Similar supposed syndromes are also called *communicated insanity, double insanity, induced insanity.* **f. du doute.** Formerly called doubting mania; now classified under anxiety neurosis, *q.v.*

fo·li·ner′in, fo·lin′er·in. A glycoside from *Nerium oleander* which, on hydrolysis, yields gitoxigenin, the same steroid aglycone as is obtained from the digitalis glycoside, gitoxin. Syn., *oleandrin.*

fo·lin′ic ac′id. 1. Collectively, a group of chemical compounds, usually occurring in liver extracts and also obtained from pteroylglutamic acid, which contains growth factors essential to the bacterium *Leuconostoc citrovorum*. 2. 5-Formyl-5,6,7,8-tetrahydrofolic acid, the form in which folic acid probably exists and is active in tissues. See *leucovorin.*

fol/li·cle. 1. Old term for a lymphatic nodule. 2. A small secretory cavity or sac, as an acinus or alveolus. 3. A small, saccular structure, as a hair follicle. —**follic′ular,** *adj.* **aggregate f.** An aggregation of lymphatic nodules situated in the mucous membrane of the lower part of the small intestine, opposite the mesenteric attachment. Also called *Peyer's glands, Peyer's patches.* **atretic f.** An involuted or degenerated ovarian follicle. Also called *corpus atreticum.* **Graafian f.** The mature ovarian follicle. Syn., *vesicular f.* **growing f.** Any stage in the maturation of an ovarian follicle between the primary follicle and the Graafian follicle. **hair f.** The tubular epithelial invagination containing the root of a hair. **ovarian f.** An ovum and the epithelial follicular cells which surround it, lying in the cortex of the ovary. **palpebral follicles.** The tarsal glands. **primary f.** An ovarian follicle in which the ovum is surrounded by a single layer of follicular cells. **sebaceous f.** A sebaceous gland of the skin.

fol/li·clis. A tuberculid involving the extremities and at times the face. The histopathology is that of tuberculosis,

and the lesions are papules or crusted pustules.

fol·lic″u·li′tis. Inflammation of a group of follicles. **f. barbae.** Inflammation of the hair follicles of the beard; sycosis.

fol·lic″u·lo′ma. A tumor originating in a Graafian follicle.

follutein. The trade-mark for a preparation of chorionic gonadotropin obtained from the urine of pregnant women.

folvite. Trade-mark for folic acid.

fo″men·ta′tion. 1. The application of heat and moisture to a part to relieve pain or reduce inflammation. 2. The substance applied to a part to convey heat or moisture.

fo′mes (fo′meez, fom′eez) (pl. *fomites*). Any substance regarded as capable of transmitting contagious disease. *Obs.*

fo′mi·tes (fo′mi·teez, fom′i·). Plural of fomes, *q.v.*

fon·tac′to·scope. An instrument for ascertaining the radioactivity of waters and gases.

fon″ta·nel′, fon″ta·nelle′. A membranous space between the cranial bones in fetal life and infancy. **anterior f.** That at the region of union of the frontal, sagittal, and coronal sutures. Closes during the second year. Also called *fonticulus major, fonticulus quadrangularis.* **great f.** See anterior *f.* **lateral fontanels.** Two membranous spaces, one in front between the parietal, frontal, great wing of the sphenoid, and temporal bones (the **anterior lateral** or **sphenoid fontanel**), and one behind between the parietal, occipital, and temporal bones (the **posterior lateral, mastoid, Casser's** or **Casserio's fontanel**). They usually close by three months after birth. **posterior f.** That at the region of junction of lambdoid and sagittal sutures. Also called *fonticulus minor, fonticulus triangularis.* **sagittal f.** One occasionally found in the sagittal suture, about midway between the anterior and posterior fontanels. **small f.** See posterior *f.*

fon″ta·nelle′. Fontanel, *q.v.*

food. Nutriment; any substance which, when taken into the body of an organism, may be used either to supply energy or to build tissue. Foods are organic substances classified in three groups: proteins, carbohydrates, and fats. All of these may occur in animal or vegetable substance.

foot. 1. The terminal extremity of the leg. It consists of the tarsus, metatarsus, and phalanges or toes. 2. A measure of length equal to 12 inches, or 30.479 cm. Abbreviated, ft. **congenital deformity of the f.** See

talipes. **frosted feet.** See *chilblain.*
shelter f. A condition resembling trench foot and immersion foot, but of less severity; it occurs in persons who are confined to cold and damp shelters; associated with some vitamin deficiency. **splay f.** Flatfoot with extreme eversion of the forefoot and tarsus. **trench f.** A condition of the feet somewhat like frostbite; it occurs in those long exposed to wet and cold. **weak f.** Chronic eversion of the foot, due usually to faulty walking habits associated with loss of muscular tone. Frequently confused with flatfoot.

foot-can'dle. The illumination received at a surface 1 foot from a standard lamp of 1 candlepower; 1 foot-candle = 1 lumen per square foot.

foot drop. A falling of the foot due to a paralysis of the dorsiflexors of the ankle.

foot'-pound'. A unit of energy; the work equal to that of raising a pound to the height of one foot. Abbreviated, ft.-lb.

foot'print". An ink impression of the sole of the foot; used for identification of infants.

fo·ra'men (pl. *foramens, foramina*). A perforation or opening, especially in a bone. **—foram'inal,** *adj.* **anterior ethmoid f.** A canal between the ethmoid and frontal bones, giving passage to the nasal branch of the ophthalmic nerve and anterior ethmoid vessels. **anterior sacral f.** One of the eight (four on each side) on the anterior surface of the sacrum, connecting with the sacral canal, and giving passage to the anterior branches of the sacral nerves. **aortic f.** Aortic hiatus. **apical f.** The orifice in the end of a root of a tooth through which pass the nerves and vessels of the pulp. **epiploic f.** An aperture of the peritoneal cavity between the liver and the stomach, bounded in front by the portal vein, hepatic artery and duct, behind by the inferior vena cava, below by the duodenum, and above by the liver. Formed by folds of the peritoneum, it establishes communication between the greater and lesser cavities of the peritoneum. Also called *f. of Winslow.* **esophageal f.** Esophageal hiatus. **f. magnum.** A large oval aperture centrally placed in the lower and anterior part of the occipital bone; it gives passage to the spinal cord and its membranes and venous plexuses, the spinal accessory nerves, and the vertebral arteries. **f. of Magendie.** A median foramen in the membranous roof of the fourth ventricle of the brain. **f. ovale of the heart.** A fetal opening between the two atria of the heart, situated at the lower posterior portion of the septum. **f. ovale**

of the sphenoid. An oval opening near the posterior margin of the great wing of the sphenoid, giving passage to the mandibular branch of the trigeminal nerve, an accessory meningeal artery, and occasionally the lesser superficial petrosal nerve. **f. rotundum.** A round opening in the great wing of the sphenoid bone for the maxillary branch of the fifth nerve. **f. of Luschka.** A small opening in each lateral recess of the fourth ventricle, allowing passage of the cerebrospinal fluid into the subarachnoid space. The free ends of the choroid plexus project through them. **f. spinosum.** A passage in the great wing of the sphenoid bone, near its posterior angle, giving passage to the middle meningeal artery and spinosus nerve. **infraorbital f.** In the maxilla, the external aperture of the infraorbital canal; it gives passage to the infraorbital nerve and artery. **internal auditory f.** One located in the petrous portion of the temporal bone; it gives passage to the auditory and facial nerves and vessels and the internal auditory vessels. **interventricular f.** That between the lateral and third ventricles of the brain. Also called *f. of Monro.* **intervertebral f.** The aperture formed by the notches opposite to each other in the laminas of adjacent vertebrae; a passage for a spinal nerve and vessels. **jugular f.** The space formed by the jugular notches of the occipital and temporal bones, divided into two portions, the posterior portion giving passage to an internal jugular vein and the anterior portion giving passage to the ninth, tenth, and eleventh cranial nerves and the inferior petrosal sinus. **mandibular f.** The aperture of the inferior dental or alveolar canal in the ramus of the mandible, which transmits the inferior dental or alveolar vessels and nerve to the lower jaw. **mastoid f.** A small foramen behind the mastoid process; it transmits a small artery from the dura and a vein opening into the sigmoid sinus. **nutrient f.** The canal which gives passage to the main blood vessels of the medullary cavity of a bone. **obturator f.** The large oval opening between the ischium and the pubis, anterior and inferior to the acetabulum, partly closed by a fibrous membrane; it gives passage to the obturator vessels and nerves. **olfactory foramens.** Numerous foramens in the cribriform plate of the ethmoid, giving passage to the olfactory nerves. **optic f.** The canal at the apex of each orbit, the anterior termination of the optic groove, just beneath the lesser wing of the sphenoid bone; it gives passage to an optic nerve and ophthalmic artery. **palatine foramens.** The orifices of the pterygopalatine canal on the posterior part of the hard palate, giving passage to branches of the descending palatine vessels and nerves. **sciatic foramens.** The **greater sciatic foramen** is the oval space between the sacrotuberous ligament and the innominate bone, conveying the piriformis muscle, the gluteal, sciatic, and pudendal vessels and nerves; the **lesser sciatic foramen** is the space included between the sacrotuberous and sacrospinous ligaments and the portion of the innominate bone between the spine and tuberosity of the ischium, giving passage to the internal obturator tendon and the internal pudendal vessels and nerves. **stylomastoid f.** One between the styloid and mastoid processes of the temporal bone; the external aperture of the facial canal. **supraorbital f.** A notch in the superior orbital margin at the junction of the middle with the inner third, sometimes converted into a foramen by a bony process or a ligamentous band; it gives passage to the supraorbital artery, veins, and nerve. **vertebral f.** The space included between the body and arch of a vertebra, giving passage to the spinal cord and its appendages.

force. 1. Strength, power; physical might, vigor. 2. That which initiates, changes, or arrests motion. 3. Binding power, validity. **—forced,** *adj.* **animal f.** Muscular energy. **electromotive f.** The force which tends to alter the motion of electricity, measured in volts. Abbreviated, **E**, emf., e.m.f., E.M.F. **psychic f.** Mental power or force generated by thinking; contrasted with physical force. **reserve f.** Energy latent within an organism or part over and above that required for usual functions. Cardiac reserve is the latent force of the heart available to meet any additional burden placed on the circulation. **vital f.** The energy or power characteristic of living organisms.

for'ceps. A surgical instrument with two opposing blades or limbs; controlled by handles or by direct pressure on the blades. Used to grasp, compress, and hold tissue, a part of the body, needles, or other surgical material. **—forcip'ial,** *adj.* **alligator f.** A type of heavy-toothed forceps. **alveolar f.** Dental forceps for biting into the alveolar processes. **artery f.** Any forceps used for seizing and compressing an artery; usually self-locking, with scissors handles. Syn., *hemostatic f.* **aural f.** A delicate dressing forceps used in aural surgery. **axis-traction f.** An obstetric forceps, the so-called high forceps instrument, equipped

with a mechanism to permit rotation of the fetal head and traction in the line of the pelvic axis. **bonecutting f.** A double-jointed or single-jointed, powerful, heavy-bladed cutting forceps, with great power derived from the leverage exerted by the long handles. **bone-holding f.** A forceps with heavy jaws and long handles, for use in holding bone during an operation. Syn., *lion-jawed f.* **bulldog f.** Forceps with strong teeth and a clasp to prevent slipping. **bullet f.** Instrument for extracting bullets. **crushing f.** A forceps, usually in the form of a clamp, for crushing heavy tissues or pedicles prior to ligation. **dental f.** Any one of a variety of forceps adapted for the extraction of teeth. **disk f.** A type used in ophthalmic surgery. **dressing f.** A two-limbed, slender-bladed instrument or spring forceps, with blunt or serrated teeth; for use in surgical dressings. **epilating f.** Special forceps used for removing the hairs of the lashes, eyebrows, or other areas where hair is not desired. **esophageal f.** A special forceps for removing foreign bodies from the esophagus. **extracting f.** Dental forceps. **hemostatic f.** See artery *f.* **high f.** An obstetric forceps applied to the fetal head which has descended into the pelvic canal, when its greatest diameter is still above the superior strait. **lion-jawed f.** See bone-holding *f.* **lithotomy f.** A special type of forceps for removing a stone from the bladder or ureter. **low f.** An obstetric forceps applied to the fetal head when it is well within the lower portion of the pelvic canal. **mid f.** An obstetric forceps applied when the presenting part is at, or immediately above, the ischial spines. **mosquito f.** A delicate, sharp-pointed hemostat. Also called *Halsted's mosquito f.* **mousetooth f.** A dressing forceps with interlocking fine teeth at the tips of the blades. **needle f.** A needle holder, *q.v.* **obstetric f.** A large, fenestrated, double-bladed traction forceps; the blades are demountable and are applied separately before interlocking at the handles, in order to fit the fetal head. Employed in difficult or delayed labor. **roller f.** A forceps equipped with small rollers; used for compressing the eyelids in cases of trachoma. **rongeur f.** Bone-gouging forceps. **sequestrum f.** Forceps designed for removing spicules or sequestra of bone. **tenaculum f.** A slender forceps with scissors handles and one or two long, overlapping teeth or hooks at the end of the blade; adapted especially for gynecologic surgery. **towel f.** A snap, clamp, or forceps with sharp hooked ends which overlap; adapted to holding towels fast to the skin during operations. Also called *towel clamp, skinholding f.* **volsella f.** A type of tenaculum forceps.

for'ci·pres"sure. Pressure exerted on a blood vessel by means of a forceps, to prevent hemorrhage.

fore-. A prefix signifying *before* (in time or place), *in front.*

fore'arm". That part of the upper extremity between the wrist and the elbow.

fore'brain". The prosencephalon.

fore'con"scious. 1. *In psychoanalysis*, that portion of the unconscious containing mental experiences which are not in the focus of immediate attention, but which may be recalled to consciousness. 2. Capable of being recalled into the conscious mind, although not in the realm of consciousness. Syn., *coconscious, preconscious.*

fore'fin"ger. The index finger.

fore'foot". Anterior part of the foot; from a clinical standpoint, that portion of the foot which includes the toes, metatarsal, cuneiform, and cuboid bones.

fore'gut". The cephalic part of the embryonic digestive tube that develops into pharynx, esophagus, stomach, part of the small intestine, liver, pancreas, and respiratory ducts.

fore'head. That part of the face above the eyes.

fore'milk". Colostrum.

fo·ren'sic. Relating to a law court.

fore'pleas"ure. *In psychoanalysis*, the erotic pleasure, both physical and emotional, accompanied by a rise in tension, which precedes the culmination of the sexual act, or end pleasure, *q.v.*

fore'skin". The prepuce.

fore'wa"ters. Hydrorrhea gravidarum.

form. The configuration, shape, or particular appearance of living things or tissues, especially when modified under particular conditions; for example, bacteria, parasites, malignant growths, etc.

form·al'de·hyde. Formic aldehyde or methanal, HCHO. A colorless gas obtained by the oxidation of methyl alcohol. It is soluble in water and in alcohol. **f. sodium sulfoxylate.** CH_2OH·$SO_2Na.2H_2O$. A white, water-soluble compound, introduced as an antidote for poisoning by mercury bichloride. Syn., *sodium formaldehyde sulfoxylate, rongolite.* Also called *sodium sulfoxylate, formaldehyde hydrosulfite.* **f. solution.** An aqueous solution containing not less than 37% by weight of formaldehyde. It is a powerful antiseptic. **para–f.** $(CH_2O)_x$. A solid polymer of formaldehyde. On heating, a portion of it is converted to formaldehyde.

formalin. A trade-mark for a formaldehyde solution.

form·am'ide, form'am·ide. 1. $HCONH_2$, the amide of formic acid. 2. A compound containing the HCONH– radical.

for'mate, for'mi·ate. A salt of formic acid.

for·ma'tion. 1. The process of developing shape or structure. 2. That which is formed; a structure or arrangement.

form'a·tive. 1. Relating to the process of development, as of tissue or of the embryo. 2. Forming, producing, originating.

for'ma·zin. Formalazin; an insoluble, white, amorphous compound formed from hydrazine sulfate and hexamethylenetetramine. In gelatin suspension, it is used in making permanent albumin standards in the life insurance method for the determination of protein in urine.

for'mic. Relating to, or derived from, ants; or pertaining to formic acid. **f. acid.** An aqueous solution containing 24 to 26% of HCOOH. **f. aldehyde.** Formaldehyde.

for"mi·ca'tion. Paresthesia; an abnormal sensation as of insects crawling in or upon the skin; a common symptom in diseases of the spinal cord and the peripheral nerves.

formin. A trade-mark for methenamine.

for'mol. A solution of formaldehyde.

for"mo·ni'trile (for"mo·nigh'tril, ·tryle). Hydrocyanic acid.

for·mox'yl. Formyl.

for'mu·la. 1. A prescribed method. 2. The representation of a chemical compound by symbols. 3. A recipe or prescription. Abbreviated, F. **dental f.** One showing the number and arrangement of teeth. **empirical f.** One that indicates only the constituents and their proportions in a molecule, as $C_6H_{12}O_6$, dextrose. **graphic f.** See structural f. **official f.** One given in an official publication. **officinal f.** A pharmaceutical formula which, though not official, is commonly followed by pharmacists. **structural f.** One which shows the arrangement and relation of every atom in a molecule. One in which the symbols are united by the bonds of affinity according to their valence, as H–O–H.

for'mu·lar"y (for"mew·lerr"ee). A collection of formulas for making medicinal preparations.

for'myl. 1. HCO–, the radical of formic acid. Also called *formoxyl.* 2. The trivalent radical, HC≡. **f. iodide.** Iodoform.

for"ni·cate. Commit fornication.

for'ni·cate. Arched.

for"ni·ca'tion. The illicit sexual intercourse of unmarried persons.

for'nix. 1. An arched body or surface;

a concavity or cul-de-sac. 2. One of the two fiber tracts beneath the corpus callosum, extending from the fimbria of the hippocampus to the mammillary body. **—fornical**, *adj.* **f. of the conjunctiva.** The cul-de-sac at the point where the bulbar conjunctiva is reflected upon the lid. **f. of the vagina.** The vault of the vagina: the upper part of the vagina which surrounds the cervix of the uterus.

fos′sa (pl. *fossae*). A depression or pit. **acetabular f.** A depression in the center of the acetabulum. **antecubital f.** One in front of the elbow. **axillary f.** The armpit. **cranial f.** Any of the three depressions, **anterior, middle,** and **posterior,** in the base of the skull. **cystic f.** A depression, on the lower surface of the right lobe of the liver, in which the gallbladder is situated. **digastric f.** (a) A deep groove on the inner aspect of the mastoid process marking the attachment of the posterior belly of the digastric muscle. (b) A depression on the inside of the mandible for the attachment of the anterior belly of the digastric muscle. **f. ovalis.** (a) An oval fossa in the interatrial septum; its floor is derived from the embryonic septum primum, and its rim from the septum secundum. (b) A fossa in the thigh which gives passage to the great saphenous vein. **glenoid f.** (a) Any shallow, oval articular facet. (b) Old term for mandibular fossa. **hypophyseal f.** A depression in the sphenoid bone, lodging the hypophysis. Also called *sella turcica, f. hypophyseos.* **ileocecal fossae.** Peritoneal recesses in the region of the ileocecal junction. **ischiorectal f.** The space on either side of the rectum, bounded laterally by the obturator internus and medially by the levator ani and coccygeus muscles. **mandibular f.** A depression in the temporal bone that receives the condyle of the mandible. **pituitary f.** The hypophyseal fossa. **rectouterine f.** The peritoneal pouch between rectum and uterus; the pouch of Douglas, or cul-de-sac. **supratonsillar f.** The upper recess of the tonsillar sinus between the faucial pillars and above the palatine tonsil; it is covered by the semilunar fold. **tonsillar f.** The depression between the glossopalatine and pharyngopalatine arches, in which the palatine tonsil is situated. It is approximately at the site of the second visceral pouch.

fos·sette′. 1. A dimple; a small depression. 2. A small, deep ulcer of the cornea.

found′ling. An infant found after being abandoned by its parents.

four·chette′ (foor-shet′). 1. A fold of mucous membrane just inside the posterior commissure of the vulva. 2. A fork used in dividing the frenulum linguae.

fo′ve·a. A small pit or depression; applied to many depressions in the body, but especially to the **fovea centralis** of the retina (the spot of most distinct vision), a small pit in the macula lutea in the visual axis. **—foveate,** *adj.* **coccygeal f.** A persistent depression near the tip of the coccyx at the site of the terminal attachment of the embryonic neural tube to the dermis. Also called *postanal dimple, f. sacrococcygea.*

fo·ve′o·la. A small fovea or depression. **—foveolate,** *adj.* **gastric f.** One of the pits or grooves in the mucous membrane of the stomach, which receive the secretions of the gastric glands.

fox′glove″. See *digitalis.*

frac′tion·al. 1. Pertaining to a fraction. 2. In chemistry, divided successively; applied to any one of the several processes for separating a mixture into its constituents through differences in solubility, boiling point, etc., such as fractional distillation, fractional sterilization, etc.

frac″tion·a′tion. 1. *In chemistry,* the separation of a mixture into its constituents, as in fractional distillation. 2. *In microbiology,* the process of obtaining a pure culture by successive culturing of small portions of a colony. Also called *fractional cultivation.* 3. *In physiology,* the phenomenon whereby maximal stimulation of a given efferent nerve produces contraction of only a fraction of the fibers in the responding muscle.

frac′ture. The breaking of a bone or cartilage. **articular f.** A fracture entering into a joint. **avulsion f.** The tearing-off of a bony prominence, as a tuberosity, by the forcible pull of its tendinous or muscular attachments. **chip f.** A minor fracture involving a bony process. **closed f.** A simple fracture. **Colles′ f.** A fracture of the distal end of the radius within one inch of the articular surface; characterized by dorsal displacement of the distal fragment, radial and dorsal deviation of the wrist and hand, and disturbance of the radioulnar articulation. **comminuted f.** A fracture in which there is splintering or fragmentation of the bone. **complete f.** One in which the continuity of the entire bone is destroyed. **complicated f.** One associated with injury of the surrounding soft parts, which will complicate treatment and/or recovery. **compound f.** One in which the point of fracture is in contact with the external surface of the body. **compression f.** One in which a surface of a bone is driven toward another surface; commonly found in vertebral bodies. **dentate f.** One in which the ends of the fragments are toothed and interlocked. **depressed f.** A fracture of the skull in which the fractured part is depressed below the normal level. **double f.** One in which there are two fractures in the same bone. **fissured f.** One in which there is an incomplete break; a crack or fissure extending into, but not through, a bone. **greenstick f.** An incomplete fracture of a long bone, seen in children; the bone is bent but splintered only on the convex side. **impacted f.** A fracture in which the harder cortical bone of one fragment has been driven into the softer cancellous bone of another fragment. **incomplete f.** One which does not extend through the entire bone. **intracapsular f.** One within the joint capsule. **intrauterine f.** A fracture occurring during fetal life, due to faulty development of the osseous matrix. **march f.** Fracture of the metatarsal bones without obvious trauma, as a result of marching. Syn., *fatigue f.*, *stress f.* **multiple f.** Two or more fractures occurring in the same or different bones. **pathologic f.** One which occurs at the site of a local disease in a bone, as carcinoma, without external violence. **Pott's f.** Fracture at the inferior tibiofibular joint; usually associated with a splitting-off of the tip of the medial malleolus, rupture of the tibial collateral ligament, and outward displacement of the foot. **puncture f.** One in which there is a loss of bone without disruption of continuity, as a hole drilled through a bone by a projectile. **simple f.** One in which there is no communication with the outside. **spontaneous f.** One occurring without apparent trauma; occurs in cases of bone atrophy or other general diseases of the bone. **ununited f.** One in which, after the normal period, there is failure of union. **fac'ture box.** A wooden case for immobilizing fractures of the leg.

fra·gil'i·tas. Brittleness. **f. crinium.** Atrophic condition of the hair in which the individual hairs split into numerous fibrils or break off. **f. ossium.** A familial disease of the long bones, characterized by abnormal brittleness and associated with blue scleras. Also called *Eddowes' disease*, *Lobstein's disease*.

fra·gil'i·ty. Quality of being easily broken or destroyed. **—frag'ile,** *adj.* **capillary f.** Weakness of the capillaries, as in purpura.

frag″men·ta'tion. 1. Division into small portions. 2. Amitosis.

fram·be'si·a (fram-bee'zhuh, ·zee-uh). See *yaws.*

fran'ci·um. Element number 87, symbol Fa, isolated in 1939 by Perey; formerly called virginium, *q.v.*

fran'gu·la. The bark of *Rhamnus frangula*, or glossy buckthorn.

fran'gu·lin. A product of the enzymatic cleavage of a glycoside in frangula.

frank'in·cense. An aromatic gum resin. See *olibanum.*

frax'in. A glycoside, $C_{15}H_{16}O_{10}$, from the bark of the European ash, *Fraxinus excelsior*; it is diuretic.

F.R.C.P. Fellow of the Royal College of Physicians.

F.R.C.S. Fellow of the Royal College of Surgeons.

free'mar″tin. An intersexual female calf, commonly sterile, twinborn with a male; produced by masculinization by sex hormones of the male twin when the placental circulations are partially fused.

free rad'i·cal. A non-ionic compound, highly reactive and of relatively short life, in which the central element is linked to an abnormal number of atoms or groups of atoms.

frem'i·tus. A palpable vibration. **echinococcus f.** The vibration felt over an echinococcus cyst. **friction f.** The vibrations produced by the rubbing together of two dry surfaces. **tactile f.** The vibratory sensation conveyed to the hand when applied to the chest of a person speaking. **tussive f.** Thrill felt by the hand when applied to the chest of a person coughing. **vocal f.** The sounds of the voice transmitted to the ear when applied to the chest of a person speaking.

fre·not'o·my. The cutting of any frenum, particularly of the frenulum of the tongue for tongue-tie.

frenquel. Trade-mark for azacyclonol hydrochloride.

fren'u·lum, frae'nu·lum (freen'-yoo·lum, fren'·). A small frenum; a slight ridge on the upper part of the anterior medullary velum. **f. of the clitoris.** One of the two folds of mucous membrane coming from the labia minora and being united under the glans of the clitoris. **f. of the lips.** One of the folds of mucous membrane in the median line uniting each lip to the corresponding gum. **f. of the prepuce.** The fold on the lower surface of the glans penis connecting it with the prepuce. **f. of the tongue.** The vertical fold of mucous membrane under the tongue.

fre'num, frae'num. A fold of integument or mucous membrane that checks or limits the movements of any organ. See *frenulum.* **—frenal,** *adj.*

fren'zy. Violent mania.

freon. Trade-mark for a group of halogenated hydrocarbons containing one or more fluorine atoms; widely used as refrigerants and propellants.

fre'quen·cy. 1. Rate of occurrences of a periodic process. 2. *In biometry*, the ratio of the number of observations falling within a classification group to the total number of observations made.

fre'quen·cy dis"tri·bu'tion. *In biometry*, a statistical table showing the frequency, or number, of observations (as test scores, ages, etc.) falling in each of certain classification groups or intervals (as 10–19, 20–29, etc.).

Freud, Sigmund [*Austrian psychiatrist*, 1856–1939]. With Breuer, is credited with the discovery of the unconscious mind. Introduced psychoanalysis, *q.v.*, for the treatment of neuroses. According to *Freud's theory*, hysteria is due to a past psychic trauma, usually of sexual character, the reaction having been repressed at the time the trauma was received.

Freud'i·an (froyd'ee·un). 1. Relating to the theories and practices of Sigmund Freud. 2. One who adheres to Freud's school of psychoanalysis.

fri'a·ble. Easily broken or crumbled.

fric'tion. 1. The act of rubbing, as rubbing the body for stimulation of the skin. 2. The resistance offered to motion between two contacting bodies.

fright. Sudden and extreme fear. **precordial f.** The precordial sensations of impending physical collapse experienced in the acute panic of an anxiety neurosis, *q.v.*

fri·gid'i·ty. Coldness; absence of sexual desire in women, probably of psychic origin.

frig"o·ther'a·py. The treatment of disease by cold.

frôle"ment' (frawl"mahn'). A succession of slow, brushing movements in massage, done with the palmar surfaces of the fingers.

fron'tal (frun'tul, fron'tul). 1. Pertaining to the anterior part or aspect of an organ or body. 2. Belonging to the forehead. See Table of Bones in the Appendix.

fron·ta'lis (frun·tah'lis, ·tal'is). The frontal portion of the epicranius muscle.

fron'to-. *In anatomy* and *zoology*, combining form denoting *anterior position* or expressing a *relation with the* forehead or frontal region.

fron"to·max·il'lar"y (frun"to·mack'si·lerr"ee). Relating to the frontal bone and the maxilla.

fron"to·na'sal. Pertaining to the frontal and nasal bones, as frontonasal suture.

fron"to·oc·cip'i·tal (frun"to·ock·sip'i·tul). Pertaining to the forehead and the occiput or to the frontal and occipital bones, as fronto-occipital muscle.

frost'bite". A condition similar to the lesions produced by burns, resulting from exposure to severe degrees of cold. The three stages of frostbite are marked by erythema, vesication, and necrosis, respectively. The parts most commonly affected are the ears, tip of the nose, fingers, and toes.

fro'zen sec'tions. Histologic sections cut from frozen tissues or organs as from those removed from the body during operation and examined immediately for possible malignancy.

F.R.S. Fellow of the Royal Society.

fruc"to·fu·ran'o·san. One of the polysaccharides of fructose.

fruc"to·fu'ran·ose. A fructose with a 2-5 butylene oxide or furanose ring.

fruc"to·fu·ran'o·side. A glycoside of fructofuranose.

fruc"to·py'ran·ose. A fructose with a 2-6 pyranose ring.

fruc'tose. Levulose.

fruc'to·side. A glycoside which yields levulose on hydrolysis.

fruc"to·su'ri·a. The presence of fructose in the urine; levulosuria.

fru·giv'o·rous (froo·jiv'o·rus, ·giv'o·rus). Fruit-eating.

fruit. The developed ovary of a plant, especially the succulent, fleshy part gathered about the same.

fru·men'tum. Wheat or other grain. **spiritus frumenti.** Whisky.

frus·tra'tion. 1. The condition that results when an impulse to act or the completion of an act is blocked or thwarted, preventing the satisfaction of attainment. 2. The blocking or thwarting of an impulse.

FSH. Prolan-A, *q.v.*

ft. 1. *In pharmacy*, fiat or fiant; let there be made. 2. Abbreviation for foot.

ft.-lb. Abbreviation for foot-pound.

fuadin. The trade-mark of sodium antimony III bis-catechol-2,4-disulfonate, proposed for use in the treatment of granuloma inguinale and of schistosomiasis.

fuch'sin (fook'sin, fook'sin). A red dyestuff occurring in two forms, acid and basic.

fuch·sin'o·phil (fook·sin'o·fil, fook·). Stainable with fuchsin.

-fuge (-fewdj). A combining form denoting *that which causes to flee*, or *drives away*.

fu'gi·tive. Wandering or transient, as a pain.

fugue (fewg). A state of amnesia of considerable duration, sometimes involving a flight from familiar surroundings. During the fugue, the patient appears to act in a conscious way and retains his mental faculties, but after recovery has no remembrance of the state.

ful·gu·rant. Synonym for fulgura-ting, q.v.

ful'gu·ra'ting, ful'gu·rant. Lightninglike; used to describe sudden excruciating pain.

ful"gu·ra'tion. Destruction of tissue, usually malignant tumors, by means of electric sparks.

fu·lig'i·nous (few-lidj'i·nus). Smoke-like; very dark; soot-colored.

ful'mi·nant, ful'mi·na"ting. Sudden, severe, and rapid in course.

Fu·ma"ri·a'ce·ae (few-mair"ee-ay'-se-ee). A family of plants including the genera Adlumia, Corydalis, Dicentra, and Fumaria. Many alkaloids are found among the plants of the Fumariaceae.

fu·mar'ic ac'id. COOH.CH:CH.-COOH. Trans-ethylene dicarboxylic acid, the trans-isomer of maleic acid. It occurs in Fumaria officinalis and in mammalian tissues as an intermediate in the metabolism of carbohydrate.

fu'ma·rine (few'muh-reen, -rin). An alkaloid, $C_{20}H_{19}O_5N$, found in opium and other Papaveraceae. It is identical with protopine and macleyine.

fu·mi·ga'cin. An antibiotic substance produced by different strains of Aspergillus fumigatus. It is identical with helvolic acid.

fu·mi·ga'tin. A maroon-colored, crystalline substance, 3-hydroxy-4-methoxy-2:5-toluquinone, $C_8H_8O_4$, isolated from cultures of Aspergillus fumigatus. It has antibacterial properties. It differs from fumigacin.

fu"mi·ga'tion. Disinfection by exposure to the fumes of a vaporized disinfectant.

fu'ming. Emitting smoke or vapor, as fuming nitric acid.

func'tion. 1. The normal or special action of a part. 2. The chemical character, relationships, and general properties of a substance. 3. Act or perform special action. **—functional,** adj.

fun'da·ment. 1. The foundation or base. 2. The buttocks.

fun·dec'to·my. Removal of a fundus, as of the uterus, or corpus uteri by abdominal operation.

fun'di·form. Shaped like a sling, or loop.

fun'dus (pl. fundi). The base of an organ; the part farthest removed from the opening of the organ. **—fundic,** adj. **f. oculi.** The posterior portion of the interior of the eye. **f. uteri.** That part of the uterus most remote from the cervix. **f. ventriculi.** The large, rounded cul-de-sac cephalad to the cardia of the stomach, when that organ is dilated. **f. vesicae.** Posterior part or base of the urinary bladder.

fun'gate (fung'gate, fun'gate). Grow up rapidly, like a fungus, as certain pathologic growths.

fun'gi (fun'jye). Plural of fungus, q.v.

fun'gi·cide. An agent that destroys fungi. **—fungici'dal,** adj.

fun'gi·form. Having the form of a mushroom, as the fungiform papillae of the tongue.

fun"gin·ert'ness. Failure to support fungous growth because of absence of the necessary nutrients; to be distinguished from fungistasis. **—fun-ginert',** adj.

fun"gi·sta'sis. The active prevention or hindrance of fungous growth by a chemical or physical agent; to be distinguished from funginertness. **—fun-gistat'ic,** adj.

fun'goid. Resembling a fungus.

fun·gos'i·ty. 1. A fungous excrescence. 2. Fungous quality.

fun'gus (pl. fungi). 1. A low form of plant life, a division of the Thallophytes without chlorophyll. The chief classes of fungi are the Phycomycetes, Ascomycetes, Basidiomycetes, and Fungi Imperfecti. Most of the pathogenic fungi belong to the last group. 2. A spongy morbid excrescence. **—fun-gous, fungal,** adj.

fu·nic"u·li'tis. Inflammation of the spermatic cord.

fu·nic'u·lus (pl. funiculi). 1. One of the three main divisions of white matter, which are named with reference to the gray matter of the cord as dorsal, lateral, and ventral. 2. Formerly used for fasciculus, q.v. 3. Old term for the umbilical or spermatic cord. **—funic-ular,** adj.

fu'nis. A cord, particularly the umbilical cord. **—funic,** adj.

fun'nel. A wide-mouthed, conical vessel ending in an open tube; for filling bottles or other containers, and as a support for filter papers.

fun'ny bone. The region of the medial condyle of the humerus, crossed superficially by the ulnar nerve. Blows upon it give a painful tingling sensation to the hand.

fur. 1. A coating of epithelial debris, as on the tongue. 2. The hairy coat of some animals. **—furred,** adj.

furacin. Trade-mark for nitrofurazone.

furadantin. Trade-mark for nitrofurantoin.

fur·al'de·hyde. See furfural.

fu'ran, fu'rane. A constituent of wood tars. Also called furfuran, furfurane.

fu'ra·nose. A sugar having a ring structure resembling that of furan.

fur'fur. Dandruff; a branny desquamation of the epidermis. **—fur-fura'ceous,** adj.

fur'fur·al. $C_4H_2O.CHO$. A liquid obtained by distillation of oat hulls and corn cobs. Also called *fural, furole, furaldehyde, furfuraldehyde.* Improperly called *furfurol.*

fur·fur·an, fur·fur·ane. Furan.

fur·fur·ol. Incorrect term for furfural.

fur·fur·yl. The monovalent radical $C_5H_3O—$ derived from furfural.

furmethide. The trade-mark for furfuryl trimethylammonium iodide, a parasympathetic nerve stimulant.

fu·ror. Madness; fury; a mania or maniacal attack. **paroxysmal f.** Unprovoked attacks of intense anger occurring in patients with epileptic psychoses, not associated with convulsions. Also called *f. epilepticus.*

fur·row. A groove. **gluteal f.** The groove between the nates. **interventricular furrows.** Two longitudinal grooves separating the two ventricles of the heart.

fu·run·cle (few′rung·kul, ·run·kul). A boil; a cutaneous abscess a few millimeters or less in size; usually the result of infection of a hair follicle or, more rarely, of ducts of cutaneous glands by pyogenic bacteria, especially by *Micrococcus aureus (Staphylococcus aureus).* —**furun′cular,** *adj.*

fu·run″cu·lo′sis. A condition marked by affection with numerous furuncles, or in which new crops of furuncles follow repeatedly after healing of preceding crops.

fu·run′cu·lus. See *furuncle.*

Fu·sa·ri·um (few·sair′ee·um, ·zair′ee·um). A genus of fungi, including species that may act as allergens, and that are pathogenic for plants.

fu′sel alcohol. Amyl alcohol.

fus′cin (fuss′in, few′sin). The brown melanin pigment of the retina.

fu′si·ble (few′zi·bul). Capable of being melted.

fu′si·form (few′zi·form, few′si·). Spindle-shaped.

Fu″si·for′mis (few″zi·for′mis, few″si·). Bacteria with the form of elongated spindles. There are aerobic and anaerobic types. **F. dentium.** A bacillus found in Vincent's angina. Syn., *Fusobacterium plauti-vincenti.* Also called *fusiform bacillus.*

fu′sion. The process of melting; the act of uniting or cohering. **atomic** [The uniting of atomic nuclei, resulting in a release of energy. **spinal** The fusion of two or more vertebra for immobilization of the spinal column. Used in the treatment of spinal deformities, tuberculosis of the spine and severe arthritis of the spine.

Fu″so·bac·te′ri·um (few″zo·back′teer′ee·um, few″so·). A genus of bacteria, including slender, Gram-negative, anaerobic, rectilinear, or incurving bacilli, which are frequently spindle-shaped and which stain irregularly. They are obligatory parasites of man and animals, and are found in necrotic areas, often in association with spirochetes. **F. plauti-vincenti.** species present in certain forms of gingivitis, in Vincent's angina, and in abscesses in the lungs and other organs. Also called *Fusiformis dentium.*

fu″so·spi″ro·che·to′sis (few″zo·spy″ro·ki·to′sis, few″so·). Infection characterized by the presence of fusiform bacilli and spirochetes. The organisms are present in certain forms of gingivitis, Vincent's angina, and in abscesses in the lungs and other organs.

G

G. 1. Gravitation constant or Newtonian constant. 2. *In aviation,* the force of acceleration is expressed as the number of pounds of force per pound of mass of the pilot; G is one gravitational unit and equals one pound of force divided by one pound of mass. Greater accelerations are expressed in multiples of G. Blackout occurs above 7G in most pilots.

g. Gram(s).

Ga. Chemical symbol for the element gallium.

gad″o·lin′i·um. Gd = 156.9. A rare earth metal.

Ga′dus. A genus of soft-finned fish. **G. morrhua.** The common cod; a

fish from the livers of which cod liver oil is obtained.

gag. 1. An instrument placed between the teeth to prevent closure of the jaws. 2. Retch.

gage. Same as *gauge.*

gait. The manner of walking. **ataxic g.** A gait in which the foot is raised high, thrown forward, and brought down suddenly, the whole sole striking the ground at once. **cerebellar g.** A staggering, lurching gait, causing a zigzag line of travel. **cow g.** A swaying movement due to knock-knee. **equine g.** That seen in peroneal nerve paralysis. Because of foot drop the leg must be raised high by flexing the thigh on the abdomen. Syn., *step-page g.* **frog g.** The hopping gait of infantile paralysis. **paraparetic g.** That observed in chronic myelitis in which the steps are short and the feet are dragged, from inability to lift them. **paretic g.** A gait in which the steps are short, the feet are dragged, and the legs are held more or less widely apart; as the disease progresses, there is uncertainty, shuffling, and staggering. **scissors g.** That seen in congenital or acquired infantile paraplegia and in certain brain tumors. The gait is spastic and the legs are adducted. **spastic g.** That resulting from lesions of the pyramidal tracts. The leg is extended at the knee and hip, the thigh adducted, and the heel raised; causes a stiff gait in which the foot is circumducted because it cannot be lifted. **tabetic g.** See *ataxic g.* **waddling g.** That of pseudohypertrophic muscular dystrophy, resembling the gait of a duck.

ga·lact'-, ga·lac'to-. A combining form meaning *milk, milky fluid.*

ga·lac''ta·cra'si·a (ga·lack″tuh·ray′zhuh, -zee·uh). Deficiency of or abnormality in mother's milk.

ga·lac'ta·gogue. An agent that induces or increases the secretion of milk.

ga·lac'tan. A complex carbohydrate made up of anhydro-galactose units and capable of forming galactose by hydrolysis.

ga·lac'tase. A soluble proteolytic enzyme present normally in milk.

gal''ac·te'mi·a, gal''ac·tae'mi·a (gal″ack·tee′mee·uh). A milky state or appearance of the blood.

ga·lact''hi·dro'sis. Sweating of a milklike fluid.

ga·lac'tic. Relating to or promoting the flow of milk.

ga·lac'tin. 1. An amorphous substance derived from milk. 2. Pituitary hormone stimulating lactation. See *prolactin.* Also called *mammotropin.*

gal''ac·tis'chi·a (gal″ack·tiss′kee·uh). Suppression of the secretion of milk.

ga·lac'to·cele. 1. A cystic tumor in the ducts of the breast. 2. Hydrocele with milky contents.

ga·lac'toid. Resembling milk.

ga·lac''to·lip'id. Any phosphorus-free nitrogenous, fatty substance which also contains galactose, such as kerasin, found in large amounts in the brain. Syn., *cerebroside.*

gal''ac·tom'e·ter. 1. Graduated glass funnel for determining the fat in milk. 2. Instrument for determining the specific gravity of milk.

gal''ac·ton'ic ac'id. $C_6H_{12}O_7.$ A pentahydroxyhexoic acid; a monobasic acid derived from galactose.

gal''ac·toph'a·gous. Subsisting on milk.

gal''ac·toph'ly·sis. 1. A vesicular eruption containing a milklike fluid. 2. Crusta lactea.

ga·lac'to·phore. A milk duct. **—ga·lactoph'orous,** *adj.*

gal''ac·toph'o·ri'tis. Inflammation of a milk duct.

gal''ac·toph'y·gous. Arresting the secretion of milk.

ga·lac''to·poi·et'ic, ga·lac''to·po·et'ic. 1. Pertaining to the formation and secretion of milk. 2. Galactagogue.

ga·lac'to·py'ra. Milk fever, *q.v.,* under *fever.* **—galactopyret'ic,** *adj.*

ga·lac''to·r·rhe'a, ga·lac''tor·rhoe'a (ga·lack″to·ree′uh). Excessive flow of milk.

ga·lac''tos·a·mine'. Galactose containing an amino group. It is widely distributed in nature.

ga·lac'tose (ga·lack′toce, -toze). $C_6H_{12}O_6.$ A sugar formed by boiling lactose sugar with dilute acids or by enzymic action.

ga·lac'to·si'dase. See *lactase.*

ga·lac'to·side. A glycoside which, on hydrolysis, yields the sugar galactose and an aglycone.

gal''ac·to'sis. The secretion of milk by the mammary glands.

gal''ac·tos'ta·sis, ga·lac''to·sta'si·a (ga·lack″to·stay′zee·uh, -see·uh). 1. Suppression of milk secretion. 2. An abnormal collection of milk in a breast.

ga·lac''to·su'ri·a. Passage of urine containing galactose.

ga·lac''to·ther'a·py. 1. The treatment of disease in suckling infants by the administration of drugs to the mother or wet nurse. 2. Milk cure. 3. Hypodermic use of milk to produce fever in fever therapy.

ga·lac''to·tox'in. A poisonous substance or ptomaine generated in milk by the growth of microörganisms.

ga·lac''to·tox'ism. Milk poisoning.

gal''ac·tot'ro·phy. Nourishing with milk only.

ga·lac''to·xy'mase (ga·lack″to·zy′mace, -maze). A ferment found in milk; capable of liquefying starch.

gal''ac·tu'ri·a. Milkiness of the urine; chyluria.

gal''e·an'thro·py (gal″ee·an′thro·pee, gay″lee·). A form of zoanthropy in which the patient believes himself to be transformed into a cat.

ga·le'na. Native lead sulfide.

Ga·len'ic (ga·len′ick, -lee′nick), **Ga·len'i·cal** (ga·len′i·kul, -lee′ni·kul). Relating to, or consistent with, the teachings of Galen.

Ga·len'i·cal. Medicine prepared from plants, according to standard formulas, as contrasted with definite chemicals.

gal″e·o·phil′i·a. Excessive love of cats.

gal″e·o·pho′bi·a. A morbid fear of cats. Also called *gatophobia, silurophobia*.

gal″e·ro′pi·a, gal″e·rop′si·a. An abnormally clear and light appearance of objects due to some defect in the visual apparatus.

gall (gawl). The bile.

gal·lac″e·to·phe·none′ (ga·lass″i·to·fi·nohn′, ·fee′nohn). Trihydroxyacetophenone, $CH_2CO.C_6H_2(OH)_2$. White to brownish powder used as 10% ointment or solution in skin diseases. Also called *alizarin yellow C*.

gal′la·mine tri″eth·i′o·dide. 1,2,3-*tris*(β-Diethylaminoethoxy) benzene triethiodide, a potent curariform drug used as an anesthetic and in shock therapy. See *flaxedil*.

gall′blad′der (gawl′blad″ur). A hollow, pear-shaped, musculomembranous organ, situated on the under surface of the right lobe of the liver, for the storage and concentration of bile and the secretion of mucus. **sandpaper g.** Roughness of the lining of the gallbladder, due to deposition of cholesterin crystals. **strawberry g.** A benign papilloma or hyperplasia of the folds lining the organ. It is a soft, friable, reddish mass containing cholesterin crystals and fat, which may fill the entire gallbladder, the color and appearance giving it the name.

gal′lic ac′id. Trihydroxybenzoic acid, occurring in white to yellowish crystals; soluble in water. Occasionally used for its astringent effect.

gal′li·um. Ga = 69.72. A gray-white metal which melts at 29.7° C.

gal′lo-. *In chemistry,* a combining form denoting *gallic acid*.

gal′lon. A standard unit of volumetric measurement. Capacity in the United States 231 cubic inches; four quarts. In the apothecaries' measure, the Latin equivalent, congius, abbreviated C., is frequently employed. **imperial g.** In Great Britain, a capacity equivalent to 1.20094 U. S. gallons.

gal″lo·tan′nic ac′id. Tannic acid.

gall′stone″ (gawl′stone″). A concretion formed in the gallbladder or the biliary ducts, composed, in varying amounts, of cholesterol, bilirubin, and other elements found in bile.

gal″va·ni·za′tion. The transmission of a direct current of low electromotive force through any part of the body for the purpose of diagnosing or treating disease. **—gal′vanize,** *v.*

gal′va·no- (gal′vuh·no-, gal·van′o-). A combining form denoting a *galvanic* or *direct current of electricity; employing* or *produced by the galvanic current.*

gal″va·nom′e·ter. An instrument for measuring relatively small electric currents.

gal″va·no·mus′cu·lar. Denoting a reaction produced by the application of a direct galvanic current to a muscle.

gal″va·no·sur′ger·y. The surgical use of direct or galvanic currents.

gal″va·no·ther′a·py. Treatment of disease through the use of direct or galvanic currents.

gal′va·no·ther″my (gal′vuh·no·thur″mee, gal·van′o·). The production of heat by direct or galvanic currents.

gal″va·not′o·nus. 1. Electrotonus. 2. The continued tetanus of a muscle between the make and break contraction of direct or galvanic current. **—galvanoton′ic,** *adj.*

gal″va·not′ro·pism. The turning movements of living structure or beings, under the influence of a direct current of electricity.

gam′bir. An aqueous extract from the twigs and leaves of *Uncaria Gambir*. Gambir yields catechutannic acid and catechin. Used as an astringent and in dyeing and tanning.

gam·boge′ (gam·bohdj′, ·boozh′). The gum resin obtained from *Garcinia Hanburyi*. It is a drastic, hydragogue cathartic.

gam′ete (gam′eet, ga·meet′, *the latter commonly in compounds*). A male or female reproductive cell capable of entering into union with another in the process of fertilization or of conjugation. In higher animals, these sex cells are the egg and sperm; in higher plants, the male gamete is part of the pollen grain, while the ovum is contained in the ovule. In lower forms, the gametes are frequently similar in appearance and their union is called conjugation.

ga·me′to·cyte (ga·mee′to·sight, gam′i·to·sight). A cell which by division produces gametes; a spermatocyte or oöcyte.

gam′ma. 1. The third letter of the Greek alphabet (Γ, γ), equivalent to English g. 2. *In chemistry,* microgram (one thousandth of a milligram). 3. *In photography,* the contrast of a negative or print, usually controlled by developing time, and expressed as a relationship between the density of the negative and the time of exposure. **g. roentgen.** A unit of radium dosage such that the same amount of ionization in air is produced as by one roentgen unit of gamma rays. Also called *gamma-ray roentgen*.

gam′ma·cism. Guttural stammering; difficulty in pronouncing guttural consonants, especially hard g and k.

gammexane. Trade-mark for gamma-hexachlorocyclohexane, $C_6H_6Cl_6$, a insecticide more powerful than DDT effective in the treatment of scabies. The chemical is also known as *666* and *benzene hexachloride*. See *lindane*.

am'o-. 1. In *biology*, a combining form denoting *sexual union*. 2. In *botany*, a combining form signifying *union* or *fusion of parts*.

am"o·ma'ni·a. Insane desire for marriage.

am"o·pho'bi·a. A morbid fear of marriage.

an'gli·a"ted (gang'glee·ay"tid, gang'lee·), **gan'gli·on·a"ted.** Supplied with ganglions.

an"gli·ec'to·my (gang"glee·eck'-to·mee, gang"lee·). See *ganglionectomy*.

an'gli·o- (gang'glee·o-, gang'lee·o-). A combining form meaning *ganglion*.

an'gli·on (gang'glee·un, gang'-ee·un) (pl. *ganglions*, *ganglia*). 1. A group of nerve cell bodies, usually located outside of the brain and spinal cord, as the dorsal root ganglion of a spinal nerve. 2. A cyst in a tendon sheath, or in a recess of a synovial cavity. —**gangliar, ganglion'ic,** adj. **acoustic g.** The embryonic ganglionic mass which separates into cochlear and vestibular ganglions. Syn., *vestibulocochlear g.* **basal ganglions.** An old term for the corpus striatum, or the corpus striatum and the thalamus considered together as the important subcortical centers. **cardiac g.** A ganglion of the superficial cardiac plexus, located between the aortic arch and the bifurcation of the pulmonary artery. Formerly called *ganglion of Wrisberg.* **celiac g.** A collateral sympathetic ganglion lying in the celiac plexus near the origin of the celiac artery. Formerly called *semilunar g.* **cervical g.** One of two or three ganglions on the sympathetic chain in the neck, named superior, middle (sometimes absent), and inferior. **collateral g.** Any one of the large peripheral ganglions of the sympathetic nervous system. **dorsal root g.** One of the sensory ganglions associated with the dorsal root of a spinal nerve. **enteric ganglions.** Small ganglions of the myenteric and submucous plexuses of the intestine. **Gasserian g.** See semilunar *g.* **inferior mesenteric g.** An outlying or collateral sympathetic ganglion lying in the inferior mesenteric plexus near the aorta at the origin of the inferior mesenteric artery. **jugular g.** (a) The superior ganglion of the vagus nerve. (b) The superior ganglion of the glossopharyngeal nerve. **nodose g.** The lower ganglion of the vagus nerve. **otic g.** That immediately below the foramen ovale of the sphenoid bone, medial to the mandibular nerve; from

it arise postganglionic parasympathetic fibers to the parotid gland. **semilunar g.** The large ganglion of the sensory root of the trigeminal nerve; from it arise the ophthalmic, maxillary, and mandibular divisions of the trigeminal nerve. Syn., *trigeminal g.* Also called *Gasserian g.* **sphenopalatine g.** One in the pterygopalatine fossa near the sphenopalatine foramen; from it arise postganglionic parasympathetic fibers to the lacrimal gland and to the mucous membrane of the nose and palate. **spinal g.** One of the sensory ganglions associated with the dorsal roots of spinal nerves. Syn., *dorsal root g.* **stellate g.** That formed by the fusion of the inferior cervical and the first thoracic sympathetic ganglions. **superior mesenteric g.** A collateral sympathetic ganglion lying in the superior mesenteric plexus near the origin of the superior mesenteric artery. **sympathetic ganglions.** The ganglions of the sympathetic nervous system, including those of the sympathetic trunk, the collateral, and the peripheral or terminal ganglions.

gan'gli·on·a"ted (gang'glee·un-ay"tid, gang'lee·). See *gangliated*.

gan"gli·on·ec'to·my. The surgical excision of a ganglion.

gan"gli·o·neu·ro'ma. A tumor derived from both ganglion cells and nerve fibers; found principally in connection with cranial or spinal nerves and may contain glial fibers.

gan"gli·o·ni'tis. Inflammation of a ganglion.

gan'gli·o·sides. Brain cerebrosides which contain a special fatty acid, called neuraminic acid, and which yield more than one equivalent of galactose.

gan·go'sa. Destructive lesions of the nose and hard palate, sometimes more extensive, considered to be a tertiary stage of yaws.

gan'grene (gang'green, gang·green'). 1. Mortification or death of a part; due to failure of the blood supply, to disease, or to injury. 2. The putrefactive changes in dead tissue. —**gangrenous,** adj. **amebic g.** An extensive destruction of the skin surrounding a drainage wound, following removal of an amebic abscess of the liver. **arteriosclerotic g.** Senile g., *q.v.* **carbolic acid g.** See chemical *g.* **chemical g.** That following burns from caustic or poisonous chemicals, as carbolic acid. **cutaneous g.** Skin gangrene. See decubital *g.* **decubital g.** A pressure gangrene of the skin and adjacent tissues; occurs in patients who are bedridden for long periods. Also called *decubitus.* **diabetic g.** A moist type occurring in the course of diabetes mellitus; often the result of slight injuries. **direct g.** That due to direct destruction of tissue from injury, pressure, burns, chemical action, etc. **dry g.** Local death of a part which does not become infected and undergoes mummification. Seen commonly following blocking of blood supply, as that due to freezing or embolism. **embolic g.** That resulting from embolism. **foudroyant g.** Infectious, fulminating, or spreading gangrene. **fusospirochetal g.** One due to infections following human bites or wounds of the neck which involve the pharynx; the organisms involved are spirochetes, fusiform bacteria, and nonhemolytic streptococci. **g. from ergot.** A dry gangrene resulting from contracted arterioles; due to the presence of ergot as a contaminant in grain or from medicinal use. **g. from thrombosis.** That resulting from occlusion of the blood supply by a thrombus; similar to embolic gangrene. Also called *atrophic g.* **g. of the appendix.** Necrosis of the appendix in appendicitis, with sloughing of the organ. **g. of the lung.** A diffuse, putrefactive necrosis of a lung or of a lobe; due to anaerobic or other bacteria; usually a termination of lung abscess in a patient with low resistance. **gas g.** A form occurring in massive wounds, where there is crushing and devitalization of tissue and contamination with earth. The organisms found are anaerobes, including *Clostridium perfringens* Type A and *Clostridium septicum.* It is marked by high fever, offensive, thin, purulent discharge from the wound, and the presence of gas bubbles in the tissues. **hemolytic streptococcus g.** A bacterial gangrene due to infection by *Streptococcus pyogenes.* **hospital g.** An infectious type especially involving amputation stumps. **line of demarcation in g.** The line of junction between living and dead tissue. **line of separation in g.** The deepening groove of ulceration and granulation which gradually separates living and dead tissue. **moist g.** Local death of a part which becomes infected, so that the signs and symptoms of infection are superimposed upon those of gangrene. **senile g.** A dry gangrene of the extremities; due to failure of the terminal circulation in elderly persons or those afflicted with arteriosclerosis. Also called *arteriosclerotic g., g. of the aged.* **white g.** Gangrene with anemia of the tissues.

gan′ja, gan′jah. Gunjah. See *cannabis.*

gan′jah See *cannabis.*

gantrisin. Trade-mark for 3,4-dimethyl-5-sulfanilamido-isoxazole, a

sulfonamide characterized by hi[g] solubility in neutral or slightly ac body fluids. See *sulfisoxazole.*

gap. Any break or opening.

Gar·cin′i·a. A genus of the Gutt ferae. **G. Hanburyi,** the Siam gar boge tree, yields the gum oleoresi gamboge. **G. mangostana** yiel the palatable fruit called mangostee

gar′gle. 1. A solution for rinsing t[h] pharynx and nasopharynx. 2. Rinse t[h] pharynx and nasopharynx.

gar′goyl·ism. A heredofamilial co[n] dition characterized by mental def ciency, defective vision, a large hea a prominent abdomen, and short e[x] tremities.

gar·rot′ing (ga-rot′ing, ga-rot′ing [). *In legal medicine,* forcible compressio[n] of a victim's neck from pressure wit[h] intent to rob or kill.

gas. The vaporous or airlike state matter. A fluid which distributes itse[lf] uniformly throughout any space which it is placed, regardless of quantity. —**gas′eous,** *adj.* **asphy[x]iating g.** Carbon monoxide. **laug[h]ing g.** Nitrous oxide. **sewer g.** T[h] mixture of gases and vapors whic emanate from a sewer. **tear g.** Su[b]stances used by civil authorities to pr duce physical discomfort without i[n] jury by causing inflammation of t[h] mucous membranes of the eyes a[n] nose, followed by lacrimation. Esp cially useful in dispersing mob **war g.** A chemical agent which, field concentrations, produces a to[x] or strongly irritant effect. May be finely dispersed liquid or solid as w as a true gas.

gas·om′e·ter. A device for holdi[ng] and measuring gas. —**gasomet′ri** *adj.*

gasp. Catch for breath; breathe spa modically with open mouth.

Gasserian ganglion. See sem lunar *ganglion.*

gas′sing. 1. In warfare, the drenchi[ng] of an area with poisonous gas. 2. T execution or attempted execution of person by means of toxic ga —**gassed,** *adj.*

-gas′ter. *In anatomy and biology,* combining form denoting *part of* or li *a stomach.*

gas′ter·o-, gaster-. A combini[ng] form denoting *pertaining to the sto[m]* ach.

Gas″ter·oph′i·lus. A genus of bo flies. The larvae are parasites of hors and occasionally infest the cutaneo and subcutaneous tissues in ma **G. hemorrhoidalis.** A speci which attacks the lower lip or ja **G. intestinalis.** A species attac ing the inner side of the legs and t sides of the abdomen. This species pr duces a cutaneous lesion in man, t hatched larvae causing an eruption similar to that produced by the *Ancylostoma braziliense*. **G. nasalis.** The chin fly, which attacks the lower lip or jaw.

gastr-. See *gastro-*.

gas″tral′gi·a. Pain in the stomach.

gas″tral·go·ke·no′sis (gas″trul·go·keh·no′sis, ga·stral″go·). Pain due to emptiness of the stomach; relieved by taking food.

gas″tra·tro′phi·a. Atrophy of the stomach.

gas·trec′ta·sis. Dilatation of the stomach.

gas·trec′to·my. Excision of the whole or a part of the stomach.

gas′tric. Pertaining to the stomach.

gas′trin. A hormone, originating in the pyloric glands of the stomach, purported to excite secretion of the fundic cells.

gas·tri′tis. Acute or chronic inflammation of the stomach. —**gastrit′ic,** *adj.* **atrophic g.** A chronic form with atrophy of the mucous membrane. **catarrhal g.** A type, usually acute, with mucinous exudate. **corrosive g.** An acute gastritis which is caused by corrosive poisons. **fibrinous g.** An acute inflammation with a large amount of fibrin in the exudate. Also called **croupous** *g.,* **diphtheritic** *g.,* **membranous** *g.,* **pseudomembranous** *g.* **hypertrophic g.** A chronic form with increased thickness of mucosa, exaggerated granulation, and larger, more numerous rugae. Polyps may develop. **infectious g.** Acute gastritis associated with infectious diseases such as measles, scarlet fever. **simple exogenous g.** The acute type often associated with enteritis and characterized by vomiting, pain, and malaise; may be due to ingested food or to an infection. **suppurative g.** Acute, purulent gastritis.

gas″tro-, gastr-. A combining form meaning *stomach* or *belly.*

gas″tro·an·as″to·mo′sis. In hourglass contraction, the formation of a communication between the two pouches of the stomach. Also called *gastrogastrostomy.*

gas″tro·cele. A hernia of the stomach.

gas″troc·ne′mi·us. A muscle on the posterior aspect of the leg, arising by two heads from the posterior surfaces of the lateral and medial condyles of the femur, and inserted with the soleus muscle, into the Achilles tendon, and through this into the back of the calcaneus.

gas″tro·col′ic. Pertaining to the stomach and the colon.

gas″tro·di′a·phane. An electric apparatus for illuminating the interior of the stomach so that its outlines can be seen through the abdominal wall. —**gastrodiaph′any,** *n.*

gas″tro·di·aph″a·nos′co·py. The examination of the stomach by means of the diaphanoscope; gastrodiaphany.

gas″tro·dis·ci′a·sis (gas″tro·dis·kigh′uh·sis). Infestation of the cecum by the fluke *Gastrodiscoides hominis,* causing inflammation and producing diarrhea.

gas″tro·du″o·de′nal (gas″tro·dew″o·dee′nul, ·dew·od′i·nul). Pertaining to the stomach and the duodenum.

gas″tro·du″o·de·ni′tis. Inflammation of the stomach and duodenum.

gas″tro·du″o·de·nos′to·my. Establishment of an anastomosis between stomach and duodenum.

gas″tro·en″ter·i′tis. Inflammation of stomach and intestine.

gas″tro·en″ter·o·a·nas″to·mo′sis. Anastomosis between the intestine and the stomach. See *gastroenterostomy, gastroduodenostomy, gastrojejunostomy.*

gas″tro·en″ter·ol′o·gist. One who specializes in diseases of the stomach and intestine.

gas″tro·en″ter·ol′o·gy. The study of the stomach and intestine and their diseases.

gas″tro·en″ter·os′to·my. The formation of a communication between the stomach and the small intestine, usually the jejunum. See *gastroduodenostomy, gastrojejunostomy.*

gas″tro·ep″i·plo′ic. Pertaining to the stomach and omentum, as the gastroepiploic artery. See Table of Arteries in the Appendix.

gas″tro·e·soph″a·gi′tis. Combined inflammation of the stomach and the esophagus.

gas″tro·gas·tros′to·my. The surgical anastomosis of one portion of the stomach with another.

gas″tro·ga′vage (gas″tro·gah″vahzh′). Artificial feeding through an opening in the stomach wall; gavage.

gas′tro·graph. An apparatus for registering the peristaltic movements of the stomach from the outside.

gas″tro·he·pat′ic. Relating to the stomach and liver, as the gastrohepatic ligament.

gas″tro·hy″per·ton′ic. Relating to morbid or excessive tonicity or irritability of the stomach.

gas″tro·in·tes′ti·nal. Pertaining to the stomach and intestine.

gas″tro·je·ju′nal. Pertaining to the stomach and to the jejunum, as gastrojejunal anastomosis.

gas″tro·je″ju·ni′tis (gas″tro·jee″jew·nigh′tis, ·jedj″oo·nigh′tis). Inflammation of both the stomach and jejunum; may occur after gastrojejunostomy.

gas″tro·je″ju·nos′to·my (·jee″-jew·nos′to·mee, ·jedj″oo·nos′to·mee). The surgical anastomosis of the jejunum to the anterior or posterior wall of the stomach; gastroenterostomy.

gas′tro·lith. A calcareous formation in the stomach.

gas″tro·li·thi′a·sis. A morbid condition associated with the formation of gastroliths.

gas·trol′o·gy. The science of the stomach and its functions and diseases.

gas·trol′y·sis. The breaking-up of adhesions between the stomach and adjacent organs.

gas″tro·meg′a·ly. Abnormal enlargement of the stomach.

gas·trom′e·lus. An individual with an accessory limb attached to the abdomen.

gas″tro·my·co′sis (gas″tro·migh·ko′sis). Gastric disease due to fungi.

gas″tro·my·ot′o·my (gas″tro·migh·ot′o·mee). Incision of the circular muscle fibers of the stomach. See *pyloromyotomy.*

gas·trop′a·thy. Any disease or disorder of the stomach.

gas″tro·pex′y, gas″tro·pex′y. The fixation of a prolapsed stomach in its normal position by suturing it to the abdominal wall or other structure.

gas″tro·pho′tor. A stomach camera which takes pictures of the inside of the stomach.

gas″tro·plas′ty, gas′tro·plas″-ty. Plastic operation on the stomach.

gas″tro·pli·ca′tion. An operation for relief of chronic dilatation of the stomach, consisting in suturing a large horizontal fold in the stomach wall; quilting of the stomach wall for redundancy due to chronic dilatation. See *gastroplasty, gastrorrhaphy.*

gas″trop·to′sis. Prolapse or downward displacement of the stomach.

gas″tro·py″lo·rec′to·my. Excision of the pyloric portion of the stomach; pylorectomy.

gas″tror·rha′gi·a. Hemorrhage from the stomach.

gas·tror′rha·phy. Surgical repair of a stomach wound by infolding of the edges and employing repeated rows of sutures.

gas″tror·rhe′a. Excessive secretion of gastric mucus or of gastric juice.

gas·tros′chi·sis (gas·tros′ki·sis). A congenital malformation in which the abdomen remains open.

gas′tro·scope. An instrument for examining the interior of the stomach. —**gastros′copy,** *n.*

gas′tro·spasm. Stomach spasm.

gas″tro·splen′ic. Relating to the stomach and the spleen.

gas″tro·stax′is. The oozing of blood from the mucous membrane of the stomach.

gas·tros′to·my. The establishing of a fistulous opening into the stomach, with an external opening in the skin; usually for artificial feeding.

gas·trot′o·my. Incision into the stomach.

gas″tro·tox′in. A cytotoxin which has a specific action on the cells lining the stomach.

gas″tro·tym″pa·ni′tes (gas″tro·tim″puh·nigh′teez, ·nigh′tis). Gaseous distention of the stomach.

gas′tru·la. An embryo at that stage of its development when it consists of two cellular layers, the primary ectoderm and entoderm, and a primitive gut or archenteron opening externally through the blastopore. The simplest type is derived by the invagination of the spherical blastula, but this is greatly modified in the various animal groups. —**gastrula′tion,** *n.*

gat′o·phil′i·a. Fondness for cats.

gat′o·pho′bi·a. A morbid fear of cats.

gauge, gage. An instrument for measuring the size of a structure, or the status of a process or phenomenon, as blood pressure.

gaul·the′ri·a. The plant, *Gaultheria procumbens,* the leaves of which yield a volatile oil. Syn., *teaberry; wintergreen.* **g. oil.** Contains 90% of methyl salicylate; used in acute rheumatism and as a local antiseptic and flavoring agent. Syn., *wintergreen oil.* **synthetic g. oil.** Methyl salicylate.

gaul·ther′o·lin. Methyl salicylate.

gaunt′let. A bandage that covers the hand and fingers like a glove.

gauze. A thin, open-meshed cloth of varying degrees of fineness, used in surgical operations and for surgical dressings. When sterilized, it is called **aseptic gauze;** when packaged for use in the operating room, the individual folded pieces are called sponges.

ga′vage′ (gah″vahzh′). The administration of liquid nourishment through a stomach tube.

Gd. Chemical symbol for gadolinium.

Ge. Chemical symbol for germanium.

Geiger, Hans [*German physicist,* 1882–1945]. Made important studies of radioactivity. See Geiger-Müller counting *circuit,* Geiger-Müller *tube,* Geiger-Müller *counter.*

Gei′ger-Mül′ler count′er. An instrument for the detection of individual ionizing particles; entry of a charged particle into the apparatus produces ionization and a momentary flow of current which is relayed to a counting device. Also called *Geiger counter.*

gei·so′ma (guy·so′muh). The eyebrows of the face, or the supraorbital ridges of the skull. Also called *geison.*

gel. A colloidal system comprising a

solid and a liquid phase which exists as a solid or semisolid mass.

ge·las'mus (jeh·laz'mus, ·lass'mus), **ge·las'ma** (jeh·laz'muh, ·lass'muh). Insane or hysterical spasmodic laughter.

gel'a·tin. The product obtained by the partial hydrolysis of collagen, derived from the skin, white connective tissue, and bones of animals. —**gelat'inoid, gelat'inous,** *adj.* **glycerinated g.** A preparation of gelatin, glycerin, and water. Used as a vehicle for suppositories and bougies. Also called *glycerinjelly.*

ge·lat'i·nase. An enzyme liquefying gelatin. It is found in various molds and yeasts.

ge·lat'i·nize. Convert into a jellylike mass.

gel·a'tion. 1. The change of a colloid from a sol to a gel. 2. Freezing.

gel'a·tose. A product of the hydrolysis of gelatin by acid, alkali, or enzyme.

gelfoam. Trade-mark for an absorbable gelatin sponge that acts as a hemostatic agent and is used to control capillary bleeding in surgery.

gel'ose (jel'oce, jeh·loce'). 1. The gelatinizing principle of agar. 2. A culture medium for bacteria. See *agaragar.*

ge·lot'o·lep"sy, gel'o·to·lep"sy. A sudden loss of muscle tone during laughter, with a transitory loss of consciousness.

gel·sem'i·cine (jel·sem'i·seen, ·sin). An alkaloid from gelsemium.

gel·sem'i·dine. An alkaloid from gelsemium.

gel'se·mine (jel'si·meen, ·min). An alkaloid, $C_{20}H_{22}O_2N_2$, from gelsemium.

gel·sem'in·ine. An alkaloid from gelsemium.

gel·se'mi·um (jel·see'mee·um, ·sem'ee·um). The dried rhizome and roots of *Gelsemium sempervirens,* used as an antispasmodic and antineuralgic. Also called *yellow jasmine root.*

gem'i·nate, gem'i·nous. 1. In pairs; coupled. 2. Double; become double. —**gemina'tion,** *n.*

gem·ma'tion. Budding; a mode of reproduction seen in low forms of animal and vegetable life characterized by the formation of a small projection from the parent organism, which is constricted off and forms another organism.

gemonil. Trade-mark for metharbital.

·gen. 1. *In chemistry,* a combining form denoting *a substance that produces or generates.* 2. *In biology,* a combining form denoting *a thing produced or generated.*

gene, gen. Any hereditary factor; the ultimate unit in the transmission of hereditary characteristics, regarded as an ultramicroscopic particle, capable of self-reproduction and imitation, which occupies a definite locus on a chromosome. Any known gene is a modifier of development and is regarded as a cellular physiologic agent which acts as a center of specific chemical activity.

gen'er·a. Plural of genus, *q.v.*

gen'er·al. Common to a class; distributed through many parts; diffuse. —**generalize,** *v.t.*

gen"er·a'tion. 1. The act or process of producing offspring. 2. A period extending from the birth of an individual to the birth of his offspring, in humans usually a third of a century. 3. The production of a gas or electric current. —**gon'erative,** *adj.;* **gen'erate,** *v.t.* **asexual g.** Reproduction without sexual union; reproduction by fission or gemmation. **sexual g.** Reproduction by the union of a male and a female gamete. **spontaneous g.** See *abiogenesis.*

gen'er·a"tor. 1. *In electricity,* a machine which transforms mechanical power into electric power. 2. *In radiology,* a machine which supplies the roentgen-ray tube with the electric energy necessary for the production of roentgen rays. 3. *In chemistry,* an apparatus for the formation of vapor or gas from a liquid or solid by heat or chemical action.

ge·ner'ic. 1. Pertaining to a genus. 2. General.

ge·nes'ic (ji·ness'ick, ji·nee'sick). Of or relating to generation or to the genital organs.

ge·ne"si·ol'o·gy (ji·nee"see·ol'o·jee, ji·nee"zee·). The science of reproduction or heredity.

gen'e·sis. The origin or generation of anything; the developmental evolution of a specific thing or type.

-gen'e·sis. A combining form signifying *origination, development, evolution of a thing or type.*

ge·net'ic. 1. Pertaining to or having reference to origin, mode of production or development. 2. Pertaining to genetics. 3. Produced by genes.

-ge·net'ic. *In biology,* a combining form meaning *of or pertaining to heredity.*

ge·net'i·cist. A specialist in genetics.

ge·net'ics. The branch of biology which deals with the phenomena of heredity and variation. It seeks to understand the causes of the resemblances and differences between parents and progeny, and, by extension, between all organisms related to one another by descent.

Ge·ne'va con·ven'tion. An agreement signed by the European powers in Geneva, Switzerland, in 1864, guaranteeing humane treatment of the wounded and those caring for them in time of war. In July, 1906, a full revised convention was adopted in Geneva. In 1907, this was again revised at The Hague Peace Conference, and was adopted as Convention X.

ge·ni·al (jee'nee·ul, ji·nigh'ul). Pertaining to the chin. Syn., *mental*.

-gen·ic. A combining form meaning *of* or *pertaining to production*.

ge·nic·u·lar. Pertaining to the knee joint, as the genicular artery. See Table of Arteries in the Appendix.

ge·nic·u·late, ge·nic·u·la"ted. Abruptly bent.

ge·nic·u·lum. A small, kneelike structure; a sharp bend in any small organ.

ge·ni·o- (jee'nee·o-, i·nigh'o-). *In anatomy*, a combining form meaning *chin, lower jaw*.

ge·ni·o·plas"ty (jee'nee·o·plas"tee, ji·nigh'o·). Plastic operation on the chin.

gen·i·tal. Pertaining to the organs of generation or to reproduction.

gen"i·ta·li·a (jen"i·tay'lee·uh, ·tal'ee·uh). The organs of generation. The male has two testes or seminal glands, with their excretory ducts, the prostate, the penis, and the urethra. The female genitalia include the vulva, the vagina, the ovaries, the uterine tubes, and the uterus.

gen·i·to-. A combining form signifying *genital*.

gen"i·to·cru'ral. Pertaining to the genitalia and the leg.

gen"i·to·fem'o·ral. Pertaining to the genitalia and the thigh; genitocrural.

gen"i·to·u'ri·nar"y (jen"i·to·yoor'i·nerr"ee). Relating to the genitalia and the urinary organs or functions; urogenital.

gen'i·us. 1. Distinctive character or inherent nature. 2. Unusual artistic or creative ability; mental superiority.

gen'o·cide. A denial of the right of existence to entire human groups just as homicide is the denial of the right to individual human beings.

gen"o·pho'bi·a. A morbid fear of sex.

gen'o·type. 1. The hereditary constitution of an organism resulting from its particular combination of genes. 2. A class of individuals having the same genetic constitution. **—genotyp'ic, genotyp'ical,** *adj.*

-gen'ous. A suffix signifying *producing* or *yielding; produced by* or *arising in*.

gen"ti·a·mar'in. A glycosidal constituent of gentian.

gen'tian. 1. The common name for species of *Gentiana*. 2. The official gentian; the dried rhizome and roots of *Gentiana lutea*. Gentian is a bitter tonic. **compound g. tincture.** A tincture of gentian, bitter orange peel,

and cardamom. **g. violet.** (a) A violet aniline dye; a mixture of the chlorides of methylated pararosanilines composed of pentamethyl and hexamethyl pararosaniline, or either of these compounds alone. It is a biologic stain. (b) Methylrosaniline chloride, *q.v.*

gen"ti·an'ic ac'id (jen"shee·an'·ick). See *gentianin*.

gen'tian·in. A constituent of gentian, chemically the 3-monomethyl ether of 1,3,7-trihydroxyflavone. Syn., *gentisin, gentianic acid*.

gen'tian·ose. A crystallizable trisaccharide from gentian root.

gen"ti·o·bi'ose. A disaccharide in several plants; on hydrolysis it yields two molecules of glucose.

gen"ti·o·pic'rin (jen"shee·o·pick'rin). A bitter, crystalline glycoside obtained from gentian.

gen·tis'ic ac'id. 2,5-Dihydroxybenzoic acid, the sodium salt of which is used as an antirheumatic agent.

gen·tis'yl al'co·hol. 2,5-Dihydroxybenzyl alcohol. A substance of slight antibacterial activity obtained as a metabolic product of *Penicillium patulum*.

ge'nu (jeen'yoo, jen'yoo) (pl. *genua*). 1. The knee. 2. Any structure like a knee, as the genu of the corpus callosum, the internal capsule, or the optic tract. **—gen'ual,** *adj.* **g. recurvatum.** The backward curving of the knee joint. **g. valgum.** The inward curving of the knee; knock-knee. **g. varum.** Bowleg.

gen"u·cu'bi·tal (jen"yoo·cue'bi·tul, jeen·yoo·). Relating to or supported by the knees and elbows.

gen"u·fa'cial (jen"yoo·fay'shul, jeen·yoo·). Relating to, or resting on, the knees and face.

gen"u·pec'tor·al. Relating to the knees and the chest, as the knee-chest posture.

ge'nus (pl. *genera*). A taxonomic group, next above the species and forming the principal subdivision of the family.

-geny. A suffix signifying *generation, production, science of the origin* and *development of*.

gen"y·chei'lo·plas"ty (jen"i·kigh'lo·plas"tee, jee"ni·). Plastic operation on both cheek and lip.

gen'y·o-, gen'y-. A combining form meaning *lower jaw*.

gen'y·plas"ty. Plastic operation on the lower jaw.

ge"o·med'i·cine. The study of diseases from the standpoint of their geographic distribution.

ge"o·met'ric mean. The antilogarithm of the arithmetic mean of the logarithms of a series of observations.

ge·oph'a·gy, ge"o·pha'gi·a, ge·oph'a·gism. The practice of eating earth or clay; chthonophagia. —**ge-oph′agous**, adj., **geoph′agist**, n.

ge·ot′ro·pism. In biology, the gravitational factor which in plants causes roots to grow downward toward the earth and shoots to grow up, and in some animals causes the climbing, swimming, or right-side-up orientation.

ge·phy″ro·pho′bi·a (ji·figh″ro·fo′-bee·uh, jef″i·ro·). A morbid fear of crossing a bridge.

ge·ra′ni·ol. $C_{10}H_{17}OH$. A colorless liquid of pleasant odor, a constituent of several volatile oils.

ge·rat′ic. Pertaining to old age; gerontic.

ger″a·tol′o·gy. The scientific study of decadence and its phenomena.

ger″i·a·tri′cian (jerr″ee·uh·trish′-un, jeer″ee·uh·). One who specializes in the treatment of the diseases of old age. Also called geriatrist.

ger″i·at′rics (jerr″ee·at′ricks, jeer″ee·). That branch of medical science which is concerned with old age and its diseases.

ger″i·o·psy·cho′sis (jerr″ee·o·sigh·ko′sis). Psychosis of old age.

germ. 1. A small bit of protoplasm capable of developing into a new individual, especially an egg, spore, or seed; any of the early stages in the development of an organism. 2. Any microorganism, especially any of the pathogenic bacteria. —**ger′minal**, adj. **dental g.** The dental sac, enamel organ, and dental papilla regarded as a unit; comprising all the formative tissues of a tooth. Also called tooth germ. **hair g.** The solid epithelial invagination of the germinal layer of the fetal epidermis that forms the primordium of the hair. Also called hair column.

germanin. See suramin.

ger·ma′ni·um. Ge = 72.60. A brittle, grayish white, metallic element.

ger′mi·cide. An agent that destroys germs. —**germici′dal**, adj.

ger′mi·dine. A highly active ester alkaloid isolated from veratrum viride; on hydrolysis it yields germine, acetic acid, and α-methylbutyric acid.

ger″mi·na′tion. The beginning of growth of a spore or seed.

ger′mi·na′tive. Having the power to begin growth or to develop.

ger′mine. An alkaloid from veratrum viride resulting from hydrolysis of the ester alkaloids germidine and germitrine.

ger′mi·trine. A highly active ester alkaloid isolated from veratrum viride; on hydrolysis it yields germine, methylethylglycolic acid, and α-methylbutyric acid.

ge·roc′o·my (ji·rock′o·mee, jerr′o·ko·mee), **ger″o·co′mi·a** (jerr″o·ko′-mee·uh, jeer″o·). The medical and hygienic care of old people. —**gero·com′ical**, adj.

ger″o·der′ma (jerr″o·dur′muh, jeer″o·). The skin of old age, showing atrophy, loss of fat, loss of elasticity, etc.

ger″o·ma·ras′mus (jerr″o·ma·raz′-mus, jeer″o·). Emaciation characteristic of extreme old age.

ger″o·mor′phism. The condition of appearing aged while still young.

ge·ron′tic, ge·ron′tal. Pertaining to decadence or old age. —**geron·tism**, n.

ger″on·tol′o·gy (jerr″on·tol′o·jee, jeer″on·). Scientific study of the phenomena of old age.

ge·ron″to·phil′i·a. Love for old people.

ge·ron″to·pho′bi·a. Fear of old age.

ge·ron″to·ther′a·py. Treatment of the aging process.

ges·ta′tion. Pregnancy. **abdominal g.** The form of extrauterine gestation in which the product of conception is developed in the abdominal cavity. **double g.** (a) Twin pregnancy. (b) The coexistence of uterine and extrauterine pregnancy. **ectopic g.** See extrauterine g. **extra·terine g.** Development of the ovum outside of the uterine cavity. See pregnancy.

ges·to′sis (pl. gestoses). Any toxemic manifestation in pregnancy.

geu″ma·pho′bi·a (gew″muh·fo′-bee·uh). A morbid fear of taste.

-geu′si·a (-gew′see·uh, -jew′see·uh). A combining form denoting a condition of the taste sense.

gi′ant. A being or organism of abnormally large size.

gib·bos′i·ty (ghi·bos′i·tee, ji·bos′i·tee). The condition of being humpbacked.

gib′bous (ghib′us, jib′us). Humpbacked; swollen, convex, or protuberant, especially on one side.

gid′di·ness. Dizziness; an unpleasant sensation of disturbed relations to surrounding objects in space; it differs from vertigo in that there is no experience of the external world or of the patient being in motion.

gi·gan′tic ac′id (jye·gan′tick). An antibiotic substance from Aspergillus giganteus; identical with aspergillin, flavacidin, flavicin, flavatin, and parasiticin.

gi·gan′tism (jye·gan′tiz·um). Abnormal size and tallness; a height in man in excess of 79 inches; due to an oversupply of growth hormone of the anterior pituitary before the fusion of the epiphyses, or to an enhanced ability of the body tissues to respond to growth stimuli. Gigantism may be *normal*, the type in which bodily proportions and sexual function are normal; or *eunuchoid*, the type in which there are eunuchoid proportions and sexual insufficiency; or *acromegalic*, the form in which features of acromegaly are superimposed on those of gigantism.

gill (ghill). A respiratory organ of water-breathing animals.

gill (jill). One-fourth of a pint.

gin'ger. The dried rhizome of *Zingiber officinale*, a carminative. See *zingerone*.

gin'ger·ol. Zingerone.

gin'gi·va (pl. *gingivae*). That part of the oral mucous membrane which surrounds the tooth distal to the alveolar crest. —**gingival,** *adj.;* **gingivally,** *adv.* **attached g.** The portion of the gingiva firmly attached to the tooth and to the periosteum of the alveolar crest. **free g.** The portion which lies occlusally or incisally to the floor of the gingival sulcus. Also called *marginal g.*

gin'gi·vae (jin'ji-vee). Plural of gingiva, *q.v.*

gin"gi·val'gi·a. Pain in the gums.

gin"gi·vec'to·my. Excision of a portion of the gums.

gin"gi·vi'tis. Inflammation of the gingiva. Acute, chronic, purulent, ulcerative, hyperplastic, are some of the types recognized.

gin"gi·vo·glos·si'tis. Inflammation of the gums and tongue; stomatitis.

gin'gly·mus (jing'gli-mus, ghing'·). A hinge joint. —**ginglymoid,** *adj.*

gin'seng. The root of several species of *Panax*. It has no medicinal virtues other than those of a demulcent.

gir'dle. A band designed to go around the body; a structure resembling a circular belt or band. **pelvic g.** The two hip bones united at the pubic symphysis; they support the trunk on the lower extremities. **shoulder g.** The system of bones supporting the upper limbs or arms; it consists of the clavicles, scapulas, and, for some authorities, the manubrium of the sternum. Also called *pectoral girdle*.

git'a·lin (jit'uh-lin, ji-tal'in). $C_{35}H_{56}O_{13}$. A glycoside from digitalis leaves. See *digitoxin, gitoxin*.

git"o·gen'in (jit"o-jen'in, ji-todj'i-nin). The steroid aglycone of gitonin.

git'o·nin (jit'o-nin, ji-to'nin). A saponin from *Digitalis purpurea*.

gi·tox"i·ge'nin (ji-tock"si-jee'nin, -jen'in). The steroid aglycone or sugar-free component of gitoxin.

gi·tox'in. $C_{41}H_{64}O_{14}$. One of the partially hydrolyzed glycosides obtained from both *Digitalis purpurea* and *Digitalis lanata*.

Gl. Chemical symbol for glucinum, an obsolete name for beryllium.

gla·bel'la. 1. The bony prominence

on the frontal bone joining the supra-orbital ridges. 2. A craniometric point found in the sagittal plane of the bony prominence joining the supraorbital ridges, usually the most anteriorly projecting portion of this region.

gla'brous. Smooth; devoid of hairs.

glair'y. Slimy; viscous; mucoid. Resembling the white of an egg.

gland. 1. A cell, tissue, or organ which elaborates and discharges a substance which is used elsewhere in the body (secretion), or eliminated (excretion). 2. Acorn-shaped termination of the penis or clitoris; see *glans clitoridis; glans penis*. 3. Obsolete term for lymph node. —**glan'dular,** *adj.* **accessory g.** A mass of gland tissue separate from the main body of a gland of similar structure. **accessory parotid g.** A small auxiliary parotid gland. Also called *socia parotidis.* **acid glands.** Glands of the stomach which secrete acid. Syn., *fundic glands.* **acinotubular g.** One with both tubular and saccular elements. **acinous g.** One in which the secretory end-pieces have the form of an acinus, *q.v.* **adipose glands.** Hibernating glands of certain mammals, containing pigmented multilocular fat cells (brown fat). **adrenal g.** An endocrine gland located immediately above the superior pole of the kidney. It consists of two portions: a *cortex*, which elaborates steroid hormones, the adrenal cortical hormones, and a *medulla*, which elaborates epinephrine. Syn., *suprarenal g.* **anal g.** Any gland of the anal region. **apocrine glands.** Glands producing sweat of a characteristic odor; larger and more deeply situated than the common sweat glands, and found in the axillary, mammary, anal, and genital areas. The gland cells lose some of their cytoplasmic substance when functioning. **areolar glands.** Glands in the areola about the nipple in the female breast. They are intermediate in character between mammary glands and apocrine sweat glands. Syn., *Montgomery's glands.* **axillary glands.** The axillary lymph nodes. **Bartholin's glands.** The major vestibular glands. **Blandin's g.** The anterior lingual gland, a mixed gland on the under surface of the tongue. Syn., *Nuhn's g.* **Bowman's glands.** Serous glands found in the olfactory mucous membrane. Also called *olfactory glands.* **bronchial glands.** (a) The mixed glands of the mucous membrane of the bronchi. (b) The chain of lymph nodes along the bronchi. **Brunner's glands.** The duodenal glands, *q.v.* **buccal glands.** The mixed glands of the mucous membrane of the cheek. **bulbourethral g.** One of two compound tubular glands situated in the urogenital diaphragm, anterior to the prostate gland. Also called *Cowper's g.* **cardiac glands.** Glands of the cardia of the stomach. **carotid glands.** Carotid bodies. See under *body.* **ceruminous glands.** Sweat glands of the external auditory meatus which secrete the watery component of the cerumen. **cervical glands.** The lymph nodes of the neck. **ciliary glands.** Modified sweat glands of the eyelids. Also called *Moll's glands.* **circumanal glands.** The anal glands, *q.v.* **Cloquet's g.** The large lymph node in the femoral sheath. Also called *Rosenmueller's g.* **closed g.** A ductless or endocrine gland. *Obs.* **coccygeal g.** A small group of arteriovenous anastomoses near the tip of the coccyx. **coil g.** Old term for sweat gland, *q.v.* **compound g.** A gland which has a branching system of ducts. **conglomerate glands.** Acinous glands. **conjunctival glands.** The accessory lacrimal glands. Also called *Krause's glands.* **convoluted g.** Sweat gland, *q.v.* **Cowper's g.** The bulbourethral gland, *q.v.* **cutaneous g.** Any gland of the skin. **cytogenic g.** A gland producing living cells, as the testis or ovary. **deep g.** A gland which has its secreting portion deep to a mucous membrane, usually in the tunica submucosa. **ductless glands.** Glands without ducts, secreting directly into the blood stream. See *endocrine g.* **duodenal glands.** The deep mucoserous glands of the first part of the duodenum. Also called *Brunner's glands.* **Ebner's glands.** The serous glands opening into the trenches of the vallate papillae of the tongue. Also called *von Ebner's glands.* **endocrine g.** One secreting hormonal substance into the blood stream; a ductless gland. See *pancreas, parathyroid, thyroid g.* See also *pituitary, suprarenal, thymus.* **epithelial g.** A group of glandular cells within an epithelial layer. **exocrine glands.** Glands which secrete onto an epithelial surface. **Fraenkel's glands.** Minute mixed glands immediately inferior to the vocal folds. **fundic glands.** Those of the corpus and fundus of the stomach. Syn., *acid glands.* **gastric glands.** Glands of the stomach, including the cardiac, fundic, and pyloric glands. **hair glands.** The sebaceous glands of hair follicles. **holocrine g.** One which forms its secretion by degeneration of its cells. Also called *holocrinous g.* **incretory g.** Endocrine gland, *q.v.* **lacrimal g.** The compound tubulo-alveolar gland secreting the tears, situated in the orbit in a depression of the frontal bone. **Lieberkühn's**

glands. The simple straight tubular glands of the intestinal mucous membrane. **Littré's glands.** The small mucous glands of the male urethra. Formerly called *glands* or *lacunas of Morgagni.* Syn., *urethral glands.* **Luschka's glands.** Aberrant bile ducts in the wall of the gallbadder. Also called *Luschka's ducts.* **mammary g.** One that secretes milk. **Meibomian glands.** Tarsal glands. **merocrine g.** One in which the secreting cells maintain their integrity in successive cycles of secretory activity. **mixed g.** One containing both serous and mucous components. **Naboth's glands.** The mucous glands of the external os of the cervix uteri. **Nuhn's glands.** The anterior lingual glands. See *Blandin's g.* **paraurethral glands.** Small vestigial glands opening into the posterior wall of the female urethra close to its orifice. The homolog of the distal prostatic glands of the male. Syn., *Skene's glands* or *tubules.* **parotid g.** One of the salivary glands in front of and below the external ear. It is a compound racemose gland. Its duct is Stensen's duct. **peptic glands.** The fundic glands of the stomach. **preputial glands.** Sebaceous glands in the prepuce of the penis. **pyloric glands.** The glands of the mucous membrane of the pyloric portion of the stomach. **racemose g.** A compound alveolar or tubuloalveolar gland. **salivary g.** One that secretes saliva, as the parotid. **sebaceous g.** One which secretes sebum, an unctuous material composed primarily of fat. **serous g.** One which secretes a watery, albuminous fluid. **simple g.** (a) A gland which is entirely composed of secretory cells, without a differentiated ductile portion. (b) A gland with but one secretory end-piece and an unbranched duct. **Skene's glands.** The paraurethral glands in the female. **sublingual g.** A complex of small salivary glands situated in the sublingual fold on each side of the oral floor. **submaxillary g.** A large salivary gland situated below each lower jaw. Also called *mandibular g., submandibular g.* **sudoriferous glands.** The sweat glands. **sudoriparous glands.** The sweat glands of the skin. **superficial g.** One lying entirely within the limits of a mucous membrane. **suprarenal g.** A gland above and medial to the kidney. Syn., *adrenal g.* **sweat g.** One of the coiled tubular glands of the skin which secrete perspiration. **tarsal glands.** Sebaceous glands in the tarsal plates of the eyelids. Also called *Meibomian glands.* **thyroid g.** One of the endocrine glands, lying in front of the trachea and consisting of two lateral lobes connected centrally by an isthmus. The organ is composed of follicles lined by epithelium, producing a colloid material. Hypertrophy of the gland (goiter) is sometimes associated with a peculiar disease known as exophthalmic goiter; hypofunction of the gland leads to cretinism or myxedema. **tubular g.** A secreting gland, tubelike or cylindrical in shape. **Tyson's glands.** Sebaceous glands of the prepuce which secrete the smegma. **urethral glands.** Small, branched, tubular mucous glands in the mucous membrane of the urethra. Syn., *Littré's glands.* **uterine g.** A gland of the endometrium. **vestibular glands.** Glands of the vestibule of the vagina. They comprise the compound tubulo-alveolar **major vestibular glands** (of Bartholin), one in each lateral wall, and the **minor vestibular glands,** which are several small branched tubular mucous glands around the urethral orifice.

glan'ders. A highly contagious acute or chronic disease of horses, mules, and asses; caused by *Malleomyces mallei.* It is communicable to dogs, goats, sheep, and man, but not to bovines. It is characterized by fever, inflammation of mucous membranes (especially of the nose), enlargement and hardening of the regional lymph nodes, formation of nodules which have a tendency to coalesce and then degenerate to form deep ulcers. In man the disease usually runs an acute febrile course and terminates fatally. Syn., *farcy, equinia.*

glans (glanz). The conical body which forms the distal end of the clitoris (**glans clitoridis**) or of the penis (**glans penis**).

glass'es. The popular term for spectacles or eyeglasses. **bifocal g.** Those that have a different refracting power in the upper part from that in the lower; the effect usually is produced by the superposition of segment lenses. **glass wool.** White, silky threads obtained by the action of a powerful blast on a falling stream of molten glass.

glau·co'ma (glaw·ko'muh). A disease of the eye marked by heightened intraocular tension; results in hardness of the globe, excavation of the optic disk, restricted field of vision, corneal anesthesia, a colored halo seen surrounding artificial lights, and lessening of the visual power; may lead to blindness. **absolute g.** The completed glaucomatous process when the eyeball is exceedingly hard and totally blind. **acute g.** The first (or the renewed) attack, with the characteristic and inflammatory symptoms. **auricular g.**

That associated with a great increase in the intralabyrinthine pressure. **congenital g.** See infantile *g.* **hemorrhagic g.** That associated with retinal hemorrhage. Also called *apoplectic g.* **infantile g.** That affecting infants or children; due to a failure of development of Schlemm's canal and a consequent lack of normal drainage for the intraocular fluid. May be very mild with low tension, or may be clinically severe with a distention and stretching of the eye due to its increased fluid contents (buphthalmia or hydrophthalmos). Syn., *congenital g., intercalary staphyloma.* **malignant g.** A grave form attended with violent pain and rapidly leading to blindness. **secondary g.** That consequent upon other ocular diseases. **simple g.** That chronic form occurring without inflammatory symptoms.

gleet. The chronic stage of urethritis, characterized by a slight mucopurulent discharge. —**gleet'y,** *adj.*

gle"no·hu'mer·al. Pertaining to the glenoid cavity and the humerus, as the glenohumeral ligament.

gle'noid. 1. Having a shallow cavity; resembling a shallow cavity or socket. 2. Specifically, the socket of the shoulder joint.

gli'a. The neuroglia. —**gli'al,** *adj.*

gli"o·blas·to'ma mul"ti·for'me. The most frequent glioma of the central nervous system, usually the brain, composed of spongioblasts that may be either stellate or unipolar. Also called *spongioblastoma.*

gli·o'ma (glye·o'muh). A tumor composed of cells and fibers representative of the special supporting tissue of the central nervous system, and derived from neuroglial cells or their antecedents; occurs principally in the brain, spinal cord, peripheral nerves, and adrenals. —**gliom'atous,** *adj.;* **gli·omato'sis,** *n.*

gli·o'sis (glye·o'sis). Proliferation of neuroglia in the brain or spinal cord, as a replacement process or due to low-grade inflammation; may be diffuse or focal. **Gliosis of the spinal cord** is the earliest pathologic change in syringomyelia.

gli"o·tox'in. An antibiotic; obtained from cultures of *Trichoderma, Gliocladium,* and *Aspergillus fumigatus.*

globe. *In ophthalmology,* the eyeball.

glo'bin. One of a class of proteins, histone in nature, obtained from the hemoglobins of various animal species.

glob"u·lar'e·tin, glob"u·la·re'tin. A hydrolysis product of globularin.

glob"u·lar'in, glob'u·lar·in. A glycoside from the leaves of *Globularia alypum.* Its action upon the heart and nervous system is similar to that of caffeine, but it diminishes the quantity of the urine.

glob'ule. A small spherical droplet of fluid or semifluid material. **milk g.** A fat drop in milk.

glob'u·li·cide", glob'u'li·cide". 1. Destructive of blood cells. 2. An agent that destroys blood cells. —**globuli·ci'dal,** adj.

glob'u·lin. A general name for a group of animal and plant proteins characterized by solubility in dilute salt solutions and differentiated from albumins by lesser solubility, more alkaline isoelectric points, larger molecular weight, faster sedimentation rates, and slower electrophoretic mobilities, α-, β-, γ-**globulins** are fractions of serum globulin separated by electrophoresis. α-**g.** contains certain seroenzymes and hormones. β-**g.** contains the blood group antibodies, prothrombin, and certain fractions of complement. γ-**g.** includes most antibodies. See Table of Normal Values of Blood Constituents in the Appendix. **immune g.** Human immune globulin; a sterile solution of antibodies extracted from the human placenta and used in the prevention, modification, and treatment of measles. **serum g.** The globulin fraction of blood serum.

glob'u·li·nu'ri·a. The presence of globulin in the urine.

glo'bus. A ball or globe. **g. hystericus.** The choking sensation, or so-called lump in the throat, occurring in hysteria.

glom'er·ate. Rolled together like a ball of thread.

glo·mer"u·lo·ne·phri'tis. A type of renal disease in which the primary important lesion is in the glomeruli. The lesion may be proliferative, degenerative, or exudative without suppuration. In a majority of cases, there is an antecedent, or associated infectious process, usually a streptococcic infection. Classified as to duration, there are acute, subacute, and chronic types. Hypertension, convulsions, edema, nitrogen retention, and acidosis may occur in the course of the disease.

glo·mer'u·lus (pl. glomeruli). 1. A small rounded mass. 2. The tuft of capillary loops projecting into the lumen of a renal corpuscle. —**glomerular, glomerulose,** adj.

glo'mus. 1. A fold of the mesothelium arising near the base of the mesentery in the pronephros, and containing a ball of blood vessels. Also called glomerule of the pronephros. 2. The part of the choroid plexus of the lateral ventricle which covers the thalamus. Also called glomus chorioideum. —**glomic,** adj. **g. body.** An arteriog-

venous anastomosis which has a special arrangement of muscle and nerve tissue; usually present in the cutis and subcutis of fingers and toes.

glon'o·in (glon'o·in, glo'no·in). Glyceryl trinitrate or nitroglycerin.

glos'sa. The tongue. —**glossal,** adj. -**glos'sa.** A combining form meaning tongue.

glos·sal'gi·a. Pain in the tongue.

glos·sec'to·my. Excision of the tongue.

-**glos'si·a.** A combining form meaning a (specified) condition of the tongue.

Glos·si'na, Glos'si·na. A genus of bloodsucking flies, known as tsetse flies; confined to tropical and subtropical Africa. The species G. fusca, G. palpalis, and G. morsitans transmit the trypanosomes of sleeping sickness in man and of nagana and the souma disease of horses, cattle, and sheep.

glos·si'tis. Inflammation of the tongue. —**glossit'ic,** adj. **atrophic g.** Hunter's glossitis. **benign migratory g.** Chronic glossitis characterized by local areas of inflammation and atrophy of filiform papillae. Such areas may change shape or location. Syn., geographic tongue. **Hunter's g.** That associated with pernicious anemia, characterized by atrophy of papillae, redness, burning sensation, and pain. Syn., atrophic glossitis. **median rhomboidal g.** A developmental anomaly, in which an oval or rhomboidal area devoid of papillae and sometimes elevated is found on the dorsum of the tongue, anterior to the vallate papillae. **Moeller's g.** Chronic glossitis of uncertain origin, characterized by irregular superficial areas of atrophy or excoriation, and sometimes coexistent with vitamin-B complex deficiency and allergy or with hormonal imbalance.

glos'so-, gloss-. A combining form meaning tongue.

glos'so·cele. Swelling, or edema, of the tongue, with consequent extrusion of the organ.

glos"so·dy"na·mom'e·ter (glos"-o·dye"nuh·mom'i·tur, ·din"uh·mom'i·tur). An apparatus for measuring the capacity of the tongue to resist pressure.

glos"so·dyn'i·a. Pain in the tongue.

glos"so·ep"i·glot'tic, glos"so·ep"i·glot·tid'e·an. Pertaining to both tongue and epiglottis.

glos'so·graph. An instrument for registering the movements of the tongue in speech.

glos"so·hy'al, glos"so·hy'oid. Pertaining to the tongue and the hyoid bone.

glos″so·kin″es·thet′ic. Relating to the motions of the tongue in speech.

glos″so·la′bi·al. Relating to the tongue and lips, as glossolabial paralysis.

glos″so·la′li·a (glos″o·lay′lee·uh, ·lal′ee·uh). Unintelligible jabbering; talk in a strange or unknown tongue; jargon.

glos·sol′o·gy. 1. The study of the tongue and its diseases. 2. The definition and explanation of terms; nomenclature.

glos″so·pal′a·tine (·pal′uh·tyne, ·tin). Relating to the tongue and the palate, as the glossopalatine arch, or anterior pillar of the fauces.

glos·sop′a·thy. Any disease of the tongue.

glos″so·pha·ryn′ge·al (glos″o·fa·rin′jee·ul, ·far″in·jee′ul). Pertaining to tongue and pharynx, as glossopharyngeal nerve. See Table of Nerves in the Appendix.

glos″so·pha·ryn′ge·us (·fa·rin′jee·us, ·far″in·jee′us). A portion of the superior constrictor muscle of the pharynx, attached to the tongue.

glos″so·plas′ty, glos″so·plas′ty. Plastic surgery of the tongue.

glos″so·ple′gi·a. Paralysis of the tongue.

glos″so·py·ro′sis (glos″o·pye·ro′sis). A burning sensation of the tongue.

glos·sor′rha·phy. Surgical suturing of the tongue.

glos·sos′co·py. Diagnostic inspection of the tongue.

glos″so·spasm″. Spasm of the tongue.

glos·sot′o·my. 1. The dissection of the tongue. 2. An incision of the tongue.

glos″so·trich′i·a (glos″o·trick′ee·uh). Hairy tongue.

glot′tis. The rima glottidis; the opening between the free margins of the vocal folds. **—glottal, glottid′ean,** adj.

glu′case. The enzyme that converts starch into glucose. Obs.

glu′cide. A group term for carbohydrates and glycosides. **—glucid′ic,** adj.

glu·ci′num. Beryllium; symbol, Gl. Obs.

glu′co-, gluc-. 1. In chemistry, a combining form signifying glucose. 2. See glyco-.

glu″co·cor′ti·coid. An adrenal cortex hormone that affects glucose metabolism; any related natural or synthetic substance that affects glucose metabolism.

glu″co·fu′ran·ose. A glucose with a 1-4 furanose ring.

glu″co·gen. See glycogen.

glu″co·ne″o·gen′e·sis. The formation of glucose by the liver from noncarbohydrate sources.

glu·con′ic ac′id. $CH_2OH(CHOH)_4$·COOH. An acid resulting from the oxidation of dextrose and other sugars.

glu″co·no·ki′nase. An enzyme present in microörganisms adapted to grow on D-gluconic acid, which catalyzes phosphorylation of the acid.

glu″co·no·lac′tone. The ring structure of D-gluconic acid.

glucophylline. Trade-mark for preparations containing a double salt of theophylline and methylglucamine.

glu″co·pro·te′in. Old term for glycoprotein, q.v.

glu″co·py′ran·ose. A glucose with a 1-5 pyranose ring.

glu″cos·a·mine′ (gloo″ko·suh·meen′, gloo·ko′suh·meen). See glycosamine.

glu′co·san. A polysaccharide which yields glucose upon hydrolysis.

glu·co′sa·zone (gloo·ko′suh·zone, ·koss′uh·zone). See phenylglucosazone.

glu′cose. 1. The crystalline monosaccharide dextrose, $C_6H_{12}O_6$, more correctly designated D-glucose. See dextrose. 2. A product which is obtained by the incomplete hydrolysis of starch, consisting chiefly of dextrose (D-glucose), dextrins, maltose, and water; being liquid, it is more correctly designated liquid glucose. See Table of Normal Values of Blood Constituents in the Appendix.

D-glucose. Glucose, 1.

glu″cose-1-phos′phate. CH_2OH·$\overset{\frown}{CH(CHOH)}_3CH.OPO(OH)_2$. The postulated first product in the breakdown of glycogen; a hexosemonophosphate. See glycophosphomutase.

glu″cose-6-phos′phate. $(OH)_2$·$OPOCH_2\overset{\frown}{CH(CHOH)}_3CHOH$. A product, resulting from a reversible change of glucose-1-phosphate, obtained in the breakdown of glycogen; a hexosemonophosphate. See glycophosphomutase.

glu′co·si·dase. 1. An enzyme which catalyzes the hydrolysis of glucosides. 2. Emulsin.

glu′co·side. 1. Any member of a series of compounds, usually of plant origin, that may be hydrolyzed into dextrose (D-glucose) and another principle; the latter is often referred to as an aglucone. 2. Formerly, any compound of plant origin which on hydrolysis yields a sugar and another principle. Now called glycoside, q.v.

glu″co·sul′fone so′di·um. p,p′-Diaminodiphenylsulfone-N,N′-di-(dextrose sodium sulfonate), used in the treatment of leprosy and as an adjunct to streptomycin therapy of tuberculosis. See promin sodium.

glu·co′sum. Glucose.

glu″co·su′ri·a. Old term for glycosuria, *q.v.*

glu″cu·ron′ic ac′id. CHO.HCOH.-HOCH.HCOH.HCOH.COOH, or D-glucuronic acid, the acid resulting from oxidation of the primary alcohol group of glucose to carboxyl, also a component of aldobionic acid. Also called *glycuronic acid.* See also *glucuronide.*

glu″cu·ron′i·dase. An enzyme which catalyzes hydrolysis of glucuronides. Also called *glycuronidase.*

glu·cu′ron·ide. A compound resulting from the conjugation of glucuronic acid with a phenol, an alcohol, or an acid containing a carboxyl group. Also called *glycuronide.*

glue. An impure gelatin prepared by boiling the skin, hoofs, and horns of animals. **fish g.** Isinglass, prepared from the swim-bladder of fishes.

glu′side. See *saccharin.*

glu·tam′ic ac′id. COOH.(CH₂)₂.CH-NH₂.COOH. An amino acid resulting from the hydrolysis of proteins. **g. a. hydrochloride.** A water-soluble glutamic acid salt which releases hydrochloric acid in the stomach.

glu·tam′i·nase. The enzyme which catalyzes the conversion of glutamine to glutamic acid and ammonia.

glu′ta·mine (gloo′tuh-meen, gloo-tam′een). The monamide of aminoglutaric acid.

glu·tar′ic ac′id (gloo-tar′ick, -tahr′-ick). COOH(CH₂)₂COOH. A crystalline acid found in sheep wool.

glu″ta·thi′one (gloo″tuh-thigh′ohn, -thigh-ohn′). A tripeptide widely distributed in plant and animal tissues.

glu·te·lin. A class of simple proteins occurring in seeds of cereals.

glu′ten. A mixture of proteins found in the seeds of cereals.

glu′ten bread. Bread made from wheat flour from which all the starch has been removed.

lu·teth′i·mide. 2-Ethyl-2-phenylglutarimide, a hypnotic and sedative. See *doriden.*

glu·te′us (gloo-tee′us). One of the large muscles of the buttock, attached to the ilium and femur. See Table of Muscles in the Appendix.

glu′tin. 1. A protein obtained from gelatin. 2. Vegetable casein.

glu′ti·nous. Viscid; gluelike.

glut′ton·y. Abnormally excessive indulgence in eating.

gly′case (glye′case, ·kayz). Old term or maltase.

gly·ce′mi·a, gly·cae′mi·a (glye-see′mee·uh). The presence of glucose in the blood. **—glycemic,** *adj.*

glyc″er·al′de·hyde (glis″er·al′de-hide). A compound that is formed by the oxidation of glycerin and that is the simplest aldose exhibiting optical activity; the D- and L- forms are used as the configurational references for carbohydrates. See also D-, L-.

glyc′er·ide (gliss′ur·ide, ·id). An ester in which glycerin provides the alcohol radical. Fats are glycerides of certain long-chain organic acids.

glyc′er·in (gliss′ur·in). 1. Trihydroxypropane. C₃H₅(OH)₃. A clear, colorless, syrupy liquid of sweet taste, obtained by the hydrolysis of fats. Syn., *glycerol.* 2. British Pharmacopoeia name for a glycerite. **g. supposi·tories.** Prepared from glycerin, sodium stearate, and water.

glyc′er·ite (gliss′ur·yte). A solution of one or more medicinal substances in glycerin.

glyc″er·o·gel′a·tin (gliss″ur·o·jel′uh·tin). One of a class of pharmaceutical preparations composed of glycerin, gelatin, water, and one or more medicinal substances.

glyc′er·ol (gliss′ur·ole, ·ol). Glycerin.

glyc″er·o·phos′pha·tase. An enzyme capable of liberating phosphoric acid from glycerophosphoric acid and certain of its derivatives.

glyc″er·o·phos′phate. A salt of glycerophosphoric acid.

glyc″er·o·phos·phor′ic ac′id. CH₂OH.CHOH.CH₂.O.PO(OH)₂. A pale yellow, oily liquid, soluble in water.

glyc′er·ose. The triose sugar resulting from oxidation of glycerin.

glyc″er·ose-3-phos′phate. Glyceraldehyde-3-phosphoric acid, CHO.-CHOH.CH₂OPO(OH)₂, an intermediate in a postulated cleavage of carbohydrates to form lactic acid.

glyc′er·yl (gliss′ur·il). The trivalent radical, C₃H₅, combining with fatty acids to form fats. **g. trinitrate.** C₃H₅(NO₂)₃. A colorless, or pale yellow, volatile liquid used in the preparation of explosives. Physiologically, it possesses the actions of the nitrites. Syn., *nitroglycerin, glonoin.*

gly′cin. A poisonous photographic developer, p-hydroxyphenylaminoacetic acid.

gly′cine (glye′seen, glye·seen′). Aminoacetic acid.

gly′ci·nin. The principal protein of the soybean.

gly′co-, glyc-. A combining form meaning *sweet,* or denoting *glycerin.*

gly″co·cho′late (glye″ko·ko′late, ·kol′ate). A salt of glycocholic acid.

gly″co·chol′ic ac′id. An acid obtained by the conjugation of cholic acid with glycine; found in bile.

gly″co·coll. Aminoacetic acid.

gly″co·cy″a·mine′. Guanidine acetic acid, COOHCH₂NHC(NH)NH₂, a product of interaction between glycine and arginine which by transmethylation is converted to creatine.

gly′co·gen. (C₆H₁₀O₅)ₙ. A carbohydrate found in many tissues and stored in the liver, where it is converted, as the system requires, into sugar (glucose). It is also known as *animal starch*.

gly″co·ge·nase″ (glye′ko·ji·nace″, glye″ko·ji·nace′). An enzyme found in the liver, which hydrolyzes glycogen to maltose and dextrin.

gly″co·gen′e·sis. Formation of sugar in the liver. —**glycogenet′ic, glycog′enous,** *adj.*

gly″co·gen′ic. Pertaining to glycogen or to glycogenesis.

gly″co·ge·nol′y·sis. The conversion of glycogen into glucose by hydrolysis.

gly″co·ge·no′sis. A disturbance of glycogen metabolism occurring in early infancy. Also called *glycogen disease, von Gierke's disease.*

gly′col. 1. An aliphatic compound containing two hydroxyl groups. 2. Ethylene glycol.

gly·col′ic ac′id (glye·kol′ick). CH_2·OH.COOH. Hydroxyacetic acid produced by the reduction of oxalic acid.

gly″co·lip′ids. Lipids which, on acid hydrolysis, liberate a carbohydrate, an alcohol, and a fatty acid.

gly·col′y·sis (glye·kol′i·sis). The hydrolysis of sugar in the body. —**gly·colyt′ic,** *adj.*

gly″co·me·tab′o·lism. The metabolism of sugar in the body. —**glyco·metabol′ic,** *adj.*

gly″co·phos″pho·mu′tase. An enzyme which catalyzes the reaction, glucose-1-phosphate $\rightleftharpoons$ glucose-6-phosphate.

gly″co·pro′te·in. One of a group of conjugated proteins which upon decomposition yield a protein and a carbohydrate, or derivatives of the same.

gly″co·pty′a·lism (gly″ko·ty′uh·liz·um). Presence of glucose in the saliva.

gly″cor·rha′chi·a (gly″ko·ray′kee·uh, ·rack′ee·uh). Glucose in the cerebrospinal fluid.

gly″cor·rhe′a, gly″cor·rhoe′a (gly″ko·ree′uh). Discharge of sugar-containing fluid from the body.

gly″cos·a·mine′ (gly″ko·suh·meen′, gly·ko′suh·meen). $C_6H_{13}O_5N$. An amino derivative of glucose; formed on hydrolysis of chitin and other glycoproteins. Syn., *glucosamine.*

gly″co·si·al′i·a (gly″ko·sigh·al′ee·uh, ·ay′lee·uh). The presence of glucose in the saliva.

gly″co·si′a·lor·rhe′a. Excessive salivary secretion containing glucose.

gly′co·side. Any plant principle which yields on hydrolysis a sugar and another substance designated as an aglycone. See also *glucoside.*

gly″co·su′ri·a. The presence of sugar in the urine. **alimentary g.** That

due to excessive ingestion of carbohydrates. **anxiety g.** A transitory form due to worry. **artificial g.** Glycosuria resulting from puncture of the floor of the fourth ventricle in the inferior part of the medulla. Formerly called *traumatic g., piqûre diabetes.* **diabetic g.** That resulting from diabetes mellitus. **renal g.** An anomalous condition characterized by a low renal threshold for sugar together with a normal blood sugar level; of little or no pathologic significance. Erroneously called *renal diabetes.* **toxic g.** That observed after poisoning by chloral, morphine, or curare, after the inhalation of chloroform or carbon monoxide, or after the ingestion of phlorhizin.

gly″co·su′ric ac′id. Homogentisic acid.

gly″u·re′sis (glick″yoo·ree′sis, gly″cue·). Excretion of sugar seen normally in the urine.

gly″cu·ron′ic ac′id. Glucuronic acid, *q.v.*

gly″cu·ron′i·dase. Glucuronidase.

gly·cu′ron·ide. Glucuronide.

gly″cu·ro·nu′ri·a. The presence of glucuronic acid in the urine.

glyc″yr·rhi′za (glis″i·rye′zuh). Licorice. The dried rhizome and roots of several varieties of *Glycyrrhiza glabra.*

glyc″yr·rhi′zic ac′id (glis″i·rye′zick). The characteristic acid of the sweet principle of glycyrrhiza. See *glycyrrhizin.*

glyc″yr·rhi′zin (glis″i·rye′zin). A very sweet, crystalline principle found in glycyrrhiza and consisting of salts of glycyrrhizic acid.

gly·ox′a·lase (glye·ock′suh·lace). An enzyme present in various body tissues which catalyzes the conversion of methylglyoxal into lactic acid.

gly·ox′a·line (glye·ock′suh·leen, ·lin). Imidazole.

gly″ox·yl′ic ac′id. (HO)$_2$CHCOOH. Dihydroxyacetic acid, used as a reagent for protein.

Gm., gm. Gram(s); gramme(s).

gnat. Any one of various dipterous insects belonging to the suborder Nematocera. Mosquitoes, black flies, biting midges, and sand flies are included.

gnath-. See *gnatho-.*

gnath·al′gi·a (na·thal′juh, ·jee·uh) Pain or neuralgia of the jaw.

gnath′ic (nath′ick, nay′thick). Pertaining to the jaw.

gnath·i′tis (na·thigh′tis). Inflammation of the jaw or cheek.

gnath′o- (nath′o-, nayth′o-), **gnath-.** A combining form signifying *the jaw.*

gnath″o·dy″na·mom′e·ter (·dye″nuh·mom′i·tur, ·din″uh·mom′i·tur). An instrument for recording the force exerted in closing the jaws.

gnath·o·dyn′i·a. Pain in the jaw, gnathalgia.

gnath'o·plas''ty. Plastic surgery of the cheek or jaw.

gnath·os'chi·sis (na·thos'ki·sis). Cleft alveolar process.

gnomy. A combining form meaning *the science* or *art of judging.*

gno'sis (no'sis). The faculty of knowing in contradistinction to the function of feeling, in respect to any external stimulus.

gnos'tic (nos'tick). Relating to discriminative or epicritic sensations in contradistinction to vital or protopathic sensations.

goi'ter, goi'tre. Enlargement of the thyroid gland. Also see *struma.* **—goitrous,** *adj.* **aberrant g.** That of a supernumerary thyroid gland. Also called *accessory g.* **acute g.** One which develops rapidly. **adenomatous g.** An asymmetric type due to isolated nodular masses of thyroid tissue (adenomas). **adolescent g.** Diffuse enlargement of the thyroid in adolescents. Also called *juvenile g.* **benign metastasizing g.** A malignant goiter, from which metastases may grow slowly, simulating benign lesions. **cancerous g.** Carcinoma of the thyroid gland. Also called *carcinomatous g.* **colloid g.** A diffuse, soft, sometimes large goiter in which many of the acinar spaces are distended with colloid. **congenital g.** One present at birth. **cystic g.** One in which a cyst, or cysts, forms by the degeneration of tissue, as within preëxisting adenomas. **diffuse g.** A type in which the thyroid gland is diffusely enlarged, in contrast to adenomatous goiter. **endemic g.** That occurring commonly in iodine-poor and mountainous areas. **exophthalmic g.** A disease caused chiefly by overproduction of the thyroid hormone; characterized by goiter, tachycardia, nervous excitability, fine involuntary tremor, exophthalmos and other ocular signs, loss of weight, muscular weakness, and a tendency to intense, acute exacerbations called thyroid crises. There is excessive excretion of nitrogen and increased excretion of calcium, leading to osteoporosis and disturbance in carbohydrate metabolism. Also called *Basedow's disease, Flajani's disease, Graves' disease, hyperthyroidism, Parry's disease, thyrotoxicosis, toxic g.* **hyperplastic g.** One characterized by an increased number of cells, particularly those lining the acini, with an accompanying increase in vascularity of the gland. Also called *parenchymatous g.* **intrathoracic g.** A goiter which has a portion lying within the thoracic cavity. **lingual g.** A tumor, composed of thyroid tissue, at the upper end of the original thyroglossal duct, near the

foramen cecum of the tongue. **malignant g.** One which is the seat of carcinoma or sarcoma. **sarcomatous g.** Sarcoma of the thyroid gland. **simple g.** A diffuse goiter, either colloid or hyperplastic in type; usually unassociated with constitutional features. **sporadic g.** Goiter which occurs in limited geographic areas. **sulfonamide g.** That due to continued administration of one of the soluble sulfonamides. **thiocyanate g.** One due to prolonged administration of a thiocyanate. **thiourylene g.** One due to administration of a thiourylene compound; as thiourea, thiouracil, thiobarbital; associated with hyperplasia of the thyroid gland and thought to be due to prevention of synthesis of thyroglobulin. **toxic g.** See *exophthalmic g.*

goi''tro·gen'ic. Producing goiter; as iodine-deficient diets or, experimentally, diets of cabbage and other brassica plants, the feeding of sulfonamides, drugs of the thiourea group, etc.

gold. Au = 197.2. A yellow metal, easily malleable and ductile. **g. and sodium thiosulfate.** Sodium aurothiosulfate. $Na_3Au(S_2O_3)_3.2H_2O$. Used in lupus erythematosus. See *sanocrysin.* **g. bromide.** Gold tribromide, auric bromide, $AuBr_3$. Used in epilepsy and in whooping cough. **g. leaf.** Pure gold in very thin, transparent sheets of blue-green color. **g. sodium thiomalate.** See *myochrysine.*

gold'en·rod''. The common name for several species of the genus *Solidago* of the Compositae. Their pollen may produce hay fever.

gom·phi'a·sis. Looseness of the teeth in their sockets; periodontosis. *Obs.*

gom·pho'sis. A form of synarthrosis, *q.v.*

gon'ad. 1. A gland or organ producing gametes; a general term for ovary or testis. 2. The embryonic sex gland before morphologic identification as ovary or testis is possible. Also called *indifferent g.* **—gonadal,** *adj.* **female g.** The ovary. **male g.** The testis.

gon''a·dec'to·my. Surgical removal of a gonad.

gon''a·do·ther'a·py. Treatment with gonadal extracts or hormones.

gon''a·do·tro'pic. Gonad-stimulating.

gon''a·do·tro'pin (gon''uh·do·tro'pin). A gonad-stimulating hormone. **anterior pituitary g.** That produced by the anterior lobe of the pituitary gland. There are thought to be three such gonadotropins: follicle-stimulating (FSH, prolan A), luteinizing (LH, prolan B), and luteotropic. **chorionic g.** That produced

by chorionic villi. It is present in the blood and urine in pregnancy. Also called *chorionic gonadotropic hormone (CH)*, *anterior pituitarylike hormone*, *pregnancy urine hormone*, *P.U.* See *A.P.L.*
equine g. That obtained from the serum of pregnant mares; a mixture of follicle-stimulating and luteinizing hormones.

gon'a·duct. Duct of a gonad; oviduct or sperm duct.

go·nag'ra (go-nag'ruh, gon'ag-ruh). Gout of the knee joint.

go·nal'gi·a. Pain in the knee joint.

gon"an·gi·ec'to·my (gon"an-jee-eck'to-mee, go-nan"jee·). Excision of part of the ductus deferens.

gon"ar·thri'tis. Inflammation of the knee joint.

gon"ar·throt'o·my. Incision into the knee joint.

go·nat'o·cele. A swelling or tumor of the knee.

gon'e·cyst, gon"e·cys'tis. A seminal vesicle. **–gonecys'tic,** *adj*.

gon"e·cys·ti'tis. Inflammation of the seminal vesicles.

gon"e·cys'to·lith. A concretion or calculus in a seminal vesicle.

gon"e·poi·e'sis. The formation of semen. **–gonepoiet'ic,** *adj*.

gon'ic. Pertaining to semen or to generation.

go"ni·om'e·ter. An instrument for measuring angles, as the angle of the mandible.

go'ni·o·scope. A special optical instrument for studying in detail the angle of the anterior chamber of the eye, and for testing ocular motility. **–gonios'copy,** *n*.

go·ni'tis. Inflammation of the knee joint.

gon"o·coc·ce'mi·a, gon"o·coc·cae'mi·a (gon"o-cock-see'mee-uh). The presence of gonococci in the blood.

gon"o·coc'cus (pl. *gonococci*). The common name for the organism causing gonorrhea; *Neisseria gonorrhoeae*. **–gonococcal, gonococcic,** *adj*.

gon"or·rhe'a. A specific infectious inflammation of the mucous membrane of the urethra and adjacent cavities, due to the *Neisseria gonorrhoeae*. The disease is characterized by pain, burning urination, a profuse mucopurulent discharge, and may be accompanied by complications: prostatitis, periurethral abscess, epididymitis, cystitis, purulent conjunctivitis. It may also cause arthritis (gonorrheal rheumatism), endocarditis, and salpingitis. **–gonorrhe'al,** *adj*.

gon"y·ba'ti·a. Walking upon the knees; a symptom in some paralytic and paretic cases.

gon"y·camp'sis. Deformity of a knee by curvation.

gon"y·on'cus. A tumor or swelling of the knee.

goose flesh. Skin marked by prominence about the hair follicles. Results from contraction of the arrectores pilorum muscles. Also called *goose skin, cutis anserina*.

gor'get (gor'jit). A channeled instrument similar to a grooved director formerly used much in lithotomy **probe g.** One whose tip is probe pointed.

Gos·syp'i·um. A genus of plants of the Malvaceae from which cotton and cotton-root bark are obtained.

gouge. A transversely curved chisel for cutting or removing bone or other hard structures.

goun'dou (goon'doo). An exostosis of the face; probably a sequela of yaws involving the nasal and adjacent bone to produce a projecting, tumorlike mass. Also called *anakhre, big nose, henpue*.

gout. A constitutional hereditary condition of uric acid metabolism, associated with a high blood level and a decreased urinary excretion of uric acid often with fever and leukocytosis. There are sudden attacks of acute painful arthritis which may last a few days to a few weeks, recurring at irregular intervals with complete remission between attacks. Usually one joint is involved, the great toe being the part most commonly affected. The joint involved may be hot, red, and tender, and the surrounding skin is shiny. Repeated attacks may result in deformity. **–gout'y,** *adj*.

gr. Grain(s).

grac·i'lis (grass'i-lis). A long, slender muscle on the medial aspect of the thigh. See Table of Muscles in the Appendix.

grac'i·lis. Long and slender, as the gracilis muscle.

gra'di·ent. 1. The rate of increase of a variable magnitude or the curve which represents it. 2. *In biology*, system of relations within the organism, or a part of it, which involve progressively increasing or decreasing differences in respect to rate of growth, rate of metabolism, or of any other structural or functional property of the cells.

grad'u·ate. A vessel, usually of glass, marked with lines at different levels used for measuring liquids.

grad'u·a"ted. Divided into units by a series of lines, as a barometer, graduate, a thermometer.

graft. A portion of tissue, such as skin, periosteum, bone, fascia, or rarely, an entire organ, used to replace a defect in the body. See *implantation, implants, transplant, transplantation.*
arterial g. See arterial bridge.
autogenous g. One taken from the

patient's body. Also called *autoplastic g.,* *autograft.* **bone g.** One composed of osseous tissue; may be cortical, cancellous, or medullary; used to repair bone defects, to afford support, or to supply osteogenic tissue. **bridging g.** One which connects the cut ends of arteries, bones, nerves, etc., where there is loss of substance and the divided ends cannot be approximated. **cable g.** *In neurosurgery,* the placing together of several sections of nerve to be transplanted, to bridge a gap in a nerve larger than the sections available for the grafting. **cartilage g.** Cartilage autograft or homograft, commonly used for replacing damaged or destroyed cartilage, or to replace bone loss. **chorioallantoic g.** A graft of tissue onto the chorioallantoic membrane of the hen's egg, which furnishes a favorable environment for growth. Also used for culturing viruses for the preparation of vaccines. **corneal g.** Corneal tissue, usually human, transplanted into a defective cornea to provide a clear window. **derma-fat-fascia g.** A tissue graft employing full-thickness skin, fat, and fascia. **dermic g.** A skin graft. **fascial g.** A strip of fascia lata or aponeurosis; used either for the repair of a defect in muscle or fascia, or for suturing. **fat g.** A portion of fat, implanted to fill a hollow and improve a contour. **free g.** A graft of any type of tissue which is cut free and transplanted to another area. **full-thickness g.** A skin graft including all layers of the skin. **heterogenous g.** Heterograft. **heteroplastic g.** One from a source other than the patient; a heterograft. **homogenous g.** Homograft. **implantation g.** See *implantation,* 1. **inlay g.** One placed beneath the tissue, as a bone graft placed in the medullary cavity of a bone, or an Esser inlay beneath the skin or mucous membrane. **mucosal g.** A graft of oral mucous membrane or of conjunctiva to repair a defect. **muscle g.** A portion of muscle sutured in place, for checking hemorrhage where a bleeding vessel cannot be secured. **nerve g.** A portion of a nerve sutured in place to restore the continuity of a severed nerve trunk where apposition cannot be secured. **omental g.** A portion of omentum transplanted to fill a defect or to check a hemorrhage, or placed over an intestinal suture line to prevent adhesions. **onlay g.** A bone graft which is laid on the surface of a bone where bone substance has been lost and where conditions are unsuited to inlay grafts. Onlay grafts are fixed in place by vitallium screws. **osteoperiosteal g.** One of bone and periosteum.

ovarian g. A portion of ovary implanted anywhere except in its normal bed, usually in the abdominal wall, for the preservation of the hormone production. **pedicle g.** See pedicle *flap.* **periosteal g.** One consisting entirely of periosteum and used for minor bone defects to promote healing or union. See bone *g.* **pinch g.** A small, full-thickness graft lifted from the donor area by a needle and cut free with a razor. Many such small deep grafts are fitted together to cover the defect. **sieve g.** A large skin graft, with openings throughout, corresponding to skin islands left on the donor area. **skin g.** A portion of skin, of any size or thickness, cut from a donor area and transferred to the recipient site where repair is needed. **surface g.** A graft applied anywhere on the surface of the body where part of the skin is missing. **tendon g.** One of tendon to bridge a gap in a tendon. Also see tendon *transplantation.* **testis g.** The grafting by implantation of an entire testis or portion to replace one lost or destroyed, for the production of hormones. **tunnel g.** A skin graft with the epithelial side inward, introduced into tissues under a contracted scar, etc. The tunnel is split later, and the epithelial surface becomes superficial or is left in place to replace a part, such as the urethra. **zoograft.** A graft of tissue taken from an animal. **zooplastic g.** A graft of tissue obtained from an animal.

grain. 1. The seed or seedlike fruit of the cereal grasses. 2. A minute portion or particle, as of sand, or of starch. 3. A unit of weight of the troy, the avoirdupois, and the apothecaries' systems of weights. Abbreviated, gr.

gram, gramme. The basic unit of mass, and of weight, in the metric system; corresponds almost exactly to the weight of a milliliter, or cubic centimeter, of water at the temperature of maximum density. Abbreviated Gm., gm., g.

-gram, -gramme. A combining form meaning *something drawn,* or *written, a drawing* or *a writing.*

gram″i·ci′din (gram″i-sigh′din). A potent germ-killing chemical obtained from cultures of soil bacilli.

gram″i·ci′din S. A heat-stable antibiotic obtained from *Bacillus brevis* and reported to be more effective than gramicidin against Gram-negative organisms but not less toxic.

gram′-me·ter, gram-me′ter. A unit of work, equal to the energy used in raising one gram to a height of one meter.

gram′mole. See *gram molecule.*

gram mol′e·cule. That weight of any substance, in grams, equivalent to its molecular weight. Syn., *grammole, mol, mole.*

Gram'-neg'a·tive. Remaining unstained by the Gram method.

Gram'-pos'i·tive. Holding the dye after being stained by the Gram method.

gra'na. Minute disks of chlorophyll in the stroma of plants.

gra·na'tum. Pomegranate. The bark of the stem and root of *Punica granatum;* contains several alkaloids, notably pelletierine. Used as a taeniacide. See *pelletierine* tannate.

gran'di·ose. *In psychiatry,* characterized by a feeling of being important, wealthy, or influential, when there is no true basis for such feeling.

grand' mal' (grahn mahl'). A complete epileptic seizure; see under *epilepsy.*

gran'u·lar lids. Trachoma.

gran'u·la"ted lids. Lay term for chronic blepharitis.

gran"u·la'tion. 1. The tiny red granules which are grossly visible in the base of an ulcer; made up of loops of newly formed capillaries and fibroblasts. 2. The process of formation of granulation tissue in or around a focus of inflammation. 3. The formation of granules. —**gran'ulated,** *adj.* **arachnoidal granulations.** Prolongations of the arachnoid layer of the cerebral meninges through the dura mater into the superior sagittal sinus and into its tributary sinuses. Also called *arachnoid villi, Pacchionian bodies.* **exuberant g.** An excess of granulation tissue in the base of an ulcer or in a healing wound. Also called *fungous g., proud flesh.* **g. tissue.** The mixture of newly formed capillaries and fibroblasts in connection with inflammation, especially of exudative character, representing the early stages of healing. Followed by a growth into exudate or destroyed tissue, the process becomes one of organization. As it progresses to cicatrization by atrophy of blood vessels and maturation of connective tissue, inflammatory foci are cicatrized, or such foci or foreign bodies are encapsulated; on surfaces, especially serous, fibrous adhesions are formed; wounds are healed.

gran'ule. 1. A minute particle or mass. 2. A small, intracellular particle, usually staining selectively. 3. A small pill. —**granular,** *adj.* **acidophil granules.** Those staining with acid dyes, such as eosin. **azurophilic granules.** Fine granules that are blue-staining with a stain containing methylene azure; they are frequently, but inconstantly, present in the cytoplasm of lymphocytes and monocytes. **basophilic granules.** Those staining with basic dyes, espe-

cially those of the methylene blue series, or hematoxylin. **neutrophil granules.** Granules which take up simultaneously both a basic and an acid dye, assuming a combination tint **sulfur g.** A characteristic mass of hyphae found in cases of actinomycosis **zymogen granules.** Secretion antecedent granules in gland cells, particularly in the pancreatic acini and the chief cells of the stomach, which are precursors of the enzyme secretion

gran'u·lo·cyte". A mature granular leukocyte; a polymorphonuclear leukocyte, either eosinophilic, basophilic, or neutrophilic. Also called *polymorph polymorphonuclear, eosinophil, basophil, neutrophil.*

gran"u·lo·cy"to·pe'ni·a. Agranulocytosis.

gran"u·lo'ma. A focalized nodule of inflammatory tissue in which the process of granulation is significant —**granulom'atous,** *adj.* **g. inguinale.** A chronic, often serpiginous, destructive ulceration of external genitalia; due to *Donovania granulomatis.* It may extend to the groin perineum, and lower abdomen, and may be complicated by suppuration in inguinal lymph nodes (bubo). **g. venereum.** See venereal *lymphogranuloma* **infectious g.** A disease, due to a specific microörganism, which in some stage exhibits the formation of a granuloma, as tuberculosis, syphilis, or leprosy.

gran"u·lo"ma·to'sis. A disease characterized by multiple granulomas

graph. A representation of statistical data by means of points, lines, surfaces or solids, their position being determined by a system of coördinates.

-graph. A combining form meaning *a writing; an instrument that transcribes or transmits.* —**graph'ic,** *adj*

graph"es·the'si·a. The sense of sensation of recognizing numbers, figures, or letters which are traced on the skin.

-graph'i·a. A combining form meaning *writing characterized by a* (specified) *abnormality.*

graph'ite. Plumbago, or black lead an impure allotropic form of carbon.

grapho·o-. A combining form denoting *pertaining to writing.*

graph·ol'o·gy. The study of the handwriting; may be used in diagnos ing nervous disorders.

graph"o·ma'ni·a. An insane desir to write. —**graphomaniac,** *n.*

graph"o·mo'tor. Relating to graphic movements or to the move ments concerned in writing.

graph"o·pho'bi·a. A morbid fear of writing.

graph"or·rhe'a. *In psychiatry,* an uncontrollable desire to write, in which pages are covered with usually unconnected and meaningless words; an intermittent condition, most often seen in manic patients.

grat·tage′ (gra·tahzh′). Brushing, scrubbing, or scraping; a method sometimes used in treatment of trachoma. A hard brush, as a toothbrush, is used to scrub the conjunctival surface of the eyelid in order to remove the granulations.

grav′el. A granular, sandlike material forming the substance of urinary calculi and often passed with the urine.

grav′id. Pregnant; heavy with child, as the gravid uterus. Used also of other than human females when carrying young or eggs. —**gravid′ity**, n.

gra′vi·da. A pregnant woman.

grav″i·do·car′di·ac. Relating to cardiac disorders due to pregnancy.

gra·vim′e·ter. An instrument used in determining the specific gravity of a substance, especially a hydrometer, aerometer, or urinometer. —**gravimet′ric**, adj.; **gravim′etry**, n.

grav″i·ta′tion. The force by which bodies are drawn together.

grav′i·ty. The effect of the attraction of the earth upon matter. **specific g.** The measured mass of a substance compared with that of an equal volume of another taken as a standard. For gases, hydrogen or air may be the standard; for liquids and solids, distilled water at a specified temperature. Abbreviated, sp. g., sp. gr.

green blind′ness. Aglaucopsia; a variety of color blindness in which green is not distinguished.

gre·ga′ri·ous·ness. The herd instinct.

grin·de′li·a. The leaves and flowering tops of various *Grindelia* species used as a stimulating expectorant.

grip, grippe. Old term for influenza.

gripe. A lay term for colic, q.v.

groin. The depression between the abdomen and thigh. Also called *inguinal region*.

groove. An elongated depression. Also see *sulcus, furrow*. —**grooved**, adj. **alveolingual g.** One between the tongue and the lower jaw. **bicipital g.** The deep groove on the anterior surface of the humerus, separating the greater and lesser tuberosities and containing the long tendon of the biceps. **branchial g.** See visceral *g*. **carotid g.** A broad groove on the superior surface of the sphenoid bone, lodging the internal carotid artery and the cavernous sinus. **costal g.** A deep furrow lying along the lower border and inner surface of a rib, for lodgment of the intercostal vessels and nerve. **nasolacrimal g.** The groove or furrow between the embryonic maxil-

lary and lateral nasal processes, the epithelium of which is said to form part of the lacrimal duct. **ventricular grooves.** Two furrows, one on the anterior, one on the posterior surface of the heart; they indicate the interventricular septum. **vertebral g.** That formed by the laminas of the vertebrae and the sides of the spinous processes; it lodges the deep muscles of the back. **visceral g.** The external groove or furrow between two embryonic visceral arches, lined by ectoderm.

ground sub′stance. The fluid, semifluid, or solid material, in the connective tissues, cartilage, and bone, which fills part or all of the space between the cells and fibers. Syn., *matrix*, in the strict sense, see *matrix*, 3; *interstitial substance*.

growth. 1. The increase in the amount of actively metabolic protoplasm, accompanied by an increase in cell number, or cell size, or both. In a broader sense, growth is the increase in the size of the organism or its parts, measured as an increase in weight, volume, or linear dimensions. 2. Any abnormal, localized increase in cells, such as a tumor, a neoplasm.

grume. A clot, as of blood; a thick and viscid fluid. —**gru′mous**, adj.

gry·po′sis (grye·po′sis, gri·po′sis). Curvature; especially abnormal curvature of the nails.

gt. *Gutta*, drop.

gtt. *Guttae*, drops.

gua″cha·ma′ca (gwah″chuh·mah′kuh, gwah″chah·mah·kah′). The bark of *Malouetia nitida* (Apocynaceae), used as a source of a type of curare.

gua′cin (gwah′sin, gway′sin). A bitter resin from guaco.

gua′co (gwah′ko). The plants *Mikania guaco* and other species of *Mikania* and *Aristolochia*.

guai′ac (gwy′ack). The resin of the wood of *Guaiacum officinale* or of *G. sanctum*.

guai′a·col. A liquid consisting principally of $C_6H_4(OH)(OCH_3)$ 1:2, usually obtained from wood creosote; or a solid, consisting almost entirely of $C_6H_4(OH)(OCH_3)$ 1:2, usually prepared synthetically. **g. carbonate.** $CO(OC_6H_4·OCH_3)_2$. Occurs in crystals which are insoluble in water; it is used as an expectorant. See *duotal*.

gua′nase (gwah′nace, ·naze). An enzyme found in the pancreas, thymus, and adrenals; it converts guanine into xanthine.

guan′i·dine (gwan′i·deen, gwah′ni·). Aminomethanamidine, $NH:C(NH_2)_2$, a normal product of protein metabolism found in the urine. Syn., *carbamidine, iminourea*. See Table of

Normal Values of Blood Constituents in the Appendix.

gua'nine (gwah'neen, ·nin). 2-Amino-6-oxypurine, a leucomaine found in the pancreas, in liver, and in muscle extract as a decomposition product of nuclein. It also occurs in guano.

gua'no (gwah'no). The excrement of sea fowl found on certain islands in the Pacific Ocean. It contains guanine and various other nitrogen bases.

gua'no·sine (gwah'no·seen, gwan'o·). A nucleoside which contains pentose sugar and guanine.

gua·nyl'ic ac'id (gwa·nill'ick). A nucleotide obtained by the hydrolysis of nucleic acid.

gua"ra·na' (gwah"rah·nah', gwah·rah'nah). A dried paste prepared from the seeds of *Paullinia cupana*, found in Brazil. It contains caffeine.

guard. An appliance placed on a knife to prevent too deep an incision.

gu"ber·nac'u·lum. A guiding structure. **g. testis.** A fibrous cord extending from the fetal testis to the scrotal swellings; it occupies the potential inguinal canal and guides the testis in its descent. See *chorda gubernaculum.*

gum. The mucous membrane and underlying connective tissue covering the alveolar processes and the necks of erupted teeth; the gingiva, *q.v.* **spongy g.** Hyperplastic gingival tissue, associated with inflammation and other gingival swelling.

gum. A concrete vegetable juice exuded from many plants. The gums consist of glycosidal acids, partly or wholly combined with calcium, potassium, or magnesium. **acacia g.** Gum arabic. See *acacia.* **British g.** Dextrin. **g. arabic.** See *acacia.* **g. benjamin.** See *benzoin.* **g. resin.** A concrete vegetable juice insoluble in water, but soluble in organic solvents. **g. tragacanth.** See *tragacanth.*

gum'boil". See alveolar *abscess.*

gum'ma. The specific lesion of tertiary or late syphilis, which may occur in almost any tissue but is observed particularly in the brain, liver, and heart. Grossly, it is a well-defined mass a few millimeters to a centimeter or more in diameter, with a tendency to encapsulation and surrounding fibrosis, and with a gelatinous, hyalinized, necrotic center which has the elastic consistency of firm rubber or gum. Microscopically, the necrotic mass is surrounded by lymphocytes, epithelioid cells, and a few Langhans' giant cells. **—gummatous,** *adj.*

gum'mic ac'id. Arabin.

gun'cot·ton. Pyroxylin. **Syn.,** *soluble guncotton.*

gun'jah. See *cannabis.*

gus·ta'tion. The sense of taste; the act of tasting.

gus'ta·to"ry. Pertaining to the sense of taste.

gut. 1. The intestine. 2. The embryonic digestive tube, consisting of *fore-gut, midgut,* and *hindgut.* 3. Short term for catgut. Also see *suture.* **blind g.** The cecum. **postanal g.** A transient part of the hindgut caudal to the cloaca.

gut'ta (pl. *guttae*). A drop. Abbreviated, gt.

gut'tae (gut'ee). Plural of gutta, *q.v.* Abbreviated, gtt.

gut"ta-per'cha. The latex of various trees of the family Sapotaceae.

gut·ta'tim. Drop by drop.

gut'ter. 1. A shallow groove. 2. Shape bone to eliminate dead spaces in an operation for chronic osteomyelitis. **Syn.,** *saucerize.* **hepatic g.** The anlage of the liver and gallbladder. See hepatic *diverticulum.*

gut'ti·form. Drop-shaped.

gut"tu·ro·tet'a·ny. A stammering due to tetanoid spasm of the laryngeal muscles.

gu·va'cine (gew·vay'seen, guh·vay'·). Tetrahydronicotinic acid, an alkaloid from seeds of *Areca Catechu,* the areca nut or betelnut.

gym·nas'tics. Systematic exercise for restoring or maintaining bodily health. **—gymnastic,** *adj.* **medical g.** Systematic muscular movements designed to bring an ailing or feeble part back to normal. **ocular g.** Regular muscular exercise of the eye by the use of prisms or other means to overcome muscular insufficiency. **Swedish g.** A system of movements made by the patient against the resistance of an attendant.

gym·ne'mic ac'id (jim·nee'mick, ·nem'ick). $C_{32}H_{55}O_{18}$. A substance obtained from the leaves of *Gymnema sylvestre.*

gym"no·pho'bi·a. A morbid fear of a naked person or a naked part of the body.

gyn'ae- (jin'i-, jy'ni-). For words beginning with *gynae-,* see under *gyne-.*

gy·nan"dro·mor'phism. An abnormality in which the individual contains both genetically male and genetically female tissue.

gyn"a·tre'si·a (jin"uh·tree'zhuh, ·shuh). Imperforation of the vagina.

gy·ne'cic, gy·nae'cic (ji·nee'sick, ·ness'ick). Relating to women or the female sex.

gyn"e·co·gen'ic (jin"i·ko·jen'ick, guy"ni·ko·). Causing or producing female characteristics; estrogenic.

gyn"e·coid (jin'i·koyd, jy'ni·, jin"i·koyd'). Resembling or like a woman.

gyn"e·col'o·gist (jin"i·kol'o·jist,

guy″ni·, jy″ni·). One who practices gynecology.

gyn″e·col′o·gy (jin″i·kol′o·jee, guy″ni·, jy″ni·). The science of the diseases of women, especially those affecting the sexual organs. —**gyne·colog′ic, gynecolog′ical,** adj.

gyn″e·co·mas′ti·a. Enlargement of the mammary gland in the male, more frequently unilateral. Microscopically, there is multiplication of ducts and proliferation of lining epithelium; increase in amount of supporting connective tissue; infiltration of lymphocytes, plasma cells, large mononuclear cells, and, sometimes, polymorphonuclear leukocytes and eosinophils. The condition may accompany outspoken endocrine disorders, especially of the adrenals and of the testes, and neoplasms such as choriocarcinoma; may follow administration of estrogenic substances; or may have no apparent cause, appearing often in adolescence. **Anisogynecomastia** is unequal enlargement of the breasts. **Pseudogynecomastia** is enlargement of the breasts due to deposition of adipose tissue. Also called *gynecomazia, gynecomasty.*

gyn″e·cop′a·thy (jin″i·kop′uth·ee, guy″ni·, jy″ni·). Any disease of, or peculiar to, women.

gyn″e·pho′bi·a (jin″i·fo′bee·uh, jy″ni·). Morbid fear of the society of women.

gyn″e·phor′ic. Pertaining to a mode of inheritance in which phenotypically normal heterozygous women transmit the recessive gene to some of their sons, as in sex-linked recessive characters (e.g., hemophilia).

Gynergen. Trade-mark for ergotamine tartrate.

gyn″i·at′rics (jin″ee·at′ricks, ·ay′tricks, jy″nee·). Treatment of the diseases of women.

gyn′o- (jin′o-, jy′no-), **gyn-.** 1. A combining form denoting *woman.* 2. *In botany and medicine,* a combining form denoting a *female reproductive organ.*

gyn″o·car′dic ac′id. An acid from the oil of *Gynocardia odorata.*

gyn″o·plas·ty, gyn″o·plas′ty. Plastic surgery of the female genitals. —**gynoplas′tic,** adj.

gyp′sum. $CaSO_4.2H_2O$. Native calcium sulfate.

gy·ra′tion (jye·ray′shun). 1. A turning in a circle. 2. Old term for arrangement of gyri in the cerebral hemisphere. —**gy′rate,** adj.

gy′ro·mele. A probe with a rotating center, fitted with various attachments for treating the stomach. *Obs.*

gy′rose. Marked with curved or undulating lines.

gy′rus (pl. *gyri*). A convolution on the surface of the cerebral hemisphere. —**gyral,** adj. **angular g.** A cerebral convolution which forms the posterior portion of the inferior parietal lobule and arches over the posterior end of the superior temporal sulcus. **ascending frontal g.** The cerebral convolution which lies between the precentral sulcus and the central sulcus and extends from the superomedial border of the hemisphere to the posterior ramus of the lateral fissure. Syn., *g. centralis anterior, precentral g., anterior central g.* **ascending parietal g.** The cerebral convolution which lies immediately posterior to the central sulcus and extends from the longitudinal fissure above to the posterior ramus of the lateral fissure below. Syn., *posterior central g., postcentral g., g. centralis posterior.* **g. of Broca.** The left inferior frontal gyrus; location of Broca's center for articulate speech. **Heschl's gyri.** Two or three gyri which cross the upper surface of the temporal lobe transversely. Syn., *transverse temporal gyri.* **inferior frontal g.** The most inferior of the three frontal convolutions, situated in relation to the horizontal and ascending branches of the Sylvian fissure. Also called *g. frontalis inferior.* **superior frontal g.** A convolution of the frontal lobe situated between the dorsal margin of the hemisphere and the superior frontal sulcus, immediately above the middle frontal gyrus. Also called *g. frontalis superior.* **superior temporal g.** A convolution of the temporal lobe lying between the lateral cerebral fissure and superior temporal sulcus. **supramarginal g.** A cerebral convolution which forms the anterior portion of the inferior parietal lobule and arches over the upturned end of the lateral cerebral fissure. **transverse temporal gyri.** Two or three gyri which cross the upper surface of the superior temporal gyrus transversely. Syn., *Heschl's gyri.* **uncinate g.** The recurved, hook-like end of the hippocampal gyrus. Also called *g. uncinatus, uncus.*

H

H. 1. Chemical symbol for hydrogen. 2. Abbreviation for hypermetropia.

h. *Hora*, hour; height; hundred.

h. Symbol for quantum constant.

H⁺ Symbol for hydrogen ion.

H¹ Symbol for protium.

H², H^D Symbol for deuterium.

H³ Symbol for tritium.

ha·be'na. Old term for frenum or bandage. —**habenar,** *adj.*

ha·ben'u·la. 1. The stalk of the pineal body, attaching it to the thalamus. 2. A ribbonlike structure. —**habenular,** *adj.*

hab'it. 1. A behavior pattern fixed by repetition. 2. The body build, as associated with a disease or a predisposition thereto; as an **apoplectic habit,** said of a stocky, thick-necked, plethoric individual, presumably liable to apoplexy. Syn., *habitus.*

hab'i·tat. The natural home of an animal or vegetable species.

ha·bit"u·a'tion. 1. A condition of tolerance to the effects of a drug or a poison, acquired by its continued use; marked by a psychic or emotional craving for it when the drug is withdrawn. 2. Drug addiction, especially a mild form in which withdrawal does not result in severe abstinence symptoms.

hab'i·tus. See *habit.*

hack'ing. Form of massage consisting of a succession of chopping strokes with the edge of the extended fingers or with the whole hand.

hack'ing cough. Lay term for a short, dry cough.

ha"de·pho'bi·a. A morbid fear of hell.

hae-. For words beginning with *hae-* not found here, see under *he-.*

Hae·man'thus (hi·manth'us). Bloodlily. A genus of the Amaryllidaceae.

Haem"a·to·ther'ma (hem"uh·to·thur'muh, hee"muh·to·). The warmblooded vertebrates: birds and mammals.

Hae"mo·spo·rid'i·a (hee"mo·spo·rid'ee·uh). An order of microörganisms of the class Sporozoa that live for a part of their life cycle within the red blood cells of their host.

Haenel's variant. Progressive muscular atrophy affecting only the upper extremities.

haf'ni·um (haf'nee·um, hahf'nee·um). Hf = 178.6. A rare earth element.

Hah'ne·mann·ism. See under *homeopathy.*

hair. A keratinized filament growing from the skin of mammals; collectively, all the filaments covering the skin.

Hair is a modified epidermal structure, consisting of a *shaft,* which is the hair itself, exclusive of its sheaths and papilla, and a *root.* The root is found in the **hair follicle,** a depression in the corium and subcutaneous connective tissue, and is expanded at its lower end into the **hair bulb.** This caps the **hair papilla,** a portion of the corium which projects upward into the center of the bulb. The epithelial parts of a hair and its sheaths are developed from the **hair column,** an epithelial ingrowth. The space in this hair column through which the developing hair shaft grows toward the surface is known as the **hair canal.**

hal'a·kone. A small cone of stiffened gauze, designed to fit the nostril; it is filled loosely with absorbent material which may be medicated, and through which inhaled air must pass.

ha·la'tion. Blurring of the visual image under a powerful direct light coming from a direction different from the line of vision.

halazone. p-Sulfonedichloramidobenzoic acid, a white, crystalline powder sparingly soluble in water; it sterilizes water.

Haldane scale. A standard for establishing hemoglobin levels in which 13.8 Gm. in 100 cc. of blood equals 100 per cent.

half-life. The time during which half of any given amount of a radioactive substance will have undergone transmutation; a constant for any given radioactive isotope.

hal'i·but liv'er oil. The fixed oil from the livers of *Hippoglossus hippoglossus;* contains vitamins A and D.

hal'ide. A binary salt in which a halogen serves as anion.

ha·lis"ter·e'sis. The loss of lime salts from previously well-calcified bone. —**halisteret'ic,** *adj.*

hal'ite. Rock salt; a native sodium chloride occurring in extensive deposits.

hal'i·to'sis. The state of having offensive breath. Syn., *bromopnea, fetor ex ore.*

hal'i·tus. A vapor, as that expired from the lung.

hal·la·chrome. A quinone intermediate in a postulated mechanism of the conversion of tyrosine to melanin.

hal·lu"ci·na'tion. A false sense perception; perception of objects which have no reality and sensations which have no external cause.

hal·lu"ci·no·gen'ic. Designating a

310

drug or agent capable of producing *hallucinations.* **—hallucinogenic,** n.

hal·lu"ci·no'sis. *In psychiatry,* the condition of being possessed by more or less persistent hallucinations.

hal'lux (pl. *halluxes*). The great toe. **—hallucal,** *adj.* **h. flexus.** A condition allied to and perhaps identical with hammertoe, or flexion of the first phalanx of the great toe. The second phalanx is usually extended upon the first, and there is more or less rigidity of the metatarsophalangeal joint. **h. valgus.** Displacement of the great toe toward the other toes. **h. varus.** Displacement of the great toe away from the other toes.

hal"ma·to·gen'e·sis. A sudden change of type from one generation to another.

hal'o-. 1. A combining form denoting *the sea, salt.* 2. *In chemistry,* a combining form signifying *of* or *pertaining to a salt* or denoting *the presence of a halogen.*

hal'o·gen. Any one of the nonmetallic elements chlorine, iodine, bromine, and fluorine.

hal'oid. Resembling, or derived from, a halogen.

halotestin. Trade-mark for fluoxymesterone.

ham. 1. The posterior portion of the thigh above the popliteal space and below the buttock. 2. The popliteal space. 3. Colloquial term for the buttock, hip, and thigh.

Ham"a·me'lis. A genus of small trees or shrubs. **H. virginiana.** The witch hazel.

ha·mar'ti·a. A nodular or localized fault of embryonal development; cells and structures natural to the part are not in normal orderly arrangement, giving rise to a hamartoma. **—hamartial,** *adj.*

ham·ar"to·blas·to'ma. A neoplasm arising from a hamartoma, *q.v.*

ham"ar·to'ma. A nodular or tumorlike mass resulting from faulty embryonal development of cells and tissues natural to the part, as exemplified in vascular birthmarks (angiomas) and nevi. Not true neoplasms but may undergo neoplastic transformation.

ham"ar·to·pho'bi·a. A morbid fear of error or sin.

ha·ma'tum. The hamate bone; the most ulnar of the distal row of carpal bones. Formerly called *unciform bone.* See Table of Bones in the Appendix.

ham'mer. 1. *In anatomy,* the malleus. See Table of Bones in the Appendix. 2. An instrument for striking. **percussion h.** A small hammer with a rubber head; used to tap the surface of the body to elicit sounds of diagnostic value. Syn., *plexor.* **reflex h.** One

used to elicit reflexes by tapping on muscles, nerves, and tendons.

ham'mer·toe". A condition of the toe, usually the second, in which the proximal phalanx is extremely extended while the two distal phalanges are flexed.

ham'ster. A short-tailed rodent with large cheek pouches, belonging to the family Cricetidae. Found in Europe, western Asia, and Africa. It is susceptible to a variety of microörganisms, and is used for laboratory purposes.

ham'string". 1. One of the tendons bounding the ham on the outer and inner side. See Table of Muscles in the Appendix. 2. Cripple by cutting the hamstring tendons. **inner h.** The tendons of the semimembranosus and semitendinosus muscles. **outer h.** The tendon of the biceps femoris muscle.

ham'u·lus. A hook-shaped process, as of the hamate bone or of the medial lamina of the pterygoid process of the sphenoid bone. **—hamular, hamulate,** *adj.*

hand. The organ of prehension; composed of the carpus, metacarpus, and phalanges. **accoucheur's h.** A characteristic cone-shaped deformity of the hand; seen in tetany with carpal spasm and muscular dystrophy. Also called *obstetrician's h.* **ape h.** An unusual shape of the hand, resembling that of apes; caused by wasting thumb muscles, as in progressive muscular atrophy. **battledore h.** The large hand seen in acromegaly. **claw h.** A deformity resulting from paralysis of the ulnar and/or median nerve. **cleft h.** A congenital deformity of the hand in which the cleft between adjacent fingers extends into the metacarpal region. **forceps h.** One which has lost the three middle fingers. **ghoul h.** A slowly developing condition of the hand in which the skin of the palm is depigmented except for scattered areas of hyperpigmentation, and is thickened, dry, and taut. It is due probably to tertiary yaws. **trailing h.** In synchronous writing of both hands, that upon which the attention, visual or central, is not fixed.

hand'ed·ness. The tendency to use the right or left hand, according to preference or habit.

hang'nail". A partly detached piece of skin of the nail fold, friction against which has caused inflammation.

hap"a·lo·nych'i·a (hap"uh·lo-nick'ee·uh). A condition in which the nails are soft, may fold, and split easily. They become atrophied due to defective nail production.

hapamine. Trade-mark for a product made from histamine and despeciated horse serum globulin; used subcutaneously in allergic conditions.

haph″al·ge′si·a (haf″al·jee′zee·uh, ·see·uh). A sensation of pain experienced upon the mere touching of an object.

haph″e·pho′bi·a. A morbid fear of being touched.

hap′lo-, hapl-. A combining form signifying *single, simple.*

hap′loid. Having the reduced number of chromosomes, as in mature germ cells, as distinguished from the diploid or full number of chromosomes in normal somatic cells.

ha·plo′pi·a. Single vision, as opposed to *diplopia.*

hap′lo·scope. An instrument for measuring the visual axes.

hap′ten, hap′tene. A partial antigen which reacts with a specific antibody in vitro only; when combined with a protein it may behave as a true antigen.

hap′tene. See *hapten.*

hap″te·pho′bi·a. Morbid fear of being touched.

hap′tics. The branch of psychology dealing with the tactile sense. —**hap′tic,** *adj.*

hap″to·dys·pho′ri·a. The disagreeable sensation aroused by touching certain objects, as velvet, a peach, or a russet apple.

hare′lip″. A cleft, or clefts, in the upper lip, so called from its resemblance to a hare's lip. **acquired h.** A cleft in the lip, due to accidental means, giving the same appearance as congenital harelip. **congenital h.** Congenital fissure of the upper lip, due to failure of fusion of embryonic facial processes, often associated with cleft palate, *q.v.* The fissure may be of varying degrees, from a notch at the vermilion border to complete separation between the median nasal process and the maxillary process, the cleft extending into the nostril. **double h.** One in which there is a cleft on both sides of the upper lip. Also called *bilateral h.* **single h.** One in which the cleft occurs on one side only. Also called *unilateral h.*

har′ma·line (hahr′muh·leen, ·lin). An alkaloid in wild rue, *Peganum harmala.*

har′mine (hahr′meen, ·min). An alkaloid from wild rue; chemically identical with banisterine from *Banisteria caapi.*

harmonyl. Trade-mark for deserpidine.

har′mo·sones, har′mo·zones. Name applied by Gley to a class of hormones which influence growth.

har″pax·o·pho′bi·a. Morbid fear of robbers.

Harrison Act. The federal law regulating the possession, sale, purchase, and prescription of habit-forming drugs.

harts′horn″. 1. Cornu cervi, the horn of a stag; formerly a source of ammonia, or hartshorn spirit. 2. A name popularly given to ammonia water, and sometimes applied to ammonium carbonate.

Harvey, William [*English physiologist,* 1578–1657]. Discovered the mechanism of the circulation of the blood; his *Exercitatio de Motu Cordis et Sanguinis in Animalibus* (*Essay on the Motion of the Heart and Blood in Animals,* 1628) has been called the most important book in the history of medicine. Also made an important study of generation.

hash′ish (hash′eesh, ·ish), **hash′eesh.** See *cannabis.*

Hassall's body. See thymic *corpuscle.*

Hass̲l's corpuscle. See thymic *corpuscle.*

Hau·dek, Martin [*Austrian roentgenologist,* 1880–1931]. Drew attention to the characteristic niche of gastric ulcer (1910); called *Haudek's niche.*

haunch. Colloquial term for the part of the body which includes the hips and the buttocks.

haus′trum (haw′strum) (pl. *haustra*). One of the pouches or sacculations of the colon. —**haustral,** *adj.*

hawk. Clear the throat by a forcible expiration.

hay fe′ver. An acute affection of the conjunctiva and upper air passages; due to a sensitivity to pollen. In common usage, the term refers to that produced by ragweed or biologically related pollens. May be caused by other allergens, as tree and flower pollens and atmospheric molds. That caused by grass pollen is known as *rose fever.* In a small percentage of cases, the etiologic factor is undetermined. Chief symptoms are coryza, sneezing, rhinorrhea, headache, and intense itching of the eyes and upper air passages. Syn., *allergic rhinitis.*

hb. Hemoglobin.

h. d. *Hora decubitus,* at the hour of going to bed.

He. Chemical symbol for helium.

head. 1. The uppermost part of the body, containing the brain, organs of sight, smell, taste, hearing, and part of the organs of speech. 2. The top, beginning, or most prominent part of anything. **aftercoming h.** The head of the fetus in a breech presentation. **floating h.** A freely movable fetal head above the pelvic brim. **h. locking.** The entanglement of the heads of twins at the time of birth. **scald h.** Any crusting disease of the scalp. *Colloquial.*

head′ache″. Pain in the head. Syn.,

cephalalgia. **bilious h.** Migraine. **blind h.** Migraine. **cyclic h.** That associated with menstruation. **histamine h.** A type of headache considered to be due to dilatation of the carotid vascular tree as the result of action by circulating histamine. It is characterized by abrupt onset, pain in the temple, neck, face, and the eye, lacrimation and congestion of the eye, stuffiness of the nostril, and swelling of the temporal vessels. **migrainous h.** The headache of migraine, *q.v.* **ocular h.** Pain in and about the head that results from organic disease or impaired function of the eyes. **posttraumatic h.** The persistent and recurrent headache which often follows head injury. **puncture h.** Headache following spinal puncture and removal of the cerebrospinal fluid. **sick h.** Migraine. **vascular dilatation h.** Headache associated with or due to dilatation of intracranial arteries.

head'band". A strap for securing a mirror to the forehead.

heal'er. 1. One who effects cures. 2. Colloquial term for a Christian Science practitioner. 3. One without formal medical education who claims to cure by some form of suggestion. **natural h.** One supposed to possess personal magnetism capable of overcoming disease.

heal'ing. The process or act of getting well or of making whole; the restoration to normal, as in the closure of an ulcer or a wound, or the union of a broken bone. **—heal,** *v.t., v.i.* **h. by first intention.** The primary union of a wound when the incised skin edges are approximated and so held that union takes place without the process of granulation. **h. by second intention.** The process of wound closure where the edges remain separated; the wound becomes closed after granulation tissue has filled the cavity to the skin level so that epithelium can grow over the unhealed area. **mental h.** Psychotherapy. Also called **spiritual h.**

health. That condition of bodily soundness in which the functions are performed normally; a state of well being and freedom from disease. **—health'y,** *adj.* **public h.** The state of health of a population, as that of a state, nation, or a particular community.

health cer·tif'i·cate. A formal or official document signed by a physician, attesting to the state of health of the individual named therein.

health of'fi·cer. A quarantine officer or an officer of a board of health; an officer of sanitation.

health phys'ics. The branch of radiology dealing with protection from harmful effects of radiation.

health so·ci'e·ty. An association which has for its objective the promotion of some phase of public health.

hear. Perceive by the ear.

hear'ing. The special sense by which the sonorous vibrations of the air are communicated to the mind. **residual h.** In the measurement of hearing loss, the amount of hearing that a person retains irrespective of temporary reductions. **visual h.** The understanding of speech by means of visual impulses. Also called *lip reading.*

hear'ing aid. An instrument that amplifies the intensity of sound waves for the benefit of those with impaired hearing. **air conduction h. a.** An electric hearing aid, the transmitter of which fits into the ear canal. **bone conduction h. a.** An electric hearing aid, the transmitter of which is held against the skin over the mastoid process. **carbon h. a.** An electric hearing aid of the carbon granule transmitter type, as the telephone. **electric h. a.** One getting its source of power from electricity. **fixed h. a.** One that is permanently installed, as in a church, school, or theater. **mechanical h. a.** One that amplifies the intensity of sound waves by some physical means other than electricity. **portable h. a.** An electric hearing aid that can be carried with relative ease. **vacuum h. a.** An electric hearing aid of the vacuum tube type, as a radio. **wearable h. a.** One that can be worn on the person.

heart. A hollow, muscular organ, whose function is to pump the blood through the vessels. It is enveloped by the pericardium and consists of two symmetrical halves, a right atrium and ventricle and a left atrium and ventricle. The right atrioventricular orifice is guarded by the tricuspid valve; the left, by a valve with two leaflets, the mitral. These valves are broad and thin and consist of two layers of the lining membrane of the heart, the endocardium, separated by a slight amount of connective tissue. To support them, thin chordae tendineae join their free margins to the papillary muscles in the wall of the ventricle. The outlet of the right ventricle into the pulmonary artery, and that of the left into the aorta, are guarded by the semilunar valves. **armored h.** The chalky deposits on the pericardium, due to chronic inflammation. **athletic h.** Generalized enlargement of the heart without disease of the valves, supposedly the result of excessive participation in sports. **boatshaped h.** That caused by aortic disease. **bony h.**

One with calcareous patches on its walls. **bovine h.** The markedly hypertrophied heart which develops as a result of aortic valvular disease. Also called *cor bovinum.* **fatty h.** A name given to two distinct pathologic conditions of the heart tissue. In the first, there is a true fatty degeneration of the cardiac muscular fibers; in the second, there is an increase in the quantity of subpericardial and intramyocardial fat, which is true fat infiltration. **fibroid h.** Extensive fibrosis of myocardium, the fibrous tissue replacing numerous foci of necrosis. **glycogenic h.** Deposits of glycogen in the heart muscles and consequent hypertrophy. **goiter h.** A condition characterized by atrial fibrillation, cardiac enlargement, and congestive cardiac failure; due to thyrotoxicosis. Also called *thyroid h., thyrotoxic h.* **hairy h.** The peculiar, shaggy appearance of the heart in acute fibrinous pericarditis, the deposited fibrin existing in long shreds. Also called *cor villosum, shaggy h.* **h. clot.** Coagulation of blood in the cardiac cavity. **h. disease.** The extrinsic form is caused by compression, angulation, and torsion of the heart, or by abnormally high pressure in either the systemic or pulmonary circulation; the intrinsic form by disease of the heart muscle, valves, or coronary arteries. **h. sac.** The pericardium. **icing h.** One whose entire surface is covered with a dense, thick, marble-white tissue. **irritable h.** Neurocirculatory asthenia, *q.v.* **kyphotic h.** Pulmono-cardiac strain and failure due to deformities of the thorax or spine. **left h.** The part which furnishes blood to the systemic and coronary vessels. **peripheral h.** An obsolete term for muscular coat of the blood vessels. **pulmonary h.** The effect of pulmonary hypertension on the right ventricle; caused by dilatation and failure of the left ventricle, mitral valve disease, massive pulmonary embolism, chronic pulmonary disease, severe chest deformity, or primary disease of the pulmonary arteries. It is acute or chronic. Also called *cor pulmonale.* **right h.** The part which furnishes blood to the lungs. **skin h.** The peripheral blood vessels. **soldier's h.** Neurocirculatory asthenia, *q.v.* **tobacco h.** A condition which is characterized by irregular action and palpitation; produced by excessive indulgence in tobacco.

heart block. The cardiac mechanism resulting from defective transmission of impulses from atrium to ventricle. The first stage is that in which the P-R interval is prolonged; in the second stage, beats are dropped; in the third

stage, the ventricular contractions are independent of the atrial. **arborization h. b.** Heart block occurring in fibers of the Purkinje system. Also called *intraventricular h. b.* **atrioventricular h. b.** That in which the impulses are blocked in the A-V node or bundle of His. May be of any stage. **bundle-branch h. b.** The blocking which occurs in one or the other branch of the bundle of His, resulting in a difference in contraction time of the two ventricles. **complete h. b.** The third stage of block, when the ventricles assume their own rhythm, about 30–40 beats per minute. **congenital h. b.** That due to defective development of the conduction system. **entrance h. b.** A term used in electrocardiography to describe the condition in which the automatic center in the ventricle is constantly operating and is not disturbed by outside stimuli. Also called *protective h. b.* **exit h. b.** A term used in electrocardiography to describe the condition in which there is a local region of abnormal unidirectional block, which prevents some of the impulses generated by an ectopic pacemaker from passing on to the rest of the heart. **incomplete h. b.** The first stage of blocking, in which the conduction time is prolonged, recognized only by the electrocardiograph. **intratrial h. b.** A type which shows on the electrocardiographic record a broad, notched P wave of longer than normal duration. **intraventricular h. b.** Arborization heart block, *q.v.* **partial h. b.** The second stage of blocking, in which beats are dropped, giving a 2: 1, 3: 1, 4: 1, etc., A-V ratio. **protective h. b.** Entrance heart block, *q.v.* **sinoatrial h. b.** A type in which the impulses originating in the sinoatrial node are partially or completely prevented from leaving it. **unidirectional h. b.** A type in which the impulses will pass out of, but not into, the area of block.

heart′burn″. A burning sensation over the precordium or beneath the sternum; usually related to esophageal spasm. Gastric pyrosis.

heart fail′ure. See *cardiac failure, circulatory failure.*

heart mur′mur. An adventitious sound heard over the heart and sometimes transmitted to areas not directly over the cardiac dullness. These sounds are described according to intensity, pitch, quality, duration, and time of their occurrence in the cardiac cycle. Also see under cardiac *murmur.*

heart rate. The number of heart beats per minute.

heart sounds. Those heard on auscultation over the heart. The first sound is deeper in pitch and longer than the second, and is attributed to ventricular systole and the closure of the A-V valves. The second sound is higher pitched, short, and of snapping quality, and is attributed to closure of the semilunar valves. Heart sounds are described according to intensity, quality, duration, and time. Occasionally a faint third sound is heard, which is supposedly due to ventricular filling.

heat. 1. A form of kinetic energy communicable from one body to another by conduction, convection, or radiation; it is that form of molecular motion which is appreciated by a special thermal sense. **2.** The periodic sexual excitement in animals. **atomic h.** The specific heat of an atom of an element multiplied by its atomic weight. **h. capacity.** The specific heat of a substance multiplied by its mass. **latent h.** The quantity of heat necessary to convert a body into another state without changing its temperature. **mechanical equivalent of h.** The mechanical energy which is required to produce a given amount of heat. One calorie is equivalent to 426.5 gram-meters, or 3.085 foot-pounds, of work. **molecular h.** The molecular weight of a compound multiplied by its specific heat. **prickly h.** See *miliaria*. **specific h.** The amount of heat required to raise the temperature of 1 Gm. of a substance 1° C.

heat pros·tra'tion. A syndrome resulting from exposure to high temperatures, seen most frequently in infants and the aged; characterized by a moist, cold skin, poor circulation, a normal mouth and elevated rectal temperature, restlessness, and anxiety. Also called *heat exhaustion*.

he″be·phre'ni·a (hee″bi·free'nee-ah, heb″i·). A type of schizophrenia, often occurring in young persons at or soon after the age of puberty. Consists of a regression to an infantile and primitive behavior and ideation. Characterized by silliness, unexplained laughter and smiling, masturbation, hallucinosis, seclusiveness, and untidiness. **—hebephren'ic,** *adj*.

Heberden, William (Senior) [English physician, 1710–1801]. First to distinguish between chickenpox and smallpox (1767). Accurately described angina pectoris, so named by him (1768), and once called *Heberden's asthma*, *Rougnon-Heberden disease*. Described a degenerative disease producing nodular enlargement about the terminal joints of the fingers; called *Heberden's arthritis*, *Heberden's disease*, *Rosenbach's disease*. The swellings are called *Heberden's nodes*.

he·bet'ic. Relating to, or occurring at, puberty or adolescence.

heb'e·tude. Dullness of the special senses and intellect. **—hebetu'dinous,** *adj*.

hec'tic. 1. Habitual. **2.** Pertaining to or having hectic fever; consumptive. **3.** Hectic fever; one suffering from hectic fever. **4.** A hectic flush.

hec'to-, hect-. A combining form signifying *one hundred*.

hec'to·gram. One hundred grams. Abbreviated, hg.

hec'to·li″ter (heck'to·lee″tur). One hundred liters. Abbreviated, hl.

hec'to·me″ter. One hundred meters. Abbreviated, hm.

he″de·o'ma (hee″dee·o'muh, hed″-ee·). American pennyroyal. The leaves and tops of *Hedeoma pulegioides*.

he·do'ni·a. Abnormal cheerfulness; amenomania.

he'don·ism (hee'dun·iz·um, hed'un-iz·um). The pursuit of pleasure; the belief that acts should be directed toward the attainment of pleasure. Consequently, an unreasoning emphasis on pleasure or on some hobby or whim.

he″do·no·pho'bi·a. A morbid fear of pleasure.

heel. The hinder part of the foot. **big h.** Epidemic enlargement of the calcaneus, a disease found on the west coast of Africa, on the coast of China, and notably in Formosa. It is marked by fever, pain, and enlargement of the heel. There are frequent remissions followed by recurrence. The etiology is unknown. **painful h.** Tenderness of the heel, causing severe pain on walking; usually due to gonococcal infection or to bony spurs.

Hegar, Alfred [German gynecologist, 1830–1914]. Devised an operation for lacerated perineum: a triangular excision is made in the posterior wall of the vagina, and the muscles and fascia are sutured in the midline. Invented metal dilators in graduated sizes for stretching the cervix of the uterus; called *Hegar's dilators*. Softening of the lower segment of the uterus is called *Hegar's sign* of pregnancy in the early stages.

he·gem'o·ny. Leadership, domination; as the supremacy of one function over a number of others.

hel'co-, helc-. A combining form meaning *an ulcer*.

hel'coid, hel·cot'ic. Resembling an ulcer; ulcerative.

he·len'a·lin. A toxic principle from *Helenium autumnale* or wild sunflower.

hel'e·nin. A stearoptene from *Inula helenium*. Syn., *alantolactone*.

he″li·an'thin, he″li·an'thine (hee″lee·an'thin, ·theen). Methyl orange, an acid-base indicator.

he″li·an'thine. See *helianthin*.

hel'i·cine (hell'i·sin, ·syne). **1.** Ascendingly spiral. 2. Pertaining to the helix.

hel'i·co-, helic-. A combining form meaning *spiral.*

hel''i·co·pod, hel''i·co·po'di·a. Circumduction; movement of the leg in a lateral arc as it scrapes the floor; the gait seen in spastic hemiplegia.

hel''i·co·tre'ma. The opening connecting the scalae tympani and vestibuli of the spiral canal of the cochlea.

he''li·en·ceph''a·li'tis. Encephalitis caused by exposure to the sun's rays.

he'li·o-, heli-. A combining form signifying *the sun.*

he'li·o·phobe''. One who is morbidly sensitive to the effects of the sun's rays.

he'li·o·stat''. A mirror moved by clockwork in such a manner as to reflect the sun's rays continuously on a given spot. **—heliostat'ic,** *adj.*

he''li·o·tax'is. A form of taxis in which there is attraction toward (**positive heliotaxis**) or repulsion from (**negative heliotaxis**) the sun or sunlight.

he''li·o·ther'a·py. The treatment of disease by exposure of the body to sunlight.

he''li·ot'ro·pism. In biology, that property of a plant or plant organ by virtue of which it bends toward or away from the sunlight. **—heliotrop'ic,** *adj.*

he'li·um. He = 4.003. A chemically inert, colorless, odorless, gaseous element, occurring in certain natural gases and in small amount in the atmosphere.

he'lix. The rounded, convex margin of the pinna of the ear.

hel'le·bore. A plant of the genus *Helleborus,* particularly *H. niger,* black hellebore. **American h.** *Veratrum viride.* **green h.** *Veratrum viride.*

hel''le·bo're·in. A poisonous glycoside from *Helleborus niger* and *H. viridis.*

hel·leb'o·rin (heh-leb'o-rin, hell'l-bor-in). A poisonous glycoside from *Helleborus niger* and *H. viridis.*

hel'le·brin. A glycoside from *Helleborus niger.*

Hellin's law. Twins occur in one of 80 pregnancies; triplets in one of 80², or 6,400; quadruplets in one of 80³, or 512,000. A recent modification of this law states that, in the U.S.A., twins are to be expected in one of 88 pregnancies, triplets in one of 88³, and quadruplets in one of 88³ (Patten).

hel'minth. Originally any parasitic worm; now includes those wormlike animals, either parasitic or free-living, of the phyla Platyhelminthes and Nemathelminthes as well as members of the phylum Annelida. **—helmin'-**

thic, helmin'thous, helmin'thoid, *adj.*

hel''min·them'e·sis. The vomiting of parasitic worms.

hel''min·thi'a·sis. The diseased condition produced by the presence of parasitic worms in the body. **h. elas'tica.** Elastic tumors of the axilla and groin due to filarial worms.

hel'minth·ism. Helminthiasis, *q.*

hel'min·tho-, helminth-. A combining form signifying *worm.*

hel''min·thol'o·gy. The study of parasitic worms. **—helmintholog'ic,** *adj.*

hel''min·tho'ma. A tumor caused by the presence of a parasitic worm.

hel·min''tho·pho'bi·a. A morbid fear of worms or of becoming infested with worms.

he'lo-. A combining form meaning *marsh.*

he'lo-. A combining form meaning *nail.*

he·lot'o·my. The cutting of a corn; surgery upon a corn.

hel·vol'ic ac'id. An antibiotic substance, now known to be identical with fumigacin.

hem-, haem-. See *hemo-.*

he'ma-, hae'ma- (hee'muh-, hem'uh-). For words beginning with *hema* or *haema-* not found here, see under *hemo-.*

he'ma·chrome, hae'ma·chrome. The coloring matter of the blood, heme.

he''ma·dy·nam'ics, hae''ma·dy·nam'ics (hee''muh·dye·nam'icks). See *hemodynamics.*

he''ma·dy''na·mom'e·ter, hae''ma·dy''na·mom'e·ter. An instrument for measuring the pressure of the blood within the arteries. **—hemadynamometry,** *n.*

he''mag·glu''ti·na'tion, hae''mag·glu''ti·na'tion. The clumping of red blood cells.

he''mag·glu'ti·nin, hae''mag·glu'ti·nin (hee''muh·glue'ti·nin, hem''uh·). A substance in normal blood serum which has the power to clump red blood cells.

he'mal, hae'mal. 1. Pertaining to the blood or the vascular system. Pertaining to that part of the body containing the heart and major blood vessels; ventral to the vertebral bodies.

he''ma·nal'y·sis. Analysis of the blood.

he·man''gi·ec'ta·sis, he·man''gi·ec·ta'si·a (hee·man''jee·eck·tay'zhuh, hem·an''·). Dilatation of blood vessels. **—hemangiectat'ic,** *adj.*

he·man''gi·o·blas·to'ma. An aggregation of blood vessels comprising a neoplastic disorder rather than a hamartoma. Most frequently found

...e cerebellum, where it may be cystic.
...he brain, retina, pancreas, and kid-
...eys may be involved.

**·man″gi·o·en″do·the″li·o′-
...ma.** A hemangioma in which there is
...onsiderable proliferation of endothe-
...um between the vascular spaces.

**·man″gi·o·ma, hae·man″gi-
...ma** (hee·man″jee·o′muh, hem·an″·).
...n angioma made up of blood vessels.

·man″gi·o·sar·co′ma. A he-
...angioma with sarcomatous compo-
...ents.

**″mar·thro′sis, hae″mar-
...hro′sis** (hee″mahr·thro′sis, hem″-
...ar·). Extravasation of blood into a
...int.

″ma·te′in, hae″ma·te′in
...ee″muh·tee′in, hem″uh·). C₁₆H₁₂O₆.
...he reddish brown substance obtained
... oxidation of hematoxylin.

**″ma·tem′e·sis, hae″ma·tem-
...sis.** The vomiting of blood.

**″mat·hi·dro′sis, hae″mat·hi-
...ro′sis** (hee″mat·hi·dro′sis, ·high-
...o′sis). An excretion of blood or blood
...gments through the glands of the
...in.

·mat′ic. Pertaining to, full of, or
...aving the color of, blood.

m′a·tin, haem′a·tin (hem′uh-
...n, hee′muh·tin). C₃₄H₃₃N₄O₄FeOH, the
...ydroxide of ferriheme in which the
...on is in the ferric state, formed by
...eating hemin with alkali.

**m″a·ti·ne′mi·a, haem″a·ti-
...e′mi·a.** The presence of heme in
...e blood.

m″a·tin′ic, haem″a·tin′ic. 1.
...elating to hematin, or heme. 2. An
...ent which tends to increase the
...emoglobin content of the blood.

m′a·tite. Ferric oxide, Fe₂O₃, con-
...ining little water of hydration; a red
...owder.

m″a·to-, haem′a·to- (hem′uh·to-,
...ee′muh·to-), **hemat-, haemat-.** A
...mbining form signifying of or per-
...ining to the blood.

m″a·to·aer·om′e·ter. A device
...r recording the pressure of gases in
...e blood.

**m″a·to·cele″, haem′a·to-
...cele″.** A tumor formed by the extrav-
...sation and collection of blood in a
...art, especially in the cavity of the
...unica vaginalis testis or the pelvis.

m″a·to·chy′lo·cele (hem″uh·to-
...gh′lo·seel, hee″muh·to·). A tumor
...rmed by the extravasation and col-
...ction of chyle and blood in a part,
...pecially in the tunica vaginalis testis.
...is a complication of filariasis.

m″a·to·chy·lu′ri·a (hem″uh·to-
...gh·lew′ree·uh, hee″muh·to·). The
...resence of blood and chyle in the
...rine.

hem″a·to·col′pos. A collection of
blood within the vagina.

hem″a·to·crit″, haem′a·to·crit″
(hem″uh·to·krit″). 1. A small centrifuge used to separate blood cells in
clinical analysis. 2. That percentage of
the whole blood volume occupied by the
blood cells after centrifuging in a special graduated tube. Also called *h. reading.* 3. A flat-bottomed graduated centrifuge tube in which the blood cells
are separated. Also called *h. tube.*

**hem″a·to·cyst″, haem′a·to-
cyst″.** A cyst containing blood.

hem″a·to·cy·tol′y·sis (hem″uh·to-
sigh·tol′i·sis, hee″muh·to·). Hemolysis;
destruction of red blood cells with setting free of the contained hemoglobin.

**hem″a·to·cy·tom′e·ter, haem″-
a·to·cy·tom′e·ter.** See *hemocytometer.*

**hem″a·to·dy·nam′ics, haem″-
a·to·dy·nam′ics** (hem″uh·to·dye-
nam′icks, hee″muh·to·). See *hemodynamics.*

hem″a·to·dys·cra′si·a (·dis·kray′-
zhuh, ·shuh). A diseased state of the
blood.

**hem″a·to·gen′e·sis, haem″a·to-
gen′e·sis.** Formation of the blood or
blood cells. —**hematogenic, hem-
atog′enous,** *adj.*

he″ma·tol′o·gist (hee″muh·tol′o-
jist, hem″uh·). One who specializes in
the study of blood.

**he″ma·tol′o·gy, hae″ma·tol′-
o·gy.** The science of the blood, its
nature, functions, and diseases. —**he-
matolog′ic,** *adj.*

**hem″a·to·lym″phan·gi·o′ma,
haem″a·to·lym″phan·gi·o′ma.**
A tumor composed of blood vessels and
lymph vessels.

hem″a·to·lym·phu′ri·a. The discharge of urine containing lymph and
blood. Sometimes occurs in filariasis.

he″ma·tol′y·sis (hee″muh·tol′i·sis,
hem″uh·). Hemolysis; destruction of
red blood cells with setting free of the
contained hemoglobin.

he″ma·to′ma, hae″ma·to′ma
(hee″muh·to′muh, hem″uh·to′muh). A
focalized extravasation of blood, which
soon clots to form a solid mass and
readily becomes encapsulated by connective tissue. Of such a size as to
constitute a visible, tumorlike swelling.
May be due to traumatic injury or to
other causes of rupture of blood vessels. May constitute a false aneurysm
between artery and vein in so-called
varicose aneurysm, a form of arteriovenous fistula. **chronic subdural h.**
A hematoma lying underneath the
dura, or slightly adherent to it, usually
resulting from head injury and giving
rise to slowly progressive symptoms
and signs of cerebral compression.

hem″a·to·me″di·as·ti′num. An

effusion of blood into the mediastinal spaces.

he″ma·tom′e·ter. An instrument to estimate the properties or constituents of blood. **—hematometry,** n.

hem″a·to·me′tra, haem″a·to·me′tra. An accumulation of blood or menstrual fluid in the uterus.

hem″a·to·my·e′li·a, haem″a·to·my·e′li·a (hem″uh·to·migh·ee′lee·uh, hee″muh·to·). Hemorrhage into the spinal cord.

hem″a·to·my″e·li′tis, haem″a·to·my″e·li′tis. An acute myelitis attended with an effusion of blood into the spinal cord.

he″ma·ton′ic, hae″ma·ton′ic (hee″muh·ton′ick, hem″uh·ton′ick). A blood tonic which increases the hemoglobin percentage of the blood.

hem″a·to·pa·thol′o·gy, haem″a·to·pa·thol′o·gy. The study of the manifestations of diseases of the blood.

he″ma·top′a·thy (hee″muh·top′uh·thee, hem″uh·). Any disease of the blood.

hem·a·to·phyte″, haem·a·to·phyte″. A vegetable organism, such as a bacterium, living in the blood.

hem″a·to·por″phy·rin. $C_{34}H_{38}O_6N_4$. Iron-free heme. A porphyrin obtained in vitro by treating hemoglobin with sulfuric acid. It is closely related to the naturally occurring porphyrins.

hem″a·to·por″phy·ri·ne′mi·a, haem″a·to·por″phy·ri·ne′mi·a (hem″uh·to·por″fi·ri·nee′mee·uh, hee″muh·to·). Presence of hematoporphyrin in the blood.

hem″a·to·por″phy·ri·nu′ri·a, haem″a·to·por″phy·ri·nu′ri·a (hem″uh·to·por″fi·ri·new′ree·uh, hee″muh·to·). The presence of hematoporphyrin in the urine.

hem″a·tor·rha′chis (hem″uh·to·ray′kis, hee″muh·to·). Hemorrhage into the spinal meninges producing irritative phenomena.

hem″a·tor·rhe′a. Copious or profuse hemorrhage.

hem″a·to·sal′pinx, haem″a·to·sal′pinx. A collection of blood in a uterine tube.

hem·a·to·scope. An instrument used in the spectroscopic examination of the blood, by means of which the thickness of the layer of the blood can be regulated.

hem·a·tose, haem·a·tose (hem′uh·toce, hee′muh·toce). Full of blood.

he″ma·to′sis (hee″muh·to′sis, hem″uh·). The process of the formation of blood; the arterialization of blood.

hem″a·to·spec′tro·scope, haem·a·to·spec′tro·scope. A spectroscope adapted to the study of the blood. **—hematospectros′copy,** n.

hem″a·to·sper′ma·to·cele″, haem″a·to·sper′ma·to·cele″ (hem″uh·to·spur′muh·to·seel″, ·spu[...] mat′o·seel). A spermatocele containi[...] blood.

hem″a·to·sper′mi·a, haem″a·to·sper′mi·a. The discharge [...] bloody semen.

hem·a·to·tym′pa·num. Bloo[...] exudation into the tympanic cavity.

he″ma·tox′y·lin (hee″muh·tock′s[...] lin, hem″uh·) (C.C.). $C_{16}H_{14}O_6$. A co[...] orless crystalline compound occurri[...] in logwood, used as a stain in micro[...] copy.

he″ma·tox′y·lon, hae″ma·tox′y·lon (hee″muh·tock′si·lon, hem[...] uh·). Logwood. The heartwood of _Ha[...] matoxylon campechianum._

hem″a·to·zo′on, hem″a·to·zo′on (pl. _hematozoa_). Any anim[...] parasite living in the blood. **—hem[...] tozoal, hematozoic,** adj.

hem″a·tu′ri·a (hem″uh·tew′ree·u[...] hee″muh·). The discharge of uri[...] containing blood. Often associated wi[...] diseases of the kidney. **false h.** T[...] passage of red urine, due to the inge[...] tion of food or drugs containing r[...] pigments.

heme (heem). $C_{34}H_{32}N_4O_4Fe$, the ferro[...] complex of protoporphyrin 9 which [...] the prosthetic component of hem[...] globin. If the iron of heme is oxidiz[...] to the ferric state, its higher valen[...] imparts a positive charge which [...] alkaline solution forms hematin, a[...] in hydrochloric acid solution form[...] hemin. See also _hemochromogen._ Sy[...] _ferroheme._

hem″er·a·lo′pi·a. Day blindne[...] frequently incorrectly used to descr[...] the condition of reduced dark adap[...] tion resulting temporarily from vi[...] min-A deficiency or permanently fr[...] retinitis pigmentosa or other perip[...] eral retinal diseases. See _night blin[...] ness._

hem″er·a·pho′ni·a. Loss of vo[...] during the day, and recovery of it [...] night; a hysterical symptom.

hem′i-. 1. A prefix signifying _half._ In _biology_ and _medicine,_ a prefix [...] noting either _the right_ or _the left h[...] of the body._ 3. In _chemistry,_ a pre[...] denoting a combining ratio of one-ha[...]

hem″i·a·geu′si·a (hem″ee·ag·yo[...] see·uh, hem″ee·a·jew′see·uh). Loss [...] diminution of the sense of taste [...] one side of the tongue, usually caus[...] by injury to the chorda tympani ner[...]

hem″i·al′bu·mose. A product [...] the digestion of certain kinds of p[...] teins. It is a normal constituent [...] bone marrow. Also called _propepto[...]_

hem″i·al·bu″mo·su′ri·a. T[...] presence of hemialbumose in the uri[...] propeptonuria.

hem″i·an″al·ge′si·a (·an″al·je[...]

ee·uh, ·see·uh). Analgesia of one lateral half of the body and limbs.

em″i·an″en·ceph′a·ly. Anencephalia in one lateral half only.

em″i·an″es·the′si·a (·an″ess·hee′zhuh, ·zee·uh). Anesthesia of either lateral half of the body. **alternate h.** That affecting one side of the head and the opposite side of the body. **cerebral h.** That due to a lesion in the internal capsule or either lenticular nucleus. **hysterical h.** Hemianesthesia as a manifestation of hysteria.

em″i·an·op′si·a. Blindness in one half of the visual field; may be bilateral or unilateral. Also called *hemiopia, hemianopia.* **bitemporal h.** Blindness on the temporal side of the visual field, due to disease of the central parts of the optic commissure. **homonymous h.** The form affecting the inner half of one field and the outer half of the other. **quadrantic h.** Blindness in one quadrant; may be bitemporal or homonymous.

em″i·a·tax′i·a. Ataxia affecting the side of the body.

em″i·ath′e·to′sis. Athetosis of the side of the body.

em″i·at′ro·phy. Atrophy confined to one side of an organ.

em″i·bal′lis′mus, hem″i·bal′ism. A form of hemichorea, characterized by sudden, violent, spasmodic movements of the extremities of one side of the body. Caused by a destructive lesion of the subthalamic nucleus. The condition ceases suddenly if a true hemiplegia intervenes.

′mic, hae′mic (hee′mick, hem′ик). Pertaining to or developed by the blood.

m″i·car′di·a. The presence of only a lateral half of the usual four-chambered heart.

m″i·ceph′a·ly. A congenital anomaly with absence of cerebrum but with rudimentary cerebellum and basal ganglions; partial anencephalia.

m″i·cho·re′a (hem″ee·kor·ee′uh). A form of chorea in which the convulsive movements are confined to one side of the body.

m″i·co·lec′to·my. Excision of a part of the colon.

m″i·cra′ni·a. 1. Pain or headache on one side of the head only. 2. Partial encephalia. 3. Migraine.

m″i·cra″ni·o′sis. Enlargement of one half of the cranium or face.

m″i·di′a·phragm. 1. A lateral half of the diaphragm. 2. A half diaphragm, designating a diaphragm in which the muscle development is deficient on one side.

m″i·fa′cial. Pertaining to one lateral half of the face.

m″i·glos·sec′to·my. Removal of the lateral half of the tongue.

hem″i·glos″so·ple′gi·a. Unilateral paralysis of the tongue with relatively minor disturbances of motility; the tongue deviates toward the palsied side upon protrusion.

hem″i·gna′thi·a (hem″ee·nayth′ee·uh, hem″ee·nath′ee·uh). Partial or complete absence of the lower jaw on one side. **—hemignath′us,** n.

hem″i·hy″pal·ge′si·a (hem″ee·high″pal·jee′zee·uh). Hypalgesia, or decreased sensitivity to pain, on one lateral half of the body.

hem″i·hy″per·es·the′si·a (·high″·pur·ess·thee′zhuh, ·zee·uh). Increased sensitivity on one lateral half of the body.

hem″i·hy″per·hi·dro′sis (·high″·pur·hi·dro′sis, ·high″pur·high·dro′sis). Excessive sweating on one side of the body.

hem″i·hy″per·to′ni·a. Increased muscular tonicity confined to one half of the body; may occur following apoplexy.

hem″i·hy·per′tro·phy. Hypertrophy of half of the body or unilateral hypertrophy of one or more bodily regions (e.g., the head, an arm).

hem″i·hy″pes·the′si·a (hem″ee·high″pes·thee′zhuh, ·zee·uh). Decreased sensitivity in one lateral half of the body.

hem″i·hy″po·to′ni·a. Partial loss of tonicity of one side of the body.

hem″i·lab″y·rin·thec′to·my. The removal of one or more of the semicircular canals while leaving the ampullated ends and the saccule.

hem″i·lam″i·nec′to·my. Laminectomy in which laminas of only one side are removed.

hem″i·lar″yn·gec′to·my (hem″ee·lar″in·jeck′to·mee). Extirpation of one lateral half of the larynx.

hem·im′e·lus. An individual with incomplete or stunted extremities.

he′min. C₃₄H₃₂N₄O₄FeCl, the chloride of ferriheme in which the iron is in the ferric state, formed by heating hemoglobin with glacial acetic acid in the presence of sodium chloride, thus producing reddish-brown (Teichmann's) crystals, which reaction is the basis for a test for blood.

hem″i·ne·phrec′to·my. Removal of part of a kidney.

hem″i·pa·re′sis, hem″i·par′e·sis. Paresis of one side of the body.

hem″i·ple′gi·a. Paralysis of one side of the body. **—hemipleg′ic,** adj. **alternate h.** Paralysis of the facial muscles or tongue on one side of the body, and of the trunk and the extremities on the other side. Also called *crossed h.,* h. cruciata. **congenital h.** A spastic type due to a birth injury. Also called *infantile h.* **facial h.** Motor paralysis of one side of the face. **spastic h.** A form characterized by rigidity of the affected extremities.

hem″i·ra·chis′chi·sis (hem″ee·ra-kis′ki·sis). Incomplete spina bifida. See *spina bifida occulta.*

hem″i·sco·to′sis. A dark spot in one half of the visual field.

hem″i·so′mus. An individual with one side of the body imperfectly developed.

hem′i·spasm. A spasm affecting only one side of the body.

hem′i·sphere. The lateral half of the cerebrum or cerebellum. **dominant h.** The cerebral hemisphere which controls certain motor activities, such as movements of speech; usually the left hemisphere in right-handed individuals.

He·mis′po·ra. A genus of fungi whose species are contaminants. **H. stellata.** A species which has been found in osteoperiostitis, cold abscesses, and sporotrichoid lesions.

hem″i·sys′to·le (hem″ee·sis′to·lee). Contraction of the left ventricle after every second atrial contraction so that for each two beats of the heart only one pulse beat is felt.

hem″i·thy″roid·ec′to·my. Removal of one lateral lobe of the thyroid gland.

hem″i·ver′te·bra. A congenital anomaly of the spine in which one of the two lateral growth centers of a vertebra fails to develop, resulting in the absence of half of the vertebra.

hem′lock. 1. Common name for the genus *Tsuga;* actually a misnomer. 2. Originally the common name for the genus *Conium* (renamed poison hemlock). See *conium.*

he′mo-, hae′mo- (hee′mo-, hem′o-). A combining form signifying *of* or *pertaining to the blood.*

he″mo·bil″i·ru′bin (·bil″i·roo′-bin). 1. Bilirubin as it occurs normally in serum before passing through the hepatic cells. 2. The form of bilirubin present normally in blood serum. Also see *cholebilirubin.*

he″mo·chro″ma·to′sis. A disease characterized by excessive deposits of iron in the body, especially in the liver, the pancreas, and the skin; it is accompanied by hepatic cirrhosis and diabetes. Also called *pigmentary cirrhosis, bronze diabetes.*

he″mo·chro′mo·gen. A compound formed by union of heme with a nitrogen-containing substance.

he″mo·chro·mom′e·ter, hae″-mo·chro·mom′e·ter. Colorimeter; an instrument for estimating the amount of hemoglobin in the blood.

he″mo·con″cen·tra′tion, hae″-mo·con″cen·tra′tion. An increase in the concentration of blood cells resulting from the loss of plasm or water from the blood stream; anhydremia.

he″mo·co′ni·a, hae″mo·co′ni·a. Minute, colorless, highly refractiv particles of fat found in the blood. Al called *blood dust, chylomicrons.*

he″mo·co″ni·o′sis, hae″mo·co″ni·o′sis. The condition of having a abnormal amount of hemoconia in th blood.

he″mo·cyte, hae′mo·cyte. A bloo cell.

he″mo·cy′to·blast, hae″mo·cy′to·blast. The cell considered by som to be the primitive stem cell, givin rise to all blood cells. Syn., *lymphoid cyte.* **—hemocytoblas′tic,** *adj.*

he″mo·cy·tom′e·ter, hae″mo·cy·tom′e·ter. An instrument f estimating the number of blood cell

he″mo·cy″to·zo′on, hae″mo·cy″to·zo′on. A protozoan parasite i habiting the red blood cells.

he·mo′di·a. Hypersensitivity of th teeth.

he″mo·di″ag·no′sis, hae″mo·di″ag·no′sis. Diagnosis by exam nation of the blood.

he″mo·di′a·stase. The amylolyt enzyme of blood.

he″mo·di·lu′tion. A condition the blood in which the ratio of bloo cells to plasma is reduced.

he″mo·drom′o·graph, hae″mo·drom′o·graph. An instrument f registering small variations in t velocity of the blood stream.

he″mo·dro·mom′e·ter, hae″mo·dro·mom′e·ter. An instrument f measuring the velocity of the bloo current.

he″mo·dy·nam′ics, hae″mo·dy·nam′ics (hee″mo·dye-nam′icks, ·o nam′icks). The study of how the phys cal properties of the blood and i circulation through the vessels affe blood flow and pressure.

he″mo·flag′el·late, hae″mo·flag′el·late (hee″mo·fladj′i·la hem″o·). Any protozoan flagellate li ing in the blood of its host.

he″mo·fus′cin, hae″mo·fus′ci (hee″mo·fuss′in, hem″o·). The yello ish brown, iron-free pigment found hemochromatosis.

he″mo·glo′bin, hem″o·glo′bi. The respiratory pigment of the r blood cells. Abbreviated, **hb.** See Tal of Normal Values of Blood Constit ents in the Appendix.

he″mo·glo″bi·ne′mi·a, hae″m glo″bi·ne′mi·a. A condition which the hemoglobin is dissolved o of the red cells, and is held in soluti in the serum.

he″mo·glo″bi·nom′e·ter, hae mo·glo″bi·nom′e·ter. An instr ment for determining the hemoglob concentration of the blood. **—hemo-globinometry,** n.

he″mo·glo″bi·nu′ri·a. The presence of hemoglobin in the urine, due either to its solution out of the red cells or to disintegration of the red cells. **—hemoglobinuric,** adj. **epidemic h.** Hemoglobinuria of the newborn; associated with jaundice, cyanosis, and nervous symptoms. Also called *Winckel's disease.* **march h.** A paroxysmal hemoglobinuria noted in soldiers after strenuous marching. **nocturnal h.** A form of hemoglobinuria which attacks at night. **paroxysmal h.** A form characterized by recurring periodic attacks following exposure to cold or, occasionally, after exertion. Usually a manifestation of late syphilis. **toxic h.** That form due to poisoning.

he′mo·gram. A differential count of the leukocytes to show the qualitative as well as the quantitative variations in the cells.

he′mo·lith. A stone or concretion within the lumen of a blood vessel, or incorporated in the wall of a blood vessel, as in the pampiniform plexus in the aged.

he·mol′y·sin, hae·mol′y·sin (hee-mol′i·sin, hee″mo·lye′sin). A substance produced in the blood which frees hemoglobin from the red cells. **bacterial h.** That formed by the action of bacteria. **immune h.** One formed by the animal body in response to the injection of erythrocytes of another species.

he·mol′y·sis (hee·mol′i·sis, hem·ol′·). The destruction of red blood cells and the resultant escape of hemoglobin. **—hemolytic,** adj.

he′mo·lyze, hae′mo·lyze. Produce hemolysis. **—hemolyzation,** n.

he″mo·ma·nom′e·ter, hae″mo·ma·nom′e·ter. A manometer used in estimating blood pressure.

he″mo·pa·thol′o·gy, hae″mo·pa·thol′o·gy. The science dealing with the diseases of the blood.

he″mo·per″i·car′di·um, hae″mo·per″i·car′di·um. An effusion of blood into the pericardial cavity.

he″mo·per″i·to·ne′um, hae″mo·per″i·to·ne′um. An effusion of blood into the peritoneal cavity.

he′mo·phage, hae′mo·phage (hee′mo·faydj, hem′o·faydj). A phagocytic cell which destroys red blood cells. **—hemophagic, hemophag′ous,** adj.

he″mo·pha′gi·a, hae″mo·pha′gi·a. 1. Ingestion of blood as a therapeutic agent. 2. Feeding on the blood of another organism. 3. Phagocytosis of the red blood cells.

he′mo·phil. Denoting an organism growing preferably on blood mediums.

he″mo·phil′i·a (hee″mo·fill′ee·uh, hem″o·). A sex-linked, hereditary disease occurring only in males but transmitted by females. It is characterized by a prolonged coagulation time and abnormal bleeding.

he″mo·phil′i·ac. One who is affected with hemophilia.

he″mo·phil′ic. 1. *In biology,* pertaining to bacteria growing well in culture media containing hemoglobin. 2. Pertaining to hemophilia. 3. Pertaining to a hemophiliac.

He·moph′i·lus. A genus of bacteria of the family Parvobacteriaceae. **H. ducreyi.** A species of small, Gram-negative bacilli tending to grow in short chains; the cause of chancroid. **H. duplex.** A species responsible for infections of the cornea and conjunctiva; pathogenic for the human eye only. Syn., *Moraxella lacunata.* **H. influenzae.** Certain strains of this species produce conjunctivitis and influenzal meningitis and have a definite invasive power, but in respiratory infections commonly follow some other microörganism. **H. pertussis.** This species is the causative agent of whooping cough. **H. suis.** This species, together with a filtrable virus, produces swine influenza.

he″mo·pho′bi·a (hee″mo·fo′bee·uh, hem″o·), **hem″a·to·pho′bi·a** (hem″uh·to·fo′bee·uh, hee″muh·to·). Morbid fear of the sight of blood.

he″moph·thal′mi·a, he″moph·thal′mos. Hemorrhage into the vitreous body.

he″moph·thi′sis (hee″moff·thigh′sis, hee·moff′thi·sis). Anemia due to undue degeneration or inadequate formation of red blood cells.

he″mo·pneu″mo·tho′rax, hae″mo·pneu″mo·tho′rax (hee″mo·new″mo·thor′acks, hem″o·). A collection of air and blood within the pleural cavity.

he·mop′ty·sis, hae·mop′ty·sis. The spitting of blood from the larynx, trachea, bronchi, or lungs.

hem′or·rhage, haem′or·rhage (hem′o·ridj, hem′ridj). An escape of blood from the vessels, either by diapedesis through intact walls or by flow through ruptured walls. **—hemorrhag′ic** (hem″o·radj′ick), adj. **antepartum h.** Bleeding from the uterus before delivery. **autogenous h.** One due to causes within the body; not traumatic. **capillary h.** Oozing of blood from the capillaries. **cerebral h.** Bleeding from blood vessels in the cerebrum, either traumatic or due to disease. **choroidal h.** Bleeding of the vessels of the choroid of the eye; discoverable by ophthalmoscopic examination. **cyclic h.** (a) Excessive menstruation. (b) Menstrual bleeding of ectopic endometrial implants, as in endometriosis. **external h.** Hemorrhage that is visible to the eye by the escape of blood to the exterior of the body from a wound or ruptured tissue. **extradural h.** Hemorrhage into the space outside of the dura mater. **internal h.** Bleeding which is concealed by escape into a cavity, as the intestine, belly, or skull. **petechial h.** Hemorrhage in the form of petechiae, rounded spots. **post-partum h.** Bleeding occurring shortly after childbirth. **primary h.** One that immediately follows any traumatism. **secondary h.** One that occurs some time after the traumatism. **splinter h.** A subungual hemorrhage resembling a splinter under the nail; found in cases of subacute bacterial endocarditis. **subarachnoid h.** Bleeding between the arachnoid and the pia mater of the brain. **subdural h.** Hemorrhage between the dura mater and the pia arachnoid. It usually results from injury to the meningeal vessels on the inner side of the dura mater.

hem″or·rhoi′dal, haem″or·rhoi′dal. 1. Pertaining to or affected with hemorrhoids. 2. Applied to blood vessels, nerves, etc., of the anal canal.

hem″or·rhoid·ec′to·my, haem″or·rhoid·ec′to·my. Surgical removal of hemorrhoids.

hem′or·rhoids. An enlarged and varicose condition of the veins of the lower portion of the rectum and the tissues about the anus. Syn., *piles*. **external h.** Those situated outside of the sphincter ani. **internal h.** Those within the anal orifice.

he″mo·sid′er·in, hae″mo·sid′er·in. An iron-containing pigment; a product of the decomposition of hemoglobin.

he″mo·sid″er·o′sis, hae″mo·sid″er·o′sis. See *hemochromatosis*.

he″mo·sta′si·a, hae″mo·sta′si·a (hee″mo·stay′zhuh, hem″o·), **he″mo·sta′sis, hae″mo·sta′sis.** 1. Stagnation of the blood. 2. Arrest of a flow of blood.

he″mo·stat, hae″mo·stat. An agent or instrument which arrests the flow of blood.

he″mo·stat′ic, hae″mo·stat′ic. 1. Arresting hemorrhage. 2. An agent that arrests hemorrhage.

he″mo·ta·chom′e·ter, hae″mo·ta·chom′e·ter (hee″mo·ta·kom′i·tur, hem″o·). An instrument for measuring the rate of flow of blood. —**he·motachometry,** n.

he″mo·ther′a·py (hee″mo·therr′uh·pee, hem″o·). The treatment of disease by means of blood or blood derivatives.

he″mo·tho′rax, hae″mo·tho′rax. An accumulation of blood in the pleural cavity.

he″mo·tox′in, hae″mo·tox′in. A cytotoxin capable of destroying re blood cells. —**hemotoxic,** adj.

he″mo·trophe, hae″mo·troph (hee′mo·troaf, hem′o·). All the nutritive substances supplied to the embry from the maternal blood stream viviparous animals having a decidua placenta. —**hemotroph′ic,** adj.

he″mo·tym′pa·num. Blood in th tympanic cavity.

he″mo·xo′in. A dark brown or re brown pigment, seen within plasmodi which has been formed from disint grated hemoglobin.

hemp. *Cannabis sativa;* the bast fib is used for textile purposes. **blac Indian h.** Apocynum. **Indian** Cannabis, *q.v.*

hen′bane″. Hyoscyamus, *q.v.*

he′par. 1. The liver. 2. An obsole designation for a substance having t color of liver, generally a compound sulfur, as *hepar sulfuris*. **h. loba tum.** A liver having numerous lob produced by deep fissures, the result contraction of connective tissue aroun cicatrized or cicatrizing syphilitic gum mas. Also called *syphilitic cirrhos* **h. siccatum.** The dried and pow dered liver of swine freed from bloo

hep′a·rin, he′pa·rin. A polysa charide substance found in the liv and other tissues; possesses the pow of preventing coagulation of blood an is used therapeutically for this effec It yields, on hydrolysis, sulfuric aci acetic acid, 2-aminoglucose (gl cosamine), and a uronic acid. —**he arinized,** adj. **heparinize,** v.

hep′a·tal′gi·a. Pain in the live —**hepatalgic,** adj.

hep′a·tec′to·my. Excision of t liver or of a part of it.

he·pat′ic. 1. Pertaining to the live 2. A hepatic medicine.

He·pat′i·ca. Liverwort; a genus ranunculaceous plants.

he·pat′i·co-. A combining form f hepatic.

he·pat″i·co·du″o·de·nos′to·m Anastomosis between the hepatic du and the duodenum.

he·pat″i·co·en″ter·os′to·my. T surgical establishment of communic tion between the hepatic duct and t intestine.

he·pat″i·co·gas·tros′to·m Anastomosis between the hepatic du and the stomach.

he·pat″i·co·li·thot′o·my. Surgic removal of a biliary calculus from t liver or any of its ducts.

he·pat″i·cos′to·my. The format of a fistula in the hepatic duct for t purpose of drainage.

he·pat″i·cot′o·my. Incision into the hepatic duct.

hep″a·tit′i·des (hep″uh·tit′i·deez). A term denoting various inflammatory diseases of the liver; the plural of hepatitis.

hep″a·ti′tis. Inflammation of the liver. **amebic h.** A diffuse inflammation of the liver due to *Endamoeba histolytica*; it may resolve or lead to hepatic abscess. **arsenical h.** Hepatitis occurring in syphilis clinics formerly attributed to injury by arsenicals, but now believed to be due to a virus; homologous serum hepatitis. **chronic interstitial h.** Cirrhosis of the liver. **epidemic h.** A transmissible systemic disease occurring either in epidemic or in endemic form with fever, chills, malaise, gastrointestinal disturbances, and usually jaundice; probably due to a virus, the essential lesions being degeneration, necrosis, and more or less marked inflammation of the liver. Also called *infectious hepatitis, epidemic jaundice.* **hemorrhagic h.** A term applied to the lesions in the liver which often accompany eclampsia. Grossly, the liver is enlarged, showing foci of necrosis and of hemorrhage. Microscopically, the necrosis is usually peripheral in the lobule but may be widespread. The widened peripheral sinusoids may contain thrombi of agglutinated erythrocytes. Hemorrhage may be slight in the periphery of the lobule, more extensive in the lobule and, rarely, may constitute a hematoma. Exudation is absent or only slight; the lesion is not primarily or principally inflammatory. **homologous serum h.** A form of viral hepatitis transmitted by the parenteral injection of human blood or blood products contaminated by the causative agent. **infectious h.** Epidemic hepatitis. **interstitial h.** A condition in which there are associated degeneration or necrosis of hepatic parenchymal cells and infiltration of lymphocytes, plasma cells, and large mononuclear cells, and sometimes polymorphonuclear leukocytes in the portal canals. Also called *acute nonsuppurative h.* **postvaccinal h.** A condition similar to epidemic hepatitis, following vaccination or yellow fever or following the use of human serum. **viral h.** Any inflammation of the liver due to viral infection.

ep″a·ti·za′tion. The conversion of tissue into a liverlike substance, as of the lungs during pneumonia. —**hep′atized,** *adj.*

ep′a·to-, hepat-. A combining form denoting *the liver, hepatic.*

ep″a·to·cho·lan″gi·o·du″o·de·nos′to·my (hep″uh·to·ko·lan″jee·o-

dew″o·di·nos′to·mee). Establishment by surgical means of communication between the hepatic duct and the duodenum.

hep″a·to·cho·lan″gi·o·en″ter·os′to·my. Anastomosis between the hepatic duct and some portion of the small intestine.

hep″a·to·cho·lan″gi·o·gas·tros′to·my. Anastomosis between the hepatic duct and stomach.

hep″a·to·cho·lan″gi·o·je″ju·nos′to·my (hep″uh·to·ko·lan″jee·o·jee″jew·nos′to·mee). The surgical establishment of communication between the hepatic duct and the jejunum.

hep″a·to·col′ic. Relating to the liver and the colon.

hep″a·to·cyst′ic. Pertaining to the liver and the gallbladder.

hep″a·to·du″o·de′nal (hep″uh·to·dew″o·dee′nul, ·dew·od′i·nul). Relating to the liver and the duodenum.

hep″a·to·fla′vin. Riboflavin, *q.v.*

hep′a·to·gram. A graphic record of the liver pulse.

hep″a·to·li·e′nal (hep″uh·to·lye·ee′nul, ·lye′i·nul). Pertaining to the liver and the spleen.

hep″a·to·li″en·og′ra·phy. Radiographic examination of the liver and spleen.

hep′a·to·lith. A calculus in the biliary passages of the liver.

hep″a·to·li·thi′a·sis. A diseased condition characterized by the formation of gallstones in the biliary passages of the liver.

hep″a·to′ma. Any tumor originating in the liver; applied more particularly to nodular foci of regeneration, to adenomas, and to that form of primary hepatic carcinoma made up of cells which, in arrangement and form, resemble the cells of the hepatic cords.

hep″a·to·meg′a·ly, hep″a·to·me·ga′li·a. Enlargement of the liver.

hep″a·to·pex″y. Surgical fixation of a movable, or ptosed, liver; usually by utilizing additional supportive power of the round and the falciform ligaments.

hep″a·top·to′sis (hep″uh·top·to′sis, hep″uh·to·to′sis). Abnormally low position of the liver in the abdomen, due to stretching of attachments to the diaphragm.

hep″a·to·re′nal. Relating to both the liver and kidney.

hep″a·tor′rha·phy. Suturing of the liver following an injury or an operation.

hep″a·tos′co·py. Inspection of the liver, as by laparotomy or peritoneoscopy.

hep″a·to′sis. 1. Enlargement of the liver due to obstructive dilatation of intrahepatic biliary passages. 2. A degeneration or inflammation of the liver which cannot be clearly distinguished clinically.

hep"a·to·sple"no·meg'a·ly. Enlargement of the liver and spleen.

hep"a·to·ther'a·py. Therapeutic use of liver or liver extract.

hep"a·tot'o·my. Incision into the liver.

hep"a·to·tox'in. 1. A poisonous or deleterious product elaborated in the liver. 2. An injurious substance, such as chloroform, phosphorus, or an arsenical, which acts especially on parenchymal cells of the liver. —**hepatotoxic,** adj.

hep"ta·bar'bi·tal. 5-(1-Cyclohepten-1-yl)-5-ethylbarbituric acid, a short-acting barbiturate. See medomin.

hep'tane. C_7H_{16}. n-Heptane. A liquid hydrocarbon of the paraffin series.

hep'tose. Any member of the division of the monosaccharides containing seven carbon atoms.

her'a·path·ite, her·ap'a·thite. Quinine iodosulfate.

herb (urb, hûrb). 1. A plant without a woody stem. 2. A plant used for medicinal purposes or for its odor or flavor.

her·biv'o·rous. Living on vegetable food.

herd in'stinct. The fundamental psychic urge to identify oneself with a group and to function in the same manner as the group; group feeling.

he·red'i·ty. The inborn capacity of the organism to develop ancestral characteristics; it is dependent upon the constitution and organization of the cell or cells which form the starting point of the new individual. In biparental reproduction this starting point is the fertilized ovum. —**hereditary,** adj.

her'e·do-. In medicine, a combining form used for hereditary. Often used erroneously in the sense of congenital, as in heredosyphilis.

her'it·age. In genetics, the sum total of the genes or characteristics transmitted from parents to their children.

her·maph'ro·dite. 1. An individual showing hermaphroditism. 2. Pertaining to or characterized by hermaphroditism. —**hermaphrodit'ic,** adj.

her·maph'ro·dit·ism (hur·maf'ro·dye·tiz·um), **her·maph'ro·dism.** A condition characterized by the coexistence in an individual of ovarian and testicular tissue. It is rare in humans (Young admits only 20 human cases), but more common in lower forms. Pseudohermaphroditism is a more common condition. See pseudohermaphrodite. **bilateral h.** That in which the individual has an ovary and testis on each side; seen in humans. **lateral h.** The form of human hermaphroditism in which there is an ovary on one side

and a testis on the other. **unilateral h.** The form in which there is an ovotestis on one side and an ovary or a testis on the other.

her·met'ic. Protected from exposure to air; air-tight.

her'ni·a. The abnormal protrusion of an organ or a part through the containing wall of its cavity, beyond its normal confines. The term applies usually to the abdominal cavity and implies the existence of a covering or sac. Syn., rupture. Also see prolapse. —**hernial,** adj. **acquired h.** A noncongenital form resulting from strain, weight lifting, or as the direct sequence of operation, muscular weakening, etc. **bladder h.** The protrusion of any part of the urinary bladder through any opening in the abdominal cavity. Syn., cystic h., vesical h. **cerebral h.** A protrusion of the brain through an acquired opening in the skull, as a result of operation, injury, or disease. Syn., h. of the brain. **complete h.** One in which the hernial sac and its contents have escaped through the opening; applied especially to inguinal hernias where the sac and its contents are to be found in the scrotum. **concealed h.** One which is not evident by ordinary manual examination. **congenital h.** One in which the defect is present in fetal life and exists at birth. This form is represented by inguinal hernias in which the processus vaginalis remains patent, leading to the early descent of intestine into the scrotum; and by diaphragmatic hernias in which abdominal organs have passed into the thoracic cavity. **diaphragmatic h.** One which passes through the diaphragm into the thoracic cavity; may be congenital, acquired, or traumatic, and may contain the stomach, small intestine, and colon. Usually a false hernia. **direct h.** An inguinal hernia in which the sac does not emerge from the internal ring but through a defect in the floor of Hesselbach's triangle, between the inferior epigastric artery and the outer edge of the rectus muscle. **diverticulum h.** A type of sliding hernia which contains a bladder diverticulum; the term is also applied to hernia of an intestinal diverticulum. **epigastric h.** A hernia in the linea alba, between the umbilicus and the xiphoid process, generally found in young adult males; the contents of the sac are usually extraperitoneal fat, lipomas, and, only rarely, bowel. Also called properitoneal h., fatty h. **false h.** One which has no sac covering the hernial contents. **femoral h.** That involving the femoral canal; the second most common hernia. Found more often in women, it is usually small and painful.

less, often remaining unnoticed. The neck lies below the inguinal ligament and lateral to the tubercle of the pubic bone. Syn., *crural h.* **foraminal h.** (a) A so-called hernia of the medulla into the foramen magnum of the skull, from increased intracranial pressure. (b) A false hernia of a loop of bowel through the epiploic foramen. **funicular h.** A variety of congenital, indirect hernia into the processus vaginalis which is closed below and open above. **h. of the lungs.** A rare, congenital anomaly associated with fissured chest, in which a portion of the lung protrudes through the opening, the swelling enlarging with each expiration. **h. of the nucleus pulposus.** Protrusion of the substance of the intervertebral disk into the spinal canal, causing pressure upon the cord or cauda equina. **hiatus h.** A form of hernia through the esophageal hiatus; usually a small, intermittent hernia of a part of the stomach. **incarcerated h.** A term applied either to an irreducible or to a strangulated hernia. **incisional h.** One occurring from an operative or accidental incision, the predisposing factors being wound infection, prolonged drainage, or interference with nerve supply. Also called *postoperative h.*, *posttraumatic h.* **incomplete h.** An inguinal hernia in which the sac has not passed far into the inguinal canal. Also called *bubonocele.* **indirect h.** An inguinal form which follows the spermatic cord into the scrotum or, in the female, the round ligament into the labium majus. The hernial sac leaves the abdomen through the internal abdominal ring, traverses the inguinal canal, and passes through the external ring. Syn., *lateral hernia, oblique hernia.* **infantile h.** A congenital, indirect, inguinal hernia in which the vaginal process is sealed high in the canal and remains open below. The sac then invaginates or passes behind the tunica vaginalis, so that two or three layers of peritoneum lie over the contents. **inguinal h.** A hernia through the inguinal canal. This variety constitutes more than four-fifths of all hernias. **inguinolabial h.** An inguinal hernia which has descended into the labium majus. **intermuscular h.** An interstitial hernia of the abdominal muscles through the fascial planes. Syn., *interparietal h.* **internal h.** One occurring within the abdominal cavity; a sac of peritoneum, containing intraabdominal contents, protrudes through a normal or abnormal opening. It may be retroperitoneal or intraperitoneal. **intersigmoid h.** A hernia involving the prolapse of a loop of bowel into

a retroperitoneal space occurring at the root of the mesosigmoid. **intraperitoneal h.** A type of false, internal hernia in which some of the intraabdominal contents pass through an anomalous opening in the mesentery, omentum, or broad ligaments. **iris h.** Prolapse of the iris after iridectomy or following trauma. **irreducible h.** A hernia which cannot be returned through the opening by manipulation; due to adhesions or blocking by fecal impaction, not to gaseous distention. **labial h.** Complete, indirect inguinal hernia into the labium majus. **lumbar h.** A hernia passing out of the abdomen through the lumbar triangle, resulting usually from operation, lumbar abscess, or injury. **masked h.** A type of ventral hernia in which the hernial sac is situated within the abdominal wall. **mesenteric h.** One in which a loop of intestine or a portion of omentum or other viscus has passed through an opening in the mesentery. **perineal h.** A hernia passing through the pelvic diaphragm to appear as a rectal hernia, vaginal hernia, or bladder hernia, *q.v.* Also called *ischiorectal h.* **rectal h.** A condition in which the small bowel, or other abdominal contents, protrudes through the rectovesical or rectouterine pouch, carrying the anterior rectal wall through the anus. **reducible h.** One whose contents can be replaced through the hernial opening. **retroperitoneal h.** Hernia into a recess of the peritoneum, as into a paraduodenal recess. Syn., *duodenojejunal h., ileoappendicular h.* **retrovesical h.** A hernia behind the bladder into the retrovesical space. **Richter's h.** A form of enterocele in which only a part of the intestinal wall is situated within the hernial sac. **sciatic h.** That through one of the sciatic notches. Also called *ischiadic h.* **scrotal h.** Any hernia which is found within the scrotum. See complete *h.*, inguinal *h.*, sliding *h.* **sliding h.** A variety of acquired, indirect, irreducible inguinal hernia in which a section of the colon, either sigmoid or cecum, has entered the sac and become a part of it by attachment. Generally a large scrotal hernia. **strangulated h.** A hernia in which the circulation of the blood and the fecal current are blocked. If unrelieved, this leads to ileus and necrosis of the intestine. **synovial h.** The protrusion of the inner lining of a joint capsule through the outer portion of the capsule. **true h.** One having a sac, usually of peritoneum, covering the hernial contents. **umbilical h.** One occurring through the umbilical ring, either early in life (infantile) from imperfect closure, or later (acquired) from diastasis of the recti, obesity, or muscular weakness. Congenital midline defects lead to hernia into the umbilical cord, or omphalocele. If liver is contained in the sac, it is called a hepatomphalocele. Syn., *annular h.* **vaginal h.** A perineal hernia which follows the course of the vagina after leaving the abdomen, and which may enter the labium majus; resembles a labial inguinal hernia. **ventral h.** A hernia of any part of the abdominal wall not involving the inguinal, femoral, or umbilical openings. It exists in three varieties: median, lateral, and postincisional. Syn., *abdominal h., epigastric h.*

her″ni·at′ed. Of or pertaining to a hernia. —**her′ni·ate,** *v.;* **hernia′tion,** *n.*

her′ni·o-. A combining form used to mean *hernia.*

her″ni·o·plas″ty. Plastic operation for the radical cure of hernia.

her″ni·or′rha·phy. Any operation which includes suturing for the repair of hernia.

her″ni·o·tome. A special knife or curved bistoury, with a blunt end, sometimes used in operations for hernia.

her″ni·ot′o·my. An operation for the relief of irreducible hernia, by cutting through the neck of the sac. Often wrongly used to indicate hernioplasty.

her′o·in. Diacetylmorphine. C₂₁H₂₃NO₅. White, odorless, bitter, crystalline powder.

her′o·in·ism. Addiction to heroin; a very prevalent form of drug addiction.

her·pan′gi·na. A mild, febrile disease characterized by vesicular, aphthous lesions of the faucial region; it occurs mainly in children and is contagious.

her′pes (hur′peez). An acute inflammation of the skin or mucous membrane, characterized by the development of groups of vesicles on an inflammatory base. —**herpet′ic,** *adj.* **h. facialis.** A type of herpes simplex occurring on the face, usually about the lips. May also occur in the mouth and pharynx. Syn., *h. febrilis, h. labialis.* Also called *coldsore.* **h. gestationis.** A type of dermatitis herpetiformis occurring during pregnancy. **h. simplex.** An acute disorder, characterized by groups of vesicles on an erythematous base. Commonly recurrent, and at times seen in the same place. Due to a virus. **h. zoster.** Herpes in which the lesions are distributed in relation to the course of a cutaneous nerve, and, as a rule, unilateral. They are often seen in the line of an intercostal nerve, but may follow in the course of any nerve. The out-

break of the eruption is often preceded and may be followed by severe neuralgic pain, referred to as herpetic neuralgia. It is a systemic infection caused by a virus; may be serious in elderly or debilitated persons. Syn. *shingles, zoster.* Also called *zona.* **h. zoster oticus.** Aural herpes associated with facial paralysis and otalgia; due to disease of the seventh cranial nerve. Also called *Hunt's syndrome.*

het″er·a·de′ni·a. Any abnormality in the formation or location of gland tissue. —**heteraden′ic,** *adj.*

het′er·o-, heter-. A combining form signifying *other, other than usual, different.*

het″er·o·ag·glu′ti·nin. An agglutinin in normal blood having the property of agglutinating foreign cells including the blood corpuscles of other species of animals.

het″er·o·al′bu·mose. A variety of albumose soluble in salt solutions, insoluble in water, and precipitated by saturation with sodium chloride or magnesium sulfate.

het″er·o·aux′in. 3-Indoleacetic acid. White, crystalline powder, insoluble in water. An activator of growth substance (auxin). Used experimentally as a plant growth stimulant.

het″er·o·aux′one (het″ur·o·awk′sohn). A growth-promoting substance. See *heteroauxin.*

het″er·o·chro′ma·tin. Originally the substance of heterochromosomes, e.g., the Y chromosome. It has been extended to include any chromatin similarly characterized by an excessive amount of desoxyribose-type nucleo protein, by a looser structure, and functionally by a more generalized metabolism, other than the more specific action of genes in the euchromatin which gives the familiar Mendelian ratio. —**heterochromat′ic,** *adj.*

het″er·o·chro′mi·a. A difference in coloration in two parts of a structure, or in two structures that are normally alike, as the iris of the eye. —**hetero chromous,** *adj.*

het″er·o·cy′clic (het″ur·o·sigh′ click, ·sick′lick). *In chemistry,* pertaining to dissimilar atoms in a ring structure. See *carbocyclic.*

het″er·o·dro′mi·a. Better conduction in one than in the other direction in a nerve.

het″er·o·er′o·tism. The direction of the sexual desire toward another person or toward any object other than oneself. —**heteroerot′ic,** *adj.*

het″er·o·ge′ne·ous. Differing in kind or nature; composed of different substances; not homogeneous. —**het erogene′ity,** *n.*

het″er·o·gen′e·sis. Alternation of generations in the complete life cycle, especially the alternation of a dioecious generation with one or more parthenogenetic generations and sometimes with an alternation of hosts, as in many trematode parasites. —**het·erogenet′ic,** adj.

het″er·og′e·nous. Of, relating to, or derived from a different species, as heterogenous graft.

het′er·o·graft″. A graft of tissue obtained from an animal of one species and transferred to the body of an animal of a different species.

het″er·o·in·tox′i·ca′tion. Intoxication by a poison not produced within the body.

het″er·o·ki·ne′si·a (het″ur·o·ki·nee′shuh, het″ur·o·kigh·). The execution of body movements which are opposite to those ordered.

het″er·ol′o·gy. Deviation from the normal in structure, organization, or time or manner of formation.

het″er·o·mor′phic. 1. Differing in size or form as compared with the normal. 2. In chemistry, crystallizing in different forms. 3. In zoology, having different forms at different stages of the life history. 4. In cytology, unlike in form or size; applied to either chromosome of a synaptic pair of unlike chromosomes, as an X and a Y chromosome. —**heteromorphism,** n.

het″er·o·mor′phous. Differing from the normal in form.

het″er·o·os′te·o·plas″ty. The grafting, by operation, of bone taken from an animal. Also see heterograft.

het′er·o·phe′my (het′ur·o·fee″mee, het″ur·off′i·mee), **het″er·o·phe′mi·a.** The unconscious saying of one thing while another is intended; heterolalia; heterophasia.

het″er·o·pho′ni·a. Abnormal quality or change of voice.

het″er·o·pho′ri·a. Any tendency of the eyes to turn away from the position correct for binocular vision; latent deviation. Actual deviation does not occur unless one eye is covered, as the desire for binocular vision is sufficient to overcome imbalance of the ocular muscles. In esophoria, the tendency is to deviate inward; in exophoria, outward; in hyperphoria, one eye tends to deviate upward; in hyperesophoria, upward and inward; in hyperexophoria, upward and outward.

het″er·oph′y·es (het″ur·off′ee·eez). A genus of trematode worms, found in Egypt and the Far East, which produces heterophyiasis in man. **H. het′erophyes.** A species which has as definitive hosts man, cats, dogs, foxes, hogs, and other fish-eating animals; as first intermediate hosts, snails, and as second intermediate hosts, mullet fish.

het″er·o·phy·i′a·sis (het″ur·o·figh·eye′uh·sis). Infestation by any fluke of the family Heterophyidae, of which the species Heterophyes heterophyes and Metagonimus yokogawai are the most important and most common to man. The flukes inhabit the small intestine but may also pass into the muscles of the heart through the lymphatics.

het″er·o·plas″ty. The operation of grafting parts taken from another species. —**heteroplas′tic,** adj.

het″er·o·pro′te·ose. One of a group of hydrolytic products, intermediate in the conversion of proteins to peptones.

het″er·op′si·a. Inequality of vision in the two eyes.

het″er·o·sex″u·al′i·ty. Sexual feeling directed toward one of the opposite sex.

het′er·o·side′. A term proposed for a class of glycosides.

het″er·o·sug·ges″ti·bil′i·ty. The state of being susceptible to influence by another.

het″er·o·to′pi·a. Displacement or deviation from natural position, as of an organ or a part; especially, congenital displacement of gray matter of the spinal cord into the white matter.

het″er·o·top′ic. Occurring in an abnormal location, as intestinal epithelial cells occurring in the gastric epithelium.

het″er·o·xan′thine (het″ur·o·zan′theen, -thin). Methyl xanthine; 7-methyl-2,6-diketo purine; a methylated purine.

HETP. Hexaethyltetraphosphate.

hetrazan. Trade-mark for N,N-diethyl-4-methyl-1-piperazinecarboxamide, a substance under clinical investigation in the treatment of filariasis.

hex″a·chlo′ro·phene. $HO.Cl_2C_6H.CH_2.C_6HCl_3.OH.$ Bis-(2-hydroxy-3,5,6-trichlorophenyl)methane, a germicide active in the presence of soap. Syn., Compound G-11.

hex″a·chro′mic. Capable of distinguishing only six of the seven spectrum colors, indigo not being distinguished.

hex′ad. An element the atom of which has a valence of six.

hex″a·dac′ty·lism. The state of having six fingers or toes.

hex″a·dec″e·no′ic ac′id. A fatty acid component of human depot fat.

hex″a·eth″yl·tet″ra·phos′phate. $(C_2H_5)_6P_4O_{13}.$ A substance having power to inhibit cholinesterase. Syn., HETP.

hex″a·hy′dric. Containing six atoms of replaceable hydrogen.

hex″a·hy·dro·hem″a·to·por′phy·rin (heck″suh·high″dro·hem″-

uh-to-por′fi·rin). A reduction product of hematin.

hex″a·me·tho′ni·um. A compound containing a methonium ion with six CH_2 groups, that possesses potent ganglion-blocking activity and is effective in reducing blood pressure. Also see *methonium.*

hex″a·meth″yl·en·a·mine′ (heck″suh-meth″il-een-uh-meen′, -am′-een). Methenamine.

hex″a·meth″yl·ene·tet″ra·mine′ (·tet″ruh·meen′, ·tet·ram′een). Methenamine.

hex′ane. Any one of the isomeric liquid hydrocarbons, C_6H_{14}, of the paraffin series.

hex″a·va′lent (heck″suh·vay′lunt, heck·sav′uh·lunt). Having a valence of six.

hexestrol. $HO.C_6H_4(C_2H_5)$ $CH.CH$ $(C_2H_5).C_6H_4.OH$. A trade name for dihydrodiethylstilbestrol, a synthetic estrogen.

hex′e·tal so′di·um. Nonproprietary name for sodium *n*-hexyl-ethyl barbiturate. See *ortal sodium.*

hex″o·bar′bi·tal (heck″so·bahr′bi·tawl, ·tal). 5-(1-Cyclohexenyl)-1,5-dimethylbarbituric acid, a rapidly acting barbiturate. Syn., *hexobarbitone.* See *evipal.* **h. sodium.** The water-soluble monosodium derivative of hexobarbital; may be administered intravenously to produce anesthesia of short duration. See *evipal sodium.*

hex″o·bar′bi·tone. British generic name for hexobarbital.

hex″o·ki′nase, hex·ok′i·nase. The enzyme which catalyzes the transfer of phosphate from adenosinetriphosphate to glucose or fructose, forming glucose-6-phosphate or fructose-6-phosphate and adenosinediphosphate.

hex′one bas′es. Term applied to the diaminomonocarboxylic acids (arginine, lysine, and histidine) which contain six carbon atoms and are basic in reaction.

hex·os″a·mine′ (heck·sohss″uh-meen′, heck′sohss·uh·meen″). A primary amino-derivative of a hexose obtained on hydrolysis of certain glycoproteins, mucins, heparin, chitin, etc.

hex′o·san. Any complex carbohydrate, such as cellulose, starch, or glycogen, which yields hexose on hydrolysis.

hex′ose. $C_6H_{12}O_6$. Any monosaccharide which contains six carbon atoms in the molecule.

hex″ose·di·phos′phate (heck″-sohss·dye·fos′fate). One of the hexosephosphates formed during the decomposition of glucose and glycogen in muscle-tissue metabolism.

hex″ose·mon″o·phos′phate. One of the hexosephosphates formed during the decomposition of glycogen in muscle-tissue action.

hex″ose·phos′phates. Any one of the phosphoric acid esters of a hexose, notably glucose, formed during the utilization of carbohydrates by mammalian tissues.

hex″u·ron′ic ac′id. The name originally given to the substance isolated from lemon juice and later identified as vitamin C.

hex′yl. The univalent radical, C_6H_{13}—.

hex′yl·caine hy″dro·chlo′ride. 1-Cyclohexylamino-2-propyl benzoate hydrochloride, a local anesthetic. See *cyclaine hydrochloride.*

hex″yl·res·or′cin·ol (heck″sil·res·or′sin·ole, ·ol). $C_6H_3C_6H_3(OH)_2$. White crystals, very slightly soluble in water. Used as germicide, as urinary antiseptic, and as anthelmintic. See *caprokol.*

Hf. Chemical symbol for hafnium.

Hg. Chemical symbol for mercury.

hg. Hectogram.

hi·a′tus (high·ay′tus). A space or opening. **—hiatal,** *adj.* **adductor h.** The tendinous hiatus. **aortic h.** An opening behind the diaphragm giving passage to the aorta. **buccal h.** Transverse facial cleft. **esophageal h.** Passage through the diaphragm for the esophagus. **facial h.** Hiatus of the facial canal. **h. of Fallopius.** Hiatus of the facial canal. **h. of the facial canal.** The opening which transmits the greater superficial petrosal nerve and the petrosal branch of the middle meningeal artery. **h. tendineus.** The tendinous hiatus. **maxillary h.** On on the inner aspect of the body of the maxilla, establishing communication between the nasal cavity and maxillary sinus. **semilunar h.** (a) A groove in the lateral wall of the middle meatus of the nasal cavity. The maxillary sinus and anterior ethmoid cells open into it. (b) An opening in the deep fascia of the arm for the passage of the basilic vein. **subarcuate h.** A depression on the petrous part of the temporal bone lodging the flocculus. **tendinous h.** [NA] The gap in the insertion of the adductor magnus muscle; the point of transition between the femoral and popliteal vessels.

hi″ber·na′tion. The dormant condition or winter sleep of certain animals.

hic′cup, hic′cough. A spasmodic contraction of the diaphragm causing inspiration, followed by a sudden closure of the glottis.

hid·rad″e·ni′tis. Inflammation of the sweat glands. **h. suppurativa.** An inflammatory disease of the apocrine sweat glands, especially those of the axillas, characterized by painful red nodules, abscesses, and sin-

...acts; partial remissions alternate
..ith acute exacerbations. Syn., *hidros-
.denitis axillaris.*

.d'ro-, hidr-. A combining form
.eaning *sweat.*

.d·ro'a (hid·ro'uh, high·dro'uh). Any
..rmal lesion associated with, or
.aused by, profuse sweating.

.d"ro·cys·to'ma (hid"ro·sis·to'-
..uh, high"dro·). A chronic condition
..aracterized by noninflammatory ves-
..les on the face.

.d"ro·poi·e'sis (hid"ro·poy·ee'sis,
..gh"dro·). The formation of sweat.
hidropoiet'ic, *adj.*

.d"ror·rhe'a (hid"ro·ree'uh,
..gh"dro·). Excessive flow of sweat.

."dros·ad"e·ni'tis (high"dro-
..ad"i·nigh'tis, hid"ro·). Inflammation
.. the sweat glands. Also called *hidra-
.enitis, hydrosadenitis.* **h. axillaris.**
..e *hidradenitis* suppurativa.

.dros'che·sis (hi·dros'ki·sis, high-
..ros'·). Retention or suppression of
..e sweat.

·dro'sis (hi·dro'sis, high·dro'sis).
.. The formation and excretion of
.veat. 2. Abnormally profuse sweating.
hi'drose, *adj.*

·drot'ic (hi·drot'ick, high·drot'-
..k). 1. Diaphoretic or sudorific. 2. A
.edicine that causes sweating.

.d"ro·to·path'ic. Relating to a
..orbid state of the perspiratory func-
.on.

."er·o·pho'bi·a. A morbid fear of
.cred things.

gh take-off. Colloquial term for
..usual elevation—more than one mil-
.meter—of the isoelectric line at
.·igin; seen in electrocardiograms in
..ses of myocardial injury, infarction,
.auma, and pericarditis.

ll'ock. A slight prominence or ele-
.ation. Also see *colliculus.* **axon h.**
..he region in a nerve cell, free from
..ssl substance, from which the axon
.kes origin.

'lum. Old term for hilus.

'lus (pl. *hili*). A pit, recess, or open-
..g in an organ, usually for the
.ntrance and exit of vessels or ducts.
.hilar, *adj.*

nd'brain". The rhombencephalon.
nd'gut". The caudal part of the
..bryonic digestive tube formed by
..e development of the tail fold.

.nton test. A macroscopic floccula-
.on test for syphilis.

.p. 1. The upper part of the thigh at
.s junction with the buttocks. 2. The
.p joint. See Table of Joints and Liga-
.ents in the Appendix. 3. The lateral
.rominence of the body at the level of
..e hip joint. **snapping h.** An ab-
..ormality caused by the presence of a
.ndinous band on the surface of the
.uteus maximus muscle. Certain

movements of the hip cause this band
to slip over the great trochanter.

hip'bone', hip'bone". The innominate bone.

hip·pan'thro·py. A delusional state
in which the patient believes he is a
horse. Also see *zoanthropy. Rare.*

Hippocrates [*Greek physician,* ca.
460–ca. 377 B.C.]. Called the father of
medicine. Best known for his astute
clinical descriptions of diseases. His
voluminous works include discussions
of epidemics, fevers, epilepsy, fractures,
instruments for reduction, and climate
and health. He knew the operations of
trephining and paracentesis. He believed that the body tends to heal itself
by natural processes, and that the role
of the physician should be ancillary to
that of nature. See also *facies* hippocratica; clubbed *finger,* also called
Hippocratic *finger* or *nail.* **oath of H.**
An oath setting forth the duties of the
physician to his patients, as follows:
I swear by Apollo the physician, and
Asclepius, and Health, and All-heal,
and all the gods and goddesses, that,
according to my ability and judgment,
I will keep this Oath and this stipulation—to reckon him who taught me
this Art equally dear to me as my
parents, to share my substance with
him, and relieve his necessities if required; to look upon his offspring in the
same footing as my own brothers, and
to teach them this art, if they shall
wish to learn it, without fee or stipulation; and that by precept, lecture, and
every other mode of instruction, I will
impart a knowledge of the Art to my
own sons, and those of my teachers,
and to disciples bound by a stipulation
and oath according to the law of medicine, but to none others. ¶ I will follow
that system of regimen which, according to my ability and judgment, I consider for the benefit of my patients,
and abstain from whatever is deleterious
and mischievous. I will give no deadly
medicine to any one if asked, nor suggest any such counsel; and in like manner I will not give to a woman a pessary
to produce abortion. With purity and
with holiness I will pass my life and
practise my Art. ¶ I will not cut persons labouring under the stone, but
will leave this to be done by men who
are practitioners of this work. Into
whatever houses I enter, I will go into
them for the benefit of the sick, and
will abstain from every voluntary act
of mischief and corruption; and, further, from the seduction of females
or males, of freemen and slaves.
¶ Whatever, in connexion with my professional practice, or not in connexion
with it, I see or hear, in the life of men,
which ought not to be spoken of abroad,
I will not divulge, as reckoning that all

such should be kept secret. While I continue to keep this Oath unviolated, may it be granted to me to enjoy life and the practice of the art, respected by all men, in all times! But should I trespass and violate this Oath, may the reverse be my lot!

hippuran. Trade-mark for sodium iodohippurate, a radiopaque agent.

hip·pu'ri·a. Excess of hippuric acid in the urine.

hip·pu'ric ac'id. $C_6H_5CONHCH_2$ COOH. Benzoylaminoacetic acid; an acid produced in the detoxication of benzoic acid. Syn., *urobenzoic acid.*

hip·pur'i·case. An enzyme found in kidney, liver, muscle, and pancreas which catalyzes the hydrolysis of hippuric acid to benzoic acid and glycine. Syn., *hippurase, histozyme.*

hip'pus. Spasmodic pupillary movement, independent of the action of light.

Hirschsprung, Harald [*Danish physician,* 1830–1916]. Known for his description of congenital megacolon or congenital dilatation of the colon; known as *Hirschsprung's disease.* Contributed to the knowledge of congenital pyloric stenosis in infants.

hir'sute (hur'suit, hur·suit'). Shaggy; hairy.

hir·su'ti·es (hur·sue'shee·eez, ·tee·eez). Excessive growth of hair; hypertrichosis.

hir'sut·ism (hur'suit·iz·um, hur·suit'iz·um). A condition characterized by growth of hair in unusual places or in unusual amounts.

hir'u·din, hi·ru'din. The active principle of a secretion derived from buccal glands of leeches. It prevents coagulation of blood.

hi·ru'di·ni·cul''ture. The artificial breeding of leeches.

Hi·ru'do. A genus of leeches of the class Hirudinea. **H. medicinalis.** The medicinal leech; formerly extensively used for bloodletting.

histadyl. Trade-mark for N,N-dimethyl-N'(2-thenyl)-N'(2-pyridyl)-ethylenediamine hydrochloride or thenylpyramine hydrochloride, a synthetic antihistaminic.

histalog. Trade-mark for betazole hydrochloride.

his·tam'i·nase, his''tam·i·nase'. An enzyme, obtainable from extracts of kidney and intestinal mucosa, capable of inactivating histamine and other diamines. Syn., *diamine oxidase.*

his'ta·mine (hiss'tuh·meen, ·min). β-Imidazolyl-4-ethylamine, $C_5H_9N_3$. An amine occurring as a decomposition product of histidine and prepared synthetically from that substance. —**his·tamin'ic,** *adj.* **h. phosphate.** Clear, colorless crystals soluble in water. Also called *histamine acid phosphate.*

his'ti·dase. An enzyme found only the liver in higher animals. It acts on upon L-histidine, with formation glutamic acid, formic acid, and ammonia.

his'ti·dine (hiss'ti·deen, ·din). C_3H $N_2.CH_2.CH(NH_2)$ COOH. β-Imidazole-alanine, an amino acid resulting fro the hydrolysis of many proteins. elimination of a molecule of carbo dioxide it is converted to histamine.

his''ti·di·nu'ri·a. A state in whic histidine is found in the urine, fr quently occurring in women after t first month of pregnancy. Attributed restricted activity of histidase in t liver.

his'ti·o-, histi-. A combining for meaning *a web, cloth, tissue.*

his'ti·o·cyte. Fixed macrophage the loose connective tissue. Histiocyte in common with other cells belongi to the reticuloendothelial system, *q.* store electively certain dyes such trypan blue or lithium carmine. Fo merly called *resting wandering cell.*

his''ti·o·cy·to'ma (hiss''tee·o·sig to'muh). A tumor containing h tiocytes.

his''ti·o·cy''to·sar·co'ma. A tum only slightly malignant, occurring dermis especially; made up of larg mononuclear cells, supposed by some be histiocytes. Others believe the ce to be fibrocytes and fibroblasts, an name the lesion a fibroma or fibr sarcoma.

his''ti·o·cy·to'sis (·sigh·to'sis). Pr liferation of histiocytes, especially lymph nodes and other organs of t hematopoietic system; sometimes occu with lipoidosis.

his'to-, hist-. 1. A combining for meaning *loom, web.* 2. *In biology,* combining form denoting *tissue.*

his'to·blast. A cell engaged in t formation of tissue.

his''to·chem'is·try. The chemist of the tissues of the body. —**histo chemical,** *adj.*

his''to·di·al'y·sis (hiss''to·dye·al i·sis). The dissolution of organic tissu

his''to·flu''o·res'cence. Fluore cence of tissues during x-ray trea ment produced by the prior administr tion of fluorescing drugs.

his''to·gen·e'sis, his·tog'e·r (hiss·todj'i·nee). Differentiation of ce and cell products from their earlie appearance to the completion of a ma ture tissue. —**histogenet'ic,** *adj.*

his·tog'ra·phy. Description of t. tissues.

his''to·hem'a·tin (hiss''to·hem'u tin, ·hee'muh·tin). Old term f cytochrome, *q.v.*

his'toid, his'ti·oid. 1. Resemblin

tissue. 2. Composed of only one kind of tissue.

his·tol'o·gist. One who is learned in histology.

his·tol'o·gy. The branch of biology which deals with the minute structure of tissues; microscopic anatomy. —**histolog'ic, histolog'ical,** *adj.,* **histolog'ically,** *adv.* **normal h.** The study of healthy tissues. **pathologic h.** The study of diseased tissues. **topographic h.** The study of the minute structure of the organs and especially of their formation from the tissues.

his·tol'y·sis. Disintegration and dissolution of organic tissue. —**histolyt'ic,** *adj.*

his·to'ma. A tumor whose cells are typical of a tissue, such as a fibroma. Also called *histioma.*

his"to·met"a·plas'tic. Causing the transformation of one tissue into another type. See *metaplasia.*

his"to·mor·phol'o·gy. The morphology of the tissues of the body; histology.

his'tone, his'ton. Any one of a group of strongly basic proteins found in cell nuclei, such as thymus histone and globin of hemoglobin.

his·ton'o·my. The laws of the development and arrangement of organic tissue.

his"to·nu'ri·a. The presence of histone in the urine.

his"to·pa·thol'o·gy. The study of minute changes in diseased tissues.

his"to·phys"i·ol'o·gy (hiss"to-fizz"ee-ol'o·jee). The science of tissue functions.

his"to·plas·mo'sis (hiss"to-plaz-mo'sis). A fatal disease caused by the fungus *Histoplasma capsulatum.* It is characterized by fever, anemia, leukopenia, and emaciation. The infection primarily involves the reticuloendothelial system. Syn., *cytomycosis.*

his'to·ry. A written account of events; a record of past events; a narrative or story. **biologic h.** The life story of any animal. **medical h.** The account obtained from a patient as to his health, past and present, and the symptoms of his disease.

his"to·ther'a·py. The remedial use of animal tissues.

his"to·throm'bin. A thrombin formed from connective tissue.

his'to·tome. An instrument for cutting tissue in preparation for microscopic study; a microtome.

his·tot'o·my. 1. The dissection of tissues. 2. The cutting of thin sections of tissues; microtomy.

his"to·tox'ic. Designating a poisonous condition of cells.

his'tri·o·nism. Dramatic action, as seen in some psychoses and psychoneuroses. —**histrion'ic,** *adj.*

hives. Urticaria, *q.v.*

Hl. Latent hypermetropia.

Ho. Chemical symbol for holmium.

hoarse. 1. Harsh, grating; used of sounds. 2. Having a harsh, discordant voice, resulting from an abnormal condition of the larynx or throat. —**hoarse'ness,** *n.*

hoar'y. Gray or white with age; said of the hair. —**hoariness,** *n.*

hob'nail" liv'er. Colloquial term for the more or less shrunken stage of Laennec's cirrhosis, in which nodules of parenchyma, a few millimeters in diameter and fairly uniform in size, project on the surface.

Hodgson, Joseph [*English physician,* 1788–1869]. Described a nonsacculated dilatation of the aortic arch (1815); called *Hodgson's disease.*

ho"do·pho'bi·a. Morbid fear of travel.

hoe. 1. A scraping instrument used in operations for cleft palate. 2. *In dentistry,* an instrument used in cavity preparation.

ho·lan'dric. Referring to genes carried by the Y chromosomes, or to characteristics inherited only through the paternal line.

holarsol. Trade-mark for dichlorophenarsine hydrochloride.

hol"er·ga'si·a (hol"ur·gay'zhuh, -shuh). *In psychobiology,* a mental disorder which disrupts the entire structure of the personality; a major psychotic reaction, as schizophrenia.

hol'mi·um (hole'mee·um, hol'mee·um). Ho = 164.94. A rare earth element.

hol'o-, hol'o-. A combining form signifying *complete, entire.*

hol"o·a·car'di·us. A placental parasitic twin (omphalosite) which lacks a heart. Syn., *acardiacus, acardius.*

hol"o·a·cra'ni·a. Complete absence of the cranial vault, with partial or complete anencephalia.

hol"o·blas'tic. Referring to an egg which divides completely into cells during cleavage.

hol'o·crine (hol'o·kryne, -krin). Designating a gland in which the secretion is formed by disintegration of the glandular cells. See *merocrine.*

hol"o·en'zyme. The complete enzyme formed from its purely protein part, or apoenzyme, and the coenzyme.

hol"o·gas·tros'chi·sis (hol"o·gas-tros'ki·sis). Celosoma involving the entire length of the abdomen.

hol"o·gyn'ic (hol"o·jin'ick, -jy'nick). Descriptive of a mode of inheritance in which a characteristic is transmitted only in the female line from mother to daughter generation after generation, as in the case of attached X chromosomes. Also see *holandric*.

hol″o·ra·chis′chi·sis (hol″o·ra·kis′ki·sis). That type of spina bifida in which the entire spinal canal is open.

hom″a·lo·ceph′a·lus. An individual with a flat head.

hom·at′ro·pine (ho·mat′ro·peen, ·pin). $C_{16}H_{21}NO_3$. An alkaloid prepared from tropine and mandelic acid. It causes dilatation of the pupil and paralysis of accommodation, as does atropine, but its effects pass off more quickly.

hom·ax′i·al, hom″ax·o′ni·al. Having all axes equal.

ho′me·o-, ho′moe·o-. A combining form meaning *like, similar*.

ho″me·o·mor′phous, ho″moe·o·mor′phous. Like or similar in form and structure.

ho″me·o·path′ic al′co·hol. Ethyl alcohol of 87% strength; used in making attenuations.

ho″me·op′a·thy, ho″moe·op′a·thy. A system of healing advocated by Hahnemann, whose motto was *Similia similibus curantur*: likes cure likes. He taught that drugs should be tested upon normal human beings; that symptoms caused by drugs in healthy persons were cured when present in illness by the same drugs; that the effectiveness of the drug was in inverse proportion to the size of the dose; and that eruptive diseases of the skin must be allowed to come out, and should not be driven in. —**homeopath′ic**, *adj.*; **ho′meopath, homeopathist,** *n.*

ho″me·os′ta·sis. The maintenance of steady states in the organism by coordinated physiologic processes which involve the brain, nerves, heart, lungs, kidneys, and spleen. —**homeostat′ic**, *adj.*

ho″me·o·ther′mal, ho·moi″o·ther′mal. Pertaining to animals that are warm-blooded, that maintain a uniform temperature despite variation in the surrounding temperature.

home′sick″ness. Nostalgia; an urgent desire to return to one's home. It may be accompanied by a morbid sluggishness of the functions of the various organs of the body, and may develop into depression and morbid anxiety.

ho″mi·chlo·pho′bi·a. A morbid fear of fog.

hom′i·cide. 1. The killing of a fellow human being; by law, it may be justifiable, excusable, or felonious; felonious homicide is murder or manslaughter. 2. One who takes the life of another. —**homici′dal**, *adj.*

Ho′mo. The genus of mammals belonging to the order Primates and whose sole representative, Homo sapiens, includes all extant races of man.

ho′mo- (ho′mo-, hom′o-), **hom-.** 1. A combining form denoting *common, like, same*. 2. *In chemistry,* a combining form designating *a homolog of a* (specified) *compound*.

ho″mo·cy′clic. Pertaining to or designating closed-chain, or ring, compounds in which all the atoms of the ring are of the same element, usually carbon. See also *carbocyclic, heterocyclic*.

ho″mo·cys′te·ine (ho″mo·sis′tee-een, ·sis·tee′in). $SH.(CH_2)_2.CHNH_2.COOH$. α-Amino-γ-thiol-n-butyric acid. A demethylated product of methionine.

ho″mo·cys′tine (ho″mo·sis′teen, ·tin). $[-S.(CH_2)_2.CHNH_2.COOH]_2.γ,γ′$-Dithiobis(α-amino-butyric acid). The oxidized, disulfide form of homocysteine, analogous to cystine, the oxidized form of cysteine.

ho′moe·o-. See *homeo-*.

ho″mo·er′o·tism, ho″mo·erot′i·cism. The direction of the libido toward a member of the same sex; may find expression in homogenitality, *q.v.*, homosexuality, *q.v.*, or may be repressed. In true homoerotism, the erotic feeling is not sexual or genital, but is well sublimated and expressed in socially acceptable behavior. —**homoerot′ic**, *adj.*, *n.*

ho·mog′e·nate. A suspension of animal tissues that is ground in the all-glass "homogenizer" described by Potter and Elvehjem in 1936.

ho″mo·ge′ne·ous (ho″mo·jee′nee-us, hom″o·). Having the same nature or qualities; of uniform character in all parts. —**homogene′ity**, *n.*

ho″mo·gen″i·tal′i·ty. A form of homoerotism in which the sexual impulses are given genital expression; that sexual perversion marked by genital relations between members of the same sex. —**homogen′ital**, *adj.*

ho″mo·ge·ni·za′tion (ho″mo·jee″ni·zay′shun, ho·modj′i·ni·zay′shun). 1. The act or process of becoming homogeneous. 2. The production of a uniform suspension or emulsion from two or more normally immiscible substances.

ho·mog′e·nous. Of, or derived from, an individual of a related or similar strain of the same species.

ho″mo·gen·tis′ic ac′id (ho″mo·jen·tiz′ick, ·jen·tiss′ick). (OH)$_2C_6H_3$-$CH_2.COOH$. Dihydroxyphenylacetic acid. Formerly called *glycosuric acid*.

hom′o·graft. A tissue graft taken from a donor of the same species as the recipient.

ho·moi′o-. See *homeo-, homo-*.

ho″mo·lat′er·al. On, or pertaining to, the same side.

ho·mol'o·gous. 1. Corresponding in structure, either directly or as referred to a fundamental type. 2. *In chemistry,* being of the same type or series; differing by a multiple, such as CH₂, or an arithmetic ratio in certain constituents. **—hom'olog, hom'ologue, homology,** *n.*

ho''mo·plas''ty. Surgery using grafts from another individual of the same species.

ho''mo·qui'nine (ho''mo·kwye'nine, ·kwi·neen'). A principle from cuprea bark; it can be decomposed into quinine and cupreine.

ho''mo·ser'ine. HOH₂C.CH₂CH-(NH₂) COOH. An amino acid formed in the breakdown of cystathionine in cysteine in animal tissues.

ho''mo·sex''u·al'i·ty. 1. The state of being sexually attracted by members of one's own sex. 2. The state of being in love with one of the same sex. 3. *In psychoanalysis,* a form of homoerotism in which the interest is sexual but sublimated, not receiving genital expression. **—homosex'ual,** *adj., n.*

ho''mo·sul'fa·nil·a·mide. Marfanil.

ho'mo·type, hom'o·type. A part corresponding to a part on the other lateral half of the body.

ho·mun'cu·lus. 1. A little man with normal proportion of parts; a dwarf; a manikin. 2. The human fetus.

Hon·du'ras bark. Cascara amarga.

hon'ey. See *mel.*

hook. A curved instrument for exerting traction. **blunt h.** An instrument for exercising traction upon the fetus in an arrested breech presentation. **squint h.** A right-angled or a curved instrument used in the operation for strabismus for exerting traction on tendons.

hook'worm''. Any nematode belonging to the superfamily Strongyloidea, particularly the *Ancylostoma duodenale* and *Necator americanus.*

hop. See *humulus.*

hora. Hour; abbreviated, h. **h. de·cubitus.** At the hour of going to bed; abbreviated, h. d. **h. somni.** Bedtime; abbreviated, h. s.

hor·de·nine (hor'di·neen, ·nin). An alkaloid from germinating barley.

hor·de·o'lum. A stye; a furuncular inflammation of the connective tissue of the lids, near a hair follicle. **external h.** A circumscribed, acute inflammation on the edge of the lid, produced by staphylococcus infection of one of the sebaceous glands of Zeis. **internal h.** An infection of a tarsal (Meibomian) gland.

hor''me·pho'bi·a. Morbid fear of shock.

hor'mone. A specific chemical product of an organ or of certain cells of

an organ, transported by the blood or other body fluids, and having a specific regulatory effect upon cells remote from its origin. **—hormo'nal, hor·mon'ic,** *adj.* **adrenal cortical h.** A steroid hormone of the adrenal cortex, which has the following biologic activity in adrenalectomized animals: maintenance of life; influence on carbohydrate and protein metabolism; protection against stress; influence on muscular efficiency. Six biologically active steroids have been isolated from the adrenal cortex. **adrenal medullary h.** Epinephrine, *q.v.* **adrenotropic h.** A hormone from the anterior pituitary, which controls the adenohypophysis; adrenotropic factor. Also called *corticotropic h.* **anterior pituitary hormones.** Protein hormones produced by the anterior lobe, the exact number of which is uncertain. The best established are somatotropin, growth-stimulating; thyrotropin, thyroid-stimulating; gonadotropin, gonad-stimulating; adrenotropin or corticotropin, stimulating the adrenal cortex; and lactogenic hormone, a regulator of mammary-gland functions. **chorionic gonadotropic h.** (CH). See chorionic *gonadotropin.* **corpus luteum-stimulating h.** (CLSH). See luteinizing *h.* **diabetogenic h.** Hormone of the anterior pituitary, provoking hyperglycemia. **estrogenic h.** A hormone, found principally in the ovary and also in the placenta, which stimulates the accessory sex structures and the secondary sex characteristics in the female; affects also the anterior pituitary. Production in pregnancy is greatly increased. **follicle-stimulating h.** (FSH). An anterior pituitary hormone which stimulates the gonads, follicular growth in the ovary, and spermatogenesis in the testis. **gonadotropic h.** Any gonad-stimulating hormone. See *gonadotropin.* **growth h.** An organic substance which promotes an increase in the size of the organism or of a part of the organism, as somatotropin. **ketogenic h.** A hormone possibly formed in the anterior pituitary; it stimulates the rate of fatty acid metabolism. Also called *fat-metabolizing h.* **lactation h.** A hormone of the anterior lobe of the pituitary which promotes lactation. See *prolactin.* **luteinizing h.** (LH). An anterior pituitary hormone which stimulates the interstitial cells of the testis and ovary and is concerned with formation of corpora lutea. Acts in concert with the follicle-stimulating hormone. Also called *interstitial-cell-stimulating h.* (ICSH), *corpus luteum-stimulating h.* (CLSH). **N h.** An adrenal factor responsible for changes similar to those induced by the male sex hormone. **ovarian hormones.** Two types of hormone are produced by the ovary: the follicular or estrogenic hormones, estradiol, estrone, and estriol, produce estrus in the spayed animal; the luteal hormone, progesterone, is produced by the corpus luteum. **posterior pituitary hormones.** Two active amino principles have been isolated from pituitrin, an extract of neurohypophysis: beta-hypophamine or pitressin, which stimulates smooth muscle of small arteries, intestine, and bladder; and alpha-hypophamine, known also as pitocin or oxytocin, which causes contraction of uterine muscle. **S h.** One of 11-oxygenated steroids; secreted by the adrenal cortex and related to the conversion of protein to glucose. Also called *sugar h.* **somatotropic h.** See *somatotropin.* **testicular hormones.** Those elaborated by the testis; the best known is testosterone, a steroid which matures and maintains the male genitalia and the secondary sex characteristics. **thyroid h.** Either iodothyroglobulin or one of its component chemical groups, the amino acid compound thyroxin, *q.v.* It accelerates the metabolism of all cells in the body, increasing oxygen consumption; stimulates growth, maturation, and differentiation of tissue; increases nervous irritability, muscular tonus, and circulation; and has a diuretic action. Without thyroid hormone, no cell in the body can function normally. **thyroid-stimulating h.** See thyrotropic *h.* **thyrotropic h.** A hormone of the adenohypophysis which controls the status of the thyroid. **wound hormones.** Substances which can stimulate growth by resumption of division in mature cells.

hor·mo"no·poi·e'sis (hor·mo"no-poy·ee'sis, hor"mo·no·). The production of hormones. **—hormonopoi·et'ic,** *adj.*

hor'mo·zone. One of the hormones which govern metabolism or maintain a stable fluid medium.

horn. 1. A substance composed chiefly of keratin. 2. Cornu, *q.v.* **—horn'y,** *adj.* **cutaneous h.** Cornu cutaneum, *q.v.* **dorsal h.** The posterior column of gray matter in the spinal cord. **lateral h.** The lateral column of gray matter in the spinal cord. **pulpal h.** The extension of the dental pulp into a cusp of a tooth. **ventral h.** The anterior column of gray matter in the spinal cord.

Horner, Johann Friedrich [*Swiss ophthalmologist,* 1831–86]. Described ptosis of the eyelid, due to section of the cervical sympathetic nerve. *Horner's syndrome,* which may result from paralysis of the nerve or from any lesion interrupting the cervical sympathetic chain, includes also constriction of the pupil and vasodilatation, and usually enophthalmos and absence of sweating on the affected side of the head and face. Also called *Bernard-Horner syndrome.*

ho·rop'ter. The sum of all the points seen singly by the two retinas while the fixation point remains stationary. **—horopter'ic,** *adj.*

horse'shoe". A metal bow for the attachment of Steinmann pins and Kirschner wires.

hos'pi·tal. A place or institution designed and equipped to furnish medical and surgical care and treatment to the sick or wounded. **army h.** New designation for "named" station or general hospital in the Zone of the Interior (U. S.). Capacity varies for either type. **station h.,** *q.v.,* furnishes definitive medical care for a post, camp, or station. **general h.,** *q.v.,* furnishes advanced definitive medical care for all military personnel. (Examples: U. S. Army Hospital, Fort Bliss, Tex.; Letterman Army Hospital, Presidio of San Francisco, Calif.) **base h.** An army hospital within the lines of communication, for receiving and caring for sick and wounded returned from field hospitals. *Obs.* **closed h.** One closed to all physicians except those on its own staff. **contagious h.** One restricted to the care of patients with communicable diseases. Syn., *isolation h.* **evacuation h.** A mobile military unit (400 or 750 beds) of a field army, equipped with canvas shelter, to furnish definitive medical and surgical care within the army or corps sector of the combat zone. (Example: 9th Evacuation Hospital.) **field h.** A mobile military unit (300 beds) established in a Theater of Operations, designed primarily to furnish definitive medical care to large troop centers or supply bases. Can be operated as three separate platoons of 100 beds each. (Example: 37th Field Hospital.) **general h.** A fixed military unit (1000 to 2000 beds), established in the Communications Zone, Theater of Operations, designed primarily to furnish advanced definitive medical and surgical care. See *army h.* (Example: 4th General Hospital.) **governmental h.** One supported and administered by a governmental subdivision; as a municipal, county, state, federal army, navy, Public Health Service, or Veterans' Administration hospital. **maternity h.** One restricted to the care of women during pregnancy and parturition. **mobile army surgical h.** A mobile military unit (60 beds) established adjacent to a division *clearing station,* designed primarily to furnish preliminary definitive medical care for all nontransportable casualties therefrom. Acts as a holding section when clearing station moves in combat. (Example: 5th Mobile Army Surgical Hospital.) **station h.** A fixed military unit (25 to 750 beds) established in a Theater of Operations, designed primarily to furnish definitive medical and surgical care in the Communications Zone, Theater of Operations. See *army h.* (Example: 23rd Station Hospital.) **veterinary h.** One for the care of animals.

hos′pi·tal cen′ter. *In military medicine,* an aggregation of one or more general hospitals, often including schools, central laboratories, and utilities, all administered under the central authority of a commanding officer, generally an officer of the Medical Department of the army or navy.

hos′pi·tal corps′man. In the U. S. Navy, an enlisted man of the Medical Department.

hos′pi·tal ship. *In military medicine,* a vessel equipped as a floating hospital for the reception of sick and wounded military personnel not likely to be returned early to combat duty. The hospital ship is used largely for evacuations to a base and does not accompany rapidly moving units, such as a task force.

hos′pi·tal train. A Medical Department railway train, consisting of ward cars and mess and kitchen car, fitted for the evacuation of sick and wounded from the war theater to the Zone of the Interior.

hos′pi·tal u′nit. *In military medicine,* any properly constituted group of Medical Department personnel organized and equipped to provide medical services, as an evacuation hospital or field hospital. **mobile h. u.** Any hospital installation whose organization and equipment permit ready movement under field or combat conditions.

host. 1. The organic body upon or in which parasites live. 2. The relatively normal twin to which a parasitic twin or part is attached. **definitive h.** One in which the sexual stages of the parasite develop. **intermediate h.** One in which the parasite passes its larval or asexual stage.

lot. Of or referring to a substance that is highly radioactive.

lot at′om. An atom with high internal energy or high kinetic energy as a result of a nuclear process.

lot lab′o·ra·tor″y. A laboratory designed with special facilities and precautions for handling large amounts of radioactive material.

Hot′ten·tot a′pron. An overgrowth of the minor lips of the vulva seen in the Hottentots.

hot′ten·tot·ism. An extreme form of stammering.

house phy·si′cian. A physician who lives in a hospital and is constantly available, as an intern.

house staff. The resident physicians and surgeons of a hospital. The term is generally understood to refer to those having the status of intern or resident.

house sur′geon. A surgeon who lives in a hospital and is constantly available.

h. s. *Hora somni;* bedtime.

H-sub′stance. A substance similar to, if not identical with, histamine; believed to play a prominent role in the response of local blood vessels to tissue damage.

Ht. Total hypermetropia.

hum. A low murmuring sound. **venous h.** A continuous blowing or singing sound heard in the large veins of the neck in some cases of anemia. Also called *humming-top murmur.*

hu′man. Pertaining to mankind.

hu′man. A human being.

hu″mer·o·ra′di·al. Pertaining to the humerus and the radius; applied to the joint between these two bones and to the ligaments joining them.

hu″mer·o·scap′u·lar. Pertaining to both the humerus and the scapula.

hu″mer·o·ul′nar. Pertaining to the humerus and the ulna; applied to the joint between these two bones and to the ligaments joining them.

hu′mer·us (pl. *humeri*). The bone of the upper arm, arm proper, or brachium. See Table of Bones in the Appendix. —**humeral,** *adj.*

hu·mid′i·ty. The state or quality of being moist; moisture; dampness. —**hu′mid,** *adj.* **absolute h.** The percentage of water vapor in the air. **relative h.** The amount of water vapor in the air as compared with the total amount the air would hold at a given temperature.

hu′mor. 1. Any fluid or semifluid part of the body. 2. *In old physiology,* one of the four cardinal body fluids, making up the four humors of Galen: the choleric, the melancholic, the phlegmatic, and the sanguine. They were said to determine a person's constitution, disposition, or temperament. 3. Disposition, temperament.

hump′back. Kyphosis.

hu′mu·lin. Lupulin, *q.v.*

hu′mu·lone, hu″mu·lon. $C_{21}H_{30}O_5$. One of the bitter constituents of humulus.

hu′mu·lus. Hops. The dried strobile *of Humulus lupulus* bearing the glandular trichomes known as lupulin.

hunch′back″. Kyphosis.

hun′ger. A sensation of emptiness of the stomach, with a longing for food.

air h. Distressing dyspnea marked by deep, labored respiration, as in acidosis of diabetic coma. Also called *Kussmaul breathing.*

hy′a·lin. A clear, structureless, homogeneous, glassy material occurring normally in matrix of cartilage, vitreous body, colloid of thyroid gland, mucin, glycogen, jelly of Wharton; occurs pathologically in degenerations of connective tissue, epithelial cells, and in the form of mucinous and colloid degenerations, glycogen infiltration, etc. **—hyaline,** *adj.*

hy″a·li·nu′ri·a. Presence of hyalin or of hyaline casts in the urine.

hy″a·li′tis. Inflammation of the vitreous body, or of the hyaloid membrane of the vitreous body.

hy′a·lo-, hyal-. 1. A combining form meaning *glass.* 2. A combining form signifying of or *pertaining to hyalin.*

hy′a·loid. Transparent; glasslike.

hy″a·lo·nyx′is. Puncture of the vitreous body of the eye.

hy″a·lo·pho′bi·a. A morbid fear of glass.

hy′a·lo·plasm. The fluid portion of the protoplasm.

hy″a·lo·se″ro·si′tis. Chronic inflammation of a serous membrane, observed principally in the capsule of the liver and of the spleen, with production of a thick layer of hyalinized, pearly gray, translucent connective tissue, said to resemble icing on a cake.

hy″a·lu·ron′ic ac′id. A viscous mucopolysaccharide occurring in connective tissues and in bacterial capsules.

hy″a·lu·ron′i·dase. An enzyme occurring in pathogenic bacteria, snake venoms, sperm, etc. It causes the breakdown of hyaluronic acid in protective polysaccharide barriers, promoting invasion of cells and tissues by the invading agent; it is a spreading factor. Syn., *invasin.*

hy′brid. The offspring of parents belonging to different species, varieties, or genotypes. **—hybridism, hybrid′ity,** *n.*

hy″brid·i·za′tion. Crossbreeding.

hy″dan·to′ic ac′id. NH₂CONHCH₂COOH. An acid resulting from the union of aminoacetic acid and carbamic acid.

hy·dan·to·in (high·dan′to·in, high″-dan·to′in). Glycolyl urea. A crystalline substance derived from allantoin and related to urea.

hydase. Trade-mark for a brand of hyaluronidase.

hy·dat′id (high·dat′id). 1. A cyst formed in tissues due to growth of the larval stage of *Echinococcus granulosus* (dog tapeworm), containing a clear watery fluid, lined by an inner germinal cellular layer and an outer laminated layer of hyaline material. Formation of scolices in the germinal layer is followed by a deposit of pinched-off scolices and of hooklets in the fluid. 2. A cystic remnant of an embryonal structure. **—hydat′ic, hydatid′iform,** *adj.* **h. of Morgagni.** A small, cystic remnant of the Müllerian duct attached by a fibrous stalk to the fimbriated end of the oviduct, or, in the male, to the head of the epididymis. **secondary h.** Echinococcus cyst due to the rupture of another cyst and deposit of germinal cells and scolices in the neighborhood. **stalked h.** See *h. of Morgagni.*

hy″da·tid′o·cele. Scrotal hernia containing echinococcus cysts.

hydeltra. A trade-mark for prednisolone.

hyd″no·car′pic ac′id. An acid, C₁₆H₂₇COOH, occurring as the glyceride in chaulmoogra oil.

hyd″no·car′pus oil. Chaulmoogra oil.

hy″dra·bam′ine phe·nox″y·meth′yl pen″i·cil′lin. Chiefly, the phenoxymethyl penicillin salt of N,N′-bis-(dehydroabietyl)ethylenediamine. See *compocillin-V hydrabamine.*

hy·drac′id (high·dras′id). An acid containing no oxygen.

hy′dra·gogue, hy′dra·gog. 1. Causing the discharge of watery fluid. 2. A purgative that causes copious liquid discharges.

hy·dral′a·zine hy″dro·chlo′-ride. 1-Hydrazinophthalazine hydrochloride, a hypotensive agent. See *apresoline hydrochloride.*

hy·dran′ge·a (high·drain′juh, high·dran′-). The dried rhizome and roots of *Hydrangea arborescens.*

hy″drar·gyr″o·pho′bi·a. A morbid fear of mercurial medicines.

hy″drar·thro′sis. An accumulation of fluid in a joint. **intermittent h.** A condition characterized by acute regularly recurring effusions of fluid into a joint cavity.

hy′drase. An enzyme which removes or adds water to a substrate without hydrolyzing it.

hy·dras′tine (high·dras′teen, ·tin). An alkaloid from hydrastis.

hy·dras′ti·nine (high·dras′ti·neen, ·nin). An oxidation product of hydrastine.

hy·dras′tis. The rhizome and roots of *Hydrastis canadensis*, which contain the alkaloids hydrastine, berberine, and canadine. Syn., *yellow root.* Also called *goldenseal.*

hy′drate. 1. A compound containing water in chemical combination, water of hydration. 2. Hydroxide. *Obs.* **—hydrated,** *adj.;* **hydra′tion,** *n.*

hy·drau′lics. The science which

deals with the mechanical properties of liquids.

hy′dra·zine (high′druh·zeen, ·zin). 1. $H_2N.NH_2$. Diamine; a colorless liquid, soluble in water, having a strong alkaline reaction. 2. One of a class of bodies derived from hydrazine by replacing one or more hydrogen atoms by a radical.

hy″dre·lat′ic. Pertaining to the secretory effect of nerves upon glands, causing them to discharge the watery part of their secretion. Also called *hydrokinetic.*

hy·dre′mi·a, hy·drae′mi·a (high-dree′mee·uh). A condition of the blood in which the fluid content is increased but the total amount of the blood does not increase proportionately. —**hy·dremic,** *adj.*

hy″dren·ceph′a·lo·cele. Protrusion, through a defect in the cranium, of a sac and brain substance in which a cystic cavity contains fluid.

hy″dren·ceph″a·lo·me·nin′go·cele. A hernia through a cranial defect of meninges and brain substance, fluid filling the space between these.

hy′dride. A compound containing hydrogen united to a more positive element or to a radical.

hy″dri·od′ic ac′id. The gas hydrogen iodide, HI, or an aqueous solution thereof.

hy·dri′on (high·dry′on, high′dree·on). Hydrogen in the ionized form.

hy′dro-, hydr-. 1. A combining form meaning *water.* 2. *In chemistry,* a combining form denoting *the presence of hydrogen or the addition of hydrogen to a compound.* 3. *In medicine,* a combining form denoting *a disease characterized by an accumulation of water or other fluid in a bodily part.*

hy·dro′a (high·dro′uh, hid·ro′uh). Any skin disease characterized by vesicles or bullae. **h. vacciniforme.** A skin disease, occurring in the summer on the exposed parts, usually in young males. It is characterized by vesicles and crusted ulcers, and gradually disappears following puberty. Also called *h. aestivale, summer prurigo.*

hy″dro·bro′mate. A hydrobromic acid salt; a hydrobromide.

hy″dro·bro′mic. Composed of hydrogen and bromine.

hy″dro·bro′mic ac′id. 1. Hydrogen bromide, HBr; a heavy, colorless gas with a pungent irritating odor. 2. An aqueous solution of HBr.

hy″dro·bro′mide. A salt of hydrobromic acid.

hy″dro·car′bon. Any compound composed only of hydrogen and carbon. **saturated h.** One that has the maximum number of hydrogen atoms; that is, without double or triple bonds between carbon atoms. **unsatu-**rated h. One that has one or more double or triple bonds between carbon atoms.

hy′dro·cele. An accumulation of fluid in the sac of the tunica vaginalis of the testis. In adults, the cause is unknown and the fluid is clear, slightly viscid, and contains 6–10% of solids, including proteins, salts, and sometimes cholesterol. **spermatic h.** Accumulation of spermatic fluid in the tunica vaginalis of the testis; caused by the rupture of a spermatocele.

hy″dro·ce·lec′to·my. Surgical removal of part of the tunica vaginalis for the cure of hydrocele.

hy″dro·ceph′a·ly. An increase in the volume of cerebrospinal fluid within the skull. The term is commonly applied to distentions of the ventricular system by cerebrospinal fluid which cannot escape into the subarachnoid space, is blocked in the subarachnoid pathways, or cannot be absorbed into the venous system. Also called *hydrocephalus.* —**hydrocephal′ic,** *adj.* **communicating h.** A form in which there is normal communication between the ventricles and the subarachnoid space. **congenital h.** A progressive form in infancy. Also called *chronic h., infantile h.* **external h.** An increased accumulation of fluid in the subarachnoid space, or rarely, in the subdural space; usually a passive process due to atrophy of the brain. **internal h.** That due to obstruction of the normal circulation of cerebrospinal fluid from the ventricles to the subarachnoid space. Also called *obstructive h., noncommunicating h.*

hy″dro·chi′none (high″dro·kigh′nohn, ·kin′ohn). See *hydroquinine.*

hy″dro·chlo′rate. An older name for salts formed by hydrochloric acid with certain organic nitrogenous bases, especially alkaloids.

hy″dro·chlo′ric ac′id. 1. Hydrogen chloride, HCl, a colorless gas of pungent odor which can be liquefied under pressure. 2. An aqueous solution containing 35% to 38% of HCl.

hy″dro·chlo′ride. Term for that formed by the reaction of hydrochloric acid with organic nitrogenous bases.

hy″dro·chol″er·e′sis (high″dro·kol′er·e′sis). Choleresis characterized by increased water output, or by bile relatively low in specific gravity, viscosity, and total solids. —**hydrocholeret′ic,** *adj.* and *n.*

hy″dro·col′li·dine (high″dro·kol′i·deen, ·din). A poisonous ptomaine from putrefying flesh, such as mackerel, horseflesh, and oxflesh.

hy″dro·con′qui·nine (high″dro·kon′kwi·neen, ·nin). Hydroquinidine.

hy″dro·cor′ti·sone. A steroid hormone isolated from adrenal cortex or prepared synthetically, used in treating rheumatoid arthritis and osteoarthritis. Also see *cortisone, glucocorticoid*. Syn., *17-hydroxycorticosterone*. See *cortef, cortril, hydrocortone*. **h. acetate.** The 21-acetate ester of hydrocortisone.

hydrocortone. A trade-mark for hydrocortisone.

hy″dro·co·tar′nine (high″dro-ko-tahr′neen, -nin). A crystalline alkaloid derived from narcotine and occurring in small amount in opium.

hy″dro·cu′pre·ine. $C_{19}H_{24}N_2O_2$. A reduction product of cupreine; employed in synthesis of ethylhydrocupreine and other similar medicinals.

hy″dro·cy·an′ic ac′id (high″dro-sigh-an′ick, high″dro-see-an′ick). Hydrogen cyanide, HCN; used as a fumigant. Syn., *prussic acid*.

hy″dro·dip″so·ma′ni·a. Periodic attacks of uncontrollable thirst; often seen in schizophrenia and epilepsy.

hy″dro·dy·nam′ics (high″dro-dye-nam′icks, -di-nam′icks). That branch of mechanics which deals with liquids.

hy″dro·er·got′i·nine (·ur-got′i-neen, -nin). Ergotoxine.

hy″dro·flu·or′ic ac′id. 1. Hydrogen fluoride, HF; a highly corrosive, colorless gas. 2. An aqueous solution containing about 50% of HF.

hy′dro·gel. A colloidal gel with water as the dispersion medium.

hy′dro·gen. H = 1.0080. A univalent, inflammable, gaseous element; the lightest element known. Three isotopes of hydrogen (namely, protium, deuterium, and tritium, having atomic masses of approximately one, two, and three, respectively) exist. **h. acceptor.** A substance which, on reduction, accepts hydrogen atoms from another substance called a hydrogen donor. See *coenzyme.* **h. arsenide.** Arsine. AsH₃. **h. bonds.** Chemical bonds resulting from the attraction of two electronegative atoms for one proton (a hydrogen nucleus). The bonds are relatively weak and are responsible for association of molecules. Syn., *h. bridges.* **h. donor.** A substance which, on oxidation, gives up hydrogen atoms to another substance called a hydrogen acceptor. **h. ion.** The positively charged nucleus of the hydrogen atom, a proton. Acids are characterized by their ability to liberate hydrogen ions when in aqueous solution. Symbol, H⁺. See *hydronium.* **h. sulfide.** H₂S. A colorless, highly toxic gas of unpleasant odor. **light h.** Protium.

hy″dro·gen·a′tion. The process of combining with hydrogen.

hy″dro·gym·nas′tics. Active exercises performed in water; the buoyancy thus obtained enables weakened muscles to move the limbs more easily.

hy″dro·hem″a·to·ne·phro′sis (high″dro-hem″uh-to-ni-fro′sis, high″-dro-hee″muh-to-). The presence of blood and urine in a dilated renal pelvis.

hy″dro·ki·net′ic (high″dro-ki-net′-ick, -kigh-net′ick). Concerning or producing water transfer during glandular secretion; hydrelatic.

hy″dro·ki·net′ics. The science of the motion of liquids.

hy′drol. The single molecule of water, H₂O. Sometimes called *monohydrol*. See *dihydrol, trihydrol*.

hy″dro·lac·tom′e·ter. An instrument used in estimating the percentage of water in milk.

hy′dro·lase (high′dro-lace, -laze). An enzyme causing hydrolysis.

hy·drol′o·gy. Knowledge of water in the widest sense.

hy·drol′y·sis. Any reaction with water, frequently of the type AB + HOH → AOH + HB, the latter being the reverse reaction of neutralization. —**hydrolyt′ic,** *adj.*; **hy′drolyze,** *v.*

hy′dro·lyte. The substance undergoing hydrolysis.

hy·drol′y·zate, hy·drol′y·sate. The product of hydrolysis.

hy″dro·me·nin′go·cele. 1. A cystic tumor of the meninges protruding through the cranium. 2. A form of spina bifida in which the sac contains cerebrospinal fluid.

hy·drom′e·ter. An instrument for determining the specific gravity of liquids. —**hydromet′ric,** *adj.*; **hy·drom′etry,** *n.*

hy″dro·mi″cro·ceph′a·ly. Microcephaly with increased cerebrospinal fluid.

hy″dro·my·e′li·a (high″dro-migh-ee′lee-uh). Dilatation of the central canal of the spinal cord which contains an increased quantity of cerebrospinal fluid. **acquired h.** That due to tumors in the cerebellum or injuries to the cord. **congenital h.** Usually a diffuse dilatation of the canal with atrophy, mainly of the gray matter.

hy″dro·my′e·lo·cele′. 1. Excessive accumulation of fluid in the central canal of the spinal cord. 2. Hydromyelia.

hy″dro·ne·phro′sis. A collection of urine in the distended pelvis of the kidney, from obstructed outflow. The pressure of the fluid in time causes atrophy of the kidney structure, and the whole organ is converted into a large cyst. —**hydronephrot′ic,** *adj.*

hy·dro′ni·um. The solvated hydrogen ion, H⁺(H₂O) or H₃O⁺, considered to be present in aqueous solutions of all acids.

hy·drop′a·thy. The internal and external use of water for the attempted cure of all diseases. —**hydropath'ic**, *adj.*

hy″dro·per″i·car·di'tis. Pericarditis accompanied by serous effusion into the pericardium.

hy·dro·per″i·car'di·um. A collection of a serous effusion in the pericardial sac.

hy″dro·per″i·to·ne'um. An accumulation of nonpurulent, watery fluid in the peritoneal cavity; ascites.

hy'dro·phil, hy'dro·phile (high'-dro·fill, ·file). A substance, usually in the colloidal state, which is capable of combining with, or attracting, water. —**hydrophil'ic**, *adj.*

hy'dro·phobe. 1. A substance, usually in the colloidal state, which lacks affinity for water. 2. One who has hydrophobia. —**hydropho'bic**, *adj.*

hy″dro·pho'bi·a. 1. Morbid fear of water. 2. Rabies, *q.v.* —**hydropho'bic**, *adj.*

hy″dro·pho″bo·pho'bi·a. An intense dread of hydrophobia; a condition sometimes producing a state simulating true hydrophobia.

hy'dro·phone. An instrument used in auscultatory percussion, the sound being conveyed to the ear through a liquid column.

hy″droph·thal'mos, hy″droph·thal'mi·a, hy″droph·thal'mus. An increase in the fluid contents of the eye, causing the organ to become distended. Syn., *buphthalmia.* See infantile *glaucoma.*

hy″dro·pneu″ma·to'sis (high″-dro·new″muh·to'sis). A collection of liquid and gas within the tissues.

hy″dro·pneu″mo·per″i·car'di·um. A collection of a serous effusion and gas in the pericardial sac.

hy″dro·pneu″mo·per″i·to·ne'um. A collection of serum and gas within the peritoneal cavity.

hy″dro·pneu″mo·tho'rax. The presence of serous fluid and gas in the pleural cavity.

hy'drops. Accumulation of the fluid of edema, or more rarely, of other watery fluids. —**hydrop'ic**, *adj.* **h. gravidarum.** Edema in pregnancy. **h. of the gallbladder.** Distention of the gallbladder by a clear, or slightly cloudy, somewhat mucinous, white or colorless thin fluid.

hy″dro·py″o·ne·phro'sis. Distention of the pelvis of the kidney with urine and pus.

hy″dro·quin'i·dine (high″dro·kwin'i·deen, ·din). An alkaloid in cinchona bark. Syn., *hydroconquinine.*

hy″dro·quin'ine (high″dro·kwin'een, ·in). An alkaloid obtained from cinchona, and frequently contaminating quinine. Also called *dihydroquinine.*

hy″dro·qui·none' (high″dro·kwi·nohn', ·kwin'ohn). 1,4-$C_6H_4(OH)_2$. Para-dihydroxybenzene.

hy″dror·rhe'a. A flow of watery liquid. **h. gravidarum.** A discharge of fluid from the vagina prior to parturition; often mistaken by the patient for amniotic fluid. The so-called forewaters.

hy″dro·sal'pinx. A distention of the uterine tube with fluid.

hy″dro·sat'ur·nism. Lead poisoning that is caused by lead in water supply.

hy'dro·sol. A colloid system in which water is the dispersion medium.

hy″dro·sol'u·ble. Soluble in water.

hy″dro·stat'ics. That branch of hydrodynamics which treats of the properties of liquids in a state of equilibrium. —**hydrostatic**, *adj.*

hy″dro·sul·fu'ric ac'id. 1. Hydrogen sulfide, H_2S. 2. Dithionic acid, $H_2S_2O_6$. 3. An organic acid of the formula R.CS.SH.

hy″dro·sy·rin″go·my·e'li·a (·si·ring″go·migh·ee'lee·uh). Dilatation of the central canal of the spinal cord by watery effusion, accompanied by degeneration and formation of cavities.

hy″dro·tax'is. Response of organisms to stimulus of moisture. Also see *hydrotropism.*

hy″dro·ther″a·peu'tics (high″-dro·therr″uh·pew'ticks). Hydrotherapy.

hy″dro·ther'a·py. The treatment of disease by means of water; hydrotherapeutics.

hy″dro·ther'mal. Pertaining to warm water; said of springs.

hy″dro·thi″o·nu'ri·a. The presence of hydrogen sulfide in the urine.

hy″dro·tho'rax. A collection of serous fluid in the pleural space. —**hydrothorac'ic** (high″dro·thor·ass'-ick), *adj.*

hy·dro'tis (high·dro'tis). Dropsy of, or effusion into, the external ear, the middle ear, or the inner ear, seldom in combination.

hy″dro·tro'pic a'gents. Emulsifying agents, colloidal or crystalloidal.

hy·drot'ro·pism (high·drot'ro·pizum, high″dro·tro'piz·um). *In botany*, the tendency of a growing plant or organ to turn either away from, or toward, moisture.

hy·drot'ro·py. *In physiology*, the property of bringing insoluble compounds into solution.

hy″dro·tym'pa·num. Serous effusion into the cavity of the middle ear.

hy″dro·u·re'ter (high″dro·yooree'tur, ·yoor'i·tur). Abnormal distention of the ureter with urine, usually due to partial obstruction.

hy'drous. Containing water.

hy·drox'ide (high·drock'side, ·sid). A compound formed by the union of a metal, or of an inorganic or organic radical, with one or more hydroxyl (OH) groups.

hy·drox'y- (high·drock'see-). *In chemistry*, a combining form indicating *the hydroxyl group —OH.*

hy·drox'y·a·ce'tic ac'id. Glycolic acid.

hy·drox'y am·phet'a·mine hy''dro·bro'mide. *p*-(2-Aminopropyl)phenol hydrobromide, a sympathomimetic agent. See *paredrine hydrobromide.*

hy·drox'y·ap'a·tite. 3Ca₃(PO₄)₂·Ca(OH)₂. The basic inorganic constituent of bone.

hy·drox'y·ben'zene. Phenol.

β-hy·drox'y·bu·tyr'ic ac'id. CH₃.CHOH.CH₂COOH. An organic acid intermediary in fat metabolism. It is a member of a group of compounds called acetone bodies or ketone bodies.

17-hy·drox''y·cor''ti·cos'te·rone. Hydrocortisone.

17-hy·drox''y-11-de·hy''dro·cor''ti·cos'te·rone. A steroid hormone with adrenal cortical activity, often effective in the treatment of rheumatoid arthritis. Syn., *Kendall's Compound E, cortisone.* See *cortone.*

17-hy·drox''y-11-des·ox''y·cor''ti·cos'te·rone. A steroid hormone possessing adrenal cortical activity.

hy·drox'y·di'one so'di·um suc'cin·ate. Sodium 21-hydroxypregnane-3,20-dione succinate, a hypnotic and general anesthetic. See *viadril.*

hy·drox'y·glu·tam'ic ac'id. HO·OCCH₂CH(OH)CH₂(NH₂)COOH. An amino acid resulting from the hydrolysis of protein.

hy·drox'yl (high·drock'sil). The univalent radical OH, the combination of which with a basic element or radical forms a hydroxide.

hy·drox'yl·a·mine' (high·drock''sil·uh·meen', ·sil·am'een). NH₂OH. A basic substance, known only in solution in water or in combination with acids.

hy·drox'y·ly'sine. Common name for the amino acid, α-ε-diamino-β-hydroxy-n-caproic acid.

hy·drox'y·pro'line (high·drock''see·pro'leen, ·lin). One of the natural amino acids.

hy·drox'y·quin'o·line (·kwin'o·leen, ·lin). Oxyquinoline.

5-hy·drox'y·tryp'ta·mine. 5-Hydroxy-3-(β-aminoethyl)indole. Syn., *serotonin.*

hy·drox'y·zine hy''dro·chlo'ride. 1-(p-Chlorobenzhydryl)-4-[2-(2-hydroxyethoxy)ethyl]piperazine dihydrochloride, a psychotherapeutic agent. See *atarax hydrochloride.*

hy·dru'ri·a (high·droor'ee·uh). The passage of large amounts of urine of low specific gravity, as in diabetes insipidus; polyuria. **—hydruric,** *adj.*

Hygeia. In Greek mythology, the goddess of health; daughter of Asclepius.

hy'giene. The science that treats of the laws of health and the methods of their observation. **—hygien'ic,** *adj.* **industrial h.** That branch concerned with the promotion of healthful conditions in industry, the prevention of occupational accidents and sickness, and measures for their emergency treatment. **mental h.** That branch of hygiene dealing with the preservation of mental and emotional health.

hy'gi·en·ist. One who specializes in the science of hygiene. **dental h.** One trained to practice dental prophylaxis.

hy'gro-, hygr-. A combining form denoting *moisture* or *humidity.*

hy·gro'ma. A cystic cavity derived from distended lymphatics and filled with lymph; a congenital malformation usually seen in young children. Also called *h. cysticum colli, cystic h., multiloculated h.* **—hygrom'atous,** *adj.*

hy·grom'e·ter. An instrument for determining quantitatively the amount of moisture in the air. **—hygrome·try,** *n.*

hy'gro·pho'bi·a. Morbid fear of liquids or of moisture.

hy'gro·scope. An instrument for indicating the humidity of the atmosphere. **—hygros'copy,** *n.*

hy''gro·sto'mi·a. Chronic salivation.

hy'lic. Of or pertaining to matter; material.

hy'lo-, hyl-. A combining form meaning *wood, material, substance, matter.*

hy''lo·pho'bi·a. Morbid fear of forests.

hy''lo·trop'ic. Denoting the capacity of a substance for changing its form without changing its composition.

hy''lo·zo'ism. The theory that all matter is endowed with life.

hy'men. A membranous partition partially blocking the orifice of the vagina. The opening may be of several forms, such as circular, crescentic, etc.; it may be multiple. The hymen may be entirely lacking, or it may be imperforate. **—hymenal,** *adj.*

hy''me·nec'to·my. Excision of the hymen.

hy''me·ni'tis. Inflammation of the hymen.

Hy''me·nol'e·pis. A genus of tapeworms. **H. nana.** A species, cosmopolitan in distribution and known as the dwarf tapeworm, which infests man.

hy''me·nor'rha·phy. 1. Suture of the hymen to occlude the vagina. 2. Suture of any membrane.

hy·men'o·tome. A surgical instrument used for cutting membranes.

hy''me·not'o·my. 1. Surgical incision of the hymen. 2. Dissection or anatomy of membranes.

hy'o-, hy-. *In anatomy,* a combining form meaning u, indicating *connection with the hyoid bone or arch.*

hy''o·ep''i·glot'tic, hy''o·ep''i·glot·tid'e·an. Relating to the hyoid bone and the epiglottis.

hy''o·glos'sal. 1. Pertaining to the hyoglossus. 2. Extending from the hyoid bone to the tongue.

hy''o·glos'sus. An extrinsic muscle of the tongue arising from the hyoid bone. See Table of Muscles in the Appendix.

hy'oid. 1. A bone between the root of the tongue and the larnyx, supporting the tongue and giving attachment to numerous muscles. See Table of Bones in the Appendix. 2. Concerned with the definitive hyoid, as the hyoid arch of the embryo.

hy'o·man·dib'u·lar. Relating to the hyoid and mandibular arches of the embryo or to the groove and pouch between them.

hy'os·cine (high'o-seen, ·sin). Scopolamine.

hy''os·cy'a·mine (high''o-sigh'uh-meen, ·min). $C_{17}H_{23}NO_3$. An alkaloid occurring in many of the Solanaceae, notably belladonna, hyoscyamus, and stramonium. It is the levorotatory component of the racemic atropine.

hy''os·cy'a·mus. Henbane. The dried leaf, with or without flowering tops, of *Hyoscyamus niger;* it yields the alkaloids hyoscyamine and scopolamine.

hyp''al·bu''mi·no'sis (hip''alb-yoo''mi·no'sis, high''palb-yoo''mi·). Diminution in the amount of albumin in the blood.

hyp''al·ge'si·a (hip''al·jee'zee-uh, high''pal·). Diminished sensitivity to pain. Also called *hypalgia.* —**hyp·algesic,** *adj.*

hyp·am'ni·on (hip-am'nee-on, high-pam'·). A small amount of amniotic fluid.

hy·paph'o·rine (high-paf'o-reen, -rin). $C_{14}H_{18}N_2O_3$; the betaine of tryptophan, occurring in various *Erythrina* species; it is a convulsive poison.

hypaque sodium. Trade-mark for diatrizoate sodium.

hy''pas·the'ni·a (high''pass-thee'nee-uh, hip''ass·). A slight loss of strength.

hy·pen''gy·o·pho'bi·a (high-pen''jee-o-fo'bee-uh). Morbid fear of responsibility.

hy'per-. 1. A prefix signifying *abnormal* or *excessive.* 2. *In anatomy* and in *zoology,* a prefix denoting *position above.*

hy''per·ab·duc'tion. Excessive abduction of a limb or part. Syn., *superabduction.*

hy''per·ac''id·am·i·nu'ri·a. The presence of an excessive amount of amino acids in the urine.

hy''per·ac·id'i·ty. Excessive acidity.

hy''per·ac·tiv'i·ty. Excessive or abnormal activity.

hy''per·a·cu'i·ty. Unusual sensory acuity or sharpness, especially of vision.

hy''per·a·cu'si·a (high''pur-a-cue'-shuh, high''pur-a-koo'·), **hy''per·a·cu'sis** (high''pur-a-cue'sis, -a-koo'sis). Abnormal acuteness of the sense of hearing; auditory hyperesthesia.

hy''per·ad'e·no'sis. Enlargement of the lymph nodes.

hy''per·ad·re'nal·ism. A condition due to hyperfunction of the adrenal gland; marked by a tendency toward increased basal metabolism, decreased sugar tolerance, glycosuria, and adrenal hyperplasia; occurs chiefly in relation to adrenal cortical tumors.

hy''per·ad·re'ni·a. Symptoms caused by overactivity of the adrenal gland.

hy''per·al·ge'si·a (high''pur-al-jee'-zee-uh, ·see-uh). Excessive sensitivity to pain. Also called *hyperalgia.* —**hyperalgesic,** *adj.*

hy''per·al''i·men·ta'tion. Overfeeding; superalimentation.

hy''per·al''i·men·to'sis. Any disease due to excessive eating.

hy''per·an''a·ki·ne'si·a (·an''uh-ki-nee'shuh, ·zhuh). Excessive activity of a part. **h. ventriculi.** Exaggerated activity of the gastric functions.

hy''per·a'phi·a. Excessive sensitivity to touch. —**hyperaph'ic,** *adj.*

hy''per·az''o·te'mi·a. The presence of an excessive amount of nitrogenous substances in the blood.

hy''per·az''o·tu'ri·a. An excess of nitrogenous matter in the urine.

hy''per·bil''i·ru''bi·ne'mi·a (·bil''i·roo''bi·nee'mee-uh, ·buy''li·). Excessive amount of bilirubin in the blood.

hy''per·bu'li·a. Exaggerated willfulness.

hy''per·cal·ce'mi·a, hy''per·cal·cae'mi·a. Excessive quantity of calcium in the blood. Syn., *calcemia.*

hy''per·cal''ci·nu'ri·a, hy''per·cal''ci·u'ri·a, hy''per·cal·cu'ri·a. An abnormally high level of calcium in the urine. **essential h.** A high level in the absence of acidosis. Also called *idiopathic h.*

hy''per·cal''ci·u'ri·a. See *hypercalcinuria.*

hy''per·cal·cu'ri·a. See *hypercalcinuria.*

hy''per·cap'ni·a. Excessive amount of carbon dioxide in the blood, causing overactivity in the respiratory center.

hy″per·ca·thar′sis. Excessive purgation of the bowels. **—hypercathartic,** *adj.*

hy″per·ca·thex′is. Excessive concentration of the psychic energy upon a particular focus.

hy″per·ce·men·to′sis. Excessive formation of cementum on the root of a tooth.

hy″per·ce″nes·the′si·a (·see″ness-thee′zhuh, ·sen″ess·). A feeling of extreme well-being; euphoria.

hy″per·chlo·re′mi·a, hy″per·chlo·rae′mi·a. An increase in the sodium chloride content of the blood.

hy″per·chlor·hy′dri·a (high″pur-klor·high′dree·uh, ·hid′ree·uh). Excessive secretion of hydrochloric acid in the stomach; may be a manifestation of neuroticism.

hy″per·cho·les″ter·e′mi·a, hy″per·cho·les″ter·ae′mi·a (·ko-les″tur·ee′mee·uh). Excess of cholesterol in the blood.

hy″per·cho′li·a (high″pur·ko′lee-uh). Excessive secretion of bile.

hy″per·chro′ma·tism. The excessive formation of the pigment of the skin.

hy″per·chy′li·a (high″pur·kigh′lee-uh). Excess of secretion; excessive formation of chyle.

hy″per·cry″al·ge′si·a (·cry″al-jee′zee·uh, ·see·uh). Abnormal sensitivity to cold. Syn., *hypercryesthesia.*

hy″per·dis·ten′tion. Forcible or extreme distention.

hy″per·dy·na′mi·a (high″pur·dye-nay′mee·uh, ·dye·nam′ee·uh). Excessive strength or exaggeration of function, as of nerves or muscles. **—hyperdynam′ic,** *adj.*

hy″per·em′e·sis. Excessive vomiting. **—hyperemet′ic,** *adj.* **h. gravidarum.** Pernicious vomiting in pregnancy. **h. lactentium.** Vomiting of nurslings.

hy″per·e′mi·a. An increased content of blood in a part, with distention of the blood vessels. Hyperemia may be active, when due to active dilatation of blood vessels, or passive, when the drainage is hindered. **Active hyperemia** occurs in physiologic activity of glands or other organs and in inflammation. **Passive hyperemia** occurs in congestive heart failure and in other conditions where veins are compressed or occluded. **—hyperemic,** *adj.*

hy″per·er′gi·a. Increased functional activity.

hy″per·er·gy. An altered state of reactivity, in which the response is more marked than usual; hypersensitivity. It is one form of allergy or pathergy.

hy″per·es·the′si·a, hy″per·aes·the′si·a (high″pur·ess·thee′zhuh,

·zee·uh). Excessive sensibility. **—hyperesthet′ic,** *adj.*

hy″per·ex·ten′sion. Overextension of a limb or part for the correction of deformity or for the retention of fractured bones in proper position and alignment.

hy″per·flex′ion. Overflexion of a limb or part of the body.

hy″per·func′tion. Excessive function.

hy″per·geu′si·a (high″pur·gew′see-uh, ·jew′see·uh). Abnormal acuteness of the sense of taste.

hy″per·glob′u·li·ne′mi·a. Increased amount of globulin in the blood plasma.

hy″per·gly·ce′mi·a, hy″per·gly·cae′mi·a (·gly·see′mee·uh). Excess of sugar in the blood. **—hyperglycemic,** *adj.*

hy″per·gly″cor·rha′chi·a (·glye″-ko·ray′kee·uh, ·rack′ee·uh). Excess of sugar in the cerebrospinal fluid.

hy″per·gly″co·su′ri·a. The presence of excessive amounts of sugar in the urine.

hy″per·gon′ad·ism. Excessive internal secretion of the sexual glands (testes or ovaries).

hy″per·he·do′ni·a. 1. An excessive feeling of pleasure in the gratification of a desire. 2. Sexual erethism. Syn., *hyperhedonism.*

hy″per·hi·dro′sis (high″pur·hi-dro′sis, ·high·dro′sis), **hy″per·i·dro′sis.** Excessive sweating; may be localized or generalized, chronic or acute; the sweat often accumulates in visible drops on the skin. Syn., *hidrosis, ephidrosis, sudatoria, polyhidrosis.*

hy″per·his″ta·mi·ne′mi·a. An increased amount of histamine in the blood.

hy″per·in″su·lin·ism. The syndrome of spontaneous, intermittent, or continuous loss of consciousness, with or without convulsions, from excessive production of insulin by the pancreatic islets.

hy″per·in″vo·lu′tion. A rapid return to less than normal size of an organ that has been enlarged, as of the uterus after delivery.

hy″per·ker″a·to′sis. 1. Hypertrophy of the cornea. 2. Hypertrophy of the horny layer of the skin, usually associated with hypertrophy of the granular and prickle-cell layers. **—hyperkeratot′ic,** *adj.*

hy″per·ke″to·nu′ri·a. The presence of an excess of ketone in the urine.

hy″per·ki·ne′mi·a. A condition marked by a greater cardiac output of blood than normal.

hy″per·ki·ne′si·a (high″pur·ki-nee′shuh, high″pur·kigh·nee′·), **hy″-**

per·ki·ne′sis (high″pur·ki·nee′sis, ·kigh·nee′sis). Excessive movement, as that associated with muscular spasm. **—hyperkinet′ic,** *adj.* **essentialh.** A condition seen in children, marked by excessive and sustained voluntary and involuntary movements; they are not, however, disorganized or dissociated as they are in the choreas and athetoses.

hy″per·lac·ta′tion. Excessive or prolonged secretion of milk.

hy″per·ley′dig·ism. Abnormally high secretion of the interstitial or Leydig cells of the testes.

hy″per·li·pe′mi·a. Excess of fat in the blood.

hy″per·li·thu′ri·a. Excess of lithic acid in the urine.

hy″per·lo′gi·a (high″pur·lo′juh, ·jee·uh). Excessive or maniacal loquacity.

hy″per·ma′ni·a. An advanced maniacal state; a mania which has progressed beyond the acute stage. Marked by extreme excitation and acceleration of activity. **—hypermanic,** *adj.,* *n.*

hy″per·mas′ti·a. Overgrowth of the mammary gland.

hy″per·ma·ture′. Overmature, overripe, as a cataract.

hy″per·men″or·rhe′a. Excessive menstrual flow. Syn., *menorrhagia.* To be distinguished from polymenorrhea, metrorrhagia, intermenstrual flow, *q.v.*

hy″per·me·tro′pi·a. The condition of the refractive media of the eye in which, with suspended accommodation, the focus of parallel rays of light is behind the retina. It is due to an abnormally short anteroposterior diameter of the eye or to a subnormal refractive power of the media. Abbreviated, H. **—hypermetrop′ic,** *adj.;* **hypermet′rope,** *n.* **absolute h.** That which cannot be corrected completely by accommodation, so that there is indistinct vision even for distance. **facultative manifest h.** That part of the manifest hypermetropia that can be concealed by the accommodation. **latent h.** That part of the total hypermetropia that cannot be overcome by the accommodation, or the difference between the manifest and the total hypermetropia. Abbreviated, Hl. **manifest h.** The amount of hypermetropia represented by the strongest convex lens which a person will accept without paralysis of the accommodation. Abbreviated, Hm. **relative h.** A high hypermetropia in which distinct vision is possible only when excessive convergence is made.

hy″per·mi″cro·so′ma. Extreme dwarfism.

hy″per·mim′i·a (high″pur·mim′ee·uh, ·my′mee·uh). Excessive emotional expression or mimetic movement.

hy″perm·ne′si·a (high″purm·nee′zhuh, ·zee·uh). **hy″perm·ne′sis.** Increased retentiveness of memory.

hy″per·mo·til′i·ty. Increased motility, as of the stomach or intestines.

hy″per·ne·phro′ma. Originally applied by Grawitz to a variety of tumors of the kidney, supposed to be derived from embryonal inclusions of adrenal in the kidney. Now applied to a tumor, of the kidney or other organ, which in its type of cell growth resembles that of the adrenal carcinoma or adenoma. If chromaffin cells are present, identification can be established. Also called *Grawitz's tumor; clear-cell carcinoma.*

hy″per·on′to·morph. *In constitutional medicine,* a person of a long, thin body type with short intestines. Also called *asthenic type, microsplanchnic type.*

hy″per·o·nych′i·a (high″pur·o·nick′ee·uh). Hypertrophy of the nails.

hy″per·os′mi·a (high″pur·oz′mee·uh, ·oss′mee·uh). An abnormally acute sense of smell.

hy″per·os″te·og′e·ny (·os″tee·odj′i·nee). Excessive development of bone.

hy″per·os·to′sis. Exostosis or hypertrophy of bony tissue.

hy″per·ox·e′mi·a. Extreme acidity of the blood.

hy″per·ox″y·gen·a′tion. A condition of the blood in which it contains more than the normal amount of oxygen. It is caused by hyperventilation, *q.v.*

hy″per·par″a·thy′roid·ism. A state produced by an increased functioning of the parathyroid glands, as ostetis fibrosa cystica and osteomalacia.

hy″per·pep·sin′i·a. Excessive secretion of pepsin in the stomach.

hy″per·per″i·stal′sis. An increase in the rate and depth of the peristaltic waves; nervous diarrhea.

hy″per·pha·lan′gism. The presence of supernumerary phalanges.

hy″per·pho′ni·a. Stammering or stuttering resulting from excessive irritability of the vocal muscles.

hy″per·pi·e′si·a (high″pur·pye·ee′zhuh, ·shuh), **hy″per·pi·e′sis.** Abnormally high blood pressure; especially, essential hypertension. **—hyperpiet′ic,** *adj.*

hy″per·pig″men·ta′tion. Excessive or increased pigmentation.

hy″per·pi·tu′i·ta·rism. Any one of a number of abnormal conditions resulting from overactivity of the cells of the adenohypophysis, such as acromegaly, gigantism.

hy″per·pla′si·a (high″pur·play′zhuh, ·shuh). Excessive formation of tissue; an increase in the size of a tissue or organ owing to an increase in the number of cells. Syn., *numerical hypertrophy.* —**hyperplas'tic,** *adj.*

hy"perp·ne'a. Increase in depth of inspiration.

hy"per·po·ro'sis. An excessive formation of callus in the union of fractured bones.

hy"per·po"tas·se'mi·a. An abnormally high level of potassium in the blood; also called *hyperkalemia, hyperkaliemia.*

hy"per·prag'i·a. An excess of thinking and feeling, commonly observed in the manic phase of manic-depressive psychoses. —**hyperprag'ic,** *adj.*

hy"per·prax'i·a. The restlessness of movement characterizing certain forms of mania; hyperactivity.

hy"per·pro"cho·re'sis (high"pur-pro"kor·ee'sis). Excessive motor action of the stomach; hyperperistalsis, *q.v.*

hy"per·pro·sex'i·a. Marked attention to one subject, as, for example, one idea or symptom.

hy"per·psy·cho'sis. Exaggerated mental activity. Syn., *hypernea. Obs.*

hy"per·py·rex'i·a (high"pur·pye-reck'see-uh). Excessively high fever, as above 106° F. —**hyperpyret'ic,** *adj.*

hy"per·re·flex'i·a. A condition in which reflexes are increased above normal; due to a variety of causes.

hy"per·res'o·nance. Full resonance of a percussion note, which is slightly lower in pitch than normal resonance, and which possesses also a tympanitic element. It gives the impression of exaggeration of normal resonance. Heard chiefly in certain cases of pulmonary emphysema and pneumothorax.

hy"per·sal"i·va'tion. Abnormally increased secretion of saliva.

hy"per·se·cre'tion. Excessive secretion.

hy"per·sen"si·tiv'i·ty. The state of being abnormally sensitive or susceptible, as to the action of allergens. See *allergy.* —**hypersen'sitive,** *adj.*

hy"per·som'ni·a. Excessive sleepiness.

hy"per·sthe'ni·a (high"pur-sthee'nee-uh, high"pur-sthen'ee-uh). A condition of exalted strength or tone of the body. —**hypersthen'ic,** *adj.*

hy"per·sus·cep"ti·bil'i·ty. Hypersensitivity, *q.v.*

hy"per·ten'sin. The pressor substance, a polypeptide, formed by interaction between an enzyme from the kidney, renin, and hypertensinogen, a globulin in the blood plasma. Syn., *angiotonin.*

hy"per·ten'sin·ase. An enzyme present in blood and tissues which destroys hypertensin. Syn., *angiotonase.*

hy"per·ten·sin'o·gen. A globulin in the blood plasma, the substrate upon which renin acts to produce hypertensin.

hy"per·ten'sion. Excessive tension, usually synonymous with high blood pressure; supertension. —**hypertensive,** *adj.;* **hypertensor,** *n.* **essential h.** High blood pressure disease of unknown etiology, *i.e.* no constant underlying disease process can be identified. **Goldblatt h.** Hypertension in man similar to experimental renal hypertension produced by permanent constriction of one or both main renal arteries. **red h.** Benign essential hypertension, associated with renal vascular disease, but without renal insufficiency. The skin of the face is frequently red. **renal h.** Hypertension resulting from hemodynamic disturbances.

hy"per·the'li·a. The presence of supernumerary nipples.

hy"per·ther"mal·ge'si·a (high"pur-thur"mal·jee'zee·uh, ·see·uh). Abnormal sensitivity to heat.

hy"per·ther'my, hy"per·ther'mi·a. 1. An abnormally high fever; hyperpyrexia. 2. The treatment of disease by the induction of fever; this can be done by inoculation with malaria, by intravenous injection of foreign proteins, or by physical means.

hy"per·thy'mi·a. 1. Mental hyperesthesia; morbid oversensitiveness. 2. Vehement cruelty or foolhardiness as a symptom of mental disease. 3. Labile or unstable emotionality, as seen in some psychopathic personalities.

hy"per·thy"mi·za'tion. Exaggerated activity of the thymus gland, with resulting toxic symptoms.

hy"per·thy'roid·ism. An abnormal condition brought about by excessive functional activity of the thyroid gland.

hy"per·to'ni·a. Excess of muscular tonicity.

hy"per·ton'ic. 1. Exceeding in strength or tension. 2. Referring to a solution whose osmotic pressure is greater than that of physiologic salt solution, or any other solution taken as a standard. —**hypertonic'ity,** *n.*

hy"per·tri·cho'sis (high"pur·tri-ko'sis), **hy"per·tri·chi'a·sis** (high"pur·tri·kigh'uh·sis). Excessive growth of normal hair; superfluous hair; abnormal hairiness. —**hypertrichot'ic,** *adj.*

hy·per·tro·phy, hy"per·tro'phi·a. An increase in size of an organ, independent of natural growth; due to enlargement or multiplication of its constituent cells; usually connotes accompanying increase in functional capacity. —**hypertroph'ic,** *adj.* **adaptive h.** That which adapts an organ to increased functional requirements, as hypertrophy of the heart associated with valvular deformities or hypertension, hypertrophy of the bladder in cases of enlarged prostate. **cicatricial h.** Overgrowth of connective tissue in a scar; increase in scar tissue. **compensatory h.** That which follows destruction or injury in another part of the same organ. **concentric h. of the heart.** An increase in the weight and volume of cardiac muscle, especially of the ventricles; accompanied by reduction in the volume of the chambers; probably due to rigor mortis rather than to a special form of cardiac hypertrophy. **eccentric h. of the heart.** Hypertrophy accompanied by dilatation, beyond that always seen in cardiac hypertrophy. **false h.** An increase in size of an organ due to an increase in amount of tissue not associated with functional activity, such as connective tissue; a hyperplasia. **numerical h.** That due to multiplication of component cells. **physiologic h.** That due to natural physiologic rather than pathologic causes, as hypertrophy of the pregnant uterus. **simple h.** That due to an increase in the size of the component cells rather than to their multiplication. **ventricular h.** A term used in electrocardiography as either **right ventricular hypertrophy** (designating abnormal right axis deviation and QRS in the limb leads possibly over 0.10 sec.) or **left ventricular hypertrophy** (designating abnormal left axis deviation, QRS in the limb leads over 0.10 sec., T flat or inverted in lead I and at times T₃ similarly changed).

hy″per·tro′pi·a. Vertical concomitant strabismus; one eye fixes upon an object and the other deviates upward.

hy″per·vas′cu·lar. Excessively vascular.

hy″per·ven″ti·la′tion. Hyperpnea or forced respiration; an increase in the quantity of air breathed (minute volume) as a result of an increase in the rate or depth of respiration, or both. Symptoms are those of hyperoxygenation of the blood and include tingling of the extremities and buzzing in the head, with occasional syncope. **involuntary h.** Occurs in hysteria as a physiologic concomitant of fear or anger, or as a result of diffuse or focal encephalopathy.

hy″per·vi″ta·min·o′sis. A condition due to the ingestion of toxic amounts of vitamins.

hy″per·vo·le′mi·a. Blood volume greater than normal.

hyp″es·the′si·a, hyp″aes·the′si·a (hip″ess·thee′zhuh, high″pess·). Impairment of sensation; lessened tactile sensibility. **—hypesthesic, hyp·esthet′ic,** adj.

hy′pha (pl. *hyphae*). One of the filaments of a mycelium.

hyp″he·do′ni·a (hip″hi·do′nee·uh, hype″hi·do′nee·uh). Diminution of pleasure sensations in acts that normally give pleasure.

hy·phe′ma, hy·phae′ma (high-fee′muh). Blood in the anterior chamber of the eye.

hy·phe′mi·a (high-fee′mee·uh). 1. Deficiency of blood. Also called *oligemia*. 2. Blood in the anterior chamber of the eye.

hyp″hi·dro′sis (hip″hi·dro′sis). Deficiency of perspiration.

hyp″i·no′sis. A deficiency of fibrin factors in the blood.

hyp″na·gog′ic (hip″nuh·godj′ick). Inducing sleep; pertaining to the inception of sleep. Applied to visions seen just preceding complete sleep.

hyp′na·gogue. Hypnotic, 3, *q.v.*

hyp·nal′gi·a. Pain recurring during sleep.

hyp′nic. 1. Pertaining to or inducing sleep. 2. An agent that induces sleep.

hyp′no-, hypn-. A combining form meaning *sleep* or denoting *hypnotism*.

hyp″no·gen′ic, hyp″no·ge·net′ic. 1. Producing or inducing sleep. 2. Inducing hypnotism. **—hypnogen′esis,** n.

hyp″no·lep″sy. Excessive or morbid sleepiness; narcolepsy.

hyp·nol′o·gy. The science dealing with sleep or with hypnotism.

hyp″no·nar·co′sis. Deep sleep induced through hypnosis.

hyp″no·pho′bi·a. Morbid dread of sleep or of falling asleep. **—hypnophobic,** adj.; **hyp′nophoby,** n.

hyp″no·phre·no′sis. A general term for all forms of sleep disturbance.

hyp″no·pom′pic. Pertaining to the state of awakening. Applied to visions seen at the moment of awakening from sleep or prior to complete awakening, as when a dream figure persists in waking life.

hyp·no′sis. A state of sleep or trance; induced artificially in a subject by means of verbal suggestion by the hypnotist or by the subject's concentration upon some object; characterized by extreme responsiveness to suggestions made by the hypnotist.

hyp″no·ther′a·py. The treatment of disease by means of hypnotism.

hyp·not′ic. 1. Inducing sleep. 2. Pertaining to hypnotism. 3. A remedy that causes sleep. 4. One who is susceptible to hypnotism; one who is hypnotized.

hyp′no·tism. 1. The act of inducing hypnosis. 2. The study of hypnosis. **—hypnotist,** n.

hyp′no·tize. Bring into a state of hypnosis. **—hypnotiza′tion,** n.

hy'po. 1. Colloquial term for hypochondriasis; also for hypodermic syringe or medication. 2. Sodium thiosulfate.

hy'po- (high'po-), **hyp-.** 1. A prefix denoting *deficiency* or *lack; under, below,* or *beneath.* 2. A prefix indicating *acids and salts having the least number of atoms of oxygen in a series of compounds of the same elements.*

hy"po·a·cid'i·ty. Deficiency in acid constituents.

hy"po·ac·tiv'i·ty. Diminished activity.

hy"po·ad·ren"al·i·ne'mi·a. A condition in which the adrenalin content of the blood is insufficient.

hy"po·ag'na·thus. An individual with no lower jaw.

hy"po·al'i·men·ta'tion. The state produced by insufficient or inadequate food.

hy"po·al"ler·gen'ic. A term applied to a preparation in which every possible care has been taken in formulation and production to insure minimum instance of allergic reactions.

hy"po·az"o·tu'ri·a. A diminished amount of urea in the urine.

hy"po·bro'mous ac'id. HBrO. An unstable acid containing bromine having a positive valence number of one.

hy"po·bu'li·a. Deficiency of will power.

hy"po·cal·ce'mi·a. Condition in which there is a diminished amount of calcium in the blood.

hy"po·cal"ci·fi·ca'tion. Reduction of the normal amount of mineral salts in calcified tissue, such as bone, dentin, or dental enamel.

hy"po·ca·thex'is. A lack of concentration of the psychic energy upon a particular object.

hy"po·chlo·re'mi·a, hy"po·chlo·rae'mi·a. Reduction in the blood chlorides.

hy"po·chlor·hy'dri·a (high"po·klor·high'dree·uh, hip"o-). A condition in which there is a diminished amount of hydrochloric acid in the gastric juice.

hy"po·chlo'rite. Any salt of hypochlorous acid, HClO.

hy"po·chlo"ri·za'tion. Reduction in the intake of sodium chloride.

hy"po·chlo'rous ac'id. HClO. An unstable compound, known only in solution.

hy"po·chlor·u'ri·a. A diminution in the amount of chlorides excreted in the urine.

hy"po·cho·les"ter·e'mi·a (·ko·les"tur·ee'mee·uh). Decrease or deficiency of the cholesterol of the blood.

hy"po·chon'dri·ac. Affected with or caused by hypochondriasis.

hy"po·chon'dri·ac. A person affected by hypochondriasis. **—hypo·chon·dri'a·cal,** *adj.*

hy"po·chon·dri'a·sis (high"po·kon·dry'uh·sis, hip"o·). A chronic condition in which the patient is morbidly concerned with his own health, and believes himself suffering from grave bodily disease; traceable to some long-standing intrapsychic conflict. In true hypochondriasis, the symptoms are focused upon one organ.

hy"po·chon'dri·um (high"po·kon'dree·um, hip"o·). The upper lateral region of the abdomen below the lower ribs.

hy"po·chro'mic. Pertaining to erythrocytes in which the hemoglobin concentration is below the mean normal. **—hypochromat'ic,** *adj.;* **hypochromia,** *n.*

hy"po·der'mic. 1. Pertaining to the region beneath the skin. 2. Placed or introduced beneath the skin. 3. Injection under the skin. 4. Syringe used in hypodermic injection.

hy"po·der·moc'ly·sis, hy"po·der"ma·toc'ly·sis. The introduction into the subcutaneous tissues of large quantities of fluids, especially saline solution.

hy"po·don'ti·a (-don'she·uh). Deficient development of the teeth.

hy"po·er'gy. An altered state of reactivity, in which the response is less marked than usual; hyposensitivity. It is one form of allergy or pathergy.

hy"po·func'tion. Diminished function.

hy"po·gas'tri·um. The lowest of the three median regions of the abdomen, above the symphysis pubis and below the umbilical region. Also called *hypogastric region.* **—hypogastric,** *adj.*

hy"po·gen'i·tal·ism. Underdevelopment of the genital system. See *eunuchoidism.*

hy"po·geu'si·a (high"po·gew'see·uh, hip"o·). Diminution in the sense of taste.

hy"po·glos'sal. Situated under the tongue.

hy"po·glos·si'tis. Inflammation of the tissue under the tongue.

hy"po·glot'tis, hy"po·glos'sis. The under part of the tongue.

hy"po·gly·ce'mi·a (·glye·see'mee·uh). The condition produced by a low level of glucose in the blood; due to excessive utilization of sugar or to interference with the formation of sugar in the liver. Symptoms, which usually appear when the blood sugar drops to 0.06–0.04%, are hunger, nervousness, profuse sweating, alternate pallor and flushing of the face, and vertigo. See *hyperinsulinism.* **—hypoglycemic,** *adj.*

hy″po·gnath′ous (high″po·nath′-us). Having the lower jaw longer than the upper.

hy″po·gon′ad·ism (high″po·gon-uh·diz·um, hip″o·). Diminished internal secretion of the testes or ovaries.

hy″po·hi·dro′sis (high″po·hi·dro′-sis, hip″o·). Deficient perspiration.

hy″po·ki·ne′si·a (·ki·nee′shuh, ·kigh·nee′·), **hy″po·ki·ne′sis** (·ki·nee′sis, ·kigh·nee′sis). Abnormally decreased muscular movement. **—hypo·kinet′ic,** adj.

hy″po·lem′mal. Lying under a sheath, as the motor end-plates under the sarcolemma or sheath of a muscle fiber.

hy″po·lo′gi·a. Poverty of speech as a symptom of cerebral disease.

hy″po·mag″ne·se′mi·a. A state of magnesium deficiency manifested by twitching and convulsions.

hy″po·ma′ni·a. A slight maniacal state, in which the patient is easily distracted and clang associations occur, but no marked behavior differences are present; a less intense form of mania. **—hypomanic,** adj.

hy″po·mas′ti·a, hy″po·ma′zi·a. Abnormal smallness of the mammary glands.

hy″po·men″or·rhe′a. A deficient amount of menstrual flow at the regular period; to be distinguished from oligomenorrhea, q.v.

hy′po·mere. The ventrolateral unsegmented mesoderm from which the coelom develops.

hy″po·me·tab′o·lism. Metabolism below the normal rate.

hy″po·mi″cro·gnath′us (high″-po·migh″kro·nath′us). An individual having an abnormally small lower jaw.

hy″pom·ne′si·a (high″pom·nee′-huh, ·zee·uh). Weakened memory.

hy″po·nan″o·so′ma. Extreme dwarfishness.

hy″po·no′ic. Pertaining to that behavior which arises from unconscious processes.

hy″po·nych′i·um (high″po·nick′-e·um, hip″o·). The thickened stratum corneum of the epidermis, which lies under the free edge of a nail. **—hypo·nychial,** adj.

hy″po·par″a·thy′roid·ism. A pathologic state due to insufficiency of the parathyroid glands.

hy″po·per″me·a·bil′i·ty. A state in which membranes have reduced permeability for electrolytes, and other solutes, or colloids.

hy″po·pha·lan′gism. Congenital absence of one or more phalanges in a finger or toe.

hy″po·pho′ri·a. A tendency of the visual axis of one eye to deviate below that of the other.

hy″po·phos′phite. A salt of hypophosphorous acid.

hy″po·phos′pho·rous ac′id (·fos′-fo·rus, ·fos·for′us). An aqueous solution containing 30–32% of HPH_2O_2.

hy″po·phre′ni·a. Feeblemindedness. **—hypophren′ic,** adj., n.

hy·poph′y·sis (high·pof′i·sis, hi-pof′·). The pituitary. **—hypophys′-eal,** adj.

hy·poph′y·sis cer′e·bri. The pituitary.

hy″po·pi·e′si·a (·pye·ee′zhuh, ·shuh), **hy″po·pi·e′sis** (·pye·ee′sis, ·pye′i·sis). Subnormal arterial pressure.

hy″po·pi·tu′i·ta·rism. Deficient production of pituitary hormones, especially those of the anterior lobe as in hypopituitary cachexia or certain pituitary tumors. There may be impotence, sterility, amenorrhea, hypoglycemia, signs of adrenal cortical failure, hypometabolism, and a tendency of the tissues and viscera to shrink.

hy″po·pla′si·a (high″po·play′zhuh, hip″o·), **hy″po·plas″ty.** Defective development of any tissue. **—hypoplas′tic,** adj.

hy″po·prax′i·a. Deficient activity; inactivity; listlessness.

hy″po·pro·sex′i·a. Inadequate attention; lack of the ability to give attention.

hy″po·pro″te·i·ne′mi·a. A lowering of the protein content in the blood plasma, due to disease or to diet deficiency.

hy″po·psel″a·phe′si·a (high″po·sel″uh·fee′zee·uh, ·see·uh). Diminution of sensitivity to tactile impressions.

hy″po·psy·cho′sis (high″po·sigh·ko′sis, hip″o·). Diminution or blunting of thought.

hy·po′py·on (high·po′pee·on, hi·po′·). A collection of pus in the anterior chamber of the eye.

hy″po·sal″i·va′tion. Pathologically insufficient secretion of saliva; formerly called *zerostomia.*

hy″po·se·cre′tion. Diminished secretion.

hy″po·sen″si·tiv′i·ty. A state of diminished sensitiveness, especially to external stimuli. **—hyposen′sitive,** adj.; **hyposen′sitiveness,** n.

hy·pos′mi·a (high·poz′mee·uh, hi-poz′·). Diminution of the sense of smell.

hy″po·som′ni·a. An insufficient number of hours of sleep.

hy″po·spa′di·as. 1. A congenital anomaly of the penis and urethra in which the urethra opens upon the ventral surface of the penis or in the perineum. 2. Term also used to denote a congenital malformation in which the urethra opens into the vagina.

hy·po·spray. A metallic device for administering injections subcutaneously; it operates on the principle that a stream of fluid ejected with high velocity through an orifice, 75 to 80 microns in diameter and held against the skin, penetrates the skin without pain and usually without leaving a readily visible mark. Also called *jet injection*.

hy·pos'ta·sis (high·pos'ta·sis, hi·pos'·). 1. A deposit which forms at the bottom of a liquid; a sediment. 2. The formation of a sediment, especially the settling of blood in dependent parts of the body.

hy"po·stat'ic. 1. Due to, or of the nature of, hypostasis. 2. *In genetics*, subject to being suppressed, as a gene whose effect is suppressed by another gene that affects the same part of the organism.

hy·pos"the·nu'ri·a (high·poss"thi·new'ree·uh, hi·poss"·). The secretion of urine of low specific gravity, due to the inability of the kidney to concentrate the urine adequately.

hy"po·sto'mi·a. A form of microstomia in which the mouth is a vertical slit opening into a pharyngeal sac.

hy"po·sul'fite. A name, recommended to be abandoned, which has been applied to salts both of thiosulfuric acid and of hydrosulfurous acid.

hy"po·tax'i·a. A condition of emotional rapport between the subject and the hypnotist existing in the beginning of hypnosis.

hy"po·tax'is. Light, hypnotic sleep.

hy"po·ten'sion. Diminished or abnormally low tension, usually synonymous with low blood pressure. —**hypotensive,** *adj.* **orthostatic h.** A fall of blood pressure which occurs when the erect position is assumed. **postural h.** That due to a sudden change from the horizontal to the upright position or from prolonged standing, causing dizziness, faintness, and sometimes syncope.

hy"po·ten'sive. A drug that lowers blood pressure, often used in treating hypertension.

hy"po·ten'sor. Any substance capable of lowering blood pressure. It implies a persistent effect, as opposed to the fleeting effect of a depressor.

hy"po·thal'a·mus. The region of the diencephalon that forms the floor of the third ventricle and including neighboring associated nuclei. —**hypothalam'ic,** *adj.*

hy"po·the'nar (high"po·thee'nur, high·poth'i·nur). Designating the fleshy eminence on the ulnar side of the palm of the hand.

hy"po·ther'mi·a, hy"po·ther"·my. Subnormal temperature of the body. —**hypother'mal,** *adj.*

hy·poth'e·sis. 1. A supposition or conjecture put forth to account for known facts. 2. A theory accepted tentatively, as, for example, **Kossel and Siegfried's protamine nucleus h.,** the theory that all proteins are built around a nucleus of the three amino acids, arginine, histidine, and lysine, and that arginine is the most important member of this triad.

hy"po·thy'mi·a. Despondency; depression of spirits; a diminution in the intensity of emotions.

hy"po·thy'roid·ism. A morbid condition due to deficiency of thyroid hormone; in advanced form expressed as cretinism or myxedema; in the mild form, a nonmyxedematous condition associated with basal metabolic rates approximating 20% below normal and to a mild degree, with other characteristics of myxedema. Also see *cretinism, myxedema.* **primary h.** That caused by primary loss of functioning thyroid tissue, such as surgical removal, infection, or atrophy. **secondary h.** That due to inadequate stimulation of the thyroid.

hy"po·ton'ic. 1. Below the normal strength or tension. 2. Referring to a solution whose osmotic pressure is less than that of physiologic salt solution or any other solution taken as standard. —**hypotonic'ity,** *n.*

hy"po·vi"ta·min·o'sis. A condition due to deficiency of one or more vitamins in the food.

hy"po·vo·le'mi·a. Low, or decreased, blood volume.

hy"po·xan'thine (high"po·zan'theen, ·thin). 6-Oxypurine, 6-keto-purine. An intermediate product resulting when adenine is transformed into uric acid and allantoin.

hy"po·xan·thyl'ic ac'id (·zan·thil'ick). Inosinic acid. A nucleotide found in muscle; formed by the deamination of adenylic acid.

hy"pox·e'mi·a. A condition of insufficient oxygen in the blood.

hy·pox'i·a (high·pock'see·uh). Oxygen want or deficiency.

hyp"so·pho'bi·a. Morbid dread of being at a great height.

hys'sop. The leaves and tops of *Hyssopus officinalis,* an aromatic stimulant.

hys"ter·al'gi·a. Neuralgic pain in the uterus. —**hysteralgic,** *adj.*

hys"ter·ec'to·my. Total or partial removal of the uterus. In **abdominal hysterectomy,** the removal is effected through an abdominal incision; in **vaginal hysterectomy,** through the vagina.

hys"ter·eu·ryn'ter (hiss"tur·yoo·rin'tur). A metreurynter used for dilating the cervix uteri.

hys·te'ri·a (hiss·teer'ee·uh, hiss·terr'·

e-uh). A psychoneurotic disorder, characterized by extreme emotionalism involving disturbances of the psychic, sensory, motor, vasomotor, and visceral functions. Frequently a result of repression of conflicts from the conscious mind. —**hyster'ic, hyster'ical,** *adj.;* **hyster'iac,** *n.* **anxiety h.** The combination of an anxiety neurosis, *q.v.,* with hysteria. **conversion h.** That in which the mechanism of conversion is predominantly used; if the physical symptoms are referred to external parts of the body, the condition is called **fixation hysteria. major h.** A hysteria marked by violent mental excitement and movements suggesting grand mal epilepsy. **minor h.** A mild form of hysteria, as in anorexia nervosa and globus hystericus.

hys·ter'ics. 1. Colloquial term for a hysterical attack. 2. A fit of laughing and crying, similar to that seen in hysteria.

hys'ter·o-, hyster-. A combining form denoting *connection with,* or *relation to, the uterus or to hysteria.*

hys'ter·o·cele". A hernia containing all or part of the uterus.

hys"ter·o·clei'sis (hiss"tur-o·kly'-sis). The closure of the uterus by suturing the edges of the external os.

hys"ter·o·cys'tic. Relating to the uterus and urinary bladder.

hys"ter·o·cys"to·clei'sis (hiss"tur-o·sis"to·kly'sis). Operation for relief of vesico-uterovaginal fistula, consisting in turning the cervix uteri into the urinary bladder and suturing it. Also called *Bozeman's operation.*

hys"ter·o·de"mon·op'a·thy. Hysteria characterized by demonomania; frequently accompanied by self-reproach and motivated by a strong sense of guilt.

hys"ter·o·dyn'i·a. Pain in the uterus.

hys"ter·o·ep'i·lep"sy. A type of hysteria associated with convulsions similar to epileptic convulsions.

hys"ter·o·fren'ic. Capable of checking an attack of hysteria.

hys"ter·og'e·ny (hiss"tur-odj'i·nee). The induction of the hysteric state or paroxysm. —**hysterogen'ic, hys'trog'enous,** *adj.*

hys"ter·og'ra·phy. Roentgenologic examination of the uterus.

hys"ter·o·lap"a·rot'o·my. Abdominal hysterectomy.

hys"ter·o·lith. A calculus in the uterus.

hys"ter·o·li·thi'a·sis. The formation of a concretion in the uterus.

hys"ter·ol'y·sis. Severing the attachments or adhesions of the uterus.

hys"ter·o·ma'ni·a. 1. A state or condition of psychomotor overactivity seen in hysteria. *Rare.* 2. Nymphomania. *Rare.*

hys"ter·om'e·ter. An instrument for measuring the length of the intrauterine cavity. —**hysterometry,** *n.*

hys"ter·o·my·o'ma (hiss"tur-o·migh-o'muh). Myoma of the uterus.

hys"ter·o·my"o·mec'to·my. Surgical removal of fibroid uterine tumor.

hys"ter·o·my·ot'o·my (hiss"tur-o·migh-ot'o·mee). Incision into the uterus for removal of a solid tumor.

hys"ter·o·o"ö·pho·rec'to·my. The surgical removal of the uterus and ovaries.

hys"ter·op'a·thy. Any disease or disorder of the uterus. —**hysteropath'ic,** *adj.*

hys"ter·o·pex"y. Fixation of the uterus by a surgical operation to correct displacement.

hys"ter·o·phil'i·a. A term applied to certain psychosomatic disturbances resembling hysteria, such as migraine, asthma, intestinal spasm, or occupational cramps.

hys"ter·op·to'sis. Falling or inversion of the uterus.

hys"ter·or·rha'phy. The closure of a uterine incision or rent by suture.

hys"ter·or·rhex'is. Rupture of the uterus.

hys"ter·o·sal"pin·gec'to·my. (·sal"pin·jeck'to·mee). Excision of the uterus and oviducts.

hys"ter·o·sal"pin·gog'ra·phy. Roentgenographic examination of the uterus and oviducts after injection of a radiopaque substance; metrosalpingography.

hys"ter·o·sal"pin"goo·o"ö·pho·rec'to·my (-o"o·fo·reck'to·mee, -o"off·o·reck'to·mee). Excision of the uterus, oviducts, and ovaries.

hys"ter·o·sal"pin"goo·o"ö·the·cec'to·my (-o"o·thi·seck'to·mee). Hysterosalpingo-oöphorectomy.

hys"ter·o·sal"pin·gos'to·my. The establishment of an anastomosis between an oviduct and the uterus.

hys"ter·o·scope". A uterine speculum, with a reflector. —**hysteros'copy,** *n.*

hys"ter·o·tome". An instrument for incising the uterus.

hys"ter·ot'o·my. 1. Incision of the uterus. 2. A Cesarean section.

hys"ter·o·tra"che·lec'to·my (·tray"ki·leck'to·mee, ·track"i·leck'to·mee). Amputation of the cervix of the uterus.

hys"ter·o·tra'che·lo·plas"ty (·tray"ki·lo·plas"tee, ·track"i·lo·plas"-tee). Plastic surgery on the cervix of the uterus.

hys″ter·o·tra″che·lor′rha·phy.
A plastic operation for the restoration
of a lacerated cervix uteri.

hys″ter·o·tra″che·lot′o·my. Surgical incision of the cervix uteri.

hys″ter·o·trau′ma·tism. Hysteric

symptoms due to or following a severe
injury.

hytakerol. A trade-mark for dihydrotacherol.

hy′ther. The effect of the atmospheric
heat and humidity on an organism.

I. The chemical symbol for iodine; symbol for permanent incisor.

I¹³¹. Symbol for iodine-131.

i. Optically inactive; iso-; deciduous
incisor.

I.A.D.R. International Association for
Dental Research.

-i′as·is. A combining form denoting *a
process, a course of action; a morbid
or a diseased condition.*

i·at′ro- (eye·at′ro-, eye·ay′tro-). A
combining form signifying *a relation
to medicine or to physicians.*

i·at″ro·chem′is·try. 1. The application of chemistry to therapeutics; the
treatment of disease by chemical
means. 2. The theory developed in the
seventeenth century that disease and
its treatment are explicable on a chemical basis.

i″bo·ga′ine (eye″bo·gay′een, i·bo′-
gay·een). An alkaloid from the roots of
Tabernanthe iboga, a plant of the
Congo.

-ic. 1. A suffix signifying *of or pertaining to.* 2. *In chemistry,* a suffix denoting *the higher of two valencies assumed
by an element* and, incidentally, in
many cases, *a larger amount of oxygen.*

ice. Water in its solid state, which it
assumes at a temperature of 0° C. or
32° F. **dry i.** Carbon dioxide in its
solid state.

ice′land spar. A crystalline form of
calcium carbonate, having doubly refracting properties.

ich′no·gram (ick′no·gram). *In legal
medicine,* the record of a footprint.

i′chor (eye′kor, eye′kur). An acrid
thin discharge from an ulcer or wound.
—ichorous, ichoroid, *adj.*

i″chor·rhe′a, i″chor·rhoe′a
(eye″ko·ree′uh). A copious flow of
ichor.

**i″chor·rhe′mi·a, i″chor·rhae′-
mi·a** (eye″ko·ree′mee·uh). The presence of purulent material in the blood.

ich′tham·mol (ick′thuh·mole, ·mol).
A reddish brown to brownish black,
viscid fluid obtained by destructive distillation of certain bituminous schists,
followed by sulfonation of the distillate
and neutralization with ammonia.

ich′thu·lin (ick′thew·lin). A variety
of protein derived from fish eggs.

ich′thy·o- (ick′thee·o-), **ichthy-.** A
combining form meaning *fish.*

ich″thy·o·col′la. Isinglass; a gelatinous substance prepared from the air
bladders of the sturgeon and other fish,
occurring in horny, translucent, white
sheets which form a jelly when combined with hot water. Used as a food,
an adhesive, and a clarifying agent.

ich′thy·oid. Resembling a fish.

ichthyol. Trade-mark for a brand of
ichthammol.

ich″thy·ol·sul·fon′ic ac′id. C₂₈
H₃₆O₆S₃. An acid produced from Tyrolean bituminous material by the
action of sulfuric acid.

ich″thy·o′sis. A congenital abnormality of cornification characterized
by dry, hard scaliness of the skin. The
disease increases in severity in cold
weather. **—ichthyot′ic,** *adj.* **i. follicularis.** See *keratosis follicularis.*
i. hystrix. A disease characterized
by warty growths, consisting of elongated and hypertrophied papillae
covered by greatly thickened epidermis;
a type of nevus. **i. simplex.** The
common form which develops in early
life, characterized by large, finely corrugated, papery scales with deficient
secretions of sebaceous glands and
sometimes of the sweat glands.

i′con. An image or model.

i″co·nog′ra·phy. 1. Graphic or
plastic representation or illustration.
2. History and theory of the technique
and styles of illustration or representation.

i·con″o·lag′ny (eye·kon″o·lag′nee,
eye·kon′o·lag″nee). Sexual stimulation
induced by the sight of statues or pictures.

ICSH. See *luteinizing hormone.*

ic′tal. Pertaining to an acute epileptic
attack.

ic·ter′ic. Pertaining to or characterized by jaundice.

**ic″ter·o·gen′ic, ic″ter·og′e·
nous** (ick″tur·odj′i·nus). Causing
icterus.

ic′ter·oid. Resembling the color of
or having the nature of, jaundice.

'ter·us. Jaundice. **diffusion i.**
hat due to the hepatic cells having
st their power of holding back the
le, which consequently diffuses into
e fluids of the body. **familial
hemolytic i.** A chronic disease,
robably hereditary, due to fragility
f erythrocytes, and accompanied by
splenomegaly. Anemia caused by the
ncreased destruction of erythrocytes
sually accompanies the jaundice,
hich is acholuric. Also called *hemo-
tic jaundice*. **i. gravis.** Acute yel-
w atrophy of the liver, a disease
aracterized by jaundice, marked
ervous symptoms, diminution in size
f the liver, and a rapid, fatal termina-
on. The urine contains bile and crys-
ls of leucine and tyrosine. **i. index.**
he index of the bilirubin content of
e blood as expressed by comparison
f the color of the serum with the color
f a 1:10,000 potassium dichromate
lution. The normal range is from 4
6. From 6 to 15 is the zone of latent
undice, in which the blood holds an
mount of bilirubin above the normal
ithout spilling it over into the scleras
r other tissues. With an icterus index
ove 15, clinical jaundice is present.
i. neonatorum. That which is
metimes observed in infants during
e first few days after birth. The
uses are various and range from
ysiologic jaundice, which has no
tereffects, through that of erythro-
astosis foetalis and septic jaundice,
the severe jaundice due to absence
the bile ducts.

tus. **1.** An acute apoplectic attack.
An epileptic attack with no aura and
sudden onset. *Obs.*

. *In psychoanalysis*, the primitive,
eformed psychic force in the uncon-
ious, which is the source of the in-
inctive energy necessary for self-pres-
vation and propagation.

. A suffix pertaining to a sensitivity
ate of the skin, which reacts to bac-
rial, fungal, or other agents emanat-
g from a distant focus of infection.
e reactive condition ending in -id, or
e secondary inflammation, is usually
ee from microorganisms, and relief is
tained only through treatment of the
imary focus.

e'a. **1.** A mental impression or
ought; a belief or object existing in
e mind or thought. **2.** *In psychology*,
mental representation of something
t actually perceived. **autochtho-
ous i.** An idea which appears to
e patient as a finished product, hav-
g originated in his unconscious. The
tient feels the idea is thrust upon
m by malevolent outside influences.
ompulsive i. One involving an
esistible urge for action. **fixed i.**
 unfounded, delusional idea which

the patient refuses to relinquish even
after its disproof, and which controls
all his actions. **imperative i.** One
which the patient dislikes, but which
persists in his consciousness and dominates his will; characteristic of the
compulsive and ruminative ideas in
psychasthenia. **ruminative i.** One
which is pondered repeatedly.

i·de″al·i·za′tion. *In psychoanalysis*,
a sexual overevaluation of the love object.

i″de·a′tion. The formation of a
mental conception; the cerebral action
by which, or in accord with which, an
idea is formed.

i·den″ti·fi·ca′tion. **1.** A method of
describing and registering a person by
certain physical characteristics. **2.** *In
psychopathology*, a mental mechanism
of defense in which one unconsciously
assumes, on the basis of love or aggression, the characteristics of another.
Bertillon system of i. That
method which uses those skeletal measurements which remain practically unchanged after adult life is reached.
Syn., *anthropometric i.* **Galton system of i.** That method based upon
fingerprints. The records used are the
printed impressions of the ten digits
placed in definite order upon a card.
palm and sole system of i. An
extension of the Galton system to include the palmar and plantar surfaces.

id′e·o- (id′ee·o-, eye′dee·o-). A combining form meaning *idea*.

id″e·ol′o·gy (id″ee·ol′o·jee, eye″-
dee-). The science of ideas.

id″e·o·mo′tor. Pertaining to nonvoluntary movement which results
from some idea.

id″e·o·mus′cu·lar. Pertaining to
nonvoluntary muscular movement produced by a mental concept.

id″e·o·pho′bi·a. A morbid fear of
ideas.

id″e·o·vas′cu·lar. Relating to a
vascular change resulting from an emotional impression.

id′i·o-. **1.** A combining form meaning
one's own, separate, distinct. **2.** *In biochemistry* and *medicine*, a combining
form meaning *self-produced*.

id″i·o·chro′mo·some. A sex chromosome.

id′i·o·cy. The lowest grade of mental
deficiency, in which the subject's mental age is under three years and the I.Q.
under 25; usually congenital, and accompanied by physical defects. **amaurotic familial i.** See *amaurotic
familial idiocy*. **hydrocephalic i.**
That due to hydrocephaly, whether
congenital or acquired. **microce-
phalic i.** That form associated with
a small head. **Mongolian i.** See
Mongolism. **moral i.** That in which

all feeling for or interest in others is entirely absent.

id″i·og′a·mist. One who is capable of coitus only with his marital partner or with a few women, and impotent with women in general.

id″i·o·glos′si·a. In psychopathology, extremely defective utterance, in which the sounds used seem to belong to no known language. —**idioglot′tic**, adj.

id″i·o·hyp′no·tism. Self-induced hypnotism.

id″i·ol′o·gism. A form of utterance peculiar to any person, especially a speech defect.

id″i·op′a·thy. A primary disease; one not a result of any other disease, but of spontaneous origin. —**idiopath′ic, idiopathet′ic**, adj.

id″i·o·psy·chol′o·gy. Psychology based upon introspective study of one's own mental acts.

id′i·o·some″, id′i·o·zome″. The central apparatus of an auxocyte, especially a spermatocyte, including the surrounding Golgi apparatus and mitochondria.

id″i·o·syn′cra·sy. 1. Any special or peculiar characteristic or temperament by which a person differs from other persons. 2. A peculiarity of constitution that makes an individual react differently from most persons to drugs or treatments. —**idiosyncrat′ic**, adj.

id′i·ot. A person afflicted with idiocy, q.v.

i·dol″o·ma′ni·a (eye·dol″o·may′-nee·uh). Exaggerated idolatry.

id′ose. A synthetic hexose sugar; isomeric with glucose.

i″ga·su′ric ac′id. An organic acid found in the seeds of nux vomica.

ig·na′ti·a. St. Ignatius' bean. The seed of *Strychnos ignati;* contains the alkaloids strychnine and brucine.

ig′ni·punc″ture. Puncture with metal needles heated to either red or white heat.

ig·ni′tion (ig·nish′un). The process of heating solids until all volatile matter has been driven off. When performed in the presence of air, oxidizable matter such as carbon is burned.

Il. Chemical symbol for illinium.

il″e·ec′to·my. Excision of the ileum.

il″e·i′tis. Inflammation of the ileum. —**ileit′ic**, adj. **regional i.** A chronic, nonspecific, granulomatous process frequently involving the terminal portion of the ileum, but occasionally extending into the colon or arising in the more proximal portions of the ileum. Also called *terminal i.*

il′e·o-. A combining form denoting *the ileum.*

il″e·o·ce·cos′to·my. The surgical formation of an anastomosis between the cecum and the ileum.

il″e·o·col′ic. Pertaining conjointly to the ileum and the colon.

il″e·o·co·los′to·my. The surgical establishment of an anastomosis between the ileum and the colon.

il″e·o·sig″moid·os′to·my. The surgical formation of an anastomosis between the ileum and the sigmoid colon.

il″e·os′to·my. The surgical formation of a fistula or artificial anus through the abdominal wall into the ileum.

iletin. Trade-mark for a brand of insulin.

il′e·um. The lower portion of the small intestine, extending from the jejunum to the large intestine. —**ileac**, adj.

il′e·us. A condition brought about by intestinal obstruction which may be *adynamic,* due to paralysis of the bowel; or *mechanical,* due to pressure upon or blockage of the gut. It is marked by abdominal distention, severe pain, vomiting which gradually becomes fecal, with rising pulse and toxemia, and ends fatally unless relieved. **acute duodenal i.** Caused by obstruction of the lumen of the duodenum following operations or resulting from external pressure. Also called *arteriomesenteric i.; gastromesenteric i.* **spastic i.** Spastic contraction of a section of the bowel, usually the colon, causing obstruction. Also called *dynamic i.*

il′i·a. Plural of ilium.

ilidar phosphate. Trade-mark for azapetine phosphate.

il′i·o-. A combining form meaning relating to the ilium; iliac.

il″i·o·coc·cyg′e·al (il″ee·o·cock′-sidj′ee·ul). Pertaining to the ilium and the coccyx, as the iliococcygeal muscle.

il″i·o·fem′or·al. Pertaining conjointly to the ilium and the femur, as the iliofemoral ligament.

il″i·o·hy″po·gas′tric. Pertaining conjointly to the ilium and the hypogastrium, as the iliohypogastric nerve. See Table of Nerves in the Appendix.

il″i·o·in′gui·nal. 1. Pertaining to the ilium and the groin. 2. Lying partly within the iliac and partly within the inguinal region, as the ilioinguinal nerve. See Table of Nerves in the Appendix.

il″i·op′a·gus. Conjoined twins united in the iliac region. Syn., *iliadelphus.*

il″i·o·pec·tin′e·al (il″ee·o·pec-tin′ee·ul, ·peck″ti·nee′ul). Pertaining conjointly to the ilium and the pubis, as iliopectineal line.

il″i·o·pso′as (il″ee·o·so′us, il″ee·o-so·us). Pertaining conjointly to the ilium and the loin, as the iliopsoas muscle.

il″i·o·tho″ra·cop′a·gus. Co

...oined twins united at their thoracic
and iliac regions.

il'i·o·xi·phop'a·gus (il"ee-o-zi-
op'uh·gus). Conjoined twins united
from the xiphoid to the iliac region.

il'i·um (pl. *ilia*). 1. The flank. 2. The
superior broad portion of the hipbone,
a separate bone in the fetus. —**iliac,**
ilial, *adj.*

ill. Not healthy; sick; indisposed.

il·laq"ue·a'tion (i·lack"wee·ay'-
shun, il"ack·). The correction of an ingrowing eyelash by drawing it with a
loop through an opening in the lid.
—**illaq'ueate,** *v.*

il·le·git'i·mate. 1. Not in accordance with statutory law. 2. Born out of
wedlock; bastard. —**illegitimacy,** *n.*

il·lic'i·um (i·liss'ee·um). Star anise.
The fruit of *Illicium verum.*

il·li·ni'tion (il"i·nish'un). A rubbing in or on; inunction.

il·lin'i·um. Il = 146 *ca.* A rare earth
element, atomic number 61, reported in
1926 by B. S. Hopkins. Prior discovery
has been claimed by Rolla and Fernandez, who named the element *florentium.*
Both claims have been challenged,
while other investigators have reported
discovery of synthetic forms of element
61 and proposed the names *cyclonium*
and *promethium.*

ill'ness. 1. The state of being ill or
sick. 2. A malady; sickness; disease;
disorder.

il·lu"mi·na'tion. 1. The lighting up
or illuminating, as of a surface or
cavity, in the examination of a patient.
2. The quantity of light thrown upon an
object. 3. *In microscopy,* the type or
direction of light thrown upon the object studied. **dark-field i.** A method
in which light enters the objective only
by reflected, refracted, or scattered by
the object, making it or its parts appear
bright against a dark background. The
central rays of light are obliterated by
a central stop, in or below the condenser; a hollow cone of peripheral rays
strikes the object obliquely from the
side. Used especially for the examination of spirochetes. **i. by transmit-**
ted light. *In microscopy,* the usual
method of illuminating an object by
sending a beam of light, concentrated
by a substage condenser, through the
object. If the beam is centered in the
optical axis, the illumination is axial;
if it strikes the objective at an angle
to the optical axis, it is a form of oblique illumination. **Köhler's method**
i. A method of microscopical illumination in which an image of the source
is focused in the lower focal plane of
the microscope condenser, and the condenser, in turn, focuses an image of the
lamp lens in the object field. **oblique i.**
Illumination of an object by throwing
light upon it, or through it, obliquely.

Also called *lateral i.* **vertical i.** Microscopical illumination in which a
beam of light is thrown on the object
from above, or from the direction of
observation. Also called *direct i.*

il·lu'mi·nism. A mental state in
which the subject imagines that he con-
verses with supernatural beings.

il·lu'sion. A false interpretation of a
real sensation; a perception which mis-
interprets the object perceived. —**illu-**
sional, *adj.*

ilotycin. Trade-mark for erythromycin.

im-. *In chemistry,* a prefix used to indicate the bivalent group NH.

i'ma. The lowest.

im'age. 1. A more or less accurate
representation of an object. 2. The picture of an object formed by a lens; a
collection of foci, each corresponding
to a point in the object. 3. *In psycho-*
analysis, see *imago,* 2. **acoustic i.**
An idea of something which has been
heard. **aerial i.** A real image formed
on a screen or any surface becomes an
aerial image, existing in space. **after-**
image. See *afterimage.* **direct i.** A
picture obtained by rays that have not
yet come to a focus. Also called *erect i.*
double i. The two images, known as
true and false, which occur when one
eye deviates, when the visual lines of
the two eyes are not directed toward
the same object. **false i.** In diplopia,
the image of the deviating eye; it is not
on the macula, but is projected to a
peripheral part of the retina. **in-**
verted i. One turned upside down;
the image on the retina is always inverted. **real i.** One formed by the
meeting of rays; an image formed of
real foci. **virtual i.** One which can
be seen only by looking through a lens
or at a mirror; formed of diverging
rays which are prolonged backward
until they meet at a point. An image
formed of virtual foci.

im·ag"i·na'tion. The picture-mak-
ing power of the mind. The faculty by
which one creates new ideas or mental
pictures by means of separate data derived from experience, ideally revivified,
extended, and combined in new forms.

i·ma'go. 1. The adult, sexually mature
stage of an insect. 2. *In psychoanalysis,*
the childhood conception of the parent
or of some loved person, which is carried into adulthood and retained in the
unconscious. The term implies that the
image is only partly based on reality.

im·bal'ance. 1. Lack of balance. 2.
Lack of muscular balance especially
between the muscles of the eyes. **auto-**
nomic i. Lack of regulation of equilibrium particularly of the peripheral
blood vessels; if severe enough may
cause either hyperemia or ischemia.

Also called *sympathetic imbalance*, *vasomotor instability*.

im'be·cile. One who is afflicted with imbecility, *q.v.*

im"be·cil'i·ty. An intermediate grade of mental deficiency, in which the subject's mental age is between three and seven years and his I.Q. between 25 and 49.

im·bed'. See *embed, implantation*, 3.

im"bi·bi'tion (im"bi·bish'un). The absorption of liquid by a solid or a gel. **—imbibe'**, *v.*

im"bri·ca'tion. *In surgery*, closing wounds or covering deficiencies with tissue arranged in layers overlapping one another. **—im·bricated**, *adj.*

im"id·az'ole (im"id·az'ole, im"id-uh·zole'). NH.CH:N.CH:CH. A substance, readily synthesized, which is of interest because of the importance of a number of its derivatives, such as histamine, histidine. Syn., *glyoxaline*.

im"id·az'o·lines. Derivatives of the compound, NH.CH:N.CH₂.CH₂. They show a variety of physiologic actions.

im'ide, im'id. Any compound of the radical NH united to a divalent acid radical.

i·mi'do- (i·mee'do-, im'i·do-). *In chemistry*, a combining form denoting *imide*.

i·min'a·zole (i·min'uh·zole, i·mee'-nuh·). Imidazole, *q.v.*

i·mi'no- (i·mee'no-, im'i·no-). *In chemistry*, a combining form designating the bivalent group NH when attached to or in nonacid radicals.

i·mi'no ac'id. An organic acid that contains the bivalent imino group (=NH).

im"i·ta'tion. *In psychology*, the performance of an act as a result of seeing another person do the same thing; behaving in the manner in which another has been seen to behave.

im"ma·ture'. Unripe; not yet adult or fully developed.

im·me'di·ate. Direct; without the intervention of anything.

im·med'i·ca·ble. That which does not yield to medicine or treatment. Incurable.

im·mer'sion. The plunging of a body into a liquid. **homogeneous i.** A fluid between the objective or condenser of a microscope, and the cover glass or slide, having about the same refractive and dispersive power as the glass.

im·mer'sion foot. A serious and disabling condition of the feet due to prolonged immersion in sea water at 60° F. or lower, but not at freezing temperature. A condition similar to trench foot.

im·mer'sion lens. A lens, usually of high power, the lower end of which is immersed in a drop of some liquid, such as oil, that has nearly the same refractive index as glass, and is placed on the cover glass of the object under examination.

im·mer'sion oil. An oil, such as cedar, especially prepared to have a refractive index of 1.515 at 18° C.

im·mis'ci·ble. Not capable of being mixed.

im·mo"bi·li·za'tion. The act of rendering motionless, such as immobilization of a joint by means of splints in surgery.

im"mor·tal'i·ty. *In psychiatry*, the belief or delusion that the person has always existed and will live forever; delusion of timelessness.

im·mune'. Safe from attack; protected against a disease by an innate or an acquired immunity.

im·mu'ni·ty. The condition of a living organism whereby it resists and overcomes infection. **acquired i.** That obtained by a living organism as the result of active or passive immunity. **active i.** That possessed by an organism as the result of disease or unrecognized infection, or that induced by immunization with bacteria or products of bacterial growth. **individual i.** The particular power of certain individuals to resist or overcome infection. **local i.** One confined to a given tissue or area of the body. Syn., *tissue i.* **nonspecific i.** One produced by the introduction of microorganisms containing group antigens. **passive i.** (a) That conferred through the parenteral injection of antibodies prepared either in animals or in other human beings. (b) May also refer to that immunity acquired by the child *in utero* by the placental transfer of antibodies from the mother. **racial i.** Apparent differences in susceptibility among different races of the same species. **tissue i.** See local i.

im"mu·ni·za'tion. The act or process of rendering immune. **—im'mu·nize,** *v.*

im·mu'no-. A combining form signifying *immune*.

im·mu"no·chem'is·try. That branch of science which deals with the chemical changes and phenomena of immunity; specifically, the chemistry of antigens, antibodies, and their reactions.

im"mu·nol'o·gist. A specialist in the science of immunity.

im"mu·nol'o·gy. That science which is concerned with the study of immunity. **—immunolog'ic,** *adj.*

im·mu"no·trans·fu'sion. Transfusion with the blood of a donor previously rendered immune by repeated inoculations with a given agent.

im·pac'tion. 1. The state of being

lodged and retained in a part or strait. **2.** *In dentistry,* confinement of a tooth in the jaw so that its eruption is prevented. **3.** *In surgery,* a condition in which a fragment of bone is firmly driven into another fragment of bone so that neither can move against the other. **—impacted,** *adj.*

im·pal'pa·ble. Not capable of being felt; imperceptible to the touch.

im'par. Without a fellow; azygous.

im·pe'dance. The apparent resistance of a circuit to the flow of an alternating electric current.

im·per'a·tive. Peremptory, absolute; compulsory; binding.

im"per·cep'tion. Defective perception.

im·per'fo·rate. Without the normal opening. **—imperfora'tion,** *n.*

im·per'me·a·ble. Not permitting a passage.

im·per'vi·ous. Not permitting a passage, especially of fluids.

im"pe·ti'go. An acute, inflammatory skin disease which may be circinate, bullous, or furfuraceous in character. **—impetig'inous, impetig'- inoid,** *adj.* **i. contagiosa.** The highly contagious form of impetigo characterized by vesicles, pustules, and crusts. It is commonly found on exposed parts of the body and heals without sequelae. **i. herpetiformis.** A rare disease of the skin characterized by the formation of superficial miliary pustules that may be discrete but tend to form circular groups. Most cases of this disease have occurred in pregnant women; it is often fatal. **i. neonatorum.** A form of bullous impetigo occurring in the newborn.

im·pin'ger (im·pin'jur). An instrument for determining the number of dust particles in the air. A measured air sample is propelled through an underwater jet against a perpendicular plate. The dust is collected in the water, which is transferred to a shallow chamber in which the suspended particles can be counted under a microscope. Other instruments used for the same purpose are the jet dust counter, konimeter, and precipitator. Also see *dust count.*

im"plan·ta'tion. 1. The act of setting in, as the transplantation of a tissue, tooth, duct, or organ from one place in the body to another, or from the body of one person to that of another, implying the placing of the tissue in depth, as distinguished from the placement of a surface graft, *q.v.* Tissue implants are sometimes used as guides or ladders for the restoration of damaged nerve trunks and tendons. **2.** The placement within the body tissues of a substance, such as tantalum, vital-

lium, wire filligree, for restoration by mechanical means; as, for example, the closure of a bone defect or the repair of a ventral hernia. **3.** The embedding of the embryo into, or on, the endometrium. **—implant',** *v.,* **im'plant,** *n.* **i. of the bile ducts.** The placement of the proximal end of the common or the hepatic duct into the wall of the duodenum, stomach, or jejunum for the cure of biliary fistula. **i. of the ureters.** The transfer of the distal ends of the ureters into the intestine or the skin after cystectomy for malignant disease and in certain cases of exstrophy. **pellet i.** Administration of hormone products by implantation of pellets of solid active material under the skin.

im'plants. 1. Small tubes or needles which are radioactive, placed deeply in tissues for therapeutic reasons. **2.** Tissue grafts placed in depth. See *graft.* **basket implant.** A fenestrated, lucite framework designed to be embedded in the eye socket after enucleation, for use as a prosthesis for an artificial eye.

im·pon'der·a·ble. Incapable of being weighed; without weight.

im'po·tence, im'po·ten·cy. Lack of power, especially inability for sexual intercourse in the man. Syn., *agonia, asynodia, invirility.* **—impotent,** *adj.* **functional i.** Impotence due to a disturbance of the nervous mechanism for the sexual act. **organic i.** Impotence due to some anatomic defect in the sexual organs; may occur in either male or female. **psychic i.** That form of impotence which is due to some mental or emotional disturbance. Also called *cerebral i.*

im·preg'nate. 1. Render pregnant. **2.** Saturate or charge with. **—impregna'tion,** *n.*

im·pres'sion. 1. A mark produced upon a surface by pressure. **2.** *In dentistry,* a mold, usually of a jaw or its parts, from which a cast is made. Materials employed commonly include plaster of Paris, wax mixtures, and hydrocolloids. **3.** An effect produced by an external force upon the senses or the mind. **maternal impressions.** The effects supposed to be produced upon the fetus in the uterus by mental impressions of a disturbing character received by the mother during pregnancy. Also called *psychic trauma.*

im'pulse. 1. A push or communicated force. **2.** A sudden mental feeling that urges onward to an action. **cardiac i.** The beat of the heart felt in the fifth intercostal space to the left of the sternum. **catabolic i.** Generalized tissue breakdown in shock. **enteroceptive impulses.** Afferent nerve impulses which derive their stimulation from internal organs. **exterocep-tive impulses.** Afferent nerve impulses which derive their stimulation from external sources. **involuntary i.** One not activated by the will of the person, as the cardiac impulse. **morbid i.** A sudden, almost uncontrollable desire to do an unlawful act. **nerve i.** A transient physicochemical change in the membrane of a nerve fiber which sweeps rapidly along the nerve fiber to its termination, where it causes excitation of other nerves, muscle cells, or gland cells, depending on the connections and functions of the nerve.

im·pul'sion. The act of driving or urging onward, either mentally or physically.

im·pu"ta·bil'i·ty. *In legal medicine,* that degree of mental soundness which makes one responsible for his own acts.

In. Chemical symbol for indium.

in-. A prefix signifying *into, within, in, toward, on.*

in-. A prefix denoting negation; *not, non-, un-.*

in-. See *ino-.*

-in. *In chemistry,* a termination applied to *neutral nitrogenous substances,* as proteins and bitter principles; *an ester,* as palmitin; *the names of glycosides* and *neutral principles.* Also see *-ine.*

in·ac'ti·vate. To render inactive; usually applied to fresh serum, heated at 56° C. for 30 minutes to destroy its complement.

in·ad'e·qua·cy. Insufficiency of function or capacity. **renal i.** The condition in which the amount of urinary solids, and often the quantity of urine itself, is considerably diminished.

in·an'i·mate. Not animate; dead; without life.

in"a·ni'tion (in"a·nish'un). A pathologic state of the body due to the lack of any foodstuff (including water) which is essential to the living organism.

in"ar·tic'u·late. 1. Not jointed or articulated. 2. Vocal sounds not capable of arrangement into syllables, or of being understood.

in"as·sim'i·la·ble. Incapable of being assimilated.

in"born". A constitutional characteristic which is inherited or implanted during intrauterine life; innate.

in"breed"ing. Any system of mating which gives a smaller number of ancestors than the maximum possible. The closest inbreeding is self-fertilization, as in plants, or brother-by-sister mating in animals.

in·car"cer·a'tion. The abnormal imprisonment of a part, as in some forms of hernia. **—incar'cerated,** *adj.*

in'cest. Sexual intercourse between persons of such close relationship that their marriage is prohibited by law.

inch. The twelfth part of a foot; 2.54 cm.

in'ci·dence. 1. The act or manner of falling upon; the way in which one body strikes another. 2. The amount or extent of occurrence, as of a disease. **angle of i.** *In optics,* the angle at which a ray of light strikes a reflecting or refracting surface. **i. rate.** The number of cases of a disease appearing per unit of population within a defined time interval. **point of i.** The point upon which a ray or projectile strikes a reflecting or refracting surface. **racial i.** The incidence rate according to race.

in'ci·dent. Falling upon.

in·cin"er·a'tion. The process of heating organic substances until all organic matter is driven off and only the ash remains; cremation.

in·cip'i·ent. Initial, commencing, as incipient tuberculosis. **—incipience, incipiency,** *n.*

in·ci'sal (in·sigh'zul). Cutting; used of the cutting edge of incisor and canine teeth.

in·cised' (in·sized'). Cut; made by cutting.

in·ci'sion (in·sizh'un). 1. A cut or wound of the body tissue. It is named according to the location, as abdominal incision; the organ to be operated on, as appendiceal; the shape, as gridiron; the direction, as vertical, oblique; or, frequently, after the surgeon who first used it, as McBurney, Cushing. 2. The act of cutting. **buttonhole i.** A small, straight cut made into an organ or cavity. **crucial i.** Two cuts at right angles, made deeply into the tissues, usually to insure free drainage. **exploratory i.** One made for the purpose of diagnosis. **muscle-splitting i.** One in which the muscles are split in the direction of their fibers in order to secure a better line of closure, as the McBurney incision. **paramedian i.** That made to one side of the median line. **rectus i.** One made through the rectus abdominis muscle or through its sheath.

in·ci'sive. 1. Cutting. 2. Pertaining to the incisor teeth.

in·ci'sor. 1. A cutting tooth; one of the four front teeth of either jaw. 2. Pertaining to the incisor teeth. **deciduous i.** One of the eight incisors of the temporary (milk) dentition. Abbreviated, **i. permanent i.** One of the eight teeth which replace the deciduous incisors in the permanent (adult) dentition. Abbreviated, **I.**

in·ci'sure. (in·sigh'zhur, in·sizh'ur). A slit or notch. Also see *notch.* **radio-**

logic i. Any indentation seen in an opaque meal radiograph of the stomach.

in"cli·na'tion. 1. A propensity; a leaning. 2. The deviation of the long axis of a tooth from the vertical.

in·clu'sion bod'y. A particle found in nuclei and cytoplasm, caused by certain filterable virus infections.

in·clu'sion con·junc"ti·vi'tis. An inflammatory disease of the conjunctiva, most commonly found in newborn infants; caused by a filtrable virus, which is transmitted to the child from the mother's genital tract during birth. Characterized by a swelling and redness of the lids, by a mucoid discharge, and by inclusion bodies in the epithelial cells.

in"co·ag'u·la·ble. Incapable of coagulation or curdling.

in"co·her'ence. The quality of being incoherent; absence of connection of ideas or of language; incongruity or inconsequence of diction.

in"com·bus'ti·ble. Incapable of being burned.

in"com·pat'i·ble. Incapable of being used or put together because of resulting chemical change or of antagonistic qualities, as two drugs or two types of blood. **—incompatibil'ity,** n.

in·com'pe·tence. 1. Insufficiency; inadequacy to perform the natural functions. 2. *In legal medicine,* incapacity; want of legal fitness, as the incompetence of a drunken man to drive a car. **—incompetent,** *adj.*
valvular i. The state or condition of failure of a heart valve to prevent regurgitation of blood; it is due to weakness or dilatation of the valve ring without the valve itself being deformed.

in"con·gru'i·ty. Absence of agreement, correspondence, or needful harmony.

in·con'ti·nence. Inability to control the natural evacuations, as the feces or the urine; involuntary evacuation.

in"co·ör"di·na'tion. Inability to bring into common, harmonious movement or action, as inability to produce voluntary muscular movements in proper order or sequence.

in'cre·ment. The amount of increase or growth in a given period of time. **—incremen'tal,** *adj.*

in·cre'tin. That fraction of secretin which, upon oral or intravenous administration, produces hypoglycemia and does not stimulate pancreatic secretion; obtained by treatment of secretin by pepsin. Also see *excretin.*

in·cre'tion. An internal secretion. **—in'cretory,** *adj.*

in"crus·ta'tion. The formation of a crust or hard coating, as from an exudate; scab, scale.

in"cu·ba'tion. 1. The act or process of hatching or developing, as eggs or bacteria. 2. The phase of an infectious disease from the time of infection to the appearance of the first symptoms. 3. The process of culturing bacteria for qualitative or quantitative growth studies, as in microbiologic assays. 4. The process of maintaining mixtures of substances in suspension or solution at definite temperatures for varying periods of time for the study of enzyme action or other chemical reactions.

in'cu·ba"tor. 1. A small chamber with controlled temperature and humidity for the care of prematurely born infants. 2. A laboratory cabinet with controlled temperature for the cultivation of bacteria or for facilitating biologic tests. 3. A device for the artificial hatching of eggs.

in·cur'a·ble. 1. Not curable. 2. A person suffering from an incurable disease.

in'cus. The middle one of the chain of ossicles in the middle ear, so termed from its resemblance to an anvil. See Table of Bones in the Appendix. **—incudal,** *adj.*

in d. *In dies;* daily.

in"da·ga'tion. 1. Close investigation. 2. Digital examination.

indalone. Trade-mark for butopyronoxyl.

in·de'cent. Not decent; obscene.

in"de·ci'sion. Morbid irresolution; want of firmness or of will; abulia. A symptom of early melancholia.

in"den·ta'tion. 1. A notch, dent, or depression. 2. A condition of being notched or serrated.

in'dex (pl. *indexes, indices*). 1. The forefinger. 2. The ratio, or the formula expressing the ratio, of one dimension of a thing to another dimension. 3. *In craniometry,* the ratio of one dimension of the skull to another dimension, usually the length, which is taken as the standard and is represented by 100. The formula is

$$i = \frac{\text{breadth} \times 100}{\text{length}}$$

cephalic i. The ratio of the greatest width of the head, taken wherever it may be found in a horizontal plane perpendicular to the sagittal plane, × 100, to the greatest length, taken in the sagittal plane between glabella and opisthocranion. Its values are classified as:

dolichocephalic	x–75.9
mesocephalic	76.0–80.9
brachycephalic	81.0–85.4
hyperbrachycephalic	85.5–x

chemotherapeutic i. The formula expressing the relationship between the toxicity of a compound for the body and for parasites, as:

$$C.I. = \frac{\text{maximal tolerated dose per kg. body wt.}}{\text{minimal curative dose per kg. body wt.}}$$

color i. The amount of hemoglobin per cell relative to normal, as:

$$C.I. = \frac{\text{per cent normal hemoglobin concentration}}{\text{per cent normal erythrocyte count}}.$$

Different workers use different normal values in this formula. **inhibition i.** The amount of an antimetabolite needed to overcome the biological effect of a unit weight of metabolite, used as a measure of the antagonism between metabolite and antimetabolite. **opsonic i.** The ratio of the phagocytic index of a patient's serum to that of pooled normal serum. **parasite i.** The percentage of individuals in a community showing parasites in the blood. **pelvic i.** The relation of the anteroposterior to the transverse diameter of the pelvis. **pelvic-inlet i.** That ratio of the sagittal diameter, or conjugata vera of the pelvic inlet, taken between the points where the sagittal plane cuts the sacral promontory and the posterior edge of the superior surface of the symphysis pubis, to the transverse diameter, taken between the points on the arcuate lines that lie farthest lateral from the midline, at right angles to the conjugata vera. When multiplied by 100, values are classified as:

platypellic   x–89.9
mesatipellic   90.0–94.9
dolichopellic   95.0–x

refractive i. The refractive power of any substance as compared with air. It is the quotient of the angle of incidence divided by the angle of refraction of a ray passing through a substance. Symbol, n. **therapeutic i.** The ratio of toxicity (measured as the lethal dose) to the therapeutic dose.

in'di·can. 1. Indoxyl glucoside, $C_{14}H_{17}NO_6.3H_2O$, occurring in indigo plants; upon hydrolysis and subsequent oxidation, it is converted to indigotin, the chief constituent of indigo. 2. Indoxyl potassium sulfate, $C_8H_6NSO_4K$, a substance occurring in urine and formed from indole.

in'di·cant. 1. Serving as an index or as an indication. 2. A fact or symptom that indicates a certain treatment.

in''di·ca'tion. Any symptom, cause, or occurrence in a disease which points out its course of treatment.

in''di·ca''tor. In chemistry, a substance used to show by a color or other change when a reaction has taken place or a chemical affinity has been satisfied.

in''di·ces. Plural of index, q.v.

in di'es. Daily. Abbreviated, in d.

in·dif'fer·ent. Neutral; undifferentiated or nonspecialized, as indifferent cells. **—indifferentism**, n.

in·dig'e·nous (in-didj'i-nus). Native; originating or belonging to a certain locality or country.

in''di·ges'tion. Lack of digestion; imperfect digestion.

in''di·glu'cin. $C_8H_{10}O_6$. A yellow syrup, one of the decomposition products of indican.

in''di·go. A blue pigment formed by the hydrolysis and oxidation of the indican contained in various species of Indigofera. **i. blue.** $C_{16}H_{10}N_2O_2$, indigotin. **i. carmine** (C.C.). A blue dye, sodium or potassium indigotindisulfonate. **i. white.** A substance obtained by the reduction of indigo blue.

in·dig'o·tin, in''di·go'tin. $C_{16}H_{10}N_2O_2$. The chief constituent of indigo. Also see indican.

in''di·go·u'ri·a. The presence of indigo in the urine; due to a decomposition of indican.

in''di·rect'. Not direct; not in a direct line; acting through an intervening medium.

in'di·um. In = 114.76. A rare metal. It is very soft, resembles lead in its properties, and is used in many alloys.

in'dole. 1-Benzazole; ketole; 2,3-benzopyrrole. C_8H_7N. A substance formed during intestinal putrefaction and in certain bacterial cultures. It is responsible, in part, for the odor of feces.

in''dole·a·ce'tic ac'id. Indole-3-acetic acid, a bacterial decomposition product of tryptophan; found in urine and feces. It possesses pronounced growth-promoting activity for leaves.

in'do·lent. Sluggish; usually applied to slowness in healing, as an indolent ulcer.

in''do·lu'ri·a. The excretion of indole in the urine.

in''do·phe'nol (in''do·fee'nole, ·nol). Any of a series of dyes derived from quinone imine.

in·dox'yl. C_8H_7ON. A yellow, crystalline oxidation product of indole and skatole. **i. glucoside.** See indican, 1. **i. potassium sulfate.** Indican. $C_8H_6NSO_4K$. The potassium salt of indoxyl, conjugated with sulfuric acid; occurs in urine. Sometimes called indoxyl sulfate.

in·dox''yl·glu''cu·ron'ic ac'id. A product formed by the detoxification of indole.

in·dox″yl·sul·fu′ric ac′id. The substance resulting from conjugation of indoxyl with sulfuric acid.

in·dox″yl·u′ri·a. The presence of indoxyl in the urine.

in·duc′tion. 1. The act of bringing on or causing. 2. The bringing about of an electric or magnetic state in a body by the proximity (without actual contact) of an electrified or magnetized body. 3. The period from the first administration of the anesthetic until consciousness is lost and the patient is stabilized in the desired surgical plane of anesthesia. 4. In embryology, the specific morphogenetic effect brought about by the action of one tissue upon another, acting through organizers or evocators.

in·duc″to·py·rex′i·a (in·duck″to-pye·reck″see·uh). Artificial fever produced by electromagnetic induction; a form of electrotherapy.

in″duc·to′ri·um. In physiology, an instrument for the generation and administration of induction shocks; it consists of a primary and a secondary coil mounted on a stand.

in·duc′to·ther″my (in·duck′to-thur″mee, in·duck″to·thur′mee). The application of energy to tissue through the agency of a high-frequency magnetic field. It is produced by means of a heavily insulated conductor wound into a coil of appropriate configuration and number of turns through which a high-frequency current is conducted from an oscillator. It is usually applied to local parts but may be used to produce general artificial fever.

in′du·lin. One of a group of dyes similar to the safranines, highly phenylated amino derivatives. The only important one in medicine is nigrosine, q.v. Also called i. black.

in″du·ra′tion. 1. The hardening of a tissue or part, resulting from hyperemia, inflammation, or infiltration by neoplasm. 2. A hardened area of tissue. —**in′durated, in′dura·tive,** adj.

-ine (-een, -in). In chemistry, a termination indicating a basic nitrogenous compound, as morphine, purine; a halogen, as bromine. Also see -in.

in·e′bri·ant. 1. Intoxicant; causing inebriation. 2. An agent that causes inebriation.

in·e″bri·a′tion. Intoxication.

in″e·bri′e·ty. Habitual drunkenness.

in·ef′fi·ca·cy. Failure to produce the desired effect.

in″e·nu′cle·a·ble. Not removable by enucleation.

in·er′ti·a. 1. Dynamic opposition to acceleration, common to all forms of matter, including electrons and quanta. 2. Lack of activity, said of the uterus when in labor the contractions have diminished or ceased entirely. Also called uterine i. —**inert′,** adj.

in ex·tre′mis. At the end; at the last; at the point of death.

in′fant. 1. A child, usually up to two years. 2. A minor; a person under legal age, according to common law, 21, though some states of the United States do not follow this rule. —**in·fancy,** n.

in·fan′ti·cide. 1. The murder of an infant. 2. The murderer of an infant.

in′fan·tile (in′fun·tile, ·til). Pertaining to infancy; like an infant in actions.

in·fan′ti·lism. 1. The persistence of infantile or childish traits and characteristics into adolescent and adult life; the condition is marked by mental, physical, and sexual underdevelopment and sometimes dwarfish stature. Also called ateliosis, Lorain syndrome. 2. In psychoanalysis, the state of infancy prolonged into adult life. **dysthyroidal i.** Infantilism resulting from impaired thyroid activity. **lymphatic i.** That form associated with lymphatism. Also called Paltauf's nanism. **myxedematous i.** The underdevelopment seen in cretinism, q.v., characterized by an infantile face, prominent lips and tongue, distended abdomen, rudimentary genitalia, arrested mental and emotional development, and delayed or absent second dentition. **pituitary i.** Dwarfism resulting from a lack of the growth-promoting and gonadotropic hormones of the pituitary body. **sex i.** Continuation of childish sex traits and development beyond puberty.

in·farct′, in′farct. A region of necrosis of tissue due to complete interference with blood flow, usually the result of occlusion of the supplying artery or, rarely, to occlusion of the draining vein. In viscera, the infarct is generally of conical form, but in extremities it occupies the region supplied by the occluded artery (ischemic necrosis). **cicatrized i.** One in which the necrotic mass is replaced or encapsulated by fibrous tissue. **healed i.** See cicatrized i. **hemorrhagic i.** See red i. **marginal i.** Zone of degeneration forming a yellowish white fibrous ring, found at term about the edge of the placenta. **red i.** One in which the necrotic focus is swollen, firm, and either bright or dark red, as the result of hemorrhage. **white i.** One in which the hemorrhage is slight, or the blood and blood pigments have been removed; that is, the infarct has become decolorized.

in·farc′tion. The process leading to the development of an infarct. Immediately following vascular occlusion, there is successive occurrence of hyperemia, cloudy swelling, fatty degeneration, and necrosis. Necrotic tissue stimulates mild inflammation, which results in the formation of a cicatrix or capsule.

in·fec'tion. 1. The introduction of pathogenic organisms into or onto the body of a host; specifically, microörganisms such as bacteria, rickettsiae, viruses, protozoa, or fungi. See also *infestation.* 2. The communication of disease from one subject to another. 3. Autoinfection. 4. The pathologic state caused by microörganisms. **—infectious, infective,** *adj.;* **infect',** *v.* **air-borne i.** The transfer of infection from one individual to another without direct contact between them by means of droplets of moisture containing the causative agent. Also called *droplet i.* **concurrent i.** Simultaneous existence of two or more forms of infection. **focal i.** One in which a bacterial disease process is limited to a definite area or focus, as in certain tissues, glands, or organs; not only may the local tissue be destroyed, but toxemia may result if the microörganism produces a soluble toxin. **food i.** Food poisoning. **mixed i.** Concurrent infection. **secondary i.** Implantation of a new infection upon one already in existence. **terminal i.** An infection occurring late in the course of another disease, causing the death of the patient.

in"fe·cun'di·ty. Sterility; barrenness.

in·fe'ri·or. Lower; applied to structures nearer the feet, as contrasted to superior, nearer the head.

in·fe"ri·or'i·ty. A state or condition of being lower, inferior, less adequate, less well-developed or adapted; it may be organic or psychic. **feeling of i.** *In psychology,* a morbid feeling of personal inadequacy; may result in timidity or submission, or, because of overcompensation, in selfish aggression. Also called *i. complex.*

in"fer·til'i·ty. Sterility.

in"fes·ta'tion. The presence, in or on a host, of animal parasites, such as ticks, lice, roundworms, or flatworms. **—infest,** *v.*

Confusion with the term infection has resulted from the fact that an infesting parasite, as a louse, may transmit an infection, such as typhus.

in·al'trate. 1. Pass into tissue spaces or cells, as fluids, cells, or other substances. 2. The material which has infiltrated.

in"fil·tra'tion. 1. A process by which cells, fluid, or other substances pass into tissue spaces or into cells. The various substances may be natural to the part or cell, but in excess; or

they may be foreign to the part or cell. 2. The material taking part in the process. 3. *In radiology,* the production in a part or organ of a change whereby radioluminescence is decreased.

in·ârm'. Weak or feeble.

in·âr'ma·ry. A hospital; an institution where ill and infirm persons are maintained during treatment period.

in·âr'mi·ty. 1. Weakness; feebleness. 2. A disease producing feebleness.

in"flam·ma'tion. The reaction of the tissues to injury. The essential process, regardless of the causative agent, is characterized clinically by local heat, swelling, redness, and pain; pathologically, by primary vasoconstriction followed by vasodilatation, with slowing of the blood current, accumulation and emigration of leukocytes, exudation of fluid, and deposition of fibrin. Some authorities include under inflammation the process of repair, the production of new capillaries and fibroblasts, organization, and cicatrization. **—inflam'matory,** *adj.;* **inflame',** *v.* **acute i.** One in which the progress is rapid and the course is short. **allergic i.** That which is excited by a localized, hyperactive response to an allergen to which the subject is hypersensitive. Also called *hyperergic i.* **chronic i.** One characterized by slow progression and long course; a progressive condition in contrast to an end stage of cicatrization. **exudative i.** That in which exudation is the conspicuous feature. **productive i.** One in which there is a considerable multiplication of fibroblasts. Also called *plastic i.* **purulent i.** One in which pus is formed. Also called *suppurative i.* **serous i.** That in which the exudate is composed largely of serum. **subacute i.** A form which has a somewhat longer progress and course than acute inflammation, with moderate proliferation of fibroblasts. **subchronic i.** Inflammation of somewhat more rapid progress and course than chronic inflammation. **suppurative i.** See purulent *i.*

in·fla'tion. Distention with air.

in·flec'tion, in·flex'ion. 1. A bending inward. 2. Modification of the pitch of the voice in speaking.

in"flu·en'za. An epidemic disease, sometimes becoming pandemic; characterized by catarrhal inflammation of the mucous membrane of the respiratory tract, accompanied by a mucopurulent discharge, fever, pain in the muscles, and prostration. At times, symptoms are mainly referred to the nervous system. The cause is an influenza virus, various strains being designated as A, B, etc. Complications are common, pneumonia being the most frequent; pleurisy, otitis media, and neuritis also may appear.

in'fra-. A prefix signifying *below* or *beneath, inferior, or within.*

in"fra·car'di·ac. Situated below or beneath the heart.

in"fra·cla·vic'u·lar. Below the collarbone.

in·frac'tion. Incomplete fracture of a bone.

in"fra·hy'oid. Situated below the hyoid bone.

in"fra·or'bit·al. Beneath or below the floor of the orbit.

in"fra·pa·tel'lar. Below the patella.

in"fra·red'. Pertaining to wave lengths of radiant energy longer than those of the red end of the visible spectrum and shorter than those of Hertzian waves.

in"fra·scap'u·lar. Below the shoulder blade.

in"fun·dib'u·li·form" (in"fun-dib'yoo·li·form", in"fun·dib·yoo'li-form"). Funnel-shaped.

in"fun·dib'u·lum. 1. A funnel-shaped passage or part. 2. The stalk of the pituitary gland. **—infundibu-lar,** *adj.* **1. of uterine tube.** The wide, funnel-shaped portion of the uterine tube at its fimbriated end.

in·fu'sion. 1. The process of extracting the active principles of a substance by means of water, but without boiling. 2. The product of such a process. 3. The slow injection of liquid into a vein.

in"fu·so'ri·a (in"few·sor'ee·uh, -zor'ee·uh). Formerly a class of Protozoa which is now called Ciliata.

in·ges'ta. Substances taken into the body, especially foods.

in·ges'tion. 1. The act of taking substances, especially food, into the body. 2. The process by which a cell takes up foreign matter, such as bacilli or smaller cells. **—ingestive,** *adj.*

in·gre'di·ent. Any substance that enters into the formation of a compound or mixture.

in'gui·nal (ing'gwi·nul). Pertaining to the inguinal region or groin.

in'gui·no- (ing'gwi·no-), **inguin-.** A combining form signifying *groin.*

in·ha'lant. 1. One who inhales. 2. That which is inhaled, as a medicine. 3. Related to, or used for, inhaling. **—inhalent,** *adj.;* **inhaler,** *n.*

in"ha·la'tion. 1. The breathing in of air or other vapor. 2. A medicinal substance to be used by inhalation. **—inhale',** *v.*

in·ha·la"tor, in"ha·la"tor. A device for facilitating the inhalation of a gas or spray. Used for providing oxygen or oxygen-carbon dioxide mixtures for respiration in resuscitation.

in·ha'ler. 1. An apparatus used for filtering air, etc., to protect the lungs against damp or cold air, dust, or gases. 2. Inhalator.

in·her'ent (in·heer'unt, in·herr'unt). Innate; natural to the organism.

in·her'it·ance. 1. The acquisition of characteristics by transmission of germ plasm from ancestor to descendant. 2. The sum total of characteristics dependent upon the constitution of the fertilized ovum; also, the total set of genes in the fertilized ovum.

in·her'it·ed. Derived from an ancestor.

in·hib'in, in'hib·in. A testicular hormone inhibiting the gonadotropic secretion of the adenohypophysis.

in"hi·bi'tion (in"hi·bish'un). 1. The act of checking or restraining the action of an organ or of a cell. 2. *In psychiatry,* an unconscious restraining of an instinctual impulse by an opposing impulse. **—inhib'itory,** *adj.;* **inhib'it,** *v.*

in·hib'i·tor. 1. A substance which checks or stops a chemical action. 2. A neuron whose stimulation stops, or suppresses, the activity of the part it innervates, or of a neuron with which it synapses.

in·i'tial. Pertaining to the beginning of a process; primary.

in·ject'. Introduce fluids into the skin, subcutaneous tissue, muscle, blood vessels, spinal canal, or any body cavity.

in·jec'tion. 1. The act of injecting or throwing in. 2. The substance injected. **hypodermic i.** Injection which is made into the subcutaneous connective tissue, by means of a syringe. **nutrient i.** Injection of nutrient fluids into the rectum or other cavity of the body. **repository i.** One containing the therapeutic agent in slowly absorbable form so as to delay its absorption and prolong the effect.

in·ju·ry. Damage or wound to the body or any body region, traumatic in origin; usually includes trauma of several tissues, organs, or systems. More general and inclusive than paralysis, hemorrhage, hematoma, and other such specific terms.

in'lay". *In dentistry,* applied to fillings first made and then inserted into a cavity with cement. **bone i.** A bone graft fitted into the two fragments and lying across a fracture or filling a gap between the fragments.

in'let. The entrance to a cavity. **i. of the pelvis.** The space within the brim of the pelvis; the superior pelvic strait.

in'nate, in·nate'. Dependent upon the genetic constitution.

in"ner·va'tion. 1. The distribution of nerves to a part. 2. The amount of nerve stimulation received by a part.

in·no·cent. Benign; not malignant; not apparently harmful.

in·noc·u·ous. Not injurious; harmless.

in·nom·i·nate. 1. Unnamed; unnamable, as innominate artery. 2. The irregular bone forming one side and anterior wall of the pelvic cavity, and composed of the ilium, ischium, and pubis; the hipbone.

in'o- (in'o-, eye'no-), **in-.** A combining form denoting *fibrous tissue* or *fibrous components of a tumor*.

in·oc"u·la'tion. The act of introducing the agent of a disease into the body. Specifically, the intentional introduction of an organism for the purpose of producing a mild form of a disease which would be severe if spontaneously introduced. This is known as **preventive inoculation.**

in·oc'u·la"tor. One who or that which inoculates; an instrument used in inoculation.

in·oc'u·lum. A small amount of bacteria-containing substance used to grow a culture of the bacteria or to infect an experimental animal.

in·op'er·a·ble. That which should not be operated upon; implies a condition in which the prognosis is unfavorable if an operation is undertaken.

in"or·gan'ic. Not organic; not produced by animal or vegetable organisms.

in·os'cu·late. Unite by small openings; anastomose.

in·os"cu·la'tion. The joining of blood vessels by direct communication.

in'o·sine (in'o·seen, eye'no·). A compound occurring in muscle which is formed by the union of hypoxanthine and ribose. It is a decomposition product of inosinic acid.

in"o·sin'ic ac'id (in"o·sin'ick, eye"no·). A nucleotide constituent of muscle; on hydrolysis with acid it yields hypoxanthine and D-ribose-5-phosphoric acid.

in·o'si·tol (in·o'si·tole, in·oss'i·). $C_6H_8(OH)_6.2H_2O$. Hexahydroxycyclohexane; a sugarlike alcohol occurring in muscle tissue, brain, red blood cells, and the tissues of the eye; also in leaves and seeds of plants.

in·o'si·tol-hex"a·phos·phor'ic ac'id. Phytin. An ester of inositol and phosphoric acid which is present in the seeds of plants.

in'quest. In legal medicine, a judicial inquiry, as a coroner's inquest, for the purpose of determining the cause of death of one who has died by violence or in some unknown way.

in"qui·si'tion (in"kwi·zish'un). An inquiry, especially one into the sanity or lunacy of a person.

in·san'i·tar"y (in·san'i·terr"ee). Not sanitary; not in a proper condition as respects the preservation of health.

in·san"i·ta'tion. Lack of proper sanitary conditions; defect of sanitation.

in·san'i·ty. 1. Loose term for any mental disorder or derangement. See *psychosis*. 2. *In legal medicine*, a mental disorder of such severity that the individual is unable to manage his own affairs and fulfill his social duties or is dangerous to himself or others. —**in·sane'**, *adj*. **circular i.** That marked by alternating manic and depressive episodes. Syn., *alternating i.* **climacteric i.** That occurring at or near the menopause. **consecutive i.** That following some disease or injury not of the brain. **cyclic i.** See circular *i.* **delusional i.** An acute condition in which delusions or hallucinations are the outstanding symptoms. **depressive i.** Melancholia. **impulsive i.** A form in which the patient possesses an uncontrollable desire to commit acts of violence. **intermittent i.** Recurrent insanity, *q.v.* **melancholic i.** Paranoid melancholia, *q.v.* **moral i.** A form marked by perversion and depravity of the moral sense, apparently without impairment of the reasoning and intellectual faculties. *Rare.* **periodic i.** Manic-depressive psychosis, *q.v.* **puerperal i.** Puerperal psychosis. **recurrent i.** A succession of attacks of the disorder. **senile i.** That due to old age. **stuporous i.** Old term for anergic stupor, *q.v.* **toxic i.** An acute form due to systemic poisoning by certain drugs.

in·scrip'tion. The body or main part of a prescription; contains the ingredients and amounts to be used.

in·scrip"ti·o'nes ten·din'e·ae (in·skrip"tee·o'neez ten·din'ee·ee). Transverse, fibrous bands between segments of the rectus abdominis muscle.

in'sect. A member of the class Insecta of the phylum Arthropoda. In the adult, the body is segmented and is divided into head, thorax, and abdomen; there are three pairs of legs and a single pair of antennae.

in·sec'ti·cide. A substance that is destructive to insects.

in·sec'ti·fuge. Any substance which repels insects.

in"se·cu'ri·ty. The state, feeling, or quality of being uncertain or unsafe; an attitude of apprehensiveness, as in respect to one's social status, circumstances, or safety.

in·sem"i·na'tion. 1. The planting of seed. 2. The introduction of semen into the vagina. 3. Impregnation. **artificial i.** The instrumental injection of semen into the vagina or uterus to induce pregnancy.

in·sen·si·ble. 1. Incapable of sensation or feeling; unconscious. 2. Incapable of being perceived or recognized by the senses. **—insensibility,** n.

in·ser·tion. 1. The act of setting or placing in. 2. That which is set in. 3. The point at which anything, as a muscle, is attached; the place or the mode of attachment of an organ to its support. The insertion of a muscle is contrasted with its origin as being the attachment to a relatively more movable part of the skeleton. **velamentous i.** The attachment of the umbilical cord to the margin of the placenta.

in·sid·i·ous. Coming on gradually or almost imperceptibly, as a disease, whose onset is gradual or inappreciable.

in·sight". In psychiatry, the patient's ability to understand his symptoms and their origin and to know that they indicate abnormalities.

in·sip·id. Tasteless.

in si·tu (in sigh'tew). In a given or natural position; undisturbed.

in·so·la·tion. 1. Exposure to the rays of the sun. 2. Treatment of disease by such exposure. 3. Sunstroke, q.v.

in·sol·u·ble. Incapable of dissolving in a liquid. **—insolubility,** n.

in·som·ni·a. Sleeplessness; disturbed sleep; a prolonged condition of inability to sleep.

in·spec·tion. In medicine, the examination of the body or any part of it by the eye.

in·spi·ra·tion. The drawing in of the breath; inhalation. **—inspire',** v.

in·spi·ra·to·ry. Pertaining to the act of inspiration.

in·spi·rom·e·ter. An instrument for measuring the amount of air inspired.

in·spis·sate. Make thick by evaporation or by removal of fluid. **—inspissated,** adj.

in·sta·bil·i·ty. 1. Lack of firmness; insecurity of support or balance. 2. Lack of fixed purpose; inconstancy in opinions or beliefs.

in·stance. In psychoanalysis, referring to the dominance or perseverance of one level of mental function in comparison to others.

in·step. The arch on the medial side of the foot.

in·stil·la·tion. The introduction of a liquid into a cavity drop by drop.

in·stil·la·tor. An apparatus for introducing, by drops, a liquid into a cavity or space.

in·stinct. 1. A precise form of behavior in which there is an invariable association of a particular series of responses with specific stimuli; an un-

conditioned compound reflex. 2. In psychoanalysis, a primary tendency, as toward life, reproduction, and death.

in·stinc·tive. Prompted or determined by instinct; of the nature of instinct.

in·stru·ment. A mechanical tool or implement. **—instrumen'tal,** adj. **stitching i.** A surgical appliance consisting of a needle holder which utilizes all varieties of surgical needles, the suture material feeding from a continuous spool supply attached to the handle.

in·stru·men·ta·tion. The use of instruments in treating a patient.

in·suf·fi·cien·cy. The state of being inadequate; incapacity to perform a normal function. **renal i.** Inadequate function of the kidney, characterized by its failure to remove urea from the blood at a normal rate.

in·suf·fla·tion. The act of blowing into, as blowing a gas, powder, or vapor into a body cavity. **endopharyngeal i.** A method of inducing anesthesia through a tube introduced through the mouth or nose to the back of the pharynx. **intratracheal i.** Insufflation through a tracheal tube introduced into the larynx. **mouth-to-mouth i.** The blowing of air into the mouth of a person, usually a newborn infant, to distend the lungs and counteract asphyxia. **perirenal i.** In roentgenography, the injection of air or carbon dioxide into the perirenal tissue to outline the adrenal glands and kidneys. **tubal i.** Used to demonstrate the patency of the uterine tubes; a gas, preferably carbon dioxide, is introduced into the uterus under pressure. Also called Rubin test.

in·suf·fla·tor. An instrument used in insufflation.

in·su·la. Portion of cortex overlying the corpus striatum; it lies hidden from view in the adult brain at the bottom of the lateral fissure. **—insular,** adj.

in·su·lin. The antidiabetic hormone arising from the beta cells of the islets of Langerhans of the pancreas. It is a protein with a molecular weight of approximately 12,000. **—insulinoid,** adj. **amorphous i.** The form of insulin obtained in commercial processes in the absence of added zinc or certain other metal ions. Also called regular i., unmodified i. **crystalline i.** The crystalline product obtained when insulin is precipitated in the presence of added zinc ion. **globin i. with zinc.** A preparation of insulin modified by the addition of globin (derived from the hemoglobin of beef blood) and zinc chloride. **histone i.** A preparation containing insulin and thymus histone which precipitates the insulin, the resulting suspension producing a prolonged hypoglycemic effect. **i. allergy.** The tissue reaction to insulin which may be represented by varying degrees of local tissue reaction, urticaria, or anaphylaxis. Local reactions may be characterized by stinging, itching, soreness, heat, and induration about the site of injection. The reaction may depend upon the animal source of the insulin. Contamination or alteration of the proteins in solution must be considered. Similar reactions may be due to substances such as protamine in the mixture injected. **i. shock.** The reaction of the body to doses of insulin which produce hypoglycemia. Common symptoms are a sense of nervous agitation, weakness, trembling, sweating, speech difficulty, pallor, listlessness, negativism, unconsciousness; in severe attacks, convulsions, vomiting, diarrhea, and incontinence. Also called *i. reaction.* **i. tolerance.** The relative degree of response of the body to insulin. **isophane i.** A preparation of protamine and insulin in their combining proportions, called the isophane ratio, of approximately 0.5 mg. of protamine for each 100 U.S.P. units of insulin. See also NPH *insulin.* **lente i.** One of a series of protein-free injectable insulins, having a varying duration of activity, obtained by mixing crystalline long-acting zinc insulin with amorphous short-acting insulin to produce a suspension in a phosphate-free saline and acetate medium of pH 7.2. **NPH i.** Neutral Protamine *Hagedorn* insulin, an isophane insulin in a buffered medium of pH 7.1 to 7.4, each injection containing 40 or 80 U.S.P. units of insulin per cc. **pectin i.** A slowly absorbed preparation of insulin in a viscous medium containing pectin. See *decurvon.* **protamine i.** A preparation of insulin combined with protamine, a protein prepared from the sperm of fishes of the trout family. **protamine zinc i.** A preparation similar to protamine insulin, but containing also zinc. **vegetable i.** Any one of several noninsulin blood-sugar-depressing plant extracts.

in″su·lin·e′mi·a. The presence of an abnormal, or dangerous, amount of insulin in the circulating blood.

in″sus·cep″ti·bil′i·ty. Absence of contagious quality; want of susceptibility.

in′take. 1. That amount of food or other susbtance which is taken into the body either orally or parenterally. See also *uptake.* 2. The act of taking in. 3. The orifice through which a substance is received.

in″te·gra′tion. 1. The process of unifying different elements into a single whole. 2. The combination of bodily activities to coöperate in the welfare of the whole organism. 3. *In neurology,* the impingement of impulses from various centers upon one final, common pathway, resulting in an adaptive response.

in·teg′u·ment. A covering, especially the skin. **—integumen′tary,** *adj.* **fetal i.** The fetal membranes. *Obs.*

in′tel·lect. The mind, the understanding, or the reasoning power.

in·tel′li·gence. 1. The understanding, intellect, or mind. 2. The ability to perceive qualities and attributes of the objective world, and to employ purposively a means toward the attainment of an end.

in·tel′li·gence quo′tient. A figure used to designate a person's intelligence; can be arrived at by dividing the mental age by the chronologic age (up to 16 years). The three grades of mental deficiency (idiocy, imbecility, and moronity) are marked by intelligence quotients of 69 or lower. Above 69, the classification is as follows: dull normal, 70–90; normal, 90–110; superior, 110–125; very superior, 125–140; and genius, 140 and above. Abbreviated, I.Q.

in·tem′per·ance. Want of moderation; immoderate indulgence, especially in alcoholic beverages. **—intemperate,** *adj., n.*

in·tense′. 1. In an extreme degree; showing to a high degree the characteristic attribute. 2. Feeling deeply.

in·ten″si·fi·ca′tion. The condition occurring in cutaneous sensory disturbances in which certain sensations are abnormally vivid.

in·ten′si·ty. 1. The state or condition of being intense. 2. Amount or degree of strength or power. **i. of x-rays.** The dose of radiation in roentgens divided by the time required to deliver it.

in·ten′tion. 1. The end or purpose. 2. A process or manner of healing, *q.v.*

in′ter-. A prefix signifying *between* or *among, mutual, intervening,* or *within.*

in″ter·a′tri·al (in″tur·a̅y′tree·ul, ·a̅t′ree·ul). Between the atria of the heart.

in·ter·ca′la″ted. Placed or inserted between, as intercalated disks of cardiac muscle.

in″ter·cap″il·lar″y glo·mer″u·lo·scle·ro′sis (in″tur·cap′i·lerr″ee). A lesion of the renal glomeruli which is accompanied by diabetes mellitus, renal edema, pronounced albuminuria, and sometimes hypertension and renal insufficiency. However, it occurs in diabetic persons without the associated phenomena mentioned and may occur in those without diabetes. Microscopically, the glomerular tufts show spherical, oval, or less well-defined foci of acellular, acidophilic, hyalinized tissue, with concentric argyrophilic laminas, situated between the capillaries. Said to be a more specific morphologic evidence of diabetes than is hyalinization of the pancreatic islets.

in″ter·cel′lu·lar. Between cells, as intercellular substance of tissue.

in″ter·cos′tal. Between the ribs, as intercostal spaces.

in″ter·coup′ler (in″tur·cup′lur). An apparatus used during the administration of an inflammable anesthetic to equalize the electric potential among anesthetist, patient, operating table, and anesthetic machine; designed to prevent explosions or fires due to static electricity.

in′ter·course. Communication; intimate connection between persons. **sexual i.** Sexual connection; coitus.

in″ter·cur′rent. Occurring or taking place between, as a disease arising or progressing during the existence of another disease in the same person.

in″ter·dic′tion. *In legal medicine,* a judicial or voluntary restraint placed upon an insane person or one suspected of insanity, preventing him from the management of his own affairs or the affairs of others.

in″ter·dig″i·ta′tion (in″tur·didj″i·tay′shun). The locking or dovetailing of similar parts, as the fingers of one hand with those of the other; or of the ends of the obliquus externus muscle with those of the serratus anterior. *In dentistry,* denoting that, in closure of the buccal teeth, the cusps of one denture strike fairly into the occluding sulci of the other denture.

in″ter·face. A surface that forms the boundary between two phases, systems, or substances.

in″ter·fer′ence. 1. *In physics,* the mutual action of two beams of light, or of two series of sound vibrations, or, in general, of two series of any type of waves when they coincide or cross. 2. The mutual extinction of two excitation waves that meet in any portion of the heart.

in″ter·fer·om′e·ter (in″tur·feer·om′i·tur). An apparatus for the production and demonstration of interference fringes between two or more wave trains of light from the same area. It is chiefly used to compare wave lengths with a standard wave length, by means of interference fringes.

in·te′ri·or. Situated within, with reference to a cavity, part, or organ.

in″ter·lo′bar. Situated between lobes, as interlobar pleurisy.

in″ter·mar′riage. 1. Marriage of blood relations. 2. Marriage between persons of different races.

in″ter·max′il·lar″y (in″tur·mack′si·lerr″ee). 1. Between the maxillary bones. 2. The os incisivum, a small bone that receives the upper incisors, situated between the maxillary bones of the fetus. Also called *premaxilla.*

in″ter·me″di·o·lat′er·al. Both lateral and intermediate, as the intermediolateral tract of the spinal cord, lying between the anterior and posterior gray columns.

in″ter·men′stru·al. Between menstrual periods.

in·ter′ment. The burial of a body.

in″ter·mit′tent. Occurring at intervals, as intermittent fever, insanity, pulse, or sterilization.

in″ter·mus′cu·lar. Situated between muscles.

in′tern. A resident physician in a hospital, usually in his first year of service.

in·ter′nal. Situated within or on the inside. —**internad,** *adv.*

in·ter′nist. A physician who specializes in internal medicine, *q.v.*

in″ter·node. The space between two nodes of a nerve fiber, as the internode between the nodes of Ranvier. Also called *internodal segment.* —**inter·no′dal,** *adj.*

in″ter·nun′ci·al (in″tur·nun′shul). Serving as a connecting or announcing medium, as internuncial neurons, nerve cells between two others in a nervous pathway.

in·ter′nus. See *internal.*

in″ter·o·cep′tor. Any one of the end-organs situated in the viscera which receive stimuli from visceral activities, such as digestion, excretion, circulation. Also called *visceroceptor.*

in″ter·o·fec′tive sys′tem. That part of the nervous system that is concerned with the regulation of the internal environment of the body; essentially, equivalent to the autonomic nervous system.

in″ter·os′se·ous. Between bones, as interosseous arteries, membranes, muscles, or ligaments.

in″ter·os′se·us. Interosseous muscle of the hand or foot, one of the small muscles inserted on the phalanges. See Table of Muscles in the Appendix.

in″ter·prox′i·mal. *In dentistry,* between two adjacent teeth, as an interproximal space.

in″ter·pu″pil·la″ry dis′tance. The distance between the centers of the pupils of the two eyes.

in″ter·sex″. An individual whose constitution is intermediate between male and female; a sex-intergrade. Syn., *hermaphrodite.* —**intersex′ual,** *adj.;* **intersexual′ity,** *n.*

in″ter·space″. An interval between the ribs, or between the fibers or lobules of a tissue or organ.

in″ter·spi′nous. Situated between spinous processes.

in·ter'sti·ces (in·tur'sti·siz). Spaces or intervals; pores.

in"ter·sti'tial (in"tur·stish'ul). 1. Situated between important parts; occupying the interspaces or interstices of a part. 2. Pertaining to the finest connective tissue of organs.

in"ter·trans"ver·sa'ri·i (in"tur·trans"vur·sah'ree·ee). Short bundles of muscular fibers extending between the transverse processes of contiguous vertebrae. See Table of Muscles in the Appendix.

in"ter·trans·verse' (·trans·vurs', ·tranz·). Connecting the transverse processes of contiguous vertebrae.

in"ter·tri'go (in"tur·try'go, ·tree'go). An erythematous eruption of the skin produced by friction of adjacent parts.

in'ter·val. 1. The time intervening between two points of time. 2. The lapse of time between two recurrences of the same phenomenon. 3. The empty space between any two things or parts of the same thing. **lucid i.** *In psychiatry,* a transitory return of the normal mental faculties, seen in psychoses or delirious conditions.

in"ter·ven·tric'u·lar. Situated between ventricles, as interventricular septum.

in"ter·ver'te·bral. Between the vertebrae, as an intervertebral disk.

in"ter·vil'lous. Situated between villi.

in·tes'tine. The part of the digestive tube extending from the pylorus to the anus. It consists of the small and large intestine. The former is about 6¾ meters (20 feet) in length, and extends from the pylorus to the junction with the large intestine at the cecum. Three divisions are described—the duodenum, 22 cm. long, the jejunum, 2.2 meters long, and the ileum, 4 meters long. The large intestine is about 1.6 meters (5 feet) long, and consists of the cecum (with the vermiform process), the colon, and the rectum. The wall of the intestine is made up of four coats, mucous, submucous, muscular, and serous. Embedded in the wall are minute glands, and projecting from the surface, in the small intestine, are the villi. —**intestinal,** *adj.*

in"tes·ti'num. See *intestine.* **i. crassum.** The large intestine. **i. tenue mesenteriale.** That portion of the small intestine which has a mesentery, namely the jejunum and ileum.

in·ti'ma. The innermost of the three coats of a blood vessel. —**intimal,** *adj.*

intocostrin. Trade-mark for a physiologically standardized curare extract or for its active component tubocurarine chloride.

in·tol'er·ance. 1. Lack of capacity to endure, as intolerance of light or pain. 2. Sensitivity, as to a drug.

in·tox'i·cant. 1. Intoxicating; capable of producing intoxication or poisoning. 2. An agent capable of producing intoxication.

in·tox"i·ca'tion. 1. Poisoning, as by a drug, a serum, alcohol, or any poison. 2. State of being intoxicated, especially the acute condition produced by overindulgence in alcohol; drunkenness. **pathologic i.** An alcoholic psychosis marked by unusual symptoms, as epileptiform seizures, confusion, illusions, anxiety, rage, violent criminal tendencies, and sometimes hallucinations; it is usually followed by amnesia for the episode. May occur in susceptible individuals after only a small amount of alcohol is consumed. **septic i.** A form of poisoning resulting from absorption of products of putrefaction. **water i.** A condition characterized by cramps, dizziness, headache, and vomiting; produced by the administration of large quantities of water with the resulting dilution of body salts. May occur in an experimental animal or in man, if certain diseases are present.

in'tra-. 1. A prefix signifying *within* or *into.* 2. *In anatomy,* a prefix denoting *situated within* a specified part.

in"tra·ab·dom'i·nal. Within the cavity of the abdomen, as intraabdominal pressure.

intracaine hydrochloride. A trade-mark for parethoxycaine hydrochloride.

in"tra·cap'su·lar. Within the fibrous capsule of a joint, as intracapsular fracture.

in"tra·cel'lu·lar. Within a cell.

in"tra·cra'ni·al. Within the skull, as intracranial pressure.

in"tra·cu·ta'ne·ous. Within the skin substance; applied to injection of substances into the skin.

in"tra·der'mal, in"tra·der'mic. Within the skin.

in"tra·lob'u·lar. Within a lobule as an intralobular vein of the liver.

in"tra·mem'bra·nous. Developed or taking place within a membrane, as intramembranous ossification.

in"tra·mu'ral. Within the substance of the walls of an organ, as intramural fibroid of the uterus.

in"tra·mus'cu·lar. Within the substance of a muscle, as intramuscular injection of drugs.

in"tra·nu'cle·ar. Within a nucleus

in"tra·oc'u·lar. Within the globe of the eye, as intraocular hemorrhage.

in"tra·o'ral. Within the mouth.

in"tra·or'bit·al. Within the orbit

in"tra·per·i·to·ne'al. Within the peritoneum, or peritoneal cavity, as intraperitoneal injection of drugs.

in″tra·tra′che·al (in″truh·tray′-kee·ul). Within the trachea, as intratracheal insufflation through a tracheal tube introduced through the larynx.

in″tra·u′ter·ine (in″truh·yōō′-tur·in, ·yōō′tuh·ryne). Within the uterus.

in″tra·vas′cu·lar. Within the blood vessels.

in″tra·ve′nous. Within, or into, the veins, as intravenous injection.

in·trin′sic. Inherent; situated within; peculiar to a part, as the intrinsic muscles of the larynx.

a′tro-. A prefix signifying *within* or *into; inward.*

in·tro′i·tus. An aperture or entrance, particularly the entrance to the vagina.

in″tro·jec′tion. 1. A mechanism by which there is possible an absorption of parts of the environment or of the personality of others into one's own personality. 2. *In psychoanalysis*, the process of transferring feeling or love from an object or person to the mental picture of the object or person.

in″tro·mis′sion. Insertion, the act of putting in, the introduction of one body into another, as of the penis into the vagina.

in″tro·mit′tent. Conveying or allowing to pass into or within, as into a cavity; refers to the penis, which carries the semen into the vagina.

in″tro·spec′tion. The act of looking inward, as into one's own mind. **mor′bid i.** The morbid habit of self-examination; irrational and obsessive dwelling upon one's own thoughts, feelings, impulses, fears, or conduct.

in″tro·ver′sion (in″tro·vur′shun, ·zhun). 1. A turning within, as a sinking within itself of the uterus. 2. *In psychopathology*, a turning inward of psychic energy in the form of introspection and subjective thinking.

in′tro·vert′. 1. One whose interests are directed inwardly upon himself and not toward the outside world. 2. Turn one's interests to oneself rather than to external things.

in″tu·ba′tion. The introduction of a tube into a hollow organ to keep it open, especially into the larynx to insure the passage of air, in edema of the glottis or in the acute stage of diphtheria.

in′tu·ba″tor. An instrument used for the introduction of an intubation tube.

in″tu·mes′cence. 1. A swelling of any character whatever, as an increase of the volume of any organ or part of the body. 2. The process of becoming swollen. Syn., *tumescence.*

in″tus·sus·cep′tion. The receiving of one part within another; especially, the invagination, slipping, or passage of one part of the intestine into another, occurring usually in young

infants. Acute intussusception is characterized by the symptom complex of paroxysmal pain, vomiting, the presence of a sausage-shaped tumor in the lower abdomen, and the passage of blood and mucus per rectum.

in″tus·sus·cep′tum. In intussusception, the invaginated portion of intestine.

in″tus·sus·cip′i·ens (in″tus·suhsip′ee·enz). In intussusception, the segment of the intestine receiving the other segment.

in′u·la. Elecampane. The root of *Inula helenium*, of the family Compositae. It contains inulin.

in′u·lase. An enzyme capable of converting inulin into levulose.

in′u·lin. ($C_6H_{10}O_5$)n. A carbohydrate from many plants of the Compositae. Yields levulose on hydrolysis.

in·unc′tion. 1. The act of rubbing an oily or fatty substance into the skin. 2. The substance used.

in u′te·ro. Within the uterus; not yet born.

in vac′u·o. In a vacuum; in a space from which most of the air has been exhausted.

in·vag″i·na′tion (in·vadj″i·nay′-shun). 1. The act of ensheathing or becoming ensheathed. 2. The process of burrowing or infolding to form a hollow space within a previously solid structure, as the invagination of the nasal mucosa within a bone of the skull to form a paranasal sinus. 3. Intussusception. 4. *In embryology*, the infolding of a part of the wall of the blastula to form a gastrula. —**invag′inate,** *adj., v.*

in·va′lid. 1. Not well. 2. One who is not well, especially one who is chronically ill or whose convalescence is slow. 3. Suitable or adapted for an invalid person, as invalid diet, invalid chair. —**invalidism,** *n.*

in·va′sion. 1. That period in the course of disease, especially an infectious disease, immediately following inception or infection, and preceding prodromal signs and symptoms. 2. The process whereby bacteria or other microörganisms enter the body; subsequent multiplication of pathogens causes disease.

inversine hydrochloride. Trademark for mecamylamine hydrochloride.

in·ver′sion (in·vur′shun, ·zhun). 1. The act of turning inward. 2. A turning upside down. 3. *In chemistry*, usually the change of a compound having optical activity into one or more other compounds conferring opposite optical activity on the product. Also the change of any compound into an isomeric form. **sexo-esthetic 1.** The adoption of the habits, manners, and costume of the opposite sex. Also see *eonism, transvestitism.* **sexual i.** *In psychiatry,* the direction of the sexual instinct toward one of the same sex; homosexuality.

in'vert. *In psychiatry,* a homosexual.

in·ver'tase (in·vur'tace, in'vur·taze). See *saccharase.*

In·ver"te·bra'ta. A division of the animal kingdom which includes all except the animals with a backbone.

in·ver'te·brate. 1. Without a spinal column; invertebral. 2. An animal without a backbone.

in·vert'in, in'vert·in. See *saccharase.*

in'ver·tose. See *invert sugar.*

in'vert sug'ar. A mixture of approximately equal parts of dextrose and levulose, obtained from the hydrolysis of sucrose. Also called *invertose.*

in·vest'ing. Enveloping, enclosing, embedding.

in·vest'ment. A sheath; a covering. **fibrous i.** General term describing an outer sheath of connective tissue found about various organs outside the proper capsule of the organ.

in·vet'er·ate. Long established, chronic, resisting treatment.

in vit'ro. In glass; referring to a process or reaction carried out in a culture dish, test tube, etc., as opposed to *in vivo.*

in vi'vo. In the living organism; used in contrast to *in vitro.*

in"vo·lu'crum. 1. The covering of a part. 2. New bone laid down by periosteum around a sequestrum in osteomyelitis.

in·vol'un·tar"y. Performed or acting independently of the will, as involuntary muscles of viscera.

in'vo·lute. *In biology,* rolled up, as the edges of certain leaves in the bud.

in"vo·lu'tion. 1. A turning or rolling inward. 2. The retrogressive change to their normal condition that certain organs undergo after fulfilling their functional purposes, as the uterus after pregnancy. 3. The period of regression or the process of decline or decay which occurs in the human constitution after middle life. —**involutional,** *adj.* **i. of the uterus.** The return of the uterus to its normal weight and condition after childbirth.

in'ward. Toward the inside or center.

iodeikon. A trade-mark for iodophthalein sodium.

i·od'ic ac'id (eye·od'ick). HIO₃. A crystalline powder, soluble in water.

i'o·dide. Any binary compound, such as a salt or ester, containing iodine having a negative valence of one.

i"o·dim'e·try. Usually, volumetric analysis by titration with an iodine solution.

i'o·dine (eye'o·dyne, -deen, -din) I = 126.92. A nonmetallic element occurring as gray-black plates or granules with metallic luster; it is only sparingly soluble in water. A local irritant and germicide. See Table of Normal Values of Blood Constituents in the Appendix.

i'o·dine-131 (-one thirty-one). A radioactive isotope of iodine, which emits beta and gamma rays, used in the form of sodium iodide in the diagnosis of thyroid disease and in the treatment of hyperthyroidism. Symbol, I¹³¹.

i·od'i·nin (eye·od'i·nin). A purple bronze antibiotic pigment produced by *Chromobacterium iodinum.*

i"o·dip'a·mide. N,N'-Adipyl-bis(3-amino-2,4,6-triiodo) benzoic acid, a roentgenographic contrast medium used in the form of sodium and methylglucamine salts. See *cholografin.*

iodipin. Trade-mark for an iodized vegetable oil.

i'o·dism. A condition arising from the prolonged use of iodine or iodine compounds; marked by frontal headache, coryza, ptyalism, and various skin eruptions, especially acne.

i'o·dized oil. An iodine addition product of vegetable oils, used for iodine therapy and as an x-ray contrast medium.

i·o'do- (eye·o'do-, eye'o·do-), **iod-** *In chemistry,* a combining form signifying iodine or an iodine compound.

i·o"do·al'phi·on'ic ac'id. β-(4-Hydroxy-3,5-diiodophenyl)-α-phenyl propionic acid, an orally administered contrast medium used in cholecystography. See *priodax.*

i·o"do·chlor"hy·drox'y·quin. C₉H₅ClINO. A brownish yellow powder, practically insoluble in water. Used in treatment of intestinal amebiasis, and as antiseptic powder with marked trichomonacidal power. See *vioform.*

i·o"do·der'ma. Skin eruptions due to iodine; generally used in reference to a pustular eruption caused by the ingestion of iodine compounds.

i·o"do·form. Triiodomethane, CHI₃. A yellow powder, only slightly soluble in water. An antiseptic and anesthetic.

i·o"do·gor·go'ic ac'id. Diiodotyrosine, *q.v.*

i·o"do·meth'ane. Methyl iodide.

i·o"do·phe'nol. 1. C₆H₄OH.I. Para iodophenol; has been used as an antiseptic. 2. A solution of 20 parts of iodine in 76 parts of fused phenol with 4 parts of glycerin.

i·o"do·phthal'ein (eye·o"do·thal'een, eye"o·do-). Tetraiodophenolphthalein. C₂₀H₁₀I₄O₄. A light yellow powder used externally as an antiseptic dusting powder.

i·o"do·phthal'ein so'di·um. C₂

$H_3I_4O_4Na_2.3H_2O$. The disodium salt of tetraiodophenolphthalein; a pale, blue-violet powder, soluble in water. It is employed to render the gallbladder opaque for roentgenologic examination. Syn., *soluble iodophthalein, tetiothalein sodium.* See *iodeikon.*

o″do·py′ra·cet in·jec′tion. The nonproprietary title for a solution of the trade-marked product *diodrast.*

i″o·dox′yl. British Pharmacopoeia title for disodium N-methyl-3:5-diiodo-4-pyridone-2:6-dicarboxylate or sodium iodomethamate, a radiopaque medium used in the diagnosis of urinary-tract affections. It is available under the trade-marked title neo-iopax.

i′on. An atom or group of atoms which has lost or gained one or more orbital electrons and has thus become capable of conducting electricity. **i. trans·fer.** The migration of ionic medication through intact skin under the influence of a direct electric current. Also called *iontophoresis.* **negative i.** Anion, *q.v.* **positive i.** Cation, *q.v.* **zwit·ter i.** An ion which contains both a positive and a negative charge. Amino acids in solution may yield such ions by a shift of a hydrogen ion from the carboxyl group, as, for example, RNH_2·COOH forming $RNH_3^+COO^-$ ion.

i·on′ic strength (eye·on′ick). Measure of the intensity of the electric field in a solution; half the sum of the activity of each ion in solution, multiplied by the square of its ionic charge.

i·o′ni·um (eye·o′nee·um). A radioactive element which emits alpha particles; an isotope of thorium and the direct parent of radium.

i′on·iz′a·ble. Capable of producing ions.

i′on·i·za′tion. The process of producing ions. **—i′onize,** *v.*

i′on·iz′ing e′vent. Any occurrence of a process in which an ion or group of ions is produced, as by passage of alpha or beta particles or of gamma rays through a gas.

i′o·none, i′o·none. A ketone, $C_{13}H_{20}O$, prepared from citral and used as a synthetic violet odor.

i·on″to·pho·re′sis (eye·on″to·fo·ee′sis). See *ion transfer.*

i·o′pax. Trade-mark for sodium 2-oxy-5-iodopyrine-N-acetate, a water-soluble compound used as a contrast medium in radiology.

i′o·phen′dyl·ate in·jec′tion. A preparation of a sterile mixture of isomers of ethyl iodophenylundecylate, used as a radiopaque medium for study of the lumbar region. See *pantopaque.*

i′o·phe·nox′ic ac′id. α-Ethyl-3-hydroxy-2,4,6-triiodohydrocinnamic acid, a roentgenographic contrast medium. See *teridax.*

i″o·pro′pane. See *iothion.*

iothion. Trade-mark for a brand of iopropane, chemically diiodohydroxy-propane.

i″o·thi′o·ur′a·cil so′di·um. Sodium 5-iodo-2-thiouracil, an antithyroid drug. See *itrumil sodium.*

ip′e·cac. The dried rhizome and roots of one of a number of *Cephaëlis* species. Used as an emetic and nauseating expectorant.

ip′e·cine (ip′i·seen, ·sin). Emetine, *q.v.*

ip″o·me′a, ip″o·moe′a (ip″o·mee′uh, eye″po·). The dried root of a plant, *Ipomoea orizabensis,* that yields cathartic resins.

ipral calcium. Trade-mark for probarbital calcium or calcium 5-ethyl-5-isopropyl barbiturate. The substance is used as a sedative and hypnotic.

ipral sodium. Trade-mark for probarbital sodium or sodium 5-ethyl-5-isopropyl barbiturate. The substance is used as a sedative and hypnotic.

i″pro·ni′a·zid. 1-Isonicotinyl-2-isopropyl hydrazide, an antituberculosis drug. See *marsilid.*

ip″si·lat′er·al. Situated on the same side, as paralytic (or similar) symptoms which occur on the same side as the cerebral lesion causing them.

I.Q. Intelligence quotient.

Ir. Chemical symbol for iridium.

i·ras″ci·bil′i·ty. The quality of being choleric, irritable, or of hasty temper. It is a frequent symptom in some psychoses and in neurasthenia.

i′ri·dal (eye′ri·dul, irr′i·dul), **i·rid′i·al** (eye·rid′ee·ul, i·rid′ee·ul), **i·rid′i·an.** Relating to the iris.

ir″i·dal′gi·a. (irr″i·dal′juh, eye″ri·). Pain referable to the iris.

ir″i·dec′to·mize. Excise a part of the iris; perform iridectomy.

ir″i·dec′to·my. The cutting out of a part of the iris.

ir″i·den·clei′sis (irr″i·den·klye′sis). See under *iridotasis.*

i·rid″e·re′mi·a. Total or partial absence of the iris; aniridia.

ir″i·des′cence. A rainbowlike display of intermingling and changing colors, as in mother-of-pearl. **—iri·descent,** *adj.*

i·rid′i·um (i·rid′ee·um, eye·rid′ee·um). Ir = 193.1. An element of the platinum family.

ir″i·di·xa′tion (irr″i·di·zay′shun, eye″ri·). The subjective appearance of an iridescent image, seen by persons affected with glaucoma.

ir′i·do- (irr′i·do-, eye′ri·do-), **irid-.** A combining form denoting the iris.

ir″i·do·cap″su·li′tis. Inflammation involving the iris and the capsule of the lens.

ir″i·do·cho″roid·i′tis (·ko″roy·dye′tis). Inflammation of both the iris and the choroid of the eye.

ir″i·do·col″o·bo′ma. A coloboma of the iris.

ir″i·do·cy·clec′to·my (·sigh·kleck′·to·mee). Excision of the iris and of the ciliary body.

ir″i·do·cy·cli′tis (irr″i·do·sigh·klye′tis, eye″ri·). Inflammation of the iris and the ciliary body. Also see *iritis*.

ir″i·do·cys·tec′to·my. An operation for making a new pupil; the edge of the iris and the capsule are drawn out through an incision in the cornea and cut off.

ir″i·do·di·al′y·sis (irr″i·do·dye·al′i·sis, eye″ri·). The separation of the iris from its attachments.

ir″i·do·do·ne′sis. Tremulousness of the iris; hippus.

ir″i·don′cus. A tumor or swelling of the iris.

ir″i·do·pa·ral′y·sis. Paralysis of the iris; iridoplegia.

ir″i·do·plat′i·num. An alloy of iridium and platinum.

ir″i·do·ple′gi·a. Paralysis of the sphincter of the iris.

ir″i·do·scle·rot′o·my. Puncture of the sclera with division of the iris.

ir″i·dot′a·sis. Stretching the iris, as in glaucoma; in place of iridotomy. The stretched iris is left in the wound, under the conjunctiva. If at the same time a piece of limbus is cut away to allow for better drainage of the aqueous into the areolar tissue of Tenon's capsule, the operation is called iridencleisis.

ir″i·dot′o·my. An incision into the iris.

I′ris. A genus of plants of the Iridaceae.

i′ris (pl. *irises, irides*). A colored, circular disk, part of the uvea of the eye, suspended in the aqueous humor from the ciliary body. Its posterior surface rests on the lens, hence it separates the anterior and posterior chambers. It surrounds the adjustable pupil. It consists of a mass of loose, vascular connective tissue, the stroma, covered anteriorly by endothelium, posteriorly by heavily pigmented epithelium, the iridial part of the retina. Two sets of smooth muscle cells control the size of the pupil; one circularly arranged in the pupillary border, forms the sphincter pupillae; the other, radially arranged, is the dilator pupillae. The color is governed by the number of melanophores in the stroma. **i. bom·bé.** A condition in which the iris bulges forward at the periphery due to an accumulation of the intraocular fluid in the posterior chamber.

i·ri′tis (eye·rye′tis, i·rye′tis). Inflammation of the iris; usually associated with inflammation of the ciliary body and often used for iridocyclitis, q.u. —**irit′ic,** *adj.*

i′ron. Fe = 55.85. A silver-white or gray, hard, ductile, malleable metal. See Table of Normal Values of Blood Constituents in the Appendix.

i′ron lung. Lay term for a respirator which induces breathing in a patient with paralyzed respiratory muscles. The patient's chest expands and contracts alternately in response to changes in air pressure in the respirator which encloses the body up to the neck. Also called *Drinker respirator*.

ir·ra′di·ate. Treat with x-rays or radium rays.

ir·ra′di·a″ting. 1. Radiating from a center, as a pain arising from a definite focus of irritation. 2. Treating with roentgen or radium rays.

ir·ra″di·a′tion. 1. A phenomenon in which, owing to the difference in the illumination of the field of vision or its background, objects appear much larger than they really are. 2. Diffusion in all directions from a common center; applied to nerve impulses, stellate fractures, pains felt in some position in an undemonstrable anatomic connection with an affected organ, etc. 3. Treatment of diseases by radiant energy such as by roentgen, radium, ultraviolet, infrared, or other rays.

ir·ra′tion·al (i·rash′un·ul). *In psychiatry,* outside the province of reason; said of mental behavior.

ir″re·du′ci·ble. Not reducible; not capable of being replaced in a normal position.

ir·reg″u·lar′i·ty. *In medicine,* deviation from a rhythmic activity.

ir″re·sus′ci·ta·ble. Not capable of being resuscitated or revived; irrevivable.

ir″re·ver′si·ble. 1. Not capable of being reversed. 2. Irrecoverable; said of a stage of shock or nerve injury from which recovery cannot be achieved. —**irreversibil′ity,** *n.*

ir″ri·ga′tion. The act of washing out by a stream of water, as irrigation of the urinary bladder. **continuous i.** A continuous stream of water washed over a surface to reduce or limit inflammation.

ir″ri·ga″tor, ir″ri·ga′tor. An apparatus, or device, for accomplishing the irrigation of a part, surface, or cavity.

ir″ri·ta·bil′i·ty. 1. A condition or quality of being excitable; the power of responding to a stimulus. 2. A condition of morbid excitability of an organ or part, when it reacts excessively to a slight stimulation.

ir′ri·ta·ble. 1. Reacting to stimuli. 2. Easily excited; susceptible of irritation.

ir′ri·tant. 1. Causing or giving rise to irritation. 2. An agent that induces irritation.

ir″ri·ta′tion. 1. A condition of undue excitement or irritability. 2. The act of irritating or stimulating. 3. The stimulus necessary to the performance of a function. **spinal i.** A form of neurasthenia characterized by pain in the back, tenderness along the spines of the vertebrae, fatigue on slight exertion, and, occasionally, numbness and tingling in the limbs. **sympathetic i.** Irritation of an organ arising from infiltration of another related organ, as sympathetic irritation of one eye from irritation of the other.

ir″ru·ma′tion. Fellatio, q.v.

i″sa′tro·pyl·co·caine′ (eye″suh-tro″pil·ko·kayn′, ·ko·kay′in). $C_{19}H_{23}$-NO_4. An amorphous alkaloid from coca leaves.

is·che′mi·a (iss·kee′mee·uh). Local diminution in the blood supply, due to obstruction of inflow of arterial blood; local anemia. This condition is seen in Raynaud's disease, in frostbite, in angina pectoris. —**ischemic,** adj.

is·che′sis (iss·kee′sis, iss′ki·sis). Retention of a discharge or secretion.

is″chi·al′gi·a. Sciatica. —**ischialgic,** adj.

is″chi·dro′sis (iss″ki·dro′sis). Suppression of the secretion of sweat. —**ischidrot′ic,** adj.

is·chi·o- (iss′kee·o-), **is·chi-.** A combining form denoting the ischium or the hip.

is″chi·o·cav″er·no′sus. A muscle covering each crus of the penis or clitoris. See Table of Muscles in the Appendix.

is·chi·op′a·gus. Conjoined twins united end-to-end by their ischial regions. The **ischiopagus tetrapus** has four legs; the **ischiopagus tripus,** three.

is″chi·o·rec′tal. Pertaining to both the ischium and the rectum.

is′chi·um (iss′kee·um). The inferior part of the os innominatum; the bone upon which the body rests in sitting. —**ischial, ischiad′ic,** adj.

is′cho- (iss′ko-), **isch-.** In medicine, a combining form denoting suppression, checking, stoppage, or deficiency.

is″cho·ga·lac′tic. 1. Suppressing the natural flow of milk. 2. An agent which suppresses the flow of milk.

is″cho·me′ni·a. Suppression of the menstrual flow.

is·chu′ri·a (isk·yoor′ee·uh). Retention or suppression of urine. —**ischuret′ic,** adj.

is′land. 1. An isolated structure; particularly, a group of cells differentiated from the surrounding tissue by staining or arrangement. 2. The insula, q.v., of the cerebral hemisphere. Formerly called i. of Reil. **blood i.** One of the masses of condensed splanchnic mesenchyme in the wall of the yolk sac that gives rise to the primitive erythrocytes of the embryo and to the vascular plexus of the yolk sac. **i. of Langerhans.** See islet of pancreas. **pancreatic i.** See islet of pancreas.

is′let (eye′lit). A small island, q.v. **i. of pancreas.** A small, irregular island of cell cords, found in the pancreas; it has no connection with the duct system, and is delimited from the acini by a reticular membrane. It is of an endocrine nature, as indicated by its great vascularity, and consists mainly of alpha and beta cells, the former secreting a hormone like lipocaic, and the latter secreting insulin. Syn., island of Langerhans.

i′so-, is-. 1. A combining form denoting equality, similarity, uniformity, or identity. 2. In bacteriology, a combining form denoting for or from different individuals of the same species. 3. In chemistry, a combining form denoting a compound isomeric with another, or a compound with a straight chain of carbon atoms at one end of which two methyl groups are attached. Symbol, i.

i″so·ag·glu′ti·nin. An agglutinin which acts upon the red blood cells of members of the same species. Also called isohemagglutinin.

i″so·al·lox′a·zine (eye″so·a·lock′suh·zeen). 1. $C_{10}H_6N_4O_2$. The three-ring compound pyrimido [4,5-b] quinoxaline-2,4(3H,10H)-dione; an isomer of alloxazine. Derivatives of the compound are widely distributed and include such substances as riboflavin and the yellow enzymes. 2. A term loosely applied to derivatives of (1).

i″so·an·dros′ter·one. $C_{19}H_{30}O_2$. 3(β)-Hydroxy-17-keto-androstane, an androgenic steroid found in the urine of men and women. See also androsterone.

i″so·an″ti·bod″ies. Antibodies, in certain members of a species, for cells of certain other members of the same species.

i″so·an′ti·gen. An antigen which is active only in serum of animals of the same species.

i′so·bar. 1. Any one of two or more atoms which have the same atomic mass but different atomic numbers. 2. In meteorology, a line drawn through points having equal barometric pressure. —**isobar′ic,** adj.

i″so·cel′lo·bi′ose. A disaccharide formed during hydrolysis of cellulose.

i″so·cho·les′ter·ol (eye″so·ko·less′-tur·ole, ·ol). A substance isolated from wool fat; originally considered to be a sterol but now believed to consist of several complex terpene alcohols.

i″so·cho′line (·ko′leen, ·kol′een). (CH₃)₃N(OH).CHOH.CH₃. An alkaloid, isomeric with choline, found in fungi of the genera *Amanita* and *Agaricus*. Syn., *amanitine*.

i″so·chro·mat′ic. Having the same color throughout.

i·soch′ro·nal (eye·sock′ro·nul, eye″so·kro′nul), **i·soch′ro·nous** (eye·sock′ro·nus). Occurring at or occupying equal intervals of time. —**isoch·ronism,** *n.*

i″so·chro′ni·a. The condition of normal nerve-impulse transference; the chronaxie of a muscle and that of its nerve are of the same order; supposedly essential for transmission of impulse from nerve to muscle.

i″so·cit′ric ac′id. HOOCCH₂CH(C-OOH)CHOHCOOH. An intermediary in the succinic and citric acid cycle concept of carbohydrate oxidation.

i·so·co′ri·a. Equality in diameter of the two pupils.

i″so·cor′tex. Those parts of the cerebral cortex exhibiting the six characteristic layers or strata, each layer having certain predominant cells and histologic features common to all isocortical areas.

i″so·cy·tol′y·sin (eye″so·sigh·tol′i-sin, ·sigh″to·lye′sin). A cytolysin from the blood of an animal, capable of acting against the cells of other animals of the same species.

i″so·e·lec′tric. Having the same electric properties throughout. **i. point.** The pH at which the net electric charge on a particle or surface is zero.

i″so·flu′ro·phate. Diisopropyl fluorophosphate, a cholinesterase inhibitor for ophthalmic use.

i″so·gam′ete (eye″so·gam′eet). A reproductive cell, similar in form and size to the cell with which it unites; found in certain protozoans and thallophytes.

i·sog′a·mous (eye·sog′uh·mus). Characterized by the conjugation of gametes, similar in size and shape. —**isogamy,** *n.*

i″so·gen′e·sis. Similarity in morphologic growth.

i·sog′e·nous. Of the same source or parentage.

i′so·graft. Homograft.

i″so·he·mol′y·sin (eye″so·hee·mol′i-sin, ·hee″mo·lye′sin). A hemolysin produced by injecting red blood cells into an animal of the same species. An isohemolysin will destroy the red blood cells of any animal of the same species except the immunized individual. Syn., *isolysin*. —**isohemolyt′ic,** *adj.*

i″so·im″mu·ni·za′tion. Immunization of a species of animal with antigens of the same species; for example, the development of anti-Rh serum may be produced by transfusing Rh-positive blood into an Rh-negative individual or by an Rh-negative woman being pregnant with an Rh-positive fetus.

i′so·late. Separate; place apart, as to separate those patients with contagious diseases from others not affected. —**isola′tion,** *n.*

i″so·leu′cine (eye″so·lew′seen, ·sin). α-Amino-β-methyl-valeric acid, C₂H₅.C-H(CH₃).CH(NH₂).COOH. An essential amino acid.

i′so·log, i′so·logue (eye′so·log). One of a series of compounds of similar structure, but having different atoms of the same valence and usually of the same periodic group.

i″so·ly′sin (eye″so·lye′sin, eye·sol′i-sin). See *isohemolysin*.

i′so·mer. One of two or more compounds having the same percentage composition but differing in the relative positions of the atoms within the molecule. See *isomerism*.

i·so′mer·ase. Enzyme involved in establishing equilibrium between glucose-6-phosphate and fructose-6-phosphate and possibly other biochemical reactions.

i″so·mer′ic. Pertaining to isomerism. Existing as an isomer of another substance.

i·som′er·ide (eye·som′ur·ide, ·id). See *isomer*.

i·som′er·ism (eye·som′ur·iz·um). The relationship between two isomers. The phenomenon wherein two or more compounds possess the same percentage composition but differ in the relative position of the atoms within the molecule and have different properties.

i″so·meth·ep′tene. 6-Methylamino-2-methylheptene, an antispasmodic agent. See *octin*.

i″so·met′ric. Of the same dimensions.

i″so·ni′a·zid. Isonicotinic acid hydrazide.

i″so·nic″o·tin′ic ac′id hy′dra·zide. C₅H₄N.CO.NH.NH₂, a therapeutic agent used in treating human tuberculosis, administered orally or intramuscularly. Syn., *isoniazid*. See *nydrazid*.

1–i″so·nic″o·tin″yl-2-i″so·pro′pyl·hy′dra·zide. The isopropyl derivative of isonicotinic acid hydrazide formerly used in chemotherapy of tuberculosis but now employed as a central nervous system stimulant of the psychomotor type. Syn., *iproniazid*. See *marsilid*.

i″so·nip′e·caine. Meperidine hydrochloride.

i″so·os·mot′ic, i″sos·mot′ic. 1. Referring or pertaining to a solution having the same osmotic pressure as that of a reference physiological fluid, particularly that enclosed in red blood cells. 2. Referring or pertaining to a solution which is also isotonic only when the immersed tissue maintains its normal state by virtue of its lack of permeability to the solutes present, or of any interaction with the solutes.

i·sop'a·thy (eye·sop'uth·ee). The treatment of a disease by the administration of the causative agent or of its products, as the treatment of smallpox by the administration of variolar matter.

i″so·pel″le·tier′ine (eye″so·pel″- i·teer′een, ·pel″et·yair′een, ·pi·let′i- reen). One of the alkaloids of pomegranate bark. See *pelletierine*.

i·so'pi·a (eye·so'pee·uh). Equal acuteness of vision in the two eyes.

i″so·plas'tic. Transplanted from one individual to another of the same species, said of a graft.

i″so·prene. $CH_2:CH.C(CH_3):CH_2$. Methyl butadiene, a hydrocarbon formed in the dry distillation of rubber.

i″so·pro′pa·mide i′o·dide. (3- Carbamoyl - 3,3 - diphenylpropyl) diisopropylmethylammonium iodide, an anticholinergic agent. See *darbid*.

i″so·pro′pa·nol. Isopropyl alcohol.

i″so·pro″pyl·a·ce′tic ac′id. Isovaleric acid.

i″so·pro′pyl al′co·hol. $(CH_3)_2CH$- OH. Dimethyl carbinol. A homolog of ethyl alcohol. Syn., *isopropanol*.

i″so·pro″pyl·ar·ter′e·nol. *a*-(Isopropylaminomethyl) protocatechuyl alcohol, a sympathomimetic amine similar in activity to epinephrine and norepinephrine but less active on smooth muscles of blood vessels. **i. hydrochloride.** $C_{11}H_{17}NO_3.HCl$, a sympathomimetic amine salt, used principally in treating asthma and heart block. Syn., *isoproterenol hydrochloride*. See *aludrine hydrochloride*.

i″so·pro·ter′e·nol hy″dro·chlo′ride. The U.S. Pharmacopeia name for isopropylarterenol hydrochloride.

i″so·quin′o·line (eye″so·kwin′o- leen, ·lin). C_9H_7N. White, hygroscopic crystals. Numerous natural and synthetic alkaloids are derivatives of this substance. Also called 2-*benzazine*, *leucoline*.

i″sos·mot′ic. Same as *isoosmotic*.

i′so·stere. One of two or more atoms or atomic groups having analogous arrangements of electrons and hence similarity in some properties.

i″so·sthe·nu′ri·a (eye″so·sthi·new′- ree·uh, eye″sos·thi·). A condition in which the kidney cannot form urine with a higher or lower specific gravity than that of protein-free plasma.

i′so·tel. A food factor capable of replacing another in a given diet for a specified species; thus, for the human species, carotene is isotelic with vita-

min A; for the cat, it is not, since the cat is incapable of converting carotene into vitamin A. —**isotel'ic,** *adj*.

i′so·therm. A graph or a curve representing the dependence of one quantity upon another, as of gas pressure upon volume, at constant temperature.

i″so·ther′mal, i″so·ther′mic. 1. Of or pertaining to an isotherm. 2. Of equal or uniform temperature; without change in temperature.

i″so·ton′ic. 1. Applied to a solution with osmotic pressure equivalent to that of another fluid taken as a standard. 2. *In physiology*, having uniform tension under pressure or stimuli.

i′so·tope. An element which has the same atomic number as another but a different atomic weight. —**isotop′ic,** *adj*. **radioactive i.** One exhibiting the property of spontaneous decomposition, usually referring to an element rendered radioactive by artificial means, as radioiodine or radiophosphorus. Syn., *radioisotope*.

i″so·trop′ic (eye″so·trop′ick, ·tro′- pick). 1. Having the same shape and appearance, from whatever point observed. 2. Being singly and uniformly refractive.

i″so·va·ler′ic ac′id (eye″so·va- lerr′ick, ·va·leer′ick). $(CH_3)_2CH.CH_2$- COOH. The valeric acid of commerce, obtained from valerian root. See *valeric acid*. Syn., *isopropylacetic acid*.

is'sue. 1. Offspring. 2. A bloody or purulent discharge from a wound or cavity.

isth·mec'to·my (iss·meck'to·mee, isth·). Excision of an isthmus; specifically, excision of the isthmus of the thyroid gland in goiter.

isth'mus (iss'mus, isth'mus). 1. The neck or constricted part of an organ. 2. The part of the brain which, situated axially, unites the forebrain, the cerebellum, and the spinal cord. —**isthmic,** *adj*. **i. of thyroid gland.** The narrow transverse part connecting the lobes of the thyroid gland. **i. of uterine tube.** That part of a uterine tube nearest the uterus. **uterine i.** The transverse constriction of the uterus, dividing it into two portions, the body and the cervix.

isuprel hydrochloride. Trademark for 1-(3′,4′dihydroxyphenyl)-2- isopropylaminoethanol hydrochloride, a synthetic sympathomimetic amine.

itch. 1. An irritating sensation in the skin. 2. Any of various skin diseases accompanied by itching, particularly scabies. **barber's i.** See *tinea barbae*. **dhobie i.** See *tinea cruris*. **frost-i.** See *pruritus hiemalis*. **washerwoman's i.** Dermatitis of the hands, a general term for various eruptions, usually a fungous infection or contact dermatitis; seen in those who have their hands frequently in water.

itch'ing. A sensation of tickling and irritation in the skin, producing the desire to scratch. Syn., *pruritus*.

itch mite. See *Sarcoptes scabiei*.

-ite. 1. *In mineralogy*, a suffix denoting *a mineral* or *rock*. 2. *In zoology*, a suffix denoting *a division of the body* or *of a part*.

-ite. *In chemistry*, a suffix denoting *the salt* or *ester* from an acid with the termination *-ous*.

i'ter (eye'tur, it'ur). A passageway.

-i'tis (-eye'tis, -ee'tis). *In medicine*, a suffix denoting *a disease*; specifically, *an inflammatory disease of a* (specified) *part*.

itrumil sodium. Trade-mark for iothiouracil sodium.

I.U. Immunizing unit; international unit.

Ix·o'des (ick·so'deez). A genus of parasitic ticks, some species of which cause tick paralysis and are important vectors of diseases of cattle, sheep, and dogs, as well as transmitters of encephalomyelitis and tularemia to man.

ix"o·di'a·sis. Lesions or disease caused by infestation by ticks.

Ix·od'i·dae (ick·sod'i·dee). A family of hard-bodied ticks, which includes the genera *Boöphilus*, *Amblyomma*, *Dermacentor*, *Haemaphysalis*, *Hyalomma*, *Ixodes*, and *Rhipicephalus*, all of some pathologic significance to man.

J

J. Symbol for Joule's equivalent, joule.

j. Used as a Roman numeral (in prescriptions) as the equivalent of 1 for one, or at the end of a number as j, ij, iij, vj, vij, etc.

jack bean. 1. The seed of *Canavalia* from which urease is prepared for use in the estimation of urea. 2. A plant of the genus *Canavalia*.

jack'et. 1. A short coat. 2. *In medicine*, a supporting, therapeutic, or restraining apparatus covering the upper part of the body. **celluloid j.** One made principally of celluloid, fashioned over a plaster mold of the patient's body. **j. crown.** An artificial restoration of the crown of a tooth; consists of a covering of metal, porcelain, or acrylic. **leather j.** One made of leather, sometimes equipped with apparatus, made over a body mold; used principally in tuberculosis of the vertebrae and in flaccid paralysis. **plaster of Paris j.** A casing applied by winding plaster of Paris bandages over padding, so as to encase the body in a hard mold from armpits to groin; used to immobilize the spine. **pneumonia j.** A padded cotton or wool coat which may contain poultices and which encases the upper part of the body; sometimes employed in the care of patients with pneumonia. **strait-j.** A restraining apparatus, not always conforming to the jacket type, used to prevent violently insane or irresponsible persons from injuring themselves or others.

jack'screw". *In orthodontia*, an appliance used for forcing apart the fragments of certain types of fractures and retaining them in a separated condition.

Jackson, Chevalier [*American bronchoesophagologist and laryngologist*, 1865–1958]. Devised various instruments and technics for peroral endoscopy. With W. W. Babcock, introduced the *Jackson-Babcock operation* for the radical removal of an esophageal diverticulum.

Jacobson, Ludwig Levin [*Danish anatomist*, 1783–1843]. Described the tympanic nerve, called *Jacobson's nerve*.

jac"ti·ta'tion. A tossing about; great restlessness; a condition at times present in grave diseases.

jac"u·lif'er·ous. Prickly, bearing spines.

Jaeger, Eduard [*Austrian ophthalmologist*, 1818–84]. Introduced a method of testing acuteness of vision by means of lines of type of different sizes printed on cards. Called *Jaeger's test types*.

Jaksch, Rudolf von [*Austrian physician in Czechoslovakia*, 1855–1947]. Described infantile pseudoleukemic anemia (1889), called *von Jaksch's anemia* or *disease*.

jal'ap. The tuberous root of *Exogonium purga*, a plant of the Convolvulaceae. Its active principle is a resin which contains a glycoside, convolvulin. Jalap is an active hydragogue cathartic

Ja·mai'ca dog'wood. See *piscidia*.

jam'bul. *Eugenia Jambolana*, the bark and seeds of which have been variously used in medicine.

Janet, Pierre Marie Félix [*French psychiatrist*, 1859–1947]. Described psychasthenia (1903), also called *Janet's disease*.

jan'i·ceps. Conjoined twins in which there is a single head exhibiting two equal, opposite faces. Also called *cephalothoracopagus disymmetros*.

Janský, Jan [*Czechoslovakian physician*, d. 1921]. Classified human blood in four groups (1907); see *blood groups*. Infantile amaurotic familial idiocy is called *Bielschowsky-Janský disease*.

jap"a·con'i·tine (jap"uh-kon'i-teen, -tin). The most poisonous of aconite alkaloids; obtained from *Aconitum japonicum*.

jar'gon. Confused, unintelligible talk; gibberish, babble. Also see *aphasia*.

Jarvis, William Chapman [*American laryngologist*, 1855-95]. Inventor of a snare used for removing polypoid growths in the nose and throat; called *Jarvis' snare*.

jaun'dice (jawn'dis, jahn'dis). Yellowness of the skin, mucous membranes, and secretions; due to bile pigments in the blood. Also see *icterus*. **acholuric j.** That without demonstrable bile pigment in the urine. **arsenical j.** That due to arsenical hepatitis. **black j.** An extreme degree of jaundice. **catarrhal j.** That due to inflammation and edema of the bile ducts. **clinical j.** Icterus with yellowing of the skin and scleras; the icterus index is above 15. **congenital j.** That appearing at, or shortly after, birth; due to defective development of the biliary passages. **constitutional j.** Physiologic hyperbilirubinemia. **dissociated j.** Selective retention of either bile pigment or bile salts; most frequently acholuric. **familial j.** (a) Hemolytic jaundice. (b) Physiologic hyperbilirubinemia. **green j.** That in which the discoloration of the skin is green or olive-colored. **hemolytic j.** A chronic, microcytic anemia, characterized by increased erythrocyte fragility, reticulocytosis, acholuric jaundice, and splenomegaly. **hepatocellular j.** That due to destruction of liver cells by toxic or infectious agents. The secreted bile escapes via the lymphatics and thence into the blood. **hepatogenous j.** That due to hepatic disease. It may be obstructive or hepatocellular. **homologous serum j.** That associated with infectious hepatitis; transmitted by inoculation of homologous serum. **hyperhemolytic j.** That due to inability of the liver to excrete the quantity of pigment presented to it as the result of excessive hemolysis. **infectious j.** Epidemic hepatitis, *q.v.* **intralobular j.** Hepatocellular jaundice, *q.v.* **j. of the newborn.** See *icterus neonatorum*. **latent j.** Increase in bile pigment in the blood, insufficient to show jaundice clinically but determinable by the icterus index (from 6 to 15). **malignant j.** Icterus gravis, *q.v.* **mechanical j.** See ob-

structive *j.* **obstructive j.** That due to interference with the outflow of bile by mechanical obstruction of the biliary passages, as by gallstones or tumor. **parenchymatous j.** Hepatocellular jaundice, *q.v.* **postvaccinal j.** That accompanying postvaccinal hepatitis, *q.v.* **regurgitation j.** That due to secretion of bile pigment into the hepatic lymph channels and thence into the blood. It may be hepatocellular or obstructive. **retention j.** That due to the inability of the liver to excrete the bile pigment presented to it. **spirochetal j.** A disease in man caused by the spirochete, *Leptospira icterohaemorrhagiae*; characterized by fever, nausea, headache, muscular pain, and jaundice. Also called *Weil's disease*. **toxic j.** That associated with hepatitis caused by toxic substances or by a toxic reaction.

jaw. Either of the two bones that form the skeleton of the mouth; the upper jaw, or maxilla, and the lower jaw, or mandible.

je"co·le'ic ac'id (jee"ko-lee'ick, jeck"o-). An acid occurring in the glycerides of cod liver oil.

je·jun'al. Of or related to the jejunum.

je"ju·nec'to·my (jee"jew-neck'to-mee, jedj"oo-). Excision of part or all of the jejunum.

je"ju·ni'tis (jee"jew-nigh'tis, jedj"-oo-). Inflammation of the jejunum.

je·ju'no- (ji-jew'no-, jedj'oo-no-), **jejun-.** In medicine, a combining form denoting *the jejunum*.

je·ju"no·co·los'to·my. The formation of a surgical anastomosis between the jejunum and the colon.

je·ju"no·il"e·i'tis. Inflammation of the jejunum and the ileum.

je·ju"no·il"e·os'to·my. The formation of a surgical anastomosis between the jejunum and the ileum.

je·ju"no·il'e·um. That part of the small intestine extending from the duodenum to the cecum.

je·ju"no·je"ju·nos'to·my (·jee"-jew-nos'to-mee, ·jedj"oo-). Surgical formation of an anastomosis between two parts of the jejunum.

je"ju·nos'to·my (jee"jew-nos'to-mee, jedj"oo-). The making of an artificial opening (jejunal fistula) through the abdominal wall into the jejunum.

je"ju·not'o·my (jee"jew-not'o-mee, jedj"oo-). Incision into the jejunum.

je·ju'num. The second division of the small intestine extending between the duodenum and the ileum, and measuring about 8 feet (2.2 meters) in length.

jel'ly. A semisolid colloidal system of a liquid suspended in a solid, as water in gelatin. **contraceptive j.** Any one of a number of viscous substances introduced into the vagina to prevent conception; designed to act both as an occlusive and as a vehicle for contraceptive chemicals. **glycerin j.** A mixture of glycerin, gelatin, and other substances, e.g. zinc oxide. **mineral j.** Petrolatum. Also called *petroleum j.* **petroleum j.** Petrolatum. **vaginal j.** Any one of a group of substances introduced into the vagina for the treatment of disease, or, more commonly, for contraceptive purposes. **Wharton's j.** The mucoid connective tissue that constitutes the matrix of the umbilical cord.

Jenner, Edward [*English physician,* 1749–1823]. Introduced inoculation with matter containing the virus of vaccinia, to produce immunity to smallpox. See smallpox *vaccine,* also called *Jennerian vaccine.*

je·quir'i·ty. The seed of *Abrus praecatorius.*

jerk. A sudden, spasmodic movement; a term often applied to certain reflexes, as the jaw-jerk reflex, knee-jerk reflex.

Jes'u·its' bal'sam (bawl'sum). Compound benzoin tincture.

Jes'u·its' bark. Old term for Peruvian bark; the bark of several species of *Cinchona.* See *cinchona.*

Jes'u·its' drops. Compound benzoin tincture.

jet dust coun'ter. An instrument for determining the number of dust particles in the air. A measured sample of air is humidified and propelled at high velocity through a narrow aperture against a perpendicular plate to which the dust particles adhere. They are then counted under a microscope. Other instruments used for the same purpose are the konimeter, impinger, and precipitator. Also see *dust count.*

jet in·jec'tion. See *hypospray.*

jig'ger. See *Tunga penetrans.*

Jim'son weed. See *stramonium.*

jock'ey strap. The popular name given to a scrotal supporter; a suspensory.

joint. Articulation, *q.v.* For joints listed by name, see Table of Joints in the Appendix. **ball-and-socket j.** See *enarthrosis.* **biaxial j.** One in which movement is around two transverse axes at right angles to each other. The two varieties are the condyloid and the saddle joint. **Charcot's j.** A neuropathic arthropathy in which articular cartilage and subjacent bone degenerate while hypertrophic changes occur at the joint edges and present an irregular deformity with instability of the joint. Most common in tabes dorsalis. **false j.** A condition of excessive mobility resulting from failure of

the fragments of a fractured bone to achieve bony union; pseudarthrosis. **flail j.** A condition of excessive mobility often following resection of a joint. **gliding j.** One which allows only gliding movements; formed by the apposition of plane surfaces, or one slightly convex, the other slightly concave. **hinge j.** See *ginglymus.* **pivot j.** One in which movement is limited to rotation; the movement is uniaxial, and in the longitudinal axis of the bones. Also called *trochoid joint.* **rotation j.** A lateral ginglymus. **saddle j.** One in which the opposing surfaces are reciprocally concavo-convex.

joint mouse. A small, loose body within a joint, derived from the synovial membrane or articular cartilage; sometimes calcified. Syn., *arthrolith.*

joule (jowl, jōōl). 1. A unit of electric energy, equivalent to the work expended when a current of one ampere flows for one second against a resistance of one ohm. 2. A unit of work, = 10,000,000 ergs. Symbol, J.

judg'ment. The capacity to judge; the ability to draw correct conclusions from the material acquired by experience.

ju'do. See *jujitsu.*

ju'gal. 1. Connecting or uniting, as by a yoke. 2. Pertaining to the zygoma, as the jugal point. **j. point.** The craniometric point which is situated at the angle that the posterior border of the frontosphenoidal process of the zygoma makes with the superior border of its temporal process.

ju'glans (jew'glanz). The dried inner bark from the roots of *Juglans cinerea.* Also called *butternut bark.*

jug'u·lar (jug'yoo-lur, jōog'yoo-lur). Pertaining to the neck above the clavicle, as jugular vein. See Table of Veins in the Appendix.

juice. 1. The liquid contained in vegetable or animal tissues. 2. Any of the secretions of the body. **gastric j.** The secretion of the glands of the stomach; a clear, colorless liquid, having an acid reaction, and a specific gravity of about 1.006, and containing about 0.5% of solid matter. It contains hydrochloric acid, pepsin, rennin, and mucin. **intestinal j.** The secretion of the intestinal glands, a pale yellow fluid, alkaline in reaction, having a specific gravity of 1.001, and possessing diastasic and proteolytic properties. It also, to a certain extent, emulsifies and decomposes fats. **pancreatic j.** The secretion of the pancreas; a thick, transparent, colorless, odorless fluid, of a salty taste, and strongly alkaline, containing proteolytic, lipolytic, and amylolytic enzymes.

ju·jit′su, jiu·jit′su. A Japanese method of physical training used also as a system of self-defense without weapons. The opponent's own weight is used to overthrow him. Syn., *judo*.

ju′jube. The fruit of the jujube tree, *Zizyphus jujuba;* used, in the form of a lozenge or syrup, for throat irrigation.

Jukes. A fictitious name given to the descendants of certain sisters in a study of the occurrence among them of crime, immorality, pauperism, and disease in relation to heredity.

ju·men′tous. Similar to that of a horse; applied to the odor of urine.

junc′tion. The point or line of union of two parts; juncture; interface. **cementoenamel j.** That between the enamel and the cementum of a tooth. **dentinocemental j.** The interface between the dentin and the cementum in the root of a tooth. **dentinoenamel j.** The interface between the enamel and the dentin in the crown of a tooth. **mucocutaneous j.** The transition from skin to mucous membrane at the body orifices. **myoneural j.** The point of junction of a motor nerve with the muscle which it innervates. **sclerocorneal j.** The boundary between the white, opaque sclera and the transparent cornea in the eye.

junc·tu′ra. 1. An articulation; a suture of bones. 2. A junction, as of tendons.

June cold. That type of hay fever caused by sensitivity to grass pollen. Syn., *hay fever.*

Jung, Carl Gustav [*Swiss psychologist and psychiatrist,* 1875–]. Pioneer in analytic psychology, *q.v.* Regarded the libido not as an expression of the sex instinct but as the will to live. Classified all individuals as either extroverts or introverts. See also feeling-

type, intuitional-type, sensational-type, and thinking-type *personality.*

jungle rot. A lay term commonly used by military men in the tropics, usually referring to a fungous infection of the skin.

ju′ni·per. 1. The fruit of *Juniperus communis,* containing a volatile oil, resin, and fixed oil. 2. Any evergreen shrub or tree of the genus *Juniperus.*

ju″ris·pru′dence. The science of law, its interpretation and application. **medical j.** Legal medicine, *q.v.*

ju′ry. A body of adult persons chosen according to law to attend a judicial tribunal and to determine the true verdict upon a matter being tried or inquired into. **coroner's j.** That jury which attends a coroner's inquest, to determine the cause of a death. **j. of inquest.** A coroner's jury.

jury mast. An iron rod fixed in a plaster jacket; used to support the head in disease or fracture of the cervical spine.

jus′to ma′jor. Greater than normal, larger in all dimensions than normal; applied to a pelvis.

jus′to mi′nor. Abnormally small in all dimensions; said of a pelvis.

ju′ve·nile (jew′vi·nil, ··nyle). 1. Young; pertaining to youth or childhood. 2. A young person.

jux′ta-. A combining form denoting *nearness, situated near.*

jux″ta-ar·tic′u·lar. Near a joint.

jux″ta-glo·mer′u·lar. 1. Next to a glomerulus. 2. Referring to epithelioid cells near a glomerulus of the kidney.

jux″ta·po·si′tion. 1. Situation adjacent to another; in close relationship; apposition. 2. The act of placing near.

jux″ta·py·lor′ic (juck″stuh·pye·lor′ick, ·pi·lor′ick). Near the pylorus.

K

K. The chemical symbol for potassium.

K$_a$. Symbol for the dissociation constant of an acid.

K$_b$. Symbol for the dissociation constant of a base.

Kaf′ir pox. A mild form of smallpox.

kai″no·pho′bi·a (kigh″no·fo′bee-uh). A morbid fear of anything new. —**kai′nophobe,** *n.*

kak′o-. See *caco-.*

kak″or·rhaph″i·o·pho′bi·a. Morbid fear of failure.

ka′la-a·zar′ (kah′lah·ah·zahr′, -ah′-

zahr, kal″uh·ay′zur, -az′ur). Visceral leishmaniasis; there are two types: the Indian type which affects older children and adults in India, Indo-China, and Sudan, and the Mediterranean type which attacks infants in countries bordering the Mediterranean. *Leishmania donovani* is the etiologic agent of both types. The chief lesion is marked by hyperplasia of the cells of the reticuloendothelial system, particularly of the spleen and liver; there is continued irregular fever, with emaciation, anemia, and leukopenia.

ka·le′mi·a, kal″i·e′mi·a. See *po-tassemia.*

ka′li·um. Potassium, *q.v.*

Kal′li·kak. A fictitious name given to the descendants of a Revolutionary War soldier in a study of the occurrence among them of feeblemindedness and immorality and of the bearing on heredity.

ka·ma′la (kuh·may′luh, kam′uh·luh), **ka·me′la** (kuh·mee′luh). Rottlera. The glands and hairs from the capsules of *Mallotus philippinensis* (kamala tree). Purgative and anthelmintic.

kan″ga·roo′ ten′don. A tendon obtained from the tail of the kangaroo; used for surgical ligatures and sutures.

ka′o·lin. A powdered native hydrated aluminum silicate, insoluble in water. Used as a protective and absorbent.

ka·ra′ya gum (ka·rah′yuh, kar′ay-uh). An exudate from trees of the *Sterculia* or *Cochlospermum* species; with water, it swells to form a bulky mass. Also called *sterculia gum.*

ka′ry·o-, ka′ry-. A combining form meaning *nut* or *kernel;* used especially in biology to denote *relation to the karyon* or *nucleus of a cell.*

ka′ry·o·blast″. The most immature cell of the erythrocyte series. Also called *megaloblast, proerythroblast.*

ka′ry·o·chrome″. 1. A nerve cell which has a high nucleocytoplasmic ratio. 2. A nerve cell in which the nucleus stains intensely.

ka″ry·og′a·my. A conjugation of cells characterized by a fusion of the nuclei. **—karyogam′ic.** *adj.*

ka″ry·o·ki·ne′sis (care″ee·o·ki-nee′sis, ·kigh·nee′sis). Mitosis or indirect cell division; especially the nuclear transformations, as opposed to *cytokinesis.* Also called *karyomitosis.* **—karyokinet′ic,** *adj.*

ka′ry·ol′y·sis. The dissolution of the nucleus of a cell. **—karyolyt′ic,** *adj.*

ka′ry·o·mere. A segment of a chromosome. See *chromomere.*

ka′ry·o·phage″. A parasite which destroys the nucleus of the infested cell.

ka′ry·o·plasm. Old term for nucleoplasm.

ka″ry·or·rhex′is. Fragmentation or splitting up of a nucleus into a number of chromatin particles which become scattered in the cytoplasm.

ka′ry·o·some″, kar″y·o·so′ma. 1. A chromatin nucleolus or false nucleolus, by differentiation from a true nucleolus or plasmosome. 2. A large, deeply staining body in the nucleus of many Protista, associated with the chromosomes or other structures. **kata-.** See *cata-.*

kat″a·did′y·mus. Duplication of the superior pole, as in diprosopia or dicephalism. Has been incorrectly used for inferior duplicity. Also called *superior duplicity.*

kat″a·ther·mom′e·ter. A double-bulbed, alcohol thermometer, graduated from 100°–90° F., which records how quickly air is cooling, thus permitting an estimate of evaporation of moisture from the body.

Kat″a·ya′ma (cat″uh·yah′muh, kah″tuh·). A genus of amphibious snails. **K. formosana.** A species found in Formosa; one of the intermediate hosts of *Schistosoma japonicum.* **K. nosophora.** A species found in Japan and along the coast of China; an intermediate host of *Schistosoma japonicum.*

kath″i·so·pho′bi·a. Morbid fear of sitting down.

kath′ode. See *cathode.*

kat′i″on. See *cation.*

kau′ri (kou′ree). The fossilized resinous exudate from the Kauri pine.

ka′va (kah′vah, kav′uh), **ka″va-ka′va.** 1. An intoxicating beverage prepared in the Hawaiian Islands from the root of *Piper methysticum.* 2. The root of *Piper methysticum.*

kef′ir. A beverage prepared, especially in certain European countries, from the milk of cows, sheep, or goats through fermentation by kefir grains, which contain unidentified species of yeast or bacterial organisms.

ke′loid. A fibrous hyperplasia usually at the site of a scar, elevated, rounded, white, sometimes pink, firm and with ill-defined borders. There is predilection for the upper trunk and face, and the condition is observed especially in young adults, females, and Negroes. Composed of parallel bundles of hyalinized connective tissue covered by thin epidermis with atrophic interpapillary epithelium.

kel′vin. A commercial unit of electricity; 1000 watt-hours.

Kel′vin scale. An absolute scale of temperature which has its zero at −273° C.

kemadrin. Trade-mark for procyclidine hydrochloride.

kemithal. Trade-mark (British) for 5-allyl-5-(Δ²-cyclohexenyl)-2-thiobarbituric acid, the sodium salt of which is used intravenously as an anesthetic.

Kendall, Edward Calvin [*American physiologist and chemist,* 1886–   ]. Isolated thyroxin (1914) and adrenal cortical hormones (1936); prepared Compound A by partial synthesis (1944); collaborated in the preparation of cortisone (Compound E) (1948). With Hench, Slocumb, and Polley first showed the influence of cortisone in rheumatic and related diseases (1948). Nobel laureate with Philip S. Hench and Tadeus Reichstein (1950).

Kenny, Elizabeth [*Australian nurse in the United States*, 1886–1952]. Introduced the *Kenny treatment* for anterior poliomyelitis. Splints are not used. In the acute stage the affected muscles are treated with hot, moist packs. Passive exercise is started very early, and is followed as soon as possible by active exercise.

ken'o-, ken-. A combining form meaning *empty*.

ken"o·pho'bi·a. A morbid fear of large, empty spaces.

ken"o·tox'in. A hypothetical poisonous substance developed in the tissues during their activity which has been said to be responsible for their fatigue and for sleep.

ker'a·sin. A cerebroside separated from the brain; contains sphingosine, galactose, and fatty acid.

ker"a·tal'gi·a. Pain in the cornea.

ker"a·tec·ta'si·a (kerr″uh-teck-ay′zhuh). A protrusion of the cornea.

ker"a·tec'to·my. Surgical excision of a part of the cornea.

ke·rat'ic. Horny.

ker'a·tin. One of a group of albuminoids characteristic of horny tissues, hair, nails, feathers, etc.

ker"a·tin·i·za'tion. 1. Development of a horny quality in a tissue. 2. Process whereby keratin is formed. 3. Coating of pills with keratin.

ke·rat'i·nous. 1. Relating to keratin. 2. Horny.

ker"a·ti'tis. Inflammation of the cornea. **annular k.** An inflammation round the periphery of the cornea. Also called *marginal k.* **band-shaped k.** An inflammation occurring in the form of a transverse band across the cornea opposite the palpebral fissure. **dendritic k.** A superficial form attributed to the virus of herpes simplex; characterized by a line of infiltration of the corneal tissue near the surface, developing later into an arborescent ulcer. Also called *furrow k., herpetic k., k. arborescens, mycotic k.* **exposure k.** Inflammation of the cornea due to trauma from excessive drying or from foreign particles. **fascicular k.** A vesicular form that is characterized by the formation of a bundle of blood vessels. **interstitial k.** A form of keratitis in which the entire cornea is invested with a diffuse haziness, almost completely hiding the iris. The surface of the cornea has a ground-glass appearance. Later, blood vessels form in the superficial layers of the cornea from ciliary injection, and produce a dulled color or the so-called salmon patch. Seen most frequently in children between 5 and 15, resulting from congenital syphilis. Syn., *syphilitic k.*

k. bullosa. The formation of blebs upon the cornea in cases of iridocyclitis, glaucoma, or interstitial keratitis. **k. hypopyon.** That accompanied by the formation of pus. Also called *serpiginous k.* **k. neuroparalytica.** Keratitis following lesion of the trigeminal nerve; caused by mechanical irritation and drying of the cornea. Syn., *trophic k.* **k. punctata.** The presence of white blood cells on the back of Descemet's membrane. Not a primary inflammation of Descemet's membrane, since the cells derive from the ciliary body as a result of its inflammation. Includes two varieties, **keratitis punctata leprosa** (that caused by leprosy), and **keratitis punctata profunda** (that of syphilitic origin). Syn., *descemetitis.* **k. pustuliformis profunda.** That accompanied by the formation of deep pustules; due to acquired syphilis. Syn., *k. punctata profunda.* **k. rosacea.** The occurrence of small, sterile infiltrates at the periphery of the cornea, which are approached but not invaded by small blood vessels. They are most frequently seen unaccompanied by acne rosacea, but are most severe in this connection. **lagophthalmic k.** That due to the failure of the eyelids to close completely; a form of exposure keratitis. **phlyctenular k.** A variety characterized by the formation of small papules or pustules, often associated with similar lesions upon the conjunctiva. It is marked by severe local congestion, lacrimation, and intense photophobia; is usually associated with childhood tuberculosis, and is frequently precipitated by acute tonsillitis or otitis media. **sclerosing k.** An interstitial form associated with scleritis. **traumatic k.** That consequent upon wounds or injury of the cornea.

ker'a·to-, kerat-. 1. A combining form meaning *horn* or denoting *horny tissue.* 2. *In anatomy, medicine, and surgery,* a combining form denoting *the cornea.*

ker'a·to·cele. A hernia of Descemet's membrane through the cornea; descemetocele.

ker"a·to·cen·te'sis. Corneal puncture.

ker"a·to·con·junc"ti·vi'tis. Simultaneous inflammation of the cornea and the conjunctiva. **epidemic k.** A virus infection, usually affecting adults; is epidemic and self-limited. **k. sicca.** That due to drying of the cornea and conjunctiva.

ker"a·to·co'nus. A conic protrusion of the cornea.

ker"a·to·der'ma. A horny condition of the skin, especially of the palms and soles. **k. climactericum.** A circumscribed hyperkeratosis of the palms and soles occurring in women during the menopause.

ker″a·to·gen′e·sis. Development of horny growths.

ker″a·to·glo′bus. A globular protrusion of the cornea.

ker″a·to·hel·co′sis. Ulceration of the cornea.

ker″a·to·hy′a·lin, ker″a·to·hy′a·line (kerr″uh·to·high′uh·lin, ·lyne). The substance of the granules in the stratum granulosum of keratinized stratified squamous epithelium; an early phase in the formation of keratin.

ker″a·to·ir′i·do·scope (·irr′i·do·scope, ·i·rid′o·). An apparatus for examining the cornea and iris.

ker″a·to·i·ri′tis (kerr″uh·to·eye·rye′tis, ·i·rye′tis). Combined inflammation of the cornea and the iris.

ker″a·to·lep·tyn′sis. Removal of the anterior thickness of the cornea and replacement of it by bulbar conjunctiva.

ker″a·to·leu·ko′ma (kerr″uh·to·lew·ko′muh). A leukoma or whitish opacity of the cornea.

ker″a·tol′y·sis. 1. Exfoliation of the epidermis. 2. A congenital anomaly in which the skin is shed periodically. **k. neonatorum.** See *dermatitis exfoliativa.*

ker″a·to·lyt′ic. 1. Pertaining to keratolysis. 2. An agent which causes exfoliation of the epidermis to a greater degree than that which occurs normally.

ker″a·to·ma·la′ci·a (kerr″uh·to·ma·lay′shee·uh). A softening of the cornea. Syn., *xerotic keratitis.*

ker′a·tome. A knife with a trowel-like blade, for incising the cornea in the operation of iridectomy.

ker″a·tom′e·ter. An instrument for measuring the curves of the cornea. —**keratometry,** n.

ker″a·to·my·co′sis (kerr″uh·to·migh·ko′sis). A fungoid growth in or on the cornea.

ker″a·to·nyx′is. Puncture of the cornea; especially, the needling of a soft cataract by puncture of the cornea.

ker′a·to·plas″ty. Plastic operation upon the cornea, especially the transplantation of a portion of cornea. —**keratoplas′tic,** adj.

ker″a·tor·rhex′is. Rupture of the cornea, due to ulceration or traumatism.

ker″a·to·scle·ri′tis. Inflammation of the cornea and the sclera.

ker′a·to·scope. An instrument for examining the cornea and testing the symmetry of its meridians of curvature.

ker′a·tose. Horny.

ker″a·to′sis. Any disease of the skin characterized by an overgrowth of the cornified epithelium. **k. blennor-**

rhagica. A disease characterized by horny growths, chiefly of the hand and feet, and occurring during the course of an attack of gonorrhea. Syn., *keratoderma blennorrhagica.* **k. follicularis.** A disease characterized by horny, prominent projections occurring about the hair follicles; they are firmly adherent and produce a roughness. Also called *Darier's disease, psorospermosis.* **k. palmaris et plantaris.** A marked, congenital thickening of the volar surfaces of the hands and feet. This condition may be complicated with painful fissures. **k. seborrheica.** Nummular and flat lesions covered with greasy scales; occurs in older people. The lesions are superficial and seldom become malignant. **k. senilis.** A patchy keratosis of the skin of old people; found chiefly on the face and dorsal surfaces of the hands and feet or those surfaces exposed to wind and sun. Some lesions may develop into epitheliomas.

ker·a·tot′o·my. Incision of the cornea.

ke′ri·on cel′si. A type of dermatophytosis of the scalp or beard, with deep, boggy infiltration. Also called *tinea kerion.*

ker·nic′ter·us (kair·nick′tair·oos, kur·nick′tuh·rus). Biliary pigmentation of gray matter of central nervous system, especially basal ganglions, accompanied by degeneration of nerve cells; occurs in icterus neonatorum.

ker′o·sene″ oil. A liquid mixture of hydrocarbons distilled from petroleum. Sometimes called *coal oil.*

ke′tene. $H_2C:CO$. A colorless gas of penetrating odor, forming acetic acid upon hydrolysis.

ke′to-, ket-. In chemistry, a combining form denoting the presence of the *ketone group.*

ke″to·cho·lan′ic ac′id (kee″to·ko·lan′ick). Cholic acid in which one or more of the secondary alcohol groups have been oxidized to ketone groups.

ke″to·gen′e·sis. The production of ketone, or acetone, bodies.

ke″to·glu·tar′ic ac′id (kee″to·glue·tarr′ick, ·tahr′ick). COOH(CH₂)CO.COOH. A dibasic keto acid, an intermediate product in the metabolism of carbohydrates and proteins.

ke″to·hep′tose. A general term for monosaccharides consisting of a seven carbon chain and containing a ketone group.

ke″to·hex′ose. A general term for monosaccharides consisting of a six carbon chain and containing a ketone group.

ke″to·hy·drox″y·oes′trin (kee″to·high·drock″see·es′trin, ·ees′trin). See *estrone.*

ke'tol. A ketone alcohol; a compound containing both a keto (=CO) and a hydroxy (—OH) group.

ke'tole. Indole.

ke·tol'y·sis. The dissolution of ketone bodies. **—ketolyt'ic,** adj.

ke'tone. An organic compound derived by oxidation from a secondary alcohol; it contains the characterizing group =CO.

ke"to·ne'mi·a. The presence of ketone bodies in the blood.

ke"to·nu'ri·a. The presence of ketone bodies in the urine.

ke"to·re·duc'tase (kee"to·ri·duck'ace, ·taze). An enzyme occurring in muscle, liver, and kidney, which converts diacetic acid into beta-oxybutyric acid.

ke'tose. A carbohydrate containing the ketone group =CO.

ke·to'sis. 1. A condition in which ketones are present in the body in excessive number. 2. The acidosis of diabetes. **k. threshold.** The critical ratio at which ketone substances can be oxidized by the tissues as they are put forth by the liver. Ketosis occurs when the ketosis threshold has been passed and the liver is spilling out ketone substances faster than they can be oxidized by the tissues.

ke"to·ster'oid (kee"to·sterr'oyd, ·teer'oyd). One of a group of neutral steroids possessing ketone substitution, which produces a characteristic red color with m-dinitrobenzene in alkaline solution. The ketosteroids are principally metabolites of adrenal cortical and gonadal steroids; also called 17-ketosteroids.

kg. Kilogram.

khel'lin. A crystalline constituent, chemically dimethoxy-methyl-furanochrome, of the umbelliferous plant Ammi visnaga, the fruits of which have been used in Egypt as an antispasmodic in renal colic and ureteral spasm. It is a coronary vasodilator. Also called khellin, chellin, visammin.

khel'li·nin. The oxyglucoside of khellin, q.v., pharmacologically inactive. Syn., khellol-glucoside.

khel'lol-glu'co·side. Khellinin.

kid'ney. One of the paired glandular organs situated retroperitoneally lateral to the spine, caudal to the spleen on the left and the liver on the right side. The kidney has a characteristic bean shape; convex laterally and concave on the medial border. The hilus on the medial border expands into a central cavity, the renal sinus, which contains the renal calyxes. The calyxes are cup-shaped tubes embracing the renal papillae. They unite to form a funnel-shaped sac, the renal pelvis. In the adult each kidney weighs about 150

Gm. and measures about 11.5 × 6 × 3.5 cm. It is covered by a fairly dense fibrous capsule and embedded in perirenal fat. The kidney consists of a medulla and cortex. The medulla consists of eight to eighteen conical masses, the renal pyramids; the apexes of the pyramids converge toward the renal sinus and project into the lumens of the minor calyxes. The cortex lies immediately beneath the capsule, and dips in between adjacent pyramids; the parts between the pyramids are called renal columns of Bertin. The kidney helps to regulate the normal concentrations of blood constituents by the excretion of water and various substances usually considered as waste products; it probably also furnishes products which have to do with control of systemic blood pressure. The filtering, excreting, and reabsorbing functions of the kidney take place in the nephrons, each composed of a renal corpuscle and tubule. The renal corpuscle consists of a tuft of capillary loops, the glomerulus, and a glomerular (Bowman's) capsule. The latter consists of a simple squamous epithelium seated on a basement membrane. It has a visceral layer fitting closely over the loops of the glomerulus and a parietal layer which is continuous with the epithelium of the renal tubule. The part of the tubule near the glomerulus is the proximal convoluted tubule, continuous with the medullary loop or loop of Henle which consists of a descending and ascending limb, the latter communicating with the distal convoluted tubule and thence with the collecting tubule. The renal artery (or arteries) enters at the hilus and divides dichotomously to provide branches for the medulla, the so-called arcuate arteries at the junction of pyramid and medulla, and the interlobar arteries of the cortex; the veins are distributed in parallel. **cystic k.** One containing cysts, usually of the congenital variety. **fatty k.** Fatty degeneration of the renal epithelium. **floating k.** See wandering k. **gouty k.** One with deposits of urates, usually in tips of pyramids. **horseshoe k.** Greater or lesser degree of congenital fusion of the two kidneys, usually at lower poles. **large white k.** Enlargement and pallor of kidney such as may be due to amyloidosis, marked nephrosis, chronic lipoid nephrosis, or chronic parenchymatous nephritis. **pelvic k.** One abnormally located in the pelvis. **surgical k.** Suppurative inflammation or tuberculosis of kidney. **wandering k.** A kidney with abnormal mobility due to lack of support by perirenal fat.

kie'sel·guhr" (kee'zul·goor"). See purified siliceous earth.

kil′o-. A prefix meaning *thousand*.

kil′o·cal″o·rie, kil·o·cal″o·ry. A large calorie; the amount of heat required to raise 1 kg. of water from 15° to 16° C.; used in the study of metabolism.

kil′o·gram. One thousand grams, or about 2.2 pounds avoirdupois. Abbreviated, kg.

kil″o·gram-me′ter, kil′o·gram-me″tre. A unit of energy; the amount of energy required to raise one kilogram one meter; approximately 7.233 foot-pounds.

kil′o·joule″ (kill′o·jōōl″). A unit of heat, equivalent to 239.1 small calories.

kil′o·li″ter, kil′o·li″tre (kill′o-lee″tur). One thousand liters, or 35.31 cubic feet. Abbreviated, kl.

kil′o·me″ter, kil′o·me″tre (kill′-o-mee″tur, ki·lom′i·tur). One thousand meters, or 1093.6 yards. Abbreviated, km.

kil′o·nem. A unit of nutriment, equivalent to 667 calories.

kil′o·watt″ (kill′o·wot″). A unit of electric power; one thousand watts. Abbreviated, kw.

kil′u·rane. A unit of radioactivity; one thousand uranium units.

ki′nase (kigh′nace, kin′ace). A substance which acts on a zymogen to form an enzyme. See *activator*.

kin″e·mat′ics. The science of motion.

kin″e·ra″di·o·ther′a·py. X-ray therapy whereby the tube is moved in relation to the patient, or the patient in relation to the stationary tube. The object is the attainment of larger depth doses without overloading the skin.

kin′e·scope. An instrument for testing the refraction of the eye; consists of a moving disk with a slit of variable width, through which the patient observes a fixed object.

ki·ne′si- (ki·nee′see-, kigh·nee′see-). A combining form meaning *movement, motion.*

ki·ne′si·a (ki·nee′shuh, kigh·nee′·). 1. Any form of motion sickness, such as seasickness. 2. A suffix implying motion or movement, as hyperkinesia.

ki·ne′si·at′rics. The treatment of disease by systematic active or passive movements. Syn., *kinesitherapy, kinetotherapy.*

ki·ne″si·es·the″si·om′e·ter. An instrument for testing the muscular sense.

kin″e·sim′e·ter, ki·ne″si·om′e·ter. An instrument for determining quantitatively the motion of a part.

ki·ne′si·ol′o·gy. The science of movements, considered especially as therapeutic or hygienic agencies.

ki·ne′sis (ki·nee′sis, kigh·nee′sis). The general term for transformation of physical forms of energy.

ki·ne′sis par″a·dox′a. The sudde[n] and violent overexertion in walking an[d] running observed in patients wit[h] paralysis agitans who, because of gen[-] eralized muscular rigidity, are ord[i-] narily inactive or sluggish. Also calle[d] *Souques' sign.*

ki·ne″so·pho′bi·a. Morbid fear o[f] motion.

kin″es·the′si·a (kin″ess-thee′zhu[h] ·zee-uh), **kin″es·the′sis.** The mus[-] cle sense; the sense of perception o[f] movement, weight, resistance, and pos[i-] tion. —**kinesthet′ic,** *adj.*

kin″es·the″si·om·e·ter. Instru[-] ment for measuring the degree of mus[-] cle sense.

ki·net′ic (ki-net′ick, kigh-net′ick[)]. Pertaining to motion; pro[-] ducing motion.

ki·ne′sic. Pertaining to motion; pro[-] ducing motion.

ki·net′ics. The science of force a[nd] producing motion.

ki′no (kee′no, kigh′no). The drie[d] juice obtained from the trunk of *Pter[o-] carpus marsupium.* Powerful astri[n-] gent.

ki′o·tome. An instrument for amp[u-] tating the uvula.

ki·ot′o·my (kigh·ot′o·mee). Surgic[al] removal of the uvula.

kl. Kiloliter.

Kleb·si·el′la. A genus of bacteria [of] the family Enterobacteriaceae; fr[e-] quently associated with infections [of] the respiratory tract and patholog[ic] conditions of other parts of the bod[y.] **K. pneumoniae.** A species of sho[rt,] plump, heavily capsulated, nonmoti[le] and Gram-negative bacteria, respons[i-] ble for a very small proportion of lob[ar] pneumonias in man.

klep″to·ma′ni·a. A morbid des[ire] to steal; obsessive stealing; a ment[al] disorder in which the objects stolen a[re] usually of symbolic value only, bei[ng] petty and useless items. —**klepto[-] maniac,** *n.*

klep″to·pho′bi·a. 1. A morbid dre[ad] of thieves. 2. A morbid dread of becom[-] ing a kleptomaniac, observed in ps[y-] chasthenia.

Kline test. A microscopic flocculati[on] test for syphilis.

kli′no-. For words beginning wi[th] *klino-,* see under *clino-.*

km. Kilometer.

knee. The articulation between t[he] femur and the tibia. Also see *genu.* S[ee] Table of Joints and Ligaments in t[he] Appendix.

knee′cap″. The patella.

knife. A cutting instrument of vary[ing] shape, size, and design, used in surge[ry] and in dissecting; a scalpel. Also [see] *bistoury.* **amputating k.** A lo[ng,] pointed, single- or double-edged instr[u-] ment, used for amputations. **ca[u-] tery k.** A knife to produce caute[ry] usually with an insulated handle and heated by electricity or in a flame. **electrosurgical k.** See radio *k.* **radio k.** One operating on a high-frequency current, which divides tissues by means of an electric spark; used in electrosurgery. **tenotomy k.** See *tenotome.*

knit'ting. A lay term to indicate the process of union in a fractured bone.

knob. A rounded prominence or protuberance.

knock'-knee". See *genu* valgum.

knot. In *surgery*, the interlacing of the ends of a ligature, suture, bandage, sling, or cord, so placed that they remain fixed without slipping or detachment. **clove-hitch k.** One formed of two contiguous loops, placed around an object, such as a limb, the ends of the cord parallel and extending in opposite directions. This knot remains firm only so long as traction is applied. **double k.** One in which the ends of the cord or suture are twisted twice around each other before tying; friction knot; surgeon's knot. It does not slip and can be adjusted. **false k.** (a) See granny *k.* (b) External knotlike bulges of the umbilical cord caused by loops in the umbilical blood vessels. **granny k.** A double knot in which unlike the square knot, in the second loop the end of one cord is over, and the other under, its fellow; the loops, not being in the same plane, tend to slip. A false knot. **square k.** A double knot in which the free ends of the second knot lie in the same plane as the ends of the first. The knot which is in most general use in surgery. **true k.** A knot of the umbilical cord formed by the fetus slipping through a loop in the cord.

knuck'le. 1. An articulation of the phalanges with the metacarpal bones or with each other. 2. The distal convex ends of the metacarpals.

Koch, Robert [*German bacteriologist*, 1843-1910]. Considered one of the founders of modern bacteriology. See the *law* of specificity of bacteria, also called *Koch's law.* Introduced improved methods of cultivating and staining bacteria. Discovered the tubercle bacillus (1882), formerly called *Koch's bacillus.* He introduced tuberculin (1890), which, though disappointing in the treatment of tuberculosis, proved useful in diagnosis. When tuberculin is injected into the skin of an animal or human being previously exposed to the tubercle bacillus, a local inflammatory reaction indicates continued hypersensitivity; called *Koch's phenomenon.* Nobel laureate (1905).

Köhler's tar'sal scaph"oid-i'tis. Osteochondritis occurring in the navicular bone of the foot.

koi"lo·nych'i·a (koy"lo·nick'ee-uh). A condition in which the outer surface of the nail is concave. Also called *spoon nail.*

koi·not'ro·py. In *psychobiology*, the state of being socialized; the condition of being identified with the common interests of the people. —**koinotrop'-ic,** *adj.*

ko'jic ac'id. $C_6H_6O_4$. 3-Hydroxy-5-hydroxymethyl-γ-pyrone, formed from glucose by the action of certain molds.

ko'la. The dried cotyledon of *Cola nitida* or of other species of *Cola* (cola nut); the chief constituent is caffeine.

kolp-. For words beginning with *kolp-* not found here, see under *colp-.*

kol'po-. See *colpo-.*

ko·ni·me'ter (ko'ni·mee"tur, ko-nim'i·tur), **ko'no·me'ter** (ko'no-mee"tur, ko·nom'i·tur). An instrument for determining the number of dust particles in the air. A measured air sample is propelled against a perpendicular surface coated with an adhesive substance to which the dust adheres. The particles are then counted under a microscope. Other instruments used for the same purpose are the impinger, jet dust counter, and precipitator. Also see *dust count.*

Koplik's sign. See under *sign.*

Koplik's spots. See *Koplik's sign.*

kop"o·pho'bi·a. Morbid fear of fatigue or exhaustion.

korotrin. Trade-mark for a brand of chorionic gonadotropin.

ko"so·tox'in. The chief active constituent of brayera, *q.v.*

Kr. Chemical symbol for krypton.

kra·me'ri·a. The dried root of *Krameria triandra*, known as Peruvian rhatany, or of *Krameria argentea*, known as Para or Brazilian rhatany. An active astringent.

krau·ro'sis. A progressive, sclerosing, shriveling process of the skin; due to glandular atrophy. **k. of vulva.** A disease of elderly women, characterized by pruritus, atrophy, and dryness of the genitalia. Stenosis of the vaginal orifice and epithelioma may develop.

kre"o·tox'in. A meat poison or ptomaine formed by bacteria.

kryp'to-. See *crypto-.*

kryp'ton. Kr = 83.7. A colorless, inert gaseous element which occurs in the atmosphere.

Kupffer cells. See under *cell.*

kur'chi (koor'chee). A bark extract used in amebic dysentery. Also called *holarrhena antidysenterica.*

Kussmaul, Adolf [*German physician*, 1822-1902]. Gave a classic description of the labored breathing associated with diabetic coma (1874); called *air hunger, Kussmaul's respiration* or *sign.*

kw. Kilowatt.

ky·es'te·in (kigh-ess'tee-in). A filmy deposit upon decomposing urine, once thought to be diagnostic of pregnancy.

ky'mo·gram. The record made on a kymograph.

ky'mo·graph. An instrument for recording physiologic cycles or actions in a patient or an experimental animal; consists of a clock- or a motor-driven cylinder, covered with paper on which the record is made. Time intervals can be recorded simultaneously with the phenomena. **—kymograph'ic,** adj.

ky·mog'ra·phy (kigh-mog'ruh-fee). Use of the kymograph. **roentgen k.** See radiokymography.

kynex. Trade-mark for sulfamethoxypyridazine.

kyn"u·re'nic ac'id (kin"yoo-ree'nick, kigh"new-). $C_{10}H_7NO_3$. γ-Hydroxy-β-quinoline carboxylic acid, a product of the metabolism of tryptophan occurring in the urine of some animals, but not in man.

ky·nur'e·nine (kigh-new'ri-neen, kin"yoo-ree'neen). An intermediate product, $C_{11}H_{12}N_2O_2$, of tryptophan metabolism isolated from the urine of certain animals, but not man.

ky"pho·ra·chi'tis (kigh"fo·ra· kigh'tis). Rachitic deformity of th thorax and spine, resulting in an an teroposterior hump. The pelvis is some times involved. **—kyphorachit'ic** adj.

ky"pho·sco"li·o·ra·chi'tis. combined kyphosis and scoliosis due t rickets. The pelvis and thorax may b involved in the deformity. **—kypho scoliorachit'ic,** adj.

ky"pho·sco"li·o'sis. Lateral curva ture of the spine with vertebral rota tion, associated with an anteroposterio hump in the spinal column. **—ky phoscoliot'ic,** adj.

ky·pho'sis (kigh-fo'sis). Angula curvature of the spine, the convexity o the curve being posterior, usually situ ated in the thoracic region, and in volving few or many vertebrae; th result of such diseases as tuberculosi osteoarthritis, or rheumatoid arthriti of the spine, or an improper postur habit. Syn., humpback, hunchback. Als see round shoulders. **—kyphot'ic** adj.

ky'to-. See cyto-.

L

L. Latin; limes.

L$_+$. Symbol for limes death.

L$_0$. Symbol for limes zero.

L-. In chemistry, a prefix, printed as a small capital letter, used to indicate the structural configuration of a particular asymmetric carbon atom, with reference to the standard substance L-glyceraldehyde, as distinguished from D-glyceraldehyde. See also D-, d- dl-, isomerism, l-.

l. Left, left eye, libra, liter, lethal.

l-. 1. In chemistry, an abbreviation used as a prefix, meaning levorotatory. See also d-, dl-. 2. In chemistry, formerly same as L-.

La. Chemical symbol for lanthanum.

Labbé, Leon [French surgeon, 1832-1916]. Labbé's triangle is that area bounded by a horizontal line along the lower border of the cartilage of the ninth rib, by the left costal arch, and by the lower edge of the liver.

la'bi·a. Plural of labium, q.v.

la'bi·al·ism. The tendency to pronounce any articulate sounds as if they were labial consonants, as b, p, or m; the addition of a labial or labiodental quality to an articulate sound.

la'bile (lay'bil, lay'bile). Unstable; readily changing; moving from place to place.

la'bi·o-. A combining form denotin the lips, labial.

la"bi·o·al·ve'o·lar. Pertaining the lip and to one or more dental a veoli.

la"bi·o·cer'vi·cal. Pertaining to lip and a neck; the labial, or bucca surface of the neck of a tooth.

la"bi·o·den'tal. Pertaining to t lips and the teeth.

la"bi·o·gin'gi·val (lay"bee·o·jir ji-vul, -jin-jy'vul). Pertaining to t lips and gums.

la"bi·o·glos"so·la·ryn'ge·a Pertaining conjointly to lips, tongu and larynx, as in labioglossolaryngo paralysis, a form of bulbar paralys

la"bi·o·men'tal. Relating to the l and chin.

la"bi·o·pal'a·tine (lay"bee·o·pal uh-tyne, -tin). Relating to the lip a palate.

la'bi·o·plas"ty. Cheiloplasty, q.v.

la'bi·um (pl. labia). 1. A lip. 2 invertebrate zoology, the lower li opposed to the labrum, the upper l See also lip. **—labial,** adj. **l. maju** One of two folds (labia majora) the female external genital orga arising just below the mons pubis, a surrounding the vulval entrance. Al called l. majus pudendi, major l

l. minus. One of the two folds (labia minora) at the inner surfaces of the labia majora. Also called *l. minus pudendi, minor lip.*

a'bor. Childbirth. **artificial l.** That effected or aided by means other than the forces of the maternal organism. **dry l.** That in which there is a deficiency of amniotic fluid, or in which there has been a premature rupture of the amniotic sac. **false l.** Painful, usually irregular uterine contractions, frequently occurring several days before normal labor, which are ineffective in achieving the first stage of labor. **induced l.** Labor brought on by artificial means. **instrumental l.** One requiring instrumental means to extract the child. **l. pains.** The pains associated with childbirth. **missed l.** Retention of the dead fetus in the uterus beyond the period of normal gestation. **postponed l.** Delayed beyond nine months. **precipitate l.** The sudden expulsion of the fetus and its appendages. **premature l.** Labor taking place before the normal period of gestation, but when the fetus is viable. **protracted l.** Labor prolonged beyond the usual limit (10–20 hours in primiparas, 2–6 hours in multiparas). **rotation stage of l.** That period in the mechanism of childbirth in which the presenting part turns about its vertical axis to accommodate itself to the birth canal. This turning may be internal, occurring before the birth of the presenting part, or external, occurring afterward. **spontaneous l.** That requiring no artificial aid. **stages of l.** Arbitrary divisions of the period of labor; the first includes the entire process of dilatation of the cervix uteri; the second ends with the expulsion of the child; the third (placental) consists in the expulsion of the placenta.

a'brum, lab'rum. 1. A liplike structure. 2. *In invertebrate zoology,* the upper lip, as opposed to the labium, the lower lip. **l. glenoidale.** The fibrocartilaginous ring that surrounds a socket in which the head of a large bone is received, such as the acetabulum or the glenoid cavity; glenoid lip.

ab'y·rinth. 1. An intricate system of connecting passageways; maze. 2. The system of intercommunicating canals and cavities that makes up the inner ear. **—labyrin'thine,** *adj.* **bony l.** That part of the inner ear consisting of canals containing perilymph and the membranous labyrinth. **ethmoid l.** That formed by the air cells in the lateral portions of the ethmoid bone. **membranous l.** Those membranous canals corresponding to the shape of the bony labyrinth, sus-

pended in the perilymph, and containing endolymph. **nasal l.** The irregular cavity formed by the turbinate bones in the nasal passages.

lab"y·rin·thi'tis. Inflammation of the aural labyrinth. Syn., *otitis interna.* **serous l.** That due to bacterial infection, toxins, or trauma, marked by increased perilymphatic pressure without suppuration. **suppurative l.** That due to bacterial invasion, characterized by all of the diagnostic evidence of infection, including production of pus cells. **traumatic l.** Inflammation of the labyrinth due to trauma, as a fractured skull or such functional labyrinthine surgery as a fenestration operation.

lab"y·rin·thot'o·my. Incision into the labyrinth.

lac. 1. Milk. 2. A term applied to various natural resins used in preparing shellac.

lac'case. 1. An oxidizing enzyme present in many plants. 2. A class of oxidases which act on phenols.

lac"er·at"ed (lass'uh-ray"tid). Torn.

lac"er·a'tion. 1. A tear. 2. The act of tearing or lacerating. **l. of perineum.** A tearing of the wall separating the lower portion of the vagina and the anal canal, occurring occasionally during childbirth.

la·cer'tus. A small bundle of fibers. **l. fibrosus.** An aponeurotic band from the biceps brachii muscle to the fascia of the forearm.

lach'ry·mal. See *lacrimal.*

la·cin'i·ate. Jagged, fringed; cut into narrow flaps, as laciniate ligament.

lac'ri·mal. 1. Pertaining to the tears, or to the organs secreting and conveying the tears. 2. The lacrimal bone. See Table of Bones in the Appendix.

lac"ri·ma'tion. Normal secretion of tears; also excessive secretion, as in weeping.

lac'ri·ma"tor. Any substance, as a gas, which irritates the conjunctiva and causes secretion of the tears; a tear gas.

lac'ri·mo·tome. A cutting instrument used in operating on the nasolacrimal duct or lacrimal sac.

lac"ri·mot'o·my. Incision of the nasolacrimal duct.

lac"tal·bu'min. A simple protein contained in milk which resembles serum albumin and is of high nutritional quality.

lac'tam. An organic compound, containing a —NH—CO— group in ring form. It is the keto form of its isomer, lactim, *q.v.*

lac·tam'ic ac'id. Alanine.

lac'tant. Suckling.

lac'tase. A soluble enzyme found in

the animal body which hydrolyzes lactose to dextrose and galactose.

lac·ta'tion. 1. The period of suckling, that during which the child is nourished from the breast. 2. The formation or secretion of milk. **—lactational,** *adj.*

lac'te·al. 1. Pertaining to milk. 2. Any one of the lymphatics of the small intestine that transport the chyle.

lac'tic. Pertaining to milk or its derivatives.

lac'tic ac'id. A mixture of $HC_3H_5O_3$ and lactic anhydride; a colorless, nearly odorless, syrupy liquid, miscible with water. Employed in infant feeding formulas, as a caustic antiseptic, and as a spermatocide. See Table of Normal Values of Blood Constituents in the Appendix.

lac·tif'er·ous. Conveying or secreting milk. Syn., *lactigerous.*

lac'tim. An organic compound, containing a —N:COH— group in ring form. It is the enol form of its isomer, lactam, *q.v.*

lac'to-, lact-. A combining form meaning *milk.*

Lac"to·ba·cil'lus. A genus of bacteria composed of microörganisms capable of producing lactic acid from carbohydrates and carbohydratelike compounds. **L. acidophilus.** A species of large bacilli producing acid but no gas from glucose, lactose, maltose, and sucrose. It coagulates milk and is used in the production of acidophilus milk. It is thought to be synonymous with Döderlein's bacillus (*Bacillus vaginalis*) which is believed to contribute to the acidity of the vaginal secretions and thus help in the defense against infection. **L. lactis Dorner.** A microörganism used in the study of B_{12} since it requires this vitamin for growth.

lac"to·fla'vin (lack"to·flay'vin, ·flav'in). Riboflavin, *q.v.*

lac'to·gen. Any agent or substance which stimulates the secretion of milk.

lac"to·glob'u·lin. One of the proteins of milk.

lac·tom'e·ter. An instrument for determining the specific gravity of milk.

lac'tone. An anhydro-ring compound produced by elimination of water from a molecule of an oxyacid.

lac·ton'ic ac'id. Galactonic acid.

lac"to·pro'te·in. A protein in milk.

lac'tose. $C_{12}H_{22}C_{11}.H_2O$. Milk sugar; a sugar in the milk of mammals. Employed in infant feeding formulas, occasionally as a diuretic; extensively used as a water-soluble inert diluent. Syn., *lactin.*

lac"to·su'ri·a. The presence of lactose in the urine.

la·cu'na. 1. A little depression or space. 2. The space in the matrix occupied by a cartilage cell or by the body of a bone cell. **—lacunar,** *adj.* **blood l.** Any one of the cavities containing maternal blood in the early syncytiotrophoblast before the development of the true villi; they become the intervillous spaces of the placenta.

la·cu'nu·la. A small or minute lacuna; an air space, as seen in a gray hair when magnified.

Ladd-Franklin, Christine [*American psychologist and logician, 1847–1930*]. Advanced a theory of color vision developed upon a basis of evolution (1892). From a primitive black-white substance operative in rod vision in retinas without cones, the first stage in the development of color vision is said to have produced yellow and blue substances and cones; in the final stage, red and green substances were produced from the yellow, finishing the series of substances for white, yellow, red, and green vision. Called *Ladd-Franklin theory of vision.*

Laehr-Henneberg hard palate reflex. In pseudobulbar paralysis contraction of the orbicularis oris and lowering of the upper lip when the hard palate is tickled.

Laennec, René Théophile Hyacinthe [*French physician, 1781–1826*]. Invented the stethoscope, and made a basic study of auscultation. Gave classic descriptions of tuberculosis, lobar pneumonia, pleurisy, bronchiectasis, pneumothorax, emphysema, and hydatid cysts of the lung. See also Laennec's *cirrhosis,* Laennec's *thrombus.*

lae've (lee'vuh). Smooth; nonvillous; as chorion laeve.

lae'vo- (lee'vo-), **laev-.** See *levo-.*

lag. The space of time between the application of a stimulus and the resulting response.

lag'am bal'sam (bawl'sum). A thick yellow liquid resembling Copaiba balsam.

la·ge'ni·form (la·jee'ni·form, lajen'i·). Flask-shaped.

lag·nei'a (lag·nigh'uh). Satyriasis or nymphomania; erotomania.

lag"neu·o·ma'ni·a. A mental disorder characterized by lustful, sadistic, lewd, and lecherous actions.

lag"oph·thal'mos. A condition in which the eyes cannot be entirely closed. **—lagophthalmic,** *adj.*

Lagrange, Pierre Félix [*French ophthalmologist, 1857–1928*]. Devised an operation combining iridectomy and sclerectomy, for the relief of glaucoma; called *Lagrange's operation.*

la grippe (lah grip). Old term for influenza.

lake. 1. A small, fluid-filled hollow

cavity; lacus. 2. A pigment prepared by precipitating a vegetable or animal coloring matter with a metallic compound. 3. Hemolyze. **blood l.** See *hematoma.* **lacrimal l.** The space at the inner canthus of the eye, near the puncta, in which the tears collect.

la'ky. Lake-colored; of a purplish red; said of blood serum which has a transparent red color after hemolysis.

al·la'tion. 1. Any unintelligible stammering of speech, as word-salad or the prattling of a baby. 2. Pronunciation of the letter r so that it sounds like *l*. **al"o·ple'gi·a.** Inability to speak, due to paralysis of the muscles concerned in speech, except those of the tongue.

Lamarck, Jean Baptiste Pierre Antoine de Monet de [*French naturalist,* 1744–1829]. One of the greatest of comparative anatomists and biologists. Classified animals as vertebrates and invertebrates. Antedated Darwin in postulating some elements of Darwin's theory of evolution.

La·marck'ism. The theory that organic evolution takes place through the inheritance of modifications caused by the environment, and of the effects of use and disuse of organs.

lamb'da. 1. The eleventh letter of the Greek alphabet (Λ, λ). 2. The point where the sagittal suture meets the lambdoid suture. 3. Microliter.

lamb'da·cism. 1. Difficulty in uttering the sound of the letter *l*. 2. Too frequent use of the *l* sound, or its substitution for the *r* sound.

lamb'doid. Resembling the Greek letter Λ, as lambdoid suture.

lam'bert. A photometric unit for describing the brightness of light reflected from a surface. One lambert is the equivalent of one lumen per sq. cm.

la·mel'la (pl. *lamellas*). 1. A thin scale or plate. 2. *In ophthalmology,* a medicated gelatin disk intended to be inserted under the eyelid. **circumferential l.** A thin layer of bone deposited under the periosteum or endosteum. **concentric l.** One of the plates of bone making up the Haversian systems in compact bone. **enamel l.** A thin organic sheet extending from the surface of the enamel toward and sometimes into the dentine of a tooth. It may be due to local developmental disturbance or a crack filled with organic matter. **ground l.** See interstitial *l.* **Haversian l.** One of the concentric layers of bone surrounding a Haversian canal. **interstitial l.** One of the layers of bone in the regions between Haversian systems. **l. of bone.** A thin layer of bone deposited during one period of osteonic activity.

la·mel'lar, lam'el·lar. Resembling a thin plate; composed of lamellas or thin plates, as lamellar cataract.

lame'ness. Limping; weakness or partial loss of function of a leg, so that the gait is abnormal, whether due to acute disease, shortening, atrophy of muscle, pain, or to any other disturbance of the member. **lame,** *adj., v.* **elbow l.** Lameness in the horse, due to disease of the elbow joint. **intermittent l.** See intermittent *claudication.*

lam'i·na. A thin plate, *q.v.,* or layer. **—laminar, laminated,** *adj.* **anterior elastic l.** The condensed, outer layer of the substantia propria of the cornea. Also called *l. elastica anterior, Bowman's membrane.* **basal l.** A homogeneous membrane covering the inner surface of the choroid. Also called *Bruch's membrane.* **choriocapillary l.** The inner layer of the choroid, consisting of a capillary plexus. **cribriform l.** See cribriform *plate.* **dental l.** The epithelial ingrowth into the jaw which gives rise to the enamel organs of the developing teeth. **external elastic l.** See external elastic *membrane.* **labiodental l.** The epithelial ingrowth which forms the labiogingival lamina and the dental lamina. **labiogingival l.** The portion of the vestibular lamina opposite the lips. Also called *labial l.* **l. affixa.** The line of union of a hemisphere with the thalamus. **l. cribrosa.** (a) That portion of the sclera which is perforated for the passage of the optic nerve. (b) The fascia covering the saphenous opening. (c) The anterior or posterior perforated space of the brain. (d) The perforated plates of bone through which pass branches of the cochlear or auditory nerve. **l. elastica.** The layer of interlacing elastic fibers in the mucous membrane of the pharynx, larynx, and respiratory tree. **l. muscularis mucosae.** The layer or layers of smooth muscle at the deep face of the mucous membrane of the digestive tube. **l. papyracea.** A thin, smooth, oblong plate of bone which closes in the ethmoidal cells and forms a large part of the medial wall of the orbit. Also called *os planum.* **l. propria.** (a) The middle or fibrous layer of the tympanic membrane. (b) See *l. propria mucosae.* **l. propria mucosae.** The connective tissue of a mucous membrane. Syn., *tunica propria mucosae.* **l. quadrigemina.** The alar plate of the midbrain from which the corpora quadrigemina are developed. **l. terminalis.** The connecting layer of gray matter between the optic chiasma and the anterior commissure where it becomes continuous with the rostral lamina. **l. vascu-**

losa chorioideae. The outer, pigmented layer of the choroid, composed of small arteries and veins. **lateral pterygoid l.** The lateral pterygoid plate, *q.v.* **medial pterygoid l.** The medial pterygoid plate, *q.v.* **osseous spiral l.** The thin shelf of bone projecting from the modiolus and partially subdividing the cochlea; the basilar membrane completes the division. **posterior elastic l.** An elastic, transparent, homogeneous membrane covering the posterior surface of the substantia propria of the cornea. Also called *Descemet's membrane.* **reticular l.** The hyaline membrane of the inner ear, extending between the heads of the outer rods of Corti and the external row of the outer hair cells. **spiral l.** A thin plate in the ear, osseous in the inner part and membranous in the outer, which divides the spiral tube of the cochlea into the scala tympani and scala vestibuli. See osseous spiral *l.* and basilar *membrane.* **vestibular l.** The vertical sheet of oral ectoderm which splits to form the vestibule of the mouth.

lam″i·nag′ra·phy. See sectional *radiography.*

lam″i·na′tion. 1. Arrangement in plates or layers. 2. An operation in embryotomy consisting in cutting the skull in slices.

lam″i·nec′to·my. The operation of removing the vertebral arches, particularly the posterior parts, with the vertebral spines.

lamp. An apparatus for furnishing artificial light or heat. **annealing l.** An alcohol lamp used by dentists for annealing gold leaf. **carbon arc l.** A source of therapeutic light, produced by an electric arc between carbon electrodes. **cold quartz mercury vapor l.** A mercury vapor lamp emitting radiations which are practically devoid of heat. **infrared l.** A source of heat rays, which emanate from a surface heated to a temperature of 300° to 800° C. The spectral emission ranges through infrared from 8000 to 150,000 angstroms. Such rays have poor penetrability for skin. **mercury vapor l.** A hollow fused quartz lamp filled with mercury vapor, producing radiations a large proportion of which have high germicidal action. **slit l.** An instrument designed for examination of the anterior segment of the eye. It produces a bright beam of parallel light and has a microscope which can be focused on any opaque structure of the cornea, iris, or lens. **sunlight l.** One which at a measured distance produces rays which imitate in range and intensity the wave lengths of sunshine.

lamp′black″. A fine black substance, almost pure carbon, made by burning oils, tars, fats, and resins in an atmosphere deficient in oxygen.

lan′a·to·side. A natural glycosid from the leaves of *Digitalis lanata* three such glycosides have been isolate and are designated **lanatoside A lanatoside B,** and **lanatoside C** formerly called digilanid A, digilani B, and digilanid C, respectively. The are cardioactive.

lance. Cut or open, as with a lance or bistoury.

lan′cet. A short, double-edged punc turing knife, once in common use fo bleeding patients and for lancing th gums of teething children. **spring l** One in which the blade is thrust ou by means of a small spring operatin on a trigger; often used to obtain sma quantities of blood for laboratory ex aminations.

lan′ci·na″ting. Tearing; shooting sharply cutting, as lancinating pains —**lancinate,** *v.*

land′marks″. Superficial marks, and eminences, lines, and depressions, tha serve as guides to, or indications of deeper parts.

Landolt, Edmond [*French oph thalmologist,* 1846–1926]. Made impor tant contributions to the knowledge of physiologic optics. Described small, elon gated bodies lying between the rods an cones at the outer nuclear layer of th retina; called *Landolt's bodies.* Th *Landolt ring* is an incomplete ring use as a test object for visual acuity.

Landouzy, Louis Théophil Joseph [*French physician,* 1845 1917]. Described spirochetal jaundic (1883), called *Landouzy's disease, Fied ler's disease, Weil's disease.* Independ ently and with Déjèrine, describe facioscapulohumeral atrophy, calle *Landouzy-Déjèrine atrophy* or type Neuralgia of the sciatic nerve wit atrophy of part or all of the affecte leg is known as *Landouzy's sciatica.* form of purpura with serious system symptoms is called *Landouzy's purpur* The *Landouzy-Grasset law,* named fo Landouzy and Joseph Grasset, state that in disease of a single cerebr hemisphere, if there are spastic symp toms, the patient's head inclines to ward the side of the affected muscles if paralysis occurs, the head is turne toward the side of the cerebral lesion

Landry, Jean Baptiste Octav [*French physician,* 1826–65]. Describe acute ascending paralysis, *q.v.,* als called *Landry's paralysis.*

Landsteiner, Karl [*America pathologist,* 1868–1943]. Established th basis of blood grouping; discovered iso agglutinins in human blood serum an isoagglutinogens in blood cells (1900) Discovered three of the four main bloo groups. The classification adopted b he Permanent Commission on Biology tandards, which designates the four roups as O, A, B, and AB, is also nown as the *Landsteiner classification*. andsteiner and Alexander S. Wiener iscovered the Rh factor, *q.v.* (1940). obel laureate (1930).

ane, William Arbuthnot [*Scottish surgeon in England*, 1856–943]. Devised steel plates of various hapes, with holes for screws, for fixing ragments in position in cases of fracure; called *Lane's plates*. Described inestinal bends or twists, called *Lane's inks; Lane's kink* usually refers to an bstructive twist of the ileum. Devised n operation of ileosigmoidostomy for he relief of chronic constipation; alled *Lane's operation*. Intestinal asis is known as *Lane's disease*.

·nette′ wax. An emulsifier, introuced in England as an ingredient of ashable ointment bases.

angenbeck, Bernhard Ruolph Konrad von [*German sureon*, 1810–87]. Made numerous contriutions to the development of orthoedic and plastic surgery. Modified the ndian method of rhinoplasty. Devised n operation for cleft palate in which losure was effected by means of periosal flaps obtained from either side and tured in the midline.

anger, Carl von [*Austrian anatmist*, 1819–87]. Plotted lines indicating he direction of skin tension; called *anger's lines*. Linear scars following he direction of skin tension usually pread little, whereas scars crossing the nsion lines have an opposite tendency. anger described an inconstantly presnt musculotendinous slip of the latisimus dorsi extending across the axilla nterior to the vessels; it is inserted in he region of the pectoralis major. alled *Langer's axillary arch*.

angerhans, Paul [*German physican and anatomist*, 1847–88]. Described he islets of the pancreas (1869), called *lets or islands of Langerhans;* see *islet f pancreas*. Described two types of cells alled *Langerhans' cells:* star-shaped lls in the stratum germinativum, and ·indle-shaped cells in the lumens of he acini of the pancreas. Also an ellate *corpuscle,* called *Langerhans' orpuscle.*

anghans, Theodor [*German anatnist and pathologist in Switzerland*, 39–1915]. Described the cytotropho·ast, called *layer* or *stria of Langhans;* he cells forming the cytotrophoblast ·e known as *Langhans' cells.* See also anghans' *giant cell.*

n′guor (lang′gur). A condition of ind and/or body caused by exhausn; lassitude.

n′o·lin. See hydrous *wool fat.*

n·os′ter·ol, lan″o·ster′ol. C₅₀

H₄₉OH. A complex terpene alcohol in wool fat.

lan′tha·num. La = 138.92. A rare metallic element.

la·nu′go. 1. The downlike hair that covers the fetus about the fifth month of gestation. 2. The fine, downy hair that appears on all parts of the body except palms of hands and soles of feet, and those parts, such as the scalp, where other varieties of hair are found. —**lanuginous,** *adj.*

lan′u·lous. Covered with short, fine hair.

la·pac′tic. 1. An evacuant. 2. Any purgative substance.

lap′a·ro-, lapar-. *In medicine and surgery,* a combining form denoting the *flank* or, more loosely, the *abdomen.*

lap″a·ror′rha·phy. Suture of the abdominal wall.

lap″a·rot′o·my. 1. An incision through the abdominal wall; celiotomy. 2. The operation of cutting into the abdominal cavity through the loin or flank.

lap″a·ro·tra″che·lot′o·my (·tray″ki·lot′o·mee, ·track″i·lot′o·mee). Low Cesarean section. The peritoneal cavity is not opened, the approach being through the cervix of the uterus.

la′pis (lay′pis, lap′is). A stone; an alchemic term applied to any nonvolatile substance. 1. **calaminaris.** Calamine. 1. **imperialis.** Silver nitrate. Also called *l. infernalis.* 1. **mitigatus.** Diluted silver nitrate. 1. **pumicis.** Pumice.

lap′pa. The root of the common burdock, *Arctium lappa,* or of *Arctium minus.*

lap′sus. A fall or slip; ptosis. 1. **linguae.** Slip of the tongue, considered by psychoanalysts to reveal an unconscious desire.

lard. The purified internal fat of the abdomen of the domestic hog. Used as an ingredient of ointment bases. **benzoinated** 1. Lard with 1% benzoin; a mild antiseptic and ointment base.

lar·da′ceous. 1. Resembling lard. 2. Containing diffuse amyloid infiltration.

lark′spur. The dried ripe seed of *Delphinium ajacis.* 1. **tincture.** Larkspur 10% w/v in alcohol; used as a pediculicide.

Larrey, Dominique Jean [*French army surgeon*, 1766–1842]. Devised numerous operations, including methods of amputation at the shoulder and hip joints. Improved the methods of treating war wounded, using advanced first-aid stations and fast ambulances.

lar′va (pl. larvae). An immature, free-living stage in the life cycle of various animals which reach the adult form by undergoing a metamorphosis. 1. **migrans.** A skin disorder characterized by a red linear eruption which extends at one end while fading at the other end; produced by burrowings of larvae. The majority of cases are caused by the larval form of *Ancylostoma braziliense*, but pig and cat nematodes of the genus *Gnathostoma* or larvae of *Gasterophilus* and *Hypoderma linearis* produce similar eruptions. Syn., *creeping eruption, sandworm disease.*

lar'vae (lahr'vee). Plural of larva, *q.v.*

lar'val. 1. Pertaining to or in the condition of a larva. 2. Pertaining to an abortive form of a disease, the full clinical syndrome not developing; as larval pneumonia, larval scarlet fever.

lar'vate. Concealed; masked; applied to diseases and conditions that are hidden by more obvious conditions, or by some peculiarity of their symptoms.

lar'vi·cide. Any agent destroying insect larvae.

la·ryn'ge·al cri'sis (la·rin'jul, lar"in·jee'ul). An acute laryngeal spasm, sometimes occurring in tabes dorsalis.

lar"yn·gec'to·my (lar"in·jeck'to-mee). Extirpation or partial excision of the larynx.

lar"yn·gis'mus (lar"in·jiz'mus, ·jis'mus). A spasm of the larynx. **—laryngismal,** *adj.* l. **stridulus.** A spasmodic affection of the larynx, seen most commonly in rachitic infants and young children; characterized by a sudden crowing inspiration followed by an arrest of respiration of several seconds' duration, with increasing cyanosis, and ending with long, loud, whistling inspirations.

lar"yn·gi'tis. Inflammation of the larynx. It may be acute or chronic, catarrhal, suppurative, croupous (diphtheritic), tuberculous, or syphilitic. **—laryngit'ic,** *adj.* **chronic catarrhal** l. The most common form of laryngitis; consists of a hypertrophic and an atrophic stage. Symptoms are hoarseness, pain, dryness of the throat, dysphagia, and cough. **dry** l. A form characterized by sensations of heat and of fatigue in the throat, persistent cough, and sometimes aphonia. Also called *l. sicca, Türck's trachoma.*

la·ryn'go- (la·ring'go-), **laryng-.** A combining form signifying *the larynx.*

la·ryn'go·cele. A saccular dilatation of the mucosa of the larynx occurring at some site between the hyoid bone and the cricoid cartilage.

la·ryn'go·fis'sure. 1. Division of the larynx for the removal of tumors or foreign bodies. 2. The aperture made in the operation of laryngofissure.

lar"yn·gol'o·gist. One who specializes in the practice or science of laryngology.

lar"yn·gol'o·gy. The science of the

anatomy, physiology, and diseases of the larynx.

la·ryn"go·pa·ral'y·sis. Paralysis of the laryngeal muscles.

la·ryn"go·phar"yn·gi'tis. 1. Inflammation of the laryngopharynx. Inflammation of the larynx and the pharynx.

la·ryn"go·phar'ynx. The inferior portion of the pharynx. It extends from the greater cornua of the hyoid bone to the inferior border of the cricoid cartilage. Also called *hypopharynx, laryngeal pharynx.*

la·ryn"gor·rhe'a, **la·ryn"gorrhoe'a** (la·ring"go·ree'uh). Excessive secretion of mucus from the larynx especially when it is used in phonation.

la·ryn'go·scope. An instrument for examining the interior of the larynx, consisting of a mirror attached to a long handle. **—laryngoscop'ic,** *adj.*

lar"yn·gos'co·py. Examination of the interior of the larynx with the laryngoscope. **suspension** l. method of laryngoscopy devised by Killian, in which the head is suspended on a combined mouth gag and tongue spatula, this is supported by a bar connected with a moving overhead crane. The advantages of the method are that it leaves both hands of the examiner free and gives excellent exposure of the larynx, as in examining laryngeal tumors.

la·ryn'go·spasm. Spasmodic closure of the glottis; laryngismus stridulus.

la·ryn'go·ste·no'sis. Contraction or stricture of the larynx.

lar"yn·gos'to·my. The establishing of a permanent opening into the larynx through the neck.

lar"yn·got'o·my. The operation of incising the larynx.

la·ryn"go·tra'che·al (la·ring"go·tray'kee·ul). Pertaining conjointly to the larynx and the trachea.

la·ryn"go·tra·che·i'tis (·tray"kee·eye'tis). Inflammation of the larynx and the trachea.

la·ryn"go·tra"che·o·bron·chi'tis (·tray"kee·o·brong·kigh'tis). Acute inflammation of the mucosa of the larynx, trachea, and bronchi.

la·ryn"go·tra"che·ot'o·my. Tracheotomy in which the cricoid cartilage and one or more of the upper rings of the trachea are divided.

lar'ynx. The organ of the voice, situated between the trachea and the base of the tongue. It consists of a series of cartilages: the thyroid, the cricoid, and the epiglottis, and three pairs of cartilages: the arytenoid, corniculate, and cuneiform. The cavity is lined by mucous membrane, and the cartilages are moved by the muscles of the larynx. The mucous membrane is, on each side thrown into two transverse folds that constitute the vocal folds, the upper being the false, the lower the true, vocal folds. By the approximation or separation of the vocal folds, the changes in the pitch of the voice are produced. The space between the vocal folds is termed the rima glottidis. **-laryn'geal,** adj.

las·civ'i·ous. Libidinous; wanton; having an unlawful desire; lustful.

las'si·tude. A state of exhaustion or weakness; debility.

la'tent. Concealed; not manifest; potential. **—latency,** n.

lat'er·ad. Toward the lateral aspect.

lat'er·al. At, belonging to, or pertaining to the side; situated on either side of the median vertical plane.

lat"er·i·ver'sion. See lateroversion.

lat'er·o-. A combining form denoting laterally, to one side.

lat"er·o·flex'ion (lat"ur·o·flek'-shun). Bending or curving to one side; the alteration in position of the uterus in which the uterine axis is bent upon itself to one side.

lat"er·o·ver'sion. The alteration in position of the uterus in which the entire uterine axis is displaced to one side.

la'tex (pl. latices). The milky juice of various trees and plants, chiefly those of Brazil, Ecuador, Central America, the East Indies, Borneo, and West Africa. Rubber and gutta-percha are products of latex.

lath'y·rism (lath'i·riz·um). An affection produced by the use of meal from varieties of vetches, chiefly Lathyrus sativus and L. cicera. It is a form of spastic paraplegia with tremor, involving chiefly the legs. Syn., lupinosis.

la·tis'si·mus. Widest, as latissimus dorsi muscle. See Table of Muscles in the Appendix.

la·trine'. A water closet or privy, especially any one of a number of types used in military installations; it may be permanent or temporary.

la'tus, -a, -um. Broad, as ligamentum latum, the broad ligament of the uterus.

Latzko, Wilhelm [Austrian obstetician, 1863–1945]. Devised an operation of low Cesarean section in which the approach is extraperitoneal, with lateral displacement of the bladder and peritoneal reflection. Called Latzko's low Cesarean, Latzko's operation.

lau'da·nine (law'duh·neen, ·nin). $C_{20}H_{25}NO_4$. One of the alkaloids of opium.

lau·dan'o·sine (law·dan'o·seen, w'dun·o·). $C_{21}H_{27}NO_4$. A crystallizable alkaloid of opium.

lau'da·num. Opium tincture.

laugh. 1. Make an audible expression

of mirth. 2. The audible expression of mirth. **canine l.** Risus sardonicus, q.v. **sardonic l.** Risus sardonicus, q.v.

laugh'ter. A succession of rhythmic, spasmodic expirations with open glottis and vibration of the vocal folds, expressing mirth. **compulsive l.** That seen in schizophrenics; it is without cause and mirthless; the patient usually does not know he is laughing. Also called obsessive l.

Laurence, John Zachariah [English ophthalmic surgeon, ca. 1829–1870]. With Moon, described familial retinitis pigmentosa associated with general defective development (1866).

lau'ric ac'id. $CH_3(CH_2)_{10}COOH$. A fatty acid derived from cherry laurel and spermaceti.

lau'ro-, laur-. In chemistry, a combining form denoting lauric acid.

Lauth, Ernest Alexandre [Alsatian anatomist and physiologist, 1803–37]. Described the venous sinus of the sclera (1829); called Lauth's canal, Schlemm's canal. See venous sinus of the sclera.

la·vage' (lah·vahzh'). The irrigation or washing out of an organ, such as the stomach, bowel, urinary bladder, or paranasal sinus.

lav'en·der. The flowers of Lavandula officinalis. The active principle is a volatile oil. **compound l. tincture.** Lavender oil, rosemary oil, cinnamon, clove, myristica, and red sandalwood in a hydroalcoholic menstruum. A popular remedy for nausea and flatulence. **l. oil.** The volatile oil distilled from the fresh flowering tops of Lavandula officinalis. Used chiefly as a perfume; sometimes as a carminative.

Laveran, Charles Louis Alphonse [French army physician and bacteriologist, 1845–1922]. Discovered malarial parasites in blood cells (1880). Nobel laureate (1907).

Lavoisier, Antoine Laurent [French chemist, 1743–94]. Called the founder of modern chemistry. Named oxygen and discovered its function in combustion; is sometimes called the discoverer of oxygen. With Laplace, demonstrated by means of an ice calorimeter that respiration is a form of combustion.

law. 1. Statement of a relation or sequence of phenomena invariable under the same conditions. 2. A rule of conduct prescribed by authority. **all-or-nothing l.** The weakest stimulus capable of producing a contraction produces the maximal contraction in cardiac muscle or skeletal muscle. Increased strength of contraction depends upon the stimulation of more muscle or nerve fibers. **l. of**

filial regression. According to Galton, children whose parents deviate from the average of the population likewise deviate from the average in the same direction as the parents, but regress by about one-third of the parental deviation toward the mean. For example, children whose parents are 3 inches above the average stature are themselves on the average about 2 inches above the mean stature of the population. **l. of independent assortment.** The members of different gene-pairs segregate at miosis independently of one another, provided they are located on different pairs of homologous chromosomes. **l. of multiple proportions.** If more than one compound is formed by two elements, the weight of one element remains constant, that of the other element varies as a multiple of the lowest amount of that element in the series of compounds. **l. of segregation.** The two members of any given pair of genes separate at meiosis so that a mature germ cell receives one or the other member of each pair of genes. **l. of specificity of bacteria.** As elucidated by Robert Koch, the microorganism must be present in every case of the disease; it must be capable of cultivation in pure culture; it must, when inoculated in pure culture, produce the disease in susceptible animals. To this has been added a fourth condition: that the organism must be recovered and again grown in pure culture. Also called *Koch's l.* **l. of the intestines.** A stimulus applied to a given point in the intestinal wall initiates a band of constriction on the proximal side and relaxation on the distal side of the stimulated point. **linkage l.** Different gene-pairs tend to segregate together if they are located on the same pair of homologous chromosomes. Linked genes may be separated with a frequency which varies from 0 to 50%, depending chiefly upon the relative linear distances between them. **Mendel's laws.** The laws of heredity. They refer to the way in which the hereditary units, the genes, pass from one generation to the next by way of the germ cells. In neo-Mendelian terms the principles may be stated as follows: Genes segregate at the time of maturation, with the result that a mature germ cell gets either the maternal or the paternal gene of any pair. Genes of different pairs segregate independently of one another, provided they are located on different pairs of chromosomes. If they are located on the same pair of chromosomes, they are linked and consequently segregate in larger or smaller blocks depending mainly on their relative distances apart

on the chromosome, i.e., on the per centage of crossing over. **periodic l** If the elements are arranged in th sequence of their atomic weights, ele ments having similar characteristic recur regularly in the series, that i. most of the physical and chemica properties of the elements are periodi functions of their atomic weights. Als called *Mendeléev's l.* **Wolff's l.** Ever change in the use or static relation of a bone leads not only to a chang in its internal structure and architec ture but also to a change in its func tion and external form.

lax'a·tive. 1. Aperient; mildly ca thartic. 2. An agent that loosens th bowels; a mild purgative.

lax'i·ty. 1. Lack or loss of tone, ten sion, or firmness. 2. Lack of strictnes or precision. **—lax,** *adj.*

lay'er. A deposited material of uni form, or nearly uniform, thickness spread over a comparatively consider able area; cover; stratum. **basal cell l.** The deepest layer of cells i the germinative layer of a stratifie epithelium. **basal l.** The nondecidu ate stratum basalis of the endome trium, containing the blind ends of th uterine glands. Syn., *stratum basali* **compact l.** The superficial layer o the endometrium during the secretor phase of the menstrual cycle; it is cha acterized by the presence of man decidual cells in pregnancy. Syn *stratum compactum.* **cuticular l** Cuticle. **external granular l.** Th second layer of the cerebral corte containing a large number of sma pyramidal and granule cells. Also calle *layer of small pyramidal cells.* **gar glionic l.** (a) The inner cell laye of the retina. (b) The deep layer large pyramidal cells in the cerebra cortex; in the motor area it contair the giant pyramidal cells. **germina tive l.** The deeper, proliferative laye of cells of the epidermis, including th basal-cell layer and the prickle-ce layer. Syn., *stratum germinativur Malpighian l.* **germ l.** One of th epithelial layers of the blastula o blastocyst from which the various o gans of the embryo are derived. S ectoderm, entoderm, mesoderm. **gra ular l.** The layer deep to the mole ular layer of the cerebellar cortex, co taining a large number of granule cell **half-value l.** *In roentgenology,* th thickness of a suitable absorber whic reduces the intensity of a given x-ra beam to half of its initial value. **inne nuclear l.** The layer of the retin made up chiefly of the cell bodies the bipolar neurons. **internal grar ular l.** The fourth layer of the cere bral cortex containing many sma multipolar cells with short axons, ar

attered small pyramidal cells. **l. of
asiform cells.** The deepest layer
the cerebral cortex, with irregular
asiform and angular cells, whose axons
ater the subjacent white matter. **l. of
enle.** The outermost layer of the
ternal root sheath of hair. **l. of
uxley.** The middle layer of the
ternal root sheath of hair. **l. of
anghans.** The inner, cellular layer
the ectoderm of the chorion. Syn.,
totrophoblast. **l. of pyramidal
ells.** The third layer of the cerebral
rtex, having a superficial stratum
th chiefly medium-sized pyramidal
lls and a deeper stratum with large
ramidal cells. **l. of rods and
ones.** Outer layer of the retina.
olecular l. (a) The outermost
yer of the cerebral or of the cerebellar
rtex, made up of neuroglia, a few
all ganglion cells, and a reticulum
myelinated and unmyelinated nerve
ers. (b) One of the two layers, inner
d outer of the retina, made up of
terlacing dendrites. Also called plexi-
rm layer. **osteogenic l.** The
eper layer of periosteum, connected
th the formation of bone. **outer
uclear l.** The layer of the retina
nich contains the rod and cone gran-
es, or cell bodies. **papillary l.** The
rface layer of the derma, extending
to the papillae formed by the uneven
ne of union of the dermis and epi-
ermis. **prickle-cell l.** The germi-
tive layer of the epidermis exclusive
the basal cells. **somatic l.** The
ternal layer of the lateral mesoderm
ter the formation of the coelom,
rming a part of the somatopleure.
lanchnic l. The internal layer of
e lateral mesoderm after the forma-
n of the coelom, forming a part of
e splanchnopleure. **spongy l.** The
ddle zone of the endometrium during
e secretory phase of the menstrual
cle, characterized by the dilated por-
n of the glands and edematous con-
ctive tissue. Syn., stratum spongi-
um.

ette'. A full outfit of garments,
dding, etc., for a newborn child.
Libra; pound (usually avoirdupois).
D. Lethal dose; the smallest dose
at kills the test animal.
D.₅₀. The dose that is lethal to 50%
test animals.
D. A. Left dorsoanterior position
the fetus.
D. P. Left dorsoposterior position
the fetus.
ch'ing. The process of washing or
tracting the soluble constituents from
oluble material.
d (led). Pb = 207.21. A soft, bluish
ay, malleable metal, occurring in
ture chiefly as the sulfide, PbS,
own as galena. Its soluble salts are

violent irritant poisons; formerly used
as local astringents. Insoluble lead
salts at one time were used as protec-
tives; however, due to the danger of
absorption, the therapeutic use of lead
compounds has been practically discontinued. **diluted l. subacetate
solution.** Lead subacetate solution
diluted with approximately 30 volumes
of water; applied externally. Syn.,
l. water. **l. acetate.** $(CH_3COO)_2$-
Pb.3H₂O. Occurs as white crystals; a
local astringent in 1-2% solution. Syn.,
sugar of lead. **l. and opium lotion.** Prepared from lead acetate,
opium tincture, and water. An embro-
cation of doubtful value for sprains
and bruises. Also called l. and opium
wash. **l. arsenate.** An agricultural
insecticide. **l. borosilicate.** A mixture of the borate and silicate of lead;
a constituent of certain optical glasses.
l. nitrate. Pb(NO₃)₂; occasionally
employed in solution as an astringent.
l. oleate. An unctuous material of
varying composition; active ingredient
of lead oleate plaster. **l. oleate
plaster.** Made by the interaction of
lead monoxide, olive oil, and lard; used
as a protective for skin inflammations.
Syn., l. plaster. Also called diachylon
plaster. **l. plaster.** See l. oleate plaster. **l. subacetate solution.** A
solution of approximately Pb₂O(CH₃-
COO)₂; an externally applied astringent
and sedative. Also called Goulard's
extract. Also see diluted l. subacetate
solution; l. water and laudanum.
l. tetraethyl. Pb(C₂H₅)₄. A colorless, inflammable toxic liquid; used as
an anti-knock ingredient in motor
fuels. **l. water.** See diluted l. subacetate solution. **l. water and
laudanum.** A mixture of lead subacetate solution with an equal volume
of opium tincture; used as an external
application to sprains and bruises.
sugar of l. See l. acetate.
lead (leed). A record taken by means
of a suitable instrument, which represents the difference in electric potential between two electrodes placed upon
the surface or within the body. Thus,
an electrocardiographic lead represents
the differences in potential between two
such electrodes, due to the electric currents that flow within the body as a
result of the beating heart, and an elec-
troencephalographic lead measures the
potential differences between two points
on the skull, resulting from cerebral
activity. Many different kinds of leads
may be used to record the electric
activity of a single organ. The standard
limb leads, universally employed in
electrocardiography, are called leads
I, II, and III, and are obtained by leading from electrodes placed upon the
right and left arms, the right arm and

left leg, and the left arm and left leg, respectively. **electrocardiogram l.** A curve of electric potential differences due to cardiac action recorded from the body surfaces. A typical normal record shows P, Q, R, S, T, and U waves. P is due to excitation of the atria; Q, R, S, to excitation of the ventricles; and T to repolarization of the ventricles. U is a diastolic wave of unknown origin. **unipolar l.** An electrocardiogram taken with one electrode on a region with potential variations of considerable magnitude and another on a region with minimal potential changes.

Leadbetter, Guy Whitman [*American orthopedic surgeon*, 1893–1945]. Devised a method of reduction in fracture of the femoral neck. The patient lies supine on a table, the anterior superior spines of the ilia being held firmly. The operator, facing the patient's feet, places his shoulder under the patient's calf to provide a fulcrum, and with both hands over the front of the leg above the ankle, exerts downward pressure on the long axis of the femur. Called *Leadbetter's procedure.*

lead′er (lee′dur). A sinew or tendon. *Obs.*

lead poi′son·ing. A form of poisoning due to the introduction of lead into the system. **Acute lead poisoning** is characterized by an immediate metallic taste and a burning sensation in the throat. Severe abdominal pain occurs, and, later, local paralysis and collapse. **Chronic lead poisoning** (saturnism or plumbism) occurs in persons long exposed to repeated absorption of small amounts of the element. There is anorexia, general lassitude, various dyspeptic symptoms, and obstinate constipation associated with violent pain. A blue line on the gums may appear, as may basophilic degeneration of the red blood cells. Various nervous symptoms may develop, such as the characteristic wrist drop.

leaf. A term occasionally employed in anatomic descriptions of certain parts of the body, as the right or left leaf of the diaphragm.

lec′i·thal (less′i-thul). Having a yolk; used especially in combination, as alecithal and telolecithal.

lec′i·thin (less′i-thin). Any one of a group of phospholipids of the general composition $CH_2OR_1.CHOR_2.CH_2OPO_2\text{-}OHR_3$ in which R_1 and R_2 are fatty acids and R_3 is choline. A colorless to yellow-brown, waxy solid widely distributed in the body. —**lecithoid,** *adj.*

lec′i·thi·nase. An enzyme which catalyzes the breakdown of a lecithin to its constituents. **l. A.** An enzyme catalyzing the removal of only one fatty acid from lecithin and yielding

lysolecithin. **l. B.** An enzyme catalyzing the removal of the fatty acid fro[m] lecithin or lysolecithin and yieldin[g] choline phosphate.

lec′i·tho·pro′te·in. A compound [of] lecithin with a protein molecule.

leech. Any parasitic annelid of th[e] class Hirudinea; some leeches ha[ve] been detrimental, and some have aide[d] medically. Infestation by leeches ma[y] be either internal or external. **medic[]inal l.** See *Hirudo medicinalis.*

Leeuwenhoek, Antonj va[n] [*Dutch naturalist*, 1632–1723]. Pionee[r] microscopist, credited with the di[s]covery of bacteria and protozoa. Ga[ve] the first description of spermatozo[a] which had been pointed out to him [as] a student, and the first reasonabl[y] accurate description of red blood cell[s.] Described the crystalline lens and th[e] rods of the retina.

left. Sinistral; opposite of right. Th[e] left-hand side. Abbreviated, l.

left′-hand′ed. Having the left han[d] stronger or more expert than the righ[t] or using the left hand in preference [to] the right.

leg. The lower extremity, especial[ly] that part from the knee to the ankl[e.] **bowleg.** Genu varum. See *bowle[g.]* **milk l.** Phlegmasia alba dolen[s.] **restless legs.** A disease of unknow[n] mechanism characterized by pare[s]thesia, pain in muscles and bone[s] and weakness, especially in the leg[s.] Relief generally is afforded by movin[g] the legs and walking around. Al[so] called *Wittmaack-Ekbom syndrom[e.]* **rider′s l.** Strain of the adducto[r] muscles of the thigh.

lei′o- (lye′o-), **li′o-.** A combinin[g] form signifying *smooth.*

lei″o·der′ma·tous. Smooth[-] skinned.

lei″o·my′o·fi·bro′ma (lye″o·my′[o-] o·figh·bro′muh). A benign tumor com[-] posed of cells of smooth muscle an[d] fibrous connective tissue.

lei″o·my·o′ma (lye″o·migh·o′muh[).] A benign tumor consisting largely [of] smooth muscle cells; may be found [in] any position where there is preëxistin[g] smooth muscle. In the uterus, the[se] tumors are usually multiple, and ma[y] reach a weight of several kilograms; [in] skin, they are usually small, thoug[h] multiple and arranged in groups, an[d] are at times painful.

lei″o·my″o·sar·co′ma. A malig[-] nant tumor composed in large part [of] smooth muscle cells, many of which a[re] poorly differentiated or of embryon[ic] form; multinucleated, neoplastic cel[ls] are frequent.

Leish·ma′ni·a (leesh·may′nee·u[h,] lyshe·). A genus of protozoa flagellat[es] whose species are morphologically sim[-] lar but differ in serologic reactions; transmitted to man by the bite of a species of *Phlebotomus*. **L. braziliensis.** That species confined largely to Central and South America. This parasite shows a predilection for the mucocutaneous borders of the nose and mouth and produces leishmaniasis americana. **L. donovani.** A species which is the etiologic agent of kalaazar, the visceral form of leishmaniasis. **L. tropica.** This species affects primarily the skin and produces oriental sore.

leish″man·i·a·sis (leesh″mun·eye′-uh·sis, lyshe″mun·). A variety of visceral and superficial infections caused by protozoan parasites of the genus *Leishmania*. Several species of biting flies belonging to the genus *Phlebotomus* are chiefly responsible for transmission. In India, man constitutes the chief reservoir, but in the Mediterranean region infected dogs are considered to be the reservoirs for the infantile form of the disease. **l. americana.** A form of leishmaniasis caused by the *Leishmania braziliensis*, differing primarily from oriental sore by the fact that in 10–20% of the cases the mucous membranes are involved, leading to extensive necrosis of the nose, mouth, and pharynx.

Lembert, Antoine. Widely known and remembered for his introduction of an interrupted approximation suture adapted to uniting divided serous layers of intestine. This is regarded as having brought about a new concept of intestinal surgery, and is considered the basis for present-day gastric and intestinal surgery. Called *Lembert's suture*.

-lem′ma. A combining form denoting a *sheath* or *envelope*.

lem·nis′ci (lem·niss′eye). Plural of lemniscus, *q.v.*

lem·nis′cus (pl. *lemnisci*). A secondary sensory pathway of the central nervous system, which usually decussates and terminates in the thalamus. **lateral l.** The secondary auditory pathway arising in the cochlear nuclei and terminating in the inferior colliculus and medial geniculate body; it crosses in the trapezoid body. **medial l.** That arising in the nucleus gracilis and nucleus cuneatus, crossing immediately as internal arcuate fibers, and terminating in the ventrolateral nucleus of the thalamus. **spinal l.** The lateral and anterior spinothalamic tracts combined as they ascend in the brain stem. **trigeminal l.** The secondary fibers from the main sensory nucleus of the trigeminal nerve and spinal nucleus of the trigeminal nerve, terminating in the ventrolateral nucleus of the thalamus.

lem′on. The fruit of *Citrus limon*.

Lempert, Julius [*American otologist*, 1891–]. Devised a one-stage fenestration operation for the improvement of hearing in otosclerosis; a permanently mobile window is formed in the lateral semicircular canal. Called *Lempert's operation*.

len′i·ceps. Obstetric forceps with short handles.

lenigallol. Trade-mark for a brand of pyrogallol triacetate.

len′i·tive. 1. Soothing, emollient, demulcent. 2. An emollient remedy or application.

lens. 1. A piece of glass or crystal for the refraction of rays of light. 2. The crystalline lens of the eye. **absorption l.** One used in spectacles, designed to prevent certain wave lengths from reaching the retina; may be a yellow or amber lens, which absorbs the upper range beyond violet (the actinic rays) which may have been said to be harmful, or may be one designed to absorb a determined amount of the entire spectrum, as in antiglare glasses or sunglasses, which, while altering the apparent color, diminish visual acuity only when illumination is reduced to threshold. **achromatic l.** A double lens, each part made of such optical glass that the one neutralizes the dispersive effects of the other, without affecting the refraction. **apochromatic l.** A compound lens corrected for spherical and chromatic aberration. **biconcave l.** A negative or minus, thick-edged lens, having concave spherical surfaces upon its opposite sides; used in spectacles in the correction of myopia. **biconvex l.** A positive or plus, thin-edged lens, having two convex surfaces; used in the correction of hyperopia. **bifocal l.** See *bifocal*. **contact l.** A lens for the correction of refractive errors, consisting of a plastic shell, the concavity of which is in contact with the globe of the eye, and a layer of liquid which is interposed between the lens and the cornea. **converging l.** A double convex or planoconvex lens that focuses rays of light. **crystalline l.** The lens of the eye, a refractive organ of accommodation; a biconvex, transparent, elastic body lying in its capsule immediately behind the pupil of the eye, suspended from the ciliary body by the ciliary zonule. **cylindrical l.** A minus or plus lens, with a plane surface in one axis and a concave or convex surface in the axis at right angles to the first. Abbreviated, *Cyl.* **decentered l.** One with the optic center not opposite to the pupil of the eye. **iseikonic l.** A temporary lens, known as a fit-over; may be of two kinds, overall or meridional. **overcor-**

rection of l. An aberration of a lens causing the light rays passing the central zones to focus at a point nearer to the lens than rays passing the outer zones. **punktal l.** One which is corrected for astigmatism in all powers throughout the entire field. **undercorrection of l.** The spherical aberration which normally exists in a simple lens. Rays from the outer zones of the source are brought to a focus closer to the lens than the rays from the central portion.

lens·om'e·ter (len-zom'i·tur). An instrument for determining the refractive power of a lens.

len"ti·co'nus. A rare, usually congenital, anomaly of the lens; marked by a conical prominence upon its anterior or, more rarely, upon its posterior surface.

len·tic'u·lar. 1. Pertaining to or resembling a lens. 2. Pertaining to the crystalline lens. 3. Pertaining to the lenticular nucleus of the brain.

len·tic"u·lo·stri'ate. Pertaining to the lenticular nucleus of the corpus striatum, as lenticulostriate artery.

len·tic"u·lo·tha·lam'ic (len-tick"yoo·lo·tha·lam'ick, ·thal'uh·mick). Extending from the lenticular nucleus to the thalamus, as the lenticulothalamic tract.

len'ti·form. Lens-shaped or lentil-shaped.

len"ti·glo'bus. A spherical bulging of the lens of the eye.

len·ti'go, len'ti·go (pl. *lentigines*). A freckle; a circumscribed patch of pigment, small in size, occurring mainly on exposed skin. **—lentig'inous** (len-tidj'i·nus), *adj.*

le"on·ti'a·sis. A lionlike appearance of the face, seen in lepromatous leprosy. **l. ossea.** An overgrowth of the bones of the face, through which the features acquire a lionlike appearance. Also called *megalocephaly*.

lep'i·do-, lepid-. A combining form meaning *a scale* or *scaly*.

Lep'i·dop'ter·a. An order of insects distinguished by featherlike scales and spirally coiled suctorial apparatus. The order includes butterflies, moths, and skippers.

lep'o·thrix. A skin condition in which masses of reddish, black, and yellow fungous material are found in nodular or diffuse distribution about the axillary or genital hair; usually seen in those who sweat freely. Also called *trichomycosis axillaris*, *trichomycosis rubra*, *trichomycosis flava nigra*.

lep·ro'ma. The cutaneous nodular lesion of leprosy. **—leprom'atous,** *adj.*

lep"ro·sar'i·um (lep"ro·sair'ee-

um). An institution for the treatment of persons affected with leprosy.

lep'ro·sin. A neutral, acid-fast, waxlike substance isolated from *Mycobacterium leprae*, consisting of a complex mixture of solid glycerides and waxes.

lep'ro·sy. Hansen's disease. **indeterminate l.** A nonspecific form with clinical manifestations of the skin and peripheral nerves. **lepromatous l.** A form marked by the occurrence of lepromas in the skin accompanied by much infiltration and with many of the causative organisms present. **tuberculoid l.** A form characterized by marked peripheral nerve involvement and tissue destruction and with few causative organisms present.

lep'rous, lep·rot'ic. Applied to lesions caused by *Mycobacterium leprae*, and to persons affected with leprosy.

lep·tan'dra. The dried rhizome and roots of *Veronicastrum virginicum*, a cathartic.

leptazol. The British Pharmacopoeia name for pentylenetetrazol. See *metrazol*.

lep'to-, lept-. A combining form signifying *thin, small, weak, fine*.

lep"to·ceph'a·lus. An individual with an abnormally small head from premature union of the frontal and sphenoid bones.

lep"to·dac'ty·lous. Characterized by slenderness of the fingers or toes, or both.

lep"to·men"in·gi'tis. Inflammation of the pia and arachnoid of the brain or the spinal cord.

Lep"to·spi'ra. A genus of spirochetes able to survive in water; characterized by sharply twisted filaments with one or both extremities hooked or recurved. These organisms are not predominantly blood parasites, but are also found in the tissues.

Lep'to·thrix. A genus of unbranched filamentous organisms of the Chlamydobacteriaceae. **L. buccalis.** A species which is a common inhabitant of the oral cavity. Pathogenic properties have been claimed for it, but its invasive power is probably slight.

lep"to·tri·cho'sis (lep"to·tri·ko'sis, ·try·ko'sis). Any disease caused by a species of *Leptothrix*. **l. of the conjunctiva.** A conjunctivitis caused by members of the genus *Leptothrix*; usually associated with swelling of the lacrimal gland and preauricular lymph nodes. Also called *Parinaud's conjunctivitis*.

leritine. Trade-mark for anileridine.

Les'bi·an·ism (lez'bee·un·iz·um, less'-). An abnormal affection between women; homosexuality between women. Syn., *Lesbian love, sapphism, tribadism*.

le'sion. 1. An alteration of structure or of functional capacity due to injury or disease. 2. *In osteopathy*, any structural perversion which produces or maintains discomfort or functional disorder, or impairs natural immunity of the body or a part. **—lesional**, *adj*. **primary l.** (a) In syphilis, the chancre. (b) In tuberculosis, the focus of the first infection, as the tuberculous, caseous mass near the hilus or periphery in the lung. **secondary l.** One which follows, and is due to, a primary lesion, as the secondary, cutaneous lesions of syphilis; the involvement of mediastinal lymph nodes following pulmonary tuberculosis.

le'thal. Deadly; pertaining to or producing death. Abbreviated, l.

leth'ar·gy. A morbid condition of drowsiness or stupor. **—lethar'gic**, *adj*.

Letterer, Erich [*German pathologist*, 1895–]. Described a form of reticuloendotheliosis (1924). The pediatrist Siwe later described the same disease from the clinical point of view. *Letterer-Siwe's disease* is nonfamilial and of variable duration. The manifestations include splenohepatomegaly, cutaneous petechiae, enlargement of the lymph nodes, bone tumor, osseous defects, and secondary anemia.

leu'cine (lew'seen, ·sin). a-Aminoisocaproic acid, an amino acid obtainable by the hydrolysis of milk and other protein-containing substances. It is essential to the growth of man. **—leucoic**, *adj*.

leu''ci·no'sis. Excessive proportion or production of leucine, as in the liver.

leu'co-, leuc-. See *leuko-*.

leu·co'ma·ine (lew·ko'may·een, ·muh·een, lew'ko·myne). The name applied to any one of the nitrogenous bases normally developed by the metabolic activity of living organisms, as distinguished from the bases developed by putrefactive processes, and called ptomaines. **—leucomain'ic**, *adj*.

Leu''co·nos'toc. A genus of saprophytic bacteria, species of which are found in milk, fermenting vegetables, and slimy sugar solutions.

leu'co·sin. A simple protein of the albumin type found in wheat and other cereals.

leu''co·tax'in. A substance which appears to be liberated by injured tissues and toward which phagocytes are positively chemotactic.

leucovorin. Trade-mark for folinic acid, 2.

leu·ke'mi·a. A disease of the blood-forming organs characterized by uncontrolled proliferation of the leukocytes. Immature leukocytes usually are present in the blood, often in large numbers. **—leukemic**, *adj*. **acute l.**

A form of leukemia with rapid onset and progress. Usually there is a high temperature, marked anemia, and enlargement of the spleen and lymph nodes. **lymphocytic l.** A form of leukemia with enlargement of the lymph nodes and spleen. The lymphocytes of the blood are usually increased. **monocytic l.** A relatively rare form of leukemia characterized pathologically by excessive proliferation of the reticuloendothelial tissues in the lymph nodes, spleen, and liver with a high blood count of apparent monocytes, and clinically by severe anemia, hemorrhagic disorders, variable lymphadenopathy and splenomegaly with fatal termination in a few weeks to a few months. **myelogenous l.** A form of leukemia in which the leukocytes of the bone marrow are primarily affected. Usually abnormal, immature cells of the myeloid series are present in the blood in large numbers. Formerly called *myeloid l.*

leukeran. Trade-mark for chlorambucil.

leu'ko-, leuk-. 1. A combining form meaning *white, colorless*. 2. *In chemistry*, a combining form denoting a *colorless* or *weakly colored* compound. 3. *In medicine*, a combining form denoting a *whitish decolorization*.

leu'ko·cyte. One of the colorless, more or less ameboid cells of the blood, having a nucleus and cytoplasm. Those found in normal blood are usually divided according to their staining reaction into **granular leukocytes**, consisting of neutrophils, eosinophils, and basophils, and **nongranular leukocytes**, consisting of lymphocytes and monocytes. Those found in abnormal blood consist of myeloblasts, promyelocytes, neutrophilic myelocytes, eosinophilic myelocytes, basophilic myelocytes, lymphoblasts, plasma cells, and Türk's irritation cells. Syn., *white blood cell, white corpuscle*. **acidophil l.** See eosinophil *l.* **basophil l.** One containing granules which stain deep purple (basic dye) with Wright's stain, and having a nucleus without distinct lobulation. **eosinophil l.** One containing coarse round granules which stain pink to bright red (acid dye) with Wright's stain and usually having a bilobed nucleus. **granular l.** One of those containing granules in their cytoplasm. Syn., *granulocyte.* **heterophil l.** See neutrophil *l.* **lymphoid l.** A nongranular leukocyte including lymphocytes and monocytes. **neutrophil l.** A highly motile and phagocytic leukocyte having numerous fine granules which do not stain definitely either blue (basic dye) or red (acid dye). Its polymorphous nucleus may be ribbonlike, bandlike, or segmented, with two to seven lobules. **nongranular l.** One with clear homogeneous cytoplasm, such as a lymphocyte or monocyte. **polymorphonuclear l.** The neutrophil leukocyte so-called because of its irregularly shaped and lobulated nucleus. Syn., *granulocyte.*

leu″ko·cy·to′sis (lew″ko-sigh-to′-sis). An increase in the leukocyte count above the upper limits of normal. It is physiologic during pregnancy and pathologic in many infections and toxemias. —**leukocytot′ic,** *adj.*

leu″ko·der′ma. A condition of defective pigmentation of the skin, especially a congenital absence of pigment in patches or bands. —**leukodermic,** *adj.* **l. colli.** A condition coincident with the appearance of the macular eruption of cutaneous syphilis; characterized by mottled skin on the neck, chin, or rarely on other parts.

leu·ko′ma. 1. An opacity of the cornea as a result of an ulcer, wound, or inflammation, which presents an appearance of ground glass. 2. Leukoplakia buccalis, *q.v.* —**leukom′atous, leukom′atoid,** *adj.*

leu·ko′ma·ine (lew-ko′may-een, -muh-een, lew′ko-myne). See *leucomaine.*

leu″ko·nych′i·a (lew″ko-nick′ee-uh). A whitish discoloration of the nails; due to the presence of air beneath them.

leu″ko·pe′ni·a. A decrease below the normal number of leukocytes in the peripheral blood. —**leukopenic,** *adj.*

leu″ko·phleg·ma′si·a (·fleg·may′-zhuh, ·shuh). 1. A condition marked by dropsy, a pale flabby skin, and general edema. 2. Phlegmasia alba dolens.

leu″ko·pla′ki·a. A disease characterized by a whitish thickening of the epithelium of the mucous membrane. —**leukoplakial,** *adj.* **l. buccalis.** One characterized by pearly-white or bluish white patches on the surface of the tongue or the mucous membrane of the cheeks, due to a hyperplasia of the epithelium. **l. vulvae.** Occurrence of irregular white patches on the mucosa of the vulva. There is thickening of the epithelium and the papillae may be hypertrophied. Also see *kraurosis* of the vulva.

leu″ko·pla′si·a (lew″ko-play′zhuh, ·zee-uh). See *leukoplakia.*

leu″ko·pro′te·ase (·pro′tee·ace, ·aze). An enzyme in leukocytes which splits protein. In inflammation it causes liquefaction of necrotic tissue.

leu·kop′sin. Visual white, produced from rhodopsin by the action of light.

leu″kor·rhe′a. A whitish, mucopurulent discharge from the female genital canal. —**leukorrheal,** *adj.*

leu″ko·sar·co″ma·to′sis. A condition characterized by multiple sarcomatous tumors associated with a leukemic blood picture.

leu″ko·tox′in. A cytotoxin obtained from lymph nodes.

leu″ko·trich′i·a (lew″ko·trick′ee-uh). Whiteness of the hair; canities. —**leukot′richous,** *adj.*

leu″ko·n″ro·bil′in (·yoor″o·bil′in, ·buy′lin). A colorless decomposition product of bilirubin.

lev·al·lor′phan tar′trate. (−)-3-Hydroxy-N-allylmorphinan tartrate, an antagonist to excessive dosage with narcotic analgesics. See *lorfan tartrate.*

Le·vant′ worm′seed. See *santonica.*

lev″ar·ter′en·ol bi·tar′trate. The U.S. Pharmacopeia name for the levorotatory form of norepinephrine hydrochloride.

le·va′tor. 1. That which raises or elevates, as levator palpebrae superioris, the muscle which widens the palpebral fissure or opens the eye. See Table of Muscles in the Appendix. 2. An instrument used for raising a depressed portion of the skull.

le′ver (lee′vur, lev′ur). A vectis or one-armed tractor, used in obstetrics.

lev″i·ga′tion. The reduction of a substance to a powder by grinding in water, followed by fractional sedimentation, in order to separate the coarser from the finer particles. —**lev′igate,** *v.*

lev″i·ta′tion. 1. The illusion of the suspension of a body in air; performed by modern magicians. 2. The subjective sense of rising into the air or being aloft without support, as in dreams or certain mental disorders.

le′vo-, lae′vo- (lee′vo-, lev′o-). 1. A combining form meaning *left, on the left side.* 2. *In chemistry,* a combining form signifying *levorotatory.*

levo-dromoran tartrate. Trademark for levorphanol tartrate.

le″vo·gy′rous. Rotating to the left, as the rotation of rays of polarized light.

le″vo·pho′ri·a. A tending of the visual lines to the left.

le″vo·ro·ta′tion. Rotation toward the left, especially of the plane of polarization of light.

le″vo·ro′ta·to″ry. Turning the rays of light to the left. Abbreviated, *l-.* Also see (−) in Table of Signs and Symbols in the Appendix.

lev·or′phan·ol tar′trate. The levorotatory form of 3-hydroxy-N-methylmorphinan tartrate, a potent synthetic analgesic related to morphine; formerly called *levorphan tartrate.* Also see *racemorphan hydrobromide.* See *levo-dromoran tartrate.*

lev·or'phan tar'trate. Levorphanol tartrate.

le″vo·tar·tar'ic ac'id (lee″vo·tahr·tar'ick, ·tahr·tahr'ick). The optical isomer of tartaric acid which rotates polarized light to the left.

lev'u·lose. $C_6H_{12}O_6$, a levorotatory monosaccharide that occurs in many fruits and is obtained also by hydrolysis of sucrose, useful for parenteral alimentation. Syn., *fructose*.

lev″u·lo·su'ri·a. Presence of levulose in the urine.

lew'is·ite. Chlorovinyldichloroarsine; an oily substance having vesicant, lacrimatory, and lung irritant effects; it was developed for use as a chemical warfare agent.

Leydig, Franz von [*German histologist, 1821–1908*]. Described the interstitial cells of the testis, thought to be the source of the male sex hormone; called *Leydig cells, Gley's cells.*

L. F. A. Left frontoanterior position of the fetus in utero.

L. F. P. Left frontoposterior position of the fetus in utero.

LH. Prolan-B, *q.v.*

Li. Chemical symbol for lithium.

lib″er·a'tion. The act of freeing. **l. of the arms.** In breech presentations, a lowering of the arms of the fetus when they have become extended along the sides of the child's head.

li·bi'do (li·buy'do, li·bee'do). 1. Sexual desire. 2. In *psychoanalysis*, the sum total of all instinctual forces; psychic energy. **—libid'inous,** *adj.*

li'bra. A pound. A weight of twelve troy ounces. Abbreviated, l. Symbol, ℔.

lice. Plural of louse, *q.v.*

li'cense. An official permit or authority conferring on the recipient the right and privilege of exercising his profession.

li·cen'ti·ate (lye·sen'shee·ate). One who practices a profession by the authority of a license.

li'chen (lye'kin, ·kun). A generic term used to describe certain lesions of the skin which consist of solid papules with exaggerated skin markings. **—lichenoid,** *adj.* **l. chronicus simplex.** The chronic stage of neurodermatitis characterized by lichenification of lesions in various regions. Also called *neurodermatitis circumscripta.* **l. nitidus.** A chronic, inflammatory skin disease characterized by groups of tiny papules which are asymptomatic; found frequently in the genital region and the flexor region of a joint. **l. planus.** A common, inflammatory skin disease with an eruption of papules, broad and angular at the base, flat and glazed at the summit; slightly umbilicated, and of a dull purplish red color. The papules may be discrete or may coalesce, and itching may be slight or severe. The disease may be either acute and widespread or chronic and localized. **l. ruber moniliformis.** A disease of unknown cause, with linear lesions of flat papules which resemble those of lichen planus; but it is probably a separate disease. **l. spinulosus.** A skin disease of children, probably due to a vitamin-A deficiency; characterized by spines protruding from follicles or follicular papules.

li″chen·if·i·ca'tion (lye″kun·if·i·kay'shun, lye·ken″if·i·). The process whereby the skin becomes leathery and hardened; often the result of chronic pruritus and the irritation produced by scratching or rubbing skin eruptions.

lic'o·rice. See *glycyrrhiza.*

li'do·caine hy″dro·chlo'ride. α-Diethylamino-2,6-acetoxylidide hydrochloride, a local anesthetic. See *xylocaine hydrochloride.*

Liebig, Justus von [*German chemist, 1803–73*]. Pioneer investigator of metabolism. Credited with discovering chloral and hippuric acid. Devised a method of estimating urea.

lie de·tec'tor. A polygraph used to reveal a repressed sense of guilt or a fear of detection in a subject who is confronted by questions pertaining to a misdemeanor or crime; it records sudden changes in pulse rate, respiration, and blood pressure.

li'en. The spleen. **—lienal** (lye'i·nul, lye·ee'nul), *adj.*

li·e'no- (lye·ee'no-, lye'i·no-), **lien-** A combining form denoting *the spleen; splenic.*

li·e″no·re'nal. Relating to the spleen and kidney, as the lienorenal ligament, a fold of peritoneum between spleen and kidney.

life. The sum of properties by which an organism grows, reproduces, and adapts itself to its environment; the quality by which an organism differs from inorganic or dead organic bodies. **change of l.** See *menopause.* **embryonic l.** The life of the embryo, *q.v.* **expectation of l.** See *expectation of life.*

life ex·pec'tan·cy. See *expectation of life.*

lig'a·ment. 1. A band of flexible, tough, dense white fibrous connective tissue connecting the articular ends of the bones, and sometimes enveloping them in a capsule. 2. Certain folds and processes of the peritoneum. For ligaments listed by name, see Table of Joints and Ligaments in the Appendix. **—ligamen'tous,** *adj.* **alar l.** Lateral synovial folds of the capsule of the knee joint. **alar odontoid l.** Any one of the broad, strong ligaments arising on each side of the apex of the odontoid process and connecting the axis with the skull. Also called *check* *l., odontoid l.* **apical dental l.** A fibrous cord extending from the summit of the dens of the epistropheus to the occipital bone near the anterior margin of the foramen magnum. Also called *apical odontoid l., suspensory l.* **arcuate l. of diaphragm.** One of the arched ligaments extending from the body of the diaphragm to the last rib and to the transverse process of the first lumbar vertebra. **arcuate l. of knee.** That which extends from the back of the head of the fibula, arching medially over the popliteal tendon to join the capsule of the knee joint. **broad l. of uterus.** A fold of peritoneum which extends laterally from the uterus to the pelvic wall and in which run the uterine blood vessels. **capsular l.** A heavy fibrous structure surrounding a diarthrosis, and lined by synovial membrane. **coronary l.** A reflection of the peritoneum between the liver and the diaphragm. Its right and left margins are called the **right triangular ligament** and the **left triangular ligament** of the liver. **cruciate ligaments of knee.** Two ligaments crossing in the middle of the knee joint, designated as anterior and posterior by their attachment to the tibia. **deltoid l.** The medial collateral ligament of the ankle joint. **dentate l.** A narrow fibrous band separating the dorsal and ventral roots of the spinal cord throughout its entire length. Along its lateral border, triangular toothlike processes are fixed at intervals to the dura mater. **falciform l. of liver.** The ventral mesentery of the liver extending from the diaphragm to the umbilicus and containing the round ligament of the liver. **fundiform l. of penis.** That arising from the front of the sheath of the rectus abdominis muscle and the linea alba, splitting into two bands to encircle the root of the penis. **gastrocolic l.** The mesentery or portion of the omentum between stomach and transverse colon produced by fusion of the embryonic mesocolon with part of the great omentum. **gastrohepatic l.** The portion of the lesser omentum extending between the liver and the stomach. **gastrosplenic l.** The fold of peritoneum passing from the stomach to the spleen. **iliofemoral l.** A strong ligament extending from the anterior inferior iliac spine to the lesser trochanter and the intertrochanteric line. Also called Y l. **inguinal l.** The lower portion of the aponeurosis of the external oblique muscle extending from the anterior superior spine of the ilium to the tubercle of the pubis and the pectineal line. Also called *Poupart's l.* **laciniate l.** A strong fibrous band extending from the

medial malleolus to the calcaneus. **lateral umbilical l.** One of two cordlike folds extending from the urinary bladder to the umbilicus representing the degenerated distal parts of the umbilical arteries. **median umbilical l.** A fold of the peritoneum extending from the umbilicus to the bladder containing vestiges of the urachus and its connective tissue. Also called *vesicoumbilical l.* **nuchal l.** An elastic ligament extending from the external occipital protuberance and middle nuchal line to the spinous process of the seventh cervical vertebra. **patellar l.** The ligament attaching the patella to the tuberosity of the tibia. **pectinate l.** Trabecular tissue from the posterior elastic lamina which extends into the substance of the iris. **round l. of femur.** A flattened band extending from the fovea on the head of the femur to attach on either side of the acetabular notch where it blends with the transverse ligament. Also called *ligamentum teres femoris.* **round l. of liver.** A fibrous cord running from the umbilicus to the notch in the anterior border of the liver. It represents the remains of the obliterated umbilical vein. Also called *ligamentum teres hepatis.* **round l. of uterus.** A ligament running from the anterior surface of the lateral border of the uterus through the inguinal canal to the labium majus. Also called *ligamentum teres uteri.* **sacrospinous l.** A thin triangular band running from the spine of the ischium medially to the lateral margin of the sacrum and coccyx. **sacrotuberous l.** A ligament extending from the sacrum, coccyx, and posterior iliac spines to the tuberosity of the ischium. **stylohyoid l.** A fibrous cord attached to the tip of the styloid process of the temporal bone and the lesser horn of the hyoid bone, derived from Reichert's cartilage. **suspensory l. of ovary.** A small peritoneal fold passing upward from the tubal end of the ovary to the peritoneum over the iliac vessels and psoas muscle. Also called *infundibulopelvic l.* **suspensory l. of penis.** Fibers from the linea alba and symphysis pubis forming a strong fibrous band which extends to the upper surface of the root to blend with the fascial sheath of the penis. **uterosacral l.** A concentric fold of peritoneum containing much fibrous tissue which passes backward from the cervix of the uterus on either side of the rectum to the posterior wall of the pelvis.

lig″a·men′to·pex″y. Suspension of the uterus by shortening or fixation of the round ligaments.

lig″a·men′tum (pl. *ligamenta*). Ligament, *q.v.* **l. arteriosum.** The remains of the fetal ductus arteriosus, extending from the pulmonary trunk to the arch of the aorta. **l. venosum.** Ligament of the liver representing the remains of embryonic ductus venosus.

li·ga'tion (lye-gay'shun). The operation of tying, especially arteries, veins, or ducts, with some form of knotted ligature. —**li'gate,** v.

lig'a·ture. 1. A cord or thread for tying vessels. 2. The act of tying or binding; ligation. **absorbable l.** One composed of animal tissue, such as catgut, which can be absorbed by the tissues. **nonabsorbable l.** One which cannot be absorbed by the tissues, such as silkworm gut.

light. Electromagnetic radiations that give rise to the sensation of vision when the rays impinge upon the retina. **axial l.** Light rays that are parallel to each other and to the optic axis. **polarized l.** Light which has undergone polarization, q.v. **refracted l.** Light rays that have passed from one medium into another and have been bent from their original course. **transmitted l.** The light passing through an object.

light'en·ing. The sinking of the fetal head into the pelvic inlet with an accompanying descent of the uterus.

light'ning pains. The lancinating pains of spinal root disease, coming on and disappearing with lightninglike rapidity, as in tabes dorsalis.

light sense test'er. Any instrument used to test the sensitivity of the eye to light. **perimetric l. s. t.** An attachment for a perimeter which may be used for determining the light threshold of the eye at any desired position or positions in the visual field.

lig"ni·fi·ca'tion. The process by which the cell wall of a plant acquires greater rigidity by deposition of lignin.

lig'nin. A modification of cellulose, constituting the greater part of the weight of most dry wood.

lig'ro·in. A liquid fraction obtained from petroleum; used as a solvent.

Lilienthal, Howard [*American surgeon, 1861–1946*]. Well known for his many contributions to the knowledge of thoracic surgery. He described low posterior mediastinotomy by resection of the ninth rib, with transillumination of the esophagus for ease of access. Described esophagogastrostomy through the posterior approach, implanting the lower end of the esophagus into the stomach wall by intussusception, using traction sutures through a secondary stomach incision; called *Lilienthal's operation.* Inventor of a guillotine type of costotome for use in removing the first rib; called *Lilienthal's costotome.*

limb. 1. One of the extremities at-

tached to the sides of the trunk and used for prehension or locomotion. 2. Elongated limblike structures, as the limbs of the internal capsule.

lim'bus (pl. *limbi*). A border; the circumferential edge of any flat organ or part. —**limbic,** *adj.* **corneoscleral l.** The edge of the cornea at its junction with the sclera. **l. alveolaris.** See alveolar crest. **l. fossae ovalis.** The thick margin of the fossa ovalis of the heart, representing the margin of the embryonic septum secundum. Syn., *annulus ovalis.*

lime. CaO, calcium oxide, q.v., under *calcium.* **chlorinated l.** The product of the chlorination of lime; consists chiefly of calcium hypochlorite and calcium chloride. Employed as a disinfectant. **l. milk.** A milky fluid consisting of calcium hydroxide suspended in water. **l. water.** An aqueous solution containing 0.14% Ca(OH)$_2$ at 25° C. Used as an antacid. **slaked l.** Lime which has been acted on by water; it consists chiefly of calcium hydroxide.

li'men (pl. *limina*). 1. A boundary line. 2. See threshold. **l. nasi.** The boundary line between the osseous and the cartilaginous portions of the nasal cavity.

li'mes death (lye'meez). The least amount of toxin which, when mixed with one unit of antitoxin and injected into a guinea pig weighing 250 Gm., kills within five days. Symbol, L$_+$.

li'mes ze'ro. The greatest amount of toxin which causes no local edema when mixed with one unit of antitoxin and injected into a guinea pig weighing 250 Gm. Symbol, L$_0$.

lim'i·nal. Pertaining to the limen or threshold, especially pertaining to the lowest limit of perception.

Lim·na'tis. A genus of aquatic leeches.

lim'o·nene. C$_{10}$H$_{16}$. A terpene constituent of various volatile oils.

li'mo·nite (lye'mo-night, lim'o-). Ferric oxide, of the approximate formula 2Fe$_2$O$_3$.3H$_2$O; a yellow powder.

limp. A halting gait. See *claudication.*

lin·al'o·öl (lin-al'o-ole, lin"uh-lool'). C$_{10}$H$_{17}$OH. An alcohol occurring in coriander, lavender, and bergamot oils.

lin"a·ma'rin, lin·am'a·rin. The toxic glycoside of flaxseed.

lin'dane. Non-proprietary name for gammexane of not less than 99 per cent purity.

line. 1. Extension of dimension having length, but neither breadth nor thickness. 2. *In anatomy,* anything resembling a mathematical line in having length without breadth or thickness; a boundary or guide-mark. 3. The ½ part of an inch. *Obs.* 4. *In genetics,* lineage;

the succession of progenitors and progeny. **abdominal lines.** Transverse lines of the abdominal wall. Also called *striae albicantes gravidarum.* **anocutaneous l.** The junction between skin and mucous membrane at the anus. **arcuate l.** (a) The iliac portion of the iliopectineal line. (b) An arched thickening of the obturator fascia from which the levator ani muscle arises. Also called *arcus tendineus.* **epiphyseal l.** The scar left at the site of the epiphyseal plate after fusion of an epiphysis with the diaphysis of a long bone. **l. of demarcation.** A line of division between healthy and gangrenous tissue. **mammillary l.** A vertical line passing through the center of the nipple. **midaxillary l.** A perpendicular line drawn from the apex of the axilla. **midclavicular l.** A vertical line parallel to, and midway between, the midsternal line and a vertical line drawn downward through the outer end of the clavicle. **midsternal l.** A vertical line through the middle of the sternum. **scapular l.** A vertical line drawn on the back through the inferior angle of the scapula. **semicircular l.** The curved lower edge of the internal layer of the aponeurosis of the internal oblique muscle, where it ceases to cover the posterior surface of the rectus muscle. Also called *linea semicircularis of Douglas.* **semilunar l.** A line, convex laterally, marking the transition of the internal oblique and transverse muscles of the abdomen to aponeuroses. Also called *linea semilunaris of Spigelius.* **subcostal l.** An imaginary transverse line drawn around the abdomen at the level of the lower border of the tenth costal cartilage. **transpyloric l.** A horizontal line drawn through a point midway between the jugular notch and the symphysis pubis.

lin′e·a (pl. *lineae*). Line, *q.v.* **l. alba.** A tendinous raphe extending in the median line of the abdomen from the pubes to the xiphoid process; it is formed by the blending of the aponeuroses of the oblique and transverse muscles. **l. aspera.** A rough longitudinal ridge on the posterior surface of the middle third of the femur serving as attachment for muscles.

lin′gua. The tongue. **—lingual,** *adj.* **l. plicata.** Fissured tongue.

lin′gu·la. 1. A small lobule between the anterior medullary velum and the central lobule of the cerebellum. 2. A tonguelike structure. **—lingular,** *adj.* **l. of the mandible.** The prominent, thin process of bone partly surrounding the mandibular foramen.

lin″guo·gin′gi·val (ling″gwo·jin′-

ji·vul, ·jin·jy′vul). Relating to the tongue and the gingiva.

lin′i·ment. A liquid intended for application to the skin by gentle friction.

li′nin. 1. A strongly purgative principle obtainable from *Linum catharticum,* or purging flax. 2. In *biology,* the substance of the achromatic network of the nucleus of a cell.

link′age. 1. In *chemistry,* the lines used in structural formulas to represent the valency of atoms: a single line represents a valency of one, a double line a valency of two, etc. 2. In *genetics,* the association of genes located in the same chromosome.

Linnaeus, Carolus (von Linné) [*Swedish physician and naturalist,* 1707–78]. Known for his work in classifying minerals, plants, and animals. Classified diseases (1763). Said to have given the first description of aphasia (1745).

lin″o·le′ic ac′id (lin″o·lee′ick, li-no′lee·ick). An acid, containing two double bonds, in the glycerides of linseed and other oils. Syn., *linolic acid.*

li·no′le·in. The glyceride of linoleic acid found in all drying oils.

lin″o·le′nic ac′id (lin″o·lee′nick, ·len′ick). An acid, containing three double bonds, occurring in the glycerides of linseed and other oils. It is essential for normal nutrition.

li·no′lic ac′id. See *linoleic acid.*

lin′seed. The dried ripe seed of *Linum usitatissimum;* it contains a fixed oil. Linseed is demulcent, emollient, and laxative. Syn., *flaxseed.* **l. oil.** The fixed oil obtained from linseed (oil that has been treated with a drier must not be used medicinally); used mostly in liniments and cerates, occasionally for its laxative effect.

lint. A loosely woven or partly felted mass of broken linen fibers, once used as a dressing for wounds.

lin′tin. Absorbent cotton rolled or compressed into sheets; used for dressing wounds.

li′o-. See *leio-.*

lip. 1. One of the two fleshy folds surrounding the orifice of the mouth. 2. One of the labia majora or labia minora. See *labium.* 3. A projecting margin; rim. **cleft l.** Harelip, *q.v.* **l. of the cervix of the uterus.** One of two surrounding the external os.

li′pa. Fat.

lip″a·ro·trich′i·a (lip″uh·ro·trick′-ee·uh). Abnormal oiliness of the hair.

li′pase (lye′pace, lip′ace). A fat-splitting enzyme contained in the pancreatic juice, in blood plasma, and in many plants. See Table of Normal Values of Blood Constituents in the Appendix. **pancreatic l.** A fat-splitting enzyme secreted by the pancreas. Syn., *steapsin*.

lip·ec'to·my. Excision of adipose tissue.

li·pe'mi·a, li·pae'mi·a (li·pee'mee·uh). The presence of a fine emulsion of fatty substances in the blood. —**lipem'ic,** *adj.*

lip'id (lip'id, lye'pid), **lip'ide** (lip'-yde, ·id, lye'pyde, ·pid). Any one of a group of fats and fatlike substances having in common the property of insolubility in water and solubility in the fat solvents. See Table of Normal Values of Blood Constituents in the Appendix. Also called *lipin.*

lip'ide. See *lipid.*

li'pin (lye'pin, lip'in). See *lipid.*

lipiodol. Trade-mark for an iodized poppy seed oil used as a substitute for inorganic iodides, or as a contrast medium for roentgenologic work.

lip'o-, lip- (lip'o-, lye'po-). 1. *In medicine and physiology,* a combining form denoting *fat, fatty.* 2. *In chemistry,* a combining form denoting a lipid.

lip″o·chon″dro·dys'tro·phy (lip″o·kon″dro·dis'tro·fee). A congenital disease characterized by dwarfism; short, kyphotic spinal column; short fingers; depression of bridge of the nose; stiffness of joints; cloudiness of cornea; and mental deficiency. There is associated lipodystrophy. Also called *gargoylism.*

lip″o·chon·dro'ma (lip″o·kon·dro'-muh). Chondroma containing fat cells.

lip'o·chrome. Any one of a group of fatlike substances containing a pigment or coloring matter, and occurring in natural fats, such as egg yolk. Also called *chromolipoid.*

lip″o·dys'tro·phy. A disturbance of fat metabolism in which the subcutaneous fat disappears over large areas of the body, but is unaffected in others. May be progressive.

lip″o·fi″bro·myx·o'ma. A mesodermal mixed tumor, containing fatty tissue, fibrous tissue, and mucoid or myxomatous tissue.

li·pog'e·nous (li·podj'i·nus). Fat-producing.

lip″o·gran″u·lo'ma. A nodule of fatty tissue, consisting of a center of degenerated and necrotic fat enclosed by granulation tissue. Due usually to trauma; may possibly be caused by faulty fat metabolism.

lip'oid (lip'oyd, lye'poyd). 1. Resembling fat or oil. 2. Having the character of a lipid; lipoidic. 3. Old term for lipid, particularly one of the intracellular lipids which contain nitrogen.

lip″oi·do'sis. A general term for various conditions in which lipoproteins or lipids are deposited in different organs, particularly in the spleen or liver. Syn., *lipoid histiocytosis.* See

xanthomatosis, Schüller-Christian disease.

lipoiodine. Trade-mark for an iodine-containing compound, used where iodide therapy is indicated and as a contrast medium in roentgen-ray examinations.

li·po'ma. A tumor, which in the gross is obviously fatty; microscopically composed of fat cells usually of mature form but occasionally in part or wholly of embryonal type. —**lipom'atous, lipom'atoid,** *adj.*

li·po″ma·to'sis. Multiple lipomas. A general deposition of fat; obesity.

lip″o·pro'te·in. One of a group of conjugated proteins consisting of a simple protein combined with a lipid.

lip″o·sar·co'ma. A sarcoma derived from fat cells of bone marrow or soft tissues. Microscopically composed largely of highly undifferentiated spindle or polygonal cells often containing droplets of fat; embryonal type of fat cells and rarely mature fat cells may be present.

lip″o·tro'pic (lip″o·tro'pick, ·trop'-ick). 1. Having an affinity for lipids, particularly fats and oils. 2. Having a preventive or curative effect on the development of fatty livers.

lip″o·vac'cine (lip″o·vack'seen, ·sin). A vaccine with a fatty or oily menstruum.

lip'ping. The perichondral growth of osteophytes which project beyond the joint margin in degenerative joint disease.

lip″pi·tu'do, lip″pi·tude. A condition of the eyes marked by ulcerative marginal blepharitis; a state of being blear-eyed.

lip read'ing. The ability to understand what a person is saying by observing the movements of his lips and other facial muscles, without hearing him speak; important in instruction of the deaf.

liq″ue·fac'tion (lick″wi·fack'shun). The change to a liquid form, usually of a solid tissue to a fluid or semifluid state.

liq'uid. A fluid or substance that flows readily.

liq″uo·gel. A gel which, when melted, yields a sol of low viscosity.

liq'uor. 1. Certain medicinal solutions; usually includes aqueous solutions of nonvolatile substances. 2. An English designation for any liquid, as dye liquor, mother liquor, etc. 3. A term applied to an alcoholic drink. **l. folliculi.** The fluid filling the follicular space about the developing ovum in the Graafian follicle.

liq″uo·rice (lick'ur·iss, lick'ur·ish). Glycyrrhiza.

Lisfranc de Saint Martin, Jacques [*French surgeon,* 1790–

1847]. Described the scalene tubercle on the upper surface of the first rib for the insertion of the scalenus anterior muscle; called *Lisfranc's tubercle*. Partial amputation of the foot by disarticulation of the metatarsal bones from the tarsus is known as *Lisfranc's amputation*.

lisp. Speak indistinctly; pronounce imperfectly the sibilant letters *s* and *z*, as by giving them the sound of *th*, and by giving the letter *l* the sound of *w*.

lis"sen·ce·pha'li·a. Agenesia of the cerebral gyri, resulting in a smooth brain.

lissephen. A trade-mark for mephenesin, *q.v.*

Lister, Joseph [*English surgeon, 1827–1912*]. Considered the founder of antiseptic surgery; established the use of antiseptics in the operating room.

Lister, Joseph Jackson [*English optician and wine merchant, 1786–1869*]. Made important improvements in microscope lenses. Discovered the law of aplanatic foci.

Lis·te'ri·a. A genus of bacteria of the family Corynebacteriaceae. Its members are small, nonspore-forming, Gram-positive rods, motile by means of a single terminal flagellum. **L. monocytogenes.** A species believed to be the etiologic agent of infectious mononucleosis in man.

li'ter (lee'tur). The metric unit of volume. One liter is the volume occupied by 1 kg. of pure water at 4° C. and 760 mm. pressure. It is equal to 1.056 United States quarts. Abbreviated, l.

lith'a·gogue (lith'uh·gog). Any agent which is supposed to expel calculi from the urinary bladder.

lith'arge (lith'ardj, li·thardj'). Lead monoxide.

lith'i·a. Li₂O. Lithium oxide. **Lithia tablets** contain lithium citrate. **Lithia water** is a mineral water containing lithium salts in solution.

lith'ic ac'id. Uric acid.

lith'i·um. Li = 6.940. A soft, silver-white metal belonging to the alkali group. **l. benzoate.** C₆H₅COOLi. Has the therapeutic effect of benzoates. **l. bromide.** LiBr. Sometimes used for its bromide effect. **l. citrate.** C₆H₄·OH·(COOLi)₃. An ingredient of lithia tablets; its effect is probably like that of other alkali citrates. **l. salicylate.** C₆H₄·OH·COOLi. Used for the effect of salicylate ion.

lith'o-, lith-. A combining form meaning *stone, calculus*.

lith"o·gen'e·sis, li·thog'e·ny (li·thodj'i·nee). The formation of calculi or stones. **—lithogenet'ic, lithog'enous** (li·thodj'i·nus), *adj.*

li·thol'a·pax"y (li·thol'uh·pack"see, lith'o·luh·). The operation of crushing

a urinary calculus in the bladder by means of the lithotrite, and then removing the fragments by irrigation, a procedure now performed by a transurethral approach.

lith"o·ne·phri'tis. Inflammation of the kidney, associated with the presence of renal calculi.

lith"o·pe'di·on. A retained fetus that has become calcified.

li·thot'o·my. The removal of a calculus, usually urinary, through an operative incision. **perineal l.** A type in which the incision is made through the membranous urethra in the middle of the perineum. The calculus is then removed by means of a lithotrite or suitable forceps. **suprapubic l.** A type in which the incision into the urinary bladder is made through the abdominal wall just above the symphysis, the stone being removed by forceps.

lith'o·trip"sy, li·thot'rip·sy. The operation of crushing calculi in the urinary bladder.

lith'o·trite. An instrument for crushing a vesical calculus. **—lith·otrit'ic,** *adj.*

lit'mus. A blue pigment obtained from *Roccella tinctoria*, a lichen; used as an indicator for acids and alkalies.

lit'ter. A stretcher or bed for carrying the sick or injured. It consists of parallel bars of wood or metal, the ends serving as handles, over which is stretched canvas for supporting the body. It may be made in the form of an open metal basket for greater safety, especially for transfer of persons from shore to ship or vice versa.

Little, William John [*English surgeon, 1810–94*]. Pioneer orthopedist. Described cerebral spastic paralysis of infants; called *Little's disease*.

Littré, Alexis [*French surgeon and anatomist, 1658–1726*]. Described the small mucous glands of the male urethra (1700); called *Littré's glands*. Described a hernia of Meckel's diverticulum; called *Littré's hernia*. In *Littré's operation* of inguinal colostomy a sigmoid loop is brought out on the left side of the inguinal ligament through a small incision parallel to the ligament.

liv'er. The largest gland or organ in the body, weighing approximately 1750 Gm. in the adult. It lies in the right upper part of the abdomen immediately under the diaphragm and is attached to it by the falciform and other ligaments. There are two principal lobes, the larger right and the smaller left; in addition there are smaller divisions of the right lobe: the quadrate lobe and caudate lobe. **l. extract.** A dry, brownish powder containing that soluble thermostable fraction of mammalian livers which increases the number of red blood cells in the blood of persons affected with pernicious anemia. **l. injection.** A sterile aqueous solution of that soluble thermostable fraction of mammalian livers which increases the number of red blood cells in the blood of persons affected with pernicious anemia. **l. solution.** A brownish liquid containing that soluble thermostable fraction of mammalian livers which increases the number of red blood cells in the blood of persons affected with pernicious anemia. **nutmeg l.** A liver the cross section of which shows a fine mottling of yellow and brown or dark red, somewhat suggestive of the cross section of a nutmeg. In marked passive hyperemia the enlarged red central zones of adjacent lobules fuse to form a network in the meshes of which are the peripheral zones, yellow because of fatty degeneration. In amyloidosis, foci of pale brown glossy amyloid are interspersed in the darker brown hepatic tissue. **syphilitic l.** Rarely, fine bands of connective tissue interlace to divide off small segments of hepatic tissue about a centimeter or two in transverse dimension, the so-called packet liver. See *hepar lobatum.*

liv'id. Of a pale lead color; black and blue; discolored, as flesh from contusion or from hyperemia. —**livid'ity,** n.

li·vid'i·ty. The state of having a black and blue discoloration. **cadaveric l.** The reddish or bluish discoloration in the dependent parts of a corpse, due to the gravitation of laked blood.

L. M. A. Left mentoanterior position of the fetus in utero.

L. M. P. Left mentoposterior position of the fetus in utero; last menstrual period.

L. O. A. Left occipitoanterior position of the fetus in utero.

lobe. A more or less rounded part or projection of an organ, separated from neighboring parts by fissures and constrictions. —**lo'bar, lo'bate,** *adj.* **anterior l. of hypophysis.** The anterior part of the hypophysis which is separated from the posterior lobe by a thin cleft and the pars intermedia. Also called *pars distalis, adenohypophysis.* **frontal l.** That part of the cerebral hemisphere that is in front of the central, and above the lateral, cerebral fissure. **occipital l.** One of the lobes of the cerebrum, a triangular area at the occipital extremity. **parietal l.** The cerebral lobe above the lateral cerebral fissure. **posterior l. of hypophysis.** The posterior part of the hypophysis which is separated from the anterior lobe by a thin cleft and by the pars intermedia. Also called *pars nervosa, neurohypophysis.* **pyramidal l.** An inconstant portion of the thyroid gland extending upward from the isthmus; it arises from the persisting caudal end of the thyroglossal duct. **temporal l.** That part of the cerebral hemisphere below the lateral cerebral fissure, continuous posteriorly with the occipital lobe.

lo·bec'to·my. Excision of a lobe of an organ or gland; specifically, excision of a lobe of the lung.

lo·be'li·a. The leaves and tops of *Lobelia inflata;* contains several alkaloids including lobeline. Lobelia is a respiratory stimulant, but unreliable.

lobelin. Trade-mark for an injectable solution of the hydrochloride of alpha-lobeline used as a respiratory stimulant.

lo'be·line (lo'bi·leen, lo·bee'·). 1. A mixture of alkaloids from lobelia; these have been separated into alpha-, beta-, and gamma- forms. 2. Alpha-lobeline, an alkaloid from lobelia having emetic, respiratory, and vasomotor actions similar to those of nicotine.

lo·bot'o·my. Section of brain tissue. **frontal l.** Operative section of the white matter (frontothalamic fibers) of the frontal lobes of the brain; used in treatment of certain mental disorders.

lob'ule. A small lobe or a subdivision of a lobe. —**lobular, lobulated,** *adj.* **anatomic l. of the liver.** A polygonal prism with a central vein running through the center of its long axis, with branches of the portal vein, the interlobular bile ducts, branches of the hepatic artery and lymph vessels running in the periphery. **physiologic l. of the liver.** That portion of the liver tissue which surrounds and is drained by an interlobular bile duct. **pulmonary l.** A respiratory bronchiole and its branches, the alveolar ducts and alveolar sacs, all with pulmonary alveoli in their walls, constituting a physiologic unit of the lung. **lob'u·lus** (pl. *lobuli*). Lobule, q.v. **l. simplex.** The most rostral part of the posterior lobe of the cerebellum, forming a broad crescentic band across the superior surface.

lo'bus (pl. *lobi*). A lobe.

lo'cal. Limited to a part or place; not general.

lo"cal·i·za'tion. The determination of the site of a lesion. 2. The limitation of a process to a circumscribed area. **cerebral l.** (a) Determination of the position of the centers in the brain that preside over certain physiologic acts. (b) Determination of the seat of pathologic conditions interfering with the normal function of these centers.

lo′cal·ized. Confined to a particular situation or place.

lo′chi·a (lo′kee·uh, lock′ee·uh). The discharge from the uterus and vagina during the first few weeks after labor. **—lochial,** adj. **l. alba.** The whitish or yellowish white flow that takes place after the seventh day after labor. **l. cruenta.** The sanguineous flow of the first few days after labor. Also called lochia rubra. **l. serosa.** The serous discharge taking place about the fifth day after labor.

lo″chio·col′pos (lo″kee·o·kol′poss, lock″ee·o·). Distention of the vagina by retained lochia.

lock′jaw′. See tetanus.

lo′co dis·ease′. A poisoning produced in livestock by eating plants which take up selenium from the soil.

lo″co·mo′tion. The act or power of moving from place to place. **—locomotive, locomotor,** adj.

lo′co weed. Those species of Astragalus which contain selenium.

loc″u·la′tion. The formation of loculi in tissue.

loc′u·li. Plural of loculus.

loc′u·lus (pl. loculi). A small space or compartment. **—loculated,** adj.

lo′cum te′nens (lo′kum ten′enz). A physician who temporarily acts as a substitute for another physician.

lo′cus (pl. loci). 1. A place, spot, or organ. 2. In genetics, the point on a chromosome occupied by a gene. **l. minoris resistentiae.** A spot of diminished resistance.

Loeb, Jacques [American biologist, 1859–1924]. Advanced the theory of tropisms (1890) and the mechanistic theory of life. Made important studies of parthenogenesis; raised fatherless frogs to maturity.

Loeb, Leo [American pathologist, 1869–1959]. Made important studies of the transplantation of tumors; analyzed the factors governing successful transplantation. Showed that the incidence of mammary cancer in mice could be reduced by oöphorectomy. Described the formation of decidual tissue in the uterus as a result of mechanical stimulation; called Loeb′s decidual reaction.

Loeffler, Friedrich August Johannes [German bacteriologist, 1852–1915]. Discovered the glanders bacillus. Gave the first full description of the diphtheria bacillus (1884), called Klebs-Loeffler bacillus. With Frosch, was first to discover a filtrable virus to be the cause of a disease of animals (foot and mouth disease, 1897). See also Loeffler′s stain for flagella.

Loef″fler·el′la mal′le·i (lef″lur·el′uh). Malleomyces mallei, the causative agent of glanders.

log″o·ma′ni·a. A form of mental disorder characterized by talkativeness.

log″o·pe′dics, log″o·pe′di·a. The study, knowledge, and treatment of defective speech.

log″o·pha′si·a (log″o·fay′zhuh, ·zee·uh). A speech disturbance characterized by loss of the ability to articulate correctly. Syn., dysarthria.

-logy. A combining form denoting a saying or a speaking; a science, theory, or doctrine.

lo·i′a·sis. Filariasis caused by Loa loa. The infestation is acquired from bites by the Chrysops dimidiata and C. silacea and involves the subcutaneous tissues, particularly those of the eye.

loin. The lateral and posterior region of the body between the so-called false ribs and the top of the pelvis.

lon·gev′i·ty. Long life; length of life.

lon·gis′si·mus. Longest; applied to muscles, as longissimus dorsi. See Table of Muscles in the Appendix.

lon″gi·tu′di·nal. Lengthwise; in the direction of the long axis of a body.

lon′gus (long′gus). Long. **l. colli.** A deep muscle of the anterior neck region. See Table of Muscles in the Appendix.

loop. 1. A bend in a cord or cordlike structure. 2. A platinum wire, in a glass handle, with its extremity bent in a circular form; used to transfer bacterial cultures.

loose′ness. 1. The state of being free, loose, or unrestrained. 2. Colloquial term for diarrhea. **l. of the teeth.** A condition of the teeth due to disease of the gums and the gradual destruction of the alveolar processes. See periodontosis.

L. O. P. Left occipitoposterior position of the fetus in utero.

lo′pho·dont (lo′fo·dont, lof′o·). Having the crowns of the molar teeth formed in crests or ridges; opposed to bunodont.

lo·phot′ri·chous (lo·fot′ri·kus). Pertaining to microörganisms characterized by a tuft of cilia or flagella at each pole.

lo·quac′i·ty (lo·kwass′i·tee). Volubility of speech; talkativeness; a condition that is frequently excessive in various forms of mental disorders.

lor·do′sis. Forward curvature of the lumbar spine. **—lordot′ic,** adj.

lorfan tartrate. Trade-mark for levallorphan tartrate.

lo·ri′ca. A protective external covering or case. **—lor′icate,** adj.

lo′ti·o (lo′shee·o, lo′tee·o). A lotion.

lo′tion. An aqueous solution or suspension for local application; a wash.

loupe (loop). A magnifying lens. **binocular l.** A binocular magnifier consisting of a combination of lenses in an optical frame, worn like spectacles.

louse (pl. *lice*). A small, wingless, dorsoventrally flattened insect which lacks true metamorphosis. An ectoparasite of birds and mammals, it is medically important as a vector of disease and as a producer of irritating dermatitis.

lous'y. Infested with lice. See *pediculosis*. **—lousiness,** *n.*

loz'enge. A medicated tablet; usually intended for throat medication; usually sweetened.

LSD. d-Lysergic acid diethylamide.

L. S. P. Left sacroposterior position of the fetus in utero.

Lu. Chemical symbol for lutetium.

lu·can'thone hy"dro·chlo'ride. 1-(2-Diethylaminoethylamino)-4-methylthiaxanthone hydrochloride, a drug effective in treating certain types of schistosomiasis.

lu·cid'i·ty. Clearness; the state of being of a clear mind.

lu·cif'u·gal. Fleeing from, or avoiding, light.

lu'cite. See *acrylics*.

Luer [*German instrument maker in France, d. 1883*]. Invented a glass syringe with a glass piston, for use in intravenous and hypodermic injections. Called *Luer syringe*.

lu'es (lew'eez). A euphemism for syphilis. Also called *l. venerea*. **—luet'ic,** *adj.*

lu'e·tin. An extract of the killed cultures of several strains of the *Treponema pallidum*; used in skin tests for syphilis.

luke'warm". Tepid; about the temperature of the body.

lum·ba'go. A general term for backache in the lumbar or lumbosacral regions.

lum'bar. Pertaining to the loins.

lum·bo-, lumb-. A combining form denoting *the loin, lumbar.*

lum"bo·cos'tal. Pertaining to the loins and ribs, as lumbocostal arch, *q.v.*

lum"bo·dor'sal. Pertaining to the lumbar and dorsal regions, as lumbodorsal fascia.

lum"bo·in'gui·nal (lum"bo·ing'-gwi·nul). Pertaining to the lumbar and inguinal regions, as the lumboinguinal nerve, a branch of the genitofemoral, distributed to the skin on the front of the thigh.

lum"bo·sa'cral. Pertaining to the lumbar vertebrae and to the sacrum, as the lumbosacral plexus, the plexus made up of the lower lumbar and upper sacral nerves.

lum'bri·cal. 1. Relating to, or resembling, an earthworm or *Lumbricus*. 2. One of four small muscles in the

hand or foot (pl. *lumbricales*). See Table of Muscles in the Appendix.

lu'men (pl. *lumens, lumina*). 1. The space inside of a tube, as the lumen of a thermometer, blood vessel, duct. 2. A measure of light flux. A source of 1 candlepower emits 4π lumens; 1 footcandle = 1 lumen per square foot; 1 lumen = 0.0015 watt, $\lambda = 555 \mu$.

lu'mi·na. Plural of lumen.

lu'mi·nal. Of or pertaining to the lumen.

luminal. Trade-mark for a brand of phenobarbital.

luminal sodium. Trade-mark for a brand of phenobarbital sodium.

lu"mi·nes'cence. An emission of light without a production of heat sufficient to cause incandescence. It is encountered in certain animals, as some protozoa and fireflies.

lu·mis'ter·ol. The first product obtained in the irradiation of ergosterol with ultraviolet light; further irradiation produces calciferol (vitamin D_2).

lump. 1. A small mass; a protuberant part. 2. Any localized swelling or tumor.

lump'y jaw. See *actinomycosis*.

lu'na·cy. 1. *In legal medicine*, mental disorder in which the individual is not legally responsible; insanity. 2. Insanity formerly supposed to be influenced by the moon. *Obs.*

lu'nar. Pertaining to the moon or to silver (*luna* of the alchemists). **l. caustic.** Toughened silver nitrate.

lu'nate. Semilunar bone, one of the carpal bones. See Table of Bones in the Appendix.

lu·na'tic. 1. Pertaining to, or affected with, lunacy. 2. A psychotic person.

lung. The organ of respiration, in which the venous blood is oxidized by the air drawn through the trachea and bronchi into the alveoli. There are two lungs, a right and a left, the former consisting of three, the latter of two, lobes. The lungs are situated in the thoracic cavity, and are enveloped by the pleura. **iron l.** A mechanical respirator; Drinker respirator; used in respiratory paralysis. Also called *artificial l.*

lung'mo"tor. An apparatus for pumping air or air and oxygen into the lungs.

lu'nu·la, lun'u·la. 1. The white, semilunar area of a nail near the root. 2. The thin, crescentic area of a semilunar valve of the heart, on either side of the nodule.

lu'pine (lew'pin, -peen). A plant of the genus *Lupinus*. One or more poisonous alkaloids have been found in various species of the genus.

lu"pi·no'sis. See *lathyrism*.

lu·po'ma. The primary nodule of lupus.

lu'pu·lin. The glandular trichomes separated from the strobiles of *Humulus lupulus*. It is reputedly antispasmodic and sedative.

lu'pu·lone, lu'pu·lon. $C_{26}H_{38}O_4$. A constituent of humulus; possesses antibiotic activity.

lu'pus. A chronic tubercular disease of the skin and mucous membranes, characterized by the formation of nodules of granulation tissue. Syn., *lupus exedens, lupus vulgaris.* —**lupoid, lupiform,** *adj.* **discoid l. erythematosus.** A usually chronic disease of the skin occurring in the exposed areas, as the face, scalp, and hands, characterized by red, scaly patches of various sizes and shapes that induce atrophy and superficial scar formation and that cause follicular plugging. Syn., *l. sebaceus, l. superficialis, ulerythema centrifugum.* Also called *l. erythematodes.* **disseminated follicular l.** A variety of lupus confined to the face, especially in the situations usually occupied by acne. The papules vary from a large pinhead to a pea in size, conical and deep red. **disseminated l. erythematosus.** A disease of unknown cause, characterized by fever, muscle and joint pains, anemia, leukopenia, and frequently by a skin eruption similar to discoid lupus erythematosus. **l. miliaris disseminatus.** A more acute form usually occurring in children and at times following measles. Many small lesions appear rapidly. May be fatal. **l. vulgaris.** True tuberculosis of the skin. A diverse and variable disease. Nodules of the apple jelly type are usually seen. It is a slowly developing, scarring, and deforming disease, often asymptomatic, and often involving the face. Syn., *tuberculosis luposa.*

lute. A pasty substance which hardens when dry; used to make joints waterproof in pharmaceutical apparatus.

lu'te·al. Of or pertaining to the corpus luteum or to its principle, as the luteal hormone.

lu'te·in. 1. A yellow pigment obtained from the corpora lutea by extraction with chloroform. 2. An internal secretion of the ovary.

lu'te·o-. 1. A combining form signifying *orange yellow* or *brownish yellow.* 2. *In botany,* a combining form denoting *yellowish.* 3. *In chemistry,* a combining form used in naming a series of yellow ammoniacal cobaltic salts.

lu''te·o'ma. An ovarian tumor of the general order of a granulosa-cell tumor, in which the cells are luteinized.

lu·te'ti·um (lew·tee'shum, ·see·um). Lu = 174.99. A rare earth metal. Formerly spelled *lutecium.*

lutocylol. Trade-mark for anhydrohydroxyprogesterone.

lux·a'tion. 1. A dislocation, *q.v.* 2. *In dentistry,* the partial or complete separation of a tooth from its socket as a result of trauma.

lux·u'ri·ant. Growing to excess, exuberant; specifically referring to the abnormal growth of certain body cells, as in granulation tissue.

ly·can'thro·py (lye·can'thro·pee). A belief that one is a wolf or some other wild beast, common among schizophrenic patients. Syn., *lycomania.* —**lycanthrop'ic,** *adj.;* **ly'canthrope,** *n.*

ly'cine (lye'seen, ·sin). See *betaine.*

ly''co·ma'ni·a. See *lycanthropy.*

ly''co·po'di·um. The spores of *Lycopodium clavatum,* occurring as a light yellowish powder. Used as a desiccant and absorbent on moist and excoriated surfaces, as an inert powder in which to embed pills. Also called *club moss, witch meal, wolf's claw.*

ly''co·rex'i·a. A wolfish or canine appetite.

lye. 1. An alkaline solution obtained by leaching wood ashes. 2. A solution of sodium or potassium hydroxide.

lymph. 1. The fluid in the lymph vessels, collected from the interstitial fluid. 2. Old term for exudate. —**lymph'oid,** *adj.* **l. gland.** [BNA] Lymph node. **l. node.** See under *node.*

lym·phad''e·nec'to·my. Excision of a lymph node.

lym·phad''e·ni'tis. Inflammation of a lymph node. **tuberculous l.** Tuberculous infection of the lymph nodes.

lym·phad''e·no'ma. A tumorlike enlargement of a lymph node, in which the architectural pattern is obliterated by proliferation of lymphocytes; it probably exists in two forms, the neoplastic and the hyperplastic.

lym·phad''e·nop'a·thy. Disease or enlargement of the lymph nodes.

lym'pha·gogue (lim'fuh·gog). 1. Stimulating the flow of lymph. 2. An agent that stimulates the flow of lymph.

lym·phan''gi·ec·ta·sis (lim·fan''jee·eck'tuh·sis), **lym·phan''gi·ec·ta'si·a** (·eck·tay'zhuh, ·shuh). Dilatation of the lymphatic vessels. It may cause elephantiasis, *q.v.* —**lymphangiectat'ic,** *adj.*

lym·phan''gi·o'ma. A dilated or varicose condition or tumor of the lymphatics. **l. circumscriptum congenitale.** A very rare skin disease of unknown cause, occurring in early life, marked by the formation of straw-yellow vesicles, deeply situated in the skin, with thick and tense walls, and connected with the lymphatics. **l. tuberosum multiplex.** A very rare skin disease; probably congenital; characterized by the formation of large, brownish red papules or tubercles, the size of lentils, not arranged in groups or clusters, but scattered indiscriminately over the trunk. See *hygroma.*

lym″phan·gi′tis. Inflammation of a lymphatic vessel; may be acute or chronic, or of tuberculous origin.

lym·phat′ic. 1. Pertaining to lymph. 2. A vessel conveying lymph. **afferent l.** A vessel conveying lymph to a lymph node. **efferent l.** A vessel conveying lymph away from a lymph node.

lym·phat′ic block·ade′. The bits of fibrinous exudate that pass into the local lymphatics and the fibrinous network thrown about a wounded part, blocking the passage of foreign bodies, notably microörganisms, to other parts of the body.

lym′pha·tism. A condition in which all the lymphatic tissues, the thymus, the spleen, and the bone marrow are hyperplastic; sudden death is said to occur, especially in surgical anesthesia. Syn., *status lymphaticus, status thymicus.*

lym′pho-, lymph-. A combining form denoting *connection with,* or *relation to, lymph* or *the lymphatics.*

lym′pho·blast. A precursor of a lymphocyte, or nongranular white blood cell.

lym″pho·blas·to′ma. A lymphosarcoma in which the predominant cell type has some of the features of lymphoblasts.

lym″pho·cyte. A lymph cell. One of the class of agranular leukocytes; small cells with large nuclei and very little cytoplasm.

lym″pho·cy·the′mi·a (lim″fo·sigh·theem′ee·uh). An excess of lymphocytes in the blood. Syn., *lymphocytosis.*

lym″pho·cy·to′ma (lim″fo·sigh·to′muh). A lymphosarcoma in which the predominant cell type closely resembles mature lymphocytes.

lym″pho·cy″to·pe′ni·a. Decrease of the normal number of lymphocytes in the peripheral blood.

lym″pho·cy″to·poi·e′sis. The genesis of lymphocytes.

lym″pho·cy·to′sis (lim″fo·sigh·to′sis). See *lymphocythemia.*

lym″pho·ep″i·the″li·o′ma. A rapidly growing tumor, usually in the nasopharynx about the orifice of the auditory tube or in the tonsils, often with metastases to cervical lymph nodes. Microscopically there is an association of cells resembling lymphocytes and larger, indistinctly outlined, mononuclear cells of epithelial character. Responds readily to irradiation but often recurs. A more distinctly alveolated type sometimes occurs in which the epithelial cells are arranged as trabeculae.

lym·phog′en·ous (lim·fodj′in·us). Producing lymph.

lym″pho·glan′du·la. BNA term for a lymph node.

lym″pho·gran″u·lo′ma. Old term for Hodgkin's disease, *q.v.* **venereal l.** A virus disease characterized by an initial lesion, usually on the genitalia, followed by regional lymph-node enlargement and, at times, systemic involvement. The Frei test is a specific skin test for this condition. A venereal disease. Also called *fourth venereal disease, l. inguinale, l. venereum, lymphopathia venereum, Nicolas-Favre disease, Durand-Nicolas-Favre disease.*

lym″pho·gran″u·lo·ma·to′sis. See Hodgkin's *disease.*

lym″pho·gran″u·lo·ma·to′sis cu′tis. A specific autonomous venereal disease which typically involves the inguinal lymph nodes in a subacute inflammation.

lym·pho′ma. Loosely, a group of malignant or premalignant conditions of lymphatic tissue in which splenomegaly and lymphadenopathy usually are present.

lym″pho·sar·co′ma. A malignant tumor of lymphatic tissue distinguished from lymphocytic leukemia only by the absence of malignant cells from the peripheral blood.

lynoral. Trade-mark for ethinyl estradiol.

ly′o-, ly-. A combining form signifying to *dissolve, loose.*

ly′o·chrome. See *flavin.*

ly″o·en′zyme. See extracellular *enzyme.*

ly′o·gel. A gel rich in liquid.

ly′o·phile (lye′o·file, ·fil), **ly″o·phil′ic.** Referring to the dispersed phase of a colloidal system when the dispersion medium is attracted to the former. Also see *lyophobe.* **l. process.** A desiccation procedure involving rapid freezing of the material to be dried followed by evaporation of the moisture at low temperature under vacuum.

ly″o·phil·i·za′tion. The process of rapidly freezing a substance (pollen, blood plasma, antitoxin, serum, etc.) at low temperature, then quickly dehydrating the frozen mass in a high vacuum. **—lyophilized,** *adj.*

ly′o·phobe, ly″o·pho′bic, ly″o·phob′ic. Denoting lack of solubility; a colloidal system in which there is lack of strong affinity between the colloid and the dispersion medium. Also see *lyophile.*

lyse. To cause or to undergo lysis, 3.

ly·ser′gic ac′id. $C_{16}H_{16}N_2O_2$. A component of ergot alkaloids.

d-ly·ser′gic ac′id di·eth″yl·a′mide. A psychotomimetic agent that produces hallucinations or other psychotic manifestations in normal persons, used in research of mental disorders. Abbreviated, LSD.

ly'si- (lye'si-, lis'i-), **lys-**. A combining form signifying *loosening*.

ly'sin. A cell-dissolving substance.
beta 1. Certain thermostable bactericidal serum constituents; similar to leukins and obtained from granulocytes and perhaps from blood platelets. The relation of these factors to immunity is not clear.

ly'sine (lye'seen, ·sin). The a-amino-e-caproic acid, an amino acid obtainable by the hydrolysis of casein and other proteins. It is essential to the growth of man.

ly'sis. 1. Gradual decline in the manifestations of a disease, especially an infectious disease. Syn., *defervescence.* 2. Gradual fall of fever. 3. The solution of a cell or tissue by the action of a lysin, as the solution of erythrocytes by chemical substances, by alteration of environment, or by action of a

specific immune hemolysin and complement.

-lysis. 1. A combining form signifying *dissolving, dissolution.* 2. In biochemistry, a combining form signifying *dissolution.* 3. In chemistry, a combining form signifying *decomposition.* 4. In medicine, a combining form denoting *relief* or *reduction, detachment,* or *paralysis.*

ly"so·gen'ic. Giving rise to lysins or producing lysis. **_lysogenesis,_** n.

ly'so·zyme. An enzyme found in tears, leukocytes, mucous secretions, egg albumin, and many plants. It exerts a strong antiseptic action, due to lysis of bacteria.

lys'sic. Pertaining to rabies; due to rabies.

ly·te'ri·an (lye-teer'ee-un). Indicative of a lysis, or of a favorable crisis terminating an attack of disease.

-lyt'ic. A suffix signifying *lysis* or *a lysin.*

M

M. 1. A symbol for metal. 2. An abbreviation for mass, permanent molar, molar (chemistry); molecular weight; *misce,* mix. 3. The Roman numeral for one thousand.

M. *Misce,* mix.

m. Meter, deciduous molar.

m-. *In chemistry,* meta-.

M. A. Master of Arts.

MA. Mental age.

Ma. Chemical symbol for masurium.

ma. Milliampere.

mac'er·ate (mass'ur·ate). Soften a solid or a tissue by steeping. **—maceration,** n.

mac'ley·ine, mac·ley'ine. See *fumarine.*

mac"ra·cu'si·a (mack"ra-cue'zhuh, mack"ra-kōō'·). A cerebral disorder simulating epilepsy, in which there is exaggerated reaction to sounds.

macro-, macr-. 1. *In anatomy and medicine,* a combining form denoting *an enlargement.* 2. *In botany and zoology,* a combining form signifying *having an unusually large or elongated part.*

mac"ro·bra'chi·a (mack"ro-bray'-kee-uh). Excessive development of the arms.

mac"ro·ce·pha'li·a, mac"ro·ceph'a·ly. Abnormal largeness of the head. **—macroceph'alous,** adj.

mac"ro·chei'li·a (mack"ro-kigh'-lee-uh). Excessive development of the lips; characteristic of certain Negro

tribes and of cretins; in the latter due to lymphangioma of lips and cheeks.

mac"ro·chei'ri·a (mack"ro-kigh'-ree-uh). Enlargement of the hands.

mac'ro·cyte. A giant red blood cell found in the blood in certain anemias, especially in pernicious anemia. **—macrocyt'ic,** adj.

mac"ro·cy·to'sis (mack"ro-sigh-to'sis). The presence of macrocytes, or abnormally large erythrocytes, in the blood.

mac"ro·dac·tyl'i·a, mac"ro·dac'ty·ly, mac"ro·dac'tyl·ism. Abnormally large fingers or toes.

mac'ro·dont. Having large teeth; megadont. **—macrodon'tia,** n.

mac"ro·ga·mete (mack"ro-ga-meet', ·gam'eet). A relatively large, nonmotile reproductive cell of certain protozoans and Thallophytes, comparable to an ovum of the metazoans.

mac"ro·gen'i·to·so'mi·a. Precocious development with large genitals.

mac"ro·glos'si·a. Enlargement of the tongue; a condition seen in cretins, due to lymphangioma.

mac"ro·gnath'ic (mack"ro-nath'ick, mack"rog-). Having long jaws; prognathous. **—macrog'nathism,** n.

mac"ro·gy'ri·a. A congenital condition of excessively large convolutions of the brain.

mac"ro·mas'ti·a. Abnormal enlargement of the breast. Also called *macromazia.*

mac″ro·me′li·a. Abnormally large size of arms or legs.

ma·crom′e·lus. An individual having excessively large limbs.

mac″ro·mo·lec′u·lar. Having large molecules.

mac″ro·nor′mo·blast. A stage in the development of an erythroblast into a red blood cell. See also *erythroblast.*

mac″ro·nu′cle·us. The vegetative or trophic nucleus of protozoa as contrasted with the micronucleus which is reproductive in function.

mac″ro·nych′i·a (mack″ro-nick′ee-uh). Excessive size of the nails.

mac′ro·phage. A phagocytic cell, not a leukocyte, belonging to the reticuloendothelial system, *q.v.* It has the capacity for storing certain aniline dyes, as trypan blue or lithium carmine, in its cytoplasm in the form of granules. **fixed m.** A nonmotile macrophage, as that found in loose connective tissue (histiocyte), or lining the sinuses in the liver (Kupffer cell), the spleen, bone marrow, or lymph nodes. **free m.** An actively ameboid macrophage found in an area of inflammation. Also called *inflammatory m.*

mac″ro·po′di·a. Abnormal size of the foot or feet.

mac″ro·pro·so′pi·a. Abnormal enlargement of the face.

mac″ro·pro·so′pus (mack″ro-pro′so-pus, ·pro·so′pus). An individual with an abnormally large face.

ma·crop′si·a, ma·crop′sy. A disturbance of vision in which objects seem larger than they are. Syn., *megalopia.*

mac″ro·scop′ic. Large enough to be seen by the naked eye; gross; not microscopic.

mac″ro·so′mi·a. Gigantism.

mac″ro·sto′mi·a. Abnormally large mouth; a mild form of transverse facial cleft.

ma·crot′i·a (ma·kro′shee·uh). Abnormal largeness of the external ear.

mac′u·la (pl. *maculas, maculae*). 1. A spot, usually upon the skin, not elevated above the surrounding level and distinguished by a discoloration. Syn., *macule.* 2. The area of most distinct vision of the retina. —**macular,** *adj.* **false m.** The point on the retina of a squinting eye which receives the same impression as the macula of the fixing eye. **m. communis.** The thickening in the medial wall of the otic vesicle, which divides to form the maculae, cristae, and organ of Corti of the internal ear. **m. corneae.** A permanent corneal opacity from an ulcer or keratitis. **m. cribrosa.** One of the perforations of the wall of the vestibule for the passage of the filaments of the auditory nerve. **macu-lae acusticae.** The terminations of the vestibular nerve in the saccule and utricle. **m. germinativa.** The nucleolus of the ovum. **m. lutea.** The yellow spot of the retina; the point of clearest vision.

mac′ule. See *macula,* 1.

mac″u·lo·pap′u·lar. Having the characteristics of a macule and a papule.

mad. 1. Colloquial term for insane. 2. Affected with rabies; rabid.

mad″a·ro′sis. Loss of the eyelashes or eyebrows. —**madarot′ic, mad′arous,** *adj.*

mad′i·dans (mad′i-danz, ·dance). Weeping, oozing.

mad′ness. Colloquial term for mental disorder.

ma·du′ra foot (mad-oor′uh, mad-yoor′uh). See *mycetoma.*

mag″en·stras′se (mah′gun-shtrah″suh). A longitudinal groove in the mucous membrane of the stomach, along the lesser curvature from the cardiac end to the pyloric end. It is associated with the direct passage of food through the stomach, and is one of the most frequent sites of gastric ulcer.

ma·gen′ta. Basic fuchsin. **acid m.** Acid fuchsin.

mag′got. The larval form of an insect, especially of the order Diptera. Maggots have been used in the healing of suppurating wounds. Also see maggot *therapy.*

mag′is·ter″y (madj′i·sterr″ee). Formerly, a preparation considered to have especial virtue as a remedy. **bismuth m.** Bismuth subnitrate. **tin m.** Precipitated stannous oxide, SnO.

mag′ma. 1. Any pulpy mass; a paste. 2. *In pharmacy,* a more or less permanent suspension of a precipitate in water.

mag·na′li·um. An alloy of aluminum and magnesium.

magnamycin. Trade-mark for carbomycin.

mag·ne′sia (mag-nee′shuh, ·shuh). Magnesium oxide; MgO. **calcined m.** Magnesium oxide prepared by ignition of the carbonate. **heavy m.** Magnesium oxide prepared by ignition of heavy magnesium carbonate. **light m.** Magnesium oxide prepared by ignition of light magnesium carbonate. **m. magma.** Milk of magnesia.

mag′ne·site. Native magnesium carbonate; used as a substitute for plaster of Paris.

mag·ne′si·um (mag-nee′zee-um, ·zhum, ·shee·um, ·shum). Mg = 24.32. A bluish white metal. Abundantly distributed throughout inorganic and organic nature and essential to life; its salts are used in medicine. See Table of Normal Values of Blood Constituents in the Appendix. —**mag·ne'sic**, *adj.* **m. car'bonate**. Basic or normal hydrated magnesium carbonate. Exists in two forms: light and heavy magnesium carbonate. Antacid and laxative. **m. hydrox'ide**. $Mg(OH)_2$. Antacid and cathartic. Also called *m. hydrate*. **m. man'delate**. $(C_6H_5CHOHCOO)_2$-Mg. A urinary antiseptic. **m. ox'ide**. MgO. Obtained by calcining magnesium carbonate. Exists in two forms: light magnesia and heavy magnesia. **m. sul'fate**. $MgSO_4.7H_2O$. Epsom salt, an active cathartic. **m. trisil'icate**. Approximately $2MgO.3SiO_2$ with varying amounts of water. Almost insoluble in water; used as an antacid and adsorbent. **triba'sic m. phos'phate**. $Mg_3(PO_4)_2$. A gastric antacid; almost insoluble in water.

mag'net. 1. Loadstone, iron that attracts iron. 2. Any body having the power to attract iron. —**magnet'ic**, *adj.* **electromag'net**. See *electromagnet*. **gi'ant m**. A large, powerful, stationary magnet for extracting particles of steel from the eye. **m. oper·a'tion**. The operation of removing foreign bodies of steel from the eye by means of a magnet. **Mel'linger m**. A type of giant magnet, with a magnetized core held in the surgeon's hand, the coil being over the patient's eye, and devised for extracting steel particles from the eyeball. **per'manent m**. One whose magnetic properties are permanent. **tem'porary m**. One which derives its magnetism from another magnet or from a galvanic current.

mag'net·ism. 1. The power possessed by a magnet to attract or repel other masses. 2. The force formerly supposed to be transmitted from man to man, an important factor in hypnotism or mesmerism. Also called *animal m*.

mag·ne"to·stric'tion. A magnetic phenomenon involving the change in length of a rod or tube of ferromagnetic material when it is exposed to a magnetic field parallel to its length.

mag·ne"to·ther'a·py. The treatment of diseases by magnets.

mag"ni·fi·ca'tion. Apparent enlargement, especially the enlargement of an object by means of lenses. —**mag'nify**, *v.*

mag'num. 1. Large, as in foramen magnum, *q.v.* 2. An old term for capitate bone (os magnum).

maid'en·head". The hymen, the allusion being to the intact organ of the maid or virgin.

ma·ieu"si·o·ma'ni·a (may·yōō"-see·o·may'nee·uh, migh·yōō"·). Puerperal psychosis. *Obs.*

ma·ieu"si·o·pho'bi·a. Morbid fear of childbirth.

ma·ieu'tic (may·yōō'tick, migh·yōō'-tick). 1. A rubber bag used for dilating the cervix uteri. 2. Obstetric.

maim. Deprive a person or animal of any part of the body; disable or cripple.

maize. Indian corn. A cereal grain; the seed of *Zea mays*.

maize oil. Corn oil.

make. *In electricity*, the establishing of the flow of an electric current.

mak'ro·. See *macro-*.

mal. Disease. **grand m**. See grand mal *epilepsy*. **m. de Cayenne'**. Elephantiasis. **m. de mer'**. Seasickness. **petit m**. See petit mal *epilepsy*.

mal-. A combining form denoting *ill, bad*.

mal'a·chite green (mal'uh·kite) (C.C.). Tetramethyl-di-p-aminotriphenylcarbinol, a triphenylmethane dye. Violet-green crystals or powder; soluble in water or alcohol. Used as a bacteriologic stain and medicinal dye.

ma·la'ci·a (ma·lay'shee·uh, ·see·uh). Softening of part of an organ or structure, the result of necrosis. Also see *encephalomalacia, osteomalacia*.

mal"ad·just'ment. A state of faulty or inadequate conformity to one's environment, due to the inability to adjust one's desires, attitudes, or feelings to social requirements.

mal'a·dy. Disease or illness.

ma·laise' (ma·layz'). A general feeling of illness, sometimes accompanied by restlessness and discomfort.

ma'lar. Pertaining to the cheek or to the zygoma.

ma·lar'i·a (ma·lair'ee·uh). An infectious, usually chronic disease caused by protozoa of the genus *Plasmodium* and transmitted by the anopheles mosquito, characterized by intermittent fever, splenomegaly, debility, and anemia, and, in its acute form, by chills, high fever, and profuse sweating in regular cycles that may recur every day, every other day, or every fourth day, alternating with periods of comparative well-being. —**mala'rial, malar'i·ous**, *adj.* **a'vian m**. Malaria of birds and poultry. **be·nign' ter'tian m**. Vivax malaria. **equine m**. Malaria in horses. **fal·cip'arum m**. A severe form caused by the species *Plasmodium falciparum* characterized by acyclic paroxysms and often by localization of the parasite in an organ, as the brain, lungs or intestinal mucosa. **o'vale m**. A form similar to vivax malaria, caused by the species *Plasmodium ovale*. **quar'tan m**. A form caused by the species *Plasmodium malariae*, characterized by short paroxysms that recur every third day. **quotid'ian m**. A form caused by the species *Plasmodium vivax*, in which paroxysms occur every day, usually due to two concomitant infections. **subtertian m.** Falciparum malaria. **tertian m.** Vivax malaria. **vivax m.** A form caused by *Plasmodium vivax*, characterized by typical paroxysms, usually occurring every second day and sometimes every third day.

ma·lar″i·o·ther′a·py. Treatment of neurosyphilis by infecting the patient with malaria.

mal″as·sim″i·la′tion. Defective assimilation.

mal″di·ges′tion. Disordered or imperfect digestion.

male. 1. Pertaining to the male or impregnating sex. 2. An individual of the male sex. The designative symbol is □, ♂ (that of the female is ○, ♀). 3. Of a double-bladed instrument, the blade which is received into a hollow of the other (female) blade. 4. *In botany*, a plant having stamens only.

ma·le′ate. Any salt of maleic acid.

ma·le′ic ac′id (ma·lee′ick, ma·lay′ick). COOH.CH:CH.COOH. Cis-ethylene carboxylic acid. A dibasic acid, the cis-isomer of fumaric acid.

mal″for·ma′tion. An abnormal development or formation of a part of the body; deformity.

mal′ic ac′id (mal′ick, may′lick). COOH.CH₂.CHOH.COOH. An acid found in apples and many other fruits.

ma·lig′nant. Virulent; threatening life, as malignant tumors. —**malignancy,** *n.*

ma·lin′ger·er (ma·ling′gur·ur). One who feigns illness or inability, usually to escape military duty or to secure benefit from an alleged injury. —**malingering,** *n.*

mal′le·a·ble. Capable of being beaten or rolled into thin sheets. —**malleability,** *n.*

mal″le·a′tion. A spasmodic action of the hands, consisting in continuously striking any near object.

mal′le·in. A fluid obtained from cultures of *Malleomyces mallei* (glanders bacillus). Has been recommended for use in the early diagnosis of glanders.

mal·le′o·lus (pl. *malleoli*). A part or process of bone having a hammerhead shape. —**malleolar,** *adj.* **lateral m.** The lower extremity of the fibula. Also called *external m.* **medial m.** A process on the internal surface of the lower extremity of the tibia. Also called *internal m.*

Mal″le·o·my′ces (mal″ee·o·migh′-seez). A genus of the family Parvobacteriaceae; composed of small, slender, Gram-negative, nonmotile, nonsporulating, rodlike bacteria sometimes developing into branched filaments. **M. mallei.** That species which is the causative agent of glanders. **M. pseudomallei.** That species which causes melioidosis in rodents and in man.

mal″le·ot′o·my. 1. Incision or division of the malleus. 2. Division of the ligaments attached to the malleoli.

mal′le·us. 1. One of the ossicles of the internal ear, having the shape of a hammer. See Table of Bones in the Appendix. 2. *In veterinary medicine*, synonym for glanders, *q.v.* —**malleal,** *adj.*

Mal·lo′tus. A genus of trees and shrubs of the Euphorbiaceae.

mal″nu·tri′tion. Imperfect nutrition.

mal″oc·clu′sion (mal″oc·clue′-zhun). Any deviation from normal occlusion of the teeth; usually associated with abnormal developmental growth of the jaws.

ma·lo′nic ac′id (ma·lo′nick, ·lon′-ick). COOH.CH₂.COOH. A dibasic acid found in many plants.

mal′o·nyl (mal′o·nyl, ·neel). $H_2C{<}^{CO-}_{CO-}$. The bivalent radical of malonic acid.

mal″po·si′tion. An abnormal position of any part or organ, as of the fetus.

mal″prac′tice. Improper medical or surgical treatment, through carelessness, ignorance, or intent.

mal″pres″en·ta′tion (mal″prez″-un·tay′shun, ·pree″zen·tay′shun). Abnormal position of the child at birth, making delivery difficult or impossible.

mal″re·duc′tion. Faulty or incomplete reduction of a fracture.

malt (mawlt). Grain, commonly of one or more varieties of barley, which has been soaked, made to germinate, and dried.

Mal′ta fe′ver (mawl′tuh). See *brucellosis*.

malt′ase (mawl′tace, ·taze). An enzyme found in the saliva and pancreatic juice which converts maltose into dextrose.

Malthus, Thomas Robert [*English political economist*, 1766–1834]. Evolved the theory that population, in the absence of such checks on its growth as epidemics and war, tends to increase more rapidly than the food supply. Advocated sexual continence as a means of limiting the birth rate. Acceptance of Malthus' doctrines is called *Malthusianism*. The term is incorrectly applied to advocacy of restriction of the birth rate by means of birth control.

mal″to·bi′ose (mawl″to·buy′oce). Maltose.

mal″to·dex′trin. A form of dextrin convertible into maltose.

malt′ose (mawl′toce). C₁₂H₂₂O₁₁.H₂O. A variety of sugar obtainable from malt and starch.

mal″to·su′ri·a. The presence of maltose in the urine.

mal·turned'. Turned abnormally; applied to a tooth so turned on its long axis as to stand in malposition.

ma'lum. Disease. m. **Aegyptia·cum.** Diphtheria. m. **coxae se·nilis.** Hypertrophic arthritis of the hip joint in the aged. m. **pilare.** Trichinosis. m. **venereum.** Syphilis.

mal·un'ion. Incomplete or faulty union of the fragments of a fractured bone.

Mal'va. The mallow; a genus of the Malvaceae.

mam'ma (pl. *mammae*). The breast; the milk-secreting gland. m. **aber·rans.** Supernumerary breast. Also called *m. erratica*. m. **virilis.** The male breast.

mam'mal. An individual of the class Mammalia.

mam·mal'gi·a. Pain in the breast.

Mam·ma'li·a. The highest class of vertebrates, including all animals that have hair and suckle their young.

mam'ma·ry. Of or pertaining to the breast or the mammary gland.

mam·mec'to·my. Excision or amputation of a breast.

mam'mi·form. Shaped like a breast or nipple.

mam·mil'la (pl. *mammillae*). A small prominence or papilla; nipple.

mam·mil·la"ted. Covered with nipplelike protuberances.

mam"mil·la'tion. A granulation, especially on some mucous surface.

mam·mil'li·form. Nipple-shaped.

mam·mil'li·plas"ty. Plastic surgery of the nipple.

mam"mil·li'tis. Inflammation of the mammilla, or nipple.

mam"mil·lo·tha·lam'ic. Connecting the mammillary body with the thalamus, as the mammillothalamic tract.

mam·mi'tis. See *mastitis*.

mam·mog'ra·phy. Radiographic examination of the breast; performed after injecting the ducts of the mammary gland with an opaque contrast medium.

mam'mose (mam'ohss, ma-mohss'). Having full or abnormally large breasts.

mam·mot'o·my. Mastotomy, *q.v.*

man. 1. The human race; mankind. 2. An adult male human being.

man·del'ic ac'id (man-del'ick, -dee'lick). C₆H₅CH(OH)COOH. Alpha-hydroxyphenylacetic acid, occurring as white crystals or powder; soluble in water. Employed, chiefly in the form of one of its salts, as a urinary antiseptic. Also called *amygdalic acid, inactive mandelic acid, racemic mandelic acid.*

man'di·ble, man·dib'u·la. The lower jawbone. See Table of Bones in the Appendix. —**mandib'ular,** *adj.*

Man·drag'o·ra. The mandrake. A genus of solanaceous plants.

man'drake. Common name for *Man·dragora.*

man'drin. A guide or stylet, *q.v.*

man"du·ca'tion. The chewing or mastication of food. —**man'duca·tory,** *adj.*

ma·neu'ver. 1. Skillful procedure or manual method. 2. Manipulate. **Prague m.** Delivery of the aftercoming head by grasping the shoulders from below with two fingers of one hand, while the other hand draws the feet up over the abdomen of the mother.

man'ga·nese (mang'guh-niece, -neez, man'guh-). Mn = 54.93. A brittle, hard, grayish white metal resembling iron in its properties.

man·gan'ic (man-gan'ick, mang-gan'ick). Referring to manganese when it has a valence of four.

man·ga·nous (mang'guh-nus, man'guh-nus). Referring to manganese when it has a valence of two.

mange (mayndj). Infestation of the skin of mammals by mange mites which burrow into the epidermal layer of the skin; characterized by multiple lesions in the skin with vesiculation and papule formation accompanied by intense itching. **follicular m.** That form produced by the *Demodex folliculorum* which parasitizes the hair follicles or sebaceous glands of man and domestic animals. **sarcoptic m.** The form most common to man, caused by the *Sarcoptes scabiei.* See *scabies.*

man'go (mang'go). The fruit of *Mangifera indica.*

ma·ni·a. 1. Excessive enthusiasm or excitement; a violent desire or passion. Also called *acute m., Bell's m.* 2. A form of mental disorder marked by a sustained elevation of mood with exaggerated feelings of well-being, flight of ideas, delusions of greatness, and psychomotor overactivity. See manic-depressive *psychosis.* Also see *hypermania, hypomania.* —**man'ic, ma'nic,** *adj.;* **maniac,** *n.* **brooding m.** A morbid mental state characterized by an impulse to prolonged and anxious meditation. **histrionic m.** Mania in which the patient assumes a dramatic manner, playing the role of an actor. *Obs.* **periodic m.** A succession of manic attacks. Also called *recurrent m.* **transitory m.** A form characterized by sudden onset and short duration (one hour to a few days).

man'ic·de·pres'sive (man'ick-di-press'iv, may'nick-). See manic-depressive *psychosis.*

Man'i·hot. A genus of the Euphorbiaceae; yields cassava.

man'i·kin. 1. A model of the body made of plaster, papier-mâché, or other material, and showing, by means of movable parts, the relations of the organs. 2. A model of a term fetus; used for the teaching of obstetrics. 3. A little man with normal proportion of parts; a dwarf; a homunculus.

man'i·oc, ma'ni·oc. The cassava plant or its product, tapioca. See *Manihot*.

ma·nip"u·la'tion. The use of the hands in a skillful manner, as in reducing a dislocation or a hernia, or in changing the position of a fetus. **conjoined m.** The use of both hands in obstetric or gynecologic procedure, one being in the vagina and the other on the abdomen.

man'na. The concrete, saccharine exudation of the flowering ash, *Fraxinus ornus*.

man'nan. See *mannosan*.

man'ni·tan. $C_6H_{12}O_5$. A sweet, syrupy substance, the anhydride of mannitol.

man'nite. See *mannitol*.

man'ni·tol. $C_6H_{14}O_6$. Mannite. A hexatomic alcohol from manna and other plant sources. **m. hexanitrate.** $C_6H_8(O.NO_2)_6$. Employed for the vasodilator effect of the nitrite ion.

man'ni·tose. See *mannose*.

man·non'ic ac'id (ma·non'ick, ma·no'nick). $CH_2OH(CHOH)_4COOH$. An acid derived by the oxidation of mannitol.

man'no·san. A polysaccharide, occurring in plants, which upon hydrolysis yields mannose. Sometimes called *mannan*.

man'nose. $C_6H_{12}O_6$. A fermentable monosaccharide obtained from manna.

ma·nom'e·ter. An instrument for measuring the pressure of liquids and gases. —**manomet'ric,** *adj.* **optical m.** Device for the accurate registration of the details of pressure pulses, in which pressure changes are led through a rigid, fluid-filled system to a tense rubber or metallic membrane on which is mounted a small mirror. The deflections of a beam of light reflected from this mirror are recorded on moving photographic paper.

ma·nu'bri·um. 1. A handle. 2. The first or upper piece of the sternum. —**manubrial,** *adj.*

man"u·duc'tion. Operation performed by the hands in surgical and obstetric practice.

ma'nus. The hand. **m. cava.** Excessive concavity of the palm of the hand. **m. curta.** Clubhand. **m. extensa.** Clubhand with a backward deviation. **m. flexa.** Clubhand with a forward deviation. **m. valga.** Clubhand with ulnar deviation. **m. vara.** Clubhand with radial deviation.

man"u·stu·pra'tion. Masturbation, *q.v.*

mapharsen. Trade-mark for oxophenarsine hydrochloride crystallized with half a molecule of alcohol.

Ma·ran'ta. See *arrowroot*.

ma·ran'tic. 1. Pertaining to marasmus. 2. Pertaining to slowed circulation.

ma·ras'mus (ma·raz'mus). A gradual wasting of the tissues of the body from insufficient, imperfect food supply, or from poor absorption of a good food supply. —**marasmic, marasmoid,** *adj.*

mar"ble·i·za'tion. The condition of being marked or veined like marble.

marc (mark, mar). The residue remaining after the extraction of the active principles from a vegetable drug, or after the extraction of the juice or oil from fruits.

march foot. See march *fracture*.

marezine. Trade-mark for cyclizine.

mar'fa·nil. 4-Amino-2-methylbenzenesulfonamide. Also called *homosulfanilamide* and *mesudin*. See *sulfamylon*.

mar·gar'ic ac'id. $CH_3(CH_2)_{15}COOH$. A fatty acid occurring naturally in certain lichens.

mar'ga·rin. The glyceryl ester of margaric acid. **m.·needles.** Fatty crystals found in putrid bronchitis and pulmonary gangrene.

mar'gin. The boundary or edge of a surface. —**marginal,** *adj.*

mar"gi·na'tion. Adhesion of leukocytes to the walls of capillaries in the early stage of inflammation.

mar'gi·no·plas"ty. Plastic surgery of the marginal portion of the eyelid.

mar'go (pl. *margines*). Margin, *q.v.*

ma'ri·hua'na (mah'ri·hwah'nuh, ·nah, marr'i·wah'nuh). See *cannabis*.

mar'jo·ram. Sweet marjoram, *Majorana hortensis* of the Lamiaceae, is a seasoning herb. **Wild marjoram** or origanum consists of the dried leaves and flowering top of *Origanum vulgare*.

mark. Birthmark, a nevus. **port-wine m.** Congenital hemangioma.

mar'row. The soft tissues contained in the medullary canals of long bones and in the interstices of cancellous bone. **primary m.** The embryonic marrow, before it becomes hematopoietic. **red m.** Marrow of all bones in early life and of restricted locations in adulthood in which active formation of blood cells (hematopoiesis) is taking place. Syn., *myeloid tissue*. **yellow m.** Marrow which has lost its hematopoietic function and become largely replaced by fat cells.

mar·ru'bi·um (ma·roo'bee·um). Horehound. The dried leaves and tops of *Marrubium vulgare* of the Lamiaceae.

Marsh's test. See under *test*.

marsh gas. The gaseous products, chiefly methane, formed from decaying, moist organic matter in marshes and mines.

marsh'mal'low. See *althea*.

marsilid. Trade-mark for iproniazid.

mar·su"pi·al·i·za'tion. A surgical procedure used for removing various types of cysts (such as hydatid, pancreatic, etc.) when extirpation of the cyst walls and complete closure are not possible. The cyst is evacuated and the walls sutured to the edges of the wound, leaving the packed cavity to close by granulation. The procedure has been used also in cases of extrauterine pregnancy where the placenta cannot be removed.

Mar'ti·us yel'low (mahr'shus, -shee-us) (C.C.). An acid nitro dye used as a stain and in preparing certain light filters for photomicrography. Also called *Manchester yellow, naphthol yellow.*

M + As. Symbol for compound myopic astigmatism.

mas'cu·line. Having the qualities of a male. —**masculin'ity,** *n.*

mas"cu·lin·i·za'tion. The induction of male secondary sex characteristics in a female or sexually immature animal.

mask. 1. A bandage applied to the face. 2. The characteristic expressionless facies seen in certain pathologic conditions, notably paralysis agitans. 3. A gauze shield, fitted with tapes, to enclose the mouth and nose during surgical operations. 4. An apparatus for covering the nose and mouth in giving anesthetics. **death m.** A plaster or other mold of a dead person's face, taken soon after death. **ecchymotic m.** The cyanotic facies of traumatic asphyxia. **m. of pregnancy.** Irregularly shaped, yellowish patches of varying size which frequently appear on the face and neck during pregnancy.

mask'ing. The interference of a given tone with the perception of other tones.

mas'o·chism" (maz'o·kiz"um, mass'o-). A sexual perversion in which pleasure is obtained in receiving cruel treatment, pain, and humiliation. —**masochist,** *n.*

mass. 1. An aggregation of particles of matter characterized by inertia. Abbreviated, M. 2. A cohesive substance that may be formed into pills. **atomic m.** Mass of an element measured on an arbitrary scale and expressed relatively to mass 16 for oxygen. Also called *atomic weight.*

mas·sage'. A method of rubbing, kneading, or stroking the superficial parts of the body with the hand or with an instrument, for the purpose of modifying nutrition, restoring power of movement, breaking up adhesions,

etc. **buttonhole method of cardiac m.** A means of resuscitation after the heart has stopped beating. A buttonhole incision is made just below the xiphoid process, between the attachments of the two sides of the diaphragm; and the thumb of the right hand is thrust through the opening. The heart can then be compressed between the thumb, within the pericardium, and the fingers, beneath the diaphragm. **electrovibratory m.** That performed by means of an electric vibrator. **vibratory m.** Light, rapid percussion either by hand or by an electric apparatus.

mas·se'ter. A muscle of mastication arising from the zygomatic arch, and inserted on the mandible. See Table of Muscles in the Appendix. —**mas·seter'ic,** *adj.*

mas·seur' (mas·sur'). 1. A man who practices massage. 2. An instrument used for mechanical massage.

mas·seuse' (mas·suz'). A woman who practices massage.

mas"so·ther'a·py. Treatment by massage.

mast"ad·e·ni'tis. Inflammation of the mammary gland. Syn., *mastitis.*

mast"ad·e·no'ma. A glandular tumor of the breast.

mas·tal'gi·a. Pain in the breast.

mast"a·tro'phi·a, mast·at'ro·phy. Atrophy of the breast.

mast cells. Cells with small, spheroid nuclei, with numerous large, metachromatic granules in their cytoplasm; widely distributed in the connective tissues.

mas·tec'to·my. Excision, or amputation, of a breast.

mas"thel·co'sis. Ulceration of the breast.

mas'tic. The resin from the bark of the *Pistacia lentiscus.*

mas"ti·ca'tion. The act of chewing.

mas'ti·ca·to"ry. 1. Pertaining to mastication or to the muscles of mastication. 2. A remedy to be chewed, but not swallowed; used for its local action in the mouth. **m. surface.** The occlusal or biting surface of a tooth.

mas'ti·che (mass'ti·kee). Old term for mastic.

Mas"ti·goph'o·ra. A class of flagellated protozoa which includes both free-living and parasitic species.

mas·ti'tis. Inflammation of the breast. **chronic cystic m.** Any one of various dysplasias of the breast. **interstitial m.** Inflammation of the connective tissue of the breast. **parenchymatous m.** Inflammation of the proper glandular substance of the breast. **puerperal m.** A complication of the early puerperium, in which part or all of the breast becomes in durated from retention of milk and engorgement of the tissues.

mas"to-, mast-. 1. A combining form denoting *the breast.* 2. A combining form denoting *mastoid*

mas"to·car"ci·no'ma. Mammary carcinoma.

mas"to·de·al'gi·a. Pain in, or over, the mastoid process.

mas"to·dyn'i·a. Pain in the breast.

mas'toid. 1. Breast-shaped, as the mastoid process of the temporal bone. 2. The mastoid process of the temporal bone. 3. Pertaining to the mastoid process, as mastoid foramen, mastoid operation.

mas"toid·ec'to·my. Exenteration of the mastoid air cells. **modified radical m.** An operation for the removal of as many potentially infected cells as is possible without disturbing hearing; a simple mastoidectomy is performed, the epitympanic air cells are exenterated without disturbing the ossicular chain, the posterior bony canal wall is partially taken down, and the perilabyrinthine cells are cleaned out. **radical m.** The complete exenteration of mastoid, epitympanic, perilabyrinthine, middle ear, and tubal air cells. The tympanic membrane, ossicular chain, middle ear mucous membrane, stapedius muscle, and tensor tympani muscle are also removed. **simple m.** Exenteration of the air cells in the mastoid process alone, without disturbing those air cells in the epitympanic space, the posterior bony canal wall, or the perilabyrinthine area.

mas"toid·i'tis. Inflammation of the mastoid cells. Formerly called *mastoid abscess.*

mas"toid·ot'o·my. Incision into mastoid cells or the mastoid antrum.

mas·ton'cus. Any tumor of the mammary gland or nipple.

mas·top'a·thy. Any disease or pain of the mammary gland.

mas'to·pex"y. Surgical fixation of a pendulous breast.

mas"to·pla'si·a (mas"to·play'zhuh, ·shuh). Hyperplasia of breast tissue.

mas'to·plas"ty. Plastic surgery on the breast.

mas"tor·rha'gi·a. Hemorrhage from the breast.

mas"to·scir'rhus (mas"to·skirr'us, ·sirr'us). Hardening, or scirrhus, of the breast; usually cancer.

mas·to'sis. Hypertrophy of the breast.

mas·tot'o·my. Incision of the breast.

mas'tous. Having large breasts.

mas"tur·ba'tion. Production of an orgasm by self-manipulation of the genitalia. Also called *self-abuse, chiromania.*

ma·su'ri·um (ma·sue'ree·um, ma·zue'·). Ma, atomic number 43; an ele-

ment reported in 1925, but its existence not established. Subsequently prepared artificially and in 1947 named technetium, *q.v.*

ma·te'ri·a al'ba. A soft, cheeselike, white deposit on the necks of teeth and adjacent gums, made up of epithelial cells, leukocytes, bacteria, and molds.

ma·te'ri·a med'i·ca. The science that treats of the sources and preparations of the substances used in medicine.

ma·ter'nal. Pertaining to the mother.

ma·ter'ni·ty. 1. Motherhood. 2. A lying-in hospital. *Colloquial.*

ma·ti'co (ma·tee'ko). The leaves of *Piper angustifolium,* of the Piperaceae.

ma'ting. The meeting of individuals for sexual reproduction.

mat"ri·ca'ri·a. German camomile; the flower tops of *Matricaria chamomilla,* of the order Compositae. Contains a volatile oil.

ma'trix, mat'rix. 1. A mold; the cavity in which anything is formed. 2. That part of tissue into which any organ or process is set, as the matrix of a nail. 3. The intercellular substance of a tissue, as of cartilage.

matromycin. A trade-mark for oleandomycin phosphate.

mat'ter. 1. Matter is described as having three states of aggregation, solid, liquid, or gaseous. 2. Pus. **gray m.** The gray substance of the central nervous system. Also called *substantia grisea.* **suspended m.** Solid particles, oils, etc., which are either insoluble or not dissolved in a liquid. **white m.** The white substance of the central nervous system. Also called *substantia alba.*

mat'u·rate. Bring to maturity; to ripen, especially to bring a boil to a head; to suppurate.

mat"u·ra'tion. 1. The process of coming to full development. 2. The final series of changes in the growth and formation of the germ cells. It includes two divisions of the cell body but only one division of the chromosomes, with the result that the number of chromosomes in the mature germ cell is reduced to one-half the original number. The term also includes the cytoplasmic changes which occur in the preparation of the germ cell for fertilization.

ma·ture'. 1. Become ripe. 2. Fullgrown, ripe.

ma·tu'ri·ty. The state or quality of being mature; full growth and development.

ma·tu'ti·nal. Occurring in the morning, as matutinal nausea.

max·il'la (pl. *maxillas*). The right or left upper jawbone. See Table of Bones in the Appendix. **—max'illary,** *adj.*

max·il″lo·fa′cial. Pertaining to the lower half of the face. *In plastic surgery*, pertaining to a subdivision called maxillofacial surgery.

max′i·mal. Pertaining to the maximum; highest; greatest.

max′i·mum (pl. *maxima*). The greatest possible degree or amount of anything; the highest point attained or attainable by anything.

may′hem. *In legal medicine*, the offense of depriving a person, by violence, of any limb, member, or organ, or causing any mutilation of the body.

maze. A network of paths, blind alleys, and compartments; used in intelligence tests and in experimental psychology for developing learning curves.

ma·zop′a·thy (may·zop′uth·ee). Any disease of the placenta.

ma′zo·pex″y. Surgical fixation of a pendulous breast; mastopexy.

M. B. *Medicinae Baccalaureus*, Bachelor of Medicine.

mc. Abbreviation for millicurie.

M. C., M. Ch. *Magister Chirurgiae*, Master of Surgery.

mcg, mcg. U.S. Pharmacopeia abbreviation for microgram.

M. D. *Medicinae Doctor*, Doctor of Medicine.

M. D. S. Master of Dental Surgery.

mean. See *arithmetic mean; geometric mean*.

mea′sles. 1. An acute, infectious disease, characterized by a morbilliform eruption and by catarrhal inflammation of the conjunctiva and of the air passages. After a period of incubation of nearly two weeks, the disease begins with coryza, cough, conjunctivitis, and the appearance of Koplik spots on the oral mucous membranes; on the third or fourth day a chill, fever, and dusky rose-red, maculopapular eruption appears, arranged in the form of crescentic groups, at times becoming confluent, usually appearing first on the face or behind the ears. In three or four days, the eruption gradually fades, and is followed by a branny desquamation. The symptoms are worse at the height of the eruption. The disease affects principally the young, is exceedingly contagious, and one attack usually confers immunity. It is caused by a virus. 2. *In veterinary medicine*, a disease of hogs, cattle, and sheep, due to the presence in the body of the larval form of the *Taenia solium* and larvae of other tapeworms. 3. Cysticerci. **black m.** A grave variety of measles in which the eruption is hemorrhagic and the constitutional symptoms are profound. **German m.** See *rubella*. **hemorrhagic m.** See *black m*. **m. vaccine.** The measles virus is grown on fertile eggs of the hen, thus attenuating the infective agent; in-

jected under the skin or placed in the nose, it causes a very mild form of measles in some individuals but causes no symptoms at all in others.

meas′ly. 1. Infected with measles; spotted, as with measles. 2. Pertaining to meat infested with encysted worms of the genus *Trichinella* or with cysticerci of the genus *Taenia*.

meas′ure. For units of measure, see Tables of Weights and Measures in the Appendix.

me·a′to-. *In surgery*, a combining form signifying *meatus* or *opening*.

me″a·tot′o·my. Incision into the urethral meatus.

me·a′tus. An opening or passage. **—meatal,** *adj.* **auditory m.** See *m. acusticus externus* and *m. acusticus internus*. **m. acusticus externus.** The external auditory canal extending from the pinna to the membrana tympani. **m. acusticus internus.** The internal auditory canal. **m. nasopharyngeus.** That part of the nasal cavity communicating with the pharynx beneath the body of the sphenoid. **m. of the nose.** The space between a turbinate bone, or concha, and the lateral wall of a nasal cavity. **m. urethrae.** The orifice of the urethra.

mebaral. A trade-mark for mephobarbital.

mec″a·myl′a·mine hy″dro·chlo′ride. 3-Methylaminoisocamphane hydrochloride, a hypotensive agent. See *inversine hydrochloride*.

mech′a·nism. 1. An aggregation of parts arranged in a mechanical way to perform the functions of a machine. 2. The manner in which a mechanical act is performed, as the mechanism of labor. **trigger m.** A focus located in a region of anoxic cardiac muscle which sets off ventricular extrasystoles or ventricular fibrillation.

mech″a·no·ther′a·py (meck″uh·no·therr′uh·pee). Treatment of injury or disease by mechanical means. **—mechanotherapist,** *n.*

me″chlor·eth′a·mine hy″dro·chlo′ride. Nitrogen methyl bis(β-chloroethyl)amine hydrochloride, a nitrogen mustard type of cytotoxic agent acting mainly on proliferating cells. See *mustargen hydrochloride*.

mecholin. See *mecholyl chloride*.

mecholyl bromide. Trade-mark for acetyl-beta-methylcholine bromide.

mecholyl chloride. Trade-mark for acetyl-beta-methylcholine chloride. See *methacholine chloride*.

me′cism. A condition marked by abnormal prolongation of one or more parts of the body.

me′cli·zine hy″dro·chlo′ride. The dihydrochloride of ᴅ-chlorobenzyl hydryl-4-*m*-methylbenzylpiperazine, drug used to prevent motion sickness. See *bonamine*.

me·com'e·ter. An instrument used in measuring newborn infants.

me''co·nal'gi·a. Pain or neuralgia when the use of opium is discontinued.

mec'on·ate (meck'o-nate, mee'ko-nate). A salt of meconic acid.

mec''o·neu''ro·path'i·a (meck'o-new''ro-path'ee-uh). Nervous disorder due to misuse of opium or its narcotic derivatives.

me·con'ic ac'id (mi-kon'ick, -ko'nick). $C_7H_4O_7$. A dibasic acid found in opium.

me·con'i·dine (mi-kon'i-deen, -din). An alkaloid of opium.

mec'o·nin, me'co·nin. A principle occurring in opium and hydrastis.

mec''o·ni·or·rhe'a. An excessive discharge of meconium.

me·co'ni·um. The pasty, greenish mass, consisting of mucus, desquamated epithelial cells, bile, lanugo hairs, and vernix caseosa, that collects in the intestine of the fetus. It forms the first fecal discharge of the newborn and is not wholly voided until the third or fourth day after birth.

meo'o·no-. A combining form signifying *opium*.

me·cys'ta·sis. A process in which a muscle increases in length but maintains its original degree of tension. Also called *mecystatic relaxation*.

me'di·a. 1. The middle coat of a vein, artery, or lymph vessel; tunica media. 2. Plural of medium. **transparent m. of the eye.** The cornea, aqueous humor, lens, and vitreous body.

me'di·ad. Toward the median plane or line.

me'di·al. Internal, as opposed to lateral (external); toward the midline of the body.

me'di·an. 1. Situated or placed in the middle of the body or in the middle of a part of the body, as the arm. 2. That value on the numerical scale of classification in a frequency distribution below which and above which half the observations fall.

ne''di·as·ti''no·per''i·car·di'tis (mee''dee-ass-tigh''no-, ·ass''ti·no-). Combined inflammation of the mediastinum and the pericardium.

ne''di·as''ti·not'o·my. Incision into the mediastinum.

ne''di·as·ti'num. 1. A partition separating adjacent parts. 2. The space left in the middle of the chest between the two pleurae, divided into the anterior, middle, posterior, and superior mediastinum. The anterior mediastinum contains the internal mammary vessels of the left side, loose areolar tissue, lymphatic vessels, and a few lymph nodes. The middle mediastinum contains the heart and pericardium,

the ascending aorta, the superior vena cava, the bifurcation of the trachea, the pulmonary arteries and veins, and the phrenic nerves. The posterior mediastinum contains a part of the aorta, the greater and lesser azygos veins, the vagus and splanchnic nerves, the esophagus, the thoracic duct, and some lymph nodes. The superior mediastinum, that part lying above the pericardium, contains the origins of the sternohyoid and sternothyroid muscles, and part of the longus colli muscles, the transverse portion of the aortic arch, the innominate, left carotid and subclavian arteries, the superior vena cava and the innominate veins, the left superior intercostal vein, the vagus, cardiac, phrenic, and left recurrent laryngeal nerves, the trachea, esophagus, and thoracic duct, the remains of the thymus, and the lymphatics. **—mediastinal**, *adj.* **m. testis.** A septum in the posterior portion of the testis, formed by a projection inward of the tunica albuginea. Formerly called *body of Highmore*.

me'di·ate. Indirect; performed through something interposed, as mediate percussion, percussion on a pleximeter.

med'i·ca·ble. Amenable to cure.

med'i·cal. Pertaining to medicine, as medical ethics, the principles of conduct which physicians follow.

med'i·cal cen'ter. 1. A medical clinic, usually serving a specific geographic area. 2. A center, incorporating all the medical specialties, for the care and treatment of patients and the diagnosis of disease, and usually providing facilities for medical education and research.

Med'i·cal Corps. In the U. S. Army and Navy Departments and the Air Force, the medical officers of the Regular Army, Navy, and Air Force, the National Guard, and the Reserve Corps, together with medical officers appointed from civil life during war.

Med'i·cal De·part'ment. In the U. S. Army and Navy Departments and the Air Force, a subdivision consisting of commissioned officers, nurses, and enlisted and civilian personnel, with a surgeon general as directing head.

med'i·cal ex·am'in·er. 1. A medical officer appointed to an office of a municipality or state, whose duty it is to determine facts concerning causes of death and to testify thereto in courts of law. The medical examiner in many states and counties replaces the former coroner or coroner's jury. 2. An officer of a corporation or bureau, whose duty it is to determine facts relating to injuries and deaths alleged to have occurred, to place responsibility on the part of the corporation or other agency, and to make recommendations as to compensation. In certain cases, as in life insurance applications, etc., the examiner is charged with passing upon the state of health of the applicant.

med'i·cal group. In the U. S. Army, a command embracing clearing companies, collecting companies, ambulance companies, and those elements required for emergency treatment and evacuation of combat casualties.

me·dic'a·ment, med'i·ca·ment. A medicinal substance.

med'i·ca"ted. Impregnated with a medicinal substance.

med"i·ca'tion. 1. Impregnation with a medicine. 2. Treatment by medicines; the administration of medicines. **hypodermic m.** Treatment by the introduction of medicines beneath the skin, usually by means of a hypodermic syringe. **preanesthetic m.** Administration of drugs, such as sedatives or anticholinergic agents, before anesthetizing a patient, to facilitate induction and to reduce the amount of the anesthetic by allaying apprehension, reducing basal metabolic rate, and lessening oral and nasal secretions.

me·dic'i·nal. Pertaining to, due to, or having the nature of, a medicine, as medicinal rashes, eruptions on the skin following the administration of certain drugs.

me·dic'i·nal. Medicine, 1.

med'i·cine. 1. Any substance used for treating disease. 2. The science of treating disease; the healing art. In a restricted sense, that branch of the healing art that deals with diseases which can be treated by a physician. **anatomic m.** That system which deals with the anatomic changes in diseased organs and their connection with symptoms manifested during life. **aviation m.** That branch of medicine concerned with the pathologic conditions and physiologic and emotional disturbances resulting from aviation flights. **clinical m.** The study of disease by the bedside of the patient. **constitutional m.** That branch of medicine which deals with the relation between a patient's constitution and his susceptibility to disease. See *constitution, 2.* **domestic m.** The treatment of disease or injuries, at home, by a layman. **experimental m.** That based upon experiments on animals by the observation of pathologic changes in diseases induced in them and the effect of drugs administered. **forensic m.** See legal *m.* **group m.** (a) Medicinal practice by a group of physicians associated together for more ready availability of consultation among specialists and for the accessibility to laboratory facilities; some-

times known as a clinic. (b) The practice of medicine carried on under a legal agreement in a community, by a body of registered physicians and surgeons; for the purpose of caring for a group of persons who have subscribed to such service by the payment of a definite sum for a specified time, which entitles each subscriber to medical care and hospitalization under definite rules and regulations. **internal m.** That branch of medicine which treats of diseases that are nonsurgical. **legal m.** Medical jurisprudence, or medicine in its relation to questions of law. Syn. *forensic m.* **military m.** That part of general medicine dealing with the character, epidemiology, prevention and treatment of diseases which are brought about by the special conditions incident to military life. Syn., *war m.* **osteopathic m.** The principles and practice of medicine as employed by osteopaths. **patent m.** (a) Medicine the manufacture of which is protected by a patent. (b) Term commonly applied to an advertised nostrum of secret composition. **physical m.** The science dealing with the treatment of disease by physical agents such as light, heat, cold, water, electricity, massage, and mechanical agents. Also called *physical therapy, physiotherapy.* **practice of m.** The practical application of the principles taught by the theory of medicine. **preventive m.** That which aims at the prevention of disease. **proprietary m.** One, the manufacture of which is limited or controlled by an owner, because of a patent, copyright, or secrecy as regards its constitution or method of manufacture. **psychosomatic m.** That branch of medicine dealing with psychic and physical components as a unit, and the interrelationship between them. **quack m.** A medicine falsely advertised to the laity as being able to cure certain diseases. **regular school of m.** A term formerly used to designate the great mass of the profession as contrasted with the homeopathic and eclectic schools. **socialized m.** State medicine, (b). **social m.** A method for the maintenance and advancement of health and the prevention, amelioration, and cure of disease based on the study of man in relation to his environment, by the medical and sociological agencies in the community. **state m.** (a) Legal medicine. (b) The control or direction of the practice of medicine by the state. Also called *socialized m., federal m.* **tropical m.** That branch of medicine, science concerned chiefly with diseases found commonly or exclusively in the tropical or subtropical regions. **veterinary m.** That branch of medicine practice which treats of the diseases and injuries of animals. **war m.** See military *m.*

med″i·co·chi·rur'gi·cal (med″i-ko·kigh·rur'ji·kul). Pertaining conjointly to medicine and surgery.

med″i·co·le'gal. Relating both to medicine and law.

med″i·co·psy·chol'o·gy. The study of mental diseases in relation to medicine.

med″i·co·sta·tis'tic. Relating to medicine as connected with statistics.

medinal. Trade-mark for a brand of barbital sodium.

me'di·o-, me'di-. A combining form meaning *middle;* used to denote *medially, relating to the middle* or *median plane,* or *intermediate.*

me″di·o·car'pal. Pertaining to the articulation between the two rows of carpal bones.

me″di·o·dor'sal. Both median and dorsal; on the median line of the back.

me″di·o·fron'tal. Pertaining to the middle of the forehead.

me″di·o·tar'sal. Pertaining to the middle articulations of the tarsal bones.

Med″i·ter·ra'ne·an fe'ver. See *brucellosis.*

me'di·um. 1. That in which anything moves or through which it acts. 2. *In bacteriology,* a substance used for the cultivation of bacteria; may be modified for certain purposes. Also see *culture.*

me'di·us. 1. The middle. 2. The middle finger.

medomin. Trade-mark for heptabarbital.

me·dul'la. 1. The marrow. 2. The medulla oblongata. 3. Anything resembling marrow in its structure or in its relation to other parts, as a fatty substance or marrow occupying certain cavities; the central parts of certain organs as distinguished from the cortex. —**med'ullary,** *adj.* **m. oblongata.** The lower part of the brain stem, extending from the spinal cord opposite the foramen magnum to the pons. **m. ossium.** Bone marrow.

med″ul·la'ted (med″uh·lay″tid, midull'ay·tid). Provided with a myelin sheath. Syn., *myelinated.*

med″ul·la'tion. The process of acquiring a myelin sheath, as in the case of many nerve fibers in the course of their development; myelinization.

med″ul·li·za'tion. Conversion into marrow, as the replacement of bone tissue in the course of osteitis.

med″ul·lo·blas·to'ma (med″uh·lo-blas·to'muh, mi·dull″o·). A malignant brain tumor with a tendency to spread in the meninges; most common in the cerebellum of children. The cells show many mitoses, are small, with scanty cytoplasm, dense spheroid or oval

nuclei, and have a tendency to form pseudo rosettes.

meg'a-, meg-. A combining form meaning *great, mighty;* used to signify *great, extended.*

meg″a·car'di·a. A large heart. Hypertrophy of the heart.

meg″a·co'lon. Congenital, hypertrophic dilatation of the colon; called *Hirschsprung's disease.*

meg'a·dont. Having abnormally large teeth; macrodont.

meg″a·du″o·de'num (meg″uh-dew″o·dee'num, ·dew·od'i·num). Idiopathic dilatation of the duodenum.

meg″a·e·soph'a·gus. An abnormally large esophagus.

meg″a·gna'thus (meg″uh·nayth'us). Large-jawed.

meg″a·kar'y·o·cyte. A giant cell of the bone marrow containing a large lobulated nucleus. Its cytoplasm is thought to fragment, thus producing the blood platelets.

meg'a·lo-, megal-. A combining form meaning *large, great;* used especially to denote *abnormal enlargement.*

meg″a·lo·blast″. A large erythroblast with a characteristic nuclear pattern, formed in marrow in liver principle deficiency anemias during relapse. The basophilic, polychromatophilic, and acidophilic (orthochromatic) forms mature to become nonnucleated megalocytes. Megaloblasts may appear in the peripheral blood. They resemble erythroblasts from embryos and fishes. Megaloblast is not synonymous with macronormoblast.

meg″a·lo·car'di·a. Auxesis; hypertrophy of the heart.

meg″a·lo·ce·phal'ic. Largeheaded; applied to a skull the capacity of which exceeds 1450 cc.

meg″a·lo·ceph'a·ly. 1. The condition of having a very large head. 2. A disease characterized by progressive enlargement of the head, face, and neck, involving both the bony and the soft tissues. Also called *leontiasis ossea.*

meg″a·lo·chei'rous (meg″uh·lo-kigh'rus). Large-handed.

meg″a·lo·cor'ne·a. An enlarged cornea.

meg″a·lo·cy·to'sis (meg″uh·lo·sigh·to'sis). The occurrence of megalocytes and megaloblasts in peripheral blood.

meg″a·lo·en'ter·on. An excessively large intestine.

meg″a·lo·gas'tri·a. Abnormal enlargement of the stomach.

meg″a·lo·ma'ni·a. The delusion of personal greatness, a symptom common in schizophrenia and other psychoses. Patient expresses and acts out ideas of exalted attainment. —**megalomanic,** *adj.;* **megalomaniac,** *n.*

meg″a·lo·me'li·a. Gigantism of one or more limbs.

meg″a·lo·ny·cho′sis (meg″uh-lo-ni·ko′sis). Universal, noninflammatory hypertrophy of the nails.

meg″a·loph·thal′mus. Excessive largeness of the eyes.

meg″a·lo·splanch′nic. Possessing large viscera, especially a large liver.

meg′a·phone. An instrument used for assisting the hearing of the deaf, by means of large reflectors of the sound waves.

meg″a·pros′o·pous. Having an unusually large face.

meg′a·volt″. A unit equal to 1,000,-000 volts.

meg′ohm″. An electric unit equal to 1,000,000 ohms.

me′grim. Old term for migraine.

Meibom, Heinrich [*German physician and anatomist*, 1638–1700]. Described the tarsal glands, *q.v.*, also called *Meibom's glands, Meibomian glands.* Chalazion is also called *Meibomian cyst.*

mei′o- (migh′o-). See *mio-*.

mei·o′sis (migh·o′sis). The nuclear changes which take place in the last two cell divisions in the formation of the germ cells. The chromosomes divide once but the cell body divides twice with the result that the nucleus of the mature ovum or sperm contains the reduced (haploid) number of chromosomes. Syn., *reduction division.* **—meiotic,** *adj.*

mel. 1. Honey; the saccharine secretion deposited in the honeycomb by the bee. 2. A preparation of honey with some medicinal substance.

mel-. *In medicine,* a combining form signifying *limb.*

mel-, mel′o-. *In medicine,* a combining form meaning *cheek.*

me·la′gra, me·lag′ra. Muscular pains in the extremities.

me·lal′gi·a. Pain or neuralgia in the extremities.

mel″an·cho′li·a, mel′an·chol″y. A form of mental disorder characterized by extreme depression, fear, brooding, and painful delusions. All activity is usually inhibited, but a melancholic patient may show psychomotor overactivity (agitated depression) or he may have many depressive ideas that shift rapidly (depressive mania). When mild, a melancholic state is called retardation. When moderate, it is called acute depression. When severe, it may become stuporous depression. **—melanchol′ic,** *adj.;* **melancho′liac,** *n.* **climacteric m.** That occurring at the menopause. **involutional m.** A form of melancholia, arising during the involutional period; characterized by agitation, anxiety, and brooding in conjunction with narrow mental horizons and lack of adaptability. See *involutional psychosis.* **m. agitata.**

(a) Old term for catatonia. (b) Agitated melancholia. A form associated with excessive motor excitement; usually implies association with manic-depressive psychosis or with involutional melancholia. **m. attonita.** The morbid state characterized by muscular rigidity. Common in catatonia. **m. simplex.** Simple depression. A mild form without delusions. **paranoid m.** The depressive phase of manic-depressive psychosis when it assumes a paranoid character. Syn., *melancholic insanity.*

mel′a·nin. A group of black or dark brown pigments; produced by metabolic activity of certain specialized cells. Occurs naturally in the choroid coat of the eye, the skin, hair, cardiac muscle, and pia mater.

mel′a·nism. Abnormal deposition of dark pigment (melanin) in tissues, in organs, or in the skin.

mel′a·no-, melan-. A combining form signifying *dark-colored,* or *relating to* melanin.

mel′a·no·blast″. An immature melanin-forming cell.

mel″a·no·blas·to′ma. Melanoma.

mel″a·no·car″ci·no′ma. Melanoma.

mel″a·no·der′ma, mel″a·no·der′mi·a. Black pigmentation of the skin. **—melanodermic,** *adj.*

mel″a·no·ep″i·the″li·o′ma. A pigmented, malignant epithelioma.

me·lan′o·gen. The colorless precursor which is transformed into melanin on oxidation. Patients, especially those with widespread melanomas, may excrete urine containing melanogen; on standing or oxidation, the urine becomes dark brown or black.

mel″a·no·gen′e·sis. The formation of melanin.

mel″a·no′ma. A malignant tumor, derived from melanophores of skin, of the choroid, of the anus, of meninges, and perhaps of adrenals, the cells of which are of immature type and which may or may not contain granules of melanin.

mel″a·no·ma·to′sis. 1. Widespread distribution of melanoma. 2. Diffuse melanotic pigmentation of the meninges.

mel″a·no·nych′i·a (mel″uh·no·nick′ee·uh). A condition in which the fingernails or toenails turn black.

mel′a·no·phore″, me·lan′o·phore. A cell of the connective tissue which bears granules of brown pigment (melanin) in its cytoplasm. Melanophores are partly responsible for color changes in many animals. Also called *dermal melanoblast.*

mel″a·no·pla′ki·a. Pigmentation of the mucous membrane of the mouth, usually in patches and occasionally with leukoplakia superimposed.

mel"a·no·sar·ce'ma. Melanoma.

mel"a·no'sis. Dark brown or brownish black pigmentation of surfaces by melanins or, in some instances, by hematogenous pigments. In the skin, melanosis is observed in such conditions as sunburn, Addison's disease, various dermatoses, and about the nipples and elsewhere in pregnancy. **—melanot'ic,** adj. **m. iridis.** The invasion of the iris by melanoblasts; a form of melanosis of the eye.

mel"a·not'ri·chous (mel"uh·not'ri·kus). Black-haired.

mel"a·nu'ri·a. The presence of black pigment in the urine, the result of oxidation of melanogen. **—melanuric,** adj.

me·le'na, me·lae'na. The discharge of stools colored black by altered blood. **m. neonatorum.** An extravasation of blood into the stomach and intestines of the newborn infant, occurring most often in the first few hours of life.

me·lex'i·tose. Trisaccharide obtained from the Douglas fir and the larch. Also called melicitose.

mel'i-. A combining form meaning honey.

mel"i·bi'ase. An enzyme from certain brewer's yeasts catalyzing the hydrolysis of melibiose.

mel"i·bi'ose. A disaccharide obtained from certain carbohydrates, notably molasses.

mel"i·lot'ic ac'id. OH.C₆H₄(CH₂)₂-COOH. An acid in Melilotus species and in coumarin.

Mel"i·lo'tus. A genus of the Leguminosae. **M. officinalis.** Yellow sweet clover.

melin. Rutin.

me"li·oi·do'sis. An infectious granuloma in rodents, similar to glanders; caused by Malleomyces pseudomallei.

Me·lis'sa. A genus of plants of the Labiatae.

me·lis'sic ac'id. CH₃(CH₂)₂₈COOH. An acid occurring in beeswax.

me·lis"so·pho'bi·a. A morbid fear of bees.

me·li'tis. Inflammation of the cheek.

mel"i·tose. See raffinose.

mel"i·tox'in. Dicoumarin.

mel"i·tri'ose. Raffinose.

mel"i·tu'ri·a. General term indicating the presence of any sugar in urine.

mel'o-. See mel-, melo-.

me·lom'e·lus. An individual with one or more rudimentary accessory limbs attached to a limb.

me·los'chi·sis (mi·los'ki·sis). A congenital cleft of the cheek.

me·lo'tus. An individual showing

congenital displacement of the ear, which lies on the cheek.

melt'ing point. The degree of temperature at which fusible solids begin to melt. Abbreviated, m.p.

mem'ber. A part of the body, especially a projecting part, as the leg or the arm.

mem'brane. A thin layer of tissue surrounding a part, separating adjacent cavities, lining a cavity, or connecting adjacent structures. **animal m.** A membrane made from animal tissues, used in dialyzing. **basal m. of Bruch.** That which forms the outer of the four layers of the choroid coat of the eye. **basement m.** The delicate, noncellular membrane on which an epithelium is seated. **basilar m.** The membranous portion of the spiral lamina separating the scala vestibuli from the scala tympani, extending from the base to the apex of the cochlea and supporting the organ of Corti. **Bowman's m.** A thin membrane which separates the corneal epithelium from the substantia propria of the cornea. **choroid m.** That part of the vascular tunic, or uvea, of the eye which extends anteriorly as far as the ora serrata. **croupous m.** The yellowish white membrane forming in the larynx in tracheobronchitis. **decidual m.** One of the membranes formed by the superficial part of the endometrium during pregnancy. See decidua basalis, decidua capsularis, decidua parietalis. **Descemet's m.** The posterior elastic lamina of the cornea which covers the posterior surface of the substantia propria. **diphtheritic m.** A fibrinous layer formed on a mucous membrane or cutaneous surface and extending downward for a variable depth. It is the result of coagulation necrosis, generally brought about by the bacillus of diphtheria. **elastic m.** One composed of elastic fibrous tissue. **external elastic m.** That of the arterial wall, forming the boundary between the tunica media and tunica adventitia. **external limiting m.** (a) In the eye, the thin layer between the outer nuclear layer of the retina and that of the rods and cones. (b) In embryology, the membrane investing the outer surface of the neural tube. **extraembryonic m.** Any of the membranes surrounding the embryo or fetus, shed at birth. See amnion, chorion, yolk sac, allantois. **fenestrated m.** One of the layers of elastic tissue in the media and intima of large arteries. **fetal m.** A name given to the chorion, amnion, or allantois. **fibroserous m.** A thin, transparent, glistening structure forming closed sacs that contain certain organs. They are the peritoneum, the two pleurae, the pericardium, the tunica vaginalis testis, the arachnoid, and synovial membranes. **hyalin m.** (a) Basement membrane. (b) The membrane between the inner fibrous layer of a hair follicle and its outer root sheath. (c) The basement membrane of a Graafian follicle. **hyaloid m.** The limiting membrane surrounding the vitreous body, and forming the suspensory ligament and zonule. **hyoglossal m.** The membrane at the posterior portion of the tongue: unites the tongue to the hyoid bone and gives attachment to the posterior fibers of the genioglossus muscle. **intercostal m.** Either of the membranes between the ribs, which replaces either intercostal muscle. **internal elastic m.** Forms the boundary between the tunica intima and the tunica media, being prominent in arteries of medium caliber. **internal limiting m.** (a) In the eye, the inner layer of the retina. (b) *In embryology,* the membrane which lines the lumen of the neural tube. **interosseous m.** (a) Of the forearm, the strong fibrous membrane between the interosseous borders of the radius and ulna. (b) Of the leg, the strong fibrous sheet between the interosseous crests of the tibia and fibula. **m. bone.** Any bone that originates, not in cartilage, but in membrane, as some of the cranial bones. **mucous m.** The membrane lining those cavities and canals communicating with the air. It is kept moist by the secretions of various types of glands. **nuclear m.** The layer of condensed protoplasm at the periphery of the nucleus. **obturator m.** (a) That of the pelvis, the fibrous membrane closing the obturator foramen. (b) That of the stapes, the thin membrane between the crura and footplate. **perineal m.** Fibrous membrane stretching across the pubic arch and dividing the urogenital triangle into a superficial and a deep portion; also called *inferior fascia of the urogenital diaphragm.* **periodontal m.** The connective tissue between the root of a tooth and the bone of the alveolar process, or extending from the root into the gingiva. Syn., *pericementum.* Once called *peridental m.* **permeable m.** One which permits the passage of water and certain dissolved substances. **placental m.** The tissues of the placenta separating the maternal and fetal blood streams. Syn., *placental barrier.* **pyogenic m.** The lining of an abscess cavity or a fistulous tract. The term should be restricted to the lining of an abscess that is spreading and in which the membrane produces pus. **quadrangular m.** The membrane of the

larynx which extends from the aryepiglottic folds above to the level of the ventricular folds below. **semipermeable m.** One which permits water to pass but which holds back salts and their ions. **serous m.** A delicate membrane covered with flat, mesothelial cells lining closed cavities of the body. **sternal m.** The periosteum ensheathing the sternum in front and behind. **suprapleural m.** The extrapleural fascia attached to the inner margin of the first rib and covering the dome of the pleura. Also called *Sibson's fascia.* **synovial m.** The lining of an articular capsule, concerned with formation of synovial fluid into the articular cavity; it is lacking over articular surfaces. **tectorial m.** A jellylike membrane covering the organ of Corti in the internal ear. **tympanic m.** The drum membrane; the membrane separating the external from the middle ear. It consists of three layers: an outer or skin layer, a fibrous layer, and an inner mucosal layer. **urogenital m.** That part of the cloacal membrane cranial or ventral to the urorectal septum; it forms the floor of the urethral groove of the phallus. **vestibular m.** A thin membrane within the semicircular ducts of the ear, stretching from the upper surface of the osseous spiral lamina to the outer wall of the cochlea, separating the cochlear duct from the scala vestibuli. **vitelline m.** A structureless cytoplasmic membrane on the surface of the ovum.

mem'brum. Member. **m. muliebre.** The clitoris. **m. virile.** The penis.

mem'o·ry. That faculty of the mind by which ideas and sensations are recalled. **anterograde m.** Memory for events in the remote past; forgetfulness for recent occurrences, or retrograde amnesia, is implied. **retrograde m.** Memory for events in the recent past, as contrasted with retrograde amnesia, the loss of memory for recent events.

me·nac'me. The period of a woman's life during which menstruation persists.

men"·a·di'ol. 2-Methyl-1,4-naphthohydroquinone or 2-methyl-1,4-naphthalenediol, the alcohol obtained from menadione. **m. sodium diphosphate.** The hexahydrate of the tetrasodium salt of menadiol diphosphate possessing vitamin-K activity and used as an antihemorrhagic agent. See *synkayvite.*

men·ad'i·one (men-ad·ee-ohn, men"·uh·dye'ohn). 2-Methyl-1,4-naphthoquinone, occurring as a bright-yellow powder; practically insoluble in water. Possesses vitamin-K activity in hemor rhagic diatheses due to prothrombin deficiency in the blood. Syn., **menaphthone,** synthetic vitamin K, vitamin K_3. See **proklot. m. sodium bisulfite.** A water-soluble compound containing 50% menadione; suited for parenteral administration.

men·aph'thone. The British Pharmacopoeia name for menadione.

men·ar'che (men·ar'kee). The time when menstruation starts. **delayed m.** Late onset of menstruation.

Mendel, Gregor Johann [Austrian botanist, 1822–84]. Discovered a principle, called *Mendel's law* or *Mendelian law,* governing the inheritance of certain characteristics: in a specific character the individual offspring is not intermediate between the parents, but is like one parent or the other, and a specific character may be dominant or recessive. For example, in crossing red and white flowers, Mendel found that the first generation of hybrids were all red, and when self-fertilized produced red- and white-flowering plants in the ratio of 3:1. See Mendelian *ratio.* In this case the red was dominant, the white recessive. When the second generation of hybrids was self-fertilized, the white bred true, as did one of each three reds; the remaining two reds produced both colors, again in the ratio of three dominant to one recessive. The term *Mendelism* applies to the body of knowledge growing out of Mendel's discovery; it refers to all inheritance through the chromosomes, in contradistinction to non-Mendelian inheritance depending on autonomous bodies in the cytoplasm. See also *Mendel's laws* under *law.*

me·nin'ge·al. Pertaining to the meninges.

me·nin'ges (mi·nin'jeez). Plural of meninx.

me·nin''gi·o'ma. A tumor situated usually in the meninges, but occasionally in other parts of the central nervous system, probably derived from cells of the meningeal primordium. Grows by expansion but may be invasive. Also called *dural endothelioma, arachnoid fibroblastoma, meningeal fibroblastoma, dural sarcoma.*

me·nin'gism, men'in·gism. 1. An acute, infectious state of meningeal irritation, usually associated with the specific fevers and pneumonias in childhood. **2.** A hysterical state simulating meningitis. Also called *meningismus.*

men''in·git'i·des (men#in·jit'i·jeez). Plural of meningitis.

men''in·gi'tis. Inflammation of the membranes of the brain or cord; that of the dura is termed *pachymeningitis;* that of the piarachnoid, *leptomeningitis,* or simply meningitis. **—menin-**

git'ic, *adj.* **acute pyogenic m.** Acute inflammation of the meninges due to the streptococcus, pneumococcus, micrococcus, or pyogenic organisms other than the meningococcus. **bacteroides m.** Meningitis due to anaerobic, Gram-negative, nonspore-bearing bacilli (*Bacteroides*). **basilar m.** Inflammation of the meninges at the base of the brain. **cerebrospinal m.** Inflammation of the meninges of the brain and spinal cord. **epidemic cerebrospinal m.** An acute purulent inflammation of the meninges of endemic and epidemic incidence caused by the *Neisseria meningitidis* (meningococcus). **gummatous m.** A granulomatous infection of the meninges occurring in the third stage of syphilis. **influenzal m.** A form of inflammation of the meninges caused by the *Hemophilus influenzae* (influenza bacillus). **m. serosa circumscripta.** Inflammation of the meninges with formation of cystic accumulations of fluid which cause symptoms of tumors. **plasmodial m.** Meningitis caused by some form of *Plasmodium.* **rickettsial m.** Meningitis caused by some member of the Rickettsiae. **serous m.** Meningitis associated with a cranial focus of infection, for example mastoiditis, without the passage of organisms into the cerebrospinal fluid. **spinal m.** Inflammation of the meninges of the spinal cord, usually secondary to osteitis of the vertebrae. **sterile m.** Meningitis without infection, usually resulting from subarachnoid injection of foreign materials such as gases, serums, or chemical compounds. **syphilitic m.** Inflammation of the meninges caused by syphilis. **traumatic m.** Meningitis resulting from the invasion of organisms after injuries to the head or spine. **tuberculous m.** Inflammation of the meninges due to the tubercle bacillus which reaches the brain from a distant focus via the blood stream; the disease occurs most commonly in children. **virus m.** Meningitis caused by a virus. **yeast m.** Meningitis caused by a form of yeast such as *Torula.*

me·nin'go- (muh·ning'go-, meh·nin'go-), **mening-.** A combining form meaning *membrane* or denoting *the meninges.*

me·nin'go·cele. A protrusion of the cerebral or spinal meninges through a defect in the cranium or vertebral column. It forms a cyst filled with cerebrospinal fluid.

me·nin''go·coc·ce'mi·a (·cock·see'mee·uh). The presence of meningococci in the blood.

me·nin''go·coc'cus. Common name for the coccus *Neisseria meningitidis.*

—meningococcal, meningococcic (-cock'sick), *adj.*

me·nin"go·cor'ti·cal. Pertaining to the meninges and the cerebral cortex.

me·nin'go·cyte. A flattened epithelioid cell lining a subarachnoid space, which may become phagocytic.

me·nin"go·en·ceph'a·li'tis. Inflammation of the brain and its membranes.

me·nin"go·en·ceph'a·lo·cele. Hernia of the brain and its meninges through a defect in the skull.

me·nin"go·en·ceph"a·lo·my"e·li'tis. Combined inflammation of the meninges, brain, and spinal cord.

me·nin"go·en·ceph"a·lop'a·thy. Disease of the brain and meninges.

me·nin"go·my"e·li'tis. Inflammation of the spinal cord and its meninges.

me·nin"go·my'e·lo·cele. A protrusion of a portion of the spinal cord and membranes through a defect in the vertebral column.

men"in·gop'a·thy. Any disease of the cerebrospinal meninges.

me·nin"go·ra·dic'u·lar. Pertaining to the meninges and nerve roots (cranial or spinal).

me·nin"go·rha·chid'i·an (·ra·kid'ee·un). Pertaining to the spinal cord and its membranes.

me·nin"gor·rha'gi·a. Hemorrhage from the meninges.

me·nin"go·vas'cu·lar. Involving both the meninges and the cerebral blood vessels, as meningovascular syphilis. See *syphilis.*

men"in·gu'ri·a. The passage, or presence, of membranous shreds in the urine.

me'ninx (pl. *meninges*). A membrane, especially one of the brain or spinal cord; the meninges covering the brain and spinal cord consist of the dura, pia, and arachnoid.

men"is·cec'to·my (men"i·seck'to·mee). The surgical excision of a meniscus or semilunar cartilage.

men"is·ci'tis (men"i·sigh'tis, ·sky'tis). An inflammation of any interarticular cartilage; specifically, of the semilunar cartilages of the knee joint.

me·nis'cus (pl. *meniscuses, menisci*). 1. A crescent or crescentic body, especially an interarticular fibrocartilage. 2. A concavoconvex lens (positive meniscus) or a convexoconcave lens (negative meniscus). 3. The curved surface of a column of liquid. **m. lateralis.** The external, semilunar fibrocartilage of the knee joint. **m. medialis.** The internal, semilunar fibrocartilage of the knee joint. **tactile m.** A form of nerve ending with a concave surface turned ectad, each concavity containing a tactile cell.

men'o-. A combining form meaning *month;* denotes *relation to the menses.*

men"o·ce'lis. Dark, erythematous or hemorrhagic spots occurring upon the skin in amenorrhea.

men'o·lip'sis. The retention or absence of the menses; amenorrhea.

men'o·pause (men'o·pawz). The physiologic cessation of menstruation usually between the forty-fifth and fiftieth years. Also called *climacteric.* **—menopausic, menopaus'al,** *adj.*

men'o·pha'ni·a. The first appearance of the menses; menarche.

men'o·pla'ni·a. A discharge of blood occurring at the menstrual period, but derived from some part of the body other than the uterus; vicarious menstruation.

men"or·rha'gi·a. See *hypermenorrhea.* To be distinguished from polymenorrhea, metrorrhagia, intermenstrual flow, *q.v.* **functional m.** Excessive menstruation due to no demonstrable anatomic or pathologic lesion; usually assumed to be due to endocrine dysfunction.

men"or·rhal'gi·a. Pelvic pain other than characteristic midline cramp at the menstrual period; characteristic of endometriosis.

men"or·rhe'a, men"or·rhoe'a. 1. The normal flow of the menses. 2. Excessive menstruation.

me·nos'che·sis (mi·nos'ki·sis, men"o·skee'sis). Retention of the menses.

men"o·sta'si·a (men"o·stay'zhuh·zee·uh), **me·nos'ta·sis.** A suppression of the menstrual flow.

men"o·stax'is. Prolonged menstruation.

mens. Mind. *Compos mentis,* of sound mind. *Non compos mentis,* of unsound mind.

men'ses (men'seez). The recurrent monthly discharge of blood from the genital canal of a woman during sexual maturity.

men'stru·ant. 1. Subject to, or capable of, menstruating. 2. One who menstruates.

men'stru·ate. Discharge the menses.

men"stru·a'tion. A periodic discharge of a sanguineous fluid from the uterus, occurring during the period of a woman's life from puberty to the menopause. **—men'strual,** *adj.* **anovular m.** That unaccompanied by the discharge of the ovum. **regurgitant m.** A backflow through the uterine tubes. **supplementary m.** A discharge of blood from some other site, accompanying menstruation. **suppressed m.** Nonappearance of the menstrual flow in patients who formerly menstruated. Syn., *menostasia.*

vicarious m. The discharge of blood at the time of menstruation from some place other than the vagina.

men'su·al (men'shoo·ul, men'sue·ul). Monthly.

men"su·ra'tion (men"shoo·ray'shun, men"sue·). The act of measuring; one of the methods of physical diagnosis.

men'tal. Pertaining to the mind.

men'tal. Pertaining to the chin. Syn., *genial.*

men'tal age. A score, derived from intelligence tests, expressed in terms of the age at which an average individual attains that score. Abbreviation, MA.

men'tal de·fi'ciency. Feeblemindedness; arrested or incomplete mental development. May be of three grades: idiocy, the lowest; imbecility, the intermediate; and moronity, the highest.

men'tal dis·or'der. A psychiatric condition or reaction, sometimes the result of impairment or disease of the brain or of difficulty or inability to adjust to environment. See also *mental deficiency.*

men·ta'lis. A muscle of the lower lip. See Table of Muscles in the Appendix.

men·tal'i·ty. Mental activity and power; intellect.

Men'tha. A genus of plants of the Labiatae; the mints. **M. piperita.** Peppermint. The dried leaves and flowering tops of *M. piperita.* **M. pulegium.** European pennyroyal. See also *hedeoma.* **M. viridis.** Spearmint. The dried leaves and flowering tops of *M. spicata.*

men'tho-, menth-. A combining form denoting *menthol.*

men'thol. $C_{10}H_{19}OH$. A solid alcohol obtained from peppermint oil or other mint oils, or prepared synthetically. Very slightly soluble in water. Used for anesthetic, counterirritant, or antiseptic effects. **camphorated m.** A liquid mixture of equal parts of menthol and camphor; used externally as a counterirritant and anodyne.

men'thone. $C_{10}H_{18}O$. The ketone of menthol; obtained from peppermint oil.

men'to-. *In anatomy,* a combining form signifying *pertaining to the chin.*

men"y·an'thes (men"ee·an'theez). The dried leaves of *Menyanthes trifoliata.* Also called *buckbean.*

mep'a·crine hy"dro·chlo'ride (mep'uh·kreen, mi·pack'reen). British Pharmacopoeia name for quinacrine hydrochloride, *q.v.*

mep'a·crine meth"ane·sul'fo·nate. The British Pharmacopoeia name for quinacrine methanesulfonate.

mep'a·zine. 10-[(1-Methyl-3-piperidyl)methyl]phenothiazine, an antiemetic and tranquilizer, used in the

form of acetate and hydrochloride salts. See *pacatal.*

me·per'i·dine hy"dro·chlo'ride (meh·perr'i·deen, mep'ur·i·deen"). The hydrochloride of ethyl 1-methyl-4-phenylpiperidine-4-carboxylate. A colorless powder, soluble in water. It exerts both the analgesic and sedative action of morphine and the antispasmodic action of atropine. See *demerol hydrochloride, dolantin, isonipecaine, pethidine.*

me·phen'e·sin, meph"e·ne'sin. $CH_2C_6H_4OCH_2.CHOH.CH_2OH$. α,β-Dihydroxy-γ-(2-methylphenoxy)-propane, colorless crystals; soluble in water. An antispasmodic. See *avosyl, lissephen, myanesin, oranizon, tolserol.*

meph"o·bar'bi·tal. 5-Ethyl-1-methyl-5-phenylbarbituric acid, a sedative. See *mebaral.*

mephyton. Trade-mark for phytonadione.

meprane dipropionate. Trademark for promethestrol dipropionate, a synthetic estrogen.

me"pro·bam'ate. 2-Methyl-2-n-propyl-1,3-propanediol dicarbamate, a psychotherapeutic agent. See *equanil, miltown.*

mEq. Milliequivalent.

me·ral'gi·a. Neuralgic pain in the thigh. **m. paresthetica.** Bernhardt's term for a paresthesia of the skin at the lower and outer aspect of the thigh in the region supplied by the lateral cutaneous nerve of the thigh. Also called *Roth-Bernhardt disease, Roth's disease.*

me·ral'lu·ride (meh·ral'yoo·ride, ·rid). A mixture of approximately molecular proportions of methoxyhydroxymercuripropylsuccinylurea and theophylline, used as a diuretic. See *mercuhydrin.*

mer·bro'min. The disodium salt of 2,7-dibromo-4-hydroxymercurifluorescein, occurring as green scales or granules forming a red solution with yellowgreen fluorescence; freely soluble in water. A surgical disinfectant. See *mercurochrome.*

mer·cap'tal, mer"cap·tal'. A product of the union of a mercaptan and an aldehyde.

mer·cap'tan, mer"cap·tan'. A derivative of an alcohol in which the oxygen is replaced by sulfur.

mer·cap"to·mer'in so'di·um. Disodium N-[3-(carboxymethylmercaptomercuri)-2-methoxypropyl]-α-camphoramate, a mercurial diuretic. See *thiomerin sodium.*

mer·cap"to·pu'rine. 6-Mercaptopurine, the analog of 6-aminopurine or adenine, a cytotoxic agent useful for treatment of leukemias. See *purinethol.*

mer"co·cre'sols. A mixture of secondary amyltricresol and o-hydroxyphenylmercuric nitrate, used as a germicide and fungicide. See *mercresin*.

mercresin. Trade-mark for a solution of mercocresols.

mercuhydrin. Trade-mark for meralluride.

mer·cu″ma·til′in. A mercurial diuretic containing 8-(2′-methoxy-3′-hydroxymercuripropyl) coumarin-3-carboxylic acid and theophylline.

mer·cu·ri-. A combining form signifying *mercury*; used in chemistry to denote *mercuric*.

mer·cu″ri·al. 1. Pertaining to or caused by mercury. 2. Any preparation of mercury or its salts.

mer·cu″ri·a′lis. An herbaceous European plant, *Mercurialis annua*. Also called *mercury herb, French mercury*.

mer·cu″ri·al·ism. Poisoning due to absorption of mercury.

mer·cu′ric. Pertaining to mercury as a bivalent element. **m. chloride.** See mercury bichloride. **m. cyanide.** Hg(CN)₂. Colorless or white crystals, soluble in water. **m. nitrate.** Hg(NO₃)₂. A white or slightly yellow deliquescent salt, soluble in water. **m. oxycyanide.** Approximately Hg(CN)₂.HgO. A white powder, soluble in water; used locally as an antiseptic. **m. salicylate.** A white powder of variable composition containing 54–59% Hg, practically insoluble in water. **m. succinimide.** C₄H₅NO₄Hg. A white powder, soluble in water; used in the treatment of syphilis. **red m. iodide.** HgI₂. A scarlet-red powder, insoluble in water, but soluble in solutions of iodides. **red m. oxide.** HgO. An orange-red powder, almost insoluble in water. **yellow m. oxide.** HgO. A yellow powder, differing from the red variety in being more finely subdivided.

mercurochrome. Trade-mark for the disodium salt of 2,7-dibromo-4-hydroxymercurifluorescein. See *merbromin*.

mercurophen. Trade-mark for sodium hydroxymercuri-o-nitrophenolate. A brick-red powder.

mer″cu·ro·phyl′line (mur″cue-ro-fill′een, ·in). The sodium salt of β-methoxy-γ-hydroxymercuripropylamide of trimethylcyclopentanedicarboxylic acid and of theophylline in approximately molecular proportions. Employed intravenously as a diuretic. See *mercuzanthin*.

mer·cu′rous, mer′cu·rous. Pertaining to compounds containing mercury as a univalent radical. **mild m. chloride.** HgCl. A white powder, insoluble in water; used as an antisyphilitic, cathartic, diuretic, and antiseptic.

Syn., *calomel*. **yellow m. iodide.** HgI. A yellow, amorphous powder, practically insoluble in water; used as an antisyphilitic.

mer′cu·ry. Hg = 200.61. A shining, silver-white, liquid, volatile metal, having a specific gravity of 13.55. **ammoniated m.** NH₂HgCl. Mercuric ammonium chloride; used chiefly locally to treat various skin conditions. Syn., *white precipitate*. **m. bichloride.** HgCl₂. Corrosive sublimate; employed for the systemic effects of mercury as well as for its germicidal property.

mercuzanthin. Trade-mark for mercurophylline injection.

me·rid′i·an. A circle surrounding a sphere and intersecting the poles. **m. of the eye.** A line drawn around the globe of the eye and passing through the poles of the vertical axis (vertical meridian), or through the poles of the transverse axis (horizontal meridian). —**meridional,** adj.

mer″in·tho·pho′bi·a (merr″in-tho-fo′bee-uh, mi-rin″tho-). A morbid fear of being bound.

me·ris′tic. Pertaining to, or divided into, segments.

mer′o-, mer-. A combining form meaning *part*.

mer″o·blas′tic. Dividing only in part, referring to an egg in which the cleavage divisions are confined to the animal pole, owing to the presence of a large amount of yolk.

mer′o·crine (merr′o-kryne, ·krin). Pertaining to glands in which the act of secretion leaves the cell intact. See *apocrine, holocrine*.

mer″o·mi″cro·so′mi·a. Abnormal smallness of some part of the body.

me·ro′pi·a. Partial blindness; obscuration of vision.

mer″o·ra·chis′chi·sis (merr″o-ra-kiss′ki-sis). Partial spina bifida.

mer″o·zo′ite, me″ro·zo′ite. Any one of the segments resulting from the splitting up of the schizont in the asexual form of reproduction of sporozoa.

mer′sa·lyl (mur′suh-lil, ·leel). The sodium salt of salicyl-(γ-hydroxymercuri-β-methoxypropyl)-amide-O-acetic acid, a white powder; soluble in water. Mersalyl was introduced as an antisyphilitic, but is now employed mainly as a diuretic. See *salyrgan*. **m. and theophylline injection.** A sterile aqueous solution of approximately 10% of mersalyl and 5% of theophylline.

merthiolate. Trade-mark for sodium ethyl mercurithiosalicylate, a light cream-colored crystalline powder, used as an antiseptic, germicide, and fungicide.

mer′y·cism. The voluntary regurgitation of food, its remastication, and swallowing a second time; occurs in certain idiots and some psychiatric patients.

mes·an'to·in. 3-Methyl-5-phenyl-5-ethyl-hydantoin, an anticonvulsant.

mes"a·or·ti'tis. Inflammation of the middle coat of the aorta.

mes·ar"te·ri'tis. Inflammation of the middle coat of an artery.

mes"a·ti·pel'lic, mes"a·ti·pel'vic (mess"uh·ti·pel'vick, mi·sat"i·). *In osteometry*, designating a pelvis in which the transverse diameter of the pelvic inlet is nearly equal to the conjugata vera; having a pelvic-inlet index of 90.0 to 94.9.

mes·cal'. An intoxicant spirit distilled from Mexican pulque, a fermented beverage. **m. buttons.** The dried tops from a species of cactus, *Lophophora williamsii*.

mes·cal'ine (mess·kal'een, ·in). An alkaloid from mescal buttons.

mes"en·ceph'a·lon. The midbrain; that part of the brain developed from the middle cerebral vesicle and consisting of the corpora quadrigemina and cerebral peduncles, and traversed by the cerebral aqueduct. **—mesen·cephal'ic,** *adj.*

mes"en·chyme (mez'un·kyme), **me·sen'chy·ma** (mee·seng'ki·muh, ·seng'kigh·muh). The portion of the mesoderm that produces all the connective tissues, most smooth muscle, the blood vessels and the blood, the entire lymphatic system, and the heart; the nonepithelial portions of the mesoderm. **—mesen'chymal,** *adj.*

mes"en·chy·mo'ma. Tumor of mesenchymal tissue.

mes"en·ter·ec'to·my. Excision of the mesentery or a part of it.

mes"en·ter"i·or·rha·phy. Surgical repair of a mesentery.

mes"en·ter"i·pli·ca'tion. Mesenteriorrhaphy; reduction of folds of redundant mesentery by overlapping and suture.

mes"en·ter"y. A fold of the peritoneum that connects the digestive tube with the posterior abdominal wall; that of the small intestine is termed mesentery proper; that of the stomach, colon, cecum, and rectum, mesogastrium, mesocolon, mesocecum, mesorectum, respectively. **—mesenter'ic,** *adj.* **dorsal m.** The mesentery of the digestive tube attached to the dorsal abdominal wall. **ventral m.** See lesser *omentum*, gastrohepatic *ligament*.

mes·en'to·derm. 1. The entodermal division of the mesoderm. 2. The indifferent tissue from which both entoderm and mesoderm are developed. 3. The portion of the mesoderm from which certain digestive-tract structures are derived.

mes"en·tor·rha·phy. Suture of the mesentery.

me'si·al (mee'zee·ul, mee'see·ul). 1. Old term sometimes used for medial. 2. *In dentistry*, toward the midline following the curve of a dental arch.

me'si·o- (mee'zee·o-, mee'see·o-). *In dentistry*, a combining form which denotes the aspect of a tooth *facing* the midline, *following* the dental arch.

me"si·o·dis'tal. Pertaining to a line or a plane between the mesial and distal surfaces of a tooth.

mes'o- (mess'o-, mee'so-), **mes-.** 1. A combining form signifying *middle*. 2. *In anatomy*, a combining form denoting *an intermediate connective part*, mesentery. 3. *In medicine*, a combining form which denotes *partial* or *secondary*.

mes"o·ap·pen'dix. The mesentery of the vermiform process.

mes'o·blast. Synonym *(O.T.)* for mesoderm, q.v. **—mesoblas'tic,** *adj.*

mes"o·co'lon. The mesentery connecting the colon with the posterior abdominal wall. It may be divided into ascending, descending, and transverse portions. **—mesocol'ic,** *adj.*

mes'o·derm. The third germ layer, lying between the ectoderm and entoderm. It gives rise to the connective tissues, skeleton, muscles, urogenital system, vascular system, and the epithelial lining of the coelom. **—mesoderm'al,** *adj.* **extraembryonic m.** The earliest mesoderm of the embryo derived from the trophoblast that forms a part of the amnion, chorion and yolk sac, and the body stalk. **intermediate m.** The unsegmented mass of mesoderm uniting the somite and the lateral mesoderm and from which the nephrogenic tissue of the embryonic and definitive kidneys is derived. Syn., *nephrotome*. **intraembryonic m.** The mesoderm of the embryo formed largely from the primitive streak. **lateral m.** The mesoderm lateral to the intermediate mesoderm. After formation of the coelom it is separated into the somatic and the splanchnic mesoderm. **paraxial m.** The medial part of the mesoderm forming a platelike mass that eventually segments to form the somites. **somatic m.** The external layer of the lateral mesoderm associated with ectoderm after formation of the coelom. **splanchnic m.** The internal layer of the lateral mesoderm associated with entoderm after formation of the coelom.

mes"o·gas'tri·um. The mesentery of the stomach. Syn., *mesogaster*.

me·sog'li·a. A type of ameboid phagocyte found in the neuroglia, probably of mesodermal origin.

mes'on. *In nuclear physics*, any of several elementary particles, having a rest mass between that of a proton and an electron, the exchange of which between nucleons is believed to constitute the force holding nucleons together in the nucleus of the atom. The various mesons are distinguished as mu, pi (two kinds), tau, V_{10}, V_{20}, $V_\pm$, chi, and kappa; all are unstable. Also see *mesotron*.

mes″o·ne·phro′ma. A term used to cover a variety of tumors and cystic structures supposed to be, but not proved to be, derived from the mesonephros (Wolffian body), and occurring in the genital tract. Included are extrauterine adenomyomas, cystic or solid tumors of the ovary situated near the hilus, and tumors resembling the adenomyosarcoma of the kidney. **m. ovarii.** A cystic malignant tumor of the ovary which microscopically contains cystic and papillary structures resembling primitive mesonephros. Its origin from the mesonephros is disputed. Also called *papilloendothelioma ovarii*.

mes″o·neph′ros (pl. *mesonephroi*). The middle kidney of higher vertebrates; functional in the embryo, it is replaced by the metanephros in reptiles, birds, and mammals. Syn., *Wolffian body*. —**mesonephric,** *adj.*

mes′o·pex″y. The surgical fixation of a mesentery.

mesopin. A trade-mark for homatropine methylbromide.

me·sor′chi·um (mee·sor′kee·um, meh·sor′-). The mesentery of the fetal testis by which it is attached to the mesonephros; represented in the adult by a fold between testis and epididymis.

mes″o·rec′tum. The narrow fold of the peritoneum connecting the upper part of the rectum with the sacrum.

mes″o·sal′pinx. A fold of peritoneum connecting a uterine tube and broad ligament.

mes″o·sig′moid. The mesentery of the sigmoid flexure of the colon.

mes″o·tar·tar′ic ac′id (mess″o·tahr·tar′ick, mes″o·). Tartaric acid which is optically inactive by reason of internal compensation.

mes″o·ten′don. The fold of synovial membrane extending to a tendon from its fibrous sheath.

mes″o·the″li·o′ma. A primary benign tumor of mesothelial structures; as the peritoneum, pericardium, or pleura, composed of sheets of cells morphologically resembling mesothelial or endothelial cells. Also called *endothelioma*.

mes″o·the′li·um. The epithelium lining the primitive and the definitive body cavity. —**mesothelial,** *adj.*

mes″o·tho′ri·um. Either of the two radioactive disintegration products, **mesothorium-1** (MsTh₁) and **mesothorium-2** (MsTh₂), formed from

thorium and ultimately converted to radiothorium.

mes′o·tron. A meson, especially the kind now known as the *mu meson*. *Obs.*

mes″o·var′i·um (mess″o·vair′ee·um, mee²·so·). A peritoneal fold connecting the ovary and the broad ligament; in the embryo connecting the ovary with the mesonephros.

mes′quite (mess′keet, mess·keet′). The tree or shrub, *Prosopis chilensis*, of the southwestern U. S., Mexico, and Hawaii. It yields a gum resembling acacia.

me·stil′bol. Monomethyl ether of diethylstilbestrol. See *monomestrol*.

mesudin. Marfanil, *q.v.*

met″a-, met-. 1. A prefix signifying *over, after, beyond, among, between, change*, or *transformation*. 2. *In chemistry*, a prefix denoting the 1,3 position of benzene derivatives. Symbol, *m-*. 3. *In medicine*, a prefix denoting *post-*. 4. *In anatomy*, a prefix denoting *dorso-*. 5. *In zoology*, a prefix denoting *a later or more highly developed form of some type*, as Metazoa.

met″a·bol′ic fail′ure. Advanced, progressive debility, characterized by rapid failure of mental and physical functions, terminating in death.

me·tab′o·lism. The phenomena of synthesizing foodstuffs into complex tissue elements (assimilation, anabolism) and complex substances into simple ones in the production of energy (disassimilation, catabolism). —**metabol′ic,** *adj.* **acid-base m.** Those physiologic activities which pertain to the relative concentrations of hydrogen and hydroxyl ions. **basal m.** The minimum amount of energy expenditure necessary to maintain cellular activity when the body is at complete rest in a warm atmosphere 12–18 hours after the intake of food. Also see *basal metabolic rate*. **energy m.** Physiologic activities concerned with the intake, interchange, and output of energy.

me·tab′o·lite. A product of metabolic change. **essential m.** A substance necessary for proper metabolism, such as vitamins.

me·tab′o·lize. Transform by means of metabolism.

met″a·bol′o·gy. Study of the metabolic processes.

met″a·car′pal. Pertaining to the metacarpus or to a bone of it.

met″a·car·pec′to·my. Excision of a metacarpal.

met″a·car″po·pha·lan′ge·al. Belonging to the metacarpus and the phalanges, as metacarpophalangeal ligaments. See Table of Joints and Ligaments in the Appendix.

met″a·car′pus. That part of the hand between the carpus and the phalanges. See Table of Bones in the Appendix.

met″a·chlo′ral. A tasteless, polymeric form of chloral.

met″a·chro·ma′sia (met″uh-kro-may′zhuh, ·shuh). The assumption of different colors or shades by different substances when stained by the same dye. —**metachromat′ic,** *adj.;* **metachro′matism,** *n.*

met″a·cre′sol. $C_6H_4(CH_3)$ OH. The meta form of cresol; a colorless liquid obtained from coal tar.

met″a·cy·e′sis (met″a·sigh·ee′sis). Extrauterine gestation.

Met″a·gon′i·mus. A genus of digenetic trematodes. **M. yokogawai.** That species found most commonly in the Far East which infests the small intestine of man, producing a mild diarrhea.

met′al. An elementary substance usually characterized by hardness, malleability, ductility, fusibility, luster, conduction of heat and electricity, and basic character of its oxides. Symbol, M.

me·tal″les·the′si·a (mi·tal″ess-thee′zhuh, meh·tal″·). The ability to distinguish between various metals by the sense of touch, presumed to occur in hysterical or hypnotized subjects.

me·tal′lic. 1. Resembling metal. 2. *In physical diagnosis,* referring to a sound similar to that produced by metal. It is high-pitched, short in duration, and possesses overtones. A form of tympany.

met′al·loid. 1. Resembling a metal. 2. An element having the physical properties of a metal and the chemical properties of a nonmetal.

met″al·lo·por′phy·rin. A compound formed by the combination of a porphyrin with a metal. Heme is a metalloporphyrin in which a porphyrin is combined with iron.

met′a·mer. One of two or more compounds having the same number and kind of atoms but with a different distribution of the component radicals.

met′a·mere. One of the linear series of more or less similar segments of the body of many animals.

met″a·mer′ic. Pertaining to a metamere or metamerism.

me·tam′er·ism. 1. The repetition of more or less similar parts or segments in the body of many animals, as exhibited especially by the Annelida, Arthropoda, and Vertebrata. 2. The relationship existing between two or more metamers.

metamine. A trade-mark for aminotrate phosphate.

met″a·mor·phop′si·a. A defect of vision in which objects appear distorted; due to disease of the retina or imperfection of the media.

met″a·mor·pho·sis (met″uh-mor′fo·sis, ·mor·fo′sis). A structural change or transformation. *In pathology,* a retrogressive change. **fatty m.** Fatty degeneration, fat infiltration, or both. **sexual m.** A variety of sexual perversion in which the individual has the tastes and feelings of, and assumes the dress and habits of, the opposite sex.

met″a·mor′phous. Amorphous, but with a tendency to crystallize.

metandren. Trade-mark for methyltestosterone, a crystalline androgen.

met″a·neph″ro·gen′ic. Capable of forming, or giving rise to, the metanephros.

met″a·neph′ros (pl. *metanephroi*). The definitive or permanent kidney of reptiles, birds, and mammals. It develops from the caudal part of the nephrogenic cord in association with the ureteric bud from the mesonephric duct. —**metanephric,** *adj.*

met·an′il yel′low. Sodium salt of *m*-sulfanilic acid-azodiphenylamine, a brownish yellow powder used as an indicator. Also called *tropaeolin G, victoria yellow.*

met′a·phase (met′uh-faze). The middle stage of mitosis when the chromosomes lie nearly in a single plane at the equator of the spindle, forming the equatorial plate. It follows the prophase and precedes the anaphase.

metaphen. Trade-mark for the anhydride of 4-nitro-3-hydroxy-mercuri-ortho-cresol, designated as nitromersol by the National Formulary.

met″a·phos·phor′ic ac′id. HPO_3. A clear, viscous liquid; the commercial product, occurring in sticks, contains about 17% Na_2O.

metaphyllin. Trade-mark for aminophylline.

me·taph′y·sis. 1. The region of growth between the epiphysis and diaphysis of a bone. Also called *epiphyseal plate.* 2. The growing end of the diaphysis.

met″a·pla′si·a (met″uh·play′zee·uh, ·see·uh). Transformation of one tissue into another without the intervention of an embryonal tissue, as the replacement of respiratory epithelium by stratified squamous epithelium. —**metaplas′tic,** *adj.*

met′a·plasm (met′uh-plaz·um). The lifeless inclusions in protoplasm collectively.

met″a·pro·te·in. A product of acid or alkaline hydrolysis of a protein.

met·ar′am·i·nol bi·tar·trate. *l*-α-(1-Aminoethyl)-*m*-hydroxybenzyl alcohol hydrogen *d*-tartrate, a vasopressor agent. See *aramine bitartrate.*

me·tas′ta·ses. Plural of metastasis.

me·tas′ta·sis. 1. The transfer of disease from a primary focus to a secondary site by the conveyance of causal agents or cells through the blood vessels or lymph channels. 2. A secondary metastatic growth of cancer. **—me·tastat'ic,** *adj.*

me·tas'ta·size. To transfer, or to be transferred to secondary sites, as a cancer.

Met"a·stron'gy·lus (met"uh-stron'ji·lus). A genus of nematode parasites.

met"a·tar·sal'gi·a. A condition characterized by pain and tenderness in the metatarsal region. **Morton's m.** A specific clinical type, described by T. G. Morton (1876), characterized by severe pain between the heads of the third and fourth metatarsal bones and due to a neurofibroma at the point of union of the digital branches from the medial and lateral plantar nerves. Also called *Morton's foot* or *toe.*

met"a·tar·sec'to·my. Excision of a metatarsal bone.

met"a·tar"so·pha·lan'ge·al. Pertaining to the metatarsus and the phalanges, as the ligaments between these bones. See Table of Joints and Ligaments in the Appendix.

met"a·tar'sus. The portion of the foot between the tarsus and the phalanges, containing five bones of the foot. See Table of Bones in the Appendix. **—metatarsal,** *adj.*

me·tath'e·sis. A chemical reaction in which there is an exchange of radicals or elements with no change in valence. **—metathet'ic,** *adj.*

Met"a·zo'a. A subdivision of the animal kingdom, which includes all the multicellular forms, and so stands in contrast to the Protozoa.

met"em·pir'ic. Not derived from experience, but implied or presupposed by it.

met"en·ceph'a·lon. The cephalic part of the rhombencephalon, giving rise to the cerebellum and pons.

me'te·or·ism. Gaseous distention of the abdomen or intestine; tympanites.

me"te·or·ol'o·gy. The science which treats primarily of atmospheric phenomena.

me'ter. 1. The basic unit of linear measure of the metric system, 39.37 inches. Abbreviated, m. 2. An instrument for measuring and recording quantities, as a roentgen meter, which measures roentgen-ray quantities in roentgens by ionization. **—met'ric,** *adj.*

meth"a·cho'line chlo'ride (meth"uh·ko'leen, ·lin). The pharmacopeial name for acetyl-β-methylcholine chloride. See *mecholyl chloride.*

meth·a·done hy"dro·chlo'ride. A nonproprietary title for amidone hydrochloride, *q.v.* Also spelled *methadon hydrochloride.*

meth"al·len·es'tril. α,α-Dimethyl-β-ethyl-6-methoxy-2-naphthalenepropionic acid, an estrogen. See *vallestril.*

meth"am·phet'a·mine hy"dro·chlo'ride. The U.S.P. name for d-desoxyephedrine hydrochloride.

meth·an'al. Formaldehyde.

meth·ane. CH₄. Marsh gas. The first member of the homologous series of paraffins having the general formula CₙH₂ₙ₊₂.

meth·a·nol. Methyl alcohol.

meth·an'the·line. Nonproprietary name for β-diethylaminoethylxanthene-9-carboxylate, a substance possessing atropine-like and autonomic ganglion blocking actions. **m. bromide.** Nonproprietary name for β-diethylaminoethylxanthene-9-carboxylate methobromide, an anticholinergic drug. See *banthine bromide.*

meth"a·pyr'i·lene hy"dro·chlo'ride. The nonproprietary name for the antihistaminic substance N,N-dimethyl-N'-(α-pyridyl)-N'-(α-thenyl)-ethylenediamine hydrochloride. See *thenylene hydrochloride.*

meth·ar·bi'tal. 5,5-Diethyl-1-methylbarbituric acid, a barbiturate that is less sedative than phenobarbital, used in treating various forms of epilepsy. See *gemonil.*

meth·e·drine. Trade-mark for d-desoxyephedrine hydrochloride or methamphetamine hydrochloride.

met·he"mo·glo'bin, met·hae"mo·glo'bin (met-hee"mo·glo'bin, met·hem″o·). The dark-brown oxidized form of hemoglobin in which the iron atom is trivalent and which cannot combine reversibly with oxygen, found in the blood after poisoning, as by chlorates, nitrates, or ferricyanides. Syn., *ferrihemoglobin.*

met·he"mo·glo"bi·ne'mi·a, met·hae"mo·glo"bi·ne'mi·a. The presence of methemoglobin in the blood, causing cyanosis, dizziness, headache, diarrhea, and anemia.

met·he"mo·glo"bi·nu'ri·a, met·hae"mo·glo"bi·nu'ri·a. The presence of methemoglobin in the urine.

me·the'na·mine (meth·ee'nuh·meen, ·min, meth″in·uh·meen'). (CH₂)₆N₄. Hexamethylenetetramine, occurring in colorless crystals or as a white powder, soluble in water. Used mainly as a urinary antiseptic. Syn., *hexamine.* See *formin, urotropin.*

meth'ene. Methylene. The bivalent group =CH₂.

meth'e·nyl. The trivalent radical, ≡CH. **m. tribromide.** Bromoform. **m. trichloride.** Chloroform. **m. triiodide.** Iodoform.

meth·er·gine. Trade-mark for N-(α-hydroxy-methyl-propyl)-d-lysergamide, an oxytocic.

me·thim′a·zole. 1-Methyl-2-mercaptoimidazole, used as an antithyroid drug. See *tapazole.*

meth·i′o·dal so′di·um. Sodium monoiodomethanesulfonate, a roentgenographic contrast medium. See *skiodan.*

meth·i′o·nine (meth-eye′o-neen, -nin). $CH_3.S.(CH_2)_2.CHNH_2.COOH.$ α-Amino-γ-methylthiol-*n*-butyric acid. A naturally occurring amino acid.

meth·it′u·ral so′di·um. 5-(1-Methylbutyl)-5-[-2-(methylthio)ethyl]-2-thiobarbiturate, an ultrashort-acting thiobarbiturate. See *neraval sodium.*

methocel. Trade-mark for methyl cellulose.

meth′od. The manner of performance of any act or operation. The term embraces open and closed operations, reduction of fractures and dislocations, maneuvers and tests performed in a definite way and according to a described and practiced plan. For methods of treatment, see under *treatment;* for methods of staining, see under *stain;* for methods of making qualitative tests, see under *test.* **alternate case m.** A method of investigating the effects of different treatments by using alternate types of treatment on alternate patients who suffer from the same disease. **alternate paired case m.** A method of investigating the effects of different treatments by pairing cases as to extent and similarity of disease, using one type of treatment on one pair and another type on the second pair. **epidermic m.** A method of administering medicinal substances by applying them to the skin. **Evans blue m.** A method for determining the volume of blood plasma. After intravenous injection of the dye (T-1824), the concentration of the dye in the plasma is determined colorimetrically. From this, plasma volume and blood volume (using hematocrit data) can be calculated. **flotation m.** A technic employed for separating ova and larvae from stool specimens. The stool is put into a salt solution where it sinks while the ova and larvae, due to their lower specific gravity, rise to the surface. **Koch-McMeekin's m.** (*for nonprotein nitrogen*). The organic matter is digested with sulfuric acid and hydrogen peroxide and the resulting solution is nesslerized. May also be used for total nitrogen of urine. **Meduna's m.** Convulsion therapy in dementia precox. **metatrophic m.** A therapeutic method of modifying the nutrition by changes in the food, with a view of administering some drug, as suppression of sodium chloride in food of epileptics in order to reinforce the action of bromides. **micromethod.** A method of laboratory examination in

which very small quantities of the substances to be examined are used.

Prague m. A method of delivery of the aftercoming head. The child's ankles are grasped above the medial malleoli with the right hand. The index finger of the left hand is flexed over one clavicle, and the remaining fingers of the same hand over the other clavicle.

me·tho′ni·um. A homologous series of compounds containing the ion $(CH_2)_3N^+(CH_2)_nN^+(CH_3)_3$, which possess therapeutic activity and which include pentamethonium, hexamethonium, and decamethonium, so designated when n is 5, 6, or 10, respectively. Used clinically in the form of one of its salts, usually the bromide or iodide.

meth″o·trex′ate. 4-Amino-N[10]-methylfolic acid, a folic acid antagonist, to which the trade-mark *amethopterin* was formerly applied.

meth·ox′a·mine hy″dro·chlo′ride. β-Hydroxy-β-(2,5-dimethoxyphenyl)isopropylamine hydrochloride, a drug possessing pressor activity and used to maintain blood pressure during anesthesia, to treat hypotension caused by myocardial infarction, and to counteract hypotensive effects of some drugs. See *vasoxyl hydrochloride.*

meth·ox′y-. A combining form denoting the univalent radical $CH_3O.$

meth·ox″y·phen′a·mine. Nonproprietary name for beta-(ortho-methoxyphenyl)isopropyl-methylamine, a sympathomimetic amine. See *orthoxine.*

meth″yl. The univalent radical $CH_3.$ —**methyl′ic,** *adj.*

meth′yl al′co·hol. $CH_3OH.$ A colorless liquid, obtained in the destructive distillation of wood and by synthesis. Syn., *carbinol, methanol, wood alcohol, wood spirit.*

meth′yl al′de·hyde. Formaldehyde.

meth″yl·am′ine (meth″il·am′een, -a-meen′). $CH_3NH_2.$ A colorless gas.

meth″yl·am·phet′a·mine. N-methylamphetamine or desoxyephedrine.

meth′yl·ate. A compound formed from methyl alcohol by the substitution of the hydrogen of the hydroxyl by a base. —**methylated,** *adj.*

meth″yl·a′tion. The process of substituting a methyl group for a hydrogen atom.

meth″yl·ben′zene. Toluene.

meth″yl·benz″e·tho′ni·um chlo′ride. Benzyldimethyl{2-[2-(*p*-1,1,3,3-tetramethylbutylcresoxy)ethoxy]ethyl}ammonium chloride, a quaternary ammonium salt with surface-active and disinfectant properties used especially as a bacteriostatic agent in diaper dermatitis. See *diaparene chloride.*

meth′yl blue. Sodium triphenyl-pararosaniline trisulfonate; an anti-septic dye.

meth′yl cel′lu·lose. A cellulose ether occurring in dry fibrous masses which form a jelly in aqueous solution. See *methocel.*

meth″yl chlo′ride. CH_3Cl. A liquid local anesthetic; when applied as a spray it volatilizes rapidly and pro-duces a localized freezing.

meth″yl·cho·lan·threne (meth″-il·ko·lan′threen). A cancer-producing hydrocarbon which may be derived from certain steroids.

meth′yl·ene. The bivalent hydrocar-bon radical, $=CH_2$.

meth′yl·ene blue. $C_{16}H_{18}ClN_3S·$ $3H_2O$. A medicinal aniline dye; it occurs as dark green crystals or powder having a bronzelike luster. Solutions have a deep blue color. It is an ingredient of many biologic stains. Syn., *methylthi-onine chloride.*

meth′yl·ene vi′o·let (C.C.). A weakly basic thiazine dye; an oxidation product of methylene blue; used as a blood stain.

meth′yl e′ther. $(CH_3)_2O$. Dimethyl oxide; a gas having anesthetic proper-ties.

meth″yl·eth″yl·a·ce′tic ac′id. See under *valeric acid.*

meth″yl·gly·ox′al. CH_3COCHO. The aldehyde of pyruvic acid, capable of transformation into glycogen by the liver.

meth′yl green (C.C.). An aniline dye; used in staining tissues.

meth′yl hy′drate. Methyl alcohol.

meth′yl hy′dride. CH_4. Methane or marsh gas.

meth″yl·hy·drox″y·ben·zo′ic ac′id (meth″il·high·drock″see·ben-zo′ick). Cresotic acid.

meth′yl i′o·dide. CH_3I. A colorless liquid, insoluble in water. Has been used as a vesicant. Syn., *iodomethane.*

meth″yl·mer·cap′tan. CH_3SH. Methyl hydrosulfide gas, found nor-mally in the intestines.

meth′yl meth·ac′ryl·ate. See *ac-rylics.*

meth″yl·meth′ane. See *ethane.*

meth″yl·mor′phine (meth″il-mor′feen, ·mor·feen′). See *codeine.*

meth′yl or′ange (C.C.). Dimethyl-aminoazobenzene sodium sulfonate, an indicator.

meth″yl·par′a·ben. $C_8H_4.OH.COO$-CH_3. Methyl parahydroxybenzoate; an antiseptic used to preserve medicinal preparations.

meth′yl par″a·hy·drox″y·ben-zo·ate (par″uh·high·drock″see·ben-zo·ate). Methylparaben.

meth″yl·phe′nol. Cresol.

meth″yl·pu′rine (meth″il·pure′een, ·in). Any compound in which one or more methyl radicals have been intro-duced into the purine nucleus.

meth′yl red. Dimethylaminoazoben-zene-o-carboxylic acid; an indicator.

meth″yl·ros·an′i·line chlo′ride (meth″il·ro·zan′i·leen, ·lin). Hexameth-ylpararosaniline chloride, usually con-taining also pentamethylpararosaniline chloride and tetramethylpararosaniline chloride. A dark green powder soluble in water to form a purple solution. Used medicinally and as a biologic stain. Also called *gentian violet, methyl violet, crystal violet.*

meth′yl sal′i·cyl″ate (sal′i·sil″-ate, sa·liss′i·late). $C_6H_4(OH)COOCH_3$, an oily liquid, used chiefly as a coun-terirritant.

meth″yl·sul′fo·nal. See *sulfoneth-ylmethane.*

meth″yl·tes·tos′ter·one. 17-Methyltestosterone. $C_{20}H_{30}O_2$. An orally effective male sex hormone. See *metan-dren, neo-hombreol-M, oreton-M.*

meth′yl the″o·bro′mine (·bro′-meen, ·min). Caffeine.

meth″yl·thi′o·nine chlo′ride (meth″il·thigh′o·neen, ·nin). Methyl-ene blue.

meth′yl vi′o·let. The U. S. Pharma-copeia synonym for methylrosaniline chloride.

meth·y·pry·lon. 3,3-Diethyl-5-meth-yl-2,4-piperidinedione, a sedative and hypnotic. See *noludar.*

meticortelone. A trade-mark for prednisolone.

meticorten. A trade-mark for pred-nisone.

met′o·don·ti′a·sis. 1. The second dentition. 2. Loosely used for abnormal-ity of teething.

me·top′ic, me·to′pic. 1. Relating to the forehead; frontal. 2. A name ap-plied to a cranium having a mediofron-tal suture.

me·to′pi·um. Expressed almond oil.

met′o·pon hy″dro·chlo′ride. Methyl dihydromorphinone hydrochlo-ride. A derivative of morphine having analgesic effectiveness.

met′o·pryl. $CH_3CH_2CH_2.O.CH_3$. n-Propyl methyl ether, a colorless liquid, isomeric with, but less volatile than, ethyl ether.

met″ra·pec′tic (met″ruh·peck′tick, mee″truh·). Referring to a disease which is transmitted through the mother, but which she herself escapes (such as hemophilia).

met″ra·to′ni·a (met″ruh·to′nee·uh, mee″truh·). Atony of the uterus.

met″ra·tro′phi·a. Atrophy of the uterus.

metraxol. A trade-mark for pentyl-enetetrazol. See *cardiazol, leptazol.*

me′tre. See *meter.*

met″rec·ta′si·a   (met″reck·tay′-

zhuh, mee"treck·). Dilatation of the nonpregnant uterus.

met"rec·to'pi·a (met"reck·to'pee-uh, mee"treck·), **me·trec'to·py.** Displacement of the uterus.

me·tre'mi·a. Congestion of the uterus.

met"reu·ryn'ter (met"roo·rin'tur, mee"troo·). An inflatable bag for dilating the cervical canal of the uterus.

met·reu'ry·sis (met·roor'i·sis). Dilatation of the uterine cervix with the metreurynter.

me·tri·a. 1. Any uterine affection. 2. Any inflammatory condition during the puerperium.

met'ric sys'tem. A system of weights and measures, originated in France about 1790, and nearly universally employed for scientific purposes. It is a decimal system based primarily on the meter as the fundamental *unit of length*. The meter is defined as the distance between two scratches on a platinum-iridium bar, deposited at the International Bureau of Weights and Measures at Sèvres, near Paris. It is equivalent to exactly 39.37 U. S. inches. The basic *unit of mass*, and of *weight*, is the gram, defined as ¹⁄₁₀₀₀ of the international kilogram, also deposited at the International Bureau of Weights and Measures. The main *unit of capacity* is the liter, which is the volume of a kilogram of water at the temperature of maximum density under normal atmospheric pressure, and which very closely approximates 1000 cubic centimeters. Multiples of the principal units are designated by the prefixes deca- meaning 10, hecto- meaning 100, and kilo- meaning 1000. For fractional units the corresponding prefixes are deci-, ¹⁄₁₀; centi-, ¹⁄₁₀₀; and milli-, ¹⁄₁₀₀₀. The following equivalents of U. S. units in metric units are close enough for most purposes:

1 inch = 2.54 centimeters
1 ounce (avoirdupois) = 28.35 grams
1 pound (avoirdupois) = 453.6 grams
1 fluidounce = 29.57 milliliters (or cubic centimeters)
1 quart = 0.9463 liter
1 minim = 0.0617 milliliter (or cubic centimeter)

Also see Tables of Weights and Measures in the Appendix.

me·tri'tis. Inflammation of the uterus.

me'tro- (mee'tro-, met'ro-), **metr-.** A combining form denoting *relation to the uterus.*

me'tro·cele. Hernia of the uterus.

me'tro·clyst. An instrument for giving uterine douches.

me"tro·col'po·cele (mee"tro·kol'po·seel, met"ro·). Protrusion or prolapse of the uterus into the vagina,

with prolapse of the anterior vaginal wall.

me"tro·cys·to'sis (mee"tro·sis·to'-sis, met"ro·). 1. The formation of uterine cysts. 2. The condition giving rise to uterine cysts.

me"tro·dy"na·mom'e·ter. An instrument for measuring the force of uterine contractions.

me"tro·dyn'i·a. Pain in the uterus.

met·rog'ra·phy. Roentgenography of the uterus through the injection of contrast mediums; uterography.

me·trol'o·gy. The science that deals with methods of measurement and units of measure.

me"tro·ma·la'ci·a (mee"tro·ma·lay'shee·uh, met"ro·). Softening of the tissues of the uterus.

me"tro·pa·ral'y·sis. Uterine paralysis, usually that which may occur immediately following childbirth.

me"tro·path'i·a hem"or·rha'gi·ca. Abnormal uterine bleeding, now generally considered to be of endocrine origin.

me·trop'a·thy. Any uterine disease. —**metropath'ic,** *adj.*

me"tro·phle·bi'tis. Inflammation of the veins of the uterus.

me"trop·to'sis. Uterine prolapse.

me"tror·rha'gi·a (mee"tro·ray'juh, met"ro·). Uterine hemorrhage independent of the menstrual period.

me"tror·rhe'a, me"tror·rhoe'a. Any pathologic discharge from the uterus.

me"tror·rhex'is. Rupture of the uterus.

me"tro·sal"pin·gi'tis. Inflammation of the uterus and oviducts.

me"tro·sal"pin·gog'ra·phy (mee"tro·sal"ping·gog'ruh·fee, met"ro·). Radiography of the uterus and oviducts after injecting an iodized oil contrast medium into the cervical canal under pressure. Same as hysterosalpingography and uterosalpingography.

me'tro·scope. An instrument for examining the uterus.

me"tro·stax'is. Slight but persistent uterine hemorrhage.

me"tro·ste·no'sis. Abnormal constriction of the cavity of the uterus.

me'tro·tome (mee'tro·tohm, met'ro·tohm). An instrument for incising the cervix uteri.

-metry. A combining form denoting *an art, process,* or *science of measuring.*

me·try"per·ci·ne'sis (mi·try"pur·si·nee'sis, mee"try·). Excessive uterine contraction.

me·try"per·tro'phi·a. Hypertrophy of the uterus.

metycaine. Trade-mark for gamma-(2-methyl-piperidino)-propyl benzoate hydrochloride, a local anesthetic.

mev. Million electronvolts. A customary unit for expressing energies of nuclear particles. 1 mev = 1.59 × 10⁻⁶ erg.

me·ze're·um. The dried bark of *Daphne mezereum* and other species of *Daphne*.

mez·quite' (mess·keet', mess·kee'tay). See *mesquite*.

Mg. Chemical symbol for magnesium.

mg. Milligram.

mg. %. Milligrams per cent.

mgh. Milligram-hour; the radium dosage obtained by the application of one milligram of radium element for one hour.

mho. The unit of electric conductance; the reciprocal of the ohm.

mi'ca. 1. A crumb. 2. A silicate mineral occurring in the form of thin, shining, transparent laminae.

mi"cra·cous'tic (migh"kruh·koos'tick). 1. Assisting in hearing very faint sounds. 2. An instrument possessing this property.

mi"cren·ceph'a·lous. Having an abnormally small brain.

mi'cro-, micr-. 1. A combining form meaning *small* or *petty*, or *one-millionth*. 2. A combining form denoting *microscopic*. 3. *In botany*, a combining form signifying *very small in a specified feature*. 4. *In chemistry*, a combining form signifying *of or pertaining to very small amounts of material*. 5. *In medicine*, a combining form signifying *abnormally small*.

mi"cro·au'di·phone. An instrument for rendering very slight sounds audible.

mi'crobe. A living organism of very small size; microörganism. Applied to bacteria, especially those of a pathogenic nature. Also see *dissociation*, 4. —**micro'bial, micro'bian, micro'bic,** adj.

mi·cro'bi·cide (migh·kro'bi·side). 1. Destructive to microbes. 2. An agent that destroys microbes. Syn., *germicide*. —**microbicidal,** adj.

mi"cro·bin·ert'ness. Failure to support microbial growth because of absence of the necessary nutrients. —**microbinert,** adj.

mi"cro·bi·ol'o·gist (migh"kro·buy·ol'o·jist). An expert in microbiology.

mi"cro·bi·ol'o·gy. The science of the nature, life, and actions of microorganisms. —**microbiolog'ic,** adj.

mi"cro·bi·ot'ic (migh"kro·buy·ot'ick). Any antibacterial substance produced by molds, bacteria, or other organisms; an antibiotic or antibacterial.

mi'cro·blast. 1. An immature blood cell. 2. A small, nucleated, red blood cell.

mi"cro·bleph'a·ron, mi"cro·ble·pha'ri·a (migh"kro·bli·fay'ree·uh), **mi"cro·bleph'a·rism.** Smallness of the eyelids.

mi"cro·bra'chi·a (migh"kro·bray'kee·uh). Abnormally (congenital) small arms.

mi"cro·bu·ret'. An apparatus for delivering or measuring small quantities of liquids or gases.

mi"cro·cal'o·rie, mi"cro·cal'o·ry. A small calorie; the quantity of heat necessary to raise the temperature of 1 Gm. of water from 15° to 16° C. Also see *calorie*.

mi"cro·car'di·a. Congenital smallness of the heart.

mi"cro·ceph'a·ly. A congenital hypoplasia of the cerebrum with a thick cranium and early closure of the fontanels, resulting in a small head. —**microcephal'ic, microcephalous,** adj.

mi"cro·chei'li·a (migh"kro·kigh'lee·uh). Abnormal smallness of the lips.

mi"cro·chem'is·try. 1. The study of chemical reactions, using small quantities of materials, frequently less than 1 mg. 2. The chemistry of individual cells and minute organisms. —**microchemical,** adj.

mi"cro·chi'ri·a (migh"kro·kigh'ree·uh). Smallness of the hand to an unnatural degree.

Mi"cro·coc'cus. A genus of bacteria of the family Micrococcaceae, **M. albus.** Synonym for *Staphylococcus albus*. **M. ascoformans.** The causative organism of botryomycosis in horses. Also called **M.** *pyogenes* var. *aureus, M. pyogenes* var. *albus, Staphylococcus aureus, S. albus.* **M. aureus.** Synonym for *Staphylococcus aureus.* **M. catarrhalis.** Bacteria found in the secretions of patients afflicted with the common cold, but not supposed to be the causative agent. **M. gonorrhoeae.** Synonym for *Neisseria gonorrhoeae.* **M. intracellularis meningitidis.** Synonym for *Neisseria meningitidis.* **M. lanceolatus.** Synonym for *Diplococcus pneumoniae.* **M. melitensis.** Synonym for *Brucella melitensis.* **M. meningitidis.** Synonym for *Neisseria meningitidis.* **M. pneumoniae.** Synonym for *Diplococcus pneumoniae.* **M. tetragenus.** A species of parasitic cocci frequently found on the mucous membranes of the upper respiratory tract; of low grade virulence; probably unable to invade human tissues. Syn., *Gaffkya tetragena.*

mi"cro·co'lon. An abnormally small colon.

mi"cro·cor'ne·a. Abnormal smallness of the cornea.

mi"cro·cou'lomb (migh"kro·koo'lom, ·koo·lom'). The one-millionth part of a coulomb, *q.v.*

mi"cro·crys'tal·line. Composed of crystals of microscopic size.

mi"cro·cu'rie. The one-millionth part of a curie or the one-thousandth part of a millicurie. Symbol, μc. See Table of Signs and Symbols in the Appendix.

mi'cro·cyst. A cyst of small size, visible only microscopically.

mi'cro·cyte. A small red blood cell.

mi"cro·cy·to'sis (migh"kro·sigh·to'-sis). A condition of the blood, characterized by abnormally small red blood cells.

mi"cro·dac·tyl'i·a. Abnormal smallness of the fingers or toes.

mi"cro·dis·sec'tion. Dissection with the aid of a microscope.

mi'cro·dont. Pertaining to abnormally small teeth.

mi"cro·e·lec"tro·pho·ret'ic. Pertaining to electrophoresis of minute quantities of solutions.

mi"cro·e·lec"tro·pho·ret'ic cells. Either flat or cylindrical cells, the flat cell containing a layer of colloidal sol 0.6 mm. in depth, and the cylindrical cell consisting of a capillary tube through which colloidal particles pass under the influence of an electric field.

mi"cro·far'ad. The one-millionth part of a farad, q.v.

mi"cro·fi·lar'i·a (migh"kro·fi·lay'-ree·uh) (pl. *microfilariae*). The embryonic or prelarval forms of filarial worms; slender motile forms, 150–300 μ in length, found in the blood stream and tissues. On ingestion by the proper blood-sucking insects the microfilariae pass through developmental stages in the body of the host and become infestive larvae. **sheathed microfilariae.** Microfilariae encased in a delicate membrane which usually protrudes beyond the ends of the parasite. The membrane is thought to be the remains of the egg shell. When the membrane or shell breaks, an unsheathed microfilaria results.

mi"cro·gam'ete (migh"kro·gam'-eet, ·ga·meet'). A male reproductive cell in certain Protozoa, corresponding to the sperm cell in Metazoa.

mi"cro·gen'e·sis. Development of an abnormally small part.

mi"cro·ge'ni·a. Abnormal smallness of the chin.

mi"cro·gen'i·tal·ism. Having extremely undersized genital organs.

mi·crog'li·a (migh·krog'lee·uh). Small neuroglia cells of the central nervous system, having long processes and exhibiting ameboid and phagocytic activity under pathologic conditions. Probably mesodermal in origin.

mi"cro·glos'si·a. Abnormal smallness of the tongue.

mi"cro·gna'thi·a (migh"kro·nay'-thee·uh, migh"krog·). Abnormal smallness of the jaws, especially of the lower jaw.

mi'cro·gram. One one-thousandth of a milligram. Sometimes called *gamma*. Symbol, μg. See Table of Signs and Symbols in the Appendix.

mi·crog'ra·phy (migh·krog'ruh·fee). 1. A description of bodies studied under the microscope. 2. Very minute writing.

mi"cro·gy'ri·a (migh"kro·jy'ree·uh, ·jirr'ee·uh). Abnormal smallness of the convolutions of the brain.

mi'crohm. One one-millionth of an ohm.

mi"cro·in·cin·er·a'tion. Reduction of thin sections to ash on a quartz slide, for microscopic study.

mi"cro·in·jec'tion. The injection of solutions into cells by means of a micropipet.

mi"cro·len'ti·a. Having an abnormally small crystalline lens.

mi"cro·leu'ko·blast (migh"kro·lew'ko·blast). A small leukoblast.

mi'cro·li'ter. A millionth of a liter, or a thousandth of a milliliter. Sometimes called *lambda*.

mi'cro·lith. A microscopic calculus.

mi"cro·ma'ni·a. A delusional state in which the patient believes himself diminutive in size and mentally inferior.

mi"cro·ma·nip'u·la"tor. A device for moving exceedingly fine instruments, under the magnification of a microscope, for dissection of cells or for other operations involving minute objects.

mi"cro·mas'ti·a. Abnormal smallness of the breasts. Syn., *micromazia*.

mi"cro·me'li·a, mi·crom'e·ly (migh·krom'i·lee). Abnormal smallness of the limbs.

mi·crom'e·lus (migh·krom'i·lus). An individual characterized by the presence of abnormally small limbs.

mi·crom'e·ter (migh·krom'i·tur). An instrument designed for measuring minute distances, or apparent diameters, as one used with a microscope or telescope. **—micrometry,** n.

mi'cro·me"ter. The millionth part of a meter; a micron, generally represented by the Greek letter μ. See Table of Signs and Symbols in the Appendix

mi"cro·meth'od. Method or test performed on small quantities of a substance.

mi"cro·mi'cron. The millionth part of a micron, generally denoted by μμ. See Table of Signs and Symbols in the Appendix.

mi'cro·mil. A micromillimeter.

mi"cro·mil'li·me"ter. The one-millionth part of a millimeter or the one-thousandth part of a micron. Incorrectly used to denote the one-thousandth part of a millimeter or the one-millionth part of a meter. Also called *millimicron*. Symbol, mμ. See Table of Signs and Symbols in the Appendix.

mi"cro·mon"o·spo'rin. An antibiotic substance produced by species of the genus *Micromonospora*.

mi"cro·mo'to·scope. An apparatus for photographing and exhibiting motile microörganisms.

mi"cro·my·e'li·a (migh"kro-migh-ee'lee-uh). Abnormal smallness of the spinal cord.

mi'cron. The one-thousandth part of a millimeter, or the one-millionth part of a meter. Generally represented by the Greek letter μ. See Table of Signs and Symbols in the Appendix.

mi"cro·nu'cle·us. 1. A small or minute nucleus. 2. *In biology*, the paranucleus, or the nucleolus. 3. The reproductive nucleus of protozoa as contrasted with the macronucleus, *q.v.*

mi"cro·nu'tri·ents. The vitamins and minerals occurring in traces essential for growth, development, and health. The essential minerals are also called trace minerals.

mi"cro·nych'i·a (migh"kro-nick'ee-uh). The presence of one or more small nails which in every other respect seem normal.

mi"cro·ör'gan·ism, mi·cro·or'gan·ism. A microscopic organism, either animal or plant, especially bacteria and protozoa. **_microorgan'ic,** *adj.* **pyogenic m.** A microörganism producing pus; usually staphylococci and streptococci, but many other organisms may also produce pus.

mi"cro·pe'nis. Abnormal smallness of the penis. Syn., *microphallus*.

mi"cro·phal'lus. Abnormal smallness of the penis. Syn., *micropenis*.

mi"cro·pho'bi·a. 1. Morbid fear of microbes. 2. Morbid fear of small objects.

mi'cro·phone. An instrument in which feeble sounds modulate an electric current which can be amplified so that the sounds become audible.

mi"cro·pho'ni·a, mi·croph'o·ny (migh-krof'o-nee). Weakness of voice.

mi"cro·pho'no·graph. A combination of microphone and phonograph used for the recording of sounds.

mi"cro·pho'no·scope. A binaural stethoscope with a membrane in the chestpiece to accentuate the sound.

mi"cro·pho'to·graph. 1. A photograph of microscopic size. 2. Photomicrograph, *q.v.*

mi"croph·thal'mus. 1. A condition in which the eyeball is abnormally small. Also called *microphthalmia*. 2. A person manifesting such a condition.

mi"cro·phys'ics. That branch of

science which deals with electrons, atoms, and molecules.

mi"cro·phyte. Any microscopic plant, especially one that is parasitic.

mi"cro·pi·pet'. An exceedingly fine pipet used in microinjection.

mi"cro·po'di·a, mi·crop'o·dy. Congenital smallness of the feet.

mi"cro·pro·jec'tion. The projection of the image of microscopic objects on a screen.

mi"cro·pro·so'pi·a. Congenital abnormal smallness of the face.

mi·crop'si·a (migh-crop'see-uh). Disturbance of visual perception in which objects appear smaller than their true size.

mi'cro·pus (migh'kro-pus, migh-kro'pus). Abnormal smallness of the feet; a congenital defect.

mi'cro·pyle. A minute opening in the investing membrane of many ova, permitting entrance of the sperm.

mi"cror·rhi'ni·a. Congenital hypoplasia or smallness of the nose.

mi"cro·ruth'er·ford. A unit equivalent to ¹⁄₁,₀₀₀,₀₀₀ of a rutherford or 1 disintegration per second. See *rutherford*. Abbreviated, μrd.

mi"cro·scel'ous (migh"kro-skell'us, migh-kros'kil·us). Short-legged.

mi'cro·scope. An apparatus through which minute objects are rendered visible. It consists of a lens, or group of lenses, by which a magnified image of the object is produced. **binocular m.** A microscope having two oculars, so that the object is seen with both eyes. **compound m.** One that consists of two or more lenses or lens systems, of which one, the objective, placed near the object, gives a large and inverted real image; the other, the ocular, acting like a simple microscope, gives an enlarged virtual image of the real image. **corneal m.** A microscope used to examine the cornea in the living patient. **electron m.** A device for directing streams of electrons by means of electric and magnetic fields so as to resolve detail fifty to one hundred times finer than the optical microscope. **fluorescence m.** A microscope with quartz lenses, which transmit ultraviolet wave lengths, or any microscope used in fluorescence studies. **Greenough binocular m.** A binocular microscope equipped with erecting prisms; it has an objective for each tube and so is truly stereoscopic. **phase m.** A compound microscope with an annular diaphragm at the front focal plane of the condenser and a diffraction plate at the back focal plane of the objective of the brightfield compound microscope. By suitable choice of diffraction plate the image contrast may be varied to give increased visibility. **reflecting m.** One using mirror pairs in the objective and thus extending the range of achromatism throughout the optical spectrum. **simple m.** One of one or more lenses or lens systems acting as a single lens. The rays of light that enter the observer's eye after refraction through these lenses proceed directly from the object itself. **television m.** A television camera fitted to a microscope; large audiences may view microscopical phenomena at one time.

mi″cro·scop'ic, mi″cro·scop'i·cal. 1. Pertaining to the microscope. 2. Visible only with the aid of a microscope. 3. Colloquial term for "of extremely small size."

mi·cros'co·pist (migh-kros'ko-pist). One who is skilled in the use of the microscope.

mi·cros'co·py, mi″cro·sco″py. The use of the microscope; examination with the microscope. **bright-field m.** Microscopy utilizing trans-illumination of the specimen with light rays in the optical axis of the microscope. **phase m.** A method for controlling the contrast in the image by means of absorption and optical path difference within the microscope. Transparent materials with small optical path differences or of low absorption contrast may be examined with phase microscopy when bright-field microscopy fails to reveal detail. Also called *phase difference m., phase contrast m.*

mi″cro·so'mi·a. Abnormal smallness of the whole body. Syn., *dwarfism, nanosomia.*

mi″cro·spec·trog'ra·phy. Spectrographic methods applied to the study of the composition of protoplasm.

mi″cro·sphyg'my. Diminished amplitude of the pulse with small oscillometric index.

mi″cro·sphyx'i·a. Weakness or smallness of the pulse.

mi″cro·spo'rin. Extract prepared from a culture of a species of *Microsporum;* used to determine sensitivity to the fungus.

Mi″cro·spo'ron. Former name for a genus of fungi. **M. audouini.** Synonym for *Microsporum audouini.* **M. furfur.** Synonym for *Malassezia furfur,* the causative agent of pityriasis versicolor. **M. minutissimus.** Synonym for *Nocardia minutissima.*

mi″cro·spo·ro'sis. Dermatophytosis caused by a species of *Microsporum.*

Mi″cro·spo'rum, Mi·cros'po·rum (migh-kros'po-rum). A genus of dermatophytes which attack only the hair and the skin. **M. audouini.** That species which is sometimes the causative agent of tinea capitis maculosus. This species produces low-grade scaling lesions. **M. canis.** That spe-

cies which causes the kerion type of tinea capitis, an inflammatory form.

mi″cro·steth'o·phone. A stethoscope which amplifies the sounds heard.

mi″cro·steth'o·scope. A stethoscope which amplifies the sounds heard.

mi″cro·sto'mi·a. Abnormal smallness of the mouth.

mi″cro·sur'ger·y. Surgery practiced on single cells, tissues, or microorganisms, using a microscope and special minute cutting instruments.

mi″cro·the'li·a. Congenital hypoplasia of the nipple of the breast.

mi·cro'ti·a (migh-kro'shee-uh). Abnormal smallness of the external ear(s).

mi'cro·tome. An instrument for cutting thin sections of tissues for microscopical examination. The tissues are usually embedded in paraffin or cellodin to prevent distortion of the thin slice. **freezing m.** One in which the tissue is frozen, in order to secure the hardness required for properly cutting sections of tissue that is fixed but not embedded in a hardening medium.

mi·crot'o·my (migh-krot'o-mee). Section cutting.

mi″cro·trau'ma. Injury resulting from repeated mechanical stimuli which individually are not recognizably injurious.

mi″cro·u'nit. A unit of minute measurements; the one-millionth part of an ordinary unit.

mi'cro·volt. One one-millionth of a volt.

mi'cro·wave. The region of the electromagnetic spectrum extending from a few tenths of a millimeter to a few meters.

mi″cro·zo'on. A microscopic animal.

mictine. Trade-mark for aminometradine.

mic'tu·rate. Urinate.

mic″tu·ri'tion (mick″choo-rish'un). The act of passing urine. Syn., *miction.*

mid-. A combining form denoting *the middle.*

mid'brain. The mesencephalon.

midge. An insect of those Diptera which comprise the family Chironomidae; small, delicate forms usually smaller than mosquitoes. The genus *Culicoides* is the most important medically.

midg'et. A dwarf; an adult who has never reached full growth. Such persons are usually well proportioned, but are low in the scale of reproductivity, especially if mated to another midget.

mid'line. The median line of a body or organ.

mid'pain″. Intermenstrual pain.

mid'riff. The diaphragm. Loosely used for the upper part of the abdomen.

mid'wife″. A woman, trained or experienced, who attends other women in labor.

mi'graine (migh'grain). A paroxysmal intense pain in the head, preceded or accompanied by characteristic sensory or motor disturbances or both, with vasomotor or psychic phenomena. The attack is probably the result of functional, vasomotor disturbances in the intracranial branches of the carotid artery. The etiology is unknown. Also called *sick headache.* —**migrain'ous**, *adj.* **abdominal m.** Recurrent attacks of abdominal pain associated with migraine. **ocular m.** An attack of migraine accompanied by amblyopia or other visual disturbances.

mi·gra'tion. A wandering. **external m.** The passage of the ovum from an ovary to the oviduct. **internal m. of the ovum.** The passage of the ovum through the oviduct into the uterus. **m. of leukocytes.** One of the phenomena of inflammation, consisting in the passage of the leukocytes through the vessel wall into the connective tissues. **m. of ovum.** The passage of an ovum from the ovary to the oviduct and uterus. **transperitoneal m.** The passage of an ovum from one ovary to the oviduct of the opposite side.

mi'kro-. See *micro-.*

mil·am'me"ter. Milliammeter, *q.v.*

mil'dew. A common name for minute fungi parasitic on plants, and also found on dead vegetable substances such as textiles, clothes, paper, etc.

mil'i·a·ri·a. An acute inflammatory skin disease, the lesions consisting of vesicles and papules, accompanied by a pricking or tingling sensation. It occurs especially in summer and in the tropics, often in the folds of the skin. Syn., *prickly heat, heat rash, strophulus, lichen tropicus.* Also called *miliaria rubra.* **m. crystallina.** A skin condition in which the sweat accumulates under the superficial horny layers of the epidermis to form small, clear, transparent vesicles. Syn., *sudamen.*

mil'i·ar"y (mil'ee·err"ee, ·air"ee). 1. Of the size of a millet seed, 1.0 to 2.0 mm., as miliary aneurysm, miliary tubercle. 2. Characterized by the formation of numerous lesions the size of a millet seed distributed rather uniformly throughout one or more organs, especially as in miliary tuberculosis.

mil'i·um. A disease of the skin characterized by the formation of small, pearly, noninflammatory elevations or globoid masses situated mainly on the face or genitalia. They often become hard and may last for years. **colloid m.** A rare skin disease characterized by the presence, especially on the face, of minute, shining, flat, or

slightly raised lesions of a pale or bright lemon color. It is a form of colloid degeneration of the skin, affecting persons of middle or advanced age.

milk. 1. The whitish fluid secreted by the mammary gland for the nourishment of the young. It is composed of carbohydrates, proteins, fats, mineral salts, vitamins, antibodies. 2. Any whitish fluid resembling milk, as cocoanut milk. 3. A suspension of certain metallic oxides, as milk of magnesia. **acidophilus m.** Milk inoculated with cultures of *Lactobacillus acidophilus;* used in various enteric disorders to produce a change of bacterial flora. **adapted m.** Milk that is modified to suit the digestive capacity of the child. **after-milk.** The stripping, or the last milk obtained at each milking. **albumin m.** Milk high in casein and fat, but poor in lactose and salts, a preparation devised by Finkelstein. **buddeized m.** Sterilization of milk by adding hydrogen peroxide (H_2O_2) and heating. **buttermilk.** That which remains after churning butter. **centrifugalized m.** Milk from which the cream has been separated by whirling it in a centrifuge. **certified m.** Milk, the purity of which is certified by a special commission of physicians, bacteriologists, or sanitarians. **condensed m.** Milk that is partially evaporated and enriched by the addition of sugar. **diabetic m.** One that contains only a small amount of lactose. **dialyzed m.** Milk with the sugar removed by dialysis through a parchment membrane. **evaporated m.** Milk treated with heat to lose about half of its water content. It is then canned and sterilized, and usually fortified by ultraviolet radiation. Popular in making infants' formulas. **fore-milk.** (a) That first withdrawn at each milking. (b) Colostrum, *q.v.* **fortified m.** That which is enriched by the addition of albumin, cream, or vitamins. **homogenized m.** Milk especially processed so that the fat globules are very minute and emulsification is so complete that the cream does not separate from the rest of the milk. **m. crust.** Seborrhea of the scalp in nursing infants; a form of eczema. **m. cure.** Treatment of disease by a diet of milk or milk products. **modified m.** One altered so that its composition approximates mother's milk. **pasteurized m.** One treated by pasteurization. **peptonized m.** Milk partially digested by the use of pepsin or pancreatic extract. **ropy m.** Milk that becomes viscid so that it may be drawn out into a stringy mass; caused by a growth of bacteria, *Alcaligenes viscosus.* **skim m.** Milk after the cream is removed. **soft**

curd m. Milk that is treated by boiling or by the addition of cream or sodium citrate, to produce a soft, flocculent curd. **sour m.** Milk containing lactic acid produced by the lactic acid bacteria normally present. **vegetable m.** Synthetic milk expressed from various vegetables, as the soybean; used to replace natural milk for those with milk allergy. **vitamin-D m.** Cow's milk fortified by the direct addition of vitamin D, by exposure to ultraviolet rays, or by feeding irradiated yeast to the animals. **witch's m.** Milk sometimes secreted from the breasts of the newborn.

milk′ing. 1. The process of expressing milk from the mammary gland, manually or mechanically. 2. Pressing a finger along a compressible tube or duct in order to squeeze out the contents.

mil′let seed. The edible seed of a grass; frequently used to designate the approximate size of small lesions or tumors, being about 2 mm. in diameter.

mil′li-. A combining form denoting *a thousand* or *a thousandth*.

mil″li·am′me″ter. An ammeter which records electric current in milliamperes.

mil″li·am′pere. One one-thousandth of an ampere. Abbreviated, ma.

mil″li·bar. Unit of atmospheric pressure, the one-thousandth part of a bar.

mil″li·cu′rie. One one-thousandth of a curie.

mil″li·cu′rie-hour′. A dosage unit of radon; the amount of radiation emitted by a millicurie of radon multiplied by time of treatment in hours.

mil″li·e·quiv′a·lent. The weight of a substance contained in, represented by, or equivalent to 1 cc. of a solution of specified normality, usually one-normal. Abbreviated, mEq.

mil′li·gram. One one-thousandth of a gram. Abbreviated, mg.

mil′li·gram-hour′. A dosage unit of radium; the amount of radiation emitted by a milligram of radium in one hour of treatment. Abbreviated, mgh.

mil″li·grams per cent. In biochemistry, indicating milligrams of a substance per 100 cc. of a fluid, as blood. Symbol, mg. %.

mil′li·li″ter. (mil′i-lee′tur). The one one-thousandth part of a liter, for all practical purposes equivalent to a cubic centimeter. Abbreviated, ml.

mil″li·me″ter. One one-thousandth of a meter. Abbreviated, mm.

mil″li·mi′cron. One one-thousandth of a micron. Also called *micromillimeter*. Symbol, mμ.

mil′li·mol. One one-thousandth of a gram molecule.

mil″li·nor′mal. Containing a thousandth part of the quantity designated as normal.

mil′li·pedes, mil″le·pedes (mil′i-peedz). Arthropods of the order Diplopoda. Some of the species have been incriminated as hosts of the *Hymenolepis diminuta*.

mil″li·ruth′er·ford. A unit of radioactivity representing 10^3 disintegrations per second. Abbreviated, mrd.

milontin. Trade-mark for N-methyl-α-phenylsuccinimide, an anticonvulsant used in treating some types of epilepsy.

mil·pho′sis. Baldness of the eyebrows.

miltown. A trade-mark for meprobamate.

mi·me′sis (mi·mee′sis, migh·mee′sis). 1. Mimicry, as of an organic disease. 2. The assumption of the symptoms of one disease by another disease. Also called *mimosis*. **—mimet′ic, mim′ic,** *adj.*

mim·ma′tion. The unduly frequent use of the sound of the letter M in speech.

mind. 1. The understanding; the reasoning and intellectual faculties considered as a whole. 2. *In psychiatry,* the psyche, *q.v.*

mind cure. The alleged cure of disease through mental influence; mental healing.

min′er·al. An inorganic chemical substance found in nature, especially one that is solid. **m. glycerin.** Petroleum. **m. oil.** Petroleum; also the liquid petrolatum used medicinally. **m. water.** Water naturally or artificially impregnated with sufficient inorganic salts to give it special properties.

min″er·al·o·cor′ti·coid. A steroid hormone secreted by the adrenal cortex, that primarily regulates mineral metabolism and, indirectly, fluid balance.

min′er·al spring. A spring reputed to be of value in restoring health, especially to persons with arthritic disease.

min′im. A unit of volume in the apothecaries' system; it equals ¹⁄₆₀ fluidrachm or about 1 drop (of water). Symbol, ♏. Abbreviated, min.

min′i·mal. Least; lowest. Of doses, the smallest quantity that is effective.

min′i·mum (pl. *minima*). The least; the lowest; the lowest intensity or level.

mi′nor. 1. Less; lesser; smaller. 2. An individual under legal age; one under the authority of parents or guardians.

mi′o-. 1. A combining form denoting *smaller, less.* 2. *In medicine,* a combining form denoting *decrease* or *contraction.*

mi″o·car′di·a. The systolic diminution of the volume of the heart.

miokon sodium. Trade-mark for sodium diprotrizoate.

mi·o′sis (migh·o′sis). Constriction of the pupil of the eye. —**miotic**, *adj.*

mi·ot′ic. 1. Pertaining to, or characterized by, miosis. 2. Causing contraction of the pupil. 3. An agent which constricts the pupil.

mir′bane oil. Nitrobenzene.

mir′ror. A polished surface for reflecting light or forming images of objects placed in front of it; used in rhinoscopy, ophthalmoscopy, laryngoscopy, dentistry, etc. **frontal m.** A head mirror. **head m.** A circular mirror with a central perforation, strapped to the head by a band, and used to throw light on parts to be examined. **laryngeal m.** A small circular mirror affixed to a long handle, used in laryngoscopy; a similar instrument is used by dentists, in the examination of the teeth. **plane m.** A mirror with a flat reflecting surface.

mir′ror writ′ing. A peculiar kind of writing in which the letters appear backward, as if seen in a mirror.

mis·an′thro·py (mi·san′thro·pee, mi·zan′·). An aversion to society; hatred of mankind. —**mis′an·thrope,** *n.;* **misanthrop′ic,** *adj.*

mis·car′riage. 1. Expulsion of the fetus before it is viable. 2. Abortion.

mis·car′ry. Give birth to a nonviable fetus.

mis′ce (miss′ee). Mix, a direction placed under the ingredients of compound prescriptions, and usually abbreviated M.

mis″ce·ge·na′tion. Intermarriage or interbreeding of different races of man.

mis′ci·ble. Capable of mixing or dissolving in all proportions.

mis′o- (miss′-, migh′so-), **mis-.** A combining form denoting *hatred, hating, aversion.*

mi·sog′a·my (mi·sog′uh·mee, migh·sog′·). Aversion to marriage. —**misog′amist,** *n.*

mi·sog′y·ny (mi·sodj′i·nee, migh·sodj′·). Hatred of women. —**misog′ynist,** *n.*

mi·sol′o·gy (mi·sol′o·jee, migh·sol′·), **mis″o·lo′gi·a.** Unreasoning aversion to intellectual or literary matters, or to argument or speaking.

mis″o·ne′ism. Hatred or horror of novelty or change. —**misoneist,** *n.*

mis″o·pe′di·a. Morbid hatred of all children, but especially of one's own.

mist. *Mistura;* mixture.

mis′tle·toe. The woody parasites *Viscum album* (European mistletoe) and *V. flavescens* (American mistletoe).

mite. Any representative of a large group of small arachnids, which together with the larger ticks constitute the order Acarina.

mith′ri·date. An old concoction believed to contain an antidote to every known poison.

mi′ti·cide. A substance destructive to mites.

mit′i·gate. Allay, make milder; moderate.

mi′tis. Mild.

mi·to′sis (mi·to′sis, my·to′sis). 1. Indirect nuclear division; usually divided into a series of stages: prophase, metaphase, anaphase, and telophase. Syn., *karyokinesis.* 2. The division of the cytoplasm and nucleus. —**mitot′ic,** *adj.*

mi′tral. 1. Resembling a bishop's miter. 2. Pertaining to the atrioventricular valve of the left side of the heart. **fish-mouth m.** Advanced degree of constriction of the mitral orifice of the heart.

mi′troid. Shaped like a miter cap.

mix′ture. *In pharmacy,* usually a preparation made by incorporating insoluble ingredients in a liquid vehicle, preferably with the aid of a suspending agent so that the insoluble substances do not readily settle out. **Basham's m.** Iron and ammonium acetate solution. **brown m.** Compound opium and glycyrrhiza mixture. **freezing m.** A mixture of salt and snow or ice, which absorbs heat in undergoing solution.

ml. Milliliter.

M. L. D. Minimum lethal dose.

mm. Millimeter.

Mn. Chemical symbol for manganese.

mne″mas·the′ni·a (nee″mass·thee′nee·uh). Weakness of memory not due to organic disease.

mne·mon′ics (nee·mon′icks). The science of cultivation of the memory by systematic methods.

Mo. Chemical symbol for molybdenum.

moan. 1. Utter a low, dull sound expressive of suffering. 2. The sound so uttered.

mo′bile op′ti·cal u′nit. A Medical Department installation, equipped to make or repair spectacles in the field; no refraction or eye examination is done.

mo·bil′i·ty. The condition of being movable.

mo″bi·li·za′tion. 1. The act of rendering an ankylosed part movable. 2. Freeing an organ during surgical operation to make it accessible. 3. The liberation of a substance stored in the body, as the mobilization of glycogen stored in the liver. —**mo′bilize,** *v.t.*

mo·dal′i·ty. 1. A method of therapy; also, the apparatus or material used in therapy. 2. Any of the forms of sensation, such as touch or vision.

mode. That value in a series of observations which occurs most frequently.

mod′el. 1. The form or material pattern of anything to be made, or aleady existing. 2. A reproduction in plaster or metal of any object, as a tooth or the dental arch; made by pouring the material into an impression, q.v., taken from that object. Also see *cast*.

o'dus. A mode or method. **m. operandi.** The method of doing something.

og"i·graph'i·a (modj"i-graf'ee-uh, ·gray"fee-uh). Writer's cramp.

og"i·la'li·a. Difficult or painful speech, as stammering or stuttering. Syn., *molilalia.*

og"i·pho'ni·a. Difficulty in speaking, excited by an effort to sing or speak loudly.

oi'e·ty. A part or portion, as of a molecule or a compound, having a characteristic chemical or pharmacological property.

oist. Damp; slightly wet; characterized by the presence of fluid.

ol. See *gram molecule.*

o'lal. Pertaining to moles of a solute per 1000 Gm. of solvent. Also see *molar.*

o'lar. A grinding tooth; a grinder. Abbreviated, M. —**molar'iform,** *adj.* **sixth-year molars.** The first of the permanent molar teeth.

o'lar. 1. Pertaining to masses, in contradistinction to molecular. 2. Pertaining to moles of solute in a definite volume of solution, usually 1 liter. Also correctly called *molal.*

o·las'ses. The syrupy residual liquid obtained in the refining of sugar.

old. 1. Make conform to a given shape, as the fetal head. 2. A cavity or form in which a thing is shaped.

old. Any one of those saprophytic fungi which form slimy or cottony growths on foodstuffs, leather, etc.

old'ing. The act of shaping or modeling, as changing the shape of a child's head in vertex presentations, resulting from pressure during labor.

ole. 1. A mass formed in the uterus of fetal membranes or a fetus, the growth of which has become arrested and which has undergone degeneration. See *nevus.* **blood m.** A mass of coagulated blood and retained fetal membranes and placenta, sometimes found in the uterus after an abortion. **false m.** One not containing any tissues derived from a fetus or fetal membranes. **fleshy m.** 1. A blood mole which has become more solid and has assumed a fleshy appearance. 2. The more or less amorphous remains of a dead fetus in the uterine cavity. **hydatidiform m.** One formed by proliferation and cystic degeneration of the chorionic villi. It may be partial or complete, involving the entire placenta. When trophoblastic proliferation

is extensive, invasion of the blood vessels of the uterine wall may occur, but metastases rarely occur. Also called *hydatid m.* **true m.** One which is the remains of a fetus or fetal membranes. **tubal m.** Remains of a fetus or fetal membranes in incomplete tubal abortion which have become infiltrated with blood.

mole, mol. A gram molecule, or formula weight expressed in grams. —*molar, adj.*

mol·ec'u·lar. 1. Of or designating a molecule. 2. Of or pertaining to a compound resulting from a more or less loose combination of molecules of two or more substances.

mol'e·cule. 1. A minute mass of matter. 2. The smallest quantity into which a substance can be divided and retain its characteristic properties; or the smallest quantity that can exist in a free state.

mo·li'men, mo'li·men (pl. *molimina*). 1. Effort. 2. *In physiology,* laborious functioning. 3. *In gynecology,* nervous or circulatory symptoms accompanying menstruation.

mol·li'ti·es (mo·lish'ee·eez). Softness.

mol·lus'cum. 1. A term applied to certain diseases of the skin. 2. A chronic skin disease with pulpy nodules. —**mollus'cous,** *adj.* **m. contagio'sum.** A chronic disease of the skin, characterized by the formation of pinhead-sized to pea-sized, rounded, sessile or pedunculated, waxlike elevations of a yellowish white or pinkish color, usually with central umbilication. The lesions on microscopical examination are found to contain peculiar ovoid, sharply defined bodies—molluscum bodies—which generally are considered to be forms of epithelial degeneration (the older idea that they are parasitic inclusion bodies has been abandoned). Syn., *m. epitheliale.*

molt, moult (mohlt). Shed skin, feathers, or hair.

mo·lyb'date. Any salt of molybdic acid.

mo·lyb'de·num (mo·lib'di·num, mol"ib·dee'num). Mo = 95.95. A heavy metallic element.

mo·lyb'dic. Containing trivalent or hexavalent molybdenum.

mo·lyb'dic ac'id. H_2MoO_4. Molybdic hydroxide. Used as a reagent.

mo·lyb'do-, molybd-. 1. A combining form meaning *lead.* 2. *In chemistry,* a combining form denoting *molybdous.* 3. *In medicine,* a combining form denoting *lead poisoning.*

mo·lyb'dous. Containing divalent molybdenum.

mo'ment. The arithmetic mean of the deviations of the observations in a frequency distribution from any selected value, each raised to the same power. First power for first moment, second power for second moment, etc.

mo·men'tum. The mass of a body multiplied by its linear velocity.

mon-. See *mono-*.

mon'ad, mo'nad. 1. A univalent element or radical. 2. Any of the small flagellate protozoa. 3. In meiosis, one of the elements of the tetrad produced by the pairing and splitting of homologous chromosomes. Each monad is separated into a different daughter cell as the result of the two meiotic divisions.

mon·am'ide. An amide formed by the replacement of a hydrogen in one molecule of ammonia by an acid radical.

mon·am'ine (mon-am'een, -in). An amine formed by the replacement of a hydrogen in one molecule of ammonia by an alkyl radical.

Mo·nar'da. A genus of labiate plants.

mon·ar'thric. Pertaining to one joint.

mon"ar·thri'tis. Arthritis affecting only a single joint.

mon"ar·tic'u·lar. Pertaining to one joint.

mon·as'ter. 1. The chromosomes in the equatorial plate at the end of the prophase of mitosis; the "mother-star." 2. The single aster formed in an aberrant type of mitosis, in which the chromosomes are doubled but the cell body does not divide.

mon"a·tom'ic. 1. Having but one atom of replaceable hydrogen, as a monatomic acid. 2. Having only one atom, as a monatomic molecule. 3. Having the combining power of one atom of hydrogen, as a monatomic radical. 4. Formed by the replacement of one hydrogen atom in a compound by a radical, as a monatomic alcohol.

mo·ne'sia (mo-nee'shuh, -zhuh). An extract from the Brazilian tree *Pradosia lactescens*.

Mon'go·lism. A type of idiocy having some similarities to myxedema and cretinism; characterized by a broad face, flat or stubby nose, obliquely set eyes, open mouth, fat and soft skin, and flaccid muscles. Also called *Mongolian idiocy*.

mo·nil'e·thrix, mon"i·leth'rix. A congenital and hereditary disease of the hair; characterized by dryness and fragility of the scalp hair with nodes regularly or irregularly along the hair shaft, giving it a beaded appearance. Also called *moniliform hair, beaded hair*.

mo·nil·i'a·sis (mo"ni·lye'uh·sis, mon"i-). A condition produced by infection with a fungus of the genus *Candida*, usually *C. albicans*. Various parts of the body may be involved: skin, mucous membrane, nails, bron-

chi, lungs, vagina, and gastrointestinal tract. Rarely, a septicemia may occur. Also see *thrush, intertrigo, onychomycosis, paronychomycosis, perlèche, erosio interdigitalis blastomycetica*.

Mo·nil"i·for'mis. A genus of acanthocephalan worms. **M. moniliformis.** A species of worms which infests some mammals and, accidentally, man.

mo·nil'i·id. A secondary eruption characterized by sterile, grouped, vesicular lesions. It is a result of hypersensitivity and hematogenous spread from the primary focus which is caused by *Candida*. Also called *levurid*.

mon'i·tor·ing. The periodic or continuous checking, as of a region or of personnel, to determine the amount of ionizing radiation or of radioactive contamination present, in order to protect health.

mon'o-, mon-. 1. A combining form meaning *single, one,* or *alone*. (mon'o-, mo'no-). *In chemistry*, a combining form denoting the presence of one atom or group of that to the name of which it is attached.

mon"o·ac'id (mon"o·ass'id, mo"no·ass'id), **mon"o·a·cid'ic** (mon"o·a·sid'ic, mo"no-). 1. Having one replaceable hydroxyl group (OH), as a monoacid base. 2. Capable of uniting directly with a molecule of a monobasic acid, or with half a molecule of a dibasic acid, etc.

mon"o·am'ine. Same as *monamine*.

mon"o·a'mine ox'i·dase. An enzyme that catalyzes oxidative deamination of monoamines, as norepinephrine and serotonin.

mon"o·bas'ic (mon"o·bay'sic, mo"no-). Having one hydrogen atom which can be replaced by a metal or positive radical, as a monobasic acid.

mon"o·ben'zone. p-Benzyloxyphenol, a melanin inhibiting agent. See *benzoquin*.

mon"o·blep'si·a, mon"o·blep'sis. 1. A condition in which either eye has a better visual power than both together. 2. The form of color blindness in which but one color can be perceived.

mon"o·bra'chi·us (mon"o·bray'kee·us). 1. An individual lacking one arm congenitally. 2. Characterizing a one-armed condition, congenital or acquired.

monocaine. Trade-mark for 2-isobutylamino-ethyl-p-aminobenzoate, a local anesthetic. See *butethamine*.

mon"o·car'di·an. Having a heart with a single atrium and ventricle.

mon"o·cel'lu·lar. Unicellular.

mon"o·cho·re'a (mon"o·ko·ree'uh). Chorea confined to a single part of the body.

mon″o·chro′ic. Having one color.

mon″o·chro′ma·sy, mon″o·chro·ma′si·a (mon″o·kro·may′zhuh, ·shuh). The perception of one color only.

mon″o·chro′mat, mon″o·chro′mate. A person in whom all the variations of color are reduced to a system of one color.

mon″o·clin′ic. Applied to crystals in which the vertical axis is inclined to one, but is at a right angle to the other, or lateral axis.

mon″o·coc′cus. A coccus occurring singly, not united in chains, pairs, or groups.

mon″o·cro′ta·line (mon″o·kro′-tuh·leen, mo″no·). A toxic alkaloid, $C_{16}H_{23}NO_6$, from *Crotalaria spectabilis* and *C. retusa*.

mon″o·crot′ic. Having but a single beat (as the normal pulse) for each cardiac systole; not dicrotic.

mon·oc′u·lar. 1. Pertaining to or affecting only one eye, as monocular diplopia; performed with one eye only, as monocular vision. 2. Having a single ocular or eyepiece, as a monocular microscope.

mon″o·cy·e′sis (mon″o·sigh·ee′sis). Pregnancy with but one fetus.

mon′o·cyte. A large, mononuclear leukocyte. **—monocyt′ic,** *adj.*

mon″o·cy·to′sis (mon″o·sigh·to′-sis). Increase in the number of large mononuclear leukocytes in the peripheral circulation.

mon″o·dac′ty·lism. The presence of only one toe or finger on the foot or hand.

mon″o·di·plo′pi·a. Double vision with a single eye.

mo·nog′a·my. Marriage with only one person at a time.

mon″o·gas′tric. Having one digestive cavity.

mon″o·ger′mi·nal. Having or developing from a single ovum, as in twins where there is but one chorionic vesicle.

mo·nog′o·ny. Asexual reproduction. Syn., *agamogony, agamocytogony.* **monogonous,** *adj.*

mon″o·hy′drate. A crystal containing one molecule of water of crystalization. **—monohydrated,** *adj.*

mon″o·hy′dric. Containing one replaceable hydrogen atom.

mon″o·i·de′ism (mon″o·eye·dee′izm). A mental condition marked by the domination of a single idea; induced by suggestion or hypnosis, wherein an elementary idea or image is left isolated and is not synthesized or associated with other ideas or impressions. Persistent and complete preoccupation with one idea.

mon″o·ma′ni·a. A form of mental disorder in which the patient's thoughts

and actions are dominated by one subject or one idea, as in paranoia. **—monomaniac,** *adj., n.*

mon″o·mel′ic. Pertaining to one limb, as monomelic hyperostosis.

mon″o·mer′ic. Consisting of a single piece or segment.

monomestrol. Trade-mark for mestilbol.

mon″o·mor′phous. Having but a single form; not polymorphous.

mon″o·neph′rous. Limited to one kidney.

mon″o·neu′ral. 1. Pertaining to a single nerve. 2. Receiving branches from but one nerve; said of muscles.

mon″o·neu·ri′tis. Neuritis affecting a single nerve. **m. multiplex.** Neuritis affecting simultaneously single nerves remote from each other.

mon″o·nu′cle·ar cell. A monocyte or a histiocyte.

mon″o·nu″cle·o′sis. A condition of the blood or tissues in which there is an increase in the number of large mononuclear leukocytes or monocytes above the normal. **infectious m.** A communicable disease of unknown etiology, with fever, sore throat, general swelling of lymph nodes, especially those of the posterior cervical area, and an increase in abnormal mononuclear cells. There may be a rubelliform eruption and enlargement of the spleen. Also called *Pfeiffer's disease, glandular fever.*

mon″o·nu′cle·o·tide. A product obtained by hydrolytic decomposition of nucleic acid; it is a compound of phosphoric acid, a hexose or pentose, and a purine or pyrimidine base.

mon″o·pa·re′sis (mon″o·pa·ree′sis, ·par′i·sis). Paresis of a single part of the body, as of one limb.

mon″o·pha′gi·a. 1. Desire for a single article of food. 2. The eating of a single daily meal.

mon″o·pha′si·a (mon″o·fay′zhuh, ·zee·uh). A form of aphasia in which speech is limited to a single syllable, word, or phrase.

mon″o·pha′sic (mon″o·fay′zick). Having a single phase.

mon″o·pho′bi·a. Morbid dread of being alone.

mon″oph·thal′mi·a. Congenital absence of one eye. Also called *unilateral anophthalmia.*

mon″o·phy·let′ic (mon″o·figh·let′-ick). Pertaining to, or derived from, a single original ancestral type; opposed to *polyphyletic.*

mon″o·phy′o·dont. Having but a single set of teeth, the permanent ones.

mon″o·ple·gi·a. Paralysis of a single limb or of a single muscle or group of muscles. It is designated as brachial, crural, or facial, when affecting the arm, the leg, or the face, respectively, and as central or peripheral, according to the site of the causal lesion.

mon'o·pus. An individual with congenital absence of one foot or leg.

mon"o·ra·dic'u·lar. Having only one root, said of teeth.

mon·or'chid (mon-or'kid). A person who has but one testis, or in whom only one testis has descended into the scrotum.

mon"or·rhi'nous. Having a single median nasal cavity.

mon"o·sac'cha·ride (mon"o·sack'-uh-ride, -rid, mo"no-). Any carbohydrate whose molecule cannot be split into simpler carbohydrates.

mon"o·so'di·um glu'ta·mate. HOOC.CH(NH$_2$)CH$_2$CH$_2$COONa. White or nearly white powder, very soluble in water; possesses a meat-like taste. Employed to impart meat flavor to foods. Syn., *sodium glutamate, MSG.*

Mon"o·spo'ri·um. A genus of the Fungi Imperfecti. The species **M. apiospermum** and **M. sclerotiale** have been isolated in cases of white-grained mycetoma.

mon"o·stra'tal. Arranged in a single layer or stratum.

mon"o·symp'to·mat'ic. Having but one dominant symptom.

mon"o·ther'mi·a. Evenness of body temperature.

mon·ot'ic, mon·ot'ic. Pertaining to or affecting but one of the ears.

mo·not'o·cous. Producing one young at a birth.

mon·ox'ide. 1. An oxide containing a single oxygen atom. 2. A popular name for carbon monoxide.

mons (pl. *montes*). *In anatomy,* an eminence. **m. pubis.** The fatty eminence in front of the body and superior ramus of the os pubis. **m. veneris.** The mons pubis of the female.

mon'ster. A fetus (rarely an adult) which, through congenital faulty development, is incapable of properly performing the vital functions, or which, owing to an excess or deficiency of parts, differs markedly from the normal type of the species; a teratism.

mon·stri·cide. The killing of a monster.

mon·strip'a·ra. A woman who has given birth to one or more monsters.

mon·stros'i·ty. 1. The condition of being a monster. 2. A monster.

mon·tic'u·lus. A small elevation.

mood. *In psychology,* a sustained emotional or affective tone, such as in mania or melancholia.

Mor"ax·el'la. A genus of the tribe Hemophileae of the family Parvobacteriaceae. **M. lacunata.** The type species of the genus. It is a nonmotile, Gram-negative, short rod, occurring singly, in pairs, or in short chains. Also called *Hemophilus duplex.*

mor'bid. Pertaining to disease or diseased parts, as morbid anatomy, an old term for pathologic anatomy.

mor·bid'i·ty. 1. The quality of disease or of being diseased. 2. The conditions inducing disease. 3. The ratio of the number of sick individuals to the total population of a community.

mor·bid'i·ty rate. The number of cases of a specific disease in a calendar year in a given place per 100,000 actual or estimated population at the middle of the year.

mor·bil'li (mor-bil'eye). Old term for measles. —**morbilliform,** *adj.*

mor'bus. Obsolete term for disease, *q.v.* **m. coeliacus.** Chronic disease usually of children, with profuse, large, pale, pasty or frothy, foul-smelling stools, delayed development, and, ultimately, bronchopneumonia. **m. cucularis.** Pertussis; whooping cough. **m. divinus.** Epilepsy. **m. gallicus.** Syphilis. **m. maculosus neonatorum.** A fatal disease occurring during the first few days of life and consisting of hemorrhages in various parts of the body. **m. magnus.** Epilepsy. **m. major.** Epilepsy. **m. medicorum.** The mania of those who seek the advice of physicians for imaginary diseases. **m. miseriae.** Any disease due to poverty. **m. regius.** Jaundice. **m. vesicularis.** Pemphigus.

mor·da'cious. Biting, pungent.

mor'dant. A substance, such as alum, phenol, or aniline oil, that fixes the dyes used in coloring textiles or in staining tissues or bacteria.

morgue. 1. A place where unknown dead are exposed for identification. A place where dead bodies are stored pending disposition.

mo·ri·a. 1. A dementia characterized by talkativeness and silliness. 2. A morbid desire to joke.

mor'i·bund. In a dying condition.

morn'ing sick'ness. Nausea and vomiting occurring on arising, an early symptom of pregnancy.

mo'ron. One afflicted with moronity, *q.v.*

mo·ron'i·ty. The highest grade of mental deficiency in which the subject's mental age is from 7 to 12 years and I.Q. between 50 and 74. Syn., *moronism.*

mor'phi·a. See *morphine.*

mor'phine (mor'feen, ·fin, mor-feen'). C$_{17}$H$_{19}$NO$_3$.H$_2$O. A colorless white crystalline alkaloid from opium to which the chief effects of the latter are due. **m. sulfate.** (C$_{17}$H$_{19}$NO$_3$)$_2$H$_2$SO$_4$.5H$_2$O; in the U.S.A. the most frequently prescribed morphine salt.

mor'phin·ism. 1. The condition caused by the habitual use of morphine. 2. The morphine habit.

or″phi·no·ma′ni·a, mor″phi·ma′ni·a. A morbid craving for orphine.

or″pho·gen′e·sis. The morphogic transformations including growth, terations of germinal layers, and fferentiation of cells and tissues during development. —**morphogenet′-**, adj.

or·phol′o·gy. The branch of biology which deals with structure and rm. It includes the anatomy, histology, and cytology of the organism any stage of its life history. —**morpholog′ic, morpholog′ical,** adj.

or·phom′e·try. The measurement the forms of organisms.

ors. Death. **m. putativa.** Apparent death. **m. subita.** Sudden eath.

or′sus. A bite.

or′tal. Liable to death or dissolution; terminating in death; causing eath; deadly.

or·tal′i·ty. 1. The quality of being ortal. 2. The death rate.

or′tar. A bowl-like vessel of porelain, iron, or glass; used for pulerizing substances by means of a estle.

or″ti·fi·ca′tion. Old term for gangrene.

or″ti·na·tal′i·ty. The stillbirth ate.

or″tu·ar″y (mor′choo-err″ee). 1. morgue. 2. Relating to death or urial.

or′vin. See mallein.

o·sa′ic. 1. In genetics, an individual ith adjacent tissues of different enetic constitution, as a result of utation, somatic crossing over, or hromosome elimination. 2. In embryology, descriptive of the development of ggs in which the cells of the early eavage stages have already a type of ytoplasm which determines their later ate. See regulative. 3. In plant pathology, descriptive of plants infected ith a virus which produces a characteristic spotting, as in tobacco mosaic isease.

o·sa′ic bone. Microscopically, bone ppearing as though formed of small eces fitted together, due to cement nes indicating regional alternating eriods of osteogenesis and osteoclasis; haracteristic of Paget's disease, q.v.

os·qui′to. An insect of the family ulicidae.

oss. Low green bryophytic plants the class Musci. **Ceylon m.** See var. 1. **club m.** See lycopodium. **Iceand m.** See Cetraria. **Irish m.** See hondrus.

oth′er. 1. A female parent. 2. The urce of anything.

oth′er. A slimy film formed on the surface of fermenting liquid, as on vinegar.

mo′tile (mo′til). Able to move; capable of spontaneous motion, as a motile flagellum.

mo·til′i·ty. Ability to move spontaneously.

mo′tion. 1. The act of changing place; movement, q.v. 2. An evacuation of the bowels; the matter evacuated. **passive m.** The movement produced by external agency and not by the person himself. **vermicular m.** Peristalsis.

mo′tion sick′ness. A syndrome characterized by nausea, vertigo, and vomiting; occurs as the result of the motion of a conveyance, as a ship, airplane, train, or automobile. See airsickness, seasickness.

mo″to·neu′ron. An efferent neuron.

mo′tor. 1. That which causes motion. 2. Concerned in or pertaining to motion, as motor cell, motor center, motor nerve. **m. end-plate.** Myoneural junction. An area of specialized structure beneath the sarcolemma where the motor nerve fiber makes functional contact with the muscle cell. **m. points.** The points on the surface of the body where the various branches of the motor nerves supplying the muscles may be excited by electric stimuli.

mot′tled en·am′el. A dappled condition of the teeth caused by hypocalcification or hypoplasia with or without later extraneous staining; chronic dental fluorosis, q.v.

mot′tling. A spotted condition.

mou″lage′ (moo″lahzh′). A mold or cast made directly from any portion of the body, used especially to show a surface lesion or defect.

mound′ing. The rising in a lump of muscle fibers when struck by a slight, firm blow. It is observed in the thin and feeble, and in certain diseases, as pulmonary tuberculosis and advanced locomotor ataxia. See myoedema.

moun′tain sick′ness. A condition occurring in those who ascend mountains to high altitudes, especially those over 15,000 feet; due to diminished atmospheric pressure. Symptoms include rapid pulse, headache, vertigo, mental dullness, loss of appetite, nausea, vomiting, cyanosis, dyspnea, muscular weakness, and euphoria; due to the rarefied air, symptoms appear at a lower altitude than in aviators affected by altitude sickness. Syn., hypobaropathy.

mouth. 1. The commencement of the alimentary canal; the cavity in which mastication takes place. In a restricted sense, the aperture between the lips. 2. The entrance to any cavity or canal. **trench m.** Vincent's stomatitis, q.v.

move'ment. The act of moving. **active m.** Movement effected without any outside help. **angular m.** The movement between two bones that may take place forward or backward, inward or outward. **associated movements.** Synergistic, coincident, or consensual movements of muscles other than the leading one, which are involuntarily connected with its action; as in reading both eyeballs move alike although one eye may be blind. **bowel m.** Lay term for: (a) the evacuation of feces; an act of defecation; (b) the feces evacuated by defecation; a stool. **Brownian m.** A physical phenomenon, a form of communicated motion observed in aggregations of minute particles, and consisting of a rapid oscillating movement without change of the relative position of the moving particles. Also called *pedesis*. **ciliary m.** A lashing movement produced by delicate hairlike processes termed cilia, as on the epithelium of the respiratory tract and in certain microorganisms. **circus m.** A rapid, circular movement or somersault, produced by injury on one side to some part of the posture-controlling mechanisms of the nervous system, as the vestibular apparatus or the cerebral peduncles. **fetal m.** The movement of the fetus in the uterus. **forced m.** Movement of the body from injury of the motor centers or the conducting paths. **gliding m.** The simplest movement that can take place in a joint, one surface gliding or moving over another, without any angular or rotatory movement. **ideomotor m.** Unconscious movement due to impulses of the mind when the attention is otherwise absorbed. **passive m.** Movement effected by the aid of some outside agency. **segmenting m. of the small intestine.** Spaced constrictions of the intestinal lumen at successive points along the intestine, acting to expose repeatedly new surfaces of the intestinal contents to the action of digestive juices. **vermicular m.** Peristalsis.

m.p. Melting point.

MPI. Multiphasic personality inventory. See *Minnesota multiphasic personality inventory* under *test*.

M. R. C. Medical Reserve Corps.

M. R. C. P. Member of the Royal College of Physicians.

M. R. C. S. Member of the Royal College of Surgeons.

mrd. Millirutherford.

M. S. Master of Surgery, Master of Science.

M. Sc. Master of Science.

mu'cic ac'id. COOH(CHOH)₄COOH. A dibasic acid resulting from the oxi-

dation of galactose or of carboh drates yielding this sugar.

mu·cif'er·ous. Producing or secre ing mucus.

mu'ci·lage (mew'si-lidj). *In pha macy*, a solution of a gum in wate —**mucilag'inous,** *adj.*

mu''ci·la'go. See *mucilage*.

mu'cin. A mixture of glycoprotei that forms the basis of mucu —**mucinous,** *adj.*

mu·cin'o·gen. The antecedent pri ciple from which mucin is derived.

mu·cip'a·rous. Secreting or produ ing mucus.

mu'co-, muc-. A combining form d noting *relation to mucus* or *muco membrane.*

mu'co·cele. 1. A mucous tumor. An enlarged lacrimal sac.

mu''co·col'pos. A collection of m cus in the vagina.

mu''co·cu·ta'ne·ous. Pertaining a mucous membrane and the skin, a to the line where these join.

mu''co·en''ter·i'tis. Inflammati of the mucous membrane of the inte tine.

mu''co·hem''or·rhag'ic (mew''h hem''o-radj'ick). Related to, or accom panied by, mucus and blood.

mu'coid. Resembling mucus.

mu'coids. A group of glycoprotein found in cartilage, in the cornea a crystalline lens, in white of egg, a in certain cysts and ascitic fluids.

mu·co'i·tin-sul·fu'ric ac'id. component of the mucin of saliva; hydrolysis, yields sulfuric acid, gl curonic acid, glucosamine, and ace acid.

mu·con'ic ac'id. HOOC.CH:C CH:CH.COOH. An oxidation product benzene resulting from detoxication the latter in the animal body.

mu''co·per''i·os'te·um. Periostee with a closely associated mucous me brane.

mu''co·pu'ru·lent. Containing m cus mingled with pus.

mu''co·pus''. A mixture of mucus a pus.

mu''co·rif'er·ous. Covered with moldlike substance.

mu·co'sa. A mucous membra tunica mucosa. —**mucosal,** *adj.*

mu''co·san·guin'e·ous (mew'' sang-gwin'ee-us). Consisting of mu and blood.

mu''co·se'rous. Mucous and sero containing mucus and serum.

mu·co'sin. A term suggested mucin from nasal, uterine, and br chial mucous membranes.

mu·cos'i·ty. Sliminess.

mu''co·stat'ics. *In dentistry,* method of obtaining an impress with minimum displacement or dist tion of the oral mucosa.

mu'cous. Relating to mucus; secreting mucus, as mucous gland; depending on the presence of mucus, as mucous rales. **mu'cro·nate.** Tipped with a sharp point.

Mu·cu'na. A genus of leguminous herbs.

mu'cus. The viscid liquid secreted by mucous glands. It consists of water, mucin, inorganic salts, with epithelial cells, leukocytes, etc., held in suspension.

mu''li·e'bri·a (mew''lee·ee'bree·uh, eb'ree·uh). The female genitals.

mu''li·eb'ri·ty. 1. Womanliness. 2. Puberty in the female. 3. Assumption of female qualities by the male.

mul·tan'gu·lum. A bone with many angles. Also called *multangular.* **m. majus.** The trapezium, lateral carpal bone of the distal row. Also called *greater multangular.* See Table of Bones in the Appendix. **m. minus.** The trapezoid bone, second carpal bone of the distal row. Also called *lesser multangular.* See Table of Bones in the Appendix.

mul'ti-. 1. A combining form meaning *many, much.* 2. *In medicine,* a combining form signifying *affecting many parts.*

mul''ti·cel'lu·lar. Having many cells.

mul''ti·cos'tate. Having many ribs. **mul''ti·cus'pid.** Having several cusps, as the molar teeth. Also called *multicuspidate.*

mul''ti·den'tate. Having many teeth or toothlike processes.

mul''ti·dig'i·tate (mul''ti·didj'i·tate). Having many digits or digitate processes.

mul''ti·fa·mil'i·al. Attacking several successive generations of a family, as certain diseases.

mul''ti·fid. Branched into many parts. **mul''ti·form.** Polymorphic.

mul''ti·glan'du·lar. Pertaining to several glands, as multiglandular secretions, a mixture of secretions from two or more glands.

mul''ti·grav'i·da. A pregnant woman who has had two or more previous pregnancies.

mul''ti·in·fec'tion. A mixed infection.

mul''ti·lo'bar, mul''ti·lo'bate. Composed of many lobes.

mul''ti·loc'u·lar. Many-celled; polycystic.

mul''ti·mam'mae (mul''ti·mam'ee). Polymastia; the presence of more than two breasts in a human being

mul''ti·nod'u·lar. Having many nodules.

mul''ti·nu'cle·ar, mul''ti·nu'cle·a'ted. Having many nuclei.

mul·tip'a·ra. A pregnant woman who has already borne one or more children.

mul''ti·par'i·ty (mul''ti·par'i·tee). The condition of having borne several children. **—multip'arous,** *adj.*

mul'ti·ple. Manifold; affecting many parts at the same time, as multiple sclerosis.

mul''ti·po'lar. Having more than one pole, as multipolar nerve cells, those having more than one process. **mul''ti·va'lent, mul·tiv'a·lent.** Capable of combining with more than one atom of a univalent element.

mum''mi·fi·ca'tion. The change of a part into a hard, dry mass; dry gangrene.

mum'mi·fied. Dried, as mummified pulp, the condition of the dental pulp when it is affected by dry gangrene.

mumps. An acute infectious disease caused by a virus; characterized by swelling of the parotid and at times of the other salivary glands as well as the pancreas, ovaries, and testes. After a period of incubation of from two to three weeks, the disease begins with fever, pain below the ear, and swelling of the parotid gland. In the course of a week, the swelling subsides without suppuration. One attack usually confers immunity. Syn., *parotitis.* **metastatic m.** Complication involving organs other than the salivary glands, such as a testis or an ovary.

mun·dif'i·cant. 1. Having the power to cleanse, purge, or heal. 2. A cleansing or healing agent.

mu'ral. Pertaining to a wall, as a mural fibroid, mural abscess, or mural pregnancy.

mu''ri·at'ic. Pertaining to brine.

mu''ri·at'ic ac'id. An old term for hydrochloric acid.

mur'mur. A blowing or rasping sound heard on auscultation. **aneurysmal m.** The murmur or bruit heard over an aneurysm. **aortic m.** One produced at the aortic orifice. **apex m.** One heard best in the area directly over the apex of the heart. Also called *apical m.* **arterial m.** The sound made by the arterial current. **attrition m.** A pericardial murmur. **cardiac m.** Any adventitious sound heard over the region of the heart. In relation to their seat of generation, cardiac murmurs are designated as mitral, aortic, tricuspid, and pulmonary; according to the period of the heart's cycle at which they occur they are divided into systolic, those occurring during systole; diastolic, those occurring in diastole; and presystolic, those occurring just before systole. **cardiopulmonary m.** One produced by the impact of the heart against the lung. **diastolic m.** A cardiac murmur occurring during diastole. **direct m.** A murmur produced by obstruction to the blood as it is passing in its normal direction. **Duroziex's m.** The double murmur heard over the femoral artery in aortic regurgitation. **endocardial m.** A murmur produced within the cavities of the heart. **exocardial m.** A murmur connected with the heart, but which is produced outside of its cavities. **Flint's m.** An apical diastolic murmur sometimes heard in aortic regurgitation. It is probably due to the fact that because of the extreme ventricular dilatation the valves cannot be forced back against the walls and produce a relative narrowing of the atrioventricular orifice. **friction m.** A sound produced by the rubbing of two inflamed serous surfaces upon each other. **functional m.** A cardiac murmur occurring in the absence of any structural change in the valves or orifices. **Graham Steell m.** A murmur of pulmonary valve incompetence: it may occur in cases of severe mitral stenosis and cardiac insufficiency. **heart m.** A cardiac murmur. **hemic m.** A murmur heard over the heart or jugular bulb in severe anemia, due to decreased viscosity of the blood. **indirect m.** One produced by blood flowing in a direction contrary to its normal current. **inorganic m.** A murmur not due to valvular lesions. A hemic or functional murmur. **machinery m.** A loud, continuous, rough cardiac murmur heard in cases of patent ductus arteriosus. **mitral m.** One produced at the mitral orifice. **muscular m.** (a) The sound heard on auscultation of a contracting muscle. (b) The first sound of the heart-beat. **musical m.** A cardiac murmur having a musical quality. **organic m.** A murmur due to structural changes in the heart. **paradox m.** A systolic murmur prolonged so as to appear to be followed by a diastolic murmur. **pericardial m.** A murmur produced in the pericardium. **placental m.** A sound attributed to the circulation of the blood in the placenta. Formerly called *placental bruit*. **presystolic m.** A cardiac murmur occurring just before systole. **pulmonary m.** One produced at the pulmonary orifice. **regurgitant m.** One due to regurgitation. **respiratory m.** The sound produced by the air entering and escaping from the lungs during respiration. **systolic m.** A cardiac murmur occurring during systole. **to-and-fro m.** A pericardial murmur heard during both systole and diastole. **tricuspid m.** One produced at the tricuspid orifice. **venous m.** One occurring in a vein. **vesicular m.** A fine inspiratory breath

sound heard over the chest during normal breathing. **whiffing m.** A humming, rushing sound heard in the veins in anemia.

Murphy, John Benjamin [*American surgeon*, 1857–1916]. Internationally known as surgeon, educator, and inventor. He exercised a great influence in many surgical fields, including orthopedic surgery. Contributed to the knowledge of ankylosed joints and their treatment. Invented (1892) the metal button used in rapid, end-to-end anastomosis of divided intestine, called *Murphy button.*

Murphy, William Parry [*American physician*, 1892–   ]. With George Richards Minot, introduced the *Minot-Murphy diet,* consisting chiefly of liver in the treatment of pernicious anemia (1926). This led to the present-day therapeutic use of liver extracts. Nobel laureate with G. R. Minot and G. H. Whipple (1934).

Mus'ca. A genus of flies of the family Muscidae. **M. domestica.** The most important species, the common house fly; carries and frequently transmits the causal agents of a number of diseases, including typhoid fever, infantile diarrhea, bacillary and amebic dysentery, cholera, trachoma, and tuberculosis.

mus'cae vol"i·tan'tes (mus'ke vol"i·tan'teez). Floating specks in the field of vision, due to opacities in the media of the eye. Also called *mouches volantes.*

mus'ca·rine (mus'kuh-reen, -rin, mus-kay'·). A poisonous alkaloid obtained from certain mushrooms, as *Agaricus muscarius.*

mus'ca·rin·ism. Mushroom poisoning.

mus'ci·cide (mus'ki-side). An agent which is poisonous or destructive to flies.

mus'cle. 1. Muscle tissue composed of individual muscle fibers or muscle cells. Classified by microscopical appearance as nonstriated (smooth) or striated; by volitional control as voluntary or involuntary; by location in the body as skeletal, cardiac, or visceral. 2. A contractile organ composed of muscle tissue, effecting the movements of the organs and parts of the body; particularly, that composed of a belly of skeletal muscle tissue attached by tendons to bone on either side of a joint effecting movements at the joint by contraction of the belly drawing the more movable attachment, the insertion, toward the more fixed attachment, the origin. For muscles listed by name, see Table of Muscles in the Appendix. **—muscular,** *adj.* **accessory m.** An anomalous muscle slip addition to a muscle which occurs constant (regularly), as scalenus minimus, a muscle inserted on the first rib in addition to the scalenus anterior. **antagonistic m.** One acting in opposition to another, as the triceps, which extends the elbow, in opposition to the biceps, which flexes the elbow. **antigravity m.** Muscles, chiefly extensors, the contraction of which supports the body against gravity, as in standing. **articular m.** A muscle inserted in part into the fibrous capsule of a joint, holding the capsule taut in sudden movements of the joint. **axial m.** One attached to the vertebral column. **bicipital m.** One having two heads or attachments of origin. **bipennate m.** A muscle whose fibers are inserted on two sides of a central tendon, thus resembling a feather. **cardiac m.** The muscle of the heart. **circumpennate m.** A muscle whose fibers are inserted on all sides of a central tendon. **cutaneous m.** One having an insertion into the skin or both origin and insertion in the skin. **dermal m.** See cutaneous m. **digastric m.** One having two muscular bellies joined by a central tendon. **extrinsic m.** One which has its origin outside, its insertion within an organ, as a rectus muscle of the eye. See intrinsic m. **fixation m.** One which holds a part from moving to allow more accurate control of a distal part, as a muscle which holds the wrist steady to allow more precise control of finger movement. **fusiform m.** A spindle-shaped muscle. **intra-aural m.** One in the ear, particularly inside the tympanic cavity; includes the tensor tympani and the stapedius muscles. **intrinsic m.** One which has both its origin and its insertion within an organ, as the transverse muscle of the tongue. See extrinsic m. **involuntary m.** One not under the control of the will; usually consists of smooth muscle tissue and lies within a viscus. **mimetic m.** One of the muscles of facial expression. **multicipital m.** One having more than two heads or attachments of origin. **multipennate m.** See circumpennate m. **m. of Treitz.** Muscle tissue sometimes associated with the suspensory ligament of the duodenum; arises from the right crus of the diaphragm and is inserted on the duodenum at the jejunal junction. **nonstriated m.** See smooth m. **papillary m.** The muscular eminences in the ventricles of the heart from which the chordae tendineae arise. **pectinate m.** One of the small muscular columns traversing the inner surface of the auricles of the heart. **pennate m.** One whose fibers are inserted on a central tendon. **postaxial m.** One on the dorsal aspect of

an extremity. **postural m.** See antigravity m. **preaxial m.** One on the anterior aspect of an extremity. **red m.** A muscle which appears red in the fresh state; in the fibers of red muscles, the longitudinal striation is more prominent and the transverse striation is somewhat irregular. The red color probably is due to muscle hemoglobin and cytochrome. **skeletal m.** One attached to a bone or bones of the skeleton and concerned in body movements. **smooth m.** One consisting of spindle-shaped, unstriped muscle cells and found in the walls of viscera and blood vessels; an involuntary muscle. Also called nonstriated m., unstriated m. **striated m.** A muscle consisting of cross-striated muscle fibers. **striped m.** See striated m. **supernumerary m.** See accessory m. **synergistic m.** One which, though not directly concerned as a prime mover in a particular act, helps some other muscle to perform the movement more efficiently. **tricipital m.** One having three heads. **twojoint m.** A muscle which crosses two joints and effects the movements at each joint. **unipennate m.** One whose fibers are inserted obliquely into one side of a tendon. See smooth m. **unstriped m.** See smooth m. **visceral m.** (a) Muscle of a viscus. (b) Muscle associated with the visceral skeleton. **voluntary m.** One directly under the control of the will. Also called skeletal m. **white m.** Skeletal muscle which appears paler in the fresh state than red muscle, q.v., and is associated with slow movements.

mus″cu·lar′is mu·co′sae (mus″-cue·lar′is mew·ko′see). The single or double thin layer of smooth muscle in the deep portion of some mucous membranes, as in most of the digestive tube. **mus″cu·lar′i·ty.** The quality of being muscular.

mus′cu·la·ture. The muscular system of the body, or a part of it.

mus′cu·lo-, muscul-. A combining form denoting relating to the muscles.

mus″cu·lo·ap″o·neu·rot′ic. Composed of muscle and of fibrous connective tissue in the form of a membrane.

mus″cu·lo·cu·ta′ne·ous. Pertaining to or supplying the muscles and skin, as the musculocutaneous nerve of the arm. See Table of Nerves in the Appendix.

mus″cu·lo·fas′ci·al (mus″cue·lo-fash′ee·ul). Consisting of both muscular and fascial elements, as in an amputation flap.

mus″cu·lo·phren′ic. Pertaining to or supplying the muscles of the diaphragm, as the musculophrenic artery. See Table of Arteries in the Appendix.

mus″cu·lo·spi′ral. 1. Old term for radial, as the musculospiral or radial nerve. 2. Referring to the radial groove on the posterior surface of the humerus.

mus″cu·lo·ten′di·nous. Pertaining to both muscle and tendon.

mu″si·co·ther′a·py. The use of music in the treatment of mental and nervous diseases.

musk. The dried secretions from the preputial glands of musk deer. **arti-ficial m.** One of several musk substitutes, as xylene musk, ketone musk, and musk ambrette, each having a characteristic composition. Used in perfumery.

mus″si·ta′tion. Speechless movement of the lips.

mus′tard. 1. A plant of the genus *Brassica.* 2. The dried ripe seed of *Brassica alba* or *B. nigra.* **black m.** The finely ground seeds of *Brassica nigra.* **m. flour.** Black and white mustard seeds mixed and pulverized. **red m.** Black mustard. **white m.** The finely ground seeds of *Brassica hirta.*

mus′tard oil. A volatile oil, chiefly allyl isothiocyanate, obtained from the dried ripe seeds of the plant *Brassica nigra* or *B. juncea,* a powerful rubefacient and blistering agent.

mustargen hydrochloride. A trade-mark for mechlorethamine hydrochloride.

mu′tant. An individual with characteristics different from those of the parental type, or the stock established from such individuals; due to a genetic constitution that includes a mutation.

mu″ta·ro·ta′tion. A change in optical rotation of solutions of certain sugars occurring while standing; equilibrium finally is attained.

mu′tase. An enzyme which simultaneously catalyzes the oxidation of one molecule and reduction of another molecule of the substrate. **alde-hyde m.** An enzyme, occurring in liver and yeast, which catalyzes conversion of two molecules of acetaldehyde to one each of acetic acid and ethyl alcohol.

mu·ta′tion. 1. A change of small or moderate extent, which represents a definite stage in the gradual evolution of an organism, such as may be recognized in a series of fossils from successive geologic strata (Waage, 1868). 2. A change in the characteristics of an organism produced by an alteration of the hereditary material. The alteration in the germ plasm may involve an addition of one or more complete sets of chromosomes, the addition or loss of a whole chromosome, or some change within a chromosome, ranging from a gross rearrangement, loss or addition of a larger or smaller section, down through minute rearrangements to a

change at a single locus. The latter are gene mutations, or simply mutation in the restricted use of the term.

mute. Unable to utter articulate speech.

mu″ti·la′tion. The act of maiming or disfiguring; depriving of a limb, member, part, or organ.

mu′tism. The condition or state of being speechless; dumbness. **deaf-m.** The condition of being both deaf and mute; the mutism may result from the deafness, which can be congenital or acquired, or the entire condition may be due to hysteria. **hysterical m.** That of psychic or hysterical origin, seen in stupors and in schizophrenic patients; there is an obstinate and voluntary silence, although the vocal organs are uninjured and there is no visible lesion of the cerebral speech centers.

muz′zle. The projecting jaws and nose of an animal; a snout.

my. Symbol for myopia.

my·al′gi·a (migh·al′juh, ·jee·uh). Pain in the muscles; muscular rheumatism. —**myalgic,** *adj.*

myanesin. A trade-mark for mephenesin.

my″as·the′ni·a (migh″ass·thee′nee·uh, ·ass·thi·nigh′uh). Muscular debility. **m. gravis pseudoparalyt′-ica.** A disease characterized by an abnormal exhaustibility of the voluntary muscles, manifesting itself in a rapid diminution of contractility, both when the muscle is activated by the will and when stimulated by electric current. It may be associated with overactivity of the lymphatic tissues of the thymus. —**myasthen′ic,** *adj.*

my″a·to′ni·a. Absence of muscular tone. Syn., *amyotonia.* **m. congen-ita.** Myatonia occurring in infants, and affecting only muscles which are innervated by spinal nerves.

my·ce′li·um. The vegetative filaments of fungi, usually forming interwoven masses. —**mycelial,** *adj.*

my·ce″to·gen′ic (migh·see″to·jen′-ick, migh·set″o·), **my″ce·tog′e-nous** (migh″si·todj′i·nus). Produced or caused by fungi.

my″ce·to′ma. A chronic affection involving usually the foot but may be found in other parts. Nodules of variable size appear in skin and subcutaneous tissues, which break down with discharge of oily serosanguineous pus in which are small granules, the color of which varies from case to case, as black, white, red, or intermediate shades. Microscopically, masses of fungi simulating actinomyces granules lie in abscesses, which are surrounded by granulation tissue and fibrosis. Occurs most frequently in tropical and subtropical regions. Due to a wide variety of fungi of the classes Schizomycetes, Ascomycetes, and Fungi Imperfecti. Syn., *madura foot, maduromycosis*.

mycifradin sulfate. A trade-mark for neomycin sulfate.

my′co-, myc-. 1. A combining form meaning *fungus*. 2. A combining form signifying *mucus* or *mucous membrane*.

my″co·an″gi·o·neu·ro′sis (migh″ko·an″jee·o·new·ro′sis). A neurosis accompanied by a hypersecretion of mucus, producing mucous colitis.

My″co·bac·te′ri·um. A genus of rod-shaped, aerobic bacteria of the family Mycobacteriaceae. Species of this genus are rarely filamentous and occasionally branch but produce no conidia. They are Gram-positive, and stain with difficulty, but are acid-fast. **M. leprae.** That species which is the causative organism of leprosy. **M. tuberculosis.** A species of bacilli which produces tuberculosis in mammals; is subdivided into the **Mycobacterium tuberculosis** var. **hominis** and **Mycobacterium tuberculosis** var. **bovis.**

my″co·ci′din. An antibiotic substance extracted from a mold of the Aspergillaceae family.

my′coid. Resembling, or appearing like, a fungus; fungoid.

my′co·in. An antibiotic believed to be identical with *Escherichia coli* factor, corylophilline, notatin, penatin, and penicillin-B.

my·col′o·gy. The science of fungi.

my″coph·thal′mi·a. Ophthalmia due to a fungus.

my·co′sis (pl. *mycoses*) (migh·ko′sis; pl. migh·ko′seez). An infection caused by a fungus. It may be a **superficial mycosis** as in tinea capitis, tinea barbae, when the fungus first invades the stratum corneum, later the hair follicle, and eventually the deeper portions of the hair; or it may be a **deep mycosis** where the infection is essentially or potentially systemic, as in actinomycosis, mycetoma, and coccidioidomycosis. **—mycot′ic,** *adj.* **m. fungoides.** A form of lymphoma with cutaneous manifestations characterized by eczematoid areas, infiltrations, nodules, tumors, and ulcerations. Syn., *granuloma fungoides*.

mycostatin. Trade-mark for nystatin.

my·cos′ter·ol. Any sterol occurring in yeast or fungi.

myc″ter·o·pho′ni·a. A nasal quality of the voice.

my·de′sis (migh·dee′sis). 1. Putrefaction. 2. A discharge of pus from the eyelids.

my·dri′a·sis (mi·dry′uh·sis, migh·dry′·). Dilatation of the pupil of the eye. **—mydriat′ic,** *adj., n.* **alter-**

nating m. Mydriasis which, by normal light and convergence reaction, attacks first one eye and then the other; due to disorder of the central nervous system. Also called *leaping m., springing m.* **paralytic m.** That due to paralysis of the oculomotor nerve. **spasmodic m.** That caused by overaction of the sympathetic or dilator nerve of the iris. Also called *spastic m.* **spinal m.** That produced by irritation of the ciliospinal center of the spinal cord.

my·ec′to·my (migh·eck′to·mee). Excision of a portion of muscle.

my·ec′to·py. The abnormal placement of a muscle.

my″e·lat′ro·phy. Atrophy of the spinal cord.

my″e·len·ceph′a·lon. The lower part of the embryonic hindbrain, from which the medulla oblongata develops. **—myelencephal′ic,** *adj.*

my·el′ic (migh·el′ick). Pertaining to the spinal cord.

my′e·lin. 1. The white, fatty substance forming a sheath of some nerve fibers, also called *white substance of Schwann.* 2. A complex mixture of lipins extracted from nervous tissue.

my″e·li·nat′ed (migh′el·i·na″ted). Medullated.

my″e·li·ni·za′tion. The process of supplying or accumulating myelin during the development, or repair, of nerves. **—myelina′tion,** *n.*

my″e·li·nop′a·thy. Any disease of the myelin.

my″e·li·no′sis. Decomposition of fat with the formation of myelin.

my″e·li′tis. 1. Inflammation of the spinal cord. 2. Inflammation of the bone marrow. See *osteomyelitis.* **—myelit′ic,** *adj.* **acute ascending m.** An ascending form of inflammation of the spinal cord, usually occurring as a manifestation of anterior poliomyelitis or of postvaccinal or postexanthematous myelitis. It may be simulated by a progressive diphtheritic polyneuritis or by the toxic effect of tick bites. Also called *Landry's paralysis.* **acute m.** Acute inflammation of the spinal cord. **apoplectiform m.** Paralysis of sudden onset, due to inflammation of the spinal cord. **funicular m.** The degenerative conditions observed in subacute combined degeneration of the spinal cord; due to nutritional deficiency. **postvaccinal m.** Inflammation of the spinal cord which sometimes follows vaccination. Also see acute ascending m. **pressure m.** Myelitis from pressure on the cord. **syphilitic m.** Inflammation of the spinal cord due to syphilis. **transverse m.** Inflammation extending across the spinal cord at a specific level.

my'e·lo-, myel-. A combining form denoting *myelin, the spinal cord,* or *bone marrow.*

my'e·lo·blast''. A free, undifferentiated stem cell or hemocytoblast of the bone marrow from which myelocytes develop.

my''e·lo·blas·te'mi·a. Presence of myeloblasts in the circulating blood.

my''e·lo·blas·to'ma. A malignant tumor composed of undifferentiated myeloid cells.

my''e·lo·blas·to'sis. A manifestation of myeloblastic leukemia characterized by the presence of myeloblasts in the circulating blood and a proliferation of myeloblasts in hematopoietic and other tissues and other viscera.

my'e·lo·cele''. Spina bifida, with protrusion of the spinal cord.

my'e·lo·cys'to·cele. A hernial protrusion, in spina bifida, in which there is accumulation of fluid in the central canal of the spinal cord.

my'e·lo·cyte''. 1. A general term for all the developmental stages of the several types of granular leukocytes in the bone marrow. 2. Specifically, a marrow cell containing characteristic granules and a large unlobulated nucleus intermediate in development between a promyelocyte and a metamyelocyte. —**myelocyt'ic,** *adj.*

my''e·lo·cy·to'ma (migh''i·lo·sigh·to'muh). A malignant tumor of bone marrow derived from granular leukocytes. See *myeloma.*

my''e·lo·cy·to'sis (-sigh·to'sis). An excess of myelocytes in the blood.

my''e·lo·dys·pla'si·a (migh''i·lo·dis·play'zhuh, -shuh). Defective development of the spinal cord, especially in its lumbosacral portion.

my''e·lo·en·ceph''a·li'tis. Inflammation of both spinal cord and brain.

my''e·lo·fi·bro'sis (migh''i·lo·figh·bro'sis). Fibrosis of the bone marrow.

my''e·lo·gen'ic, my''e·log'e·nous (migh''i·lodj'i·nus). Produced in, or by, bone marrow, as in myelogenic leukemia, leukemia due to disease of the bone marrow.

my'e·lo·gram. Radiograph of the spinal cord, made after the injection of a contrast medium into the subarachnoid space.

my''e·log'ra·phy. Roentgenographic demonstration of the spinal subarachnoid space, after the introduction of contrast mediums such as lipiodol, air, or pantopaque.

my'e·loid. Pertaining to bone marrow.

my''e·lo·lym'pho·cyte. A small lymphocyte formed in the bone marrow.

my''e·lo'ma. A primary malignant tumor of bone marrow, usually in multiple foci, derived from specific cells of the marrow. Ewing recognizes plasma-cell myeloma, myelocytoma, lymphocytoma, and erythroblastoma, the first being the most frequent. He excludes lymphosarcoma and endothelial myeloma, the latter a true tumor of bone. Myeloma is rarely primary in tissues other than bone marrow.

my''e·lo·ma·la'ci·a (migh''i·lo·ma·lay'shee·uh, -see·uh). Softening of the spinal cord.

my''e·lo·ma·to'sis. Multiple myeloma.

my''e·lo·men''in·gi'tis. Inflammation of the spinal cord and its meninges.

my''e·lo·me·nin'go·cele''. Spina bifida with protrusion of a meningeal sac containing elements of the spinal cord or cauda equina.

my'e·lo·mere''. A segment of the spinal cord; a neuromere.

my''e·lo·mon'o·cyte''. A monocyte developing in the bone marrow.

my''e·lo·neu·ri'tis (migh''i·lo·new·rye'tis). Multiple neuritis combined with myelitis.

my''e·lo·pa·ral'y·sis. Spinal paralysis.

my''e·lop'a·thy. Any disease of the spinal cord, or of myeloid tissues.

my''e·lop'e·tal. Moving toward the spinal cord.

my''e·loph'thi·sis. 1. Synonym for tabes dorsalis. 2. Aplastic anemia, *q.v.*

my''e·lo·plast''. A leukocyte of the bone marrow.

my''e·lo·ple'gi·a. Paralysis of spinal origin.

my''e·lo·poi·e'sis. The process of formation and development of the blood cells in the bone marrow. **ectopic m.** The formation in the adult of erythrocytes and granulocytes in regions other than bone marrow. Also called *extramedullary m.*

my''e·lo·ra·dic''u·li'tis. Inflammation of the spinal cord and roots of the spinal nerves.

my''e·lo·ra·dic''u·lo·dys·pla'si·a (-dis·play'zhuh, -shuh). Congenital abnormality of the spinal cord and roots of the spinal nerves.

my''e·lo·ra·dic''u·lop'a·thy. Disease of the spinal cord and roots of the spinal nerves.

my''e·lor·rha'gi·a. Hemorrhage into the spinal cord.

my''e·lo·sar·co'ma. Myeloma, *q.v.*

my''e·los'chi·sis. Complete or partial failure of the neural plate to form a neural tube, resulting in a cleft spinal cord.

my''e·lo·scin'to·gram (migh''el·o·sin'toe·gram). A myelogram using human serum albumin containing radioactive iodine as a tracer.

my''e·lo·scin·tog'raph·y. The technique of introducing human serum albumin containing radioactive iodine as the tracer into the subarachnoid space, in order to determine the distribution of the albumin and the profile of the tissue by means of a scintiscanner.

my"e·lo·scle·ro'sis. Sclerosis of the spinal cord.

my"e·lo'sis. 1. Myelocytosis. 2. The formation of myeloid tumors.

my·en'ta·sis (migh·en'tuh·sis). The extension or stretching of a muscle.

my"en·ter'ic. Relating to the muscular coat of the intestine.

my·en'ter·on. The muscular coat of the intestine.

my"es·the'si·a (migh"ess·thee'zhuh, ·zee·uh). Muscle sense; the perception of a muscular contraction.

my·i'a·sis (migh·eye'uh·sis). Invasion by the larvae of flies. The type of disease produced depends upon the area or cavity invaded; may be aural, nasal, intestinal, ophthalmic, cutaneous, etc.

myleran. Trade-mark for busulfan.

my'lo-, myl-. A combining form denoting *molar*.

my·lo'dus (pl. *mylodontes*). A molar tooth. *Obs*.

my"lo·hy'oid. Pertaining to the region of the lower molar teeth and the hyoid bone, as mylohyoid muscle. Also called *mylohyoidean*.

my'o-, my-. *In medicine*, a combining form denoting *muscle*.

my"o·arch"i·tec·ton'ic (migh"o-ark"i·teck·ton'ick). Pertaining to the structure and arrangement of muscle fibers.

my'o·blast. A cell developing into a muscle fiber. **—myoblas'tic,** *adj*.

my"o·blas·to'ma. A tumor of the tongue, lip, or neck, or occasionally elsewhere; it is generally benign and is composed largely of cells resembling myoblasts. The cells are rounded, with one or more dense or vesicular nuclei and with a fairly rich cytoplasm in which are tiny rods. Ewing favors the view that the cells are degenerated striated muscle fibers, but others think they are true myoblasts.

my"o·car'di·al in"suf·fi'cien·cy. See *cardiac failure*.

my"o·car·di'tis. Inflammation of the myocardium.

my"o·car'di·um. The muscular tissue of the heart. **—myocardial,** *adj*.

my"o·car·do'sis. Any noninflammatory disease of the myocardium.

myochrysine. Trade-mark for a solution of gold sodium thiomalate.

my"o·clo'nus (migh"o·klo'nus, migh·ock'lo·nus). Clonic spasm of a muscle or of various muscles. **—myoclonic,** *adj*. **palatal m.** Rhythmic contractions of the palate seen in patients with

lesions in the brain stem when these lesions involve the olives or their connections with the tegmentum. Also called *palatal nystagmus*. **Unverricht's familial m.** A hereditary form of myoclonic epilepsy most frequently affecting the tongue, pharynx, and diaphragm; occurs mainly in girls about 10 years of age.

my'o·cyte. A muscle cell.

my"o·dys·to'ni·a. A condition in paralysis agitans marked by the rapid response of the muscles to faradic stimulation, followed by relaxation and then several recontractions.

my"o·dys'tro·phy. Degeneration of muscles.

my"o·e·de'ma. Edema of a muscle.

my"o·e·las'tic. Pertaining to the layer of intimately interrelated smooth muscle cells and elastic fibers in bronchi and bronchioles.

my"o·ep"i·the'li·al. Referring to contractile cells of ectodermal origin.

my"o·fas'ci·al (migh"o·fash'ee·ul). Pertaining to the fasciae of muscles, as myofascial inflammation.

my"o·fas·ci'tis (migh"o·fa·sigh'tis). A term, both anatomic and descriptive, indicating low back pain of obscure etiology, with symptoms severe enough to indicate probable inflammatory origin.

my"o·ge·lo'sis. A hardened region in a muscle.

my"o·gen'ic. Of muscular origin; used in myogenic contraction of muscle, as opposed to neurogenic contraction.

my"o·glo'bin. Myohemoglobin, muscle hemoglobin; the form of hemoglobin occurring in the muscle fibers. It differs somewhat from blood hemoglobin in showing a displacement of the spectral absorption bands toward the red, a higher oxygen affinity, and a hyperbolic dissociation curve, a smaller Bohr effect, a lower affinity for carbon monoxide, and a lower molecular weight. It serves as a short-time oxygen store, carrying the muscle from one contraction to the next.

my'o·gram. The tracing made by the myograph.

my'o·graph. An instrument for recording the phases of a muscular contraction. **—myograph'ic,** *adj*.

my"o·he"mo·glo'bin (·hee"mo·glo'bin, ·hem"o·). The red pigment of muscle formed by combination of heme with muscle globulin. Also called *myoglobin, q.v.*

my"o·in·o'si·tol. Inositol, especially as distinguished from its other possible stereoisomers.

my"o·ki'nase, my·ok'i·nase. An enzyme present in muscle tissue.

my"o·ky'mi·a (migh"o·kigh'mee·uh,

·kim'ee·uh). Constant quivering of a muscle. See *myoclonus*.

my·ol'o·gy (migh·ol'o·jee). The science of the nature, structure, functions, and diseases of muscles.

my·o'ma (migh·o'muh). A tumor derived from muscle. When it is derived from smooth muscle, it is called a **lei·omyoma;** when derived from striated muscle, it is called a **rhabdo·myoma. —myom'atous,** *adj.* **m. telangiectoides.** A myoma with many blood vascular spaces, often cavernous. Also called *angiomyoma*.

my"o·ma·la'ci·a (migh"o·ma·lay'·shee·uh, ·see·uh). Degeneration, with softening, of muscle tissue. **m. cordis.** Softening of a portion of the heart muscle, usually resulting from thrombosis or embolism.

my"o·mec'to·my. Excision of a uterine or other myoma.

my"o·me·tri'tis. Inflammation of the uterine muscular tissue.

my"o·me'tri·um. The uterine muscular structure.

my"o·neu'ral. 1. Pertaining to both muscle and nerve. 2. Relating to the nerve endings in muscle tissue.

my"o·pal'mus. Twitching of the muscles.

my"o·pa·ral'y·sis. Paralysis of a muscle or muscles.

my"o·pa·re'sis (migh"o·pa·ree'sis, ·par'i·sis). Slight paralysis of muscle.

my"o·path'i·a ra·chit'i·ca (ra·kit'i·kuh). The muscular atonia of rachitic infants.

my"o·path'ic. Depending upon or relating to disease of the muscles.

my·op'a·thy, my"o·path'i·a. Any disease of the muscles.

my'ope. A person affected with myopia.

my"o·per"i·car·di'tis. A combination of pericarditis with myocarditis.

my·o'pi·a (migh·o'pee·uh). Nearsightedness; an optical defect, usually due to too great length of the antero-posterior diameter of the globe, whereby the focal image is formed in front of the retina. Symbol, my. **—myop'ic,** *adj.* **malignant m.** Rapidly progressing myopia. **progressive m. of children.** Continuous increase of myopia, due to increasing growth of the eyeball.

my"o·plas"ty. Plastic surgery on a muscle or group of muscles.

my"o·por·tho'sis. The correction of myopia.

my"o·psy·chop'a·thy (migh"o·sigh·kop'uth·ee). A disease of the muscles associated with feebleness or defect of mind. Syn., *myopsychosis*.

my·or'rha·phy (migh·orr'uh·fee). Suture of a muscle.

my"o·sar·co'ma. A sarcoma derived from muscle.

my"o·scle·ro'sis. Fibrous myositis.

my'o·sin. One of the principal proteins occurring in muscle. Its coagulation after death is the cause of rigor mortis.

my'o·sin·ase". The enzyme involved in the conversion of myosinogen to myosin.

my"o·sin'o·gen. One of the proteins of muscle protoplasm; the antecedent of myosin.

my"o·si'tis. Inflammation of muscle, usually referring to voluntary muscle. **—myosit'ic,** *adj.* **fibrous m.** Chronic myositis with formation of fibrous tissue. **interstitial m.** Inflammation of the stroma of muscle. **ischemic m.** Inflammatory reaction in muscle due to marked reduction of blood supply, as by prolonged tight bandaging for a fracture. **m. ossificans.** Myositis with formation of bone. It includes a circumscribed form, with bone formation in a scar; a traumatic form with bone formation in the injured part of the muscle; and a multiple progressive form, characterized by bone formation in many foci in muscles, tendons, ligaments, etc., beginning in early life and progressively increasing. **parenchymatous m.** Inflammation affecting the muscle fibers.

my"o·stat'ic. Referring to a muscle of fixed length in relaxation, as in myostatic contracture.

my"o·su'ture. Suture of a muscle; myorrhaphy.

my"o·tac'tic. Relating to muscular sense.

my·ot'a·sis (migh·ot'uh·sis). Stretching of a muscle. **—myotat'ic,** *adj.*

my"o·ten"o·si'tis. Inflammation of a muscle and its tendon.

my"o·te·not'o·my. Surgical division of a muscle and its tendon.

my'o·tome. 1. An instrument for performing myotomy. 2. That part of a somite that differentiates into striated muscle. Syn., *muscle plate*.

my·ot'o·my (migh·ot'o·mee). Division of a muscle, particularly through its belly.

my"o·to'ni·a. Tonic muscular spasm. **m. congenita.** A congenital and usually hereditary disease characterized by tonic spasms in the voluntarily moved muscles. Also called *Thomsen's disease*.

myr'i·a·gram. Ten thousand grams.

myr·ri'ca. The dried bark of the root of *Myrica cerifera* and *M. pennsylvanica*. Also called *bayberry bark*.

myr'i·cin. Myricyl palmitate, $C_{30}H_{61}$·$O_2C_{15}H_{31}$, a constituent of beeswax.

myr'i·cyl. The univalent hydrocarbon radical, $C_{30}H_{61}$. **m. alcohol.** $C_{30}H_{61}OH$; a constituent of beeswax.

myr·in'ga. The tympanic membrane.

myr″in·gi′tis (mirr″in·jy′tis, my=rin·). Inflammation of the tympanic membrane.

my·rin″go·dec′to·my. Excision of a part or of the whole of the tympanic membrane.

my·rin″go·my·co′sis (mi·ring″go·migh·ko′sis). An exudative inflammation of the eardrum and external auditory canal; caused by a fungus. Also called *otomycosis, mycotic otitis externa.*

my·rin′go·plas″ty. A plastic operation on the tympanic membrane. —**myringoplast′ic,** *adj.*

my·rin′go·tome. Instrument used in incising tympanic membrane.

myr″in·got′o·my. Incision of the tympanic membrane.

my·ris′ti·ca (mi·ris′ti·kuh, migh·ris′·). Nutmeg, *q.v.*

my·ris′tic ac′id (mi·ris′tick, migh·ris′tick). $CH_3(CH_2)_{12}COOH$. A fatty acid occurring in the glycerides of many fats.

my·ris′tin. $(C_{14}H_{27}O_2)_3C_3H_5$. Glyceryl trimyristate, a component of sperma-ceti, nutmeg butter, and other fats.

my·ron′ic ac′id (migh·ron′ick, mi·ron′ick). $C_{10}H_{19}NS_2O_{10}$. The acid component of the glycoside, sinigrin, found in black mustard, which on hydrolysis yields allyl isothiocyanate.

myr′o·sin (mirr′o·sin, migh′ro·sin). An albuminous ferment found in mustard seed; liberates mustard oil from potassium myronate.

myrrh (mur). A gum resin obtained from *Commiphora molmol, C. abyssinica,* or other species of *Commiphora.*

myr′tle. The dried leaves of *Myrtus communis.*

mysoline. Trade-mark for primidone.

my″so·pho′bi·a. Abnormal dread of contamination or dirt.

my′ta·cism. Excessive or faulty use of the letter *m,* and its substitution for other sounds. Syn., *mutacism.*

myth″o·ma′ni·a. A morbid tendency to lie or to exaggerate; a condition seen in certain psychiatric patients.

myth″o·pho′bi·a. A morbid dread of stating what is not absolutely correct.

myt″i·lo·tox′ism. Mussel poisoning, with paralysis of the central and peripheral nervous system.

myx·ad″e·ni′tis. Inflammation of a mucous gland. **m. labia′lis.** Inflammation of the mucous membrane of the lips; characterized by painless papules.

myx″e·de′ma. A constitutional disorder, occurring usually in adults or older children; due to decrease or absence of thyroid hormone resulting from atrophy, removal, lack of normal stimulation, inhibition of hormone formation, or prevention of hormone utilization, as with drugs. It is charac-terized by a sallow, puffy appearance, especially of the face and hands, low basal metabolic rate (−25 to −40%), increased sensitivity to cold, dryness of skin and absence of sweating, dryness and sparseness of the hair, brittleness of the nails, paresthesia, apathy, lethargy, delayed cerebration, retarded reflexes, slow, thick, coarse speech, anemia, increased glucose tolerance, change in plasma protein levels, hypercholesterolemia, cardiac dilatation, bradycardia, and low-voltage electrocardiogram. It is completely controlled by the continued administration of a sufficient dose of desiccated thyroid orally or thyroxin intravenously. Also called *Gull's disease, athyrea, athyreosis.* —**myxedem′atous,** *adj.*
operative m. That arising as a result of removal of a large part of the thyroid gland. Syn., *cachexia strumipriva.* **pituitary m.** A rare type of myxedema developing in association with, and probably resulting from, pituitary deficiency, as in pituitary adenoma.

myx·id′i·o·cy. Cretinism.

myx′o-, myx-. A prefix meaning *relating to mucus or mucoid.* A combining form meaning *mucus;* denotes a *mucous gland* or *mucous tissue.*

myx″o·ad″e·no′ma. An adenoma with a myxomatous component; an adenoma of a mucous gland.

myx″o·chon′dro·fi″bro·sar·co′ma (mick″so·kon″dro·). A malignant tumor composed of a mixture of myxomatous, chondromatous, and fibromatous elements.

myx″o·chon·dro′ma (mick″so·kon·dro′muh). A combination of myxoma and chondroma. More often mucoid degeneration of a chondroma, that is, chondroma myxomatodes.

myx″o·chon″dro·sar·co′ma. A malignant tumor composed of a mixture of myxomatous and chondromatous elements. Often occurs as mucoid degeneration in a chondrosarcoma, as in chondrosarcoma myxomatodes.

myx′o·cyte. A large cell, polyhedral or stellate, found in mucoid tissue.

myx″o·fi·bro′ma (mick″so·figh·bro′muh). A fibroma with a myxomatous component.

myx″o·fi″bro·sar·co′ma. A malignant tumor composed of myxomatous and fibrosarcomatous elements. Often mucoid degeneration in a fibrosarcoma, that is, fibrosarcoma myxomatodes.

myx″o·gli·o′ma (mick″so·glye·o′muh). A gelatinous form of glioma.

myx′oid. Like mucus.

myx″o·li·po′ma. A combination of myxoma and lipoma. Often occurs as mucoid degeneration of the connective tissue of lipoma, that is, lipoma myxomatodes.

myx·o′ma. A connective-tissue tumor, probably derived from embryonal tissue, which has its prototype in mucoid tissue. The cells, of stellate and spindle form, and their processes, are separated by mucoid, the mucinous material produced by connective tissue. Often a mucoid degeneration of another connective-tissue tumor such as fibroma. —**myxom′atous,** *adj.* **cystic m.** One with an accumulation of mucoid so as to resemble cysts. Also called *cystoid m.* **telangiectatic m.** One with a rich vascular component. Also called *m. telangiectodes, vascular m.*

myx″o·ma·to′sis. The presence of numerous myxomas.

Myx″o·my·ce′tes (mick″so-migh-see′teez). A division of fungi, known as the slime molds, none of which is pathogenic to man; they resemble protozoa in some respects.

myx″o·neu·ro′ma. 1. A neuroma, or more often a neurofibroma, with a myxomatous component, occurring in peripheral nerves. 2. Mucoid form of meningioma. 3. A gelatinous form of glioma.

myx″or·rhe′a. A copious discharge of mucus.

myx″o·sar·co′ma. A sarcoma with a myxomatous component.

N

N 1. Chemical symbol for nitrogen. 2. Abbreviation for normal.

N-. *In chemistry,* a symbol prefixed to a radical to show that it is attached to a nitrogen atom.

n. 1. A unit of neutron dosage corresponding to the roentgen. 2. Symbol for refractive index. 3. Abbreviation for nasal.

N. A. Numerical aperture.

NA. Abbreviation for Nomina Anatomica, the anatomic nomenclature adopted in Paris, 1955, by the Sixth International Congress of Anatomists. Also see *Basle anatomical nomenclature.*

Na. Chemical symbol for sodium.

na′cre·ous (nay′kree′us, nack′ree-us). Resembling mother-of-pearl.

N. A. D. No appreciable disease.

nae′paine   hy″dro·chlo′ride (nee′pain). 2-Amylaminoethyl p-aminobenzoate hydrochloride, a local anesthetic. See *amylsine hydrochloride.*

na·ga′na. A trypanosomiasis of domestic animals, chiefly horses, in East Africa, which is transmitted by the tsetse fly.

nagamol. Trade name for suramin.

nail. 1. The horny structure that covers the dorsal aspect of the terminal phalanx of each finger or toe. 2. *In surgery,* a device shaped like a pin, usually of metal, used to anchor bone fragments. See Küntscher *nail.* **ingrowing n.** An overlapping of the nail by the adjacent tissues, often attended by painful ulceration and exuberant granulations. It is most common in the great toe. **Küntscher n.** A stainless steel rod used for intramedullary fixation of fractures of long bones, especially the femur, tibia, humerus, radius,

and ulna. **n. bed.** The vascular tissue, corresponding to the corium and the germinative layer of the skin, on which a nail rests. **n. en raquette.** A dystrophy in which a nail, usually that of the thumb, appears wider than normal, its transverse curvature diminished so that it appears flat. The effect is that of a miniature tennis racket. **n. fold.** The fold of skin bounding the sides and proximal portion of a nail. **n. groove.** The sulcus between the nail fold and the nail bed. **n. root.** The part of the body of the nail covered by the proximal nail fold. **parrot-beak n.** A nail curved like a parrot's beak. **spoon n.** A nail with the lateral edges raised and the central part hollowed out. **turtle-back n.** A nail curved in all directions; a condition seen in certain trophic disturbances.

nail bit′ing. Onychophagia; a nervous affliction or neurosis developing in adolescents and children, manifested by the habit of biting the fingernails down to the quick. The habit is difficult to break and frequently persists into middle age.

na′ked. Unclothed; nude.

nalline   hydrochloride. Trademark for nalorphine hydrochloride.

nal·or′phine   hy″dro·chlo′ride. N-Allylnormorphine hydrochloride, a morphine derivative with little or no analgesic effect and with antagonism to narcotic analgesics such as morphine, meperidine, and methadone, used in treating narcotic overdosage and in combating extreme narcosis produced by morphine. See *nalline hydrochloride.*

na′nism (nay′niz·um, nan′iz·um). Ab-

nano·ceph'a·lus (nay"no·sef'uh-lus, nan"o·). A fetus with a dwarfed head; microcephalus.

nano·noid (nay'noyd, nan'oyd). Dwarf-like.

nano·nom'e·lus. An individual characterized by undersized limbs; micromelus.

nano·so'ma, na"no·so'mi·a. Dwarfism. **nanosomia pituitaria.** Pituitary dwarfism.

nano·so'mus. An individual with a dwarfed body.

na'nus (nay'nus, nan'us). 1. A dwarf. 2. Dwarfed; stunted. —**nanous**, *adj*.

nape. The back of the neck; the nucha.

na·pel'line (na·pel'een, ·in). An alkaloid of *Aconitum Napellus*.

na'pex. That portion of the scalp just below the occipital protuberance.

naph·az'o·line hy"dro·chlo'-ide (naf·az'o·leen, ·lin). 2-(1-Naphthylmethyl)imidazoline hydrochloride, a local vasoconstrictor used as a nasal decongestant. See *privine hydrochloride*.

naph'tha (naf'thuh). 1. Formerly, any strong-smelling, inflammable, volatile liquid. 2. A mixture of low-boiling hydrocarbons distilled from petroleum and bituminous shale. **coal tar n.** A fraction distilled from coal tar; contains benzene, toluene, xylene, and similar hydrocarbons. **petroleum n.** The more volatile part of petroleum collected during distillation and known as crude naphtha, or again separated by distillation into gasoline, benzene, and refined naphtha. **shale n.** Naphtha distilled from bituminous shale. **wood n.** Mainly methyl alcohol and acetone obtained by the distillation of wood.

naph'tha·lene. $C_{10}H_8$. A hydrocarbon crystallizing in large rhombic plates, insoluble in cold water, commonly used as a moth repellent.

naph"tha·lene·a·ce'tic ac'id. $C_{10}H_7CH_2COOH$. A substance having plant-growth-regulating properties.

naph'tho-, naphth-. A combining form denoting *relationship to naphthalene or its ring structure*.

naph'thol. $C_{10}H_7OH$. A substance found in coal tar existing in two isomeric forms, **alphanaphthol** and **betanaphthol**.

naph'thyl. $C_{10}H_7$. The radical of naphthalene.

naph'tol. Naphthol, *q.v*.

naphuride sodium. Trade-mark for suramin sodium.

na'pi·form (nay'pi·form, nap'i·). Turnip-shaped.

nar'ce·ine (nahr'see·een, ·in). $C_{23}H_{27}O_8N.3H_2O$. An alkaloid contained in opium.

nar·cis'sine (nahr·sis'een, ·in). An alkaloid obtained from the daffodil *Narcissus pseudonarcissus*.

nar·cis'sism. 1. Self-love, frequently without genitality as an object. 2. In psychoanalysis, fixation of the libido upon one's own body. Syn., *ego erotism, narcism*. —**narcissis'tic**, *adj*.; **nar·cissist**, *n*.

narco-. A combining form signifying *narcosis, numbness*, or *stupor*.

nar"co·hyp'ni·a. Waking numbness; a peculiar state in which the patient feels numb on awaking.

nar"co·hyp·no'sis. A state of deep sleep induced by hypnosis. Also called *hypnonarcosis*.

nar'co·lep'sy. An uncontrollable tendency to attacks of deep sleep of short duration. Has been observed in epilepsy, encephalitis, and in tumors of the third ventricle and hypothalamus. —**narcolep'tic**, *n*.

nar·co'ma. Stupor from the use of a narcotic. —**narcom'atous**, *adj*.

nar"co·ma'ni·a. A morbid craving for narcotics (medicinal or psychologic) in order to escape painful stimuli. —**narcomaniac**, *n*.

narconumal. Trade-mark for N-methyl alurate, a hypnotic recommended as a surgical anesthetic and general nerve sedative.

nar"co·pep'si·a. Old term for slow or torpid digestion.

nar·co'sis. A state of profound stupor, unconsciousness, or arrested activity.

nar'co·spasm. Spasm accompanied by stupor.

nar"co·syn'the·sis. A form of treatment applied to psychoneuroses, especially to the war neuroses. A hypnotic drug is injected intravenously to induce the bringing forth of emotionally charged material and this is followed by a discussion (synthesis).

nar·cot'ic. 1. Producing stupor. 2. A drug that produces stupor, complete insensibility, or sleep, as opium, chloral, and cannabis. There are three main groups: the opium group which produces sleep, the belladonna group which produces illusions and delirium, and the alcohol group which produces exhilaration and sleep. 3. An individual addicted to the use of narcotics.

nar·cot'i·co-. A combining form meaning *narcotic*.

nar·cot'i·co-ac'rid. Both narcotic and irritant. Also called *narcotico-irritant*. See *acronarcotic*.

nar'co·tine (nahr'ko·teen, ·tin). $C_{22}H_{23}NO_7$, an alkaloid occurring in opium. Syn., *noscapine*.

nar'co·tism. The condition resulting from the use of a narcotic.

nar'co·tize. Put under the influence

of a narcotic; render unconscious by means of a narcotic.

na'res (nair'eez). Plural of naris, q.v.

na·rin'gin. The bitter glycoside of grapefruit rind.

na'ris (pl. *nares*). A nostril. One of a pair of openings at the anterior part (anterior nares) or at the posterior part (posterior nares) of the nasal cavities.

na'sal (nay'zul). 1. Pertaining to the nose. Abbreviated, n. 2. The nasal bone. See Table of Bones in the Appendix.

nas'cent (nass'unt, nay'sunt). Pertaining to gaseous substances at the moment of their liberation from chemical combination.

na″si·o·al·ve·o·lar (nay″zee·o·, nay″see·o·). Relating to, or connecting, the nasion and the alveolar point.

na'si·on (nay'zee·on, nay'see·on). The craniometric point where the sagittal plane intersects the nasofrontal suture.

na'so- (nay'zo-). *In anatomy*, a combining form denoting *connection with*, or *relation to, the nose*.

na″so·cil′i·ar″y (nay″zo·sil′ee·err″ee). Applied to a nerve distributed to the nose, the ethmoid sinuses, and the eyeball. See Table of Nerves in the Appendix.

na″so·fron′tal. Pertaining to the nasal and frontal bones or regions.

na″so·gen′i·tal. Pertaining to a correlation that exists between functional changes in the reproductive organs and changes in the nasal mucosa.

na″so·la·bi·al. Pertaining to the nose and lip.

na″so·lac′ri·mal. Pertaining to the nose and the lacrimal apparatus, as the nasolacrimal duct.

na″so·pal′a·tine (nay″zo·pal′uh·tyne, ·tin). Pertaining to both the nose and the palate, as the nasopalatine nerve. See Table of Nerves in the Appendix.

na″so·pha·ryn′go·scope. An electrically lighted instrument for inspecting the nasopharynx.

na″so·phar′ynx. The space behind the posterior nares and above a horizontal plane through the lower margin of the palate. Also called *epipharynx.* —**nasopharyn′geal,** *adj.*

na″so·spi·na′le (nay″zo·spy·nah′lee). A craniometric point where the sagittal plane meets a line joining the lowest points on the nasal margins. If this falls within the substance of the anterior nasal spine, a point on the left side wall of the nasal spine is used for taking measurements.

na'sus. The nose. **n. aduncus.** Hook nose. **n. cartilagineus.** Cartilaginous part of the nose. **n. externus.** The external nose. **n. incurvus.**

Saddle nose. **n. osseus.** The bony part of the nose. **n. simus.** Pug nose.

na'tal. 1. Native; connected with one's birth. 2. Referring to the nates.

na·tal'i·ty (nay·tal'i·tee). *In medical statistics,* the birth rate.

na·tal'o·in. $C_2H_{25}O_{11}$. The aloin derived from Natal aloes.

na'tant. Swimming or floating on the surface of a liquid.

na'tes (nay'teez). Old term for buttocks. —**natal,** *adj.*

Na′tion·al For′mu·lar″y (for′mew·lerr″ee). A formulary published by the American Pharmaceutical Association. Abbreviated, N. F.

Na′tion·al In′sti·tutes of Health. A division of the U. S. Public Health Service that is devoted to research in public health and the disease of man. It controls the manufacture and sale of biologic products by li... censure.

na'tive. Of indigenous origin o growth; occurring in its natural state not artificial, as native albumins, class of proteins occurring ready formed in the tissues.

na'tri·um. See *sodium.*

na'tron. Native sodium carbonate $Na_2CO_3.10H_2O$.

na'trum. Sodium.

nat'u·ral. Not abnormal or artificia

nat'u·ral se·lec'tion. Darwin theory of evolution, according to whic organisms tend to produce progeny fa above the means of subsistence; struggle for existence ensues which re sults in the survival of those wit favorable variations. Since the favor able variations accumulate as the ger erations pass, the descendants tend t diverge markedly from their ancestor and to remain adapted to the cond tions under which they live.

na′tur·o·path′ (nay′chur·o·path nach′ur·o·). One who practices natu opathy, *q.v.*

na″tur·op′a·thy (nay″chur·op uth·ee, nach″ur·). A therapeutic sy tem embracing a complete physia thropy employing nature's agencie forces, processes, and products, exce major surgery.

nau'se·a. A feeling of discomfort the region of the stomach, with ave sion to food and a tendency to vom —**nauseous,** *adj.* **creatio n.** Mo bid aversion to meat.

nau'se·ant. 1. Producing nausea. Any agent that produces nausea.

Na'val Med′i·cal Cen'ter. An i stallation of the United States Na similar in character and purpose to t Army Medical Center, *q.v.*

na'vel. The umbilicus.

na·vic'u·lar. Boat-shaped. **n. foss** (a) A depression between the vagi...

aperture and the fourchette. (b) The dilated distal portion of the urethra in the glans penis.

na·vic·u·lar. 1. [NA] The boat-shaped bone of the tarsus. 2. [BNA] The scaphoid bone of the carpus.

Nb. Chemical symbol for niobium, formerly known as columbium.

N. C. A. Neurocirculatory asthenia.

Nd. Chemical symbol for neodymium.

Ne. Chemical symbol for neon.

near point. The punctum proximum; the point nearest the eye at which an object can be seen distinctly. **absolute n. p.** That near point for either eye alone at which no effort at accommodation is made. **relative n. p.** That near point for both eyes at which accommodation is brought into play.

ne″ar·thro′sis. A new and abnormally produced articulation as a sequence of a fracture, dislocation, or disease of the bone.

neb′u·la. 1. A faint, grayish opacity of the cornea. 2. A spray, a liquid intended for use in an atomizer.

neb′u·lize. Convert into a spray or vapor.

neb′u·li″zer. Atomizer.

Ne·ca′tor. A genus of nematode hookworms. **N. americanus.** That species widely distributed in the tropical regions of the Western Hemisphere and throughout southern United States; produces the infestation necatoriasis, q.v.

nec″a·to·ri′a·sis. Infestation of man with the American hookworm, *Necator americanus*, whose infestive larvae enter the skin usually at the interdigital regions and may produce a ground itch and vesicular lesions. The adult parasite is found in the small intestine of man and during the larval migration to the intestine damage to the lungs is commonly incurred.

neck. 1. The constricted portion of the body connecting the head with the trunk. 2. The narrow portion of any structure serving to join its parts. 3. The line of junction of the crown and root of a tooth. **anatomic n.** The constricted portion of the humerus, just below the superior articular surface, serving for the attachment of the capsular ligament. **n. of the bladder.** That portion of the urinary bladder immediately surrounding the internal ureteral orifice. **n. of the gallbladder.** The constricted S-shaped portion of the gallbladder between the fundus and the cystic duct. **surgical n.** The constricted part of the humerus just below the tuberosities.

Ne″cro·ba·cil′lus. A highly pleomorphic, nonspore-forming, Gram-negative anaerobe found in feces, in abscesses of various organs, and in chronic ulcerative colitis. Also called

Bacterium necrophorum, *Actinomyces necrophorus*.

nec″ro·bi·o′sis (neck″ro-buy-o′sis). Physiologic death of a cell or group of cells, in contrast to necrosis or pathologic death of cells, and to somatic death or death of the entire organism. **—necrobiot′ic,** adj. **n. lipoidica diabeticorum.** A cutaneous disease, characterized by multiple yellow to red plaques generally seen on the extremities. Occurs mostly in female diabetics. There is also connective-tissue necrosis with an accumulation of macrophages containing lipids. Also called *Oppenheim-Urbach disease*.

nec″ro·cy·to′sis (neck″ro-sigh-to′sis). Death of cells.

nec″ro·cy″to·tox′in. A toxin produced by the death of cells.

nec″ro·gen′ic, ne·crog′e·nous (neh-krodj′i-nus). Originating from dead substances.

nec″ro·ma′ni·a. 1. A morbid desire for death or attraction to dead bodies. 2. See *necrophilism*.

nec″ro·mi·me′sis. 1. A delusional state in which the patient believes himself to be dead. 2. Simulation of death by a deluded person.

ne·croph′a·gous, ne·croph′a·gic. Pertaining to the eating of carrion, or putrid meat.

nec″ro·phil′i·a, ne·croph′il·y. 1. Necrophilism, q.v. 2. A longing for death.

ne·croph′il·ism. Sexual perversion in which dead bodies are violated; insane sexual desire for a corpse. **—nec′rophile,** n.

ne·croph′i·lous. Subsisting on dead matter; used in qualifying certain bacteria.

nec″ro·pho′bi·a. 1. Insane dread of dead bodies. 2. Thanatophobia; extreme dread of death.

nec′rop·sy. The examination of a dead body; autopsy; post-mortem examination.

ne·crose′ (neh-krohss′, neck′rohss). Undergo necrosis or tissue death.

nec′ro·sin. A substance isolated from inflamed areas; said to be capable of injuring body cells.

ne·cro′sis. The pathologic death of a cell or group of cells in contact with living cells. **—necrot′ic,** adj. **aseptic n.** That without infection and inflammation. Also called *anemic n.*, *avascular n.*, *bland n.*, *quiet n.*, *simple n.*, *spontaneous n.* **caseation n.** That occurring typically in tuberculosis, with formation of a cheesy substance. **coagulation n.** A variety characterized by cell death in situ with preservation of cell form and arrangement; most frequent in infarction. **diphtheritic n.** Necrosis of the mucous membrane; characterized by the formation of a tough, leathery membrane composed of coagulated cells and fibrin. **embolic n.** Coagulation necrosis in an anemic infarct following embolism. **fat n.** A type of necrosis of peripancreatic fat due to acute destructive disease of the pancreas. **ischemic n.** Death of tissue due to occlusion of an artery supplying the region. **liquefactive n.** A type resulting in liquefaction of the involved tissue. **medial (muscle) n.** The death of cells located in the muscular coat of the walls of arteries. **phosphorus n.** A necrosis of bone, especially of the lower jaw, occurring in those exposed to the fumes of yellow phosphorus.

nec′ro·sper′mi·a. Sterility due to loss of motility of the spermatozoa.

nec′ro·tize. Produce necrosis.

nec′ro·xo·o·sper′mi·a. A condition in which spermatozoa are present but are immobile and without evidence of life.

nectadon. A trade-mark for noscapine.

nee′dle. A sharp-pointed steel instrument, used for puncturing or for sewing tissue; of various shapes, sizes, and edges, the sewing needle having an eye for carrying suture material through the parts. **aneurysm n.** One fixed on a handle, half curved and at a right angle to the handle, with an eye at the point; used for passing a ligature about a vessel. **aspirating n.** A hollow needle for withdrawing fluid from a cavity. **cataract n.** One used for operating upon a cataract or its capsule. **curved n.** One with a curve of any degree up to a full semicircle. **cutting n.** One with a sharp edge, either curved or straight. **discission n.** One used for inserting into the capsule of the lens for breaking up a cataract. **exploring n.** A hollow needle, or a trocar with a grooved side, which allows the passage of fluid along it after it is plunged into a part where fluid is suspected. **hypodermic n.** A hollow needle, used with a hypodermic syringe. **radium needles.** Steel or platinum-iridium-walled, needle-shaped containers filled with radium salt and used in radium therapy. **round n.** Any needle which is circular in cross section without a cutting edge; may be either curved or straight. **spinal n.** A hollow needle equipped with obturator, used for spinal or sacral anesthesia or lumbar puncture. **surgical n.** Any sewing needle used in surgical operations.

nee′dle hold′er. A handle, usually in the form of a self-locking forceps, for clasping a surgical needle.

nee′dling. Discission with a nee-

dle, as of a cataract, to afford entrance to the aqueous humor and cause absorption of the lens. **n. in aneurysm.** A method of treatment, formerly in use, by the passage of needles into the sac of an aneurysm. **n. of the heart.** The aspiration of an overdistended right atrium; cardiocentesis. **n. of the kidney.** Puncture of the kidney substance for locating a stone. *Obs.*

neg′a·tive. 1. Denying; contradicting; opposing. 2. Of quantities, less than nothing. 3. *In physics,* opposed to a quality termed positive. Symbol,–.

neg′a·tiv·ism. A symptom of mental illness, usually schizophrenia, characterized by a state of markedly reduced activity in which the subject ignores inner stimuli or is indifferent, and even resistant, to suggestions and commands. **active n.** That in which the individual does the opposite of what he is asked to do. **passive n.** That in which the individual does not do what he is expected to do.

Negri, Adelchi [*Italian physician and pathologist,* 1876–1912]. Remembered for his discovery of the inclusion bodies noted in the Purkinje cells and cells of the hippocampus which are diagnostic of rabies; called *Negri bodies.*

Neis·se′ri·a (nigh-seer′ee-uh, nigh-serr′ee-uh). A genus of Gram-negative anaerobic cocci of the family Neisseriaceae. **N. catarrhalis.** A specie found in the respiratory tract; appear to excite catarrhal inflammation and sometimes pneumonia in man. **N. discoides.** An anaerobic species of unknown pathogenicity found in the intestinal and genitourinary tracts. **N. flavescens.** A species found i the spinal fluid in certain cases o clinical meningitis. **N. gonorrhoeae.** The type species of th genus; the causative agent of gonor rhea. **N. meningitidis.** Specie which causes epidemic cerebrospina meningitis. **N. orbiculata.** A anaerobic species found in the respira tory tract; of unknown pathogenicity **N. reniformis.** An anaerobi species found in the respiratory trac of unknown pathogenicity. **N. sicca** A species which apparently is th causative agent of kidney infection found in the blood stream in cases o clinical endocarditis.

Nélaton, Auguste [*French su geon,* 1807–73]. Introduced a soft ru ber catheter called *Nélaton's cathete* and a probe tipped with rough porc lain for locating bullets, called *Nél ton's probe.* Described pelvic hem tocele. Subastragalar disarticulatio usually with wedging between tibia a

bula, is called *Nélaton's disarticulation*. A line drawn from the anterior
superior iliac spine to the tuberosity of
the ischium is called *Nélaton's line*. In
dislocated hip the tip of the greater
trochanter of the femur is above this
line.

em″a·thel·min'thes (nem″uh-
nel·min'theez, nee″muh·). The phylum of the roundworms, which includes
the true roundworms or nematodes, the
hair snakes, and acanthocephalan
worms.

em″a·to'da (nem″uh·to'duh, nee″-
uh·). A class of the phylum Nema-
helminthes; the true roundworms.
Members of the class are bilaterally
symmetrical, unisexual, without a
roboscis, and have a body cavity not
ined with epithelium.

em'a·tode (nem'uh·toad, nee'-
uh·). Any worm of the class Nema-
oda.

em″a·tol'o·gy (nem″uh·tol'o·jee,
ee″muh·). That portion of the science
parasitology concerned with the
udy of nematode worms.

mbutal. Trade-mark for pento-
arbital sodium.

'o-, ne-. 1. A combining form mean-
g *new* or *recent*. 2. In biology, a com-
ning form signifying an *immature
rm*, a recently formed part, or an
normal new formation. 3. In chemis-
y, a combining form denoting a *new
mpound*.

o-antergan. Trade-mark for the
tihistaminic substance pyrilamine or
-p-methoxybenzyl-N'-N'-dimethyl-N-
pyridylethylene diamine.

″o·ars″phen·a·mine' (nee″o-
s″fen·uh·meen', ·in). Chiefly sodium
3'-diamino-4:4'-dihydroxyarsenoben-
ne-N-methylenesulfoxylate. A yellow
wder, very soluble in water; used as
antisyphilitic. See *neosalvarsan.*
so called *novarsenobenzol, arsphen-
ine-S*.

″o·ar·thro'sis. A false joint, *q.v.*

″o·blas'tic. Pertaining to, or of
e nature of, new tissue.

ocaine. Trade-mark for procaine
drochloride.

″o·cal'a·mine (nee″o·kal'uh-
en, ·min). A mixture of red ferric
ide, yellow ferric oxide, and zinc
ide.

″o·cer″e·bel'lum. The part of
e cerebellum which is phylogeneti-
ly most recent in development, con-
sing the lateral lobes, the medial
as, and the lobulus simplex.

″o·cin'cho·phen (nee″o·sing'ko-
). C₁₉H₁₇O₃N. The ethyl ester of
nethyl-2-phenylquinoline-4-carbox-
acid; a white powder, nearly in-
uble in water. See *tolysin.*

″o·dym'i·um. Nd = 144.27. A rare
earth metal occurring in cerium and
lanthanum minerals.

ne″o·gen'e·sis. Regeneration of tissues. —**neogenet'ic,** *adj.*

neo-hombreol. A trade-mark for
testosterone propionate, a male sex
hormone derivative.

neo-hombreol-M. A trade-mark for
methyltestosterone.

neohydrin. Trade-mark for chlor-
merodrin.

neo-iopax. A trade-mark for iodoxyl.

neolin. A trade-mark for benzathine
penicillin G.

ne·ol'o·gism. *In psychiatry*, meaningless, or newly coined, words uttered
by the insane.

ne″o·mem'brane. A new or false
membrane.

ne″o·mor'phism. *In biology*, the
development of a new form.

ne″o·my'cin. An antibiotic substance
produced by a *Streptomyces* species isolated from soil.

ne'on. Ne = 20.183. A chemically inert,
gaseous element occurring, in small
amounts, in air.

neonal. Trade-mark for 5-*n*-butyl-5-
ethylbarbituric acid, a hypnotic and
sedative. See *butethal.*

ne″o·na'tal. Newborn, *q.v.*

ne″o·na'tal mor·tal'i·ty rate.
The number of deaths reported among
infants under one month of age in a
calendar year per 1,000 live births reported in the same year and place.

ne″o·na·to'rum. Pertaining to the
newborn.

ne″o·na'tus, ne'o·nate. A newly
born infant. —**neona'tal,** *adj.*

ne·oph'il·ism. Morbid or undue desire for novelty.

ne″o·pho'bi·a. Dread of new scenes
or of novelties.

ne″o·phren'i·a (nee″o·fren'ee·uh,
·free'nee·uh). Mental deterioration in
early youth.

ne'o·pine (nee'o·peen, ·pin). An alkaloid, isomeric with codeine, occurring
in opium.

ne″o·pla'si·a (nee″o·play'zhuh,
·shuh). 1. Formation of new tissue. 2.
Formation of tumors or neoplasms.

ne'o·plasm. Any new growth; usually
applied to a tumor, an aberrant new
growth. —**neoplas'tic,** *adj.* **metastatic n.** A metastatic tumor, *q.v.*

ne'o·prene. Generic name for synthetic rubber made by polymerization
of 2-chloro-1,3-butadiene.

neoprontosil. A trade-mark for
disodium 4'-sulfamidophenyl-2-azo-7-
acetylamino-1-hydroxynaphthalene-3,-
6-disulfonate, a red, medicinal dye.
*Prontosil soluble, prontosil red, strep-
tozon-S,* and *azosulfamide* are other
trade-marks for the same drug.

ne″o·quas'sin. See *quassin.*

ne″o·sal′var·san. A name given by Ehrlich to neoarsphenamine, *q.v.*

neo·silvol. Trade-mark for a compound of silver iodide with a soluble gelatin base.

neostam stibamine glucoside. A brand of stibamine glucoside, a pentavalent organic antimony compound employed in kala-azar.

neostibosan. Trade-mark for a mixture of pentavalent organic antimony compounds used in the treatment of filariasis. See *ethylstibamine*.

ne″o·stig′mine (nee″o·stig′meen, -min). The dimethylcarbamic ester of 3-hydroxyphenyl-dimethylamine, used to prevent atony of the intestinal and bladder musculature, and for symptomatic control of myasthenia gravis. **n. bromide.** A salt which, because of its lesser hygroscopicity, is suited for use in tablets. See *prostigmin bromide*. **n. methylsulfate.** The salt used for hypodermic injection. See *prostigmin methylsulfate*.

ne″o·stri·a′tum (nee″o·stry·ay′tum). The caudate nucleus and putamen combined. Also called *corpus striatum*.

neo-synephrine hydrochloride. Trade-mark for phenylephrine hydrochloride.

neph′a·lism. Total abstinence from alcoholic liquors.

neph″e·lom′e·ter. An apparatus for ascertaining the number of bacteria in a suspension, or the turbidity of a fluid.

neph″e·lom′e·try. The determination of the degree of turbidity of a fluid.

nephr-. See *nephro-*.

ne·phral′gi·a. Pain in a kidney.

ne″phrec·ta′si·a (nee″freck·tay′zhuh, nef″reck-). Dilatation of a kidney.

ne·phrec′to·mize. Remove a kidney.

ne·phrec′to·my. Excision of a kidney. **abdominal n.** Nephrectomy performed through an abdominal incision. **lumbar n.** Nephrectomy through an incision in the loin.

neph′ric. Pertaining to the kidney; renal.

ne·phrit′ic. Pertaining to nephritis.

ne·phri′tis. Inflammation of the kidney. If the inflammation is primarily of the glomeruli, the disease is called **glomerulonephritis**, *q.v.* Nephritis caused by an infection ascending from the ureter is called pyelonephritis, *q.v.* **chronic parenchymatous n.** Chronic glomerulonephritis with marked changes in the renal tubules, as fibrosis, atrophy, cloudy swelling, hydropic or fatty degeneration, and dilatation with formation of cystic spaces. **interstitial n.** Nephritis marked by foci of exudation in the interstitial connective tissue. **scarlatinal n.** The acute catarrhal nephritis arising in the course of, or during the convalescence from, scarlatina. **tubular n.** Nephritis involving chiefly the renal tubules of the *kidney*.

nephro-, nephr-. A combining form meaning *kidney*.

neph″ro·ab·dom′i·nal. Pertaining to the kidneys and abdomen.

neph″ro·cal″ci·no′sis. Renal calcinosis, marked by the precipitation of deposits of calcium phosphate in the kidney tubules.

neph″ro·cap·sec′to·my, neph″ro·cap″su·lec′to·my. Excision of the capsule of a kidney.

neph″ro·cap″su·lot′o·my. Incision of the renal capsule.

neph″ro·car′di·ac. Pertaining to the kidneys and heart.

neph″ro·col″o·pex′y (·kol′o·peck·see, ·ko′lo·peck″see). The surgical anchoring of a kidney and the colon by means of the nephrocolic ligament.

neph″ro·co″lop·to′sis. Downward displacement of a kidney and the colon.

neph″ro·cys″tan·as″to·mo′sis. The surgical formation of an opening between a kidney and the urinary bladder.

neph″ro·cys·ti′tis. Inflammation of both urinary bladder and kidney.

neph″ro·gen′ic. 1. Having the ability to produce kidney tissue. 2. Of renal origin.

neph′roid. Kidney-shaped; reniform; resembling a kidney.

neph′ro·lith. A calculus of the kidney.

neph″ro·li·thi′a·sis. The formation of renal calculi, or the diseased state that leads to their formation.

neph″ro·lith′ic. Pertaining to, affected with, a nephrolith.

neph″ro·li·thot′o·my. An incision of the kidney for the removal of a calculus.

ne·phrol′y·sin, neph″ro·ly′sin. A toxic substance capable of disintegrating kidney cells.

ne·phrol′y·sis. 1. The disintegration of the kidneys by the action of a nephrolysin. 2. The operation of loosening a kidney from surrounding adhesions. —**nephrolyt′ic,** *adj.*

neph·ro′ma. A malignant tumor of the kidney cortex common in adults. Some believe that nephromas are really adenocarcinomas.

neph′ron (pl. *nephrons, nephroi*). The renal unit, consisting of a glomerulus and its capsule and the attached uriniferous tubule.

neph′ro·pex″y. Surgical fixation of a floating kidney.

neph″ro·poi′e·tin (nef″ro·poy′i·tin, ·poy·ee′tin). A substance supposed to stimulate growth of renal tissue.

neph″rop·to′sis, neph″rop·to′-si·a (nef″rop·to′shuh, ·zhuh). Prolapse of a kidney.

neph″ro·py″e·li′tis. Inflammation of the pelvis of the kidney; pyelonephritis.

neph″ro·py′e·lo·plas″ty. A plastic operation on the pelvis of the kidney.

neph·ror′rha·phy. 1. The stitching of a floating kidney to the posterior wall of the abdomen or to the loin. 2. Suturing a wound in a kidney.

neph″ro·scle·ro′sis. Involvement of the kidneys in hypertensive vascular disease. Gives rise to disturbances in renal function and a clinical picture identical with that of chronic glomerulonephritis. **arterial n.** Arteriosclerosis of the kidneys, causing a reduction in blood supply and atrophy of the parenchyma, with resulting fibrosis of the kidneys. Often accompanies arteriosclerosis in the aged. Also called *senile* sclerosis in the aged. Also called *senile arteriosclerotic n.* **arteriolar n.** Diffuse fibrosis of the kidneys due to arteriolar disease. **malignant n.** Nephrosclerosis characterized by rapidly progressive renal disease and marked interference with renal function; associated with malignant hypertension. There is sclerosis or hyaline necrosis of renal arterioles, or sometimes acute exudative arteriolitis.

e·phro′sis. Any degeneration of the kidneys without signs of inflammation.

·nephrot′ic, *adj.* **acute n.** That which accompanies an acute infectious disease, or an intoxication or poisoning. **chronic lipoid n.** A condition seen usually in children and associated with disturbances of protein metabolism, characterized by albuminuria, cylindruria, and lipoid droplets in the urine. **chronic n.** A slowly progressing degeneration associated with metabolic diseases, such as gout or diabetes.

e·phros′to·my. The formation of a fistula leading to the pelvis of the kidney.

e·phrot′o·my. Incision of a kidney. **abdominal n.** One through an abdominal incision. **lumbar n.** One through an incision in the loin.

eph″ro·tox′ic. 1. Pertaining to nephrotoxin. 2. Destructive to the kidney cells; nephrolytic.

eph″ro·tox′in. A cytotoxin which has a supposedly specific action on the cells of the kidney.

eph″ro·tu·ber′cu·lo′sis. Disease of the kidney due to the tubercle bacillus.

eph″ro·u·re·ter·ec′to·my. The excision of a kidney and whole ureter at one operation.

ep·tu′ni·um. Np = 239 ca. An element, atomic number 93, obtained by bombarding ordinary uranium with neutrons. Undergoes transformation into plutonium, *q.v.*

neraval sodium. Trade-mark for methitural sodium.

ne″re·an′tin. See *nerianthin.*

ne″ri·an′thin, ne″re·an′tin. A crystalline glycoside obtained from the leaves of *Nerium oleander.*

ne′ri·in. A glycoside from the bark and leaves of *Nerium oleander.*

ne″ri·o·do′re·in. A glycoside from *Nerium oleander.* See *nerium.*

ne′ri·um. The leaves and bark of *Nerium oleander.*

nerve. A bundle of nerve fibers, usually outside the brain or spinal cord; the nerve fibers are held together by connective tissue called endoneurium inside the nerve bundle and perineurium, the enclosing sheath. A collected bundle of nerve fibers within the brain and spinal cord is usually called a fiber tract. For nerves listed by name, see Table of Nerves in the Appendix. **accelerator n.** A cardiac sympathetic nerve, stimulation of which causes acceleration of the heart's action. **adrenergic n.** A postganglionic sympathetic fiber which, upon stimulation, releases an adrenergic substance at its termination. **afferent n.** One that transmits impulses from the periphery to the central nervous system; a sensory nerve. **autonomic n.** A nerve of the autonomic nervous system. **cerebrospinal n.** Any nerve taking origin from the brain or spinal cord. **cranial n.** Any of the nerves arising directly from the brain stem and making their exit to the periphery via openings in the skull. They are designated by number or name as follows: I, olfactory; II, optic; III, oculomotor; IV, trochlear; V, trigeminal; VI, abducens; VII, facial (including nervus intermedius); VIII, acoustic (cochlear and vestibular); IX, glossopharyngeal; X, vagus; XI, accessory; XII, hypoglossal. See also Table of Nerves in the Appendix. **depressor n.** One which, upon stimulation, lowers the blood pressure either in a local part or throughout the body. **effector n.** Efferent nerve. **efferent n.** One conducting impulses from the central nervous system to the periphery, as to a muscle. **excitoreflex n.** A visceral nerve, excitation of which brings about a reflex action. **extrinsic n.** One which conveys nervous impulses to an organ from the central nervous system or from the ganglionated chain of the sympathetic nervous system. It may synapse with a secondary neuron which lies within the organ. See *intrinsic n.* **inhibitory n.** Any nerve which, upon stimulation, lowers the activity of a center or organ.

intrinsic n. One which innervates the muscles, glands, or mucous membrane of an organ. It may be the nerve fiber of a sensory neuron or of a postganglionic neuron of the autonomic nervous system. **mixed n.** A nerve composed of both afferent and efferent fibers. **motor n.** Any nerve composed chiefly or wholly of motor fibers. **n. avulsion.** Operation of tearing a nerve from its central origin by traction. **n. block.** The interruption of the passage of impulses through a nerve, as by chemical, mechanical, or electric means. **n. ending.** The termination of a nerve at the periphery or in the nerve centers. **n. grafting.** The transplantation of a portion of a nerve to reëstablish the continuity of a severed nerve. **n. tract.** A bundle of nerve fibers having the same general origin and destination within the nervous system; as a rule, all fibers of a nerve tract serve the same or a very similar function. See *tract.* **parasympathetic n.** A nerve of the parasympathetic nervous system. **peripheral n.** (a) Specifically, one whose distribution is to the skin or to superficial structures of the body. (b) Often used to denote any nerve which is a branch of the central nervous system. **pilomotor n.** A nerve causing contraction of one of the arrectores pilorum muscles. **pressor n.** An afferent nerve, stimulation of which excites the vasomotor center. **respiratory n.** One of two nerves supplying important muscles of respiration: the external is the long thoracic, the internal is the phrenic nerve. **secretory n.** An efferent nerve, stimulation of which causes increased activity of the gland to which it is distributed. **sensory n.** A nerve which conducts afferent impulses from the periphery to the central nervous system, as those mediating sensations of pain, touch, and temperature. **somatic n.** One of the nerves supplying somatic structures, as voluntary muscles, skin, tendons, joints, and parietal serous membranes. **spinal n.** A nerve arising from the spinal cord and making its exit through an intervertebral foramen. There are 31 pairs of spinal nerves distributed as 8 cervical, 12 thoracic, 5 lumbar, 5 sacral, and 1 coccygeal. **sudomotor nerves.** The nerves which excite the sweat glands to activity. **sympathetic n.** A nerve of the sympathetic nervous system. **vasomotor nerves.** Those concerned with controlling the caliber of blood vessels. They are of two types: those which cause constriction of the blood vessel or **vasoconstrictor nerves,** and those which cause dilation of the blood vessel or **vasodilator nerves.** Ordinarily vasomotor is synonymous with vasoconstrictor. **visceral n.** Any nerve supplying a visceral structure.

nerve tracing. A method used by chiropractors for locating nerves and studying their pathology. It depends on the patient's reports about areas of tenderness or pain when adjoining areas are pressed upon by the operator.

ner′vi (nurv′eye). Plural of nervus, *q.v.*

ner′vone. A cerebroside occurring in brain tissue; its characteristic fatty acid is nervonic acid.

ner·von′ic ac′id. $C_8H_{45}COOH$. An unsaturated acid, related to lignoceric acid, believed to exist in nervone.

ner·vos′i·ty. Excessive nervousness.

nerv′ous ex·haus′tion. A state of fatigue and discomfort due to emotional causes. See *neurasthenia.*

nerv′ous·ness. A popular term denoting excessive excitability of the nervous system; characterized by shaken mental poise, muscle tremors or weakness, and an uncomfortable awareness of self.

nerv′ous sys′tem. 1. The entire nervous apparatus of the body, including the brain, brain stem, spinal cord, cranial and peripheral nerves, and ganglions. 2. A functional or anatomic part of the nervous apparatus of the body. **autonomic n. s.** The nervous system supplying, and exerting a regulatory influence over, involuntary muscle, glands, viscera, etc.; divided into sympathetic and parasympathetic nervous systems. **central n. s.** The brain and spinal cord. **cerebrospinal n. s.** The brain, spinal cord, and cranial and spinal nerves. **craniosacral autonomic n. s.** The parasympathetic system composed of those nerves whose preganglionic fibers exit from the central nervous system by way of the third, seventh, ninth, and tenth cranial nerves, and the second third, and fourth sacral nerves. **involuntary n. s.** Old term for autonomic nervous system. **parasympathetic n. s.** The craniosacral division of the autonomic nervous system consisting of preganglionic nerve fibers carried in cranial and sacral nerves, outlying ganglions, postganglionic fibers, and associated afferent nerve fibers; in general, innervating the same structures and having a regulatory function opposite to that of the sympathetic nervous system. **peripheral n. s.** The autonomic nervous system and the cerebrospinal nerves, the peripheral portions of the nervous system conducting impulses to and from the central nervous system. **somatic n. s.** That part of the nervous system exercising control over skeletal muscle and relating the organism to i environment. **sympathetic n. s.** (a) The entire autonomic nervous system. (b) The thoracolumbar division of the autonomic nervous system; the ganglionated sympathetic trunk, sympathetic plexuses, and the associated preganglionic, postganglionic and afferent nerve fibers. **thoracolumbar autonomic n. s.** The sympathetic nervous system composed of those nerves whose preganglionic fibers exit from the spinal cord by way of the thoracic and upper lumbar spinal nerves.

ner'vus (pl. *nervi*). Nerve, *q.v.* **nervi nervorum.** Nerve filaments going to the nerve sheaths. **nervi vasorum.** Small nerves which innervate the walls of the blood vessels. **n. erigens.** Sacral parasympathetic fibers which pass through the pelvic plexus to terminal ganglions in the pelvic viscera and are concerned with the emptying mechanisms of the urinary bladder and rectum, and with erection of the genital organs. **n. furcalis.** The fourth lumbar nerve which forks to send fibers to both the lumbar and sacral plexus. **n. intermedius.** The sensory and autonomic components of the facial nerve.

nest. A group, as of ova or insects. **cell n.** An isolated mass of epithelial cells surrounded by connective tissue, as in carcinoma.

nes"ti·at'ri·a (nes"tee-at'ree-uh, -ay'tree-uh). Treatment by fasting; the hunger-cure.

nes'tis. 1. Fasting. 2. The jejunum.

nethamine. A trade-mark for *l*-N-ethylephedrine.

net'tle rash. See *urticaria*.

net'work". The arrangement of fibers or vessels in a reticulum. See *rete*.

neu'ral. Pertaining to nerves or nervous tissue.

neu·ral'gi·a. Severe paroxysmal pain along the course of a nerve; not associated with demonstrable structural changes in the nerve. According to their anatomic situation, the following forms of neuralgia are described: trigeminal neuralgia, tic douloureux, or prosopalgia; supraorbital neuralgia; cervico-occipital neuralgia; cervicobrachial and brachial neuralgia; intercostal neuralgia, sciatica, or ischialgia; coccygodynia; visceral neuralgia (as hepatic, gastric, intestinal, uterine, ovarian neuralgia). The pain of neuralgia is sharp, stabbing, and paroxysmal, lasting usually but a short time; tenderness is often present at the points of exit of the nerve (points douloureux), and the paroxysm can be produced by contact with specific areas (trigger zones). Intercostal neuralgia is at times associated with herpes zoster. —**neuralgic**, *adj.* **articular n.** Neuralgia of a joint. **ciliary n.** Neuralgic

pain of the eye, brow, or temple. **facial n.** Neuralgia over the region of facial distribution of the trigeminal nerve. Also called *trifacial n.*, *trigeminal n.* **Seeligmueller's n.** Bilateral neuralgia of the auriculotemporal nerves with pain extending over the vertex, characteristic of neurosyphilis. **sphenopalatine n.** Sluder's neuralgia. Neuralgia caused by infection of the nasal sinuses, which is referred to the root of the nose, the upper teeth, the eyes, and even to the ears, the mastoid regions and the occiput. **trifacial n.** Old term for trigeminal neuralgia. See *facial n.*

neu·ral'gi·form. Resembling neuralgia.

neur"a·min'ic ac'id. A fatty acid believed to exist in certain brain cerebrosides.

neu"ra·poph'y·sis. Either one of the two apophyses on each vertebra which blend and form the neural arch, or the dorsal wall of the spinal foramen.

neu"ra·prax'i·a. A brief suspension of function in peripheral-nerve fibers, brought about by compression, drugs, or cold, and causing a temporary motor and sensory paralysis.

neu"ras·the'ni·a. A group of symptoms formerly ascribed to debility or exhaustion of the nerve centers. The symptoms include fatigability, lack of energy, various aches and pains, and disinclination to activity. Some individuals have many symptoms, in others the symptoms center upon some particular organ or region. **abdominal n.** That in which gastrointestinal symptoms predominate. **professional n.** That manifested in the individual's total or partial inability to use the organ or organs commonly employed in his occupation, as the inability of a writer to write due to a spasm or a painful feeling of fatigue in his arm.

neu"rax·i'tis. 1. Inflammation of an axon. 2. Encephalitis.

neu"reo·ta'si·a (new"reck·tay'zhuh, -shuh), **neu·reo'ta·sis.** Nerve stretching.

neu·rec'to·my. Excision of a part of a nerve.

neu"rec·to'pi·a, neu·rec'to·py. Displacement, or other abnormality, of the distribution of a nerve.

neu'ri-. A combining form denoting a nerve.

neu·ri'a·try. The study and treatment of nervous diseases.

neu·ri·dine (new'ri-deen, -din). A basic substance said to be present in brain tissue, identical with spermine, *q.v.*

neu"ri·lem'ma. The sheath encasing a nerve fiber; the sheath of Schwann. See nerve *fiber*.

neu″ri·lem·mi′tis. Inflammation of the neurilemma.

neu″ri·lem·mo′ma. A tumor of a peripheral nerve, derived from the supporting tissues. Authorities differ as to whether it is derived from endoneurium or neurilemma. Also called *neurinoma, perineurial fibroblastoma, peripheral glioma, schwannoma*.

neu′rine (new′reen, ·rin). (CH₃)₃N-(OH)CH=CH₂. A product of bacterial decomposition of lecithin.

neu″ri·no′ma. A neurofibroma; neurilemmoma. Also called *schwannoma*.

acoustic n. An intracranial neoplasm involving the acoustic nerve sheath. There is an associated tinnitus in the ear and deafness on the affected side in late stages.

neu′rit, neu′rite. Old term for the axis cylinder process of a nerve cell.

neu·ri′tis. Lesions of a nerve or nerves; either degenerative or inflammatory, with pain, hypersensitivity, anesthesia or paresthesia, paralysis, muscular atrophy, and lost reflexes in the part supplied. There are numerous forms, according to cause, pathology, location, and number of nerves involved. **—neurit′ic,** *adj.* **adventitial n.** That affecting the nerve sheath. **alcoholic n.** Neuritis associated with chronic alcoholism, presumably due to thiamine deficiency resulting from insufficient food intake. **ascending n.** That extending from the periphery of a nerve to the brain or cord. **axial n.** A form affecting the central part of the nerve. **degenerative n.** That involving the nerve fibers; usually multiple neuritis, *q.v.* **descending n.** Neuritis extending from the brain or cord to the periphery of the nerve. **disseminated n.** Segmental neuritis. **endemic n.** Beriberi. **infectious n.** An acute multiple neuritis, probably due to a virus disease. **interstitial n.** The form involving the connective tissue of a nerve. **mononeuritis.** Involvement of a single nerve. **multiple n.** Simultaneous involvement of several nerves, usually symmetrical; due to poisons such as alcohol, arsenic, lead, or mercury, or to diseases such as diphtheria, typhoid, or syphilis. Also called *polyneuritis*. **nutritional n.** That caused by vitamin-B deficiency. **parenchymatous n.** Degenerative neuritis. **retrobulbar n.** Inflammation of the optic nerve posterior to the eyeball. **sciatic n.** Due to involvement of the sciatic nerve; sciatica. **segmental n.** Neuritis affecting a segmental nerve. **toxic n.** That due to some poisonous substance. See

multiple *n.* **traumatic n.** Neuritis due to trauma.

neu′ro-, neur-. A combining form denoting *a nerve, nervous tissue,* or *the nervous system*.

neu″ro·a·nas′to·mo′sis. Surgical anastomosis of nerves.

neu″ro·a·nat′o·my. The anatomy of the nervous system.

neu″ro·ar′thri·tism. A combined nervous and gouty diathesis.

neu″ro·ar·throp′a·thy. Manifestations of disease in both joints and nervous system.

neu″ro·bi·ol′o·gy. Biology of the nervous system.

neu″ro·blast. A formative cell of a neuron, derived from ectoderm of the neural plate.

neu″ro·blas·to′ma. A malignant tumor arising in some part of the autonomic nervous system; composed of small cells of a type resembling primitive neuroblasts or medulloblasts, pseudorosettes, and delicate fibrils, the nature of which is not certain. Syn., *sympathoblastoma*.

neu″ro·cal″o·rim′e·ter. An instrument for measuring the heat of a nerve.

neu″ro·ca·nal′. The central canal of the spinal cord. O.T.

neu″ro·cele. The system of cavities and ventricles in the central nervous system. O.T.

neu″ro·chem′is·try. The chemistry of nervous tissue.

neu″ro·cho″ri·o·ret″i·ni′tis (·kor″ee·o·ret″i·nigh′tis). Choroidoretinitis combined with optic neuritis.

neu″ro·cho″roid·i′tis (new″ro·kor″oy·dye′tis). Combined inflammation of the choroid body and optic nerve.

neu″ro·cir′cu·la·to′ry. Concerned with both the nervous and the vascular systems, as neurocirculatory asthenia, *q.v.*

neu·roc′la·dism. A theoretical, neurotropic phenomenon in which regeneration of injured neuraxons is considered to occur by the production of collateral or terminal branches in response to the attraction of external, mechanical, or chemical stimuli.

neu″ro·cra′ni·um. The brain case, or cranial portion of the skull.

neu″ro·cu·ta′ne·ous. Pertaining to the innervation of the skin.

neu″ro·cyte″. A nerve cell; a neuron; the essential element of nervous structures. Neurons are cells specialized as conductors of impulses.

neu″ro·cy·to′ma (new″ro·sigh·to′muh). A comprehensive term which includes various forms of cellular tumors of the central nervous system and autonomic nervous system, such as sympathoblastoma (neuroblastoma), pheochromocytoma, ganglioneuroma, neuroepithelioma.

neu"ro·de·al'gi·a. Retinal pain.

neu"ro·der"ma·ti'tis. A skin disorder characterized by localized, often symmetrical, patches of pruritic dermatitis with lichenification. It appears characteristically on the neck, antecubital and popliteal spaces in women of nervous temperament. *N. circumscripta* is also called *lichen chronicus simplex.*

neu"ro·der"ma·to·my"o·si'tis. A disease of inflammatory or infectious nature, manifested by neuritic pain with induration of the skin, subcutaneous tissue and underlying muscles.

neu"ro·der"ma·to'sis. A neurotic skin affection.

neu"ro·der"ma·tro'phi·a. Atrophy of the skin from nervous disturbance.

neu"ro·di·as'ta·sis (new"ro-dye-ass'tuh·sis). Stretching of nerves; neurectasia.

neu"ro·dy·nam'i·a (new"ro-dye-nam'ee·uh). Nervous strength or energy. —**neurodynamic,** *adj.*

neu"ro·e·lec"tro·ther"a·peu'tics. The treatment of nervous affections by means of electricity.

neu"ro·en·ceph"a·lo·my"e·lop'a·thy. Acute or subacute demyelinating disease, involving the optic nerves and chiasma and the spinal cord. Also called *Devic's disease, optic neuromyelitis.*

neu"ro·ep"i·the·li·o'ma. A tumor derived from primitive neuroepithelium, containing cells of small cuboidal or columnar form with a tendency to form true rosettes. Occurs in the retina, central nervous system, and occasionally in peripheral nerves.

neu"ro·ep"i·the'li·um. The highly specialized epithelial structures constituting the terminations of the nerves of special sense, as the rod and cone cells of the retina, the olfactory cells of the nose, the hair cells of the internal ear, the gustatory cells of the taste buds. —**neuroepithelial,** *adj.*

neu"ro·fi'bril. A fibril of a nerve cell, usually extending from the processes and traversing the cell body.

neu"ro·fi·bro'ma (new"ro·figh-bro'muh). A tumor of peripheral nerves, essentially fibrous in nature, which may show palisading of nuclei or loose reticular structure or both. Authorities differ as to whether it is derived from endoneurium or cells of the neurilemma. Also called *neurilemmoma, perineurial fibroblastoma, schwannoma.*

neu"ro·fi·bro·ma·to'sis (·figh-bro"muh·to'sis). A condition characterized by the presence in the skin, or along the course of peripheral nerves, of neurofibromas. Usually the tumors are multiple, from a few to hundreds, gradually increasing in both number and size, and are painless. There is a hereditary tendency and, occasionally, malignancy supervenes. Also called *molluscum fibrosum, von Recklinghausen's disease, Smith-Recklinghausen's disease, molluscum pendulum.*

neu"ro·fi"bro·sar·co'ma. The malignant form of neurofibroma. Syn., *neurogenic sarcoma.*

neu"ro·fi"bro·si'tis. A fibrositis which involves fibers of a nerve and also of muscle.

neu"ro·gas'tric. Relating to the nerves and the stomach.

neu"ro·gen'e·sis. The formation of nerves.

neu"ro·gen'ic. 1. Of nervous origin, as neurogenic tumors. 2. Stimulated by the nervous system, as neurogenic muscular contractions.

neu·rog'e·nous (new·rodj'i·nus). Originating in the nervous system.

neu·rog'li·a. 1. A general term for the fibrous and cellular, nonnervous, supporting elements of the nervous system, chiefly derived from ectoderm. Includes the ependyma, the epithelial lining of the choroid plexuses, neuroglia proper, microglia; also, in the peripheral nervous system, the neurilemma sheath cells of nerves and the satellite cells of ganglions. 2. Specifically neuroglia proper, comprising the astrocytes and the oligodendroglia cells of the central nervous system.

neu·rog"li·o'ma. A tumor composed of neuroglial tissue; a glioma. **gan·gli·o'nar n.** A glioma containing ganglion cells.

neu·rog"li·o'sis. A condition of multiple neurogliomas developing diffusely throughout the nervous system.

neu'ro·gram. *In psychiatry,* Morton Prince's term for the record of theoretic changes imprinted on the brain by life's experiences.

neu"ro·his·tol'o·gy. The histology of the nervous system.

neu"ro·hu'mor. The chemical excitor in a neuron which, supposedly, activates a neighboring neuron or a muscle. Chemical substances are liberated at the visceral endings of stimulated nerves; thus sympathin is produced by stimulation of postganglionic sympathetic fibers, whereas acetylcholine is produced at the endings of stimulated parasympathetic nerves.

neu"ro·hy·poph'y·sis. The neural portion of the pituitary gland, developing as a downward evagination from the floor of the diencephalon.

neu'roid. Resembling a nerve or nerve substance.

neu″ro·in·duc′tion. Suggestion.

neu·rol′o·gist. One versed in neurology, usually a physician who specializes in the diagnosis and treatment of disorders of the nervous system.

neu·rol′o·gy. The study of the anatomy, physiology, and pathology of the nervous system. **—neurolog′ic,** *adj.*

neu″ro·lu′es (new″ro·lew′eez). Neurosyphilis, *q.v.*

neu·rol′y·sis. 1. Exhaustion of a nerve by overstimulation. 2. Nerve stretching to relieve excessive tension. 3. The loosening of adhesions binding a nerve. 4. The disintegration of nerve tissue. **—neurolyt′ic,** *adj.*

neu·ro′ma. A term used by Virchow to designate tumors of the nervous system, which since then have been classified, histologically, into special groups. Also see *pseudoneuroma.* **—neurom′atous,** *adj.* **appendical n.** A tumorlike growth of nerve fibers, and often of ganglion cells, in chronic fibrotic lesions of the vermiform process. **n. cutis.** A cutaneous neurofibroma. **n. telangiectodes.** One with a rich content of blood vessels, often cavernous in type. **plexiform n.** A tumor or tumorlike mass of whorls of myelinated and unmyelinated nerve fibers and of connective tissue. Occurs in early life and probably is congenital. There is doubt as to whether it is neoplasm, anomaly, or hamartoma.

neu″ro·mech′a·nism. The correlated structure and function of the nervous system in relation to a bodily activity.

neu′ro·mere. An embryonic segment of the brain or spinal cord.

neu″ro·mi·me′sis (new″ro·mi·mee′sis, ·migh·mee′sis). A group of hysterical phenomena resembling true organic disease. **—neuromimet′ic,** *adj.*

neu″ro·mus′cu·lar. Pertaining jointly to nerves and muscles, as neuromuscular junction.

neu″ro·my″e·li′tis. Inflammation of the spinal cord and of nerves. **n. optica.** A morbid process, probably due to a virus or an infectious toxic agent, involving the optic nerve and the white and gray matter of the cord. It is closely allied to other demyelinating diseases, such as multiple sclerosis and encephalomyelitis disseminata.

neu′ron, neu′rone. The complete nerve cell, including the cell body or perikaryon, axon, and dendrites; specialized as a conductor of impulses. **—neuron′al,** *adj.* **n. pathway.** The successive neurons over which a given impulse is transmitted. **n. pattern.** The theoretic pathways which determine an instinct, reflex, sensation, or other nervous response.

neu″ro·ni′tis. Inflammation of a neuron or nerve cell. **infective n.** See Guillain-Barré *syndrome.*

neu·ro″no·pha′gi·a. The destruction of neurons by phagocytes.

neu′ro·path. One who is predisposed to disorders of the nervous system.

neu″ro·path′ic. 1. Characterized by a diseased or imperfect nervous system. 2. Depending upon, or pertaining to, nervous disease.

neu″ro·path′ic es′char (es′kahr). Bedsore; decubitus ulcer.

neu·rop′a·thist. Neurologist.

neu″ro·pa·thol′o·gy. Pathology of the nervous system.

neu·rop′a·thy. Any nervous disease.

neu″ro·pho′ni·a. A rare choreic disease of the larynx and muscles of expiration, characterized by the utterance of sharp, spasmodic cries.

neu″ro·phys″i·ol′o·gy. The physiology of the nervous system.

neu′ro·pil. A region of the nervous system consisting mainly of nerve-cell processes; a region of synapses between axons and dendrites; gray matter with few nerve-cell bodies.

neu′ro·plasm. The cytoplasm filling the interstices of the fibrils of nerve cells.

neu′ro·plas″ty. A plastic operation on the nerves.

neu″ro·pleg′ic. Of, or pertaining to, a drug or an agent capable of diminishing the intensity of nerve function. **—neuroplegia,** *n.*

neu′ro·pore. The anterior or posterior terminal aperture of the embryonic neural tube before complete closure occurs (about the 20–25-somite stage).

neu″ro·psy·chi′a·try. The branch of medical science dealing with both nervous and mental diseases.

neu″ro·psy·chol′o·gy. A system of psychology based on neurology.

neu″ro·psy·chop′a·thy (new″ro·sigh·kop′uth·ee). A mental disease based upon, or manifesting itself in, nervous disorders or symptoms. **—neuropsychopath′ic,** *adj.*

neu″ro·re·lapse′. Acute syphilitic meningitis, occurring usually during the treatment of early syphilis. Syn., *neurorecidive, neurorecurrence.*

neu″ro·ret″i·ni′tis. Inflammation of both the optic nerve and the retina.

neu·ror′rha·phy. The operation of suturing a divided nerve.

neu″ro·sar·co′ma. A sarcoma of the general order of a neuroma.

neu″ro·se·cre′tion. The process of elaboration and discharge of colloidlike granules and masses by nerve cells which, during phases of such activity, assume the appearance of gland cells.

neu·ro'sis (pl. *neuroses*). A disorder of the psyche or psychic functions. See *psychoneurosis*. —**neurosal,** *adj.* **anxiety n.** *In psychoanalysis,* a psychoneurosis characterized by emotional instability, irritability, apprehension, and a sense of utter fatigue; caused by incomplete repression of emotional problems. It is associated with visceral phenomena such as tachycardia, palpitation, nausea, a sense of suffocation, diarrhea, tremors, and perspiration. Also called *anxiety state.* Also see anxiety *hysteria.* **blast n.** (a) A nervous disorder developing after rapid and extreme changes in atmospheric pressure without producing any external evidence of injury. (b) A disorder caused by detonation of explosives; often terminated by sudden death, necropsy showing multiple brain hemorrhages. **combat neuroses.** War neuroses. **compulsion n.** A mental disorder characterized by an irresistible impulse to perform some act contrary to the conscious will of the individual. See *obsession.* **occupational n.** (a) One in which the occupation of the individual appears to be the precipitating cause. (b) A disorder affecting groups of muscles used in the performance of special movements. Syn., *copodyskinesia, professional neurasthenia.* **traumatic n.** One in which an injury is the precipitating cause. **vasomotor n.** Angioneurosis. **war n.** Any one of many mental disorders, such as hysteria, neurasthenia, or psychasthenia, following exhaustion or emotional stress in warfare.

neu'ro·spasm. Nervous spasm or twitching of a muscle.

neu''ro·sur'geon. One who specializes in surgery of the brain and the nervous system.

neu''ro·sur'ger·y. Surgery of the nervous system.

neu''ro·su'ture. The suture of a nerve.

neu''ro·syph'i·lis. Syphilitic infection of the nervous system.

neu''ro·the·ci'tis. Inflammation of a nerve sheath.

neu''ro·ther'a·py. The treatment of nervous diseases. Also called *neurotherapeutics.*

neu·rot'ic. 1. Pertaining to or affected with a neurosis. 2. Pertaining to the nerves. 3. An emotionally unstable individual.

neu·rot'i·ca. Functional nervous disorders.

neu·rot'i·cism. A neurotic condition, character, or trait.

neu·rot''i·za'tion. 1. The regeneration of a divided nerve. 2. Surgical implantation of a nerve into a par-

alyzed muscle. 3. Providing an anatomic structure with a nerve supply.

neu''ro·tol'o·gy. That branch of medical science dealing with the structure and functions of the internal ear, its nervous connections with the brain, and the central pathways within the brain.

neu'ro·tome. 1. An instrument for the division or dissection of a nerve. 2. One of the segments of the embryonic neural tube. Also called *neuromere.*

neu·rot'o·my. The surgical division or dissection of some or all of the fibers of a nerve.

neu''ro·tox'in. A toxin capable of destroying nerve tissue. —**neurotoxic,** *adj.*

neu''ro·trau'ma (new''ro·traw'-muh). Injury to a nerve.

neu''ro·trip'sy. The crushing of a nerve.

neu''ro·troph'ic, neu''ro·tro'phic. Relating to the influence of nerves upon the nutrition and maintenance of normal condition in tissues.

neu''ro·trop'ic. That which turns toward, or has an affinity for, nervous tissue.

neu''ro·var'i·co'sis. A varicosity on a nerve fiber, or the formation of one.

neu''ro·vas'cu·lar. Pertaining to both the nervous and vascular structures.

neu'ru·la. *In embryology,* the stage following the gastrula stage in Amphibia. It is characterized by the development of the neural plate and axial embryonic structures and corresponds to the somite stage in human development.

neu'tral. 1. Inert; on neither one side nor the other. 2. Neither alkaline nor acid; bland and soothing, inactive.

neu''tra·li·za'tion. 1. That process or operation that counterbalances or cancels the action of an agent. 2. *In medicine,* the process of checking the operation of any agent that produces a morbid effect. 3. *In chemistry,* a change of reaction to that which is neither alkaline nor acid.

neu'tral·ize. Render neutral; render inert; counterbalance an action or influence.

neu'tral red (C.C.). Dimethyl-diaminotoluphenazine hydrochloride, a dye used as an indicator and in staining as a vital stain. Also called *toluylene red.*

neu·tri'no (new·tree'no). An atomic particle having the mass of the electron but without an electric charge.

neu'tron. An atomic nuclear particle with mass = 1 and charge = 0. A constituent of all atomic nuclei except $_1H^1$. (Isotopes differ from one another solely by the number of neutrons in their nuclei.)

neu″tro·pe′ni·a. A decrease below the normal standard in the number of neutrophils in the peripheral blood.

neu′tro·phil. 1. Stained readily by neutral dyes. 2. Any histologic element readily stainable with neutral dyes. 3. The polymorphonuclear leukocyte of the blood, which contains neutrophil granules in its cytoplasm.

neu″tro·phil′i·a. 1. An affinity for neutral dyes. 2. Great increase of neutrophilic leukocytes in the blood or tissues.

ne′vi (nee′vye). Plural of nevus.

ne′vose. Spotted, having nevi.

ne′vus (pl. *nevi*). 1. A circumscribed area of pigmentation or vascularization on the skin, usually manifest at, or shortly after, birth; a birthmark. 2. An angioma of the skin, usually congenital. **—nevoid,** *adj.* **blue n.** One composed of a mass of melanin-forming cells in the deeper parts of the derma. **linear n.** A verrucous type which occurs in bands or streaks. **n. acneiformis unilateralis.** A type of linear nevus in which folliculitis, perifolliculitis, and ulceration occur, followed by scar formation. Also called *n. comedonicus.* **n. araneus.** Vascular dilatation with minute central tumor and radiating capillaries. Also called *stellar n., spider n.* **n. flammeus.** Port-wine mark; a diffuse, very slightly raised, deep red or purple variety of capillary nevus often involving the face. **n. lipomatodes.** A large, soft mole containing a quantity of fat and loose connective tissue. **n. pigmentosus.** A pigmented mole; a circumscribed congenital pigmentary deposit in the skin, varying in color from light fawn to blackish, which sometimes undergoes malignant change. **n. pilosus.** A pigmented type having one or more coarse hairs, usually small but occasionally covering a large area. Also called *hairy n., hairy mole.* **n. vascularis fungosus.** A cavernous angioma marked by formation of red or bluish erectile tumors. **port-wine n.** A congenital capillary hemangioma. Also called *n. flammeus, port-wine mark.* **spider n.** A type of telangiectasis characterized by a central, elevated, tiny red dot, pinhead in size, from which blood vessels radiate like spokes of a wheel. Syn., *nevus araneus.* **verrucous n.** A type characterized by a warty appearance; it is hairless.

new′born′. A term applied to infants up to two or three days of age. Syn., *neonatal.*

new growth. A circumscribed, new formation of tissue, characterized by abnormality of structure or location. Syn., *neoplasm.*

nex′us. A tying or binding together, as the grouping of several causes which bring about an infectious disease; an interlacing.

N. F. National Formulary.

Ni. Chemical symbol for nickel.

ni′a·cin. Nicotinic acid.

nib′ble. Gnaw; eat in small bits.

nic′co·lum. Nickel.

niche (nitch). A recess.

nick′el. Ni = 58.69. A metal of silver-white luster, resembling iron in physical properties.

nic″o·tin·am·ide (nick″o·tin·am′-ide, ·id, nick″o·tin′uh·mide, ·mid). Nicotinic acid amide, occurring as a white, crystalline powder; soluble in water. It is a specific for pellagra. Syn., *niacinamide.*

nic′o·tine (nick′o·teen, ·tin). A liquid, poisonous alkaloid found in the leaves of tobacco.

nic″o·tin′ic ac′id. Beta- or 3-pyridinecarboxylic acid; occurs as a white, crystalline powder; soluble in water. A specific for the treatment of pellagra. Also called *niacin, P.P. factor.*

nic′ti·ta″ting. Winking, as nictitating membrane, a vestigial fold in the human eye.

nic″ti·ta′ti·o (nick″ti·tay′shee·o). A clonic form of eyelid spasm.

nic″ti·ta′tion. Abnormal frequency of winking.

ni·da′tion (nigh·day′shun, ni·-). The implantation of the fertilized ovum in the endometrium (decidua) of the pregnant uterus.

ni′dus (pl. *nidi*). 1. A focus of infection. 2. Old term for a nucleus in the central nervous system. **—nidal,** *adj.*

night blind′ness. The condition of reduced dark adaptation, resulting temporarily from vitamin-A deficiency or permanently from retinitis pigmentosa or other peripheral retinal diseases. Syn., *nyctalopia.*

night cry. A shrill cry uttered by a child during sleep; sometimes symptomatic of physical disorders, as in the early stages of hip disease; sometimes of psychic origin.

Nightingale, Florence [*English nurse,* 1820–1910]. Immortalized as the founder of modern nursing service and famous throughout the world for her devotion to the English soldiers in the Crimean War. She created a woman's nursing service at Scutari and Balaklava (1860). From funds donated, she organized a school of nursing bearing her name. She was known far and wide as The Lady with the Lamp.

night′mare″. A terrifying dream which usually awakens the sleeper; characterized by great distress and a sense of oppression or suffocation.

night pain. Pain, usually in the hip or knee, occurring during muscular relaxation of the limb in sleep; often a symptom of disease of the joint.

night pal'sy (pawl'zee). Numbness of the extremities occurring during the night, or on waking in the morning, affecting women about the period of the menopause.

night'shade. A name applied to plants of the family Solanaceae. **deadly n.** A poisonous plant, *Atropa belladonna.* See *belladonna.*

night sweat. Profuse nocturnal sweating. A frequent accompaniment of any diurnal fever and, by tradition, associated especially with pulmonary tuberculosis.

night vi'sion. The ability to see at night. Nocturnal visual efficiency is determined by the ability to perform visual tasks at light intensities below the cone threshold, that is, at scotopic levels of illumination.

ni·gran'i·line (nigh-gran'i·leen, -lin). Aniline black, a black dye obtained by the oxidation of aniline. Used as a stain in microscopy. Also called *nigrosine.*

ni·gri'ti·es (nigh-grish'ee·eez). Black, hairy tongue.

ni'gro·sine (nigh'gro·seen, -sin). Any one of several black or dark blue aniline dyes; variously used in bacteriologic and histologic technics.

NIH. National Institutes of Health.

ni'hil·ism (nigh'hi·liz·um, nigh'l·). 1. Pessimism in regard to the efficacy of drugs. 2. *In psychiatry,* the content of delusions encountered in depressed or melancholic states. The patient insists that his inner organs no longer exist, and that his relatives have passed away.

ni·keth'a·mide. The diethylamide of nicotinic acid, occurring either as an oily liquid, or as a crystalline solid, soluble in water. Stimulates medullary centers; used as an analeptic, and for its respiratory stimulant effects. See *coramine.*

Nile blue A (C.C.). A basic oxazine dye, of value as a fat stain.

ninhydrin. Trade name of triketohydrindene hydrate. A water-soluble substance which gives a color reaction with proteins and amino acids.

ni·o'bi·um (nigh·o'bee·um). Nb = 92.91. Chemical element No. 41, a steel gray, lustrous metal, formerly called *columbium.*

niph''a·blep'si·a. Snow blindness.

niph''o·typh·lo'sis. Snow blindness.

nip'pers. An instrument for seizing small bodies. **bone n.** An instrument for grasping small bits of bone; a small bone-trimming forceps.

nip'ple. The conical projection in the center of the mamma, containing the outlets of the milk ducts. Also called *papilla.* **cracked n.** One in which the epidermis is broken. **n. line.** A vertical line drawn on the surface of the chest through the nipple. **n. protector.** A device worn by nursing women to protect the nipple. Also called *nipple shield.* **retracted n.** A nipple drawn below the surrounding level.

nir'va·nol (nur'vuh·nole, ·nol). $C_{11}H_{13}O_2N_3$. Phenylethylhydantoin, a sedative and soporific.

nisentil hydrochloride. Trademark for prisilidine hydrochloride.

nisulfazole. Trade-mark for 2-(p-nitrophenylsulfonamido)-thiazole, a drug for the treatment of ulcerative colitis.

ni'sus. 1. Any strong effort or struggle. 2. The periodic desire for procreation manifested in the spring season by certain species of animals; called **nisus formativus.** 3. The contraction of the diaphragm and abdominal muscles for the expulsion of feces, urine, or a fetus.

nit. The egg or larva of a louse.

ni'ter. Potassium nitrate or saltpeter. **Chile n.** Sodium nitrate. **cubic n.** Sodium nitrate. **sweet spirit of n.** Ethyl nitrite spirit. An alcoholic solution of ethyl nitrite.

ni'ton. Radon, *q.v.* Symbol, Nt.

ni'tra·gin. A nitrifying bacterial ferment obtained from the root tubercles of leguminous plants.

ni'tra·mine (nigh'truh·meen, ·min, nigh·truh·meen'). See *tetryl,* 2.

ni'trate. A salt of nitric acid.

ni·tra'tion. The process of combining or reacting with nitric acid.

nitrazine. Trade-mark used for a dye, sodium dinitrophenylazo-naphthol disulfonate, used as an indicator.

ni'tre. Niter, *q.v.*

nitretamin. A trade-mark for aminotrate phosphate.

ni'tric ac'id. A liquid containing 67-71% HNO_3, the remainder being water. **fuming n. a.** Nitric acid containing more or less nitrogen tetroxide.

ni''tri·fi·ca'tion. The oxidation of ammonium to nitrites and nitrates in the soil.

ni'tri·fi''er. A microörganism that participates in the process of nitrification; bacteria of the genus *Nitrosomonas* oxidize ammonium to nitrite; bacteria of the genus *Nitrobacter* oxidize nitrite to nitrate.

ni'trile (nigh'trile, ·tril). An organic compound containing the monovalent CN group.

ni'trite. A salt of nitrous acid.

ni''tri·tu'ri·a. The presence of nitrates or nitrites, or both, in the urine when voided.

nitro-, nitr-. 1. A combining form denoting *the presence of the mono-*

valent radical NO₃. 2. A combining form denoting *combination with nitrogen.*

ni″tro·ben′zene. C₆H₅NO₂, an oily, sweetish liquid.

ni″tro·ben′zol. Nitrobenzene.

ni″tro·cel′lu·lose. See *pyroxylin.*

ni″tro·chlo′ro·form. See *chloropicrin.*

ni″tro·er′y·throl. C₄H₆(NO₃)₄. Erythrityl tetranitrate; it explodes on percussion. It is used in the same manner as nitroglycerin.

ni″tro·fur·an′toin. N-(5-Nitro-2-furfurylidene)-1-aminohydantoin, a broad-spectrum antibacterial active against Gram-negative and Gram-positive organisms, used in treating bacterial infections of the urinary tract. See *furadantin.*

ni″tro·fur′a·zone. C₉H₆N₄O₄. 5-Nitro-2-furaldehyde semicarbazone, a derivative of furfural possessing bacteriostatic and bactericidal properties. See *furacin.*

ni′tro·gen. N = 14.008. A gaseous element existing free in the atmosphere, of which it constitutes about 77% by weight. See Table of Normal Values of Blood Constituents in the Appendix. **blood urea n.** Nitrogen in the form of urea found in whole blood or serum. Abbreviated, BUN. **n. balance.** The difference between the nitrogen intake (as protein) of an individual and his total nitrogen excretion. **n. dioxide.** N₂O₂. A toxic gas resulting from the decomposition of nitric acid. **n.-lag.** The time elapsing between the ingestion of a protein and the appearance in the urine of an amount of nitrogen equal to that taken in. **n. monoxide.** Nitrous oxide. **n. mustard.** One of a series of nitrogen analogs of dichlorodiethylsulfide (*q.v.*), of which *tris* (β-chloroethyl)amine, N(CH₂CH₂Cl)₃, and methyl-*bis* (β-chloroethyl)amine, CH₃N(CH₂CH₂Cl)₂, in the form of water-soluble hydrochloride salts, have been found useful in the treatment of neoplastic diseases. **n. pentoxide.** The solid substance N₂O₅; reacts with water to form nitric oxide. **n. tetroxide.** N₂O₄. A toxic gas resulting from oxidation of nitrogen dioxide. Also called *n. peroxide.* **nonprotein n.** The fraction of nitrogen in the blood, tissues, urine, and excreta, not precipitated by the usual protein precipitants such as sodium tungstate. Symbol, N. P. N.

ni·trog′e·nous (nigh·trodj′i·nus). Containing nitrogen.

ni″tro·glyc′er·in (nigh″tro·gliss′-ur·in). C₃H₅(NO₃)₃. Glonoin, glyceryl trinitrate; a colorless, oily liquid. A powerful explosive; physiologically, has the actions of the nitrites.

ni″tro·hy″dro·chlo′ric ac′id. Prepared by mixing 1 volume of nitric

acid and 4 volumes of hydrochloric acid; contains the component acids together with nitrosyl chloride and chlorine. Syn., *nitromuriatic acid.*

ni″tro·mer′sol. The anhydride of 4-nitro-3-hydroxy-mercuri-ortho cresol, containing about 57% of mercury; it is a brownish yellow to yellow powder, employed as a germicide. See *metaphen.*

ni·trom′e·ter (nigh·trom′i·tur). An apparatus for collecting and measuring nitrogen or other gas evolved during a chemical reaction.

ni″tro·mu″ri·at′ic ac′id. See *nitrohydrochloric acid.*

ni·tro′so- (nigh·tro′so-). A combining form signifying *combination with nitrosyl,* the univalent NO.

ni·tro′so·ni′tric ac′id. Fuming nitric acid containing nitrous acid gas.

ni·tro′syl (nigh·tro′sil, nigh″tro·seel′ nigh′tro·sil). The univalent radical NO.

ni′trous. 1. Containing nitrogen as a trivalent positive element. 2. Pertaining to or derived from nitrous acid. **n. ether.** C₂H₅NO₂. Ethyl nitrite, a very volatile liquid having properties similar to those of amyl nitrite. **n. oxide.** N₂O. A colorless gas; used as a general anesthetic in dentistry and in surgery. Also called *hyponitrous oxide, laughing gas, nitrogen monoxide.* **ni′trous ac′id.** HNO₂. An unstable solution prepared by passing N₂O₃ into water.

nizin. Trade-mark for a brand of zinc sulfanilate.

NK. *Nomenklatur Kommission;* the committee appointed to revise the BNA. The recommendations of this committee, published in 1935, have not been widely adopted.

N. L. N. E. National League of Nursing Education.

N. N. D. Abbreviation for *New and Nonofficial Drugs,* a book describing therapeutic, prophylactic, and diagnostic agents evaluated by the Council of Drugs of the American Medical Association. Formerly, *N. N. R.*

N. N. R. Abbreviation for *New and Nonofficial Remedies.*

No. *Numero,* number, to the number of.

Nobel, Alfred Bernard [Swedish manufacturer of munitions, 1833-96]. The inventor of dynamite, he provided (1895) for a yearly distribution of prizes for noteworthy advances in literature, chemistry, physics, and medicine, as well as in the cause of international peace. The recipient is known as *Nobel laureate* or *prizeman.*

no′ble gas′es. The inert gases helium, neon, argon, krypton, xenon and radon, so called because they w

ot enter into chemical combination
with any other element.

o·car'di·a. A genus of aerobic fungi
of the family Actinomycetaceae.
N. asteroides. A species which is
an aerobic and acid-fast actinomycete;
causes pulmonary, brain, and subcutaneous lesions, usually without granules.
N. madurae. A species which is one
of the causes of white-grained mycetoma. **N. minutissima.** A species
which causes the chronic infection of
the stratum corneum known as ery-
thrasma. **N. somaliensis.** A species
which is one of the causes of white-
grained mycetoma. **N. tenuis.** A
species which is the causative agent of
trichomycosis axillaris.

o'car·di·o'sis. Actinomycosis
caused by certain species of the aerobic
actinomycetes, *Nocardia.* The disease
is indistinguishable from that caused
by *Actinomyces bovis.*

o'ci·cep'tive. Referring to sensory
nerves which mediate impulses stimulated by trauma; pain receptors.

o'ci·fen'sor. A term introduced by
Lewis to denote efferent fibers which
release chemical substances at their
terminals, which stimulate the pain
endings.

o'ci·per·cep'tion. Perception of
pain by the central nervous system.

o'ci·per·cep'tor. One of the peripheral nerves concerned in the reception of pain stimuli.

oc"tal·bu"mi·nu'ri·a. Excretion
of albumin in night urine only.

oc·tam"bu·la'tion. Sleep walking.

oc"ti·pho'bi·a. Morbid fear of
night.

oc·tu'ri·a. 1. Nocturnal enuresis. 2.
Frequency of urination at night. Syn.,
nycturia.

oc·tur'nal. Pertaining to night, as
nocturnal emission, discharge of semen
without coitus during sleep.

oc'u·ous. Noxious; hurtful; venomous.

od. 1. Drop the head forward with a
quick motion. 2. The motion so made.

ode. 1. A knob, or protuberance. 2.
A point of constriction. 3. A small,
rounded organ. **—nod'al,** *adj.*

trioventricular n. A small mass
of interwoven Purkinje fibers of the
conduction system in the central fibrous body of the heart. **lymph n.**
A usually small, bean-shaped aggregation of lymph nodules and cords between which lymph from afferent vessels flows in lymph sinuses to an efferent
vessel. **signal n.** Metastatic tumor in
a supraclavicular lymph node, usually
on the left side, and most frequently
secondary to primary carcinoma in the
abdomen or thorax. Also called *Virchow's n., Virchow's signal n.* **sing-**

er's n. Inflammatory nodule of the
vocal cords. **sinoatrial n.** A dense
network of Purkinje fibers of the conduction system at the junction of the
superior vena cava and the atrium.
syphilitic n. A localized exostosis
on a bone due to syphilitic periostitis.

no'dose. Characterized by nodes;
jointed or swollen at intervals.

nod'ule. 1. A small node. 2. A small
aggregation of cells. **—nod'ular,** *adj.*
lymph n. A small mass of dense
lymphatic tissue in which new lymphocytes are formed.

no'dus. A node.

no"e·mat'ic. Pertaining to thought
or to any mental process.

noludar. Trade-mark for methy-
prylon.

no'ma. A stomatitis, often fatal, starting in debilitated children during convalescence from disease, usually one of
the exanthemas. It begins in the mucous membrane, becomes gangrenous,
and ulcerates through the cheek. Also
called *cancrum oris, gangraena oris,
gangrenous stomatitis.* **n. pudendi.**
An ulceration similar to that described
above, occurring about the genital
region of female children. Also called
n. vulvae.

no·mad'ic. Spreading; said of ulcers.

no'men·cla·ture. A systematic
arrangement of the distinctive names
employed in any science. See *BNA, BR.*

nom'o·graph. A graph on which
appear graduated lines for all variables
in a formula, arranged in such a manner that the value of one variable can
be read on the appropriate line from a
knowledge of the values of the other
variables; as the DuBois nomograph
for estimation of surface area.

non-. A prefix meaning *not.*

non"ad·he'rent. Not connected to
an adjacent organ or part.

non"al·ler'gic. Unrelated to allergy.

no'nan. Having an exacerbation every
ninth day.

non·a'que·ous (non·ay'kwee·us,
-ack'wee·us). Not consisting of, or pertaining to; water; said of organic solvents.

non com'pos men'tis. Of unsound
mind.

non"con·duc'tor. Any substance
not transmitting electricity or heat.

no"ni·grav'i·da (no"ni·grav'i·duh,
non"i·). A woman pregnant for the
ninth time.

no·nip'a·ra. A woman who has been
in labor nine times.

non"lu·et'ic. Not due to syphilitic
infection.

non"ma·lig'nant. Lacking any features of malignant disease, usually referring to tumors. Syn., *benign.*

non·mo'tile (non-mo'til). Not having the power of spontaneous motion.

non'ose. A monosaccharide which contains nine carbon atoms in the molecule.

non·pro'te·in. Not derived from protein, as nonprotein nitrogen; not containing protein, as nonprotein fraction of an extract.

non·pro'te·in ni'tro·gen. The total nitrogen of the blood less that of the blood proteins.

non"py·o·gen'ic (non"pye-o-jen'-ick). Not inducing the formation of pus.

non"re·frac'tive. Not possessing properties permitting the refraction of light rays.

non·re·straint'. The treatment of insanity without any forcible means of compulsion.

non·sex'u·al. Asexual, q.v.

non"spe·cif'ic. Referring to relations that are not specific, but general.

non·sup'pu·ra"tive. Uninfected; surgically clean; not forming pus.

non·vi'a·ble. Incapable of living.

no'ö·psy"che (no'o-sigh"kee). Mental or reasoning processes.

N. O. P. H. N. National Organization for Public Health Nursing.

nor-. A prefix indicating the *parent compound* from which another is derived.

nor"e·phed'rine hy"dro·chlo'-ride. Phenylpropanolamine hydrochloride.

nor·ep"i·neph'rine (nor-ep"i-nef'-reen, ·rin). 3,4-Dihydroxyphenylamino-ethanol. $C_6H_3(OH)_2CHOH.CH_2.NH_2$. A demethylated epinephrine formed at sympathetic nerve endings as a mediator of functional activity; it probably is the postulated *sympathin E.* Syn., *arterenol.*

nor·leu'cine (nor-lew'seen, ·sin). $CH_3(CH_2)_3CH(NH_2)COOH$. Alpha-amino-caproic acid, a component of many proteins.

norm. A standard.

nor'ma (pl. *normae*). *In anatomy,* a view or aspect, essentially of the skull.

nor'mal. 1. Perfect according to some ideal standard. 2. Well; not handicapped by symptoms of disease. 3. Pertaining to the central values of a homogeneous group. 4. Referring to solutions containing the equivalent weight of a substance, in grams, in a liter. Abbreviated, N.

norm·er'gy. *In allergy,* a normal degree of capacity to react.

nor'mo·blast. The smallest of the precursors of the erythrocyte, having almost a full complement of hemoglobin and a small pycnotic nucleus.

nor"mo·chro'mi·a. The condition

of the blood with normal hemoglobi content.

nor'mo·cyte. A red blood cell normal size (7.5 μ). —**normocyt'i** adj.

nor·nic'o·tine (nor-nick'o-tee-tin). A minor alkaloid occurring tobacco.

nor·val'ine. $CH_3(CH_2)_2CH(NH_2$ COOH. α-Amino-n-valeric acid. A amino-acid component of casein, gl bin, and the protein of horn.

nos'ca·pine. Narcotine. See *necta* *don.*

nose. The prominent organ in the cen ter of the face; the upper part (reg olfactoria) constitutes the organ smell, the lower part (regio respir toria) the beginning of the respirato tract, in which the inspired air warmed, moistened, and deprived impurities. **bridge of n.** The prom nence formed by the junction of t nasal bones. **saddle n.** One with depression in the bridge due to the lo of the nasal septum.

nose'bleed". A hemorrhage from t nose. Syn., *epistaxis.*

nose clip. A rubberized, spring-ste device worn by swimmers and divers prevent the passage of water into t nose.

nose drops. A preparation containi medicaments, which is administered placing drops in the nose.

nos'o-, nos-. A combining form si nifying *disease.*

nos"och·tho·nog'ra·phy (noss ock-tho-nog'ruh-fee). Geography endemic diseases; medical geograp

no·sog'e·ny (no-sodj'i-nee). The velopment of diseases. —**nosogene** ic, adj.

no·sol'o·gy. The science of the clas fication of diseases. —**nosolog'i** adj.

nos"o·ma'ni·a. 1. A morbid dread disease. 2. A delusion that one is suf ing from disease.

nos"o·pho'bi·a. The exagger fear of disease.

No"sop·syl'lus. A genus of fle N. fasciatus. A species of rat fl which may transmit plague.

nostal. Trade-mark for 5-isoprop 5-β-bromallyl barbituric acid, a b notic. See *propallylonal.*

nos·tal'gi·a. Homesickness. —**n** talgic, adj.

nos"to·ma'ni·a. Nostalgia amou ing to monomania.

nos'tras. Denoting a disease belo ing to the country in which it is scribed, in contradistinction to a si lar disease originating elsewhere, cholera nostras as distinguished f Asiatic cholera.

nos'trate. Endemic.

nos'tril. One of the external orifices of the nose. Syn., *naris.*

nos'trum. A quack medicine; a secret medicine.

nostyn. Trade-mark for ectylurea.

no·ta'tin. An antibiotic from *Penicillium notatum.* Also called *corylophilline, Escherichia coli factor, mycoin, penatin, penicillin-B.*

notch. A deep indentation. —**notched,** *adj.* **acetabular n.** A notch in the lower border of the acetabulum. **angular n.** A notch in the lesser curvature of the stomach formed at the junction of its body and the pyloric portion. Also called *angular incisure.* **cardiac n.** A notch in the anterior border of the left lung, occupied by the heart within the pericardium. **greater sciatic n.** A notch between the spine of the ischium and the posterior inferior iliac spine; it is converted into a foramen by the sacrospinous and sacrotuberous ligaments. **jugular n. of the sternum.** The depression on the superior border of the manubrium between the two clavicles. **lesser sciatic n.** The notch below the spine of the ischium which is converted to a foramen by the sacrotuberous and sacrospinous ligaments; it transmits the tendon of the obturator internus and the internal pudendal vessels and pudendal nerve. **suprasternal n.** The jugular notch of the sternum.

note. A sound. **amphoric n.** A low-pitched, hollow sound, obtained over a large cavity of the chest, or over pneumothorax. **cracked-pot n.** A note with a peculiar clinking quality, heard on percussion over a superficial pulmonary cavity. **percussion n.** The sound elicited on percussion, usually described as flat, dull, resonant, or tympanitic.

no″ten·ceph'a·lus. An individual with occipital encephalocele, or more usually hydrencephalocele.

no'ti·fi″a·ble. Pertaining to a disease which must be made known to health authorities.

no'to·chord (no'to·kord). An elongated cord of cells enclosed in a structureless sheath, which is the primitive axial skeleton of the embryo. It serves as a focal axis about which the vertebral bodies develop and persists as the nuclei pulposi of the intervertebral disks. Also called *chorda dorsalis.* —**notochord'al,** *adj.*

novatrin. A trade-mark for homatropine methylbromide.

novatropine. Trade-mark for the methylbromide of the alkaloid homatropine.

no″vo·bi'o·cin. An antibiotic from *Streptomyces niveus* or from *S. sphe-* *roides,* used in the form of calcium and sodium salts. See *albamycin, cathomycin.*

novocain. Trade-mark for a brand of procaine hydrochloride.

nox'ious (nock'shus). Harmful; poisonous or deleterious.

Np. Chemical symbol for neptunium.

NPH. Designation for an insulin of intermediate duration of action, the *N* referring to neutral, the *P* to protamine, and the *H* to Hagedorn, in whose laboratory the product was originally developed.

N. P. N. Nonprotein nitrogen.

n-rays. A nonluminous radiation of lower wave length than visible light. Emitted by an x-ray tube, the sun, or a Welsbach burner; passes through thin metals, and increases the luminosity of phosphorescent bodies. Discovered by Blondlot.

Nt. Chemical symbol for niton.

nu'bile (new'bil). Marriageable; of an age for childbearing. —**nubil'ity,** *n.*

nu'cha (new'kuh). The nape of the neck. —**nuchal,** *adj.*

nu'cle·ar. Pertaining to, or resembling, a nucleus.

nu'cle·ar fis'sion. *In chemistry* and *in physics,* the splitting of certain heavy nuclei into two large fragments, accompanied by the emission of neutrons and the release of large amounts of energy.

nu'cle·ar re·ac'tor. An apparatus in which nuclear fission is sustained by a chain reaction and which contains fissionable material, or fuel, such as plutonium or uranium; a moderating material such as carbon, beryllium, or heavy water; and a reflector to conserve escaping neutrons.

nu'cle·ase (new'klee·ace, ·aze). An enzyme capable of splitting nucleic acids to nucleotides, nucleosides, or the components of the latter.

nu'cle·i (new'klee·eye). Plural of nucleus.

nu·cle'ic ac'id. One of a group of compounds found in nuclei and cytoplasm and distinguished by a prefix to indicate the specific source. They generally contain four molecules of phosphoric acid combined with four glycoside molecules from which latter the bases adenine, guanine, cytosine, and either uracil (from the nucleic acid of yeast) or thymine (from the nucleic acid of thymus) may be derived; the sugar component is generally either ribose or desoxyribose. Syn., *nucleinic acid.*

nu'cle·ide. A compound of nuclein with some metal, as iron, copper, silver, mercury, etc.

nu'cle·in. Any one of a group of ill-defined complexes of protein and nucleic acid occurring in the nuclei of cells.

nu'cle·in·ase (new"klee·in·ace, ·aze). An enzyme which resolves nucleic acid into nucleotides.

nu"cle·in'ic ac'id. See *nucleic acid*.

nu'cle·o-, nucle-. A combining form signifying *relating to a nucleus*.

nu"cle·o·al·bu'min. A compound of nucleic acid and albumin.

nu"cle·o·his'tone. A basic protein from cell nuclei.

nu·cle'o·lus. A small spherical body within the cell nucleus. Syn., *plasmosome.* —**nucleolar,** *adj.*

nu'cle·on. A collective term for protons and neutrons.

nu"cle·on'ics. Nuclear physics.

nu"cle·o·pro'te·id. See *nucleoprotein*.

nu"cle·o·pro'te·in. A protein constituent of cell nuclei, consisting of nucleic acid and a basic protein. On hydrolysis, nucleoproteins yield purine bases, pyrimidine bases, phosphoric acid, and a carbohydrate.

nu"cle·o·si'dase (new"klee·o·sigh'-dace, ·dace, new"klee·oss'i·). An enzyme that catalyzes the hydrolysis of a nucleoside into its component pentose and purine or pyrimidine base.

nu·cle'o·side. A glycoside resulting from the removal of phosphate from a nucleotide. It is a combination of a sugar (pentose) with a purine or pyrimidine base.

nu"cle·o·ti'dase (new"klee·o·tye'-dace, ·daze, new"klee·ot'i·). One of a group of nucleophosphatases which split phosphoric acid from nucleotides, leaving nucleosides.

nu'cle·o·tide. The combination of a purine or pyrimidine base with a sugar and phosphoric acid. The basic structural unit of nucleic acid. **phospho-pyridine nucleotides.** See *phosphopyridine nucleotides*.

nu"cle·o·tox'in. A toxin derived from cell nuclei; any toxin affecting the nuclei of cells.

nu'cle·us (pl. *nuclei*). 1. The differentiated central protoplasm of a cell; its trophic center. 2. A collection of nerve cells in the central nervous system concerned with a particular function. 3. A stable and characteristic complex of atoms to which other atoms may be attached. 4. The center around which the mass of a crystal aggregates. 5. The center of an atom consisting of protons and neutrons. **n. cuneatus.** The collection of nerve cells lying in the dorsal aspect of the medulla oblongata in which the fibers of the fasciculus cuneatus terminate. **n. gracilis.** A nucleus in the dorsal aspect of the medulla oblongata in which the fibers of fasciculus gracilis terminate.

n. pulposus. The pulpy body in the center of an intervertebral disk.

nu'clide. A species of atom characterized by the constitution of its nucleus, in particular by the number of protons and neutrons in the nucleus.

nud'ism. 1. *In phychiatry,* a more or less complete intolerance of clothing; a morbid tendency to remove the clothing. 2. The practice of a cult, nudists, who profess to believe in the benefits of a society in which clothes are discarded.

nui'sance. *In legal medicine,* that which is noxious, offensive, or troublesome; applied to persons or things.

nujol. A trade-mark for liquid petrolatum.

nul·lip'a·ra. A woman who has never borne a child. —**nulliparous,** *adj.*; **nullipar'ity,** *n.*

Numa Pompillus [*second legendary king of Rome,* 715–673 B. C.]. Known medically for his law ordering the operation of abdominal incision for women dying in late pregnancy or childbirth, in order to save the child; called *lex regia.* Under the Caesars the lex regia became known as *lex caesaria.*

numb. Having impaired cutaneous sensibility.

num'ber. 1. The total count of units. 2. A numeral, designating place in a series. Abbreviated, No. Symbol, #. **atomic n.** The total number of protons in an atom. Each element has a characteristic atomic number. **Avogadro's n.** The number of molecules of a substance in one gram-molecular weight; it is 6.06×10^{23}.

numb'ness. Partial, or local, anesthesia with torpor; deficiency of sensation. Obdormition.

nu·mer'i·cal·ap'er·ture. The product of the sine of half the angular aperture of a lens, and the index of the medium through which the light passes. A mathematical relationship discovered by Abbe between the resolving power of an objective and its aperture. Microscope objectives and condensers are largely designated by the numerical aperture (generally abbreviated N. A.) value.

num'mi·form. Having the form of a coin.

num'mu·lar. Resembling a coin in form, as nummular sputum; resembling rouleaux or rolls of coin.

nun·na'tion. The frequent, or abnormal, use of the *n* sound.

nupercaine hydrochloride. Trade-mark for a water-soluble derivative of cinchoninic acid used as a local anesthetic.

nurse. 1. Suckle an infant. 2. Care for a sick person. 3. One who cares for an infant or young child, also called a nursemaid. **4.** One who cares for a sick person, often under the supervision of a physician. **attending n.** One who visits patients in their homes. **community n.** One employed by a subdivision of the government to assist in the medical care and supervision of health in a locality. **general duty n.** One assigned to a ward or division of a hospital and performing many different duties for all the patients. **graduate n.** One who has been graduated from a recognized school of nursing. **head n.** One who is in charge of a ward or division of a hospital. **hospital n.** One who works for a hospital rather than one special patient or physician. **practical n.** One skilled in the care of the sick but who has not been graduated from a regular nursing school or passed an examination to qualify as a graduate nurse. **private n.** One who works exclusively for one patient at a time and is employed by him whether in a hospital or a home. **probationer n.** A girl who has recently entered nurses' training and is still under probation. This usually lasts three months, at the successful conclusion of which the girl becomes a student nurse. **public health n.** A graduate nurse working for a public health official or public health agency, as the Visiting Nurse Association, to assist in safeguarding the health of the people in her district. She gives instruction and actual care to the people in their homes and helps in the prevention and spread of disease. **registered n.** A graduate nurse who has passed her state board examination and is thus qualified to be a nurse. She is legally entitled to add R.N. to her name. **school n.** A graduate nurse who visits the children in one or more schools, assisting the school physician in his duties. **scrub n.** One who is part of an operating team, being scrubbed, gowned, and surgically clean so that she can assist the operating surgeon. **special n.** (a) A private nurse taking special care of one patient. (b) One well trained in a particular specialty. **student n.** A girl who is still in nurses' training school. **visiting n.** See community n. **wet n.** A woman who furnishes breast feeding to an infant not her own.

nurse corps. The women nurses in the Army and Navy, who have ranks, titles, and status as officers, corresponding to the officer component of the Armed Services.

nurs'ing. 1. Obtaining milk from a breast by an infant. **2.** Giving milk to an infant from a breast. **3.** Caring for the sick. **n. bottle.** A bottle fitted with a rubber tip or nipple for feeding infants not nursed from the breast.

nurs'ling. An infant that is nursed.

nut'gall'' (nut'gawl''). Galls. The excrescence on young twigs of *Quercus infectoria;* caused by the deposition of eggs of the insect *Cynips tinctoria.* Nutgall contains gallotannic acid, an astringent.

nut'meg. 1. Any plant of the genus *Myristica.* **2.** The dried ripe seed of *Myristica fragrans* deprived of its covering (mace). A spice.

nu·tri·ent. 1. Affording nutrition. **2.** A nourishing food.

nu'tri·lite. A substance which, in small amounts, functions in the nutrition of microörganisms. *Obs.*

nu'tri·ment. Anything that nourishes.

nu·tri'tion. 1. The sum of the processes concerned in the growth, maintenance, and repair of the living body as a whole, or of its constituent parts. **2.** Nourishment; food. **—nutritional,** *adj.*

nu'tri·ture. Nutritional status.

nux (pl. *nuces*). Musky nut. The nutmeg; myristica. **n. vomica.** The seed of *Strychnos nux-vomica,* an Indian tree of the Loganiaceae. Contains several alkaloids, the most important being strychnine and brucine.

nyc·tal'gi·a. Pain, which occurs chiefly during the night.

nyc'ta·lope. One who cannot see at night. See *night blindness.*

nyc'ter·ine (nick'tur·een, ·in). **1.** Occurring in the night. **2.** Obscure.

nyc''to·phil'i·a. Preference for night or darkness.

nyc''to·pho'bi·a. A morbid fear of night and of darkness.

nyc''to·pho'ni·a. The hysterical loss of the voice during the day, in one who is capable of speaking during the night.

nyc''to·typh·lo'sis. Night blindness, *q.v.*

nydrazid. A trade-mark for isoniazid.

ny'li·drin hy''dro·chlo'ride. 1-(*p*-Hydroxyphenyl)-2-(1-methyl-3-phenylpropylamino)propanol hydrochloride, a peripheral vasodilator. See *arlidin hydrochloride.*

nym'pha (pl. *nymphae*). A minor lip of the vulva.

nym·phec'to·my. Surgical removal of one or both minor lips.

nym·phi'tis. Inflammation of the minor lips.

nym'pho·lep'sy. Ecstasy of an erotic type.

nym''pho·ma'ni·a. Excessive sexual desire on the part of a woman. **—nymphomaniac,** *adj., n.*

nym·phot'o·my. Incision of one or both minor lips.

nys·tag'mus. An oscillatory movement of the eyeballs. It may be congenital or dependent on intracranial disease, as meningitis or multiple sclerosis. **—nystagmic,** *adj.* **lateral n.** Oscillation of the eyes in the horizontal meridian. **miners' n.** That occurring in men who work in cramped quarters with insufficient illumination. **oscillatory n.** That which occurs when vision in both eyes has long been extremely poor, as an occupational disorder such as miners' nystagmus, and as a congenital defect. Also called *pendulous n.* **rotatory n.** An oscillatory, partial rolling of the eyeball around the visual axis. **vertical n.** Oscillatory movement in the vertical meridian.

ny·stat'in. An antibiotic from *Streptomyces noursei,* effective in treatment of moniliasis. See *mycostatin.*

○

O. 1. Chemical symbol for oxygen. 2. Abbreviation for *oculus,* eye; *octarius,* a pint; opening of an electric circuit; occiput.

o-. *In chemistry,* ortho-.

oak. A genus of trees, *Quercus,* of the Fagaceae.

oa'kum (o'kum). The loose fiber made by picking old hemp rope to pieces. Oakum was formerly used as a dressing for wounds.

o·ar'i·o-. For words beginning with *oario-,* see under *ovario-* or *oöphor-.*

o·a'sis. *In surgery,* an isolated spot of normal tissue situated in a pathologic area.

ob-. A prefix signifying *on, against, in front of,* or *toward.*

ob"ce·ca'tion (ob"si·kay'shun). Partial blindness.

ob"dor·mi'tion (ob"dor·mish'un). Numbness of a part due to interference with nervous function; the state of a part when it is said to be asleep.

ob·duc'tion. A post-mortem examination; an autopsy; a necropsy. *Obs.*

o·bese'. Extremely fat; corpulent. **—obesely,** *adv.;* **obeseness,** *n.*

o·be'si·ty (o·bee'si·tee, o·bess'i·tee). A condition in which excessive fat is stored in the body, due to a positive energy balance. **endocrine o.** That due to dysfunction of the endocrine glands. **hypothalamic o.** That resulting from a disturbance of function of the appetite-regulating centers of the hypothalamus.

ob"fus·ca'tion. Mental confusion.

ob·jec'tive. 1. Pertaining to an object or to that which is contemplated or perceived, as distinguished from that which contemplates or perceives. 2. Pertaining to those relations and conditions of the body perceived by another, as objective signs of disease. 3. The lens of a microscope nearest the object.

ob"li·gate. Constrained; bound; not facultative, as an obligate anaerobe, one that can live only as an anaerobe.

ob·lique' (o·bleek', o·blike'). 1. Not direct; aslant; slanting. 2. *In botany,* unequal-sided. 3. *In anatomy,* an oblique muscle, as the external or internal oblique of the abdomen, or the superior or inferior oblique of the eye.

ob·liq'ui·ty. The state of being oblique. Particularly, *in obstetrics,* a term used for a theory of the mechanism of labor.

ob·lit"er·a'tion. 1. The complete removal of a part by disease or surgical operation; extirpation. 2. Complete closure of a lumen. 3. The complete loss of memory or consciousness of certain events.

ob"mu·tes'cence. Aphonia; loss of voice. *Rare.*

ob·nu"bi·la'tion. A form of mental haze preceding loss of consciousness.

ob·ses'sion. An idea or emotion that persists in an individual's mind in spite of any conscious attempts to remove it an imperative idea, as in psychoneurosis. **—obsessive,** *adj.*

ob·ses"sive ru'mi·na"tive state. A condition marked by a compulsion to entertain imperative ideas; morbid preoccupation with trivial or inconsequential ideas or acts. A compulsive-obsessive form of psychoneurosis.

ob"so·les'cence. The state of becoming old or obsolete.

ob"ste·tri'cian (ob"steh·trish'un). One who practices obstetrics.

ob·stet'rics. The branch of medicine that cares for women during pregnancy, labor, and the puerperium. **—obstetric, obstetrical,** *adj.*

ob·struc'tion. 1. The state of being occluded or stenosed, applied especially to hollow viscera, ducts, and vessels. 2. The act of occluding or blocking. 3. An obstacle. **—obstructive,** *adj.* **intestinal o.** Any hindrance to the passage of intestinal contents. **mitral o.** See mitral *stenosis.* **partial o.** Incomplete obstruction. **ureteral o.**

Any hindrance to the flow of urine through the ureter to the bladder. **uri·nary o.** Any hindrance to the passage of urine through the urinary system, specifically to the evacuation of urine from the bladder.

b·stru·ent. 1. Obstructive; tending to obstruct. 2. Any agent closing the orifice of vessels or ducts.

b·tund´. Blunt or dull; lessen, as to obtund sensibility.

b·tund´ent. Soothing, quieting; a remedy that relieves or overcomes irritation or pain. *Obs.*

b″tu·ra´tion. 1. The closing of an opening or passage. 2. A form of intestinal obstruction in which the lumen of the intestine is occupied by its normal contents or by foreign bodies. *Rare.*

b″tu·ra″tor. 1. Closing an opening. 2. That which closes an opening. 3. Pertaining to the obturator membrane, muscles, etc. See Table of Muscles in the Appendix. 4. A solid wire or rod which is contained within a hollow needle or cannula. Obturators may be bayonet-pointed for piercing tissues, or obliquely faced at the end for fitting, exactly, large aspirating needles. The term is also applied to the metal carriers within urethroscopes and cystoscopes, etc. 5. An appliance which closes a cleft or fissure of the palate.

b·tuse´. 1. Blunt. 2. Of angles, greater than 90°.

b·tu´sion (ob·tew´zhun). The blunting or weakening of normal sensation, a symptom of certain diseases.

o·cip´i·tal (ock·sip´i·tul). 1. Pertaining to, or in relation with, the occiput. 2. The occipital bone. See Table of Bones in the Appendix.

o·cip´i·to- (ock·sip´i·to-). *In anatomy,* a combining form denoting occipital.

o·cip″i·to·an·te´ri·or. Having the occiput directed toward the front, as the occipitoanterior position of the fetus in the uterus.

o·cip″i·to·pos·te´ri·or. Having the occiput directed backward, as the occipitoposterior position of the fetus in the uterus.

o´ci·put (ock´si·put). The back part of the head.

·clu´si·o. Closure. **o. pupillae.** obliteration of the pupil. **o. pupillae lymphatica.** Obliteration of the pupil by a false membrane.

·clu´sion (o·clue´zhun). 1. A closing or shutting up. 2. The state of being closed or shut. 3. The absorption, by a metal, of gas in large quantities, as of hydrogen by platinum. 4. The full meeting or contact in a position of rest of the masticating surfaces of the upper and lower teeth; erroneously called articulation of teeth. **coronary o.**

Occlusion of a branch of the arterial system that supplies blood to the heart muscle. **puerperal tubal o.** The agglutination of mucosal folds of the uterine tube occurring about one week after labor, presumably from a mild gonococcus infection and producing one-child sterility. **tubal o.** Loss of patency of the oviduct.

oc·cult´, oc´cult. Hidden; concealed; not evident, as occult blood, the blood in excrement or secretion not clearly evident to the naked eye, or occult disease, any disease the nature of which is not readily determined.

oc″cu·pa´tion·al dis·ease´. One caused by the occupation of the patient. It may be organic, as lead poisoning, or functional. See occupational *neurosis.*

oc″cu·pa·tion·al ther´a·py. The teaching of trades and arts as a means for the rehabilitation of patients handicapped physically or mentally.

och″lo·le´sis (ock·lee´sis). A morbid condition produced by crowding many people together in a small space with a lack of ventilation.

och″lo·pho·bi·a (ock″lo·fo´bee·uh). Morbid fear of crowds.

o·chrom´e·ter. An instrument for measuring the capillary blood pressure.

o″chro·no´sis, o·chron·o·sis. A blue or brownish blue pigmentation of cartilage and connective tissue, especially around joints, by a melanotic pigment. The condition is frequently accompanied by alkaptonuria and may occur in those who have had phenol, in large quantities, applied to skin or mucous membrane for a long time. A disturbed metabolism of aromatic compounds is associated with this condition. —**ochron·ot´ic,** *adj.*

O″co·te´a (o″ko·tee´uh, o·ko´tee·uh). A large genus of tropical trees of the order Lauraceae.

oc´ta-, oct-. A combining form meaning *eight.*

oc´ta·caine. β-Octyl-2-amino-β,β-dimethylethyl *p*-aminobenzoate hydrochloride. A local anesthetic.

oc´tad. 1. An octavalent element or radical. 2. Having a valence of eight.

oc″ta·meth´yl py″ro·phos″phor·am´ide. Bis[bisdimethylamino-phosphonous]anhydride, a systemic insecticide; also, a potent anticholinesterase agent used in treating myasthenia gravis. Abbreviated, OMPA.

oc´tan. Returning every eighth day, as an octan fever.

oc´tane. C_8H_{18}. The eighth member of the paraffin or marsh gas series.

oc·ta´ri·us. An eighth part of a gallon; a pint. Abbreviated, O.

oc″ta·va´lent, oc·tav´a·lent. Having a valence of eight.

oc´tene. See *octylene.*

oc'ti·grav'i·da. A woman pregnant for the eighth time.

octin. Trade-mark for isometheptene.

oc·tip'a·ra. A woman who has been in labor eight times.

oc"ti·va'lent. See *octavalent*.

oc'to-, oct-. A combining form meaning *eight*.

oc"to·roon'. The offspring of a white person and a quadroon; a person who has one-eighth part of Negro blood.

oc'tyl. The radical C_8H_{17}—.

oc'tyl·ene. One of a group of liquid unsaturated hydrocarbons of the formula C_8H_{16}.

oc'u·lar. 1. Pertaining to or in relation with the eye. 2. The lens assembly of a microscope, telescope, or other optical instrument that is nearest the eye; an eyepiece.

oc"u·len'tum. An ointment for use in the eye.

oc'u·list. See *ophthalmologist*.

oc'u·lo-, ocul-. A combining form denoting *the eye* or *ocular*.

oc"u·lo·gy·ra'tion (ock"yoo·lo·jye·ray'shun). Movement of the eyeballs.

oc"u·lo·gy'ric. Referring to movements of the eyes.

oc"u·lo·mo'tor. 1. Pertaining to the movement of the eye, as the oculomotor nerve. See Table of Nerves in the Appendix. 2. Pertaining to the oculomotor nerve, as the oculomotor nucleus.

oc"u·lo·my·co'sis (ock"yoo·lo·migh·ko'sis). Any disease of the eye or its appendages, due to the presence of a fungus.

oc'u·lus (pl. *oculi*). An eye. Abbreviated, O. **o. cae'sius.** Glaucoma. **o. dex'ter.** The right eye. Abbreviated, O. D. **o. duplex.** A bandage covering both eyes. **o. sinister.** The left eye. Abbreviated, O. S. **o. uterque.** Each eye. Abbreviated, O. U. Also called *o. unitas*.

o"cy·o·din'ic (o"see·o·din'ick, o"sigh·o-). Oxytocic; hastening the delivery of the fetus.

O. D. *Oculus dexter*, right eye.

o"dax·es'mus (o"dacks·es'mus). The biting of the tongue, lip, or cheek, during an epileptic seizure.

o"don·tal'gi·a. Toothache. **phantom o.** Pain felt in the space from which a tooth is absent.

o"don·tal'gic. 1. Relating to toothache. 2. A remedy for toothache.

o"don·tec'to·my. Surgical removal of a tooth.

o·don'ti·a. Any abnormality of the teeth. **o. deformis.** Deformity of the teeth, arising either from error of shape or position, or from malformation of the jaws or alveolar border. **o. incrustans.** Tartar of the teeth.

o"don·ti'a·sis. Dentition; the cutting of teeth.

o"don·ti·a·try, o·don"ti·at'ri·a

(o·don"tee·at'ree·uh, o·don"tee·uh tree'uh). Treatment of the diseases o the teeth. **—odontiatrist,** *n.*

o"don·ti'tis. Inflammation of th teeth.

o·don'to-, odont-. A combining form meaning *tooth*.

o·don"to·blas·to'ma. A tumor developing from the mesenchymal portion of the tooth germ.

o·don"to·chi·rur'gi·cal (·kigh rur'ji·kul). Pertaining to dental surgery.

o"don·tog'e·ny (o"don·todj'i·nee) The origin and development of teeth.

o"don·tog'ra·phy. The descriptive anatomy of the teeth. **—odonto graph'ic,** *adj.*

o·don"to·hy"per·es·the'si·a (·high"pur·ess·thee'zhuh, ·zee·uh). Hy persensitiveness of dentine or nerves the teeth.

o·don'toid. Resembling a tooth toothlike, or pertaining to the dens o the axis, as odontoid ligament.

o·don'to·lith. Dental calculus, *q.v.*

o"don·tol'o·gist. A dental surgeon

o"don·tol'o·gy. The branch of sc ence dealing with the anatomy an diseases of the teeth.

o"don·to'ma. A tumor or tumorlik hyperplasia which develops from on or more parts of a tooth germ. Th resulting tissue may be soft, calcifie or a mixture of both.

o·don"to·ne·cro'sis. Necrosis or de cay of the tissues of the teeth; dent caries.

o·don"to·neu·ral'gi·a. Neuralg due to diseased teeth.

o·don"to·par"al·lax'is. Irregular ity of the teeth; deviation of one more of the teeth from the natur position.

o"don·top'a·thy. Any disease of th teeth.

o·don"to·pho'bi·a. Morbid fear teeth (usually animals' teeth).

o·don"to·pri'sis (o·don"to·pry's o"don·top'ri·sis). Grinding of the teet See *bruxism*.

o·don"tor·rha'gi·a. Hemorrha from the socket of a tooth.

o·don'to·scope. 1. A dental mirr used for inspecting the teeth. 2. magnifying device for inspection tooth surfaces.

o"don·tot'o·my. Cutting into tooth. **prophylactic o.** The oper tion of opening and filling structur imperfections of the enamel to preve dental caries.

o'dor. A scent, smell, or perfume; fragrance.

o"dor·if'er·ous. Emitting an odor

o·dyn"a·cou'sis (o·din"uh·koo's **o·dyn"a·cu'sis** (o·din"uh·cue' ·koo'sis). Pain caused by noises.

-o·dyn′i·a, -o·dy′ni·a. A combining form meaning *state of pain.*

o·dyn″o·pho′bi·a. Morbid dread of pain; algophobia.

oe-. For words beginning with *oe-* not found here, see under *e-*.

oe·de′ma (i·dee′muh). See *edema.*

oed′i·pism. See *edipism.*

Oed′i·pus com′plex. See under *complex.*

oes·tra′di·ol (es·tray′dee·ole, ·ol, ·awl, es·trad′ee·, es″truh·dye′·). See *estradiol.*

Oes′tri·dae (es′tri·dee). A family of botflies (warble flies), some species of which produce larvae which live under the skin of cattle, causing a characteristic swelling called the warble. Also see *warbles.*

oes′trin (es′trin). Estrin.

oes′tri·ol (es′tree·ole, ·ol, ·awl). Estriol.

oes″tro·gen′ic (es″tro·jen′ick). Estrogenic.

oes′trone (es′trone). Estrone.

oes′trus. Estrus.

of′fal. Refuse of any kind.

of·fi′cial. Referring to medicines recognized by, and conforming to the standards of, the United States Pharmacopeia or the National Formulary.

of·fic′i·nal. On sale without prescription.

ohm. The unit of electric resistance. The **international ohm,** adopted 1893, is the resistance of a column of mercury 106.3 centimeters long and weighing 14.4521 grams at 0° C. Its cross section is 1 mm.²

ohm′-am′me″ter. A combined ohmmeter and ammeter.

ohm′me″ter. Apparatus for measuring electric resistance in ohms.

-oid. A suffix signifying *like* or *resembling.*

oi·kol′o·gy. 1. The science of home. 2. Old term for ecology.

oi″ko·pho′bi·a. Morbid fear of home, or of a house.

oil. Any of a large class of carbon-containing substances, usually liquid and unctuous, which are insoluble in water but soluble in ether and in chloroform. The three principal groups are **fixed oils** that consist chiefly of glyceryl esters having a high proportion of unsaturated fatty acids obtained from plant or animal sources; **mineral oils** that are hydrocarbons obtained from petroleum; and **volatile oils** (also called **essential oils**) that consist of a great variety of chemical compounds, such as alcohols, ethers, and ketones, and sulfur and nitrogen compounds, obtained from plants. See under specific name for definition of an oil.

oil of vit′ri·ol. Sulfuric acid.

oi·no·ma′ni·a. 1. A form of mental disorder characterized by an irresistible craving for, and consequent indulgence in, drink. 2. Delirium tremens.

oint′ment. A semisolid preparation used for a protective and emollient effect or as a vehicle for the local or endermic administration of medicaments.

-ol. 1. A suffix denoting an alcohol or a phenol, as in ethan*ol.* 2. Formerly, sometimes same as *-ole.*

O. L. A. *Occipito laevo anterior;* left occipitoanterior position of the head of a fetus in labor.

-ole. A suffix denoting: (a) a five-membered heterocyclic ring, as in pyrr*ole;* (b) names of certain ethers, as in anis*ole,* $C_6H_5OCH_3$.

o′le·a. Plural of *oleum, q.v.*

o″le·ag′i·nous (o″lee·adj′i·nus). Oily.

o″le·an′der. See *nerium.*

o″le·an′do·my′cin. An antibiotic from species of *Streptomyces antibioticus,* used in the form of the phosphate salt in treatment of infections caused by Gram-positive coccal organisms. See *matromycin.*

o″le·an′drin. See *folinerin.*

o′le·ate. 1. A salt of oleic acid. 2. A pharmaceutical preparation made by a solution of medicinal ingredients in oleic acid.

o″le·cra″nar·thri′tis (o″li·kray″·nahr·thry′tis, o·leck″ran·ahr·thry′tis). Inflammation of the elbow joint.

o″le·cra″nar·throc′a·ce (o″li·kray″nahr·throck′uh·see, o·leck″ran·ahr·). Inflammation of the elbow joint.

o″le·cra″nar·throp′a·thy (o″li·kray″nahr·throp′uth·ee, o·leck″ran·ahr·). A disease of the elbow joint.

o·lec′ra·non, o″le·cra′non. The large process at the upper extremity of the ulna. —**olecranal,** *adj.*

o·lef′i·ant gas (o·lef′ee·unt, o·lee′fee·unt). Old term for ethylene.

o′le·fine (o′li·feen), **ol′e·fin** (ol′i·fin). Any member of the ethylene series of hydrocarbons; unsaturated compounds of the general formula C_nH_{2n}.

o·le′ic ac′id (o·lee′ick, o′lee·ick). An unsaturated acid, $CH_3(CH_2)_7CH:CH-(CH_2)_7COOH$, obtained from fats and fixed oils. Brownish yellow, oily liquid insoluble in water. **o. a. series.** Unsaturated fatty acids having one double bond and corresponding to the general formula, $C_nH_{2n-1}COOH$.

o′le·in. Glyceryl oleate, $(C_{17}H_{33}COO)_3$·C_3H_5, the chief constituent of olive oil and occurring in varying amounts in most other fixed oils. A colorless or yellowish, tasteless, and odorless oil; insoluble in water. Syn., *triolein.*

o′le·o·. 1. A combining form meaning *oil.* 2. In chemistry, a combining form signifying *olein, oleic.*

o″le·o·mar′ga·rine (o″lee·o·mahr′juh·reen, ·rin, ·mahr′guh·reen, ·rin). A butter substitute made by hydrogenation of a mixture of vegetable oils.

o″le·op′tene. See *eleoptene*.

o″le·o·res′in (o″lee·o·rez′in). A substance consisting chiefly of a mixture of an oil, either fixed or volatile, and a resin, sometimes with other active constituents, extracted from plants by means of a volatile solvent.

o″le·o·ther′a·py. The treatment of disease by the administration of oils. Also called *eleotherapy*.

o″le·o·tho′rax. A condition in which a lung is compressed, in tuberculosis, by using injections of sterile oil.

o″le·o·vi′ta·min. A solution of a vitamin in oil.

o·le′um (pl. *olea*). 1. Oil, *q.v.* 2. Fuming sulfuric acid; a solution of sulfur trioxide in concentrated sulfuric acid.

ol·fac′tion. The function of smelling or perceiving odors. —**olfactory,** *adj*.

ol″fac·tom′e·ter. An instrument for determining the power of smell.

o·lib′a·num. A gum resin produced by various species of *Boswellia*. Syn., *frankincense*.

ol″i·ge′mi·a (ol″i·ghee′mee·uh). A state in which the total quantity of the blood is diminished. See *hydremia*.

ol″i·ger·ga′si·a (ol″i·ghur·gay′-zhuh, ·shuh). *In psychiatry*, Adolf Meyer's term for all types of feeblemindedness and mental deficiency.

ol″ig·hid′ri·a (ol″ig·hid′ree·uh, ol″i·ghid′ree·uh), **ol″ig·id′ri·a** (ol″i·ghid′ree·uh, ·jid′ree·uh). Deficiency of perspiration.

ol″ig·hy′dri·a (ol″ig·high′dree·uh, ol″i·ghid′ree·uh). Deficiency of the fluids of the body.

ol′i·go-, olig-. A combining form meaning *few, scant*; used in medicine to denote *deficiency*.

ol″i·go·blen′ni·a. A deficient secretion of mucus.

ol″i·go·cho′li·a (ol″i·go·ko′lee·uh). A deficiency of bile.

ol″i·go·chro·ma′si·a (·kro·may′-zhuh, ·shuh). A decreased amount of hemoglobin in the red cells, which present a pale appearance.

ol″i·go·chro·me′mi·a. Deficiency of hemoglobin in the blood.

ol″i·go·chy′li·a (ol″i·go·kigh′lee·uh). Deficiency of chyle.

ol″i·go·cy·the′mi·a (ol″i·go·sigh·thee′mee·uh). A reduction in the total quantity of erythrocytes in the body.

ol″i·go·cy·the′mic nor″mo·vo·le′mi·a (ol″i·go·sigh·thee′mick, ·themm′ick). A normal blood volume with a decrease in red cells.

ol″i·go·dac′ry·a. Deficiency of the tears.

ol″i·go·dac·tyl′i·a. A condition

characterized by a deficiency of fingers or toes. See *ectrodactylia*.

ol″i·go·den·drog′li·a. Small supporting cells of the central nervous system, located about nerve cells, between nerve fibers, and along blood vessels, and characterized by spheroidal or ovoid nuclei and fine cytoplasmic processes with secondary divisions. Syn., *oligodendrocyte, oligoglia*.

ol″i·go·den″dro·gli·o′ma (ol″i·go·den″dro·glye·o′muh, ·den″drog·lee·o′muh). A slowly growing glioma of the cerebrum, rarely of the septum lucidum, fairly large and well defined, with a tendency to focal calcification. Microscopically, most of the cells are small, with richly chromatic nuclei and scanty, poorly staining cytoplasm without processes of neuroglia. Astrocytes in various stages of differentiation are often present.

ol″i·go·ga·lac′ti·a (ol″i·go·ga·lack′tee·uh, ·shee·uh). Deficiency in the secretion of milk.

ol″i·go·hy·dram′ni·os (ol″i·go·high·dram′nee·os). Deficiency of the amniotic fluid.

ol″i·go·hy·dru′ri·a (ol″i·go·high·droor′ee·uh). Urine with a relative diminution of water content; highly concentrated urine.

ol″i·go·me′li·a. Excessive congenital thinness of the limbs, or a deficiency in their number.

ol″i·go·men″or·rhe′a. Abnormally infrequent menstruation; to be distinguished from hypomenorrhea, *q.v.*

ol″i·go·phos″pha·tu′ri·a. A decrease in the amount of phosphates in the urine.

ol″i·go·phre′ni·a. Feeblemindedness; mental deficiency, *q.v.* —**oligophren′ic,** *adj*.

ol″i·gop·noe′a (ol″i·gop·nee′uh, oli·gop′nee·uh). Respiration diminished in depth or frequency.

ol″i·gop·ty′a·lism (ol″i·gop·ty′uh·liz·um, ol″i·go-). Deficient secretion of saliva.

ol″i·go·py′rene. A term descriptive of abnormal sperm cells which contain only a part of the full complement of chromosomes.

ol″i·go′ri·a. An abnormal apathy or indifference to persons or to environment, as in melancholia.

ol″i·go·si·a′li·a (ol″i·go·sigh·ay′-lee·uh, ·see·ay′lee·uh). Deficiency of saliva.

ol″i·go·sper′mi·a. Scarcity of spermatozoa in the semen.

ol″i·go·trich′i·a (ol″i·go·trick′ee·uh). Scantiness or thinness of hair.

ol″i·go·zo″o·sper′mi·a. Deficiency in the number of spermatozoa in the spermatic fluid.

ol″i·gu′ri·a. A diminution in the quantity of urine excreted.

ol'ive. 1. The oil tree, *Olea europaea*, or its fruit from which olive oil is expressed. 2. The inferior olive, or olivary body, a convoluted mass of gray matter with an inner core of white fibers, situated in the lateral part of the medulla oblongata between the pyramidal tract and the spinocerebellar tracts, and extending from the pons caudad for a distance of about 1.25 cm. Also called *oliva, inferior olive, olivary body, inferior olivary nucleus.* 3. An oval eminence on the anterior, ventrolateral surface of the medulla oblongata, which marks the location of the inferior olivary nucleus, which lies just beneath the surface. **—olivary,** *adj.*

ol'ive oil. A fixed oil obtained from the ripe fruit of the tree *Olea europaea*, chiefly glyceryl esters of oleic and palmitic acids, used as a nutrient, laxative, and emollient and as an ingredient of liniments, ointments, and plasters. Syn., *sweet oil.*

ol"o·pho'ni·a. Abnormal speech due to malformation of the vocal organs.

O. L. P. Abbreviation for *occipito laevo posterior*, or the left occipitoposterior position of the head of the fetus during parturition.

-o'ma. A suffix signifying *a morbid affection*, usually a tumorlike nodule or swelling.

o·ma'gra (o·may'gruh, o·mag'ruh). Gout in the shoulder.

o"mar·thral'gi·a. Pain in the shoulder joint.

o"mar·thri'tis. Inflammation of the shoulder joint.

om"bro·pho'bi·a. A morbid fear of rain.

o"men·tec'to·my. Excision of a portion of the omentum; omentumectomy.

o·men'to·pex·y. The surgical operation of suspending the great omentum, especially by suturing it to the abdominal wall.

o"men·tor'rha·phy. Suture of an omentum.

o·men'tum. Apron; a fold of the peritoneum connecting the abdominal viscera with the stomach. **—omental,** *adj.* **great o.** A fold of peritoneum attached to the greater curvature of the stomach above and, after dipping down over the intestine, returning to fuse with the transverse mesocolon. Between the ascending and descending folds is the cavity of the great omentum. Also called *gastrocolic o.* **lesser o.** A fold of peritoneum passing from the lesser curvature of the stomach to the transverse fissure of the liver. On the right its edge is free and enclses all the structures issuing from or entering the transverse fissure of the liver; portal vein, hepatic artery, bile duct, nerves and lymphatics. Behind the free edge is the epiploic foramen. Also called *gastrohepatic o.*

o·men"tum·ec'to·my (o·men"tuh·meck'to·mee). The surgical excision of any portion of the great omentum; omentectomy.

om·niv'o·rous. Subsisting on all kinds of food.

o'mo-, om-. A combining form meaning *the shoulder.*

o"mo·hy'oid. Pertaining conjointly to the scapula and the hyoid bone, as the omohyoid muscle, which is attached to these bones. See Table of Muscles in the Appendix.

OMPA (oh·em·pee·ay). Abbreviation for octamethyl pyrophosphoramide.

om"pha·lec'to·my. Excision of the navel.

om·phal'ic. Pertaining to the umbilicus, as the omphalic duct or vitelline duct: that which connects the yolk sac with the fetal intestine during the first three months of intrauterine life.

om"pha·li'tis. Inflammation of the navel.

om"pha·lo-, omphal-. A combining form meaning *the navel, umbilicus.*

om"pha·lo·mes"en·ter'ic (om"fuh·lo·mess"en·terr'ick, ·mez"en·terr'ick). Pertaining conjointly to the umbilicus and mesentery, as the omphalo-mesenteric artery.

om"pha·lo·prop·to'sis. Abnormal protrusion of the navel.

om·pha·los. The umbilicus.

om·phal'o·tome. An instrument for dividing the umbilical cord.

om"pha·lot'o·my. The cutting of the umbilical cord.

om"pha·lo·trip"sy. Separation of the umbilical cord by a crushing instrument.

o'nan·ism. 1. Incomplete coitus; coitus interruptus. 2. Masturbation. **—o'nan·ist,** *n.*

on'cho- (ong'ko-). See *onco-*.

On"cho·cer'ca. A genus of filarial worms. **O. caecutiens.** Synonym for *O. volvulus.* **O. volvulus.** A species which infests man, forming fibrous nodular tumors with encapsulation of the adult worms in the subcutaneous connective tissue.

on"cho·cer·ci'a·sis (ong"ko·sur·sigh'uh·sis, ·kigh'uh·sis). Infestation with the filarial worm *Onchocerca volvulus;* produces tumors of the skin, papular dermatitis, and ocular complications in man.

on'co-, oncho-. A combining form meaning *bulk;* used in medicine to denote *a tumor.*

on·col'o·gy. The study or science of neoplastic growth.

On"co·me·la'ni·a. A genus of amphibious snails. **O. hupensis.** A species found in the Yangtze basin; one of the intermediate hosts of *Schistosoma japonicum*. **O. hydrobiopsis.** A species found in Leyte and other of the Philippine Islands; an intermediate host of *Schistosoma japonicum*.

on·com'e·ter. An instrument for measuring variations in the volume of an organ, as of the kidney or spleen, or of an extremity.

on·co'sis. Any condition marked by the development of tumors. —**oncot'·ic**, *adj*.

-one. A suffix applied in organic chemistry to denote a *ketone*.

o·nei"ro·dyn'i·a (o·nigh"ro·din'ee·uh). Disquietude of the mind during sleep; painful dreaming; nightmare.

o"nei·rol'o·gy. The science, or scientific view, of dreams.

o"nei·ron'o·sus. Disorder manifesting itself in dreams; morbid dreaming.

o"nei·ros'co·py. Diagnosis of mental conditions by the analysis of dreams.

o"ni·o·ma'ni·a. A mania for buying.

on'ion (un'yun). The *Allium cepa* and its bulb. The latter contains a volatile oil resembling garlic oil and consisting principally of allyl sulfide (C_3H_5)$_2$S.

on"o·mat"o·ma'ni·a. An irresistible impulse to repeat certain words.

on"o·mat"o·pho'bi·a. Morbid fear of hearing a certain name, usually a commonplace word.

on"o·mat"o·poi·e'sis. 1. The formation of words in imitation of a sound. 2. *In psychiatry*, the extemporaneous formation of words on the basis of sound association; frequently a symptom of schizophrenia.

O·no'nis. A genus of leguminous plants.

on"to·gen·e'sis, on·tog'e·ny (on·todj'i·nee). The origin and development of the individual organism from fertilized egg to adult, as distinguished from phylogenesis, the evolutionary history of the race or group to which the individual belongs. —**ontogenet'ic**, *adj*.

on"y·chal'gi·a ner·vo'sa (on"i·kal'juh, o"ni·). Extreme sensitivity of apparently normal nails. Also called *hyperesthesia unguium*.

on"y·cha·tro'phi·a (on"i·kuh·tro'fee·uh, o"ni·kuh·), **on"y·chat'ro·phy.** 1. Atrophy of nails. 2. Failure of development of the nail.

on"y·chaux'is (on"i·kawk'sis, o"ni·). Hypertrophy of the nail.

on"y·chec'to·my (on"i·keck'to·mee, o"ni·). Excision of a fingernail or toenail.

on"y·chex"al·lax'is (on"i·keck"suh·lack'sis). Degeneration of nails.

o·nych'i·a (o·nick'ee·uh). Inflammation of the nail matrix. **o. craquelé.** Fragility and fracture of the nail.

o. maligna. A form occurring in debilitated persons; characterized by an ulcer in the matrix of the nail, which becomes discolored and is thrown off. **o. punctata.** A nail characterized by numerous small, punctiform depressions. **o. simplex.** Onychia without much ulceration, with loss of the nail and its replacement by a new one.

on'y·cho- (on'i·ko-), **onych-.** A combining form meaning *a nail*, or *claw*.

on"y·choc'la·sis (on"i·cock'luh·sis). Breaking of a nail.

on"y·cho·cryp·to'sis. Ingrowing of the nail. Syn., *unguis incarnatus*.

on"y·cho·dys'tro·phy. Any distortion of a nail; a symptom seen in several diseases.

on"y·cho·gry·po'sis (on"i·ko·grye·po'sis, ·gri·po'sis). A thickened, ridged, and curved condition of a nail.

on"y·cho·hel·co'sis. Ulceration of the nail.

on"y·cho·het"er·o·to'pi·a. An anomaly consisting of the presence of abnormally situated nails, as on the lateral aspect of the terminal phalanges. Most often occurs on the little finger.

on'y·choid (on'i·koyd). Resembling a fingernail in form or texture.

on"y·chol'y·sis (on"i·kol'i·sis). A slow process of loosening of a nail from its bed, beginning at the free edge and progressing gradually toward the root.

on"y·cho'ma (on"i·ko'muh). A tumor of the nail bed.

on"y·cho·ma·de'sis. Spontaneous separation of a nail from its bed beginning at the proximal end and progressing rapidly toward the free edge until the nail plate falls off. Syn., *defluvium unguium*.

on"y·cho·ma·la'ci·a (on"i·ko·ma·lay'shee·uh, ·see·uh). Abnormally soft nails.

on"y·cho·my·co'sis (on"i·ko·migh·ko'sis). A disease of the nails due to fungi.

on"y·cho·pac'i·ty (on"i·ko·pas'i·tee). White spots within the nail. Syn., *leukonychia*.

on"y·cho·path'y (on"i·cop'uth·ee). Any disease of the nails. —**onychopath'ic**, *adj*.

on"y·cho·pha'gi·a. The habit of biting the nails at the free edge.

on"y·choph'a·gist (on"i·kof'uh·jist). One addicted to biting the fingernails.

on"y·chor·rhex'is (on"i·ko·reck'sis). Longitudinal striation of the nail plate, with or without the formation of fissures.

on"y·chor·rhi'za. The root of the nail.

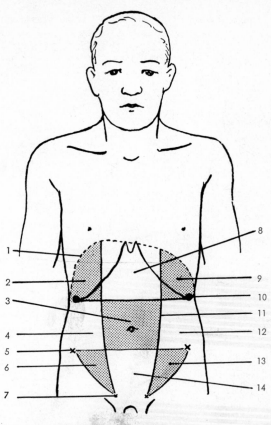

REGIONS OF ABDOMEN

, Level of diaphragm. **2,** Right hypochondrium. **3,** Umbilical region. **4,** Right umbar region. **5,** Anterior superior iliac spine. **6,** Right iliac region. **7,** Lateral order of rectus muscle, at lateral pubic spine. **8,** Epigastrium. **9,** Left hypo- hondrium. **10,** Level of 10th rib. **11,** Lateral border of rectus muscle (semilunar ne). **12,** Left lumbar region. **13,** Left iliac region. **14,** Hypogastrium.

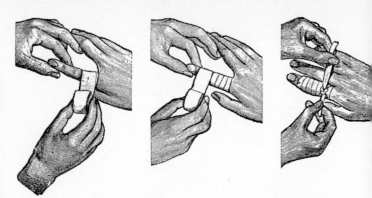

Spiral bandage for finger (or toe).

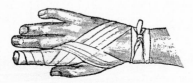

Spiral bandage to cover end of finger.

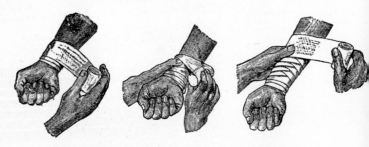

Spiral reverse bandage for limbs.

(From American Red Cross: "First Aid Textbook." Copyright, The American National Red Cross.)

TYPES OF BANDAGES

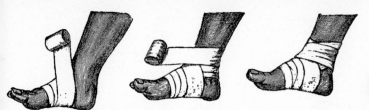

Figure-of-eight bandage of ankle.

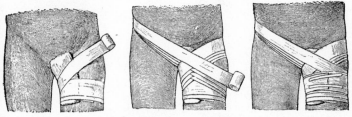

Spica bandage of groin.

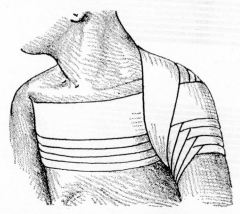

Ascending spica of shoulder.

TYPES OF BANDAGES—(Continued)

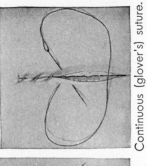

Continuous (glover's) suture.

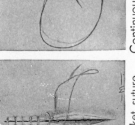

Blanket suture.

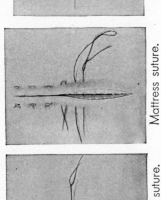

Mattress suture.

Interrupted suture.

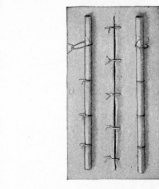

Relaxation sutures over dental rolls.

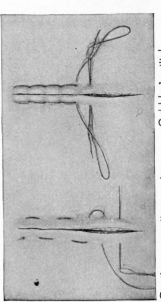

Cobbler's stitch.

Continuous mattress suture.

SUTURES

4

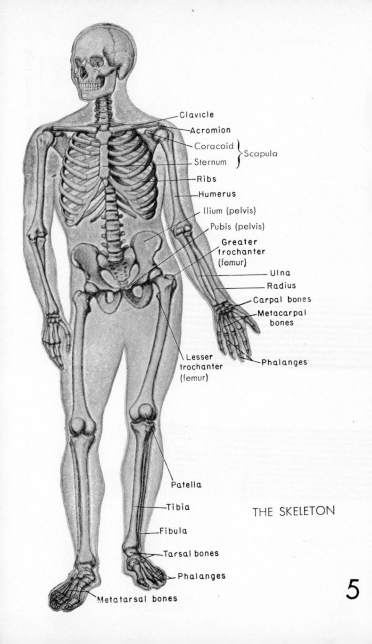

Clavicle
Acromion
Coracoid ⎫
Sternum ⎬ Scapula
Ribs
Humerus
Ilium (pelvis)
Pubis (pelvis)
Greater
trochanter
(femur)
Ulna
Radius
Carpal bones
Metacarpal
bones
Phalanges
Lesser
trochanter
(femur)
Patella
Tibia
Fibula
Tarsal bones
Phalanges
Metatarsal bones

THE SKELETON

5

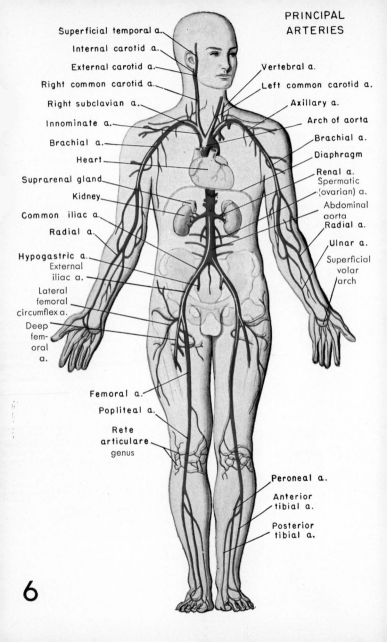

PRINCIPAL ARTERIES

Superficial temporal a.
Internal carotid a.
External carotid a.
Right common carotid a.
Right subclavian a.
Innominate a.
Brachial a.
Heart
Suprarenal gland
Kidney
Common iliac a.
Radial a.
Hypogastric a.
External iliac a.
Lateral femoral circumflex a.
Deep femoral a.

Vertebral a.
Left common carotid a.
Axillary a.
Arch of aorta
Brachial a.
Diaphragm
Renal a.
Spermatic (ovarian) a.
Abdominal aorta
Radial a.
Ulnar a.
Superficial volar arch

Femoral a.
Popliteal a.
Rete articulare genus

Peroneal a.
Anterior tibial a.
Posterior tibial a.

6

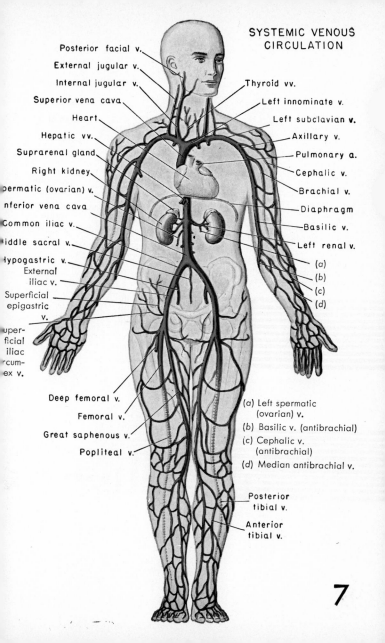

SYSTEMIC VENOUS
CIRCULATION

Posterior facial v.
External jugular v.
Internal jugular v.
Superior vena cava
Heart
Hepatic vv.
Suprarenal gland
Right kidney
Spermatic (ovarian) v.
Inferior vena cava
Common iliac v.
Middle sacral v.
Hypogastric v.
External iliac v.
Superficial epigastric v.
Superficial iliac circumflex v.

Thyroid vv.
Left innominate v.
Left subclavian v.
Axillary v.
Pulmonary a.
Cephalic v.
Brachial v.
Diaphragm
Basilic v.
Left renal v.
(a)
(b)
(c)
(d)

Deep femoral v.
Femoral v.
Great saphenous v.
Popliteal v.

(a) Left spermatic (ovarian) v.
(b) Basilic v. (antibrachial)
(c) Cephalic v. (antibrachial)
(d) Median antibrachial v.

Posterior tibial v.
Anterior tibial v.

7

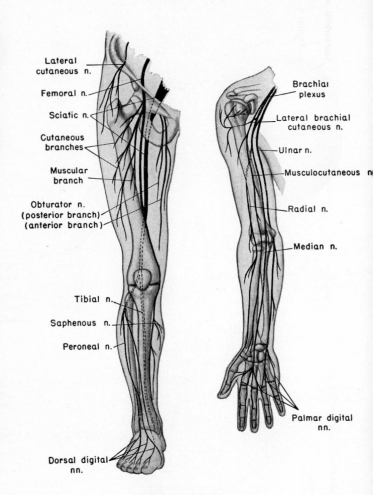

Lateral
cutaneous n.

Femoral n.

Sciatic n.

Cutaneous
branches

Muscular
branch

Obturator n.
(posterior branch)
(anterior branch)

Tibial n.

Saphenous n.

Peroneal n.

Dorsal digital
nn.

Brachial
plexus

Lateral brachial
cutaneous n.

Ulnar n.

Musculocutaneous n

Radial n.

Median n.

Palmar digital
nn.

PRINCIPAL NERVES OF
LEG AND ARM

8

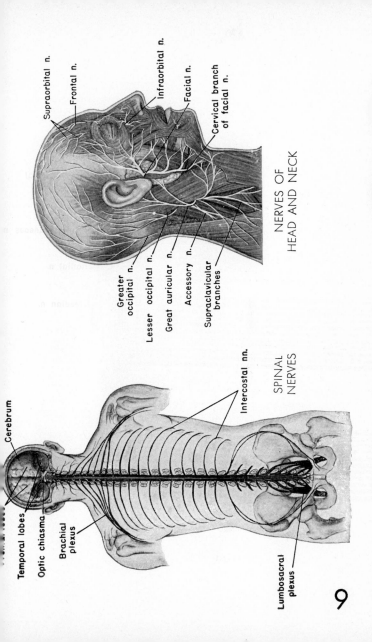

NERVES OF HEAD AND NECK

Supraorbital n.
Frontal n.
Infraorbital n.
Facial n.
Cervical branch of facial n.

Greater occipital n.
Lesser occipital n.
Great auricular n.
Accessory n.
Supraclavicular branches

SPINAL NERVES

Cerebrum
Temporal lobes
Optic chiasma
Brachial plexus
Intercostal nn.
Lumbosacral plexus

9

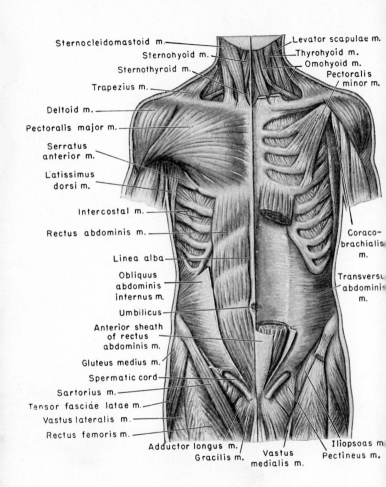

Sternocleidomastoid m.
Sternohyoid m.
Sternothyroid m.
Trapezius m.
Deltoid m.
Pectoralis major m.
Serratus anterior m.
Latissimus dorsi m.
Intercostal m.
Rectus abdominis m.
Linea alba
Obliquus abdominis internus m.
Umbilicus
Anterior sheath of rectus abdominis m.
Gluteus medius m.
Spermatic cord
Sartorius m.
Tensor fasciae latae m.
Vastus lateralis m.
Rectus femoris m.

Levator scapulae m.
Thyrohyoid m.
Omohyoid m.
Pectoralis minor m.
Coraco-brachialis m.
Transversus abdominis m.
Iliopsoas m.
Pectineus m.

Adductor longus m.
Gracilis m.
Vastus medialis m.

MUSCLES OF SHOULDER, TRUNK, AND HIP

10

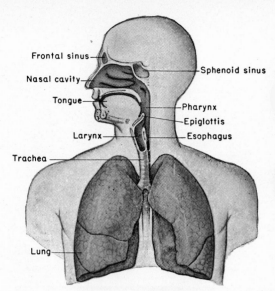

RESPIRATORY TRACT
(SCHEMATIC)

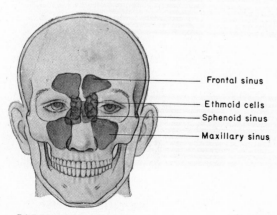

PARANASAL SINUSES
(ANTERIOR VIEW) (SCHEMATIC)

11

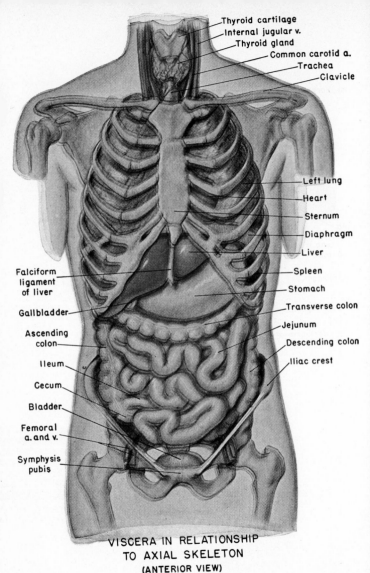

Thyroid cartilage
Internal jugular v.
Thyroid gland
Common carotid a.
Trachea
Clavicle

Left lung
Heart
Sternum
Diaphragm
Liver
Spleen
Stomach
Transverse colon
Jejunum
Descending colon
Iliac crest

Falciform ligament of liver
Gallbladder
Ascending colon
Ileum
Cecum
Bladder
Femoral a. and v.
Symphysis pubis

VISCERA IN RELATIONSHIP
TO AXIAL SKELETON
(ANTERIOR VIEW)

12

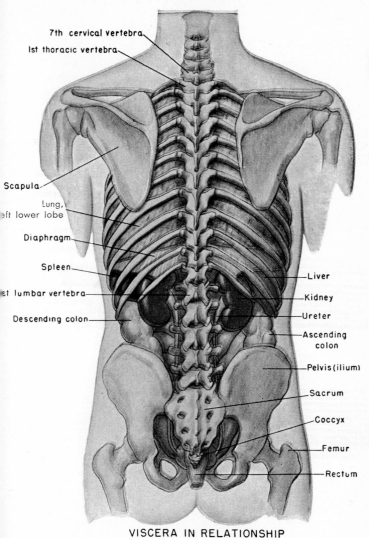

VISCERA IN RELATIONSHIP
TO AXIAL SKELETON
(POSTERIOR VIEW)

13

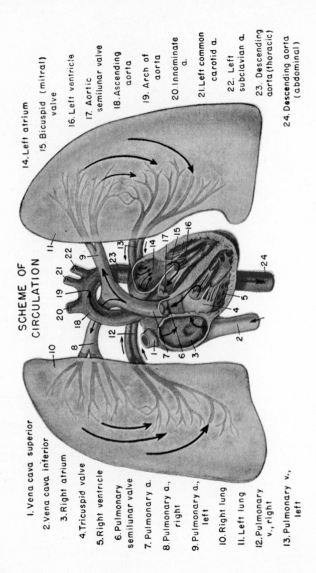

SCHEME OF CIRCULATION

1. Vena cava superior
2. Vena cava inferior
3. Right atrium
4. Tricuspid valve
5. Right ventricle
6. Pulmonary semilunar valve
7. Pulmonary a.
8. Pulmonary a., right
9. Pulmonary a., left
10. Right lung
11. Left lung
12. Pulmonary v., right
13. Pulmonary v., left
14. Left atrium
15. Bicuspid (mitral) valve
16. Left ventricle
17. Aortic semilunar valve
18. Ascending aorta
19. Arch of aorta
20. Innominate a.
21. Left common carotid a.
22. Left subclavian a.
23. Descending aorta (thoracic)
24. Descending aorta (abdominal)

14

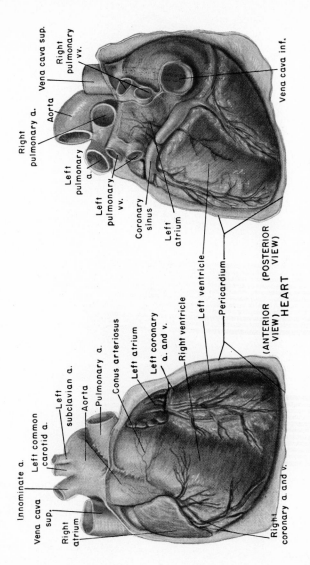

Innominate a.

Left common carotid a.

Left subclavian a.

Aorta

Pulmonary a.

Conus arteriosus

Left atrium

Left coronary a. and v.

Right ventricle

Vena cava sup.

Right atrium

Right coronary a. and v.

(ANTERIOR VIEW)

Right pulmonary a.

Aorta

Vena cava sup.

Right pulmonary vv.

Left pulmonary a.

Left pulmonary vv.

Coronary sinus

Left atrium

Left ventricle

Pericardium

Vena cava inf.

(POSTERIOR VIEW)

HEART

15

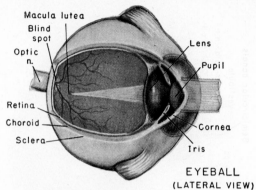

Macula lutea
Blind spot
Optic n.
Retina
Choroid
Sclera
Lens
Pupil
Cornea
Iris

EYEBALL
(LATERAL VIEW)
(A SEGMENT OF LATERAL WALL HAS BEEN
REMOVED TO SHOW STRUCTURES WITHIN)

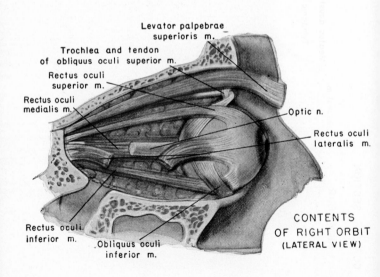

Levator palpebrae
superioris m.
Trochlea and tendon
of obliquus oculi superior m.
Rectus oculi
superior m.
Rectus oculi
medialis m.
Optic n.
Rectus oculi
lateralis m.
Rectus oculi
inferior m.
Obliquus oculi
inferior m.

**CONTENTS
OF RIGHT ORBIT**
(LATERAL VIEW)

CORONAL SECTION
OF
RIGHT EAR

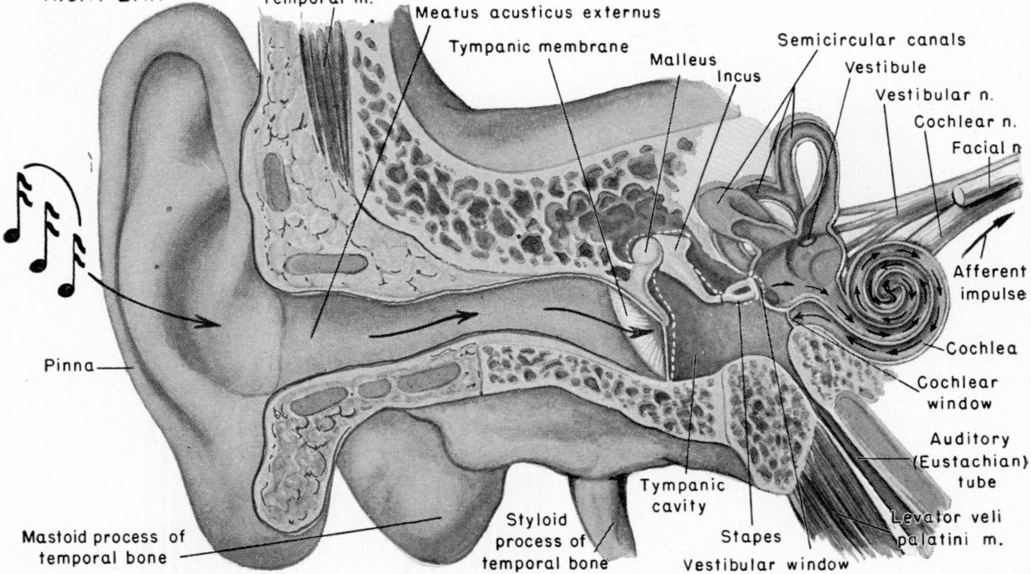

Temporal m.

Meatus acusticus externus

Tympanic membrane

Malleus

Incus

Semicircular canals

Vestibule

Vestibular n.

Cochlear n.

Facial n.

Afferent impulse

Cochlea

Cochlear window

Auditory (Eustachian) tube

Levator veli palatini m.

Vestibular window

Stapes

Tympanic cavity

Styloid process of temporal bone

Mastoid process of temporal bone

Pinna

17

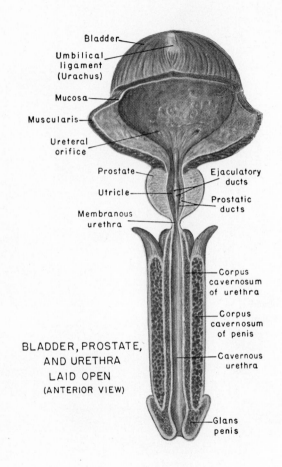

Bladder

Umbilical ligament (Urachus)

Mucosa

Muscularis

Ureteral orifice

Prostate

Utricle

Membranous urethra

Ejaculatory ducts

Prostatic ducts

Corpus cavernosum of urethra

Corpus cavernosum of penis

Cavernous urethra

Glans penis

BLADDER, PROSTATE, AND URETHRA LAID OPEN (ANTERIOR VIEW)

18

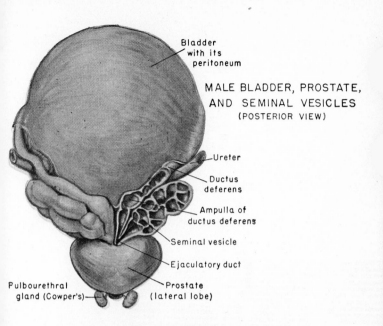

Bladder
with its
peritoneum

MALE BLADDER, PROSTATE,
AND SEMINAL VESICLES
(POSTERIOR VIEW)

Ureter

Ductus
deferens

Ampulla of
ductus deferens

Seminal vesicle

Ejaculatory duct

Pulbourethral
gland (Cowper's)

Prostate
(lateral lobe)

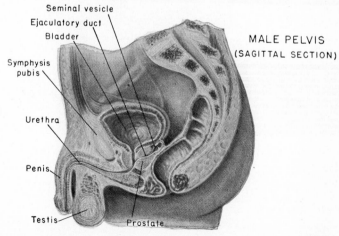

Seminal vesicle

Ejaculatory duct

Bladder

MALE PELVIS
(SAGITTAL SECTION)

Symphysis
pubis

Urethra

Penis

Testis

Prostate

19

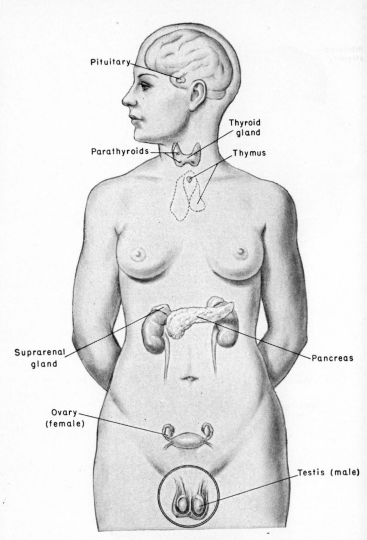

ENDOCRINE GLANDS
(SCHEMATIC)

20

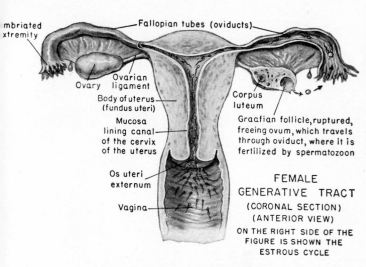

mbriated xtremity

Fallopian tubes (oviducts)

Ovarian ligament

Ovary

Body of uterus (fundus uteri)

Mucosa lining canal of the cervix of the uterus

Os uteri externum

Vagina

Corpus luteum

Graafian follicle, ruptured, freeing ovum, which travels through oviduct, where it is fertilized by spermatozoon

FEMALE GENERATIVE TRACT

(CORONAL SECTION)
(ANTERIOR VIEW)

ON THE RIGHT SIDE OF THE FIGURE IS SHOWN THE ESTROUS CYCLE

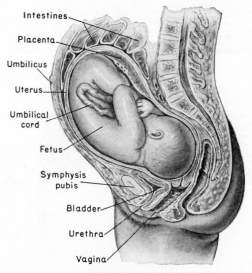

Intestines

Placenta

Umbilicus

Uterus

Umbilical cord

Fetus

Symphysis pubis

Bladder

Urethra

Vagina

PREGNANT UTERUS AT TERM

21

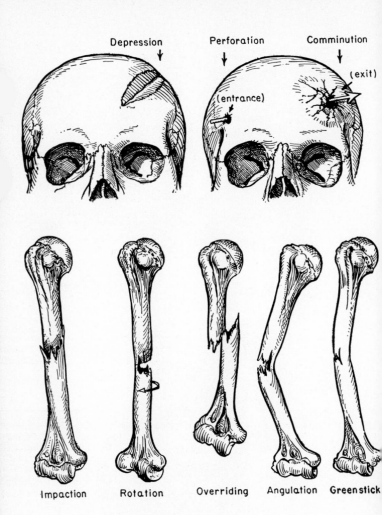

Depression   Perforation   Comminution

(exit)

(entrance)

Impaction   Rotation   Overriding   Angulation   Greenstick

TYPICAL FRACTURES

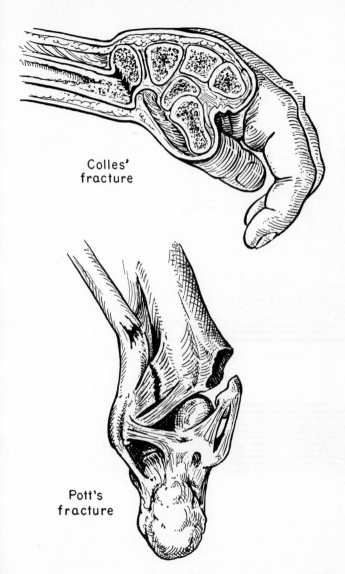

Colles'
fracture

Pott's
fracture

23

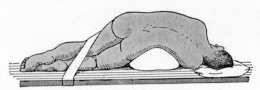

Nephrectomy position

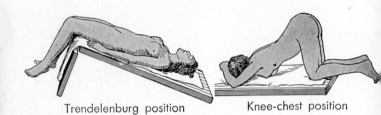

Trendelenburg position

Knee-chest position

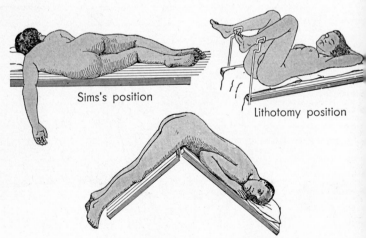

Sims's position

Lithotomy position

Reversed Trendelenburg position

OPERATIVE POSITIONS

24

on″y·cho·stro′ma. The matrix or bed of the nail.

on″y·chot″il·lo·ma′ni·a (on″i-cot″i·lo·may′nee·uh). The neurotic picking at a nail until it is permanently altered.

on″y·chot′o·my (on″i·cot′o·mee). Surgical incision into a fingernail or toenail.

on′yx (on′icks). 1. A nail of the fingers or toes. 2. A collection of pus between the corneal lamellas at the most dependent part.

o′ö- (o′o-). A combining form meaning *an egg.*

o′ö·cyst. The encysted zygote in the life history of some sporozoa. See *oökinete.*

o′ö·cyte. An egg cell before the completion of the maturation process. Its full history includes its origin from an oögonium, a growth period, and the final miotic divisions.

o″ö·gen′e·sis. The process of the origin, growth, and formation of the ovum in its preparation for fertilization. **—oögenet′ic,** *adj.*

o″ö·go′ni·um. A cell in an ovarian follicle which, by division, gives rise to oöcytes.

o″ö·ki·ne′te (o″o·ki·neet′, -kin′eet, o′o·kin·eet). The elongated, motile zygote in the life history of some sporozoan parasites; as that of the malarial parasite as it bores through the epithelial lining of the mosquito's intestine, in the wall of which it becomes an oöcyst. **—oökinet′ic,** *adj.*

o″ö·pho·rec′to·my (o″o·fo·reck′to·mee, o·off″o-). Excision of an ovary.

o″ö·pho·ri′tis. Inflammation of an ovary.

o·öph′o·ro-, oöphor-. A combining form denoting *an ovary* or *ovarian.*

o·öph″o·ro·cys·tec′to·my. Removal of an ovarian cyst.

o·öph″o·ro·cys·to′sis. The formation of ovarian cysts.

o·öph″o·ro·hys″ter·ec′to·my. Removal of the uterus and ovaries.

o·öph″o·ro·path′i·a. Any disease of the ovary.

o·öph′o·ro·pex″y. Surgical fixation of an ovary in a new position.

o·öph″o·ro·sal″pin·gec′to·my. Excision of an ovary and oviduct.

o·öph″o·ro·sal″pin·gi′tis. Inflammation of an ovary and oviduct.

o″ö·phor′rha·phy. Operation of suturing an ovary to the pelvic wall.

o″ö·por′phy·rin. A porphyrin occurring in the pigment from the eggshells of certain birds.

o·ös′po·ra. A genus of fungi which reproduce by mycelial fragmentation. **O. madurae.** Synonym for *Nocardia madurae.* **O. minutissima.** Synonym for *Nocardia minutissima.*

o″ö·the′co-. For words beginning with *oötheco-,* see under *ovario-* or *oöphoro-.*

o·pac′i·ty (o·pas′i·tee). 1. The condition of being impervious to light. 2. An opaque spot, as opacity of the cornea or lens.

o″pal·es′cent. Showing a play of colors; reflecting light; iridescent.

o·paque′. Dark; obscure; not transparent; impervious to light.

o·pei′do·scope (o·pye′do·scope). An instrument for studying the vibrations of the voice.

o′pen. 1. Exposed to the air, as an open wound. 2. Interrupted, as an open circuit, one through which an electric current cannot pass.

o′pen·ing. An orifice; a hole or gap.

op″er·a·bil′i·ty. Possessing the qualities or being in a state which will permit surgical operation without the expectation of a fatal result.

op′er·a·ble. Admitting of an operation; referring to a condition where operation is not contraindicated.

op″er·a′tion. 1. Anything done or performed, especially with instruments; a surgical procedure by a surgeon in which the method follows a definite routine. 2. The mode of action of anything; the specific action of a drug. **ablative o.** One in which a part is removed. **anastomotic o.** One where two hollow organs, vessels, or ducts are joined by suture so that their contents may flow from one to the other. **bloodless o.** One performed with little or no loss of blood. **capital o.** One which may threaten life; a grave or serious operation. **compensating o.** *In* ophthalmology, tenotomy of the associated antagonist in cases of diplopia from paresis of one of the ocular muscles. **cosmetic o.** A surgical operation to improve the appearance of a defective or unsightly part. **crescent o.** For lacerated perineum, involving the vaginal entrance only; a crescent-shaped denudation is made from the vulvovaginal entrance, the angles of which extend into the vulvovaginal sulci. **elective o.** One in which the time for operation may be set in advance, as a tonsillectomy. **emergency o.** One which must be done at once to save the patient from an extension of the disease or from death. **exploratory o.** One performed for the purpose of diagnosis, often an abdominal operation. **fenestration o.** *In* otology, the establishment of a window in the horizontal semicircular canal, for the treatment of otosclerosis. **high o.** The application of forceps to the fetal head at the superior strait. **interval o.** One done between acute attacks of a disease, as an interval appendectomy. **major o.** A capital operation. **minor o.** An operation which does not threaten life; one in which there is little or no danger. **palliative o.** One designed to make the patient more comfortable when the condition cannot be cured. **plastic o.** A reconstructive operation. **prophylactic forceps o.** The routine delivery by forceps in head presentations as soon as the head has come to rest on the pelvic floor. **radical o.** One which seeks to extirpate or remove the causative factor of the disease or condition. **reconstructive o.** One done to repair a defect, either congenital or acquired. **shelf o.** An arthroplastic procedure in the open reduction of a congenitally displaced hip, in which a bony shelf is inserted, by bone grafting, into the upper portion of the acetabulum so as to hold the femoral head and prevent its slipping out of the shallow joint cup.

op'er·a"tor. 1. A surgeon. 2. One who gives treatments, especially those involving mechanotherapy. 3. An expert technician, as in roentgenology.

o·phid"i·o·pho'bi·a. Morbid fear of snakes.

o'phid·ism. Poisoning from snake venom.

oph'i·o'sis. Circumscribed baldness with scaliness.

oph·ry·i'tis. Inflammation of the eyebrow.

oph·ry·o'sis. Spasm of the eyebrow.

oph"ryph·thei·ri'a·sis (off"rif-thigh-rye'uh·sis). Pediculosis of the eyebrows and eyelashes.

ophthaine. Trade-mark for proparacaine hydrochloride.

oph·thal"ma·cro'sis. Enlargement of the eyeball.

oph"thal·ma'gra (off"thal·may'gruh, ·mag'ruh). Painful ophthalmic symptoms attributable to an attack of gout.

oph"thal·mal'gi·a. Neuralgia of the eye.

oph"thal·mec"chy·mo'sis (off"-thal·meck"i·mo'sis). An effusion of blood into the conjunctiva.

oph"thal·mec'to·my. Excision, or enucleation, of an eye.

oph·thal'mi·a. Inflammation of the eye, especially one in which the conjunctiva is involved. **catarrhal o.** Simple conjunctivitis; a hyperemia of the conjunctiva with a mucopurulent secretion. **caterpillar hair o.** Inflammation of the conjunctiva or of the cornea, the result of penetration of the tissues by caterpillar hairs. Syn., o. nodosa. **gonorrheal o.** An acute and severe form of purulent conjunctivitis, caused by infection by the *Neisseria gonorrhoeae*. Syn., *gonorrheal conjunc-*

tivitis. **granular o.** See *trachoma*. **o. electrica.** Conjunctivitis due to intense electric light. **o. neonatorum.** A gonorrheal or purulent ophthalmia of the newborn. Also called *acute infectious conjunctivitis*. **phlyctenular o.** Conjunctivitis characterized by phlyctenules or small vesicles situated in the epithelial layer of the conjunctiva or cornea; a manifestation of childhood tuberculosis. **purulent o.** Conjunctivitis with a purulent discharge. **sympathetic o.** A severe destructive inflammation, a form of iridocyclitis secondary to injury or disease of the fellow eye. **varicose o.** That associated with a varicose state of the veins of the conjunctiva.

oph·thal'mic. Pertaining to the eye.

oph"thal·mi'tis. Inflammation of the eye. **—ophthalmit'ic,** *adj.* **sympathetic o.** That following injury of the fellow eye.

oph·thal'mo-, ophthalm-. A combining form meaning *eye*.

oph·thal"mo·blen"nor·rhe'a. Blennorrhea of the conjunctiva.

oph·thal"mo·cen·te'sis. Surgical puncture of the eye.

oph·thal"mo·co'pi·a. Fatigue of visual power; asthenopia.

oph·thal"mo·dyn'i·a (off·thal"mo·din'ee·uh, ·dye'nee·uh). Neuralgic pain referred to the eye.

oph"thal·mog'ra·phy. Descriptive anatomy of the eye.

oph·thal"mo·gy'ric. Pertaining to or causing, movements of the eye.

oph·thal"mo·lith". A calculus of the eye or lacrimal duct.

oph"thal·mol'o·gist. One skilled or specializing in ophthalmology.

oph"thal·mol'o·gy. The science of the anatomy, physiology, and disease of the eye. **—ophthalmolog'ic,** *adj.*

oph·thal"mo·ma·cro'sis. Enlargement of the eye.

oph·thal"mo·ma·la'ci·a (off·thal"mo·ma·lay'shee·uh, ·see·uh). Abnormal softness or subnormal tension of the eye.

oph·thal"mo·mel"a·no'ma. A melanotic tumor, usually sarcoma, of the eye.

oph·thal·mom'e·ter. 1. An instrument for measuring refractive error, especially astigmatism. 2. An instrument for measuring the capacity of the chambers of the eye. 3. An instrument for measuring the eye as a whole.

oph·thal"mo·my·co'sis (off·thal"mo·migh·ko'sis). Any disease of the eye or its appendages due to the presence of a fungus.

oph·thal"mo·my'i·a·sis (·migh·yuh·sis, ·migh·eye'uh·sis). The invasion of the eye by the larvae of flies.

oph·thal"mo·my·i'tis (·migh·eye-tis). Inflammation of the ocular muscles.

oph·thal″mo·my·ot′o·my (ofthal″mo-migh-ot′o-mee). Division of a muscle or muscles of the eye.

oph·thal″mo·neu·ri′tis. Inflammation of the ophthalmic nerve.

oph″thal·mop′a·thy. Any disease of the eye. **external o.** An affection of the eyelids, cornea, conjunctiva, or muscles of the eye. **internal o.** Any disease affecting the eyeball proper.

oph·thal″mo·phth′i·sis (off″thalmof′thi·sis, off·thal″mo·tye′sis). Shrinking of the eyeball.

oph·thal″mo·phy′ma. Swelling of the eyeball.

oph·thal″mo·plas″ty. Plastic surgery of the eye or accessory parts. —**ophthalmoplas′tic,** adj.

oph·thal″mo·ple′gi·a. Paralysis of the ocular muscles. —**ophthalmo-pleg′ic,** adj. **o. externa.** Paralysis of the extrinsic ocular muscles. **o. interna.** Paralysis of the intrinsic muscles of the eye—those of the iris and ciliary body. **progressive o.** A form in which all of the muscles of both eyes gradually become paralyzed. **total o.** That form involving the intrinsic muscles, as well as the extrinsic muscles, of the eyeball.

oph·thal″mop·to′sis. Protrusion of the eyeball; exophthalmos.

oph·thal″mor·rha′gi·a. Hemorrhage from the eye.

oph·thal″mor·rhe′a. A watery or sanguineous discharge from the eye.

oph·thal″mor·rhex′is. Rupture of the eyeball.

oph·thal″mo·scope. An instrument for examining the interior of the eye. It consists essentially of a mirror with a hole in it, through which the observer looks, the interior of the eye being illuminated by light reflected from the mirror into the eye and seen by means of the rays reflected from the eye ground back through the hole in the mirror. The ophthalmoscope is fitted with lenses of different powers that may be revolved in front of the observing eye, and these neutralize the ametropia of either the patient's or the observer's eye, thus rendering clear the details of the fundus oculi. Many ophthalmoscopes now in use are of the portable type and are fitted with a battery in the handle so that bedside examinations may be made. —**ophthalmoscop′ic,** adj. **stereo-o.** An ophthalmoscope with two eyepieces.

oph″thal·mos′co·py. The examination of the interior of the eye by means of an ophthalmoscope. **direct o.** The method of the erect or upright image, the observer's eye and the ophthalmoscope being brought close to the eye of the patient. **indirect o.** The method of the inverted image; the observer's eye is placed about 16 inches from that of the patient, and a 20 D. biconvex lens is held about two inches in front of the observed eye, thereby forming an aerial inverted image of the fundus.

oph·thal″mo·spasm. Ocular spasm.

oph·thal″mo·spin′ther·ism. A condition of the eye in which there is a visual impression of luminous sparks.

oph″thal·mos′ta·sis. Fixation of the eye during an operation upon it.

oph·thal″mo·ste·re′sis. Loss or absence of one or both eyes.

oph·thal″mo·syn′chy·sis (offthal″mo-sin′ki·sis). Effusion into the interior chambers of the eye.

oph″thal·mot′o·my. The dissection or incision of the eye.

oph·thal″mo·vas′cu·lar. Pertaining to the blood vessels of the eye.

oph·thal′mu·la. A scar of the eye.

-o′pi·a, -o′py. A combining form denoting a defect of the eye.

o″pi·an′ic ac′id. An acid, $C_{10}H_{10}O_5$, obtained from narcotine.

o″pi·an′ine (o″pee-an′een, -in). Old term for narcotine.

o′pi·ate. A preparation of opium; a substance that brings on rest or inaction; that which quiets uneasiness or dulls the feelings.

o″pi·o·ma′ni·a. A morbid desire for opium; opium habit. —**opiomaniac,** n.

o″pi·o·pha′gi·a, o″pi·oph′a·gism, o″pi·oph′a·gy. The eating of opium.

o′pi·o·phile. An addict, or eater, of opium; an opium smoker.

op″is·thog′na·thism (op″iss-thog′nuh-thiz·um, ·thohn/uh·thiz·um). Recession of the lower jaw.

o·pis″tho·po·rei′a (o·pisth″o-po-rye′uh). Involuntary walking backward in an attempt to go forward; occurs in Parkinsonism.

Op″is·thor′chis (op″iss·thor′kis, o″pis·). A genus of trematodes or flukes. **O. felineus.** A species naturally parasitic in cats, dogs, foxes, and hogs, and accidentally in man. Produces hepatic lesions and extensive hyperplasia of the bile ducts.

op″is·thot′o·nos (op″iss-thot′o·nos, o″pis·). A condition in which, from a tetanic spasm of the muscles of the back, the head and lower limbs are bent backward and the trunk is arched forward. —**opisthoton′ic, opisthot-onoid,** adj.

o′pi·um. The air-dried juice from unripe capsules of Papaver somniferum, or its variety album. It contains a number of alkaloids, of which morphine is the most important. **camphorated o. tincture.** Contains opium, anise oil, benzoic acid, and camphor. Syn., *paregoric.* **compound o. and glycyrrhiza mixture.** Contains camphorated opium tincture, glycyrrhiza fluidextract, antimony potassium tartrate, ethyl nitrite spirit, glycerin, and water. Also called *brown mixture, compound glycyrrhiza mixture.* **granulated o.** A coarse powder containing from 10–10.5% of anhydrous morphine. **ipecac and o. powder.** Contains 10% each of ipecac and opium. Syn., *Dover's powder.* **o. extract.** Prepared by maceration or percolation with hot water, contains 20% of anhydrous morphine. **o. tincture.** Contains 1% of anhydrous morphine. Also called *laudanum, deodorized opium tincture.* **powdered o.** Contains 10–10.5% of anhydrous morphine.

o'pi·um hab'it. The habitual use of opium or its derivatives.

op'o-. In pharmacology, a combining form meaning *juice.*

op"o·ceph'a·lus. A monster characterized by fusion of the ears, one orbit, and absence of mouth and nose.

op"o·del'doc. A soap liniment. **liquid o.** Camphor and soap liniment. **solid o.** Solid soap liniment. Also called *camphorated soap liniment.*

op"pi·la'tion. 1. Obstruction; a closing of the pores; that which causes constipation. 2. A constipating agent or remedy. *Obs.*

op·po'nens (o·po'nenz). Opposing; applied to certain muscles that bring one part opposite another, as opponens pollicis, a muscle placing the thumb opposite the little finger. See Table of Muscles in the Appendix.

-ops. In botany and zoology, a combining form meaning *-eyed.*

-op'si·a, -op'sy. A combining form denoting a *condition of vision.*

op·sig'e·nes (op·sidj'i·neez). Born late, referring to certain body tissues which come into use long after birth, as the wisdom teeth.

op"si·o·no'sis (op"see·o·no'sis, -on'o·sis). Disease of the eye, or of vision.

op"so·ma'ni·a. Intense craving for dainties or some special food. **—opsomaniac,** *n.*

op'so·nin, op·so'nin. A substance occurring in blood serum which is necessary to prepare bacteria for phagocytosis. It occurs normally and may be increased by immunization. **—opson'ic,** *adj.* **immune o.** A thermolabile opsonin in the serum resulting from infection or inoculation with dead bacteria of the same species. It is active only against the microörganism that stimulated its formation. See *bacteriotropin.*

op·son"o·ther'a·py. The treatment

of disease by increasing the opsonic power of the blood.

op"tes·the'si·a (op"tess·thee'zhuh, ·zee·uh). Visual sensibility.

op'tic. Pertaining to the eye.

op'ti·cal. 1. A synonym for optic, *q.v.* 2. Pertaining to light and the science of optics.

op'ti·cal flat. A glass or quartz plate or disk, ground flat until any remaining unevenness can be measured only by interferometric methods.

op'ti·cal glass. An especially fine glass made under the most carefully controlled conditions. There are many kinds, some with low index and high dispersion values and some with high index and low dispersion.

op·ti'cian. A maker of optical instruments or lenses. **dispensing o.** One who retails spectacles and ophthalmic lenses.

op"ti·co·cil'i·ar"y. Pertaining to the optic and ciliary nerves.

op"ti·co·pu'pil·lar"y. Pertaining to the optic nerve and the pupil.

op'tics. That branch of physics treating of the laws of light, its refraction and reflection, and of its relation to vision. **electron o.** A method of controlling electron beams by means of properly adjusted electric and magnetic fields, the electron beams thus behaving like rays of light in optical instruments. Also see electron *microscope.*

op'ti·mum. The temperature or other conditions at which vital processes are carried on with the greatest activity. Between the minimum and maximum temperatures or other conditions. **—optimal,** *adj.*

op'to-. A combining form denoting *vision* or *optic.*

optochin. Trade-mark for ethylhydrocupreine, a potent pneumococcide.

op·tom'e·ter. An instrument for determining the strength of vision, especially the degree of refractive error that is to be corrected.

op·tom'e·trist. One who measures the degrees of visual powers, usually without the aid of a cycloplegic or mydriatic; a refractionist.

op·tom'e·try. Measurement of the visual powers.

op"to·my·om'e·ter (op"to·mighom'i·tur). An instrument for measuring the strength of the extrinsic muscles of the eye.

op'to·type. A test type used in testing the acuity of vision.

o'ra. Margin. **o. serrata.** The serrated margin of the sensory portion of the retina, behind the ciliary body.

o'ral. Pertaining to the mouth.

o'ral char'ac·ter. A Freudian term applied to persons who, during the developmental period, have undergone an unusual degree of oral stimulation through poor feeding habits and otherwise and who thereby have laid the basis for a particular type of character, usually characterized by a general attitude of carefree indifference and by dependence on a mother or mother substitute to provide for their needs throughout life with little or no effort of their own.

r'ange G (C.C.). An acid monoazo dye; used as a counterstain with nuclear stains.

r'ange II (C.C.). An acid monoazo dye; used in histologic staining.

ranixon. A trade-mark for mephensin, *q.v.*

r·bic'u·lar. Circular; applied to circular muscles, as the orbicular muscle of the eye (orbicularis oculi) or of the mouth (orbicularis oris).

r'bit. The bony cavity containing the eye, which is formed by the frontal, sphenoid, ethmoid, nasal, lacrimal, maxillary, and palatal bones. —**or'bital,** *adj.*

r"bi·ton·om'e·ter. A device used to measure the repressibility of the eye into the orbit in cases of exophthalmic goiter.

r"bi·tot'o·my. Incision into the orbit.

r'ce·in, or·ce'in (C.C.). $C_{28}H_{24}N_2O_7$. Brownish red, crystalline powder synthesized from orcin; insoluble in water, soluble in alcohol. Used in microscopy as a stain.

r·ches"tro·ma'ni·a (or·kes"tro-may'nee-uh). Dancing mania; chorea, or St. Vitus' dance.

r'chi- (or'ki-). See orchio-.

r'chic (or'kick). Pertaining to the testis.

:"chi·dop'a·thy. Disease of a testis.

··chid'o·plas"ty. Orchioplasty; plastic surgery of a testis.

r"chi·dot'o·my. Incision into a testis.

r"chi·ec'to·my. Surgical removal of one or both testes; castration.

r"chi·ep"i·did'y·mi'tis. Inflammation of both testis and epididymis.

r'chi·o- (or'kee·o-), **or'chi-.** A combining form meaning *testis*.

r"chi·o·ca·tab'a·sis. The normal descent of the testes into the scrotum.

r'chi·o·cele. *In surgery,* a term sometimes used to denote a complete scrotal hernia.

r"chi·op'a·thy. Any disease of the testis.

r'chi·o·pex"y (or'kee·o·peck"see, r'kee·o·peck'see). Surgical fixation of testis, as in a plastic operation for relief of an undescended testis.

r'chi·o·plas"ty. Any plastic operation on a testis.

or·chi'tis (or·kigh'tis). Inflammation of the testis. —**orchit'ic,** *adj.*

or'cin (or'sin), **or'cin·ol.** 3,5-Dihydroxytoluene. White crystals, reddened by exposure to air, freely soluble in water, ether, or alcohol. Prepared from many species of lichens. A reagent.

or'der. 1. Systematic arrangement. 2. *In biology,* the taxonomic group below a class and above a family.

or'der·ly. A male hospital attendant.

or'di·nate. The vertical line of the two coördinates used in plotting the interrelationship of two sets of data. The horizontal one is called the abscissa.

oreton. Trade-mark for testosterone propionate.

oreton-F. Trade-mark for testosterone.

oreton-M. Trade-mark for methyltestosterone.

or'gan. A differentiated part of an organism adapted for a definite function. **sex organs.** Those pertaining entirely to the sex of the individual; in the male, the external generative organs, the penis and testes, and the internal, the prostate, deferential ducts, and seminal vesicles; in the female, the external generative organs, the vulva, vagina, and clitoris, and the internal, the uterus, uterine tubes, and ovaries. In woman the breasts are considered as secondary sex organs.

or·gan'ic. 1. Having, pertaining to, or characterized by organs; pertaining to living substances; affecting the structure of organs. 2. *In chemistry,* of or pertaining to compounds of carbon.

or'gan·ism. Any living thing, plant or animal, having regard especially to the fact that it consists of differentiated parts with specialized functions, so related to one another as to form a unified whole.

or"gan·i·za'tion. 1. The systematic interrelationships of the structurally and functionally differentiated parts to form an integrated whole. 2. The process of repair in wounds; especially, the changes occurring in the blood clot.

or'gan·i"zer. Spemann's term for the region of the dorsal lip of the blastopore, comprising chordamesoderm, that is self-differentiating and capable of inducing the formation of medullary plate in the adjacent ectoderm. Also, any living part of the embryo exerting a morphogenetic stimulus on an adjacent part or parts. Also called *organizator, organization center.*

or'ga·no-. 1. A combining form meaning *organ.* 2. *In chemistry,* a combining form signifying *organic.*

or·gan'o·gel. A hydrogel in which

the dispersion medium is an organic liquid instead of water.

or″ga·nol′o·gy. The science that treats of the organs of plants and animals.

or″ga·nos′co·py. The examination of an organ with a special lens system, such as a cystoscope, esophagoscope, or laryngoscope.

or″ga·no·ther′a·py. The treatment of diseases by means of animal organs or their extracts. —**organothera-peu′tic,** *adj.*

or″ga·no·troph′ic (or ″guh·no-trof′ick, ·tro′fick). Relating to the nutrition of living organs.

or″ga·no·trop′ic. 1. Pertaining to substances which act on the organs of the body. 2. Having affinity for the tissues. —**organot′ropism, organot′ropy,** *n.*

er′gasm (or′gaz·um). Intense excitement, especially that occurring during sexual intercourse; the culmination or climax of the sexual act, followed by ejaculation of the seminal fluid or, in the female, by relaxation and detumescence. —**orgas′tic,** *adj.*

o″ri·en′tal sore. A form of cutaneous leishmaniasis caused by infection with *Leishmania tropica* and transmitted by some species of *Phlebotomus.* It is characterized by ulcerated granulomatous lesions of the skin which lead to hypertrophy of the stratum corneum and hypertrophy and proliferation of the papillae. Necrosis and ulceration occur as well as secondary infections with bacteria. Syn., *Delhi boil, Aleppo boil, tropical sore, Biskra button, Bagdad boil, Kandahar sore, Delhi sore, Tashkend ulcer.*

o″ri·en·ta′tion. 1. The act of determining one's relation to time (**temporal orientation**) to space (**spatial orientation**), or one's relation to other individuals (**personal orientation**). Sometimes referred to as subjective and objective orientation. 2. The relative position of the substitution elements or radicals in the benzene ring.

or′i·fice. An opening, an entrance to a cavity or tube. —**orif′icial,** *adj.*

or′i·gin. The beginning or starting point of anything. **o. of a muscle.** The end of attachment of a muscle which remains relatively fixed during contraction of the muscle.

orinase. Trade-mark for tolbutamide.

or′ni·thine (or′ni·theen, ·thin). NH₂.(CH₂)₂.CHNH₂.COOH. α,δ-Diaminovaleric acid.

or′o-. See orrho-.

o′ro-. A combining form meaning *mouth* or *oral.*

o″ro·phar′ynx. The oral pharynx, situated below the level of the lower

border of the soft palate and above the larynx, as distinguished from the naso-pharynx and laryngopharynx. —**oro-pharyn′geal,** *adj.*

or′phan. Any one of a number of intestinal viruses, now known as ECHO virus.

or·phen′a·drine hy″dro·chlo′-ride. N,N-Dimethyl-2-(o-methyl-α-phenylbenzyloxy)ethylamine hydrochloride, a parasympatholytic agent. See disipal.

or′phol. Bismuth betanaphthol.

or′pi·ment. Native arsenic trisulfid.

or′rho-, or′o-. A combining form meaning *serum.*

or″rho·men″in·gi′tis. Inflammation of a serous membrane. *Obs.*

or′ris. The peeled and dried rhizome of *Iris germanica florentina* or *Iris pallida.* **o. root.** A powder from certain varieties of iris; used in various cosmetics, toothpastes, etc.

ortal sodium. Trade-mark for a brand of sodium n-hexyl-ethyl barbiturate, used as a short-acting sedative and hypnotic. See *hexetal sodium.*

or′tho-, orth-. 1. A combining form denoting *straight, normal,* or *true.* In *chemistry,* a prefix indicating the neighboring or 1,2 positions on the benzene ring. Symbol, *o-.* See *meta-, para-.*

or″tho·caine. British Pharmacopoeia title for the methyl ester of m-amino-p-hydroxybenzoic acid, HO.C₆H₃(NH₂)COOCH₃, a local anesthetic. See ortho-form.

or″tho·chlo″ro·phe′nol. C₆H₄Cl·OH. A compound of high germicidal activity and high toxicity.

or″tho·cho·re′a (orth″o·ko·ree′uh). Choreic movements in the erect posture.

or″tho·chro·mat′ic. A term originally used in photography to denote correctness in the rendering of color; orthochromatic emulsions are not sensitive to red, and may be developed under a red safe light.

or″tho·cre′sol. CH₃.C₆H₄.OH. One of the isomers of cresol, *q.v.* It has the weakest germicidal activity of the three isomers.

or″tho·dac′ty·lous. Having straight digits.

er″tho·di′a·gram. A tracing of the outer contours and exact size of an organ, usually the heart; made by illuminating the edge of the organ with parallel x-rays through a small, movable aperture and marking the outer edge of the shadow cast upon a fluoroscopic screen.

or″tho·di·ag′ra·phy. Determining by the aid of roentgen rays the exact dimensions of an internal organ, especially the heart, by the shadow which it throws upon the fluorescent screen.

or″tho·don′tics. The branch

dentistry concerned with the treatment of malocclusion.

or'tho·dont'ist. A practitioner of orthodontics.

orthoform. A trade-mark for methyl m-amino-p-hydroxybenzoic acid. See orthocaine.

or'tho·grade. Walking or standing in the upright position.

or·thom'e·ter. An instrument for measuring the relative degree of protrusion of the eyes. Also called exophthalmometer.

or'tho·pe'dics. That branch of surgery concerned with corrective treatment of deformities, diseases, and ailments of the locomotor apparatus, especially those affecting limbs, bones, muscles, joints, and fasciae, whether by apparatus, manipulation, or open operation. Formerly devoted to the correction and treatment of deformities in children.

or'tho·pe'dist. One who practices orthopedic surgery; a specialist in orthopedics.

or'tho·phe·nan'thro·line (-fi-nan'thro-leen, -lin). $C_{12}H_8N_2.H_2O$. A white, crystalline powder which forms a complex with ferrous ions and is used as an indicator.

r'thop·ne'a. A condition in which there is need to sit up to breathe more easily. It usually indicates cardiac dyspnea, and is often lacking in other kinds of dyspnea. **—orthopneic,** adj.

c'tho·prax'is. Correction of the deformities of the body.

r'tho·psy·chi'a·try (orth"o-sigh-kigh'uh-tree). A subdivision of psychiatry primarily concerned with the prevention and treatment of behavior disorders. Mental hygiene and preventive methods are the main interests of orthopsychiatry.

r·thop'tics. The science of rendering visual reactions and responses right and efficient, usually by some form of exercise or training. These measures include the treatment of amblyopia, the education of stereopsis, and the treatment of muscle imbalances and strabismus.

r·thop'to·scope. An instrument used in orthoptic training.

r'tho·scope. 1. An instrument for examination of the eye through a layer of water, whereby the curvature, and hence the refraction, of the cornea is neutralized, and the cornea acts as a plane medium. 2. An instrument for use in drawing the projections of skulls.

r·tho'sis. The straightening of a deformity. **—orthot'ic,** adj.

r'tho·stat'ic. Pertaining to, or caused by, standing upright, as orthostatic albuminuria, which occurs when the patient stands on his feet or exer-

cises for long periods of time, but which disappears after a period of rest in bed.

or'tho·tast. A device for straightening curvatures of long bones. It has also been used as a tourniquet.

or"tho·ter'i·on (orth"o-teer'ee-on). An apparatus for straightening curved limbs.

or·thot'o·nus. Tetanic cramp in which the body lies rigid and straight.

orthoxine. Trade-mark for beta-(ortho-methoxyphenyl) isopropyl-methylamine, a sympathomimetic amine available as the hydrochloride salt. See methoxyphenamine.

o·ryx'a·min. Thiamine hydrochloride.

or'y·zen'in. A glutelin from rice.

O. S. Oculus sinister, left eye.

Os. Chemical symbol for osmium.

os (pl. ora). A mouth. **o. uteri externum.** The external opening of the cervix of the uterus. Also called o. uteri. **o. uteri internum.** The opening at the junction of the cervix and body of the uterus.

os (pl. ossa). A bone. **o. calcis.** Old term for calcaneus, the bone of the heel. **o. magnum.** Old term for the capitate, the third bone of the second row of the carpus.

o'sa·zone (o'suh-zone, o"suh-zone'). A compound formed by reaction of a sugar with phenylhydrazine.

os'che·o- (oss'kee-o-), **os'che-.** A combining form meaning the scrotum.

os"cil·la'tion. A swinging or vibration; also any tremulous motion.

os·cil·la'tor. A vibratory apparatus used in mechanical therapeutics.

os'cil·lo·graph". An apparatus for recording oscillations. **—oscillographic,** adj. **cathode ray o.** An instrument in which a pencil of electrons, striking a fluorescent screen, will trace a graph of any two variables that have been converted into electric equivalents.

os'cil·lom'e·ter. An instrument for measuring oscillations, as those seen in taking blood pressures. **—oscillometric,** adj.

os"cil·lom'e·try. Measurement or detection of oscillations of any type, especially circulatory, usually by means of a string galvanometer.

os"cil·lop'si·a. Oscillating nystagmus of disseminated sclerosis, usually occurring only during walking.

os·cil'lo·scope. A vacuum tube so constructed as to portray the deflections or oscillations of electromotive forces. Also called cathode ray o.

os"cu·la'tion. 1. The union of vessels by their mouths. 2. Kissing.

os'cu·lum. A small aperture.

-ose. 1. A suffix denoting carbohydrate.

2. A suffix denoting a *substance derived by hydrolysis of a protein.*

-o′sis. 1. A suffix signifying a *condition* or *state;* used in pathology to denote a diseased condition. 2. A suffix denoting a *disease caused by a fungus.*

os′mate (oz′mate, os′mate). A salt of osmic acid.

os·mat′ic (os·mat′ick, oz·mat′ick). Characterized by a keen sense of smell.

os″mes·the′si·a (oz″mess-thee′-zhuh, os″mess·). Olfactory sensibility.

os′mic ac′id (oz′mick, os′mick). OsO_4. A crystalline substance employed as a histologic stain and reagent.

os′mics (oz′micks). The science of smell.

os″mi·dro′sis (oz″mi·dro′sis, os″·mi·). The secretion of a malodorous perspiration; bromhidrosis.

os′mi·um (oz′mee·um, os′·). Os = 190.2. A heavy metallic element belonging to the platinum group.

os′mo-. A combining form meaning 1. *smell, odor;* 2. *osmosis.*

os″mo·dys·pho′ri·a. Intolerance of certain odors.

os·mol′o·gy (os·mol′o·jee, oz·). The science of odors and the sense of smell.

os·mol′o·gy. That part of physical science treating of osmosis.

os·mom′e·ter (os·mom′i·tur, oz·). 1. An instrument for testing the sense of smell; an olfactometer. 2. An apparatus for measuring osmosis, *q.v.*

os″mo·pho′bi·a. A morbid fear of odors.

os″mo·reg″u·lar′i·ty. Affecting or regulating the extent and rate of osmosis.

os·mo′sis (os·mo′sis, oz·). The passage of a solvent through a membrane from a dilute solution into a more concentrated one. **—osmot′ic,** *adj.*

os′sa. Plural of os (meaning "bone").

os′se·in, os′se·ine (oss′ee·in). 1. Collagen. 2. The organic framework of osseous tissue.

os′se·ine. See ossein.

os″se·o·car″ti·lag′i·nous (oss″·ee·o·kahr″ti·ladj′i·nus). Pertaining to or composed of both bone and cartilage.

os″se·o·mu′coid. A mucin or glycoprotein obtained from bone.

os′se·ous. Bony; composed of or resembling bone.

os′si·cle. A small bone; particularly, one of three small bones in the tympanic cavity: the malleus, incus, and stapes.

os″si·cu·lec′to·my. The removal of one or more of the ossicles of the middle ear.

os″si·cu·lot′o·my. Surgical incision involving the tissues about the ossicles of the ear.

os·sif′er·ous. Containing or producing bone tissue.

os·sif′ic. Producing bone.

os″si·fi·ca′tion. The formation o bone; the conversion of tissue int bone. **pathologic o.** Bone develop ment in unusual sites, or abnorma bone formation. Metaplastic or hetero plastic bone may be observed in sof tissues.

os·sif′lu·ent. Breaking down an softening bony tissue, as an ossifluen abscess.

os′si·fy (oss′i·figh). Turn into bone.

os·tal′gi·a. Pain in a bone. **—os talgic,** *adj.*

os″tal·gi′tis. Inflammation of a bon attended by pain.

os″te·al′le·o′sis. A metamorphosi of the substance of bone, as exempli fied in osteosarcoma.

os″te·an″a·gen′e·sis. Regeneratio of bone. *Obs.*

os″te·a·naph′y·sis. The reproduc tion of bone tissue. Syn., *osteano genesis. Obs.*

os·tec′to·my, os″te·ec′to·my. Ex cision of a bone or a portion of a bon

os·tec′to·py. Bone displacement. *Ob*

os″te·i′tis. Inflammation of bon **—osteit′ic,** *adj.* **condensing o.** form usually involving both marrow an periosteum, and resulting in the fillin of the medullary cavity with a dens bony mass; new bone usually forms o the surface, so that the bone become heavier and denser than normal. **gum matous o.** A chronic form due t syphilis and characterized by the for mation of gummas in the cancellou tissue of the epiphysis, in the shaft o a bone, or in the periosteum. **o. fi brosa cystica.** Hyperparathyroid ism: a disease due to hyperplasia o adenoma of the parathyroid gland re sulting in an abnormal calcium an phosphorus metabolism. It is charac terized clinically by thinning of th bony skeleton, often in the form o cysts. Also called *von Recklinghausen' disease.* **o. interna.** Osteomyelitis o the alveolar process resulting from in fection of a tooth.

os·tem′bry·on. An ossified fetus.

os″tem·py·e′sis (os″tem·pye·ee′sis ·pee·ee′sis). Suppuration of bone.

os′te·o-, os′te-. A combining forr meaning bone.

os″te·o·an′eu·rysm (os″tee·o·an yoo·riz·um). Aneurysm of the bloo vessels of a bone; a pulsating tumor o a bone.

os″te·o·ar·threc′to·my. Surgica excision or partial excision of the bon portion of a joint.

os″te·o·ar·throp′a·thy. Any dis ease of bony articulations. **hyper trophic pulmonary o.** A diseas characterized by a bulbous enlargemen of the terminal phalanges of the finger and toes, a thickening of the articula ends of the bones, and a peculia curvature of the nails. The disease usually is associated with disease of the lungs or pleura resulting in cyanosis. The most probable cause is local increase of flow of blood and arterial pressure.

os"te·o·blast". Any one of the cells of mesenchymal origin concerned in the formation of bony tissue. **—osteoblast/ic,** *adj.*

os"te·o·blas·to'ma. Osteosarcoma.

os"te·o·car"ci·no'ma. An ossifying carcinoma; carcinoma of bone.

os"te·o·car"ti·lag'i·nous (os"tee-o-kahr"ti-ladj'i-nus). Pertaining to or composed of both bone and cartilage.

os"te·o·chon'dral,   os"te·o·chon'drous. Composed of both bone and cartilage, as an osteochondral callus.

os"te·o·chon·dri'tis (-kon-dry'tis). A process involving ossification centers, chiefly during periods of rapid growth, characterized by aseptic necrosis followed by slow regeneration. Sometimes called *osteochondrosis.* **o. deformans juvenilis.** A disease of the upper femur, affecting children between five and ten years of age. Syn., *Legg-Calvé-Perthes disease, coxa plana.* **o. dissecans.** A condition of a joint, usually of the knee, characterized by the partial detachment of a fragment of cartilage and underlying bone from the articular surface.

os"te·o·chon"dro·dys·pla'si·a (-kon"dro-dis-play'zhuh, -shuh). A general term used to indicate abnormal development of bony and cartilaginous structures.

os"te·o·chon·dro'ma (-kon-dro'-muh). A tumor originating in bone or cartilage, occasionally in another structure, which histologically contains both bone and cartilage; not malignant but tends to recur after surgical removal.

os"te·o·chon"dro·sar·co'ma. A malignant tumor of the same general structure as osteochondroma, but less well differentiated.

os"te·o·chon·dro'sis (-kon-dro'-sis). Osteochondritis.

os"te·o·cla'sis. 1. The fracture of a long bone without resort to open operation, for the purpose of correcting deformity. 2. The destruction of bony tissue; the resorption of bone.

os"te·o·clast". 1. A powerful surgical apparatus or instrument through which leverage can be brought to bear at the point desired to effect osteoclasis or the forcible fracture of a long bone. 2. One of the large multinuclear cells found in association with the resorption of bone. **—osteoclas'tic,** *adj.*

os"te·o·clas·to'ma. Giant cell tumor of bone.

os"te·o·cys·to'ma. A cystic bone tumor.

os"te·o·cyte". A bone cell.

os"te·o·den'tine (os"tee-o-den'teen, -tin). A tissue intermediate in structure between bone and dentine.

os"te·o·der"ma·to·plas'tic. Pertaining to the formation of osseous tissue in dermal structures.

os"te·o·der'mi·a. Bony formations in the skin.

os"te·o·dyn'i·a. A chronic pain in a bone.

os"te·o·dys·tro·phi·a, os"te·o·dys'tro·phy. General term for defective bone formation. It includes such bone defects as are seen in rickets, dwarfism, etc. See *dystrophy.* **o. deformans.** A disease of late life, affecting one or more bones, with deformity from abnormal nutrition or growth. The cause is not known. Syn., *osteitis deformans, Paget's disease.*

os"te·o·fi"bro·li·po'ma. A tumor with bony, fibrous, and fatty components.

os"te·o·fi·bro'ma (os"tee-o-figh-bro'muh). An osteoma with a rich fibrous component; a fibroma with osseous metaplasia.

os"te·o·fi·bro'sis (-figh-bro'sis). Fibrosis of bone; a change involving mainly the red bone marrow.

os'te·o·gen. The substance from which osteogenic fibers are formed.

os"te·o·gen·e·sis. The development of bony tissue; ossification; the histogenesis of bone. **o. imperfecta.** A defect of bone formation and calcification, of unknown cause, but often hereditary, characterized by bone fragility, blue scleras, and sometimes deafness. Multiple fractures may occur before birth, in infancy, or later in childhood. Also called *fragilitas ossium, osteopsathyrosis, Lobstein's disease, Eddowes' disease.*

os"te·o·hy"per·troph'ic. Pertaining to overgrowth of bone.

os'te·oid. 1. The young hyaline matrix of true bone in which the calcium salts are deposited. 2. Resembling bone.

os"te·o·lith. A petrified or fossil bone.

os"te·ol'o·gy. The science of anatomy and structure of bones.

os"te·ol'y·sis. 1. Resorption of bone. 2. Degeneration of bone.

os"te·o'ma. A tumor which contains the various elements of bone in disorderly arrangement; difficult to distinguish from exostosis and enostosis. **—osteomatoid,** *adj.*

os"te·o·ma·la'ci·a (os"tee-o-ma-lay'shee-uh, -see-uh). Osteoporosis resulting from lowered calcium absorption from the intestine, due usually to vitamin-D deficiency. Occurs chiefly in adults, particularly during pregnancy and lactation. **—osteomalacial, osteomalac'ic,** *adj.*

os"te·om'e·try. The study of the proportions and measurements of the skeleton. **—osteomet'ric,** *adj.*

os"te·o·my'e·li'tis. Inflammation of the marrow of bone.

os"te·o·my'e·log'ra·phy. Roentgenography of bone marrow and marrow spaces.

os"te·o·ne·cro'sis. Necrosis of bone in mass.

os"te·o·path, os"te·op'a·thist. One who practices osteopathy.

os"te·op'a·thy. A school of healing which teaches that the body is a vital mechanical organism whose structural and functional integrity are coördinate and interdependent, the perversion of either constituting disease. Its major effort in treatment is in manipulation, but surgery and the specialties are also included. **—osteopath'ic,** *adj.*

os"te·o·pe'di·on. A calcified fetus. Syn., *lithopedion.*

os"te·o·per''i·os·ti'tis. Combined inflammation of bone and its periosteum.

os"te·o·pe·tro'sis. A rare developmental disorder in which most or all bones have excessive radiologic density, and in which sclerotic changes and fibrosis of the marrow occur. Also called *Albers-Schönberg disease, marble bones, osteosclerosis.*

os"te·oph'o·ny. The transmission of sound through bone.

os"te·o·phyte". A bony outgrowth.

os"te·o·plaque" (os'tee·o·plack"). A layer of bone; a flat osteoma.

os"te·o·plas'tic. 1. Pertaining to the formation of bone tissue. 2. Pertaining to reparative operations upon bone.

os"te·o·plas"ty. Plastic operations on bone.

os"te·o·po·ro'sis. An enlargement of the spaces of bone (Haversian canals) whereby a porous appearance is produced. The loss of bony substance results in brittleness or softness of the bones. **—osteoporot'ic,** *adj.*

os"te·op·sath''y·ro'sis (os"tee·op·sath''i·ro'sis, os"tee·o·sath''i·). Osteogenesis imperfecta.

os"te·o·ra''di·o·ne·cro'sis. Bone necrosis due to irradiation by roentgen or radium rays.

os"te·o·sar·co'ma. A sarcoma derived from cells of bone and containing bony structures. **—osteosarcomatous,** *adj.*

os"te·o'sis. Abnormal bone formation.

os"te·o·spon"gi·o'ma (os"tee·o·spon"jee·o'muh, ·spun"jee·o'muh). A tumor consisting of cancellous bone.

os"te·o·stix'is. Surgical puncturing of a bone.

os"te·o·syn'o·vi'tis (os"tee·o·sin"o·vy'tis, ·sigh"no·vy'tis). Synovitis

complicated with osteitis of adjacent bones.

os"te·o·syn'the·sis. Fastening the ends of a fractured bone together by mechanical means, such as a plate.

os"te·o·ta'bes (os"tee·o·tay'beez). Bone degeneration beginning with the destruction of the cells of the bone marrow, which disappears in parts and is replaced by soft gelatinous tissue; later the spongy bone diminishes, and lastly the compact bone.

os"te·o·throm·bo'sis. Thrombosis of the veins of a bone.

os"te·o·tome". An instrument for cutting bone. Specifically, an instrument somewhat similar to a chisel but without the beveled edge, used for cutting long bones, generally with the aid of a surgical mallet.

os"te·o·to"mo·cla'si·a (os"tee·o·to"mo·clay'zhuh, os·tee·ot"o·mo·). **os"te·o·to·moc'la·sis** (os"tee·o·to·mock'luh·sis, os·tee·ot"o·). The correction of a pathologically curved bone by forcible bending following partial division by the osteotome.

os"te·ot'o·my. 1. The division of a bone. 2. Making a section of a bone for the purpose of correcting a deformity. **cuneiform o.** An ostectomy in which a wedge of bone is removed. **linear o.** A simple division of a bone. **subcutaneous o.** Osteotomy, usually by Macewen's technic, in which a small incision is made in the skin over the bony area to be divided, the bone itself being unexposed, and the operation completed by the sense of touch.

os"te·ot'ro·phy. Nutrition of bony tissue.

os'ti·um (pl. *ostiums, ostia*). A mouth or aperture. **—ostial,** *adj.* **o. abdominale.** The orifice of the oviduct communicating with the peritoneal cavity. **o. internum.** The uterine opening of the oviduct. **o. pharyngeum.** The pharyngeal opening of the auditory tube. **o. tympanicum.** The tympanic opening of the auditory tube. **o. vaginae.** The external orifice of the vagina.

os"tre·o·tox·is'mus (os"tree·o·tock·siz'mus). Poisoning due to eating diseased or deteriorated oysters.

O.T. 1. *In anatomy,* old term, in opposition to BNA term. 2. Original, or old, tuberculin. Also abbreviated T.O.

o·tal'gi·a. Earache. **—otalgic,** *adj.*

o"tan·tri'tis. Inflammation of the mastoid antrum.

o·the"ma·to'ma (o·theem"uh·to'muh, o·them"uh·). Hematoma of the external ear, usually the pinna.

ot"hem·or·rha'gi·a (oath"em·o·ray'juh, ·radj/uh). Hemorrhage from the ear.

ot"hem·or·rhe'a (oat"hem·o·ree'uh·

path″em·o·). A sanguineous discharge from the ear.

ʺtic. Pertaining to the ear.

ʺti·co·din′i·a. Vertigo from ear disease.

·ti′tis. Inflammation of the ear.

—otit′ic, *adj.* **aeroötitis.** An occupational affection of the ears of aviators. **furuncular o.** The formation of furuncles in the external auditory meatus. **o. externa.** Inflammation of the external ear. **o. interna.** Inflammation of the internal ear. **o. labyrinthica.** Inflammation of the labyrinth. **o. mastoidea.** Inflammation confined to the mastoid cells; mastoid disease. **o. media.** Inflammation of the middle ear. **o. parasitica.** Inflammation caused by a parasite. **o. sclerotica.** Inflammation of the inner ear with hardening of the tissues. See *otosclerosis*.

ʺto-, ot-. A combining form meaning the ear.

ʺto·blen″or·rhe′a. Any discharge of mucus from the ear.

ʺto·clei′sis (o″to·kly′sis). Occlusion of the ear.

ʺto·dyn′i·a. Pain in the ear.

ʺto·gen′ic, o·tog′e·nous (o·todj′·nus). Originating or arising within the ear.

ʺto·hem″1·neur″as·the′ni·a. A condition in which hearing is limited exclusively to one ear, without the evidence of any material lesion of the auditory apparatus.

ʺto·lar″yn·gol′o·gist. One skilled in the practice of otology, rhinology, and laryngology.

ʺto·lar″yn·gol′o·gy. A medical specialty including otology, rhinology, laryngology, and, usually, peroral endoscopy.

ʺto·lith. One of the calcareous concretions within the membranous labyrinth of the ear, especially the large ear stones of fishes.

·tol′o·gist. One versed in otology.

·tol′o·gy. The science of the ear, its anatomy, functions, and diseases. **—otolog′ic, otolog′ical,** *adj.*

ʺto·my″as·the′ni·a. 1. Weakness of the muscles of the ear. 2. Defective hearing due to a paretic condition of the tensor tympani or stapedius muscle.

ʺto·my′ces (o″to·migh′sees). Fungous growth within the ear.

ʺto·my·co′sis (o″to·migh·ko′sis). The growth of fungi within the ear, or the diseased condition caused thereby.

ʺto·neur″as·the′ni·a. A condition of deficient tone of the auditory apparatus.

ʺto·pha·ryn′ge·al (o″to·fa·rin′·ul, ·far″in·jee′ul). Pertaining to the ear and the pharynx.

ʺto·plas″ty. Plastic surgery of the external ear.

o″to·pol′y·pus. A polyp occurring in the ear.

o″to·py″or·rhe′a. A purulent discharge from the ear.

o″to·py·o′sis (o″to·pye·o′sis). Suppuration within the ear.

o″to·rhi·nol′o·gy (o″to·rye·nol′o·jee). Literally, the study of diseases of the ears and the nose only. The terms most frequently employed for the study of the diseases of the ear, nose, and throat are otolaryngology or otorhinolaryngology.

o″tor·rha′gi·a. A discharge of blood from the external auditory meatus.

o″tor·rhe′a. A discharge from the external auditory meatus.

o″to·scle·ro′sis. A clinical entity, the symptom being progressive impairment of hearing. The end result of the pathologic process is the laying down of new bone around the oval window, the cochlea, or both. Erroneously thought to be new bone growth around any one of the ossicles. **—otosclerot′ic,** *adj.*

o′to·scope. An apparatus designed for examination of the ear and for rendering the tympanic membrane visible.

o·tos′co·py. Visualization of the auditory canal and tympanic membrane by means of the otoscope. **—otoscop′ic,** *adj.*

o·tot′o·my. Dissection of the ear; incision of any tissues of the external auditory meatus or the ear proper.

O. U. *Oculus uterque*, each eye.

ona·ba′in (wah·bah′in, ·bay′in). C₂₉H₄₀O₁₂. A crystalline glycoside obtained from *Strophanthus gratus*.

ou′loid (oo′loyd). Resembling a scar.

ou″lor·rha′gi·a (oo″lo·ray′juh, ·jee·uh). Hemorrhage from the gums.

ounce. A unit of measure or weight. See Tables of Weights and Measures in the Appendix. **avoirdupois o.** The sixteenth part of the avoirdupois pound, or 437.5 gr. (28.35 Gm.). Abbreviated, oz. **fluidounce.** One-sixteenth of a pint; 8 fluidrachms (U.S.P.); 29.57 cc. **troy o.** The twelfth part of the troy pound, or 480 gr. (31.10 Gm.). Symbol, ℥.

ou′ro- (oor′o-). See *uro-*.

-ous (-us). 1. A suffix meaning *full of* or *having*. 2. In chemistry, a suffix denoting the *lower* of two valences assumed by an element.

ont′flow. In neurology, the transmission of efferent impulses, particularly of the autonomic nervous system; these are divided into thoracolumbar and craniosacral outflows.

out′let. The lower aperture of the pelvic canal.

out′pa″tient. A hospital patient who does not occupy a bed in the institution.

o′va. Plural of ovum, an egg.

o'val. 1. Having the outline of an egg. 2. Pertaining to an ovum.

o''val·bu'min. The albumin of the egg white.

o·va''ri·al'gi·a. Neuralgic pain in the ovary. Also called *oarialgia*.

o·va'ri·an. Pertaining to the ovary.

o·va'ri·ec'to·my. Excision of an ovary; oöphorectomy.

o·va'ri·o-, ovari-. A combining form denoting *an ovary* or *ovarian*.

o·va'ri·o·cele'. Tumor of the ovary; hernia of an ovary. **vaginal o.** A condition in which an ovary is in contact with the vaginal wall.

o·va''ri·o·cen·te'sis. Puncture of an ovary or of an ovarian cyst.

o·va''ri·o·cy·e'sis (o·vair''ee·o·sigh·ee'sis). Ovarian pregnancy.

o·va''ri·o·dys·neu'ri·a. Ovarian neuralgia.

o·va''ri·o·gen'ic. Arising in the ovary.

o·va''ri·o·hys''ter·ec'to·my. Surgical removal of the ovaries and uterus.

o·va''ri·o·lyt'ic. Disorganization of ovarian tissue.

o·va''ri·or·rhex'is. Rupture of an ovary.

o·va''ri·ot'o·my. Literally, incision of an ovary. As generally used, removal of an ovary; oöphorectomy.

o·va''ri·o·tu'bal. Pertaining to an ovary and oviduct.

o'va·ry. 1. One of a pair of glandular organs giving rise to ova. It consists of a fibrous framework or stroma, in which are embedded the ovarian follicles, and is surrounded by a serous covering derived from the peritoneum. 2. The dried, undefatted, and powdered ovary of cattle, sheep, or swine; one part represents approximately six parts by weight of fresh glands. Syn., *desiccated ovarian substance.*

o'ver·bite. The extent to which the upper anterior teeth overlap the lower when the jaws are at rest.

o'ver·de·ter''mi·na'tion. *In psychoanalysis*, the state of having more than one etiologic factor.

o''ver·ex·ten'sion. Extension beyond the normal point or line.

o'ver·flow''. The escape of liquid from a filled vessel or viscus.

o'ver·growth''. Hypertrophy or hyperplasia.

o''ver·ly'ing. A cause of death in infants sleeping with adults; suffocation occurs when one of the adults lies upon the child.

o''ver·rid'ing. The slipping of an end of a fractured bone over the other fragment. Said also of toes which overlap.

o'ver·strain''. 1. Strain to excess. 2. A condition resulting from exhausting effort.

o'ver·tone''. A harmonic tone hea[...] above the fundamental tone. **psy** **chic o.** An associated impression co[...] tributing to a mental image.

o'ver·weight''. Exceeding norm[...] weight, usually meaning an excess more than 10%.

o'vi-. A combining form meaning *eg* used to denote *ovum*.

o'vi·duct. The duct serving to tran[...] port the ovum from the ovary to t[...] exterior, or to an organ such as th[...] uterus. In mammals, the oviduct is al[...] called the uterine or Fallopian tub[...] —**ovidu'cal, oviduc'tal,** *adj.*

o''vi·fi·ca'tion. The production [...] ova.

o·vig'e·nous (o·vidj'i·nus). Produ[...] ing ova, as the ovigenous layer, th[...] outer layer of the ovary, in which th[...] follicles containing the ova are sit[...] ated.

o·vip'a·rous. Laying eggs; bringi[...] forth young in the egg stage of develo[...] ment. —**ovipara,** *n.*

o'vo-. See *ovi-*.

o''vo·fla'vin (o''vo·flay'vin, ·flav'in [...] A flavin separated from eggs; it is ide[...] tical with riboflavin.

o'void. Egg-shaped.

o''vo·tes'tis. A rare form of aberra[...] development in which an ovary and [...] testis are combined.

o''vo·vi·tel'lin (o''vo·vye·tel'in, ·v[...] tel'in). A protein contained in egg yo[...]

o''vu·la'tion. The maturation a[...] escape of the ovum.

o'vum (pl. *ova*). 1. A female germ ce[...] an egg cell; a cell which is capable [...] developing into a new member of t[...] same species, in animals usually on[...] after maturation and fertilization. T[...] human ovum is a large, spheroidal ce[...] containing a large mass of cytoplas[...] and a large nucleus (germinal vesicle[...] within which is a nucleolus (germin[...] spot). 2. The early human embryo fro[...] the time of fertilization until the [...] laminar blastodisk is formed.

ox-. *In chemistry*: 1. Short for *oxal-*[...] Combining form denoting *presence* [...] *oxygen.*

ox'a-. *In chemistry*, a combining for[...] denoting the *presence of oxygen* [...] place of carbon.

ox'al-, ox'al·o-. *In chemistry*, a co[...] bining form denoting *oxalic.*

ox''al·a·ce'tic ac'id. HOOC.CH[...] CO.COOH. A metabolic product in carb[...] hydrate metabolism. Also called *oxa[...] acetic acid.*

ox'a·late. Any salt or ester of oxa[...] acid.

ox''a·le'mi·a. Excess of oxalates [...] the blood.

ox·al'ic ac'id. HOOC.COOH.2H₂O[...] poisonous dibasic or dicarboxylic ac[...] occurring in many plants.

ox'a·lism. Poisoning by oxalic acid or potassium binoxalate. It is characterized by gastroenteritis with nephritis, collapse, cyanosis, mydriasis, labored breathing, and dyspnea.

ox"a·lu'ri·a. The presence of oxalic acid or oxalates in the urine.

ox"a·lu'ric ac'id. $NH_2.CO.NH.CO.COOH$. An acid occasionally found in traces in normal human urine.

ox'a·tyl. Carboxyl, *q.v.*

ox"a·zol'i·dine. The heterocyclic compound $O.CH_2.NH.CH_2.CH_2$, from which medicinal derivatives have been prepared. See *trimethadione*.

ox bile. The fresh bile of the ox, *Bos taurus*. See *bile*. **o. b. extract.** Contains sodium salts of ox bile acids standardized to be equivalent to not less than 45% of cholic acid.

ox gall (gawl). Ox bile.

ox'i·dant. An oxidizing agent.

ox'i·dase (ock'si·dace, ·daze). Any enzyme which promotes an oxidation reaction. **amino acid o.** An enzyme capable of causing the oxidation of amino acids; **D-amino acid oxidase** occurs in most animal tissues and is specific for the oxidation of D-amino acids to keto acids; **L-amino acid oxidase** also occurs in animal tissues and is specific for the oxidative deamination of the naturally occurring L-amino acids. **choline o.** An enzyme causing the oxidation of choline. **indophenol o.** A heme-containing enzyme in living cells which, in the presence of oxygen and cytochrome C, oxidizes p-aminodimethylaniline so that it will form indophenol blue with α-naphthol. The enzyme is probably identical with Warburg's respiratory enzyme and with cytochrome oxidase. **monophenol o.** A copper-containing protein enzyme which catalyzes the oxidation of monophenols, including tyrosine. It is probably identical with tyrosinase and perhaps also with polyphenol oxidase. **polyphenol o.** A copper-containing protein enzyme which catalyzes the oxidation of polyphenols. It is probably identical with tyrosinase and perhaps also with monophenol oxidase. **xanthine o.** A flavoprotein enzyme catalyzing the oxidation of certain purines.

ox"i·da'tion. 1. An increase in the positive valence, or a decrease in the negative valence, of an element, resulting from the loss of electrons which are taken on by some other element. Also see *reduction*, 1. 2. Originally, the process of combining with oxygen. **beta o.** Oxidation of the carbon atom which is in the beta position with reference to a functional group in the molecule. **omega o.** The oxidation of a fatty acid at the end of a chain opposite to where the carboxyl group occurs, thereby forming a dicarboxylic acid.

ox'ide. A binary compound of oxygen and another element or radical.

ox'i·dize. Produce an oxidation or increase in positive valence (or decrease in negative valence) through the loss of electrons.

ox'imes (ock'seemz, ·simz). A series of compounds resulting from the action of hydroxylamine upon aldehydes and ketones; they contain the radical, —CH:NOH.

ox·im'e·ter. An instrument for measuring the per cent-saturation of the blood hemoglobin with oxygen. It consists of an earpiece, control box, and galvanometer.

ox"o·i·som'er·ase. An enzyme which catalyzes the interconversion of glucose-6-phosphate and fructofuranose-6-monophosphate.

ox"o·phen·ar'sine hy"dro·chlo'ride (ock"so·fen·ahr'seen, ·sin). 3-Amino-4-hydroxyphenylarsinoxide hydrochloride, $(NH_2)(OH)C_6H_3AsO.HCl$, employed as an antisyphilitic.

ox'y-. 1. A combining form meaning *sharp, acid, acute, shrill, quick.* 2. In *botany*, a combining form signifying *pointed* or *smooth.* 3. In *medicine*, a combining form denoting *acuteness of perception, swift, sharp in pitch,* or *acute.* 4. A prefix meaning *oxygen;* used to denote *one oxygen atom united to two different atoms.* 5. A prefix denoting *the presence of the hydroxyl group.*

ox"y·a·can'thine (ock"see·a·can'theen, ·thin). $C_{27}H_{40}N_2O_6$. An alkaloid of berberis.

ox'y·ac'id. Any acid containing oxygen.

ox"y·a'phi·a (ock"see·ay'fee·uh, ·af'ee·uh). Abnormal acuteness of the sense of touch.

ox"y·blep'si·a. Acuteness of vision.

oxycel. A trade-mark for oxidized cellulose.

ox"y·ceph'a·ly. A condition in which the head is roughly conical in shape. Caused by premature closure of the coronal or lambdoid sutures, or both, which induces compensatory development in the region of the bregma. Is also caused by pressure on the frontal and occipital regions of the heads of infants to alter the shape. Commonly known as *sugar loaf head.*

ox"y·chlo'ride. Any compound containing both —OH and —Cl attached to the same element; a compound containing the —OCl radical.

ox"y·chro'ma·tin. That part of the chromatin having an affinity for acid dyes.

ox"y·den'dron. The leaves of the sorrel tree, *Oxydendrum arboreum.*

ox"y·es·the'si·a (ock"see·ess·thee'-zhuh, ·zee·uh). A condition of increased acuity of sensation.

ox'y·gen. O = 16.0000. A colorless, tasteless, odorless gas, constituting one-fifth of the atmosphere, eight-ninths of water, and about one-half the crust of the globe; it supports combustion, and is essential to life of animals.

ox'y·gen ac'id. An acid which contains oxygen.

ox'y·gen·ase. An enzyme that enables atmospheric oxygen to be utilized by the organism or in the system in which it occurs.

ox"y·ge·na'tion. The saturation of a substance with oxygen, either by chemical combination or by mixture. —**ox'ygenated,** *adj.*

ox'y·gen ca·pac'i·ty. The maximum amount of oxygen absorbed by a given amount of blood when it is equilibrated with an excess of oxygen expressed in volume per cent (cc. per 100 cc.). See Table of Normal Values of Blood Constituents in the Appendix.

ox'y·gen con'tent. Oxygen in volume per cent present in blood at a given moment. See Table of Normal Values of Blood Constituents in the Appendix.

ox'y·gen tent. An airtight chamber enclosing the patient's head and shoulders in which the oxygen content of the atmosphere can be maintained at a higher than normal level.

ox"y·geu'si·a (ock"si·gew'see·uh, ·jew'see·uh). Marked acuteness of the sense of taste.

ox"y·hem'a·tin (ock"si·hem'uh·tin, ·hee'muh·tin). $C_{34}H_{32}N_4O_7Fe$. The coloring matter of oxyhemoglobin; on oxidation, it yields hematinic acid; on reduction, hematoporphyrin.

ox"y·hem"a·to·por'phy·rin. A pigment sometimes found in urine; it is related to hematoporphyrin.

ox"y·he"mo·glo'bin (ock"si·hee"-mo·glo'bin, ·hem"o·glo'bin). Oxidized hemoglobin; that found in arterial blood.

ox"y·la'li·a (ock"si·lay'lee·uh, ·lal'-ee·uh). Rapid speech.

ox'y·mel. 1. A mixture of honey, water, and vinegar or dilute acetic acid. 2. Any preparation containing honey and vinegar (or acetic acid) as a vehicle.

ox"y·ner'vone, ox"y·ner'von. A galactolipin, isolated from nerve tissue, reported to contain oxynervonic acid.

ox"y·ner·von'ic ac'id. $C_{23}H_{44}.OH.-COOH$. An unsaturated acid, the hydroxy derivative of nervonic acid, reported to exist in oxynervone.

ox"y·neu'rine (ock"si·new'reen ·rin). See *betaine.*

ox·yn'tic. Secreting acid, formerl[y] applied to the parietal cells of th[e] stomach.

ox"y·o'pi·a. Increased acuity of vi[-] sion.

ox"y·os·phre'si·a (ock"see·os·free' zhuh, ·shuh). Marked or abnorma[l] acuteness of sense of smell.

ox"y·phe·non'i·um bro'mide Diethyl (2 - hydroxyethyl) methyl - am monium bromide α-phenylcyclohexane glycolate, an anticholinergic agen[t] used in treating peptic ulcer and gas trointestinal spasm. See *antrenyl bro mide.*

ox'y·phil, ox'y·phile. Pertainin[g] to histologic elements that attract aci[d] dyes. Syn., *acidophil, eosinophil.*

ox"y·pho'ni·a. Shrillness of voice

ox"y·pol"y·gel'a·tin. An oxidized polymerized gelatin used experimentally as a blood plasma substitute.

ox"y·pro'line. Hydroxyproline, *q.v*

ox"y·quin'o·line (ock"si·kwin'o leen, ·lin). 8-Hydroxyquinoline, C_9H_7NO Used as a chemical reagent in precipi tation of metals. **o. benzoate.** A germicide and fungicide for the treat ment of infectious skin diseases. **o. sul fate.** A bacteriostatic agent in 1:100[0] to 1:3000 solution; used as nasal spray douche, gargle, eyewash. See *chinoso[l]*

ox"y·tet"ra·cy'cline. An antibi otic from *Streptomyces rimosus,* ac tive against a number of Gram-posi tive and Gram-negative bacteria, rick ettsiae, and viruses. See *terramycin*

ox"y·to'ci·a (ock"si·to'shee·uh, ·see uh). Rapid childbirth.

ox"y·to'cic. 1. Hastening parturition 2. A drug that hastens parturition.

ox"y·to'cin. The water-soluble oxy tocic hormone of the neurohypophysis Syn., *alpha-hypophamine.* See *pitocin*

Ox"y·u'ris ver·mic"u·la'ris Synonym for *Enterobius vermicularis*

oz. Ounce (avoirdupois).

o·ze'na. A chronic disease of the nos[e] accompanied by a fetid discharge. It i[s] due to atrophic rhinitis, syphilitic ul ceration, or caries.

o"zo·chro'ti·a (o"zo·kro'shuh, ·see uh). An offensive odor of the skin —**ozoch'rotous,** *adj.*

o'zone. O_3. An allotropic form of oxy gen, the molecule of which consists o[f] three atoms; a common constituent o[f] the atmosphere. It is a powerful oxidiz ing agent.

o'zo·nide. A compound of ozone wit[h] certain unsaturated organic substances

o"zos·to'mi·a. A foul odor of th[e] breath of oral origin.

P

P. 1. Chemical symbol for phosphorus. 2. Abbreviation for pharmacopeia; position; *pugillus*, handful; *punctum, proximum*, near point, premolar.

P³². Symbol for phosphorus-32.

p-. *In chemistry,* para-.

Pa. Chemical symbol for protactinium.

PABA. Para-aminobenzoic acid.

pab′u·lum. Food; any nutrient.

pacatal. Trade-mark for mepazine.

pace′mak″er. That portion of the right atrium of the heart, normally the sinoatrial node, where the stimulus for the heart beat originates.

pach′y- (pack′ee-). A combining form meaning *thick*.

pach″y·ac′ri·a. A condition marked by clubbing of the fingers and toes, and thickening of the skin of the extremities. Formerly called *acropachyderma, pseudoacromegaly*. See hypertrophic pulmonary *osteoarthropathy*.

pach″y·bleph′a·ron. Thickening of the eyelids.

pach″y·bleph″a·ro′sis. Chronic thickening and induration of the eyelids.

pach″y·chi′li·a, pach″y·chei′li·a (pack″i·kigh′lee-uh, ·kil′ee-uh). Increased thickness of one or both lips.

pach″y·dac′tyl′i·a, pach″y·dac′ty·ly. A condition characterized by great thickness of the fingers.

pach″y·der′ma·tous. Abnormally thick-skinned.

pach″y·der′mi·a, pach″y·der′ma. 1. Abnormal thickening of the skin. 2. Elephantiasis. **—pachyder′mial**, *adj*.

pach″y·glos′si·a. Thickness of the tongue.

pach″y·hem′a·tous. Referring to thickening of the blood.

pach″y·lo′sis. A thick, dry, harsh, and scaly skin, especially of the legs.

pach″y·men″in·gi′tis (pack″i·men″in·jy′tis). Inflammation of the dura. **pachymeningit′ic**, *adj*. **epidural p.** Inflammation of the epidural space and the external aspect of the dura, usually resulting from tuberculosis of the spine. **hypertrophic cervical p.** A localized or diffuse, gummatous or granulomatous thickening of the dura in the cervical region, causing symptoms of irritation of spinal nerve roots and compression of the spinal cord.

pach″y·men″in·gop′a·thy. Disease of the dura mater, or pachymeninx.

pach″y·me′ninx. The dura mater.

pa·chyn′sis (pa·kin′sis). A thickening, as of a membrane. **—pachyntic**, *adj*.

pach″y·o·nych′i·a (pack″ee·o·nick′ee-uh). Thickening of the nails.

pach″y·o′ti·a (pack″ee·o′shuh, ·shee-uh). Thickness of the ears.

pach″y·pel″vi·per″i·to·ni′tis. Pelvic peritonitis with a fibrous deposit over the uterus.

pach″y·per″i·os·to′sis. Pathologic alteration of the long bones in which the periosteum is greatly thickened.

pach″y·per″i·to·ni′tis. Thickening of the peritoneum by inflammation.

pa·chyp′o·dous (pa·kip′o-dus). Having thick feet.

pach″y·rhi′nic, pach′y·rhine (pack″i·rye′nick). Having a thick or unusually broad and flat nose.

pach″y·sal·pin·go-o″va·ri′tis. Inflammation of the ovary and oviduct with thickening of the parts.

pach′y·tes (pack′i·teez). Pachyblepharon, *q.v.*

pa·chyt′ic (pa·kit′ick). Thick.

pach″y·vag″i·ni′tis (pack″i·vadj″i·nigh′tis). Vaginitis accompanied by thickening of the vaginal walls.

pac′i·fi″er. Any article, such as a rubber nipple, placed in the mouths of irritable or teething children to quiet or pacify them.

Pacini, Filippo [*Italian anatomist,* 1812–83]. Described the lamellar corpuscle (1835); called *Pacini's corpuscle, Pacinian corpuscle, corpuscle of Vater-Pacini.* See Pacinian corpuscle.

pack. A blanket, either dry or soaked in hot or cold water, and wrapped about the body. **cold p.** A blanket wrung out of cold water and wrapped about the body. **hot p.** A blanket wrung out of hot water and wrapped about the body. **wet p.** A blanket wrung out of warm or cold water.

Packard, Francis Randolph [*American otolaryngologist,* 1870–1950]. Widely known for his interest in historical medicine. Author of *History of Medicine in the United States.*

pack′er. A tapered surgical instrument equipped with a point ending in a shoulder, for inserting gauze or other dressings into a cavity; used generally in conjunction with an aural, vaginal, or other speculum.

pack′ing. 1. The act of filling a wound or cavity with gauze or other material. 2. The material used for filling the cavity.

pad. 1. A small cushion stuffed with

501

cotton, hair, etc., for supporting any part of the body. 2. Compress, *q.v.* **dinner p.** A removable pad of felt, cotton, or other material placed over the abdomen prior to the application of a plaster jacket, to allow for normal distention after eating. **fat p.** In anatomy, any mass of fatty tissue. **p. of corpus callosum.** The splenium of the callosum. **sucking p.** A fatty mass situated between the masseter and the buccinator muscles, well developed in infancy; the buccal fat pad.

Padgett, Earl Calvin [*American surgeon*, 1893–1946]. Made many contributions to plastic surgery. Devised an operation for reconstruction of the lip using transplanted tubular grafts from the scalp and neck; called *Padgett's operation.* Especially known for his invention of an instrument for cutting a uniform sheet of skin of any given thickness, for grafting. The skin is attached by rubber cement to a semicircular drum held by a central handle. An adjustable knife is set against the periphery. Called *Padgett's dermatome.*

pae-. For words beginning with *pae-*, see under *pe-*.

Pagenstecher, Alexander [*German ophthalmologist*, 1828–79]. Introduced an ophthalmic ointment of yellow oxide of mercury and petrolatum, called *Pagenstecher's ointment.* Inventor of a special type of suture made of flax or linen thread coated with celluloid; called *Pagenstecher's suture.* Assisted by his brother, Hermann, devised several operations. An operation for cataract in which the lens is removed in a closed capsule using pressure on the cornea is called *Pagenstecher's operation.*

Paget, James [*English surgeon*, 1814–99]. Able writer on surgical pathology. Described carcinoma simplex of the nipple (1874); also called *Paget's disease of the nipple.* Described osteitis deformans (1882); also called *Paget's disease.* The disease of the nipple associated with his name is now recognized as a distortion due to a true dermal carcinoma, accompanied by a chronic inflammation. Occasionally duct-type carcinoma is present.

pagitane hydrochloride. Trademark for cycrimine hydrochloride.

pa″go·plex′i·a. Numbness from cold; frostbite.

-pa·gus. 1. A suffix expressing union in conjoined twins (diplopagi). 2. A suffix used by I. Geoffroy Saint-Hilaire to express anterior and posterior duplicity in conjoined twins.

pain. 1. A disturbed sensation causing suffering or distress. 2. A rhythmic contraction of the uterus during labor; labor pain. **—pain, v. bearing-down p.** A feeling of distress with a sensation of dragging of the pelvic organs; occurs during labor and in pelvic inflammatory disease. **boring p.** A severe feeling of distress simulating the action of a drill or other piercing instrument. **dilating p.** That accompanying the stretching of the cervix in the first stage of labor. **excentric p.** Radiating pain symptomatic of spinal disease, due to irritation of the posterior nerve roots; it is felt to be in peripheral areas, thus accounting for the name. **expulsive p.** A bearing-down sensation accompanying the last two stages of labor. **false p.** Mild, recurring lower abdominal cramps, occurring late in pregnancy, but not followed by labor. **fulgurant p.** The intense darting pain affecting principally the limbs of patients suffering from tabes dorsalis. Also called *lancinating p.*, *lightning p.*, *shooting p.* **girdle p.** A painful sensation as of a cord tied about the waist; it is a symptom of organic disease of the spinal cord. **growing p.** Soreness about the joints at puberty, often an evidence of rheumatism. **heterotopic p.** See referred *p.* **homotopic p.** Soreness felt at the site of trauma. **intermenstrual p.** Lower abdominal pain occurring between menstrual periods, apparently associated with ovulation. Also called *Mittelschmerz.* **lancinating p.** See fulgurant *p.* **osteocopic p.** The boneache that characterizes syphilis. **p. joy.** Hysterical enjoyment of suffering. **phantom limb p.** Pain which seems to the individual to be located in an amputated limb. **referred p.** Pain whose origin is not in the area in which it is felt; for example, pain felt under the right scapula due to gallbladder disease. **starting p.** Pain caused by a spasmodic contraction of the muscles just before the onset of sleep. It occurs in individuals with an inflammatory joint disease. **terebrating p.** See boring *p.*

pain′ful. Characterized by pain.

pain′less. Without pain.

pa′lae-o-. See *paleo-*.

pal′ate. The roof of the mouth. It is composed of the **hard palate**, formed by the palatal processes of the maxillary bones and the palatine bones with their covering mucous membranes, and the **soft palate**, or velum palati, consisting of an aggregation of muscles, the tensor palati, levator palati, azygos uvulae, palatoglossus, and palatopharyngeus, and their covering mucous membrane. **—palatine** (pal′uh·tyne, ·tin), **palatal**, *adj.* **cleft p.** A congenital deformity characterized by incomplete closure of the lateral halves of the palate. The soft palate and the uvula, the hard palate, or all together, may be involved. It may or may not be associated with cleft lip or cleft alveolar process.

pal'ate-hook''. A surgical instrument for retracting the uvula.

pal'a·tine. 1. Pertaining to the palate. 2. The palatine bone. See Table of Bones in the Appendix.

pal''a·ti'tis. Inflammation of the palate.

pal'a·to-. A combining form denoting *relation* to the palate.

pal''a·to·glos'sus. The muscle within the anterior pillar of the fauces; it connects the soft palate with the tongue; the glossopalatinus. See Table of Muscles in the Appendix.

pal''a·to·pha·ryn'ge·al (-fa·rin'jul, ·far''in·jee'ul). Pertaining conjointly to the palate and the pharynx, as the palatopharyngeal muscle or arch.

pal''a·to·pha·ryn'ge·us (pal''uh-to·fa·rin'jee·us, ·far''in·jee'us). The muscle in the posterior pillar of the fauces, connecting the soft palate with the lateral wall of the pharynx below; the pharyngopalatinus. See Table of Muscles in the Appendix.

pal'a·to·plas''ty. Plastic surgery of the palate.

pal''a·to·ple'gi·a. Paralysis of the soft palate.

pal''a·tor'rha·phy. Suture of a cleft palate.

pal''a·tos'chi·sis (pal''uh·tos'ki-sis). Cleft palate.

pal'a·tum (pl. *palata*). The palate. **p. du'rum.** Hard palate. **p. fis'sum.** Cleft palate. **p. mo'bile.** The soft palate. Also called *p. molle*.

pa'le·o-, pa'lae·o-. A combining form meaning *old, ancient;* used to denote *early, primitive, long ago.*

pa''le·o·cer''e·bel'lum. Phylogenetically old parts of the cerebellum: the anterior lobe, composed of lingula, centralis, and culmen, and the posterior part of the posterior lobe, composed of pyramid, uvula, and paraflocculus; may include the flocculonodular lobe.

pa''le·o·ki·net'ic (pay''lee·o·ki·net'-ick, ·kigh·net'ick). Referring to motor nervous mechanisms of submammals; represented in mammals by the extrapyramidal systems, which are the pathways concerned with postural and automatic associated movements.

pa''le·on·tol'o·gy. That branch of science which is based upon the study of fossil remains of organisms that lived in past geologic periods.

pa''le·o·pa·thol'o·gy. A branch of pathology dealing with diseases of ancient times demonstrated in human and animal remains.

pa''le·o·stri·a'tum (pay''lee·o-strye·ay'tum). The globus pallidus, a representative of the primitive corpus striatum of lower vertebrates.

pal''i·ki·ne'si·a (pal''i·ki·nee'shuh, pal''i·kigh·), **pal''i·ki·ne'sis** (pal''-i·ki·nee'sis, ·kigh·nee'sis). Constant and involuntary repetition of movements.

pal''i·la'li·a. Pathologic repetition of words or phrases.

pal''in·dro'mi·a. Recurrence or growing worse of a disease; a relapse. —**palindrom'ic,** *adj.*

pal''in·gen'e·sis. The development of characteristics during ontogeny which are regarded as inherited from ancestral species; opposed to *cenogenesis*. See recapitulation *theory.*

pal''i·phra'si·a (pal''i·fray'zhuh, ·zee·uh). Pathologic repetition of words or phrases.

pal''ir·rhe'a, pal''ir·rhoe'a. 1. The recurrence of a mucous discharge. 2. Regurgitation.

pal·la'di·um. Pd = 106.7. Silver-white, fairly ductile, hard metal, belonging to the platinum group of metals.

pal''an·es·the'si·a (pal''an·ess-thee'zhuh, ·zee·uh). Absence of pallesthesia.

pal''les·the'si·a (pal''ess·thee'-zhuh, ·zee·uh). Sensation similar to that felt when a vibrating tuning fork is touched; the sense of vibration.

pal''li·a'tion. Alleviation; the act of soothing or moderating, without really curing. —**palliate,** *v.*

pal''li·a''tive (pal'ee·ay''tiv, pal'ee·uh·tiv). 1. Relieving or alleviating suffering. 2. A drug relieving or soothing the symptoms of a disease without curing it.

pal'li·dum. The globus pallidus, medial pale portion of the lenticular nucleus of the brain. —**pallidal,** *adj.*

pal'lor. Paleness, especially of the skin and mucous membranes.

palm. 1. The inner or flexor surface of the hand; the hollow of the hand. 2. A palm tree. —**pal'mar,** *adj.*

pal·ma'ris. One of two muscles, palmaris longus and palmaris brevis, inserted into the fascia of the palm. See Table of Muscles in the Appendix.

pal'ma·ture. Union of the fingers; may be congenital or due to burns, wounds, or other trauma.

pal'min. Palmitin, *q.v.*

pal'mi·ped. Having webbed feet.

pal'mi·tate. A salt or ester of palmitic acid.

pal·mit'ic. 1. Relating to or derived from palm oil. 2. Relating to palmitin.

pal·mit'ic ac'id. $CH_3(CH_2)_{14}COOH$. A saturated acid occurring in the glycerides of many fats and oils.

pal'mi·tin. $C_3H_5(C_{16}H_{31}O_2)_3$; glyceryl

tripalmitate or glyceryl palmitate; an ester of glycerin with palmitic acid; found in vegetable and animal fats and oils.

pal'mi·tyl. The radical, $C_{15}H_{31}CO-$, of palmitic acid.

pal"mo·plan'tar. Pertaining to both the palms of the hands and the soles of the feet. Syn., *volar*.

pal'mus. 1. A convulsive tic, with echolalia and abulia; frequently a manifestation of hysteria or schizophrenia. 2. Palpitation, throbbing, pulsation, twitching, jerkiness. 3. The heartbeat.

pal'pa·ble. 1. Capable of being touched or palpated. 2. Evident.

pal·pa'tion. In physical diagnosis, the laying of the hand on a part of the body or the manipulation of a part with the hand for the purpose of ascertaining its condition or that of underlying organs. —**pal'pate**, v. **bimanual p.** The use of the two hands in examining an organ.

pal"pa·to·per·cus'sion. Combined palpation and percussion.

pal'pe·bra (pal'pi·bruh, pal·pee'bruh) (pl. *palpebrae*). The eyelid. —**palpebral**, adj. **p. inferior.** The lower eyelid. **p. superior.** The upper eyelid.

pal'pe·brae (pal'pi·bree, pal·pee'bree). Plural of palpebra, q.v.

pal'pe·brate. 1. Furnished with eyelids. 2. Wink.

pal'pe·bra'tion. The act of winking; nictitation.

pal'pi·tate. Flutter, tremble, or beat abnormally fast; applied especially to the heart.

pal"pi·ta'tion. A fluttering or throbbing, especially of the heart; any heart action of which the patient is conscious.

pal'sy (pawl'zee). A synonym for paralysis used to designate special types. For terms not found here, see under *paralysis*. **Bell's p.** Peripheral paralysis of the facial nerve. **birth p.** A paralysis due to injury sustained during parturition; the common form is the Erb-Duchenne syndrome, or obstetric paralysis with deltoid involvement from injury to the brachial plexus. Also used as a synonym for spastic diplegia. **brachial birth p.** Paralysis of the arm due to injury of the brachial plexus during birth. It may involve the entire arm, the upper arm (Erb-Duchenne type), or the forearm (Klumpke type). **bulbar p.** Progressive degeneration of motor conduction pathways in the bulbar region of the brain. See progressive bulbar *paralysis*. **cerebral p.** Paralysis due to a lesion of the brain. Also used as a synonym for spastic diplegia. **congenital cerebral p.** Spastic diplegia. **crutch p.** Paralysis of the arm

due to pressure of the crutch in the axilla. **diver's p.** Caisson disease. **drummer's p.** Paralysis of the extensor of the distal phalanx of the thumb occurring in drummers. **Erb's p.** See Erb-Duchenne *paralysis*. **hod-carrier's p.** Paralysis of the long thoracic nerve, from continuous muscular effort with the arms above the shoulder or from carrying heavy objects on the shoulder, characterized by unilateral "winging" of the scapula. **infantile cerebral p.** Cerebral spastic infantile paralysis. See spastic *diplegia*. **lead p.** Weakness of the hand grasp and paralysis of the extensors of the wrist and fingers resulting from degenerative changes in the posterior interosseous branch of the radial nerve produced by lead poisoning. **painter's p.** Lead palsy. **pressure p.** Paralysis due to pressure on a nerve. **printer's p.** A rare form of paralysis due to polyneuritis in chronic antimony poisoning occurring in printers. **progressive bulbar p.** See progressive bulbar *paralysis*. **pseudobulbar p.** See pseudobulbar *paralysis*. **scriveners' p.** Writers' cramp. **shaking p.** Paralysis agitans. Also called *Parkinson's disease*. **wasting p.** Progressive muscular atrophy, q.v.

paludrine hydrochloride. A trade-mark for chloroguanide hydrochloride.

pam'a·quine naph'tho·at (pam'uh·kween, ·kwin). $C_{18}H_{25}N_3O$. The methylene-bis-β-hydroxynaphthoate of 6-methoxy-8-(1-methyl-4-diethylamino)butylaminoquinoline; a yellow powder; insoluble in water. Used as an antimalarial. Also called *aminoquin naphthoate*. See *plasmochin*.

pam·pin'i·form. Having the form of a tendril, used particularly for the pampiniform plexus of veins in the spermatic cord.

pan. A low, flat-bottomed vessel. **bed p.** A large, flat, oval pan, usually of agate or enameled ware or stainless steel, serving as a receptacle for the fecal discharges and urine of patients confined to bed. **brain p.** The skull.

pan-. A combining form meaning all, every; used in medicine to signify general or affecting all or many parts.

pan"a·ce'a. A cure-all; a quack remedy.

pan"ar·te·ri'tis. 1. Inflammation of all the coats of an artery. 2. Inflammation of several arteries at the same time.

pan"ar·thri'tis. Inflammation of many joints.

pa·nat'ro·phy. 1. Atrophy affecting every part of a structure. 2. General atrophy.

pan″car·di′tis. General inflammation of the heart.

pan′cre·as (pan′kree·us, pang′kree-us) (pl. *pancreata*). A compound racemose gland, from six to eight inches in length, lying transversely across the posterior wall of the abdomen. Its right extremity, the head, lies in contact with the duodenum; its left extremity, the tail, is in close proximity to the spleen. It secretes a limpid, colorless fluid that digests proteins, fats, and carbohydrates. The secretion is conveyed to the duodenum by the pancreatic duct. It furnishes an important internal secretion, insulin, from the islets of Langerhans. —**pancreat′ic,** *adj.* **accessory p.** A small mass of glandular structure similar to the pancreas and adjacent to it. **annular p.** An anomalous pancreas encircling the duodenum. **lesser p.** A small, partially detached portion of the gland, lying posteriorly to its head, and occasionally having a separate duct that opens into the pancreatic duct proper.

pan″cre·a·tec′to·my. Excision of the pancreas.

pan″cre·at″i·co·du″o·de′nal (pan″kree·at″i·ko·dew″o·dee′nul, ·dew·od′i·nul). Pertaining to the pancreas and the duodenum, as the pancreaticoduodenal arteries. See Table of Arteries in the Appendix.

pan″cre·at″i·co·en″ter·os′to·my. The surgical anastomosis of the pancreatic duct or a pancreatic fistulous tract with the small intestine.

pan″cre·at″i·co·gas·tros′to·my. The surgical anastomosis of a pancreatic fistulous tract with the pyloric portion of the stomach.

pan″cre·at″i·co·je″ju·nos′to·my (·jee″jew·nos′to·mee, ·jedj″oo·nos′to·mee). Anastomosing the pancreatic duct with the jejunum.

pan″cre·at″i·co·li·thot′o·my. The surgical removal of a stone in the pancreatic duct.

pan′cre·a·tin. A substance containing enzymes, principally pancreatic amylase (amylopsin), trypsin, and pancreatic lipase (steapsin), obtained from the fresh pancreas of the hog, *Sus scrofa,* var. *domesticus,* or of the ox, *Bos taurus;* it is a cream-colored amorphous powder.

pan″cre·a·ti′tis. Inflammation of the pancreas. The acute form may be hemorrhagic, suppurative, or gangrenous. The onset of acute pancreatitis is usually sudden, with severe abdominal pain, vomiting, tympanites, and tenderness of the abdomen. Chronic pancreatitis may be interlobular, with an increase of interlobular connective tissue, or interacinar, in which the interacinar spaces are invaded and the islets of Langerhans involved. —**pancreat′ic,** *adj.*

pan″cre·a·to·du″o·de·nos′to·my. The anastomosis of a portion of the pancreas, especially a fistulous tract with the duodenum.

pan″cre·a·to·en″ter·os′to·my. Anastomosing the pancreatic duct with some part of the small intestine.

pan″cre·a·tog′e·nous (pan″kree-uh·todj′i·nus, pang″kree·). Arising in the pancreas.

pan″cre·a·to·li′pase. Lipase found in the pancreatic juice.

pan″cre·at′o·lith. A calculus of the pancreas. Syn., *pancreolith.*

pan″cre·a·to·li·thec′to·my. Surgical removal of a pancreatic calculus.

pan″cre·a·to·li·thot′o·my. Operative removal of calculus from the pancreas. Also called *pancreolithotomy.*

pan″cre·a·tol′y·sis, pan″cre·ol′y·sis. Destruction of the pancreas. —**pancreatolyt′ic,** *adj.*

pan″cre·a·tot′o·my. Incision of the pancreas.

pan″cre·a·tro′pic, pan″cre·a·to·to′pic. Pertaining to a postulated hormone of the anterior pituitary gland, which stimulates the cells of the pancreatic islets.

pan″cre·op′a·thy, pan″cre·o·path′i·a. Disease of the pancreas.

pan·de′mi·a, pan′de·my. An epidemic that attacks all persons.

pan·dem′ic. Epidemic over a wide geographic area.

pan·dic″u·la′tion. The act of stretching the limbs, especially on waking from sleep, accompanied by yawning.

pan″e·lec′tro·scope. An inspection apparatus for use in proctoscopy, esophagoscopy, urethroscopy, etc. It throws concentrated light through the whole tube, thus illuminating the spot that is to be inspected.

pan″es·the′si·a (pan″ess·thee′zhuh, ·zee·uh). General or total sensation; cenesthesia. —**panesthet′ic,** *adj.*

pang. A momentary, sharp pain. **breast p.** Angina pectoris.

pan·gen′e·sis. Darwin's comprehensive theory of heredity and development, according to which all parts of the body give off gemmules which aggregate in the germ cells. During development they are sorted out from one another and give rise to parts similar to those of their origin.

pan·glos′si·a. Excessive or psychotic garrulity.

pan″hi·dro′sis. Generalized perspiration.

pan·hy′grous. Damp as to the entire surface.

pan″hys·ter·ec′to·my. Total extirpation of the uterus.

pan·hys″ter·o·col·pec′to·my. Complete removal of the uterus and vagina.

pan·hys″ter·o·o″ö·pho·rec′to·my. Excision of the entire uterus and one or both ovaries.

pan·hys″ter·o·sal″pin·gec′to·my (·sal″pin·jeck′to·mee). Excision of the entire uterus and the oviducts.

pan·hys″ter·o·sal·pin″go·o″ö·pho·rec′to·my. Excision of the uterus, oviducts, and ovaries.

pan′ic. An extreme anxiety attack during which the person may become temporarily incapacitated.

pan″im·mu′ni·ty. General immunity to disease.

pa·niv′o·rous. Subsisting on bread.

pan·mne′si·a (pan·nee′zhuh, ·zee·uh). A potential remembrance of all impressions.

panmycin. A trade-mark for tetracycline, 3.

pan″my·e·loph′thi·sis (pan″migh·i·lof′thi·sis, pan·migh″i·lof·thigh′sis). A general wasting of the bone marrow. O.T.

pan″my·e·lo′sis (pan″migh·i·lo′sis). Proliferation of all the constituents of bone marrow.

pan·my″e·lo·tox″i·co′sis. A condition in which all elements of the bone marrow are affected.

pan·nic″u·li′tis. Inflammation of the panniculus adiposus. **nodular nonsuppurative p.** That form characterized by the formation of painful nodules in the subcutaneous fat. Also called *Weber-Christian's disease.*

pan·nic′u·lus. A membrane or layer. **p. adiposus.** The layer of subcutaneous fat. **p. carnosus.** The layer of muscles contained in the superficial fascia. It is well developed in the lower animals, but in man is represented mainly by the platysma.

pan′nus. 1. Vascularization and connective-tissue deposition beneath the epithelium of the cornea. 2. Chloasma. 3. Connective tissue overgrowing the articular surface of a diarthrodial joint.

pan″oph·thal·mi′tis. Inflammation of all the tissues of the eyeball. Also called *panophthalmia.* **p. purulenta.** A severe form, with great protrusion of the eyeball and formation of pus, usually resulting in blindness.

pan″os·te·i′tis. An inflammation of all parts of a bone.

pan″o·ti′tis. A diffuse inflammation of all parts of the ear, usually beginning in the internal ear.

panparnit. Trade-mark for caramiphen hydrochloride.

pan″scle·ro′sis. Complete hardening of a part.

pan·si″nus·i′tis (pan·sigh″nuh·sigh′tis, ·sigh″new·sigh′tis). Inflammation of all the air sinuses of the nose or head.

pant. Breathe hard or quickly.

pan″ta·mor′phi·a. General deformity. **—pantamorphic,** *adj.*

pan″ta·pho′bi·a. Total absence of fear.

pan″ta·som′a·tous (pan″tuh·som′uh·tus, ·so′muh·tus). Involving the entire body.

pan″ta·tro′phi·a, pan·tat′ro·phy. Complete or general atrophy.

pan·ther′a·pist. One who treats upon the basis of any available remedial agent.

pan′to-. See *pan-.*

pan′to·caine. A term occasionally applied to tetracaine hydrochloride.

pan′to·graph″. An instrument for the mechanical copying of diagrams, etc., upon the same scale, or upon an enlarged or a reduced scale.

pantopaque. A proprietary compound, ethyl iodophenylundecylate, which is opaque to the x-ray and is used in roentgenographic visualization.

pan″to·pho′bi·a. Morbid fear of everything; a symptom present in some cases of psychasthenia.

pantopon. Trade-mark for a preparation containing all the alkaloids of opium in the form of hydrochlorides, and in the relative proportion in which they occur in the whole gum.

pan″top·to′sis. A condition in which several viscera are prolapsed.

pan″to·then′ic ac′id. $CH_2OH.-C(CH_3)_2CHOH.CONH.CH_2.CH_2COOH.$ $\alpha,-\gamma$-Dihydroxy-β,β-dimethylbutyryl-$\beta′$-alanide. A factor of the vitamin-B complex.

pan″to·then′yl al′co·hol. $\alpha-\gamma$-Dihydroxy-N-(3-hydroxypropyl)-β,β-dimethylbutyramide, a substance which is converted in the body to pantothenic acid and which, because of its greater stability, is sometimes used in place of the acid.

pan″toyl·tau′rine. $HOCH_2.-C(CH_3)_2.CHOH.CO.NH.CH_2.CH_2.SO_3H.$ A substance antagonistic to pantothenic acid for a variety of microörganisms but not to those which can synthesize pantothenic acid. Also called *thiopanic acid.*

pa′nus. An inflamed, nonsuppurating lymph node.

pap. A soft, semiliquid food for infants.

pa·pa′in (pa·pay′in, pay′puh·in). An enzyme obtained from the juice of the fruit and leaves of *Carica papaya.* Used as a digestive enzyme. Also called *papayotin.*

Pa·pa′ver. A genus of herbs of the Papaveraceae; the poppy. See *opium.*

pa·pav′er·ine (pa·pav′ur·een, ·in,

pa·pay'vur·). $C_{20}H_{21}O_4N$. An alkaloid obtained from opium. **p. hydrochloride.** $C_{20}H_{21}O_4N.HCl$, the hydrochloride of an alkaloid obtained from opium; occurs as white crystals, or powder; soluble in water. Papaverine relaxes smooth muscle.

pa·paw'. 1. The seed of *Asimina triloba*; has been used as an emetic. **2.** See *papaya*.

pa·pa'ya (pa-pah'yuh, pa-pay'uh). Melon tree; papaw; *Carica papaya*, a tree of the Passifloraceae. The unripe fruit yields a milky juice containing papain.

pap''a·yo'tin (pa-pah'yo-tin, papay'o-tin). See *papain*.

pa'per. A processed material pressed into thin sheets; made from wood pulp, cloth, or other substances. **mustard p.** A mixture of powdered black mustard and an adhesive spread on paper or a thin cloth. When applied to the skin, it acts as a rubefacient. Syn., *charta sinapis*.

pa·pil'la (pl. *papillae*). **1.** A small, nipplelike eminence. **2.** A pimple or pustule. —**pap'illary,** *adj.* **filiform p.** Any one of the papillae occurring on the dorsum and margins of the oral part of the tongue, consisting of an elevation of connective tissue covered by a layer of epithelium. Variously divided to appear shredded. **foliate p.** One of the papillae, similar in structure to the vallate papillae, found on the posterolateral margin of the tongue of many mammals, but vestigial or absent in man. **fungiform p.** One of the low, broad papillae scattered over the dorsum and margins of the tongue. **gustatory p.** A papilla of the tongue which is furnished with taste buds. **incisive p.** The oval or pear-shaped thickening of the palatine mucous membrane overlying the incisive fossa and containing vestiges of the nasopalatine ducts. Also called *palatine p.*, *incisive pad*. **lacrimal p.** A small, conical eminence on the eyelid at the inner canthus pierced by the lacrimal punctum. **mammary p.** The nipple of the breast. **vallate p.** One of the large, flat papillae, each surrounded by a trench, in a group anterior to the sulcus terminalis of the tongue. Syn., *circumvallate p.* **vascular p.** A dermal papilla containing capillary loops.

pap'il·late. Having small papillary or nipplelike projections.

pap''il·leo'to·my. Surgical removal of a papilla or papillae.

pa·pil''le·de'ma. Edema of the optic nerve. If severe, it may result in choked disk or papillitis.

pap''il·li'tis. Inflammation of the optic disk. Also called *optic neuritis*.

pap''il·lo'ma. A neoplastic growth of surface epithelium, supported on cores or papillae of vascularized connective tissue. May arise from skin, mucous membranes, or glandular ducts, such as those of mammary glands, glandular acini, and acinar spaces of adenomas and adenocarcinomas. Similar growths may arise from serous surfaces and are covered with mesothelial cells. The epithelial papillomas are benign, but tend to recur unless completely eradicated. They may be caused by a virus, as those of the skin. Others, as those of the bladder, may be due to chemical factors such as the products of anilines. —**papillomatous,** *adj.*

pap''il·lo''ma·to'sis. The widespread formation of papillomas; also the state of being affected with multiple papillomas. **verrucose p. of mouth.** Warty vegetations in the mouth that are very difficult to cure. Growths appear similar to the condyloma acuminatum seen on the genitalia.

pap''il''lo·ret''i·ni'tis. Inflammation of the optic disk and retina.

pap'pose. Covered with fine downy hair.

pap'pus. The fine downy hair first appearing on the cheeks and chin.

pa·pri'ka (pa-pree'kuh, pap'ri-kuh). The dried pulverized capsules of *Capsicum annum*. Also called *Spanish pepper*, *Turkish pepper*.

pap''u·la'tion. The stage, in certain eruptions, marked by papule formation.

pap'ule, pap'u·la. A small, circumscribed, solid elevation of the skin, varying in size from that of a pin point to that of a split pea. —**papular,** *adj.*

pap''u·lif'er·ous. Covered with papules.

pap''u·lo·er''y·them'a·tous (pap''yoo-lo-err''ith-em'uh-tus, -eem'uh-tus). Having a papular eruption superimposed on a generalized erythema.

pap''u·lo·pus'tu·lar. Characterized by both papules and pustules.

pap''u·lo·squa'mous. Characterized by both papules and scales.

pap''u·lo·ve·sic'u·lar. Characterized by both papules and vesicles.

pap''y·ra'ce·ous (pap''i·ray'shus, -see-us). Resembling paper, as the papyraceous plate of the ethmoid bone.

par'a-, par-. 1. A prefix signifying *beyond, beside, near*. **2.** *In chemistry,* a prefix (to a derivative of the benzene ring) indicating the substitution of two atoms of hydrogen situated opposite each other, in the 1,4-position. Symbol, p-. **3.** *In medicine,* a prefix denoting *a faulty or abnormal condition, associated in an accessory capacity, remotely or indirectly related to, or almost, closely resembling*.

par″a-ac″et·phe·net′i·din (par″-uh-ass″et-fi-net′i-din, par″uh-a-set″·). See *acetphenetidin*.

par″a-a·mi″no·ben·zo′ic ac′id (par″uh-a-mee″no-ben-zo′ick, par″uh-am″i-no·). $C_6H_4NH_2COOH$. A yellowish red, crystalline substance. It inhibits the action of sulfonamides, and is considered to be essential for the metabolism of bacteria. Syn., *PABA*. Also called *vitamin H′, vitamin B_x*.

par″a-a·mi″no·sal″i·cyl′ic ac′id. $C_6H_3(NH_2)(OH)(COOH)$. 4-Aminosalicylic acid or 4-amino-2-hydroxybenzoic acid, a white, crystalline substance, soluble in water. It is bacteriostatic against tubercle bacilli. Also designated as *PAS, PASA*.

par″a-an″al·ge′si·a (par″uh-an″-al·jee′zee-uh, ·see·uh). Analgesia limited to the lower half of the body.

par″a-an″es·the′si·a (-an″ess-thee′zhuh, ·zee-uh). Anesthesia of the body below the waist.

par″a-ap·pen″di·ci′tis. Inflammation of the connective tissue adjacent to that part of the appendix not covered with the peritoneum.

par″a·bi·o′sis (par″uh-buy·o′sis). The experimental fusing together of two individuals or embryos so that the effects of one partner upon the other may be studied. —**parabiot′ic,** *adj.*

par″a·blep′sis. False or perverted vision.

par″a·bu′li·a. Abnormality of volitional action.

par·ac″an·tho′ma. A new growth affecting the prickle-cell layer of the epidermis.

par″a·ca′se·in. A digestion product of casein, formed through the action of rennin.

par″a·cen·te′sis. Puncture; especially the puncture or tapping of the wall of a cavity by means of a hollow needle or trochar, to draw off the contained fluid. **abdominal p.** Puncture of the abdominal wall with an abdominal trochar and cannula, usually for the relief of ascites. **p. bulbi.** Surgical puncture of the eye. **p. oculi.** Surgical puncture of the eye. **p. of the bladder.** The puncture of the urinary bladder wall with a vesical trochar to relieve obstruction or to provide constant drainage. **p. of the chest.** The insertion of a needle or trochar into the pleural cavity for the relief of pleural effusion. **p. of the pericardium.** The insertion of a hollow needle into the pericardium in pericarditis with effusion. **p. of the tympanum.** The insertion of a paracentesis needle or knife through the tympanic membrane, for the relief of otitis media.

par″a·chlo″ro·phe′nol. $C_6H_4(Cl)$-

OH. A substitution product of phenol. It is antiseptic and disinfectant.

par″a·cho′li·a (par″uh·ko′lee-uh) 1. Any abnormality in the secretion o bile. 2. The prodrome of disturbed liver-cell activity, in consequence of which bile is present in the blood and lymph.

par″a·chro′ma. Change in color, a of the skin.

par″a·chro′ma·tism. False, or in-correct, perception of color. It is no the same as true color blindness, which it may approach more or less completely.

par″a·chro′mo·phore. Pigment excreted or retained either withir cells or in the capsule surrounding the cell. It is not an integral part of the cytoplasm of the cell. The term is ap-plied to bacteria and fungi. —**para-chromophor′ic, parachromo-phor′ous,** *adj.*

par·ac′me (par·ack′mee). 1. The de-generation or decadence of a group o organisms after they have reached their acme of development. 2. Th period of decline of a disease.

Par″a·coc·cid″i·oi′des (par″uh cock·sid″ee·oy′deez). A genus of yeast-like fungi. **P. brasiliensis.** A specie which is the etiologic agent of paracoc-cidioidomycosis. It reproduces by mul-tiple budding cells and thereby differ from the singly budding cells of th *Blastomyces dermatitidis.*

par″a·coc·cid″i·oi″do·my·co′ sis (par″uh·cock·sid″ee·oy″do·migh ko′sis). A disease clinically similar to blastomycosis and coccidioidomycosis caused by *Paracoccidioides brasiliensis* It is a chronic granulomatous diseas of the skin which may involve th lymph nodes and viscera; usually fatal Syn., *South American blastomycosis paracoccidioidal granuloma.*

par″a·co·li′tis. Inflammation of th tissue adjacent to the colon, not cov ered by peritoneum.

par″a·co′lon. A group of bacteri intermediate between the *Escherichia Aerobacter* genera and the *Salmonella Shigella* group. Culturally, these or ganisms may be confused with the non lactose-fermenting pathogenic bacteri found in the intestinal tract. Some o the paracolon bacilli probably produc disease.

par″a·col·pi′tis. Inflammation o the connective tissue about the vagin

par″a·col′pi·um. The connectiv tissue about the vagina.

par″a·co′to. A South American tre *Ocotea pseudocoto* of the Lauracea the bark of which contains a neutr substance, paracotoin.

par″a·co′to·in (par″uh·ko′to·i ·ko·to′in). $C_{12}H_8O_4$. A crystalline su stance obtained from paracoto bark.

par″a·cre′sol. C_7H_8O. One of the three isomeric forms of cresol, *q.v.*

par″a·cu′si·a (par″a·cue′zhuh, par″a·koo′·), **par″a·cu′sis** (par″a·cue′sis, -koo′sis). Any perversion of the sense of hearing. **p. acris.** Excessively acute hearing, rendering the person intolerant of sounds. **p. duplicata.** A condition in which all or only certain sounds are heard double. **p. imaginaria.** Tinnitus. **p. localis.** Difficulty in estimating the direction of sounds, met with in unilateral deafness, or when the two ears hear unequally. **p. obtusa.** Difficulty in hearing. **p. Willisii.** A condition of deafness in which the hearing is better in a noisy place, as in a train or factory.

par″a·cy·e′sis (par″uh·sigh·ee′sis). Extrauterine pregnancy.

par″a·cys′tic. Situated near, or alongside, the urinary bladder.

par″a·cys·ti′tis. Inflammation of the connective tissue surrounding the urinary bladder.

par″a·cy′tic (par″uh·sigh′tick). Lying among cells.

par″a·de·ni′tis. Inflammation of the areolar tissue about a gland.

par″a·den′tal. Near, or beside, a tooth.

par″a·did′y·mis. The atrophic remains of a few tubules of the caudal mesonephros, which separate from the mesonephric duct and lie near the convolutions of the epididymal duct. Also called *organ of Giraldès.*

par″a·dox′i·a sex″u·al′is. Sexual excitement occurring independently of the period of the physiologic processes in the generative organs; the abnormal exhibition of sexual instincts in childhood, prior to puberty, or in the senile years.

par″a·du′o·de′nal (par″uh·dew′-o·dee′nul, ·dew·od′i·nul). On either side of the duodenum, as paraduodenal mesenteric recess.

par″a·dys′en·ter″y. A mild form of dysentery.

par″a·ep′i·lep″sy. An abortive epileptic attack, consisting only of the aura.

par′af·fin. 1. Any saturated hydrocarbon having the formula C_nH_{2n+2}. These compounds constitute the **paraffin series.** Also called *alkane.* 2. A purified mixture of solid hydrocarbons obtained from petroleum; occurs as a white, more or less translucent, mass. **chlorinated p.** A liquid paraffin which has been treated with chlorine; occurs as a light yellow to light amber, clear, thick, oily liquid; immiscible with water. See *chlorcosane.* Also see *parresine.* **light liquid p.** See light liquid *petrolatum.* **liquid p.** See liquid *petrolatum.*

par″af·fi·no′ma. A nodular mass of inflammatory, granulation, or scar tissue, due to injection of paraffin into the tissues.

par″a·floc′cu·lus. A small lobule of the cerebellum found in mammals other than man.

par″a·form·al′de·hyde. $(CH_2O)_n$. A polymer of formaldehyde, or, more properly, a mixture of polyoxymethylenes; occurs as a white, friable mass or a white powder, slowly soluble in cold water. It is employed for generating small quantities of formaldehyde. Also called *paraform, trioxymethylene.*

par″a·fuch′sin (par″uh·fook′sin, ·fook′sin). See *pararosaniline.*

par″a·gam′ma·cism, par″a·gam″ma·cis′mus. Inability to pronounce the hard *g* and *k*, other consonants being substituted.

par″a·gan″gli·o′ma. A tumor derived from the chromaffin cells of ganglions and endocrine glands. In adrenals, it is usually called pheochromocytoma or chromaffinoma. Paraganglioma is applied especially to tumors of other chromaffin tissues, such as chromaffin bodies. Also called *paraganglioneuroma.*

par″a·gan′gli·ons. Groups of paraganglionic or chromaffin cells scattered along the ventral surface of the aorta, especially in the fetus. Also called *abdominal paraganglions of Zuckerkandl.*

par″a·geu′si·a (par″ug·yoo′see·uh, par″uh·jew′see·uh), **par″a·geu′sis** (par″ug·yoo′sis, par″uh·jew′sis). Perversion of the sense of taste. —**parageusio,** *adj.*

par″ag·glu″ti·na′tion. Agglutination of colon bacilli and cocci with the serum of patients infected with or recovering from infection with dysentery bacilli. The property of paragglutination disappears when the bacteria are subcultured.

par″a·glos′sa. Swelling of the tongue; a hypertrophy of the tongue, usually congenital.

par″a·glos′si·a. Inflammation of the muscles and connective tissues under the tongue.

par″a·gom·pho′sis. Impaction of the fetal head in the pelvic canal.

Par″a·gon′i·mus. A genus of trematode worms. **P. westermani.** Species of lung flukes which in the adult stage cause tissue destruction, inflammation, and hemorrhage.

par″a·gram′ma·tism. Aphasia marked by inability to speak grammatically, or by the use of improper words.

par″a·graph′i·a (par″uh·graf′ee·uh, ·gray′fee·uh). 1. Perverted writing; a form of aphasia in which letters or words are misplaced or improperly used. 2. A loss of ability to express ideas in writing, usually the result of a brain lesion. **—paragraphic,** *adj.*

par″a‧hep″a‧ti′tis. Inflammation of structures about or near the liver.

par″a‧hex′yl. Synhexyl, *q.v.*

par″a‧hy‧drox″y‧ben‧zo′ic ac′id (par″uh‧high‧drock″see‧). C_6H_4.-OH.COOH. An isomer of salicylic acid; its esters are powerful antiseptics.

par″a‧hyp‧no′sis. Abnormal sleep, as that of hypnotism or of narcosis.

par″a‧in″flu‧en′za. 1. Similar to influenza; conditions due to influenza. 2. *In bacteriology,* organisms having all but a few of the growth characteristics of *Hemophilus influenzae.* **—parainfluenzal,** *adj.*

par″a‧ker″a‧to′sis. The retention of nuclei in the stratum corneum of the epidermis. Usually associated with some inflammation in the prickle-cell layer, resulting in a disturbance in the process of keratinization. Occurs normally in the stratified squamous epithelium of true mucous membranes.

par″a‧la′li‧a. Disturbance of the faculty of speech, characterized by distortion of sounds.

par‧al′de‧hyde. (CH_3COH)₃. A polymer of acetaldehyde, occurring as a colorless, transparent liquid, soluble in water. Used as a somnifacient where rapid action is desired. Syn., *paracetaldehyde.*

par″a‧lep‧ro′sis. Attenuated or modified form of leprosy.

par″a‧le‧re′ma. Mild delirium or delirious utterance.

par″a‧le‧re′sis. Mild delirium, or moderate mental disturbance.

par″a‧lex′i‧a. Disturbance in reading, marked by the substitution or transposition of words or syllables. **—paralexic,** *adj.*

par″al‧ge′si‧a (par″al‧jee′zee‧uh, ‧see‧uh). An abnormal, painful sensation; painful paresthesia. **—paralgesic,** *adj.*

par‧al′gi‧a. Any perverted and disagreeable cutaneous sensation, as of formication, cold, or burning.

par‧al′lax. The apparent displacement of an object, caused by a change in the position of the observer, or by looking at the object alternately first with one eye and then with the other. **—parallactic,** *adj.*

pa‧ral′ler‧gy. Sensitivity to nonspecific proteins, induced by specific sensitization.

par″a‧lo′gi‧a. Difficulty in thinking logically. **thematic p.** A condition in which the thought is unduly concentrated on one subject.

pa‧ral′o‧gism. *In logic,* the error of considering effects or unrelated phe-

nomena as the cause of a conditi... **—paralogis′tic,** *adj.*

pa‧ral′y‧sis. Loss of muscle functi... or of sensation, caused by injury ... nerves or by destruction of neuron... A slight loss of function is called pals... *q.v.* **abducens p.** Paralysis of t... abducens nerve. **abductor p.** Para... ysis of the posterior cricoaryteno... muscle. Also called *posticus* p. a... **commodation p.** Paralysis of t... ciliary muscle of the eye. **acute a... cending p.** A syndrome of vari... etiology, characterized by flaccid para... ysis beginning in the muscles of the le... and spreading upward to involve t... arms and other parts of the bod... It may occur in anterior poliomyelit... postvaccinal or postexanthematous m... elitis. Also called *Landry's* p. **alc... holic p.** That due to alcoholic ne... ropathy. **alternating p.** Paralys... of various cranial nerves or their nucl... on one side, with a contralater... hemiplegia. **ambiguospinoths... lamic p.** A unilateral paralysis of t... soft palate and larynx with contr... lateral loss of deep sensibility and... pain and temperature. Also call... *Avellis' syndrome.* **amyotrophic p...** That seen in muscular atrophy. **a... apeiratic p.** A neurosis in whi... the subject believes he is paralyz... from excessive use of his limbs. **a... terior spinal p.** Anterior poliomy... litis. **arsenical p.** Paresthesia a... peripheral neuritis developing in t... later stages of arsenic poisonin... **ascending p.** Paralysis progressi... upward, due to involvement of spin... nerves or the spinal cord. **assoc... ated p.** A common paralysis or spas... of associated muscles. **axillary** ... Paralysis of the axillary nerve resul... ing in the loss of function of the de... toid muscle; usually due to fracture ... dislocation of the humerus, or to pre... sure from a crutch. **basal gangl... onic p.** One due to destruction ... cells in the basal ganglions. **Bell's** ... Peripheral paralysis of the facial nerv... **birth p.** Paralysis caused by inju... of the brain or brachial plexus duri... birth. **brachial p.** Paralysis of t... arm. **brachiofacial p.** Paralys... involving the face and arm. **Brow... Séquard's p.** Ipsilateral motor p... ralysis and contralateral loss of sens... tion for pain and temperature, due ... a unilateral lesion of the spinal co... such as tumor compression or tra... matic hemisection. **bulbar p. S... progressive bulbar p. capsular** ... That due to an injury of the intern... capsule. **central p.** Paralysis due ... a lesion of the brain or spinal co... **cerebral p.** That due to a lesion ... the brain. **cerebral spastic i... fantile p.** See spastic *diplegia.* **ci...**

cumflex p. See axillary p. **compression p.** That caused by pressure on a nerve. **crossed p.** Paralysis of the arm and leg of one side, associated with contralateral paralysis of facial or ocular muscles. **crural p.** Paralysis involving chiefly the thigh. **crutch p.** Paralysis of the muscles of the upper extremity, due to traumatic neuritis of the brachial plexus and especially of the radial nerve from pressure of the crutch head. **diphtheritic p.** That due to the effect of diphtheria toxin upon some part of the nervous system, usually the motor components of the cranial nerves or the motor nerves to the extremities. **diver's p.** See caisson disease. **epidural ascending spinal p.** A low-grade inflammation of the dura associated with thrombophlebitis of the meningorachidian veins; characterized by pain in the back, chest, or legs, followed by paralysis, loss of sensibility, and incontinence. Also called *Spiller's syndrome.* **Erb-Duchenne p.** Paralysis of the fifth and sixth cervical nerve roots, involving chiefly the functions of the biceps, deltoid, brachialis, and brachioradialis muscles. **essential p.** Paralysis without characteristic anatomic lesions. **extraocular p.** That involving the extrinsic muscles of the eye. **facial p.** Paralysis of the muscles of expression of the face. There are two types, the central or supranuclear type, and the peripheral or infranuclear type. **familial periodic p.** A hereditary disease of unknown etiology; characterized by periodic attacks of flaccid muscular paralysis, which develop abruptly and last from a few hours to several days. **flaccid p.** A condition in which the muscle manifests loss of muscular tone, diminished or absent tendon reflexes, and, eventually, atrophy and the electric reaction of degeneration. **functional motor p.** See hysterical p. **functional p.** See hysterical p. **general p.** See general p. of the insane. **general p. of the insane.** A form of neurosyphilis involving chiefly the cortex of the frontal and temporal lobes; characterized clinically by mental changes, tremors, disturbances of speech, apoplectiform and epileptiform seizures, and pupillary changes. Now called *dementia paralytica, general paresis, general paralysis.* **glossolabial p.** Paralysis of the tongue and lips in bulbar paralysis. **glossolabiopharyngeal p.** One involving the tongue, lips, and pharynx, occurring in bulbar palsy. Also called *labioglossopharyngeal p.* **hysterical p.** Muscle weakness or paralysis without loss of reflex activity, in which no organic nerve lesion can be demon-

strated. **infantile p.** Acute anterior poliomyelitis, a virus infection of the nervous system involving chiefly the anterior horn cells of the spinal cord and, occasionally, the motor nuclei of the medulla oblongata. Characterized by an acute febrile onset with flaccid paralysis and atrophy of muscle groups. **infantile spastic p.** See spastic diplegia. **infranuclear p.** Paralysis of the motor function of a cranial nerve, due to a lesion of the nerve peripheral to its nucleus. **ischemic p.** That of a part due to stoppage of the circulation, as in certain cases of embolism or thrombosis, or in Volkmann's paralysis. **jake p.** Paralysis due to peripheral neuritis, caused by the ingestion of Jamaica ginger. **Jamaica ginger p.** See jake p. **juvenile p.** General paralysis in young persons. **Landry's p.** See acute ascending p. **lead p.** One due to peripheral neuritis from lead poisoning. **mimetic p.** Paralysis of the facial muscles. **mixed p.** Associated motor and sensory paralysis. **motor p.** The loss of voluntary control of skeletal muscle, due to functional or organic interruption at any point in the motor pathway from the cerebral cortex to, and including, the muscle fiber. **myopathic p.** That in which the interruption of voluntary control is in the muscle. **nuclear p.** Paralysis from lesions of the nuclei of origin of the nerves. **obstetric p.** One due to injury of some part of the nervous system at birth. **occupational p.** Muscular weakness and paralysis due to nerve compression or overexertion in certain occupations. **ocular p.** Paralysis of the extraocular muscles, of the optic nerve, or of the ciliary muscle. **oculomotor p.** Paralysis of the oculomotor nerve. **oculophrenicorecurrent p.** That of the recurrent laryngeal and phrenic nerves with associated Horner's syndrome, such as may occur in cancer of the lung with mediastinal extension. **p. agitans.** A disturbance of motor function characterized chiefly by slowing and weakness of emotional and voluntary movement, muscular rigidity, and tremor; it is due to degeneration of the ganglion cells of the corpus striatum. Also called *Parkinsonism, Parkinson's disease.* **periodic p.** A recurrent paralysis. Also see familial periodic p. **peripheral p.** Paralysis due to any disease of peripheral nerves. **phonetic p.** Paralysis of the vocal folds. **pressure p.** That due to pressure on a nerve trunk. **progressive bulbar p.** Progressive and symmetrical paralysis of the muscles of the tongue, throat, face, and sometimes of the larynx, due to degenerative changes in the motor nuclei of the medulla oblongata. **pseudobulbar p.** Symmetrical disease of both cerebral hemispheres, involving the centers or paths of the tracts to cranial nerves in the brain stem; resembles disease of the medulla oblongata and causes voluntary paralysis of swallowing, articulation, and chewing movements, with retention of bulbar reflexes. **pseudohypertrophic muscular p.** Loss or diminution of the power of motion, accompanied by enlarged, and apparently hypertrophied, muscles. The most important type is progressive muscular dystrophy, also called *Landouzy-Déjèrine p.* **Saturday night p.** Paralysis due to compression of the radial nerve against the humerus during sleep, or when the arm is hung over the edge of a chair or bench during alcoholic stupor. **sensory p.** Loss of sensation due to disease of sensory nerves, pathways, or centers in the nervous system. **spastic p.** A condition in which a group of muscles manifests increased tone, exaggerated tendon reflexes, depressed or absent superficial reflexes, and, sometimes, clonus. **spinal p.** A central paralysis caused by injury to the spinal cord. **supranuclear p.** That of the motor function of a nerve, due to a lesion in pathways or centers above its nucleus or cells of origin. **tick p.** A flaccid type of paralysis occurring in animals and occasionally in children during the attachment of a tick. The paralysis will disappear a few hours after removal of the tick. The cause is unknown, but it is thought to be a toxin generated in the tick. **Todd's p.** A temporary paralysis which sometimes follows a focal Jacksonian convulsive seizure. **tourniquet p.** Pressure paralysis caused by too long application of a tourniquet to a limb while checking hemorrhage. It is most common in the nerves of the arm. **vasomotor p.** Paralysis of the vasomotor mechanism with resultant atony and dilatation of the blood vessels. **Volkmann's p.** Paralysis of a hand due to constriction of the blood supply when tight splints or casts are applied to the forearm. See *ischemic p.* **writer's p.** Writer's cramp, a form of occupational neurosis.

par″a·lyt′ic. 1. Pertaining to, or affected with, paralysis. 2. A person affected with paralysis.

par′a·ly″zant, par′a·ly″sant (par″ih-lye″zunt). 1. Causing paralysis. 2. An agent or drug that induces paralysis.

par′a·ly″zer. 1. Anything that will produce paralysis. 2. Any agent which will inhibit a chemical reaction.

par″a·mag·net′ic. Exhibiting a magnetic permeability greater than unity.

par″a·mag′net·ism. The phenomena exhibited by paramagnetic substances.

par″a·mas·ti′tis. Inflammation of the connective tissue about the mammary gland.

par″a·mas″toid·i′tis. Inflammation of the squamous portion of the temporal bone, from extension following mastoiditis.

par″a·me′ni·a. Difficult or disordered menstruation.

pa·ram′e·ter. An arbitrary constant which characterizes a mathematical expression by its values.

par″a·met′ric (par″uh·met′rick, ·mee′trick). Pertaining to the tissues about the uterus.

par″a·met′rism. Pain in tissues about the uterus.

par″a·me·tri′tis. Inflammation of the connective tissue about the uterus, pelvic cellulitis. —**parametrit′ic,** *adj.* **p. anterior.** That in which the inflammation is limited to the loose, vesicouterine connective tissue, or to that between the symphysis and the bladder. The swelling is anterior, and the pus generally tracks into the bladder, vagina, or inguinal region. **p. chronica atrophicans.** Inflammatory hypertrophy of the connective tissue of the pelvis, progressing to cicatricial atrophy. **p. chronica posterior.** Chronic, inflammatory processes in the rectouterine ligaments causing fixation of the uterus at the level of the internal os, anteflexion by shortening of the ligaments, and torsion of the uterus when only one ligament is shortened. **remote p.** Parametritis marked by formation of abscesses in places more or less remote from the focus of the disease.

par″a·me′tri·um. The connective tissue surrounding the uterus. —**parametrial,** *adj.*

par″a·me·trop′a·thy. Disease of the parametrium.

par″a·mim′i·a. A form of aphasia characterized by the faulty use of gestures.

par″am·ne′si·a (par″am·nee′zhuh, ·zee·uh). Perversion of memory, in which experiences and phantasies are confused.

par″a·mor′phine (par″uh·mor′feen, par″uh·mor·feen′). See *thebaine.*

par″a·mor′phism. *In chemistry,* change of molecular structure without alteration of chemical constitution, as when a mineral changes from one modification to another. —**paramorphic,** *adj.*

par″a·mu′si·a (par″uh·mew′zhuh ·zee·uh). A form of aphasia in which there is perversion of the musical sense, resulting in the production of improper notes and intervals.

par″a·my·oc′lo·nus mul′ti·plex (par″uh·migh·ock′lo·nus, ·migh″o·klo′nus). A rare degenerative disease occurring in adult life manifested by irregular rapid muscular twitching (myoclonic shocks). The seat of the disease is in the basal ganglions.

par″a·my″o·to′ni·a con·gen′i·ta. A rare, heredofamilial condition characterized by persistent contraction of the muscles of the neck, face, and extremities when the body is exposed to cold. Also called *Eulenburg's disease.*

par″a·na′sal (par″uh·nay′zul). Located next to, or near, the nasal cavities.

par″a·ne·phri′tis. 1. Inflammation of the adrenal gland. 2. Inflammation of the connective tissue adjacent to the kidney.

par″a·neu′ral. Beside or near a nerve, as paraneural analgesia, analgesia resulting from injection of an analgesic solution into the immediate vicinity of a nerve trunk.

par″a·noi′a. A psychosis characterized by well-systematized delusions of persecution and frequently hallucinations, usually of an auditory nature. —**par′anoid,** *adj.;* **paranoiac,** *adj.,* n. **litigious p.** That in which the main symptom is a desire to initiate lawsuits which have no rational basis.

par″a·noid·ism. The condition of a person affected with paranoia.

par″a·nu′cle·in. A compound of nucleic acid and protein, derived either by partial degradation of nucleoproteins or by direct combination. Syn., *nucleoalbumin, paranucleoprotein, pseudonuclein.*

par″a·nu′cle·us. 1. An irregular, spherical body lying in the cytoplasm of a cell near the nucleus, and perhaps extruded by the latter. 2. A mitochondrial aggregation of a spermatid, which becomes drawn out to form the envelope of the axial filament. Also called *nebenkern.* —**paranuclear, para·nucleate,** *adj.*

par″a·pan″cre·at′ic (par″uh·pan″kree·at′ick, ·pang″kree·at′ick). Situated beside or near the pancreas, as parapancreatic abscess.

par″a·pha′si·a (par″uh·fay′zhuh, ·zee·uh). A form of aphasia in which words are spoken freely but are inappropriate in translating ideas. —**paraphasic,** *adj.*

par″a·phe″ne·tol·car·bam′ide (·kahr·bam′ide, ·kahr′buh·mide). See *dulcin.*

par″a·phen″yl·ene″di·am′ine. $C_6H_4(NH_2)_2$. A crystalline substance

used in the manufacture of certain hair dyes.

par″a·phi·mo′sis (par″uh·figh·mo′sis, ·fi·mo′sis). Retraction and constriction, especially of the prepuce behind the glans penis. **p. oculi.** Retraction of the eyelid behind the eyeball.

par″a·pho′bi·a. A slight degree of phobia; phobia which the person can control by effort.

par″a·pho′ni·a. Any abnormal condition of the voice. **p. puberum.** The harsh, deep, irregular voice noticed in boys at puberty.

pa·raph′o·ra. 1. Slight mental derangement or distraction. 2. Unsteadiness due to intoxication.

par″a·phra′si·a (par″uh·fray′zhuh, ·zee·uh). A form of aphasia characterized by incoherence of speech. **p. ve·sana.** Jumbling of words and ideas.

par″a·phre·ni′tis. Inflammation of the tissues adjacent to the diaphragm.

par″a·plasm. 1. Hyaloplasm, *q.v.* 2. Malformed substance.

par″a·plas′tic. 1. Of the nature of paraplasm. 2. Having morbid formative powers. 3. Misshapen.

par″a·plec′tic. Pertaining to, or afflicted with, paraplegia.

par″a·ple·gi′a. Paralysis of the lower limbs. —**paraplec′tic, para·pleg′ic, paraplegiform,** *adj.* **alcoholic p.** Paralysis of the legs resulting from alcoholic neuritis. **ataxic p.** A slowly progressive degeneration of the posterior and lateral columns of the spinal cord; characterized clinically by spasticity, weakness, and incoördination of the legs. **cerebral p.** Paralysis of both legs due to a bilateral cerebral lesion, as in meningioma of the falx, thrombosis of the superior sagittal sinus, or congenital cerebral lesions. **congenital spastic p.** Spastic paralysis of the legs or arms due to a congenital lesion of the brain. Also called *infantile spastic p., cerebral diplegia, Little's disease.* **flaccid p.** Paralysis of both legs with muscular hypotonia and diminished, or absent, tendon reflexes. **hysterical p.** A psychogenic form, due to an emotional upset. **infantile spasmodic p.** Congenital, spastic paraplegia with athetoid movements; due to defective development of the lenticular nuclei. **p. in extension.** Paraplegia with extension of the legs; seen following incomplete transverse lesions of the spinal cord. **p. in flexion.** Paraplegia with flexion of the legs; seen following complete transection of the spinal cord. **peripheral p.** That due to disease of the peripheral nerves. **progressive spastic p.** A progressive heredofamilial condition characterized by spastic paralysis of the legs and weakness; due to spinal-cord lesions of the crossed pyramidal tracts. **senile p.** Spastic paralysis of the legs due to arteriosclerosis of the arteries supplying the spinal cord. **spastic p.** Paralysis of the legs with increased muscular tone and hyperactive tendon reflexes; commonly seen in multiple sclerosis and other diseases involving the pyramidal tracts of the spinal cord, and after birth injury.

par″a·pneu·mo′ni·a. A disease presenting the symptoms of lobar pneumonia, but not due to the pneumococcus.

pa·rap′o·plex″y. A masked or slight form of apoplexy.

par″a·prax′i·a. A condition in which certain intentional acts are imperfectly accomplished, as a slip of the tongue.

par″a·proc·ti′tis. Inflammation of the connective tissue about the rectum.

par″a·proc′ti·um (par″uh-prock′shee-um, -prock′tee-um). The connective tissue that surrounds the rectum.

par″a·pros′ta·ti′tis. Inflammation of tissues surrounding the prostate gland.

par″a·pso·ri′a·sis (par″uh-so-rye′uh-sis). A group of rare skin diseases characterized by red, scaly lesions resembling lichen planus or psoriasis. All types are resistant to treatment and usually present no subjective symptoms.

par″a·psy·chol′o·gy. The psychology that studies telepathy, clairvoyance, and other extrasensory phenomena.

par″a·rec′tal. Beside, or near, the rectum.

par″a·ro·san′i·line (par″uh-ro-zan′i-leen, -lin). A basic dyestuff of the triphenylmethane group.

par″a·sa′cral. Beside, or near, the sacrum.

par″a·sal″pin·gi′tis. Inflammation of the tissues around an oviduct.

par″a·se·cre′tion. Any abnormality of secretion; any substance abnormally secreted.

par′a·site. 1. An organism that lives on or in another organism known as the host, from which it obtains nourishment during all or part of its existence. 2. *In teratology*, a fetus or fetal parts attached to or included in another fetus. **—parasit′ic**, *adj.* **facultative p.** One capable of being free-living as well as parasitic. **incidental p.** One that establishes itself in a host in which it does not ordinarily live. **obligate p.** One incapable of living without a host. **permanent p.** One which remains in or on the body of the host until maturity and sometimes for its entire life. **specific p.** One which always lives on its present

host. **temporary p.** One which free-living during part of its life.

par″a·sit′i·cide. 1. Destructive parasites. 2. An agent capable of destroying parasites, especially the parasites living upon or in the skin.

par″a·sit′i·cin. See *flavicin*.

par″a·sit·ism (par″uh-sigh-tiz-um Relation a parasite bears to its ho state of being infested or infected wit parasites.

par″a·si·tize (par′uh-sigh-tize, par uh-si-tize). Infest; invade as a parasit

par″a·sit′o-. A combining form sign fying *parasite*.

par″a·si·tol′o·gist (par″uh-sigh tol′o-jist). A specialist in parasitolog

par″a·si·tol′o·gy (par″uh-sigh-tol o-jee). The study of parasites.

par″a·si″to·pho′bi·a. Morbid drea of parasites.

par″a·si·to′sis (par″uh-sigh-to′si ·si·to′sis). Any disease dependent up the presence of parasites.

par″a·si″to·trop′ic. 1. Having special affinity for parasites. 2. A su stance, such as a drug or a chemic agent, with an affinity for parasite **—parasi′totrope**, *adj.*, *n.*; **para sitot′ropy**, *n.*; **parasitot′r pism**, *n.*

par″a·small′pox. A mild form smallpox.

par″a·spa′di·as. An acquired co dition in which the urethra opens o one side of the penis.

par″a·spasm. Spasm involving th lower extremities, as in spastic para plegia.

par″a·sprue′. A dietary disea characterized by chronic watery dia rhea, weight loss, a sore red tongu and macrocytic anemia. It differs fro true sprue in that it shows less emaci tion, no swollen lower abdomen, no d skin, no dysphagia, and in having pal frothy stools with the fat content abo 40 per cent.

par″a·sym·pa·thet′ic. Of or rela ing to the craniosacral portion of t autonomic nervous system.

par″a·sym″pa·tho·lyt′ic. Desi nating or pertaining to a blocking the action of parasympathetic ner fibers.

par″a·sym″pa·tho·mi·met′i Designating or pertaining to dru having an effect similar to that pr duced by stimulating the parasymp thetic nerves.

par″a·te·re″si·o·ma′ni·a. mania for observing, or seeing ne sights; peeping mania.

par″a·thi′on. O,O-diethyl-O-p-n trophenyl thiophosphate, a liquid i secticide having pronounced choline terase-inhibiting action.

par″a·thor′mone. A hormone fro the parathyroids. See *parathyrin*.

par"a·thy'mi·a. Perversion of mood in which the emotions are out of harmony with the real situation.

par"a·thy'rin. A hormone produced in the parathyroid glands, which regulates phosphorus and calcium metabolism. Also called *parathormone, parathyroid hormone.*

par"a·thy'roid. 1. One of several (usually four) small endocrine glands which lie posterial to the capsule of the thyroid gland, or embedded in the gland, and near the superior and inferior thyroid arteries. Their hormone has a powerful effect on the rate of renal phosphorus excretion and the level of blood calcium. Complete removal of them causes tetany and death. 2. Lying beside the thyroid.

par"a·thy'roid·ec'to·my. Excision of a parathyroid gland.

par"a·thy'roid in·jec'tion. A sterile solution in water of the water-soluble principle or principles of the parathyroid glands. Also called *solution of parathyroid, parathyroid extract.*

par"a·thy'ro·pri'val. Pertaining to the condition due to loss of function, or removal, of the parathyroid glands.

par"a·thy"ro·tro'pic hor'mone. The anterior pituitary hormone which has a governing effect upon the activity of the parathyroid glands.

par"a·thy"ro·tro'pic prin'ci·ple. Principle obtained from the adenohypophysis, which is claimed to have a stimulative action on the parathyroid gland.

par"a·thy'ro·tro'pin. See *parathyrotropic hormone.*

par"a·ton'sil·lar. Near, or around, the tonsil, as paratonsillar abscess.

par"a·tri·cho'sis (par"uh·tri·ko'sis, ·try·ko'sis). A condition in which hair is either imperfect in growth or develops in abnormal places.

pa·rat'ro·phy. Perverted or abnormal nutrition.

par"a·typh·li'tis. Inflammation of the connective tissue near the cecum.

par"a·ty'phoid. An acute generalized disease of man caused by the paratyphoid bacteria, *Salmonella schottmuelleri* and *S. choleraesuis.* The disease resembles typhoid fever both clinically and pathologically but tends to be less severe.

par"a·vac·cin'i·a (par"uh·vack-sin'ee·uh). An eruption consisting of small vesicles outside the vaccinated area, which are not vaccinial.

par"a·vag"i·ni'tis (par"uh·vadj"-i·nigh'tis). Inflammation of the connective tissue surrounding the vagina.

par"a·ver'te·bral. Occurring or situated near the spinal column, as paravertebral analgesia, which is induced by the injection of a local anesthetic around the spinal nerves as they emerge from the intervertebral foramens.

par"a·ves'i·cal. Situated near the urinary bladder.

par"a·xan'thine (par"uh·zan'-theen, ·thin). $C_7H_8N_4O_2.$ 1,7-Dimethylxanthine. A crystalline substance found in normal urine and isomeric with theobromine.

par·ax'i·al. 1. Lying near the axis of the body. 2. Referring to the space or rays closely surrounding the principal axis of a lens system.

parch'ment crack'ling. The peculiar sound elicited by pressure on the cranial bones in rachitic and syphilitic children. It is due to localized thinning of the bones.

parch'ment skin. An atrophic type of epidermis seen in xeroderma pigmentosum, senile skin, and in some skins exposed to the wind and sun.

paredrine hydrobromide. Trademark for hydroxyamphetamine hydrobromide.

par"e·gor'ic (par"i·gorr'ick, ·gor'-ick). See camphorated *opium* tincture.

pa·rei'ra (pa·ray'ruh, pa·rair'uh). The root of *Chondodendron tomentosum,* formerly called pareira brava, containing the alkaloids bebeerine (pelosine), *d*-tubocurarine, and curine.

pa·ren'chy·ma (pa·reng'ki·muh). The essential or specialized part of an organ as distinguished from the supporting connective tissue. **—parenchymal, parenchym'atous,** *adj.*

par'ent. A father or mother.

par·en'ter·al. Outside of the intestine; not via the alimentary tract, as subcutaneous, intravenous, or intrasternal injection.

par"ep·i·thym'i·a (par"ep·i·thim'-ee·uh, ·thigh'mee·uh). A morbid desire or craving.

par"er·ga'si·a (par"ur·gay'zhuh). *In psychiatry,* Meyer's term for psychoses manifesting withdrawal, deep regression, delusions, and hallucinations, as schizophrenia and paranoia.

pa·re'sis, par'e·sis. A slight paralysis; incomplete loss of muscular power; weakness of a limb. **—paret'ic,** *adj.* **general p.** See general *paralysis* of the insane.

par"es·the'si·a (par"ess·thee'zhuh, ·zee·uh). A perverted sensation of tingling, crawling, or burning of the skin, such as occurs in peripheral neuritis and spinal-cord lesions. **—paresthet'ic,** *adj.*

par"eth·ox'y·caine hy"dro·chlo'ride. 2-Diethylaminoethyl *p*-ethoxybenzoate hydrochloride, a local anesthetic. See *intracaine hydrochloride.*

pa·reu'ni·a (pa·rōō'nee·uh). Coitus.

par·fo'cal. Pertaining to microscopical oculars and objectives which are so constructed or so mounted that, in changing from one to another, the image will remain in focus.

par″hi·dro′sis (par″hi·dro′sis, ·high·dro′sis), **par″i·dro′sis.** Any abnormal condition of the secretion of sweat.

pa′ri·es (pair′ee·eez) (pl. *parietes*). An enveloping or investing structure or wall.

pa·ri′e·tal. 1. Forming or situated on a wall, as the parietal layer of the peritoneum. 2. The parietal bone. See Table of Bones in the Appendix. 3. Pertaining to, or in relation with, the parietal bone of the skull, as the parietal foramen.

pa·ri′e·tes (pa·rye′i·teez). Plural of paries, *q.v.*

pa·ri′e·to-. *In anatomy*, a combining form signifying *parietal*.

pa·rig′e·nin (pa·ridj′i·nin, par″i·jee′nin). See *parillin*.

Par′i·glin. See *parillin*.

pa·ril′lin. A saponin obtained from sarsaparilla. Syn., *parigenin, pariglin*. Also called *parillinic acid*.

Par′is green. $Cu(C_2H_3O_2)_2.3Cu(AsO_2)_2$. Copper acetoarsenite; occurs as an emerald green powder; insoluble in water. It is used as an insecticide. Also called *imperial, Schweinfurth, Vienna* or *parrot green*.

par′i·ty. Condition of a woman with regard to the number of children she has borne.

par′i·ty. Similarity approaching equality.

Parkinsonism. Paralysis agitans.

par″o·don·ti′tis. Inflammation of the tissues near, or surrounding, a tooth.

par″o·ni′ri·a (par″o·nigh′ree·uh, ·nirr′ee·uh). Morbid dreaming.

par″o·nych′i·a (par″o·nick′ee·uh). A suppurative inflammation about the margin of a nail. —**paronychial**, *adj.* **mycotic p.** An inflammatory process at the base of the nails usually associated with *Candida albicans* infection.

par″onych″o·my·co′sis (par″o·nick″o·migh·ko′sis). A fungous infection around the nails.

par′o·ny·cho′sis (par″o·ni·ko′sis). 1. A diseased condition of the structures about the nails. 2. Growth of a nail in unusual places.

par″o·öph″o·ri′tis. 1. Inflammation of the parovarium. 2. Inflammation of the tissues about the ovary.

par″oph·thal′mi·a. Inflammation about the eye.

par″oph·thal·mon′cus. A tumor near the eye.

pa·ro′pi·a. The angle of the eyelid toward the temple.

par·op′si·a, par·op′sis. Disordered or false vision.

par·op′tic. Pertaining to colors produced by the diffraction of light rays.

par″o·ra′sis. Any perversion of vision or of color perception; a hallucination.

par″o·rex′i·a. A perverted appetite.

par·os′mi·a (par·oz′mee·uh, par·os′·). A perversion of the sense of smell. May be present in organic brain disease, in schizophrenia (olfactory hallucinations), or in psychoneurotic conditions.

par″os·ti′tis. Inflammation of the tissue adjacent to the periosteum.

par″os·to′sis. The abnormal formation of bone outside of the periosteum, or in the connective tissue surrounding the periosteum.

pa·ro′tic (pa·ro′tick, ·rot′ick). Situated near, or about, the ear.

pa·rot′id. 1. Situated near the ear, as the parotid gland. 2. Pertaining to, or affecting, the parotid gland.

pa·rot″id·ec·to·my. Excision of a parotid gland.

pa·rot″i·do·scle·ro′sis. Fibrous induration of the parotid gland.

par″o·ti′tis. Inflammation of the parotid gland, as in mumps; inflammation of the lymph node overlying the parotid (parotid bubo). Syn., *mumps* —**parotit′ic**, *adj.* **metastatic p.** That secondary to disease elsewhere; it occurs in infectious fevers, as typhoid fever, and usually goes on to suppuration. **phlegmonous p.** One which is the seat of pus formation. Also called *suppurative p.*

par′ous. Having borne one or more children.

par″o·va′ri·an (par″o·vair′ee·un) 1. Situated near the ovary. 2. Pertaining to the parovarium.

par″o·va″ri·ot′o·my. Excision of a parovarian cyst.

par″o·va′ri·um (par″o·vair′ee·um) The remnant of the mesonephros of the female; the homolog of the caput epididymidis in the male. Also called *epoöphoron, organ of Rosenmueller*.

par′ox·ysm. 1. The periodic increase or crisis in the progress of a disease; a sudden attack, a sudden reappearance of symptoms, or a sudden increase in the intensity of existing symptoms. 2. A spasm or fit; a convulsion.

parpanit. See *panparnit*.

Parr turbidimeter. A turbidimeter designed for the determination of sulfur.

parresine. Trade-mark for a protective dressing composed of paraffin, gum elemi, japan wax, asphalt, and eucalyptol.

par′rot fe′ver. See *psittacosis*.

pars (pl. *partes*). A part. **p. buc·calis.** The anterior lobe of the hypophysis. Also called *p. distalis*, *p. anterior*, *p. glandularis*. **p. cavernosa urethrae.** The cavernous or spongy portion of the male urethra. **p. intermedia.** (a) The intermediate part of the hypophysis. (b) Term formerly used for *nervus intermedius*. **p. iridica retinae.** The uveal tract. **p. membranacea urethrae.** The membranous portion of the male urethra. **p. posterior.** The posterior lobe of the hypophysis. Also called *p. neuralis*, *p. nervosa*, *processus infundibuli*, *neurohypophysis*.

parsidol hydrochloride. Trademark for ethopropazine hydrochloride.

pars'ley. *Petroselinum crispum*, a plant of the Umbelliferae, containing a volatile oil.

Parthe'ni·um. A genus of herbs of the Compositae.

par'tial. Incomplete; finished in part only.

par'ti·cle. A small portion or piece of a substance. **alpha p.** A particle, carrying two positive charges, ejected from the nucleus of a radioactive atom. When ejected in a stream, these particles are known as alpha rays. Each alpha particle is equivalent to the nucleus of a helium atom. **beta p.** An electron, usually given off in disintegration of radioactive elements. **colloid p.** One, smaller than particles visible under the optical microscope, which forms colloid solutions. **p. accelerator.** Any device for accelerating atomic particles.

par·tic'u·late. Composed of particles.

par·tu'ri·en·cy. The state of being in labor.

par·tu'ri·ent. 1. Being in labor; giving birth. 2. Traversed during birth, as the parturient canal.

par·tu''ri·fa'cient (pahr·tew''ri·fay'shunt). 1. Promoting labor. 2. An agent that induces labor.

par·tu''ri·om'e·ter. An instrument to determine the progress of labor by measuring the expulsive force of the uterus.

par''tu·ri'tion (pahr''tew·rish'un, pahr''chew·). The act of giving birth to young.

par'tus. The bringing forth of offspring; labor. **p. agrippinus.** Labor with breech presentation. **p. caesareus.** Cesarean section. **p. difficilis.** Dystocia. **p. immaturus.** Premature labor. **p. maturus.** Labor at term. **p. precipitatus.** Precipitate labor. **p. serotinus.** Labor unduly prolonged. **p. siccus.** Dry labor.

pa·ru'lis. 1. Abscess of the gum. 2. Incorrectly, a gumboil.

par''vi·cel'lu·lar. Pertaining to, or composed of, small cells.

par'vule. A small pill or pellet; a granule.

PAS. Para-aminosalicylic acid.

pass. 1. Go, or put through or by. 2. Discharge from the intestinal canal. 3. Void. 4. Introduce an instrument into a cavity or channel.

pas'sage. 1. A channel or lumen. 2. The act of passing from one place to another. 3. The introduction of an instrument into a cavity or channel. 4. An evacuation of the bowels. **air passages.** The nares, nasal cavities, pharynx, mouth, larynx, trachea, and bronchi.

pas''si·flo'ra. The rhizome of *Passiflora incarnata* (passionflower); has been used as a sedative and anodyne.

pas'sion. 1. Pain; suffering. *Obs.* 2. An intense emotion of the mind; fervid desire, overpowering emotion. 3. A specific intense excitement, as rage or ardent affection. —**passional**, *adj*.

pas'sive. Not active; not performed or produced by active efforts, but by causes coming from without.

pas'siv·ism. A form of sexual perversion in which one person submits to the will of another in unnatural erotic acts. —**passivist**, *n*.

paste. An ointmentlike preparation of medicinal substances, made into a smooth mixture with bases such as glycerin, soft soap, lard, petrolatum, or other fats.

Pasteur, Louis [*French scientist and bacteriologist*, 1822–95]. Generally regarded as the founder of modern bacteriology. His study of wine fermentations disclosed causative organisms, and disposed finally of the theory of spontaneous generation. With Joubert, discovered *vibrion septique*, the first pathogenic anaerobe to be identified. This led to Pasteur's distinction between aerobic and anaerobic bacteria. Experimented with attenuated virus in chicken cholera. Confirmed Koch's work on anthrax, and, with Chamberland and Roux, developed the first attenuated bacterial culture to be used therapeutically. With the same workers discovered the rabies virus in the blood (1884), and first used attenuated vaccine as a prophylactic (1885). See also *rabies*. The Pasteur Institute in Paris was established for his investigations.

Pas''teur·el'la (pas''tur·el'uh). A genus of bacteria of the tribe Pasteurelleae and of the family Parvobacteriaceae. Species are small, Gramnegative, bipolar staining, often ovoid, and are parasites of man, birds, and other higher animals. **Past. pestis.** Species known as the plague bacillus; is pathogenic to man and produces bubonic or glandular plague and plague pneumonia. **Past. tularensis.** The causative organism of tularemia, a disease of rodents, and of rabbits in particular, which is transmitted to man.

pas'teur·i·xa'tion (pas"tur·i·zay'shun, pas"choor·). Arresting the process of fermentation in milk, wine, and other organic fluids by heating them at 60° or 70° C. for about 40 minutes. Destroys the common pathogens found in milk.

pas'til (pas'til), **pas·tille'** (pas·teel', ·til'). 1. A small mass composed of aromatic substances and employed in fumigation. 2. A troche. 3. A paper disk, chemically coated, which changes color on exposure to x-rays; used to determine the dosage.

past point'ing. A test in which the patient is asked to point at a fixed object alternately with the eyes open and closed. A constant error with the eyes closed indicates a brain lesion. Also called *Bárány's pointing test*.

patch. An irregular spot or area. **butterfly p.** A patch of lupus erythematosus on the cheeks and nose. A similar patch is often the site of erysipelas. **mucous p.** A characteristic lesion of secondary syphilis, occurring as a whitish papule or superficial ulcer on mucous membranes and at mucocutaneous junctions. Syn., *condyloma latum, moist papule*. **soldier's patches.** Opaque white spots on the epicardium, of unknown origin, probably due to friction. Also called *soldier's plaques*.

pate. Old term for the crown or top of the head.

pa·tel'la. A sesamoid bone in front of the knee, developed in the tendon of the quadriceps femoris muscle. See Table of Bones in the Appendix. —**patellar**, *adj.*

pat'el·lec'to·my. The surgical removal or excision of a patella.

pa'ten·cy. The state of being open.

pa'tent, pat'ent. Open; exposed.

path"er·ga'si·a (path"ur·gay'zhuh, ·shuh). In psychiatry, a term applied by Adolf Meyer to personality maladjustments associated with organic or structural changes in the body or with gross functional disturbances.

path'er·gy, path·er'gi·a. 1. An unusually intense response to an allergen, in which the individual becomes sensitive not only to the specific substance but to others; hyperergy. 2. A subnormal response to an allergen; hypoergy.

-pathia. Same as *-pathy*.

path'o-, path-. A combining form denoting *disease, pathologic*.

path"o·don'ti·a. The branch of dental science which treats of the diseases of the teeth.

path'o·gen. Any agent which is capable of producing disease. The term is usually restricted to living agents.

path"o·gen'e·sis. The course of development of disease, including the sequence of processes or events from inception to the characteristic lesion or disease.

path"o·gen'ic. Pertaining to the capacity to produce disease, as a pathogenic microörganism.

pa·thog"no·mon'ic. Characteristic of a disease, distinguishing it from other diseases.

pa·thol'o·gist. A person trained and experienced in the study and practice of pathology.

pa·thol'o·gy. That branch of biological science which deals with the nature of disease, through study of its causes, its process, and its effects, together with the associated alterations of structure and function. —**pathologic, patholog'ical**, *adj.* **cellular p.** The study of changes in cells as the basis of disease. **chemical p.** The study of diseased structures and processes by the application of chemical methods. **comparative p.** That which compares disease in various animals, including man, to arrive at resemblances and differences which may clarify disease as a phenomenon of nature. **dermal p.** The pathology of diseases of the skin. **experimental p.** That which utilizes experimental methods for the study of disease in animals and in man. **geographic p.** Distribution of diseases and their manifestations in various parts of the world. **gynecologic p.** The pathology of the female sexual organs and associated structures. **special p.** Application of the laws of general pathology to individual organs or systems.

pa·thom'e·try. Estimation of the number of people suffering from a disease and the conditions which increase or decrease this number. **pathomet'ric**, *adj.*

path"o·mi·me'sis (path"o·mi·mee'sis, ·migh·mee'sis). Imitation of the symptoms and signs of a disease; occurs in hysteria and in malingering. Syn., *pathomimicry*.

path"o·phor'ic. Carrying or transmitting disease, said of certain insects.

path"o·psy·chol'o·gy. That branch of science dealing with the mental processes during disease, from the viewpoint of general, rather than medical, psychology. See *psychopathology*.

pa·tho'sis. A diseased condition, abnormality, or pathologic finding.

-pathy, -pathia. A combining form meaning *feeling, suffering; a disease of a (specified) kind; a method of treating a disease*. —**pathic**, *adj.*

pa'tient. A person under the care of a physician; a sick person.

pat″ri·lin′e·al. Pertaining to descent through the male line.

pat′ten. A metal support serving as a high sole and attached to the shoe on the sound leg, to prevent weight bearing in hip disease and to permit the employment of traction apparatus on the affected leg.

pat′tern. Example, model, design.

pat′u·lin. An antibacterial substance originally prepared from *Penicillium patulum*. See *clavacin*.

pat′u·lous. Expanded; open.

Paul·lin′i·a. A genus of woody vines. The seeds of **P. cupana** are the source of guarana.

pau″lo·car′di·a. A subjective sensation of intermission or momentary stoppage of the heartbeat.

paunch. Colloquial term for the abdominal cavity and its contents.

pause. A temporary stop or rest. **compensatory p.** Any pause which, immediately succeeding a premature beat, compensates by its length for the prematurity of the beat. Also called *returning cycle*.

pau″si·me′ni·a (paw″si·mee′nee·uh, paw″zi·). See *menopause*.

pa′vaex (pay′vex). See *pavex*.

pavatrine. Trade-mark for β-di-ethylaminoethyl fluorene-9-carboxylate hydrochloride, an antispasmodic.

pave′ment·ing. A stage in the process of tissue inflammation in which the blood stream in the capillaries becomes slowed, the leukocytes gravitating out of the central current to become adherent to the vessel walls.

pa′vex, pa′vaex [*passive vascular exercise*]. A positive-negative pressure apparatus for passive vascular exercise in the treatment of thromboangiitis obliterans.

Pavlov, Ivan Petrovich [*Russian physiologist*, 1849–1936]. Celebrated throughout the world for his important contributions to our knowledge of the physiology of digestion. His investigations (1897) are of great importance, ranking after those of William Beaumont (1833). Established gastric and pancreatic fistulas experimentally. Contributed important work on conditioned reflexes (1928). A small portion of the stomach communicating with the exterior, which has been completely segregated experimentally from the main stomach but retains its innervation, is sometimes called *Pavlov's pouch*. Nobel laureate (1904).

pa′vor. Fright; fear. **p. nocturnus.** Night terrors; nightmare.

paw′paw. Papaw. See *papaya*.

Pb. Chemical symbol for lead.

P. B. E. A tuberculin prepared from bovine tubercle bacilli; similar to Koch's new tuberculin.

P. D. Doctor of Pharmacy.

Pd. Chemical symbol for palladium.

pea′nut oil. A refined fixed oil obtained from seed kernels of one or more cultivated varieties of peanuts, used as a vehicle for injections. Syn., *arachis oil.*

pearl. A rounded aggregation of squamous epithelial cells, concentrically arranged, seen in certain carcinomas. Also called *epithelial p.*

peat. The product of the spontaneous decomposition of plants, especially swamp plants, in many cases mixed with sand, loam, clay, lime, iron pyrites, or ocher.

pec′tase. An enzyme, found associated with pentose in fruits, which converts the pectose into pectin.

pec′ten. 1. Old term for os pubis. 2. The middle third of the anal canal. **p. ossis pubis.** The pectineal line of the pubis, a continuation of the ileopectineal line.

pec″te·no′sis. Induration of the pecten, or middle third of the anal canal.

pec′tic ac′id. A complex acid, partially demethylated, obtained from the pectin of fruits.

pec′tin. A purified carbohydrate product obtained from the dilute acid extract of the inner portion of the rind of citrus fruits, or from apple pomace. It consists chiefly of partially methoxylated polygalacturonic acids. It is almost completely soluble in water, forming a viscous, opalescent colloidal solution. **pec′tin·ase.** The enzyme capable of transforming pectin.

pec′ti·nate. Arranged like the teeth of a comb.

pec·tin′e·us, pec″ti·ne′us. A muscle arising from the pubis and inserted on the femur. See Table of Muscles in the Appendix.

pec′tin·ose. See *arabinose.*

pec″ti·za′tion. *In colloid chemistry*, the transformation of sols into gels. *Obs.* See *coagulation, flocculation.*

pec′to·ral. Pertaining to the chest, as the pectoral muscles, which connect the arm and the chest.

pec″to·ra′lis (peck″to·rah′lis, ·ray′-lis). One of two muscles, major and minor, on the anterior aspect of the chest. See Table of Muscles in the Appendix.

pec″to·ril′o·quy. Exaggerated bronchophony, in which there is distinct transmission of articulate speech in addition to increased intensity of the voice sounds. Heard over consolidations which are either large in extent or located in proximity to a major air passage. **whispered p.** The transmission of whispered voice sounds having the same characteristics and the same significance as above.

pec′tose. The water-insoluble pectin

substance occurring in various unripe fruits. It is converted into the water-soluble pectin by the enzyme pectase. Also called *pectinogen, protopectin*.

pec′tus. The chest or breast. **p. cari-natum.** A narrow chest projecting anteriorly in the region of the sternum. Syn., *chicken breast*. Also called *cari-nate breast*. **p. excavatum.** A congenital deformity of the thorax in which the sternum is depressed toward the spine. Syn., *funnel breast*.

pe″dar·throc′a·ce (pee″dahr-throck′uh-see, ped″ahr-). A necrotic ulceration or caries of the joints of children.

pe·dat′ro·phy, pe″da·tro′phi·a. 1. Any wasting disease of childhood. 2. Tabes mesenterica.

ped′er·as″ty. Sexual intercourse through the anus; practiced on boys. See also *sodomy*. **—pederast,** *n*.

ped″i·al′gi·a (ped″ee-al′juh, pee″dee·). Pain in the foot.

pe″di·a·tri′cian (pee″dee-uh-trish′-un, ped″ee·). See *pediatrist*.

pe″di·at′rics (pee″dee-at′ricks, ped″ee·). The branch of medicine dealing with children's diseases. **—pedi-atric,** *adj*.

pe″di·at′rist (pee″dee-at′rist, pi-dye′uh-trist). A specialist in children's diseases.

ped′i·cle. A slender process acting as a foot or stem, as the pedicle of a tumor.

pe·dic′te·rus. Jaundice of the newborn; icterus neonatorum.

pe·dic′u·lar. Lousy; pertaining to lice.

pe·dic′u·li·cide. An agent which destroys lice.

pe·dic″u·lo·pho′bi·a. Morbid dread of infestation with lice.

pe·dic″u·lo′sis. A skin disease due to infestation by lice, characterized by intense pruritus and cutaneous lesions. **p. capitis.** Infestation of the scalp with the species *Pediculus humanus* var. *capitis* occurring chiefly in women and girls with long hair. **p. corporis.** Infestation of the skin of the body with the species *Pediculus humanus* var. *corporis*. In cases of long standing the chronic scratching gives rise to pigmentation and lichenification of the skin, the so-called vagabond's disease. **p. pubis.** An infestation of the pubic hair with the *Phthirius pubis*, the crab louse; may spread over the body and involve the axillas, eyebrows, and eyelashes.

pe·dic′u·lous. Infested with lice.

Pe·dic′u·lus. A genus of small parasitic insects known as lice, whose species produce dermatitis and transmit diseases, such as typhus fever, trench fever, and relapsing fever. **P. humanus** var. **capitis.** The head louse; important as a vector of disease and produces pediculosis capitis, *q.v.* **P. humanus** var. **corporis.** The body louse; important as a vector of disease and causes pediculosis corporis, *q.v.*

ped′i·cure. Care of the feet.

pe″do·don′tics. The branch of dentistry which treats abnormal oral and dental conditions occurring in childhood. Syn., *pedodontia, pedodontology*.

pe″do·don′tist. One who specializes in pedodontics.

pe·dol′o·gist. A specialist in pediatrics.

pe·dol′o·gy. The science, or sum of knowledge, regarding childhood, its diseases, hygiene, etc.

pe·dom′e·ter. An instrument for weighing and measuring a newborn child. **—pedometry,** *n*.

pe·dom′e·ter. An instrument which registers the number of footsteps in walking. **—pedometry,** *n*.

pe·dop′a·thy. Disease of the foot.

pe″do·phil′i·a. Fondness for children; usually, love of children by adults for sexual purposes.

pe″do·pho′bi·a. Morbid dislike or fear of children.

pe·dun′cle (pi-dung′kul, ped′ung-kul). A narrow part acting as a support. **—peduncular, pedunculate, pedunculated,** *adj*.

peel′ing. A term applied to the process of desquamation, as after any inflammation of the skin. It is a result of disturbed keratinization of epidermis.

peg. 1. A pointed pin of wood, metal or other material. 2. A wooden leg **bone p.** A peg or screw fashioned of beef bone, used in bone operations to secure immobility.

peg′a·nine (peg′uh-neen, -nin) l-Peganine. An alkaloid, $C_{11}H_{12}N_2O$, from the leaves of *Adhatoda vasica* and *Peganum harmala*. Syn., *vasicine*.

peganene. Trade-mark for ethotoin.

pel′age. The hairy covering of the body.

pel″ar·gon′ic ac′id. The fatty acid, $CH_3(CH_2)_7COOH$; formed by oxidation of oleic acid.

pel″i·o′sis (pel″ee-o′sis, pee″lee-) Purpura. **p. rheumatica.** Rheumatic purpura; a disease characterized by a purpuric rash, with arthritis and fever.

pel·la′gra (puh-lag′ruh, puh-lay′-gruh). A syndrome resulting from nicotinic acid deficiency, characterized by dermatitis of surfaces exposed to the sun, glossitis and stomatitis, and diarrhea, and in severe cases by disturbances of the central nervous system **—pellagrous,** *adj*.

pel·la′grin (puh-lag′rin, puh-lay′-grin). One who is afflicted with pellagra.

pel′let. A small pill.

pel″le·tier′ine (pel″i·teer′een, ·in, pel″et·yair′·). A liquid alkaloid obtained together with isomeric isopelletierine, also a liquid alkaloid, from pomegranate bark. These are also called *punicine* and *isopunicine*. **p. tannate.** A mixture in varying proportions of the tannates of several alkaloids obtained from pomegranate, *Punica granatum* Linné. Used as an anthelmintic.

pel′li·cle. 1. A thin membrane, or cuticle. 2. A film on the surface of a liquid. —**pellic′ular, pellic′ulous, pellic′ulate,** adj.

pel·lic′u·la. Epidermis.

pel′lo·tine (pel′o·teen, ·tin). $C_{13}H_{19}$-NO_3. An alkaloid from the Mexican cactus, *Lophophora williamsii*.

pel·lu′cid. Transparent; translucent; not opaque.

pe·lop′si·a. A defect of vision characterized by illusions of abnormal nearness of objects.

pel′o·sine (pel′o·seen, pi·lo′seen). An alkaloid derived from *Cissampelos pareira*. Syn., *bebeerine*.

pel′vic ham′mock. A canvas sling, generally attached to an overhead bed frame, used to suspend the lower part of the trunk and pelvis in pelvic fractures.

pel″vi·en·ceph″a·lom′e·try. Measurement of the maternal pelvis and fetal skull by means of radiographic examination.

pel·vim′e·ter. An instrument for measuring the pelvic dimensions.

pel·vim′e·try. The measurement of the dimensions of the pelvis.

AVERAGE MEASUREMENTS OF THE ADULT FEMALE PELVIS COVERED BY THE SOFT PARTS

Between iliac spines	26	cm.
Between iliac crests	29	"
External conjugate diameter	20¼	"
Internal conjugate diagonal	12¾	"
True conjugate, estimated	11	"
Right diagonal	22	"
Left diagonal	22	"
Between trochanters	31	"
Circumference of pelvis	90	"

digital p. Measurement of the pelvis by means of the hand. **external p.** Measurement of external diameters of the pelvis, to estimate the dimensions of the internal parts. **internal p.** Measurement of the internal dimensions of the pelvis by the hand or by the pelvimeter.

pel″vi·o·li·thot′o·my. Removal of a kidney stone from the renal pelvis.

pel″vi·ot′o·my. Incision of the renal pelvis.

pel′vis (pl. *pelves*). 1. A basin or basin-shaped cavity, as the pelvis of

the kidney. 2. The bony ring formed by the two innominate bones and the sacrum and coccyx. 3. The cavity bounded by the bony pelvis. The cavity consists of two parts: the true pelvis and the false pelvis, which are separated by the iliopectineal line. The entrance of the true pelvis, corresponding to this line, is known as the inlet or superior strait; the outlet or inferior strait is bounded by the symphysis pubis, the tip of the coccyx, and the two ischia. —**pelvic,** adj. **android p.** A female pelvis with a deeper cavity and more conical shape, similar to the normal male pelvis. **brachypellic p.** Oval type of pelvis having a transverse diameter more than one and less than three centimeters greater than the anteroposterior diameter. **brim of the p.** The pelvic inlet. **contracted p.** One having one or more major diameters reduced in size, interfering with parturition. **flat p.** Deformity of the pelvis in which all anteroposterior diameters are shortened but the transverse diameters are practically normal. **funnel p.** A deformity in which the usual external measurements are normal while the outlet is contracted, the transverse diameter of the latter being eight centimeters or less. **generally contracted p.** One having all diameters symmetrically shortened; a small normally shaped pelvis. **generally enlarged p.** One having all diameters symmetrically enlarged; a large normally shaped pelvis. **gynecoid p.** A female pelvis in which the inlet is circular instead of oval or blunt heart-shaped. **kyphorachitic p.** A deformity of the pelvis associated with rickets in which changes are slight because the effect of kyphosis tends to counterbalance that of rickets. **kyphoscoliotic p.** A deformity of the pelvis varying in character with the predominance of the kyphosis or scoliosis of the vertebral column. **kyphotic p.** One characterized by increase of the conjugata vera, but decrease of the transverse diameter of the outlet, through approximation of the ischial spines and tuberosities. Associated with kyphosis of the vertebral column. **Naegele p.** An obliquely contracted pelvis with ankylosis of one sacroiliac synchondrosis, underdevelopment of the associated sacral ala, and other distorting defects producing an obliquely directed conjugata vera. **osteomalacic p.** A distorted pelvis characterized by a lessening of the transverse and oblique diameters, with great increase of the anteroposterior diameter. **platypelloid p.** Flat pelvis. Also called *platypellic p.* **simple flat p.** One in which the only deformity consists in a shortening of the anteroposterior diameter. **split p.** A form in which there is congenital separation of the pubic bones at the symphysis, often associated with exstrophy of the bladder. **spondylolisthetic p.** A deformity resulting from a forward displacement of the centrum of the last lumbar vertebra.

pem'phi·gus (pem'fi·gus). An acute or chronic disease of the skin characterized by the appearance of bullae which develop in crops or continuous succession. —**pemphigoid,** adj. **p. acutus.** A type once thought to be associated with septic wounds and vaccination, and now considered to be an acute bacterial infection with septicemia. **p. erythematosus.** A benign type with bullae occurring in patches of dermatitis which clinically resemble lupus erythematosus. **p. foliaceus.** A rare type characterized by crops of flaccid blebs which recur and rupture, producing a marked scaliness and generalized exfoliation. **p. vegetans.** A form characterized by oral lesions followed by skin eruptions which rupture, leaving a raw surface on which vegetative or papillary growths develop. **p. vulgaris.** A form that is usually chronic, characterized by successive crops of blebs which leave pigmented spots when they are healed.

pen''al·ge'si·a (pen''al·jee'zee·uh, ·see·uh). Reduction in the number of pain and touch spots in trigeminal neuralgia.

pen'a·tin. An antibiotic from *Penicillium notatum*; it is identical with corylophilline, *Escherichia coli* factor, mycoin, notatin, and penicillin-B.

pen'du·lous. Hanging down loosely.

pen'e·tra''ting. Entering beyond the surface, as a penetrating wound, one that pierces the wall of a cavity or enters an organ.

pen''e·tra'tion. 1. The act of penetrating or piercing into. 2. Of a microscope, the focal depth. 3. The entrance of the penis into the vagina.

pe·nic'i·din (peh·nis'i·din, pen''i·sigh'din). An antibiotic from species of *Penicillium*.

pen''i·cil'lase. See *penicillinase*.

pen''i·cil'late. Ending in a tuft of hairs.

pen''i·cil'lic ac'id. An antibiotic from species of *Penicillium*, particularly *P. puberulum*.

pen''i·cil'li·form. Penicillate; ending in a tuft of hairs.

pen''i·cil'lin. An antibacterial produced from strains of *Penicillium notatum*. Several penicillins are known, having the formula $C_9H_{11}O_4SN_2R$. In penicillin-F (known in Britain as penicillin-I), R is the Δ^2-pentenyl (—CH_2·CH=CHCH$_2$CH$_3$) group; in penicillin-G

(penicillin-II), R is benzyl ($C_6H_5CH_2$—); in penicillin-X (penicillin-III), R is p-hydroxybenzyl ($C_6H_4OHCH_2$—); in penicillin-K, R is n-heptyl (CH_2CH_2·$CH_2CH_2CH_2CH_2CH_3$—). **p.-B.** An antibiotic identical with corylophilline, *Escherichia coli* factor, mycoin, notatin, and penatin. **p.V.** Phenoxymethyl penicillin. **procaine p.** A crystalline salt representing the combination of one molecule each of penicillin and procaine. Injected into tissue, it slowly releases penicillin, maintaining therapeutic levels for prolonged periods.

pen''i·cill'lin·ase. An enzyme which destroys penicillin.

pen''i·cil''li·o'sis. Lesions of the ear, skin, and occasionally the lungs, caused by certain species of *Penicillium*.

Pen''i·cil'li·um. A genus of fungi of the Ascomycetes in which the fruiting organs have a brushlike form. The species **Penicillium chrysogenum, P. citrinum, P. claviforme, P. notatum, P. patulum, P. puberulum, P. spinulosum** are used in the production of antibiotics. Species of this genus are also common allergens.

pen''i·cil·lo'ic ac'id. Any one of the dicarboxylic acids formed when the lactam ring in a penicillin is opened by the action of alkalies or penicillinase.

pen''i·cil'lus (pl. *penicilli*). One of the tufts of fine twigs into which the arteries of the spleen subdivide.

pe·nil'lic ac'id. Any one of the dicarboxylic acids resulting when a penicillin is subjected to a mild acid treatment; the penillic acids are isomeric with the corresponding penicillins.

pe'nis. The male organ of copulation. Its essential parts consist of the corpus cavernosum urethrae which encloses the urethra and forms the glans and the two corpora cavernosa, all covered by fascia and skin. —**penile,** adj.

pen'nate. Like a feather.

pen'ni·form. Shaped like a feather; said of certain muscles.

pen''ny·roy'al. *Mentha pulegium*. See *hedeoma*.

pen''ny·weight''. A weight of 24 grains. Abbreviated, dwt.

pe·nol'o·gist. One who makes a study of crime, its cause and prevention.

pe·nol'o·gy. The science treating of crime, its punishment and prevention; the study of the management of prisons. —**penologic,** adj.

pe''no·scro'tal. Pertaining to the penis and the scrotum.

pen'ta-, pent-. A combining form meaning *five*.

pen''ta·dac'tyl. Having five fingers or toes upon each hand or foot.

pen″ta·eryth′ri·tyl tet·ra·ni′-trate. A vasodilator, chemically $(CH_2NO_3)_4C$, similar in action to, but usually more effective than, erythrityl tetranitrate, used sometimes in preventing attacks of angina pectoris and in treating intermittent claudication.

pen″ta·hy·drox″y·hex·o′ic ac′id. Galactonic acid.

pen′tal. C_5H_{10}. See *amylene hydrate*.

pen″ta·me·tho′ni·um. A compound containing a methonium ion with five CH_2 groups, that possesses ganglion-blocking activity and reduces blood pressure. Also see *methonium*.

pen″ta·meth″yl·ene·tet′ra·zol. Pentylenetetrazol.

pen·tam′i·dine (pen-tam′i-deen, -din). A diamidine, 4:4′-diamidino-1:5 diphenoxypentane or 4,4′-[pentamethylene dioxy]dibenzamidine. Active against pathogenic trypanosomes, also inhibits growth of bacteria in wounds.

pen′tane. Chemical name for one of the three isomeric hydrocarbons of the paraffin series, having the formula C_5H_{12}. All are liquids.

pen′ta·quine (pen′tuh-kween, -kwin). 6-Methoxy-8-(5′-isopropylaminopentyl-amino)-quinoline, an effective remedial agent in malaria. Introduced as *SN 13,276*.

pen″ta·vac′cine. A vaccine composed of five different kinds of organisms.

pen″ta·va′lent, pen·tav′a·lent. Having a valence of five.

pen′tene. 1. Chemical name for one of the isomeric hydrocarbons of the olefin series, having the formula C_nH_{2n}, of which five are possible. 2. See *amylene hydrate*.

pen″to·bar′bi·tal so′di·um (pen″to-bar′bi-tawl, -tal, -tol). Sodium ethyl-(1-methyl-butyl) barbiturate, a white powder, freely soluble in water and alcohol. One of the more rapidly acting hypnotics. Also called *soluble pentobarbital*. See *nembutal*.

pen′to·san. A complex carbohydrate capable of forming a pentose by hydrolysis.

pen·to′sa·zone (pen·to′suh·zone, pen′to·say′zone). A reaction product of pentose and phenylhydrazine, used to identify pentoses.

pen′tose. Any one of a class of carbohydrates containing five atoms of carbon.

pen′to·side (pen′to·side, ·sid). A nuclein containing a pentose.

pentothal sodium. Trade-mark for the monosodium salt of 5-ethyl-5-(1-methylbutyl) thiobarbituric acid, known also as *thiopental sodium* and *thiopentone sodium*.

pent·ox′ide. An oxide containing five atoms of oxygen.

pen′tyl. Chemical name for the univalent radical of five carbon atoms. The name amyl is used interchangeably.

pen″tyl·ene·tet′ra·zol. Generic name for pentamethylenetetrazol, a central nervous system stimulant. See *cardiazol, leptazol, metrazol*.

pen·vee. A trade-mark for phenoxy-methyl penicillin.

pe′po. Seed of the pumpkin, *Cucurbita pepo*; it is a taeniafuge.

pep′per. The dried, unripe fruit of various species of *Piper*.

pep′per·mint. Consists of the dried leaf and flowering top of *Mentha piperita*, yielding a volatile oil.

pep′per·mint oil. A volatile oil distilled from the overground parts of the flowering plant *Mentha piperita*, containing menthyl acetate and menthol, used as a carminative and a flavoring.

pep′si·gogue. Referring to the secretagogue effect of substances which stimulate the discharge of pepsin in the gastric secretion; contrasted with the effect of histamine, which stimulates the secretion of hydrochloric acid but not of pepsin.

pep′sin. A substance containing a proteolytic enzyme obtained from the glandular layer of the fresh stomach of the hog, *Sus scrofa* var. *domesticus*; occurs as transparent or translucent scales, granular or spongy masses, yellow to light brown in color; freely soluble in water. Pepsin is useful to secure the digestion of protein food in the stomach.

pep·sin′o·gen. The antecedent substance or zymogen of pepsin, present in the cells of the gastric glands, which during digestion is converted into pepsin.

pep′tic. 1. Pertaining to pepsin. 2. Pertaining to digestion, as peptic ulcer. See peptic *ulcer*.

pep′ti·dase. An enzyme which splits peptides to amino acids.

pep′tide. A compound of two or more amino acids containing one or more peptide groups, —CO.NH—. An intermediate between the amino acids and peptones in the synthesis of proteins.

pep″ti·do·lyt′ic. Causing the digestion or splitting up of peptides into amino acids.

pep″ti·za′tion. 1. The liquefaction of a gel to a sol. 2. The bringing of a solid material into colloidal suspension.

pep′tone. A derived protein produced by the hydrolysis of natural protein either by an enzyme or by an acid. Complete hydrolysis of protein yields amino acids. Peptones, as well as proteoses, which are similar to peptones, are intermediate compounds between proteins and amino acids. Also called meat peptone, beef peptone. **—pep-ton'ic,** adj.

pep''to·ne'mi·a. The presence of peptone in the blood.

pep''to·nu'ri·a. The presence of peptones in the urine. **enterogenous p.** Peptonuria due to disease of the intestine. **hepatogenous p.** That accompanying certain liver affections. **nephrogenous p.** Peptonuria of renal origin. **puerperal p.** That of the puerperal state. **pyogenic p.** That produced by suppuration in the body.

per-. 1. A prefix signifying *throughout, completely, thoroughly, over,* or *very, extremely.* 2. *In chemistry,* a prefix denoting the highest valence of a series.

per''a·cid'i·ty (pur''a·sid'i·tee). Excessive acidity.

perandren. Trade-mark for the propionic acid ester of synthetic testosterone in oil.

per a'num. By the anus, said of the administration of certain drugs or nutrient substances.

per''a·to·dyn'i·a. Pain at the cardiac extremity of the stomach.

peraxil. Trade-mark for chlorcyclizine, an antihistaminic.

per·bo'rate (pur·bor'ate). A salt of perboric acid.

per·bo'ric ac'id. The hypothetical acid, HBO_3, from which perborates are derived.

per·ca'ine (pur·kay'een, ·in, pur'kay-een, ·in). See *nupercaine hydrochloride.*

per cent. *In biochemistry,* indicating milligrams of a substance per 100 cc. of a fluid, as blood; more properly *milligrams per cent.*

per·cen'tile (pur·sen'tile, ·til). A point on a frequency scale below which falls a designated percentage of the observations.

per·cep'tion. Recognition in response to sensory stimuli; the act or process by which the memory of certain qualities of an object is associated with other qualities impressing the senses, thereby making possible recognition of the object. **—perceptive,** adj. **depth p.** The ability to estimate depth or distance between points in the field of vision. **space p.** Knowledge, through the senses, of the area, dimensions, or position occupied, of any space. **stereognostic p.** The recognition of objects by touch.

per''cep·tiv'i·ty. The faculty or capability of receiving impressions.

per·chlo'rate. A salt of perchloric acid.

per·chlo'ric ac'id. $HClO_4$. A powerful oxidizing acid used in chemical analysis.

per·clu'sion. Inability to execute any movement.

per'co·late. 1. Submit to the process of percolation. 2. The solution obtained by percolation.

per''co·la'tion. The process of extracting the soluble constituents of a substance by allowing a suitable solvent to pass through a column of the powdered substance placed in a long, conical vessel, the percolator, *q.v.*

per'co·la''tor. A long, conical vessel with a delivery tube at the lower extremity; used for extracting the soluble constituents of a substance, packed in the percolator, by means of a suitable solvent passing through it.

per·co·morph. A fish of the order Acanthopteri (Percomorphi), which includes the genera *Thunnus, Xiphias, Stereolepis, Scomber,* and others. **p. liver oil.** A mixture containing the fixed oils from the fresh livers of the percomorph fishes and not more than 50% of other fish liver oil. It contains vitamins A and D. It is marketed under the trade-mark oleum percomorphum.

percorten. A trade-mark for desoxycorticosterone acetate.

per·cus'sion. The act of firmly tapping the surface of the body with a finger or a small hammer to elicit sounds, or vibratory sensations, of diagnostic value. **auditory p.** That in which attention is concentrated upon the character of the sounds produced. **auscultatory p.** That in which the sound is received through a stethoscope, the bell of which is placed on the skin, while the examiner either scratches the skin surface or percusses lightly in the near vicinity. **definitive p.** Percussion whose purpose is to outline the borders of a viscus. **direct p.** Striking the skin directly with the pads of one or two fingers without the interposition of a pleximeter. Also called *immediate p.* **indirect p.** That effected by placing a pleximeter against the skin surface to receive the taps. Also called *mediate p.* **orthopercussion.** The use of a cylindrical pleximeter, placed with its long axis perpendicular to the surface of the body, for the purpose of sharply demarcating the border of an internal organ, especially the heart. The two distal phalanges of a finger flexed at a right angle, or a glass rod or other mechanical object may be used as pleximeter. **palpatory p.** Direct percussion, in which attention is concentrated upon the sensation of resistance detected by the one or two fingers used as a pleximeter. **qualitative p.** That used to determine the physical state of the underlying tissues. **threshold p.** The termination of the border of a viscus by the transition from no sound to that least audible sound, when percussion strokes of minimum force are used.

pe·rei'rine (peh·ray'reen, ·rin, peh·rye'·). An amorphous alkaloid found in the bark of *Geissospermum laeve*.

per'fo·ra"ted. Pierced through, as perforated substance, a part of the base of the brain pierced with many small holes for the passage of blood vessels. The *anterior perforated substance* is a small triangular area on the under surface of the brain situated lateral to the anterior part of the interpeduncular fossa; the *posterior perforated substance* lies between the mammillary bodies in front, the pons behind, and the crura cerebri on either side.

per"fo·ra'tion. 1. The act or occurrence of piercing or boring into a part, especially into the wall of a hollow organ or viscus. 2. A hole made through a part or wall of a cavity, produced by a variety of means.

per'fo·ra"tor. An instrument for perforating, especially one for performing craniotomy on the fetus.

per·fu'sion. 1. A pouring of fluid. 2. The passage of a fluid through spaces. 3. The introduction of fluids into tissues by their injection into arteries.

perhydrol. Trade-mark for a 30 per cent solution of hydrogen peroxide.

peri-. A prefix signifying *about*, *beyond*, *around*, *near*; especially, *enclosing a part* or *affecting the tissues around a part*.

per"i·ad"e·ni'tis. Inflammation of tissues surrounding a gland or lymph node. **p. mucosa necrotica recurrens.** A disorder characterized by recurring necrotic or ulcerative lesions occurring on the buccal and pharyngeal mucosa. Begins as a small, smooth, hard nodule that sloughs, leaving a deep crateriform depression. May occur on the tongue or genitalia as well.

per"i·a·lien·i'tis (perr"ee·ayl·en·eye'tis, ·ay"lee·en·eye'tis). Noninfectious inflammation due to a foreign body. Also called *foreign-body reaction*, *erizenitis*.

per"i·a'nal. Situated or occurring round the anus.

per"i·an"gi·i'tis. Inflammation of the outer coat of, or the tissues surrounding, an artery, vein, or lymphatic vessel.

per"i·an"gi·o·cho·li'tis (perr"ee·an"jee·o·ko·lye'tis). Inflammation of the tissues surrounding the biliary ducts.

per"i·a"or·ti'tis. Inflammation of the tissues surrounding the aorta.

per"i·ap'i·cal. Around an apex.

per"i·ap·pen"di·ci'tis. Inflammation of the tissue around the vermiform

process, or of the serosal region of the appendix.

per"i·ar"te·ri'tis. Inflammation of the adventitia of an artery and the periarterial tissues. **p. nodosa.** An acute arteritis of unknown cause, involving all layers of the arterial wall, with the production of inflammatory nodules along the outer wall. The focal lesions show degeneration, necrosis, exudation, and, ultimately, organization. Also called *polyarteritis acuta nodosa*.

per"i·ar·thri'tis. Inflammation of the tissues about a joint. **scapulohumeral p.** Fixation of the shoulder joint resulting from bicipital tenosynovitis, tendinitis, or adherent subacromial bursitis.

per"i·ar·tic'u·lar. About a joint.

per"i·a'tri·al. Situated around the atria of the heart.

per"i·au·ric'u·lar. Around the external ear.

per"i·ax'i·al. Surrounding an axis.

per"i·blep'sis. The wild look of a patient in delirium. Also called *periblepsia*.

per"i·bron·chi'tis. Inflammation of the tissues around bronchi.

per"i·bro'sis. Ulceration at the canthus of the eyelid.

per"i·car"di·ec'to·my. Excision of a part of the pericardium.

per"i·car"di·o·cen·te'sis. Puncture of the pericardium.

per"i·car"di·o·pleu'ral (perr"i·kahr"dee·o·ploor'ul). Relating to the pericardium and to the pleura.

per"i·car"di·or'rha·phy. The suturing of a wound in the pericardium.

per"i·car"di·os'to·my. The establishing by surgical means of an opening into the pericardium, for repair of wounds of the heart or for drainage of the pericardial sac.

per"i·car"di·ot'o·my. Incision of the pericardium.

per"i·car·di'tis. Inflammation of the pericardium. The symptoms are slight fever, precordial pain and tenderness, cough, dyspnea, and rapid pulse. In the early stage, there is a distinct friction sound on auscultation, and sometimes a fremitus on palpation. In the stage of effusion, there are bulging of the precordia and a triangular area of dullness, the base of which is downward; the heart sounds are muffled. In chronic pericarditis with adhesions, there is often systolic retraction of the precordia. The causes of pericarditis are rheumatic fever, tuberculosis, septicemia (as in pneumonia), nephritis, or extension of infection from neighboring parts. **—pericardit'ic,** *adj.* **acute p.** An acute inflammation of the pericardium, characterized by serous, fibrinous, purulent, or hemorrhagic exudate. **ad-hesive p.** That in which the two layers of pericardium tend to adhere by means of fibrous adhesions, usually the result of the organization of acute exudate. **carcinomatous p.** That due to carcinoma of the pericardium. **dry p.** A form without effusion. **external p.** That affecting the outer layer of the parietal pericardium. **fibrinous p.** A form in which the membrane is covered with a fibrinous exudate, first soft and buttery in consistence, but later organizing. **hemorrhagic p.** A form in which the fluid is hemorrhagic; found most often in tuberculous pericarditis. **localized p.** A form giving rise to white areas, the so-called milk spots. **moist p.** That attended by an effusion. **p. obliterans.** A form leading to obliteration of the cavity by the adhesions of the layers. **purulent p.** A variety in which the effused fluid becomes purulent. **rheumatic p.** An inflammation of the pericardium due to rheumatic fever. **serofibrinous p.** A form in which there is but little fibrin, but a considerable quantity of serous fluid.

per''i·car'di·um. The closed membranous sac enveloping the heart. Its base is attached to the central tendon of the diaphragm; its apex surrounds, for a short distance, the great vessels arising from the base of the heart. It consists of an outer fibrous coat, derived from the cervical fascia, and an inner serous coat. The serosa normally contains from 5–20 Gm. of clear, serous liquid. The part in contact with the heart (visceral pericardium) is termed the epicardium; the other is the parietal pericardium. **—pericardiac, pericardial,** *adj.* **shaggy p.** A pericardium upon which, as the result of fibrinous pericarditis, thick, loose, shaggy layers of fibrin are deposited.

per''i·ce·ci'tis. Inflammation of the serosa of the cecum. Syn., *perityphlitis.*

per''i·ce''men·ti'tis (perr''i·see''-men·tye'tis, ·sem''en·tye'tis). Inflammation of the periodontal membrane; periodontitis.

per''i·ce·men''to·cla'si·a (·si-men''to·clay'zhuh, ·shuh). Breaking down of the periodontium with absorption of the alveolar bone.

per''i·ce·men'tum. See periodontal *membrane.*

per''i·cha·rei'a (perr''i·kah·rye'uh). Sudden vehement or abnormal rejoicing; a symptom in certain psychoses, such as mania or general paresis.

per''i·chol''an·gi'tis (perr''i·kol''-an·jy'tis, ·ko''lan·jy'tis). Inflammation in the tissues around the bile ducts. Syn., *periangiocholitis.*

per''i·chol''e·cys·ti'tis (·kol''i·sis-tye'tis, ·ko''li·). Inflammation of the

serosa or tissues around the gallbla der.

per''i·chon·dri'tis (perr''i·ko dry'tis). Inflammation of perich drium. **—perichondrit'ic,** *adj.*

per''i·chon·dri·um (perr''i·kor dree·um). The fibrous connective tiss covering cartilage, except articu surfaces. **—perichondral,** *adj.*

per''i·chon·dro'ma. A tumor of perichondrium.

per''i·col'ic. Surrounding or ab the colon.

per''i·co·li'tis. Inflammation of peritoneum or tissues around the col Also called *pericolonitis.*

per''i·cys·ti'tis. Inflammation the peritoneum or other tissue su rounding the urinary bladder.

per''i·den·ti'tis. Inflammation the tissues about a tooth; periodontos

per''i·di''ver·tic''u·li'tis. Infla mation of the structures surroundin diverticulum.

per''i·du''o·de·ni'tis. Inflamm tion, acute, chronic, or with fibr adhesions, in the tissues surround the duodenum.

per''i·en·ceph''a·li'tis. Inflamm tion of the pia mater and the cort of the brain.

per''i·en·ter·i'tis. Inflammation the intestinal peritoneum.

per''i·e·soph''a·gi'tis. Inflamm tion of the tissues that surround esophagus.

per''i·fol·lic''u·li'tis. Inflamm tion around the hair follicles.

per''i·gas·tri'tis. Inflammation the serosa of the stomach.

per''i·gnath'ic (perr''i·nath' ·nay'thick). Situated about the ja

per''i·hep''a·ti'tis. Inflammation the peritoneum covering the liver.

per''i·hys·ter'ic. Around the uter periuterine.

per''i·je''ju·ni'tis (perr''i·jee''je nigh'tis, ·jedj''oo·nigh'tis). Inflamm tion of the peritoneal coat or tiss around the jejunum.

per''i·kar'y·on. 1. The cell body a neuron, containing the nucleus an well-defined nucleolus. 2. A circum clear cytoplasmic mass.

per''i·ker·at'ic. Surrounding cornea.

per''i·lab''y·rin·thi'tis. Infla mation in the osseous labyrinth of internal ear.

per''i·lar''yn·gi'tis. Inflammat of the areolar tissue surrounding larynx.

per''i·lymph. The fluid separat the membranous from the osseous la rinth of the internal ear.

per''i·lym''phan·gi'tis. Infl mation of the tissues surroundin lymphatic vessel.

per″i·mas·ti′tis. Inflammation of the fibroadipose tissues around the mammary gland.

per·im′e·ter. 1. Circumference or border. 2. An instrument for measuring the extent of the field of vision. It consists ordinarily of a flat, narrow, metal plate bent in a semicircle, graduated in degrees, and fixed to an upright at its center by a pivot, on which it is movable. Variously colored disks are moved along the metal plate, and the point noted at which the person, looking directly in front of him, distinguishes the color.

per″i·me·tri′tis. Inflammation of the tissues about the uterus. —**perimetrit′ic,** adj.

per″i·me′tri·um. The serous covering of the uterus.

per″i·met″ro·sal″pin·gi′tis. A collective name for periuterine inflammations.

per·im′i·try. 1. The removal of a strip of conjunctival and subconjunctival tissue from about the cornea for the relief of pannus. 2. The cutting of the conjunctiva at the corneoscleral limbus prior to enucleation. Formerly called *peridectomy, peritomy.*

per″i·my″e·li′tis. 1. Inflammation of the pia mater of the spinal cord. 2. Inflammation of the endosteum.

per″i·my″o·si′tis. Inflammation of the connective tissues around muscle.

per″i·mys′i·um (perr″i·miz′ee·um, miss′ee·um). The connective tissue enveloping bundles of muscle fibers. —**perimysial,** adj.

per″i·ne′o-. A combining form denoting *relating to the perineum.*

per″i·ne′o·cele. Perineal hernia.

per″i·ne″o·col″po·rec″to·my″·o·mec′to·my. Excision of a myoma by incision of the perineum, vagina, and rectum. *Obs.*

per″i·ne·o·plas′ty. Plastic operation upon the perineum.

per″i·ne·or′rha·phy. Suture of the perineum, usually for the repair of a laceration occurring during labor.

per″i·ne″o·syn′the·sis. A plastic operation upon the perineum in which a graft of vaginal mucosa is made to cover the wound; a variety of perineorrhaphy. *Obs.*

per″i·ne·ot′o·my. Incision into the perineum.

per″i·neph′ric. Situated or occurring around a kidney, as perinephric abscess.

per″i·ne·phri′tis. Inflammation of the tissues surrounding a kidney.

per″i·neph′ri·um. The connective and adipose tissue surrounding a kidney. —**perinephrial,** adj.

per″i·ne′um. 1. That portion of the body included in the outlet of the pelvis, bounded in front by the pubic arch, behind by the coccyx and sacrotuberous ligaments, and at the sides by the tuberosities of the ischium. In the male it is occupied by the anal canal, membranous urethra, and root of the penis; in the female by the anal canal, urethra, root of the clitoris, and vaginal orifice; in both sexes by the muscles, fasciae, vessels, and nerves of these structures. 2. The region between the anus and the scrotum in the male; between the anus and the posterior commissure of the vulva in the female. —**perineal,** adj. **primary p.** A temporary perineum, present in the embryo after rupture of the cloacal membrane, formed by the caudal end of the urorectal septum with its endodermal covering. Also called *primitive perineal body.*

per″i·neu′ral an″al·ge′si·a (an″al·jee′zee·uh, -see·uh). Analgesia resulting from injection of an analgesic solution into the immediate vicinity of a nerve trunk to the area.

per″i·neu·ri′tis. Inflammation of the perineurium. **retrobulbar p.** Inflammation of the sheath of the orbital part of the optic nerve.

per″i·neu′ri·um. The connective-tissue sheath investing a fasciculus or primary bundle of nerve fibers. —**perineurial,** adj.

pe′ri·od. Duration; measure of time. The space of time during which anything is in progress or an event occurs. **childbearing p.** The time of life, from puberty to the menopause, during which a woman is capable of reproduction. **gestation p.** The period of pregnancy. The average length of human gestation is taken as ten lunar months (280 days) from the onset of the last menstrual period with a variation between 250 and 310 days. See Table of the Duration of Pregnancy in the Appendix. **incubation p.** The time required for an infective agent to produce symptoms. **last menstrual p.** Abbreviated, L.M.P. See gestation p., menstrual p. **latent p.** (a) Incubation period. (b) In *physiology,* the time intervening between the application of a stimulus and the appearance of the resulting phenomenon. **menstrual p.** The menses. Also called *monthly p.* **reaction p.** The time required for the body to respond to some form of stimulation or injury. **respiratory p.** The interval between two successive inspirations. **safe p.** The nonovulatory phase of the menstrual cycle, when conception cannot occur. Since the time of ovulation is variable, the safe period is also variable.

per·i′o·date (pur·eye′o·date). A salt of periodic acid.

per″i·od′ic ac′id (pur″eye·od′ick). $HIO_4.2H_2O$. A colorless, crystalline acid used as an oxidizing agent.

pe″ri·o·dic′i·ty. Recurrence at regular intervals.

pe′ri·od of ges·ta′tion. The duration of pregnancy; in woman, this is usually about 280 days or ten lunar months. To estimate the date of confinement, count back three months from the first day of the last menstrual period and add seven days. See Table of the Duration of Pregnancy in the Appendix.

per″i·o·don′tal, per″i·o·don′-tic. 1. Surrounding a tooth, as the periodontal membrane, which covers the cementum of a tooth. 2. Pertaining to the periodontium or to periodontia.

per″i·o·don′ti·a. That branch of dentistry dealing with the science and treatment of periodontal disease. Also called *periodontics.*

per″i·o·don·ti′tis. Inflammation of the periodontal membrane. **chronic periapical p.** Localized nodule of organising and cicatrizing inflammation at or near the apex of a tooth.

per″i·o·don′ti·um (perr″ee·o·don′-shee·um). The investing and supporting tissues surrounding a tooth; namely, the periodontal membrane, the gingiva, and the alveolar bone.

per″i·o·don″to·cla′si·a (perr″ee·o·don″to·clay′zhuh, ·zee·uh). Periodontosis, *q.v.*

per″i·o·don·tol′o·gy. The science and study of the periodontium and periodontal diseases.

per″i·o·don·to′sis. Degenerative destruction of the periodontium, characterized by noninflammatory degeneration of connective tissue of the periodontal membrane, leading to bone resorption, epithelial proliferation, migration of teeth, pocket formation, and ultimately exfoliation of teeth.

pe″ri·od′o·scope. A calendar in the form of a movable dial, used in determining the probable date of confinement.

per″i·o·dyn′i·a. Severe general pain throughout the body.

per″i·om·phal′ic. Around, or near, the umbilicus.

per″i·o·nych′i·a (perr″ee·o·nick′ee·uh). Inflammation around the nails.

per″i·o·nych′i·um (perr″ee·o·nick′ee·um). The border of epidermis surrounding an entire nail.

per″i·o″ö·pho·ri′tis. Inflammation of the peritoneum, ovary, and the adjacent connective tissues.

per″i·o·öph″or·o·sal″pin·gi′tis. Inflammation of the tissues surrounding an ovary and oviduct.

per″i·op·tom′e·try. The measurement of the limits of the visual field.

per″i·or′al. Surrounding the mouth; circumoral.

per″i·or′bit, per″i·or′bi·ta. The periosteum of the orbit. **—periorbital,** *adj.*

per″i·os″te·ot′o·my. An incision into periosteum.

per″i·os′te·um. A fibrous membrane investing the surfaces of bones, except at the points of tendinous and ligamentous attachment and on the articular surfaces, where cartilage is substituted. **—periosteal,** *adj.*

per″i·os·ti′tis. Inflammation of periosteum. It may be acute or chronic, the latter being the more frequent form. It is caused by trauma or infection. The exudative forms show serous, fibrinous, leukocytic, or purulent exudate. The proliferative forms are characterized by local or diffuse formation of collagenous fibrous tissue or bone. **—periostit′ic,** *adj.*

per″i·os·to′ma. Any morbid osseous growth occurring on or surrounding bone.

per″i·os·to′sis. An osseous formation on the exterior of a bone.

per″i·o′tic (perr″ee·o′tick, ·ot′ick). 1. Situated about the ear. 2. Of or pertaining to the parts immediately about the internal ear.

per″i·pach″y·men·in·gi′t[is] (perr″i·pack″i·men″in·jy′tis). Inflammation of the connective tissue outside the dura mater.

per″i·pan″cre·a·ti′tis. Inflammation of the tissues around the pancreas.

per″i·pap′il·lar″y (perr″i·pap′i·lerr″ee). Occurring or situated around the circumference of a papilla, and especially of the optic disk.

per″i·phak′us (perr″i·fack′us, ·fa′kus). The capsule surrounding the crystalline lens.

pe·riph′er·al ref′er·ence. The condition in which, from 10 to 14 weeks following section of a peripheral sensory nerve, tactile and painful stimuli and stimuli of cold, applied within the originally anesthetic area, elicit mixed sensations at the edge of the area sensory change. This gradually disappears as the true stimulated point becomes perceptible.

pe·riph′er·a·phose″ (peh·rif′uh·fohz″, perr″i·ferr′uh·fohz). An aphose originating in the peripheral organs of vision (the optic nerve or the eyeball).

pe·riph″er·o·phose″ (peh·rif′uh·fohz″). A phose originating in the peripheral organs of vision (the optic nerve or the eyeball).

pe·riph′er·y. Circumference; the external surface. **—peripheral,** *adj.*

per″i·phle·bi′tis. Inflammation of the tissues about a vein. **—periphlebit′ic,** *adj.*

per″i·pleu·ri′tis (perr″i·ploor·eye′-is). Inflammation of the tissues outside the parietal pleura.

pe·rip′lo·cin, per″i·plo′cin. C₃₀H₄₈O₁₃. An amorphous glycoside from the bark of *Periploca graeca*.

per″i·por′tal. Surrounding the portal vein and its branches.

per″i·proc′tal, per″i·proc′tic. Surrounding the anus or rectum.

per″i·proc·ti′tis. Inflammation of the areolar tissue about the rectum or anus.

per″i·pros″ta·ti′tis. Inflammation of the tissue situated around the prostate.

per″i·py″le·phle·bi′tis. Inflammation of the tissues surrounding the portal vein.

per″i·rhi′nal. Situated about the nose or nasal fossae.

per″i·sal″pin·gi′tis. Inflammation of the tissue surrounding a uterine tube.

per″i·sal′pinx. The peritoneum covering a uterine tube.

per″i·sig″moid·i′tis. Inflammation of the tissues, especially the peritoneum, covering the sigmoid flexure of the colon.

per″i·si″nus·i′tis (·sigh″nuh·sigh′-tis, ·sigh″new·). Inflammation of the tissues around a sinus, especially a dural sinus.

per″i·sper″ma·ti′tis. Inflammation around the spermatic cord, with an effusion of fluid; a funicular hydrocele.

per″i·sple·ni′tis. Inflammation of the peritoneum covering the spleen. **p. cartilaginea.** Hard, inflammatory overgrowth of the capsule of the spleen. Also called *hyalin capsulitis.*

per″i·spon″dy·li′tis. Inflammation of the tissues around the vertebrae.

per″i·stal′sis. A progressive wave of contraction seen in tubes provided with longitudinal and transverse muscular fibers. It consists in a narrowing and shortening of a portion of the tube, which then relaxes, while a distal portion becomes shortened and narrowed. By means of this movement the contents of this tube are forced toward the opening. —**peristal′tic,** *adj.* **reversed p.** Peristaltic movement opposite to the normal direction.

per″i·stal′tic. Pertaining to, or resembling, peristalsis. **p. rush.** An exaggerated peristaltic wave that sweeps extensively over the small intestine.

per″i·staph″y·li′tis. Inflammation of the tissues surrounding the uvula.

per″i·sta′sis. According to Ricker's hypothesis, the early stage of the vascular changes in inflammation. The inactivity of vasoconstrictors leads to hy-

peremia in arterioles, venules, and capillaries. Subsequently, vasoconstriction in the distal segments of the arterioles leads to increased slowing of the blood current, the stage of prestasis. As more proximal segments of arterioles become constricted, the current is further slowed or stopped, the stage of rubrostasis. As arteriolar constriction is subsequently reduced, circulation is resumed, the stage of poststasis or postrubrostasis. This theory supposes a neurogenic basis for these vascular changes. Syn., *peristatic hyperemia.*

per″i·tec′to·my. Excision of a ring of conjunctiva around, and near to, the cornea.

per″i·ten″di·ni′tis. Inflammation of the sheath and tissues around a tendon. Syn., *peritenonitis.* **p. calcarea.** Calcific deposits in tendons and regional tissues which cause pain and limit motion of the parts.

per″i·ten′on. Sheath of a tendon.

per″i·the″li·o·ma. A tumor with cells arranged compactly around blood or lymph vessels, supposed to originate in perithelial cells.

per″i·the′li·um. The connective tissue accompanying the capillaries and smaller vessels. —**perithelial,** *adj.*

per″i·thy″roid·i′tis. Inflammation of the capsule of the thyroid gland.

pe·rit′o·my. 1. Excision of a strip of conjunctiva around the cornea, for the treatment of pannus. 2. Obsolete term for circumcision.

per″i·to·ne″o·cen·te′sis. Puncture of the peritoneal cavity, as for the removal of ascitic fluid.

per″i·to·ne′o·pex″y. Fixation of the uterus by the vaginal route in the treatment of retroflexion of this organ.

per″i·to·ne′o·scope. A long, slender telescope, equipped with sheath, obturator, biopsy forceps, sphygmomanometer bulb and tubing, scissors, syringe, for the visualization of the gas-inflated peritoneal cavity. It is introduced into the peritoneal cavity through a small incision in the abdominal wall and permits diagnosis of abdominal and pelvic tumors, biliary disease, and other intraabdominal diseases. —**peritoneos′copy,** n.

per″i·to·ne·ot′o·my. Incision into the peritoneum.

per″i·to·ne′um. The serous membrane lining the interior of the abdominal cavity and surrounding the contained viscera. —**peritoneal,** *adj.*

per″i·to·ni′tis. Inflammation of the peritoneum. **acute p.** That with an abrupt onset and rapid course, characterized by abdominal pain, tenderness, vomiting, constipation, and fever. May be due to irritation or bacterial infection, the latter being the more serious. **adhesive p.** That characterized by the formation of fibrous bands between peritoneal surfaces. **aseptic p.** A type due to irritation of the peritoneum by chemicals, either occurring naturally, as from bile, or introduced from without, as by antiseptic solutions, by x-ray or radium, or by mechanical means, as during the course of an operation. **chronic p.** That due to infection of the peritoneum by tuberculosis or actinomycosis, or occurring as a residual peritonitis from an acute attack. **diffuse p.** A type in which the inflammation is widespread over all, or almost all, of the peritoneum. Also called *generalized* p. **localized p.** That in which only a part of the peritoneum is involved, as a local area of inflammation associated with appendicitis. **pelvic p.** That which involves only the pelvic peritoneum, frequently associated with infection of the uterine tubes in women. **primary p.** One in which the infection is carried to the peritoneum by the blood or lymph stream. **puerperal p.** One following childbirth; associated with infection of the uterus and adnexa. **purulent p.** That characterized by the formation of pus. **secondary p.** The most usual type of peritonitis, due to extension of infection from neighboring parts, the rupture of a viscus or an abscess, trauma, or as a result of irritation.

per·i·to·nize. Cover with peritoneum by operative procedures.

per″i·ton′sil·lar. About a tonsil.

per″i·ton″sil·li′tis. Inflammation of the tissues surrounding a tonsil.

per″i·tra″che·i′tis (·tray″kee·eye′tis). Inflammation of the connective tissue about the trachea.

per″i·trich′i·al (perr″i·trick′ee·ul). Surrounding a hair follicle.

per″i·trun′cal. Perivascular and peribronchial conjointly, as peritruncal carcinoma of the lung.

per″i·um·bil′i·cal. Surrounding the umbilicus.

per″i·un′gual. Around a nail.

per″i·u·re″ter·i′tis. Inflammation of the tissues around a ureter.

per″i·u″re·thri′tis. Inflammation of the connective tissue about the urethra.

per″i·vas′cu·lar. About a vessel.

per″i·vas″cu·li′tis. Inflammation of the perivascular sheaths, including the adventitia.

per″i·ves′i·cal. Situated about, or surrounding, the urinary bladder.

per″i·ve·sic″u·li′tis. Inflammation around a seminal vesicle.

per″i·vis″cer·i′tis. Inflammation around a viscus or viscera.

per″i·xe·ni′tis (perr″i·zi·nigh′tis). Inflammation around a foreign body embedded in the tissues.

perle (purl). A capsule for administ[ration] tion of medicine.

per·lèche′ (pur·lesh′, perr·lesh′). [A] superficial, inflammatory condition [oc-] curring at the angles of the mouth w[ith] resultant fissuring. It is more prevale[nt] in children, but is also seen in adul[ts.] Although it has been regarded as [an] infection, it is often a symptom of ri[bo-] flavin deficiency.

per′ma·nent. Lasting; fixed; end[ur-] ing, as permanent teeth, the teeth [of] the second dentition.

per·man′ga·nate. A salt of p[er-] manganic acid.

per″man·gan′ic ac′id. HMnO₄, [a] monobasic acid known chiefly in [the] form of its salts.

permapen. A trade-mark for ben[za-] thine penicillin G.

per″me·a·bil′i·ty. In *physiolo[gy,]* the property of plasma membra[ne] which permits transit of molecu[les] and ions by solution in, or adsorpti[on] to, membranes, and by mechani[cal] passage through fine pores. **capil- lary p.** The permeability of the capil- lary wall to proteins of high molecu[lar] weight.

per′me·a·ble. Affording passa[ge;] pervious.

per″me·a′tion. The extension of [a] malignant tumor, especially carcinom[a,] by continuous growth through ly[m-] phatics.

permutit. Trade-mark for cert[ain] synthetic solid substances used for [the] purpose of exchanging a compon[ent] ion, such as sodium, for other io[ns] such as calcium and magnesium, pr[es-] ent in water or an aqueous solution [in] contact with the solid.

per·ni′cious. Highly destructive; [of] intense severity; fatal.

per′ni·o. Chilblain.

per″ni·o′sis. Any dermatitis result[t-] ing from chilblain.

pernoston. Trade-mark for 5-se[c-] butyl-5-β-bromallyl barbituric ac[id.] The substance is used as a hypno[tic] and sedative. See *butallylonal.*

pe″ro·bra′chi·us (peer″o·bra[ch′i-] kee·us). A developmental defect [in] which the forearms and hands are m[al-] formed or wanting.

pe″ro·chi′rus, pe″ro·chei′r[us] (peer″o·kigh′rus). Congenital abse[nce] or stunted growth of the hand.

pe″ro·cor′mus. Congenital def[ect] of the trunk.

pe″ro·dac·tyl′i·a. Defective de[vel-] opment of the fingers or toes.

pe″ro·dac′ty·lus. An individ[ual] having congenitally defective and p[ar-] tially absent fingers and/or toes.

pe″ro·me′li·a. Teratic malformat[ion] of the limbs.

pe·rom′e·lus. An individual w[ith]

congenitally deficient, stunted, or misshapen limbs.

pe·rom'e·ly. Congenital deficiency or malformation of the limbs.

per"o·ne'al. Pertaining to the fibular side of the leg, as peroneal nerve. See Table of Nerves in the Appendix.

per"o·ne'o- (perr"o·nee'o-). A combining form denoting *connection with* or *relation to the fibula.*

pe·ro'ni·a. Mutilation; malformation.

pe"ro·pla'si·a (peer"o·play'zhuh, ·shuh). A malformation due to abnormal development.

pe'ro·pus. An individual with congenitally malformed feet.

per·o'ral (pur·or'ul). Passed or performed through the mouth.

per os. By way of, or through, the mouth, as in the administration of medicines.

pe·ro'sis. The condition of abnormal or defective formation.

pe"ro·splanch'ni·ca (peer"o·splangk'ni·kuh). Malformation of the viscera.

per·os'se·ous (per·os'ee·us). Through bone.

per·ox'i·dase (per·ock'si·dace, ·daze). 1. An enzyme of vegetable origin that splits hydrogen peroxide into water, or metal peroxides into the corresponding oxide and oxygen. 2. A substance which activates peroxides. See *catalase.*

per·ox'ide (per·ock'side). That oxide of any base which contains the most oxygen.

per·ox'i·dize. Oxidize completely.

per"pen·dic'u·lar. Pertaining to a line or plane forming a right angle with another line or plane.

per·phen'a·zine. 2-Chloro-10-{3-[4-(β-hydroxyethyl) piperazinyl] propyl}-phenothiazine, an antiemetic and tranquilizer. See *trilafon.*

per pri'mam. By first intention, said of normal wound healing.

per rec'tum. By way of the rectum.

per'salt". A salt which contains the maximum amount of the acid radical.

per·sev"er·a'tion. Persistent repetition of words or some activity.

per'sic oil. A fixed oil expressed from apricot or peach kernels, consisting chiefly of glycerides of the higher fatty acids, possessing emollient properties.

per'son·al. Pertaining to a person, as personal equation, the peculiar difference of individuals in their relation to various orders of stimuli.

per"son·al'i·ty. 1. The totality of traits and the habitual modes of behavior of the individual as they impress others; the physical and mental qualities peculiar to the individual, and which have social connotations. Re-

garded by psychoanalysts as the resultant of the interaction of the instincts and the environment. 2. *In psychiatry,* an individual with a special type of personal qualities. **alternating p.** One which allows the individual to live alternatingly as two different persons. **cycloid p.** One which is characterized by recurring states of increased mental and motor activity, alternating with periods of reduced animation bordering on depression. **dissociated p.** See split p. **dual p.** See alternating p. **extroverted p.** One in which instinctual energy or libido is directed from the individual and toward the environment. **feeling-type p.** One in which the total attitude or reaction i dictated by feeling or emotional tone, one of Jung's functional types of personality. **introverted p.** One in which instinctual energy is weak and thus inadequate libido is directed inwardly upon the individual himself. **intuitional-type p.** One directed by unconscious indications or by vaguely conscious stimuli; one of Jung's functional types of personality. **multiple p.** One which is capable of dissociation into several or many other personalities at the same time, whereby the delusion is entertained that the one person is many separate persons; a symptom in schizophrenic patients. **neurotic p.** One which exhibits symptoms or manifestations intermediate between normal character traits and true neurotic features. **paranoid p.** The tendency to project hostile feelings so as to be or easily become suspicious of others and to feel persecuted and jealous, often with related features of a schizoid personality. **psychopathic p.** One characterized by emotional immaturity with marked defects of judgment, prone to impulsive behavior without consideration of others and without evidence of learning by experience. **schizoid p.** One given to seclusiveness, emotional rigidity, introversion, and unsocial behavior. **sensational-type p.** One in which sensation, rather than reflective thinking or feeling, dictates action or attitude; Jung's fourth functional type of personality. **split p.** One in which there is a separation of various components of the normal personality unit, and each segregation functions as an entity apart from the remaining personality structure; commonly observed in hysteria and schizophrenia. **syntonic p.** One in which there is harmony and appropriateness of thinking, feeling, and action; one which is in harmony with the environment. **thinking-type p.** One in which actions and attitudes are ruled predominantly by deliberation and reflective thought rather than by feeling, intuition, or sensation; the first of the four functional types of personality according to Jung.

per'son·al'i·ty-for·ma'tion. In *psychoanalysis,* the arrangement of the basic constituents of personality.

per'spi·ra'tion. 1. The secretion of sweat. 2. The sweat. **insensible p.** That which takes place constantly, the fluid being evaporated as fast as excreted. **sensible p.** Visible drops or beads of sweat.

per·sul'fate. A salt of persulfuric acid, $H_2S_2O_8$, an acid obtained by electrolytic oxidation of sulfuric acid.

per·sul'fide. A sulfide that contains more atoms of sulfur than are required by the normal valence of sulfur, as, for example, in Na_2S_3.

per'tur·ba'tion. Restlessness or disquietude; great uneasiness.

per·tus'sal. Like whooping cough. Also called *pertussoid.*

per·tus'sis. See *whooping cough.*

Pe·ru'vi·an bark. Old term for cinchona.

per·ver'sion (pur·vur'zhun, ·shun). 1. The state of being turned away from the normal or correct. 2. In *psychopathology,* deviation from the normal or average in sexual practices, as homogenitality or fellatio. **—per'vert,** *n.*

pervitin hydrochloride. Trademark for *d*-desoxyephedrine hydrochloride.

pes (pl. *pedes*) (payz, pace, pl. pee'deez). A foot or footlike structure. For other terms concerning pes, see *talipes.* **p. anserinus.** (a) The radiate branching of the facial nerve after its exit from the facial canal. (b) The junction of the tendons of the sartorius, gracilis, and semitendinosus muscles. **O.T. p. contortus.** Clubfoot; talipes, *q.v.* **p. gigas.** Macropodia. An abnormally large foot. **p. pedunculi.** See *basis pedunculi.* **p. planus.** Flatfoot.

pes·sa'ry. 1. An appliance of varied form placed in the vagina. 2. Any suppository or other form of medication placed in the vagina for therapeutic purposes. *Obs.* **cradle p.** A cradle-shaped pessary once commonly used in the correction of uterine displacements. **cup p.** A type of pessary for uterine prolapse in which the cervix rests in a cup held in by a belt and straps. **diaphragm p.** The occlusive diaphragm for contraception. **doughnut p.** A ring pessary for uterine prolapse. **prolapse p.** Any of several types of rings or cups inserted into the vagina for the purpose of holding up the uterus. **retroversion p.** Any type of pessary, such as the Smith-Hodge, used to correct a retroverted uterus. **ring p.** A round or ring-shaped pessary.

stem p. A device for insertion into the cervical canal, to prevent conception or to stimulate an infantile uterus.

pes'su·lus, pes'sum. A pessary.

pest. 1. A plague; pestilence. 2. Anything destructive or annoying, such as insects.

pest'house. A hospital for persons sick with pestilential diseases.

pes'ti·cide. A substance that is destructive to pests, especially insect pests.

pes'tle (pess'ul). The device for rubbing substances in a mortar.

pe·te'chi·a (peh·tee'kee·uh, peh·teck'ee·uh) (pl. *petechiae*). A minute, rounded spot of hemorrhage on a surface such as skin, mucous membrane, serous membrane, or on a cross-sectional surface of an organ. **—petechial,** *adj.*

peth'i·dine (peth'i·deen, ·din). Meperidine hydrochloride.

pe·tit' mal' (puh·tee' mal'). See *petit mal epilepsy.*

pet'ri·fac'tion. The process of changing to stone, as petrifaction of the fetus. See *lithopedion.*

pé'tris·sage' (pay'tri·sahzh'). Kneading massage; the muscles are manipulated by lifting, squeezing, or rolling action.

pet'ro·la'tum. A purified, semisolid mixture of hydrocarbons obtained from petroleum. Occurs as an unctuous mass, varying in color from yellowish to light amber; insoluble in water. Used as a bland, protective dressing and as a base for ointments. Also called *petroleum jelly, yellow petrolatum.* **light liquid p.** A mixture of liquid hydrocarbons obtained from petroleum. Used in sprays for the nose and throat. Also called *light liquid paraffin, light white mineral oil.* **liquid p.** A mixture of liquid hydrocarbons obtained from petroleum; a colorless, oily liquid, insoluble in water. Used as a vehicle for medicinal agents and for its mechanical action in constipation. Also called *liquid paraffin, white mineral oil, heavy liquid petrolatum.* **white p.** Petrolatum wholly or nearly decolorized. Used the same as petrolatum.

pe·tro'le·um. A complex mixture of hydrocarbons consisting chiefly of the paraffins and cycloparaffins or of cyclic aromatic hydrocarbons. Occurs as a dark-yellow to brown or greenish gray, oily liquid; insoluble in water. **p. jelly.** See *petrolatum.*

pe·tro'sa. The petrous portion of the temporal bone. **—petrosal,** *adj.*

pet'ro·si'tis. Inflammation of the petrous portion of the temporal bone, usually from extension of mastoiditis or from middle-ear disease.

pet'ro·squa'mous. Pertaining to

the petrous and squamous portions of the temporal bone.

pet'rous (pet'rus, pee'trus). Stony; of the hardness of stone.

pe·trox'o·lin. A liquid or solid preparation made with a vehicle or base composed of light liquid petrolatum with soft ammonia soap and alcohol and containing medicinal substances. Petroxolins are intended for external application. **solid p.** Solid petrox, a yellowish brown solid containing yellow wax, light liquid petrolatum, oleic acid, ammonia, lavender oil, and alcohol. It is used as a base for application of various medicinal substances.

-pex'y, -pex'i·a. *In surgery,* a combining form denoting *fixation.*

P. G. *Pharmacopoeia Germanica,* German Pharmacopoeia.

pH. Symbol introduced by Sørensen; used in expressing hydrogen-ion concentration. It signifies the logarithm, on the base ten, of the reciprocal of the hydrogen-ion concentration.

pha·cen'to·cele. Displacement of the crystalline lens into the anterior chamber of the eye.

pha·ci'tis (fa·kigh'tis). Inflammation of the lens of the eye.

phac'o- (fack'o-, fay'ko-), **phac-.** A combining form denoting *a lens or the lens of the eye.*

phac''o·an''a·phy·lax'is. Anaphylaxis to the crystalline lens. If extracapsular cataract extraction has been performed on one eye, the patient may become sensitized to the lens protein, so that breakage of the other lens capsule, with release of lens protein, allows anaphylactic reaction due to the previous sensitization.

phac'o·cyst. The capsule of the crystalline lens.

phac''o·cys·tec'to·my. Excision of a part of the capsule of the crystalline lens.

phac''o·er'i·sis. An operation for cataract employing suction.

phac''o·hy''men·i'tis. Inflammation of the capsule of the crystalline lens.

pha'coid (fay'koyd, fack'oyd). Lens-shaped.

pha·col'y·sis. 1. Dissolution or disintegration of the crystalline lens. 2. An operation for the relief of high myopia, consisting in discission of the crystalline lens followed by extraction. —**pha·colyt'ic,** *adj.*

phac''o·ma·to'sis. One of a group of diseases, hereditary and developmental in origin, which produce a host of symptoms but which are all characterized by the presence of spots, tumefactions, and cysts joined to other congenital malformations in various parts of the body, especially in the central

nervous system. Three distinct syndromes can be recognized: Tuberous sclerosis (phacomatosis of Bourneville), von Hippel-Lindau's disease (angiophacomatosis retinae et cerebelli), and von Recklinghausen's disease (neurofibromatosis, neurofibro-phacomatosis).

phac''o·met''a·cho·re'sis (fack''-o·met''uh·kor·ee'sis, fay''ko·). Dislocation of the crystalline lens.

phac''o·met''e·ce'sis. Displacement of the crystalline lens into the anterior chamber of the eye.

pha·com'e·ter. An instrument for determining the refractive power of lenses. Usually called *lensometer.*

phac''o·pla·ne'sis. Displacement of the crystalline lens of the eye from the posterior to the anterior chamber and back again.

phac''o·scle·ro'sis. Hardening of the crystalline lens.

phac'o·scope. An instrument for observing the accommodative changes of the lens. —**phacos'copy,** *n.*

phac''o·sco·tas'mus. Clouding of the crystalline lens.

-phage (-faydj), **-phag.** A combining form denoting *an eater;* used especially to denote *a phagocyte, q.v.* See also *bacteriophage.*

phag''e·de'na, phag''e·dae'na (fadj''i·dee'nuh). A rapidly spreading destructive ulceration of soft parts. —**phageden'ic,** *adj.* **sloughing p.** Gangrene.

phag'o·cyte. A cell having the property of engulfing and digesting foreign or other particles or cells harmful to the body. **Fixed phagocytes** include the cells of the reticuloendothelial system and fixed macrophages (histiocytes). **Free phagocytes** include the leukocytes and free macrophages. —**phagocy'tal, phagocyt'ic,** *adj.*

phag''o·cy·to'sis (fag''o·sigh·to'sis). Ingestion of foreign or other particles, principally bacteria, by certain cells.

phag''o·dy''na·mom'e·ter. An apparatus for estimating the force exerted in chewing.

phag''o·ma'ni·a. An insatiable craving for food.

phag''o·ther'a·py. Treatment by superalimentation; overfeeding.

phak'o-. See *phaco-.*

phal''a·cro'sis. Baldness; alopecia. *Rare.* —**phalacrot'ic, phalac'rous,** *adj.*

phal''an·gec'to·my (fal''an·jeck'-to·mee). Surgical excision of a phalanx of a finger or toe.

pha·lan'ges (fay·lan'jeez, fa·lan'-jeez). Plural of phalanx, *q.v.* See Table of Bones in the Appendix.

phal''an·gi'tis. Inflammation of a phalanx or phalanges.

pha·lan''gi·za'tion. A plastic operation in which a metacarpal bone is separated from its fellows and surrounded with skin, thus forming a substitute for a finger or thumb.

pha·lan″go·pha·lan′ge·al (fa-lang″go-fa·lan′jul, ·jee-ul). Pertaining to the successive phalanges of the digits, as in phalangophalangeal amputation, removal of a finger or toe at the first or second phalangeal joints.

pha′lanx (fay′langks, fal′angks) (pl. *phalanges*). 1. One of the bones of the fingers or toes. See Table of Bones in the Appendix. 2. One of the delicate processes of the headplate of the outer rod of Corti projecting beyond the inner rod. **—phalan′geal,** *adj.*

phal′lic. Pertaining to the penis. See *phallus.*

phal′lus. 1. The penis. 2. The indifferent embryonic structure derived from the genital tubercle that, in the male, differentiates into the penis, and, in the female, into the clitoris. **—phallic, phalliform, phalloid,** *adj.*

phan″er·o·gen′ic. Having a known cause; the opposite of *cryptogenic.*

phan″er·o·ma′ni·a. A neurotic condition in which a person pays undue attention to or cannot resist the impulse to touch some external part or growth, such as a pimple, a hair, or a hangnail; a form of compulsion.

phan″er·o′sis. The act of passing from a transparent to a visible state.

phanodorn. Trade-mark for a rapidly eliminated hypnotic and sedative, cyclohexenylethylbarbituric acid or cyclobarbital.

phan′tasm. An illusive perception of an object that does not exist; an illusion or hallucination. **—phantas′mic,** *adj.*

phan·tas″ma·to·mo′ri·a (fan-tas″muh·to·mor′ee·uh). Childishness, or dementia, with absurd fancies or delusions.

phan·tas″mo·sco′pi·a. The seeing of phantasms; hallucinations involving ghosts.

phan′ta·sy. 1. Visionary imagination; the faculty of reproducing unreal, phantasmic notions or sensuous impressions. 2. An image. 3. Fantasy.

Phar. D. *Pharmaciae Doctor,* Doctor of Pharmacy.

phar′ma·cal. Pertaining to pharmacy.

phar″ma·ceu′tic (fahr″muh·sue′tick), **phar″ma·ceu′ti·cal.** Pertaining to pharmacy.

phar″ma·ceu′ti·cal. See *pharmaceutic.*

phar″ma·ceu′tist. See *pharmacist.*

phar′ma·cist. An apothecary, a druggist.

phar′ma·co-. A combining form denoting *drug.*

phar″ma·co·dy·nam′ics (fahr″-muh·ko·dye·nam′icks, ·di·nam′icks). The science of the action of drugs. **—pharmacodynamic,** *adj.*

phar″ma·cog′no·sist. One versed in pharmacognosy.

phar″ma·cog′no·sy. The science of crude drugs.

phar″ma·col′o·gist. A specialist in pharmacology.

phar″ma·col′o·gy. The science of the nature and properties of drugs, particularly their actions. **—pharmacolog′ic, pharmacolog′ical,** *adj.*

phar″ma·co·ma′ni·a. A morbid craving for medicines, or for self-medication.

phar″ma·co·pe′ia (fahr″muh·ko-pee′uh). A collection of formulas and methods for the preparation of drugs, especially a book of such formulas recognized as a standard, as the United States Pharmacopeia. Also spelled *pharmacopoeia.* Abbreviated, P. **—pharmacopeial,** *adj.*

phar″ma·co·pho′bi·a. Morbid dislike or fear of medicine.

phar″ma·co·psy·cho′sis (fahr″-muh·ko·sigh·ko′sis). Psychosis associated with drugs.

phar″ma·co·ther′a·py. The treatment of disease by means of drugs.

phar′ma·cy. 1. The art of preparing, compounding, and dispensing medicines. 2. A drug store.

pharmagel. Trade-mark for a brand of gelatin particularly designed for the preparation of emulsions and available in two types, A and B, based upon the method of manufacture.

phar″yn·gal′gi·a. Pain in the pharynx.

phar″yn·gec′to·my (far″in·jeck′to·mee). Excision of a part of the pharynx.

phar″yn·gem·phrax′is (far″in·jem·frack′sis). Obstruction of the pharynx.

phar″yn·gis′mus. Spasm of the pharynx.

phar″yn·gi′tis. Inflammation of the pharynx. **—pharyngit′ic,** *adj.* **acute p.** A form due to exposure to cold, to the action of irritant substances, or to certain infectious causes, and characterized by pain on swallowing, by dryness, later by moisture, and by congestion of the mucous membrane. Also called *catarrhal p.* **atrophic p.** A form attended by atrophy of the mucous membrane. **chronic p.** A form that is generally the result of repeated acute attacks, and is associated either with hypertrophy of the mucous membrane (**hypertrophic pharyngitis**) or with atrophy (**atrophic pharyngitis**). **diphtheritic p.** That characterized by the presence of a false membrane, the product of the action of the diphtheria bacillus. Also called *croupous* p. **granular p.** A form of chronic pharyngitis in which the mucous membrane has a granular appearance. Also called *clergyman's sore throat.* **p. sicca.** The atrophic form characterized by a dry state of the mucous membrane.

pha·ryn'go- (fa·ring'go-), **pha·ryng-.** A combining form meaning *pharynx.*

pha·ryn'go·cele. A hernia or pouch of the pharynx projecting through the pharyngeal wall.

pha·ryn''go·dyn'i·a. Pain referred to the pharynx.

pha·ryn''go·e''so·phag'e·al (fa·ring''go·ee''so·fadj'ul, ·ee''so·fuh·jee'ul). Pertaining to the pharynx and esophagus.

pha·ryn''go·ker''a·to'sis. Thickening of the mucous lining of the pharynx with formation of a tough and adherent exudate.

pha·ryn''go·lar''yn·gi'tis. Simultaneous inflammation of the pharynx and larynx.

pha·ryn'go·lith. A calcareous concretion in the walls of the pharynx.

phar''yn·gol'o·gy. The science of the pharyngeal mechanism, functions, and diseases.

pha·ryn''go·max'il·lar''y (·mack'si·lerr''ee). Relating to the pharynx and the maxilla.

pha·ryn''go·my·co'sis (fa·ring''go·migh·ko'sis). Disease of the pharynx due to the action of fungi.

phar''yn·gop'a·thy. Any disease of the pharynx.

pha·ryn'go·plas''ty. Plastic surgery of the pharynx.

pha·ryn''go·ple'gi·a (fa·ring''go·plee'juh, far''ing·go·). Paralysis of the muscles of the pharynx.

pha·ryn''go·rhi·ni'tis (fa·ring''go·rye·nigh'tis). Pharyngitis with rhinitis; inflammation of the pharyngeal and nasal mucosa.

pha·ryn''gor·rha'gi·a (fa·ring''go·ray'juh, far''ing·go·). Hemorrhage from the pharynx.

pha·ryn''gor·rhe'a. A mucous discharge from the pharynx.

pha·ryn'go·scope. An instrument for use in examining the pharynx. **—pharyngos'copy,** *n.*

pha·ryn''go·spasm. Spasmodic contraction of the pharynx.

pha·ryn''go·ste'ni·a. Narrowing or stricture of the pharynx. **—pharyngos'tenous,** *adj.*

pha·ryn'go·tome. An instrument for incising the pharynx.

phar''yn·got'o·my. Incision into the pharynx. **anterior p.** An approach to the oral pharynx by an incision above the hyoid bone and a separation of the suprahyoid structures. **lateral p.** Incision into one side of the pharynx.

pha·ryn''go·ton''sil·li'tis. Inflammation of the pharynx and tonsils.

pha·ryn''go·xe·ro'sis (fa·ring''go·zi·ro'sis). Dryness of the pharynx.

phar'ynx. The musculomembranous tube situated back of the nose, mouth, and larynx, and extending from the base of the skull to a point opposite the sixth cervical vertebra, where it becomes continuous with the esophagus. It is lined by mucous membrane, covered in its upper part with pseudostratified ciliated epithelium, in its lower part with stratified squamous epithelium. On the outside of this is a layer of fibrous tissue, the **pharyngeal aponeurosis.** This in turn is surrounded by the muscular coat. The upper portion of the pharynx, communicating with the nose through the posterior nares, the **nasopharynx,** functionally belongs to the respiratory tract; the lower portion, divided into the **oropharynx** and **laryngopharynx,** is common to the respiratory and digestive tracts. The pharynx communicates with the middle ear by means of the auditory tube. **—pharyn'geal** (fa·rin'jul, ·jee·ul, far''in·jee'ul), *adj.* **primitive p.** The embryonic pharynx with its characteristic visceral arches, grooves, and pouches.

phase (faze). 1. The condition or stage of a disease or of biologic, chemical, and physiologic functions at a given time. 2. A solid, liquid, or gas which is homogeneous throughout and physically separated from another phase by a distinct boundary.

pha·se'o·lin (fa·see'o·lin). A simple protein of the globulin type which occurs in kidney beans.

pha'sic ir·reg''u·lar'i·ty (fay'zick). A disorder consisting of a periodic slowing of the heart for a few seconds, unrelated to the respiratory cycle; occurs in convalescence from acute fevers, and sometimes during the administration of digitalis. Its manner of production is unknown, but the fact that it is abolished by atropine shows that it is a vagal effect.

phat''nor·rha'gi·a. Hemorrhage occurring from a tooth socket.

phel'lan·drene. A hydrocarbon found in oil of fennel and that of certain other plants.

phemerol chloride. Trade-mark for benzethonium chloride.

phen-, phe'no- (fee'no-, fen'o-). A combining form denoting *derivation from benzene.*

-phen. A combining form for *phene.*

phen'a·caine hy''dro·chlo'ride (fen'uh·cane, fee'nuh·cane). Ethenyl-p-diethoxydiphenylamidine hydrochloride; white crystals or powder; soluble in water. Used as a local anesthetic.

phe·nac'e·tin (fĭ-nass'ĭ-tin). Acetophenetidin.

phe·nac''e·tu'ric ac'id. C₆H₅CH₂·CO.NH.CH₂COOH. Glycine conjugate of phenylacetic acid, one form in which the latter is excreted following ingestion by animals.

phe·nam'i·dine (fĭ-nam'ĭ-deen, ·din). A diamidine, 4':4'-diamidino diphenyl ether. Active against pathogenic trypanosomes, also inhibits growth of bacteria in wounds.

phe·nan'threne. C₁₄H₁₀. A hydrocarbon isomeric with anthracene, and found with it in coal tar.

phenarsen. A trade-mark for dichlorophenarsine hydrochloride.

phe·nar'sone sulf·ox'y·late. Sodium 3-amino-4-hydroxyphenylarsonate-N-methanal sulfoxylate, a pentavalent arsenical employed medicinally. See *aldarsone.*

phe'nate, phen'ate. A compound of phenol and a base; a carbolate.

phen'a·zone. Antipyrine.

phene (feen). *In chemistry,* benzene.

phenergan hydrochloride. Trade-mark for promethazine hydrochloride.

phe·net'i·din. NH₂.C₆H₄.OC₂H₅. Aminoethoxybenzene, of which three isomers exist. The para-isomer frequently appears in the urine following administration of acetophenetidin.

phe·net'sal, phen'et·sal. Acetyl-p-aminophenyl salicylate. White, odorless crystals. Used as an antirheumatic, antipyretic, and analgesic. See *salophen.*

phen''go·pho'bi·a. A morbid fear of daylight.

phe'nic ac'id (fee'nick, fen'ick). See *phenol.*

phe'nic al'co·hol. Phenol, *q.v.*

phe·nin'da·mine (fĭ·nin'duh·meen, ·min). C₁₉H₁₉N. 2-Methyl-9-phenyl-2,3,-4,9-tetrahydro-1-pyridindene, an antihistaminic substance. See *thephorin.*

phen''in·di'one. 2-Phenylindane-1,3-dione, an anticoagulant effective when administered orally. See *danilone.*

phen·meth'y·lol. Benzyl alcohol.

phen·met'ra·zine hy''dro·chlo'ride. Generic name for 2-phenyl-3-methyltetrahydro-1,4-oxazine hydrochloride, a sympathomimetic drug. See *preludin.*

phe''no·bar'bi·tal (fee''no·bahr'bi·tawl, ·tal, fen''o·). Phenylethylbarbituric acid; white crystals; slightly soluble in water. Used as a hypnotic and sedative. Syn., *phenylethylmalonylurea, phenobarbitone.* See *luminal.* **p. sodium.** The sodium derivative of phenobarbital; very soluble in water.

Also called *soluble phenobarbitone, soluble phenobarbital.* See *luminal sodium.*

phe''no·bar'bi·tone. See *phenobarbital.*

phe'no·din. Hematin, *q.v.*

phe'nol (fee'nole, ·nol, fĭ·nole'). 1. C₆H₅OH. Hydroxybenzene; obtained from coal tar or prepared synthetically; colorless to light pink, needle-shaped crystals; soluble in water. Used as an antiseptic, germicide, disinfectant, escharotic, and local anesthetic. Also called *carbolic acid, phenyl alcohol, phenyl hydrate.* 2. Any hydroxy derivative of aromatic hydrocarbons which has the OH group directly attached to the ring. **camphorated p.** (*camphor-phenol*). Contains 30% of phenol and 60% of camphor in liquid petrolatum. **liquefied p.** (*liquefied carbolic acid*). Phenol maintained in the liquid condition by the presence of 10% of water. **p. coefficient.** A figure representing the relative strength of an antiseptic, as compared with phenol acting on the same organism and for the same length of time. **p. red.** See *phenolsulfonphthalein.*

phe'no·late. A compound of a phenol in which the hydrogen of the hydroxyl group is replaced by a univalent metal.

phe''nol·phthal'ein (fee''nole·thal'een, ·thal'ee·in, fee''nol·, fee''nawl·). (C₆H₄OH)₂CO.C₆H₄CO; a white or faintly yellowish powder; almost insoluble in water. Used as a laxative. **yellow p.** An impure form of phenolphthalein, having a canary yellow color; is two or three times as active as the white form.

phe''nol·phthal'in. 4',4''-Dihydroxytriphenylmethane-2-carboxylic acid, prepared from phenolphthalein. Used as a reagent for detecting presence of blood.

phe''nol·sul'fo·nate. A salt or ester of phenolsulfonic acid.

phe''nol·sul''fone·phthal'ein. Phenolsulfonphthalein.

phe''nol·sul·fon'ic ac'id. C₆H₄.OH.SO₂H. Of the three isomers, ortho-, meta-, and para-, the last is used, in the form of salts, as an intestinal antiseptic. Syn., *sulfocarbolic acid.*

phe''nol·sul''fon·phthal'ein. C₁₉H₁₄O₅S; bright-red to dark-red, crystalline powder; soluble in water. Used for determining the functional activity of the kidneys.

phe''nol·tet''ra·chlo''ro·phthal'ein. A dye used intravenously in the form of the sodium salt for the determination of the functional activity of the liver.

phe''nol·tet''ra·i·o''do·phthal'ein so'di·um (fee''nole·tet''ruh·eye·o''do·thal'een). See *phentetiodophthalein sodium.*

phe″no·lu′ri·a. The presence of phenols in the urine.

phe·nom′e·non (pl. *phenomena*). An event or manifestation, generally of an unusual character. **rebound p.** Sudden withdrawal of strong resistance to a movement causes marked rebound; ipsilateral to cerebellar lesion.

phe″no·thi′a·zine (fee″no·thigh′-uh·zeen, ·zin). $C_{12}H_9NS$. Thiodiphenylamine; occurs as a greenish powder; insoluble in water. Used chiefly by veterinarians for its vermifuge action.

phe′no·type. 1. The sum total of visible traits which characterize the members of a group. 2. A group of individuals who look alike, but differ in their genetic make-up. **—phenotyp′ic,** *adj.*

phen·ox′y-. A combining form denoting *the presence of C_6H_5O-*.

phe·nox″y·benz′a·mine   hy″dro·chlo′ride. N-Phenoxyisopropyl-N-benzyl-β-chloroethylamine, an adrenergic blocking agent used in treating peripheral vascular diseases and, sometimes, certain types of hypertension. See *dibenzyline*.

phe·nox″y·meth′yl   pen″i·cil′lin. A biosynthetic penicillin in which the R group is phenoxymethyl (C_6H_5·OCH_2-). Syn., *penicillin V.* See *penvee, v-cillin.*

phen·tet″i·o·thal′e·in   so′di·um (fen·tet″eye·o·thal′ee·in, ·thal′een, ·thay′lee·in). $NaO:C.C_6L.C:C_6H_4OC_6$-H_4ONa. The disodium salt of a dye, phenoltetraiodophthalein. Bronze-purple, odorless granules; soluble in water. Used for the roentgenologic examinations and for test of hepatic function. Syn., *phenoltetraiodophthalein sodium.*

phen·tol′a·mine. 2-[(m-Hydroxy-N-p-tolylanilino)-methyl]-2-imidazoline, used in diagnosis and control of hypertension resulting from pheochromocytoma. See *regitine.*

phen″yl·a·ce″tyl·glu′ta·mine. $H_2N.CO(CH_2)_2(CHNHOCCH_2C_6H_5)$-COOH. A conjugated form of phenylacetic acid excreted in man.

phen′yl   a·ce″tyl·sal″i·cyl′ate. $C_6H_4(OCH_3CO)COOC_6H_5$. A white powder, insoluble in water; hydrolyzed in the intestines. An analgesic, antipyretic and mild intestinal antiseptic.

phen″yl·al′a·nine (fen″il·al′uh·neen, ·nin, fee″nil·). $C_6H_5CH_2CH(NH_2)$-COOH. α-Amino-β-phenylpropionic acid, an amino acid essential in human nutrition.

phen′yl   al′co·hol. See *phenol.*

phen″yl·am′ine (fen″il·am′een, ·in, fee″nil·). See *aniline.*

phen″yl·bu′ta·zone. 3,5-Dioxo-1,2-diphenyl-4-n-butylpyrazolidine, a drug used in the treatment of arthritis and allied disorders. See *butazolidin.*

phen″yl·car′bi·nol. Benzyl alcohol.

phen″yl·cin″cho·nin′ic   ac′id (·sin″ko·nin′ick). Cinchophen.

phen′yl·ene (fen′i·leen, fee′ni·leen). The bivalent radical, C_6H_4.

phen″yl·eph′rine   hy″dro·chlo′ride. l-1-(m-Hydroxyphenyl)-2-methylaminoethanol hydrochloride, a sympathomimetic agent. See *neo-synephrine hydrochloride.*

phen″yl·eth″yl·a·mine′ (C_6H_5)-$C_2H_4NH_2$. A decarboxylation product of phenylalanine.

phen″yl·eth″yl·bar″bi·tu′ric   ac′id. See *phenobarbital.*

phen″yl·eth″yl·mal″o·ny·lu′re·a. See *phenobarbital.*

phen″yl·glu·co·sa′zone. $C_{18}H_{22}$-N_4O_4. A yellow, crystalline compound produced in the phenylhydrazine test for glucose.

phen″yl·hy′dra·zine (fen″il·high′druh·zeen, ·zin, fee″nil·). $C_6H_5.NH$·NH_2. A colorless to red-brown liquid, sparingly soluble in water. Used as a reagent for sugars, aldehydes, and ketones, and for other chemical reactions. **p. hydrochloride.** $C_6H_5.NH.NH_2$·HCl, occurs as white leaflets; soluble in water. Used in the treatment of polycythemia.

phen″yl·hy′dra·zone. The product resulting from the interaction of phenylhydrazine with an aldehyde or ketone.

phe·nyl′ic   ac′id. Phenol.

phen″yl·ke″to·nu′ri·a. The presence of a phenylketone in the urine.

phen″yl·mer·cu′ric   ac′e·tate (ass′i·tayt). $C_6H_5.Hg.C_2H_3O_2$; occurs as white prisms; soluble in water. Used as an antiseptic, germicide, and fungicide.

phen″yl·mer·cu′ric   chlo′ride. C_6H_5HgCl; occurs as white crystals, practically insoluble in water. Used as an antiseptic, germicide, and fungicide.

phen″yl·mer·cu′ric   ni′trate. $C_6H_5Hg.OH.C_6H_5.HgNO_3$, basic phenylmercuric nitrate; occurs as a white or grayish white powder; soluble in water. Used as an antiseptic, germicide, and fungicide.

phen′y·lon. Antipyrine, *q.v.*

phen″yl·pro″pa·nol′a·mine   hy″dro·chlo′ride. 1-Phenyl-2-aminopropanol hydrochloride, used as a nasal decongestant, antiallergic, and appetite suppressant. Syn., *norephedrine hydrochloride.* See *propadrine hydrochloride.*

phen″yl·pro″pyl·meth′yl·a·mine. Nonproprietary title for the nasal vasoconstrictor substance available under the trade-marked name *vonedrine.*

phen″yl·py·ru′vic   ac′id (fen″il·pye·roo′vick,   ·pi·roo′vick,   fee″nil·).

$C_6H_5CH_2.CO.COOH$. A metabolic product of phenylalanine.

phen"yl·quin"o·line-car"box·yl'ic ac'id (fen"il·kwin"o·leen-, -lin-, fee"nil-). Cinchophen.

phen'yl sal'i·cyl"ate. $OH.C_6H_4.COO.C_6H_5$. A white powder; very slightly soluble in water. Hydrolyzed in the small intestine by pancreatic juice, yielding phenol and salicylic acid. For this reason it is used as an internal antiseptic. Syn., *salol.*

phen"yl·sul'fate. A salt of phenylsulfuric acid.

phen"yl·sul·fur'ic ac'id. $C_6H_5O·SO_2H$. A phenol ester of sulfuric acid.

phen'y·toin so'di·um. Diphenylhydantoin sodium.

phe"o·chro"mo·cy·to'ma (fee"o-kro"mo·sigh·to'muh). A tumor of the sympathetic nervous system, found most often in the adrenal medulla but occasionally in other sites such as chromaffin bodies and in the thorax. It is made up largely of pheochromocytes, or chromaffin cells, derivatives of the primitive neurocytes, with a strong affinity for taking up chrome salts. May be accompanied by the adrenalsympathetic syndrome of spasmodic hypertension. Syn., *chromaffinoma, paraganglioma.*

phe"o·phy'tin. The product formed by replacement of magnesium in chlorophyll by hydrogen. The corresponding copper and iron derivatives of chlorophyll, which may be considered **magnesium pheophytin**, are called **copper pheophytin** and **iron pheophytin.** They are sometimes referred to simply as chlorophylls. See *chlorophyll.*

Ph. G. Graduate in Pharmacy; German Pharmacopoeia.

-phil'i·a. A combining form meaning *love of;* used to denote a *tendency toward* or a *craving for.* Also see *-phobia.*

-phile, -phil. A combining form denoting *one* or *that which has an affinity for* a specific substance or person.

phil"o·ne'ism. Abnormal love of novelty; the reverse of misoneism.

phil'trum. The depression on the surface of the upper lip immediately below the septum of the nose.

phi·mo'sis (figh·mo'sis, fi·mo'sis). Elongation of the prepuce and constriction of its orifice, so that the foreskin cannot be retracted to uncover the glans penis. —**phimot'ic,** *adj.*

phleb-. See *phlebo-.*

phleb·an"gi·o'ma. A venous aneurysm.

phleb"ar·te"ri·ec·ta'si·a. Varicose aneurysm.

phleb"ar·te"ri·o·di·al'y·sis (fleb"ahr·teer"ee·o·dye·al'i·sis). Arteriovenous aneurysm.

phleb"ec·ta'si·a (fleb"eck·tay'zhuh, -shuh), **phle·bec'ta·sis.** Dilatation of a vein; varicosity.

phle·bec'to·my. Excision of a vein or a portion of a vein.

phleb"em·phrax'is. Plugging of a vein.

phleb"ep·a·ti'tis. Inflammation of veins within the liver.

phleb"ex·ai·re'sis (fleb"ecks·eye·ree'sis). The excision of a vein.

phle·bis'mus (fli·biz'mus). Undue prominence or swelling of a vein.

phle·bi'tis. Inflammation of a vein; is generally suppurative (**suppurative phlebitis**), and is the result of the extension of suppuration from adjacent tissues. It leads to the formation of a thrombus within the vein (**thrombophlebitis**), which may break down and cause the distribution of septic emboli to various parts of the body. When not due to a suppurative process (**plastic, adhesive,** or **proliferative phlebitis**), it may give rise to obliteration of the vein. Symptoms are pain and edema of the affected part, redness along the course of the vein, the latter appearing as a hard, tender cord. —**phlebit'ic,** *adj.* **pelvic p.** Inflammation of the veins in the pelvis. **sclerosing p.** A type in which the veins become permanently occluded by scar formation. **sinus p.** Phlebitis of the sinuses of the dura mater.

phleb'o-, phleb-. A combining form meaning *vein.*

phleb"o·car"ci·no'ma. Extension of carcinoma to the walls of a vein.

phle·boc'ly·sis (fli·bock'li·sis, fleb"o·kly'sis). The injection of a saline solution into a vein.

phleb'o·gram. 1. A roentgenogram of a vein after radiopaque injection. 2. A tracing of the venous pulse by the sphygmograph.

phleb'o·graph. An instrument for recording a venous pulse.

phle·bog'ra·phy. The anatomy and physiology of veins.

phleb'o·lith. A hard concretion sometimes found in veins, produced by calcareous infiltration of a thrombus. —**phlebolith'ic,** *adj.*

phleb"o·ma·nom'e·ter. An apparatus for the direct measurement of venous pressure.

phleb"o·phle·bos'to·my. An operation in which an anastomosis is made between veins.

phleb'o·plas"ty. Plastic operation for the repair of veins.

phleb"or·rha'gi·a. Venous hemorrhage.

phle·bor'rha·phy. Suture of a vein.

phleb"or·rhex'is. Rupture of a vein.

phleb″o·scle·ro′sis. 1. Sclerosis of a vein. 2. Chronic phlebitis.

phle·bos′ta·sis. The temporary removal of some of the blood from the general circulation by means of compression of proximal parts of the extremities. Syn., *bloodless phlebotomy.*

phleb″o·ste·no′sis. Constriction of a vein.

phleb″o·strep′sis. Torsion, or twisting, of a vein.

phleb″o·throm·bo′sis. Formation of a thrombus in a vein.

phleb′o·tome. A cutting instrument used in phlebotomy.

phle·bot′o·mist. One who lets blood. *Obs.*

Phle·bot′o·mus. A genus of small blood-sucking sandflies of the family Psychodidae. The species **P. argentipes** transmits the flagellates of kala-azar in India, **P. chinensis** in China; **P. papatasii** is the vector of pappataci fever, sandfly fever of the Balkans. **P. verrucarum** transmits verruca peruviana in South America.

phle·bot′o·my. The opening of a vein for the purpose of bloodletting.

phlegm (flem). 1. A viscid, stringy mucus, secreted by the mucosa of the air passages. 2. One of the four humors of the old writers.

phleg·ma′si·a (fleg·may′zhuh, ·zee-uh). Inflammation. **p. alba dolens.** Milk leg, a painful swelling of the leg beginning either at the ankle and ascending, or at the groin and extending down the thigh, its usual cause being infection after labor.

phleg·mat′ic. 1. Of the nature of phlegm. 2. Characterized by an apathetic, sluggish temperament.

phleg′mon. Suppurative inflammation of a part, especially the connective tissues. **—phlegmonous,** *adj.*

phlo′em. *In botany,* that portion of a fibrovascular bundle lying beneath the epidermis which consists of sieve tubes, companion cells, and associated fibers or parenchyma. Also see *xylem.*

phlor·e′tin, phlo·re′tin. $C_{15}H_{14}O_5$. A product of the hydrolysis of phlorhizin.

phlo·rhi′zin (flo·rye′zin, flor′i·zin). $C_{21}H_{24}O_{10}.2H_2O$. A glycoside derived from the bark and root of apple, cherry, pear, and other trees. Also called *phlorizin, phloridzin, phlorrhizin.*

phlo·rid′zin. See *phlorhizin.*

phlor′i·zin (flor′i·zin, flo·rye′zin). See *phlorhizin.*

phlor″o·glu′ci·nol. $C_6H_6O_3.2H_2O$. Used as a reagent for hydrochloric acid in gastric juice, for lignin, pentosans, pentoses, etc.

phlor·rhi′zin. See *phlorhizin.*

phlox′ine (flock′seen, ·sin) (C.C.). A red acid dye of the xanthine series;

used as a counterstain with blue nuclear dyes.

phlyc·ten′ule (flick·ten′yool, flick′ten·yool″), **phlyc·ten′u·la.** A minute phlyctena; a little vesicle or blister. **—phlyctenular,** *adj.*

-phobe. A combining form denoting *one having a phobia.*

pho′bi·a. A specific neurotic fear, symbolic of a neurotic conflict and its resulting anxiety.

-pho′bi·a. A combining form denoting *fear* or *dread.* Also see *-philia.*

pho″bo·pho′bi·a. A morbid dread of being afraid.

pho″co·me′li·a, pho·com′e·ly. Absence of or markedly imperfect development of arms and forearms, thighs and legs, but with hands and feet present.

pho′nal, phon′ic (fon′ick, fo′nick). Pertaining to the voice or to sound.

pho″nas·the′ni·a. Weakness of voice, especially that resulting from bodily exhaustion.

pho·na′tion. The production of vocal sound or articulate speech.

pho′neme. An auditory hallucination of hearing words.

pho·net′ic. 1. Pertaining to sounds. 2. Pertaining to the voice.

pho·net′ics. The science dealing with the mode of production of sounds.

pho″ni·at′rics, pho·ni·a·try (fo·nigh′uh·tree, fo″nee·at′ree). The study and treatment of the voice.

pho′no-, phon-. A combining form meaning *sound* or *voice.*

pho″no·car′di·o·graph″. An instrument for registering the sounds of the heart. **—phonocardiograph′ic,** *adj.*

pho″no·car″di·og′ra·phy. The graphic recording of heart sounds and murmurs by electric reproduction, using microphone, amplifier, and galvanometer, or by transmission of the vibrations to a delicate membrane, the oscillations of which are optically recorded, as in the Wiggers and Dean method. Syn., *stethography.*

pho·nol′o·gy. The science and study of vocal sound. Phonetics.

pho″no·mas·sage′. Stimulation and exercise of tympanic membrane and ossicular chain, by alternating pressure and suction in the external auditory meatus.

pho″no·my·oc′lo·nus (fo″no·migh·ock′lo·nus, ·migh″o·klo′nus). A condition in which a sound is heard on auscultation over a muscle, denoting fibrillary contractions; these latter may be so fine as to be invisible.

pho″no·pho′bi·a. 1. A fear of speaking; fear of one's own voice. 2. Morbid dread of any sound or noise.

-pho′ri·a. *In ophthalmology,* a combining form meaning *bearing;* used to denote *turning of the visual axis*, as in exophoria.

phor'o·scope. An apparatus for testing vision, consisting of a trial frame for lenses, fixed to a bench or table.

phor'o·tone. An apparatus for exercising the eye muscles.

phose (fohz). The subjective sensation of light or color, as scotoma scintillans of migraine. Also see *aphose, centraphose, centrophose, chromophose, cyanophose, erythrophose, peripheraphose, peripherophose.*

phos'gene. COCl₂. Carbonyl chloride; a colorless gas used in chemical warfare and in chemical syntheses.

phosphaljel. Trade-mark for an aluminum phosphate gel containing 4% of aluminum phosphate.

phos'pha·tase (fos'fuh·tace, ·taze). A type of enzyme that catalyzes the hydrolysis of esters of phosphoric acid. Numerous phosphatases are known to exist. See Table of Normal Values of Blood Constituents in the Appendix.

phos'phate. A salt of phosphoric acid. **acid p.** One in which only one or two of the hydrogen atoms of phosphoric acid have been replaced by metals. **normal p.** One in which the three hydrogen atoms of phosphoric acid are substituted by metals. **p. cycle.** A cycle of continuous phosphorylation and dephosphorylation reactions which provides for conversion of energy derived from certain metabolic processes to useful cellular work.

phos'pha·te'mi·a. The presence of phosphates in the circulating blood.

phos'pha·tide. See *phospholipid*.

phos'pha·tu'ri·a. A condition in which an excess of phosphates is passed in the urine.

phos'phene. A subjective, luminous sensation caused by pressure upon the eyeball. Also called *pressure p.*

phos'phide. A compound containing phosphorus in its lowest valence state (−3).

phos'phine (fos'feen, ·fin). 1. Hydrogen phosphide, PH₃, a poisonous gas of garlic-like odor. 2. A substitution compound of PH₃, bearing the same relation to it that an amine does to ammonia.

phos'pho-, phosph-. A combining form denoting *phosphorous* or *phosphoric.*

phos"pho·a·mi"no·lip'id (fos"fo·a·mee"no·lip'id, ·lye'pid, fos"fo·am"i·no·). A compound lipid that contains phosphorus and an amino group.

phos"pho·ar'gi·nine (fos"fo·ahr'ji·neen, ·nin). Arginine phosphate. A phosphoric acid derivative of arginine which contains an energy-rich phosphate bond.

phos"pho·cre'a·tine (fos"fo·kree'uh·teen, ·tin). C₄H₁₀O₅N₃P. Phosphagen.

Creatine phosphate. Creatinephosphoric acid. A phosphoric acid derivative of creatine which contains an energy-rich phosphate bond.

phos"pho·di·es'ter·ase. An enzyme catalyzing hydrolysis of one ester linkage in phosphoric acid esters containing two ester linkages.

phos"pho·glu"co·mu'tase. The enzyme which catalyzes the conversion of glucose-1-phosphate to glucose-6-phosphate.

phos"pho·glyc"er·al'de·hyde. CHO.CHOH.CH₂OPO₃H₂. An intermediate product in carbohydrate metabolism.

phos"pho·gly"co·pro'te·in. See *nucleoprotein, nucleoalbumin.*

phos"pho·hex"o·i·som'er·ase (·eye·som'ur·ace). The enzyme which catalyzes the conversion of glucose-6-phosphate to fructose-6-phosphate.

phos"pho·lip'id (fos"fo·lip'id, ·lye'pid). A type of lipid compound which is an ester of phosphoric acid and contains, in addition, one or two molecules of fatty acid, an alcohol, and a nitrogenous base. See Table of Normal Values of Blood Constituents in the Appendix. Syn., *phosphatide, phospholipin.*

phos"pho·lip'in. See *phospholipid.*

phos"pho·mo·lyb'dic ac'id. H₃PO₄.12MoO₃.12H₂O. A yellow solid used as a reagent.

phos"pho·mon"o·es'ter·ase (fos"fo·mon"o·ess'tur·ace, ·aze, fos"fo·mo"no·). An enzyme catalyzing hydrolysis of phosphoric acid esters containing one ester linkage.

phos·pho'ni·um. The hypothetical univalent radical PH₄; it is analogous to ammonium, NH₄.

phos"pho·nu'cle·ase (fos"fo·new'klee·ace, ·aze). An enzyme which splits nucleotides into nucleosides and phosphoric acid. Also called *nucleotidase.*

phos"pho·pro'te·in. A conjugated protein consisting of a compound of protein with a phosphorus-containing substance other than nucleic acid or lecithin.

phos"pho·pyr'i·dine nu'cle·o·tides (fos"fo·pirr'i·deen, ·din). Complex compounds containing nicotinic acid amide, a pentose, adenine, and phosphoric acid. **diphosphopyridine nucleotide.** Coenzyme I. **triphosphopyridine nucleotide.** Coenzyme II.

phos"pho·py·ru'vic ac'id. CH₂:CO(PO₃H₂)COOH. An intermediate substance obtained in the breakdown of glycogen to lactic acid and the resynthesis of glycogen from lactic acid.

phos"pho·res'cence. 1. The prolonged emission of light from a substance without any apparent rise in temperature, produced after exposure to heat, light, or electric discharges. 2. The faint green glow of white phosphorus exposed to air, due to its slow oxidation. **—phosphorescent,** *adj.*

phos·phor'ic ac'id. H_3PO_4. Orthophosphoric acid; occurs as a colorless liquid of syrupy consistence and contains 85% of H_3PO_4; miscible with water.

phos'pho·rism. Chronic phosphorus poisoning.

phos·pho'rous ac'id (fos·for'us, fos'for·us). H_3PO_3. A yellow, crystalline acid used as a reducing agent and as a reagent.

phos'pho·rus. P = 30.98. A nonmetallic element occurring in two allotropic forms, white or yellow phosphorus and amorphous or red phosphorus. See Table of Normal Values of Blood Constituents in the Appendix.

phos'pho·rus-32. A radioactive isotope of phosphorus, which emits beta rays, used in the form of sodium phosphate for locating tumors and in treating polycythemia vera and leukemia. Symbol, P^{32}.

phos·phor'yl·ase. An enzyme widely distributed in animals, plants, and microorganisms. It is specific for the formation of glucose-1-phosphate (Cori ester) from glycogen and inorganic phosphate.

phos″pho·ryl·a'tion. The term used for the esterification of compounds with phosphoric acid.

phos″pho·ryl·cho'line (fos″fo·ril·ko'leen, ·lin, ·kol'een, ·in). An ester of choline and phosphoric acid which constitutes a portion of the lecithin molecule.

phos″pho·tri'ose i·som'er·ase. Triose isomerase, an enzyme in the Meyerhof cycle, catalyzing the interconversion of 3-phosphoglyceraldehyde and phosphodihydroxyacetone.

phos″pho·tung'stic ac'id. Approximately $P_2O_5.24WO_3.25H_2O$. A white or yellowish green crystalline acid used as a reagent.

pho·tal'gi·a. Pain arising from too great intensity of light.

pho·tau″gi·o·pho'bi·a (fo·taw″-jee·o·fo'bee·uh). A shrinking from the glare of light.

phote. A unit of intensity of illumination.

photelometer. Trade-mark for a photoelectric colorimeter.

pho″tes·the'si·a, pho″taes·the'si·a (fo″tess·thee'zhuh, ·zee·uh). 1. Sensitiveness to light. 2. Photophobia.

pho'tism. A visual sensation, as of color or light, produced by hearing, taste, smell, touch, or temperature, or even by the thought of some object, person, or general conception.

pho·to-. A combining form meaning light.

pho″to·chem'i·cal. Pertaining to chemical action produced directly or indirectly by means of radiation.

pho″to·chem'is·try. The study of chemical reactions produced directly or indirectly by means of radiation.

pho″to·col″or·im'e·ter. A colorimeter consisting of one or more photoelectric cells as indicators, and various colored filters, for examining certain parts of the spectrum.

pho″to·dyn'i·a. Pain arising from too great intensity of light; extreme photophobia.

pho″to·dys·pho'ri·a. Intolerance of light; photophobia.

pho″to·e·lec'tric. Pertaining to electric effects of various types of radiations, in particular to the release of photoelectrons from certain metals by suitable radiations.

pho″to·e·lec'tric col″or·im'e·ter. A colorimeter for determining the concentration of the colored component of a solution, consisting of one or more combinations of calibrated filters and photoelectric cells for measurement of the color.

pho″to·e·lec″tric'i·ty. Electricity produced under the influence of light or other radiations, such as ultraviolet and x-rays. When irradiated by such radiations, certain metals give off photoelectrons, *q.v.*

pho″to·e·lec'tron. An electron set into swift motion by the impact of a photon, and to which the primary photon transmits all of its energy.

pho″to·flu″or·os'co·py. Fluoroscopy permitting recording of fluoroscopic images on photographic film. Also called *fluororoentgenography, photofluorography.*

pho·tol'y·sis. Decomposition by the action of light.

pho'to·lyte. A substance that is decomposed by the action of light.

pho″to·mag'net·ism. Magnetism produced in certain substances by the action of light.

pho″to·ma'ni·a. 1. The increase of maniacal symptoms under the influence of light. 2. A morbid desire for light.

pho·tom'e·ter. 1. An instrument for measuring the intensity of light. 2. An instrument for testing the sensitiveness of the eye to light, by determining the minimum illumination in which the object is visible.

pho·tom'e·try. The measurement of the intensity of light.

pho″to·mi'cro·graph. A photograph of a minute or microscopic object, usually made with the aid of a microscope, and of sufficient size for observation with the naked eye. **—pho·tomicrog'raphy,** *n.*

pho'ton. A quantum of energy of

visible light or any other electromagnetic radiation.

pho·ton'o·sus. A diseased condition arising from continued exposure to intense or glaring light, as snowblindness.

pho"to·pho'bi·a. Intolerance or morbid fear of light. See *phengophobia.* —**photophobic,** *adj.*

pho"toph·thal'mi·a. Inflammation of the eyes due to excessively strong light, as a welder's arc light or sunlight on snow.

pho·top'si·a. Subjective sensations of sparks or flashes of light occurring in certain pathologic conditions of the optic nerve, the retina, or the brain. —**photoptic,** *adj.*

pho"top·tom'e·ter. An instrument for determining visual acuity.

pho"to·sen"si·tiv'i·ty. 1. The capacity of an organ or organism to be stimulated to activity by light. 2. The absorption of a certain portion of the spectrum by a chemical system. —**photosen'sitive,** *adj.*

pho"to·sen"si·ti·za'tion. Abnormal condition of the skin, making it hyperreactive to exposure to ultraviolet radiation or natural sunlight. It may be produced by the ingestion of fluorescent dyes, endocrine products, or heavy metals.

pho"to·syn'the·sis. The process by which simple carbohydrates are synthesized from carbon dioxide and water by the chloroplasts of living plant cells in the presence of light.

pho"to·ther'a·py. Treatment with light rays, including the invisible infrared and ultraviolet radiations.

pho"to·ti'mer. A clocklike device used in medical or other photography, especially in roentgenology, pathology, and laboratory processes to provide a proper interval of time for photographic plate or film exposures.

pho'to·tube. A radio tube which furnishes a current of about 2×10^{-8} amp. which, through a resistance of 1 megohm, provides an input to the amplifier of 2×10^{-2} volts in the operation of a photoelectric plethysmograph.

pho·tu'ri·a. The passage of phosphorescent urine.

phren"as·the'ni·a. Mental defect; feeblemindedness.

phren"em·phrax'is. Crushing of the phrenic nerve with a hemostat to produce temporary paralysis of the diaphragm. A form of collapse therapy used in the treatment of pulmonary tuberculosis.

-phre'ni·a. A combining form denoting *mental disorder.*

phren'ic. 1. Pertaining to the diaphragm, as phrenic nerve, phrenic artery. 2. Pertaining to the mind.

phren"i·cec'to·my (fren"i·seck'to-

mee). Resection of a section of the phrenic nerve or removal of the entire phrenic nerve.

phren"i·co·ex·er'e·sis. Avulsion of the phrenic nerve.

phren"i·cot'o·my. Surgical division of the phrenic nerve in the neck for the purpose of causing a one-sided paralysis of the diaphragm, with consequent immobilization and compression of a diseased lung.

phren"i·co·trip'sy. Crushing of the phrenic nerve.

phre·ni'tis. 1. Inflammation of the brain. 2. Inflammation of the diaphragm. 3. Acute delirium. —**phren'ic, phrenit'ic,** *adj.*

phren'o-, phren-. A combining form denoting *relation to the diaphragm.*

phren"o·car'di·a. A neurasthenic condition associated with dyspnea and pain in the region of the heart. A symptom-complex in anxiety neurosis.

phren"o·glot·tis'mus. Spasm of the glottis ascribed to disease of the diaphragm.

phre·nol'o·gy. The theory that the various faculties of the mind occupy distinct and separate areas in the brain cortex, and that the predominance of certain faculties can be predicted from modifications of the parts of the skull overlying the areas where these faculties are located. *Obs.*

phren"o·ple'gi·a. Paralysis of the diaphragm.

phren'o·sin. A nitrogenous substance obtained from brain tissue; a cerebroside whose fatty acid is cerebronic acid. Also called *cerebron.*

phren"o·sin'ic ac'id. $C_{25}H_{50}O_3$. Cerebronic acid. A hydroxy fatty acid which is a component of the glycolipid (cerebroside) phrenosin.

phron"e·mo·pho'bi·a. A morbid dread of thinking.

phro·ne'sis. Soundness of mind, or of judgment.

phryn"o·der'ma (frin"o·dur'muh, fry"no-). Dryness of the skin with follicular hyperkeratosis; due to a vitamin-A deficiency.

phthal-. See *phthalo-.*

phthal'ic ac'id (thal'ick). C_6H_4(COOH)$_2$. A colorless crystalline acid used in organic syntheses.

phthal'ic an·hy'dride. C_6H_4(CO)$_2$O. The anhydride of phthalic acid. Can act as an allergen.

phthal'i·dyl (thal'i·dil, -deel). 3-(2-Aminopropyl)-phthalide hydrochloride, a substance having analgesic properties.

phthal'o- (thal'o-), **phthal-.** In chemistry, a combining form for *phthalic.*

phthal"yl·sul"fa·thi'a·zole. The phthalyl derivative of sulfathiazole, a drug especially effective in the treatment of diseases of the colon. See *sul-fathalidine*.

phthei·ri·a·sis (thigh·rye'uh·sis). See *pediculosis*.

phthi·o·col (thigh'o·coal, ·kol, ·kawl). A yellow, crystalline chemical compound isolated from human tubercle bacilli. It is 2-methyl-3-hydroxy-1,4-naphthoquinone and has vitamin-K activity.

phthi·o·ic ac·id (thigh·o'ick). A cyclic fatty acid produced by the tubercle bacillus.

phthi·ri·a·sis (thigh·rye'uh·sis, thi·rye'·). Pediculosis pubis; infestation by the pubic louse *Phthirius pubis*.

phthir"i·o·pho·bi·a (thirr"ee·o·fo'bee·uh, thigh"ree·o·). Morbid dread of lice.

phthi·sis (tye'sis, thigh'sis). 1. Old term for tuberculosis, especially pulmonary tuberculosis. 2. Old term for any disease characterized by emaciation and loss of strength, especially diseases of the lungs. —**phthis'ic, phthis'i·cal**, *adj.* **fibroid p.** Chronic, slowly progressive, pulmonary tuberculosis with extensive fibrosis and mild symptoms.

phy·co·chrome. The complex blue-green pigment that masks the green of the chlorophyll in certain algae.

phy"co·cy'a·nin. In *biology*, a blue pigment, characteristic of the Cyanophyceae, blue-green algae. Active in photosynthesis.

Phy"co·my·ce'tes (figh"ko·migh·see'teez). A class of fungi, with a generally nonseptate mycelium. This group includes the common black bread mold and water mold.

phys"o·ga·lac'tic. 1. Stopping the secretion of milk. 2. An agent that checks the secretion of milk.

phy·lax'is (figh·lack'sis). The activity of the body in defending itself against infection.

phyl"lo·qui·none'. $C_{31}H_{46}O_2$. 2-Methyl-3-phytyl-1,4-naphthoquinone, the form of vitamin K occurring in the green leaf or other chlorophyll-containing portions of plants. Syn., *vitamin K_1*.

phy"lo·gen·e·sis, phy·log'e·ny (figh·lodj'i·nee). The evolution of a group or species of animals or plants from the simplest form; the evolution of the species, as distinguished from ontogenesis, the evolution of the individual. —**phylogenet'ic**, *adj.*

phy'ma. 1. A tumor or new growth of varying size, composed of any of the structures of the skin or subcutaneous tissue. 2. A localized plastic exudate larger than a tubercle; a circumscribed swelling of the skin. —**phymatoid**, *adj.*

phy"ma·to'sis. Any disease charac-

terized by the formation of phymas or nodules.

Phys"a·lop'te·ra. A genus of nematode worms of the family Strongylidae. **P. caucasica.** This is the only species infesting man, commonly found in natives of tropical Africa.

phys"i·an·thro·py. The study of the constitution of man, his diseases, and their remedies.

phys"i·at'rics. Physical medicine.

phys"i·at'rist (fiz·eye'at·rist, fiz"ee·at'rist). A physician who specializes in physical medicine.

phys'ic. 1. The science of medicine. 2. A medicine, especially a cathartic. 3. Administer medicines; purge.

phys'i·cal. 1. Pertaining to nature; pertaining to the body or material things. 2. Pertaining to physics.

phy·si'cian. One who is authorized to practice medicine.

phys'i·cist. One skilled in physical science.

phys"i·co·chem'i·cal (fizz"i·ko·kem'i·kul). Pertaining to the borderland area where physics and chemistry overlap.

phys"i·co·py·rex'i·a (fizz"i·ko·pye·reck'see·uh). Artificial fever produced by physical means for its therapeutic effect.

phys'ics. The science of the phenomena and laws of nature, especially that treating of the properties of matter and of the forces governing it.

phys"i·og'no·my (fizz"ee·og'no·mee). 1. The countenance. 2. The science of determining character by a study of the face.

phys"i·o·log'ic (fizz"ee·o·lodj'ick), **phys"i·o·log'i·cal.** 1. Pertaining to physiology. 2. Pertaining to natural or normal processes, as opposed to those that are pathologic.

phys"i·ol'o·gist. One versed in physiology.

phys"i·ol'o·gy (fizz"ee·ol'o·jee). The science that treats of the functions of living organisms or their parts, as distinguished from morphology, etc. **applied p.** Physiologic knowledge used in interpretation of problems arising in medical practice, public health, or industry. **aviation p.** The study of physiologic problems in flying. **comparative p.** The comparative study of the physiology of different animals and plants. **pathologic p.** The study of disordered functions or of functions modified by disease.

phy·sique'. Physical structure or organization; body build.

phy"so·hem"a·to·me'tra (figh"so·hem"uh·to·mee'truh, ·hee"muh·to·mee'truh). An accumulation of gas, or air, and blood in the uterus, as in decomposition of retained menses, or placental tissue.

phy″so·hy″dro·me′tra. An accumulation of gas and fluid in the uterus.

phy″so·me′tra. A distention of the uterus with gas.

phy″so·py″o·sal′pinx. Pyosalpinx with formation of gas in the uterine tube.

phy″so·stig′mine (figh″so·stig′-meen, ·min). $C_{15}H_{21}O_2N_3$. An alkaloid obtained from the seeds of *Physostigma venenosum;* slightly soluble in water; occurs as white crystals, becoming red on exposure to air and light. Extremely poisonous. Syn., *eserine.* **p. salicyl-ate.** The salicylate of an alkaloid usually obtained from the dried ripe seed of *Physostigma venenosum;* white or slightly yellow crystals, becoming red on long exposure to light and air; soluble in water. Used as a parasympathetic stimulant. Also called *eserine salicylate.*

phy′tic ac′id. $C_6H_6O_6(H_2PO_3)_6$. Inositol-hexaphosphoric acid, a constituent of cereal grains. By forming an insoluble salt, it is said to prevent utilization of calcium in the cereal.

phy′tin. The calcium or magnesium salt of inositol-hexaphosphoric acid; a constituent of cereal grains. Also a trade-mark for same.

phy′to-, phyt-. A combining form meaning *plant;* used to denote *vegetation* or a *vegetable parasite.*

phy″to·be′zoar (figh″to·bee′zor, ·bez′or). A bezoar or ball of vegetable fiber sometimes found in the stomach; food ball.

phy″to·chem′is·try. Vegetable or plant chemistry.

phy·tog′e·nous (figh·todj′i·nus). Produced by plants.

phy′tol. An aliphatic alcohol, $C_{20}H_{39}OH$; existing in chlorophyll as an ester.

phy″to·lac′ca. The dried root of *Phytolacca americana,* containing a saponin, and a resinlike material.

phy″to·lac′cin (figh″to·lack′sin). A resinoid, or the precipitate from a tincture of the root of *Phytolacca decandra.*

phy·tom′e·lin (figh·tom′i·lin). See *rutin.*

phy″to·mon′ic ac′id. $C_{20}H_{40}O_2$. A liquid saturated fatty acid isolated from the lipid fraction extracted from *Phytomonas tumefaciens.*

phy″to·na·di′one. 2-Methyl-3-phytyl-1,4-naphthoquinone, used to promote formation of prothrombin. Syn., *phylloquinone, vitamin K_1.*

phy·toph′a·gous (figh·tof′uh·gus). 1. Plant-eating. 2. Vegetarian.

phy″to·phar″ma·col′o·gy. That branch of pharmacology concerned with the effects of drugs on plant growth.

phy″to·pneu″mo·no·co″ni·o′-sis. A condition marked by inflammatory nodules in the lungs, caused by the inhalation of vegetable particles.

phy·to′sis (figh·to′sis). 1. Any disease due to the presence of vegetable parasites. 2. The production of disease by vegetable parasites. 3. The presence of vegetable parasites.

phy·tos′ter·ol (figh·tos′tur·ole, ·ol, figh″to·steer′-). Any sterol occurring in a plant oil or fat.

phy·tos′ter·ol·in. A glycoside of phytosterol.

phy″to·throm″bo·kin′ase (·kin′-ace, ·aze, ·kigh′nace, ·naze). A thrombokinase prepared from yeast or plant sources.

phy″to·tox′in. A toxin derived from a plant, such as abrin, ricin, and crotin.

phy″to·vi·tel′lin (figh″to·vi·tel′lin, ·vye·tell′in). A vegetable protein resembling vitellin.

pi′a, pi′a ma′ter. The vascular membrane enveloping the surface of the brain and spinal cord, and consisting of a plexus of blood vessels held in a fine areolar tissue. —**pial,** *adj.*

pi″a·a·rach′noid (pee″uh·a·rack′-noyd). See *piarachnoid.*

pi″a·rach′noid (pee″uh·rack′noyd). The pia and arachnoid considered as one structure. Also called *leptomeninx, leptomeninges.*

pi′ca (pye′kuh). 1. A desire for strange foods; may occur in chlorosis and during pregnancy. 2. A craving to eat strange articles, as hair, dirt, or sand; the recurrence in later life of the infantile tendency of bringing everything to the mouth.

Pic′e·a (pis′ee·uh, pye′see·uh). A genus of coniferous trees; spruces.

pic″ra·don′i·din. A glucoside obtained from adonis. It has a digitalis-like action.

Pic·rae′na (pick·ree′nuh). See *Picrasma.*

pic·ram′ic ac′id. $NH_2 \cdot C_6H_2(NO_3)_2 \cdot OH$. A detoxication product of picric acid resulting from reduction of the latter in the animal body.

Pic·ras′ma (pick·raz′muh). A genus of the Simarubaceae. The wood of **P. excelsa** is the source of Jamaica quassia, containing α-picrasmin and β-picrasmin.

pic·ras′min (pick·raz′min). $C_{22}H_{30}O_5$. The bitter principle of *Picrasma excelsa* or Jamaica quassia.

pic′rate. A salt of picric acid.

pic′ric ac′id. Trinitrophenol.

pic″ro·car′mine (pick″ro·kahr′-min, ·meen, ·myne). One of a variety of mixtures of carmine, ammonia, and picric acid, used as a stain for tissues.

pic″ro·tox′in. $C_{30}H_{34}O_{13}$. A glycoside obtained from the seed of *Anamirta* *cocculus*; occurs as crystals or a microcrystalline powder; affected by light. Soluble in water. Picrotoxin is a stimulant to apparently all the efferent centers of the cerebrospinal axis. Also called *cocculin*.

pie′dra (pee-ay′drah, pyay′drah). A nodular growth on the hair of the scalp, beard, or mustache. The type known as **black piedra** is found in tropical regions and is caused by the fungus *Piedraia hortai*, which infests only the hair shafts of the scalp. **White piedra**, a rarer form, occurs in temperate regions and is caused by the fungus *Trichosporum beigelii* which infests the hair of the beard and mustache. Also called *tinea nodosa*, *Beigel's disease*, *piedra nostros*.

pi·e″zo·e·lec′tric ef·fect′ (pye-ee″zo·i·leck′trick). The development of electric charges by certain crystals when subjected to strain.

pi′geon toed. Walking with the feet turned in.

pig′ment. 1. A dyestuff; a coloring matter. **2.** Any organic coloring matter of the body. **3.** Any stain used in microscopical work. **4.** Any medicinal agent applied externally to the skin, like paint. —**pigmented**, *adj.* **bile pigments.** Pigments found in bile or derived from it. They include bilirubin, urobilinogen, urobilin, and biliverdin. **blood pigments.** Pigments normally found in blood. See *hemoglobin, bilirubin.* **hematogenous p.** Any pigment derived from hemoglobin. Hematogenous pigments include heme, hemosiderin, methemoglobin, and bile pigments.

pig″men·ta′tion. Deposition of or discoloration by pigment.

pig·men′to·phage. A phagocyte which destroys pigment, especially that of hairs.

pig·men′tum ni′grum. The dark coloring matter which lines the choroid coat of the eye.

pil. *Pilula*, pill.

pile. A hemorrhoid. **blind p.** One which does not bleed. **external p.** A hemorrhoid which is located outside the anal sphincter. **internal p.** A hemorrhoid which is located inside the anal sphincter. **sentinel p.** The thickened wall of the anal pocket at the lower end of an anal fissure.

pile. A battery. **thermoelectric p.** A number of bars or plates in which two kinds of metal are conjoined (thermocouples). When the junctions are heated, an electric current is generated by which temperature can be measured.

piles. See *hemorrhoids.*

pi′li·gan (pee′li·gahn). The plant *Lycopodium saururus*, found in South America and Africa. It contains the al-

kaloids saururine, sauroxine, and piliganine.

pil′i·ga·nine (pill′i·guh·neen, pye·lig′uh·). An alkaloid obtained from *Lycopodium saururus*. See *piligan*.

pi″li·mic′tion. The passing of urine containing hairlike filaments.

pill. A small, solid body, of a globular, ovoid, or lenticular shape, containing one or more medicinal substances and used for internal administration.

pil′lar. A columnar structure acting as a support.

pil′let. A little pill, or pellet.

pil′le·us, pil′le·um. The caul or membrane which sometimes covers a child's head during birth.

pi′lo-, pil-. A combining form meaning *hair*.

pi″lo·car′pine (pye″lo·kahr′peen, ·pin, pill″o·). $C_{11}H_{16}N_2O_2$. An alkaloid obtained from various species of *Pilocarpus (Jaborandi)*; occurs as a colorless to yellow, viscid liquid or crystals; freely soluble in water and alcohol. It usually is employed in the form of the hydrochloride or nitrate salt.

pi″lo·car′pus (pye″lo·kahr′pus, pill″o·). The dried leaflets of *Pilocarpus Jaborandi*, or of *Pilocarpus microphyllus* and other species of *Pilocarpus*. A number of alkaloids have been obtained from various species of pilocarpus, the principal one being pilocarpine. Syn., *jaborandi*.

pi″lo·ni′dal. Containing an accumulation of hairs in a cyst.

pi·lo′sis (pye·lo′sis). The abnormal or excessive development of hair.

pil′ule. A small pill.

pim″e·li′tis (pim″i·lye′tis, pye″mi·lye′tis). Inflammation of any adipose tissue; also, inflammation of connective tissue in general.

pim″e·lo·pte·ryg′i·um (pim″i·lo·teh·ridj′ee·um, pye″mi·lo·). A fatty outgrowth on the conjunctiva.

pim″e·lor·rhe′a. 1. An excessive fatty discharge. **2.** Diarrhea with excessive fat in the stools.

pim″e·lor·thop′ne·a (pim″i·lor·thop′nee·uh, ·lor·thop·nee′uh). Orthopnea due to obesity.

pim″e·lu′ri·a. The excretion of fat in the urine.

pi·men′ta. The nearly ripe fruit of *Pimenta officinalis*, an evergreen tree. Syn., *allspice*.

pi·men′to. See *pimenta*.

pim″pi·nel′la. The dried rhizome and roots of *Pimpinella saxifraga* or other species.

pim′ple. Lay term for a small pustule or papule.

pim″a·cy′a·nol. A basic xanthine dye of the cyanine group, used as a supravital stain for mitochondria, and for the staining of frozen sections.

pince″ment′ (pans″mahng′). In

massage, a pinching or nipping of the tissues.

pine. A general name for coniferous trees. Various species of these trees yield many substances, as turpentine, resin, tar, pitch, and a variety of volatile oils. **white p.** The dried inner bark of *Pinus strobus*. It contains a glycoside, coniferin, together with tannin and some mucilage and oleoresin. Also called *white pine bark*.

pin′e·al. Referring to the pineal body. **p. body.** A small cone-shaped structure attached to the roof of the diencephalon, which appears to be a rudimentary gland of unknown function. Also called *epiphysis cerebri, pineal gland*.

pin″e·a·lec′to·my. Surgical removal of the pineal body.

pi′nene. $C_{10}H_{16}$. 2.7.7-Trimethyl-Δ^2-bicyclo (1.1.3) heptene. A terpene or hydrocarbon found in many essential oils.

pin″e·o·blas·to′ma. A blastoma of the pineal body; most often found in young males.

pine tar. A product obtained by the destructive distillation of the wood of *Pinus palustris*, or other species of *Pinus*; a very viscid, blackish brown, noncrystalline liquid, with an empyreumatic, terebinthinate odor; it is slightly soluble in water. The composition is largely phenolic. Also called *pix liquida*.

pin·guec′u·la. A small, yellowish white patch situated on the conjunctiva, between the cornea and the canthus of the eye; it is composed of connective tissue.

pin′guid. Fatty; unctuous.

pink′eye″. 1. A contagious, mucopurulent conjunctivitis occurring especially in horses. 2. Acute contagious conjunctivitis in man. Also called *Koch-Weeks conjunctivitis*.

pink′root″. See *Spigelia*.

pin′na. The projecting part of the external ear; the auricle. —**pinnal**, *adj*.

pi″no·cy·to′sis (pye″no·sigh·to′sis, pin″o·). Drinking by cells, as opposed to phagocytosis, eating by cells. Used to indicate microscopically visible "drinking" or engulfing of globules of fluid by pseudopodia.

pint. The eighth part of a gallon; 16 fluidounces. Symbol, O. (*octarius*). Abbreviated, pt. An **imperial pint** contains 20 fluidounces.

pin′worm. An intestinal nematode, *Enterobius vermicularis*, more commonly found in children.

pi″one′mi·a. The presence of an emulsion of fine oil globules in the blood, sometimes found in diabetes; a form of lipemia, *q.v.*

pi″or·thop·ne′a. Orthopnea due to obesity.

Pi′per. A genus of Piperaceae. See *pepper*.

pi·per′a·zine (pi·perr′uh·zeen, ·zin, pip′ur·uh·zeen, ·zin). Diethylenediamine. The anhydrous base occurs as colorless, volatile crystals; freely soluble in water.

pi·per′i·dine (pi·perr′i·deen, ·din, pye·perr′i·, pip′ur·i·deen, ·din). $C_5H_{11}N$. A volatile, liquid base produced by alkaline hydrolysis of piperine.

pip″er·i·do′late hy″dro·chlo′ride. 1-Ethyl-3-piperidyl diphenylacetate hydrochloride, an anticholinergic agent with peripheral atropine-like effects. See *dactil*.

pip′er·ine (pip′ur·een, ·in, pye′pur·). $C_{17}H_{19}O_3N$. An alkaloid from black pepper; occurs as white or slightly yellowish crystals; slightly soluble in water.

pip′er·o·nal (pip′ur·o·nal, pye·perr′o·nal). Dioxymethylene-protocatechuic aldehyde, $CH_2OO.C_6H_3.CHO$. A pediculicide in 5% solution with castor oil and alcohol. Also called *heliotropin, piperonyl aldehyde*.

pip″er·o′va·tine (pip″ur·o′vuh·teen, ·tin, pye″pur·). $C_{16}H_{21}O_2N$. An alkaloid from the fruits of *Piper ovatum;* occurs as colorless crystals, soluble in alcohol, insoluble in water.

pip″er·ox′an hy″dro·chlo′ride. Nonproprietary name for 2-(1-piperidylmethyl)-1,4-benzodioxan hydrochloride, an adrenergic-blocking agent. See *benodaine hydrochloride*.

pi·pet′, pi·pette′ (pi·pet′, pi·pet′). A graduated open glass tube used for measuring or transferring definite quantities of liquids.

pip″to·nych′i·a (pip″to·nick′ee·uh). Shedding of the nails.

pir′i·form, pyr′i·form. 1. Pear-shaped. 2. The piriformis, a muscle arising from the front of the sacrum and inserted on the greater trochanter of the femur.

pis·cid′i·a. The dried bark of *Piscidia piscipula (P. erythrina)*. Syn., *Jamaica dogwood*.

pi′si·form (pis′i·form, pye′si·). 1. Pea-shaped. 2. A small bone on the inner and anterior aspect of the carpus. See Table of Bones in the Appendix.

pit. 1. A depression, as the pit of the stomach; the armpit. 2. Indent by pressing. **gastric p.** One of the depressions in the gastric mucosa into which open the gastric glands. **olfactory p.** One formed about the olfactory placode in the embryo by the growth of the median and lateral nasal processes; the anlage of part of the nasal cavity. **p. of the stomach.** A name popularly given to that part of the abdomen just below the sternum and between the cartilages of the false ribs. Also called *scrobiculus cordis*.

pitch. A heavy liquid or dark residue obtained by the distillation of tar; as, pine pitch, burgundy pitch, coal tar pitch. **black p.** The black residue obtained by distilling pine tar. It consists of rosin and empyreumatic products of rosin. **Burgundy p.** The resinous exudation obtained from the stem of *Picea abies;* occurs as a reddish brown or yellowish brown solid. **Canada p.** The resinous exudation from *Tsuga canadensis (Abies canadensis).* It is a hard, brittle, opaque, dark reddish brown substance.

pitch. That quality of sound which depends upon the rapidity of the vibrations that produce the sound.

pith'i·a·tism, pi·thi'a·tism. 1. A condition caused by suggestion. See *hysteria.* 2. Treatment of disease by suggestion, *q.v.* **—pithiat'ic,** *adj.*

pitocin. Trade-mark for an aqueous solution of oxytocin.

pitressin. Trade-mark for an aqueous solution containing the pressor and diuretic-antidiuretic principle of the neurohypophysis (vasopressin). **p. tannate in oil.** A suspension in vegetable oil of a water-insoluble tannate of the pressor and diuretic-antidiuretic principle of the neurohypophysis.

pit'ted. Marked by indentations or pits, as from smallpox.

pit'ting. 1. The formation of pits. 2. The indentation that remains for a short time after releasing pressure, as by a finger.

pi·tu'i·tar'y (pi·tew'i·terr″ee). 1. Secreting mucus or phlegm. 2. Pertaining to, or designating, the pituitary body. 3. The pituitary body or gland; the hypophysis cerebri. The human pituitary is a small, rounded, reddish gray organ averaging about 0.57 Gm. in weight. It lies in the sella turcica and is attached by a stalk to the floor of the brain. The important anatomic divisions of the pituitary body are the pars glandularis, the pars intermedia, the pars tuberalis, all derived embryologically from Rathke's pouch of buccal ectoderm, and the pars neuralis, derived from the infundibular process of the diencephalon. The terms anterior lobe, pars anterior, and pars distalis ordinarily refer to the pars glandularis, but may include part of the pars tuberalis; the term pars buccalis usually includes all the structures arising from Rathke's pouch; the terms posterior lobe and pars posterior usually include the pars neuralis and the pars intermedia; the terms intermediate lobe and intermediary lobe are applied to the pars intermedia. The name pituitary as given to this organ because it was erroneously thought to secrete the mucus of the nose; it is now recognized as a most important gland of internal

secretion. The hormones produced by its anterior lobe regulate growth of all bodily tissues, control the development and function of the thyroid, the suprarenal cortex, the gonads, and probably the parathyroids, and induce lactation. Principles of the posterior lobe affect blood pressure, contractility of smooth muscle, and renal function. The intermediate lobe elaborates a melanophore-dispersion hormone the function of which in mammals is not at present definitely known.

pituitrin. Trade-mark for a brand of posterior pituitary injection.

pit'y·ri'a·sis. A fine, branny desquamation of the skin. **p. capitis.** Dermatitis seborrheica. **p. lichenoides et varioliformis acuta.** A noncommunicable, acute or subacute skin eruption characterized by vesicles and pustules that form crusts and later scars; usually runs a course of one to three months. **p. linguae.** Transitory benign plaques of the tongue. **p. rosea.** A self-limited skin disease of the trunk, usually acute; characterized by pale red patches with fawn-colored centers. The etiologic agent is unknown. Also called *p. circinata, herpes tonsurans maculosus.* **p. rubra.** A chronic, inflammatory skin disease usually involving the whole body. The skin is deep red and covered by whitish scales. The disease varies in duration from months to years and is generally fatal. **p. rubra pilaris.** A chronic, mildly inflammatory skin disease in which firm, acuminate papules form at the mouths of the hair follicles with horny plugs in these follicles. By coalescence scaly patches are formed. **p. simplex.** Dermatitis seborrheica. **p. steatoides.** Dermatitis seborrheica when large waxy scales are formed, usually associated with pruritus and alopecia. **p. versicolor.** A chronic skin disease characterized by yellowish brown desquamating macules; involves principally the trunk and is caused by the fungus *Malassezia furfur.*

pit'y·roid. Branny.

Pit″y·ro·spor'um (pit″i·ro·spor'-um, ·ros'por·um). A genus of fungi which is yeastlike in character. **P. ovale.** A species found in the hair follicles and on the skin in seborrheic dermatitis; of unknown pathogenicity.

piv'ot. *In dentistry,* old term for dowel.

piv'ot clack. An old method for attaching a crown to the root of a decayed tooth.

piv'ot·ing. The fixation of an artificial crown to a tooth by a dowel.

pK. The negative logarithm of the dissociation constant of an acid or a base.

Place, Edwin Hemphill [*American physician,* 1880–   ]. The first to report Haverhill fever, with Lee Sutton and Otto Willner (1926).

pla·ce'bo. A medicine having no pharmacologic effect, but given for the purpose of pleasing or humoring the patient.

pla·cen'ta. The organ on the wall of the uterus to which the embryo is attached by means of the umbilical cord and through which it receives its nourishment. It is developed, about the third month of gestation, from the chorion of the embryo and the decidua basalis of the uterus. The villi of the chorion enlarge and are received into depressions of the decidua. Around them form blood sinuses into which, by diffusion, the waste materials brought from the fetus by the umbilical arteries pass, and from them the blood receives oxygen and food material being transported to the fetus by the umbilical vein. At term the placenta weighs one pound, is one inch thick at its center, and seven inches in diameter. The lay term is *afterbirth.* —**placental, placentoid,** *adj.* **abruption of p.** Premature detachment of the placenta. **accessory p.** An auxiliary piece of placenta situated apart from the main structure. **adherent p.** One that fails to separate from the uterine wall after childbirth. **annular p.** One extending around the interior of the uterus in the form of a belt. **battledore p.** One in which the insertion of the cord is at the margin of the placenta. **bipartite p.** A placenta with two divisions. **circumvallate p.** A placenta with an irregular elevation on the fetal surface close to the circumference. **discoid p.** One shaped like a disk. **duplex p.** See bipartite p. **epitheliochorial p.** One, as in the sow, in which the endothelial, epithelial, and connective tissue layers are present in both the uterus and chorion. **fundal p.** One attached at the fundus. **horseshoe p.** In twin pregnancy, a condition in which two placentas are joined. **incarcerated p.** One retained by irregular contraction of the uterus. **maternal p.** The external layer developed from the decidua basalis. **p. accreta.** A placenta which has grown into the wall of the uterus and which cannot be separated from it. **p. cirsoides.** One in which the umbilical vessels have a varicose arrangement. **p. fenestrata.** An irregular, four-sided variety of placenta with an opening near the center. **p. membranacea.** One abnormally thin. **p. previa.** A placenta superimposed upon and about the internal os, a condition producing serious hemorrhage during labor. **p. previa centralis.** A condition in which the cen-

ter of the placenta is directly above th internal os. **p. previa marginali** A condition in which the edge of t placenta meets, but does not overla the internal os. **p. previa pa tialis.** A condition in which the ed of the placenta overlies, but does n completely obstruct, the internal o **retained p.** One not expelled by th uterus after labor. **velamentous** A placenta with the umbilical co springing from the outer border.

plac"en·ta'tion (plass"en·tay shun). Formation and mode of attac ment of the placenta.

plac"en·ti'tis (plass"en·ty'tis). I flammation of the placenta.

plac"en·tog'ra·phy. Roentgeno raphy of the placenta after deliver using a contrast medium.

plac"en·to'ma. A neoplasm sprin ing from a retained portion of t placenta.

pla·cen"to·ther'a·py. The remed use of preparations of the placenta animals.

placidyl. Trade-mark for ethchlo vynol.

plac'ode. A platelike epithelial thic ening, frequently marking, in the e bryo, the anlage of an organ or pa **auditory p.** The dorsolateral ect dermal anlage of the internal e **lens p.** The ectodermal anlage of t lens of the eye; its formation is i duced by the presence of the underly optic vesicle.

plad"a·ro'ma. A soft wart or tum of the eyelid.

pla"gi·o·ce·phal'ic, pla"gi ceph'a·lous. Designating a type pronounced oblique deformation of t skull.

pla"gi·o·ceph'a·ly. A type strongly asymmetric cranial deform tion, in which the anterior portion one side and the posterior portion the opposite side of the skull are d veloped more than their counterpar so that the maximum length of t skull is not in the midline but on diagonal. Due to a number of caus such as prenatal, developmental (d ordered sequence of suture closur mechanical (intentional or uninte tional).

plague. 1. Any contagious, maligna epidemic disease. 2. A contagious d ease endemic in eastern Asia, and former times occurring epidemically Europe and Asia Minor. It is an ac febrile disease characterized by infla mation of the lymphatics, with the p duction of buboes, primary or secor ary pneumonia, petechiae and diff hemorrhages, and a high mortal Caused by *Pasteurella pestis*. Primar a disease of rodents, transmitted man by fleas. **black p.** The plague which decimated the European nations in the 14th century, so called because of the high incidence of hemorrhages. **bubonic p.** The usual form of plague, characterized by bubo formation, formerly prevalent in various parts of the world. **p. vaccine.** One used for active immunization against plague; may be of either killed or attenuated living cultures of the organism. **pneumonic p.** An extremely virulent type with lung involvement and a high mortality rate.

Planck, Max [*German physicist,* 1858–1947]. Known for his contributions which form the basis of the quantum theory. Nobel laureate (1918). **P. constant.** Mathematically, 6.55×10^{-27}, a constant associated with the quantum theory and represented by h. The value $h\nu$ is the unit of energy emitted by a body, where ν equals the frequency of the atomic or molecular vibration.

plane. Any flat, smooth surface, especially any assumed or conventional surface, whether tangent to the body or dividing it. For subentries not found here, see under *planum*. **Frankfort horizontal p.** An anthropometric plane for orienting heads of the living as well as skulls in a definite position, so that measurements and contours of a series will be comparable. The F-H was proposed at the Craniometric Congress held in Munich in 1877, and was formally adopted by the International Congress of Anthropologists in Frankfurt-am-Main in 1884, whence its name. The plane was defined as being determined by *four* points, viz. the two *poria* and the two *orbitalia*. In anthropometric practice, only the two *poria* and left orbitale are the *three* points used to determine the plane, since only in perfectly symmetrical heads or skulls would four points fall in the plane. The plane was adopted because it can be determined easily on the living, making comparison between head and skull possible, and it approximates quite closely the position in which the head is carried during life. **subcostal p.** A horizontal plane passing through the lowest points of the costal arch or the lowest points of the tenth costal cartilages. This plane usually lies at the level of the third lumbar vertebra. **transpyloric p.** A horizontal plane through the body at the level of the second lumbar vertebra; the pylorus lies in this plane. **planim'e·ter.** An instrument which measures the area of a plane surface by tracing the periphery.

plan'o-, plan-. A combining form signifying *wandering*.

pla'no-. A combining form signifying *flat* or *level*.

pla"no·con'cave. Concave on one surface and flat on the opposite side.

pla"no·con'ic. Having one side flat and the other conical.

pla"no·con'vex. Plane on one side and convex on the other.

plan"o·ma'ni·a. A morbid desire for wandering; an impulse to throw off social restraints and live in the wilds.

plan'ta. The sole of the foot.

Plan·ta'go. Plantain. A genus of weeds, some of which are used medically.

plan·ta'go seed. The cleaned, dried, ripe seed of *Plantago psyllium* or of *P. indica*, known in commerce as Spanish or French psyllium seed; or of *P. ovata*, known in commerce as blonde psyllium or Indian plantago seed. It contains a mucilaginous principle and is used almost exclusively in medicine in chronic constipation. Also called *psyllium seed*, *plantain seed*.

plan'tain (plan'tin). See *Plantago*.

plan'tar. Pertaining to the sole of the foot, as plantar fascia, the dense triangular-shaped aponeurosis occupying the sole of the foot beneath the integument.

plan'tar flex'ion. Bending the foot downward. See also *dorsiflexion*.

plan·ta'ris (plan·tar'is, plan·tay'ris). A small muscle of the calf of the leg. See Table of Muscles in the Appendix.

plan'tar wart. A type of verruca, usually multiple, occurring on the bottom of the foot; may become quite painful, as the wart cannot grow out from the surface because of pressure. Also called *verruca plantaris*.

plan·ta'tion. A general term including *implantation*, *replantation*, and *transplantation*.

plan'ti·grade. Walking on the entire sole of the foot, as man and the bear.

pla'num (pl. *plana*). A plane, or level surface. For subentries not found here, see under *plane*. **p. temporale.** A relatively flat area lying below the linea temporalis inferior and composed of portions of the frontal and parietal bones, great wing of the sphenoid, and squama temporalis.

plaque (plack, plahk). A patch. **dental p.** A thin, transparent film on the surfaces of a tooth, made up of mucin, bacteria, and colloidal material secreted by the salivary glands.

plasm (plaz'um). 1. Plasma, *q.v.* 2. Old term for a part of the substance of a cell. **germ p.** The material basis of inheritance; it is located in the chromosomes.

plas'ma (plaz'muh). The fluid portion of the blood. Composed of a mixture of many proteins in a crystalloid solution and corresponds closely to the interstitial fluid of the body. **citrated normal human p.** The sterile plasma obtained by pooling approximately equal amounts of the liquid portion of citrated whole blood from eight or more healthy humans. **p. cell.** One of the cells, derived from lymphocytes, found in chronically inflamed connective tissue. See also *plasmocyte.*

plas'ma·cyte. Plasmocyte. —**plas·macyt'ic,** *adj.*

plas"ma·cy·to'ma (plaz"muh-sigh-to'muh). A type of myeloma of bones, in which the cells are mostly plasma cell types. A similar tumor originates in the soft tissues of the nasopharynx.

plas"ma·pher'e·sis (plaz"muh-ferr'i-sis, -feer'i-sis). The operation of venesection into sodium citrate solution, centrifugalization, washing the blood cells in physiological salt solution and returning them (without the plasma) into the donor's circulation.

plas"ma·ther'a·py. Treatment, as for shock, by the intravenous injection of blood plasma.

plas'mo- (plaz'mo-), **plasm-.** A combining form meaning *plasma.*

plasmochin. Trade-mark for a brand of pamaquine naphthoate.

plas'mo·cyte (plaz'mo-sight). A mononuclear cell of distinctive appearance, normally present in the bone marrow and increased in number in plasma-cell myeloma (multiple myeloma). This cell is considered by some to be an abnormal form of lymphocyte, and by others to be an independent cell series. Also present in other tissues of the body in variable numbers. —**plasmocyt'ic,** *adj.*

plas"mo·cy·to'ma (plaz"mo-sigh-to'muh). Myeloma made up largely of plasma cells.

Plas·mo'di·i·dae (plaz-mo'dee-i-dee). A family of the Haemosporidia; contains the genus *Plasmodium* which includes the malaria plasmodia of man, birds, and lower animals.

Plas·mo'di·um. A genus of protozoa that causes malaria in birds, lower animals, and man. —**plasmodial,** *adj.* **P. falciparum.** That species which is the cause of estivo-autumnal or malignant tertian malaria. **P. malariae.** That species which is the etiologic agent of malariae malaria or quartan malaria. **P. ovale.** The species of protozoa which causes tertian or ovale malaria. **P. vivax.** That species which causes vivax or benign tertian malaria.

plas·mol'y·sis. Shrinkage of a cell or its contents, due to withdrawal of water by osmosis. —**plasmolyt'ic,** *adj.*

plas"mo·trop'ic. Producing exces-

sive hemolysis in the liver, spleen, and bone marrow.

plas'ter. 1. Substance intended for external application, made of such materials and of such consistency as to adhere to the skin. **2.** Calcined gypsum or calcium sulfate. **p. of Paris.** Calcium sulfate.

plas'tic. 1. Formative; concerned with building up tissues, restoring lost parts, repairing or rectifying malformations or defects, etc., as plastic surgery, plastic operation, plastic repair. **2.** Capable of being molded. **3.** Material such as celluloid, proteins, resins, etc., which can be molded during processing by heat or pressure. **p. lymph.** The inflammatory exudate that covers wounds or inflamed serous surfaces and becomes organized by the development in it of blood vessels and connective tissues.

plas·tic'i·ty (plas-tiss'i-tee). The quality of being plastic.

plas'tics. *In dentistry,* those filling materials, such as amalgam, gutta-percha, and various cements, which are soft at the time of insertion, and may then be shaped and molded.

-plasty. A combining form denoting *plastic operation.*

plate. 1. A flattened part, especially a flattened process of bone. **2.** A thin piece of metal or some other substance to which artificial teeth are attached. **3.** *In microbiology,* a shallow, cylindrical, covered culture dish. The term is also applied to such a dish containing solid cultural medium suitable for the growth of microörganisms. Also called *Petri dish.* **chorionic p.** The chorionic membrane of the placental region, formed externally by the trophoblast layer and internally by a fibrous lining layer of mesoderm. **cribriform p.** The horizontal plate of the ethmoid bone, part of the floor of the anterior cranial fossa, and perforated for the passage of the olfactory nerves. **epiphyseal p.** (a) The broad articular surface with slightly elevated rim on each end of the centrum of a vertebra. Syn., *epiphyseal disk.* (b) The thin cartilage mass between an epiphysis and the shaft of a bone; the site of growth in length. It is obliterated by epiphyseal union. **equatorial p.** The compressed mass of chromosomes aggregated at the equator of the nuclear spindle during karyokinesis. **lateral pterygoid p.** A broad, thin plate whose lateral surface forms part of the medial wall of the infratemporal fossa and gives attachment to the external pterygoid muscle, and whose medial surface forms part of the pterygoid fossa and gives attachment to the internal pterygoid muscle. **medial pterygoid p.** A long, narrow plate whose lateral surface forms part of the pterygoid fossa and whose medial surface constitutes the lateral boundary of a choana. Its lower extremity forms a hook, the pterygoid hamulus, for the tendon of the tensor veli palatini. **motor p.** Motor end-plate; a small mass of sarcoplasm formed beneath the sarcolemma at the junction of nerve and muscle fibers. It receives the terminal ramifications of the naked axis cylinder of a somatic motor nerve. **tarsal p.** A thin, elongated plate of dense connective tissue which contributes to the form and support of an eyelid. **terminal p.** The thin plate of bone of an epiphysis laid down on the metaphyseal surface preceding epiphyseal union.

pla·teau′. In operating Geiger counter tubes, the voltage range over which the number of impulses recorded is nearly constant.

plate cul′ture. A method of obtaining pure cultures of bacteria by pouring the inoculated culture medium upon sterile glass plates and allowing it to solidify.

plate′let. See *blood* platelets, *thrombocyte.*

pla′ting. In *microbiology*, the inoculation of solid cultural medium in a dish with microörganisms. The inoculum may be distributed over the surface of the medium or incorporated within it.

pla·tin′ic. Referring to a compound containing platinum as a tetravalent element.

pla′ti·nous. Referring to a compound containing platinum as a divalent element.

pla·ti·num. Pt = 195.23. A silver-white metal occurring natively or alloyed with other metals. It is fusible only at very high temperatures, and is insoluble in all acids except nitrohydrochloric.

lat″o·nych′i·a (plat″o-nick′ee-uh). Rare dystrophy of the nail; consisting of a modification of its greatest curvature, which, instead of being transverse, as normally, is lengthwise.

lat′y-, plat-. A combining form meaning *broad, flat.*

lat″y·ba′si·a (plat″i-bay′see-uh). A developmental deformity of the occipital bone and upper cervical spine, in which the foramen magnum is small and misshapen, the atlas is occipi-alized, and the odontoid process of the axis impinges on the brain stem. It is accompanied by neurologic symptoms and signs referable to changes in the medulla, cervical spinal cord, and lower cranial nerves.

lat″y·ce·phal′ic. Characterizing a person having a skull with a flat vertex.

lat″yc·ne′mic. Designating a tibia

with a marked mediolateral flattening. Having a saber shin.

plat″y·co·ri·a,   plat″y·co·ri′a·sis. Expansion of the pupil; mydriasis.

Plat″y·hel·min′thes (plat″i-hel-minth′eez). A phylum of flatworms characterized by bilaterally symmetrical, many-celled, leaf-shaped bodies lacking a body cavity and usually containing both sexual elements. Includes the medically important classes Trematoda and Cestoidea.

plat″y·mer′ic (plat″i-merr′ick, ·meer′ick). In *osteometry*, designating a femur with a moderate anteroposterior compression and an increased mediolateral diameter in the proximal portion of the diaphysis; having a platymeric index, *q.v.*, of 75.0 to 84.9.

plat″y·pel′lic. In *osteometry*, designating a pelvis with a transverse diameter considerably greater than the conjugata vera, having a pelvic-inlet index, *q.v.*, of 89.9 or less.

plat″yr·rhine (plat′i-ryne, ·rin). 1. In *somatometry*, having a broad and flat nose with a height-breadth index of 85.0 or more. 2. In *craniometry*, having a wide bony nasal aperture with a nasal index of 51.0 or more. 3. In *taxonomy*, pertaining to the platyrrhina or New World monkeys, so named because of their broad nasal septum and wide space between the nostrils. The term is practically replaced in its application to the human nose by chamaerrhine, to avoid confusion with its taxonomic implications.

pla·tys′ma (pla·tiz′muh). A subcutaneous muscle in the neck, extending from the face to the clavicle. Formerly called *platysma myoides.* See Table of Muscles in the Appendix.

pledg′et. A small, flattened compress of cotton, gauze, etc.

-plegia. A combining form denoting *a stroke, paralysis,* or *palsy.*

plei′o- (ply′o-), **pleo-.** A combining form meaning *more.*

ple·och′ro·ism (plee-ock′ro-iz-um). The property possessed by some bodies, especially crystals, of presenting different colors when viewed in the direction of different axes. **—pleochroit′ic, pleochromat′ic,** *adj.*

ple″o·cy·to′sis (plee″o-sigh-to′sis). Increase of cells in the cerebrospinal fluid.

ple″o·mas′ti·a,   ple″o·ma′zi·a. The condition of having more than two mammae.

ple″o·mor′phism. The occurrence of widely different forms of the same species; applied especially to bacteria. **—pleomorphic, pleomorphous,** *adj.*

ple′o·nasm (plee′o-naz-um), **ple″o·nas′ty.** Any deformity marked by superabundance of certain organs or parts. —**pleonas′tic**, adj.

ple″o·nex′i·a. 1. Excessive desire to have or to possess. 2. Increased body resistance.

ple″on·os″te·o′sis. Excessive or premature ossification.

ple·ro′sis. 1. The restoration of lost tissue. 2. Plethora.

ple″si·o′pi·a (plee″see·o′pee·uh, pless″ee·). Increased convexity of the crystalline lens, producing myopia.

pless″es·the′si·a (pless″ess·thee′-zhuh, ·zee·uh). Palpatory percussion performed by placing the left middle finger firmly against the body surface and percussing with the index finger of the right hand, allowing it to remain in contact with the left finger for a few seconds.

pleth′o·ra, ple·tho′ra. A state characterized by excess of blood in the body. —**plethor′ic**, adj. **p. apocop′tica.** A temporary increase in the volume of the blood in other parts of the body, caused by forcing blood from a part to be amputated.

ple·thys′mo·graph (pli·thiz′mo-graf, ·thiss′mo·graf). A device for ascertaining the change in volume of an organ or part, through an increase in the quantity of the blood therein.

pleur-. Same as *pleuro-.*

pleu′ra (pl. *pleurae*). The serous membrane enveloping the lung (**pulmonary** or **visceral pleura**), and lining the internal surface of the thoracic cavity (**parietal pleura**). —**pleural**, adj. **diaphragmatic p.** The reflection of the pleura upon the upper surface of the diaphragm. **mediastinal p.** A continuation of the parietal pleura covering the side of the mediastinum. **pericardiac p.** The portion of the pleura contiguous to the pericardium.

pleu′ra·cot′o·my. Incision of the thoracic wall and pleura, usually exploratory. Also called *thoracotomy.*

pleu·ral′gi·a. Pain in the pleura or in the side; intercostal neuralgia. —**pleuralgic**, adj.

pleu·rec′to·my. Excision of any portion of the pleura.

pleu′ri·sy. Inflammation of the pleura; pleuritis. **acute p.** A type with a sudden onset in which the exudate may be fibrinous, fibrinoserous, purulent, putrid, or hemorrhagic. It may develop in the course of bacteremia, bacteria occasionally being recovered, or originate from infection of the underlying lung as a part of pneumonia, or from inflammatory processes in the mediastinum or other neighboring structures. Characterized by fever, pain with breathing, and crepitation or friction sounds on auscultation. **adhesive p.** That in which there are

fibrinous attachments between vis‐ceral and parietal pleural surfaces **chronic p.** A slowly developing type usually adhesive, as that seen in tuber‐culosis. **diaphragmatic p.** Pleuris of the upper surface of the diaphragm **encapsulated p.** Walled-off pocke of exudate in the pleural space. **inter lobar p.** Localized inflammation o pleural surfaces between the lobes o the lung. **purulent p.** Empyema **serous p.** Pleurisy with effusion **suppurative p.** Empyema.

pleu·ri′tis. Pleurisy. —**pleurit′ic** adj.

pleu′ro-, pleur-. A combining form denoting *connection with the pleura* o *with a side or rib.*

pleu″ro·cen·te′sis. Puncture of th pleura. Also called *thoracentesis.*

pleu″ro·chol″e·cys·ti′tis (·kol*s*sis·tye′tis, ·ko″li·). Inflammation o the gallbladder, with involvement o the pleura.

pleu″ro·cu·ta′ne·ous. In relatio with the pleura and the skin, as pleuro cutaneous fistula.

pleu″ro·dyn′i·a (ploor″o·din′ee·u ·dye′nee·uh). A sharp pain in the inter costal muscles. **epidemic p.** A acute epidemic disease with fever an pain in the chest, epigastrium, an costovertebral region. Also calle *Bornholm disease, devil's grip.*

pleu″ro·hep·a·ti′tis. Inflammatio of the liver and diaphragmatic part o the pleura.

pleu′ro·lith. A calculus in the pleur or the pleural space.

pleu″ro·per″i·car′di·al. Pertain ing to both pleura and pericardium.

pleu″ro·per″i·car·di′tis. Pleuris associated with pericarditis.

pleu″ro·pul″mo·nar′y (ploor″ pul′mo·nerr″ee). Pertaining to th pleura and the lungs.

pleu′ro·spasm. Cramp, or spasm the side, of pleural origin.

pleu″ro·thot′o·nos. A form tetanic spasm of the muscles in whic the body is bent to one side.

pleu·rot′o·my. Incision into th pleura.

pleu″ro·vis′cer·al. Pertaining the pleura or side, and to the viscera.

plex′i·form. Resembling a networ or plexus.

plex·im′e·ter. 1. A finger, usually th left third finger, held firmly again the skin to receive the stroke in ind rect percussion. 2. A small, thin, oblor plate of hard but flexible material, suc as ivory or rubber, used for the sam purpose. Also called *plessimeter.*

plex′or. 1. A finger, when used to ta the surface of the body in performi percussion. 2. A small hammer wit rubber head used for the same purpos Also called *percussion hammer.*

plex′us. A network of interlacing nerves or anastomosing blood vessels or lymphatics. See Tables of Nerves and of Veins in the Appendix. —**plexal,** *adj.* **aortic p.** A network of sympathetic nerves surrounding the aorta; continuous around both the thoracic and abdominal portions of the aorta through the aortic opening in the diaphragm. **Auerbach's p.** See myenteric p. **brachial p.** A plexus of nerves located in the neck and axilla and composed of the anterior rami of the lower four cervical and first thoracic nerves. **cardiac p.** A network of nerves situated at the base of the heart. The superficial part lies beneath the arch of the aorta just anteriad to the right pulmonary artery. The deep part of the cardiac plexus lies anterior to the bifurcation of the trachea between it and the arch of the aorta. Each portion contains nerve fibers of both sympathetic and vagal origin. **celiac p.** A large autonomic plexus lying in front of the aorta around the origin of the celiac artery. It is formed by fibers from the splanchnic and vagus nerves and is distributed to the abdominal viscera. **choroid p.** A vascular plexus found in each of the ventricles of the brain. That of the third and fourth ventricles occupies an invagination of the ependyma of the roof of each ventricle. The choroid plexus of each lateral ventricle is a prolongation of the plexus of the third ventricle through the interventricular foramen. **hypogastric p.** A large sympathetic nerve plexus lying just in front of the promontory of the sacrum. Also called *presacral nerve.* **lumbosacral p.** A network formed by the anterior branches of lumbar, sacral, and coccygeal nerves which for descriptive purposes are divided into the lumbar, sacral, and pudendal plexuses. **myenteric p.** A nerve plexus situated between the circular and longitudinal muscle layers of the digestive tube. Also called *Auerbach's p.* **pampiniform p.** A network of veins in the spermatic cord in the male; in the broad ligament near the ovary in the female. **pelvic p.** A nerve plexus situated at the side of the rectum and bladder and distributed to the pelvic viscera. **prevertebral p.** The collateral ganglions and nerve fibers of the sympathetic nervous system, such as the cardiac, celiac, and hypogastric plexuses. **pterygoid p.** A plexus of veins which accompanies the internal maxillary artery between the pterygoid muscles. See Table of Veins in the Appendix. **pulmonary p.** A nerve plexus composed chiefly of vagal fibers situated on the anterior and posterior aspects of the bronchi and accompany-

ing them into the substance of the lung. **sacral p.** A nerve plexus formed by part of anterior ramus of fourth lumbar nerve and anterior rami of fifth lumbar and first three sacral nerves. **submucous p.** A nerve plexus lying in the submucosa of the digestive tube. Also called *Meissner's p.* **sympathetic p.** A general term used to describe branches of sympathetic nerves surrounding organs or vessels. Each is named from the structure with which it is associated. **tympanic p.** A nerve network formed by the tympanic branch of the glossopharyngeal, the lesser superficial petrosal and tympanopetrosal branches of the facial, and sympathetic nerves derived from the internal carotid plexus.

pli′ca (pl. *plicae*). A fold. For terms not listed here, see under *fold.* —**plicate,** *adj.;* **plica′tion** (pligh-kay′-shun, pli-kay′shun), *n.* **alar p.** One of the fringelike folds of the synovial membrane of the knee joint, on either side of the articular surface of the patella. **duodenojejunal p.** An inconstant fold of peritoneum extending to the left from the duodenojejunal flexure to the posterior abdominal wall; it may contain the main stem of the inferior mesenteric vein. **gastropancreatic p.** A fold of peritoneum on the posterior wall of the omental bursa, extending from the pancreas to the right side of the cardia of the stomach. It contains the left gastric artery. **patellar synovial p.** A fold of synovial membrane in the knee joint which extends from the infrapatellar fatty mass to the anterior part of the interchondyloid notch; its free margins form the alar plicae. **rectouterine plicae.** Two folds of peritoneum extending from the cervix of the uterus on either side of the rectum to the sacrum, and forming the lateral boundaries of the mouth of the rectouterine pouch. See uterosacral *ligament.* **rectovesical p.** A peritoneal fold extending from the posterior part of the bladder to the rectum and sacrum. Also called *sacrogenital fold.*

plomb (plum). Any plastic material, usually paraffin, used as an extrapleural tampon to close a tuberculous pulmonary cavity.

plom·bage′ (plawm·bahzh′). The extrapleural compression of a tuberculous pulmonary cavity by the use of any plastic material, usually paraffin. A form of collapse therapy. *Obs.*

plug. 1. Something that occludes a circular opening or channel, as a tooth filling. 2. Fill a tooth cavity.

plug′ger. An instrument for the insertion and impaction of fillings in tooth cavities. **foil p.** One used for condensing gold foil in a prepared cavity of a tooth.

plum·ba'go. Native graphite. Black lead. Used in the manufacture of pencils, crucibles, and as a lubricant.

plum'bic. Describing a compound of tetravalent lead.

plum'bism (plum'biz·um). Lead poisoning.

plum'bite. A salt derived from lead hydroxide, $Pb(OH)_2$, of the types, $MHPbO_2$ or M_2PbO_2.

plum'bum. See *lead*.

plump'er. Formerly, one of a pair of pads worn in the cheeks to give them a rounded appearance; artificial dentures are now sometimes built up to produce the same effect.

plu"ri·grav'i·da. A woman during her third and subsequent pregnancies; multigravida.

plu·rip'a·ra. A woman who has given birth to several children; a multipara.

plu"ri·par'i·ty. The condition of having borne several children.

plu"to·ma'ni·a. A false belief that one is the possessor of great wealth; greed for wealth.

plu·to'nism. A disease caused by exposure to plutonium, manifested in experimental animals by graying of the hair, liver degeneration, and tumor formation. There is no record of occurrence of the disease in a human being.

plu·to'ni·um. Pu = 239 *ca.* An element, atomic number 94, obtained from neptunium, *q.v.*, and capable of undergoing fission with the release of large amounts of energy.

Pm. Symbol for promethium, *q.v.*

-pnea, -pnoea. A combining form denoting *breath* or *a type of breathing.*

pne"o·dy·nam'ics (nee"o·dye·nam'icks, ·di·nam'icks). The dynamics of respiration.

pneu'ma- (new'muh-), **pneum-.** A combining form meaning *wind* or *air.*

pneu"mar·thro'sis (new"mahr·thro'sis). The presence of air or gas in a joint cavity.

pneu·mat'ics (new·mat'icks). The branch of physics treating of the dynamic properties of air and gases.

pneu'ma·to- (new'muh·to-). 1. A combining form meaning *air;* used to denote *respiration.* 2. *In medicine,* a combining form denoting the presence of air or gas in a part.

pneu"ma·to·car'di·a. The presence of air or gas in the chambers of the heart.

pneu'ma·to·cele", pneu·mat'o·cele". A sac or tumor containing gas; especially the scrotum filled with gas. Syn., *pneumonocele, pneumocele.*

pneu"ma·to·dysp·ne'a (new"muh·to·disp·ne'uh, ·disp'nee·uh). Emphysematous dyspnea.

pneu"ma·to·gram", pneu·mat'o·gram". A tracing showing the fre[quency], duration, and depth of th[e] respiratory movements.

pneu"ma·tol'o·gy. 1. The scienc[e] of respiration. 2. The science of gases[;] also their use as therapeutic agent[s.]

pneu"ma·tom'e·try. 1. The mea[s]urement of the force in respiration. [It] is used as a means of diagnosis. 2. Th[e] treatment of pulmonary and circula[tory] diseases by means of a pne[u]matic apparatus.

pneu"ma·tor'a·chis (new"muh·tor'uh·kis). The presence of air in th[e] spinal canal.

pneu·ma·to'sis. Air or gas in ab[normal] situations in the body. **p. cys[·]toides intestinalis.** Cystlike dila[·]tations of the lymph spaces of th[e] intestinal wall due to gas-formin[g] organisms.

pneu"ma·tu'ri·a. Voiding uri[ne] containing free gas.

pneu'ma·type. Breath picture. T[he] deposit formed upon a piece of gla[ss] by the moist air exhaled through t[he] nostrils when the mouth is closed. [It] is employed in the diagnosis of nas[al] obstruction. Slate paper may be use[d,] pulverized sulfur or boric acid bein[g] blown upon the moistened surface [to] make a permanent record.

pneu'mo- (new'mo-). A combinin[g] form meaning *air* or *lung.* See al[so] *pneumono-, pneumato-.*

pneu"mo·ar·throg'ra·phy. Rad[i]ographic examination of joints in[to] which air has been injected.

pneu"mo·bul'bar. Pertaining [to] the lungs and to the respiratory cent[er] in the medulla.

pneu"mo·cen·te'sis. Puncture [of] a lung with needle or trocar; usual[ly] done to obtain tissue or exudate f[or] diagnostic study, or to establish com[·]munication with a cavity.

pneu"mo·ceph'a·lus. The presen[ce] of air or gas within the cranial cavi[ty.]

pneu"mo·coc·ce'mi·a (new"m[o·]cock·see'mee·uh). The presence [of] pneumococci in the blood.

pneu"mo·coc·co·su'ri·a. Presen[ce] of pneumococci in the urine.

Pneu·mo·coc'cus. Old term for *Di[p·]lococcus pneumoniae.*

pneu·mo·coc'cus (pl. *pneumococc[i]*). A bacterium, *Diplococcus pneumoni[ae,]* the causative agent of many types [of] pneumonia.

pneu"mo·co'lon. Distention of t[he] colon with gas as a diagnostic proc[e·]dure.

pneu"mo·co"ni·o'sis. Pneumo[·]coniosis.

pneu"mo·cra'ni·um. Presence [of] air or gas beneath the dura or with[in] the ventricles of the brain.

pneu"mo·cys'to·gram. Radiograph of the urinary bladder following its injection with air.

pneu"mo·der'ma. Air or gas collected under, or in, the skin.

pneu"mo·en·ceph'a·lo·gram". Roentgenographic examination of the brain after the replacement of cerebrospinal fluid with air or gas, which has been injected through a needle into the spinal subarachnoid space.

pneu"mo·en"ter·i'tis. Inflammation of the lungs and of the intestine.

pneu·mog'ra·phy. 1. Roentgenography of the lung. 2. The recording of the respiratory excursions.

pneu"mo·he"mo·per"i·car'di·um. (·hee"mo·perr"i·kahr'dee·um, ·hem"o·). The presence of air and blood in the pericardial cavity.

pneu"mo·hy"dro·per"i·car'di·um. An accumulation of air and fluid in the pericardial sac.

pneu"mo·hy"po·der'ma. Subcutaneous emphysema.

pneu'mo·lith. A calculus or concretion occurring in a lung.

pneu"mo·li·thi'a·sis. The occurrence of calculi or concretions in a lung. Also called *pneumonolithiasis.*

pneu"mo·me"di·as·ti'num. The presence of air in the mediastinal tissues.

pneu'mon·. See *pneumono-.*

pneu"mo·nec'to·my. Excision of an entire lung. **cautery p.** The removal of a lung by cautery.

pneu·mo'ni·a. Inflammation of the lungs; pneumonitis. **aspiration p.** That resulting from the inhalation of a foreign body, usually fluids or food particles, from the pharynx into the air passages of the lungs, usually in the course of a general anesthesia. **bronchial p.** Bronchopneumonia. **chronic p.** Long-standing lung infection. **double p.** Involvement of both lungs. **hypostatic p.** Infection of dependent parts of lungs which are hyperemic due to staying in one position for long periods of time, usually seen in elderly patients. **interstitial p.** Infection particularly of the stroma of the lungs including the peribronchial tissues and the septa between alveoli. It may originate from the pleura or mediastinum. **lipid p.** That due to aspiration of oily substances, particularly from nose drops, mineral oil, or cod liver oil. More common in children or in adults when the cough reflex is impaired. The inflammation is often chronic and is mostly in lower lobes. **lobar p.** An acute febrile disease involving one or more lobes of the lung, due to infection by one of the pneumococci. Characterized by abrupt onset, fever, dyspnea, pain, cough, rusty sputum, and general toxic symp-

toms. Typically, the fever drops by crisis after about a week. The involved lung is consolidated, gradually returning to normal by resolution. **massive p.** One which involves a large area of a lung, or an entire lung. **metastatic p.** A type due to the presence in the lungs of infected emboli. **migratory p.** Pneumonic infection which seems to shift from one part of the lungs to another. **primary atypical p.** Bronchopneumonia of unknown etiology, not secondary to any other acute infectious disease. Suspected of being caused by any one of several different strains of filtrable virus. Typically endemic, but may appear in mild epidemic form. Characterized clinically by failure to respond to sulfonamides and penicillin, absence of characteristic blood changes, tendency to protracted course and delayed resolution, and a generally good prognosis. **rheumatic p.** In the acute stage of rheumatic fever, patients may show pneumonic consolidation; lesions, focal necrosis, thromboses of interalveolar capillaries, and Masson bodies may be present. **terminal p.** That occurring in the course of other diseases and resulting in death. **tuberculous p.** An exudative reaction in the lung caused by the tubercle bacillus. Usually it is an extensive lesion which clinically and roentgenologically simulates pneumonia caused by other organisms. It is often designated *tuberculous bronchopneumonia, bronchopneumonic tuberculosis, tuberculous lobar pneumonia,* or *lobar pneumonic tuberculosis,* depending on its distribution in the lung. **virus p.** See primary atypical p.

pneu·mon'ic (new·mon'ick). 1. Pertaining to pneumonia. *Obs.* 2. Pertaining to the exudative form of pulmonary tuberculosis, when sufficiently extensive to simulate either lobar pneumonia or bronchopneumonia.

pneu"mo·ni'tis (new"mo·nigh'tis). Pneumonia.

pneu·mo'no· (new'mo·no-, new·mo'no-), **pneumon·.** A combining form meaning lung.

pneu"mo·no·coc'cic types (·cock'sick). Subdivisions of *Diplococcus pneumoniae,* based on their polysaccharide haptene or specific soluble substance (SSS). At present, over 30 such types have been distinguished.

pneu"mo·no·co"ni·o'sis. Chronic inflammation of the lungs caused by the inhalation of dust. All of the recognized forms are due to mineral dusts. (Neither irritations of the bronchial tree nor acute infections resulting from inhalation of organic dusts are classed as pneumonoconioses.) The predominant reaction is fibrosis, which varies in type with the etiologic dust. Silicosis and asbestosis are the main forms of pneumonoconiosis known to cause disability. Other forms, known as benign pneumonoconioses, in which the reaction is limited to the stromal tissues, are anthracosis, due to carbon dust, siderosis, due to iron dust, calcicosis, due to marble dust, and baritosis, due to barium dust. Also see *berylliosis*.

pneu·mo·nol′y·sis. The loosening of any portion of lung adherent to the chest wall; a form of collapse therapy used in the treatment of pulmonary tuberculosis. **extrapleural p.** The separation of an area of parietal pleura from the chest wall. Also see *apicolysis*. **intrapleural p.** The severance of adhesion bands between the visceral and parietal layers of pleura. May be closed when performed by the use of a thoracoscope, and open when an incision is made through the chest wall to permit direct vision.

pneu″mo·no·my·co′sis (·migh·ko′sis). Any disease of the lungs due to infestation by a fungus.

pneu″mo·nop′a·thy. Any abnormality of the lungs.

pneu·mo′no·pex″y (new·mo′no·peck″see, new·mo″no·peck′see). Fixation of lung tissue to the chest wall.

pneu″mo·nor′rha·phy. Suture of a lung.

pneu″mo·no′sis. Any noninfective degenerative disease of the lungs. **traumatic p.** *In aviation medicine*, acute noninflammatory pathologic changes produced in the lungs by large momentary deceleration. The principal changes are hemorrhage, emphysema, and laceration. These changes, in accordance with their location, type, and magnitude, may cause sudden death or variable clinical pulmonary signs and symptoms.

pneu″mo·not′o·my. Surgical incision of a lung.

pneu·mop′a·thy. Any abnormality of the lungs.

pneu″mo·per″i·car·di′tis. Pericarditis with the formation of gas in the pericardial sac.

pneu″mo·per″i·car′di·um. The presence of air in the pericardial sac. It is due to traumatism or to communication between the pericardium and the esophagus, stomach, or lungs, and is marked by tympany over the precordial region and peculiar, metallic heart sounds.

pneu″mo·per″i·to·ne′um. 1. The presence of gas in the peritoneal cavity. 2. Injection of a gas into the peritoneal cavity, as in special radiography of the abdomen.

pneu″mo·per″i·to·ni′tis. Peritonitis with the presence of gas in the peritoneal cavity.

pneu″mo·py′e·lo·gram″. A pyelogram in which air or oxygen is used as the contrast medium instead of an opaque solution.

pneu″mo·py″o·per″i·car′di·um. The presence of air, or gas, and pus in the pericardial sac.

pneu″mo·ra′chis (new″mo·ray′kis, new·mor′uh·kis). A collection of gas in the spinal canal, accidental or by injection of air for diagnostic purposes.

pneu″mo·ra″di·og′ra·phy. Radiography of a region, as of a joint or of the abdomen, following the injection of air into a cavity.

pneu″mo·scle·ro′sis. Fibrosis of the lungs.

pneu″mo·tax′is. Pertaining to the control of respiration.

pneu″mo·tho′rax. The presence of air or gas in a pleural cavity. May occur from perforating wounds of the chest, accidental or operative, by the rupture of an abscess or cavity of the lung, or the rupture of an air sac or bronchiole. **artificial p.** The production of a pneumothorax by the introduction into a pleural cavity, through a needle, of air or other gas to produce collapse and immobility of a lung, with obliteration of cavities. Used in the treatment of pulmonary tuberculosis. **extrapleural p.** One in which the parietal pleura is stripped from the thoracic wall, and the air or gas introduced within the space so formed, as in apicolysis, *q.v.* **spontaneous p.** The pneumothorax occurring from causes other than the introduction of air or gas into a pleural cavity from without.

pneu″mo·ty′phus. 1. Typhoid fever beginning with pneumonia dependent upon the typhoid bacillus. 2. Pneumonia occurring in the course of typhoid fever.

pneu″mo·ven·tric″u·log′ra·phy. A method of depicting the ventricular system of the brain by roentgenography, after the fluid content has been removed and air has been injected. Also called *ventriculography*.

pneu′sis (new′sis). Respiration.

pni″go·pho′bi·a (nigh″go·fo′bee·uh). The fear of choking that sometimes accompanies angina pectoris.

-pnœa. Same as *-pnea*.

Po. Chemical symbol for polonium.

pock. A pustule of an eruptive fever, especially of smallpox.

pocked. Pitted; marked with pustules.

pock′et. *In anatomy*, a blind sac, or sac-shaped cavity. A diverticulum communicating with a cavity. **intra·oral p.** An artificially created pocket within the mouth, lined with grafted skin, used to hold a prosthetic appliance in the restoration of facial contours due to the loss of half or more of the mandible. **periodontal p.** An abnormally deep gingival sulcus, associated with periodontosis, whose extension apically is at the expense of detached periodontal fibers and resorbed bone of the alveolar process.

po·dag′ra, pod′a·gra. Gout, especially of the great toe or joints of the foot.

po·dal′gi·a. Pain in the foot.

po·dal′ic. Pertaining to the feet, as podalic version, the operation of changing the position of the fetus in the uterus to bring the feet to the outlet.

pod″ar·thri′tis. Inflammation of the joints of the feet.

po·dar′thrum. *In biology*, the foot joint or metatarsophalangeal articulation. *Obs.*

pod″e·de′ma. Edema of the feet.

po·di′a·trist, po″di·at′rist. A specialist in treating diseases of the feet.

po·di′a·try. Treatment of disorders of the feet; chiropody. Unofficial synonym for chiropody.

pod″o·brom″hi·dro′sis (pod″o-brohm″hi·dro′sis, pod″o·brom″·). Offensive sweating of the feet.

pod″o·dyn′i·a (pod″o·din′ee-uh, -dye′nee-uh). Pain in the foot, especially a neuralgic pain in the heel unattended by swelling or redness.

po·dom′e·ter. An instrument which registers the number of footsteps in walking; preferably called *pedometer*.

pod″o·phyl′lin, pod·oph′yl·lin. See *podophyllum* resin.

pod″o·phyl″lo·res′in (·rez′in). See *podophyllum*.

pod″o·phyl″lo·tox′in. See *podophyllum*.

pod″o·phyl′lum. Consists of the dried rhizome and roots of *Podophyllum peltatum*. Podophyllum contains a crystallizable substance called podophyllotoxin, and an amorphous resinous substance, podophylloresin. It is a cathartic. Also called *mandrake, may apple*. **p. resin.** A light brown to greenish yellow powder, obtained by pouring an alcoholic extract of podophyllum into acidified cold water. Also called *podophyllin*.

poe-. For words beginning with *poe-*, see under *pe-*.

·poi·et′ic. A combining form denoting *making* or *producing*.

poi′ki·lo·cyte″. A large, red blood cell of irregular shape.

poi″ki·lo·cy·the′mi·a (poy″ki·lo-sigh·thee′mee·uh). The presence of poikilocytes in the blood.

poi″ki·lo·der′ma. A skin syndrome characterized by pigmentation, telangiectasia, and, usually, atrophy. **p. vasculare atrophicans.** A widespread cutaneous disease with atrophy, telangiectasia, pigmentation, and purpura. It may occur in association with, or as an end result of, other cutaneous diseases. **reticulated pigmented p.** A pigmented erythroderma arranged in a network, commonly seen on the neck, shoulders, and sides of the face. Also called *Riehl's melanosis*.

poi″ki·lo·der″ma·to·my″o·si′tis. Poikiloderma in association with muscular sclerosis.

poi″ki·lo·ther′mic. Varying in body temperature according to the surroundings; cold-blooded. Also called *poikilothermal, poikilothermous*.

poi″ki·lo·throm′bo·cyte. A blood platelet of abnormal shape.

point. 1. The sharp end of an object, especially one used to pierce anything. 2. The limit at which anything occurs, as the melting point, freezing point. 3. A mark made by a sharp object; a minute spot or area. 4. Of an abscess, to come to the surface. **boiling p.** The temperature at which a liquid has a vapor pressure equal to the barometric pressure. **cardinal p.** (a) *In obstetrics*, one of the four points of the pelvic inlet toward which the occiput of the fetus may be directed in a case of pregnancy with head presentation; the four points are the two sacroiliac articulations and the two ileopectineal eminences. (b) *In ophthalmology*, the six optical points that determine the direction of the rays entering or emerging from a series of refracting mediums. **fixation p.** That of sharpest vision in the retina; the point where the visual axis meets the retina. **freezing p.** The temperature at which a pure liquid is in equilibrium with its solid form, or at which the solid form of the solvent is in equilibrium with a solution. **isoelectric p.** The pH at which the net electric charge on a particle or surface is zero. **McBurney's p.** A point halfway between the umbilicus and the anterior superior iliac spine. A point of extreme tenderness in appendicitis. **melting p.** The temperature at which a fusible solid begins to melt. Abbreviated, m.p. **triple p.** The temperature and pressure at which the solid, liquid, and vapor phases of a substance may coexist.

point′ing. The coming to a point. **p. of an abscess.** The process whereby pus forms or collects near the surface.

poi′son. A substance that, being in solution in the blood or acting chemically on the blood, either destroys life or impairs seriously the functions of one or more of the organs of the body. Also see *poisoning*. **capillary poisons.** Substances such as peptones and foreign proteins which increase the flow of lymph, presumably by an injurious effect on the capillaries. **cellular poisons.** Cytolysins. **poi'son·ing.** The condition caused by a poison. Also see *poison*. **acetanilid p.** Symptoms: collapse, cyanosis. Treatment: evacuation, warmth, stimulants, artificial respiration. **acetophenetidin p.** Similar to acetanilid poisoning, *q.v.* **acetylsalicylic acid p.** See *p.* from salicylates. **aconite p.** Symptoms: sudden collapse, slow, feeble, and irregular pulse and respirations, tingling in the mouth and extremities, giddiness, great muscular weakness, sometimes pain in the abdomen, marked anesthesia of skin, clear mind, convulsions at times. Treatment: tannic acid solution for washing out stomach, digitalis, stimulants, absolute quiet in recumbent position. **aconitum napellus p.** See aconite *p.* **alcohol p.** Symptoms: confusion of thought, giddiness, tottering gait, slight cyanosis, narcosis from which patient can be aroused, full pulse, deep, stertorous breathing, injection of eyes, low temperature; convulsions may occur. Treatment: stomach evacuation, coffee, stimulants. **alkali p.** Ammonia, lye, washing soda, and quicklime poisoning fall into this category. Symptoms: intense gastroenteritis, often with bloody vomiting and purging, swollen lips and tongue covered with detached epithelium, violent dyspnea, characteristic odor. Treatment: dilution, vegetable acids (lemon juice or diluted vinegar), demulcents. **aniline p.** A poisoning occurring commonly in industry. Symptoms: methemoglobin formation, headache, cyanosis, dyspnea, convulsions, and collapse. Treatment: warmth, stimulants, artificial respiration. **antimony p.** Symptoms: metallic taste, violent vomiting which may become bloody, feeble pulse, pain and burning in the stomach, violent serous purging which becomes bloody, cramps in the extremities, thirst, great debility, sometimes prostration, collapse, unconsciousness, and convulsions without vomiting or purging. Treatment: tannic acid, demulcent drinks, opium, alcohol, external heat. **antipyrine p.** Symptoms: headache, nausea, vomiting, a rash like that of measles, vertigo, drowsiness, deafness, confusion of ideas, cyanosis, collapse. Treatment: recumbent position, warmth, stimulants, oxygen, artificial respiration. Also called *phenazone p.* **apomorphine p.** Symptoms: violent vomiting, paralysis of motor and sensory nerves, delirium, depression of respiration and of heart. Treatment: cardiac and respiratory stimulants. **arsenic p.** Symptoms: violent, burning pain in the stomach, retching, thirst, purging of blood and mucus with flakes of epithelium, tenesmus, suppression of urine, sense of constriction in throat, small and frequent pulse. Treatment: iron hydroxide, emetics, castor oil, demulcents, dimercaprol. **aspirin p.** See *p.* from salicylates. **atropine p.** Symptoms: heat and dryness of the mouth and throat, widely dilated pupils, scarlet rash, noisy delirium, quick pulse (at first corded, later feeble), rapid respirations (early strong, late shallow and feeble), retention of urine, sometimes convulsions, collapse, and paralysis. Treatment: tannic acid, stimulants, coffee, pilocarpine, artificial respiration, stomach and bladder evacuation. Also called *homatropine p.* **barbiturate p.** See *p.* from barbiturates. **barium sulfide p.** That occurring from the use of certain depilatories. Symptoms: violent intestinal colic, cardiac irregularity. Treatment: gastric lavage, magnesium sulfate. **belladonna p.** That caused by the deadly nightshade. See atropine *p.* **benzene p.** If taken by mouth, symptoms: pyrexia, excitement followed by narcosis, paralysis, gastrointestinal irritation, aspiration pneumonia. Treatment: dilution with oil, evacuation. If from the toxic fumes, symptoms: the initial stage resembles alcoholic intoxication followed by narcosis, convulsions, and paralysis. Treatment: stimulants, artificial respiration. **borax p.** See boric acid *p.* **boric acid p.** Symptoms: profound depression, hepatitis. Treatment: evacuation, fluid, dextrose intravenously. **brucine p.** See strychnine *p.* **caffeine p.** Symptoms: burning pain in the throat, giddiness, faintness, nausea, numbness, abdominal pain, great thirst, dry tongue, tremor of extremities, diuresis, weak pulse, cold skin, collapse. Treatment: emetics, stimulants, warmth. **calabarbean p.** See physostigma venenosum *p.* **camphor p.** Symptoms: characteristic odor, giddiness, disturbance of vision, delirium, cyclic convulsions, clammy skin, smarting on urination, quick and weak pulse. Treatment: stomach evacuation. **cannabis indica p.** Symptoms: pleasurable intoxication, heavy sleep. Treatment: stomach evacuation. Also called *Indian hemp p.* **cantharis vesicatoria p.** See *p.* from cantharides. **carbolic acid p.** See phenol *p.* **carbona p.** See carbon tetrachloride *p.* **carbon disulfide p.** Symptoms: vomiting, weakness, convulsions, coma. Treatment: evacuation, artificial respiration. **carbon monoxide p.** Symptoms: headache, giddiness, loss of muscular power, unconsciousness, dilated pupils, labored breathing, coma, cherry-red skin color. Treatment: fresh air, artificial respiration, stimulants, oxygen, coffee, bleeding and replacement with healthy blood. **carbon tetrachloride p.** Symptoms: unconsciousness, asphyxial convulsions, cardiac fibrillation, hepatitis. Treatment: evacuation, artificial respiration, dextrose intravenously. **chloral hydrate p.** Symptoms: deep sleep, loss of muscular power, lividity, diminished reflexes, weak pulse, slowed respirations, contracted pupils during sleep, but dilated on waking, low temperature. Treatment: stomach evacuation, application of heat to the extremities, massage, coffee by rectum, strychnine, amyl nitrite, artificial respiration. **chlorinated lime p.** That caused by the poisonous component of Labarraque's solution, Javelle water, or bleaching fluid. Symptoms: local irritation, gastrointestinal and pulmonary. Treatment: evacuation, sodium thiosulfate in water, milk and raw eggs. **chloroform p.** Symptoms: excitement and intoxication followed by anesthesia and unconsciousness, later profound narcosis, progressively or suddenly failing pulse and respirations. Treatment: draw tongue forward, artificial respiration; if chloroform has been taken by mouth, evacuation of stomach. **chromic acid p.** See chromium trioxide p. **chromium trioxide p.** Symptoms: dark yellow stains, abdominal pain, vomiting and purging, collapse. Treatment: stomach evacuation, chalk, milk, or albumin, demulcent drinks. **coal gas p.** See carbon monoxide p. **coal oil p.** See benzene p. **coal tar p.** See phenol p. **cocaine p.** Symptoms: faintness, giddiness, nausea, small, rapid, and intermittent pulse, dilated pupils, severe prostration, slow and feeble respiration. Treatment: stimulants, amyl nitrite, artificial respiration. **codeine p.** See opium p. **colchicum autumnale p.** Symptoms: not unlike those of malignant cholera; griping pain in the stomach, vomiting and continuous purging of seromucous material, intense thirst, muscular cramps, great prostration, collapse, dilated pupils, pain in the extremities. Treatment: stomach evacuation, tannic acid, morphine. **conium maculatum p.** Symptoms: weakness of the legs, gradual loss of all voluntary power, nausea, ptosis, dilatation of pupils, inability to speak or swallow. Treatment: stomach evacuation, tannic acid, stimulants, warmth, artificial respiration, atropine. **creosote p.** See phenol p. **cresol p.** See phenol p. **croton tiglium p.** Symptoms: intense pain in abdomen, vomiting, purging, watery stools,

pinched face, small and thready pulse, moist skin, collapse. Treatment: stomach evacuation, demulcent drinks, morphine, poultices to abdomen. Also called *croton oil p.* **cyanogen p.** See hydrocyanic acid p. **Datura stramonium p.** Symptoms and treatment similar to those of atropine poisoning, *q.v.* **depilatory p.** See barium sulfide p. **digitalis p.** Symptoms: purging, with severe pain, violent vomiting, vertigo, feeble pulse (although heart action is tumultuous), delirium, and asphyxial convulsions. Treatment: stomach evacuation, tannic acid, recumbent position. **food p.** A type of poisoning due to food contaminated by bacterial toxins or by certain living bacteria, particularly those of the *Salmonella* group, and staphylococci. The term is also used to include symptoms due to foods naturally poisonous, such as fungi (see mushroom *p.*), botulism, *q.v.*, mussel poisoning, and poisoning due to chemicals or allergens in food. Of the food poisonings, that due to bacterial contamination is the most frequent, but botulism is the most serious; two-thirds of the victims die. In food poisoning due to bacterial contamination of the food, the symptoms are: violent diarrhea, retching, prostration, dizziness, and cramps in the abdomen; symptoms generally appear from two to six hours after the food is eaten. Treatment: evacuation of stomach; fasting for at least 24 hours, then liquid diet for two days, bed rest. **foxglove p.** See digitalis p. **gasoline p.** See benzene p. **gelsemium sempervirens p.** Symptoms: appear in about twenty minutes; great muscular weakness, diplopia, ptosis, squint, widely dilated pupils, dimness of vision, labored respiration, weak pulse. Treatment: evacuation of stomach, atropine, stimulants, artificial respiration. **green hellebore p.** See veratrum p. **hellebore p.** See veratrum p. **hemlock p.** See conium maculatum p. **hydrochloric acid p.** Symptoms: pain throughout digestive tract, vomiting, feeble pulse, clammy skin, collapse, eschars externally, yellow stains on clothing, but none on skin. Treatment: demulcent drinks, oil, stimulants (intravenous injection). Also called *muriatic acid p.* **hydrocyanic acid p.** Symptoms: sudden unconsciousness, slow, labored respirations, slow pulse, staring eyes, purple face, general convulsions, then relaxation and collapse, odor of peach kernels; death may be almost instantaneous. Treatment: stomach tube if possible, alternate cold and warm effusions, artificial respiration. **hyoscyamus p.** See atropine p. **Indian to-**

bacco p. See lobelia inflata p. **iodine p.** Symptoms: pain in throat and stomach, vomiting, purging, vomit yellow from iodine, or blue if starch is present in stomach, giddiness, faintness, convulsive movements. Treatment: stomach evacuation, starch, morphine. **iodoform p.** Symptoms: slight delirium, drowsiness, high temperature, rapid pulse. Treatment: gastric lavage. **jaborandi p.** See pilocarpine p. **Jamestown weed p.** Symptoms and treatment similar to those of atropine poisoning, q.v. **kerosene p.** See benzene p. **laudanum p.** See opium p. **lead p.** Symptoms: sweet metallic taste, vomiting of white matter, great thirst, pain in abdomen, usually rigid abdominal muscles, constipation or diarrhea with black stools, cramps in the legs, paralysis of the extremities, convulsions; in the chronic forms, a blue line at the margin of the gums, basophilic stippling of the red cells. Treatment: stomach evacuation, Epsom or Glauber's salts, milk, morphine. **lobelia inflata p.** Symptoms: severe vomiting, with intense depression and prostration, giddiness, tremors, convulsions, collapse. Treatment: stomach evacuation, tannic acid, warmth, recumbent position. **manganese p.** That which results from the inhalation of manganese dust or fumes. Symptoms: resemble paralysis agitans. Treatment: preventive. **meadow-saffron p.** See colchicum autumnale p. **mercury bichloride p.** Symptoms: acrid metallic taste, burning heat in throat and stomach, vomiting, diarrhea with bloody stools, white and shriveled lips and tongue, small and frequent pulse, nephritis and colitis, death in coma or convulsions. Secondary symptoms: hectic fever, coppery taste, fetid breath, gums swollen, salivation. Treatment: albumin in some form, raw white of egg or flour; immediate stomach evacuation; reducing agents, sodium formaldehyde sulfoxylate, calcium sulfide, sodium hypophosphite or thiosulfate. **metal p.** That due to inhalation of fumes of molten brass or zinc. Symptoms: chill, sweating, nausea, thirst, fever, leukocytosis. Treatment: emetics, laxatives, milk, and sodium bicarbonate. **methyl alcohol p.** See wood alcohol p. **methyl salicylate p.** See p. from salicylates. **monkshood p.** See aconite p. **morphine p.** See opium p. **mushroom p.** Symptoms with most poisonous species: delayed gastroenteritis and hepatitis. Treatment: evacuation, dextrose injection. **naphtha p.** See benzene p. **narceine p.** See opium p. **nicotine p.** See tobacco p. **nitric acid p.** Symptoms: yellow stains on skin; otherwise similar to sulfuric acid poisoning, q.v. Treatment: alkalies, soap, demulcents, stimulants. **nitrobenzene p.** A type of poisoning important in industrial medicine with symptoms and treatment similar to aniline poisoning, q.v. **nitroglycerin p.** Symptoms: throbbing headache, pulsation over entire body, dicrotic pulse, flushed face, mental confusion, anxiety, sudden collapse. Treatment: recumbent position. **nux vomica p.** See strychnine p. **opium p.** Symptoms: preliminary mental excitement, followed soon by weariness, sensation of weight in the limbs, sleepiness, diminished sensibility, pin-point pupils, slow and strong pulse and respiration; patient can be roused with difficulty; later, rousing becomes impossible; slow, irregular, and stertorous respiration, rapid and feeble pulse. Treatment: evacuate stomach with mustard or stomach tube, arouse patient to maintain respiration by exercise, with cold and hot ablutions alternately, or stimulate by atropine or coffee if pulse fails, and apply external heat. **oxalic acid p.** Symptoms: hot, acrid taste, burning, vomiting, collapse, sometimes general paralysis, numbness, and stupor. Treatment: lime or chalk. **Paris green p.** See arsenic p. **phenacetin p.** Acetophenetidin poisoning; similar to acetanilid poisoning, q.v. **phenol p.** Symptoms: immediate burning pain from mouth to stomach, giddiness, loss of consciousness, collapse, partial suppression of urine, which is smoky in color; characteristic odor; white, corrugated patches in mouth. Treatment: gastric lavage with dilute alcohol. **phosphorus p.** Symptoms: vomiting and pain; vomit may be luminous in the dark; characteristic odor; after several days deep jaundice, coffee-colored vomit, hepatic tenderness, albuminuria, marked fall in temperature, coma, failure of pulse and respiration. Treatment: copper sulfate as an emetic, then as an antidote in small doses with opium; liquid paraffin. **physostigma venenosum p.** Symptoms: giddiness, prostration, loss of power in the lower limbs, muscular twitching, contracted pupils, clear mind. Treatment: stomach evacuation, atropine. **pilocarpine p.** Symptoms: copious sweating, dizziness, salivation, vomiting, diarrhea, myopia, pupils much contracted. Treatment: stomach evacuation, stimulants, atropine. **p. from antimony compounds.** See antimony p. **p. from arsenic compounds.** See arsenic p. **p. from barbiturates.** Symptoms: narcosis, sometimes preceded by excitement; prolonged sleep, stupor or coma. Treatment: gastric lavage, picrotoxin or metrazol. **p. from bromides.** Symptoms: vomiting, lethargy, hebetude, profound sleep, cramps, acne, mania. Treatment: sodium chloride. **p. from cantharides.** Symptoms: burning in mouth and stomach, vomiting and purging, soon becoming bloody, tenesmus, salivation, aching pains in the back, strangury, priapism, unconsciousness only very late; convulsions at times. Treatment: stomach evacuation, demulcent drinks, morphine, hot bath for the strangury; anesthetics may be necessary for the pain. **p. from cyanogen compounds.** See hydrocyanic acid p. **p. from hypnotics.** See p. from barbiturates. **p. from iodine compounds.** See iodine p. **p. from lead salts.** See lead p. **p. from salicylates.** Symptoms: nausea and vomiting, deafness, delirium, confusion, dyspnea, coma, collapse. These are complicated with local irritation for salicylic acid, acetylsalicylic acid, and methylsalicylate. The acids also produce acidosis. Treatment: evacuation, alkalies. **p. from sulfonamides.** Symptoms: nausea and vomiting, fever, delirium, skin eruptions, hemolysis, nephritis, granulocytopenia, cyanosis. Treatment: fluids. **prussic acid p.** See hydrocyanic acid p. **ptomaine p.** Incorrect term for food poisoning, *q.v.* **roach poison p.** See sodium fluoride p. **salicylic acid p.** See p. from salicylates. **santonin p.** Symptoms: disturbance of color vision; objects first assume a bluish tinge, then yellow; tinnitus, dizziness, pain in the abdomen, failure of respiration, convulsions, stupor. Treatment: evacuate stomach, mitigate convulsions with ether. **savin p.** Symptoms: pain, vomiting, bloody stools and tenesmus, disordered respirations, coma, convulsions, and collapse. Treatment: evacuation of stomach, castor oil in large doses. **selenium p.** A form of poisoning, seldom if ever acute in man, which is due to the ingestion of selenium in water and plant foods during a long period of years and characterized by general debility with degenerative changes in the liver and kidneys. Also called *alkali disease, loco disease.* **silver salts p.** Symptoms: pain, vomiting, and purging; vomit white and cheesy, rapidly turning black in the sunlight; vertigo, coma, convulsions, paralysis, and marked disturbance of respiration. Treatment: salt and water, stomach evacuation, a large amount of milk. **sodium fluoride p.** That due to a poison found in roach powder. Symptoms: violent gastroenteritis. Treatment: gastric lavage, calcium salts. **Spanish fly p.** See p. from cantharides. **stramonium p.** See

atropine p. **strophanthus p.** See digitalis p. **strychnine p.** Symptoms: tetanic convulsions in paroxysms at intervals varying from five minutes to half an hour; opisthotonos during paroxysm; prominent eyeballs; pupils dilated, impeded respiration, feeble and rapid pulse, anxiety. Treatment: evacuate stomach; tannic acid followed by an emetic; keep patient quiet; ether or barbiturates to control convulsions; artificial respiration if indicated. **sulfuric acid p.** Symptoms: vomiting, often of tarry matter, black stains, pain throughout digestive tract, feeble pulse, clammy skin, profuse and bloody salivation. Treatment: chalk, magnesia, soap, demulcent drinks. **thornapple p.** Symptoms and treatment similar to those of atropine poisoning, *q.v.* **tobacco p.** Symptoms: nausea, vomiting, weakness, weak pulse, cold and clammy skin, collapse, contracted pupils, then dilated. Treatment: stomach evacuation, tannic acid, recumbent position, artificial respiration. **veratrum p.** That caused by both the white (album) and the green (viride) varieties of veratrum, which have the same effect. Symptoms: pain and burning in the alimentary tract, vomiting and diarrhea, slow, weak pulse, labored respiration, sometimes convulsions. Treatment: stomach evacuation, opium, stimulants, coffee, warmth, recumbent position. **white hellebore p.** See veratrum p. **wintergreen oil p.** See p. from salicylates. **wood alcohol p.** Symptoms: inebriation, gastroenteritis, prolonged coma, blindness. Treatment: gastric lavage, fluids, dextrose intravenously. **yellow jasmine p.** See gelsemium sempervirens p.

poi'son i'vy. A climbing vine, *Toxicodendron radicans* (also called *Rhus toxicodendron* and *Rhus radicans*); contains an oleoresin (urushiol) which causes a form of dermatitis venenata.

poi'son nut. Nux vomica.

poi'son oak. *Toxicodendron quercifolium* (also called *Rhus toxicodendron* Linné but not the *R. toxicodendron* of American authors, which is poison ivy); produces a contact dermatitis similar to that produced by poison ivy. **Western poison oak** is the *Toxicodendron diversilobum* (also known as *Rhus diversiloba*).

poi'son-ous. Having the properties of a poison; venomous.

poi'son su'mac. A smooth shrub, *Toxicodendron vernix* (also called *Rhus vernix* and *Rhus venenata*); contains an oil which makes the plant poisonous to the touch; produces eruptions resembling poison ivy dermatitis.

poke'ber"ry. See *phytolacca*.

po'ker back. Complete stiffness of

the spine, usually due to ankylosing spondylitis or rheumatoid arthritis of the spine.

poke′root″. See *phytolacca*.

po′lar bod′ies. The two minute cells given off successively by the ovum during the maturation divisions. They mark the animal pole. Also called *polar cells, polocytes, polar globules.*

po″lar·im′e·ter. An instrument for making quantitative studies on the rotation of polarized light by optically active substances.

po″lar·im′e·try. The use of the polarimeter.

po·lar′i·scope. An instrument for studying the polarization of light; a polarimeter.

po·lar′i·ty. 1. The state or quality of having poles or points of intensity with mutually opposite qualities. 2. The electrically positive or negative condition of a battery or other electric terminals. 3. Demonstration of sedation of a nerve sensation at or near the positive electrode, and of irritation at or near the negative electrode; of anelectrotonus of muscular contraction near the positive electrode and of catelectrotonus near the negative electrode.

po″lar·i·za′tion. 1. The act of polarizing or the state of being polarized. 2. A condition produced in a ray of light such that the vibrations are restricted to planes or curves. 3. The deposit of gas bubbles (hydrogen) on the electronegative plate of a galvanic battery, whereby the flow of the current is impeded. 4. Acquisition of electric charges of opposite sign, as across semipermeable membranes in polarization of cell membranes in living tissues.

po′lar·ize. Endow with polarity; place in a state of polarization.

po′lar·i″zer. An object, such as a Nicol prism, by means of which light is polarized.

po·lar′o·gram. The current-voltage curve obtained in polarographic analysis.

po·lar′o·graph. An instrument used in polarography.

po″lar·og′ra·phy. A method of chemical analysis based on the interpretation of the current-voltage curve characteristic of a solution of an electrooxidizable or electroreducible substance when it is electrolyzed with the dropping mercury electrode. **—polarograph′ic,** *adj.*

polaroid. Trade-mark for a specially prepared cellulose film containing oriented iodoquinine sulfate crystals, mounted between two glass plates. Used as a substitute for Nicol prisms, in polariscopes, and for microscopes, reading glasses, and windshields to avoid glare.

pole. 1. Either extremity of the axis of the body, as of the fetus, the crystalline lens, etc. 2. One of two points at which opposite physical qualities, for example, of electricity or of magnetism, are concentrated; specifically, the electrodes of a galvanic battery, or of other generators of electricity. **animal p. (a)** The formative pole of an ovum distinguished by having more cytoplasm, pigment, etc. (b) In the mammalian blastocyst, the pole containing the inner cell mass. **negative p.** The active pole of a battery; the electropositive element. Also called *cathode*. **positive p.** The inactive pole of a source of electricity, as a battery, consisting of an electronegative element. Also called *anode*.

po′li·o (po′lee·o). Short for poliomyelitis, *q.v.*

po′li·o-, po′li-. A combining form meaning *gray;* used to denote *relation to the gray matter of the brain.*

po″li·o·en·ceph″a·li′tis. Inflammation of the gray matter of the brain.

po″li·o·en·ceph″a·lo·me·nin″go·my″e·li′tis. Inflammation of the gray matter of the brain and spinal cord and of their meninges.

po″li·o·en·ceph″a·lo·my″e·li′tis. Any inflammation of the gray matter of the brain and spinal cord, more specifically anterior poliomyelitis with encephalitis.

po″li·o·en·ceph″a·lop′a·thy. Any disease of the gray matter of the brain.

po″li·o·my″e·len·ceph″a·li′tis. Poliomyelitis and polioencephalitis existing together.

po″li·o·my″e·li′tis. Inflammation of the gray matter of the spinal cord. **—poliomyelit′ic,** *adj.* **acute anterior p.** An acute inflammation of the anterior horns of the gray matter of the spinal cord. It is most common in children, producing a paralysis of certain muscle groups or of an entire limb. The onset is sudden, with fever, gastrointestinal complaints, and pain in the affected muscles, and the paralysis is usually most extensive in the beginning, a certain amount of improvement taking place subsequently. The affected muscles atrophy rapidly, the reflexes in them are lost, and reaction of degeneration develops. From contraction of antagonistic muscles, deformities occur later in life. The disease is endemic with epidemic flare-ups. Some cases do not show paralysis, the diagnosis being made only by spinal fluid examination. Also called *infantile paralysis, epidemic paralysis, acute wasting paralysis, Heine-Medin's disease.* **anterior spinal p.** Anterior poliomyelitis, acute or chronic. **ascending p.** A type similar to Landry's paralysis. The paralysis starts in the toes, rapidly extends to the legs, thighs, trunk, and finally to the muscles of respiration. **metallic p.** A form of toxic neuritis due to metal poisoning where the paralysis is so severe that it simulates poliomyelitis.

po″li·o·my″e·lop′a·thy. Disease of the gray matter of the spinal cord and medulla oblongata.

po″li·o′sis. A condition characterized by the absence of pigment in the hair. Syn., *canities.*

po·litz″er·i·za′tion (po·lit″sur·i·zay′shun, po″lit·sur·). The production of sudden increased air pressure in the nasopharynx to inflate the middle ear, by means of compression by a Politzer bag.

pol″la·ki·u′ri·a (pol″uh·kee·yoor′ee·uh, ·kigh·yoor′ee·uh). Abnormally frequent micturition.

pol·lan′tin. A hay-fever antitoxin obtained from the blood of horses inoculated with pollen extract. Also called *Dunbar's serum.*

pol′len. The fecundating element produced in the anthers of flowering plants.

pol′le·no′sis. Hay fever or asthma caused by contact with pollen to which the patient is specifically sensitive.

pol′lex. The thumb. —**pollicar,** *adj.* **p. valgus.** A thumb abnormally bent toward the ulnar side. **p. varus.** A thumb abnormally bent toward the radial side.

pol·lu′tion. 1. The act of defiling or rendering impure, as pollution of drinking water. 2. The discharge of semen without sexual intercourse, as in nocturnal emission.

po·lo′ni·um. Po = 210 *ca.* A radioactive element isolated by Pierre and Marie Curie from pitchblende in 1898.

pol·toph′a·gy. Complete chewing of the food before swallowing it.

pol′y-. 1. A combining form meaning *much* or *many.* 2. *In medicine,* a combining form denoting *excessive, affecting many parts,* or *of diverse origin.*

pol″y·ac′id (pol″ee·ass′id). Applied to a base or basic radical capable of yielding two or more hydroxyl groups, as $Ba(OH)_2$, $Fe(OH)_3$.

pol″y·am′ine (pol″ee·am′in, pol″ee·uh·meen′). Nonspecific term referring to compounds possessing two or more amine groups.

pol′y·an′dry. A social state in which is recognized the marriage of one woman with more than one man at the same time.

pol″y·ar″te·ri′tis. Inflammation of a number of arteries at the same time.

pol″y·ar′thric. Pertaining to many joints.

pol″y·ar·thri′tis. Inflammation of many joints, sometimes used to mean acute rheumatic fever.

pol″y·a·tom′ic. 1. Containing several atoms. 2. Having several hydrogen atoms replaceable by bases.

pol″y·ba′sic. Applied to an acid having several hydrogen atoms replaceable by bases.

pol′y·blast. A free macrophage of inflamed connective tissue.

pol″y·bleph′a·ron. A supernumerary eyelid. Also called *polyblepharia, polyblephary.*

pol″y·chei′ri·a (·kigh′ree·uh). The state of having a supernumerary hand.

pol″y·cho′li·a (·ko′lee·uh). Excessive secretion of bile.

pol″y·chro·mat′ic. Many-colored.

pol″y·chro″ma·to·phil′ (·kro″muh·to·fill″, ·kro·mat′o·fill″). An erythrocyte which has lost its affinity for acid stain and which with mixtures of acid and basic dyes is stained atypically by either or both dyes.

pol″y·chro″ma·to·phil′i·a. The presence in the blood of polychromatophils. Also called *polychromophilia.*

pol″y·chro′mi·a. Increased or abnormal pigmentation.

pol″y·chro′mo·phil. See *polychromatophil.*

pol″y·chy′li·a (·kigh′lee·uh). Excessive formation of —**polychylic,** *adj.*

pol″y·clin′ic. A hospital in which many diseases are treated.

pol″y·clo′ni·a. An affection said to be distinct from tic and chorea but marked by clonic spasms.

pol″y·co′ri·a. The existence of more than one pupil in an iris.

pol″y·cy·e′sis (·sigh·ee′sis). Multiple pregnancy.

pol″y·cys′tic. Containing many cysts.

pol″y·cy·the′mi·a (·sigh·thee′mee·uh). Erythrocytosis.

pol″y·dac′ty·ly. The existence of supernumerary fingers or toes.

pol″y·de·fi′cien·cy. Deficiency of more than one vitamin or other food factor.

pol″y·dip′si·a. Excessive thirst. Syn., *anadipsia.*

pol″y·e′mi·a. An excess of blood over the normal amount in the body.

pol′y·ene. A compound in which three or more double bonds join the carbon atoms.

pol″y·es·the′si·a (pol″ee·ess·thee′zhuh, ·zee·uh). An abnormality of sensation in which a single touch is felt in two or more places at the same time.

pol″y·es′trous. Characterizing mammals that are in estrus more than once annually.

pol″y·eth′y·lene. A long-chain plastic polymer containing 200 to 1000 or more ethylene units per molecule. See *polythene.* **p. glycol.** A condensation polymer of ethylene oxide and water, represented by $H(OCH_2CH_2)_n$-OH, in which n varies from 5 to nearly 200; several are used in formulation of lotions and ointments.

Po·lyg'a·la. A genus of herbaceous or shrubby plants of some 260 species. **P. senega.** A species of North America; therapeutically the most important. See *senega*.

pol″y·ga·lac'ti·a (·ga·lack'tee·uh, ·shee·uh). Excessive secretion of milk.

pol″y·gal'ic ac'id. An active glycosidal principle from senega.

po·lyg'a·lin. A glycosidal saponin derived from senega. Polygalic acid.

po·lyg'a·mous. 1. Pertaining to the social state of having more than one wife or husband at one time, more particularly the former. 2. Having both unisexual and hermaphrodite flowers on one plant.—**polygamy,** *n.*

pol″y·gas'tri·a. Excessive production of gastric juice.

pol'y·graph. An instrument for recording pulsations simultaneously, such as the radial and jugular pulses. There are photographic registration and inkwriting models.

pol″y·gyr'i·a (pol″i·jirr'ee·uh, ·jye'ree·uh). The existence of an excessive number of convolutions in the brain.

pol″y·hy·dram'ni·os (·high·dram'nee·os). An excessive production of amniotic fluid.

pol″y·hy·dru'ri·a (·high·droor'ee·uh). A large increase in fluid content of the urine.

pol″y·in·fec'tion. Infection resulting from the presence of more than one type of organism.

pol″y·lep'tic. Characterized by numerous remissions and exacerbations.

pol″y·mas'ti·a. The presence of more than two breasts.

pol″y·me'li·a. The presence of more than the normal number of limbs.

pol″y·me'lus,   pol″y·me'li·us. Having more than the normal number of limbs.

pol″y·me'ni·a (·mee'nee·uh, ·men'ee·uh). Menorrhagia.

pol″y·men'or·rhe'a. Bleeding between menstrual periods. Syn., *metrorrhagia, intermenstrual flow.* To be distinguished from hypermenorrhea and menorrhea, *q.v.*

pol'y·mer. The product resulting when two or more molecules of the same substance combine.

pol″y·me'ri·a. The presence of extra or supernumerary parts of the body.

pol″y·mer'ic. 1. Exhibiting polymerism. 2. Applied to muscles which are derived from two or more myotomes.

po·lym'er·ide. One of a series of polymeric compounds. Syn., *polymer.*

po·lym'er·ism, pol″ym·er·ism. 1. The existence of more than a normal number of parts. 2. A form of isomerism

in which the molecular weights of certain substances, called polymers, are multiples of the molecular weights of simpler substances from which they are produced.

pol'y·mer·ize,   po·lym'er·ize. Form a compound from several single molecules of the same substance, the molecular weight of the new compound being a multiple of the molecular weight of single molecules which have combined.—**polymeriza'tion,** *n.*

pol″y·mor'phic,   pol″y·mor'phous. Having or occurring in several forms, as of a substance crystallizing in several forms.

pol″y·mor'pho·nu'cle·ar. Having a nucleus which is lobated, the lobes being connected by more or less thin strands of nuclear substance; for example, the nucleus of a neutrophil leukocyte.

pol″y·my″o·si'tis. Simultaneous inflammation of many muscles.

pol″y·myx'in. A mixture of related antibiotic substances, designated polymyxins A, B, C, D, and E, isolated from cultures of *Bacillus polymyxa.* See *aerosporin.*

pol″y·neu·ral'gi·a. Neuralgia in which many nerves are involved.

pol″y·neu·ri'tis. See multiple *neuritis,* Guillain-Barré *syndrome.*—**po.yneurit'ic,** *adj.* **diabetic p.** A slowly progressive polyneuritis occurring in diabetes. It first affects the legs, then the arms, with paresthesias, muscular weakness, and loss of deep reflexes accompanied by dryness and scaling of the skin. It is believed to be due to a metabolic disorder.

pol″y·neu″ro·my″o·si'tis. A disease in which there is concurrent inflammation in several peripheral nerves and muscles.

pol″y·neu·rop'a·thy. An affection of several nerves, as in alcoholism and thiamin deficiency; polyneuritis. See multiple *neuritis.*

pol″y·nu'cle·ot'i·dase. An enzyme which depolymerizes nucleic acid to form mononucleotides.

pol″y·nu'cle·o·tide. A nucleic acid composed of four mononucleotides.

pol″y·o·don'ti·a. The presence of supernumerary teeth.

pol″y·o'pi·a,   pol″y·op'si·a. A condition in which more than one image of an object is formed upon the retina.

pol″y·or'chid·ism (pol″ee·or'kid·iz·um). The presence of more than two testes in one person.

pol″y·o·rex'i·a. Excessive hunger or appetite; bulimia.

pol″y·or'ga·no·sil·ox'ane. An synthetic polymer consisting of a chain of alternate links of silicon atoms and oxygen atoms, the two other bonds the tetravalent silicon atom being attached to an organic group, represented by the general formula:

$$\begin{array}{ccccc} & R & & R & & R \\ & | & & | & & | \\ -Si & -O & -Si & -O & -Si- \\ & | & & | & & | \\ & R & & R & & R \end{array}$$

used especially as a water repellant and in its semisolid state as a putty for therapeutic hand and finger exercises. See *silicone*.

pol″y·o′ti·a. A congenital defect in which there is more than one auricle on one or both sides of the head.

pol′yp. A pedunculated nodule composed of neoplastic tissue or other structure, found especially on mucous membranes, as that of the nose, bladder, stomach, large intestine, or uterus. —**polypous,** *adj.*

pol″y·pa·re′sis (·pa·ree′sis, ·par′i-sis). General progressive paralysis of the insane, or paralytic dementia.

pol″y·path′i·a. The presence of several diseases at one time, or the frequent recurrence of disease.

pol″y·pep′ti·dase. One of the enzymes which hydrolyze proteins and molecular fragments of proteins.

pol″y·pep′tide. A compound containing two or more amino acids united through the peptide linkage. —CO.NH—.

pol″y·pep″ti·de·mi·a. The presence of polypeptides in the blood.

pol″y·pha′gi·a. Excessive eating; increased intake of food; bulimia.

pol″y·pha·lan′gism. An extra phalanx in a finger or toe.

pol″y·phar′ma·cy. The prescription of many drugs at one time; the excessive use of drugs.

pol″y·pho′bi·a. Morbid fear of many things.

pol″y·phy·let′ic (·figh·let′ick). Referring to origin from many lines of descent; opposed to *monophyletic*.

pol″y·phy′le·tism. In *hematology*, the theory that blood cells are derived from more than one type of stem cell.

pol″y·phy′o·dont. Having more than two successive sets of teeth at intervals throughout the life of the individual.

pol″yp·ne′a, pol″yp·noe′a. Very rapid respiration; panting.

pol″y·po′di·a. The condition of having supernumerary feet.

Pol″y·po′di·um. A genus of ferns of several species which are asserted to have medicinal virtues.

po·lyp′o·rous. Having many small openings; cribriform.

pol″y·po′sis. Affected with polyps. **p. coli.** Multiple polyps of the large intestine. **p. ventriculi.** Multiple polyps of gastric mucosa. When associated with chronic atrophic gastritis may be called état mamelonné.

pol″y·sac′cha·ride (·sack′uh·ride, ·rid). A carbohydrate which is formed by the condensation of two or more, usually many, monosaccharides. Examples are cellulose and starch. **bacterial p.** A substance of polysaccharide nature elaborated by bacteria. **capsular p.** A polysaccharide found in the capsule of bacteria, for example, of a pneumococcus, determining its type specificity.

pol″y·sce′li·a (·see′lee·uh). Excess in the number of legs.

pol″y·se″ro·si′tis. Widespread, chronic, fibrosing inflammation of serous membranes, especially in the upper abdomen. This may be associated with persistent ascites of chronic passive hyperemia. Syn., *multiple serositis*.

pol″y·si″nus·i′tis. Simultaneous inflammation of several air sinuses.

pol″y·so′mus. A general term embracing all grades of duplicity, triplicity, etc. It includes monochorionic twins, conjoined twins, equal or unequal, placental parasitic twins, and all grades of double monsters.

pol″y·sor′bate. A complex mixture of polyoxyethylene ethers of mixed partial esters of sorbitol anhydrides, used for emulsifying, dispersing, or solubilizing.

pol″y·sor′bate 80. The U.S.P. name for a complex mixture of polyoxyethylene ethers of mixed partial oleic esters of sorbitol anhydride.

pol″y·sper′mi·a,   pol″y·sper′mism. The secretion and discharge of an excessive quantity of seminal fluid.

pol″y·sper′my, pol″y·sper′my. Impregnation of an ovum by more than one spermatozoon.

pol″y·sphyg′mo·graph. An instrument by means of which tracings can be taken simultaneously of the cardiac movements, the arterial pulse, and the respiration.

pol″y·stich′i·a (·stick′ee·uh). A condition in which the eyelashes are arranged in more than the normal number of rows.

pol″y·stom′a·tous (·stom′uh·tus, ·sto′muh·tus). Having many mouths or apertures.

pol″y·sty′rene. A clear, lightweight plastic prepared by reaction and polymerization of ethylene and benzene. Marketed as *styron*, *lustron*, *laolin*, *bakelite polystyrene*.

pol″y·sus·pen′soid. A colloid system in which there are several phases in different degrees of dispersion.

pol″y·the′li·a,   pol″y·the′lism (pol″i·theel′iz·um,   pol″ith·i·liz·um). The presence of supernumerary nipples.

polythene. A trade-mark for polyethylene.

pol″y·trich′i·a (·trick′ee·uh), **pol″-**

y·tri·cho'sis (·tri·ko'sis). Excessive development of hair. Syn., *hypertrichosis.*

pol''y·tro'phi·a, po·lyt'ro·phy. Abundant or excessive nutrition.

pol''y·u'ri·a. The passage of an excessive quantity of urine. **—polyuric,** *adj., n.*

pol''y·va'lent, po·lyv'a·lent. Multivalent; used especially in polyvalent serum, one obtained either by immunizing animals with different strains of the same bacterium, or by mixing serums derived from different animals immunized with various strains.

pol''y·vi'nyl al'co·hol (·vy'nil, ·vin'il). (CH₂:CHOH)n; a cream-colored powder, soluble in water and insoluble in most organic solvents.

pol''y·vi''nyl·pyr·rol'i·done. A synthetic polymer of high molecular weight, formed by interactions of formaldehyde, ammonia, hydrogen, and acetylene, used as a nonantigenic plasma expander and in preparing repository forms of certain drugs with which it combines loosely. Abbreviated, PVP.

po·made' (po·mayd', po·mahd'). A perfumed ointment for applying to the scalp.

pome'gran''ate (pom'gran''it, pum·gran'it). See *pelletierine tannate.*

pom'pho·lyx. A skin disease characterized by vesicles and bullae on the palms of the hands and soles of the feet. Lesions recur in crops with a tendency to chronicity, and are usually deep-seated. The disease is not rare as formerly was taught; its cause is unknown. Also called *chiropompholyx, dyshidrosis.*

pon·der·a·ble. Having weight.

pon'o·graph, po'no·graph. An apparatus for determining and registering sensitiveness to pain, or to fatigue.

pon''o·pal·mo'sis (pon''o·pal·mo'sis, po''no·). Condition in which slight exertion produces palpitation of the heart.

pons (ponz) (pl. *pontes*). 1. A process or bridge of tissue connecting two parts of an organ. 2. The pons, a convex white eminence situated at the base of the brain. It consists of fibers and nuclei which receive impulses from the cerebral cortex, and send fibers to the contralateral side of the cerebellum by way of the brachium pontis. **—pon'tile, pon'tine** (pon'tyne), *adj.*

pon''to·bul'bar. Pertaining to the pons and to the medulla oblongata.

pontocaine hydrochloride. Trade-mark for a brand of tetracaine hydrochloride.

pop'lar bud (*populi gemma*). The air-dried, closed, winter leaf bud of *Populus candicans,* known in commerce as balm of Gilead buds, or of *Populus tacamahacca* (*Populus balsamifera*), known in commerce as balsam poplar buds.

pop·lit·e'al. Related to the popliteus, 1.

pop·lit·e'us, pop·lit'e·us. 1. The ham or hinder part of the knee joint. 2. A muscle on the back of the knee joint. See Table of Muscles in the Appendix.

pop'py. See *opium.*

pore. 1. A minute opening on a surface. 2. Opening of the duct of a sweat gland. Also see *porus.* **alveolar p.** One of the minute openings in the walls of the pulmonary alveoli, affording communication between neighboring alveoli. **taste p.** The minute opening through which project the gustatory bristles of a taste bud. Also called *gustatory p.*

po·ren''ce·pha'li·a, po''ren·ceph'a·ly. Congenitally deficient development of the cerebral cortex and gray matter so that the lateral ventricles communicate with the brain surface and are lined by a continuation of the piarachnoid. **—porenceph'alous, porencephal'ic,** *adj.*

po''ren·ceph''a·li'tis. Encephalitis with a tendency to form cavities.

po''ri·o·ma'ni·a. Uncontrollable impulse to wander away from home; fugue.

po'ri·on (pl. *poria*). The point on the upper margin of the porus acusticus externus. The two poria and the left orbitale define the Frankfort horizontal plane.

por·nog'ra·phy. 1. A treatise on prostitution. 2. Obscene writing, painting, etc.

por''o·ceph''a·li'a·sis. Infestation of the lungs, liver, trachea, and nasal cavities of man with any of the varieties of *Porocephalus.*

por''o·ker''a·to'sis. A rare skin condition that is inherited, chronic, and progressive. It is characterized by a collar of elevated hyperkeratosis about an irregular patch of depressed atrophic skin. Syn., *hyperkeratosis excentrica.*

po·ro'sis. Rarefaction; increased roentgen translucency; formation of vacuoles or pores; cavity formation.

po·ros'i·ty. The condition or quality of being porous.

po'rous. Having pores.

por'phin ring. A heterocyclic structure consisting of four pyrrole rings united by methylene groups, in the center of which may or may not be a metal (Fe or Mg). It is a structural part of chlorophyll, hemoglobin, the cytochromes, and other substances.

por"pho·bi'lin. A product derived from hemoglobin which may be excreted in urine.

por"pho·bi·lin'o·gen (por"fo-buy-lin'o·jen). One of the derivatives of hemoglobin which makes the urine a Burgundy-red color.

por·phy'ri·a. The presence of porphyrin in the blood resulting from a metabolic defect. The cause is often unknown. Rarely, it is congenital.

por·phy'rin. The iron-free, porphin-ring-containing derivative found in heme, cytochromes, iron-containing protein enzymes, etc.

por"phy·ri·nu'ri·a (por"fi-ri-new'-ree·uh, por"figh-ri··). The excretion of porphyrin in the urine, causing a dark-red discoloration. Also called *porphyruria*.

por"phyr·u'ri·a. The presence of porphyrin in the urine.

por'poise heart. A preponderance of the right ventricle, seen in underwater swimmers, not evidence of disease.

por'ta (pl. *portae*). The hilus of an organ through which the vessels enter. **p. hepatis.** The transverse fissure of the liver through which the portal vein enters the organ.

por'tal. 1. Pertaining to the porta or hilus of an organ. 2. The porta or hilus of an organ. **intestinal p.** The opening of the fore-gut or of the hind-gut into the midgut or yolk sac.

por'ti·o (por'shee·o, por'tee·o) (pl. *portiones*). 1. Portion. 2. Portio vaginalis uteri, the vaginal portion of the uterus.

por"to·ca'val. Pertaining to the portal vein and the inferior vena cava.

port'-wine' mark. A type of vascular nevus that is purple-red or violet in color. Usually seen on the face and only slightly elevated. Also called *birthmark, nevus flammeus, tache de feu, port-wine stain*.

po'rus (pl. *pori*). A pore, foramen. **p. acusticus externus.** The opening of the external auditory canal. **p. acusticus internus.** The opening of the internal auditory canal into the cranial cavity. **p. opticus.** The opening in the center of the lamina cribrosa transmitting the central artery of the retina. **p. sudoriferus.** A sweat pore.

po"si·o·ma'ni·a (po"see·o·may'nee-uh, pos"ee·o·). Dipsomania.

po·si'tion. Place; location; attitude; posture. Abbreviated, P. **anatomic p.** Attitude of a person standing erect with arms at the sides and palms forward. **apparent p.** *In ophthalmology*, the position in space to which the mind projects a visual image. **bronchoscopic p.** Posture of the patient in which he lies supine with head hyperextended to bring larynx and trachea in a straight line so as to permit introduction of the bronchoscope. **dorsal p.** Attitude of a person lying on his back. **dorsosacral p.** The posture of a patient lying on the back with the legs flexed on the thighs and the thighs flexed on the abdomen and abducted. **Fowler's p.** The posture which the recumbent patient assumes when the head of the bed is raised 18 to 20 inches, or a similar position achieved by the use of a back rest. **knee-chest p.** A position assumed by a patient resting on knees and chest as an exercise after childbirth, or for the purposes of examination and treatment. **knee-elbow p.** Posture in which the patient lies upon the knees and elbows, the head resting upon the hands. **lithotomy p.** Dorsosacral position. **mentoanterior p.** A presentation of the fetus *in utero* in which the head is sharply extended so that the occiput of the fetus is in contact with its back, and the face looks downward and anteriorly. **mentoposterior p.** A face presentation of the fetus in which the head is sharply extended so that the occiput is in contact with the back, and the face looks downward and posteriorly. **p. of the fetus.** The relation of the presenting part of the fetus to the cardinal points. For the vertex, the face, and the breech there are four positions each: a right anterior, a right posterior, a left anterior, and a left posterior. For each of the shoulders there is an anterior and a posterior position. In order to shorten and memorize these positions, the initials of the chief words are made use of, as follows: for vertex presentations the word occiput is abbreviated O., and preceded by the letter R. or L. for right or left, and followed by A. or P. according to whether the presenting part is anterior or posterior. We thus have the initials L.O.A., left occipito-anterior, to indicate that the presenting occiput is upon the anterior left side. In the same way are derived the terms L.O.P., R.O.A., R.O.P. For facial presentations we have in the same way L.F.A., left frontoanterior, L.F.P., R.F.A., R.F.P. For breech or sacral presentations, L.S.A., L.S.P., R.S.A., R.S.P., and for shoulder or dorsal presentations, L.D.A., L.D.P., R.D.A., R.D.P. **Simon's p.** The dorsal posture with the legs and thighs flexed, the hips elevated, and the thighs abducted. **Sims's p.** Posture of a patient lying on the left side with the right knee and thigh drawn up, the left arm placed along the back, and the chest inclined forward. Also called *semi-prone p*. **Trendelenburg's p.** The posture of a patient lying on a table which is tilted upward 45 degrees, with the legs and feet hanging over the upper end of it. **Walcher's p.** Posture of a patient lying on the back with the thighs and legs hanging over the edge of the table. Used during a difficult delivery to lengthen the true conjugate.

pos'i·tron (poz'i·tron). A positively charged particle having the same mass and the same charge as the electron but opposite in sign.

po·sol'o·gy. That branch of medical science dealing with the dosage of medicines.

post-. A prefix denoting *after, behind,* or *subsequent.*

post·a'nal. Situated behind the anus.

post"ap·o·plec'tic. Coming on, or occurring, after a stroke of apoplexy, as postapoplectic coma, the coma that often succeeds an apoplectic stroke.

post·ax'i·al. Situated behind the axis: in the arm, behind the ulnar aspect; in the leg, behind the fibular aspect.

post·bra'chi·al (pohst·bray'kee·ul, ·brack'ee·ul). Situated posterior to the arm.

post·ca'va. The inferior or ascending vena cava. —**postcaval,** *adj.*

post·cen'tral. 1. Situated behind a center. 2. Situated behind the central sulcus of the brain, as the postcentral gyrus.

post·co'i·tal. After sexual intercourse.

post"con·nu'bi·al. Coming on, or occurring, after marriage.

post"con·vul'sive. Coming on after a convulsion.

pos·te'ri·or. Situated behind or to the back; designating the hinder part, as of an organ. —**posteriorly, posteriad,** *adv.*
In human adult anatomy, *posterior* is usually used instead of *dorsal.*

pos'ter·o-. A combining form signifying *posterior.*

pos"ter·o·an·te'ri·or. From the back to the front of the body, as in describing the direction of x-rays traversing the patient. Also see *dorsoventral.*

pos"ter·o·ex·ter'nal. Occupying the outer side of a back part, as the posteroexternal column of the spinal cord. —**posteroexternad,** *adv.*

pos"ter·o·in·ter'nal. Occupying the inner side of a back part, as the posterointernal column of the spinal cord. —**posterointernad,** *adv.*

pos"ter·o·lat'er·al. Situated behind and at the side of a part. —**posterolaterad,** *adv.*

post·feb'rile (·feb'ril, ·fee'bril). Occurring after a fever.

post"gan·gli·on'ic (·gang·glee·on'-

ick, ·gang·lee·). Situated behind, or after, a ganglion.

pos·thet'o·my. Circumcision.

pos·thi'tis. Inflammation of the pre puce.

post'hu·mous (pos'chew·mus). 1. Occurring after death. 2. Born afte the death of the father, or by Cesarean section after the death of the mother 3. Published after the writer's death

post"hyp·not'ic. Succeeding the hypnotic state; acting after the hyp notic state has passed off, as posthyp notic suggestion.

post·ic'tal. Following an epileptic attack.

post·ic·ter'ic. Of, relating to, or designating the period or condition following jaundice.

post"-mor'tem. 1. Occurring after death. 2. An examination of the body after death; an autopsy. —**postmor tal,** *adj.*

post·na'sal. Situated behind the nose, or in the nasopharynx.

post·na'tal. Subsequent to birth, a a postnatal disease.

post"ne·crot'ic. 1. Occurring after death. 2. Occurring after the death o a tissue or a part.

post·op'er·a"tive. Occurring after an operation, as insanity, hernia; following closely upon an operation.

post·pal'a·tine (·pal'uh·tyne, ·tin) Behind the uvula.

post·par'tum. Following childbirth as post-partum hemorrhage.

post·pran'di·al. After a meal.

post"pu·bes'cent. Occurring subsequent to puberty.

post"trau·mat'ic. Pertaining to any process, such as inflammation, following traumatic injury to a part.

post"trau·mat'ic per"son·al'i ty dis·or'der. A psychosis resulting from direct injury to the head or brain Symptoms include headache, emotiona instability, fatigability, and sometime convulsions.

pos'tu·late. 1. A proposition assumed without proof. 2. A condition which must be fulfilled, as **Koch's postu late,** a law stating that the specificity of a microörganism is not demonstrated unless the following conditions obtain the microörganism must be present in all cases of the disease, it must be cul tivated in pure culture, its inoculation must produce the disease in susceptible animals, and from such animals it mus be obtained and cultivated again in pure culture.

pos'tur·al. Pertaining to posture or position; performed by means of a spe cial posture, as postural treatment.

pos'ture. Position or bearing, espe cially of the body. **jackknife p.** One in which the patient reclines on hi back with shoulders elevated, leg flexed on thighs, and thighs at right angles to abdomen; the posture assumed when the upper and lower planes of a surgical bed are elevated.

post·vac′ci·nal (pohst-vack′si-nul). Following vaccination.

po′ta·ble. Drinkable; fit to drink.

pot″a·mo·pho′bi·a. Morbid fear of sheets of water.

pot′ash″. Potassium carbonate, q.v. **caustic p.** See *potassium hydroxide*. **p. lye.** See *potassium hydroxide*. **sulfurated p.** A solid mixture composed chiefly of potassium polysulfides and potassium thiosulfate. Also called *liver of sulfur*.

po·tas′sa. Potassium carbonate, q.v.

pot″as·se′mi·a. 1. Potassium in the blood. 2. Abnormally high blood potassium level; hyperpotassemia.

po·tas′si·um. K = 39.096. Light, malleable, ductile lumps, rods, or spheres. Reacts violently with water. A small amount of potassium in the blood is essential for proper function of the various organs of the body. See Table of Normal Values of Blood Constituents in the Appendix. **dibasic p. phosphate.** K₂HPO₄. Occurs as white granules; very soluble in water. Also called *dipotassium phosphate, dipotassium hydrogen phosphate.* **monobasic p. phosphate.** KH₂PO₄. Occurs as colorless crystals or powder; soluble in water. Also called *p. biphosphate, p. acid phosphate, p. dihydrogen phosphate, monopotassium phosphate.* **p. acetate.** CH₃COOK. Occurs as colorless crystals or powder; soluble in water. **p. arsenite solution.** Represents 1% of arsenic trioxide. Also called *Fowler's solution*. **p. bicarbonate.** KHCO₃. Colorless crystals or powder; soluble in water. **p. bismuth tartrate.** See *bismuth and potassium tartrate*. **p. bitartrate.** KHC₄H₄O₆. Occurs as slightly opaque crystals or powder; soluble in water. Also called *cream of tartar, acid p. tartrate.* **p. bromide.** KBr. White cubical crystals or granular powder; soluble in water. **p. carbonate.** K₂CO₃·1½H₂O. White granular powder; soluble in water. **p. chlorate.** KClO₃. Colorless, odorless, lustrous crystals or powder; soluble in water. **p. chloride.** KCl. Colorless crystals or a white, granular powder; soluble in water. **p. citrate.** K₃C₆H₅O₇·H₂O. Transparent crystals or a white, granular powder; soluble in water. **p. cyanide.** KCN. White amorphous pieces or white, granular powder; soluble in water. **p. dichromate.** K₂Cr₂O₇. Orange-red crystals, granules or powder; soluble in water. **p. guaiacolsulfonate.** C₆H₃.OH.OCH₃.SO₃K. White crystals or a crystalline powder; soluble in water. **p. hydroxide.**

KOH; occurs as white or nearly white lumps, small pellets or rods; soluble in water; very caustic to tissue. Syn., *caustic potash.* **p. iodide.** KI; transparent crystals or a white, granular powder; soluble in water. **p. mercuric iodide.** K₂HgI₄; occurs as yellow crystals, deliquescent in air; soluble in water. **p. nitrate.** KNO₃; occurs as colorless prisms or a white, crystalline powder; soluble in water. Syn., *saltpeter.* **p. permanganate.** KMnO₄; occurs as dark purple crystals; soluble in water. **p. sodium tartrate.** Occurs as colorless crystals or white crystalline powder; soluble in water. Syn., *Rochelle salt.* **p. sulfate.** K₂SO₄. Occurs as white granules or powder; soluble in water. **p. tartrate.** (K₂C₄H₄O₆)₂H₂O. White crystals, very soluble in water. Syn., *sal vegetabile.* **p. thiocyanate.** KSCN. Occurs as colorless, transparent crystals; soluble in water. Also called *potassium sulfocyanate, potassium rhodanate.* **tribasic p. phosphate.** K₃PO₄. Occurs as white granular powder; very soluble in water. Also called *tripotassium phosphate.*

po′ten·cy. 1. Power of the male to perform the sexual act. 2. *In homeopathy,* the degree of dilution of a drug.

po·ten′tial. 1. Capable of acting or doing work, as potential energy. 2. *In electricity,* a state of tension or of difference in energy capable of doing work. **bio-electric p.** The difference of electric potential between the inside and the outside of a cell. **critical p.** The point at which the electrokinetic or zeta potential between the immobile and mobile ionic layers is lowered by addition of electrolytes so that the double layers of colloidal particles collapse, and the particles aggregate and precipitate. **disease p.** The sum of adverse health factors present in a community, which has a bearing upon the probable incidence of disease to be anticipated. **electrochemical p.** The potential drop across all of the ionic layers from the surface of the particle to the solution. Also called *epsilon p.* **electrokinetic p.** A potential at the interface between the semipermeable membrane and a solution on either side. See bio-electric *p.* Also called *zeta p.* **ground p.** Electric potential of the earth, arbitrarily used as a standard reference point for all electric measurements. **ionization p.** The lowest potential that removes an electron from an atom. **Nernst p.** The total drop of potential (at a standard state) across the interface, dependent solely on the activity of the ions in the external medium. **Stern p.** The potential between the immobile ion layer and the particle sur-

po'tion. A drink or draught.

Pott, Percival [*English surgeon*, 1714–88]. Best known for his description of the spinal curvature or kyphosis of the spine resulting from tuberculosis (1779); called *Pott's disease*. The eponym has persisted to this day, although Pott did not recognize the tuberculous nature of the disease. Described fracture of the fibula occurring three inches above the ankle, sometimes accompanied by a splitting of the medial malleolus (1765); called *Pott's fracture.*

pouch. A sac or pocket. **abdominovesical p.** One formed by the reflection of the peritoneum from the anterior abdominal wall onto the distended bladder; it contains the lateral and medial inguinal fossae. **laryngeal p.** A blind pouch of mucosa opening into the lateral part of the ventricle of the larynx. **rectouterine p.** That part of the peritoneal cavity between the rectum and the posterior surface of the uterus. Also called *p. of Douglas.* **rectovesical p.** That part of the peritoneal cavity between the bladder and the rectum in the male. Also called *rectovesical excavation.*

poul'tice (pole'tiss). A soft, semiliquid mass made of some cohesive substance mixed with water, and used for application to the skin for the purpose of supplying heat and moisture or acting as a local stimulant.

pound. A unit of measure of weight. The **troy pound** contains 12 ounces, or 5760 grains, or 372.96 grams. Symbol, ℔. The **avoirdupois pound** contains 16 ounces, or 7000 grains, or 453.6 grams. Abbreviated, ℔. For a tabulation of weights and measures, see Tables in the Appendix. **foot-pound.** The force necessary to raise one pound through the height of one foot.

pow'der. 1. A group of pharmaceutical preparations of definite formula, official in the United States Pharmacopeia or National Formulary, and consisting of intimate mixtures of finely divided medicinal substances. 2. *In pharmacy,* a single dose of medicine placed in powder paper; or may mean a dusting powder, douche powder, or other bulk powder to be administered by the teaspoonful or used externally, all being prepared extemporaneously.

pow'er. 1. Ability to produce an effect. 2. *In optics,* the magnification given by a lens or prism.

pox. 1. Any vesicular or pustular disease. 2. Common term for syphilis.

P.p. *Punctum proximum,* near point.

P.P.D. Purified protein derivative; form of tuberculin which is a dr[y] powder, dry diluted with lactose, an[d] is relatively constant in its activity.

P.P. factor. Goldberger's term fo[r] the pellagra preventive factor prese[nt] in vitamin-B complex; identical wit[h] niacin (nicotinic acid).

ppt. Precipitate.

Pr. 1. Abbreviation for presbyopia. Chemical symbol for praseodymium.

P.r. *Punctum remotum,* far point.

prac'tice. 1. The routine applicatio[n] of the principles of medicine to th[e] diagnosis and treatment of disease. [2.] Perform the duties of a physician.

prae-. See *pre-.*

prag"mat·ag·no'si·a (prag"ma[t] ag·no'see·uh, ·zee·uh). Inability t[o] recognize an object. **visual p.** Ob[-] ject blindness.

prag"mat·am·ne'si·a (·am·nee[-] zhuh, ·zee·uh). Loss of the ability to re[-] member the appearance of an objec[t.] **visual p.** A mental condition marke[d] by a loss of ability to call up the visu[al] image of an object.

pranone. Trade-mark for anhydr[o] hydroxyprogesterone.

prantal methylsulfate. Trad[e] mark for diphemanil methylsulfate.

pra"se·o·dym'i·um (pray"zee·[o·] dim'ee·um, pray"see·o·, prass"ee·o·[)] Pr = 140.92. A rare earth metal. Th[e] principal valency is three, and its sal[ts] are generally green in color.

pra·tique' (prah·teek', prat'ick). Th[e] bill of health given to vessels by [a] health officer.

-prax'i·a. A combining form mea[n-] ing *action, doing.*

prax"i·ol'o·gy. The science of co[n-] duct.

pre-. A prefix signifying *before.*

pre·ag'o·nal. Immediately precedi[ng] the death agony.

pre·ax'i·al. Situated in front of th[e] axis of the body or of a limb.

pre·can'cer·ous. Pertaining to a[ny] pathologic condition of a tissue th[at] may develop into cancer.

pre·cap'il·lar'y (pre·cap'i·lerr[·] ee). An arteriole with weakly develope[d] media preceding capillaries.

pre·car'di·ac (pree·kahr'dee·ack[).] Anterior to the heart.

pre·ca'va (pree·kay'vuh). The sup[e]rior, or descending, vena cava.

pre·cen'tral (pree·sen'trul). Sit[u]ated in front of the central fissure [of] the brain.

pre·cip'i·tant. Any reagent causi[ng] precipitation.

pre·cip'i·tate. 1. An insoluble co[m]pound deposited in a solution of a su[b]stance on the addition of a reage[nt] which produces a chemical reaction [or] otherwise decreases solubility. Abbrev[-] ated, ppt. 2. The product of the reaction between precipitinogen and precipitin. 3. Throw down in an insoluble form. 4. Headlong; hasty, as precipitate labor. **red p.** Red mercuric oxide. **white p.** Ammoniated mercury. **yellow p.** Yellow mercuric oxide.

pre·cip'i·ta'ted chalk. See precipitated *calcium* carbonate.

pre·cip'i·ta'tion. The process of making substances insoluble by the addition of a reagent, evaporation, freezing, or electrolysis. **co-precipitation.** The simultaneous precipitation of more than one compound. **fractional p.** The separation of substances by precipitating them in increasing order of solubility.

pre·cip'i·ta'tor. A type of instrument used for determining the number of dust particles in the air. In the **electric precipitator,** a high electric potential is created between two surfaces. When a measured sample of air is passed through this field, the dust particles adhere to one of the surfaces. In the **thermal precipitator,** a heated wire is suspended in a narrow slot between two cooled glass cover slips, and the dust particles from an air sample passed through the slot adhere to the cover slips. The collected particles are counted under a microscope. Other instruments used for the same purpose are the konimeter, impinger, and jet dust counter. Also see *dust count.*

pre·cip'i·tin. An antibody to a soluble antigen. A precipitate is formed when the soluble antigen is layered over the antibody or mixed with it.

pre·clin'i·cal (pre-klin'i-kul). 1. Occurring prior to the period in which recognized symptoms or signs make diagnosis possible. 2. Referring to medical studies undertaken before the study of patients.

pre·co'cious. Developing at an age earlier than usual.

pre·coc'i·ty (pri-kos'i-tee). Early development or maturity; applied especially to great development of the mental faculties at an early age.

pre''col·lag'e·nous (pree''ko-ladj'i-nus). Characterizing an incomplete stage in the formation of collagen.

pre''con·vul'sant. Relating to the stage of a disease preceding convulsions.

pre''con·vul'sive. Referring to the period just prior to the occurrence of a convulsion, as an epileptic seizure.

pre·cor'di·a. The area of the chest overlying the heart. Syn., *precordium.* —**precordial,** *adj.*

pre·cor'di·um. See *precordia.*

pre·cos'tal (pree-kos'tul). Situated in front of the ribs.

pre''di·gest'ed (pree''di-jest'id, -dye-

jest'id). Partly digested by artificial means before being taken into the stomach.

pre''di·ges'tion (pree''di-jes'chun, -dye-jes'chun). The partial digestion of food before it is eaten.

pre''dis·po'sing (pree''dis-po'zing). Rendering the body susceptible to a disease, as predisposing cause.

pre''dis·po·si·tion (pree''dis-po-zish'un). The state of having special susceptibility to a disease or condition.

pred·nis'e·lone. $\Delta^{1,4}$-Pregnene-3,20-dione-11β, 17a, 21-triol, a dehydrogenated analogue of hydrocortisone about as potent as prednisone. See *deltacortef, hydeltra, meticortelone.*

pred'ni·sone. $\Delta^{1,4}$-Pregnadiene-17a 21-diol-3, 11, 20-trione, a dehydrogenated analogue of cortisone having qualitatively similar actions, but quantitatively more potent. See *deltasone, deltra, meticorten.*

pre''dor·mi'tion (pree''dor-mish'un). Applied to the stage of unconsciousness immediately preceding actual sleep.

pre''e·clamp'si·a. A state of toxemia in the pregnant woman, associated with edema, headache, albuminuria, and increased blood pressure, but not accompanied by convulsions. Also see *eclampsia.*

pre·fron'tal lo·bot'o·my. A method of treating mental disorders, particularly melancholia and psychasthenia, by severing the white fibers connecting the prefrontal and frontal lobes with the thalamus.

pre''gan·gli·on'ic (pree''gang-glee-on'ick, -gang-lee-on'ick). Situated in front of, or preceding, a ganglion.

preg'nan·cy. Being with child; the state of the woman from conception to childbirth. The duration of pregnancy in woman is approximately 280 days. To estimate the date of confinement, take the first day of the last menstrual period, count back three months, and add one year and seven days. See Ely's Table of the Duration of Pregnancy in the Appendix. **abdominal p.** Gestation with the fetus lying within the peritoneal cavity. **ampullar p.** Gestation in the outer portion of the uterine tube. **bigeminal p.** Twin pregnancy. **cervical p.** A rare condition in which, from atrophy of the decidual membranes, the impregnated ovum is implanted in the cervical canal, where it develops until the uterus expels it. **cornual p.** Gestation occurring in one horn of a two-horned uterus. **ectopic p.** Extrauterine gestation. **extrauterine p.** Gestation outside of the cavity of the uterus. **heterotopic p.** Double gestation, with one fetus inside and the other outside the uterine cavity. **hydatid p.**

Gestation in which the chorionic sac degenerates into a hydatidiform mole. **interstitial p.** Gestation in the uterine part of a uterine tube. Also called *intramural p.* **intraligamentary p.** Gestation within the broad ligament. **membranous p.** Gestation in which there has been a rupture of the amniotic sac and the fetus is in direct contact with the wall of the uterus. **molar p.** Gestation in which the ovum has been converted into a fleshy tumor mass. **multiple p.** Gestation with two or more fetuses present within the uterus. **ovarian p.** Gestation within the ovary. **parietal p.** Interstitial gestation. **phantom p.** Enlargement of the abdomen and often other symptoms simulating gestation, usually due to hysteria. Syn., *pseudocyesis.* **sarcofetal p.** Gestation with the presence of both a fetus and a mole. **sarcohysteric p.** False pregnancy due to a mole. **signs of p.** The three so-called absolute signs are ballottement, fetal movements, and fetal heart sounds. **tubal p.** Gestation within an oviduct. **tubo-abdominal p.** Gestation which develops in the ampulla and extends into the peritoneal cavity. **tuboligamentary p.** Gestation arising in an oviduct with extension into the broad ligament. **tuboovarian p.** Gestation arising in an oviduct and extending into the ovary. **twin p.** Gestation with two fetuses. **utero-abdominal p.** Gestation with one fetus in the uterus and another within the peritoneal cavity. **utero-ovarian p.** Gestation with one fetus in the uterus and another in the ovary. **utero-tubal p.** Gestation with one fetus in the uterus and another in an oviduct.

preg′nan·cy rate. The number of pregnancies actually experienced in relation to the number of ova that theoretically might have been fertilized.

preg·nane′di·ol (preg-nan′dee-ole, ·dye-ole, ·ol, ·awl). $C_{21}H_{36}O_2$. A metabolite of progesterone, found in the urine during the progestational phase of the menstrual cycle and in pregnancy urine.

preg′nant. With child; gravid.

preg″nen·in′o·lone (preg″nen-in′o-loan, preg″neen·). Anhydrohydroxyprogesterone, *q.v.*

preg·nen′o·lone. 5-Pregnen-3-beta-ol-20-one, a steroid oxidation product of cholesterol and stigmasterol, effective in reducing fatigue and formerly believed of some value as an antiarthritic substance.

pre·hal′lux (pree-hal′ucks). A supernumerary digit attached to the great toe on its medial aspect.

pre″hem·i·pleg′ic (pree″hem-i-

pledj′ick, ·plee′jick). Occurring before an attack of hemiplegia, as prehemiplegic chorea.

pre·hen′sion. The act of grasping or seizing.

pre″lo·co·mo′tion. The movements of a child who has not yet learned to walk, which indicate the intention of moving from one place to another.

preludin. Trade-mark for phenmetrazine hydrochloride.

pre′lum. A press. **p. abdominale.** The squeezing of the abdominal viscera between the diaphragm and the rigid abdominal wall, as in the processes of defecation, micturition, and parturition.

pre″ma·lig′nant. Precancerous.

pre″ma·ni′a·cal. Previous to, or preceding, an attack of insanity.

premarin. Trade-mark for a preparation of conjugated estrogens, chiefly in the form of sodium estrone sulfate.

pre″ma·ture′. Occurring before the proper time, as premature labor.

pre″ma·ture′ beat. *In cardiology,* a beat occurring before the next expected impulse and followed usually by a pause which may or may not be compensatory.

pre″med·i·ca′tion. The administration of drugs before an operation, primarily to quiet the patient and to facilitate the administration of the anesthetic.

pre·men′stru·al (pree-men′strooul). Preceding menstruation.

pre·mo′lar (pree-mo′lur). In each quadrant of the human dentition, one of the two teeth between the canine and the first molar; a bicuspid. The term is often used incorrectly to signify a deciduous molar. The premolars replace the deciduous molars.

pre″mo·ni′tion. A warning of some future experience or event, usually tragic; a foreboding.

pre·mon′i·to·ry. Giving previous warning or notice, as in premonitory symptoms, the nonspecific signs of impending illness before specific indications begin. Also called *prodromal.*

pre″mu·ni′tion (pree″mew-nish′un). An immunity which depends upon a persistent latent infection, such as an immunity in malaria due to long-continued quiescent infection.

pre″nar·co′sis. Preliminary, light narcosis produced prior to general anesthesia.

pre·na′tal (pree-nay′tul). Existing or occurring before birth.

pre″ne·o·plas′tic. Before the development of a definite tumor.

prep″a·ra′tion. 1. The act of making ready. 2. Anything made ready, especially, in anatomy, any part of the body prepared or preserved for illustrative or other uses. 3. *In pharmacy,* any compound or mixture made after a formula. **cover glass p.** One used in examining cells of blood or of any other fluid. A small drop of blood or other fluid is placed on a thin, square cover glass. A second cover glass is dropped on the first. As soon as the fluid has stopped spreading, the two cover glasses are pulled apart horizontally; after air drying, the material is stained with an appropriate stain and studied under the microscope. **hanging-drop p.** A preparation using a special slide containing a circular concavity, or a regular slide with a petroleum jelly ring, in which a drop of solution to be examined microscopically can be suspended without spreading over the slide.

pre·pa·tel'lar. Situated in front of the patella, as prepatellar bursa.

pre·pol'lex. A supernumerary digit attached to the thumb on its radial aspect.

pre·pon'der·ance. 1. The state of being greater in weight or force. 2. A term used in electrocardiography as either (a) **left preponderance,** designating the effect of left ventricular hypertrophy due to a variation in the normal $\frac{Right}{Left}$ ventricular weight ratio (normal 1.4–2.0): abnormal left axis deviation, increased duration of QRS, and sometimes inversion of T_1 and T_3; or (b) **right preponderance,** designating the effect of right ventricular hypertrophy: abnormal right axis deviation, deep S_1, tall R_3, and $R_3 > R_2$, and sometimes increased duration of QRS.

pre·pu'ber·al (pree-pew'bur-ul). Prior to puberty.

pre'puce. The foreskin of the penis, a fold of skin covering the glans penis; also, the similar fold over the glans clitoridis. **—prepu'tial,** adj.

pre''pu·cot'o·my. An incision into the prepuce; an incomplete circumcision.

pre''ra·chit'ic (pree''ra·kit'ick). Pertaining to the interval previous to the time when rickets becomes obvious.

pre''re·pro·duc'tive. Relating to the period of life preceding puberty.

pres''by·at'rics (prez''bee-at'ricks, press''bee-). That branch of medicine which deals with the diseases of old age. Syn., geriatrics.

pres''by·cu'sis (prez''bi-cue'sis, -kōō'sis), **pres''by·cou'sis** (prez''bi-kōō'sis, press''bi-). The lessening of the acuteness of hearing that occurs with advancing age.

pres''by·o·phre'ni·a (prez''bee-o-free'nee-uh, ·fren'ee-uh). Failure of the sense of location and memory in the aged, frequently the normal condition

of old age; the general concomitant of senility. **—presbyophren'ic,** adj.

pres''by·o'pi·a (prez''bee·o'pee-uh, press''bee-). The condition of vision in the aged, due to diminished power of accommodation from impaired elasticity of the crystalline lens, whereby the near point of distinct vision is removed farther from the eye. Abbreviated, Pr. **—presbyop'ic,** adj.; **pres'byope,** n.

pres·byt'ic. Suffering from presbyopia, q.v.

pre''schiz·o·phren'ic (pree''skiz-o-fren'ick). Pertaining to symptoms and personality characteristics which usually precede a schizophrenic psychosis. See schizoid personality.

pre''scle·ro'sis. The vascular condition which precedes arteriosclerosis. **—presclerot'ic,** adj.

pre·scribe'. Give instructions concerning the use of a remedy.

pre·scrip'tion. Written instructions designating the preparation and use of substances to be administered. See Table of the More Common Latin or Greek Terms and Abbreviations Used in Prescription Writing in the Appendix.

pre''se·nil'i·ty. Premature old age. **—presen'ile,** adj.

pres''en·ta'tion (prez''un·tay'shun, pree''zen-). That part of the fetus which is palpated through the cervix uteri at the beginning of labor. The relation of the part of the fetus to the birth canal determines the type of presentation. **breech p.** The presentation of the buttocks and/or the feet first at the cervix; called double breech or complete breech if both buttocks and feet appear first; frank breech if the buttocks alone are the presenting part, the legs being bent so that the feet lie against the face. **brow p.** That in which the brow of the child presents at the cervix. **cephalic p.** That in which any part of the head is the presenting part. **compound p.** Prolapse of an extremity of the fetus alongside the presenting part. **face p.** The presentation of the face with the chin leading at the cervix during labor. **footling p.** Presentation with the feet foremost. **p. of cord.** Descent of the umbilical cord between the presenting part and the membranes at the beginning of labor. **transverse p.** That in which the child is turned with its long axis across that of the birth canal; the presenting part may be the shoulder, back, or abdomen. **vertex p.** The most usual type of presentation with the occiput the presenting part.

press·om'e·ter. A manometer for measuring pressure in the uterus and kidneys after injection of radiopaque media in doing pyelography and uterosalpingography (hysterosalpingography).

pres′sor. Producing a rise in blood pressure.

pres″so·re·cep′tor. A nerve ending, as in the carotid sinus, which is stimulated by changes in the blood pressure.

pres″so·sen′si·tive. Stimulated by changes in blood pressure, as nerve endings in the carotid sinus.

pres′sure. Force, weight, or tension. **abdominal p.** Pressure upon the viscera, as when the diaphragm is contracted while the belly wall muscles are contracted, as in urination and defecation. Also called *strain, squeeze, bearing down, prelum abdominale.* **arterial p.** The tension of the arterial wall due to the pressure of the blood within the arteries. **atmospheric p.** The pressure of the atmosphere; it equals about fifteen pounds to the square inch at sea level. **bipolar p.** Pressure on the two ends of a bone. It is used in differentiating fractures from contusions, producing pain in the case of the former. **blood p.** The pressure of the blood against the walls of the vessels or of the heart. It is measured by means of the manometer. Also see *blood pressure.* **hydrostatic p.** A pressure created in a fluid system by the energy of muscular contraction not utilized in motion, as blood pressure created by the heart beat. A fluid system may also exert such pressure as a result of the effect of gravity. **imbibition p.** Pressure due to the increase in volume of a gel as a result of the imbibition of liquid. **intracranial p.** The pressure of the contents of the cranium upon its walls. **osmotic p.** The pressure developed when a solution and its solvent component are separated by a membrane permeable to the solvent only, or when two solutions of different concentration of the same solute are similarly separated. **venous p.** The tension of the blood within the veins.

pre·sup′pu·ra′tive. Pertaining to an early stage of inflammation, prior to suppuration.

pre″sys·tol′ic. Preceding the systole of the heart, as the presystolic murmur, presystolic thrill; usually refers to the time immediately preceding the first heart sound.

pre·u″re·thri′tis. Inflammation of the vestibule of the vagina, around the urethral orifice.

prev′a·lence. The number of cases of a disease existing in a population at any given time.

pre″ven·to′ri·um. A sanatorium devoted to the care of children who

are thought to be predisposed to tuberculosis because of positive tuberculin tests and poor home environment.

pre″ver·tig′i·nous (pree″vur·tidj′i·nus). Dizzy, with a tendency to fall prone.

pre·ves′i·cal (pree·vess′i·kul). Situated in front of the bladder.

pre′vi·a. Coming before, or in front of, as placenta previa.

pri′a·pism. Persistent erection of the penis, usually unaccompanied by sexual desire.

prick′ly heat. See *miliaria.*

pri′ma·ry. First, immediate, as primary union, healing by first intention.

Pri′mates (pry′mates). The highest order of the vertebrate class Mammalia; includes man, apes, monkeys, and lemurs.

pri′mi·done. 5-Phenyl-5-ethylhexahydropyrimidine-4,6-dione, an anticonvulsant. See *mysoline.*

pri″mi·grav′i·da. A woman who is pregnant for the first time.

pri·mip′a·ra (pry·mip′uh·ruh). A woman bearing, or giving birth to, her first child. **—primiparous,** *adj.*

pri·mi′ti·ae (pry·mish′ee·ee). The part of the amniotic fluid discharged before the extrusion of the fetus at birth.

prim′i·tive. First-formed; original, as primitive groove.

pri·mor′di·al (pry·mor′dee·ul). Existing in the beginning; first-formed; primitive; original; of the simplest character.

pri·mor′di·um (pry·mor′dee·um). The earliest discernible indication of an organ or part, as **acoustico-facial primordium,** the mass of neural crest tissue that differentiates into the ganglions of the seventh and eighth cranial nerves. Syn., *anlage.*

prin′ceps. First, original, or main.

prin′ci·ple. 1. A constituent of a compound representing its essential or characteristic properties. 2. A rule or basis of action.

priodax. Trade-mark for iodoalphionic acid.

priscoline hydrochloride. Trademark for tolazoline hydrochloride.

pri·sil′i·dene hy″dro·chlo′ride. dl-Alpha-1,3-dimethyl-4-phenyl-4-propionoxypiperidine hydrochloride, a synthetic analgesic. Also called *alphaprodine hydrochloride.* See *nisentil hydrochloride.*

prism. 1. A solid whose bases or ends are similar plane figures and whose sides are parallelograms. 2. *In optics,* a transparent solid with triangular ends and plane converging sides. It breaks up white light into its component colors, and bends the rays of light toward the side opposite the angle (the base of the prism), and is used to measure or correct imbalance of the ocular muscles. **Nicol p.** One prepared from two obliquely bisected parts of a rhombohedron of calcite; used for production and analysis of polarized light.

pris·mat'ic (priz·mat'ick). Prism-shaped; produced by the action of a prism, as prismatic colors.

privine hydrochloride. Trademark for naphazoline hydrochloride.

p. r. n. Pro re nata; according as circumstances may require.

pro-. A prefix signifying for, before, in front of.

pro·ac"ti·no·my'cin. An antibiotic from Nocardia gardneri.

pro'bang. A rod of whalebone or other flexible material, used for making local applications to the esophagus or larynx or for removing foreign bodies. **ball p.** A probang having an ivory bulb attached to one end. **bristle p.** One having on the end a sheath of bristles or horsehair that can be made to spread like an umbrella as the instrument is drawn out. Also called horse hair p. **sponge p.** One with a small sponge at one end.

pro-banthine bromide. Trademark for propantheline bromide.

pro·bar'bi·tal cal'ci·um. The nonproprietary name for calcium 5-ethyl-5-isopropyl barbiturate. See ipral calcium.

pro·bar'bi·tal so'di·um. The nonproprietary name for sodium 5-ethyl-5-isopropyl barbiturate. See ipral sodium.

probe. 1. A slender, flexible rod, for exploring or dilating a natural channel, as a lacrimal duct, or for following a sinus or the course of a wound. 2. A stiff rod, usually pointed at one end, used for separating tissues in dissection. 3. The act of using a probe.

pro·ben'e·cid. p-(Di-n-propylsulfamyl)-benzoic acid, a drug that inhibits renal tubular secretion of penicillin, para-aminosalicylic acid, and phenol red; a premedication that increases the blood levels of penicillin and para-aminosalicylic acid when they are subsequently administered; a therapeutic agent in gout, presumably by blocking reabsorption of urates. See benemid.

pro·bos'cis (pro·bos'iss). The cylindrical projection from the face, above or below the orbit, with or without a cavity, which represents the nose in various grades of cyclopia.

pro'caine (pro'cane, pro'kay·een, -in, pro·cane'). 1. The base p-aminobenzoyl-diethylaminoethanol. 2. A synonym for procaine hydrochloride.

pro'caine am'ide hy"dro·chlo'ride. p-Amino-N-(2-diethylaminoethyl) benzamide hydrochloride, used in treatment of cardiac arrhythmias. See pronestyl hydrochloride.

pro'caine hy"dro·chlo'ride. p-Aminobenzoyl-diethylaminoethanol hydrochloride; occurs as white crystals or powder; soluble in water. Procaine exhibits an aggregate of simultaneous pharmacologic effects. Syn., procaine.

pro·cal'lus. The organized blood clot which forms in an early stage of repair of a fractured bone.

pro"ce·phal'ic. In biology, pertaining to the front of the head.

proc'ess, pro'cess. 1. A course of action; a group of phenomena, as an inflammatory process. 2. A prominence or outgrowth, as the spinous process of a vertebra, the axis cylinder process of a nerve. 3. In chemistry, a method of procedure; reaction; test. **alar p.** One of a pair of processes arising from the lower part of the anterior border of the cribriform plate of the ethmoid, articulating with the frontal bone and completing the cecal foramen of the frontal bone. **alveolar p.** (a) The border of the maxilla in which the alveoli, or bony sockets of the upper teeth, are embedded. (b) The border of the mandible in which the alveoli of the lower teeth are embedded. **anterior clinoid p.** A prominent process that juts backward from the medial extremity of the lesser wing of the sphenoid bone behind the optic foramen. **ciliary p.** Circularly arranged choroid foldings continuous with the iris in front. **coracoid p.** A beak-shaped process of the scapula. **coronoid p. of the mandible.** A thin, flattened process projecting from the anterior portion of the upper border of the ramus of the mandible, and serving for the insertion of the temporal muscle. **frontonasal p.** The anterior region of the embryonic head that later develops into the frontal, median nasal, and lateral nasal processes. Also called nasofrontal p. **Hickman molecular distillation p.** A commercially important process for the concentration of vitamin A from fish liver oils by distillation under high vacuum with a short path between the surface of the oil and the condenser. **mammillary p.** One of the tubercles on the posterior part of the superior articular processes of the lumbar vertebrae. **olecranon p.** A bony eminence on the upper and back part of the ulna. In extension of the forearm it fits into the olecranon fossa of the humerus. **posterior clinoid p.** One of the two short bony extensions from the superior angles of the dorsum sellae which give attachment to the tentorium cerebelli. **pterygoid p. of the sphenoid bone.** One descending perpendicularly from the point of junction of the body with the greater wing of the sphenoid bone, and consisting of a lateral and a medial plate. **spinous processes of the ilium.** The spines of the ilium, anterior and posterior superior, and anterior and posterior inferior. **styloid p. of the temporal bone.** A sharp spine about an inch in length, descending downward, forward, and inward from the inferior surface of the petrous portion of the temporal bone. **styloid p. of the ulna.** A projection from the inner and posterior portion of the lower extremity of the ulna. **vaginal p. of the peritoneum.** A tube of peritoneum which evaginates through the inguinal canal into the scrotum (or labium majus) during embryonic life. In the male the distal portion persists as the tunica vaginalis testis. In the female a portion occasionally persists, forming the canal of Nuck. **vermiform p.** A tubular diverticulum of the cecum. Also called *vermiform appendix.* **xiphoid p.** The elongated process projecting caudad from the lower end of the sternum between the cartilages of the seventh ribs. It usually becomes osseous after the age of 50. **zygomatic p. of the temporal bone.** A long projection from the lower part of the squamous portion of the temporal bone, articulating with the zygomatic bone.

pro·ces″so·ma′ni·a. A mania for litigation.

pro·chei′lon (pro·kigh′lon). Prominence in the middle of the upper lip.

pro″chlor·per′a·zine. 2-Chloro-10-[3-(1-methyl-4-piperazinyl)propyl]phenothiazine, an antiemetic and tranquilizer, used in the form of the base and as ethanedisulfonate and maleate salts. See *compazine*.

procholon. Trade-mark for dehydrocholic acid, an oxidation product of cholic acid derived from natural bile acids.

proc″i·den′ti·a (pross″i·den′shuh, pro″si·). The falling or sinking down of a part. Prolapse, prolapsus, *q.v.*

pro′cre·ate. Beget.

proc·ta′gra (prock·tay′gruh, prock·tag′ruh). Sudden pain in the anal region.

proc·tal′gi·a. Neuralgic pain in the anus or rectum.

proc″ta·tre′si·a (prock″ta·tree′zhuh, ·shuh). An imperforate condition of the anus or rectum.

proc″tec·ta′si·a (prock″teck·tay′zhuh, ·shuh), **proc·tec′ta·sis.** Dilatation of the anus or rectum.

proc·tec′to·my. Excision of the anus and rectum, usually through the perineal route.

proc·ten′cli·sis (prock·teng′kli·sis,

prock″ten·kly′sis). Stricture of the rectum or anus.

proc″teu·ryn′ter (prock″tew·rin′tur). An instrument for dilating the anus or rectum.

proc·ti′tis. Inflammation of the anus or rectum.

proc′to-, proct-. A combining form meaning *anus;* used to denote *the rectum.*

proc′to·cele. The extroversion or prolapse of the mucous coat of the rectum. **vaginal p.** A hernia of the rectum appearing in the vagina.

proc·toc′ly·sis. The slow instillation of a liquid into the rectum.

proc″to·co·li′tis. Inflammation of the rectum and colon.

proc″to·co″lon·os′co·py. Inspection of the interior of the rectum and lower colon.

proc″to·col′po·plas″ty. Closure of a rectovaginal fistula.

proc″to·de′um. A pitlike, ectodermal depression formed by the growth of the anal hillocks surrounding the anal part of the cloacal membrane. Upon rupture of the latter, it forms part of the anal canal. Also called *anal pit, primitive anus.*

proc″to·dyn′i·a. Pain about the anus or in the rectum.

proc·tol′o·gist. One versed in diseases of the anus and rectum.

proc·tol′o·gy. The science of the anatomy, functions, and diseases of rectum and anus. —**proctolog′ic,** *adj.*

proc″to·pa·ral′y·sis. Paralysis of the external anal sphincter.

proc″to·pex″y. The fixation of the rectum by anchoring it into the hollow of the sacrum by means of sutures passing across the sacrum. Also called *rectopexy.*

proc″to·pho′bi·a. A morbid dread or apprehension of pain common in persons with diseases of the rectum.

proc′to·plas″ty. Plastic surgery of the anus.

proc·tor′rha·phy. The plaiting of the enlarged and prolapsed rectal walls by suture, to reduce the circumference.

proc″tor·rhe′a. Escape of mucus through the anus.

proc′to·scope. An instrument for inspecting the anal canal and rectum.

proc·tos′co·py. Ocular inspection of the anal canal and rectum with the aid of special instruments.

proc″to·sig″moid·ec′to·my. The abdominoperineal excision of the anus and rectosigmoid, with the formation of an abdominal colostomy.

proc′to·spasm. Spasm or tenesmus of the rectum.

proc·tos′ta·sis. Constipation due to nonresponse of the rectum to the defecation stimulus.

proc″to·ste·no′sis. Stricture of the anus or rectum.

proc·tos′to·my. The establishment of a permanent artificial opening into the rectum.

proc·tot′o·my. Incision into the rectum or anus, especially for stricture or imperforate anus. The operation is described as external if the incision is below the external sphincter, and internal if the incision is above the sphincter.

pro·cur′sive. Running forward, as procursive epilepsy, a form in which the patient runs during the epileptic attack.

pro″cur·va′tion. Forward inclination of the body.

pro·cy′cli·dine hy″dro·chlo′ride. 1-Cyclohexyl-1-phenyl-3-pyrrolidino-1-propanol hydrochloride, a parasympatholytic agent. See *kemadrin.*

pro·dig″i·o′sin (pro·didj″ee·o′sin). A red antibiotic substance produced by *Bacillus prodigiosus.*

prod′ro·mal, pro·dro′mal. Relating to early manifestations or symptoms; premonitory.

pro′drome (pl. *prodromata*). An early manifestation of impending disease, before the specific symptoms begin. **—prod′romal** (prod′ro·mul, pro·dro′mul), **prod′romous** (prod′ro·mus, pro·dro′mus), **prodrom′ic** (pro·drom′ick, pro·dro′mick), *adj.*

prod′uct. 1. Effect; result; that which is produced. 2. *In chemistry,* the compound formed by a reaction.

pro·duc′tive. Forming or capable of forming new tissue.

pro·en′zyme. The substance in a living cell from which an enzyme is formed.

pro·es′tro·gen. A substance, in itself weakly estrogenic, which is converted to a more active estrogen in the body.

pro·es′trus. A phase of the estrous cycle in mammals preceding heat; characterized by growth of the endometrium and follicular development in the ovary.

pro·fes′sion·al. 1. Pertaining to a profession; in keeping with ethics. 2. Produced by the practice of a profession, as professional neuritis (writers' cramp, etc.).

pro·fla′vine (pro·flay′veen, ·vin). $C_{18}H_{11}N_3$. 2,8-Diaminoacridine. Its salts are used for their antiseptic effect in the treatment of wounds, urethritis, gingivitis, gonorrheal conjunctivitis, and other conditions requiring the use of a germicide.

pro·fun′da. Deep-seated; a term applied to certain arteries and veins.

pro·gen′er·ate. One endowed with superior faculties; a genius.

pro·gen′i·tor. An ancestor.

prog′e·ny (prodj′i·nee). Offspring; descendants.

pro·ge′ri·a. Premature senility; a morbid state showing symptoms both of infantilism and senility. Also called *Hutchinson-Gilford disease.*

pro·ges′ter·one (pro·jes′tur·ohn). $C_{21}H_{30}O_2$. A diketone having the composition of pregnene-3-20-dione. It is the hormone found in the corpus luteum; occurs as a white, crystalline powder. It is available under various trade-marked names, including *progestin, progestone,* and *proluton.*

progestin. Trade-mark for a brand of progesterone.

progestone. Trade-mark for a brand of progesterone.

progestoral. Trade-mark for anhydrohydroxyprogesterone.

prog′na·thism. The condition of having projecting jaws. **—prognath′ic, prognathous,** *adj.*

prog·no′sis. A prediction of the duration, course, and termination of a disease, based on all information available in the individual case and knowledge of how the disease behaves generally. **—prognos′tic,** *adj.*

prog″nos·ti′cian (prog″nos·tish′un). One who is versed in prognosis.

pro·gran′u·lo·cyte″. Promyelocyte.

pro·grav′id. Referring to the lutein phase or second growth phase of the endometrium; the glands become tortuous and irregularly sacculated, and the secretion contains glycogen. In pregnancy the progravid changes progress for six to eight weeks; in the nonpregnant uterus for about ten days. Syn., *progestational.*

pro·gres′sion. The act of advancing or moving forward. **backward p.** A backward walking, a rare symptom of certain nervous lesions, such as Parkinsonism.

pro·gres′sive. Gradually extending.

pro″in·va′sin I. An enzyme which accompanies and protects the hyaluronidase of pathogenic bacteria and snake venoms. It acts by destroying antinvasin I, an enzyme in blood plasma which is capable of destroying hyaluronidase, and thereby interferes with this defense mechanism of the host against the action of hyaluronidase.

pro″i·o′ti·a (pro″ee·o′shee·uh), **pro″i·o′tes** (pro″ee·o′teez). Sexual precocity.

pro·jec′tion. 1. The act of throwing forward. 2. A part extending beyond its surroundings. 3. The referring of impressions made on the organs of sense to the position of the object producing them. 4. *In psychopathology,* a mental dynamism whereby a person overcomes his feeling of inadequacy or guilt by transferring to other persons or to objects the responsibility for such inadequacy. The most prominent mental mechanism in paranoia.

pro·ki'nase (pro·kigh'nace, ·naze, pro·kin'ace, ·aze). A proteolytic enzyme found in extracts of the pancreas.

proklot. Trade-mark for a brand of menadione.

pro·la'bi·um. 1. Exposed part of the lip. 2. Central prominence of the lip.

pro·lac'tin. The lactogenic hormone from the anterior pituitary gland. The substance is used to initiate lactation in agalactia or to stimulate increased milk secretion in nursing mothers. Syn., *galactin, lactogenic hormone, mammotrophin, mammotropin.*

pro·lam'ine (pro·lam'een, ·in, pro'luh·meen, ·min). Gliadin, a vegetable protein.

pro'lan-A. A follicle-stimulating hormone which has been isolated from hog pituitary. Syn., FSH, *thylakentrin.*

pro'lan-B. A luteinizing hormone which has been isolated from swine and sheep pituitaries. Syn., LH, *metakentrin.*

pro·lapse'. The falling or sinking down of a part. **frank p.** Complete displacement downward of the uterus and inversion of the vagina, with both structures hanging outside the vulva. **p. of the cord.** Premature expulsion of the umbilical cord during parturition. **p. of the iris.** Protrusion of the iris through a corneal wound.

pro·lap'sus. Prolapse, *q.v.* **p. ani.** Extrusion of the lower division of the intestinal tract through the external sphincter of the anus. **p. uteri.** Displacement of the uterus downward, sometimes outside the vulva.

pro·lep'sis. In a periodic disease, the return of an attack or paroxysm before the expected time or at progressively shorter intervals. —**proleptic,** *adj.*

pro·lif'er·ate. To multiply rapidly, as by cellular division; to reproduce. —**prolifera'tion,** *n.*

pro·lif'ic. Fruitful.

pro·lig'er·ous (pro·lidj'ur·us). Germinating; producing offspring.

pro'lin·ase. The enzyme which hydrolyzes proline peptides to proline and simpler peptides.

pro'line (pro'leen, ·lin). $C_5H_9O_2N$. Alpha- or 2-pyrrolidine carboxylic acid, an amino acid resulting from the hydrolysis of proteins.

pro·li'pase. Inactive form of steapsin found in pancreatic juice.

proluton. Trade-mark for a brand of progesterone.

pro·lym'pho·cyte. 1. A cell of the lymphocyte series intermediate in maturity between the lymphoblast and the lymphocyte. A peroxidase negative cell more than 15 μ in diameter with a

spheroidal nucleus of coarser chromatin structure than the lymphoblast. 2. A large lymphocyte.

pro·ma·zine hy"dro·chlo'ride. 10-(3-Dimethylaminopropyl)phenothiazine hydrochloride, a neuropsychiatric agent. See *sparine hydrochloride.*

pro·meth'a·zine hy"dro·chlo'ride. 10-(2-Dimethylaminopropyl)-phenothiazine hydrochloride, an antihistaminic. See *phenergan hydrochloride.*

pro"me·thes'trol di·pro'pi·o·nate. Nonproprietary name for dimethylhexestrol dipropionate; a synthetic estrogen. See *meprane dipropionate.*

pro·me'thi·um. Pm. A name proposed for a synthetic form of element 61. See also *cyclonium, florentium, illinium.*

promin sodium. Trade-mark for glucosulfone sodium.

prom'i·nence. 1. A projection, especially on a bone. 2. The state of projecting or standing out.

promizole. Trade-mark for thiazolsulfone.

prom'on·to·ry. A projection or prominence.

pro·mox'o·lane. 2,2-Diisopropyl-1,3-dioxolane-4-methanol, a skeletal muscle relaxant. See *dimethylane.*

pro·my'e·lo·cyte. The earliest myelocyte stage derived from the myeloblast; it contains a few granules characteristic of the type of granulocyte into which it develops.

pro'nate. 1. Turn the forearm so that the palm of the hand is down or toward the back. 2. In the foot, *evert* is the preferred term; the sole is turned outward and the lateral margin of the foot is elevated.

pro·na'tion. 1. The condition of being prone; the act of placing in the prone position. 2. The turning of the palm of the hand downward.

pro·na'tor. That which pronates, as pronator teres and pronator quadratus, muscles of the forearm attached to the ulna and radius. See Table of Muscles in the Appendix.

prone. Lying with the face downward; the opposite of *supine.*

pro·neph'ros (*pl. pronephroi*). The primitive or head kidney formed by the most cephalic part of the nephrogenic tissue of the embryo. Vestigial in mammals, its duct is taken over by the mesonephros.

pronestyl hydrochloride. Trademarked name for procaine amide hydrochloride.

pro'no·grade. Walking or standing on all fours, as the quadrupeds.

pron'to·sil. $(NH_2)_2C_6H_3.N:N.C_6H_4.SO_2.NH_2$, 2,4-Diaminoazobenzene-4'-sulfonamide. A reddish crystalline powder; forerunner of the sulfonamides.

rontosil album. See *sulfanila-mide.*

rontosil soluble. See *neopronto-sil.*

roof gal'lon. A gallon of proof spirit.

roof spir'it. A mixture of ethyl alcohol and water containing 50% by volume of C_2H_5OH.

ro·o'tic (pro·o'tick, ·ot'ick). In front of the ear.

ropadrine hydrochloride. Trade-mark for phenylpropanolamine hydrochloride.

rop'a·gate. Produce offspring. —**propaga'tion,** *n.*

rop'al·lyl·o·nal. Nonproprietary title for 5-isopropyl-5-β-bromallyl barbituric acid. See *nostal.*

ro·pam'i·dine (pro·pam'i·deen, ·din). *p,p′*-(Trimethylenedioxy) dibenzamidine. NH:C(NH₂).C₆H₄.O.(CH₂)₃O.-C₆H₄C(NH₂):NH. A diamidine derivative used as a surgical antiseptic.

ro'pane. C_3H_8. A hydrocarbon, the third member of the marsh gas series, occurring in petroleum.

ro·pan'the·line bro'mide. β-Diisopropylmethylaminoethyl 9-xanthenecarboxylate bromide, a parasympatholytic agent. See *pro-banthine bromide.*

ro·par'a·caine hy''dro·chlo'-ide. 2-Diethylaminoethyl 3-amino-4-ropoxybenzoate hydrochloride, a topical anesthetic. See *ophthaine.*

ro'pene. Propylene.

ro·pe·nyl, prop'e·nyl. 1. The monovalent radical $CH_3.CH:CH-$, derived from propylene. 2. The trivalent glyceryl radical $-CH_2.CH.CH_2-$.

ro·pep'sin. The zymogen of pepsin, found in the cells of the gastric glands.

ro·pep'tone. Hemialbumose, *q.v.* See also *peptone.*

ro''pep·to·nu'ri·a. The presence of propeptone in the urine.

ro·per'din. A euglobulin representing less than 0.03% of total serum protein found in the serum of higher animals, including man, apparently a nonspecific antibody-like substance which destroys certain bacteria and viruses, lyses certain red blood cells, and requires magnesium ion and serum factors resembling complement for its action.

ro'phase (pro'fayz). The first stage of mitosis, in which the chromosomes are organized from nuclear materials as elongate spiremes.

ro''phen·pyr·id'a·mine, pro''-hen·pyr''i·dam'ine. 1-Phenyl-1-(2-pyridyl) -3 -dimethylaminopropane, an antihistaminic substance. See *tri-seton.*

pro''phy·lac'tic. A remedy or agent that prevents the development of disease.

pro''phy·lax'is. Prevention of disease; measures preventing the development or spread of disease. —**prophylac'tic,** *adj.* **dental p.** The prevention of dental and oral diseases by preventive measures, especially the mechanical cleansing of the teeth.

pro'pi·o·nate. A salt of propionic acid.

pro''pi·on'ic ac'id (pro''pee·on'ic, ·o'nick). $CH_3.CH_2.COOH$. A liquid acid of pungent odor; in the form of its calcium and sodium salts, it is used as a mold preventive or fungicide.

pro''pi·on'o- (pro''pee·on'o-, ·o'no-), **propion-.** *In chemistry,* a combining form signifying *propionic.*

pro·pri·e·tar'y. Any chemical, drug, or similar preparation used in the treatment of diseases, if such an article is protected against free competition as to name, product, composition, or process of manufacture, by secrecy, patent, copyright, or any other means.

pro''pri·o·cep'tion. Appreciation of position, balance, and changes in equilibrium on the part of the muscular system, especially during locomotion.

pro''pri·o·cep'tive im'pul·ses. Afferent nerve impulses originating in receptors in muscles, tendons, joints, and vestibular apparatus of internal ear. Their reflex functions are concerned with locomotion and maintenance of posture.

pro''pri·o·cep'tor. A receptor located in a muscle, tendon, joint, or vestibular apparatus, whose reflex function is locomotor or postural.

prop·to'sis (prop·to'sis, pro·to'sis). 1. A falling downward. 2. Prolapse. 3. Exophthalmos.

pro·pul'sion. 1. Act of pushing or driving forward. 2. A falling forward in walking, as observed in paralysis agitans.

pro'pyl. C_3H_7. The radical of propane.

pro''pyl·a·ce'tic ac'id. The normal valeric acid, *q.v.*

pro''pyl·ene, prop'yl·ene. 1. C_3H_6; the unsaturated hydrocarbon, $CH_3CH:CH_2$, a homolog of ethylene and isomer of cyclopropane; a colorless gas. 2. The monovalent radical, $CH_2CH:CH-$. 3. The bivalent radical, $-CH(CH_3)CH_2-$.

pro·pyl·ene gly'col. $CH_3CHOHCH_2-OH$; 1,2-dihydroxypropane; occurs as a colorless, viscous liquid; completely miscible with water. Used as a solvent for many medicinals.

pro''pyl·hex'e·drine (pro''pil-hex'eh·dreen, ·drin). 1-Cyclohexyl-2-methylaminopropane, a volatile sympathomimetic amine used as a nasal decongestant. See *benzedrex.*

pro"pyl·par'a·ben. $C_6H_4.OH.$-COOC$_3H_7$. Propyl parahydroxybenzoate, a white powder, soluble in water; a bacteriostatic to preserve medicinal preparations.

pro"pyl·thi"o·u'ra·cil. The 6-*n*-propyl derivative of thiouracil, *q.v.*, used like the latter but more effective and less toxic in therapeutic doses.

pro re na'ta. According to the circumstances of the case. Abbreviated, p. r. n.

pro·ren'nin. The zymogen of rennin or chymosin.

pro·se'cre·tin. The precursor of secretin; it is secreted by the epithelium of the small intestine.

pro·sec'tor. One who prepares subjects for anatomic dissection or to illustrate didactic lectures.

pros"en·ceph'a·lon. The forebrain or anterior brain vesicle of the embryo that divides into telencephalon and diencephalon. From it are derived the cerebral hemispheres, olfactory lobes, corpus striatum, and various parts of the thalamus, as well as the third and the lateral ventricles.

pro·sep'ta·zine (pro·sep'tuh·zeen, ·zin). $C_6H_3CH_3.NH.C_6H_4.SO_2.NH_2$. Benzyl sulfanilamide; occurs as a white powder, slightly soluble in water. Also called *chemodyn, septazine.*

pros"o·dem'ic. Pertaining to disease spread by individual contact, as opposed to one spread by general means such as the water or milk supply.

pros"o·pal'gi·a. Neuralgic pain in the distribution of the trigeminal nerve. Also called *facial neuralgia, tic douloureux.* —**prosopalgic,** *adj.*

pros·op'ic. 1. *In craniometry,* designating a facial skeleton that is convex or projects anteriorly in the midline; having an orbitonasal index of 110.0 or more. 2. *In somatometry,* designating a face that is convex or projects anteriorly in the midline; having an orbitonasal index of 113.0 or more.

pros"o·po"di·ple'gi·a (pross"o-po"dye·plee'jee·uh, pross"o·pod"i·). Bilateral facial paralysis.

pros"o·po·dyn'i·a. Facial pain, or neuralgia.

pros"o·po·ple'gi·a. Facial palsy; it may be unilateral (monoplegia facialis) or bilateral (diplegia facialis). —**prosopoplegic,** *adj.*

pros"o·pos'chi·sis (pross"o·poss'ki·sis). Congenital facial cleft, from mouth to orbit (oblique facial cleft), or from the mouth to just in front of the auditory meatus (transverse facial cleft).

pros'o·pus va'rus. Congenital hemiatrophy of the face and cranium, resulting in marked facial obliquity.

pros'tate. The organ surrounding the neck of the bladder and beginning of the urethra in the male (prostatic urethra). It consists of two lateral lobes and a middle lobe, and is composed of muscular and glandular tissue; a distinct capsule surrounds it. The prostate often becomes enlarged in advanced life, and may then interfere with the emptying of the bladder. —**prostatic,** *adj.*

pros"ta·tec'to·my. Excision of part or all of the prostate. It includes transurethral prostate resection of the median lobe or lateral lobes by electrocoagulation, by the use of various punches and resectoscopes (punch operation). **perineal p.** The removal of the prostate by a U-shaped or V-shaped incision in the perineum, using a special prostatic retractor or modification. **suprapubic p.** Removal of prostate by incision in bladder through abdominal (suprapubic) route in a one- or two-stage operation.

pros'ta·tism. The condition caused by chronic disorders of the prostate, especially chronic, nonmalignant prostatic enlargement.

pros"ta·ti'tis. Inflammation of the prostate gland. —**prostatit'ic,** *adj.*

pros"ta·to·cys·ti'tis. Inflammation of the prostate and urinary bladder.

pros·tat'o·lith. A prostatic calculus.

pros"ta·to·li·thot'o·my (pross"-tuh·to·li·thot'o·mee, pro·stat"o·). Removal of a stone or calculus from the prostate gland.

pros"ta·tor·rhe'a. A thin urethral discharge coming from the prostate gland.

pros"ta·tot'o·my. Incision into the prostate gland.

pros"ta·to·ve·sic"u·li'tis. Inflammation of the seminal vesicles combined with prostatitis.

pros·the·sis (pl. *prostheses*). 1. Replacement or substitution. 2. An artificial substitute for a missing part, as a denture, hand, leg, eye. —**prosthetic,** *adj.* **dental p.** An appliance to replace missing teeth, as a denture, crown, or bridgework. **maxillofacial p.** A substitute for a jaw, nose, or cheek, when the loss is too extensive for surgical repair alone. **temporary p.** An artificial limb used early following amputation and in preparation for the permanent apparatus.

pros·thet'ic group. 1. The group formed by a substance that is combined with a simple protein to form a complex protein, as the chromophore group in chromoproteins. 2. The group formed by an organic radical not rived from an amino acid, that enters into the complex molecule of a conjugated protein, *q.v.* 3. The nonprotein component, or coenzyme, of certain enzyme systems.

pros·thet'ics. The branch of surgery which deals with prostheses.

pros'the·tist. One who makes artificial limbs, artificial dentures, or external organs or parts.

pros"tho·don'tist. A dentist who specializes in prosthetic dentistry.

prostigmin. Trade-mark for neostigmine. **prostigmin bromide** and **prostigmin methylsulfate** being available commercially.

pros"ti·tu'tion. The condition or act of using the body indiscriminately for illicit sexual intercourse for a monetary consideration.

pros'trate. Lying at full length.

pros'trat·ed (pross'tray·tid). Exhausted; stricken down.

pros·tra'tion. 1. The condition of being prostrate. 2. Extreme exhaustion. **heat p.** Exhaustion due to exposure to excessive heat, as from the sun or from heated rooms.

pro"tac·tin'i·um. Pa = 231. A radioactive element occurring in pitchblende and yielding actinium on disintegration. Atomic number, 91.

pro'ta·mine (pro'tuh·meen, ·min, pro·tam'een, ·in). 1. One of a group of simple proteins occurring in the sex cells of fishes, as salmine, sturine, *q.v.* 2. An amine isolated from spermatozoa and fish spawn; $C_{16}H_{32}O_4N_9$. **p. insu·lin.** A combination of insulin hydrochloride and protamine from the trout, exerting a more prolonged action than insulin alone. **p. sulfate.** The sulfate salt of protamine, 2; used as a heparin antagonist.

pro"tan·o'pi·a. Defective red vision; green-sightedness. **—protanop'ic,** *adj.*

pro·tar'gin (pro·tahr'jin). See mild *silver* protein and strong *silver* protein.

protargol. Trade-mark for a strong silver protein.

pro'te·an (pro'tee·un, pro·tee'un). 1. Taking on many shapes, as a protean disease, protean eruption. 2. One of a group of derived proteins, insoluble products due to the action of water or enzymes.

pro'te·ase (pro'tee·ace, ·aze). An enzyme which digests proteins.

pro·tec'tive. 1. Affording defense or immunity. 2. A covering or shield which protects. 3. A specific dressing, as oiled silk or rubber, used to prevent ingress of water.

pro'te·in (pro'tee·in, pro'teen). One of a group of complex nitrogenous substances of high molecular weight which are found in various forms in animals and plants and are characteristic of living matter. On hydrolysis they yield amino acids. See Table of Normal Values of Blood Constituents in the Appendix. **adequate proteins.** Those proteins which furnish the body with all nitrogenous compounds necessary for maintenance and growth. **conjugated p.** A protein combined with a nonprotein group, other than a salt of a simple protein. **denatured p.** A protein whose structure and properties have been altered, mainly by the action of physical agents. **derived p.** A synthetic protein, a polypeptide, or any product obtained from proteins by the action of acids, alkalies, enzymes, or heat. **foreign p.** A protein which differs from the proteins of the animal or person into whom it is introduced. **globular p.** One of the supposed closed cyclic molecules of certain types in which an imaginary polyhedron surface holds a definite number of hexagonal configurations. **iron-porphyrin p.** One of a large group of proteins which contain iron and porphyrin; these include hemoglobin, the cytochromes, cytochrome oxidase, catalase, peroxidase, etc. **native p.** A protein in its original state; a protein which has not been altered in composition or properties. **plasma proteins.** The proteins present in blood plasma consisting of fibrinogen, albumins, and globulins. **serum proteins.** The proteins present in the serum from clotted blood, differing from plasma proteins only in the absence of fibrinogen. See Table of Normal Values of Blood Constituents in the Appendix. **silver p.** See *protein silver*. **simple p.** One of the class of albumins which includes globulins, glutelins, prolamines, histones, and protamines. **specific p.** One possessing capabilities of acting as an allergen. **tissue p.** That part of the body protein present in the solid tissues as distinguished from the circulating blood protein.

pro'te·in·ase (pro'tee·in·ace, ·aze). One of the subgroups of proteases or proteolytic enzymes which act directly on the native proteins in the first step of their conversion to simpler substances.

pro"te·in·o'sis. The accumulation of protein in the tissues.

pro'te·in sil'ver. Any combination of silver and protein. Also called *silver protein.* See mild *silver* protein, strong *silver* protein.

pro"te·in·u'ri·a. The presence of protein in the urine.

pro"te·o·me·tab'o·lism. The processes of digestion, absorption, and utilization of proteins. —**proteometabol'ic**, *adj.*

pro·te·o·pep'tic. Pertaining to protein digestion.

pro'te·ose. One of a group of derived proteins intermediate between food proteins and peptones. Soluble in water, not coagulable by heat, but precipitated by saturation with ammonium or zinc sulfate.

Pro'teus. A genus of the tribe Proteae belonging to the family Enterobacteriaceae. Species of this genus, **Pr. hydrophilus, Pr. mirabilis,** and **Pr. vulgaris,** have been associated with a variety of pathologic conditions, such as pleuritis, peritonitis, cystitis, and suppurative abscesses. The species **Pr. morganii** has been isolated in cases of summer diarrhea of infants.

prothricin. Trade-mark for an isotonic buffered solution of tyrothricin and propadrine used in the symptomatic treatment of nasal congestion.

pro·throm'bin. A substance present in plasma and essential for the clotting of blood. In the presence of thromboplastin and calcium ions, it is converted to thrombin which, in turn, converts fibrinogen to fibrin. Formed in liver by the action of vitamin K. Also called *thrombogen, prothrombase.* **fraction A p.** That portion of prothrombin which disappears when citrated or oxalated plasma or blood stands in contact with air. **fraction B p.** That portion of prothrombin which disappears in the animal body when there is vitamin-K deficiency.

pro·throm"bi·ne'mi·a. An excess of prothrombin in the blood plasma.

pro·throm"bi·no·pe'ni·a. Decrease in the prothrombin content of the blood. Syn., *hypoprothrombinemia.*

pro·thy'mi·a. Intellectual alertness.

pro·ti'o·dide. A salt containing the least amount of iodine of the iodides of the same base.

pro'ti·um. The predominant constituent of ordinary hydrogen; the atom consists of one proton and one electron and therefore has an atomic weight of approximately one. Symbol, H^1. Sometimes called *light hydrogen.*

pro'to-, prot-. 1. A combining form meaning *first.* 2. *In chemistry,* a combining form meaning the *lowest of a series of compounds of the same elements.*

pro"to·chlo'ride. See *proto-,* 2.

pro'to·col. 1. The original notes or records of an experiment, autopsy, or clinical examination. 2. The records from which a document is prepared.

pro"to·con'id, pro"to·co'nid. The mesiobuccal cusp on a molar tooth of the lower jaw.

pro"to·i'o·dide. See *protiodide.*

pro·tol'y·sis. Any reaction in whi a proton, or hydrogen ion, is tran ferred, as:

$$HCl + H_2O = H_3O^+ + Cl^-.$$

pro'ton. A subatomic particle iden cal with the nucleus of the hydrog atom, having a positive electric char numerically equal to the negative char on the electron, with a mass equal 6×10^{-22} Gm.

pro"to·path'ic. Designating prim tive sensibility, as opposed to more d criminating, or epicritic, sensation.

pro'to·plasm. The viscid materi constituting the essential substance living cells, upon which all the vi functions of nutrition, secretio growth, reproduction, irritability, a motility depend.

pro"to·por'phy·rin. $C_{33}H_{33}N$ (COOH)₂, any of the 15 metal-fr porphyrins having as substituents methyl, 2 vinyl, and 2 propionic ac groups, of which protoporphyrin 9 o curs in hemoglobin.

pro"to·pro'te·ose. Primary prot ose; further digestion changes it in deuteroproteose.

pro"to·tox'in. A dissociation produ of toxins differing from deuterotox and tritotoxins in having a strong affinity than either for the antitoxin

pro"to·ver'a·trine. Either of t hypotensive alkaloids, **protover trine A** and **protoveratrine** from certain *Veratrum* species.

Pro"to·zo'a. A zoologic phylum unicellular organisms. This phylum subdivided into the subphylum Pla modroma which contains the medica important classes Rhizopoda, M tigophora, and Sporozoa, and into t subphylum Ciliophora which conta the class Ciliata.

pro"to·zo'an. 1. Of or pertaining members of the phylum Protozoa. 2. protozoon.

pro"to·zo·i'a·sis. Infection by p tozoa.

pro"to·zo·ol'o·gy. The study protozoa.

pro"to·zo'on (pl. *protozoa*). A member of the phylum Protozoa.

pro·trude'. Project. Assume an a normally prominent position, as a to which is thrust forward out of line.

pro·tru'sion. The condition of ing thrust forward, as the protrus of the incisor teeth.

pro·tu'ber·ance. A knoblike pr jecting part.

proud flesh. Exuberant granulat tissue.

pro·vi'ta·min. A precursor of a vi min. That which assumes vitamin tivity upon activation or chemi change within the body, as ergoster which upon ultraviolet irradiation is converted in part to calciferol (D_2); or β-carotene, which in the liver is hydrolyzed to vitamin A.

pro·voc'a·tive. Tending to excite or provoke; arousing signs, symptoms, or reactions, similar to those of a disease phenomenon.

prox'i·mal. 1. Nearest to the body or the median line of the body, or to some other point considered as the center of a system. 2. In dentistry, the proximal surface of a tooth is that portion next to the adjacent tooth.

prox'i·mate (prock'si·mit). Nearest; immediate, as proximate cause.

prox"i·mo·a·tax'i·a. Lack of coördination in the muscles of the proximal part of the limbs; in opposition to croataxia.

prox. luc. Prozima luce; the day before.

pro·zy'mo·gen. An intracellular substance which becomes zymogen.

pru·ri'go. A chronic inflammatory disease of the skin characterized by small, pale papules and severe itching. The papules are deeply seated and are most prominent on the extensor surfaces of the limbs. The disease begins in early life. There are two forms of the disease: **prurigo mitis** which is comparatively mild and **prurigo geia** or **ferox** which is severe. **prurig'inous,** adj. p. **nodularis.** A chronic skin disease which occurs chiefly in women and is characterized by pruritic, nodular, and verrucous lesions. It is regarded as an atypical nodular form of neurodermatitis circumscripta, unrelated to the prurigos. Syn., lichen obtusus corneus.

pru·ri'tus. Itching; especially, that due to irritation of a peripheral sensory nerve. **prurit'ic,** adj. **bath p.** A burning sensation varying from a slight pricking to an intense itching experienced by some persons after a bath. **p. ani.** A common itching condition in and about the anus, especially in men; may be due to several causes. p. **hiemalis.** A form affecting certain persons only in winter, especially in dry climates. Syn., frost-itch, winter itch. **p. senilis.** The pruritus of the aged, probably caused by a lack of oil in the skin; accompanies the atrophy of the skin in old age. **p. vulvae.** Intense or mild itching of the vulva and at times adjacent parts. May lead to atrophy, lichenification, and even malignancy. Etiology is varied. **punctate p.** Patchy areas of itching with no cutaneous lesions; occurs especially over bony prominences.

Prus'sian blue. $Fe_4[Fe(CN)_6]_3$. Ferric ferrocyanide; occurs as dark blue powder or lumps; insoluble in water. Also called Berlin blue.

prus'si·ate (prush'ee·ate, pruss'-). 1. Any salt of prussic or hydrocyanic acid; a cyanide. 2. Particularly a ferricyanide or ferrocyanide.

prus'sic ac'id (pruss'ick, prōō'sick). Hydrocyanic acid.

psam'mism. The treatment of disease with sand baths. Syn., ammism, ammotherapy.

psam·mo'ma (sam·o'muh). A firm, fibrous tumor found in the membranes of the brain, the choroid plexus, and in other parts; characterized by the presence of concentrically laminated calcareous nodules.

psam"mo·sar·co'ma. A psammoma with sarcomatous features, or a sarcoma containing psammoma bodies.

psam'mous. Sandy or sabulous.

psel'lism (sel'iz·um), **psel·lis'mus.** 1. Stuttering or stammering. 2. Defective speech due to harelip or to cleft palate. **psellismus mercurialis.** The unintelligible, hurried, jerking speech accompanying mercurial tremor.

pseud-. See pseudo-.

pseu·dac"ro·meg'a·ly. Enlargement of the face and extremities without any involvement of the pituitary gland.

pseu"da·cu'sis (sue"da·cue'sis, -koo'sis). A disturbance of hearing in which the person's own voice sounds strange or peculiar, being altered in pitch and quality.

pseu"da·graph'i·a (sue"da·graf'ee·uh, -gray'fee·uh). 1. Incomplete agraphia, in which a person can copy correctly but is unable to write independently of an original. 2. The form of agraphia in which meaningless words are written.

pseu"dan·ky·lo'sis. A false joint; a false or fibrous ankylosis.

pseu"dar·thro'sis. A false joint.

pseu"des·the'si·a (sue"dess·thee'-zhuh, -zee·uh). An imaginary sensation for which there is no corresponding object, as a sensation referred to parts of the body that have been removed by accident or surgical operation. Ghost or phantom sensations.

pseu"di·a'ter (sue"dee·ay'tur). A quack, or charlatan.

pseu'do- (sue'do-), **pseud-.** 1. A combining form meaning false, deceptive resemblance to a disease or condition. 2. In chemistry, a combining form meaning resemblance to or isomerism with a compound.

pseu"do·al·bu"mi·nu'ri·a. False albuminuria; the presence in the urine of protein derived from blood, pus, or special secretions and mixed with the urine during its transit through the urinary passages.

pseu"do·a·ne'mi·a. Pallor and appearance of anemia without blood changes to support the diagnosis. Also called *apparent anemia*.

pseu″do·an·gi′na (sue″do·an·jy′-nuh, ·an′ji·nuh). A mental disorder characterized by pain in the chest at the apex of the heart and at times radiating down the left arm, with no evidence of organic disease. A psychosomatic complex in a neurotic person with precordial anxiety.

pseu″do·an″gi·o′ma. 1. Recanalized thrombus of the portal vein. 2. The formation of a temporary angioma, as is sometimes seen in healing stumps.

pseu″do·an″o·rex′i·a. Rejection of food because of gastric distress.

pseu″do·ap′o·plex″y. A condition resembling apoplexy, but unaccompanied by cerebral hemorrhage.

pseu″do·ap·pen″di·ci′tis. A condition simulating appendicitis, but with no lesion of the vermiform process.

pseu″do·ath″er·o′ma. Multiple sebaceous cysts; soft, painless tumors in or beneath the skin.

pseu″do·a·tro″pho·der′ma col′li. A rare skin disease characterized by depigmented areas surrounded by hyperpigmented skin. Often found about the neck but may occur elsewhere. Skin in center of lesion appears atrophic.

pseu″do·blep′si·a, pseu″do·blep′sis. A visual hallucination; a distorted visual image.

pseu″do·chan′cre (sue″do·shang′kur). An indurated sore simulating chancre.

pseu″do·cho″li·nes′ter·ase (·ko″li·nes′tur·ace, ·aze). An enzyme which catalyzes the hydrolysis of acetylcholine but which differs from cholinesterase in that it is nonspecific and hydrolyzes esters other than choline esters.

pseu″do·chrom″es·the′si·a (sue″do·krohm″ess·thee′zhuh, ·zee·uh). A condition in which each of the vowels of a word (whether seen, heard, or remembered) seems to have a distinct visual tint. See *photism*.

pseu″do·chrom″hi·dro′sis (sue″do·krohm″hi·dro′sis, ·high·dro′sis). A form of colored sweat in which the color changes occur after the sweat is excreted, possibly as a result of action by chromatogenous microörganisms.

pseu″do·chro′mi·a. A false or incorrect perception of color.

pseu″do·cir·rho′sis (sue″do·si·ro′sis). A condition characterized by enlargement of the liver, due to obstruction of the hepatic vein, inferior vena cava, or adhesive pericarditis. Also called *Pick's syndrome*.

pseu″do·col′loid. A mucoid material, found particularly in ovarian cysts. **p. of the lips.** A condition of

yellow-orange tumors in the lips a[...] mucosa of the mouth.

pseu″do·cri′sis. A false crisis; sudden fall of temperature resembl[...] the crisis of a disease, but subsequen[...] followed by a rise of temperature a[...] a continuation of the fever. It is co[...]mon in pneumonia.

pseu″do·croup″. False croup; lar[...] gismus stridulus.

pseu″do·cy·e′sis (sue″do·sigh·[...]sis). Phantom pregnancy; the belief, [...] the part of a woman, in the existe[...] of pregnancy when none exists. A [...]ease due to a disorder of metaboli[...] growth, or nutrition.

pseu″do·cyl′in·droid. A band [...] mucus or any substance in the ur[...] simulating a renal cast.

pseu″do·cyst″. A saclike space c[...]taining liquid, semiliquid, or gas [...] without a definite lining membran[...]

pseu″do·de·men′ti·a. A condit[...] of apathy resembling dementia, [...] without the mental degenera[...] changes.

pseu″do·e·de′ma. A condition s[...]ulating edema.

pseu″do·en″do·me·tri′tis. A co[...]dition resembling endometritis ma[...] by changes in the blood vessels, hyp[...]plasia of the glands, and atrophy [...]

pseu″do·ep′i·lep″sy. A disor[...] simulating epilepsy.

pseu″do·geu″ses·the′si·a (su[...] do·gew″sess·thee′zhuh, sue″do·jew[...] A condition in which color sensati[...] accompany the sense of taste.

pseu″do·geu′si·a (sue″do·gew′s[...]uh, ·jew″see·uh). A false perception [...] hallucination, of taste, which r[...] often be an aura in some types of fo[...] epilepsy.

pseu″do·glob′u·lin. A glob[...] fraction soluble in distilled water [...] well as in dilute salt solutions. A[...] see *euglobulin*.

pseu″do·gon″or·rhe′a. A sim[...] nonspecific urethritis.

pseu″do·he″mo·phil′i·a (sue[...] hee″mo·fill′ee·uh, ·hem″o·fill′ee·u[...] A condition characterized by prolon[...] bleeding time but without the dela[...] coagulation time of true hemoph[...] The platelets are normal in number [...] impaired in quality.

pseu″do·her·maph′ro·dite. [...] individual with congenitally malfor[...] external genitalia resembling one [...] while the gonads are those of the op[...] site sex. **pseudohermaprhodi[...]ic,** *adj.*; **pseudohermaph[...]ditism,** *n.*

pseu″do·hy″dro·ne·phro′s[...] The presence of a cyst near the kid[...] which resembles hydronephrosis.

pseu″do·hy″dro·pho′bi·a. [...] dread of hydrophobia, often produc[...]

a condition resembling the disease. Syn., *cynophobia, lyssophobia.*

pseu"do·hy·per'tro·phy (sue"do-high·pur'tro·fee). False hypertrophy; increase in the size of an organ on account of overgrowth of an important tissue. It is accompanied by diminution in function.—**pseudohypertroph'ic,** *adj.*

pseu"do·il'e·us. 1. An acute attack of severe abdominal pain with distension, resembling obstructive ileus but without apparent morphologic change. 2. Acute dilatation of the stomach.

pseu"do·jaun'dice (sue"do·jawn'dis, ·jahn'dis). Yellow discoloration of the skin from causes other than hepatic disease.

pseu"do·leu·ke'mi·a (sue"do·lew·kee'mee-uh). A condition with a blood picture which resembles leukemia. **in·fantile p.** A form of anemia occurring in young children, usually dependent on a rachitic diathesis, and associated with mild leukocytosis; also called von *Jaksch's disease.*

pseu"do·li·thi'a·sis. A condition in which the symptoms point to the existence of a calculus in the biliary or urinary passages but where no stone can be demonstrated.

pseu"do·lo'gi·a fan·tas'ti·ca. A syndrome marked by a single, elaborate phantasy, of which the patient gives full details. The phantasy includes real occurrences added to a fantastic basis.

pseu"do·mal'a·dy. An imaginary or simulated illness.

pseu"do·ma'ni·a. 1. A mental disorder in which the patient accuses himself of crimes of which he is innocent. 2. A mania characterized by lying. 3. An excited mental state in hysteria which simulates true mania.

pseu"do·men"stru·a'tion. Bloody vaginal discharge in newborn infants, ceasing after a few days.

pseu"do·mo'nas. A genus of bacteria of the family Pseudomonadaceae; members are small, motile, aerobic, and gram-negative. **Ps. aeruginosa.** A species of bacteria pathogenic to man; it is the causative agent of various suppurative infections in man. Also called *Ps. pyocyanea.* **Ps. cyanogenes.** Motile rods which form a blue pigment. Formerly called *Bacillus lactis cyanogenes.*

pseu"do·mor'phine (sue"do·mor'feen, ·fin). $C_{34}H_{38}O_8N_2.3H_2O$. A product resulting from condensation of two molecules of morphine with elimination of two hydrogen atoms. It is identical with the substances which have been called dehydromorphine, oxymorphine, oxydimorphine, and phormin.

pseu"do·mu'cin. A substance allied to mucin, found in proliferative cysts. —**pseudomucinous,** *adj.*

pseu"do·myx·o'ma. An epithelial tumor which contains much mucus, but so interspersed with tissue that grossly it suggests myxoma. **p. peritonaei.** (a) A widespread implantation in the peritoneum of secondary nodules from mucinous cystadenocarcinoma of the ovary. (b) A condition marked by the presence of mucus in the peritoneal cavity from rupture of a mucocele of the vermiform process.

pseu"do·ne'o·plasm. 1. A phantom tumor. 2. A temporary swelling, generally of inflammatory origin. —**pseudoneoplas'tic,** *adj.*

pseu"do·neu·ro'ma. A whorled mass of nerve fibers, usually myelinated, occurring in amputation stumps due to regenerating fibers of severed nerves; not a neoplasm. Also called *amputation neuroma.*

pseu"do·nu'cle·in. See *paranuclein.*

pseu"do·nys·tag'mus. Symptoms resembling nystagmus but without the regular rhythmic movements of true nystagmus.

pseu"do·os"te·o·ma·la'ci·a (sue"do·os"tee·o·ma·lay'shee-uh, ·see-uh). Rachitis in which the pelvis is distorted and resembles in form that of osteomalacia.

pseu"do·po'di·um, pseu'do·pod. 1. A temporary protrusion of a portion of the cytoplasm of an ameboid cell, as an aid to locomotion or for engulfing particulate matter. 2. *In allergy,* an irregular projection of the margin of a wheal.

pseu"do·re·ac'tion. A nonspecific reaction. A localized reaction following the intracutaneous inoculation of a test substance, due to impurities contained in the material. The reaction may be of an allergic nature and is frequently observed in the Schick test for immunity to diphtheria.

pseu·dos'mi·a (sue·doz'mee-uh, sue·dos'·). Perversion of the sense of smell; an olfactory hallucination. A disorder frequently observed in the uncinate type of epilepsy.

pseu"do·strat'i·fied. Characterizing an epithelium in which the cells all reach the basement membrane, but are of different lengths, with their nuclei lying at different levels, thus producing the appearance of several layers of cells.

pseu"do·ta'bes (sue"do·tay'beez). 1. A disease simulating tabes dorsalis or tabes mesenterica. 2. The ataxic form of alcoholic multiple neuritis.

pseu"do·tu·ber"cu·lo'sis. A general term for a pulmonary infection caused by a variety of fungi or bacteria other than the tubercle bacillus; found in man and lower animals.

pseu″do·vom′it·ing. Passive regurgitation of material from the stomach, without expulsive effort.

psi′caine (sigh′kane, sigh′kay-een, -in). (COOH.COOH) ₂NCH₃.C₇H₁₀(CO-OCH₃)O.COC₆H₅. d-ψ-Cocaine bitartrate; occurs as white crystals; soluble in water. Used as a local anesthetic.

psi·lo′sis (sigh·lo′sis). 1. Old term for sprue, q.v. 2. Falling out of the hair. **—psilot′ic,** adj.

psit″ta·co′sis (sit″uh·ko′sis). An acute febrile disease caused by a polytropic virus. Characterized in man by pneumonia and in parrots and related species by enteritis.

pso′as (so′us). One of two muscles, **psoas major** and **psoas minor**. Psoas major arises from the bodies and transverse processes of the lumbar vertebrae and is inserted on the lesser trochanter of the femur. Psoas minor has a similar origin and is inserted on the pubis. See Table of Muscles in the Appendix.

pso·i′tis (so·eye′tis). Inflammation of the psoas major muscle.

pso″mo·pha·gi·a (so″mo·fay′juh, ·jee·uh), **pso·moph′a·gy** (so·mof′-uh·jee). The swallowing of food without thorough chewing. **—psomophag′ic,** adj.

pso·ri·a·sis (so·rye′uh·sis). A chronic inflammatory skin disease characterized by the development of reddish patches covered with silvery-white imbricated scales. The disease affects especially the extensor surfaces of the body and the scalp. **p. diffusa.** A form in which there is coalescence of large contiguous lesions affecting large areas of the body. **p. discoidea.** A form in which the patches are the size of small coins. Also called p. nummularis. **p. follicularis.** A form in which scaly lesions are located at the openings of sweat and sebaceous glands. **p. gyrata.** Psoriasis with a serpentine arrangement of the patches. **p. inveterata.** One with persistent infiltrated lesions which often fissure and become covered with heavy scales. **p. palmaris.** A form affecting the palms of the hands. **p. punctata.** A form in which the lesions consist of minute red papules which rapidly become surmounted by pearly scales. **p. rupioides.** A variety in which large conical crusts marked by concentric rings occur. **p. universalis.** A form in which the lesions are all over the body. **pustular p.** A variety in which pustules and vesicles occur; involves mainly the palms and soles. It is a chronic recalcitrant eruption, and opinion is divided as to its relation to psoriasis.

pso″ri·at′ic (sor″ee·at′ick). Pertaining to or affected with psoriasis.

pso″roph·thal′mi·a (sor″off·thal′mee·uh). Blepharitis ciliaris.

P. S. P. Phenolsulfonphthalein test.

psy′cha·go″gy (sigh′kuh·go″jee). reëducational, psychotherapeutic pr cedure which stresses the proper socie ization of the individual. **—psych gog′ic,** adj.

psy·chal′gi·a (sigh·kal′jee·uh). Pai in the head, ascribed by depressed p tients to anxiety, or to some psych rather than a physical cause.

psy″chas·the′ni·a (sigh″kass·thee nee·uh, ·thi·nigh′uh). A term coined Janet which applies to all psychone roses containing compulsive, obsessiv and phobic tensions. A nervous sta characterized by an urge to think, fee or do something which at the same tin is recognized by the patient as beir senseless, silly, or irrational. Ra **—psychasthen′ic,** adj.

psy″cha·tax′i·a. Impaired power mental concentration; mental conf sion or groping.

psych·au·di·to″ry (syke·aw′di·to ree). Pertaining to the conscious or i tellectual interpretation of sounds.

psy′che (sigh′kee). The mind as functional entity, serving to adjust t total organism to the needs or deman of the environment.

psy′che·ism (sigh′kee·iz·um). Me merism; animal magnetism.

psy″chen·to′ni·a (sigh″ken·to′ne uh). Mental strain or overwork.

psy·chi′a·ter (sigh·kigh′uh·tur). alienist; a psychiatrist.

psy″chi·at′ric (sigh″kee·at′ric sick″ee·at′rick). Pertaining to psych atry.

psy″chi·at′rics. The theory or pra tice of psychiatry.

psy·chi′a·trist (sigh·kigh′uh·tri si·kigh′·). A specialist in psychiatr

psy·chi′a·try (sigh·kigh′uh·tree, kigh′·). The treatment of diseases the mind.

psy′chic, psy′chi·cal. 1. Pertainir to the mind or psyche. 2. Sensitive nonphysical forces.

psy′cho- (sigh′ko-), **psych-.** A co bining form denoting mind, ment processes, psychologic methods.

psy″cho·a·nal′y·sis (sigh″ko·a al′i·sis). 1. The method developed Sigmund Freud for the exploration a synthesis of patterns in emotion thinking and development; a techni used in the treatment of a wide varie of emotional disorders, particularly t neuroses. Relies essentially upon t free associations of the patient to pr duce valuable information of which t patient was formerly unaware, bringing to conscious manipulatio ideas and experiences from the unco scious divisions of the psyche. 2. T body of data and theory based on t discoveries of this method; concerned chiefly with the conflict between infantile instinctual striving and parental or social demand, and the manner in which this conflict affects emotional growth, character development, and the formation of mental and emotional disorders.

psy″cho·an′a·lyst (sigh″ko·an′uh·list). One who practices psychoanalysis.

psy″cho·bi·ol′o·gist (sigh″ko·buy·ol′o·jist). One who specializes in psychobiology.

psy″cho·bi·ol′o·gy. The study of the total biologic and psychic development of the individual, with particular emphasis upon the relationship of the individual to his environment. —**psychobiolog′ic,** adj.

psy″cho·di″ag·nos′tics. The evaluation of the personality, as furnished by the Rorschach test.

psy″cho·dy·nam′ics (sigh″ko·dye·nam′icks, ·di·nam′icks). The study of psychology from the point of view of the causative factors in mental activity. —**psychodynam′ic,** adj.

psy″cho·gal″va·nom′e·ter. A device for recording electrodermal responses to various mental stimuli which provoke emotional reactions. Its practical application is the lie detector, which indicates the emotional reactions of one who is suppressing the truth.

psy″cho·gen′e·sis. 1. The development of mental characteristics. 2. The process by which activities or ideas originate in the mind, or psyche. 3. The origin of psychic activity contributing to a psychosis. —**psychogen′ic, psychogenet′ic,** adj.

psy″cho·geu′sic (sigh″ko·gew′sick, ·jew′sick). Pertaining to perception of taste.

psy′cho·gram. A chart or table of personality traits.

psy″cho·graph′ic. 1. Relating to a chart of the personality traits of an individual. 2. In psychiatry, relating to the natural history of the mind.

psy″cho·ki·ne′si·a (sigh″ko·ki·nee′shuh, sigh″ko·kigh·), **psy″cho·ki·ne′sis** (sigh″ko·ki·nee′sis, ·kigh·nee′sis). Explosive or impulsive maniacal action; a lack of inhibition of primitive instincts leading to violent and hasty actions.

psy″cho·log′ic screen′ing. The use of psychologic tests, usually for large groups, as a means of determining general fitness for any specific duty, such as army service.

psy·chol′o·gist. One who specializes in psychology.

psy·chol′o·gy. The science which studies the functions of the mind, such as sensation, perception, memory, thought, and, more broadly, the behavior of an organism in relation to its environment. —**psycholog′ic, psycholog′ical,** adj. **abnormal p.** The study of the irregular and pathologic mental phenomena, such as hallucinations and delusions, which occur in mental illnesses. **applied p.** That branch of psychology which emphasizes practical rather than theoretical objectives. It includes medical, industrial, educational, clinical, and similar branches of psychology. Refers also to the interpretation of data in history, literature, and such fields according to psychologic principles. **depth p.** That relating to all unconscious mental activity. **dynamic p.** 1. In psychiatry, refers to the Freudian concepts which ascribe to the energy of the libido a potent role in mental symptoms. 2. In psychology, an approach which emphasizes the cause-and-effect relations between conscious and unconscious phenomena and stresses the process nature of personality. **experimental p.** The study of psychologic phenomena by experimental methods. **individual p.** A system developed by Alfred Adler. The individual is regarded as an indivisible unit of human society; his individual traits are compared, in terms of a striving for superiority which is assumed to exist in everyone, and then restated to provide a composite picture of a single tendency expressed in many ways. **industrial p.** Psychology applied to problems in industry dealing chiefly with the selection and mental health of personnel. **physiologic p.** That branch of psychology which investigates the structure and functions of the nervous system and bodily organs in their relationship to behavior.

psy·chom′e·try (sigh·kom′i·tree), **psy″cho·met′rics.** The measurement of the duration and intensity of psychic processes. Frequently applied to mean the measurement of intelligence. —**psychomet′ric,** adj.

psy″cho·mo′tor. Pertaining to or designating the area of the brain related to motor function; also, pertaining to voluntary movements controlled by the motor area.

psy″cho·neu·ro′sis. A term applied to a large group of clinical disorders all of which are on a functional, non-organic basis and which result in only a partial disorganization of the psyche. All varieties of psychoneurosis are characterized by emotional states of anxiety and fear, by preoccupation, obsession, and psychosomatic tension in different organ systems.

psy″cho·neu·rot′ic. Relating to, or affected by, a psychoneurosis.

psy″cho·nom′ics. That science dealing with the laws of the mind; psychology. —**psychonomic**, *adj.*

psy"cho·path. A morally irresponsible person; one who continually comes in conflict with accepted behavior and the law.

psy"cho·path'i·a. Psychopathy. **p. chirurgicalis.** A mania for being operated upon. **p. sexualis.** Psychopathic perversion of sexual functions.

psy"cho·pa·thol'o·gist. One who specializes in the pathology of mental diseases.

psy"cho·pa·thol'o·gy. The pathology of mental diseases.

psy"chop'a·thy (sigh·cop'uth·ee). Any disease of the mind. —**psychopath'ic**, *adj.*

psy"cho·phar"ma·col'o·gy. The branch of pharmacology concerned with psychological effects of drugs. —**psychopharmacolog'ic**, *adj.*

psy"cho·pho"nas·the'ni·a. A speech difficulty of mental origin.

psy"cho·phys'ics. 1. The study of mental processes by physical methods. 2. The study of the relation of stimuli to the sensations which they produce, especially the determination of the differences of stimulus required to produce recognizable differences of sensation; experimental psychology. —**psychophysical**, *adj.*

psy"cho·phys"i·ol'o·gy. Physiologic psychology; mental physiology.

psy"cho·ple'gic. A drug which lessens excitability and suppresses receptivity.

psy"cho·rhyth'mi·a (sigh"ko·rith'mee·uh, ·rith'mee·uh). A mental condition in which there is involuntary repetition of previous volitional behavior.

psy"cho·sen'so·ry. Pertaining to perception of sensory impulses at conscious levels.

psy"cho·sex'u·al. Relating to the mental and emotional aspects of sexuality as contrasted with the strictly physical or endocrine manifestations.

psy·cho'sin (sigh·ko'sin). A cerebroside derivative representing a combination of sphingosine and galactose.

psy·cho'sis (sigh·ko'sis) (pl. *psychoses*). A mental disorder characterized by disintegration of the personality and its break with reality. See also *neurosis.* —**psychot'ic**, *adj.* **alcoholic p.** Psychosis caused by alcoholism; chronic delirium tremens. **climacteric p.** A psychic reaction associated with menopause. **degenerative p.** A psychosis in which puerilism is exhibited. **exhaustive p.** Essentially the same as collapse delirium, but a more severe mental disorder. **famine p.** See *p. induced by starvation.* **gestational p.** One arising during pregnancy.

involutional p. A psychosis due to senility. See climacteric p., senile p. **manic-depressive p.** One characterized by states of mania or melancholia or both. Syn., *affective-reaction* p. **organic p.** A psychosis associated with demonstrable organic disease such as brain tumor, paresis, pellagra, and traumatic encephalopathy. **postinfectious p.** Mental disturbance following acute disease, such as pneumonia or typhoid fever. **p. induced by starvation.** A psychosis seen in war-torn countries when starvation is severe and widespread. **puerperal p.** A psychosis associated with the puerperium. **reactive p.** A psychosis which is supposed to be precipitated by an environmental condition. Also called *situational* p. **senile p.** A psychosis occurring in old age.

psy"cho·so·mat'ic. Of or pertaining to the mind and body, as in affections with an emotional background having both mental and bodily components. Especially relating to a system of medicine which emphasizes the interdependence of mental processes and physical or somatic functions.

psy"cho·sur'ger·y. Frontal lobotomy, or operative section of the frontothalamic fibers of the brain; used in the treatment of certain mental disorders.

psy"cho·ther"a·peu'tic. 1. Of or pertaining to psychotherapy. 2. Designating a drug, as an ataraxic, used in mental or clinical disorders to reduce tension and anxiety.

psy"cho·ther'a·py. 1. The treatment of disease by suggestion. 2. The treatment of mental diseases.

psy"cho·to·mi·met'ic. Capable of producing temporary psychotic symptoms, as hallucinations.

psy"cho·trop'ic. Capable of altering brain function through stimulation or sedation.

psy·chral'gi·a (sigh·kral'jee·uh). **psy"chro·al'gi·a.** A condition characterized by a painful subjective sense of cold.

psy'chro-. A combining form meaning *cold.*

psy"chro·es·the'si·a (sigh"kro·es·thee'zhuh, ·zee·uh). Subjective sensation of cold.

psy"chro·lu'si·a. Cold bathing.

psy·chrom'e·ter (sigh·krom'i·tur). A hygrometer for determining atmospheric moisture by observing the difference in the indication of two identical thermometers, the bulb of one being kept dry, and the other wet.

psy"chro·pho'bi·a. 1. Morbid fear of cold. 2. Morbid sensibility to cold.

psy'chro·phore. An instrument for applying cold to deeply seated parts, as a double-current catheter for applying cold to the posterior part of the urethra.

psy"chro·ther'a·py. The treatment of disease by the use of cold.

psy'co·sin, psy·co'sin. The galactoside of sphingol.

psyl'li·um seed (sil'ee·um). See *plantago* seed.

Pt. Chemical symbol for platinum.

pt. Pint.

ptar'mic (tahr'mick). 1. Pertaining to the act of sneezing; sternutative. 2. A substance that produces sneezing.

ptar'mus (tahr'mus). Sneezing.

pter'i·on (terr'ee·on, teer'ee·on). The region (not a point) surrounding the sphenoparietal suture where the frontal bone, parietal bone, squama temporalis, and greater wing of the sphenoid bone come together most closely.

pter'o- (terr'o-). A combining form meaning *feather, wing*.

pter"o·yl·glu·tam'ic ac'id. Folic acid.

pte·ryg'i·um (teh·ridj'ee·um, ti·ridj'·). 1. A triangular patch of mucous membrane growing on the conjunctiva, usually on the nasal side of the eye. The apex of the patch points toward the pupil, the fan-shaped base toward the canthus. 2. Eponychium. 2. 3. Any fold of skin extending abnormally from one part of the body to another. **—pterygial,** *adj.*

pter'y·go- (terr'i·go-). A combining form denoting *connection with,* or *relation to, the pterygoid process.*

pter'y·goid (terr'i·goyd). 1. Wing-shaped, as the pterygoid process of the sphenoid bone. 2. Pertaining to the pterygoid canal, pterygoid process, pterygoid plexus, etc.

pter"y·go·max'il·lar'y (terr"i·go·mack'si·lerr"ee). Pertaining to the pterygoid process and the maxilla.

pter"y·go·pal'a·tine (terr"i·go·pal'uh·tyne, ·tin). Situated between the pterygoid process of the sphenoid bone and the palatine bone, as the pterygopalatine canal.

pter"y·go·pha·ryn'ge·us. The part of the superior constrictor of the pharynx which arises from the medial pterygoid plate.

pti·lo'sis (ti·lo'sis). Falling out of the eyelashes.

P. T. O. Perlsucht tuberculin original; a tuberculin prepared from bovine tubercle bacilli, in the same manner as Koch's original tuberculin. Also called *Klemperer's tuberculin.*

pto'maine (to'mayn, to·mayn', to'may·een, ·in). An amino compound which results from the decomposition of proteins or dead animal matter by microörganisms.

pto'sis (to'sis). Prolapse, abnormal depression, or falling down of an organ; applied especially to drooping of the upper eyelid, due to paralysis or atrophy of the levator palpebrae superioris. **—ptosed, ptot'ic,** *adj.* **congenital p.** An anomaly of drooping upper eyelids due to absent or incomplete innervation of the levatores palpebrarum muscles.

-pto'sis. A combining form meaning *a lowered position of an organ.*

P. T. R. Perlsucht tuberculin rest; a tuberculin prepared from bovine tubercle bacilli.

pty·al'a·gogue (tye·al'uh·gog). A medicine producing a flow of saliva. Syn., *ptyalogogue.*

pty"a·lec'ta·sis (tye"uh·leck'tuh·sis). Dilatation of the duct of a salivary gland, either spontaneous or produced surgically.

pty'a·lin. A diastatic enzyme found in saliva, having the property of hydrolyzing starch to dextrin, maltose, and glucose, and hydrolyzing sucrose to glucose and fructose. Also called *ptyalase, salivary diastase.*

pty"a·lin'o·gen. The zymogen of ptyalin.

pty'a·lism. Salivation.

pty·al'o·gogue (tye·al'o·gog). A medicine causing a flow of saliva. Syn., *ptyalagogue.*

pty'a·lo·lith. A salivary calculus.

pty"a·lo·li·thi'a·sis (tye"uh·lo·li·thigh'uh·sis). The formation, or presence, of a salivary calculus.

pty"a·lor·rhe'a. Excessive flow of saliva.

pty'a·lose (tye'uh·loce). A sugar found in saliva. Syn., *maltose.*

ptys'ma·gogue (tiz'muh·gog). A drug that promotes the secretion of saliva.

P. U. Pregnancy urine, signifying the chorionic gonadotropic hormone found in such urine.

Pu. Chemical symbol for plutonium.

pu'ber·ty. The period at which the generative organs become capable of exercising the function of reproduction; signalized in the boy by a change of voice and discharge of semen, in the girl by the appearance of the menses. **—puberal,** *adj.*

pu·ber'u·lic ac'id. $C_8H_6O_6$. An antibiotic from *Penicillium puberulum.*

pu·ber"u·lon'ic ac'id. $C_8H_6O_6$. An antibiotic from *Penicillium puberulum.*

pu'bes (pew'beez). 1. The hairy region covering the mons pubis. 2. The two pubic bones considered together; that portion of the hipbones forming the front of the pelvis.

pu·bes'cence. 1. Hairiness; the presence of fine, soft hairs. 2. Puberty, or the coming on of puberty. **—pubescent,** *adj.*

pu"bi·ot'o·my. The operation of dividing the pubic bone to facilitate delivery in cases of pelvic malformation. *Obs.*

pu′bis. Os pubis; the pubic bone, that portion of the hipbone forming the front of the pelvis. See Table of Bones in the Appendix.

Pub′lic Health Serv′ice. A bureau of the United States Government, maintained to safeguard the public health through sanitation, hygiene, and preventive medicine.

pu′bo-. *In anatomy,* a combining form denoting *relation to the pubes or pubis.*

pu″bo·cap′su·lar. Pertaining to the os pubis and the capsule of the hip joint. Used to denote a collateral ligament of the hip joint.

pu″bo·fem′o·ral. Pertaining to the os pubis and the femur, as the pubofemoral ligament, a collateral ligament of the hip joint capsule.

pu″den·dag′ra (pew″den·dag′ruh, ·day′gruh). Pain in the genital organs.

pu·den′dum (pl. *pudenda*). The external genital organs, especially of the female. **—pudendal,** *adj.*

pu′dic. Old term for pudendal.

pu·er·i·cul″ture (pew′ur·i·kul″- chur, pew·err′i·). The specialty of child training.

pu′er·il·ism. Childishness. **—puer- ile,** *adj.*

pu″er·i′ti·a (pew″ur·ish′ee·uh). Second childhood.

pu·er′per·a (pew·ur′pur·uh). A woman who is in labor or has recently been delivered.

pu·er′per·al (pew·ur′pur·ul). Pertaining to, caused by, or following childbirth, as puerperal convulsions, puerperal eclampsia.

pu·er′per·al·ism. The state brought about by pathologic conditions of pregnancy.

pu″er·pe′ri·um (pew″ur·peer′ee- um). 1. The state of a woman in labor, or of one who has just been delivered. 2. The period from delivery to the time when the uterus has regained its normal size, which is about six weeks.

puff′ball″. Any of the fungi Lycoperdaceae which discharge their ripe spores like dust when struck. Many are edible when unripe.

Pu′lex. A genus of fleas. **P. irri- tans.** The human flea; a species which is the intermediate host and transmitter of *Dipylidium caninum* and *Hymenolepis diminuta,* and may spread plague. It is parasitic on the skin of man and also infests hogs, dogs, and other mammals.

pu″li·ca′ti·o (pew″li·kay′shee·o). The state of being infested with fleas.

pu′li·cide. An agent capable of killing fleas.

pul′mo-. A combining form meaning *lung.*

pul′mo·nar″y (pul′mo·nerr″ee, pool′mo·). Pertaining to, or affecting, the lungs or any anatomic component of the lungs. Syn., *pulmonic.*

pul″mo·nec′to·my. Pneumonectomy.

pul′mo″tor (pul′mo″tur, pool′mo″- tur). An apparatus for resuscitating persons who have been asphyxiated; it expels the gas from the lungs, introduces oxygen, and automatically establishes artificial respiration.

pulp. 1. The soft, fleshy part of fruit. 2. The soft part in the interior of an organ, as the pulp of the spleen, the pulp of a tooth. **—pulp′al, pulp′ar** *adj.* **dental p.** The soft vascular tissue which fills the pulp chamber and the root canals of a tooth and is responsible for its vitality. It consists of connective tissue, blood vessels, and nerves. A superficial layer of cells, the odontoblasts, supplies branching processes which occupy tubules in the dentine. Also called *tooth p.*

pul·pal′gi·a. Pain in the dental pulp.

pulp″i·fac′tion. Conversion into a pulpy substance.

pulp·i′tis. An inflammation of the dental pulp.

pulp·ot′o·my. The surgical removal of the whole or a part of the pulp of a tooth.

pul′sate. Beat or throb.

pul′sa·tile (pul′suh·til). Pulsating throbbing.

pul″sa·til′la. The dried herb of *Anemone pulsatilla, A. pratensis,* or *A. patens.* The drug yields a volatile oil from which can be separated pulsatilla camphor or anemonin. Also called *pasqueflower.*

pul·sa′tion. A beating or throbbing.

pulse. The intermittent change in the shape of an artery due to an increase in the tension of its walls following the contraction of the heart. The pulse is usually counted at the wrist (radial pulse), but may be taken over an artery that is palpable, as the temporal, brachial, femoral, dorsalis pedis, etc. **alternating p.** A variety in which there are alternations in amplitude of pulse waves, that is, large pulsations alternating with small ones in cycles of equal length. A sign of cardiac failure. **angry p.** Wiry pulse, *q.v.* **ardent p.** One with a quick, full wave which seems to strike the finger at a single point. **bigeminal p.** One in which the beats occur in pairs, so that the longer pause follows every two beats. **capillary p.** An intermittent filling and emptying of the capillaries of the skin. It is common in aortic regurgitation, and is seen under the fingernail or on the forehead. **di crotic p.** One in which the dicrotic wave or recoil wave is exaggerated. It is observed when the arterial tension is low, and gives to the finger the impression of two beats. **febrile p.** That characteristic of fever: full, soft, and frequent, and exhibiting a well-marked dicrotism. **filiform p.** A small, thready, almost imperceptible pulse. **full p.** One in which the artery is filled with a large volume of blood and conveys a feeling of being distended. **funic p.** The arterial tide in the umbilical cord. **hard p.** One characterized by high tension and rigidity. **high-tension p.** One due to increase of the peripheral resistance, together with a corresponding increase in the force of the ventricular systole. It is gradual in its impulse, long in duration, slow in subsiding, with difficulty compressible, and the artery between the beats feels like a firm round cord. **infrequent p.** One which has a slower rate than normal. **intermittent p.** One in which one or more beats is dropped. **intricate p.** A pulse that is irregular, small, and infrequent. **irregular p.** One in which the beats occur at irregular intervals, or in which the force, or both rhythm and force, varies. **jerky p.** A pulse in which the artery is suddenly and markedly distended, as in aortic regurgitation. **jugular p.** Pulsation of the jugular veins in the neck. **paradoxic p.** One that is weaker during inspiration, a condition sometimes observed in acute and chronic cardiac compression. **pressure p.** The recorded pressure variations in a given heart chamber or blood vessel during the cardiac cycle; pressure curve. **Quincke's p.** A capillary pulse due to a high pulse pressure; seen classically in aortic regurgitation and elicited clinically by applying light pressure to a fingernail. See capillary p. **respiratory p.** The modification in the pulse produced by respiration. **running p.** A very weak, frequent pulse with low tension in the arteries, one pulse wave running into the next with no apparent interval; it is observed after hemorrhage. **thready p.** One that is scarcely perceptible, feeling like a thread under the finger. **unequal p.** A pulse unequal in symmetrical arteries. **venous p.** A pulse observed in a vein. **water-hammer p.** The pulse observed in aortic regurgitation, characterized by a rapid rise and fall, combined with large amplitude. **wiry p.** A small, rapid, tense pulse, which feels like a cord. Observed in acute peritonitis.

pulse curve. The tracing of the pulse, called a sphygmogram and made by the sphygmograph.

pulse cycle. The period between the beginning and end of a pulse wave.

pulse/less. Devoid of pulse or pulsation.

pul·sim'e·ter. An instrument for determining the rate or force of the pulse.

pul/sus. The pulse, q.v. **p. celer.** A quick, short pulse. **p. debilis.** A weak pulse. **p. durus.** A hard, incompressible pulse. **p. irregularis perpetuus.** The pulse of atrial fibrillation which is perpetually irregular in rate and amplitude. **p. parvus.** A pulse small in amplitude. **p. tardus.** A pulse with a gradual ascent to the peak.

pul·ta'ceous. Having the consistence of pulp; mushy; soft.

pulv. Pulvis; powder.

pul'ver·ize. Reduce a substance to a powder. —**pulveriza'tion,** n.

pul'vis. Abbreviated, pulv. See powder.

pu'mex. See pumice.

pum'ice (pum'iss). A substance of volcanic origin, consisting chiefly of complex silicates of aluminum, potassium, and sodium; occurs as a very light, hard, rough, porous gray mass, or as a gritty, gray-colored powder.

pump. An apparatus which draws up a fluid into a hollow chamber, or, after sucking up the fluid, forcibly ejects it from one end. **air p.** One used to exhaust the air from a chamber, or to force more air into a chamber already containing air. **breast p.** A pump for removing milk from the breast. **stomach p.** One for removing the contents of the stomach in cases of poisoning.

pump'kin seed. The dried, ripe seed of several varieties of Cucurbita pepo. The active constituents are resinous in character. It is used as an anthelmintic and taeniafuge.

punch. A surgical instrument for perforating or cutting out a disk or segment of resistant tissue, as cartilage, bone.

punch drunk. A postconcussional syndrome occurring in prize fighters.

punc'ta. Plural of punctum, q.v.

punc'tate, punc'tat·ed (punk'-tay-tid). Dotted; full of minute points.

punc·tic'u·lum. A small point.

punc'to·graph. A radiographic instrument for the surgical localization of foreign bodies, as bullets embedded in the tissues.

punc'tum (pl. puncta). Point, q.v. **puncta vasculosa.** Minute red spots studding the cut surface of the white central mass of the fresh brain. They are produced by the blood escaping from divided blood vessels. **p. dolorosum.** Tender or painful points at the exit or in the course of nerves; the seat of neuralgia. **p. proximum.** Near point. Abbreviated, P., P.p. **p. remotum.** Far point. Abbreviated, P.r.

punc′ture. 1. A hole made by the piercing of a pointed instrument. 2. The procedure of making a puncture. **ex-ploratory p.** The puncture of a cyst or cavity for removal of a portion of the contents for examination. **lum-bar p.** Puncture of the spinal canal, usually between the third and fourth lumbar vertebrae, for the removal of fluid or the introduction of drugs or se-rums. **sternal p.** Puncture of the manubrium with a hollow needle to ob-tain bone marrow specimens in disease of the hematopoietic system. **tibial p.** A puncture method used in children to secure smears of marrow cells. A sternal puncture needle is used in the middle of the shaft of the tibia. **ven-tricular p.** Puncture into one of the lateral ventricles of the brain to intro-duce air in ventriculography.

punc′tured. Produced by a prick, or a piercing instrument, weapon, or missile, as a punctured wound.

pun′gent. Acrid; penetrating; pro-ducing a painful sensation.

Pu′ni·ca. A genus of polypetalous plants. **P. granatum.** See under *pelletierine* tannate.

pu′ni·cine (pew′ni·seen, ·sin). See *pelletierine*.

punk′to·graph. Same as *puncto-graph*.

pu′pa. The stage, usually quiescent, in the life history of some insects, which follows the larval period and precedes the adult imago. —**pupal**, *adj.*

pu′pil. The aperture in the iris of the eye for the passage of light. —**pupillary**, *adj.* **Adie′s p.** An anomaly of the pupil which includes abnormality in the size of the pupil (usually eccentrically dilated) and im-pairment in, but not loss of, the re-action of the pupil either to light or in accommodation. Sometimes called *tonic pupil*. See Adie′s *syndrome*. **arti-ficial p.** An aperture made by iri-dectomy when the normal pupil is oc-cluded. **pinhole p.** Contraction of the iris until the pupil is scarcely larger than a pin′s head. It is seen in opium poisoning, after the use of miotics, in certain cerebral diseases, and in locomotor ataxia. Also called *pinpoint p.*

pu″pil·lom′e·ter. An instrument used for measuring the pupil of the eye.

pu″pil·lo·sta·tom′e·ter (pew″pil-lo·sta·tom′i·tur, pew·pill″o·). An in-strument for measuring the exact dis-tance between the centers of the two pupils.

pure. 1. Free from mixture or contact with that which weakens or pollutes; containing no foreign or extraneous material. 2. Chaste.

pur·ga′tion. 1. The evacuation of the bowels by means of purgatives. Cleansing.

pur′ga·tive. 1. Producing purgatio[n]. 2. A purge, *q.v.*

purge. 1. Cause free evacuation of t[he] bowel. 2. A drug that causes free evac[u]ation of the bowel.

purg′ing. A condition in which the[re] is rapid and continuous evacuation [of] the bowels.

pu′ri·fied. Cleansed; freed fro[m] extraneous matter.

pu′rine (pure′een, ·in). The synthet[ic] substance $C_5H_4N_4$, having the followi[ng] structure:

Various derivatives of this structur[e] generically called *purines* and inclu[d]-ing the xanthines and uric acid, a[re] widely distributed in nature.

purinethol. Trade-mark for me[r]-captopurine.

purodigin. A trade-mark for di[gi]-toxin.

pu″ro·hep″a·ti′tis. Suppurative i[n]-flammation of the liver.

pu″ro·mu′cous. Consisting [of] mucus mixed with pus; mucopurulen[t].

pur′pu·ra. A condition in whi[ch] hemorrhages occur in the skin, muco[us] membranes, serous membranes, a[nd] elsewhere, either without definite cau[se] or due to slight injury. The hemo[r]-rhages may be in the form of petechi[ae,] macules, or large patches. —**purpu-ric**, *adj.* **hemorrhagic p.** S[ee] idiopathic thrombocytopenic p. **id[i-] opathic thrombocytopenic [p.]** A systemic disease with petechiae [or] larger hemorrhages in the skin, usua[lly] appearing first in the extremities a[nd] then in successive crops over a lar[ge] part of the surface. Bleeding into a[nd] from mucous membranes, serous ca[vi]-ties, and elsewhere may occur. There [is] prolonged bleeding time, failure of t[he] clot to retract fully, and reduction [in] the number of platelets in the blo[od.] Also called *land scurvy, morbus mac[u-] losis Werlhofii, Werlhof′s disease.* **no[n-] thrombopenic p.** A type w[ith] bleeding from the intestinal tract a[nd] accompanied by abdominal pain, vom[it]-ing, and diarrhea. Also called *Henoc[h′s] p.* **p. annularis telangiectode[s.]** An eruption of purpuric spots, group[ed] in ring form and accompanied by tela[n]-giectasis. **p. fulminans.** A gra[ve] form, occurring principally in childr[en] with acute infectious disease, of sh[ort] duration, and usually fatal. **p. si[m]-plex.** A mild form of purpu[ra]

p. urticans. That associated with urticaria. See *urticaria* hemorrhagica.

rheumatic p. A form associated with acute arthritis. Also called *Schönlein's p.* **symptomatic p.** That which may accompany acute infectious diseases or chronic diseases such as malignant tumors, nephritis, and blood dyscrasias, and following administration of certain drugs. Also called *secondary p.*

pur'pu·rin. $C_{14}H_8O_5$. 1. A dye present with alizarin in madder-root, but also prepared artificially. 2. Uroerythrin, a red pigment sometimes present in urinary deposits.

pur'pu·ri·nu'ri·a. The presence of purpurin in the urine; porphyruria.

purr. A low-pitched murmur.

pur'ring thrill. A fine, trembling vibration like the purring of a cat, perceived by palpation over the precordia. It may be due to aneurysm or to mitral stenosis.

pu'ru·lence (pure'yoo·luns). The quality or state of containing pus. Also called *purulency.*

pu'ru·lent (pure'yoo·lunt). Containing, consisting of, or forming pus.

pu'ru·loid (pure'yoo·loyd). Resembling pus; puriform.

pus. A semifluid, creamy, yellow or greenish yellow product of inflammation composed mainly of leukocytes and serum. The color varies with the causative organism.

pus'tule. A small, circumscribed elevation of the skin containing pus. —**pustular, pustulose, pustulous,** *adj.*

pus"tu·lo·der'ma. Any skin disease characterized by the formation of pustules.

pu"tre·fac'tion. The decomposition of organic matter under the influence of microörganisms, accompanied by the development of disagreeable odors. The products include gases, as ammonia, hydrogen sulfide, methane, and others; acids, as acetic, lactic, butyric, and others; and toxic substances, as indole, skatole, phenol, and others. Cadaverine and putrescine are toxic products known as ptomaines.

pu"tre·fac'tive. Pertaining to or causing putrefaction.

pu'tre·fy. Render putrid.

pu·tres'cine (pew·tress'een, ·in). $C_4H_{12}N_2$. Tetramethylenediamine. A poisonous ptomaine.

pu'trid. Rotten; characterized by putrefaction.

pu"tro·maine (pew'tro·mayn, pew"tro·may'een, ·in). A ptomaine developed in putrefactive processes.

PVP Abbreviation for polyvinylpyrrolidone.

py"ar·thro'sis. Suppuration of a joint.

pyc·nom'e·ter. An instrument for the determination of the specific gravity of fluids.

pyc"no·phra'si·a (pick"no·fray'zhuh, ·zee·uh). Thickness of speech.

pyc·no'sis. 1. Thickening; inspissation. 2. A degenerative change in cells whereby the nucleus is condensed and shrinks to a dense, structureless mass of chromatin. —**pycnot'ic,** *adj.*

py·ec'chy·sis (pye·eck'i·sis). Effusion of pus.

py"e·lec·ta'si·a (pye"i·leck·tay'zhuh). Dilatation of a renal pelvis.

py"e·li'tis. Inflammation of the pelvis of a kidney. —**pyelit'ic,** *adj.* **calculous p.** That due to calculi.

py'e·lo-. A combining form denoting relation to *the pelvis of the kidney.*

py"e·lo·cys·ti'tis. Pyelitis with cystitis.

py'e·lo·gram". A roentgenogram of the renal pelvis and ureter.

py"e·log'ra·phy. Roentgenography of a renal pelvis and ureter which have been filled with an opaque solution.

py"e·lo·li·thot'o·my. Removal of a renal calculus through an incision into the pelvis of a kidney.

py"e·lo·ne·phri'tis. Inflammation of a kidney and its pelvis, usually an infection ascending from the ureter. —**pyelonephrit'ic,** *adj.*

py'e·lo·plas"ty. Plastic repair of the renal pelvis.

py"e·lo·pli·ca'tion (pye"i·lo·plye·kay'shun, ·pli·kay'shun). Reducing an enlarged renal pelvis by plicating or suturing the infolded walls.

py"e·los'co·py. Fluoroscopic examination of the pelvis of a kidney.

py"e·los'to·my. Incision into the renal pelvis.

py"e·lot'o·my. Incision of the renal pelvis.

py·em'e·sis (pye·em'i·sis). Vomiting of pus.

py·e'mi·a (pye·ee'mee·uh). A disease due to the presence of pyogenic microörganisms in the blood and the formation, wherever these organisms lodge, of embolic or metastatic abscesses. —**pyemic,** *adj.* **arterial p.** That produced by disorganization of a cardiac thrombus and the dissemination of emboli through the arterial circulation. **cryptogenic p.** A condition in which the primary suppuration occurs in the deeper tissues of the body. **otogenous p.** Pyemia originating in the ear.

py"en·ceph'a·lus. Suppuration within the brain.

py·gal'gi·a (pye·gal'juh, ·jee·uh). Pain in the buttocks.

pyg·ma'li·on·ism. The psychopathic condition in which an individual falls in love with a creation of his own.

pyg'my. A small person or dwarf.

py·gop'a·gus (pye·gop'uh·gus). Conjoined twins united in the sacral region.

py'in. An albuminous substance of complex constitution occurring in pus. It may be separated by adding sodium chloride and filtering.

pyk'nic. Referring to a constitutional body type marked by roundness of contour, amplitude of body cavities, and considerable subcutaneous fat.

pyk'no-. For words beginning *pykno-* not found here, see under *pycno-*.

pyk'no·lep"sy. A very mild form of epileptic variant, resembling petit mal. It appears as a fleeting mental blankness associated with a momentary stare. There are no tonic seizures, no falls, and no convulsions or true losses of consciousness. Electroencephalogram shows large, slow, delta waves.

py"le·phle·bec'ta·sis, py"le·phleb"ec·ta'si·a (pye"li·fleb"eck·tay'zhuh, ·shuh). Dilatation of the portal vein, usually caused by some obstruction in the liver, but it may be due to relaxation of the vessel walls from some disturbance of innervation.

py"le·phle·bi'tis. Inflammation of the portal vein. The condition is usually secondary to disease of the intestine, is generally suppurative in character, and gives rise to the symptoms of pyemia.

py"le·throm"bo·phle·bi'tis. Inflammation and thrombosis of the portal vein.

py"le·throm·bo'sis. Thrombosis of the portal vein.

py"lo·ral'gi·a. Pain in the region of the pylorus.

py"lo·rec'to·my. Excision of the pylorus; partial gastrectomy.

py·lor"i·ste·no'sis (pye·lor"i·sti·no'sis, pi·lor"i·). Constriction of the pylorus.

py"lor·i'tis. Inflammation of the pylorus.

py·lor'o- (pye·lor'o-, pi·lor'o-), **py·lor-.** A combining form meaning *relating to the pylorus*.

py·lor"o·col'ic. Pertaining to the pyloric end of the stomach and the transverse colon.

py·lor"o·di'la·tor (pye·lor"o·dye'lay·tur, ·dye·lay'tur). An appliance for dilating the pyloric orifice of the stomach.

py·lor"o·gas·trec'to·my. Resection of the pyloric end of the stomach; pylorectomy.

py·lor"o·my·ot'o·my (pye·lor"o·migh·ot'o·mee, pi·lor'o·). The division, anteriorly, of the pyloric muscle, without incision through the mucosa; for congenital pyloric stenosis in infants.

Also called *Ramstedt's operation, Fredet-Ramstedt operation.*

py·lor'o·plas"ty. An operation upon the pylorus, usually for stenosis due to ulcer, which may involve removal of portion of the pylorus but which, in principle, divides the pylorus on the gastric and duodenal sides transversely the wound being closed by sutures which convert it into a transverse incision. It provides a larger opening from stomach to duodenum. Also see *pylorotomy.*

py·lor"op·to'sis, py·lor"op·to'si·a. Downward displacement of the pylorus.

py·lor"o·sche'sis (pye·lor"o·skee'sis, pye"lo·ros'ki·sis). Obstruction of the pylorus.

py"lor·os'co·py. Inspection of the pylorus.

py·lor"o·spasm". Spasm of the pylorus.

py·lor"o·ste·no'sis. Stenosis, or stricture, of the pylorus.

py"lor·os'to·my. Incision into the pylorus, as in the formation of a gastric fistula.

py"lor·ot'o·my. An incision into or through the pylorus in the axis of the canal, converting it by sutures from a longitudinal to a transverse wound. Also called *pyloroplasty, Finney's operation, Heineke-Mikulicz operation, gastroduodenostomy.*

py·lo'rus (pye·lor'us, pi·lor'us). The circular opening of the stomach into the duodenum. 2. The fold of mucous membrane and muscular tissue surrounding the aperture between the stomach and the duodenum. 3. The final portion of the stomach, preceding the duodenum. —**pylor'ic,** *adj.*

py'o-, py-. A combining form meaning *suppuration, accumulation of pus,* or *related to pus formation.*

py'o·cele. Accumulation of pus in the tunica vaginalis testis.

py"o·ceph'a·lus. Pus within the cranium, especially in the cerebral ventricles.

py"o·che'zi·a (pye"o·kee'zee·uh). Discharge of pus with or in the stool.

py"o·col'po·cele. A suppurative cyst of the vagina.

py"o·col'pos. An accumulation of pus within the vagina.

py"o·cy'a·nase (pye"o·sigh'uh·nace, ·naze). An antibiotic from *Pseudomonas aeruginosa.*

py"o·cy·an'ic (pye"o·sigh·an'ick). Pertaining to blue pus, or to pyocyanin.

py"o·cy'a·nin. An antibiotic from *Pseudomonas aeruginosa;* soluble in chloroform.

py"o·cy"a·nol'y·sin (pye"o·sigh"uh·nol'i·sin, ·sigh·an"o·lye'sin). A hemolysin produced in broth cultures by *Pseudomonas aeruginosa.*

py″o·cyst″. A cyst containing pus.

py″o·der′ma. Any pus-producing skin lesion or lesions, used in referring to groups of furuncles, pustules, or even carbuncles. **p. faciale.** An intensely red or cyanotic erythema of the face with superficial and deep abscesses and cystic lesions. **p. gangrenosum.** A pyogenic ulceration, usually of the trunk, often with large irregular ulcers; usually associated with ulcerative colitis.

py″o·der″ma·ti′tis. A skin disease produced by infection with pyogenic organisms.

py″o·der″ma·to′sis. An inflammation of the skin in which pus formation occurs.

py·og′e·nes (pye·odj′i·neez). Pus-producing.

py″o·gen′e·sis. The formation of pus. —**pyogenic, pyogenet′ic, pyog′enous,** *adj.*

py″o·he″mo·tho′rax (pye″o·hee″mo·thor′acks, ·hem″o·thor′acks). 'Pus and blood in the pleural cavity.

py′oid. Resembling pus.

py′oktanin. Trade-mark for methylrosanilin chloride.

py″o·lab″y·rin·thi′tis. Suppurative inflammation of the labyrinth of the ear.

py″o·me′tra. A collection of pus in the uterus.

py″o·my″o·si′tis. Suppurative myositis.

py″o·ne·phri′tis. Suppurative inflammation of a kidney.

py″o·neph″ro·li·thi′a·sis. The presence of pus and calculi in a kidney.

py″o·ne·phro′sis. An accumulation of pus in the pelvis and calyces of a kidney. —**pyonephrot′ic,** *adj.*

py″o·o·va′ri·um. Ovarian abscess.

py″o·per″i·car·di′tis. Suppurative pericarditis.

py″o·per″i·car′di·um. The presence of pus in the pericardium.

py″o·per″i·to·ne′um. The presence of pus in the peritoneal cavity.

py″o·per″i·to·ni′tis. Suppurative inflammation of the peritoneum.

py″o·pha′gi·a. The swallowing of pus.

py″oph·thal′mi·a. Purulent ophthalmia.

py″o·phy·lac′tic. A defense against pus or pus formation.

py″o·phy″so·me′tra. The presence of pus and gas in the uterus.

py″o·pneu″mo·per″i·car·di′tis (pye″o·new″mo·perr″i·car·dye′tis, ·pye″op·). Pericarditis complicated by the presence of pus and gas in the pericardium.

py″o·pneu″mo·per″i·car′di·um. Pus and air or gas in the pericardium.

py″o·pneu″mo·per″i·to·ne′um. Pus and gas in the peritoneal cavity.

py″o·pneu″mo·per″i·to·ni′tis. Suppurative inflammation of the peritoneum associated with gas in the abdominal cavity.

py″o·pneu″mo·tho′rax (pye″o·new″mo·thor′acks, pye″op·). An accumulation of air or gas and pus in the pleural cavity.

py″o·poi·e′sis. Pus formation. —**pyopoiet′ic,** *adj.*

py·op′ty·sis (pye·op′ti·sis). The expectoration of pus.

py″or·rhe′a, py″or·rhoe′a. A purulent discharge. **alveolar p.** Periodontosis, *q.v.*

py″o·sal″pin·gi′tis. Purulent inflammation of a uterine or an auditory tube.

py″o·sal·pin″go·o″ö·pho·ri′tis. Combined suppurative inflammation of an ovary and oviduct.

py″o·sal′pinx. An accumulation of pus in an oviduct.

py·o′sis (pye·o′sis). Suppuration; pus formation.

py″o·stat′ic. 1. Preventing the formation of pus. 2. An agent arresting the formation of pus.

py″o·ther′a·py. The use of pus in the treatment of disease. *Obs.*

py″o·tho′rax. Empyema.

py″o·u·ra′chus (pye″o·yoo·ray′kus). The presence of pus in or about the urachus.

py″o·u·re′ter (pye″o·yoor·ee′tur, ·yoor′i·tur). An accumulation of pus in a ureter.

py″o·xan′thin (pye″o·zan′thin), **py″o·xan′those** (pye″o·zan′thoce). A yellow pigment sometimes found in pus, and resulting from the oxidation of pyocyanin.

py″ra·hex′yl (pye″ruh·heck′sil, pirr″uh·). Synhexyl, *q.v.*

pyr′a·mid. Any conical eminence of an organ; especially of a body of longitudinal nerve fibers on each side of the anterior median fissure of the medulla oblongata. —**pyram′idal,** *adj.*

pyramidon. Trade-mark for a brand of aminopyrine.

py′ran. The six-membered heterocyclic compound C_5H_6O, of which three isomers are possible. Certain natural compounds are often characterized as derivatives of a pyran and the pyranose form of certain sugars indicates structural relationship of the latter to a pyran.

py″ra·nis′a·mine. An earlier designation for the antihistaminic substance pyrilamine.

py′ra·nose. The isomeric form of certain sugars and glycosides structurally analogous to a pyran. See also *furanose.*

pyr″a·zin·am′ide (pyr″a·zin·am′-ide, -zin′a·mide). Pyrazine-carboxylic acid amide, a therapeutic agent for human tuberculosis.

py·rec′tic (pye·reck′tick). Pyretic, feverish.

py·re′thrum (pye·reeth′rum). The root of *Anacyclus pyrethrum*.

py·re′thrum flow′ers. The flower heads of *Chrysanthemum cinerariae-folium, C. coccineum (C. roseum),* and *C. Marschallii*. Should not be confused with pyrethrum, the root. Pyrethrum flowers are used as insect powder. The insecticidal power is probably due to two related compounds, pyrethrin I and pyrethrin II.

py·ret′ic (pye·ret′ick). Pertaining to or affected with fever.

pyr′e·to- (pirr′i·to-, pye′ri·to-). A combining form meaning *fever*.

py·ret′o·gen (pye·ret′o·jin). Any agent which induces fever.

pyr″e·to·ge·ne′si·a (pirr″i·to·ji-nee′zee·uh, pye″ri·to·), **pyr″e·to·gen′e·sis.** The origin and process of fever.

pyr″e·to·gen′ic, pyr″e·tog′e·nous (pirr″i·todj′i·nus, pye″ri·). Causing or producing fever.

pyr″e·tol′o·gist. A specialist in fevers.

pyr″e·tol′o·gy (pirr″i·tol′o·jee, pye″ri·). The science of the nature of fevers.

pyr″e·tol′y·sis. Reduction of a fever.

pyr″e·to·ther′a·py. Treatment of disease by the induction of fever in the patient.

pyr″e·to·ty·pho′sis (pirr″i·to·tye-fo′sis, pye″ri·to·). Old term for delirium in fever.

py·rex″e·o·pho′bi·a (pye″reck″see-o·fo′bee·uh). A morbid fear of fever; febriphobia.

py·rex′i·a (pye·reck′see·uh). Elevation of temperature above the normal; fever. **—pyrexial,** adj.

pyribenzamine. Trade-mark for tri-pelennamine, most commonly used in the form of its hydrochloride salt.

pyr′i·dine (pirr′i·deen, ·din). C_5H_5N. A heterocyclic compound, first of a series of homologous bases, occurring as a colorless liquid with a persistent odor; miscible with water in all proportions.

pyridium. Trade-mark for phenyl-azo-α,α-diaminopyridine monohydro-chloride used in acute and chronic urogenital infections.

pyr″i·dox′al. The 4-aldehyde of pyridoxine, an essential component of enzymes concerned with amino-acid decarboxylation and with transamination, and therefore with amino-acid synthesis.

pyr″i·dox′a·mine. The amine of pyridoxine in which NH_2 replaces the OH group in position 4; obtained in transamination of pyridoxal.

pyr″i·dox′ic ac′id. 2-Methyl-3-hy-droxy-4-carboxy-5-hydroxymethyl pyridine, a decomposition product occurring in urine following ingestion of pyridoxine by man.

pyr″i·dox′ine (pirr″i·dock′seen ·sin). $C_8H_{11}O_3N$. 2-Methyl-3-hydroxy-4,-5-di(hydroxymethyl)-pyridine; the term pyridoxine is synonymous with vitamin B_6; the hydrochloride occurs as a white, crystalline powder with a saline taste; soluble in water.

py·ril′a·mine. The antihistaminic substance N-p-methoxybenzyl-N′-N′-di-methyl-N-α-pyridylethylene diamine. Originally called *pyranisamine.* See *neo-antergan.*

pyr″i·meth′a·mine. 2,4-Diamino-5-p-chlorophenyl-6-ethylpyrimidine, a drug used in the treatment of malaria. See *daraprim.*

py·rim′i·dine (pye·rim′i·deen, pi-rim′·). 1. Any six-membered cyclic compound containing four carbon and two nitrogen atoms in the ring, the nitrogen atoms being separated by one carbon atom. To this group belong barbituric acid and its derivatives, the nucleic acid hydrolysis products thymine, uracil, and cytosine, and many other compounds of physiologic or therapeutic importance. 2. $C_4H_4N_2$. 1,3-Diazine, a solid melting between 20° and 22° C.; soluble in water.

pyr″i·thi′a·mine. The pyridine analog of thiamine, obtained by replacing the —S— group in the thiazole ring of thiamine by —CH=CH—. Pyrithiamine is inhibitory to the growth of certain microörganisms which require an exogenous supply of thiamine for growth.

py′ro- (pye′ro-, pirr′o-), **pyr-.** 1. A combining form signifying *fire* or *heat.* 2. *In chemistry,* a combining form denoting *a substance derived by the action of heat.* 3. *In medicine,* a combining form denoting *fever.*

py″ro·bor′ic ac′id. $H_2B_4O_7$. An acid obtained from boric acid by heating. Also called *tetraboric acid.*

py″ro·cat′e·chin. See *pyrocatechol.*

py″ro·cat′e·chol (pye″ro·cat′i·coal ·kol, ·kawl). $C_6H_4(OH)_2$. o-Dihydroxy benzene; occurs as colorless leaflets soluble in water. Also called *pyrocate chin, catechol, oxyphenic acid.*

py″ro·gal′lic ac′id. Pyrogallol.

py″ro·gal′lol (pye″ro·gal′ole, ·ol ·awl, ·ga·lole′). $C_6H_3(OH)_3$. 1,2,3-Trihy droxybenzene; occurs as white, or nearly white crystals, soluble in water Used as an application in various skin diseases, especially psoriasis. Also called *pyrogallic acid.* **p. monoace tate.** $(OH)_2C_6H_3O.CO.CH_3$; available only in the form of a solution in ace tone, a reddish brown syrupy liquid. It is used only in the most obstinate cases of psoriasis. See *eugallol.* **p. triacetate.** $C_6H_3(COOCH_3)_3$; occurs as a white, crystalline powder; soluble in water. It is used in various skin diseases. Also called *triacetyl pyrogallol.* See *lenigallol.*

py·ro·gen. The protein organic matter or complex polysaccharides of a fever-producing nature which are found frequently in sterile water. It is produced by a certain group of bacteria which enter and develop in the water during distillation and subsequent storage and are killed during sterilization, thus leaving their bodies and products of decomposition in the solution.

py″ro·gen′ic. Producing fever.

py″ro·lag′ni·a. Sexual gratification attained by the sight of fires; sexual excitement accompanying pyromania.

py″ro·lig′ne·ous. Pertaining to the destructive distillation of wood.

py″ro·lig′ne·ous ac′id. The crude acid obtained by the destructive distillation of wood; it contains acetic acid.

py″ro·lu′site (pye″ro·lew′sight, pyerol′yoo·sight). MnO_2. A native manganese dioxide.

py·rol′y·sis (pye·rol′i·sis). The decomposition of organic substances by heat. **—pyrolyt′ic,** *adj.*

py″ro·ma′ni·a. A monomania for incendiarism. **—pyromaniac,** *n.*

py·rom′e·ter (pye·rom′i·tur). An instrument for measuring temperatures too high to be estimated by the ordinary thermometer.

py′ro·nin (C.C.). Tetraethyldiaminoxanthene; used as a histologic stain. Includes **pyronin B** and **pyronin G.**

py″ro·pho′bi·a. Morbid dread of fire.

py″ro·phos′phate. A salt of pyrophosphoric acid.

py″ro·phos·phor′ic ac′id. $H_4P_2O_7$. A crystalline acid, certain salts of which, notably iron, have been used medicinally.

py·rop″to·thy′mi·a (pye·rop″tothigh′mee·uh). A form of mental disorder in which the person imagines himself enveloped in flame.

py′ro·punc″ture. Puncturing with hot needles; ignipuncture.

py″ro·ra·ce′mic ac′id. Pyruvic acid.

py″ro·ra·ce′mic al′co·hol. See *acetyl* carbinol.

py′ro·scope. Instrument used in determining high temperatures.

py·ro′sis (pye·ro′sis). An affection of the stomach characterized by a burning sensation, accompanied by eructations of an acrid, irritating fluid; heartburn.

py″ro·tox′in. A toxic agent generated in the course of the febrile process.

py·rox′y·lin (pye·rock′si·lin, pye″rock·sil′in). A product obtained by the action of a mixture of nitric and sulfuric acids on cotton; consists chiefly of cellulose tetranitrate ($C_{12}H_{16}O_6$-$(NO_3)_4$); occurs as a yellowish white, matted mass of filaments, resembling raw cotton in appearance. It is used as a protective covering in the form of collodion. Also called *soluble guncotton.*

pyr·role′ (pi·role′, pirr′ole).

$NH.CH:CH.CH:CH.$ A colorless liquid occurring in bone oil and to a slight extent in coal tar. Many complex natural compounds, such as hemoglobin and chlorophyll, contain pyrrole molecules in their structure. See also *porphin ring, porphyrin.*

py·ru′vic ac′id (pye·roo′vick, piroo′vick). $CH_3.CO.COOH.$ An organic acid which is a normal intermediate in carbohydrate and protein metabolism. Excess quantities of pyruvic acid accumulate in blood and tissues in thiamine deficiency.

pyr·vin′i·um chlo′ride. 6-Dimethylamino-2-[2-(2,5-dimethyl-1-phenyl-3-pyrryl) vinyl]-1-methylquinolinium chloride dihydrate, a cyanine dye used as an anthelmintic. See *vanquin.*

py·u′ri·a (pye·yoor′ee·uh). The presence of pus in the urine.

Q

Q_{co2}. The rate of evolution of carbon dioxide, measured in microliters given off in 1 hour by 1 mg. (dry weight) of tissue.

Q_{o2}. The oxygen consumption in terms of the number of microliters consumed in 1 hour by 1 mg. (dry weight) of tissue; by convention, the consumption of oxygen is given a negative value.

Q fe´ver. See under *fever.*

q. h. *Quaque hora;* every hour. **q. 2 h.** *Quaque secunda hora;* every second hour. **q. 3 h.** *Quaque tertia hora;* every third hour.

q. i. d. *Quater in die;* 4 times a day.

q. l. *Quantum libet;* as much as is desired.

q. p. *Quantum placet;* as much as you please.

q. s. *Quantum sufficit;* as much as suffices.

qt. Quart.

quack. A pretender to medical skill; a medical charlatan.

quack´er·y. The practice of medicine by a quack.

quad·ran´gu·lar (kwod-rang´gew-lur). Having four angles, as the quadrangular lobe, the square lobe of the cerebellum.

quad´rant (kwod´rant). 1. The fourth part of a circle, subtending an angle of 90°. 2. One of the four regions into which the abdomen may be divided for purposes of physical diagnosis.

quad´´ran·ta·no´pi·a (kwod´´ran-tuh-no´pee-uh), **quad´´ran·ta·nop´si·a.** Loss of vision in about one-quarter of the visual field.

quad´rate. Square, four-sided, as quadrate cartilages, small, quadrangular, cartilaginous plates often found in the alae of the nose.

quad·ra´tus. Squared; having four sides, as the quadratus lumborum, a muscle of the back, attached to the crest of the ilium and the twelfth rib. See Table of Muscles in the Appendix.

quad´ri-. A combining form meaning four.

quad´ri·ceps. 1. Four-headed, as a quadriceps muscle. 2. The large extensor muscle of the thigh. See Table of Muscles in the Appendix.

quad´´ri·gem´i·nal. Fourfold; consisting of four parts, as the corpora quadrigemina, *q.v.*

quad·rip´a·ra. A woman who is bearing, or has borne, her fourth child. —**quadriparous,** *adj.*

quad´´ri·ple´gi·a. Paralysis affecting the four extremities of the body.

quad´´ri·tu·ber´cu·lar. Having four tubercles or cusps.

quad´´ri·va´lent (kwod´´ri·vay´lunt, kwod-riv´uh-lunt). *In chemistry,* having a combining power equivalent to that of four hydrogen atoms. —**quadrivalence,** *n.*

quad·roon´. The offspring of a white person and a mulatto.

quad´ru·ped. A four-footed animal. —**quadru·pedal,** *adj.*

quad´ru·plet (kwod´roo-plet, kwod-roo´plet). Any one of four children born at one birth.

qual´i·ta´´tive. Pertaining to quality.

quan´ta. Plural of quantum.

quan·tim´e·ter (kwon-tim´i-tur). An instrument for measuring the quantity of roentgen rays.

quan´ti·ta´´tive. Pertaining to quantity.

quan´tum (pl. *quanta*). 1. As much as. 2. A discrete portion of energy, of definite amount. **q. libet.** As much as is desired. Abbreviated, q.l. **q. pla·cet.** As much as you please. Abbreviated, q.p. **q. sufficit.** As much as suffices. Abbreviated, q.s. **q. vis.** As much as you wish. Abbreviated, q.v.

quar´an·tine. 1. The limitation of freedom of movement of such susceptible persons or animals as have been exposed to communicable disease, for a period of time equal to the longest usual incubation period of the disease to which they have been exposed. 2. The place of detention of such persons. 3. The act of detaining vessels or travelers from suspected ports or places for purposes of inspection or disinfection. **shotgun q.** The extemporized and unauthorized establishment of a cordon against a place suspected of being the seat of an epidemic of a communicable disease.

quart. In the U.S.A., the fourth part of a gallon; 0.9463 liter. Abbreviated, qt. An **imperial quart** contains about 20% more than the **U. S. quart.**

quar´tan (kwor´tun). 1. Recurring on the fourth day. 2. A form of intermittent malarial fever in which the paroxysms occur approximately every 72 hours, that is, on the first, fourth, seventh days, etc.

quar´ter. 1. *In veterinary anatomy,* that part of the horse's hoof between the heel and the toe. 2. The fourth part of a slaughtered animal.

quar·tip´a·ra (kwor-tip´uh-ruh). A woman who has borne four children. —**quartiparous,** *adj.*

598

quartz. A crystalline silicon dioxide, SiO_2; when pure, in colorless hexagonal crystals. Used in chemical apparatus and for optical and electric instruments.

quas'si·a (kwosh'ee-uh, kwosh'uh). The wood of *Picrasma excelsa*, known as **Jamaica quassia**, or of *Quassia amara*, known as **Surinam quassia**. An infusion is used as an enema against seatworms, *Enterobius vermicularis*. Also called *bitter wood*.

quas'sin (kwoss'in, kwass'in). The bitter principle of *Quassia amara*. The commercial article consists of two isomeric substances, quassin and neoquassin. See *picrasmin*.

qua·ter·na·ry. 1. Consisting of four elements or substances, as quaternary solutions. 2. Fourth in order or stage. 3. Referring to compounds in which four similar atoms of a radical, as the hydrogen atoms in the ammonium radical, have been replaced by organic radicals.

quat'tu·or. Four.

que·bra'chine (kay·brah'cheen, ·keen). An alkaloid of quebracho probably identical with yohimbine.

que·bra'cho (kay·brah'cho, ·ko). The name of several hard-wooded trees of South America. The **white quebracho** is *Aspidosperma quebracho-blanco*. It contains aspidospermine and quebrachine, the latter probably being identical with yohimbine.

queen's'-de·light'. See *stillingia*.

queen's'root". See *stillingia*.

quer'ce·tin (kwur'si·tin). A tetrahydroxyflavanol, $C_{15}H_{10}O_7.H_2O$, present in many fruit rinds and a product of the hydrolysis of quercitrin. Also called *meletin, flavin*.

quer'ci- (kwur'si-). A combining form meaning *an oak*.

quer'cin. A bitter, crystallizable carbohydrate, $C_6H_{12}O_6$, from acorns and oak bark.

quer"ci·tan'nic ac'id. The tannic acid from oak bark.

quer"ci·tan'nin. Quercitannic acid, *q.v.*

quer'cite. $C_6H_7(OH)_5$. Pentahydroxy-cyclohexane. White, sweet crystals; found in acorns. Also called *quercitol, acorn sugar*.

quer'ci·tol. See *quercite*.

quer'ci·trin. $C_{21}H_{20}O_{11}.2H_2O$. A glycoside found in the bark of *Quercus tinctoria* and in many other plants.

quer'cus. The dried inner bark of *Quercus alba*. See *oak*.

quick. 1. A vital, tender part, as the bed of a nail. 2. Pregnant, and able to feel the movements of the fetus.

quick'en·ing. The first feeling on the part of the pregnant woman of fetal movements, occurring between the fourth and fifth months of pregnancy.

quick'lime". Calcium oxide; unslaked lime.

quick'sil"ver. Mercury, *q.v.*

Quil·la'ja (kwi·lay'yuh, ·juh), **Quil·la'ia.** A genus of trees of the family Rosaceae.

quil·la'ja. The dried inner bark of *Quillaja saponaria*. It contains a saponin, quillain (quillaic acid), which is very toxic. Also called *soapbark, Panama bark*.

quin-, quin'o-. A combining form denoting *quina* (cinchona bark) or *quinine*.

quin'a·crine hy"dro·chlo'ride (kwin'uh-kreen, ·krin). $C_{23}H_{30}ClN_3O.2$-$HCl.2H_2O$. A bright yellow, crystalline powder; soluble in water. An acridine derivative, which destroys the asexual forms (trophozoites) of the malarial organism. Syn., *mepacrine hydrochloride*. See *atabrine dihydrochloride, chinacrin hydrochloride*.

quin'a·crine meth"ane-sul'fon-ate. A salt used like quinacrine hydrochloride but preferred over the latter for parenteral administration because of its greater solubility in water. See *mepacrine methanesulfonate*.

qui·nal'dine (kwi·nal'deen, ·din). $C_{10}H_9O$. Methylquinoline. An antipyretic similar to quinoline.

qui·nam'i·dine (kwi·nam'i·deen, ·din). $C_{19}H_{24}N_2O_2$. An alkaloid from various species of *Cinchona*.

qui·nam'ine (kwi·nam'een, kwin'uh-meen). $C_{19}H_{24}N_2O_2$. An alkaloid of the cinchonas.

quince seed. See *cydonium*.

qui·ne'tum. Totaquine, *q.v.*

quin·hy'drone (kwin·high'drone, kwin'hi·drone). A substance representing equimolecular concentrations of quinone and hydroquinone.

quin'ic ac'id. $C_7H_{12}O_6$. Hexahydro-tetrahydroxybenzoic acid, found in cinchona bark and in several other plants.

quin'i·cine (kwin'i·seen, ·sin). A cinchona alkaloid, isomeric with quinine.

quin'i·dine (kwin'i·deen, ·din). C_{20}-$H_{24}N_2O_2$. An alkaloid of cinchona bark isomeric with quinine. Used chiefly to restore normal rhythm in atrial fibrillation. **q. sulfate.** $(C_{20}H_{24}N_2O_2)_2$-$H_2SO_4.2H_2O$. Fine white crystals; soluble in water.

qui'nine (kwye'nyne, kwi·neen', kwin'een). $C_{20}H_{24}N_2O_2.3H_2O$. An alkaloid obtained from cinchona. A white, microcrystalline powder of intensely bitter taste, slightly soluble in water. Quinine kills the asexual forms (trophozoites) of the malarial organisms, and effectively arrests the malarial attacks. It is also analgesic and antipyretic. **q. acid sulfate.** See *q. bisulfate.* **q. and urea hydro-**

chloride. A double salt. $C_{20}H_{24}N_2O_2 \cdot HCl.CO(NH_2)_2 \cdot HCl.5H_2O$. Contains 58–65% of anhydrous quinine. White, crystalline powder soluble in water.

q. bisulfate. $C_{20}H_{24}N_2O_2 \cdot H_2SO_4 \cdot 7H_2O$. White, crystalline powder soluble in water. Syn., *q. acid sulfate.* **q. dihydrochloride.** $C_{20}H_{24}N_2O_2 \cdot 2HCl$. White powder; soluble in water. **q. ethylcarbonate.** $C_{22}H_{28}N_2O_4$. Fine, white needles; only slightly soluble in water. Also called *euquinine.* **q. hydrobromide.** $C_{20}H_{24}N_2O_2 \cdot HBr.H_2O$. Small, white crystals. Soluble in water. **q. hydrochloride.** $C_{20}H_{24}N_2O_2 \cdot HCl.2H_2O$. White needles. Soluble in water. **q. sulfate.** $(C_{20}H_{24}N_2O_2)_2 \cdot H_2SO_4.2H_2O$. Fine needles; soluble in water. The most popular salt of quinine.

qui·nin·ism (kwye′nyne-iz-um, kwi-neen′-, kwin′een-), **qui·nism** (kwye′-niz-um, kwin′iz-um). Cinchonism.

quin′o·chromes. Blue, fluorescent products formed by the oxidation of vitamin B_1. Also see *thiochrome.*

quin′o·line (kwin′o-leen, -lin). A tertiary liquid amine, C_9H_7N, occurring in coal tar. It is antiseptic.

qui·none′ (kwi-nohn′, kwin′ohn). 1. $C_6H_4O_2$. Ortho- or para-dioxybenzene, especially the latter. Also called *benzoquinone.* 2. A group of yellow compounds characterized by structures similar to those cited in definition 1.

quin″o·tan′nic ac′id. See *cinchotannin.*

quin″o·tox′ine (kwin″o-tock′seen, -sin). Quinicine, *q.v.*

qui·no′va·tine (kwi-no′vuh-teen, -tin). An alkaloid, $C_{23}H_{26}N_2O_4$, occurring in the bark of *Cinchona cordifolia* var. *Pelletieriana.* Also called *aricine.*

qui·no′vic ac′id. $C_{30}H_{46}O_5$. A complex acid occurring in cinchona bark.

quin′o·vin, qui·no′vin. $C_{33}H_{52}O_{11}$. Kinovin, a bitter glycoside found in the bark of cinchona and other Rubiaceae.

quin′sy (kwin′zee). Acute inflammation of a palatine tonsil and peritonsillar tissue, usually tending to suppuration. Syn. *peritonsillar abscess.* **lingual q.** Quinsy originating in the lingual tonsil and involving the tongue.

quin′tan. 1. Recurring on the fifth day. 2. An intermittent fever, the paroxysms of which recur every 96 hours; that is, on the fifth, ninth, thirteenth days, etc.

quin′ta·ry. Fifth in order or stage.

quin·tip′a·ra. A woman who has borne five children, or who is in labor for the fifth time.

quin·tu·plet, quin·tu′plet. One of five children who have been born at one birth.

quotane hydrochloride. Trademark for dimethisoquin hydrochloride.

quo·tid′i·an. 1. Recurring every day. 2. An intermittent fever, the paroxysms of which recur daily. **double q.** A fever having two paroxysms a day, usually differing in character.

quo′tient. The result of the process of division. **accomplishment q.** *In psychology,* the ratio of achievement age to mental age. Also called *achievement q.* Abbreviated, AQ. **blood q.** The result obtained by dividing the quantity of hemoglobin in the blood by the number of erythrocytes, expressed in each case as a percentage of the normal amount. **developmental q.** The mathematical expression of the relation between developmental age and actual or chronologic age. To keep the related factors clear for easy reference, it is often expressed as a fraction,

$$\frac{\text{developmental age}}{\text{actual (chronologic) age}}$$

rather than worked out as a quotient. Developmental age may be determined by serial x-ray pictures leading to standards for epiphyseal development, body measurement (height, weight, etc.), mental and motor tests, or the grid method (Wetzel). **D/N q.** The ratio of glucose to nitrogen in the urine. **intelligence q.** See *intelligence quotient.* **QO_2.** The oxygen consumption in terms of the number of microliters consumed in 1 hour by 1 mg. (dry weight) of tissue; by convention, the consumption of oxygen is given a negative value. **respiratory q.** Abbreviated, R. Q. (a) The ratio of the volume of carbon dioxide evolved by respiring cells or tissues to the volume of oxygen consumed in the same time. (b) The result obtained by dividing the carbon dioxide expired by the oxygen absorbed. This is normally

$$\frac{4.5}{5} = 0.9$$

q.v. 1. *Quantum vis;* as much as you wish. 2. *Quod vide;* which see.

R

R. Réaumur, resistance (electric), right.
℞. Symbol indicative of registered trade-mark status for a name.
. Symbol for roentgen.
℞. *Recipe,* take; used in prescription writing.
- R. Rinne's test negative. See Rinne's *test.*
- R. Rinne's test positive. See Rinne's *test.*
R₁, *In chromatography,* a symbol for the ratio of the distance traveled by a substance undergoing diffusion to the distance traveled by the solvent, the ratio being characteristic of the substance.
Ra. Chemical symbol for radium.
ab″e·la′i·sin. A glycoside from *Lophopetalum toxicum;* its action is similar to that of digitalis.
abellon. Trade-mark for a tablet containing belladonna alkaloids.
ab′id. Affected with rabies; pertaining to rabies.
a′bies (ray′beez, ray′bee·eez). An acute infectious disease of animals caused by a filtrable virus transmitted to other animals and man by the bite of an infected animal. Many animals are subject to the disease, but it occurs most frequently in the wolf, the cat, and the dog, and is chiefly propagated by the last. The virus has a special affinity for the nervous system, and is found in secretions, particularly in the saliva. In man there are usually three stages of the disease; the first or preliminary, marked by restlessness, apprehension, and obvious ill health; the second or furious stage, in which the patient is hyperactive and has spasms of the muscles of swallowing and respiration; and the third or paralytic stage, which is marked in the beginning by drooling saliva, due to poor muscular control, and terminates fatally with a general paralysis ascending the spinal cord. **r. prophylaxis.** The daily inoculation of an exposed person with emulsions of spinal cord from infected rabbits. The first injection is made with cord which has been dried for 14 days, successive inoculations being from progressively fresher cord. Other methods have been employed to inactivate the vaccine, such as chloroform and phenol. Also called *Pasteur treatment.*
r. vaccine. An emulsion made from the spinal cords of rabbits infected with rabies. Also see r. prophylaxis, *Flury strain.*
ace. A poorly defined minor subdivision of a species. **—ra′cial,** *adj.*

ra·ce′mic (ra·see′mick, ·sem′ick). Composed of equal parts of dextrorotatory and levorotatory forms of optical isomers and, therefore, optically inactive.
rac″e·mor′phan hy″dro·bro′mide. Racemic 3-hydroxy-N-methyl-morphinan hydrobromide, a potent synthetic analgesic related to morphine, the available salt of which is levorphanol tartrate. Formerly called *methorphinan hydrobromide.* See *levo-dromoran tartrate.*
rac′e·mose (rass′i·mose). Resembling a bunch of grapes.
racephedrine. Trade name for racemic ephedrine. Also called *d-l-ephed-rine.*
race su′i·cide. The gradual extinction of a human population through widespread limitation of family size.
ra′chi-. See *rachio-.*
ra′chi·cele (ray′ki·seel). Hernial protrusion of the contents of the spinal canal in spina bifida. It includes spinal meningocele, myelomeningocele, and myelocystocele (syringomyelocele).
ra″chi·cen·te′sis. Puncture into the subarachnoid space; lumbar puncture, *q.v.*
ra·chid′i·al (ra·kid′ee·ul). Of, or relating to, the spine.
ra·chil′y·sis (ra·kil′i·sis). A method of treating lateral curvature of the spine by mechanical counteraction of the abnormal curves.
ra′chi·o- (ray′kee·o-), **ra′chi-.** A combining form meaning *the spine.*
ra″chi·o·camp′sis. Curvature of the spine.
ra″chi·o·dyn′i·a (ray″kee·o·din′-ee·uh, ·dye′nee·uh). Spasmodic pain in the spinal column.
ra″chi·om′e·ter. An instrument used to measure the degree of spinal deformities.
ra″chi·o·ple′gi·a. Spinal paralysis.
ra″chi·o·sco″li·o′sis (ray″kee·o·sko″lee·o′sis, ·skol″ee·o′sis). Lateral curvature of the spine.
ra′chi·o·tome″. A cutting instrument used in operations upon the vertebrae.
ra″chi·ot′o·my. The operation of cutting into the vertebral column.
ra′chis (ray′kis). The vertebral column. **—rachid′ial, rachid′ian,** *adj.*
ra·chis′chi·sis (ra·kiss′ki·sis). Synonym for spina bifida.
ra·chit′ic. Affected with, resembling, or produced by, rickets.

601

ra·chit'ic ro'sa·ry. The row of nodules appearing on the ribs at the junctions with their cartilages; often seen in rachitic children. Also called *beading of the ribs, rachitic beads.*

ra·chi'tis (ra·kye'tis). Rickets, *q.v.*

rach"i·to·gen'ic (rack"i·to·jen'-ick). Producing rickets, as a vitamin-D deficient diet.

rad. *Radix,* root.

ra'di·al. 1. Radiating; diverging from a common center. 2. Pertaining to, or in relation to, the radius, a bone of the forearm, as the radial artery. See Table of Arteries in the Appendix.

ra"di·a'lis (ray"dee·ah'lis, ·ay'lis). Pertaining to the radius; a term applied to various arteries, nerves, and muscles, as flexor carpi radialis.

ra'di·ant. Emitting rays, as radiant energy, energy traveling in the form of electromagnetic waves.

ra'di·a'tion. 1. The act of radiating or diverging from a central point, as radiation of light; divergence from a center, having the appearance of rays. 2. The therapeutic use of roentgen rays or radium. 3. *In neurology,* certain groups of fibers that diverge after leaving their place of origin. **audi-tory r.** A large bundle of fibers in the posterior part of the internal capsule, running from the medial geniculate body to the superior and transverse temporal gyri. Also called *temporothal-amic r., acoustic r.* **fractiona-tion r.** Method of administration of roentgen rays or radium in fractions of the total dose spread over a period of days. **interstitial r.** Radiation by inserting radium or radon directly into the tissue. **irritative r.** Ultra-violet radiation to the point of producing erythema. **mitogenetic r.** A kind of radiation said to be produced in cells and tissues, which induces or is induced by the process of mitosis. Also called *Gurvich r.* **optic r.** The genic-ulocalcarine tract, connecting the lat-eral geniculate body with the calcarine occipital area of the cortex. **photo-chemical r.** Radiation which is part of the spectrum that produces chem-ical reactions. **protraction r.** De-crease of the rate of application of a given dose of roentgen rays or radium rays. **solar r.** Radiation from the sun. **thalamic r.** Tracts of nerve fibers running from the thalamus to the cere-bral cortex. **ultraviolet r.** Ra-diation comprising ultraviolet wave lengths.

rad'i·cal. 1. Belonging to a root; going to the root, or attacking the cause, of a disease; the opposite of con-servative. 2. A group of atoms that acts as a unit, but is incapable of existence in the free state, as NH_4,

ammonium, or C_6H_5, phenyl. 3. The haptophore group of an antibody.

rad'i·cle. 1. A little root, as the rad-icle of a nerve, one of the ultimate fibrils of which a nerve is composed or a radicle of a vein, one of the minute vessels uniting to form a vein. 2. See *radical,* 2, 3.

ra·dic'u·lar. Pertaining to a root or to a radicle; specifically, pertaining to the roots of the spinal nerves.

ra·dic"u·lec'to·my. Excision or re-section of a spinal nerve root.

ra·dic"u·li'tis. Inflammation of a nerve root.

ra·dic"u·lo·my"e·lop'a·thy. Dis-ease of the spinal cord and roots of the spinal nerves.

ra·dic"u·lo·neu·ri'tis. Inflamma-tion of a spinal nerve root.

ra·dic"u·lo·neu·rop'a·thy. Dis-ease of the peripheral spinal nerves and their roots.

ra·dic"u·lop'a·thy. Disease of the roots of spinal nerves.

ra'di·o-. 1. A combining form meaning pertaining to *radiant energy* or to *ra-dium.* 2. A combining form meaning *relating to the radius.*

ra"di·o·ac·tin'i·um. A radioactive product of actinium. It gives off alpha rays and disintegrates into actinium x.

ra"di·o·ac'tive. Emitting radiant energy.

ra"di·o·ac·tiv'i·ty. A property of certain substances of spontaneously emitting alpha particles, beta particles, or gamma rays from the nucleus of the atom. **—radioac'tive,** *adj.* **arti-ficial r.** That produced artificially by bombardment with high-velocity par-ticles, as in a cyclotron or betatron or by other means. Also called *induced r.*

ra"di·o·au'to·graph. A direct photographic record of the distribution of radioactive material in a specimen, such as a histologic section.

ra"di·o·bi·ol'o·gy. That branch of science devoted to the study of the results of radiation upon the body.

ra"di·o·chem'is·try. That branch of chemistry which deals with radio-active phenomena.

ra"di·o·co'balt. Any radioactive isotope of cobalt, especially cobalt-60, used in treating cancer.

ra"di·o·cys·ti'tis. Cystitis following x-ray or radium therapy.

ra'di·ode. An electric attachment for the application of radium.

ra"di·o·di"ag·no'sis. The diagno-sis of disease by means of radiographs or radioscopy.

ra"di·o·don'ti·a. Radiography of the teeth and adjacent tissues.

ra"di·o·don'tist. A specialist in radiography of the teeth and adjacent tissues.

ra″di·o·el′e·ment. An element with radioactive properties.

ra′di·o·graph″. 1. Make a photograph on a sensitive film by projection of roentgen rays through a part of the body to be examined. 2. A roentgen-ray photograph. Also called *roentgenogram.*

ra″di·og′ra·pher. One skilled in radiography; an x-ray technician.

ra″di·og′ra·phy. The practice or act of making radiographs. —**radiographic,** *adj.* **sectional r.** The technic of making radiographs of plane sections of solid objects; its purpose is to show detail in a predetermined plane of the body, while blurring the images of structures in other planes. The methods used differ slightly and have been designated stratigraphy, tomography, planigraphy, x-ray focusing, vertigraphy, laminagraphy, and body-section roentgenography. In all, the radiographs are produced by movement of the film during exposure in a direction reciprocal and proportional to the simultaneous movement of the tube.

a″di·o·hu′mer·al. Pertaining to the radius and the humerus.

a″di·o·i′o·dine (ray″dee·o·eye′o-dyne, -deen, -din). Radioactive isotope of iodine, produced artificially by bombardment with high energy positively charged atomic particles or with neutrons.

a″di·o·i′ron. Radioactive isotope of iron, produced artificially by bombardment with high energy positively charged atomic particles or with neutrons.

a″di·o·i′so·tope. A radioactive isotope.

a″di·o·ky·mog′ra·phy (ray″dee·o·kigh·mog′ruh·fee). A method of obtaining a graphic record of movement of the silhouette of an organ or tissue on a single film.

a″di·ol′o·gist. A physician specializing in the use of roentgen and/or radium rays in the diagnosis and treatment of disease.

a″di·ol′o·gy. That branch of medicine which deals with the diagnostic and therapeutic application of radiant energy, including roentgen rays and radium. —**radiolog′ic,** *adj.*

a″di·o·lu′cent. Partly or wholly transparent to roentgen rays or other forms of radiation. —**radiolu-cency,** *n.*

a″di·o·lu″mi·nes′cence. That luminescence brought about by radioactive rays striking an obstacle or screen treated with a suitable substance.

a″di·o·mag·ne′si·um (ray″dee·o-mag·nee′zee·um, -zhum). Radioactive isotope of magnesium, produced artificially by bombardment with high

energy positively charged atomic particles or with neutrons.

ra″di·om′e·ter. 1. An instrument for measuring the intensity of thermal radiation. 2. An instrument for measuring the quality or penetration of x-rays.

ra″di·o·ne·cro′sis. Destruction or ulceration of tissues caused by radiation treatment.

ra″di·o·neu·ri′tis. A form of neuritis due to exposure to x-rays or radium rays.

ra″di·o·ni′tro·gen. Radioactive isotope of nitrogen, produced artificially by bombardment with high energy positively charged atomic particles or with neutrons.

ra″di·o·paque′ (ray″dee·o·payk′). Not transparent to the x-ray; not permitting the passage of radiant energy. —**radiopac′ity,** *n.*

ra″di·o·par′ent. Transparent to the x-ray; permitting the passage of radiant energy. —**radiopar′ent,** *n.*

ra″di·o·pa·thol′o·gy. Study of tissue changes brought about by radiation.

ra″di·o·pel·vim′e·try. Radiographic procedure for making accurate measurements of the maternal pelvis and fetal skull. Also called *pelvicephalometry.*

ra″di·o·phos′pho·rus. Radioactive isotope of phosphorus, produced artificially by bombardment with high energy positively charged atomic particles or with neutrons.

ra″di·o·prax′is. The use of radiant energy either in therapy or for other purposes.

ra″di·os′co·py. The process of securing an image of an object upon a fluorescent screen by means of radiant energy.

ra″di·o·sen″si·tiv′i·ty. Sensitivity of tissues or organisms to various types of radiations, such as x-rays or rays from radioactive materials. —**radiosen′sitive,** *adj.*

ra″di·o·sil′i·con. Radioactive isotope of silicon, produced artificially by bombardment with high energy positively charged atomic particles or with neutrons.

ra″di·o·so′di·um. Sodium isotope made artificially radioactive by bombardment with high energy positively charged atomic particles or with neutrons.

ra″di·o·ster″e·os′co·py. The application of the principle of the stereoscope, obtaining a viewpoint for the left eye and one for the right by corresponding displacement of the x-ray tube along the plane of the film, and duplication of these geometric conditions in viewing the two radiographs in a properly constructed stereoscopic view box.

ra'di·o·stron'ti·um (ray"dee-o-stron'shee-um, -tee-um). A radioactive isotope of strontium, produced artificially by bombardment with high energy positively charged atomic particles or with neutrons.

ra'di·o·sur'ger·y. The use of radium in surgical therapy.

ra'di·o·tel·lu'ri·um. A radioactive product of tellurium; same as polonium.

ra'di·o·ther"a·peu'tic (ray"dee-o-therr"uh-pew'tick). Referring to therapeutic use of radiant energy.

ra'di·o·ther'a·py. The treatment of disease by means of x-rays, radium rays, and other radioactive substances.

ra'di·o·ther'my. 1. Treatment by radiant heat. 2. Short-wave diathermy.

ra'di·o·tho'ri·um. A radioactive element of the thorium family, formed from mesothorium.

ra'di·o·tox·e'mi·a. Toxemia induced from overexposure to any radioactive substance.

ra'di·o·trans·par'ent. Permitting the passage of radiations; used notably in connection with x-rays. The opposite of radiopaque.

ra'di·o·ul'nar. Pertaining to the radius and ulna.

ra'di·um. Ra = 226.05. A highly radioactive metallic element. Discovered in 1898 by Pierre and Marie Curie, who separated it from pitchblende by a tedious process. The chloride or bromide of radium is usually used. Radium salts emit continuously heat, light, and three other distinct kinds of radiation (alpha particles, beta particles, and gamma rays).

ra'di·um can'non. In radiology, a tube resembling a gun barrel, allowing radiation only in a straight line; used in deep therapy.

ra'di·um·i·za'tion. Exposure to radium rays.

ra'di·us. The outer of the two bones of the forearm. See Table of Bones in the Appendix. **r. fixus.** A line drawn from the hormion to the inion.

ra'dix (pl. *radices*). A root. For special terms, see under *root*. Abbreviated, rad.

ra'don. Rn = 222. A decay product of radium; a colorless, gaseous, radioactive element. Also called *radium emanation*.

ra'don seed. A small capillary tube, of glass, containing radon, suitable for implantation in tissues; the tube may be placed inside a small gold or platinum tube.

raf'fin·ase. An enzyme which hydrolyzes raffinose with the splitting-off of fructose. Probably identical with saccharase.

raf'fin·ose. $C_{18}H_{32}O_{16}.5H_2O$. A trisaccharide found in sugar beets, cotton seed meal, and molasses. On hydrolysis it yields glucose, fructose, and galactose.

rag'pick"er's dis·ease'. Anthrax occurring in ragpickers.

rag'weed". Any of several species of the genus *Ambrosia*; its pollen is the most important allergen in the central and eastern United States. Its pollinating period is from the middle of August to the time of frost.

Rail"li·e·ti'na (rye"lee·i·tye'nuh, -tee'nuh). A genus of tapeworm. **R. celebensis.** A species of tapeworms; infestation of man reported in Tokyo and in Formosa. **R. madagascariensis.** A species which infests man. **R. quitensis.** A species which infests man; reported from Ecuador.

rail'way" sick'ness. Car sickness; a form of motion sickness occurring as a result of the movement of a train. See *airsickness*.

rale (rahl). An abnormal sound arising within the lungs or air passages and heard on auscultation over the chest. There is no agreement among authorities concerning a classification of these sounds. A very large number of descriptive terms have been used in the past, many of them based on fanciful considerations of the physical conditions held responsible for their production. The modern tendency is to discard most of the qualifying adjectives formerly used and to characterize rales by such simple and self-explanatory terms as coarse, medium (moderate), coarse), and fine. The adjectives moist and dry are also widely used, but in a descriptive sense only. They are not intended to imply that the sound has originated in a moist or dry physical environment. Some authors hold that all rales originate in the presence of abnormal moisture. No type of rale is pathognomonic of a specific disease such as pneumonia, tuberculosis, bronchiectasis, etc., or of a physical condition such as pulmonary cavity or consolidation. There is fairly general, though not complete, agreement regarding the significance of the following terms. **consonating r.** A moderately coarse rale which sounds unusually loud and close to the ear, as though it were reinforced by transmission through the area of consolidated lung with which it is usually associated. **crepitant r.** A fine, dry, crackling sound, simulated by the rubbing together of hairs, or by the sprinkling of salt on a hot stove; often heard as a transient phenomenon around the inferior margins of normal lungs during the first few forced inspirations. **post-tussive r.** That form not heard during either natural or forced breathing, but elicited only by the use of a short cough delivered at the end of a forced expiration. **rhonchus r.** An extremely coarse type of rale which originates only in the larger air passages and sets up vibrations which usually can be palpated on the surface of the chest in addition to being heard with a stethoscope. **sibilant r.** A dry, high-pitched, hissing or whistling sound heard most often in cases of bronchiolar spasm. **sonorous r.** A dry, low-pitched, resonant, snoring sound heard most often in cases of bronchiolar spasm. **subcrepitant r.** A crackling sound similar to crepitant rale, but coarser and lower pitched. **vesicular r.** Crepitant rale, q.v.

ra'mi (ray'migh). Plural of ramus, q.v.

ram″i·fi·ca'tion. 1. The act or state of branching. 2. A branch.

ram'i·fy (ram'i·figh). Form branches; branch.

ram″i·sec'tion, ram'i·sec″tion. Surgical division of the rami communicantes of the sympathetic nervous system.

ram″i·sec'to·my. See *ramisection*.

ra'mose. Having many branches; branching.

ra'mous. Having many branches; branching.

ram'u·lus (pl. *ramuli*). A small branch, or ramus.

ra'mus (pl. *rami*). 1. A branch, especially of a vein, artery, or nerve. 2. A slender process of bone projecting like a branch or twig from a large bone, as the ramus of the mandible, or the superior or inferior ramus of the pubis. —**ramal,** adj. **gray r. communicans.** A communicating branch of the sympathetic trunk connecting it with a peripheral nerve. Also called *postganglionic r.* **r. anastomoticus.** A branch of a nerve which communicates with a neighboring nerve or with a plexus. Also, a communicating artery between two neighboring arteries. **r. caroticus.** A branch of the glossopharyngeal nerve to the carotid sinus. **r. communicans.** An anastomotic branch of a nerve, applied especially to the white and gray rami communicantes, q.v. **white r. communicans.** A communicating nerve connecting the sympathetic trunk with the dorsal and ventral roots of a spinal nerve. Also called *preganglionic r.*

ran'cid. Having the characteristic odor of decomposing fat, due chiefly to the liberation of butyric and other volatile fatty acids.

** range.** The difference between the

lowest and the highest values in a series of observations.

ra'nine (ray'nyne, ·nin). Pertaining to a ranula or to the region in which a ranula occurs.

ran'u·la. A retention cyst of the anterior lingual gland or of the sublingual gland. —**ranular,** adj.

rape. 1. Sexual intercourse by violence or without the woman's consent. Technically, a rape may be committed by stealth or deceit, as where impersonation is practiced. 2. *In veterinary medicine*, the forcible sexual intercourse of the male while the female is not in heat. **statutory r.** The violation of a female under the age of consent as fixed in the state or country in which the attack occurs.

rape seed oil. The semidrying oil from the seeds of *Brassica campestris, B. napus,* and other species.

ra'phe (ray'fee, raf·ay'). A seam or ridge, especially one indicating the line of junction of two symmetrical halves. **buccal r.** The scarlike vestige of the union of the parts of the cheek derived respectively from the maxillary and mandibular processes. **r. of the pharynx.** A fibrous band in the median line of the posterior wall of the pharynx. **r. of the scrotum.** A median ridge dividing the scrotum into two lateral halves; it is continuous posteriorly with the raphe of the perineum, anteriorly with the raphe of the penis. **r. of the tongue.** That beneath the median furrow on the dorsal surface of the tongue corresponding to the fibrous septum which divides it into symmetrical halves.

rap'tus. Any sudden attack or seizure; rape. **r. haemorrhagicus.** A sudden hemorrhage. **r. maniacus.** Transient frenzy. **r. melancholicus.** Sudden and vehement melancholy. **r. nervorum.** Cramp or spasm.

rar″e·fac'tion (rair″i·fack'shun, rar″i·fack'shun). The act of rarefying or of decreasing the density of a substance, especially the air. **r. of bone.** The process of rendering bone more radiolucent by a decrease in the mineral content.

rar'e·fy (rair'i·figh, rar'i·figh). Make less dense or more porous.

rar'i·tas. Rarity. **r. dentium.** Fewness of teeth; less than the usual number of teeth, with or without interspaces between them.

rash. A lay term used for nearly any skin eruption but more commonly for acute inflammatory dermatoses. **canker r.** Scarlet fever, q.v. **serum r.** A dermatosis coincident with serum sickness; a result of injection of antitoxin. **vaccination r.** A rash which sometimes follows vaccination; it is usually transitory but sometimes assumes an eczematous or erythematous form. **wandering r.** Benign migratory glossitis.

ra'sor·ite. A native hydrate of borax, $Na_2B_4O_7.4H_2O$; an important source of this chemical.

rasp. A sharp-toothed instrument similar to a file.

ras'pa·to"ry. A rasp or file for trimming rough surfaces or margins of bone or for removing periosteum.

rasp'ber"ry. The fruit of *Rubus idaeus,* a plant of the Rosaceae.

rat. A rodent which lives in close proximity to man, in homes, barns, wharves, ships, garbage dumps, etc. Rats are notorious disease carriers, harboring many varieties of intestinal parasites and being responsible especially for the transmission of bubonic plague, as well as a distinct septic disease, rat bite fever, *q.v.*

rate. A method of measuring a frequency or speed against a standard. **basal metabolic r.** The amount of energy expended per unit of time under basal conditions, usually expressed as large calories per square meter of body surface (or kilograms of body weight) per hour. **case fatality r.** The number of deaths from a specific disease per 100 persons suffering from the same disease. **infant mortality r.** The number of deaths reported among infants under one year of age in a calendar year per 1000 live births reported in the same year and place. **maternal mortality r.** The number of deaths reported as due to puerperal causes in a calendar year per 1000 live births reported in the same year and place. **morbidity r.** The number of cases of a disease per year for a certain number of the population. **pregnancy r.** The number of pregnancies actually experienced in relation to the number of ova that theoretically might have been fertilized. **prevalence r.** The number of cases of a disease occurring per unit of population at any given time. **pulse r.** The number of pulsations of an artery per minute. **reproduction r.** The number of total births to women of reproductive age (15 to 49 years) divided by the number of women of the same age in the population. **sedimentation r.** The rate at which red cells settle out of citrated blood; the rate is somewhat more rapid in females than in males. Increases in sedimentation rate occur during menstruation, pregnancy, and in a number of pathologic states. ESR is the abbreviation for erythrocyte sedimentation rate.

ra'tio. A proportion. **absorption r.** The ratio between the amount of light-absorbing substance in a solution an[d] the coefficient of light extinction (th[e] amount of light of a specific wav[e] length absorbed by a 1% solution of [a] substance in a layer 1 cm. thick) [in] that solution. **albumin-globu[-] lin r. (A/G).** The ratio of the albu[-] min to the globulin concentration [in] blood serum. Normal value = 1.3–1.[8.] Values below 1.0 are said to be inverte[d] and are associated with various patho[-] logic processes. **birth-death r.** Th[e] number of births per 100 deaths re[-] ported in the same population durin[g] the same calendar year. **body weight r.** Body weight in gram[s] divided by height in centimeters. **concentration r.** The ratio of the con[-] centration of a substance in the urin[e] to its concentration in the blood o[r] blood serum. **D:N r. (dextrose[-] nitrogen r.).** The ratio of the dex[-] trose to the nitrogen in the urine. I[n] the totally diabetic animal, the averag[e] value is 3.65, which is approached [in] severe human diabetes. It is considere[d] as a measure of the conversion of pro[-] tein to carbohydrate in the absence o[f] carbohydrate intake. **G:N r.** Se[e] D:N r. **isophane r.** The proportio[n] in which insulin and protaine combin[e] in preparations containing both. Als[o] see isophane *insulin.* **Mendelian r**[.] The approximate numerical relatio[n] between various types of progeny [in] crosses involving sharply contraste[d] characters that conform to Mendel[ian] law of heredity; the typical ratios fo[r] the F_2 generation are 3:1 for one pa[ir] of characters, 9:3:3:1 for two pair[s]. **monocyte-lymphocyte r.** Th[e] ratio between monocytes and lymph[o] cytes in the blood; has been used as [a] diagnostic criterion in the study of t[u] berculosis. **nucleocytoplasmic r**[.] The ratio between the measured cros[s] sectional area or the estimated volum[e] of the nucleus of a cell to its cytoplasm[.] **sex r.** The relative number of mal[es] and females in the population, usual[ly] stated as the number of males per 1[00] females. **therapeutic r.** The rat[io] of the therapeutically effective dose [to] the lethal dose per kilogram of bo[dy] weight as determined on experiment[al] animals, usually expressed by dividi[ng] the effective dose by the lethal dos[e.] The curative ratio is a correspondi[ng] fraction of the curative dose divide[d] by the lethal dose. These ratios mea[s] ure the margins of safety.

ra'tion (rash'un, ray'shun). A dai[ly] allowance of food or drink. In t[he] armed services, the term usually mea[ns] the complete subsistence for one m[an] for one day. **A r.** See field r. **B r.** T[he] overseas hospital ration. **C r.** An eme[r] gency ration of canned goods. **D r.** [An] emergency ration of chocolate ba[rs]

Obs. **emergency r.** One of concentrated foods of little bulk which can be carried when troops are separated from field kitchens. **field r.** A complete ration corresponding to the garrison ration, and served to troops in wartime. **K r.** A complete emergency ration for three meals put up in pocket size.

ra'tion·al (rash'un·ul). 1. Based upon reason; reasonable. 2. *In therapeutics,* opposed to empirical.

ra"tion·al·i·za'tion. A mode of adjustment to difficult and unpleasant situations; characterized by an attempt to justify or defend an unacceptable attitude or trait, its mode of expression, or its consequences or sequelae by withholding, misrepresenting, or falsifying essential facts, by blaming an incidental cause, or by comparing oneself with others in such manner as to excuse oneself.

rats'bane". 1. Arsenic trioxide. 2. A name given to any rat poison containing arsenic.

rat'tle. A rale.

raudixin. Trade-mark for a drug extracted from the powdered root of *Rauwolfia serpentina,* used as a sedative and tranquilizer.

rauwiloid. Trade-mark for alseroxylon.

Rau·wol'fi·a (raw·wol'fee·uh). A genus of toxic plants of the Apocynaceae. A species, *R. serpentina,* is the source of reserpine.

rau·wol'fine (raw·wol'feen, ·fin). An alkaloid from *Rauwolfia serpentina.*

ray. 1. A beam of light or other radiant energy. 2. A stream of discrete particles, such as alpha rays or beta rays. 3. Radial streak of different color in an organ, as medullary rays of the kidney. See *kidney.* **actinic rays.** See *chemical rays* under *ray.* **alpha rays.** Positively charged helium nuclei emitted from radioactive substances. **Becquerel rays.** Rays emitted from uranium. **beta rays.** Electrons with high velocities emitted from radioactive substances. **cathode r.** The stream of electrons emanating from the cathode of a Crookes tube and passing in straight lines regardless of the anode. They are capable of deflection with a magnet, and produce fluorescence and heat wherever they impinge. **chemical rays.** Solar rays that produce chemical change. **gamma rays.** Highly penetrating electromagnetic waves emitted from radioactive substances, situated between cosmic rays and the softer x-rays in the spectrum. **grenz rays.** Electromagnetic radiations of about two angstrom units, useful in roentgen-ray therapy of the skin because of their limited power of penetration. They are on the borderline or limit of utilizable and chemically

employable roentgen wave lengths. **hard rays.** Roentgen rays from a tube operated on a high potential. They have short wave lengths and high penetrating powers. Also see *soft rays* under *ray.* **Hertzian rays.** Radiant energy having longer wave lengths than infrared; used for radio transmissions. **infrared rays.** Radiant heat with wave lengths between visible light and Hertzian waves. **Millikan rays.** Cosmic rays, composed of high-energy photons and electrons. **monochromatic r.** Radiation of a single sharply defined wave length. **neutron r.** A stream of neutrons obtained by bombardment in a cyclotron. **photographic rays.** See *ultraviolet rays* under *ray.* **roentgen rays.** The radiant energy of short wave lengths discovered by Röntgen, and named x-rays by him. A vacuum tube of glass (called a Geissler tube, a Hittorf, a Crookes, or a Coolidge tube) is used with two wires sealed through the glass. These wires are connected with the two poles of a high-voltage generator, and Röntgen found that the rays had peculiar penetrative powers through matter opaque to other ether rays, and that by means of these rays photographs (shadowgrams) may be taken of bones, metallic substances, etc., situated in the tissues; they readily traverse living tissues; they have no appreciable effect on the vitality of bacteria, but are effective in certain diseases. **scattered r.** The roentgen ray which has been scattered from its original path by a reflecting collision. **secondary r.** See *secondary electron.* **soft rays.** Rays coming from a tube operated on a relatively low voltage; they are readily absorbed. Also see *hard rays* under *ray.* **ultraviolet rays.** Light waves too short to affect the retina. They can be reflected, refracted, and polarized; they will not traverse many bodies that are pervious to the rays of the visible spectrum; they produce photographic and photochemical effects, and rapidly destroy the vitality of bacteria. **x-rays.** See *roentgen rays* under *ray.*

Rb. Chemical symbol for rubidium.

R. D. Reaction of degeneration.

rd. Rutherford.

R. D. A. The right dorsoanterior position of the fetus.

R. D. P. The right dorsoposterior position of the fetus.

R. E. Right eye.

Re. Chemical symbol for rhenium.

re-. A prefix signifying *back* or *again.*

re"ac·quired'. Acquired a second time.

re·ac'tion. 1. A response to stimulus. 2. *In chemistry,* the interaction of two or more chemical substances; or, the result of a test of the hydrogen-ion concentration of a solution by means of an indicator, classified as neutral, acid, or alkaline. For reactions not listed here, see under *test, method, reflex.* **affective r.** *In psychiatry,* moods of abnormal elation, disharmony, or depression characteristic of certain psychotic states, as involutional melancholia, manic-depressive psychosis. **agglutination r.** The clumping of cellular antigens, as bacteria, upon mixture with immune serum. **alarm r.** The totality of nonspecific phenomena following a sudden exposure of a large portion of the body to stimuli to which the organism is not adapted. Among the phenomena elicited are hypotension, nervous-system depression, deranged capillary and cell-membrane permeability, electrolyte disturbances, leukopenia followed by leukocytosis, eosinopenia, adrenalin release, and corticotropin and corticosteroid release. The reaction pattern to pain as distinguished from the perception of pain; the reaction includes anxiety, distress, or perspiration. **allergic r.** A reaction based on hypersensitivity to an antigen. **anaphylactic r.** Antigen-antibody reaction in hypersensitive host. See *anaphylaxis.* **anaphylactoid r.** A reaction similar to anaphylaxis elicited by introduction into the host of a substance which has not been used to produce a hypersensitive state. The reaction is not so severe nor so generalized as true anaphylaxis. **antigen-antibody r.** A combination of an antigen with its specific antibody. See *antibody, antigen.* **Aschheim-Zondek r.** Follicular growth and luteinization produced by substances in the urine of pregnant women, while the urine following oöphorectomy and the menopause contains only the follicle growth-stimulating substance. Also see Aschheim-Zondek *test.* **bufo r.** A biologic pregnancy test; when urine, containing chorionic gonadotropic hormone, from a pregnant woman is injected into a male toad, spermatozoa migrate from the testes to the bladder and can be demonstrated in the toad's urine. **complement-fixation r.** An antigen-antibody combination with complement. Also see *fixation* of complement, complement-fixation *test.* **constitutional r.** An immediate or delayed reaction following the administration of an allergen and occurring at sites other than that of its administration (local reaction) and other than that of the original symptoms (focal reaction). Usually associated with local or focal reactions or both. **cutaneous r.** Reaction of skin to an antigen produced by either hypersensitivity or insufficient amount of circulating antibody. **decidual r.** The reaction of tissue especially the endometrium, to pregnancy; marked by the development of characteristic decidual cells from fibroblasts. **delayed r.** An inflammatory lesion of the skin or other phenomenon occurring hours or days after contact between allergen or atopen and hypersensitive tissue cells. Such a reaction may be either local at the site of contact, or systemic, or constitutional **dopa r.** (*for melanoblasts*). A reaction involving 3,4-dihydroxyphenylalanine, which stains melanoblasts black when used under special conditions. **early r.** A response becoming clinically manifest and reaching its maximum within several minutes after sensitive tissue is exposed to an excitant. It usually refers to wheal and flare reactions, to scratch or intracutaneous tests, or to an anaphylactic or anaphylactoid reaction. **false-negative r.** An erroneous or deceptive negative reaction due to faulty technic or evaluation. **focal r.** A response (exacerbation or recurrence) at the site of an active, quiescent, or healed lesion distant from the place of introduction or the point of origin of the exciting agent. **id r.** A secondary skin reaction occurring at a distance from an area of skin infection. It is believed to be an immune reaction. It occurs almost exclusively in infections conferring tuberculin type of skin sensitivity. **immune r.** A reaction which demonstrates the presence of an antibody **local r.** The phenomena or lesions occurring at the site of application of an exciting agent. **nuclear r.** A process in which an atomic nucleus reacts with another nucleus, an elementary particle, or a photon to produce one or more other nuclei and possibly neutrons or photons. **paranoid r.** A form of paranoia characterized by persistent delusions, usually of persecution or grandeur, but, ordinarily, without hallucinations. **peroxidase r.** The appearance of dark granules in the cytoplasm of the myeloid series when treated with special stains. This reaction is not given by cells of the lymphoid series. **r. of degeneration.** The reaction of a degenerated muscle to a direct current in which the anodal closing contraction becomes first equal to the cathodal closing contraction and later, greater than it. Abbreviated, R. D. **r. velocity.** Velocity directly proportional to the active masses of reactant (raised to the power equal to the number of molecules of reactant) present at a time, t. **Rh r.** The result of Rh testing; namely, either Rh positive or Rh negative. **shortening r.** Reflex contraction of extensor muscles when flexed limb is extended by some external agent, acting to maintain the joints of the limb under a certain degree of tension. **skin r.** A test or examination performed by exposure of the skin to an excitant. Typical examples are (a) the scratch test, (b) the intracutaneous test, and (c) the patch test. **specific r.** In allergy, phenomena produced by an agent which is identical with or immunologically related to one that previously produced alteration in capacity to react. **symptomatic r.** A reaction following testing or therapeutic injection of an allergen or atopen and characterized by the occurrence or reproduction of the original symptoms under investigation or treatment. **transfusion r.** The complex of symptoms resulting from a transfusion of incompatible blood with consequent intravenous agglutination of red blood cells and hemolysis of the agglutinated cells. **tuberculin r.** A localized inflammation of tissues when subjected to contact with tuberculin. It consists usually of hyperemia and induration. In severe reactions, known as the Koch phenomenon, necrosis and sloughing occur. A positive tuberculin reaction indicates that the body has been sensitized by the presence of tubercle bacilli. **wheal r.** The occurrence of a wheal at the site of a cutaneous test.

re·ac'tion for·ma'tion. *In psychoanalysis*, the development of conscious, socially acceptable activity which is the antithesis of repressed or rejected unconscious desires.

re·ac'tion time. The interval between the application of a stimulus and the beginning of the response.

re·ac'ti·vate. Render active again, as by the addition of fresh normal serum containing complement to an immune serum which has lost its complement through age, heat, etc. Also, restore complementary activity to a serum, deprived of one or several of its C' components, by the addition of these components.

re''ac·ti·va'tion. Rendering active again by the addition of complement, or one or several of its components, to a serum which has become inactive.

re·a'gent. 1. Any substance involved in a chemical reaction. 2. A substance used for the detection or determination of another substance by chemical or microscopical means. **Benedict's qualitative r.** A solution containing 17.3 Gm. of crystallized copper sulfate, 173 Gm. of sodium or potassium citrate, 200 Gm. of crystallized sodium carbonate, and distilled water to make 1000 cc., used for qualitative urine sugar determination. **Benedict's quantitative r.** A solution containing 18 Gm. of copper sulfate, 200 Gm.

of crystallized sodium carbonate, 200 Gm. of sodium or potassium citrate, 125 Gm. of potassium sulfocyanate, 5 cc. of 5% potassium ferrocyanide, and distilled water to make 1000 cc., used for the quantitative determination of urine sugar. **benzidine r.** A mixture of equal parts of a saturated solution of benzidine and 3% hydrogen peroxide used in testing for the presence of occult blood. **Fehling's r.** Two solutions, one containing 34.64 Gm. of crystalline copper sulfate in water to 500 cc., the other containing 173 Gm. of Rochelle salt and 100 Gm. of potassium hydroxide in water to 500 cc., used as a qualitative test for urine dextrose. **Haines's r.** A solution containing 2 Gm. of pure copper sulfate, 16 cc. of distilled water, 16 cc. of pure glycerin, and 156 cc. of 5% potassium hydroxide, used to test for urine sugar. **Millon's r.** A solution of mercuric nitrate and nitrite in a mixture of the corresponding acids prepared by dissolving metallic mercury in concentrated nitric acid. On heating, it gives a red color with proteins containing the tyrosine group and with substances, other than proteins, containing the hydroxy-phenyl group. **Nadi** (*naphthol, dimethyl*) **r.** A mixture of β-naphthol with dimethyl-para-phenylene diamine, used as a test for indophenol oxidase. **Töpfer's r.** A 0.5% solution of dimethyl-aminoazo-benzene in 95% alcohol, most commonly used as an indicator to detect free hydrochloric acid in the gastric contents.

re'a·gin. 1. One of a group of special antibodies in serum which react with the allergens or atopens responsible for the specific manifestations of hypersensitivity in man, as hay fever, asthma. 2. The antibodylike substance in serum and cerebrospinal fluid concerned with the flocculation of the alcohol-soluble lipids of normal tissue in the complement-fixation and flocculation reactions in syphilis.

re·al'gar. Arsenic disulfide, As_2S_2; a pigment.

ream'er. A surgical instrument used for gouging out holes or enlarging those already made. Used especially in bone operations.

re''am·i·na'tion. The introduction of an amino group into a compound from which an amino group had previously been removed.

re''am·pu·ta'tion. An amputation upon a member on which the operation has already been performed.

re·an'i·mate. Revive; resuscitate; restore to life, as a person apparently dead.

re·bound'. In reflex activity, a sudden contraction of a muscle following its relaxation; associated with a variety of forms of reflex activity. Seen most typically following the cessation of an inhibitory reflex.

re·cal″ci·fi·ca′tion (ree-kal″si-fi-kay′shun). The restoring to tissues of the lime salts which they have lost.

re″ca·pit″u·la′tion. The summarizing of the main points of a subject; the repetition of the steps of a process, as recapitulation theory, *q.v.*

re·ceiv′er. 1. The vessel receiving the products of distillation. 2. In an air pump, the jar in which the vacuum is produced.

re·cep′tive. Having the quality of, or capacity for, receiving.

re·cep′tor. 1. A name given by Ehrlich to the atomic lateral chain or haptophorous group, which, existing in each cell in addition to its nucleus, combines with intermediary bodies such as toxins, food molecules, and foreign substances. Also see side-chain *theory.* 2. Peripheral nerve endings in the skin and special sense organs.

re·cess′, re′cess. A fossa, ventricle, or ampulla; an anatomic depression. **costodiaphragmatic r.** A potential space formed by apposition of the costal and diaphragmatic layers of the parietal pleura. **duodenojejunal r.** A pouch of the mesentery on the right side of the jejunum and near its union with the duodenum. Also called *duodenojejunal fossa.* **epitympanic r.** The attic of the tympanic cavity. **ileocecal r.** The ileocecal fossa. **lateral r.** The lateral extension of the fourth ventricle in the angle between the cerebellum and the medulla oblongata. **paraduodenal r.** An occasional small pouch of peritoneum situated to the left of the last part of the duodenum. **peritoneal recesses.** Pockets behind or around organs in the peritoneal cavity, as paraduodenal recesses. **pharyngeal r.** A lateral mucosal diverticulum of the pharynx situated behind the opening of the auditory tube. Also called *Rosenmueller's r.* **piriform r.** A small space lateral to the laryngeal orifice which is bounded laterally by the thyroid cartilage and hyothyroid membrane and medially by the aryepiglottic fold. Syn., *pyriform r., piriform sinus.* **r. of tympanic cavity.** (a) Anterior and posterior pouches of the mucous membrane covering the lateral wall of the tympanic cavity and found on either side of the manubrium of the malleus. Also called *r. of Tröltsch.* (b) A superior recess situated between the flaccid part of the tympanic membrane and the neck of the malleus. Also called *Prussak's space.* **retrocecal r.** An occasional pouch of peritoneum extending upward between the cecum and posterior abdominal wall. **retroduo-**

denal r. An occasional small pouch of peritoneum situated behind the transverse portion of the duodenum extending upward from below. **sacciform r. of the wrist.** An elongation of synovial membrane extending between the radius and ulna at their distal articulation.

re·ces′sion. The gradual withdrawal of a part from its normal position, as the recession of the gums from the necks of the teeth.

re·ces′sive. 1. *In biology,* a characteristic of one of the parents of a hybrid which is expressed in the minority of the offspring, in contrast to the dominant characteristic of the other parent. 2. Pertaining to such a characteristic. See recessive *character; dominant; Mendel's law* under *Gregor Johann Mendel.*

re·ces′sus. See recess.

re·cid″i·va′tion. 1. The relapse of a patient recovering from a disease. 2. *In criminology,* a relapsing into crime.

re·cid′i·vism. The repetition of criminal or delinquent acts; bad behavior.

re·cid′i·vist. 1. A patient who returns to a hospital for treatment, especially an insane person who so returns. 2. *In criminology,* a confirmed, relapsed, or habitual criminal.

rec″i·div′i·ty (ress″i·div′i·tee). Tendency to return or to relapse.

rec′i·pe (ress′i·pee). 1. The heading of a physician's prescription, signifying *take.* Symbol, ℞. 2. The prescription itself.

re·cip′i·ent. One who receives blood or other tissue from a donor.

rec″li·na′tion. An operation for cataract, in which the lens was pushed back into the vitreous chamber. Obs. Also called *couching.*

re″com·po·si′tion. Reunion of parts or constituents after temporary disolution.

re″com·pres′sion. Resubjection to increased atmospheric pressure; a procedure used in treating caisson workers or divers who develop symptoms of caisson disease on returning to normal pressures.

re″con·stit′u·ent. A medicine which promotes continuous repair of tissue waste or makes compensation for its loss.

re·con″sti·tu′tion (ree-kon″sti·tew′shun). Continuous repair of progressive destruction of tissues.

re·cov′er·y. Restoration from illness.

rec′re·ment. A substance secreted from a part of the body, as a gland, and again absorbed by the body. —**recremen′tal, recrementi′tial, recrementi′tious,** *adj.*

re″cru·des′cence. An increase in

the symptoms of a disease after a remission or a short intermission.

rec·tal'gi·a. Pain in the rectum; proctalgia.

rec"ti·fi·ca'tion. 1. A straightening, as rectification of a crooked limb. 2. The redistillation or fractional distillation of liquids to obtain a product of higher purity or greater concentration of the desired constituent.

rec'to-. A combining form denoting *the rectum* or *rectal*.

rec'to·cele. Prolapse of the rectum into the vagina.

rec'to·cly·sis. The slow instillation of a liquid into the rectum.

rec"to·co·li'tis. Inflammation of the mucosa of the rectum and colon combined.

rec"to·cys·tot'o·my. Incision of the bladder through the rectum. *Obs.*

rec"to·pex"y, rec"to·pex'y. Fixation of the rectum to the pelvic wall by suturing.

rec"to·rec·tos'to·my. Surgical anastomosis between two parts of the rectum.

rec"to·ro·man'o·scope. A speculum used in examining the rectum and the sigmoid flexure.

rec'to·scope. A rectal speculum. —**rectos'copy,** *n.*

rec"to·sig'moid. The rectum and sigmoid portion of the colon considered together.

rec"to·sig"moid·os'co·py. Ocular inspection of the rectum and sigmoid flexure of the colon with the aid of special instruments.

rec"to·ste·no'sis. Stenosis of the rectum.

rec"to·u'ter·ine (reck″to·yōō′turin, ·yne). Pertaining to the rectum and the uterus.

rec"to·vag'i·nal (·vadj′i·nul, ·vajye′nul). Pertaining to the rectum and the vagina.

rec"to·vag"i·no·ab·dom'i·nal (·vadj″i·no·ab·dom′i·nul). Pertaining to a method of combined examination in the female.

rec"to·ves'i·cal. Pertaining to the rectum and the bladder.

rec'tum. The lower part of the large intestine, extending from the sigmoid flexure to the anal canal. It begins opposite the third sacral vertebra, passes downward and forward more or less in the midline, pierces the pelvic diaphragm and terminates in the anal canal. —**rectal,** *adj.*

rec'tus. Straight; applied to anything having a straight course, as rectus abdominis muscle.

re·cum'ben·cy. The reclining position.

re·cum'bent. Leaning back; reclining.

re·cu'per·ate. Regain strength or health.

re·cur'rence. 1. The return of symptons or a disease. 2. Reappearance of a neoplasm after apparently complete removal.

re·cur'rent. 1. Returning. 2. *In anatomy,* turning back in its course, as recurrent laryngeal nerve.

re"cur·va'tion. The act or process of bending backward.

Red Cross So·ci'e·ty. An international organization whose primary purpose was to care for the wounded, the sick, and prisoners in wartime. A more recent function is the relief of human suffering from catastrophe or any other cause.

re'di·a (pl. *rediae*). *In parasitology,* the second larval stage of a trematode, which results from the development of a parthenogenetic egg of the first larval stage.

red. in pulv. *Redactus in pulverem;* reduced to powder.

red·in"te·gra'tion. 1. The complete restitution of a part that has been injured or destroyed. 2. See *reintegration.*

red'out. A condition met with by combat flyers, in which acceleration is centripetal and the blood is driven toward the head. There is a bursting headache, and vision is blurred as by a red mist.

re'dox. A reduction-oxidation reaction, state, or system.

re·duce'. 1. Restore a part to its normal relations, as to reduce a hernia or fracture. 2. *In chemistry,* bring back to the metallic form; deprive of oxygen. 3. Lose weight by dietetic regimen.

re·duced'. 1. Restored to the proper place. 2. *In chemistry,* having undergone reduction, that is, accepted electrons. 3. Diminished in size.

re·duc'tant. A reducing agent.

re·duc'tase (ri·duck′tace, ·taze). An enzyme causing reduction. *Obs.* **cyto-chrome C r.** A flavoprotein enzyme system isolated from yeast; the oxidized form of flavoprotein is highly active in oxidizing reduced coenzyme II, while the reduced form of the flavoprotein readily reduces oxidized cytochrome C.

re·duc'tion. 1. *In chemistry,* an increase in the negative valence, or a decrease in the positive valence, of an element, resulting from the gain of electrons which are taken from some other element. See also *oxidation,* 1. 2. Originally, the process of separation from oxygen, or of combining with hydrogen. 3. The restoration of a dislocated joint or fractured bone to its normal place or condition by means of surgery or manipulation. **closed r.** Reduction of a part or a limb without performing open surgery. **open r.** Reduction of a part or a limb by means of open surgery.

re·duc'tone. A substance, probably HOCH:C(OH)CHO, the enolic form of hydroxymalonic dialdehyde. It is a strong reducing agent.

re·du"pli·ca'tion. A doubling. **r. of the heart sounds.** A doubling of either the first or the second sound of the heart. It occurs in hypertension, increased pulmonary pressure, and myocardial disease, but may also occur without clinical significance.

Reed, Walter [*American Army surgeon,* 1851–1902]. Chairman of the celebrated United States Army Yellow Fever Board. His *Experimental Yellow Fever* (1901) published the proof that yellow fever is caused by a filtrable virus transmitted to man by a mosquito, *Aëdes aegypti.*

re"ed·u·ca'tion. The development of the processes of adjustment in an individual who has acquired these processes and then lost them.

re"ev·o·lu'tion. Hughlings Jackson's term for a symptom following an epileptic attack, which consists of three stages: suspension of power to understand speech (word deafness); perception of words and echolalia without comprehension; return to conscious perception of speech with continued lack of comprehension.

re·fec'tion. The phenomena of vitamin B-complex synthesis by the bacterial flora of the intestine. With diets of certain composition, the amount of bacterial synthesis of vitamins is sufficiently increased so that rats can grow and reproduce on a diet devoid of vitamin B-complex. Man's dietary requirement for certain vitamins and other nutrients may be controlled to a considerable extent by the nature and extent of refection.

re·fine'. Purify a substance, extract it from raw material, or remove impurities from it.

re·flect'ed. 1. Cast or thrown back. 2. *In anatomy,* turned back upon itself, as visceral peritoneum from the surface of an organ to become parietal peritoneum.

re·flec'tion. 1. A bending or turning back; specifically, the turning back of a ray of light from a surface upon which it impinges without penetrating. 2. In membranes, as the peritoneum, the folds which are made in passing from the wall of the cavity over an organ and back again to the wall which bounds such cavity.

re·flec'tor. A device for reflecting light or sound.

re'flex. An involuntary, invariable, adaptive response to a stimulus. **abdominal r.** Contraction of the abdominal muscles, induced by friction on the corresponding side of the abdominal wall. **accommodation r.** The occurrence of constriction of the pupils, convergence of the eyes, and increased convexity of the lens when the eyes adjust for near vision. **Achilles tendon r.** Plantar flexion of the foot, produced by contraction of the calf muscles when the Achilles tendon receives a sharp blow. **acquired r.** Conditioned reflex. **acromial r.** Flexion of the forearm and slight medial rotation of the hand induced by a sharp blow upon the acromion. **adductor r.** Contraction of the adductors of the thigh, produced by tapping the medial condyle of the femur or any point along the inner side of the thigh. **allied reflexes.** Those elicited from different regions, producing common or reinforced protagonistic actions. **anal r.** Contraction of the external anal sphincter in response to a scratch upon the skin in the perianal region. **ankle clonus r.** Clonic contractions of the calf muscles in response to pressure against the sole of the foot. **attitudinal reflexes.** Reflex adjustments of the skeletal muscles to keep the trunk and limbs in a proper relationship to the position of the head. **audito-oculogyric r.** Movement of the eyes toward the source of a sudden sound. **auditory r.** Brief closure of the eyes resulting from eighth nerve stimulation by the sudden production of a sound. **auriculopalpebral r.** Closure of the eyelids induced by tactile or thermal stimulation of the inner part of the external auditory canal and ear drum. Also called *Kisch's r., Kehrer's r.* **axon r.** One occurring without involvement of a nerve cell body; results from a stimulus applied to a terminal branch of a sensory nerve and gives rise to an impulse that ascends to a collateral branch down which it is conducted to an effector organ; believed to be important in the local regulation of blood vessels. **Babinski r.** An abnormal reflex characterized by extension of the great toe upon stroking of the sole of the foot. Also called *Babinski's sign.* **Bainbridge r.** A reflex acceleration of the heart and rise of arterial pressure due to rise of pressure in the right atrium and roots of great veins. Also called *cardiovascular r., right heart r.* **Bekhterev's r.** (a) Facial contraction on the same side as irritation of the nasal mucosa. Syn., *nasal r.* (b) Dilatation of the pupil on exposure to light, occasionally seen in tabes and dementia paralytica. Syn., *paradoxical pupillary r.* (c) Plantar flexion of the foot induced by tapping the dorsum of the foot; seen in pyramidal tract disease. (d) Extension of the foot with flexion of the knee and hip on the same side upon release of a foot passively bent in a plantar direction; seen in pyramidal tract disease. (e) A normal response characterized by contraction of the lower abdominal muscles on stroking of the skin of the inner surface of the thigh. Syn., *hypogastric r.* **Bekhterev-Mendel r.** Dorsal flexion of the second to fifth toes induced by percussion of the dorsum of the foot in normal individuals; plantar flexion occurs in the presence of pyramidal tract disease. Syn., *Mendel's dorsal r. of the foot, dorsocuboidal r., cuboidodigital r.* **biceps r.** Contraction of the biceps brachii muscle induced by percussion of its tendon. **body-righting r.** A righting reflex initiated by asymmetrical stimulation of pressure receptors on the surface of the body. **bone r.** A reflex presumed to be elicited by stimulus applied to a bone, but really a muscle stretch reflex. **Brudzinski's r.** (a) Flexion of the ankle, knee, and hip when the head of the patient is flexed in meningitis. (b) Flexion of one leg when the opposite leg is passively flexed at the hip joint in meningitis. **bulbocavernosus r.** Contraction of the bulbocavernosus muscle, induced by tapping the dorsum of the penis. **Capps's pleural r.** Shock induced by mechanical irritation, as with a trocar, of an inflamed pleura. **carotid sinus r.** That consisting of reflex effects on heart, blood vessels, and respiration, induced by changes in pressure, or in chemical composition, of blood in the carotid sinus. **Chaddock's r.** (a) Extension of the great toe on stimulation around the lateral malleolus, seen in pyramidal tract lesions. (b) Flexion of the wrist and extension and fanning of the fingers caused by irritation of the ulnar aspect of the lower forearm in hemiplegia. **chain r.** A series of consecutive reflexes, each of which is initiated by the preceding one, resulting in an integrated action. **chin r.** A clonic movement of the jaw, induced by a stroke on the lower jaw while it hangs passively open. Syn., *jaw-jerk r.* **ciliary r.** The normal constriction of the pupil in accommodation of the eye. **ciliospinal r.** Dilatation of the ipsilateral pupil on pinching the skin on one side of the neck. **conditioned r.** A reflex acquired as a result of repeated association and training, as opposed to a natural reflex. **consensual light r.** Reflex contraction of the pupil in one eye when the pupil of the other eye is exposed to light. Also called *consensual pupillary r.* **consensual r.** A response on

one side of the body produced by stimulation of the other side. Syn., *crossed r.* **contralateral r.** An overflow response on the opposite side when a reflex is elicited on one side of the body. **convulsive r.** Incoördinated convulsive muscular contractions. **coördinated r.** A coördinated reaction of several muscles in orderly progression. **corneomandibular r.** Deflection of the lower jaw to the opposite side when the cornea of one eye is irritated, the mouth being open. **cough r.** A cough caused by irritation of the laryngeal mucosa. **cremasteric r.** Retraction of the testis on the same side induced by stimulation of the skin on the front and inner surface of one thigh. **crossed extension r.** The extension of the limb opposite to that in which a flexor reflex is induced. **crossed r.** A response on one side of the body induced by stimulation of the other side. Syn., *consensual r.* **cuboidodigital r.** On percussion of the dorsum of the foot the normal reaction is extension of all but the great toe; the abnormal reaction is flexion. **cutaneous pupillary r.** Dilatation of the pupil in response to pinching of the skin of the neck or face. Also called *ciliospinal r.* **cutaneous r.** Wrinkling or gooseflesh in response to irritation of the skin. **dartos muscle r.** Wormlike contraction of the dartos muscle when cold is applied suddenly to the perineum. **deep r.** Any muscle stretch reflex, including the so-called tendon reflexes and periosteal reflexes. **delayed r.** A reflex occurring an abnormally long while after the stimulus. **depressor r.** A reflex fall in blood pressure or vasodilatation, which may be evoked by a variety of stimuli, as increased pressure in the carotid sinus. **digital r.** Sudden flexion of the terminal phalanx of the thumb and of the second and third phalanges of some other finger, elicited by snapping the terminal phalanx of the patient's middle or index finger. Also called *Hoffmann's sign.* **direct light r.** Contraction of the sphincter pupillae induced by a ray of light thrown upon the retina. Also called *direct pupillary r.* **eyeball compression r.** Slowing of the heart caused by pressure on the eyeball. Syn., *oculocardiac r.* **eye closure r.** (a) Closure of the eyelids on tapping the supraorbital nerve. (b) Closure of the eyelids on stimulation of the external ear canal. Syn., *Kisch's r.* **femoral r.** Extension of the knee and flexion of the toes induced by irritation of the skin over the upper anterior surface of the thigh. **flexion r.** Flexion or withdrawal of a limb in response to a noxious stimulus. **Gault's r.** Contraction of the orbicularis oculi nearest the source of a sudden and unexpected sound; seen in normal persons. Syn., *cochleopalpebral r.* **Geigel's r.** Contraction of muscle fibers above the inguinal ligament, induced by stimulation of the skin over the upper and inner aspect of the thigh in the female. **gluteal r.** Contraction of the gluteal muscles induced by stimulation of the overlying skin. **Gonda r.** Extension of the great toe when the last two toes are snapped between the examiner's fingers; indicative of a pyramidal tract lesion. **Gordon's r.** Extension of the great toe produced by squeezing the calf muscles, indicative of pyramidal tract disease. Syn., *paradoxic flexor r.* **great-toe r.** A comprehensive term, signifying extension of the great toe, and including the Babinski, Chaddock, Gordon, and Oppenheim reflexes. **Hoffmann's finger r.** See Hoffmann's *sign,* digital *r.* **hypothenar r.** Contraction of the palmaris brevis muscle upon stimulation of the pisiform bone. **infraspinatus r.** Extension of the elbow and lateral rotation of the arm induced by a sudden sharp tap over the infraspinatus muscle. **inguinal r.** Contraction of muscle fibers above the inguinal ligament, induced by stimulation of the skin over the upper and inner aspect of the thigh in the female. Syn., *Geigel's r.* **intestinal r.** Contraction of the intestine above and relaxation below a portion of the intestine that is stimulated, through the influence of the myenteric nerve plexus. This action occurs in peristalsis. Syn., *myenteric r.* **Jacobsohn's r.** Flexion of the fingers induced by a mild tap on the lower end of the radius or in its neighborhood on the dorsal side of the forearm, formerly considered to indicate pyramidal tract disease, but now considered to be essentially normal, although more distinct in cases of reflex hyperirritability, of functional or organic nature. **jaw-jerk r.** Clonic contraction of the muscles of mastication and elevation of the mandible, elicited by striking the relaxed and dependent jaw with a percussion hammer, the mouth being open. Observed in disease of the upper motor neurons. **knee-jerk r.** An involuntary jerk of the leg due to sudden contraction of the quadriceps muscle when the patellar tendon (ligamentum patellae) is quickly struck with a percussion hammer. **Kocher's r.** Contraction of the abdominal muscles when a testis is compressed. Syn., *testicular compression r.* **laryngeal r.** A cough resulting from irritation of the larynx.

light r. (a) Of the tympanic membrane: a cone of light on the anterior and inferior part of the tympanic membrane, with its apex directed toward the umbo. (b) Of the retina: a circular area of light reflected from the retina during retinoscopic examination. (c) Of the pupil: contraction of the pupil in response to light. **lip r.** A reflex movement of the lips of sleeping babies induced by a sudden tap over the angle of the mouth. **mass r.** A complex reflex phenomenon induced by stimulation below the level of a complete transverse lesion of the spinal cord and characterized by flexor spasms of the legs, involuntary evacuation of the bladder, and sweating below the level of the lesion. **Mendel's dorsal r. of foot.** Extension of the second to fifth toes in response to percussion o the dorsum of the foot in normal individuals; flexion of these toes occurs in certain organic diseases of the nervou system. Syn., *Bekhterev-Mendel r., dorsocuboidal r., cuboidodigital r.* **middle ear disease r.** A reflex phenomenon used to explain the temperature variations which both adults and children occasionally exhibit with mild grades of tympanic inflammation probably depending on the individual differences in stability of central nervous control. **myenteric r.** A respons to stimulation of a segment of the intestine, characterized by contraction of the bowel above the level of stimulation and relaxation of the bowel below the level of stimulation. Syn., *intestinal r.* **nasomental r.** Contraction of the mentalis muscle with consequen elevation of the lower lip and wrinklin of the skin of the chin in response t a light tap on the side of the nose with a percussion hammer. **oculocardiac r.** Slowing of the heart rate i response to pressure upon the eyeballs a normal reaction when the rate i decreased by 5 to 13 beats per minute **oculocephalogyric r.** The associated movements of the eye, head, an body in the process of focusing visua attention upon an object. **oculopharyngeal r.** Rapid movements o deglutition and spontaneous closing o the eyes without apparent contractio of the orbicularis muscle, in respons to stimulation of the bulbar conjunctiva. **Onanoff's r.** Contraction of th bulbocavernosus muscle in response t compression of the glans penis. **Oppenheim r.** Extension of the grea toe upon stroking downward along th medial side of the tibia, a sign o corticospinal-tract lesion. **optica righting r.** Righting reflex initiate by the visual perception of an impprope orientation of the body in reference t the horizon or to familiar objects.

orbicularis oculi r. Bilateral contraction of the orbicularis oculi muscle by any of a great variety of stimuli—auditory, visual, or muscle stretching. **palatal r.** (a) Elevation of the soft palate in response to a touch. (b) Swallowing produced by irritation of the palate. **paradoxic ankle r.** An ankle reflex in which percussion over the flexor surface induces an extensor response, and vice versa. **paradoxic patellar r.** Contraction of the hamstring muscles in response to tapping of the patellar tendon (ligamentum patellae); sometimes observed in tabes, poliomyelitis, lesions of the femoral nerve, and other lesions affecting the arc of the patellar reflex. **patellar clonus r.** Clonic contraction and relaxation of the quadriceps muscle in response to sharp firm pressure against the upper margin of the patella; observed in lesions of the pyramidal tract. **patellar r.** Contraction of the quadriceps muscle with extension of the leg at the knee in response to a quick tap against the patellar tendon (ligamentum patellae). Also called *knee jerk, knee kick, quadriceps r., patellar tendon r.* **pilomotor r.** Erection of the papillae of the skin (goose flesh) in response to chilling or irritation of the skin or to an emotional stimulus. **plasticity r.** The reflex property of maintaining a spastic limb in the position of flexion or extension in which it has been placed; a resistance to change, either lengthening or shortening. **protective r.** Any response to defend the body from harm, as winking caused by an object rapidly approaching the eye. **psychogalvanic r.** A variation in the electric conductivity of the skin in response to emotional stimuli. Due to changes in blood circulation, secretion of sweat, and skin temperature changes. **pupillary r.** (a) Contraction of the pupil in response to stimulation of the retina by light. (b) Contraction of the pupil on accommodation for close vision and dilatation of the pupil on accommodation for distant vision. Syn., *accommodation r.* (c) Reflex contraction of the pupil of one eye in response to stimulation of the other eye by light. Syn., *consensual light r.* (d) Contraction of the pupil on attempted closure of the eye. Syn., *Westphal's pupillary r.* Also called *Westphal-Pilcz r.* **purposive reflexes.** Those which provide the mechanism for the preservation of the individual. **quadriceps r.** Contraction of the quadriceps muscle with extension of the leg at the knee in response to a quick tap against the patellar tendon (ligamentum patellae). Also called *knee jerk, knee kick, patellar r.* **quadrupedal extensor r.**

An associated movement of extension of the flexed arm in hemiplegia which is sometimes evoked by causing the patient, when standing or kneeling, to lean forward and throw his weight on to the observer's supporting hand placed beneath his chest. **radial r.** A muscle stretch reflex characterized by flexion of the forearm and occasionally by flexion of the fingers in response to a light blow against the lower end of the radius. **rectum r.** The mechanism by which the accumulated feces are evacuated from the rectum, characterized by peristaltic contraction of the rectal musculature and relaxation of the internal and external sphincters of the anus. **righting r.** Any of a chain of reflexes which operate to bring, or to maintain, an animal right side up; included are labyrinthine righting reflexes, body righting reflexes acting upon the head, body righting reflexes acting upon the body, neck righting reflexes, and optical righting reflexes. **Rossolimo's r.** A stretch reflex of the plantar muscles of the foot, characterized by flexion of the second to fifth toes in response to tapping of the plantar surfaces of the toes; its intensity varies with the degree of muscle tonus present. **scratch r.** Reflex scratching movements designed to remove an irritating agent from the surface of the skin; the ease with which this reflex may be initiated in experimental animals has made it one of the most commonly studied forms of reflex activity. **segmental r.** A reaction evoked by afferent impulses entering the spinal cord at the level from which the motor impulses emerge. **simple r.** An uncomplicated reflex, as one acting on a single muscle. **spinal r.** Any reflex whose arc connects with a center in the spinal cord. **Stookey's r.** Flexion of the leg in response to tapping the tendons of the semimembranosus and semitendinosus muscles while the leg is semiflexed at the knee. **sucking r.** Sucking movements of the lips, tongue, and jaw in infants in response to contact of an object with the lips. **supinator jerk r.** Contraction of the supinator muscle when the styloid process of the radius is struck a blow; a stretch reflex. **suprapatellar r.** A sudden upward movement of the patella produced by contraction of the quadriceps muscle in response to a sharp blow upon a finger which is placed against the upper border of the patella, with the leg extended. **suprapubic r.** Deflection of the linea alba toward the stroked side when the abdomen is stroked above the inguinal ligament. **swallowing r.** The chain of reflexes involved in the mechanism of deglutition which may be evoked by stimulation of the palate or pharynx. See palatal r. **tendo Achillis r.** See Achilles tendon r. **testicular compression r.** Contraction of the abdominal muscles in response to compression or squeezing of a testis. Syn., *Kocher's r.* **vagopressor r.** Reflex rise in blood pressure resulting from the stimulation of afferent fibers of the vagus nerve. The afferents probably include nerve fibers that are normally stimulated by changes in distention of the great veins. **vasomotor r.** Constriction or dilatation of a blood vessel in response to psychic or physical stimulation. Syn., *vascular r.* **vestibulo-ocular r.** A statokinetic reflex, observed as a rotation of the eyes in the opposite direction when the head is quickly rotated. **visceral r.** Any reflex induced by some irritation of an internal organ. **visceromotor r.** Tenseness of skeletal muscles evoked by painful stimuli originating in the viscera. **viscerosensory r.** A form of referred pain in which irritating stimuli within the viscera give rise to a painful sensation in some superficial region of the body. **Westphal's pupillary r.** Contraction of the pupil in response to attempted closure of the eyelids. **winking r.** Sudden closure of the eyelids in response to the unexpected appearance of any object within the field of vision. **zygomatic r.** Movement of the lower jaw toward the percussed side when the zygoma is tapped with a percussion hammer.

re·flex″o·gen′ic. Causing or increasing a tendency to reflex action; producing reflexes.

re·flex′o·graph″. An instrument for graphically recording a reflex.

re″flex·om′e·ter. An instrument used to measure the force required to produce myotatic movement.

re·flex′o·ther′a·py. A form of therapeutics based on stimulation by manipulation, anesthetization, or cauterization of areas more or less distant from the affected lesion. Also called *zone therapy, spinal therapeutics.*

re′flux. A return flow, as in a reflux condenser, which returns the condensate to the original fluid. **pancreatic r.** The flow of pancreatic fluid in reverse direction through the common duct so that pancreatic fluid is present in the biliary tract. Also called *biliary-pancreatic r.*

re·fract′. 1. Bend back. 2. Change direction by refraction. 3. Estimate the degree of ametropia, heterophoria, and strabismus present in an eye.

re·frac′ta do′si (ri·frack′tah do′sigh, do′see). In broken or divided doses.

re·frac′tion. 1. The act of refracting or bending back. 2. The deviation of a ray of light from a straight line in passing obliquely from one transparent medium to another of different density. 3. The state of refractive power, especially of the eye; the ametropia, emmetropia, or muscle imbalance present. 4. The act or process of correcting errors of ocular refraction. **angle of r.** The angle formed by a refracted ray of light with the perpendicular at the point of refraction. **coefficient of r.** The quotient of the sine of the angle of refraction into the sine of the angle of incidence. **double r.** Birefringence. The property of having more than one refractive index, according to the direction of the traversing light. **errors of r.** Departures from the power of producing a normal or well-defined image upon the retina, because of ametropia. **r. of the eye.** The influence of the ocular media upon a cone or beam of light, whereby a normal or emmetropic eye produces a proper image of the object upon the retina.

re·frac′tion·ist. One who measures errors of ocular refraction.

re″frac·tom′e·ter. 1. An instrument for measuring the refraction of the eye. 2. An instrument for the determination of the refractive indexes of liquids.

re·frac′to·ry. 1. Resisting treatment. 2. Resisting the action of heat; slow to melt. 3. Resisting stimulation, said of a muscle or nerve immediately after responding to a stimulation.

re·frac′ture (ree·frack′chur). The breaking again of fractured bones that have united by faulty union.

re·fran″gi·bil′i·ty. Capability of undergoing refraction. **—refran′gible,** *adj.*

re·fresh′. In *surgery*, give to an old lesion the character of a fresh wound. Also see *debridement.*

re·frig′er·ant (ri·fridj′ur·unt). 1. Cooling; lessening fever. 2. A medicine or agent having cooling properties or lowering body temperature.

re·frig″er·a′tion. The act of lowering the temperature of a body by conducting away its heat to a surrounding cooler substance.

ref′use. Waste from manufacturing or other establishments, or any discarded matter.

re·fu′sion. Injection of blood into the circulation after its removal from the same patient.

re·gen′er·ate. Form anew; reproduce, grow anew.

re·gen″er·a′tion. 1. The new growth or repair of structures or tissues lost by disease or by injury. 2. In *chem-*

istry, the process of obtaining from the by-products or end products of an operation a substance which was employed in the earlier part of the operation.

reg′i·men (redj′i·men). A systematic course or plan including food, sanitary arrangements, and medication, to maintain or improve health.

re′gion. One of the divisions of the body possessing either natural or arbitrary boundaries. —**regional,** *adj.* **abdominal r.** One of the nine regions of the abdomen artificially formed by two horizontal and two parasagittal lines. The horizontal lines are tangent to the cartilages of the ninth ribs and iliac crests, respectively, while the parasagittal lines are drawn vertically on each side from the middle of the inguinal ligament. The regions are, from above: the right hypochondriac region, the epigastric region, the left hypochondriac region, the right lumbar region, the umbilical region, the left lumbar region, the right inguinal region, the hypogastric region, and the left inguinal region. **axillary r.** A region upon the lateral aspect of the thorax, extending from the axilla to a line drawn from the lower border of the mammary region to that of the scapular region. **ciliary r.** The zone around the cornea of the eye, corresponding to the position of the ciliary body. **deltoid r.** The proximal part of the lateral aspect of the upper arm. **gustatory r.** The tip, margins, and root of the tongue in the neighborhood of the vallate papillae; also the lateral parts of the soft palate and the anterior surface of the glossopalatine arches. **infraclavicular r.** The area bounded superiorly by the lower border of the clavicle, inferiorly by the lower border of the third rib, on one side by a line extending from the acromion to the pubic spine, and on the other side by the edge of the sternum. **inframammary r.** The area immediately below each breast and above the costal margin. **inguinal r.** The right and left inguinal or iliac regions are two of the nine abdominal regions. The right includes the abdominal surface covering the cecum and the vermiform process, the ureter, and the spermatic vessels; the left, that covering the sigmoid flexure of the colon, the ureter, and the spermatic vessels. Also called *iliac r.* **ischiorectal r.** The region corresponding to the posterior part of the pelvic outlet, between the ischium and the rectum. **parotid r.** The area of the face anterior to the ear lying over the parotid gland. **scapular r.** The region of the back corresponding to the position of the scapula, the spine of which divides it into a supraspinous

and an infraspinous region. **submaxillary r.** The region between the mandible and the anterior and posterior bellies of the digastric muscle. The triangle so bounded contains the submaxillary or submandibular gland. Also called *submandibular triangle.* **supraclavicular r.** The space between the upper margin of the clavicle, and the lower borders of the omohyoid and sternocleidomastoid muscles. **suprainguinal r.** That bounded by the rectus abdominis muscle, the inguinal ligament, and a horizontal line through the iliac crest. **supraspinous r.** The region corresponding to the supraspinous fossa of the scapula.

reg′is·ter. The compass of a voice; also a subdivision of its compass, consisting of a series of tones produced in the same way and of a like character.

reg′is·trar. 1. An official custodian of records. 2. An officer in charge of hospital registry office.

reg″is·tra′tion. The act of recording, as of deaths, births, etc.

reg′is·try. Office listing nurses available for general or special services.

regitine. Trade-mark for phentolamine.

reg″le·men·ta′tion. The legal restriction or regulation of prostitution.

re·gres′sion. 1. A turning back. 2. The tendency for children to deviate less from the average of the population than their parents. Also called *filial r.* 3. *In psychology,* a mental state and a mode of adjustment to difficult and unpleasant situations, characterized by behavior of a type that had been satisfying and appropriate at an earlier stage of development but which no longer befits the age and social status of the individual. A terminal state in some forms of schizophrenia. 4. *In mathematics,* the tendency for a group equated in one trait to have a mean value closer to the general mean in a related trait. 5. See *retrogression.*

re·gres′sive. Going back to a former state; subsiding, said of symptoms.

reg′u·lar. 1. According to rule or custom. 2. Colloquial term for menstruating at normal time.

reg″u·la′tion. The ability of a developing organism to continue normal development in spite of experimental interference such as ablation, implantation, or transplantation.

reg′u·la″tive. *In embryology,* descriptive of development of eggs in which the cells of the early stages can be affected by inducing agents from the surrounding parts; opposed to mosaic development. See *mosaic,* 2.

re·gur″gi·ta′tion. 1. A backflow of blood through a heart valve that is defective. 2. The return of food from the stomach to the mouth soon after eating, without the ordinary efforts at vomiting. **aortic r.** That of the blood through the aortic orifice, due to incompetence of the aortic valve. **duodenal r.** The return of chyme from the duodenum into the stomach. **functional r.** A form of mitral or tricuspid regurgitation, due to dilatation of the fibrous rings surrounding the respective valves. **mitral r.** Imperfect closure of the mitral valve during the cardiac systole, permitting blood to be forced back into the left atrium.

re"ha·bil'i·ta·tion. The rendering of a physically or mentally handicapped person fit to engage in a remunerative occupation.

re"ha·la'tion. Rebreathing; the inhalation of air which has been inspired previously; sometimes used in anesthesia.

rei'neck·e salt (rye'neck·ee). Ammonium reineckate, $NH_4[Cr(NH_3)_2(SCN)_4].H_2O$. Dark-red crystals or powder, moderately soluble in cold water. Used as a reagent.

re"in·fec'tion. A second infection with the same kind of organism.

re"in·force'ment. 1. The act of reinforcing. 2. Any augmentation of force.

re"in·fu'sion. The reinjection of blood serum, or cerebrospinal fluid.

re"in·ner·va'tion. Nerve grafting where the motor nerve supply to a muscle has been lost.

re"in·oc'u·la'tion. Inoculation a second time with the same kind of organism.

re·in"te·gra'tion. In psychiatry, the restoration to harmonious mental functioning after disintegration of the personality by mental illness.

re"in·ver'sion (ree"in·vur'shun, ·zhun). The act of reducing an inverted uterus by the application of pressure to the fundus.

re·ju"ve·nes'cence. 1. A renewal of youth; a renewal of strength and vigor; specifically a restoration of sexual vigor. 2. In biology, a method of cell formation in which the entire protoplasm of an old cell escapes by rupture of the cell wall and then develops a new cell wall.

re·lapse'. Return of symptoms of a disease after convalescence has begun.

re·laps'ing fe'ver. Any one of a group of specific infectious diseases caused by spirochetes, Borrelia recurrentis and Borrelia duttonii being the most common, and transmitted to man by lice or ticks. Both varieties are widespread and resemble each other in having an acute onset with chills, fever, pain in the back and legs, enlargement of the spleen, delirium, and sometimes convulsions; a rapid disappearance of symptoms by crisis is followed after an

interval of a week or more by another paroxysm. This cycle may be repeated from two to six times. Also called famine fever, remittent fever, spirillum fever, tick fever, louse fever.

re·la'tion. 1. Interdependence; mutual influence or connection between organs or parts. 2. Connection by consanguinity; kinship. 3. In anatomy, the position of parts of the body as regards each other.

re·lax'. 1. Loosen or make less tense. 2. Cause a movement of the bowels.

re"lax·a'tion. A diminution of tension in a part; a diminution in functional activity, as relaxation of the skin.

re·lax'in. A water-soluble hormone having diverse effects, found in human serum and in serums of certain other animals during pregnancy.

re·lief'. The partial removal of anything distressing; alleviation of pain or discomfort.

re·lieve'. Free from pain, discomfort, or distress.

re·me'di·al. Having the nature of a remedy; relieving; curative.

rem'e·dy. Anything used in the treatment of disease.

Re·mij'i·a (ri·midj'ee·uh). A genus of shrubs and trees of the Rubiaceae closely related to cinchona. Some yield quinine and related alkaloids.

re"min·er·al·i·za'tion. Restoring the body's lost mineral constituents, or those of any tissue.

re·mis'sion. 1. Abatement or subsidence of the symptoms of disease. 2. The period of diminution thereof.

re·mit'tence. Temporary abatement or cessation of symptoms. **—remittent,** adj.

ren (pl. renes). The kidney. **—ren'iform,** adj. **r. mobilis.** Wandering kidney. **r. unguiformis.** Horseshoe kidney.

re'nal. Pertaining to the kidneys.

re'nes (ree'neez). Plural of ren, q.v.

re'nin, ren'in. A kidney protein which acts as a protease on renin substrate, to liberate angiotonin. In vivo intravenously injected, it exhibits pressor activity. **r. substrate.** A constituent of the a₂ globulin of plasma which is the substrate on which the enzyme renin works. Also called hypertensinogen, renin-activator.

ren'i·punc"ture (ren'i·punk"chur, ren"i·punk'chur). Puncture of the capsule of a kidney.

ren'net. 1. Rennin. 2. A preparation of the lining of the calf stomach used as a source of rennin.

ren'nin. The milk-coagulating enzyme found in the gastric juice of the fourth stomach of the calf.

ren·nin'o·gen, ren'no·gen. The zymogen of rennin, found in the wall of the fourth stomach of the calf. Also called *prorennin*.

•en'no·gen. See *renninogen*.

•en"o·va'tion. The repair or renewal of that which has been impaired.

•e"or·gan·i·za'tion. Healing by the development of tissue elements similar to those lost through some morbid process.

•ep. *Repetatur;* let it be repeated.

•e·pair'. Restoration to a normal state after injury.

•e·pel'lent. 1. Driving back. 2. Causing resolution of morbid processes.

•e·pel'lents. Various chemicals used to repel or kill external parasites, such as mosquitoes, chiggers, ticks.

•e"per·cus'sion. 1. Ballottement. 2. A driving in, or dispersion of, a tumor or eruption.

•e·ple'tion. The condition of being, or the act of making, full. —**replete'**, *adj.*

e·po"lar·i·za'tion (ree-po"lur-i-zay'shun, -eye-zay'shun). Restoration of the polarized state in a nerve or muscle fiber during recovery from the conduction of an excitatory process.

•e"po·si'tion (ree"po-zish'un, rep"-o-zish'un). The return of an abnormally placed part, organ, or fragment to its proper position.

•e·pos'i·to·ry. Of or pertaining to an injectable form of medicinal agent prepared with a vehicle that favors prolongation of therapeutic effect.

•e·pres'sion. *In psychopathology,* a psychic mechanism whereby shameful impulses or experiences are forcibly dismissed from consciousness, and the psychic energy with which they are loaded becomes part of the unconscious.

e"pro·duc'tion. A fundamental property of protoplasm by which organisms give rise to other organisms of the same kind.

•e·pul'sion. Act of repelling or driving back or apart.

RES. Reticuloendothelial system, *q.v.*

•e·sar'u·rin (ri-zazh'ur-in) (C.C.). A deep red dye used in histologic staining. Also called *diazoresorcinol*.

•es·cin'na·mine. $C_{35}H_{42}N_2O_9$, a hypotensive and sedative alkaloid present in *Rauwolfia serpentina*, closely related to reserpine.

•e·sect'. 1. Cut out a portion of a tissue or organ. 2. Cut away the end of one or more of the bones entering into a joint.

•e·sec'tion. The operation of cutting out, as the removal of a section or segment of an organ. **window r.** Submucous resection of part of the nasal septum.

•e·sec'to·scope. A tubelike instrument by means of which small structures may be divided within a body

cavity without an opening other than that made by the instrument itself.

re·ser'pine. An alkaloid, chemically $C_{33}H_{40}N_2O_9$, derived from species of *Rauwolfia*, especially from *R. serpentina*, that reduces blood pressure, slows pulse rate, and has sedative and tranquilizing properties. See *serpasil*.

re·serve' (ri-zurv'). A remainder; a capacity or potentiality, retained as an additional store. **alkali r.** The components of the blood which are capable of neutralizing acids. These include sodium bicarbonate, dipotassium phosphate, and proteins. **cardiac r.** Ability of the heart to do more work in pumping larger amounts of blood per beat. **diminished cardiac r.** Condition in which a cardiac patient develops dyspnea on performing ordinary muscular effort but has none at rest.

res'i·dent phy·si'cian. A physician living in the hospital for further training after an internship. Also called *resident*.

re·sid'u·al. 1. Pertaining to that which cannot be evacuated or discharged, as residual air in the lungs, residual urine in the bladder. 2. A remainder.

res'i·due. That which remains after a part has been removed; remainder.

re·sid'u·um (pl. *residua*). Latin for *residue*.

re·sil'i·ence. The quality of being elastic or resilient.

res'in (rez'in). 1. One of a class of vegetable substances exuding from various plants; generally soluble in alcohol and in ether, and insoluble in water; readily fusible and inflammable. 2. A class of pharmaceutical preparations made by extracting resin-containing drugs with alcohol, concentrating the liquid and adding it to water, whereby the resin and other water-insoluble principles precipitate and may be collected and dried. —**resin-ous**, *adj.* **acrylic r.** A synthetic resin, usually a polymer of methyl methacrylate. Used in dentistry and medicine for the manufacture of artificial dentures, artificial eyes, or splints. See *acrylics.* **ion exchange r.** A synthetic polymer containing fixed ionizable groups which exchange ions of the opposite charge.

res'in·oid (rez'i-noyd). 1. Resembling a resin. 2. A substance which has some of the properties of a resin.

re·sist'ance. 1. Opposition to force or external impression. 2. *In electricity,* the opposition offered by a conductor to the passage of the current. Abbreviated, R. 3. *In psychoanalysis,* the reluctance of the subject to give up habitual patterns of thinking, feeling, and acting to take on less neurotic and newer modes of adaptation.

res″o·lu′tion. 1. The subsidence of inflammation; as in pneumonia, the stage of dissolving the exudate due to proteolytic enzymes. 2. The ability of the eye or a lens to register small detail, the resolution of the human eye being 1 minute of arc.

re·solve′ (ri-zolv′). 1. Return to the normal state after some pathologic process. 2. Separate anything into its component parts.

re·sol′vent (ri-zol′vunt). 1. Causing solution or dissipation of tissue. 2. An agent causing resolution.

re·solv′ing pow′er. The capability of a lens to make clear the finest details of an object.

res′o·nance (rez′o-nuns). 1. The attribute of relatively long duration possessed by certain sounds. 2. Normal resonance; in physical diagnosis, the prolonged, nonmusical, composite sound which results from vibration of the normal chest. It consists of a mixture of fundamental tones, most of which are within the range of 90 to 130 vibrations per second, and hence varies but little in pitch. **amphoric r.** A tympanitic percussion note containing overtones which give it the sound of air blown across the mouth of an empty bottle or jar. **cracked-pot r.** A characteristic clinking sound which can be elicited occasionally by percussion over tuberculous cavities, especially when the percussion is forcible and the patient's mouth is open. Also called *cracked-pot sound.* **tympanitic r.** (a) The prolonged musical sound heard on percussion over the stomach, colon, or other air-containing cavity with flexible walls. In contrast with normal resonance, its sounds vary widely in pitch. (b) A percussion note which exhibits in varying proportion the characteristics of both resonance and tympany. Also called *bandbox r., hyperresonance, Skoda's r.*

res′o·nant. Possessing, or capable of producing, resonance.

res′o·na″tor (rez′o-nay″tur). Any physical body capable of being set into vibration in unison with another vibrating body. The thoracic cage, lung, and other human structures possess this capacity in limited degree.

re·sorb′ent. 1. Absorbing. 2. A drug which aids in the process of resorption.

re·sor′cin (ri-zor′sin). Resorcinol, *q.v.*

re·sor′cin·ol (ri-zor′sin·ole, ·ol). $C_6H_6O_2$. Meta-dihydroxybenzene; white crystals, soluble in water.

re·sorp′tion. The removal by absorption.

re·spir′a·ble (ri-spy′ruh·bul, res′pi·ruh·bul). Capable of being inspired and expired; capable of furnishing the gaseous interchange in the lungs nece sary for life. **—respirabil′ity,** n.

res″pi·ra′tion. 1. The interchan of gases of the living and the gases the medium in which they live, throu any channel, as cutaneous respiratic 2. The act of breathing with the lun the taking of air into, and its expulsi from, the lungs. It consists of two act inspiration, or the taking in of t atmospheric air, and expiration, or t expelling of the modified air. Expir air contains less oxygen and more ca bon dioxide than inspired air. T volume of air taken into the lungs a given out during an ordinary respir tion (tidal air) is 500 cc.; the volu that can be inspired in addition by forcible inspiration (complemental a is 1500 cc.; that which can be e haled after a normal expiration (r serve or supplemental air) is 1500 c the amount remaining in the che after the most complete expirati (residual air) is from 1200 to 1600 c The volume of air that can be forcib expelled after the most forcible inspir tion is termed vital or respirato capacity and is equal to the tidal a complemental air, and reserve air, about 3500 cc. **—respir′atory,** a **abdominal r.** Respiration effect by contraction of the diaphragm a the elasticity of the abdominal muscle **amphoric r.** A blowing respirati engendered in large cavities with fi walls. Its peculiar character is due an echo from the walls of the cavi **artificial r.** Artificial production the normal respiratory movements. S *artificial respiration.* **cavernous** A blowing respiration of low pitch, c cumscribed, alternating with gurgli and deriving its chief character fr the nature of the cavity in which it generated. **cerebral r.** A shalle blowing respiration seen often in t presence of fever. **Cheyne-Stokes** Periods of stertorous respiration inte rupted by periods of apnea seen in cer bral arteriosclerosis, senility, heart d ease, and a few other similar conc tions. **costal r.** Respiration in whi the chest movement predominates ov the diaphragmatic movement. **exter nal r.** The interchange of gases b tween the atmosphere and the air the lungs and between the air in lun and pulmonary capillaries. **fetal** The interchange of gases between t fetal and the maternal blood throu the medium of the placenta. **inter nal r.** The exchange of gases betwe the systemic blood and tissues. **Kus maul's r.** The deep gasping respir tion characteristic of severe acidos **labored r.** Respiration in whi owing to lack of ability on the part the ordinary muscles of respiration aerate the blood sufficiently, the auxiliary muscles of respiration are called into play. **paradoxical r.** In open pneumothorax, a condition in which the lung on the side of the pleural opening fills on exhalation and empties on inhalation. **stertorous r.** The sound produced by breathing through the nose and mouth at the same time, causing vibration of the soft palate between the two currents of air.

es'pi·ra"tor. A device for producing artificial respiration. Except for the head, the body is hermetically enclosed in a cabinet and respiratory movements are produced by introducing alternately pressure and suction. **Both r.** A cabinet of wood enclosing the body, except for the head, with a rubber collar about the patient's neck. A small motor drives a bellows connected with the chamber by a flexible pipe. By means of a valve the bellows produces suction, alternately withdrawing and admitting air. **Drinker r.** A power-driven breathing apparatus similar in type to the Both respirator, the cabinet being of metal.

e·spire'. Breathe.

es"pi·rom'e·ter. A device to determine the character of respiration.

e·sponse'. The reaction or movement of a muscle or other part due to the application of a stimulus. **triple r.** Thomas Lewis' term for three stages of normal vasomotor reaction resulting when a pointed instrument is drawn heavily across the skin. They are: reddening of the area stimulated, wide spreading of flush to adjacent skin, and development of wheals. The response is due to a histaminelike substance liberated from tissue by a noxious stimulus.

e·spon"si·bil'i·ty. 1. In legal medicine, the accountability for professional acts. 2. The capacity to differentiate right from wrong.

est. 1. Cessation of labor or action; repose. 2. An epithelial remnant persisting after its developmental activity has ceased. Also called epithelial debris. **bed r.** (a) A device to support patients in bed. (b) The keeping of a patient in bed continually. **epithelial r.** One of the cords of cells in the periodontal membrane representing remnants of the epithelial sheath of the enamel organ.

es"ti·tu'tion. 1. The act of restoring. 2. In obstetrics, a rotation of the fetal head immediately after its birth. **es"to·ra'tion.** The return to a state of health or a normal condition.

e·stor'a·tive. 1. Pertaining to restoration. 2. A remedy that is efficacious in restoring health and strength.

re·straint'. 1. Hindrance of any action, physical, moral, or mental. 2. The state of being controlled; confinement. **mechanical r.** Restraining the insane by mechanical means. **medicinal r.** The use of narcotics and sedatives in quieting the mentally deranged.

re·strin'gent. An astringent or styptic.

re"sub·li·ma'tion. The process of subliming a drug for the second time.

re·su'pi·nate. Turned in a direction opposite to normal, as an ovary with its apex downward.

re·sus"ci·ta'tion. The prevention of asphyxial death by artificial respiration. **—resus'citate,** v. **Drinker-Collins r.** The use of a negative pressure cabinet where respiration is to be maintained over a long period. **Flagg r.** The use of controlled suction and insufflation through a laryngoscope; using the Flagg machine.

re·sus"ci·ta'tion cage. An electrically heated metal cage or cradle which covers at least three-quarters of the patient; used in surgical shock.

re·sus'ci·ta"tor. A device for forcing oxygen or oxygen-carbon dioxide mixtures into the lungs for resuscitation.

re·su'ture (ree-sue'chur). Secondary suture; suture of a wound some time after a first suture has been made.

retch. Strain, as in vomiting. **—retch'ing,** n.

re'te. (ree'tee) (pl. retia). Any network or decussation and interlacing, especially of capillary blood vessels.

re'tene, ret'ene. $C_{18}H_{18}$. 1-Methyl-7-isopropylphenanthrene. Occurs in the higher boiling fractions of wood tar.

re·ten'tion. 1. The act of retaining or holding back, as the holding of urine in the bladder due to some hindrance to urination. 2. In dentistry, holding moved teeth in their new positions until stability of their investing tissues is established.

re·tic'u·lar. Resembling a net; formed by a network, as reticular tissue, which forms the finest framework of such organs as lymph nodes, liver, kidney, etc.

re·tic'u·lin. A protein isolated from the connective fibers of reticular tissue.

re·tic'u·lo·cyte". 1. An erythrocyte containing a granular or filamentous network demonstrable with brilliant cresyl blue; indicative of immaturity. Normally they constitute 1% of the erythrocytes of the blood. Also called reticulated erythrocyte or erythroplastid. 2. A cell of reticular tissue. Syn., reticular cell.

re·tic"u·lo·cy"to·pe'ni·a. Decrease of reticulocytes in the circulating blood.

re·tic″u·lo·cy·to′sis (ri·tick″yoo-lo·sigh·to′sis). Condition in which reticulocytes are present in excess in the peripheral blood.

re·tic″u·lo·en″do·the′li·al. Pertaining to cells which are grouped under the reticuloendothelial system, *q.v.*

re·tic″u·lo·en″do·the″li·o′sis. Condition of hyperplasia of the reticuloendothelial system.

re·tic″u·lo′sis. Reticuloendotheliosis. **aleukemic r.** A rare, acute, fatal disease; characterized by fever, progressive anemia, hyperplasia of reticuloendothelial system, leukopenia, general lymphadenopathy, splenomegaly.

re·tic′u·lum (pl. *reticula*). 1. A fine network. 2. *In veterinary medicine*, the second division of the ruminant stomach. **—reticulose,** *adj.*

ret′i·na. The light-receptive layer and terminal expansion of the optic nerve in the eye. It extends from the point of exit of the nerve forward to the ora serrata. It consists of the following layers, named from behind forward: the pigment layer; the neuroepithelial layer, comprising the layer of rods and cones (bacillary layer), the outer limiting membrane, and the outer nuclear layer; the outer reticular layer (outer granular layer), the inner nuclear layer, the inner reticular layer (inner granular layer), the ganglionic layer, the nerve fiber layer. These layers are united and supported by neuroglial elements, most prominent of which are the radial fibers of Müller. **—retinal,** *adj.* **detachment of r.** Separation of the retina from the choroid.

ret′i·nac′u·lum (pl. *retinacula*). A special fascial thickening which holds back an organ or part. Also called *r. tendineum.* **extensor r.** A thickening of deep fascia on the dorsum of the wrist and forearm attached to the radius laterally and the ulna, carpus, and medial ligament of the wrist medially. It overlies the compartments which transmit the extensor tendons of the wrist and fingers. **flexor r. of the ankle.** The fibrous band that stretches between the medial malleolus and medial tubercle of the calcaneus, binding down the tendons of the tibialis posterior, the flexor digitorum longus, and the flexor hallucis longus. **flexor r. of the wrist.** A thickened band of deep fascia on the volar surface of the hand and forearm, attached laterally to the navicular and greater multangular bones and medially to the pisiform and hamate bones. It binds down the tendon of the flexor pollicis longus and the flexor tendons of the fingers.

ret′i·nal cor″re·spond′ence. T relation in the two eyes of the reti areas at which associated retinal i ages are formed. **abnormal r. c** condition found in concomitant strab mus, in which the retinal image form at the macula of the fixing eye is sociated with the image formed at extramacular area of the retina of squinting eye. Also called *binocu false projection, retinal incongru* **normal r. c.** The normal condit in which the retinal image formed the macula of one eye is associa with that formed at the macula the other eye.

ret′i·nene. A pigment of the rods the retina, chemically vitamin A al hyde, which in white light is form from rhodopsin, or visual purple, a in the dark is converted to rhodops

ret″i·ni′tis. Retinal inflammati **central punctate r.** That se most often in the aged. A great num of striae or white spots are visible the fundus. **chorioidoretinitis.** form of retinitis with cellular infiltra tion, exudation, atrophy, and prolifer tion of the pigment epithelium in choroid, between the choroid and r ina, and in the retinal layers. **di betic r.** The form of retinitis occ ring in diabetes. **leukemic r.** A fo characterized by pallor of the reti vessels and optic disk, the boundary the latter being indistinct. Hemorrha appear at various points of the me brane, while numerous white patc and round bodies are visible about disk in the retina. **r. gravidarur** A form occurring in pregnant wom **r. nephritica.** That due to neph tis, usually chronic. Syn., *r. albu nurica, renal r.* **r. paralytic** Retinitis caused by paralysis affect the optic nerve. **r. pigmentosa.** affection involving all the layers of retina, and consisting in a slowly p gressing proliferation of connect tissue and pigment cells of the ent membrane, with wasting of its ne elements.

ret″i·no·blas·to′ma. Neuroepith lioma of the retina.

ret″i·no·cho″roid·i′tis (ret″i· kor″oy·dye′tis). Inflammation of retina and choroid.

ret″i·no·pap″il·li′tis. Inflamm tion of the retina and the optic disk

ret″i·nop′a·thy. Any morbid con tion of the retina.

ret″i·nos′co·py. An object method of determining the refract of the eye by observation of the mo ments of the shadow phenomena p duced and observed by means of an strument called the retinoscope (a called the skiascope). The principle that of conjugate foci, whereby image-point is conjugate with the object-point. If rotation of the illuminated mirror of the retinoscope causes the shadow in the *illuminated* pupil to move "with" the retinoscope, the patient's retina is conjugate with a point beyond the instrument (the emergent rays are divergent) and the eye is hyperopic. The dioptric strength of the lens selected to abolish motion of the shadow is the amount of the hyperopia. If the reflex moves "against" (opposite in direction to) the mirror, the conjugate focus is between the retinoscope and the patient's eye (the emergent rays are convergent) and the eye is myopic. The dioptric strength of the lens selected to abolish motion of the shadow is the amount of the myopia. Also called *skiascopy.*

re·tort'. A distilling vessel consisting of an expanded globular portion and a long neck.

ret"o·the"li·o'ma. A neoplasm, usually malignant, derived from reticuloendothelial cells and composed of cells of the same order. Syn., *reticuloendothelial sarcoma.*

re·tract'. Draw back; contract; shorten.

re·trac'tion. The act of retracting or drawing back, as a retraction of the muscles after amputation.

re·trac'tor. A surgical instrument for holding back the edges of a wound to give access to deeper parts or regions. It consists ordinarily of a handle with a right-angle flange. **abdominal r.** A large, heavy instrument, often with a curved flange, to give greater retractive power. **block tin r.** A flexible instrument which can be bent to a desired shape. **nerve r.** A delicate instrument adapted to isolating nerves during operations. **periosteal r.** A toothed instrument for holding periosteum. **self-retaining r.** A special instrument having two retractor arms clamped to a bar and adjusted by means of setscrews. Some are equipped with a third arm for retraction of the pubic portion of the bladder during bladder and prostatic operations. **toothed r.** A retractor having sharp or blunt teeth.

et"ro-, re"tro-. A combining form meaning *back, backward,* or *behind.*

et"ro·ac'tion. Reverse action.

et"ro·an'ter·o·grade. Reversing the usual order of a succession.

et"ro·bul'bar. 1. Situated or occurring behind the eyeball. 2. Caudal to the medulla oblongata.

et"ro·col'ic. Behind the colon.

et"ro·de"vi·a'tion. Any backward displacement; a retroflexion or retroversion.

et"ro·dis·place'ment. Backward displacement of a part or organ, especially uterine displacement. See *retroversion.*

ret"ro·flex. Turn back abruptly.

ret"ro·flexed". Bent backward; in a permanent, backward malposition, as in retroflexion of the uterus.

ret"ro·flex'ion. The state of being bent backward. **r. of the uterus.** A condition in which the uterus is bent backward upon itself, producing a sharp angle in its axis.

ret"ro·grade. Going backward; undoing.

re·trog'ra·phy. Backward writing; mirror writing.

ret"ro·gres'sion. 1. *In biology,* the passing from a higher to a lower type of structure in the development of an animal. 2. *In medicine,* a going backward; degeneration, involution, or atrophy, as of tissue. 3. The subsidence of a disease or its symptoms.

ret"ro·in·fec'tion. Infection of the mother by the fetus. *Obs.*

ret"ro·jec'tion. The washing out of a cavity from within outward.

ret"ro·jec'tor, ret"ro·jec"tor. An instrument for washing out the uterus.

ret"ro·lin'gual. Relating to that part of the pharynx back of the tongue.

ret"ro·mor'pho·sis (ret"ro·mor·fo'sis, ·mor·fo'sis). Catabolism; retrograde metamorphosis; catabolic change.

ret"ro·na'sal (ret"ro·nay'zul, ree"tro-). Situated behind the nose or nasal cavities; postnasal.

ret"ro·per"i·to·ne'al. Situated behind the peritoneum.

ret"ro·per"i·to·ni'tis. Inflammation of the retroperitoneal structures.

ret"ro·phar"yn·gi'tis. Inflammation of the retropharyngeal tissues.

ret"ro·phar'ynx. The posterior portion of the pharynx.

ret"ro·pla·cen'tal. Behind the placenta.

ret"ro·pla'si·a (ret"ro·play'zhuh, ree"tro-). Retrograde change in a tissue; degeneration.

ret"ro·posed (ret"ro·pozed, ree"tro-). Displaced backward.

ret"ro·po·si'tion. Backward displacement of the uterus without flexion or version.

ret"ro·pul'sion. 1. A driving or turning back, as of the fetal head. 2. A running backward; a form of walking sometimes seen in paralysis agitans.

ret"ro·stal'sis. Reversed peristalsis; peristaltic action that tends to drive the intestinal contents cephalad instead of caudad.

ret"ro·ver"si·o·flex'ion (·vur"sho·fleck'shun, ·vur"see·o·fleck'shun). Combined retroversion and retroflexion.

ret"ro·ver'sion (ret"ro·vur'shun, ree"tro-). A turning back. **r. of**

uterus. A condition in which the uterus is tilted backward without curvature of its axis.

ret″ro·vert′ed (ret″ro·vur′tid, ret′-ro·vur″tid). Tilted or turned backward, as a retroverted uterus.

re·trude′. Force inward or backward, as to correct protruding teeth.

re·tru′sion. 1. *In dentistry*, the act or process of pressing teeth backward. 2. That condition which is characterized by backward or retroposed teeth, particularly the anterior teeth.

re·un′ion. In fractures, the securing of union following its interruption by violence or disease.

re·ver″ber·a′tion. A repetitive discharge of impulses due to the development of transient automaticity of ventral horn cells. The impulses pass in circuits from cell to cell.

rev′er·ie. A state of dreamy abstraction; visionary mental or ideational movement, the mind itself, at least so far as volition is concerned, being passive.

re·ver′sal. 1. *In psychoanalysis*, the change from a love instinct to one of hate; a change of the content of an instinct. 2. The change of the object of an instinct into its opposite, as from sadism into masochism.

re·verse′. In bandaging, a half-turn employed to change the direction of a bandage.

re·ver′sion (ri·vur′shun, ·zhun). The reappearance of long-lost ancestral traits; a throwback.

re″vi·tal·i·za′tion (ree″vye·tul·i-zay′shun, ree·vye″tul·). The act or process of refreshing.

re·vive′. Return to life after seeming death; return to consciousness or strength. **—revival,** *n.*

re·viv″i·fi·ca′tion. Restoration of life after apparent death.

rev′o·lute. Turned backward or downward.

re·vul′sant. Revulsive.

re·vul′sant. A medicine or agent that, by irritation, draws the blood from a distant part of the body.

re·vul′sive. Causing extreme aversion.

re·vul′sive. A revulsant agent.

R. F. A. Right frontoanterior position of the fetus.

R. F. P. Right frontoposterior position of the fetus.

Rh. 1. Chemical symbol for rhodium. 2. See *Rh factor, Rh genes, Rh sensitization, Rh testing, Rh typing.* Also see *Rh blood types* under *blood.*

rhab″do·my·o′ma (rab″do·migh·o′-muh). A rare tumor of striated muscle usually classified as malignant, but considered by some to be benign. See *rhabdomyosarcoma.* **congenital r. of the heart.** A nontu-

morous developmental anomaly, char⸗ terized by myocardial lesions w⸗ large vacuolated cells containing g⸗ cogen and often showing radial⸗ transverse striation of their periphe⸗ cytoplasm. **embryonal r.** A mes⸗ chymoma. **r. uteri.** A maligna⸗ polypoid, mesodermal, mixed tumor⸗ the vagina in children and of⸗ cervix of the uterus in adults,⸗ which the striated muscle may rep⸗ sent metaplasia of connective-tis⸗ cells.

rhab″do·my″o·sar·co′ma. ⸗ malignant form of rhabdomyoma.

Rhab″do·ne′ma. A genus of pa⸗ sitic roundworms.

rhab″do·pho′bi·a. A morbid dre⸗ of being beaten; unreasoning f⸗ aroused by the sight of a stick.

rha′chi·o- (ray′kee·o-), **rha′ch⸗** See *rachio-.*

rha′cous. Wrinkled; lacerated;⸗ sured.

rhag′a·des (rag′uh·deez). Lin⸗ cracks or fissures of the skin; occur⸗ skin that has lost its elasticity throu⸗ infiltration and thickening. Obser⸗ in syphilis, intertrigo, keratoderm⸗ and other affections. Also called *crac⸗ rimae, fissures.*

rha·gad′i·form. Fissured.

-rha′gi·a. See *-rrhagia.*

rhag′oid. Resembling a grape.

rham′ne·gin. A glycoside, C₃₆H₃₈⸗ found in buckthorn berries. Also cal⸗ *rhamnoxanthin, xanthorhamnin.*

rham′ni·tol. CH₃(CHOH)₄CH₂OH.⸗ alcohol resulting from the reduction⸗ the sugar rhamnose. See *inositol.*

rham″no·ca·thar′tin. A glycosi⸗ C₂₇H₃₀O₁₄.½H₂O, found in buckth⸗ berries.

rham′nose (ram′nose, ·noze).⸗ methyl pentose, C₆H₁₂O₅.H₂O, obtai⸗ from quercitrin, a glycoside of c⸗ bark, or other glycosides. It is a wh⸗ crystalline powder, soluble in wat⸗ Also called *isodulcite, isodulcitol.*

rham″no·xan′thin (ram″no·za⸗ thin). See *frangulin.*

Rham′nus. A genus of trees a⸗ shrubs which yield cascara (**R. p⸗ shiana**), buckthorn bark (**R. fra⸗ gula**), and buckthorn berries (**R. c⸗ thartica**).

rha·pon′tic. Pertaining to rhuba⸗

rhat′a·ny. See *krameria.*

rhe″bo·sce′li·a (ree″bo·see′lee·u⸗ The condition of being bowlegg⸗ **—rhe″bo·sce′lic,** *adj.*

rheg′ma. A rupture of the walls o⸗ vessel or of the containing membr⸗ of an organ or region, as the coats⸗ the eye, or the peritoneum. Also,⸗ bursting of an abscess. *Rare.*

rhem·bas′mus (rem·baz′mus). M⸗ tal distraction or wandering; inde⸗ sion.

he'ni·um. Re = 186.31. An element of the manganese group; occurs as a minor constituent in many ores.

he'o-. A combining form denoting *pertaining to a current.*

he'o·base. The minimum electric potential necessary for stimulation.

he·om'e·ter. 1. A galvanometer. 2. An apparatus for measuring the velocity of the blood current.

he'o·nome. An instrument for the application to excitable tissues of electric currents of different intensity.

he'o·stat. An instrument introduced into an electric circuit and offering a known resistance, for the purpose of altering the intensity of the current.

he"o·ta·chyg'ra·phy (ree"o-ta-kig'ruh·fee). The registration of the curve of variation in electromotive action of muscles.

he"o·tax'is. The reaction of a body to mechanical stimulation by a current of fluid, whereby that body is induced to move either with or against the current of the fluid.

he'o·tome. An instrument used for breaking and making a galvanic circuit.

he'o·trope. An apparatus for reversing the direction of an electric current. Also called *commutator.*

he'um. See *rhubarb.*

heu·mat'ic. Pertaining to, of the nature of, or affected with, rheumatism. **heu·mat'ic fe'ver.** See under *fever.*

heu'ma·tism. 1. A general term indicating diseases of muscle, tendon, joint, bone, or nerve, resulting in discomfort and disability. It is often used to include rheumatoid arthritis, degenerative joint disease, spondylitis, bursitis, fibrositis, myositis, neuritis, lumbago, sciatica, and gout. 2. Acute rheumatic fever. **acute articular r.** Acute rheumatic fever. **acute r.** Acute rheumatic fever. **chronic r.** Chronic form of any of the above-mentioned types, but usually one of those leading to joint deformity such as rheumatoid arthritis, degenerative joint disease, or chronic gout. **gonorrheal r.** Arthritis due to the gonococcus. **palin-dromic r.** An acute arthritis and periarthritis occurring in multiple, afebrile, irregularly spaced attacks lasting only a few hours or days and disappearing completely. There are pain, swelling, redness, and disability of usually only one joint. It attacks adults of either sex. The cause is not known. **tuberculous r.** Arthritis due to infection of joint tissues with tubercle bacilli.

heu'ma·toid. Resembling rheumatism.

hex'is. Rupture of a blood vessel or of an organ.

Rh fac'tor. An agglutinogen first found in the red blood cells of the rhesus monkey, hence the name. Rh positive and Rh negative are terms denoting the presence or absence of this factor. It can cause antibody formation only in Rh negative blood. About 15% of individuals are Rh negative and following injection of positive antiserums, as in transfusions, will produce anti-Rh agglutinins so that subsequent transfusions of Rh positive blood will cause transfusion reactions. Also see *erythroblastosis foetalis* for the effect of this factor in pregnancy.

Rh genes. The series of allelic genes which determine the various sorts of Rh agglutinogens and Rh blood types. There are six standard genes: rh, Rh', Rh", Rh₀, Rh₁, and Rh₂. When discussing only the results of tests with the standard anti-Rh₀ serums, dividing persons into two types—Rh positive and Rh negative—only a pair of genes need be considered, Rh and rh. Rh positive persons may be either homozygous (genotype RhRh) or heterozygous (Rh-rh), while Rh negative persons are always homozygous (rhrh).

rhic·no'sis. A wrinkling of the skin, the result of muscular or subdermal elastic-tissue atrophy.

rhin-. See *rhino-.*

rhi'nal. Pertaining to the nose.

rhi·nal'gi·a (rye-nal'juh, ·jee-uh). Pain in the nose.

rhi"nan·tral'gi·a. Pain in the cavities of the nose.

rhi·nel'cos (rye-nel'koss). A nasal ulcer.

rhi"nen·ceph'a·lon. That portion of the cerebrum concerned with reception and integration of olfactory impulses, and with regulation of appropriate motor activities in response to such impulses. It comprises the archipallium (hippocampal formation) and paleopallium (olfactory lobe or piriform lobe). —**rhinencephal'ic,** *adj.*

rhi"neu·ryn'ter. A distensible bag or sac which is inflated after insertion into a nostril.

rhin"he·ma·to'ma (rine"hee-muh-to'muh, ·hem"uh-to'muh). An effusion of blood around the nasal cartilages.

rhin'i·on. The point at the distal end of the internasal suture.

rhi'nism, rhi·nis'mus (rye-niz'mus). A nasal quality of the voice.

rhi·ni'tis (rye-nigh'tis). Inflammation of the nasal mucous membrane. **acute r.** Coryza; cold in the head; the common cold. **allergic r.** Rhinitis which may be caused by any allergen, but which is frequently called hay fever. **atrophic r.** That followed by atrophy of the mucous membrane. **chronic r.** A form usually due to repeated attacks of acute rhinitis, and producing in the early stages hypertrophy of the mucous membrane (hypertrophic rhinitis) and in the later stages atrophy (atrophic rhinitis), and the presence of dark, offensive-smelling crusts. **fibrinous r.** A rare form of rhinitis characterized by the development of a false membrane in the nose. **hypertrophic r.** That marked by hypertrophy of the nasal mucous membrane. **periodic r.** Allergic rhinitis. **syphilitic r.** A chronic form due to syphilis, and usually attended by ulceration and caries of the bones and an offensive discharge (ozena). **tuberculous r.** That due to the tubercle bacillus; it is usually associated with ulceration and caries of the bones. **vasomotor r.** (a) Allergic rhinitis. (b) Hay fever. Also called *vasomotor catarrh.*

rhi″no-, rhin-. A combining form meaning *the nose.*

rhi″no·an·tri′tis. Inflammation of the mucous membrane of the nose and the maxillary sinus.

rhi″no·by′on (rye″no-buy′on, rye-no′bee·on). A nasal plug or tampon.

rhi″no·chei′lo·plas″ty (rye″no-kigh′lo·plas″tee). Surgery of the nose and upper lip.

rhi″no·clei′sis (rye″no·klye′sis). Nasal obstruction.

rhi″noc·nes′mus (rye″nock·nez′-mus). Itching of the nose.

rhi″no·dac′ry·o·lith. A calculus in a nasolacrimal duct.

rhi″no·dyn′i·a (rye″no-din′ee-uh, -dye′nee·uh). Any pain in the nose.

rhi·nog′e·nous (rye-nodj′i·nus). Having its origin in the nose.

rhi″no·ky·pho′sis (rye″no-kigh-fo′sis). The condition of having a nose with a prominent bridge.

rhi″no·la′li·a. A nasal tone in the voice due to undue closure (**rhinolalia clausa**) or to undue patulousness (**rhinolalia aperta**) of the choanae.

rhi″no·lar″yn·gi′tis. Simultaneous inflammation of the mucosa of the nose and larynx.

rhi″no·lar″yn·gol′o·gy. The science of the anatomy, physiology, and pathology of the nose and larynx.

rhi′no·lith. A nasal calculus.

rhi″no·li·thi′a·sis. The formation of nasal calculi.

rhi·nol′o·gist (rye-nol′o·jist). A specialist in the treatment of diseases of the nose.

rhi·nol′o·gy (rye-nol′o·jee). The science of the anatomy, functions, and diseases of the nose. **—rhinolog′ic,** *adj.*

rhi″no·mi·o′sis (rye″no-migh·o′-sis). Operative shortening of the nose.

rhi″nom·mec′to·my. Excision of the inner canthus of the eye.

rhi″no·my·co′sis (rye″no-migh-ko′sis). The presence of fungi in the mu-cous membrane and secretion of t.. nose.

rhi″no·ne·cro′sis. Necrosis of t.. nasal bones.

rhi·nop′a·thy (rye-nop′uth·ee). A.. disease of the nose.

rhi″no·pha·ryn′ge·al (rye″no-f.. rin′jul, ·far″in·jee′ul). Pertaining the nose and pharynx, or to the nas.. pharynx.

rhi″no·phar″yn·gi′tis. Inflamm.. tion of the nose and pharynx, or of t.. nasopharynx.

rhi″no·pha·ryn′go·lith. A nas.. pharyngeal calculus.

rhi″no·pho′ni·a. A nasal tone.. the speaking voice.

rhi″no·phy′ma. A form of ac.. rosacea of the nose characterized by marked hypertrophy of the blood ve.. sels, sebaceous glands, and connecti.. tissue, producing a lobulated appea.. ance of the end of the nose. May .. markedly disfiguring. Also called *toper.. nose, whisky nose.*

rhi′no·plas″ty. A plastic operatic.. upon the nose. This may be accor.. plished in a variety of ways, such .. the so-called Italian method of rotati.. bone and skin-lined pedicle flap fro.. the forehead, by flaps from the cheek.. by the transplantation of costal ca.. tilage, etc. **—rhinoplas′tic,** *adj.*

rhi″no·pol′yp, rhi″no·pol′y.. pus. Polyp of the nose.

rhi″nor·rha′gi·a. Hemorrhage fro.. the nose. Syn., *epistaxis.*

rhi·nor′rha·phy (rye-nor′uh·fee.. A plastic reduction in the size of t.. nose, in which redundant nasal tiss.. is removed by section, followed by a.. proximation and suture of the wou.. edges.

rhi″nor·rhe′a. A mucous dischar.. from the nose.

rhi·nos′chi·sis (rye-nos′ki·sis). Cle.. nose.

rhi″no·scle·ro′ma. A new grow.. of almost stony hardness, affecting t.. anterior nares and adjacent parts. T.. disease commences in the skin of t.. nasal vestibule and about the nares, t.. lesions consisting of flat, isolated, .. coalescent nodules.

rhi′no·scope. An instrument for e.. amination of the nasal cavities.

rhi″no·si″nus·o·path′i·a. T.. diseases of the nose and parana.. sinuses.

rhi″no·spo·rid″i·o′sis. An infe.. tion caused by the fungus *Rhinospor.. dium seeberi.* It affects the muco.. membranes of the nose, eyes, ears, la.. ynx, and occasionally the genitali.. characterized by the formation of pe.. sistent polyps.

Rhi″no·spo·rid′i·um. A genus

fungi pathogenic to man. **R. kinealyi.** Synonym for *Rhinosporidium seeberi*. **R. seeberi.** That species which is the causative agent of rhinosporidiosis.

rhi″no·ste·no′sis. Permanent constriction of the nose or nasal cavity.

rhi·not′o·my (rye-not′o-mee). Incision of the nose.

Rhi″pi·ceph′a·lus (rye″pi·sef′uhlus, rip″i·). A genus of ticks of the superfamily Ixodoidea. Many species act as vectors of such diseases as spotted fever, Q fever, and tularemia to man and lower animals. **R. sanguineus.** The most common species incriminated in the transmission of disease.

rhi′zo-, rhiz-. A combining form meaning *root*.

rhi′zoid. 1. Like a root. 2. Slender, rootlike filaments, the organs of attachment in many cryptogams. 3. A bacterial plate culture of an irregular branched or rootlike character.

rhi″zo·nych′i·a (rye″zo·nick′ee-uh), **rhi″zo·nych′i·um** (rye″zo·nick′eeum). The root of a nail. *Obs.*

Rhi·zop′o·da (rye·zop′o-duh). A class of the Protozoa which includes those amebas, characterized by the possession of pseudopodia, which parasitize man.

rhi·zot′o·my (rye·zot′o-mee). Surgical division of any root, as of a nerve or tooth.

rho′dal·line (ro′duh-leen, ro·dal′een). See *thiosinamine*.

rho′da·nate. A thiocyanate.

rho″de·o·re′tin. See *convolvulin*.

rho′di·um. Rh = 102.91. A rare metal of the platinum group.

rho′do·phane. Red pigment in the retinal cones.

rho·dop′sin. Visual purple; a retinal substance the color of which is preserved by darkness, but bleached by daylight. It is contained in the retinal rods.

rhom″ben·ceph′a·lon. The caudalmost of the three primary brain vesicles of the embryo; it divides into myelencephalon and metencephalon. Syn., *hindbrain*.

rhom′boid. Having a shape similar to that of a rhomb, a quadrilateral figure with opposite sides equal and parallel and oblique angles; said of the rhomboid ligament and rhomboid muscle. **—rhomboidal,** *adj.*

rhom·boi′de·us. Either of the rhomboid muscles, arising from the spines of the lower cervical and upper thoracic vertebrae, and inserted on the vertebral margin of the scapula. See Table of Muscles in the Appendix.

rhon′chus (rong′kus) (pl. *rhonchi*). A coarse, snoring type of rale, caused by secretions in the larger bronchi or in the trachea, sometimes palpable, as

fremitus. **—rhonchial, rhonchal,** *adj.*

Rh sen″si·ti·za′tion. The act of becoming sensitive to the Rh factor. This may occur in one of two ways; namely, as a result of a transfusion of Rh positive blood or as the result of pregnancy with an Rh positive fetus. Natural sensitivity to the Rh factor does not occur; and only 1 in 25 to 50 Rh negative persons, exposed to the Rh antigen by transfusion or pregnancy, becomes sensitized.

Rh test′ing. Examination of blood for the Rh factor, using either anti-Rhesus serum or anti-Rh₀ serum alone.

Rh typ′ing. Classification of individuals within one of the eight Rh types with the aid of anti-Rh₀, anti-Rh′, and anti-Rh″ serums. Differentiation should be made between "Rh typing" and "Rh testing," *q.v.*

rhu′barb. The dried rhizome and roots of *Rheum officinale, R. palmatum*, or other species growing in China and Tibet. A purgative.

Rhus. Sumac, a genus of shrubs or small trees of the Anacardiaceae. Poison ivy, poison oak, and poison sumac were formerly classified under this genus.

rhy·poph′a·gy (rye·pof′uh-jee). The eating of filth or excrement.

rhy″po·pho′bi·a. A morbid dread of filth.

rhy·se′ma (rye·see′muh). A wrinkle or corrugation.

-rhy′sis. A combining form meaning *flowing out*.

rhythm. 1. Action recurring at regular intervals. 2. A method of contraception, in which continence is practiced during the ovulatory phase of the menstrual cycle. **alpha r.** *In electroencephalography*, the dominant rhythm from the adult cortex. The oscillations are smooth, regular, and occur at a rate of 8–12 per second; they are best obtained from the occipital region with the subject at rest. The discharges tend to disappear when the subject concentrates. Syn., *Berger r., Berger wave, alpha wave*. **Berger r.** See alpha r. **beta r.** *In electroencephalography*, low potential fast waves, 18 to 35 cycles per second, that are more constant in the frontal lobes of the brain, related to the sensory-motor system. **cardiac r.** The normal regularity in the recurrence of heart sounds; also, recognized abnormalities of this regularity. **delta r.** *In electroencephalography*, a succession of slow waves with a frequency of six or less per second. Observed frequently during normal sleep. **gallop r.** The cadence produced when three loud sounds recur in successive cardiac cycles. The extra heart sound may occur in systole or diastole.

The protodiastolic third sound is usually of greater significance. **gamma r.** In *electroencephalography*, very fast waves whose functional significance is unknown; 40 to 50 per second recorded from the anterior head regions. **nodal r.** A succession of systoles arising from the atrioventricular node at a rate normally between 50 and 60 per minute. The P wave of the electrocardiogram is inverted in leads 2 and 3, and may occur before, during, or after the QRS deflections, depending upon whether the excitation reaches the atria before, during, or after it has reached the ventricles. **reciprocal r.** In *electrocardiography*, retrograde atrial excitation in A-V nodal rhythm, followed by ventricular excitation when the R-P interval is sufficiently long.

rhyth′mic. Pertaining to or having the quality of rhythm, as rhythmic segmentations, Cannon's term for repetitive localized contractions occurring in the small intestine during digestion.

rhyth·mic′i·ty (rith-miss′i-tee, rith-). The property of rhythmic recurrence, as of symptoms in undulant fever or malaria.

rib. One of the 24 long, flat, curved bones forming the wall of the thorax. See Table of Bones in the Appendix. **abdominal ribs.** (a) The floating ribs. (b) Ossifications of the inscriptiones tendineae. **asternal ribs.** The false ribs. **cervical ribs.** Occasional rib-like processes extending ventrally from the cervical vertebrae. **false r.** One of the five lower ribs on each side not attached to the sternum directly. **floating r.** One of the last two ribs which have the anterior end free, not attached to the sternum. **slipping r.** Excessive mobility of the lower intercostal joints. **sternal ribs.** The true ribs. **true r.** One of the seven upper ribs on each side that are attached to the sternum. **vertebrochondral ribs.** The highest three false ribs on each side; they are united in front by their costal cartilages.

ri″bo·des′ose (rye″bo-dess′oce, rye-bo′dess-oce). Desoxyribose; a pentose sugar present in thymonucleic acid.

ri″bo·fla′vin (rye″bo-flay′vin, rib″-o-). 6,7-Dimethyl-9-(d-1′-ribityl)-iso-alloxazine ($C_{17}H_{20}N_4O_6$), a member of the vitamin-B complex. Orange yellow, crystalline powder; soluble in water. Syn., *vitamin B₂, lactoflavin, vitamin G.*

ri″bo·nu′cle·ase. An enzyme present in various body tissues which depolymerizes ribonucleic acid (yeast nucleic acid) to give mononucleotides.

ri″bo·nu·cle′ic ac′id. A nucleic acid occurring in cell cytoplasm and the nucleolus and present in all ani-mal and plant cells. Abbreviated, RNA. Also see *deoxyribonucleic acid.*

ri′bose. $C_5H_{10}O_5$. A pentose sugar which occurs in yeast nucleic acid, riboflavin, and certain nucleotides.

rice. A plant, *Oryza sativa*, of the Gramineae; also its seed. Used as a food and, occasionally, as a demulcent.

ri′cin (rye′sin, ris′in). A highly toxic albumin in the seed of *Ricinus communis.*

ric′i·nine (ris′i-neen, -nin). A toxic alkaloid, $C_8H_8N_2O_2$, in the seeds and leaves of the castor plant, *Ricinus communis.*

ric′in·ism (ris′in-iz-um). Poisoning from the seeds of *Ricinus communis*. It is marked by hemorrhagic gastroenteritis and icterus.

ric″in·o·le′ic ac′id (ris″i-no′lee-ick, ris″in-o-lee′ick). $CH_2(CH_3)_5.CH-OH.CH:CH(CH_2)_7COOH$. The characteristic acid of the glycerides of castor oil.

ric″in·o·le′in (ris″i-no′lee-in). Glyceryl ricinoleate, the chief constituent of castor oil.

Ric′i·nus (ris′i-nus). A genus of the Euphorbiaceae. **R. communis** is the source of castor oil.

rick′ets. A vitamin D deficiency disease of children marked by disordered ossification. Syn., *rachitis*. **fetal r.** See *achondroplasia*. **renal r.** Rickets resulting from the failure of the kidney to maintain a normal ratio of calcium to phosphate in the blood. Also called *renal osteodystrophy.*

Rick·ett′si·a. A genus of microörganisms smaller than bacteria but larger than the filtrable viruses, usually found in the arthropods, ticks, fleas, and lice. **R. akari.** That species which is the causative agent of rickettsialpox. **R. burnetii.** A species which is the etiologic agent of Q fever. Synonym for *Coxiella burnetii.* **R. nipponica.** Synonym for *Rickettsia tsutsugamushi.* **R. orientalis.** The etiologic agent of tsutsugamushi disease. Syn., *R. tsutsugamushi.* **R. prowazekii mooseri.** That species which is the causative agent of murine typhus. **R. prowazekii prowazekii.** That species which is the causative agent of louse-borne typhus. **R. rickettsii.** That species which is the causative agent of Rocky Mountain spotted fever. **R. tsutsugamushi.** The etiologic agent of tsutsugamushi disease. Also called *R. orientalis.*

rick·ett′si·a (pl. *rickettsiae*). Any member of the family Rickettsiaceae. **—rickettsial,** *adj.*

Rick·ett″si·a′ce·ae (-a′see-ee). The family to which rickettsial organisms belong.

rick·ett′si·al·pox″. A disease

caused by *Rickettsia akari* characterized by regional lymphadenopathy, fever, chills, headache, secondary rash, and leukopenia following an initial papule at the locale of the bite of the mite *Allodermanyssus sanguineus*, which is the vector. The reservoir is the house mouse, *Mus musculus*. No deaths or sequelae have been recorded.

rick′et·y. Affected with or distorted by rickets; rachitic.

rid′er's bone. An osseous deposit in the adductor muscles of the leg, from long-continued pressure of the leg against the saddle.

ridge. An extended elevation or crest. **alveolar r.** The ridge left after resorption of the alveolar process in an edentulous jaw. **genital r.** A medial ridge or fold on the ventromedial surface of the mesonephros in the embryo produced by growth of the peritoneum; the primordium of the gonads and their ligaments. **interosseous r.** The sharp ridge along the shaft of a bone such as the ulna or fibula, for the attachment of the interosseous ligament. Also called *interosseous crest*. **mesonephric r.** A ridge or fold of the dorsal coelomic wall in the embryo lateral to the mesentery produced by growth of the mesonephros. **supraorbital r.** The curved prominential margin forming the upper boundary of the orbit. **urogenital r.** The longitudinal peritoneal fold in the embryo produced by growth of the mesonephros and gonad. Syn., *Wolffian r.* **Wolffian r.** See urogenital r.

ri′ding of bones. *In surgery*, the displacement of the fractured ends of bones which are forced past each other by muscular contraction, instead of remaining in end-to-end apposition.

Riedel, Bernhard Moritz Carl Ludwig [German surgeon, 1846-1916]. Described a tongue-shaped process of the liver extending downward, occurring infrequently; called *congenital abnormal lobulation of the liver*, *Riedel's process or lobe*.

right. Dextral. Abbreviated, R.

rig′id. Stiff, hard.

ri·gid′i·tas. Stiffness; rigidity. **r. articulorum.** Spurious ankylosis. **r. cadaverica.** Rigor mortis.

ri·gid′i·ty. Stiffness; inflexibility; immobility; tonic contraction of muscles. **anatomic r. of the cervix uteri.** Rigidity in which the cervix, though neither edematous nor tender, is not wholly effaced in labor, but retains its length and dilates only to a certain extent, beyond which the contractions of the uterus are without effect. **cerebellar r.** Rigidity of the spinal muscles, due to lesion of the middle lobe of the cerebellum. The head is drawn backward, the spine curved, and the arms and legs made rigid. **clasp-knife r.** A spastic condition of a limb, as a result of which extension is completed with a spring, as in a knife blade. It is met in the cerebral palsies of children. **cogwheel r.** The rigidity or rhythmic contractions noted on passive stretching of the muscles in paralysis agitans. **decerebrate r.** An exaggerated postural tone in the antigravity muscles resulting from interruption of extrapyramidal axons from the motor and premotor areas of the cerebral cortex, or from destruction of cortical neurons in those areas. **hemiplegic r.** Spastic rigidity of the paralyzed limbs in hemiplegia.

rig′or. Chill. **r. mortis.** Stiffening and rigidity of muscle, particularly skeletal and cardiac, which occurs after death. Cessation of circulation in the muscle causes increase in content of acids, especially sarcolactic, with resultant swelling of muscle colloid and precipitation of insoluble myosin in the substance of the muscle.

ri′ma (ree′muh) (pl. *rimae*). A chink or cleft. **r. glottidis.** The cleft between the true vocal folds; the glottis. **—rimal,** *adj.* **r. oris.** The line formed by the junction of the lips. **r. pudendi.** The fissure between the labia majora.

ri′mose (rye′moce, rye·moce′). *In biology*, marked by many crevices or furrows.

ring. 1. A circular opening or the structure surrounding it. Also see *annulus.* 2. A line, band, or structure resembling a circle. **abdominal inguinal r.** The deep inguinal ring. **deep inguinal r.** The abdominal opening of an inguinal canal. **external inguinal r.** The subcutaneous inguinal ring. **internal inguinal r.** The deep inguinal ring. **Kayser-Fleischer r.** A ring of golden brown or brownish green pigment behind the limbic border of the cornea, observed in hepatolenticular degeneration (Wilson's disease) and the pseudosclerosis of Westphal. **subcutaneous inguinal r.** The external opening of an inguinal canal; an obliquely placed, triangular opening in the aponeurosis of the external oblique muscle, giving passage to the ilioinguinal nerve and to the spermatic cord in the male, or to the round ligament of the uterus in the female. **tympanic r.** Before and at the time of birth, an incomplete osseous ring which later becomes the tympanic part of the temporal bone. **umbilical r.** The margin of the opening in the ventral body wall of the fetus; the line of attachment of the umbilical cord.

ring com'pound. A compound in which the atoms form a ring or closed chain.

ring'worm". An infestation of the skin, hair, or nails, produced by various fungi. Also called *dermatomycosis, tinea, trichophytosis.* **Burmese r.** Tinea imbricata.

ripe. Mature, completed.

ri·so'ri·us (ri·sor'ee·us, rye·). A muscle of the cheek inserted into the angle of the mouth. See Table of Muscles in the Appendix.

ris"to·ce'tin. A mixture of antibiotic substances from *Nocardia lurida,* that is active against pathogenic Gram-positive cocci. See *spontin.*

ri'sus. A grin or laugh. **r. sardoni·ous.** The sardonic grin, a peculiar grinning distortion of the face produced by spasm of the muscles about the mouth, seen in tetanus.

ri'val·ry. A struggle for supremacy. **r. of contours.** A rivalry of the contours of two objects, one of which is presented to each eye, when they overlap in the binocular field of vision.

rivanol. Trade-mark for a bactericide, chemically ethoxydiaminoacridine lactate.

riz'i·form. Resembling grains of rice.

ri'xine (rye'zeen). Rice that has been acted upon by superheated steam.

R. M. A. Right mentoanterior position of the fetus.

R. M. P. Right mentoposterior position of the fetus.

R. N. Registered Nurse.

Rn. Chemical symbol for radon.

RNA Abbreviation for ribonucleic acid.

R. O. A. Right occipitoanterior position of the fetus.

rob'o·rant (rob'o·runt, ro'bo·runt). 1. Tonic, strengthening. 2. A tonic or strengthening remedy.

Roc·cel'la (rock·sel'uh). A genus of lichens of the Parmeliaceae. Several species yield coloring principles.

Ro·chelle' salt (ro·shell'). Potassium sodium tartrate, *q.v.*

rock oil. Petroleum.

Rock'y Moun'tain spot'ted fe'ver. A form of fever with a characteristic rash occurring throughout the Western Hemisphere; formerly thought to be limited to the Rocky Mountain area. The causative organism is *Rickettsia rickettsii,* and it is transmitted to man by several varieties of ticks, principally *Dermacentor andersoni* and *D. variabilis* in the United States.

rod. One of numerous, slender, bacillary structures, as in the retina. **rods of the retina.** One of the two types of photosensitive cells in the retina. Also called *rod cells.*

ro·den'ti·cide. A preparation that is poisonous to, or destroys, rodents. Usually used for an agent against rats or mice.

ro"do·nal'gi·a. Erythromelalgia.

roent'gen (rent'gen, runt'gen). Roentgen unit, *q.v.* Symbol, *r.*

roent'gen·ize. Subject to the action of roentgen rays.

roent"gen·ky·mog'ra·phy (rent"ghin·kigh·mog'ruh·fee). A roentgenographic procedure for recording changes in the size of the heart by interposing an impermeable sheet of metal, with slits, between the patient and the film, the latter moving at right angles to the slits during exposure.

roent'gen·o·gram". A roentgenray photograph.

roent"gen·og'ra·phy. Radiography, *q.v.* —**roentgenograph'ic,** *adj.*

roent"gen·o·ky·mog'ra·phy. Same as *roentgenkymography.*

roent"gen·ol'o·gist. A physician specializing in the practice of roentgenology.

roent"gen·ol'o·gy. The branch of medical science which deals with the diagnostic and therapeutic application of roentgen rays. Also called *radiology.* —**roentgenolog'ic,** *adj.*

roent"gen·om·e·try. Measurement of the quality and quantity of roentgen rays.

roent"gen·os'co·py. Examination with roentgen rays by means of a fluorescent screen. —**roent'geno·scope,** *n.*

roent'gen rays. See under *ray.*

roent"gen·ther'a·py. The treatment of disease by means of roentgen rays.

Rolando, Luigi [*Italian anatomist,* 1773–1831]. *Rolando's area* is the motor area in the cerebral cortex. See also central *sulcus;* formerly called *fissure of Rolando.*

rolicton. Trade-mark for amisometradine.

ron"geur' (rawn"zhur'). A bonecutting forceps.

Röntgen, Wilhelm Konrad [*German physicist,* 1845–1923]. Discovered x-rays (1895) and laid the foundation for the sciences of roentgenology and radiology. See also *roentgen rays* under *ray.* Nobel laureate (1901).

root. 1. The descending axis, as of a plant. 2. The part of an organ embedded in tissue, as of a tooth or a nail. 3. The beginning or proximal portion of a structure, especially one of two bundles of nerve fibers, the posterior and anterior, emerging from the central nervous system and joining to form a nerve trunk. **anterior r.** A bundle of efferent nerve fibers emerging from the anterior part of the spinal cord to form a spinal nerve. Syn., *motor r.*, *ventral r.* **dorsal r.** See *posterior r.* **motor r.** See *anterior r.* **posterior r.** A bundle of afferent nerve fibers arising from the nerve cells in a spinal ganglion and passing to the central nervous system. Syn., *dorsal r.*, *sensory r.* **r. of the lung.** The axis formed by the bronchus, pulmonary vessels, lymphatics, and nerves in the hilus, connecting the lung with the heart and trachea. Also called *radix pulmonis.* **r. of the mesentery.** The parietal attachment of the mesentery extending from the duodenojejunal flexure to the ileocecal junction. Also called *radix mesentericus.* **r. of the nail.** The small proximal region of the nail plate covered entirely by the nail wall. Also called *radix unguis.* **r. of the nose.** The part at the forehead between the eyes, from which emerges the dorsum of the nose. Also called *radix nasi.* **sensory r.** See posterior *r.* **ventral r.** See anterior *r.*

root ca·nal′. A small channel running from the pulp chamber to the apex of a tooth, normally filled with pulp tissue.

R. O. P. Right occipitoposterior position of the fetus.

Rorschach, Hermann [*Swiss psychiatrist, 1884–1922*]. Described a test which measures the more qualitative, nonintellectual traits of personality, based on the subject's interpretation of 10 ink blots of varying designs and colors. See Rorschach *test.*

Ro′sa (ro′zuh). See *rose.*

ro·sa′ce·i·form″. Resembling acne rosacea. Having a dusky red, telangiectatic appearance.

ro·sa′li·a (ro·say′lee·uh). 1. Scarlet fever. 2. Measles. 3. Erythema.

ros·an′i·line (ro·zan′i·lin, ·leen). $C_{20}H_{21}N_3O$. Brownish red crystals, slightly soluble in water. Used as a stain and in the manufacture of dyes. **r. hydrochloride.** Red crystals, soluble in water. See *fuchsin.*

rose. Any plant or flower of the genus *Rosa.* **attar of r.** Rose oil. **r. water ointment.** A popular emollient and vehicle sometimes referred to as cold cream.

rose ben′gal (beng′gawl, ben′gawl) (C.C.). Dichlortetraiodofluorescein, or tetrachlortetraiodofluorescein; used as a bacterial stain. Also used for a liver function test.

rose cold. An allergic manifestation due to sensitivity to rose pollens. It is a form of hay fever, *q.v.*

rose fe′ver. A form of hay fever, *q.v.*

rose hips. The ripe fruit of the dog rose, *Rosa canina.*

ro·se·in (ro′zee·in, roz′ee·in), **ro′se·ine** (ro′zee·een, ·in, roz′ee·). Fuchsin, *q.v.*

rose′mar″y. *Rosmarinus officinalis,* a plant of the Labiatae.

Rosenmueller, Johann Christian [*German anatomist, 1771–1826*]. Described the parovarium, *q.v.*, also called *organ of Rosenmueller.*

ro·se·o′la (ro·zee′o·luh). 1. A name given to any rose-colored eruption. 2. See *rubella.* **epidemic r.** Rubella. **r. syphilitica.** An eruption of rose-colored spots appearing early in secondary syphilis. **r. typhosa.** The eruption of typhoid or typhus fever. **r. vaccinia.** A general rose-colored eruption occurring about ten days after vaccination. It is of short duration.

ro·se′o·lous (ro·zee′o·lus). Having the character of roseola.

ro·sette′ (ro·zet′). Groups of cells from the neuroepithelial layer of the retina described by Wintersteiner as a characteristic of glioma of the retina. They correspond to the external limiting membrane of the retina, with rudimentary rods and cones projecting into the central cavity.

ros′in (roz′in). The residue left after the volatile oil is distilled from turpentine. It consists chiefly of various modifications of anhydrides of abietic acid with varying quantities of hydrocarbons. Also called *colophony.*

ro·sol′ic ac′id (ro·zol′ick, ·sol′ick). A mixture of triphenylmethane derivatives occurring as a reddish brown powder with green luster. Insoluble in water, soluble in alcohol. An acid-base indicator. Also called *aurin, corallin.*

ros′tral. 1. Pertaining to, or resembling a rostrum. 2. Cephalic.

ros′trum (pl. *rostra*). A beak; a projection or ridge.

rot. 1. Suffer putrefactive fermentation. 2. Decay; decomposition. 3. A disease of the feet of sheep in which the hoofs are destroyed. **grinder's r.** Fibrosis of the lungs occurring in grinders, especially knife grinders. Also called *grinder's asthma.*

ro′ta·me″ter. A device for the measurement of mean blood flow in arteries or veins.

ro·ta·ting (ro′tay·ting). Revolving, as rotating devices, appliances for correcting torsion of teeth.

ro·ta′tion. 1. The act of turning about an axis passing through the center of a body, as rotation of the eye, rotation of the head. 2. *In dentistry,* the operation by which a malturned tooth is turned or twisted into its normal position. 3. The phenomenon whereby every third or fourth impulse is carried over the cochlear nerve when the exciting impulse is above

1800 cycles. See *alternation, 2. 4. In obstetrics*, part of the process of labor, consisting of a rotary movement of the fetal head or other presenting part, whereby it is accommodated to the birth canal. It may be internal, occurring before the birth of the presenting part, or external, occurring afterward.

optical r. (a) Optical activity. (b) The number of degrees of rotation of the plane of vibration of polarized light produced by the substance under examination. **specific r.** The optical rotation, expressed in angular degrees, of a solution representing 1 Gm. of solute in 1 cc. of solution, and referred to a tube 1 decimeter in length.

ro·ta'tion ther'a·py. Radiation therapy during which either the patient is rotated before the source of radiation or the source is revolved around the patient, thereby providing a larger dose of radiation at the center of rotation than on any area of the skin.

ro·te·none (ro'ti·nohn, rot'i·nohn). $C_{23}H_{22}O_6$. An insecticidal principle derived from derris root and other plant roots; insoluble in water, soluble in ether. Harmless to birds and mammals.

rot'ler·a (rot'lur·uh). See *kamala*.

rot'ler·in. A bitter principle from kamala; used as an anthelmintic.

rough'age. Food residue in the colon, usually composed for the most part of cellulose.

rou·leau' (roo·lo'). A roll of red blood cells resembling a roll of coins.

round shoul'ders. Faulty posture in which sagging of the shoulders and increased convexity of the thoracic spine are conspicuous, the postural abnormalities not being limited to the shoulder girdle and chest.

round'worm''. A worm, free-living or parasitic, of the class Nematoda; commonly used to refer to a worm of the genus *Ascaris*.

R. Q. Respiratory quotient.

-rrha'gi·a. *In medicine,* a combining form signifying *abnormal* or *excessive discharge.*

-rrha'phy. A combining form meaning *sewing, suturing.* **—rrha·phia,** *n.*

-rrhea, -rrhoea. A combining form denoting *flow, discharge.*

-rrhexis. A combining form meaning *a breaking; rupture.*

-rrhin'i·a. A combining form denoting *a* (specified) *nasal condition.* **—rrhiny,** *n.*

R. S. A. Right sacroanterior position of the fetus.

R. S. P. Right sacroposterior position of the fetus.

R. T. Registered technician; certificate awarded to qualified x-ray technicians

by the American Registry of X-Ray Technicians.

Ru. Chemical symbol for ruthenium.

rub'ber. The prepared milk juice, chemically an unsaturated hydrocarbon, of several species of trees. Also called *caoutchouc, India rubber, Pará rubber.*

ru·be'do. Any diffuse redness of the skin.

ru''be·fa'cient (roo''bi·fay'shunt). 1. Causing redness of the skin. 2. An agent that causes redness of the skin.

ru''be·fac'tion. 1. Redness of the skin due to the action of an irritant. 2. The act of causing redness of the skin.

ru·bel'la. German measles. An acute, contagious, eruptive disease, of short duration and mild character. After a period of incubation varying from one to three weeks, the disease sets in abruptly with sore throat and slight fever. The eruption appears at the end of the first day, and consists of red maculopapular lesions, and disappears usually without desquamation in about three days. The disease is associated with enlargement of the superficial cervical and posterior auricular lymph nodes. Also called *epidemic roseola, French measles, German measles.*

ru·be'o·lin. A name given to the so-called specific toxin of measles.

ru·bes'cence. The state or quality of redness; a flushed or blushing countenance. **—rubescent,** *adj.*

ru·bid'i·um. Rb = 85.48. An alkali metal resembling potassium. It reacts violently with water and is kept under a liquid hydrocarbon.

ru·big'i·nous (roo·bidj'i·nus). Rust-colored.

ru''bi·jer'vine (roo''bi·jur'veen, ·vin). $C_{26}H_{43}NO_2 \cdot H_2O$. An alkaloid of *Veratrum viride, V. album,* and other plants of the Liliaceae.

ru'bin. Basic fuchsin.

ru'bor. Redness due to inflammation.

ru·bres'e·rine (roo·bress'ur·een, roo''bri·seer'een). A red decomposition product of physostigmine.

ru'bri·blast. A cell, in the earliest stage of formation of red blood cells, in which the chromatin is fine and stippled.

ru'bri·cyte. A cell, in the formative stages of red blood cells, with a definite chromatin pattern, but no nucleolus.

ruc·ta'tion. Eructation; belching.

ruc'tus. A belching of gas from the stomach. **r. hyster'icus.** Hysteric belching, the gas escaping with a loud, sobbing, gurgling noise.

ru'di·ment. That which is only partly developed. **—rudimen'tary,** *adj.*

ru"di·men'ta·ry. Undeveloped; unfinished; incomplete.

rue. A plant, *Ruta graveolens*, of the family Rutaceae, yielding a volatile oil.

ru'fous. Reddish; ruddy.

ru'ga (pl. *rugae*). A wrinkle, fold, elevation, or ridge, as in the mucosa of the stomach, vagina, and palate.

ru'gae (roo'jee). Plural of ruga, *q.v.*

ru·gi'tus (roo-jye'tus, roo'ji·tus). Rumbling of the intestines.

ru'gose, ru·gose'. Characterized by many folds.

ru·gos'i·ty. A condition exhibiting many folds in a tissue or integument.

ru'gous. See *rugose*.

rule. An established guide for action or procedure.

rum'bling. See *borborygmus*.

ru'men. First compartment of the stomach of a ruminant, where food is temporarily stored while undergoing fermentation prior to regurgitation and remastication. Also called *paunch*.

ru"men·ot'o·my. A laparotomy operation in which the rumen is exposed and incised for the correction of certain diseases of the organ.

Ru'mex. A genus of plants of the Polygonaceae. Yellow dock, the root of **R. crispus,** is a mild laxative and astringent.

ru'mi·nant. One of an order of mammals possessing an arrangement of the fore-stomach whereby food is regurgitated for remastication. An animal which chews the cud.

ru"mi·na'tion. 1. A characteristic of ruminants in which food is regurgitated and remasticated in preparation for true digestion. Syn., *merycism.* 2. *In psychiatry,* an obsessional preoccupation with a single idea or system of ideas which dominates the mind despite all efforts to dislodge it. Observed in anxiety states and in psychasthenia.

rump. The region near the end of the backbone; the buttocks or nates.

run. *In pathology,* discharge pus or purulent matter from a diseased part.

run'·a·round". A paronychia extending completely around a nail.

ru'pi·a. A form of eruption characterized by the formation of large, dirty-brown, stratified, conic crusts, that resemble oyster shell. Commonly used to describe a type of eruption seen in syphilis. —**rupial,** *adj.*

rup'ti·o (rup'shee·o). Rupture of a vessel or organ.

rup'ture. 1. A forcible tearing of a part, as rupture of the uterus, rupture of the bladder. 2. Hernia.

rup'tured. Burst; broken; forcibly torn; affected with hernia.

Rus'sian oil. A liquid petrolatum obtained originally from Russia, but now available in the U.S., consisting chiefly of naphthene derivatives of cyclopentane and cyclohexane, and which emulsifies readily.

rut. A period of heat or sexual excitement in animals, accompanied by ovulation. Also called *heat, estrus.*

Ru·ta'ce·ae (roo-tay'see·ee). A family including herbs, trees, and shrubs. The genus *Citrus* belongs to this group.

Rut'gers 612. Ethohexadiol.

ru·the'ni·um. Ru = 101.7. A rare metal of the platinum group.

ruth'er·ford (ruth'ur·furd). A unit of radioactivity representing 10^6 disintegrations per second. Abbreviated, rd.

ru'tin. $C_{27}H_{30}O_{16}.3H_2O$. A rhamno-glycoside of quercetin which occurs in several plants; occurs as a bright yellow powder; difficultly soluble in water. It decreases capillary fragility in some cases of increased fragility. Also called *eldrin, melin, myrticolorin, osyritin, phytomelin, violaquercitrin.*

ru'tin·ose. $C_{12}H_{22}H_{10}$. A disaccharide produced by enzymatic or controlled acid hydrolysis of rutin or hesperidin. Rutinose yields one molecule each of glucose and rhamnose on hydrolysis.

ry·an'o·dine. An alkaloid isolated from the stem and root of *Ryania speciosa* Vahl., having a high degree of insecticidal activity.

rye. The plant *Secale cereale* and its grain. The grain is used for making bread and whiskey.

S

s. 1. Chemical symbol for sulfur. **2.** Abbreviation for *signa*, sign; used in prescriptions to mean "write." **3.** Abbreviation for spherical or spherical lens.

s. 1. *Sinister*, left. **2.** *Semis*, half.

Sa. Chemical symbol for samarium.

sab″a·dil′la. The dried ripe seeds of *Schoenocaulon officinale* (*Asagraea officinalis*). Contains the alkaloids cevadine (crystallized veratrine), cevine (sabadinine), veratridine (amorphous veratrine), cevadilline (sabadilline), and sabadine. Syn., *cevadilla*.

sa·bad′i·nine (sa·bad′i-neen, ·nin). See *cevine*.

sab′al, sa′bal. See *serenoa*.

Sab·ba′ti·a (sa-bay′shee-uh, sa-bat′-ee-uh). A genus of the Gentianaceae. **S. angularis.** The American centaury; has been used as a febrifuge.

sab′u·lous. Gritty; sandy.

sac. A pouch; a baglike covering of a natural cavity, hernia, cyst, or tumor. **alveolar s.** A terminal group of pulmonary alveoli; one of the branches of an alveolar duct. **aortic s.** The saclike dilatation distal to the bulbus arteriosus from which the aortic arches arise; more or less comparable to a ventral aorta. **conjunctival s.** That formed by reflection of the palpebral conjunctiva. **dental s.** The connective tissue that encloses the developing tooth. Also called *dental follicle*. **endolymphatic s.** The bulblike terminal enlargement of the endolymphatic duct. **hernial s.** The pouch or protrusion of peritoneum containing a herniated organ or part, formed gradually by pressure against a defect in the containing wall or present at birth. **lacrimal s.** The dilated upper portion of the nasolacrimal duct. **lesser s.** The omental bursa; that part of the peritoneal sac located behind the stomach, lesser omentum, and the caudate lobe of the liver and within the great omentum; it communicates with the greater sac through the epiploic foramen. **omental s.** The sac formed between the ascending and descending portions of the great omentum. **peritoneal s.** That formed by the peritoneum. **yolk s.** An extraembryonic membrane composed of endoderm and splanchnic mesoderm enclosing the yolk mass in reptiles, birds, and monotremes, or a cavity in higher mammals. Also called *umbilical vesicle, saccus omphaloentericus*.

sac′cha·rase (sack′uh·race, ·raze). An enzyme occurring in plants and microörganisms, and capable of hydrolyzing disaccharides to monosaccharides; more specifically the enzyme which is responsible for hydrolysis of sucrose to dextrose and levulose. Also called *invertase, invertin, sucrase, β-h-fructosidase*.

sac′cha·rate (sack′uh·rate). A salt of saccharic acid.

sac′cha·ra′ted. Containing sugar.

sac″char·eph″i·dro′sis. A form of hyperhidrosis, characterized by the excretion of sugar in the sweat.

sac·char′ic ac′id (sa·kar′ick). CO-OH.(CHOH)₄.COOH. A dibasic acid resulting from oxidation of dextrose and some other sugars.

sac′cha·ride. A compound of a base with sugar. A sucrate.

sac·char″i·fi·ca′tion. The act of converting into sugar.

sac·char′i·fy (sa·kar′i·figh). **1.** Make sweet. **2.** Convert into sugar.

sac″cha·rim′e·ter. An apparatus for determining the amount of sugar in solutions.

sac′cha·rin. C₇H₅O₃NS; anhydro-o-sulfaminebenzoic acid; occurs as white crystals or powder; soluble in water. It is used as a sweetening agent. Also called *benzosulfimide, gluside, garantose, saccharinol, saccharinose, saccharol, sykose*. **s. sodium.** C₇H₄O₃-NSNa.2H₂O. The sodium salt of saccharin; occurs as white crystals or powder; soluble in water. Also called *soluble saccharin, soluble gluside, sodium benzosulfimide*.

sac′cha·ro- (sack′uh·ro-), **sac-char-.** A combining form denoting *sugar* or *saccharine*.

sac″cha·ro·bi′ose (C₁₂H₂₂O₁₁). A disaccharide.

sac″cha·ro·ga·lac″tor·rhe′a. The secretion of milk which contains an excess of sugar.

sac′cha·roids. Sugarlike substances. The term is generally applied to polysaccharides of high molecular weight which do not ferment, but which yield fermentable sugars on hydrolysis.

sac″cha·ro·me·tab′o·lism. The metabolism of sugar. —**saccharo-metabol′ic,** *adj.*

Sac″cha·ro·my′ces (sack″uh·ro-migh′seez). A genus of yeasts which includes baker's and brewer's yeasts.

sac″cha·ro·my·co′sis (sack″uh·ro-migh·ko′sis). A pathologic condition due to yeasts or *Saccharomyces*.

sac″cha·ror·rhe′a. Glycosuria.

sac″cha·rose (sack′uh·roce, ·roze). **1.** Sucrose, cane sugar. C₁₂H₂₂O₁₁. **2.** A term used in the classification of carbohydrates as: **monosaccharose,** a simple carbohydrate of formula $C_6H_{12}O_6$; **disaccharose,** a carbohydrate of formula $C_{12}H_{22}O_{11}$ formed from two monosaccharose units with the elimination of a molecule of water.

sac'cha·ro·su'ri·a. The presence of saccharose in the urine.

sac'cha·rum. See *sucrose.*

sac'ci·form (sack'ĭ·form). Resembling a sac.

sac'cu·la"ted. Divided into or having small sacs.

sac"cu·la'tion. 1. The state of being sacculated. 2. The formation of small sacs.

sac'cule. 1. A small sac. 2. The smaller of two vestibular sacs of the membranous labyrinth of the ear. Also called *sacculus labyrinthi.*

sac"cu·lo·coch'le·ar (sack"yoo·lo·cock'lee·ur). Relating to the saccule of the vestibule and the cochlea.

sac'cu·lus. 1. A saccule. 2. The saccule of the vestibule.

sac'cus (pl. *sacci*). Sac, q.v.

sa"cral·i·za'tion. Fusion of the fifth lumbar vertebra to the sacrum.

sa·crec'to·my. Excision of part of the sacrum.

sa'cro- (say'kro-). A combining form meaning *relating to the sacrum.*

sa"cro·an·te'ri·or. A fetal position, with the sacrum directed forward.

sa"cro·coc·cyg'e·al (say"kro·cock·sidj'ee·ul). Pertaining to the sacrum and the coccyx.

sa"cro·coc·cyg'e·us (·cock·sidj'ee·us). One of two inconstant thin muscles extending from the lower sacral vertebrae to the coccyx.

sa"cro·dyn'i·a (say"kro·din'ee·uh). Pain in the sacrum.

sa"cro·il'i·ac (say"kro·il'ee·ack). Pertaining to the sacrum and the ilium, as sacroiliac disease, an inflammation of the sacroiliac joint, characterized by pain and tenderness over the joint, and thought to produce sciatica. See Table of Joints and Ligaments in the Appendix.

sa"cro·lum'bar. Pertaining to the sacrum and the loins. Syn., *lumbo-sacral.*

sa"cro·pos·te'ri·or. A fetal position with the sacrum directed backward.

sa"cro·sci·at'ic (say"kro·sigh·at'ick). Pertaining to the sacrum and the ischium, as the sacrosciatic notch, sacrosciatic ligaments. *O.T.*

sa"cro·spi·na'lis (say"kro·spy·nah'lis)[BNA]. Erector spinae. See Table of Muscles in the Appendix.

sa'crum (pl. *sacra*). A curved triangular bone composed of five united vertebrae, situated between the last lumbar vertebra above, the coccyx be-

low, and the innominate bones on each side, and forming the posterior boundary of the pelvis. See Table of Bones in the Appendix. —**sacral,** *adj.*

sad'dle·back. Lordosis.

sa'dism, sad'ism. Sexual perversion in which pleasure is derived from inflicting cruelty upon another. —**sadis'tic,** *adj.*

sa'dist, sad'ist. One affected with sadism.

saf'fron. Crocus.

saf'ra·nine (saf'ruh·neen, ·nin), **saf'ra·nin.** A basic aniline dye of the azine group, used as a biologic stain. The commonest form is **safranin O,** C.C., which is used as a nuclear stain, and as a counterstain in Gram's stain for bacteria.

sage. See *salvia.*

sage'brush". Any of several members of the genus *Artemisia.*

sage femme' (sahzh fahm'). A midwife.

sag'it·tal (sadj'ĭ·tul). 1. Arrowlike, as the sagittal suture of the skull. 2. Pertaining to the anteroposterior median plane of the body.

sa'go. A starch derived from the pith of certain East Indian and Malaysian palms; used as a food and as a demulcent.

Saint Agatha's disease. Disease of the female breast.

Saint Agnan's disease. Ringworm, tinea.

Saint Aman's disease. Pellagra.

Saint Anthony's dance. Chorea.

Saint Anthony's fire. Erysipelas or gangrene; ergotism.

Saint Blaize's disease. Quinsy.

Saint Guy's dance. Chorea.

Saint Valentine's disease. Epilepsy.

Saint Vitus' dance. Chorea.

sajodin. Trade-mark for a brand of calcium iodobehenate.

sal. 1. Salt. 2. Any substance resembling salt. **s. aeratus.** (a) Sodium bicarbonate. (b) Potassium bicarbonate. **s. ammoniac.** Ammonium chloride. **s. Glauberi.** Sodium sulfate. **s. kissingense.** A salt obtained from the mineral springs of Kissingen, in Bavaria. **s. marinum.** Sodium chloride. **s. mirabile.** Sodium sulfate. **s. prunella.** (a) A fused mixture of potassium nitrate, 128 parts, and sulfur, 1 part. (b) Fused potassium nitrate. Also called *s. prunelle.* **s. seignette.** Potassium sodium tartrate. **s. soda.** Sodium carbonate. **s. vegetabile.** Potassium tartrate. **s. volatile.** Ammonium carbonate.

sa·la'cious. Lustful. —**salac'ity,** *n.*

sal'ep, sa'lep. The dried tubers of various species of the genus *Orchis* and the genus *Eulophia.* Used as a food, like sago and tapioca, or as a demulcent.

sal″e·ra′tus. Potassium bicarbonate or sodium bicarbonate. Syn., *sal aeratus.*

sal′i·cin. $C_{13}H_{18}O_7$; a glycoside of orthohydroxybenzyl alcohol found in several species of willow and poplar; a white, crystalline powder; soluble in water.

sal′i·cyl. $C_7H_5O_2$. The radical, C_6H_4·OH.CO—, of salicylic acid. **s. alcohol.** $C_6H_4OHCH_2OH$; o-hydroxybenzyl alcohol; occurs as a white, crystalline powder; soluble in water and alcohol. It has marked local anesthetic powers. See *saligenin, salicyloid.*

sal′i·cyl-. See *salicylo-.*

sal″i·cyl·am′ide. o-Hydroxybenzaldehyde, an analgesic, antipyretic, and antirheumatic.

sal′i·cyl″ate (sal′i·sil″ate, sa·liss′i·late, sal″i·sil′ate). A salt of salicylic acid.

sal″i·cyl·a′zo·sul″fa·pyr′i·dine. 5-[p-(2-Pyridylsulfamyl)phenylazo]salicylic acid, an antibacterial agent. See *azulfidine.*

sal″i·cyl′ic ac′id. C_6H_4·OH.COOH. o-Hydroxybenzoic acid; occurs as white crystals or powder; soluble in water. Salicylic acid is used only for its local effect.

sal′i·cyl·ism. A toxic condition, produced by full doses of salicylates; characterized chiefly by tinnitus, hebetude, nausea, and vomiting.

sal″i·cyl′o-, salicyl-. *In chemistry,* a combining form denoting *salicylic.*

sal″i·cy·lu′ric ac′id. C_6H_4·OH.CO.NH.CH_2COOH. A detoxication product of salicylic acid found in the urine.

sal′i·fi″a·ble. Forming a salt by union with an acid.

saligenin. Trade name for salicyl alcohol.

saligenol. Trade name for salicyl alcohol.

sa·lim′e·ter. A hydrometer used to determine the density of salt solutions.

sa′line (say′lyne). 1. Saltlike in character. 2. Containing sodium chloride.

sa′lines. Salts of the alkalies or of magnesium; used as hydragogue cathartics. Magnesium sulfate and citrate, sodium sulfate, and Rochelle salt are examples.

salipyrin. A brand of antipyrine salicylate, *q.v.*

sa·li′va. The mixed secretions of the parotid, submaxillary, sublingual, and other glands of the mouth. It is opalescent, tasteless, and weakly alkaline. Its most important constituent is ptyalin. The functions of saliva are to moisten the food and lubricate the bolus, to dissolve certain substances, to facilitate tasting, to aid in deglutition and articulation, and to digest starches,

which it converts into maltose, dextrin, and glucose. **—sal′ivary, salivous,** *adj.*

sal′i·vant. 1. Stimulating the secretion of saliva. 2. A drug which increases the flow of saliva.

sal″i·va′tion. An excessive secretion of saliva; a condition produced by mercury, pilocarpine, and by nervous disturbances. In severe cases of mercurial salivation, ulceration of the gums and loosening of the teeth may occur. **—sal′ivate,** *v.*

sal′i·va″tor. An agent causing salivation. **—saliva′tory,** *adj.*

sal″i·vo·li·thi′a·sis. Presence of a salivary calculus.

sa′lix. The bark of several species of *Salix* (willow). The active constituent of all species of *Salix* is salicin.

sal′mine (sal′meen, ·min). A protamine obtained from the spermatozoa of salmon.

sal′mone. A histone obtained from the spermatozoa of salmon.

Sal″mo·nel′la. A genus of bacteria of the tribe Salmonelleae, family Enterobacteriaceae. They are nonlactose fermenting, nonsporogenous, aerobic, motile (with rare exceptions), Gram-negative rods. Almost all ferment glucose to acid and gas. Pathogenic species cause gastrointestinal symptoms, as in typhoid fever, paratyphoid fever, acute gastroenteritis, diarrhea of domestic animals, etc. **S. aertrycke.** Synonym for *S. typhimurium.* **S. choleraesuis.** A species occasionally found in epidemics of acute gastroenteritis. Syn., *Bacterium cholerae-suis.* Also called *hog cholera bacillus.* **S. enteritidis.** A species causing diarrhea of newborn calves. **S. gallinarum.** A species causing fowl typhoid, a diarrhea of domestic fowl, especially adult birds. **S. icteroides.** A bacillus isolated from yellow fever cadavers. Formerly called *Bacillus icteroides, Bacterium icteroides, Sanarelli's bacillus.* **S. oranienburg.** A species isolated from feces of normal carriers, from feces of food poisoning cases, and from abscesses; often found in dried egg products. **S. paratyphi A.** A species which produces paratyphoid fever in man. Syn., *Bacterium paratyphosum A.* **S. paratyphi B.** That species which causes paratyphoid fever in man. Syn., *Bacterium paratyphosum B.* Also called *S. schottmuelleri.* **S. paratyphi C.** A species isolated in enteric fevers in British Guiana, Asia, Africa, and southeastern Europe. Also called *S. hirschfeldii.* **S. pullorum.** A species causing pullorum disease or bacillary white diarrhea of chicks. Transmission can occur through the egg. **S. schottmuelleri.** That species which causes paratyphoid fever in man. **S. sp.** Any serotype that has not yet been assigned to a definite species. **S. suipestifer.** A species found commonly in hogs and at one time thought to be the cause of hog cholera. It occasionally causes enteritis in man. Syn., *S. choleraesuis.* **S. typhimurium.** A species commonly causing diarrhea in mice, rats, and birds and gastroenteritis in man. The most commonly isolated bacterium in outbreaks of food poisoning in the United States and Great Britain. **S. typhosa.** The causative agent of typhoid fever, the symptoms being produced largely by endotoxins liberated upon destruction of the organisms. In culture glucose is fermented to acid but not gas. Also called *Bacterium typhosum, Eberthella typhosa, S. typhi.*

sal″mo·nel·lo′sis. Infection with the genus *Salmonella;* food poisoning. Also called *diarrheal disease.*

sal′ol. Phenyl salicylate, *q.v.*

salophen. Trade-mark for a brand of phenetsal.

sal″pin·gec′to·my. Excision of a uterine tube.

sal″pin·gem·phrax′is. Closure of an auditory or uterine tube.

sal″pin·gi′tis. 1. Inflammation of a uterine tube. 2. Inflammation of an auditory tube. —**salpingit′ic,** *adj.* **chronic parenchymatous s.** Chronic interstitial inflammation and thickening of the muscular coat of a uterine tube. **chronic vegetating s.** Excessive hypertrophy of the mucosa of a uterine tube. **gonococcic s.** Gonococcal infection of a uterine tube. **interstitial s.** That marked by excessive formation of connective tissue. **purulent s.** Salpingitis with secretion of pus instead of mucus or serum. **tuberculous s.** That marked by the infiltration of the lining membrane and walls of a uterine tube with tuberculous nodules.

sal·pin′go- (sal·ping′go-, sal′ping-go-), **salping-.** A combining form meaning *a trumpet;* used to denote *relation to an auditory tube* or *to a uterine tube.*

sal″pin″go·cath′e·ter·ism. Catheterization of an auditory tube.

sal·pin′go·cele. Hernia of an oviduct.

sal·pin″go·cy·e′sis (sal·ping″go-sigh·ee′sis). Tubal pregnancy.

sal″pin·gol′y·sis. The breaking down of adhesions of a uterine tube.

sal·pin″go-o″ö·pho·rec′to·my (-o″o·fo·reck′to·mee, -o″off·o·reck′to-mee). Excision of a uterine tube and an ovary.

sal·pin″go-o″ö·pho·ri′tis. Inflammation of the uterine tubes and the ovaries.

sal·pin″go-o·öph′o·ro·cele (-o·off′o·ro·seel, -o″o·for′o·seel). Hernial protrusion of an ovary and oviduct.

sal·pin″go·per″i·to·ni′tis. Inflammation of the peritoneum and uterine tube.

sal·pin′go·pex″y. Operative fixation of one or both uterine tubes.

sal·pin″go·pha·ryn′ge·al (sal·ping″go·fa·rin′jul, ·far″in·jee′ul). Pertaining to the auditory tube and the pharynx, as the salpingopharyngeal muscle.

sal·pin′go·plas″ty. Surgery of an oviduct, or uterine tube.

sal″pin·gor′rha·phy. Suture of a uterine tube.

sal″pin·gos′to·my. 1. The operation of making an artificial fistula between a uterine tube and the body surface. 2. Any plastic operation for opening the uterine tube.

sal″pin·got′o·my. The operation of cutting into a uterine tube.

sal″pin·gys″ter·o·cy·e′sis (sal″pin·jis″tur·o·sigh·ee′sis). Interstitial pregnancy.

sal′pinx. A tube, especially the auditory or the uterine tube.

salt. 1. Sodium chloride. 2. A group of substances that result from the reaction between acids and bases; a compound of a metal or positive radical and a nonmetal or negative radical. 3. A mixture of several salts, as artificial salt and effervescent salt. **acid s.** A salt that contains unreplaced hydrogen atoms of the acid from which the salt was formed, as $NaHCO_3$. **amphoteric s.** A salt that has both acid and basic properties. **artificial s.** A mixture of the more important chemical salts naturally present in several of the well-known mineral springs of Europe. **basic s.** A salt that contains unreplaced hydroxyl groups of the base from which it was formed. **buffer s.** The salt of a weak acid and strong base, or of a strong acid and a weak base which, in solution, tends to resist a change in reaction upon addition of acid or alkali, respectively. **complex s.** A salt made up of more than one simple acid or metallic radical, but which ionizes in solution into only two types of ions; as $K_4Fe(CN)_6$. **effervescent s.** A mixture of one or more active chemical salts with an effervescent base. The base usually consists of sodium bicarbonate, citric and tartaric acids. **Epsom s.** Magnesium sulfate. **Mohr's s.** Ferrous ammonium sulfate. **Monsel's s.** Ferric subsulfate. **neutral s.** A salt whose solution has a neutral reaction, as sodium chloride. **normal s.** A salt of an acid and base that have completely neutralized each other. The reaction in solution may be neutral, acid, alkaline, or amphoteric. **rock s.** Sodium chloride as obtained in the solid form by mining.

sal·ta'tion. Dancing or leaping as in chorea.

salt'ing out. A method of precipitating proteins and other substances by the use of aqueous solutions of neutral salts.

salt"pe'ter, salt"pe'tre. Potassium nitrate. **Chile s.** Sodium nitrate.

salts. A saline cathartic, especially magnesium sulfate, sodium sulfate, or Rochelle salt.

sa·lu'bri·ty. The state or quality of being wholesome, conducive to physical well-being. **—salubrious,** *adj.*

sal'u·tar"y (sal'yoo·terr"ee). Promoting health.

salvarsan. Trade-mark for a brand of arsphenamine.

salve. Ointment.

sal'vi·a. The dried leaf of *Salvia officinalis*. Both the leaves and flowering tops contain a volatile oil. Also called *garden sage.*

salyrgan. Trade-mark for a brand of mersalyl.

Sam"a·de'ra, Sa·mad'er·a. A genus of old-world trees of the Simarubaceae. **S. indica.** Produces a niepa bark which has been used as a bitter tonic.

sa·ma'ri·um. Sa (or Sm) = 150.43. A metallic element belonging to the didymium group.

sam·bu'cus. The air-dried flower of *Sambucus canadensis*, or of *Sambucus nigra*. The flowers yield a volatile oil. It also contains rutin. Also called *elder flowers.*

sam'ple. A specimen or part to show the quality of the whole. **random s.** A finite number of individuals, cases, or measurements chosen from a larger group in such a manner that each individual, case, or measurement has an equal and independent chance of being selected.

san"a·to'ri·um. An establishment for the treatment of the chronic diseases; especially, a private hospital or place having conditions which are natural therapeutic agents.

san'dal·wood". 1. White sandalwood. The heartwood of *Santalum album*, which contains a volatile oil. Also called *white saunders, white santal.* 2. Red sandalwood. The heartwood of *Pterocarpus santalinus*. It contains a coloring principle called santalin. Also called *red saunders, red santal.*

san'da·rac. A white, transparent resin produced by *Callitris quadrivalvis*, a tree of North Africa. **s. varnish.** *In dentistry*, a solution of sandarac in alcohol used as a separating medium in making plaster casts.

sane. Of sound mind.

san·guic'o·lous (sang·gwick'o·lus). Living in the blood, as a parasite.

san·guif'er·ous. Carrying, or conveying, blood.

san"gui·fi·ca'tion. The formation of blood; conversion into blood.

san"gui·na'ri·a (sang"gwi·nair'ee-uh). The dried rhizome of *Sanguinaria canadensis*. Also called *bloodroot.*

san·guin'a·rine (sang·gwin'uh·reen, sang"gwi·nair'een). An alkaloid found in sanguinaria.

san'guine (sang'gwin). 1. Resembling blood; bloody. 2. Hopeful, active, as sanguine temperament.

san·guin'o·lent. Tinged with blood.

san'guis. Blood.

san"gui·suc'tion. Abstraction of blood by suction, as by a leech or other parasite.

sa'ni·es (say'nee·eez). A thin, fetid, greenish, seropurulent fluid discharged from an ulcer, wound, or fistula. **—sanious,** *adj.*

san"i·ta'ri·an. One skilled in sanitary science and matters of public health.

san"i·ta'ri·um. Same as *sanatorium.*

san'i·tar"y. Pertaining to health.

san"i·ta'tion. The act of securing a healthful condition; the application of sanitary measures.

san'i·ty. Soundness of mind.

sanocrysin. Trade-mark for gold and sodium thiosulfate.

san'tal. Sandalwood.

san'ta·lol. $C_{15}H_{26}O$. A constituent of the oil from sandalwood.

san'ta·lum. See under *sandalwood.*

san·ton'i·ca. The unexpanded flower heads of several species of *Artemisia*. The most important constituent is santonin. Also called *wormseed, Levant wormseed.*

san·ton'ic ac'id. $C_{15}H_{20}O_4$. An acid obtained by heating santonin with alkali; it is isomeric with santoninic acid.

san'to·nin. $C_{15}H_{18}O_3$. The inner anhydride of santoninic acid; occurs as colorless crystals or powder, almost insoluble in water. Used as a vermifuge, especially against the ascarids.

san"to·nin'ic ac'id. $C_{15}H_{20}O_4$. The acid of which santonin is the inner anhydride.

san'ton·ism. Poisoning from overdosage of santonin. Symptoms: yellow vision, gastrointestinal, renal, and vesical irritation, weakness, hallucinations, convulsions, coma.

sap. Plant juice. The watery solution which circulates through the vascular tissues of a plant.

sa·phe'na. One of two large veins of

the leg—the great or long and the small or short saphena.

sa·phe'nous, saph'e·nous. Apparent; superficial; manifest; applied to two veins of the lower limb, the great or long saphenous vein and the small or short saphenous vein, situated just beneath the surface; also applied to the nerves accompanying these veins. See Tables of Nerves and of Veins in the Appendix.

sap'id. Capable of being tasted.

sa'po. Soap.

sa·pog'e·nin (sa·podj'i·nin, sap"o·jen'in). The nonsugar or aglycone component of a saponin.

sap"o·na'ceous. Having the nature of soap.

sa·pon"i·fi·ca'tion. The conversion of an ester into an alcohol and a salt; in particular, the conversion of a fat into a soap and glycerin by means of an alkali. **—sapon'ify,** v.

sa·pon'i·form. Soaplike in appearance and consistency.

sap'o·nin, sa·po'nin. 1. A glycoside usually obtained from *Quillaja* or *Saponaria*. The commercial saponin occurs as a white to brownish, amorphous powder. 2. One of a group of glycosidal principles which have the property of foaming when shaken with water and dissolving red blood cells. Saponins are widely distributed in nature.

sap"o·tox'in. A name sometimes given to the more toxic saponins.

sap'phism (saf'iz·um). Female homosexuality.

sa·pre'mi·a, sa·prae'mi·a. The intoxication produced by absorption of the products of putrefaction.

sap'ro-, sapr-. A combining form meaning *rotten;* used to denote *dead* or *decaying organic matter* or *saprophytic.*

sap'ro·gen. A putrefactive microorganism.

sap"ro·gen'ic, sa·prog'e·nous (sa·prodj'i·nus). 1. Causing putrefaction. 2. Produced by putrefaction.

sa·proph'a·gous. Subsisting on decaying matter.

sap'ro·phyte. An organism living on dead organic matter. **—saprophyt'ic,** adj.

sap"ro·xo'ic. Characterizing an animal which lives upon decaying organic matter.

sar'a·pus. A flat-footed person.

Sar·ci'na. A genus of the family Micrococcaceae. Cell division occurs in three planes forming cubical groups.

sar·ci'tis. Inflammation of fleshy tissue; especially inflammation of muscle.

sar'co-, sarc-. A combining form meaning *flesh.*

sar"co·bi'ont. Living on flesh.

sar'co·blast. A cell developing into a muscle cell or fiber. Syn., *myoblast.*

sar'co·cele. A tumor of the testis resembling muscle.

Sar"co·cys'tis. A genus of Sarcosporidia, parasitic in muscles of higher vertebrates.

Sar"co·di'na. A class of protozoa moving and feeding by means of pseudopodia.

sar"co·gen'ic. Producing muscle.

sar"co·hy'dro·cele. A sarcocele complicated with hydrocele of the tunica vaginalis.

sar'coid. 1. Resembling flesh. 2. The characteristic lesion seen in sarcoidosis.

sar"coid·o'sis. A disease of young adults and sometimes of older persons, of unknown etiology; characterized by granulomatous lesions, somewhat resembling true tubercles, affecting lymph nodes, skin, lungs, bones in distal parts of the extremities, and other structures. Iridocyclitis and uveoparotid fever may occur. Usually shows periods of activity, and recovery may take place. Also called *Boeck's sarcoid, Besnier-Boeck disease, Besnier-Boeck-Schaumann disease, lupus pernio of Besnier, lymphogranulomatosis of Schaumann.*

sar"co·lac'tic ac'id. $CH_2 \cdot CHOH \cdot COOH$. An isomeric form of lactic acid occurring in muscle. Also called *paralactic acid.*

sar"co·lem'ma. The delicate sheath enveloping a muscle fiber. **—sarcolemmic,** adj.

sar·co'ma. A malignant neoplasm derived from nonepithelial tissues, such as connective tissue, muscle, or bone, and named after the tissue of origin, for instance, fibrosarcoma, osteosarcoma, liposarcoma. **giant-cell s.** (a) Giant-cell tumor of bone, usually benign. (b) Epulis in malignant form. (c) Synovial sarcoma. **Jensen's s.** A transmissible spindle-cell type of neoplasm which grows in a high percentage of inoculated rats and recedes in a large proportion after a few weeks' growth. **multiple idiopathic hemorrhagic s.** A multiple tumor, difficult to classify, consisting of elevated pigmented, vascular nodules which may heal spontaneously with considerable scarring. The tumors usually arise in an extremity, later involve the gastrointestinal tract, and terminate fatally. Also called *Kaposi's sarcoma.* **neurogenic s.** Neurogenous sarcoma, the malignant form of neurofibroma. **reticuloendothelial s.** A malignant neoplasm derived from cells of the reticuloendothelial system. Syn., *retothelioma.* **spindle-cell s.** A malignant connective-tissue tumor composed of spindle-shaped cells.

sar·co"ma·to'sis. The formation of

multiple sarcomatous growths in various parts of the body.

sar'co·mere. One of the segments into which a muscle fibril appears to be divided by Z disks.

sar"co·my'ces (sahr"ko·migh'seez). A fleshy growth of a fungous appearance.

Sar"co·phag'i·dae (sahr"ko·fadj'i-dee). A large cosmopolitan family of the Diptera, commonly known as flesh flies, blowflies, and scavenger flies. They normally deposit their eggs or larvae on the decaying flesh of dead animals, but sometimes also in open wounds and sores of man. The important genera are *Sarcophaga* and *Wohlfahrtia*. The maggots of *W. vigil* are known to cause cutaneous myiasis in young children. *W. magnifica* is said to be a great pest to wounded soldiers in Europe and Asia.

sar'co·plasm. The hyaline or finely granular interfibrillar material of muscle tissue; the term is opposed to the myofibrils or contractile substance. —**sarcoplas'mic,** *adj.*

Sar·cop'tes (sahr·cop'teez). A genus of minute, rounded, short-legged, flattened mites which cause scabies in man and mange in many kinds of animals. **S. scabiei.** The itch mite of man.

Sar"cop·toi'de·a. A superfamily of the parasitic mites; the mange and itch mites of the genus *Sarcoptes* are included.

sar'co·sine (sahr'ko·seen, ·sin). Methyl glycine, methylaminoacetic acid. CH₂NH.CH₂.COOH. **dimethyl s.** Betaine.

Sar"co·spo·rid'i·a. An order of the class Sporozoa, including the genus *Sarcocystis.*

sar"co·spo·rid"i·o'sis. A disease of warm-blooded animals caused by sporozoa of the order Sarcosporidia; it is rare in man. The parasites usually encyst in striated muscles and produce few symptoms.

sar'cous. Pertaining to flesh or muscle.

sar"sa·pa·ril'la. The dried root of *Smilax aristolochiaefolia, Smilax regelii,* or of undetermined species of *Smilax.* The most important principles in sarsaparilla are three saponins: smilasaponin, sarsasaponin, and parillin.

sar·to'ri·us. The tailor's muscle, so called from being concerned in crossing one leg over the other. See Table of Muscles in the Appendix.

sas'sa·fras. The dried bark of the root of *Sassafras albidum.* Contains a volatile oil.

sas'so·lin. Old term for boric acid extracted from the deposits in lagoons of Tuscany.

sas'sy bark. The bark of *Erythrophleum.* Syn., *casca bark.*

sat. Saturated.

sat"el·li·to'sis (sat"i-lye·to'sis, ·li-to'sis). *In neuropathology,* a condition in which there is an accumulation of satellite cells around the nerve cells of the ganglions in inflammatory and degenerative diseases. These satellite cells usually represent phagocytic neuroglia cells.

sa·ti'e·ty. Fullness beyond desire; a condition of gratification beyond desire or need.

sat. sol. Saturated solution.

sat'u·ra"ted. 1. Having all the atoms of molecules linked so that only single bonds exist. 2. Having sufficient substance, either solid or gaseous, dissolved in a solution so that no more of that substance can be dissolved. Abbreviated, sat. **s. compound.** An organic compound with no free valence, and in which there are neither double nor triple bonds.

sat'ur·nine (sat'ur·nyne). 1. Pertaining to or produced by lead. 2. Of gloomy nature.

sat'ur·nism. Chronic lead poisoning; plumbism.

sat"y·ri'a·sis. 1. Excessive venereal desire in man. Also called *satyromania.* See *priapism.* 2. Old term for leprosy.

sau'cer·ize. Shape bone cavity in the operation for chronic osteomyelitis, in order to eliminate sharp angles and overhanging walls, thus permitting soft parts to fill it completely during the process of healing. Also called *gutter.*

sau·ri'a·sis. Ichthyosis.

Sau·rop'si·da. A superclass of vertebrates comprising the birds and reptiles.

sau·rox'ine (saw·rock'seen, ·sin). An alkaloid obtained from *Lycopodium saururus.* See *piligan.*

sau·ru'rine (saw·roor'een, ·in). An alkaloid obtained from *Lycopodium saururus.* See *piligan.*

sau'sar·ism. 1. Paralysis of the tongue. 2. Dryness of the tongue.

sa·vin. The evergreen shrub *Juniperus Sabina,* from the tops of which a volatile oil may be obtained.

sa'vo·ry. Having a pleasant odor or flavor.

saw. An instrument having a thin blade with sharp teeth on one edge, and used for dividing bones and other hard substances. **Adams's s.** A small straight saw with a long handle. **Albee's s.** An electrically operated, double rotary circular saw with adjustable blades, for use in preparing bone grafts. **Butcher's s.** One in which the blade can be fixed at any angle. **chain s.** One in which the teeth are set in links movable upon each other, the saw being moved by pulling alternately upon one and the other handle. **crown s.** See *trephine*. **Gigli's s.** A flexible wire saw operated by handles at either end, which pass through loops. Adapted to cranial and other bone operations. **Hey's s.** A serrated disk affixed to a handle, and used for enlarging an opening in a bone. **nasal s.** A small, narrow instrument used for removing nasal spurs and turbinate bones.

saw pal·met'to. See *serenoa*.

sax'i·frage. Any plant of the genus *Saxifraga*. *S. crassifolia* and other species contain a crystalline bitter principle, bergenin.

Sb. Chemical symbol for antimony.

Sc. Chemical symbol for scandium.

scab. 1. Dried exudate covering an ulcer or wound. Syn., *crust*. 2. A disease of sheep caused by a mite.

sca'bi·cide. Any agent or drug which kills *Sarcoptes scabiei*, the causative organism of scabies.

sca'bi·es (skay'bee-eez, skay'beez). A contagious disorder of the skin caused by *Sarcoptes scabiei*; characterized by multiform lesions with intense itching which occurs chiefly at night. The female insect, burrowing beneath the epidermis to lay eggs, causes the irritation. Also called *itch, seven year itch*. **s. papuliformis.** A form marked by papular efflorescence. Also called *rank itch*, **s. papulosa. s. pustulosa.** That in which there is formation of large pustules resembling those of smallpox, occurring on the wrists and buttocks of children. Seen more commonly in warm weather.

sca"bi·o·pho'bi·a. Morbid fear of scabies.

sca·bri'ti·es (ska·brish'ee-eez). Roughness; scabbiness.

sca'la (pl. *scalae*). A subdivision of the cavity of the cochlea; especially, one of the perilymphatic spaces.

scald. The burn caused by hot liquids or vapors.

scald'ing. Burning pain in urination.

scale. 1. An instrument bearing marks or graduations at regular intervals and used as a standard in measuring, as barometric scale, thermometric scale. 2. The dry, semiopaque lamina of horny epidermis that is shed from the skin, usually as a result of imperfect cornification, a secondary skin lesion. Also called *squama*. **Haldane s.** A standard for establishing hemoglobin levels in which 13.8 Gm. in 100 cc. of blood equals 100 per cent.

sca·lene (skay·leen', skay'leen). Having unequal sides, as scalene muscle.

sca"le·nec'to·my. Excision of the scalene muscles, particularly the scalenus anterior, still commonly called the scalenus anticus by surgeons.

sca"le·not'o·my. Severing of some of the fibers of a scalene muscle.

sca·le'nus. One of three muscles in the neck, arising from the transverse processes of the cervical vertebrae, and inserted on the first two ribs. See Table of Muscles in the Appendix.

sca'ler. 1. An instrument for removing calcareous deposits from the teeth. 2. An electronic instrument for counting and recording electrical impulses produced by radioactive substances when detected by such devices as the Geiger-Müller tube.

sca'ling. 1. Desquamating; producing scales. 2. A pharmaceutical process consisting of drying concentrated solutions of drugs on glass plates.

sca'ling cir'cuit. One which permits mechanical recording of rapid counting rates with a Geiger counter by recording only every second, fourth, eighth, or 2^n impulse.

scalp. The hairy integument covering the cranium.

scal'pel. A surgical knife with a short blade, a convex or straight cutting edge, rounded or pointed at the end.

sca'ly. 1. Resembling scales; characterized by scales. 2. Covered with, or possessing scales.

scan'di·um. Sc = 45.10. A rare metal belonging to the aluminum group.

sca'pha [BNA]. The furrow of the auricle between the helix and antihelix.

scaph"o·ceph'a·ly (skaf"o·sef'uh-lee, skay"fo-). A condition of the skull, characterized by a projecting, keel-like sagittal suture, due to its premature ossification. —**scaphocephal'ic, scaphocephalous,** *adj*.

scaph'oid. Boat-shaped.

scaph'oid. 1. [NA] The boat-shaped bone of the carpus. 2. [BNA] The navicular of the carpus.

scaph"oid·i'tis. Osteochondritis of the navicular.

scap'u·la. The shoulder blade, the large, flat, triangular bone forming the back of the shoulder. See Table of Bones in the Appendix. —**scapular,** *adj*.

scap"u·lal'gi·a. Pain in the region of the scapula.

scap"u·leo'to·my. Surgical removal of a scapula.

scap'u·lo-. A combining form denoting *relation to the shoulder* or *scapula*.

scap"u·lo·pex"y (skap'yoo·lo·peck"-see, skap"yoo·lo·peck'see). Fixation of the scapula to the ribs, as in cases of paralysis of scapular muscles.

scar. A permanent mark resulting from a wound or disease process in tissue, especially the skin.

scar"a·bi'a·sis (skar"uh·buy'uh-sis). A condition occurring usually in children in which the intestine is invaded by the dung beetle. Characterized by anorexia, emaciation, and gastro-intestinal disturbances. Also called *beetle disease*.

scarf"skin". The epidermis or cuticle.

scar"i·fi·ca'tion. The operation of making numerous small, superficial incisions in skin or other tissue. **—scar'i·fy,** *v.*

scar'i·fi·ca"tor. An instrument used in scarification, consisting of a number of small lancets operated by a spring.

scar"la·ti'na (skahr"luh-tee'nuh). Scarlet fever, *q.v.* **—scarlatinal** (skahr"luh-tee'nul, skahr-lat'i-nul), **scarlatinous** (skahr"luh-tee'nus, skahr-lat'i-nus), *adj.*

scar"la·ti'noid (skahr"luh-tee'-noyd, skahr-lat'i-noyd). A disease simulating scarlet fever.

scar'let fe'ver. An acute, contagious, febrile disease, having a period of incubation varying from several hours to a week, setting in with vomiting or chill, which is followed by high fever, rapid pulse, sore throat, cervical adenitis, and the appearance of a punctiform, scarlet-red eruption from one to five days thereafter. The tongue, at first heavily coated and red at the tip and edges, soon shows prominence of the papillae, which are red and swollen (strawberry tongue). The eruption, at the appearance of which all the symptoms become intensified, gradually fades after five or six days, and is followed by a scaly desquamation. A peculiarity of scarlet fever is its tendency to involve the kidneys. The causal agent is a hemolytic streptococcus. See Dick *test*. Also called *scarlatina*. **latent s. f.** Scarlet fever without eruptions. **malignant s. f.** A form characterized by an abrupt onset, high fever, convulsions, coma, and death, often before the appearance of the eruption. **pustular s. f.** Scarlet fever with a pustular eruption.

scar'let red. $C_{24}H_{20}N_4O$. An azo dye, *o*-tolyl azo-*o*-tolyl azo-*β*-naphthol; occurs as a dark, brownish red powder; almost insoluble in water. It is used to promote the growth of epithelium in the treatment of burns, wounds, chronic ulcers, etc. Also called *s. r., medicinal; Biebrich s. r.* **s. r. sulfonate.** The sodium salt of azobenzenedisulfonic acid azobetanaphthol; the sulfonic acid derivative of scarlet red. It differs from scarlet red in that the two CH_3 groups are replaced by the SO_3Na group; occurs as a dark, brownish red powder, soluble in water. Also called *soluble s. r.*

scat'ol, sca'tol. See *skatole*.

scat"o·log'i·a, sca·tol'o·gy. The study of excreta. **—scatolog'ic,** *adj.*

sca·to'ma. A mass of fecal matter in the colon resembling, on palpation, an abdominal tumor.

sca·toph'a·gy. The eating of excrement.

sca·tos'co·py. Inspection of the excreta.

scat'ter. 1. The spreading of rays, as x-rays. 2. *In psychology*, the range of levels through which an individual passes on an intelligence test.

scav'en·ger. A macrophage. Also called *scavenger cell*.

Sc. D. Doctor of Science.

Sc. D. A. Right scapuloanterior position of the fetus.

Sc. D. P. Right scapuloposterior position of the fetus.

scent. An effluvium from any body capable of affecting the olfactory sense; odor; fragrance.

sche'ma (skee'muh). 1. A simple design to illustrate a complex mechanism. 2. An outline of a subject. **—schemat'ic,** *adj.*

sche'mo·graph (skee'mo·graf). An apparatus for tracing the outline of the field of vision; the measurement of the field is made with the perimeter.

sche·ro'ma (ski·ro'muh). Xerophthalmia, *q.v.*

Schick, Bela [*Austrian pediatrician, 1877–*]. Widely known for his development of a reliable skin test for the determination of susceptibility to diphtheria (1913). See Schick *test*.

schin"dy·le'sis (skin"di·lee'sis). A form of articulation in which a plate of one bone is received into a fissure of another.

–schisis. A combining form meaning *cleft, split, fissure*.

schis'to- (skis'to-). A combining form meaning *split, fissured*.

schis"to·ce'li·a. Celosoma.

schis"to·cys'tis. Fissure of the bladder. Also called *vesical ectopia, exstrophy of the bladder*.

schis"to·glos'si·a. Cleft tongue.

schis·tom'e·lus. An individual with a cleft extremity.

schis·tom'e·ter. A device for measuring the distance between the vocal folds.

schis"to·pro·so'pi·a, schis"to·pros'o·py. Congenital fissure of the face. **—schistopros'opous,** *adj.*

schis"to·pros'o·pus (skis"to·pros'-o·pus, ·pro·so'pus). An individual having a fissure of the face.

schis·tor'rha·chis, schis·tor'ra·chis (skis·tor'uh·kis). Spina bifida; rachischisis.

schis·to'sis. Fibrosis of the lungs occurring in slate cutters. Also see *silicosis*.

Schis"to·so'ma. The genus of blood flukes infesting man. **S. haema·tobium.** The adults are found in the

essels of the urinary bladder; common
n Africa. **S. japonicum.** The adults
re found in the mesenteric veins;
videly distributed in Japan and China.
S. mansoni. The adults are found
n the mesenteric veins and portal
ein; found in parts of Africa, South
America, and the West Indies.

his″to·so·mi′a·sis. 1. Infestation
vith *Schistosoma.* Syn., *bilharziasis.* 2.
papular and pustular dermatitis occurng on the skin of persons wading or
wimming in fresh-water lakes of the
orthern United States and Canada. A
elf-limited disease caused by the pene-
ration of one of the cercarial larvae
hich are parasites of snails. Also
alled *swimmer's itch, swamp itch.*

his″to·so′mus. A monster in
hich there is a lateral or median
ventration extending the whole length
f the abdomen, one or both lower ex-
emities being absent or rudimentary.

his″to·ster′ni·a. Sternal fissure.

his″to·tho′rax. Fissure of the
horax.

his″to·tra·che·lus (skis″to-
ay′ki·lus, ·tra·kee′lus). Cervical fis-
ure. Also called *tracheloschisis.*

hiz′o- (skiz′o-), **schiz-.** A combin-
g form denoting *split* or *cleft.*

hiz″o·ble·pha′ri·a. Fissure of
he eyelid.

hiz″o·gen′e·sis. Reproduction by
ssion.

hiz″o·gnath′ism (skiz″o-nath′iz-
m). Cleavage of the jaw.

hi·zog′o·ny (ski·zog′o·nee, sky·).
Schizogenesis. 2. Multiple division in
hich the contents of an oöcyst even-
ally split into swarm spores.
schizogon′ic, *adj.*

hiz″o·gy′ri·a (skiz″o·jye′ree·uh,
irr′ee·uh). Cerebral deformity marked
y partial separation of the gyri.

hiz′oid. 1. Resembling schizo-
hrenia. 2. *In psychiatry,* an individual
ith inadequate affect or feeling and
ith a poorly socialized personality.

hiz″o·ma′ni·a. A mental disorder
resenting features of both schizo-
hrenia and mania.

hiz″o·my·ce′tes (skiz″o·migh-
e′teez). A class of fungi; the fission
ungi or bacteria.

hiz″o·my·co′sis (skiz″o·migh·ko′-
s). A disease due to schizomycetes; a
sease caused by bacteria.

hiz′ont. A stage in the asexual life
cle of *Plasmodium,* covering the
eriod from beginning of division of
uclear material until the mature
erozoites are formed.

hiz″o·nych′i·a (skiz″o·nick′ee-
). Disease of the nails characterized
y irregular splitting.

hiz″o·pha′si·a (skiz″o·fay′zhuh,
ee·uh). Word-salad; scrambled speech
hich may occur in schizophrenia.

schiz″o·phre′ni·a. Bleuler's term
for dementia precox, *q.v.* A psychosis
characterized by lack of affect, inappropriate mood, unpredictable behavior,
and disintegration. Frequently terminates in mental regression, total withdrawal from reality into phantasies,
and paranoid formulations. —**schizo-
phren′ic,** *adj.*

schiz″o·thy′mic. Having a schizoid
personality or temperament. See *schizoid.* —**schizothymia,** *n.*

schiz″o·trich′i·a (skiz″o-trick′ee-
uh). Splitting of the hair.

schiz″o·tryp″a·no·so·mi′a·sis
(skiz″o·trip″uh·no·so·my′uh·sis, skiz″-
o·try″puh·no·). Infection with *Trypanosoma cruzi.*

sci·age′ (see·ahzh′, see′ahzh). A saw-
ing movement in massage, practiced
with the ulnar border, or with the
dorsum of the hand.

sci·ap′o·dy (sigh·ap′o·dee). Gigantism
of the foot. Also called *macropodia, pes
gigas.*

sci·as′co·py. See *retinoscopy.*

sci·at′ic (sigh·at′ick). 1. Pertaining to
the ischium, as the sciatic notch. 2.
Pertaining to the sciatic nerve, as sciatic neuralgia. See Table of Nerves in
the Appendix.

sci·at′i·ca (sigh·at′i·kuh). A disease
characterized by neuralgic pain along
the course of the sciatic nerve. It is dependent upon inflammation or injury
to the nerve. In addition to pain, there
are numbness, tingling, and tenderness
along the course of the nerve, and
eventually wasting of the muscles innervated by it.

sci′ence. Systematized and classified
knowledge.

sci″en·tif′ic. Relating to science.
That which is based upon science.

sci′en·tist. One versed in science.

scil′la. See *squill.*

scillaren. Trade-mark for a mixture
of the natural glycosides, **scillaren-A** and **scillaren-B,** occurring in fresh squill, *Urginea maritima,*
in the proportions in which they exist
in the fresh crude drug.

scil′le·nin. See under *squill.*

scil″li·di″u·ret′in. See under *squill.*

scil″li·mar′in. See under *squill.*

scil′lin. See under *squill.*

scil″li·pic′rin (sil″i·pick′rin, ·pye′-
krin). See under *squill.*

scil′lism. Poisoning from preparations of squill; characterized by vomiting, retarded pulse, cardiac arrhythmia,
and ventricular fibrillation.

scil″li·tin. See under *squill.*

scil″li·tox′in. See under *squill.*

scil″lo·ceph′a·ly. Congenital deformity of the head, in which it is small
and conically pointed.

scin′ti·gram. A printed or penned
record made by a scintiscanner.

scin·til·la·scope. An instrument for observing minute flashes of light upon a fluorescent screen struck by alpha particles, emitted from a small source of radioactive material.

scin″til·la'tion. 1. An emission of sparks. 2. A subjective visual sensation, as of sparks. 3. A flash of light produced in certain substances by radioactive radiation.

scin'ti·scan″ner. An instrument used to trace radioactive material as it is distributed in the body for therapeutic or for diagnostic reasons, and simultaneously to record its findings on a scintigram.

scir'rhous (skirr'us, sirr'us). Hard.

scir'rhus (skirr'us, sirr'us). A hard carcinoma.

scis'sors. An instrument consisting of two blades held together on a pivot, and crossing each other so that in closing they cut the object placed between them. The blades may be straight, angular, or curved, blunt, sharp, or probe-pointed. **canalicular s.** Delicate scissors, one blade of which is probe-pointed; used in slitting the lacrimal duct. **craniotomy s.** A strong S-shaped instrument used in craniotomy for perforating the skull and cutting away portions of bone. **iris s.** One having flat blades bent in such a manner that they may be applied to the eyeball. **Smellie's s.** Craniotomy scissors.

scis·su'ra. A fissure; a splitting.

scle'ra. The sclerotic coat of the eye; the firm, fibrous, outer layer of the eyeball, continous with the sheath of the optic nerve behind and with the cornea in front. **—scleral,** adj.

scler″ec·ta'si·a (sklerr″eck·tay'-zhuh, skleer″eck·). Localized bulging of the sclera.

scle·rec″to·ir″i·dec'to·my. Excision of a portion of the sclera and of the iris, for glaucoma.

scle·rec'to·my. Excision of a portion of the sclera.

scler″e·de'ma a″dul·to'rum (sklerr″i·dee'muh, skleer″i·dee'muh). An affection characterized by indurated edema, often beginning on the head and later involving larger areas of the body surface. Terminates after weeks or months, leaving no sequela. Often follows some acute general infection. Also called *Buschke's scleredema.*

scle·re'ma. Sclerosis, or hardening, especially of the skin. **s. edematosum.** A generally fatal form of edema of the skin with induration, impairment of muscular action, and subnormal temperature. **s. neonatorum.** A disease of the newborn characterized by a hardening of the subcutaneous tissue, especially of the legs and feet. Dryness

of the skin is marked, so that little flu exudes on incision.

scle″ren·ce·pha'li·a, scle″re ceph'a·ly. Sclerosis of brain tiss

scle·ri'tis. Inflammation of the sc rotic coat of the eye. It may exist alo (simple scleritis or episcleritis), or volve the cornea, iris, or choroid.

scle″ro- (skleer'o-, sklerr'o-). 1. combining form meaning *hard.* 2. combining form denoting *connect with the sclera.*

scle″ro·a·troph'ic. Pertaining fibrosis associated with atrophy.

scle″ro·cat″a·rac'ta. A hard ca ract.

scle″ro·cho″roid·i'tis (skleer″ kor″oy·dye'tis, sklerr″o·). Inflamm tion of the choroid and sclerotic co of the eye.

scle″ro·con·junc″ti·vi'tis. S multaneous conjunctivitis and sclerit

scle″ro·dac·tyl'i·a, scle″r dac'ty·ly. Scleroderma of the finge It is often symmetrical, occurs chie in women, and leads to marked defor ity.

scle″ro·der'ma. A disease chara terized by induration of the skin localized patches or diffuse areas, a associated with atrophy of the e dermis and pigmentation. Vasomo disturbances, myosclerosis, and cal nosis may occur. It may be diffuse localized. Also called *scleriasis, derm tosclerosis, chorionitis.* Also see *ac sclerosis.*

scle″ro·der″ma·ti'tis. Inflamm tory thickening and hardening of t skin.

scle'roid. Hard or bony in texture.

scle″ro·i·ri'tis (skleer″o·eye·rye' sklerr″o·). Inflammation of the scle and the iris.

scle″ro·ker″a·ti'tis. Inflammat of the sclera and cornea.

scle″ro·ker″a·to·i·ri'tis (·kerr uh·to·eye·rye'tis). Combined inflamm tion of the sclera, cornea, and iris.

scle·ro'ma. Abnormal hardness or duration of a part.

scle″ro·ma·la'ci·a (skleer″o·m lay'shee·uh, sklerr″o·). Softening the sclera.

scle″ro·nych'i·a (skleer″o·nick' uh, sklerr″o·). Induration and thicke ing of the nails.

scle″ro·nyx'is. Operative puncture the sclera.

scle″ro·o″ö·pho·ri'tis (·o″o· rye'tis, ·o″off·o·rye'tis). Sclerosis the ovary.

scle'ro·plas″ty. Plastic surgery the sclera.

scle·ro'sis. Hardening, especially o part by overgrowth of fibrous tiss applied particularly to hardening of t nervous system from atrophy or generation of the nerve elements and hyperplasia of the interstitial tissue; also to a thickening of the coats of arteries, produced by proliferation of fibrous connective tissue and deposit of lipids and calcium salts. **amyo-trophic lateral s.** A degenerative disease of the pyramidal tracts and lower motor neurons, characterized by motor weakness and a spastic condition of the limbs associated with muscular atrophy, fibrillary twitching, and final involvement of nuclei in the medulla. **arteriolar s.** That involving arterioles, producing irregularly distributed hardening of the affected arterioles with uneven reduction of the caliber of the lumens. See generalized arteriolar *s.* **combined s.** Simultaneous sclerosis of the posterior and lateral columns of the spinal cord. **diffuse s.** One extending through a large part of the brain and spinal cord. **generalized arteriolar s.** That affecting the arterioles of the kidney, liver, brain, meninges, gastrointestinal tract, skeletal muscle, adrenal, pancreas, and other organs; more frequent and severe in hypertensive subjects. Also called *diffuse arteriolar s., diffuse hyperplastic s.* **hereditary cerebellar s.** A progressive disease marked by a reeling, ataxic gait, nystagmus, and a pendulous knee jerk, due to lesions in the cerebellum. Also called *Marie's ataxia.* **hereditary spinal s.** A progressive familial disease beginning in childhood; characterized by ataxia, paralysis, and contractures; due to lesions in the spinal cord. Also called *Friedreich's ataxia.* **multiple cerebral s.** Multiple sclerosis affecting only the brain. **multiple cerebrospinal s.** Multiple sclerosis affecting both the brain and the spinal cord. **multiple s.** Chronic induration occurring in patches in different parts of the nervous system. The principal symptoms are scanning speech, nystagmus, muscular weakness, and tremor of arms and legs upon essaying voluntary action. **postero-lateral s.** Degeneration of the spinal cord affecting principally the posterior columns and pyramidal tracts and characterized by a combination of motor and sensory disturbances such as ataxia, paresthesia, spasticity, etc., with signs of pernicious anemia. **primary lateral s.** A sclerotic disease of the crossed pyramidal tracts of the cord, characterized by paralysis of the limbs, with rigidity, increased tendon reflexes, and absence of sensory and nutritive disorders. A peculiar characteristic jerking gait is produced, and clonus of the lower limbs may be readily excited. It is usually a spinal form of multiple sclerosis. **progres-**

sive muscular s. See pseudohypertrophic muscular *paralysis.*

scle″ro·ste·no′sis. Hardening with contracture of a part or closure of an orifice.

scle·ros′to·my. Making an artificial opening in the sclera for the relief of glaucoma.

scle·ro·thrix. Abnormal brittleness of the hair.

scle·rot′ic. 1. Hard; indurated. 2. Pertaining to the outer coat of the eye, as the sclerotic coat, or sclera. 3. Related to or derived from ergot.

scle·rot″i·cec′to·my. The removal of a part of the sclera.

scle·ro·tome. 1. A knife used in sclerotomy. 2. The fibrous tissue separating successive myotomes in certain of the lower vertebrates. 3. That part of a mesodermal somite which enters into the formation of the vertebrae. **—scle-rotom′ic,** *adj.*

scle·rot′o·my. The operation of incising the sclera.

scle″ro·to·nyx′is. An operation for cataract formerly practiced, in which a broad needle was introduced into the sclera, behind the ciliary region, passed between the iris and the lens, and the latter depressed into the vitreous body.

scle″ro·trich′i·a (skleer″o·trick′ee-uh, sklerr″o·). A harsh and dry state of the hair.

scle′rous. Hard; indurated.

sco′bi·nate. Having a rough surface.

scol′e·coid, sco′le·coid. Vermiform.

sco′lex (pl. *scolices*). The head of a tapeworm by means of which it attaches to the intestinal wall.

sco″li·o·lor·do′sis. Combined scoliosis and lordosis.

sco″li·o′sis. Lateral curvature of the spine, named according to location and direction of the convexity, as right thoracic. Usually there are two curves, the original and a compensatory curve, as an original right thoracic with a compensating left lumbar curve. **—scoli-ot′ic,** *adj.*

sco″li·o·som′e·ter. An instrument for measuring the amount of deformity in scoliosis.

sco′li·o·tone″. An apparatus for elongating the spine and lessening the rotation in lateral curvature.

scom′brine (skom′breen, ·brin). A protamine obtained from mature spermatozoa of mackerel.

scom′brone. A histone obtained from spermatozoa of mackerel.

scoop. An instrument resembling a spoon, for the extraction of bodies from cavities, as an ear scoop, lithotomy scoop.

sco·pa′ri·us. The dried tops of *Cytisus scoparius*, a shrub of the family

Leguminosae; they contain the alkaloid sparteine, and a glycoside, scoparin. Also called *broom-tops*.

-scope. A combining form denoting *an instrument for seeing* or *examining*.

sco·po·la, sco·po·la. The dried rhizome of *Scopolia carniolica*. It contains alkaloids, of which about 80% is hyoscamine and the rest scopolamine and nor-hyoscyamine.

sco·pol'a·mine (sko·pol'uh·meen, sko·po'luh·). $C_{17}H_{21}NO_4$. An alkaloid obtained from various plants of the Solanaceae. **s. hydrobromide.** $C_{17}H_{21}NO_4.HBr.3H_2O$. The hydrobromide of levorotatory scopolamine obtained from plants of the Solanaceae; occurs as colorless or white crystals or powder; soluble in water. Scopolamine paralyzes the peripheral endings of the parasympathetic nerves. It also appears to act frequently as a cerebral depressant and tends to promote sleep. It has slight analgesic properties, but greatly enhances the effect of other narcotics. Also called *hyoscine hydrobromide*.

sco·pom'e·try. A branch of nephelometry; matching colors or turbidities by comparing an illuminated line against a field of constant intensity.

sco''po·pho'bi·a. Morbid dread of being seen.

-scopy. A combining form denoting *inspection* or *examination*.

scor''a·cra'ti·a (skor''uh·kray'shee-uh). Involuntary evacuation of feces.

scor·bu''ti·gen'ic. Causing scurvy.

scor''di·ne'ma. Yawning.

scot''o·din'i·a (skot''o·din'ee·uh, sko''to·). Vertigo associated with the appearance of black spots before the eyes.

scot'o·gram (skot'o·gram, sko'to·). An image made on a photographic plate by a radioactive substance without the intervention of an opaque object.

sco·to'ma. A dark spot in the visual field. **—scotom'atous,** *adj.* **absolute s.** Scotoma with perception of light entirely absent. **annular s.** A partial or complete area of blindness in the form of a ring. Also called *ring s.* **central s.** One limited to the region of the visual field corresponding to the macula lutea. **color s.** Color blindness limited to a part of the visual field; may exist without interruption of the field for white light. **negative s.** A defect not noticeable to the patient but found on examination of the visual field. **positive s.** A scotoma perceptible to the patient as a dark spot before his eyes. **relative s.** A scotoma within which perception of light is only partially impaired. **scintillating s.** A scotoma with serrated margins extending peripherally and producing a large defect in the visual field.

sco·to'ma·graph. An instrument for recording the size and shape of a scotoma.

sco·tom'e·ter. An instrument for detecting, locating, and measuring scotomas.

sco''to·pho'bi·a (skot''o·fo'bee·uh, sko''to·). A morbid fear of darkness.

sco·to'pi·a. The ability to see in the dark; dark adaptation. **—scotop'ic** *adj.*

scra'per. An instrument used to produce an abrasion.

screen. That which cuts off, shelters or protects. **fluorescent s.** A screen covered with substances which become fluorescent on exposure to rays which are normally invisible to the eye. **intensifying s.** A sheet of cardboard coated with a fluorescent material, such as calcium tungstate, placed in contact with an x-ray film. When roentgen rays pass through film and screen, the fluorescent light from the screen supplements the effect of the roentgen rays on the film, thus reducing the necessary exposure time.

scrive'ner's pal'sy (skriv'nur, pawl'zee). See writer's *cramp*.

scrof'u·la. Tuberculosis of cervical lymph nodes. **—scrofulous,** *adj.*

scrof''u·lo·der'ma. Lesions of the skin produced by the local action of the tubercle bacillus by direct extension from some structure beneath the skin usually on the neck from draining lymph nodes, resulting in ulceration, draining sinuses, and scar formation.

scro·tec'to·my. Resection of the scrotum or a part of it.

scro''to·plas''ty. Plastic surgery on the scrotum.

scro'tum. The pouch containing the testes, consisting of skin, dartos, external spermatic fascia, cremasteric fascia, internal spermatic fascia, and parietal tunica vaginalis. **—scrotal** *adj.*

scru'ple. A unit of apothecaries' weight represented by the symbol ℈ and equal to 20 grains.

scru''pu·los'i·ty. An overprecision or morbid conscientiousness as to one's thoughts, words, and deeds. A prominent personality trait in those persons predisposed to psychasthenia or compulsive neurosis, and to schizophrenia.

scurf. A branlike desquamation of the epidermis, especially from the scalp; dandruff.

scur'vy. A nutritional disorder caused by deficiency of vitamin C; characterized by extreme weakness, spongy gums, and a tendency to develop hemorrhage under the skin, from the mucous membranes, and under the periosteum. **in**

fantile s. An acute form, characterized by subperiosteal hemorrhage, especially of the long bones, with painful swellings.

scu″tel·la′ri·a. The dried underground portion of *Scutellaria lateriflora.* It contains a yellow, crystalline substance, scutellarin. Also called *skullcap.*

cu·tel′la·rin, scu″tel·la′rin. See under *scutellaria.*

cu′tu·late. Shaped like a lozenge.

cyb′a·lum (sib′uh·lum) (pl. *scybala*). A mass of abnormally hard fecal matter. **—scybalous,** *adj.*

cy′phi·form (sigh′fi·form). Cupshaped.

sD. Abbreviation for streptodornase.

Se. Chemical symbol for selenium.

ea′sick″ness. A condition produced in some persons by the rolling of a ship; characterized by vertigo, nausea, retching, and prostration. A similar state may be induced by riding in cars, elevators, airplanes.

eat′worm. The pinworm, *Enterobius vermicularis.*

e′ba. Plural of sebum, *q.v.*

e·ba′ceous. Pertaining to sebum; secreting sebum.

e·bac′ic ac′id (si·bas′ick, si·bay′sick). COOH(CH₂)₈COOH. A dibasic acid obtained from olein.

e·bip′a·rous. Secreting sebum.

eb′o·lith. A concretion in a sebaceous gland.

eb″or·rhe′a, seb″or·rhoe′a. A functional disease of the sebaceous glands, characterized by an excessive secretion or disturbed quality of sebum, which collects upon the skin in the form of an oily coating or of crusts or scales. **—seborrheic, seborrheal,** *adj.* **s. ichthyosis.** A variety characterized by the formation of large, platelike crusts. **s. oleosa.** A form characterized by an excessive oiliness of the skin, especially about the forehead and nose.

e′bum (pl. *seba*). The secretion of the sebaceous glands. It is composed of fat, keratohyalin granules, keratin, and cellular débris.

e·cern′ing. Secreting; applied to the function of a gland. **—secernment,** *n.*

e·clu′sion of pu′pil. Annular or posterior synechia, *q.v.* under *synechia.*

e″co·bar′bi·tal so′di·um. Nonproprietary title for the barbiturate introduced as seconal sodium, *q.v.*

econal sodium. Trade-mark for monosodium 5-allyl-5-(1-methylbutyl) barbiturate or secobarbital sodium, a short-acting hypnotic and sedative.

ec′ond·ar″y. 1. Second in the order of time or development, as the secondary lesions of syphilis. 2. Second in relation; subordinate; produced by a cause considered primary.

se·cre′ta. The substances secreted by a gland, follicle, or other organ; products of secretion.

se·cre′ta·gogue (si·kree′tuh·gog), **se·cre′to·gogue.** A substance promoting or causing secretion, as certain hormones.

se·crete′. Separate; specifically, to separate from blood, or form out of materials furnished by the blood, a certain substance termed secretion. **—secreting,** *adj.*

se′cre·tin. A hormone produced in the epithelial cells of the duodenum by the contact of acid. It is absorbed from the cells by the blood and excites the pancreas to activity.

se·cre′tin·ase. An enzyme present in blood serum which inactivates the hormone secretin.

se·cre′tion. 1. The act of secreting or forming, from materials furnished by the blood, a certain substance which is either eliminated from the body (excretion) or used in carrying on special functions. 2. The substance secreted. **external s.** A secretion thrown out upon any epithelial surface of the body. **gastric s.** The secretion of the glands of the stomach. **internal s.** A secretion that is not thrown out upon a surface, but is absorbed into the blood. **paralytic s.** That occurring in a gland or organ after denervation, as in the stomach after vagotomy.

se·cre′to·gogue (si·kree′to·gog). See *secretagogue.*

se·cre′to·ry, se′cre·to″ry. Pertaining to secretion; performing secretion.

sec·ta′ri·an. Old term for one who, in the practice of medicine, follows a dogma, tenet, or principle based on the authority of its promulgator to the exclusion of demonstration and experience.

sec′tile (seck′tyle, ·til). Capable of being cut.

sec′tion. 1. A cutting or dividing. 2. A cut or slice. 3. Cut through or divide. **abdominal s.** Incision into the abdominal cavity. **frozen s.** In the teaching of anatomy, one of a series of divisions of the body or a part which has been frozen before being sectioned. Also see *frozen sections.* **sagittal s.** One made in the sagittal suture and hence in the median plane of the body, dividing it into equal halves.

sec·to′ri·al. Having cutting edges, as the molar teeth of carnivorous animals.

se·cun″di·grav′i·da. A woman pregnant the second time.

sec′un·dines (seck′un·dynz, ·deenz, si·kun′dynz). The placenta and membranes discharged from the uterus after birth. Also called *afterbirth.*

sec″un·dip′a·ra (seck″un·dip′uh-ruh, see″kun·). A woman who has borne two children not twins. —**secundiparous**, *adj.;* **secundiparity**, *n.*

se·cun′dum ar′tem. In the approved professional manner. *Obs.*

se·da′tion. 1. A state of lessened functional activity. 2. Production of a state of lessened functional activity.

sed′a·tive. 1. Quieting function or activity. 2. An agent which quiets activity.

sed′en·tar′y. Occupied in sitting. Pertaining to the habit of sitting.

sed′i·ment. The material settling to the bottom of a liquid. —**sedimen′tary**, *adj.*

sed″i·men·ta′tion. The process of producing the deposition of a sediment, especially the rapid deposition by means of a centrifugal machine. See sedimentation *rate.*

sed″i·men·tom′e·ter. An apparatus for recording the sedimentation rate of blood.

sedormid. Trade-mark for allylisopropyl-acetyl-carbamide; $(CH_3)_2$-$CH.(CH_3:CH.CH_2).CO.NH.CO.NH_2$, a sedative and hypnotic.

seed. A fertilized and ripened ovule produced by flowering plants, along with reserve nutritive material and protective covering. It is primarily a sporophyte in a resting stage. **radon s.** A small capillary tube, of glass, containing radon, suitable for implantation in tissues; the tube may be placed inside a small gold tube.

seg′ment. 1. A small piece cut along the radii of anything regarded as circular; a part bounded by a natural or imaginary line. 2. A natural division, resulting from segmentation; one of a series of homologous parts, as a myotome; the part of a limb between two consecutive joints. A subdivision, ring, lobe, somite, or metamere of any cleft or articulated body. **body s.** A somite or a division of the body derived from an embryonic somite. Syn., *metamere.* **bronchopulmonary s.** The portion of lung supplied by any bronchus.

seg·men′tal. 1. Pertaining to a segment; made up of segments. 2. Undergoing or resulting from segmentation.

seg″men·ta′tion. 1. The process of cleavage or cell division, especially as applied to the fertilized ovum and blastomeres. 2. The division of an organism into somites or metameres.

seg″re·ga′tion. The reappearance of contrasted Mendelian characters in the offspring of heterozygotes, or the separation of the paired maternal and paternal genes at miosis in the formation of gametes.

seg′re·ga″tor. An instrument by means of which urine from each kidney

may be secured without danger of ad mixture.

Seid′litz pow′ders (sed′lits, side′lits). Compound effervescent powder.

sei″es·the′si·a (sigh″ess·thee′zhuh ·zee·uh). Perception of concussion.

seis′mo·ther′a·py (size″mo·therr′ uh·pee, sice″mo·). The therapeutic us of mechanical vibration.

seitz filter. A bacterial filter utilizin a matted asbestos filtering pad or dish the unit being used with either vacuu or pressure.

sei′zure. 1. The sudden onset of a dis ease or an attack. 2. *In surgery,* th grasping of a part to be operated upor **larval seizures.** *In electroenceph alography,* subliminal seizures whic produce no clinical symptoms but whic are recognized by abnormal brain wav discharges.

se·junc′tion. *In psychology,* the in terruption of the continuity of asso ciation complexes, tending to break u personality.

se″la·pho′bi·a. Morbid fear of flashing light.

se·lec′tion. *In biology,* choosing fo survival or elimination. **artificial s** Process in which man, for his own pur poses, picks out some individuals in group of organisms for survival, othe for elimination. **natural s.** Darwin theory of evolution, according to whic organisms tend to produce progeny fa above the means of subsistence; struggle for existence ensues which re sults in the survival of those wit favorable variations. Since the favor able variations accumulate as the ge erations pass, the descendants tend diverge markedly from their ancestor and to remain adapted to the cond tions under which they live. **sexual** The view that the differences betwe males and females, other than the pre ence of ovaries or testes, have orig nated as the result of preferential ma ing, regarded usually as a preferen of the females for the males showi the differentiated traits.

se·lec′tor. A device for selecting separating.

se·le′ne (si·lee′nee). The white sp sometimes occurring on the fingernal Also see *lunula,* 1.

se·le′ni·ate (si·lee′nee·ate, si·len′e ate). A salt of selenic acid.

se·le′nic (si·lee′nick, si·len′ick). compound of hexavalent (sometim tetravalent) selenium.

se·le′nic ac′id. H_2SeO_4. A crystalli acid, soluble in water, forming a corr sive liquid.

sel″e·nif′er·ous. Containing se′ nium.

se·le′ni·ous ac′id. H_2SeO_3. The ac formed by tetravalent selenium.

sel'e·nite, se'le·nite. 1. A salt of selenious acid. 2. A translucent form of calcium sulfate.

se·le'ni·um. Se = 78.96. A poisonous element resembling sulfur. Plants grown in seleniferous soil may prove fatal to cattle feeding upon them.

se·le'ni·um sul'fide. A mixture of selenium monosulfide, selenium, and sulfur, used in treatment of seborrhea. See *selsun sulfide.*

self'-hyp·no'sis. Hypnosis by auto-suggestion; autohypnosis.

self'-lim'it·ed. Denoting a disease which runs a definite course in a specific time.

self'-sus·pen'sion. Suspension of the body by the head for the purpose of stretching or making extension on the vertebral column.

sel'la (pl. *sellae*). A saddle. **—sellar,** *adj.* **s. turcica.** The superior portion of the body of the sphenoid bone that surrounds the hypophyseal fossa.

sel·sun sul'fide. A trade-mark for selenium sulfide.

se·man'tics. The branch of linguistic science that treats of problems of meaning, both current and historical. **general s.** A study or theory of living which stresses a scientific approach to problems and life; emphasizes the way in which language is used as an important factor in adjustment; used in treating certain psychologic mal-adjustments.

se'men. 1. A seed. 2. The fluid pro-duced by the male reproductive organs, carrying the male germ cells or sper-matozoa. **—sem'inal,** *adj.*

sem'i-. A prefix denoting *half.*

sem''i·ca·nal'. A canal open on one side; a sulcus or groove.

sem''i·car''ti·lag'i·nous (·kahr''-ti·ladj'i·nus) Gristly; partly cartilag-inous.

sem''i·co'ma. A condition of mild or partial coma.

sem''i·com'a·tose (·kom'uh·toce, ·ko'muh·). Partially comatose.

sem''i·con'scious. Half conscious; partially conscious.

sem''i·lu'nar. 1. Resembling a half moon in shape. 2. One of the carpal bones. Old term for *lunate.* See Table of Bones in the Appendix.

sem''i·mem''bra·no'sus. One of the hamstring muscles, arising from the ischial tuberosity, and inserted on the tibia. See Table of Muscles in the Appendix.

sem''i·mem'bra·nous. Partly mem-branous, as semimembranous muscle.

sem'i·nal. Pertaining to the semen.

sem'i·nal ve·sic'u·lo·gram. A radiograph of the seminal vesicles, made by injecting a radiopaque sub-stance into them by way of the ejacu-latory ducts.

sem''i·na'tion. The intromission of semen into the uterus or vagina. Also called *insemination.*

sem''i·nif'er·ous (sem''i·nif'ur·us, see''mi·). Producing or carrying semen, as the seminiferous tubules of the testis.

sem''i·no'ma. A testicular tumor of low malignancy, made up of charac-teristic large, uniform cells with clear cytoplasm, which resemble spermato-gonia. Also called *seminal carcinoma.*

sem''i·nor'mal. Half-normal, as seminormal solution, a solution which contains one-half of an equivalent weight of the active reagent, in grams, in one liter of solution. It is written 0.5 N or N/2.

sem''i·nu'ri·a (sem''i·new'ree·uh, see''mi·). The discharge of semen in the urine.

sem''i·pro·na'tion. The assumption of a semiprone or partly prone position; an attitude of semisupination. **—semi-prone,** *adj.*

sem''i·pto'sis (sem''i·to'sis). Par-tial ptosis.

se'mis. Half; abbreviated to prescrip-tions to ss, which is placed after the sign indicating the measure. Sometimes abbreviated, s.

sem''i·som'nus. Coma. **—semi-somnous,** *adj.*

sem''i·so'por. Partial coma.

sem''i·spi·na'lis (sem''i·spy·nah'lis, ·nay'lis). One of the longitudinal mus-cles of the back, attached to the verte-brae. See Table of Muscles in the Ap-pendix.

se·mis'sis. Semis, *q.v.*

sem''i·ten''di·no'sus. One of the hamstring muscles, arising from the ischium and inserted on the tibia. See Table of Muscles in the Appendix.

Semmelweis, Ignaz Philipp [*Hungarian obstetrician,* 1818–65]. The first to recognize the septicemic char-acter of puerperal fever, and to at-tribute its spread to contamination by the hands of attending physicians.

sem''per·vi'rine. An alkaloid from gelsemium.

Se·ne'ci·o (si·nee'shee·o, ·see·o). Groundsel; a genus of composite-flow-ered plants, said to contain 960 species, many of which have been used me-dicinally.

se·ne'ci·o·nine (si·nee'shee·o·neen, si·nee'see·o·). An alkaloid, $C_{18}H_{25}NO_5$, from various species of South African *Senecio.*

se·nec'ti·tude. Old age.

sen'e·ga. The dried root of *Polygala senega.* The active principles of senega belong to the group of saponins. The names senegin and polygalic acid have been applied to them. Used as an ex-pectoral. Also called *seneca-snakeroot*.

sen'e·gin. See under *senega*.

se·nes'cence. A growing old; aging. —**senescent,** *adj.*

se'nile (see'nile, ·nil). Pertaining to, caused by, or characteristic of, old age or the infirmities of old age. —**senil'ity,** *n.*

se'nil·ism (see'nigh·liz·um, see'ni·). Senility, especially when premature.

se'ni·um. Old age. **s. precox.** Premature senility.

sen'na. The dried leaflets of *Cassia acutifolia*, or of *C. angustifolia*. Contains rhein, aloe-emodin, sennanigrin, sennoside A, and sennoside B; also sennacrol, sennapicrin, sennarhamnetin, kaempferol and its glycoside kempferin, and a small amount of volatile oil. Also called *senna leaves*.

se·no'pi·a. The change of vision in the aged, in which persons formerly myopic acquire what seems to be normal vision because of presbyopia.

sen·sa'tion. A feeling or impression produced by the stimulation of an afferent nerve. Also see *sensibility*. **cutaneous s.** A sensation produced through the medium of the skin. **kinesthetic sensations.** Sensations of motion. **psychovisual sensations.** Those of sight without the stimulation of the retina; visions.

sense. Any one of the faculties by which stimuli from the external world or from within the body are received and transformed into sensations. The faculties receiving impulses from the external world are the senses of sight, hearing, touch, smell, and taste, which are the special senses, and the muscular and dermal senses. Those receiving impulses from the internal organs, the visceral senses, are the hunger sense, thirst sense, and others. **body s.** Impressions from somatic structures which orient with regard to the body or its parts in space or which concern contacts or degrees of contact. **color s.** *In ophthalmology*, the faculty of distinguishing light of various wave lengths. **light s.** *In ophthalmology*, the faculty of perceiving gradations of intensity of light. **posture s.** The capability of recognizing (without seeing) the position in which a limb has been placed. **s. organs.** Structures capable of detecting the presence of some specific type of agent in the environment of the body and reacting to this agent by sending impulses by their afferent nerves to the central nervous system. **temperature s.** The sense by which differences in temperature are appreciated, consisting of a sense for cold, cryesthesia, and a heat sense, thermesthesia. These are represented on the surface by different

nerve-endings, the so-called cold an hot points.

sen·sib'a·mine (sen·sib'uh·meer sen"si·bam'een). A name given to a alkaloid of ergot, but later found to b an equimolecular mixture of ergotamin and ergotaminine.

sen"si·bil'i·ty. 1. The ability to re ceive and feel impressions. 2. The abil ity of a nerve or end organ to receiv and transmit impulses. **deep s.** Per ception of pressure, tension, and pai in the muscles, joints, tendons, an deep layers of the skin, as contraste with sensations derived from the super ficial layers of the skin. **epicritic s** The ability to discriminate and local ize fine degrees of stimuli, such a light touch, pain, and temperature.

sen'si·ble. Perceptible by the senses as sensible perspiration; capable of re ceiving an impression through th senses; endowed with sensation.

sen·sim'e·ter. An instrument for de termining the sensitiveness of the skin

sen'si·tive. 1. Capable of feeling capable of transmitting sensation. 2 Reacting to a stimulus. —**sensitiv' ity,** *n.*

sen"si·ti·za'tion. 1. Rendering cell sensitive by the action of an ambocep tor. 2. The process of rendering a individual sensitive to a given protein **Rh s.** The state of becoming sensitiv to the Rh factor, which may occur a a result of a transfusion of Rh positiv blood or as the result of pregnanc with an Rh positive fetus. Natura sensitivity to the Rh factor does no occur; and only 1 in 25 to 50 Rh nega tive persons exposed to the Rh antige by transfusion or pregnancy become sensitized.

sen'si·tized. Rendered sensitive t subthreshold stimuli or ordinarily in effective agents, as in allergy.

sen"so·ri·mo'tor. Both sensory an motor; concerned with the perceptio of sensory impulses and with moto impulses, as sensorimotor centers.

sen·so'ri·um. A center for sensa tions, especially the part of the brai which receives and combines impres sions conveyed to the individual sensory centers. Also called *perceptorium*.

sen'so·ry. Pertaining to, or conveying sensation.

sen'su·al·ism. The condition o character of one who is controlled b the more primitive instincts or emo tions.

sen'sus. Sense; feeling.

sen'tient (sen'shunt, ·shee·unt). Hav ing sensation; capable of feeling.

sen'ti·ment. *In psychology*, a menta attitude characterized by feeling; a emotional disposition toward some ob ject or objects.

p'a·ra"tor. 1. Anything that separates, especially an instrument for parating the teeth. 2. An instrument r detaching the pericranium or periteum. Also called *periosteal elevator.*

p'aine (sep'seen, ·sin). A poisonous omaine obtained from decomposed east and blood.

p'sis. A general reaction, usually brile, the result of action of bacteria their products or both; the organms may be parasites or saprophytes. **as s.** That due to presence of *Clostrium welchii* or other gas-forming haerobes. **puerperal s.** That occurng as a complication or sequel of egnancy; due to infection, usually reptococcal, in the birth canal, especally in the uterus.

p·tec'to·my. Excision of part of ae nasal septum.

p'tic. Relating to sepsis; affected by athogenic organisms or their toxins.

p"ti·ce'mi·a. A systemic disease oduced by microörganisms and their oisonous products in the blood stream. **septicemic,** *adj.* **puerperal s.** A febrile state caused by infection of ae blood stream of the mother through ae genital tract before, during, or folwing delivery. Also called *puerperal psis.*

p"ti·co·phle·bi'tis. Inflammaon of veins secondary to infection of e blood stream.

p'tic tank. In sewage disposal, a osed chamber through which sewage asses slowly to permit bacterial action.

p"ti·grav'i·da. A woman who is egnant for the seventh time.

p"ti·me·tri'tis. Pathogenic infecon of the uterus.

p·tip'a·ra. A woman who has borne ven children.

p·tom'e·ter. 1. An instrument for termining the thickness of the nasal ptum. 2. An apparatus for determing organic impurities in the air.

p'to·tome. An instrument for cutng the nasal septum.

p·tot'o·my. The operation of cutng the nasal septum.

p'tu·lum (pl. *septula*). A small sepm. **septula testis.** The interlobu-r septums of the testis.

p'tum (pl. *septums, septa*). A parton; a dividing wall between two aces or cavities. **—septile, septal,** *dj.* **atrial s.** The septum between ae right and left atria of the heart. **ronchial s.** The ridge at the bi-rcation of the trachea. **bulboure-hral s.** A partial median fibrous sep-m of the urethral bulb. **intermus-ular s.** A connective-tissue septum tween muscles, particularly one from hich the muscles take origin, as the ptum between the brachialis and the

triceps muscles in the arm. **inter-ventricular s.** The wall between the ventricles of the heart, largely muscular, partly membranaceous. Syn., *ventricular s.* **lingual s.** The vertical median partition of the tongue which divides the muscular tissue into halves. **nasal s.** The septum between the two nasal cavities. **orbital s.** A membranous sheet attached to the anterior edge of the orbit where it is continuous with the periosteum. **rectovagi-nal s.** The tissue forming the partition between the rectum and the vagina. **s. primum.** The first, incomplete interatrial septum in the embryonic heart. **s. secundum.** The second incomplete interatrial septum of the embryo containing the foramen ovale; it develops to the right of the septum primum and fuses with it to form the adult atrial septum.

sep'tu·plet, sep·tu'plet. One of seven offspring born from a single gestation.

sep'ul·ture. The disposal of the dead by burial.

se·que'la, se·quel'a (pl. *sequelae*). An abnormal condition following a disease upon which it is directly or indirectly dependent.

se'quence. 1. The order of occurrence, as of symptoms. 2. A sequela. **—sequen'tial,** *adj.*

se·ques'ter·ing a'gent. Any substance capable of inactivating a metallic ion in solution, as by formation of a complex compound, and of keeping the compound in solution.

se"ques·tra'tion. 1. The formation of a sequestrum. 2. The isolation of persons suffering from disease for purposes of treatment or for the protection of others.

se"ques·trec'to·my. The operative removal of a sequestrum.

se·ques'trum (pl. *sequestrums, sequestra*). A detached or dead piece of bone within a cavity, abscess, or wound. **—sequestral,** *adj.* **primary s.** That entirely detached and requiring removal. **secondary s.** One that is partially detached, and that, unless very loose, may be pushed into place. **tertiary s.** One which is cracked or partially detached and remaining firmly in place.

se"ral·bu'min. Serum albumin, the albumin fraction of serum.

se·rem'pi·on. A form of epidemic measles occurring in the West Indies, which causes great mortality, especially among children.

ser"e·no'a. The partially dried ripe fruit of *Serenoa repens*, containing an oil. Also called *saw palmetto berries, sabal.*

ser'i·ceps. A device made of loops of

ribbon for making traction upon the fetal head. *Obs.*

se'ries. 1. A succession or a group, as of compounds, objects, or numbers, arranged systematically according to a rule. 2. *In taxonomy*, the sample of a population, used as the basic working unit in modern classification. 3. *In hematology*, the succession of cell types in the development of a cell of the circulating blood. Classification and terminology vary widely among investigators in the field. There may be considered to be five series: (a) the **myeloid** or **granulocytic series** composed of the myeloblast, myelocyte, unsegmented or nonfilamentous polymorphonuclear leukocyte, and the neutrophil, eosinophil, or basophil granulocyte; (b) the **lymphoid** or **lymphocytic series** composed of the lymphoblast, young lymphocyte, and adult lymphocyte; (c) the **monocytic series** composed of the monoblast, immature monocyte, and adult monocyte; (d) the **erythrocytic series**, the megaloblast, erythroblast, normoblast, reticulocyte, and adult erythrocyte; and (e) the **blood platelet** or **thrombocytic series**, the megakaryoblast, megakaryocyte, and blood platelet or thrombocyte. **acetylene s.** Straight-chained hydrocarbons with a triple linkage. **aliphatic s.** The series of organic compounds in which the linkages of successive carbon atoms are terminated, as in an open chain. **aromatic s.** The series of organic compounds derived from benzene and characterized by the presence of a number of the carbon atoms arranged in the form of a closed chain. **closed chain s.** A series of organic compounds characterized by linkages between successive atoms as in a closed chain. **homologous s.** A group of compounds differing from one another by a definite radical or group, as CH_2. **lyotropic s.** An arrangement of the ions in the order of their behavior, such as their effect in salting-out of proteins, or on the viscosity of colloids. Also called *Hofmeister s.* **open chain s.** A series of organic compounds characterized by linkages between successive atoms as in an open chain.

ser'i·flux, se'ri·flux. Any serous or watery discharge, or a disease characterized by such a discharge. *Obs.*

ser'ine, se'rine. $CH_2OH.CHNH_2.$ $COOH.$ α-Amino-β-hydroxypropionic acid; hydroxyalanine, an amino acid; occurs as a colorless, crystalline powder; soluble in water. A constituent of many proteins.

se·ro-, ser-. A combining form denoting *relating to serum or serous*.

serobacterin. Trade-mark for emulsions of killed bacteria which have been sensitized by treatment with a specific immune serum and which more rapidly produce immunity.

se'ro·cul'ture. A bacterial culture on blood serum.

se"ro·der"ma·ti'tis. An inflammatory skin affection attended with serous effusion.

se"ro·der"ma·to'sis. A skin disease characterized by serous effusion into or onto the skin.

se"ro·di"ag·no'sis. Diagnosis based upon the reaction of blood serum of patients.

se"ro·en"ter·i'tis. Inflammation of the serous covering of the small intestine. *Obs.*

se"ro·fi'brin·ous. 1. Composed of serum and fibrin, as a serofibrinous exudate. 2. Characterized by the production of a serofibrinous exudate, as a serofibrinous inflammation.

se·rol'o·gist. One versed in serology.

se·rol'o·gy. That branch of science which deals with serum. **—serologic, serolog'ical,** *adj.*

se·rol'y·sin, se"ro·ly'sin. Bactericidal substance contained in normal blood serum.

se"ro·mu'cous. Having the nature of, or containing, both serum and mucus, as a glandular cell which has the characteristics of both a serous cell and a mucous cell. Also called *mucoserous*.

seromycin. Trade-mark for cycloserine.

se"ro·prog·no'sis. Prognosis of disease as determined by seroreactions.

se"ro·pu'ru·lent. Composed of serum and pus, as a seropurulent exudate.

se"ro·re·ac'tion. A reaction performed with serum.

se·ro'sa. 1. A serous membrane composed of mesothelium and subjacent connective tissue, lining the pericardial, pleural, and peritoneal cavities and covering their contents. Also called *tunica s.* 2. The chorion of birds and reptiles.

se·ro"sa·mu'cin. A protein resembling mucin found in ascitic fluid.

se"ro·san·guin'e·ous. Having the nature of, or containing, both serum and blood.

se"ro·si'tis. Inflammation of a serous membrane.

se"ro·syn"o·vi'tis (seer"o·sin"-vy'tis, ·sigh"no·vy'tis). A synovitis with increase of synovial fluid.

se"ro·ther'a·py. The treatment of disease by means of human or animal blood serum containing antibodies.

ser"o·to·nin. 5-Hydroxytryptamine, an amino acid derivative found many tissues, which has diverse physiologic and pharmacologic activity.

se'rous. 1. Pertaining to, characterized by, or resembling serum. 2. Producing serum, as a serous gland; containing serum, as a serous cyst.

se'ro-zyme. Thrombogen, *q.v.*

ser'pasil. Trade-mark for reserpine.

ser"pen-ta'ri-a. The dried rhizome and roots of *Aristolochia serpentaria* or of *A. reticulata*. It contains a volatile oil.

ser'pen-tine (sur'pin-teen, -tyne). Sinuous; snakelike.

ser-pig'i-nous (sur-pidj'i-nus). Creeping; having an irregular but arched and serpentine shape; applied to skin lesions.

ser-ra'tus. Serrated; said of muscles arising or inserted by a series of processes like teeth of a saw, as serratus anterior muscle, a muscle arising by digitations from the first eight ribs and inserted on the vertebral margin of the scapula. See Table of Muscles in the Appendix.

se'rum (pl. *serums, sera*). 1. The amber-colored fluid which exudes from coagulated blood as the clot shrinks. 2. A serum with antigenic properties used therapeutically. Serum is of a complex nature and is made up of water, albumin, globulins, metabolites, catabolites, lipids, hormones, salts, enzymes, etc. Serum proteins are antigenic and may be toxic for members of different species. Serum carries agglutinating, precipitating, neutralizing, opsonic, bactericidal, hemolytic, bacteriolytic, complementary, vasoconstrictive, sensitizing, and other properties. Serum proteins have been designated by Tiselius as albumin, α-globulin, β-globulin, and γ-globulin on the basis of their electrophoretic mobilities. In human serum, the albumin comprises about 55% to 60% of the total serum proteins, the α-globulin about 10% to 15%, the β-globulin varies from 7% to 13%, and the γ-globulin from 9% to 12%. The fact that the serums of immunized animals and of man contain antibodies, etc., has resulted in extensive use of serums for diagnosis, prophylaxis, and therapy. See Table of Normal Values of Blood Constituents in the Appendix. **—serous, serumal,** *adj.* **antimeningococcic s.** A serum obtained from the blood of an animal immunized with cultures of the several types of meningococci (*Neisseria meningitidis*) which prevail in the United States. It has been supplemented or supplanted by the newer chemotherapeutic agents. Also called **antimeningococcus s., meningococcus s., meningitis s. convalescent s.** Blood serum taken from a person who is convalescing from some acute, in-

fectious disease. It is injected as a prophylactic or curative measure. **normal human s.** The sterile serum obtained by pooling approximately equal amounts of serum from eight or more healthy humans. Its chief use is in the treatment of bacterial infections, in the treatment of surgical and traumatic shock, and in the treatment of burns. Also called *human s.* **pregnant mare's s.** The source for the manufacture of various sex hormones.

se'rum ur"ti-ca'ri-a. An anaphylactic reaction to the injection of a serum.

ser'vo-mech'an-ism. A control system whereby small continuous mechanical displacements involving small expenditures of power by the controller will cause proportionate displacements involving large amounts of power in the distant device.

ses'a-me (sess'uh-mee). An herb, *Sesamum indicum;* yields sesame oil, *q.v.*

ses'a-me oil. A fixed oil obtained from one or more varieties of cultivated sesame seeds, used as a vehicle for medicinals, especially injections. Syn., *benne oil, teel oil.*

ses'a-moid. Resembling a sesame seed, as in sesamoid bone, a small bone developed in a tendon subjected to much pressure (see Table of Bones in the Appendix) and sesamoid cartilages, small cartilages in the alae of the nose.

ses"a-moid-i'tis. An inflammation of a sesamoid bone which may involve the articular surfaces and cause lameness.

ses'qui-. A combining form indicating *one and one-half, the proportion of two* of one radical or element *to three* of another.

ses"qui-chlo'ride. A compound of chlorine and another element containing three parts of chlorine to two of the other element, as Fe_2Cl_3.

ses"qui-ho'ra. An hour and a half.

ses"qui-ox'ide. A compound of three parts of oxygen to two of another element, as Al_2O_3.

ses"qui-salt. A salt containing one and one-half times as much of the acid as of the radical or base, as $Fe_2(SO_4)_3$.

ses"qui-ter'pene. One of a group of terpenes of the general formula $C_{15}H_{24}$.

ses'sile (sess'il). Attached by a broad base; not pedunculated, as a sessile tumor.

set. 1. Reduce the displacement in a fracture and apply suitable bandages. 2. Harden; solidify, as a cement, amalgam, or plaster.

se'ton. A thread or skein of threads drawn through a fold of the skin, so as to produce a fistulous tract; used as a counterirritant.

se·vip′a·rous. Sebiparous; fat-producing.

se′vum. Suet.

sew′age. The heterogeneous substances constituting the excreta and waste matter of domestic economy and the contents of drains.

sew′er. A channel for the removal of sewage.

sew′er·age. 1. The collection and removal of sewage. 2. The system of pipes, etc., for the removal of sewage.

sex. The state or condition of an organism which comes to expression in the production of ova, as in the female, or of sperm cells, as in the male, or both ova and sperm cells, as in certain hermaphroditic invertebrates.

sex-. A combining form meaning *six.*

sex chro′mo·some. An odd or accessory chromosome having a special relation to determining whether a fertilized egg develops into a male or a female. The X and Y chromosomes. When other conditions are normal, a fertilized egg with two X′s becomes a female; one with the XY combination becomes a male.

sex de·ter″mi·na′tion. The process which determines the sex of an individual. See *sex chromosome.*

sex″i·dig′i·tal (seck″si·didj′i·tul), **sex″i·dig′i·tate** (seck″si·didj′i-tayt). Having six fingers or six toes.

sex′-lim′it·ed. Appearing in, or affecting, one sex only.

sex′-linked″. Applied to genes located on the X chromosome, and to the characteristics, which may occur in either sex, conditioned by such genes.

sex′o·es·thet′ic in·ver′sion. The adoption of the habits, manners, and costume of the opposite sex. Also see *eonism, transvestitism.*

sex·ol′o·gy. The science or study of sex and sex relations. —**sexolog′ic,** *adj.*

sex re·ver′sal. A change of characteristics in an individual of one sex to those of the opposite sex.

sex″ti·grav′i·da. A woman who is pregnant for the sixth time.

sex·tip′a·ra. A woman who has borne six children.

sex′tu·plet, sex·tu′plet. One of the six offspring of a single gestation.

sex′u·al. Pertaining to or characteristic of sex, as the sexual organs. —**sexual′ity,** *n.*

S. G. O. Surgeon General's Office.

SH. Sulfhydryl, *q.v.*

shaft. The trunk of any columnar mass, especially the diaphysis of a long bone. **hair-s.** A hair, particularly that portion of it imbedded in the hair follicle.

sha′king. A type of massage imparting a vibration to the tissues.

sham rage. Paroxysms of reactio in decorticate animals, giving the appearance of rage, which are evoked very mild stimuli. The reactions, su as erection of hairs, dilatation of t pupils, protrusion of claws, struggli and biting, are in considerable p those which are controlled by the au nomic nervous system.

shank. The leg from the knee to t ankle; the tibia.

sheath. 1. An envelope; a covering. *In anatomy,* the connective tiss covering vessels, muscles, nerves, te dons, etc. **carotid s.** The fibro sheath about the carotid arteries a associated structures. **myelin s.** glistening white sheath of myelina nerve fibers, immediately around t axis cylinder. Consists of a comp lipoid mixture and is a poor elect conductor. **tendon s.** In particul the synovial sheath surrounding a te don crossing the wrist or ankle joir

shed. Throw off.

shel·lac′. See *lac,* 2.

shell′shock″. Battle fatigue.

shield. 1. A protective structure apparatus. 2. *In biology,* a protecti plate, scute, lorica, or carapace. 3. structure having the shape of a shie **nipple s.** A protective covering f sore nipples.

shift. A change of direction or po tion. **chloride s.** The movement chloride ions from plasma into the r blood cells when the blood is giving oxygen and receiving carbon dioxi When hemoglobin is reduced it becom more basic, therefore a shift of neg tive ions into the cell is required maintain ionic equilibrium. The ch ride shift frees base (Na⁺) in t plasma. This unites with part of t CO_2 entering the blood to form bic bonate which together with carbo acid constitutes an acid-salt buffer pa The buffers prevent serious changes pH with respiratory gas exchanges the tissues and the lungs.

Shiga, Kiyoshi [*Japanese bacte ologist,* 1870–1957]. Collaborated wi Paul Ehrlich. Studied leprosy, berib tuberculosis. Especially known for l work on bacillary dysentery. *Shigella dysenteriae, Shiga bacillus.*

Shi·gel′la (shi·jel′uh, shi·ghel′u The genus of the dysentery bacillus the family Enterobacteriaceae, tri Salmonelleae. They are non-lactose f menting, nonmotile, Gram-negati rods. **S. ambigua** (Schmitz's bac lus), **S. madampensis, S. so nei,** and the strains of **S. parad senteriae** (Flexner, Strong, a Hiss) have been isolated from hum cases of dysentery. **S. dysenteria** Shiga bacillus, is the most virulent, these organisms elaborate a neu

...ropic exotoxin in addition to the endo-
...oxin common to all members of the
Shigella group.

...i″gel·lo′sis (shy″ji·lo′sis, shig″i-
...′sis). Bacillary dysentery caused by
...acteria of the genus *Shigella*.

...in. The sharp anterior margin of the
...ibia. **saber s.** A condition seen in
...ongenital syphilis, in which the an-
...erior border of the tibia has a sharp
...onvex edge; due to periosteal pro-
...feration.

...in′gles. See *herpes zoster*.

...iv′er. A slight tremor or shaking of
...he body due to cold, etc.

...ock. 1. The clinical manifestation
...f an inadequate volume of circulating
...lood accompanied by physiologic ad-
...ustments of the organism to a pro-
...ressive discrepancy between the ca-
...acity of the arterial tree and the vol-
...me of blood to fill it. Signs are
...arked decrease in blood pressure,
...eak thready pulse, pale cold skin
...ith cyanosis, and thirst relieved only
...y transfusion. Shock may be classified
...ccording to mechanism, as cardio-
...enic, vasogenic, hematogenic, or neu-
...ogenic. Also called *peripheral circula-
...ory failure, shock syndrome.* 2. A
...hysical or emotional trauma. 3. *In
...hysiology*, subject to an electric dis-
...harge to produce a response. **ana-
...hylactic s.** The syndrome follow-
...ng the reintroduction of an antigen in
...n animal previously sensitized to it.
...ee *anaphylaxis*. **electric s.** (a) The
...udden violent effect of the passage of
...n electric current through the body.
...) A therapeutic measure in psychosis.
...lso see electroshock *therapy*. **in-
...ulin s.** Hypoglycemia with coma as
...result of overdosage of insulin in
...iabetes or as a therapeutic measure
...n psychoses. Also see insulin shock
...herapy. **irreversible s.** A late
...tage of shock from which recovery
...annot be achieved by any known form
...f therapy. **osmotic s.** Undergone
...y certain bacteriophages. When the
...alt solution medium is rapidly diluted,
...smotic pressure is suddenly reduced,
...nd the bacteriophage may swell and
...urst; only the outer membranes can
...hen be demonstrated. **serum s.** An
...naphylactic reaction resulting from
...he injection of a serum into a sensitive
...ndividual. It may be in the nature of
...n accident, with death (serum acci-
...ent, *q.v.*); or a reaction, with cyanosis,
...eeble pulse, fall in blood pressure, cold
...ammy skin, chills, and high fever.
...ometimes adenitis, urticarial rashes,
...oint pains, etc., occur in a protein-
...ensitive individual after being given
...he homologous protein to which he is
...ensitive.

...oul′der. The region where the arm
...oins the trunk, formed by the meeting

of the clavicle, scapula, and humerus
and the overlying soft parts. See Table
of Joints and Ligaments in the Appendix. **frozen s.** A chronic tenosynovitis of unknown cause associated with
increased vascularity, degeneration,
and fibrosis in and about the shoulder
joint and characterized by pain and
limitation of motion. Also called *adhesive capsulitis, periarthritis of the
shoulder.* **slipped s.** A dislocated
humerus.

show. A bloody discharge from the
birth canal prior to labor or to a menstrual flow.

shreds. Slender strands of mucus visible grossly in urine, denoting inflammation of the urethra, bladder, or
prostate.

shriv′el. Shrink in bulk and wrinkle.

shud′der. A convulsive momentary
tremor, caused by fright, disgust, or
nervous shock.

Si. Chemical symbol for silicon.

si″a·go·nag′ra (sigh″uh·go·nag′ruh,
·nay′gruh). Gouty pain in the maxilla.

si·al′-, si·al′o-. A combining form denoting saliva.

si·al′a·den (sigh·al′uh·den). A salivary gland.

si″al·ad′e·ni′tis. Inflammation of
a salivary gland.

si·al′a·gogue (sigh·al′uh·gog), **si-
al′a·gog.** 1. Producing a flow of
saliva. 2. A drug producing a flow of
saliva. **—sialagog′ic,** *adj., n.*

si″al·a·po′ri·a. Deficiency in the
amount of saliva.

si″a·li·thot′o·my. Incision of a
salivary gland or duct for removal of a
calculus.

si″a·lo·ad″e·nec′to·my. Surgical
removal of a salivary gland.

si″a·lo·ad″e·not′o·my. Incision of
a salivary gland.

si″a·lo·a″er·oph′a·gy. The habit
of constantly swallowing and thus taking saliva and air into the stomach.

si″a·lo·an·gi′tis. Inflammation of a
salivary duct.

si″a·lo·do·chi′tis (sigh″uh·lo·do-
kigh′tis). Inflammation of a salivary
duct.

si″a·lo·do′cho·plas″ty (·do′ko·
plas″tee). Plastic surgery of a salivary
gland duct.

si″a·log′e·nous (sigh″uh·lodj′i·nus).
Generating saliva.

si·al′o·gram (sigh·al′o·gram). Roentgenogram of a salivary duct.

si″a·log′ra·phy. Radiographic examination of a salivary gland following
injection of an opaque substance into
its duct.

si·al′o·lith″ (sigh·al′o·lith″, sigh′uh·
lo·lith″). A salivary calculus.

si″a·lo·li·thi′a·sis. The presence of
salivary calculi.

si"a·lo·li·thot'o·my. Surgical incision into a salivary duct or salivary gland for the removal of a calculus.

si"a·lor·rhe'a, si"a·lor·rhoe'a. Salivation.

si"a·los'che·sis (sigh"uh-los'ki-sis). Suppression of the secretion of saliva.

si"a·lo·ste·no'sis. Stricture of a salivary duct.

si"a·lo·syr'inx (sigh"uh-lo-sirr'inks, -sigh'rinks). 1. A salivary fistula. 2. A syringe for washing out the salivary ducts. 3. A drainage tube for a salivary duct.

sib. One of a group of children of the same parents; a brother or sister. Syn., *sibling*.

sib'i·lant. Hissing or whistling, as a sibilant rale.

sib"i·la'tion. Pronunciation in which the *s* sound predominates.

sib"i·lis'mus (sib"i-liz'mus). 1. A hissing sound. 2. A sibilant rale.

sib'i·lus. A sibilant rale.

sib'ling. A brother or sister. Syn., *sib*.

sib'ship. All the brothers and sisters in a family regarded as a single group.

sic'cant, sic'ca·tive. 1. Drying; tending to make dry. 2. A drying agent or medicine.

sic'ca·tive. See *siccant*.

sic·cha'si·a (si-kay'zhuh, -zee-uh). Nausea.

sic'cus. Dry.

sick. Ill; not well. Also used colloquially for nauseated.

sick call. *In military medicine*, the assembly of the sick at a dispensary, hospital, or other point for examination and disposition by the military surgeon in charge; a term used in the United States Army.

sick'le-cell" a·ne'mi·a. See under *anemia*.

sick·le'mi·a (sick-lee'mee-uh, sick"-ul-ee'mee-uh). See *sickle-cell anemia*.

sick list. A list of persons, especially in military or naval service, who are disabled by sickness.

sick'ness. Disease. The condition of being unwell. **altitude s.** Nausea, vomiting, and dizziness occurring in rarefied atmospheres due to anoxemia. **bleeding s.** Hemophilia. **falling s.** Epilepsy. **green s.** Chlorosis. **morning s.** Nausea of early pregnancy. **motion s.** Vertigo, nausea, and vomiting occurring during travel by auto, airplane, or train. **mountain s.** See altitude *s*. **radiation s.** (a) Illness due to the effects of therapeutic irradiation with roentgen rays or radium and comprising symptoms of nausea, vomiting, headache, cramps, and diarrhea. (b) The effect of radiant energy following the explosion of an atomic bomb, the resultant effects of which include alopecia, loss of teeth, decrease in red and white blood cells, and hemor-

rhage from prolonged bleeding tir[...] **serum s.** An anaphylactic reacti[...] following serum therapy, characteri[...] by urticaria, arthritis, edema, fev[...] and prostration. **sleeping s.** E[...] demic encephalitis or trypanosomias[...]

Si'da. A genus of plants of the M[...] vaceae.

side. The lateral aspect of any body organ.

sid'er·ism. The curative influen[...] long supposed to be exerted over [...] body by the lodestone. *Obs.*

sid"er·o·dro"mo·pho'bi·a (sid[...] ur·o·dro"mo·fo'bee·uh, -drom"o[...] Morbid dread of traveling by railw[...] fear of trains.

sid"er·o·pe'ni·a. Deficiency of ir[...] especially in the blood.

sid'er·o·scope". An instrument [...] the detection of particles of iron [...] steel in the eyes.

sid"er·o·sil"i·co'sis. Diffuse fib[...] sis of the lungs due to the prolonged [...] halation of dusts containing silic[...] dioxide and iron salts.

sid"er·o'sis. Chronic inflammati[...] of the lungs due to prolonged inha[...] tion of dust containing iron sa[...] occurs in iron miners and arc welde[...] It is characterized by inflammat[...] tissue reaction mainly in the lympha[...] tissues of the lungs and by diffu[...] nodular shadows in the x-ray film. A[...] called *arc-welder's disease, arc-welde[...] nodulation*. **—sider·ot'ic,** *adj.*

sig. Abbreviation for *signa*, label [...] *signetur*, let it be labeled.

sigh. A prolonged and deep inspirat[...] followed by a shorter expiration. A[...] called *suspirium*.

sight. 1. The act of seeing. 2. T[...] special sense concerned in seei[...] **aging s.** Presbyopia. **far s.** H[...] permetropia. **short s.** Myopia.

sigmodal. A trade-mark for secon[...] ary amyl-β-bromallylbarburic ac[...]

sig'moid. 1. Shaped like the letter [...] 2. Pertaining to the sigmoid flexure[...] the colon, as the sigmoid artery ([...] Table of Arteries in the Appendix), [...] sigmoid mesocolon.

sig"moid·ec'to·my. Excision of [...] part or all of the sigmoid flexure of [...] colon.

sig"moid·i'tis. Inflammation of [...] sigmoid flexure of the colon.

sig·moi'do-, sigmoid-. A comb[...] ing form meaning *sigmoid*.

sig·moi'do·pex"y. An operation [...] prolapse of the rectum; colopexy; fi[...] tion of the sigmoid colon by obliterat[...] the intersigmoid fossa and shorten[...] the mesosigmoid by suture, through [...] abdominal incision.

sig·moi"do·rec·tos'to·my. F[...] mation by surgical means of an a[...]

ficial anus at the sigmoid flexure of the descending colon, at its junction with the rectum; sigmoidostomy; low colostomy.

ig·moi'do·scope. An appliance for the inspection, by artificial light, of the sigmoid flexure; it differs from the proctoscope in its greater length and diameter. **—sigmoidos'copy,** *n.*

ig″moid·os'co·py. Visual inspection of the sigmoid flexure, with the aid of special instruments.

ig·moi″do·sig″moid·os'to·my. Surgical anastomosis between two portions of the sigmoid colon.

ig″moid·os'to·my. The formation of an artificial anus in the sigmoid flexure of the colon; sigmoid colostomy.

ig″moid·ot'o·my. Incision into the sigmoid colon.

ign. 1. A mark or objective evidence; in a restricted sense, a physical manifestation of disease. 2. A conventional character used in printing, pharmacy, or otherwise. See Table of Medical Signs and Symbols in the Appendix. **Allis's.** When the neck of the femur is fractured, the fascia between the greater trochanter and the crest of the ilium is less tense than normally. **Babinski's s.** A sign for lesions of the corticospinal tract in which the response to plantar stimulation shows extension of the great toe with flexion and fanning of the other toes. **Ballance's s.** A sign for rupture of the spleen in which the dullness in the right flank will shift with position but not that on the left. **Broadbent's s.** A systolic retraction in the back at the eleventh or twelfth rib on the left side; seen when there are adhesions between the pericardium and the diaphragm. **Brudzinski's s.** A sign for meningeal irritation in which raising the recumbent patient's head passively causes flexion of the thighs. **Bryant's s.** When the humerus is dislocated, the anterior and posterior boundaries of the axillary fossa are lowered. **Chvostek's s.** A sign for tetany in which tapping of the face in front of the ear produces spasm of the facial muscles. **Crowe's s.** In patients with sinus thrombosis, the retinal vessels are engorged if the internal jugular vein is compressed on the normal side. **diaphragmatic s.** The movement of the diaphragm during respiratory excursions causing an altered contour of the chest wall. If the patient is observed by means of oblique illumination, a shadow is seen moving up or down the side of the chest. Also called *Litten's shadow.* **Goodell's s.** Softening of the cervix of the uterus, considered to be evidence of pregnancy. **Hicks's s.** A sign of pregnancy after the third month in which rhythmic uterine contractions can be detected. **Hoffmann's s.** A test for overactive tendon reflexes in which tapping the nail of the index or middle finger causes flexion of the thumb. Syn., *digital reflex.* **Joffroy's s.** A sign for exophthalmic goiter in which the forehead does not wrinkle when the patient looks up with the head bent down. **Kernig's s.** A sign for meningeal irritation in which an attempt to completely extend the leg at the knee with the thigh flexed at a right angle causes pain or meets resistance. **Koplik's s.** Small red spots surrounded by quite white areas seen in the mucous membrane of the mouth in the prodromal stage of measles. Also called *Koplik's spots.* **Kussmaul's s.** Air hunger seen in patients with severe diabetes. **Larrey's s.** A sign for sacroiliac joint disease in which pain in the joint is felt when the patient sits down abruptly on a hard seat. **McBurney's s.** A sign for early acute appendicitis in which the area of maximum tenderness is over McBurney's point. **Macewen's s.** Increased resonance on combined percussion and auscultation of the skull in certain gross lesions of the intracranial contents, as in cerebral abscess or overdistended lateral ventricles. **Möbius' s.** Inability to maintain convergence of the eyes in exophthalmic goiter. **Murphy's s.** A sign for cholecystitis in which the thumb presses over the area of the gallbladder and on expiration causes pain and catching of the breath. **objective s.** One apparent to the observer. **physical s.** One of the phenomena observed on inspection, palpation, percussion, auscultation, mensuration, or combinations of these methods. **Queckenstedt's s.** In normal individuals, a rapid rise in spinal-fluid pressure when the internal jugular veins are compressed. In individuals with a block in the vertebral canal, the spinal-fluid pressure does not change with compression of the veins. **Romberg's s.** (a) A sign for obturator hernia in which there is pain radiating to the knee. (b) A sign for tabes dorsalis in which the patient cannot maintain equilibrium when standing with feet together and eyes closed. **Stellwag's s.** A sign for exophthalmic goiter in which the upper eyelid is retracted. **Strümpell's s.** Dorsal flexion of the foot when the thigh is flexed; seen in paralysis. Also called *tibialis s.* **subjective s.** One recognized only by the patient. **Tinel's s.** A sign to indicate nerve regeneration in which tapping the nerve below the point of injury causes a tingling sensation in the distal parts. **Wernicke's s.** A reaction obtained in some cases of hemianopsia in which a pencil of light thrown on the blind side of the retina gives rise to no movement in the iris, but, when thrown upon the normal side, produces contraction of the iris. It indicates that the lesion producing the hemianopsia is situated at, or anterior to, the geniculate bodies.

sig'na. 1. Plural of signum, q.v. 2. Used in prescriptions to mean "write"; abbreviated, S., sig.

sig'na·ture. 1. The part of the prescription that is placed on the label, containing directions to the patient. 2. A distinguishing character. **doctrine of signatures.** A theory that the medicinal uses of a plant can be determined from its fancied physical resemblance to normal or diseased organs (liverwort, lungwort, orchis).

sig·nif'i·cant dif'fer·ence. A difference between two statistical constants, calculated from two separate samples, which is of such magnitude that it is unlikely to have occurred by chance alone. Usually this probability must be less than 0.05 (5%) before a difference is accepted as significant. The smaller the probability, the more significant is the difference.

sig'num (pl. *signa*). A mark, sign, or indication.

sil'i·ca. Silicon dioxide, SiO_2, occurring in nature in the form of quartz, flint, and other minerals.

sil"i·ca·to'sis. Chronic inflammation of the lungs caused by the prolonged inhalation of dust containing silicates. A form of pneumoconiosis. The only recognized example is asbestosis, q.v.

si·li'ceous, si·li'cious (si-lish'us). Having the nature of, or containing, silicon.

si·lic'ic ac'id (si-liss'ick). Approximately H_2SiO_3. A white, amorphous powder.

si·li'cious. Siliceous, q.v.

sil"i·co·flu'o·ride. A compound of silicon and fluorine with some other element.

sil'i·con. Si = 28.06. A nonmetallic element of the carbon group. It occurs in several allotropic modifications. Like carbon, it forms many complex compounds that are an essential part of the earth's surface. **s. dioxide.** SiO_2; silica. See purified siliceous *earth*.

silicone. Trade-mark for a class of polymers having the composition of a polyorganosiloxane.

sil"i·co'sis. Diffuse fibrosis of the lungs caused by the inhalation, through a period of years, of dust having a significant content of silicon dioxide particles less than 10μ in diameter. A form of pneumoconiosis. Also called *chalicosis, lithosis, schistosis, miner's phthi-*

sis, *miner's asthma, grinder's asthm* *grinder's rot, potter's asthma, potter* *rot, potter's consumption.* **conglom erate s.** That form in which, in add tion to discrete nodules, there ar single or multiple fibrous masses larger size. It is also known as silicos with infection, based on the concep that infection, either obsolete, laten or active, is an essential etiologic facto in the development of the conglomerat masses. Conglomerate silicosis may b indistinguishable from tuberculosili sis, q.v. **simple s.** Fibrosis in th form of discrete nodules, usually no exceeding 5 mm. in diameter and tend ing toward uniformity in size and distribution.

sil"i·co·tu·ber"cu·lo'sis. Silicos with tuberculosis; any manifestation o tuberculous infection in a silicotic lun

sil"i·co·tung'stic ac'id. $SiO_2.12$ $WO_3.26H_2O$. In white or yellowish crys tals, used as a reagent for alkaloids.

sil'ver. Ag = 107.880. A white, sof ductile, and malleable metal. Metalli silver is insoluble in water and mos acids in the cold, but dissolves in dilut nitric acid. Silver compounds are use in medicine to secure caustic, astrin gent, and antiseptic effects. **ammo niacal s. nitrate solution.** Se under *solution.* **colloidal s. iodide** See *neo-silvol.* **mild s. protein** Silver rendered colloidal by the pres ence of, or combination with, protei It contains between 19% and 23% silver; occurs as dark brown or almos black, shining scales or granules; free soluble in water. Used in medicin especially in the treatment of infectiou conditions of the mucous membrane Also called *mild protein s., mild pr targin.* **s. nitrate.** $AgNO_3$. Occurs colorless or white crystals; soluble water. It is used locally as an astrin gent and germicide, especially in in fections of the mucous membrane **s. picrate.** $C_6H_2(OAg)(NO_2)_3.H_2($ Silver trinitrophenolate; occurs as ye low crystals; sparingly soluble in wate It is used locally in the treatment gonorrhea and vaginitis. **s. trinitro phenolate.** Silver picrate. **stron s. protein.** Contains from 7.5% 8.5% of silver; occurs as a brown, odor less powder; freely soluble in water. is used in the same conditions fo which the mild compound is used. Als called *strong protein s., strong pr targin.* **toughened s. nitrate** Silver nitrate toughened by the addi tion of a small proportion of hydro chloric acid, sodium chloride, or potas sium nitrate; occurs in the form white, hard pencils or cones. Used as means of applying silver nitrate locall Also called *molded s. nitrate, fused nitrate, s. nitrate pencils, lunar causti*

silvol. Trade-mark for a brand of mild silver protein.

Sim'a·ru·ba. A genus of trees of the family Simarubaceae. The bark of the root of **S. officinalis** has been used as a simple bitter.

sim'i·an. Apelike; pertaining to or characteristic of apes or monkeys.

si·mil'i·a si·mil'i·bus cu·ran'tur. Likes are cured by likes; a sophism formulated by Hippocrates, then by Paracelsus (simile similis cura, non contrarium), and later by Samuel Christian Friedrich Hahnemann, the founder of homeopathy. It is the basic doctrine of homeopathy, that the cure of disease is accomplished through remedies which produce somewhat the same effects as the disease itself.

si·mil'i·mum. The homeopathic remedy which will produce the symptom complex most like that of a given disease.

sim'ple. 1. Not complex; consisting of but one substance, or containing only one active substance; not compound. 2. Wanting in intellect. 3. A medicinal plant.

Simpson, James Young [*Scottish obstetrician*, 1811–70]. The first to promote the use of chloroform in England, especially in obstetrics (1847). Inventor of a number of obstetric and gynecologic instruments including a forceps called *Simpson's forceps.*

Sims, James Marion [*American surgeon*, 1813–83]. Noted for his distinguished contributions to gynecology and to general surgery. Developed a successful operation for the closure of vesicovaginal fistula, in which he used sutures of silver wire (1858). Introduced his operation for amputation of the uterine cervix (1861). Performed cholecystectomy for hydrops of the gallbladder (1870). Invented the duckbill vaginal speculum, called *Sims's speculum.* See also Sims's *position.*

i'mul. At once; at the same time.

im"u·la'tion. The feigning or counterfeiting of disease; malingering.

si·mu'li·um. A genus of small, robust, humpbacked Diptera with short legs and broad wings, commonly called black flies or buffalo gnats. They are world wide in distribution. The females are vicious bloodsuckers. **S. pecu·arum.** A small black fly which is an important scourge of man and cattle in the Mississippi Valley. **S. venus·tum.** A small black fly of northern New England, New York, and Canada, most vexing to man in June and July.

in·al'bin. A glycoside found in white mustard, which on enzymatic hydrolysis yields glucose, parahydroxybenzylisothiocyanate, choline, and sinapinic acid.

i·na'pis. Mustard.

sin"a·pis'co·py. The use of mustard as a test of sensory disturbances.

sin'a·pism. A mustard plaster.

sin'ci·put (sin'sip·ut). Old term for the superior and anterior part of the head. Also, the top of the head; the bregma. —**sincip'ital,** *adj.*

sin'ew (sin'yoo). A tendon, *q.v.*

sin·gul'tus. A hiccup. —**singul·tous,** *adj.;* **singulta'tion,** *n.*

sin'i·grin. $KC_{10}H_{16}O_9NS_2.H_2O$; potassium myronate, a glycoside found in black mustard, *Brassica nigra.* Under the influence of myrosin, an albuminous ferment which is also in black mustard, the glycoside is hydrolyzed, yielding allyl isothiocyanate, acid potassium sulfate, and glucose.

sin'is·ter (sin'is·tur, si·nis'tur). **si·nis'tra, si·nis'trum.** Left. Abbreviated, s.

sin·is·trad, sin·is'trad. Toward the left.

sin·is·tral, sin·is'tral. 1. On the left side. 2. Showing preference for the left hand, eye, or foot for certain acts or functions. 3. A left-handed individual. —**sinistral'ity,** *n.*

sin"is·trau'ral. Left-eared; the opposite of *dextraural.*

sin'is·tro- (sin'is·tro-, si·nis'tro-), **sinistr-.** A combining form denoting *left* or *toward the left side.*

sin"is·troc'u·lar. Left-eyed; the opposite of *dextrocular.*

sin"is·tro·man'u·al. Left-handed.

sin"is·tro'sis. Shellshock.

sin"is·tro·tor'sion. A twisting or turning toward the left; the opposite of *dextrotorsion.*

sin·is'trous, sin·is'trous. Awkward; unskilled; the reverse is dextrous, skilled, expert.

sink'a·line (sink'uh·leen, ·lin), **sink'o·line** (sink'o·leen, ·lin). See *choline.*

si'no-. A combining form denoting *sinus.*

si"no·a'tri·al. Pertaining to the region between the atrium and the sinus venosus, as the sinoatrial node.

si"no·au·ric'u·lar. See *sinoatrial.*

sintrom. Trade-mark for acenocoumarol.

sin'u-. A combining form signifying *sinus.*

sin'u·ous. Wavy; applied especially to tortuous fistulas and sinuses.

si'nus. 1. A hollow or cavity; a recess or pocket. 2. A large channel containing blood, especially venous blood. 3. A suppurating tract. 4. A cavity within a bone. —**sinal, sinusal,** *adj.* **aor·tic s.** One of the pouchlike dilatations of the aorta opposite the cusps of the semilunar valves. Also called *s. of Valsalva.* **carotid s.** A slight dilatation of the common carotid artery at its bifurcation, the walls of which are innervated by a branch of the glossopharyngeal nerve. Its function is concerned with the regulation of systemic blood pressure. **cavernous s.** An irregularly shaped sinus of the dura mater located on the side of the body of the sphenoid bone, and extending from the superior orbital fissure in front to the apex of the petrosa behind. See Table of Veins in the Appendix. **circular s.** A sinus consisting of the two cavernous sinuses and their communications across the median line by means of the anterior and posterior intercavernous sinuses, all of which surround the hypophysis. **coronary s.** A venous sinus which drains most of the cardiac veins, opens into the right atrium, and is located in the lower part of the atrioventricular sulcus of the heart. It is derived from the transverse portion of the embryonic sinus venosus. See Table of Veins in the Appendix. **frontal s.** The paranasal sinus situated in the frontal bone. **lactiferous s.** A dilatation of a lactiferous duct where milk may accumulate. **lymph s.** One of the tracts of diffuse lymphatic tissue in a lymph node. **marginal s.** (a) An enlarged venous sinus incompletely encircling the margin of the placenta. (b) One of the bilateral, small sinuses of the dura which skirt the edge of the foramen magnum, usually uniting posteriorly to form the occipital sinus. **maxillary s.** The paranasal sinus in the maxilla. Also called *antrum of Highmore.* **oblique s. of the pericardium.** An arched reflection of pericardium forming a pocket that extends upward on the posterior aspect of the atria. **occipital s.** A sinus of the dura running in the attached margin of the falx cerebelli from the foramen magnum to the confluence of the sinuses. See Table of Veins in the Appendix. **paranasal sinuses.** Air cavities lined by mucous membrane which communicate with the nose. They are the ethmoid, frontal, sphenoid, and maxillary sinuses. **petrosal s.** A sinus of the dura mater, one situated in the inferior and the other in the superior border of the petrosa in the middle cranial fossa. **phrenicocostal s.** Bilateral space between the reflection of the costal pleura upon the diaphragm into which the inferior edge of the lung advances on inspiration. **pilonidal s.** A congenital anomaly in the sacral region which may be cystic, consisting of a tract leading to the exterior. Also called *pilonidal cyst.* **piriform s.** The space lateral to the laryngeal orifice which is bounded laterally by the thyroid car-

tilage and thyrohyoid membrane, and medially by the aryepiglottic fold. Syn. *piriform s., piriform recess.* **s. of the dura.** Any endothelially lined, venous blood space situated between the periosteal layer and meningeal layer of the dura mater. One of the channels by which blood is conveyed from the cerebral veins, and from some of the veins of the meninges and diploë, into the neck. **s. venosus.** (a) The chamber of the lower vertebrate heart to which the veins return blood from the body. (b) The chamber in the embryonic mammalian heart into which empty the umbilical and omphalomesenteric veins. **straight s.** A sinus of the dura running from the inferior sagittal sinus along the junction of the falx cerebri and tentorium to the transverse sinus. See Table of Veins in the Appendix. **superior sagittal s.** A sinus of the dura which runs along the upper edge of the falx cerebri, beginning in front of the crista galli and terminating at the confluence of the sinuses. See Table of Veins in the Appendix. **transverse s.** (a) A sinus of the dura running from the internal occipital protuberance, following for part of its course the attached margin of the tentorium cerebelli, then over the jugular process of the occipital bone to reach the jugular foramen. Also called *lateral s.* See Table of Veins in the Appendix. (b) A dorsal communication between the right and left sides of the pericardial cavity between the reflections of the epicardium at the arterial and venous attachments of the heart, passing behind the aorta and pulmonary artery and in front of the superior vena cava and left atrium. **venous s. of the sclera.** A canal in the sclera close to the sclerocorneal junction running circularly around the periphery of the cornea. It gives rise to the anterior ciliary veins. Also called *Schlemm's canal.*

si″nus·i′tis (sigh″nuh-sigh′tis, sigh″new·). Inflammation of a sinus. May affect any of the paranasal sinuses, as **ethmoidal sinusitis, frontal sinusitis,** or **maxillary sinusitis.**

si′nus·oid. 1. Resembling a sinus. 2. One of the relatively large spaces of tubes constituting part of the venous circulatory system of the suprarenal gland, liver, and other viscera.

si″nus·oi′dal. 1. Varying in proportion to the sine of an angle or of time function. 2. Pertaining to a sinus.

si″nus·ot′o·my (sigh″nus·ot′o·mee, sigh″new·sot′o·mee). The production of an artificial opening into a paranasal sinus, to promote drainage.

si′phon. A tube bent at an angle, one arm of which is longer than the other, used for the purpose of removing liquids from a cavity or vessel, by means of atmospheric pressure.

si'phon·age. The action of a siphon, such as washing out the stomach, drainage of wounds, by the use of atmospheric pressure.

Si"pho·nap'ter·a. An order of insects, commonly called fleas. They have small, hard, laterally compressed bodies without wings, and the mouth parts are adapted for piercing and sucking. They feed exclusively upon the blood of birds and mammals and so become important disease vectors. The important genera are *Ctenocephalides, Echidnophaga, Pulex, Tunga,* and *Xenopsylla.*

Si·phun"cu·li'na (sigh-funk"yoo-lye'nuh). A genus of flies found in India. **S. funicola.** The common eye fly of India which is responsible for transmitting conjunctivitis.

Sippy, Bertram Welton [*American physician,* 1866–1924]. Widely known for his advocacy of a diet adapted to the treatment of gastric and duodenal ulcer. The *Sippy* diet consisted of alternately taking Sippy's powders (q.v. under *powder,* 2), and a milk-cream mixture.

si'ren. *In teratology,* sirenomelus, q.v.

si"ren·om'e·lus. A monster whose lower extremities are intimately fused, the feet being absent. Also called *sympus apus.*

site. Situation. **placental s.** The area to which the placenta is attached.

si·tol'o·gy (sigh·tol'o·jee). The science of foods; dietetics.

si"to·ma'ni·a. An abnormal craving for food.

si"to·pho'bi·a. Morbid aversion to food; morbid fear of eating.

si"to·ther'a·py. Dietotherapy, q.v.

si'tus. A position. **s. inversus.** Reversed location or position. **s. inversus viscerum.** An anomaly in which the viscera are changed from the normal to the opposite side of the body. Also called *s. mutatus, s. transversus.* **s. perversus.** Malposition of one or more of the viscera.

SK. Abbreviation for streptokinase.

skat'ole, ska'tole. C₉H₉N, methyl indole. A nitrogenous decomposition product of proteins, formed from tryptophane in the intestine. Contributes to the typical, disagreeable odor of feces.

skat·ox'yl. C₉H₉ON. A product of the oxidation of skatole.

ske·lal'gi·a. Pain in the leg.

skel'e·tal trac'tion. Traction exerted directly upon the long bones themselves by means of pins, wire, tongs, and other mechanical devices which are attached to, or passed through, the bones by operative procedures.

skel"e·ti·za'tion. The process of converting into a skeleton; gradual wasting of the soft parts, leaving only the skeleton.

skel'e·to-. A combining form meaning *skeleton.*

skel'e·ton. A supporting structure, especially the bony framework supporting and protecting the soft parts of an organism. **—skeletal,** *adj.* **appendicular s.** The skeleton of the pectoral and pelvic girdles and limbs. **axial s.** The skeleton of the head and trunk. **dermal s.** The exoskeleton.

Skene, Alexander Johnston Chalmers [*American gynecologist,* 1838–1900]. Remembered for his description of the tubular mucous glands in the female urethra opening just within the urinary meatus (1880); called *Skene's glands, paraurethral glands.* The duct of each gland is known as *Skene's duct.*

ske·nei'tis, ske·ni'tis. Inflammation of the paraurethral glands, or Skene's ducts.

skene'o·scope" (skee'no·scope"). An endoscope for use in examining Skene's glands.

skew de"vi·a'tion. A condition in which one eyeball is deviated upward and outward, the other inward and downward; sometimes observed in cerebellar disease.

skiabaryt. Trade-mark for barium sulfate and for mixtures of barium sulfate, sugar, and tragacanth suitable for use in roentgen examinations.

ski'a·gram. The finished, printed roentgen-ray picture.

ski·ag'ra·phy. Radiography.

ski·am'e·try (sky·am'i·tree). 1. Shadow mensuration applied to a method of determining the density of x-ray shadow. 2. The measurement of x-ray intensity, for the determination of exposure time. 3. The measurement of accommodation by retinoscopy. **dynamic s.** Refraction in which retinoscopy is performed with the accommodation active but controlled.

ski·as'co·py (sky·ass'ko·pee). 1. Examination with a retinoscope. 2. Examination with a fluoroscope.

skin. The covering of the body, composed of the epidermis (**scarfskin**), or cuticle, and the corium (**true skin**), or derma. The epidermis consists of a deep layer, the stratum germinativum, and three superficial layers: the stratum granulosum, the stratum lucidum, and the stratum corneum. The corium, derma, or true skin consists of a papillary and reticular layer (stratum papillare and stratum reticulare), the former projecting upward in the form of papillae. The true skin is made up of fibroelastic connective tissue and, in some regions, smooth muscle (the arrectores pilorum). The subcutaneous tissue consists of fibroelastic and adipose tissue, blood vessels, and sweat glands in its upper portion. The appendages of the skin are the nails, hairs, and sweat, sebaceous and mammary glands, which are derivatives of the epithelial layer of the skin. In the skin are also placed terminal nerve organs subserving the senses of touch, pain, and temperature. **anserine s.** Goose flesh; cutis anserina. **atrophic s.** A wasting or retrogressive change in the skin. Also called *dermatrophia.* **edematous s.** Effusion of serum into connective tissue of the skin. Also called *dermatoclysis.* **glossy s.** A peculiar shiny skin seen in conditions in which the trophic nerve supply to the skin is cut off, as after injury to a nerve. **parchment s.** Atrophy of the skin. **pigmentation of the s.** Coloration of the skin due to natural body pigments, or to the deposition of foreign substances in the skin. Natural pigments include melanin, hemosiderin, carotene, and bile salts. Foreign pigments include atabrine and silver salts.

skin graft'ing. The application of portions of the skin, either the outer layers or the full thickness, to a granulating wound to promote healing, to fill a defect, or to replace scar tissue for plastic repair. Also see *graft.*

skin'ny. 1. Cutaneous. 2. Emaciated.

skin trac'tion. Traction exerted by direct attachment to the skin, using adhesive plaster or linen or gauze strips cemented to the skin.

skiodan. Trade-mark for methiodal sodium.

skull. The entire bony framework of the head, consisting of the cranium and the face. The cranium is made up of the occipital, frontal, sphenoid, and ethmoid bones, and the two parietal and two temporal bones. The face is composed of two nasal, two lacrimal, two zygomatic, two palate, and two inferior turbinate bones, two maxillas, the vomer, and the mandible. Sometimes loosely used to include only the fixed bones, excluding the face. See Table of Bones in the Appendix. **fenestrated s.** Osteoporosis of the skull, as from osteomyelitis.

skull'cap". 1. The bones comprising the vault of the skull; calvaria. 2. See *scutellaria.*

slake. 1. Quench or appease. 2. Disintegrate by the action of water.

slav'er. Drivel; saliva, especially that which is discharged involuntarily.

sleep. The periodic state of rest in which there is diminution of consciousness and activity.

slide. A piece of glass on which objects are examined by use of the microscope.

sling. A bandage, usually slung from the neck, to support the arm or wrist.

sling and swathe. A dressing for fractures of the humerus at the upper end. It consists of a three-cornered handkerchief sling holding the arm at the side, the forearm flexed at 90°, with an axillary pad, the swathe passing about the body and arm from shoulder to elbow and secured by pins.

slit. A narrow opening; a visceral cleft; the separation between any pair of lips. **genitourinary s.** The urogenital opening.

slough (sluff). A mass of necrotic tissue in, or separating from, living tissue, as in a wound or ulcer.

sludge. Sewage deposit.

slum'ber. 1. Sleep lightly. 2. Light sleep.

Slye, Maud [*American pathologist,* 1879–]. Noted for her work on cancer and heredity (1928). Her selective breeding of mice, both resistant to and capable of developing cancer, has had great influence upon our present concept of susceptibility to the disease.

Sm. Chemical symbol for samarium.

small'pox". A contagious infectious disease, often fatal, ushered in with severe febrile symptoms, which, in the course of two or three days, are followed by a papular eruption appearing over all parts of the body. The eruption passes successively through the states of maculation, vesiculation, pustulation, and later crust formation; after this a pitted appearance of the skin (pock-marks) is produced. The period of incubation is twelve to twenty-one days. The papules appear about the third day, pustules the sixth day, crusting the twelfth day. **hemorrhagic s.** Smallpox in which hemorrhage occurs into the vesicles, which gives them a blackish appearance. **malignant s.** A severe hemorrhagic type with high mortality.

smear. Preparation of secretions or blood for microscopical study, made by spreading them on a glass slide.

smeg'ma. Sebum. **—smegmatic,** *adj.* **s. clitoridis.** The substance secreted by the sebaceous glands of the clitoris and labia minora. **s. praeputii.** The substance secreted by the sebaceous glands of the prepuce.

smell. 1. The perception of odor. 2. Odor.

smell brain. The rhinencephalon.

Smellie, William [*English obstetrician,* 1697–1763]. Devised several types of obstetric forceps, some with lock and curved blades, called *Smellie's forceps.*

smell'ing salts. A preparation containing ammonium carbonate and stronger ammonia water, usually scented with aromatic substances.

smi′la·cin. A saponinlike glycoside from sarsaparilla. Also called *parillin*.

smi′lax. See *sarsaparilla*.

Smith-Petersen, Marius Nygaard [*American physician*, 1886–1953]. Devised a flanged metal nail used for intracapsular fractures of the neck of the femur, called *Smith-Petersen′s nail*.

smudg′ing. A form of defective speech in which the difficult consonants are dropped.

smut. 1. A fungous disease of plants involving the grains wheat, rye, oats, and corn. 2. A fungus producing such a disease; a common allergen.

Sn. Chemical symbol for tin.

snake. An elongate reptile covered with scales and without limbs, external ears, or functional eyelids; a serpent. **cottonmouth s.** A thick-bodied pit viper found in or near water; the water moccasin. **poisonous snakes.** The venom-producing snakes, which are divided into four families: Elapidae, the cobras and coral snakes; Hydrophidae, the sea snakes; Crotalidae, the pit vipers; and Viperidae, the true vipers. All have large, hypodermic-like front fangs by which venom is injected.

snake′root″. Any of various plants with long wavy roots, such as species of *Asarum* or *Cimicifuga racemosa* or *Eupatorium rugosum*.

snap. A short, abrupt sound heard in auscultation of the heart in certain cardiac diseases. Also applied to the sound made by the action of a tendon on contraction of its muscle.

snare. An instrument designed to hold a wire loop which can be constricted by means of a mechanism in the handle, and used to remove tonsils, polyps, and small growths having a narrow base or pedicle.

sneeze. A sudden, noisy, spasmodic expiration through the nose. It is caused by irritation of nasal nerves or overstimulation of the optic nerve by a very bright light.

sneez′ing. The act of expelling air violently through the nose.

Snellen, Hermann [*Dutch ophthalmologist*, 1834–1908]. Introduced a number of ophthalmic procedures, including operations for ectropion and entropion. An operation for ptosis in which he shortened the levator tendon by section or tucking is called *Snellen′s operation*. An ophthalmologic test chart which measures the degree of visual acuity is called the *Snellen chart*. See also test *type*, Snellen *test*.

snore. Breathe through the nose in such a manner as to cause a vibration of the soft palate, thereby producing a rough, audible sound.

soap. A salt of one or more of the higher fatty acids with a metal. Soaps may be divided into two classes, soluble and insoluble. The soluble soaps are the detergent or cleansing soaps, and usually are prepared from the alkali metals, sodium and potassium. The insoluble soaps are salts of the fatty acids and metals of other groups. **castile s.** A hard soap usually prepared from sodium hydroxide and olive oil. Much commercial castile soap contains coconut oil soap to increase its lathering quality. **curd s.** A soap usually made from sodium hydroxide and animal fats and oils. **disinfectant s.** A soap containing some form of disinfectant. **floating s.** A soap in which air bubbles have been incorporated. **green s.** See medicinal soft *s*. **hard s.** A soap made with sodium hydroxide. **hard water s.** Marine soap. **liquid s.** A solution of soap used as an economical and sanitary substitute for soap in public places. **marine s.** A soap for use with sea water or with water containing calcium or magnesium salts. Marine soaps usually contain coconut or palm kernel oil. Also called *salt water soap*. **medicinal soft s.** A potassium soap made by the saponification of vegetable oils, excluding coconut oil and palm kernel oil, without the removal of glycerin; occurs as a soft, unctuous, yellowish white to brownish or greenish yellow mass. Also called *green s., soft s.* **potash s.** A soft soap. See medicinal soft *s*. **soda s.** See hard *s*. **transparent s.** Soap made transparent by the presence of glycerin, alcohol, or sucrose.

sob. A convulsive inspiration due to contraction of the diaphragm and spasmodic closure of the glottis.

so·cal′o·in. Aloin obtained from Socotrine aloes.

so′cial. Gregarious; growing near, or together.

so″ci·ol′o·gy. The science of mutual relations of people and of social organization.

so″ci·o·med′i·cal. Referring to the relationship between social welfare and medicine.

sock′et. The concavity into which a movable part is inserted. **dry s.** Alveolitis after tooth extraction; without suppuration, but associated with pain.

so·cor′di·a. Hallucination.

so′da. Sodium carbonate. **baking s.** Sodium bicarbonate. **caustic s.** Sodium hydroxide. **chlorinated s. solution.** Sodium hypochlorite solution. **sal s.** Sodium carbonate. **s. ash.** Commercial sodium carbonate; essentially anhydrous but containing more or less impurity. **s. lime.** A mixture in granular form of calcium hydroxide with sodium hydroxide or potassium hydroxide or both; occurs as white or grayish white granules. Used to absorb carbon dioxide. **s. lye.** Sodium hydroxide. **s. niter.** Sodium nitrate. **s. water.** Water charged with carbon dioxide gas. **washing s.** Sodium carbonate.

so'di·o·. A combining form denoting *a compound containing sodium.*

so'di·um. Na = 22.997. A metallic element of the alkali group of metals. Light, silver-white, and lustrous when freshly cut, but rapidly oxidizes when exposed to air, becoming dull and gray. Sodium violently decomposes water, forming sodium hydroxide and hydrogen. See Table of Normal Values of Blood Constituents in the Appendix. **diluted s. hypochlorite solution.** Each 100 cc. contains 0.45–0.50 Gm. of NaOCl, equivalent to 0.43–0.48 Gm. of available Cl; occurs as a colorless or faintly yellow liquid. This solution possesses powerful germicidal action and is applied by a method of continuous irrigation. Also called *modified Dakin's solution.* **s. acetate.** NaC₂H₃ O₂.3H₂O. Occurs as colorless, transparent crystals or powder; soluble in water. **s. acetrizoate.** Sodium 3-acetamido-2.4.6-triiodobenzoate, a roentgenographic contrast medium. See *urokon sodium.* **s. acid phosphate.** Sodium biphosphate. **s. alginate.** The sodium salt of alginic acid. A gelatinous substance obtained from various seaweeds. In cold water it dissolves to form a mucilage. **s. ascorbate.** C₆H₇O₆Na. The sodium salt of ascorbic acid. **s. barbital.** Barbital sodium. **s. benzoate.** C₆H₅.COONa. Occurs as a white, granular salt or powder; soluble in water. **s. benzosulfimide.** Saccharin sodium. **s. borate.** Sodium borate. **s. bicarbonate,** NaHCO₃. Occurs as a white, crystalline powder; soluble in water. Used as a mild alkali. **s. biphosphate.** NaH₂PO₄.H₂O. Occurs as colorless crystals or powder; freely soluble in water. Also called *s. dihydrogen phosphate, monosodium orthophosphate, s. acid phosphate.* **s. bismuth iodide.** Sodium iodobismuthite. **s. bismuthyl tartrate.** Bismuth and sodium tartrate. **s. borate.** Na₂ B₄O₇.10H₂O. Occurs as colorless, transparent crystals or powder; soluble in water. Syn., *borax, s. tetraborate.* **s. bromide.** NaBr. Occurs as white crystals or powder; soluble in water. **s. cacodylate.** Na(CH₃)₂AsO₂.3H₂O. Sodium dimethylarsonate; occurs as white crystals or powder; soluble in water. Its uses are similar to those of arsenic. **s. carbonate.** (a) Na₂CO₃. 10H₂O. Usually in colorless, transparent, efflorescent crystals; soluble in water. Syn., *soda, washing soda, sal soda.* (b) Na₂CO₃.H₂O. Monohydrated

sodium carbonate. (c) Na₂CO₃. Anhydrous or exsiccated sodium carbonate. **s. cevitamate.** Sodium ascorbate. **s. chloride.** NaCl. Occurs as colorless crystals or powder; soluble in water. **s. citrate.** Na₃C₆H₅O₇.2H₂O. Occurs as colorless crystals or powder; soluble in water. **s. deficit.** A deficit of water and of some electrolytes results if sodium chloride is withdrawn from the diet. **s. dehydrocholate.** The sodium salt of dehydrocholic acid; occurs as a fine, colorless, crystalline powder; soluble in water. It is useful for its ability to increase the volume of the bile. **s. diethylbarbiturate.** Barbital sodium. Also called *s. diethylmalonylurea.* **s. dihydrogen phosphate.** Sodium biphosphate. **s. diphenylhydantoin.** Diphenylhydantoin sodium. **s. diprotrizoate.** Sodium 3,5-dipropionamide-2,4,6-triiodobenzoate, a roentgenographic contrast medium. See *miokon sodium.* **s. estrone sulfate.** An oral estrogenic hormone. **s. fluoroacetate.** A rodenticide. Also called *compound 1080.* **s. formaldehyde sulfoxylate.** CH₂OHSO₂Na.2H₂O. Occurs as a white, crystalline powder; soluble in water. Used as an antidote for poisoning by bichloride of mercury. **s. glutamate.** Monosodium glutamate. **s. glycerophosphate.** Na₂C₃H₇ (OH)₂PO₄.5½H₂O. Occurs as white, scalelike crystals or powder; soluble in water. **s. gold thiosulfate.** Gold and sodium thiosulfate. **s. hydroxide.** NaOH. Occurs as fused masses, small pellets, flakes, or sticks; soluble in water. Syn., *caustic soda.* **s. hypochlorite solution.** Contains 5% of NaOCl; occurs as a pale, clear, greenish yellow liquid. This solution possesses the germicidal value of its available chlorine. **s. hypophosphite.** NaH₂ PO₂.H₂O. Occurs as white plates or scales or powder; soluble in water. **s. hyposulfite.** Sodium thiosulfate. **s. indigotindisulfonate.** Indigo carmine. **s. iodide.** NaI. Occurs as colorless crystals or powder; soluble in water. **s. iodobismuthite.** A compound formed by the interaction of bismuth chloride and sodium iodide, consisting essentially of hydrated sodium iodobismuthite, Na₃BiI₆. It is claimed to be of value in nerve syphilis. Syn., *s. bismuth iodide.* **s. iodohippurate.** See *hippuran.* **s. lactate.** CH₃.CH OH.COONa. Occurs as a clear or faintly yellow, viscous liquid, containing about 70% of sodium lactate; soluble in water **s. lauryl sulfate.** Chiefly CH₃ (CH₂)₁₀CH₂OSO₃Na. Occurs as white crystals; soluble in water. Used as a wetting agent and substitute for soap. See *duponol C.* **s. levothyroxine.** The sodium salt of the levo isomer of thyroxin (tetraiodothyronine). See *synthroid sodium*. **s. liothyronine.** The sodium salt of the levo isomer of triiodothyronine. See *cytomel*. **s. morrhuate.** A mixture of the sodium salts of the saturated and unsaturated fatty acids occurring in cod liver oil; occurs as a pale, yellowish, granular powder; soluble in water. It is a sclerosing agent. **s. nitrate.** NaNO₃. Colorless, transparent crystals, white granules or powder; soluble in water. Syn., *Chile saltpeter, soda niter*. **s. nitrite.** NaNO₂. Occurs as a white to slightly yellow, granular powder; soluble in water. Used to dilate the general arterial system. **s. para-aminosalicylate.** NH₂.C₆H₃.OH.COONa.2H₂O, a bacteriostatic agent against tubercle bacilli used in treating tuberculosis. **s. pentothal.** See *pentothal sodium*. **s. perborate.** NaBO₃.4H₂O. Occurs as white, crystalline granules or powder; soluble in water. It is used for its antiseptic action. **s. peroxide.** Na₂O₂. The sodium compound analogous to hydrogen peroxide; occurs as a white or yellowish powder; it is soluble in water, with decomposition and evolution of heat, forming an alkaline solution and liberating oxygen. A powerful oxidizing agent. Also called *s. superoxide*. **s. phosphate.** Na₂HPO₄.7H₂O. Occurs as a colorless or white, granular salt; soluble in water. Also called *dibasic s. phosphate, disodium hydrogen phosphate*. **s. potassium bismuthyl tartrate.** A basic water-soluble sodium potassium bismuth tartrate; occurs as a white, heavy powder. Used as a means of obtaining the systemic effects of bismuth in the treatment of syphilis. **s. propionate.** CH₃CH₂COONa. Occurs as colorless crystals or powder; soluble in water. Possesses antibacterial and fungicidal properties. **s. rhodanate.** Sodium thiocyanate. **s. ricinate.** A mixture of the sodium salts of the fatty acids from castor oil, chiefly ricinoleic; occurs as a white or yellowish powder; soluble in water. Has the property of detoxifying bacterial toxins. Also called *s. ricinoleate, s. oleoricinate*. **s. salicylate.** C₆H₄.OH.COONa. Occurs as a white powder; it has not more than a faint pink tinge; soluble in water. It is used as an antirheumatic, antipyretic, and analgesic. **s. stearate.** A mixture of varying proportions of sodium stearate (NaC₁₈H₃₅O₂) and sodium palmitate (NaC₁₆H₃₁O₂). Occurs as a fine, white power; it is slightly soluble in cold water. **s. sulfate.** Na₂SO₄.10H₂O. Occurs as large, colorless, transparent crystals or powder; soluble in water. Also called *Glauber's salt*. **s. sulfocyanate.** Sodium thiocyanate. **s. superoxide.**

Sodium peroxide. **s. tetraborate.** Sodium borate. **s. thiocyanate.** NaSCN. Occurs as white or colorless crystals; it is hygroscopic; soluble in water. Used in hypertension. Syn., *s. sulfocyanate, s. rhodanate*. **s. thiosulfate.** Na₂S₂O₃.5H₂O. Occurs as large, colorless crystals or a coarse, crystalline powder; soluble in water. Also called *s. hyposulfite*. **sulfobromophthalein s.** C₂₀H₈Br₄O₁₀S₂Na₂. The disodium salt of phenoltetrabromophthalein disulfonic acid; occurs as a white, crystalline powder; soluble in water. In aqueous solution it is used as a test of the functional capacity of the liver. Also called *brometragnost*. See also *bromsulphalein*. **tribasic s. phosphate.** Na₃PO₄.12H₂O. Occurs as colorless or white crystals; soluble in water.

sod′om·y. 1. Sexual intercourse by the anus, usually considered as between males. 2. Bestiality, *q.v.*

sof′ten·ing. The act of becoming less cohesive, firm, or resistant. **anemic s.** Disintegration and liquefaction of the brain substance from lack of blood supply. **gray s.** An inflammatory softening of the brain or cord with a gray discoloration. **green s.** A purulent softening of nervous matter. **hemorrhagic s.** The softening of parts involved in a hemorrhage. **red s.** That of the brain when hemorrhage accompanies the ischemic softening, and the products of disintegration of the blood mingle with the nerve substance, giving it a red hue. **s. of the bones.** Osteomalacia. **s. of the brain.** Encephalomalacia. **s. of the heart.** Myomalacia cordis. **s. of the spinal cord.** Various stages in myelitis. **s. of the stomach.** Gastromalacia, consequent upon highly acid contents with a feeble circulation in the walls, but usually a post-mortem phenomenon.

sol. 1. A colloidal solution. A sol consists of a suitable dispersion medium, which may be gas, liquid, or solid, and the colloidal substance, the disperse phase, which is distributed throughout the dispersion medium. The disperse phase may be gas, liquid, or solid. 2. Abbreviation for solution.

so·lan′i·dine (so-lan′i-deen, -din). An alkaloid obtained by decomposing solanine.

sol′a·nine (sol′uh-neen, so′luh·). An alkaloid found in various species of *Solanum*.

So·la′num. A genus of the Solanaceae, including the tomato, potato, bittersweet, and black nightshade.

so′lar·i·za′tion. The application of solar or electric light for therapeutic purposes.

so′lar·ize. Expose to the sun's rays.

so′lar plex′us. Celiac plexus, *q.v.*

sole. The plantar surface of the foot.

so′le·us, so′le′us. A flat muscle of the calf. See Table of Muscles in the Appendix.

sol′id. 1. Firm; dense; not fluid or gaseous. 2. Not hollow.

so·lid″i·fi·ca′tion. The act of becoming solid.

sol′ip·sism. The doctrine that any organism can know only itself and its own conception of its environment.

sol′i·tar″y. Single; existing separately; not collected together, as solitary fasciculus, a strand of nerve fibers in the medulla, the central processes of the sensory fibers of the seventh, ninth, and tenth cranial nerves; and solitary follicles, minute lymphatic nodules in the mucous membrane of the intestine.

Sollmann, Torald Hermann [American pharmacologist, 1874–]. Described the carotid sinus depressor reflex (1912).

sol″u·bil′i·ty. The extent to which a substance (solute) dissolves in a liquid (solvent) to produce a homogeneous system (solution).

sol′u·bil·ize. To make soluble.

sol′u·ble. Capable of mixing with a liquid (dissolving) to form a homogeneous mixture (solution). **s. gluside.** Saccharin sodium. **s. saccharin.** Saccharin sodium.

sol′u·ble gun′cot·ton. Pyroxylin.

so′lum tym′pa·ni (tim′puh-nigh). The floor of the tympanic cavity.

sol′ute (sol′yōōt). The dissolved substance in a solution.

so·lu′tion. A homogeneous mixture of a solid, liquid, or gaseous substance (the solute) in a liquid (the solvent) from which the dissolved substance can be recovered by crystallization or other physical processes. Abbreviated, sol. **ammoniacal silver nitrate s.** An aqueous solution of silver diammino nitrate. Prepared from silver nitrate 70.4 Gm., distilled water 24.5 cc., strong ammonia solution about 68 cc., to make about 100 cc. Occurs as a clear, colorless, almost odorless liquid. Used by dentists to deposit silver in exposed dentine or to fill up minute crevices in the teeth. Also called *Howe's ammoniacal silver nitrate.* **Benedict's s.** A solution containing an easily reduced copper salt; used for the determination of glucose. **buffer s.** A solution which resists any appreciable change in pH on the addition of small amounts of acid or alkali or by dilution with water. **Burow's s.** Aluminum acetate solution. **colloidal s.** A macroscopically homogeneous system consisting of either single, large molecules or aggregations of smaller molecules (the dispersed phase) suspended in a liquid (the continuous phase). Colloidal dis-

persions are frequently called sols. **Dobell's s.** Compound sodium borate solution. **Fehling's s.** A solution containing an easily reduced copper salt; used for the determination of glucose. **hypertonic s.** A solution which has an osmotic pressure greater than that of blood serum. A hypertonic solution of sodium chloride contains more than 0.9 Gm. of sodium chloride in each 100 cc. **hypotonic s.** A solution having an osmotic pressure less than that of blood serum. A hypotonic solution of sodium chloride contains less than 0.9 Gm. of sodium chloride in each 100 cc. **isohydric s.** A solution having the same hydrogen-ion concentration as another so that no change in the concentration of this ion takes place when the solutions are mixed. **isoosmotic s.** A solution having the same osmotic pressure as that of a selected reference solution; often, a synonym for *isotonic solution*, but only when there is no diffusion of solute across the membrane of a tissue immersed in the solution. **isotonic sodium chloride s.** An isotonic solution containing 0.9 Gm. of NaCl in each 100 cc. Also called *normal saline solution, physiological salt solution.* **isotonic s.** A solution which causes no change in the form of a tissue, as erythrocytes, immersed in it. See also isoosmotic *solution.* **Locke-Ringer's s.** Sodium chloride 9 Gm.; potassium chloride 0.42 Gm.; calcium chloride 0.24 Gm.; magnesium chloride 0.2 Gm.; sodium bicarbonate 0.5 Gm.; dextrose 0.5 Gm.; water, recently distilled, to make 1000 cc. **molal s.** A solution which contains one gram-molecular weight or mole of reagent dissolved in 1000 Gm. of solvent. **molar s.** A solution which contains a gram-molecular weight or mole of reagent in 1000 cc. of solution. **Monsel's s.** Ferric subsulfate solution. **normal saline s.** Isotonic sodium chloride solution. **normal salt s.** Isotonic sodium chloride solution. **normal s.** One containing one gram-equivalent weight of reagent in 1000 cc. of solution. **physiological salt s.** Isotonic sodium chloride solution. **Ringer's s.** Contains sodium chloride 8.6 Gm., potassium chloride 0.30 Gm., calcium chloride 0.33 Gm., and distilled water a sufficient quantity to make 1000 cc. Also called *isotonic solution of three chlorides.* **saturated s.** One that normally contains the maximum amount of substance able to be dissolved. Abbreviated, sat. sol. **s. pressure.** The tendency of the molecules or ions to leave the surface of a solute and pass into the solvent. It varies in different solute-solvent combinations. **standard s.** One that contains a definite amount of substance, as a molar or normal solution. **supersaturated s.** One that contains a greater quantity of solid than can normally be dissolved at a given temperature. It is an unstable system. **test s.** A reagent solution. Abbreviated, T. S. **Tyrode s.** A solution containing sodium chloride 8 Gm., calcium chloride 0.2 Gm., potassium chloride 0.2 Gm., sodium bicarbonate 1 Gm., glucose 1 Gm., magnesium chloride 0.1 Gm., sodium diphosphate 0.05 Gm., and distilled water to make 1000 cc. **volumetric s.** A standard solution containing 1, ½, ⅒, etc., gramequivalent of a substance in 1000 cc. of solution. Used in volumetric analysis. Abbreviated, V. S.

ol′vate. A compound formed between solute and solvent in a solution.

ol·va′tion. The process of forming a solvate.

ol′vent. 1. That component of a homogeneous mixture which is in excess. 2. A liquid which dissolves another substance (solute), without any change in chemical composition, as sugar or salt in water. 3. A liquid which reacts chemically with a solid and brings it into solution, as acids which dissolve metals.

o′ma. 1. The entire body with the exclusion of the germ cells. 2. A term used loosely for the body without the limbs. **—somal,** adj.

o″mas·the′ni·a. Old term for bodily deterioration and exhaustion.

o″ma·tes·the′si·a (so″muh-tess-thee′zhuh, -zee-uh). Bodily sensation, the consciousness of the body.

o·mat′ic. 1. Pertaining to the body. 2. Pertaining to the framework of the body and not to the viscera, as the somatic musculature, the muscles of the body wall or somatopleure, as distinguished from those of the splanchnopleure, the splanchnic musculature. **o·mat″i·co·vis′cer·al.** Relating to the body and the viscera.

o′ma·tist. A psychiatrist who regards any psychoneurosis or psychosis as of physical origin.

o″ma·tog′e·ny (so″muh·todj′i·nee). The acquirement of bodily characters, especially the acquirement of characters due to environment. **—somatogen′ic,** adj.

o″ma·tol′o·gy. The study of the development, structure, and functions of the body. **—somatolog′ic,** adj.

o″ma·to·meg′a·ly. Gigantism.

o″ma·tom′e·try. Measurement of the human body with the soft parts intact. **—somatomet′ric,** adj.

o″ma·to·path′ic. Disordered in body.

o′ma·to·plasm″ (so″muh·to·plaz″-im, so·mat′o·). The protoplasm of the body cells; that form of living matter

which composes the mass of the body, as distinguished from germ plasm, which composes the reproductive cells.

so″ma·to·pleure″ (so″muh·to·ploor″, so·mat′o·). The body wall composed of ectoderm and somatic mesoderm, as contrasted with splanchnopleure. **—somatopleur′al,** adj.

so″ma·to·psy′chic (so″muh·to·sigh′kick). Pertaining to both the body and mind.

so″ma·to·to′ni·a. In constitutional medicine, the motivational drive in personality related to functions of the somatic structures—particularly the muscular system—and expressed in bodily assertiveness and directness of manner. The second component of temperament.

so″ma·to·tro′pin. The growth hormone secreted by the adenohypophysis.

so′ma·to·type″. The body type; the quantification of the primary components determining the morphologic structure of an individual. A series of three numerals, each expressing the approximate strength of one of the primary components in a physique.

-some. A combining form meaning body.

so″mes·the′si·a (so″mess·thee′zhuh, -zee·uh). Sensibility to bodily sensations.

-somia, -somus. A combining form denoting a (specified) type of body, used especially in teratology.

so′mite. A segment of the body of an embryo; one of a series of paired segments of the paraxial mesoderm composed of dermatome, myotome, and sclerotome. **—somit′ic,** adj.

som·nam′bu·lism. 1. The condition of half-sleep, in which the senses are but partially suspended; sleepwalking, a condition in which the individual walks during sleep. 2. The type of hypnotic sleep in which the subject is possessed of all his senses, often having the appearance of one awake, but his consciousness is under the control of the hypnotizer.

som·nam·bu·lis′me pro·vo·qué′ (sohm·nam·bew·leess′muh pro·vo·kay′). Sleepwalking induced by hypnotism.

som·nam′bu·list. One who walks in his sleep.

som″ni·fa′cient. 1. Producing sleep. 2. A medicine producing sleep; a hypnotic.

som·nif′er·ous. Producing sleep.

som·nif′u·gous. Driving away sleep.

som·nil′o·quism. The act of talking during sleep.

som·nil′o·quist. One given to talking during sleep.

som″no·cin″e·mat′o·graph. Apparatus for recording, experimentally, movements made during sleep.

som'no·lent. Sleepy. **—somno-lence,** n.

som"no·len'ti·a (som"no·len'shee-uh). 1. Sleep-drunkenness, a condition of incomplete sleep in which a part of the faculties are abnormally excited, while the others are in repose. 2. Somnolence.

som"no·les'cent. 1. Drowsy. 2. Inducing drowsiness.

som'no·lism. Hypnotism.

som'nus. Sleep.

-somus. Same as -somia.

sone. The unit of loudness.

so·nom'e·ter. An instrument for determining the pitch of sounds and their relation to the musical scale.

so·phis"ti·ca'tion. The adulteration or imitation of a substance.

soph"o·ma'ni·a. Megalomania in which an individual believes himself to excel in wisdom.

So·pho'ra. A genus of the Leguminosae; grows mainly in warm regions. Yields poisonous seeds.

soph'o·rine (sof'o·reen, so'fo·). $C_{11}H_{14}ON_2$. A paralyzant, poisonous alkaloid which exists in the seeds of some species of *Sophora, Cytisus,* and *Baptisia.*

so'por. Sleep, especially the profound sleep symptomatic of a morbid condition.

so"po·rif'ic, sop"o·rif'ic. 1. Producing sleep. 2. A sleep producer. 3. Narcotic.

sop'o·rose, so'po·rose. Sleepy; characterized by morbid sleep.

sor'bi·tol. $C_6H_{14}O_6$. D-Sorbitol, a hexahydric alcohol isomeric with mannitol; occurs as colorless or white, sweet crystals; soluble in water. Used as an osmotic dehydrating agent and diuretic.

D-sor'bose. $C_6H_{12}O_6$. A ketohexose obtained from the juice of fruits containing sorbitol, after oxidation by *Bacterium xylinum.*

sor'des (sor'deez). Filth, dirt, especially the crusts that accumulate on the teeth and lips in continued fevers.

sor'did. In biology, of a dull or dirty color.

sore. 1. Painful; tender. 2. An ulcer or wound. **canker s.** Small ulceration of the mucous membrane of the mouth. Some may be due to a food allergy. **coldsore.** Herpes facialis. **primary s.** The initial lesion, chancre, of syphilis. Also called *hard s.* **venereal s.** See *chancre.*

Sørensen, Søren Peter Lauritz [Danish chemist, 1868–1939]. Introduced the symbol pH, used in expressing hydrogen-ion concentration; called Sørensen's symbol. *Sørensen's indicators* are the indicators of hydrogen-ion concentration.

sor'ghum. A group of annual fodder grasses of the family Gramineae from which a sugar and syrup are obtained

so·ro'che (so·ro'chay). Altitude sickness, q.v.

so·ro"ri·a'tion. The development which takes place in the female breast at puberty.

sor'rel. A plant of the genus *Rumex* containing oxalates. **salt of s.** Potassium binoxalate.

S. O. S. *Si opus sit,* if necessary.

souf'fle (soo'ful). A blowing sound; an auscultatory murmur. **fetal s.** An inconstant murmur heard over the uterus during pregnancy. **funic s.** A hissing sound, synchronous with the fetal heart sounds, heard over the abdomen of a pregnant woman, and supposed to be produced in the umbilical cord.

sou'ma. A trypanosomiasis of domestic hoofed animals in Africa, transmitted by tsetse flies and marked by serous exudates into the body cavity.

sound. The sensation produced by stimulation of the auditory nerve by vibrations transmitted by the endolymph. **bell s.** That produced in pneumothorax by striking a coin placed flat upon the chest, with another coin. It can be heard through a stethoscope placed over the affected side. Also called *bell tympany, coin s.* **cracked-pot s.** A form of tympanitic resonance indicative of a cavity. **fetal heart sounds.** The sounds produced by the beating of the fetal heart, best heard near the umbilicus of the mother. **friction s.** The sound heard in auscultation, as a result of the rubbing together of adjacent parts, as of the pleurae, the pericardium, or the peritoneum, when the layers are dry or are roughened. **heart sounds.** The two sounds heard over the cardiac area. The first, dull and prolonged, is said to sound like *lubb,* and is isochronous with the systole of the ventricles. The second, sharp and short, is said to sound like *dup,* and is isochronous with the closure of the semilunar valves. **kettle-singing s.** A chest sound sometimes heard in incipient pulmonary tuberculosis. It resembles the sound of water boiling in a kettle. **to-and-fro s.** The friction sound of pericarditis and pleuritis.

sound. An instrument for introduction into a channel or cavity, for determining the presence of constriction, foreign bodies, or other morbid conditions, and for treatment. **esophageal s.** A long, flexible sound for examination of the esophagus. **lacrimal s.** A fine sound for exploring or dilating the lacrimal duct. **urethral s.** An elongated steel instrument, usually slightly conical, for examination and dilatation of the urethra. **uterine s.** A graduated probe for measurement of the uterine cavity.

our'wood". *Oxydendrum arboreum,* a tree of the Ericaceae. The leaves have a sour taste; has been used as a diuretic.

oy'bean", so'ya bean. The seed of *Glycine soja* (*Glycine hispida, Soja hispida*), a legume native to Asia but now cultivated in other regions, particularly the United States, because of the high food and commercial value of its seeds. The bean contains protein, fixed oil, carbohydrates, crude fiber, and several enzymes. Also called *soja bean.*

o"zo·i·od'o·late (so"zo-eye-od'o-late, ·eye'o-da-late). A salt of sozoiodolic acid.

o"zo·i"o·dol'ic ac'id. $C_6H_2I_3(SO_3H)OH$. A crystalline, odorless powder used as an antiseptic, disinfectant, and parasiticide, chiefly in the form of its salts. Also called *sozoiodole.*

p. *Spiritus,* spirit.

pa. A mineral spring, especially one having medicinal value and visited as a health resort.

pace. A delimited area or region. **—spa'tial,** *adj.* **dead s.** (a) A cavity left after the closure of a wound. (b) That space in the trachea, bronchi, and air passages in general which contains air that does not reach the alveoli during respiration, the amount of air being about 140 cc. **intervillous spaces.** Spaces within the placenta developed from the trophoblastic lacunas and the dilated maternal veins, with which the maternal vessels communicate. **ischiorectal s.** See ischiorectal *fossa.* **midpalmar s.** A deep fascial space beneath the flexor tendons on the ulnar side of the palm. Syn., *medial palmar s.* **palmar spaces.** The lateral and medial potential fascial spaces in the hand between the thenar and hypothenar areas, separated by a fibrous septum and filled with areolar tissue. **perilymphatic spaces.** Small, irregular cavities filled with perilymph, between the membranous and bony labyrinths of the internal ear. **peritoneal spaces.** Potential spaces within the peritoneum formed by the various reflections from the parietes and abdominal viscera. **perivascular spaces.** Fluid-filled spaces between the adventitia of the blood vessels of the brain-substance and the pial limiting membrane, lined with endothelial cells, connecting with the subarachnoid space. Also called *spaces of Virchow-Robin.* **rectovesical s.** The rectovesical pouch; the space between the bladder and the rectum. **retroperitoneal s.** That behind the peritoneum, but in front of the spinal column and lumbar muscles; in it lie

the kidneys, the aorta, the inferior vena cava, and the sympathetic trunk. **retropharyngeal s.** That behind the pharynx, containing areolar tissue. **semilunar s.** A percussion area on the left anterior portion of the thorax, overlying the stomach. Also called *Traube's s.* **subarachnoid s.** The space between the arachnoid and the pia proper, containing subarachnoid trabeculae and filled with cerebrospinal fluid. **subdural s.** The space between the dura and the arachnoid which normally contains only a capillary layer of fluid. **subphrenic s.** One of the two spaces, right and left, between the diaphragm and the liver, on either side of the falciform ligament. **suprasternal s.** The triangular space above the manubrium, enclosed by the layers of the deep cervical fascia which are attached to the front and back of this bone. Formerly called *s. of Burns.* **thenar s.** A deep fascial space beneath the flexor tendons of the index and, occasionally, of the middle finger and overlying the second metacarpal bone. Syn., *lateral midpalmar s.*

spa·gyr'ic. Pertaining to the obsolete chemical, alchemistic, or Paracelsian school of medicine. **—spag'yrist,** *n.* **spag'y·rism** (spadj'i-riz-um). The Paracelsian, or spagyric, school or doctrine of medicine.

Span'ish wind'lass. An improvised tourniquet consisting of a handkerchief knotted about a limb and tightened by means of a stick which is twisted.

spans. Trade-mark for a series of long chain fatty acid partial esters of hexitol anhydrides such as those of sorbitol and mannitol. The substances are used as wetting agents, emulsifiers, and solubilizing agents. See *tweens.*

spar'a·drap. A plaster spread on cotton, linen, silk, leather, paper; adhesive plaster.

spar"ga·no'sis. Infestation with *Sparganum,* which is a larval stage of the fish tapeworms.

Spar·ga'num, Spar'ga·num (pl. *Spargana*). A generic name applied to the plerocercoid larva of *Diphyllobothrium,* especially if the adult form is unknown. **S. mansoni.** A species seen in the Far East, which is frequently found in the eye. Infestation probably follows contact with freshly killed frogs. **S. mansonoides.** A species which infests mice and has also been reported in the muscles and subcutaneous tissues of man. **S. proliferum.** A species which proliferates in the tissues of the host by branching and budding off large numbers of spargana. The adult form is unknown.

spar·go'sis. Enlargement or distention, as of the breasts due to accumulation of milk.

sparine hydrochloride. Trademark for promazine hydrochloride.

spark. A light flash, usually electric in origin, as that emanating from an electrode through which a current is passing.

spar′te·ine (spahr′tee-een, ·in, spahr′teen). (C₁₅H₂₆N₂). A liquid alkaloid obtained from *Cytisus scoparius*; slightly soluble in water. **s. sulfate.** C₁₅H₂₆N₂.H₂SO₄.5H₂O; occurs as colorless crystals or powder; soluble in water. Has been used chiefly in the treatment of irregularities of the heart.

spasm. A sudden muscular contraction. **Bell′s s.** Convulsive facial tic. **bronchial s.** Asthma. **cadaveric s.** Early, or at times immediate, appearance of rigor mortis; seen after death from certain causes. The muscle spasm actually causes movements of the limbs. **carpopedal s.** A spasm of the hands and feet, or of the thumbs and great toes; associated with tetany. **clonic s.** (a) A spasm broken by relaxations of the muscles. (b) In the area of the accessory nerve it is called spasmodic torticollis, *q.v.* (c) In the area of the facial nerve it is called painless tic, *q.v.* **cynic s.** A contraction of the facial muscles upon one side, so as to expose the teeth. **facial s.** A peculiar clonic contraction of the muscles surrounding the eye, or else involving one entire side of the face. **fatigue spasms.** A group of affections characterized by spasmodic contractions, either clonic or tonic, brought about by voluntary movement, the exciting cause being limited to some particular action. Also called *business spasms, coördinated business neuroses, functional spasms, handicraft spasms, movement spasms, occupational spasms, professional spasms.* **fixed s.** Permanent or continuous tetanic rigidity of one or more muscles. **habit s.** Half voluntary spasmodic movements, the result of habit, sometimes called *habit chorea.* **histrionic s.** A condition in which local involuntary twitchings of the face, acquired in childhood, persist during adult life, and are increased by emotional causes. **inspiratory s.** A spasmodic contraction of nearly all the inspiratory muscles. **laryngeal congenital s.** A peculiar stridor developing at birth, and disappearing after one or two years. **lock s.** A form of writer's cramp in which the fingers become locked on the pen. **mimic s.** Facial tic. **mobile s.** Slow, irregular movements following hemiplegia. **myopathic s.** One attending a disease of muscles. **nodding s.** One characterized by nodding of the head. **phonic s.** A spasm of the laryngeal muscles occurring on attempting to speak. **retrocollic s.**

Spasm of the muscles at the back [of] the neck, causing retraction of t[he] head. **salaam s.** Clonic spasm cau[s]ing bowing movements. **saltatory s[.]** A clonic spasm that causes the patie[nt] to leap or jump when he attempts [to] stand. **sewing s.** An occupation[al] spasm seen in tailors, seamstresse[s] and shoemakers. **smith′s s.** An occ[u]pational spasm with associated hem[i]plegia. Also called *hephestic hemipl[e]gia.* **s. of accommodation.** Spas[m] of the ciliary muscles, in attempti[ng] accommodation for objects nearb[y]. **synclonic s.** Tremulous agitatio[n.] **tailor′s s.** An occupational neuros[is] occurring in tailors, characterized [by] spasm of the muscles of the arm a[nd] hand. Also called *tailor's cram[p.]* **tonic s.** A spasm that persists with[.] out relaxation for some time. **toxic [s.]** One due to poison. **winking s.** [A] habit tic of spasmodic twitching [or] blinking of the eyelids. Also call[ed] *spasmus nictitans.*

spasmalgin. Trade-mark for a tab[let] or injection containing papaverine h[y]drochloride, pantopon, and atrinal. T[he] preparations are used as an analge[sic] and antispasmodic.

spas′mo- (spaz′mo-). A combini[ng] form denoting *pertaining to a spasm.*

spas·mod′ic (spaz-mod′ick). Pertai[n]ing to, or characterized by, spasm.

spas·mol′o·gy (spaz-mol′o-jee). T[he] sum of scientific knowledge of t[he] nature and the causes of spasms a[nd] convulsions.

spas″mo·phil′i·a. A morbid ten[d]ency to convulsions, and to ton[ic] spasms, such as those observed [in] tetany. **—spasmophilic,** *adj.*

spas′mus (spaz′mus). A spas[m.] **s. nictitans.** Spasmodic action [of] the orbicularis oculi muscle, causing [a] winking movement of the lid. **s. n[u]tans.** Rhythmic nodding and eye jer[k]ing in infants.

spas′tic. Pertaining to, or characte[r]ized by, spasm; produced by spasm.

spas·tic′i·ty (spas-tiss′i-tee). An i[n]creased tonus or tension of a mus[cle] which is associated with an exagger[a]tion of deep reflexes, and frequent[ly] with clonus and a partial or comple[te] loss of voluntary control. **clas[p-]knife s.** The resistance of a mus[cle] to passive extension followed by a su[d]den relaxation, like the snapping of [a] clasp-knife blade.

spa′ti·um (spay′shee-um). Space, *q[.v.]*

spat′u·la. A flexible blunt blade; us[ed] for spreading ointment. **—spatulat[e,]** *adj.*

spay. Remove the ovaries.

spear′mint. Consists of the dr[ied] leaf and flowering top of *Ment[ha] spicata* (*Mentha viridis*). Contains [a] volatile oil. **s. oil.** A volatile oil o[f]

tained from the overground parts of the flowering plant *Mentha spicata*, containing carvone, used as a flavoring.

pe'cial·ist. One who limits his practice to certain diseases, or to the diseases of a single organ or class, or to a certain type of therapy. —**specialize,** *v.*

pe'cial·ty. The branch of medicine or surgery pursued by a specialist.

pe'cies (spee'sheez). 1. A group of individuals, similar in certain morphologic and physiologic characteristics which distinguish them from other groups with which they may be united on the basis of other characters into a higher group, the genus; the species also may fall into groups of minor rank, as subspecies, varieties, races. 2. A name sometimes applied to certain mixtures of herbs used in making decoctions and infusions.

pe·cif'ic. 1. Of or pertaining to a species, or to that which distinguishes a thing or makes it of the species to which it belongs. 2. A medicine that has a distinct curative influence on a particular disease, as quinine on malaria or mercury on syphilis. 3. Produced by a certain microörganism, as a specific disease; in a restricted sense, syphilitic.

pec''i·fic'i·ty (spess*''*i·fiss'i·tee). The quality of being specific. **species s.** The difference in physiologic response to one or more compounds by different species of animals.

pec'ta·cles. Framed or mounted lenses for aiding vision where there are optical or muscular defects of the eye. See *lens*. **prismatic s.** Spectacles with prismatic lenses, either alone or combined with spherical or cylindrical lenses. **protective s.** Lenses that shield the eyes from light, dust, heat. **pec'tro-.** A combining form denoting relating to a *spectrum*.

pec''tro·col''or·im'e·ter (·kul''ur·im'i·tur). Combination of spectroscope and ophthalmoscope for the detection of color blindness to one spectral color.

pec'tro·graph. A spectroscope which records a spectrum on a photographic plate. **mass s.** An instrument used for determining the mass of atoms or molecules by producing charged ions and measuring their deflection in a magnetic field.

pec·trom'e·ter. A spectroscope provided with equipment for measuring the deviations of light and other electromagnetic rays and therewith the wave lengths of spectral lines. —**spectrometry,** *n.*

pec''tro·pho·tom'e·ter. Combination of spectrometer and photometer for making quantitative measurements

in various parts of the visible, ultraviolet, or infrared spectrum. —**spectrophotometry,** *n.*

spec''tro·po''lar·im'e·ter. Combination of a spectrometer and polariscope; used for measuring optical rotation produced by certain solutions.

spec'tro·scope. An instrument for dispersing radiations by various methods, such as a prism, diffraction gratings, and crystals, and for observing the resultant spectrum. —**spectroscop'ic,** *adj.;* **spectros'copy,** *n.*

spec'trum (pl. *spectrums, spectra*). 1. The series of images resulting when a beam of electromagnetic waves (such as electric waves, infrared, visible light, ultraviolet, or x-rays), is dispersed and the constituent waves are arranged according to their frequencies or wave lengths. 2. Figuratively, any series of entities arranged according to the quantitative variation of a given property. 3. Figuratively, range. —**spectral,** *adj.* **absorption s.** Spectrum of radiation, which has passed through some selectively absorbing substance, as white light after it has passed through a vapor. **antibiotic s.** The range of activity of an antibiotic against different bacteria. Also called *antibacterial s., bacteriostatic s.* —**comparison s.** The arrangement side by side of the spectrums of two different substances. **continuous s.** A spectrum without sudden variations, representing a continuous variation of wave lengths from one end to the other. **emission s.** Spectrum of the radiation which a substance emits. The opposite of absorption spectrum, *q.v.* **solar s.** The spectrum afforded by the refraction of sunlight.

spec'u·lum. An instrument for dilating the opening of a cavity of the body in order that the interior may be more easily visible, as vaginal speculum, rectal speculum, nasal speculum, aural speculum. **anal s.** An instrument of varying design similar to a nasal speculum, but with longer blades which allows examination of the lower portion of the rectum. **aural s.** A small, hollow instrument with an expanded end, which may be introduced into the ear for examination of the external auditory canal and the tympanic membrane. **duckbill s.** A bivalve vaginal speculum with flat, broad blades. **eye s.** An instrument for retracting the eyelids. **nasal s.** A small bivalve instrument with handles, which dilates the nostril and allows examination of the nasal passages.

speech. 1. The faculty of expressing thought by spoken words; the act of speaking. 2. The words spoken. **ataxic s.** The intermittent, explosive speech resulting from cerebellar disorders.

bulbar s. The thick speech occurring when the nuclei of the medulla concerned with speech are damaged or when there is injury to both corticobulbar tracts. **interjectional s.** The expression of emotions by inarticulate sounds. **mirror s.** Defective speech characterized by pronouncing words or syllables backward. **scanning s.** A slow and measured form of speech with pauses between syllables. Characteristic of diffuse lesions of the cerebellum and brain stem, particularly common in multiple sclerosis. **slurred s.** The tremulous, feeble, careless speech which is characteristic of lesions of the basal ganglions. **syllabic s.** A form of dysphasia with halting, stumbling articulation.

sperm. 1. A spermatozoon; the mature male germ cell. Syn., *sperm cell.* 2. An inexact term for the seminal fluid.

sper″ma·cet′i (spur″muh·set′ee, ·see′tee). A waxy substance obtained from the head of the sperm whale, *Physeter macrocephalus.* The chief constituent is cetyl palmitate or cetin. Used chiefly to add firmness to ointment bases.

sperm as′ter. The radiating structure which precedes the sperm nucleus as it advances within the egg.

sper″ma·ta·cra′si·a (spur″muh·tuh·kray′zhuh, ·zee·uh). Deficiency or decrease of spermatozoa in the semen. Also called *spermacrasia.*

sper·mat′ic. 1. Pertaining to the semen. 2. Conveying the semen, as the spermatic cord. 3. Pertaining to the spermatic cord, as the spermatic fascia.

sper″ma·ti·ci′dal. Destructive to spermatozoa.

sper′ma·to-, spermat-. A combining form meaning *seed, germ.*

sper″ma·to·cele (spur′muh·to·seel″, spur·mat′o·). Cystic dilatation of a duct in the head of the epididymis or in the rete testis. Rupture into the tunica vaginalis produces spermatic hydrocele.

sper″ma·to·ce·lec′to·my. Excision of a spermatocele, or cyst of the epididymis.

sper″ma·to·ci′dal. Destructive to spermatozoa.

sper″ma·to·cys·ti′tis. Inflammation of the seminal vesicles.

sper″ma·to·cys·tot′o·my. Surgical incision of a seminal vesicle.

sper″ma·to·cyte″ (spur′muh·to·sight″, spur·mat′o·). A cell of the last or next to the last generation of cells which divide to form mature male germ cells. **primary s.** A developing sperm cell in the growth phase preceding the first meiotic division. **secondary s.** One of the two cells produced by the first meiotic division.

sper″ma·to·gen′e·sis. The phenomena involved in the production of mature male germ cells, sometimes restricted to denote the process of meiosis in the male.

sper″ma·to·go′ni·um (pl. *spermatogonia*). One of the primitive male germ cells. The primary spermatocytes arise from the last generation of spermatogonia by an increase in size.

sper′ma·toid. Resembling a sperm cell.

sper″ma·tol′y·sin (spur″muh·tol′i·sin, spur″muh·to·lye′sin). A substance causing dissolution of sperm cells.

sper″ma·top′a·thy. Disease of the sperm cells or of their secreting mechanism.

sper″ma·tor·rhe′a, sper″ma·tor·rhoe′a. Involuntary discharge of semen without orgasm.

sper″ma·to·xo′a. Plural of spermatozoon, q.v.

sper″ma·to·zo′on (pl. *spermatozoa*). The mature male germ cell —**spermatozoal,** adj.

sper″ma·tu′ri·a. The presence of semen in the urine.

sperm cen′ter. The centrosome which precedes the sperm nucleus as it advances within the egg. In flagellate spermatozoa it arises from the middle piece.

sperm·ec′to·my. Resection of part of the ductus deferens.

sperm head. The head of a spermatozoon.

sper′mi·cide. An agent that destroys spermatozoa. Syn., *spermatocide.*

sper′min, sper′mine. Diamino propyltetramethylene-diamine, H_2N $(CH_2)_3NH(CH_2)_4NH(CH_2)_3NH_2$, found in the form of a phosphate in semen and other animal fluids and tissues; its exact function is unknown. Has been used in the treatment of nervous disorders.

sper′mo·lith. A calculus in a ductus deferens or seminal vesicle.

sp. g. Specific gravity.

sp. gr. Specific gravity.

sph. Spherical or spherical lens.

sphac″e·la′tion (sfass″i·lay′shun). Necrosis, gangrene, mortification —**sphac′elate,** v.

sphac′e·lism (sfass′i·liz·um). The condition of being affected by sphacelus.

sphac″e·lo·der′ma (sfass″i·lo·dur′muh). Gangrene of the skin from any one of many different causes.

sphac′e·lus (sfass′i·lus). A slough —**sphac′eloid, sphac′elous,** adj.

spha″gi·as′mus (sfay″jee·az′mus). Epileptic spasm of the muscles of the neck.

spha·gi′tis. 1. Inflammation of jugular vein. 2. Sore throat.

sphe´no-, sphen-. A combining form meaning *wedge*; used to denote *pertaining to the sphenoid bone.*

sphe´´no·ceph´a·ly. The condition of having a wedge-shaped head.

sphe´noid. 1. Wedge-shaped, as the sphenoid bone. 2. The sphenoid bone. See Table of Bones in the Appendix.

sphe´noid·i´tis. Inflammation of the sphenoid sinus.

sphe´´noid·ot´o·my. Incision into the sphenoid sinus.

sphe´´no·pal´a·tine (sfee´´no·pal´uh·tyne, ·teen). Pertaining to the sphenoid bone and the palate, as the sphenopalatine foramen.

sphe·no´sis. The wedging of the fetus in the pelvis.

sphe´´no·tre´si·a (sfee´´no·tree´shuh, ·shuh). A variety of craniotomy in which the basal portion of the fetal skull is perforated.

sphe´no·tribe. An instrument for crushing the basal portion of the fetal skull.

sphere. 1. A ball or globe. 2. A space. —**spher´ic, spher´ical,** *adj.*

sphe´´res·the´si·a, sphe´´raes·the´si·a (sfeer´´ess·thee´zhuh, ·zee·uh). Perverted feeling, as of the contact of a ball or globe-shaped body.

sphe´ro·cyte. An erythrocyte which is spherical in form rather than biconcave.

sphe´´ro·cy·to´sis (sfeer´´o·sigh·to´sis). Anemia in which the red cells are changed to a more or less spherical shape.

sphe´roid. 1. Resembling a sphere. 2. A solid resembling a sphere.

sphe·rom´e·ter. An instrument for determining the degree of curvature of a sphere or part of a sphere, especially of optical lenses, or of the tools used for grinding them.

spher´ule. A minute sphere.

sphinc´ter. A muscle surrounding and closing an orifice. See Table of Muscles in the Appendix. —**sphinc·ter´ic,** *adj.* **anal s.** Either of the sphincter ani muscles. **cardiac s.** The circular muscle fibers around the cardiac end of the esophagus. **pyloric s.** The thickened, ringlike band of the circular layer of smooth muscle at the lower end of the pyloric canal of the stomach. **s. pupillae.** The circular band of smooth muscle of the iris which decreases the size of the pupil of the eye. **s. urethrae.** (a) The **sphincter urethrae membranaceae,** composed of bundles of voluntary muscle which surround the membranous portion of the urethra in the male; in the female the analogous muscle fibers surround the proximal portion of the urethra. See Table of Muscles in the Appendix. (b) The **sphincter vesicae,** composed of

bundles of smooth muscle which are a part of the tunica muscularis of the bladder; the fibers are looped around the neck of the bladder, thus forming an involuntary urethral sphincter.

sphinc´´ter·al´gi·a. Pain in the sphincter ani muscle, or about the anus.

sphinc´´ter·ec´to·my. Oblique blepharotomy; Stellwag's operation for the dilatation of the palpebral fissure, or for blepharospasm.

sphinc´´ter·is´mus (sfink´´tur·iz´mus). A spasmodic contraction of the sphincter ani muscle, usually attendant upon fissure or ulcer of the anus, but occasionally occurring independently of such lesion.

sphinc´´ter·i´tis. Inflammation of a sphincter, especially the anal sphincter.

sphinc´´ter·ol´y·sis. The operation of freeing the iris in anterior synechia.

sphinc´ter·o·plas´´ty. A plastic or reparative operation on a sphincter muscle.

sphinc´´ter·ot´o·my. The operation of incising a sphincter.

sphin´gol. Sphingosine, *q.v.*

sphin´go·my´e·lin. A phospholipid occurring in brain, kidney, liver, and egg yolk. It is composed of choline, sphingosine, phosphoric acid, and a fatty acid.

sphin´go·sine (sfing´go·seen, ·sin). A basic, unsaturated amino-alcohol occurring in sphingomyelin and the cerebrosides. Syn., *sphingol.*

sphyg´mo-. A combining form meaning *pulse.*

sphyg´´mo·bo·lom´e·ter. An instrument for measuring and recording the force of the pulse. —**sphygmobolometry,** *n.*

sphyg´´mo·chron´o·graph (sfig´mo·kron´o·graf, ·kro´no·graf). A registering sphygmograph.

sphyg´´mo·chro·nog´ra·phy. The registration of the extent and oscillations of the pulse wave.

sphyg·mod´ic (sfig·mod´ick, ·mo´dick). Like the pulse; throbbing.

sphyg´´mo·dy´´na·mom´e·ter (·dye´´na·mom´i·tur, ·din´uh·). An instrument for measuring the force of the pulse.

sphyg´mo·graph´´. An instrument for recording graphically the features of the pulse and the variations in blood pressure. —**sphygmograph´ic,** *adj.*

sphyg·mog´ra·phy. A description of the pulse, its pathologic variations and their significance.

sphyg´moid. Resembling or having the nature of continuous pulsation.

sphyg´´mo·ma·nom´e·ter. An instrument for measuring the tension of the blood current or arterial pressure. —**sphygmomanometry,** *n.*

sphyg´´mo·os´´cil·lom´e·ter. A form of sphygmomanometer in which the systolic and diastolic blood pressures are indicated by an oscillating device.

sphyg″mo·pal·pa′tion. The palpation of the pulse.

sphyg′mo·phone. A sphygmograph in which the vibrations of the pulse produce a sound.

sphyg′mo·scope. A pulse pressure recorder in which the force of arterial pressure is made visible. There are numerous mechanical devices for accomplishing this result.

sphyg″mo·sys′to·le (sfĭg″mo·sĭs′to·lee). That part of the sphygmogram produced under the influence of the cardiac systole upon the pulse.

sphyg″mo·tech′ny (sfĭg″mo·teck″nee, sfĭg″mo·teck′nee). The art of diagnosis and prognosis by means of the pulse.

sphyg″mo·to·no·graph. An instrument which records pulsations from an inflatable rubber cuff; systolic and diastolic pressures are read by this means.

sphyg″mo·to·nom′e·ter. An instrument for measuring blood pressure.

sphyg′mus. The pulse; a pulsation. **—sphygmous,** adj.

spi′ca. 1. A spike or spur. 2. A spiral bandage with reversed turns.

spice. An aromatic vegetable substance used for flavoring; a condiment.

spic′u·la, spic′ule. 1. A small spike-shaped bone or fragment of bone. 2. A needle-shaped body; a spike. **—spicular,** adj. **bony s.** A needle-shaped bone or fragment of bone.

spi′der. An animal of the order Araneida of the class Arachnida, characterized by having four pairs of legs, usually eight eyes, and an unsegmented abdomen. **black widow s.** The species *Latrodectus mactans,* a black spider with globose abdomen. The adult has an hourglass-shaped red or yellow spot on the ventral side. The female is about 0.5 in. long, the male about half as big as the female. Its bite has been fatal in about 5% of the reported cases. Also called *knoppie s.*

Spies, Tom Douglas [*American physician,* 1902–1960]. Distinguished for contributions in the field of vitamins and vitamin deficiency diseases. Demonstrated that folic acid is an erythrocyte maturation factor (1945–46).

Spi·ge′li·a (spy·jee′lee·uh). Pinkroot, a genus of plants of the family Loganiaceae.

spike′nard (spike′nurd, ·nard). 1. A name given to the rhizome of various species of *Valeriana* or closely related genera. 2. American spikenard.

spill. An overflow, especially that of blood. Also applied to certain forms of cellular metastasis in malignant disease.

spi′lus. A mole or colored mark on the skin; nevus.

spi′na (pl. *spinae*). A sharp projection. See *spine.* **s. bifida.** A congenital defect in the closure of the spinal canal with hernial protrusion of the meninges of the cord. The hernial sac contains cerebrospinal fluid and sometimes nervous tissue. Most common in the lumbosacral region. Also called *rachischisis.* **s. bifida occulta.** A defect in the closure of the spinal canal without hernial protrusion of the meninges usually diagnosed only by x-ray.

spi′nal cord. See under *cord.*

spi′nal man. A patient in a prolonged state of spinal shock, following complete transection of the spinal cord.

spin′dle. 1. A tapering rod. A fusiform shape. 2. That part of the achromatic figure in mitosis between the centrosomes or asters, consisting of modified cytoplasm and spindle fibers. **neuromuscular s.** Small fusiform sensory end-organs found in almost all the muscles of the body. **s. cataract.** A form of cataract characterized by spindle-shaped opacity extending from the posterior surface of the anterior portion of the capsule to the anterior surface of the posterior portion of the capsule, with a central dilatation. **tendon s.** A specialized, encapsulated sensory nerve end-organ in tendon adjacent to muscular tissue. Also called *neurotendinal s.*

spin′dle-leg″ged. Having long, thin legs.

spine. 1. A sharp process of bone. 2. The backbone or spinal column. Also see *tubercle.* **—spi′nous, spi′nal,** adj. **bifid s.** A complete or incomplete congenital cleft of the vertebral column; a posterior fusion defect of the vertebral arches. Also called *spina bifida.* **iliac spines.** Four spines of the ilium. The anterior extremity of the iliac crest forms the **anterior superior iliac spine;** the posterior extremity, the **posterior superior iliac spine.** The **anterior inferior iliac spine** is that on the anterior border of the ilium, and the **posterior inferior iliac spine** is that on the posterior border, separated from the respective superior spine by a notch. **occult bifid s.** A simple variety of spinal non-union in the lumbar or thoracolumbar region, with few or no symptoms. Often revealed only by the presence of a dimple in the skin. Also called *spina bifida occulta.* **s. of ischium.** A pointed eminence on the posterior border of the body of the ischium. It forms the lower border of the greater sciatic notch. Also called *ischial s.* **s. of the scapula.** The strong, triangular plate of bone attached obliquely to the dorsum of the scapula and dividing it into two un-equal parts, the supraspinous and in-fraspinous fossae.

spi″no·gal″va·ni·za′tion. Galvanization of the spinal cord.

spi′no·graph″. A radiograph of the spine.

spin′ther·ism. Sensation of sparks before the eyes. See scintillating *scotoma.*

spin″u·lo′sin, spin′u·lo·sin. An antibiotic substance from *Penicillium spinulosum* and *Aspergillus fumigatus.*

spi·rad″e·no′ma (spy·rad″i·no′-muh). Adenoma of the sweat glands.

spi′ral. 1. Winding screwlike, as a spiral bandage. 2. A curve having a spiral course.

Spi·ril′le·ae (spy·ril′ee·ee). A tribe of the family Pseudomonadaceae which includes the genus *Vibrio.*

spir″il·li·ci′dal (spirr″il·i·sigh′dul, spy·ril″i·). Capable of destroying spiral bacilli.

spir″il·lo′sis (spirr″i·lo′sis, spy″ri·). A disease caused by infection with one of the spiral bacilli. See rat bite *fever, Spirillum.*

Spi·ril′lum (spy·ril′um). A genus of spiral bacilli of the tribe Spirilleae and of the family Pseudomonadaceae. **S. minus.** The causative agent of rat bite fever.

spir′it. 1. An alcoholic solution of a volatile principle, formerly prepared by distillation but now generally prepared by dissolving the volatile substance in alcohol. 2. Any distilled liquid. Abbreviated, sp. **cologne s.** Ethanol. **colonial s.** Methanol. **columbian s.** Methanol. **methylated s.** Denatured ethanol.

spi′ro-, spir-. 1. A combining form meaning *a coil;* used to denote *spiral.* 2. A combining form denoting *respiration.*

Spi″ro·chae′ta (spy″ro·kee′tuh). A genus of spiral microörganisms of the family Spirochaetaceae. **S. morsus muris.** See *Spirillum minus.* **S. obermeieri.** See *Borrelia recurrentis.* **S. pallida.** See *Treponema pallidum.*

Spi″ro·chae·ta′ce·ae (spy″ro·ki·tay′see·ee). A family of spiral microorganisms which includes the genera *Spirochaeta, Saprospira,* and *Cristospira.* The family is nonpathogenic for man; a few species of *Cristospira* are parasites of crustaceans, all other species are free-living forms.

Spi″ro·chae·ta′les (spy″ro·ki·tay′leez). An order of spiral microörganisms which includes the families Spirochaetaceae and Treponemataceae.

pi′ro·chete (spy′ro·keet). Any of the spiral microörganisms belonging to the order Spirochaetales. **—spiro·che′tal,** *adj.*

spi″ro·che·te′mi·a (spy″ro·ki·tee′-mee·uh). The presence of spirochetes in the blood.

spi″ro·che′ti·cide (spy″ro·kee′ti-side). An agent which kills spirochetes.

spi″ro·che·tol′y·sis (spy″ro·ki·tol′-i·sis). Destruction of spirochetes by lysis.

spi″ro·che·to′sis. Any of the diseases caused by infection with one of the spirochetes, such as syphilis, relapsing fever, spirochetal jaundice. **—spirochetot′ic,** *adj.*

spirocid. Trade-mark for a brand of acetarsone.

spiroform. Trade-mark for phenyl acetylsalicylate.

spi′ro·gram″. A recorded tracing of the movements and excursion of the chest in respiration.

spi′ro·graph″. An instrument for registering respiration.

spi·rom′e·ter (spy·rom′i·tur). An instrument for measuring the vital capacity or volumes of inhaled and exhaled air. **—spiromet′ric,** *adj.;* **spirometry,** *n.*

splanch′na (splank′nuh). 1. The intestines. 2. The viscera.

splanch″nec·to′pi·a (splank″neck-to′pee·uh). The abnormal position or dislocation of a viscus.

splanch″nem·phrax′is. Obstruction of the intestine.

splanch″nes·the′si·a (splank″-ness·thee′zhuh, ·zee·uh). Visceral sensation. **—splanchnesthet′ic,** *adj.*

splanch″neu·rys′ma (splank″-new·riz′muh). Distention of the intestine.

splanch′nic. Pertaining to, or supplying, the viscera.

splanch″ni·cec′to·my. The surgical excision of the splanchnic nerves or their ganglions.

splanch″ni·cot′o·my. Surgical division of a splanchnic nerve.

splanch′no- (splank′no-), **splanchn-.** A combining form denoting *pertaining to the viscera.*

splanch″no·cele. A protrusion of any abdominal viscus.

splanch″no·di·as′ta·sis (·dye-ass′tuh·sis). Displacement or separation of the viscera.

splanch·nog′ra·phy. The descriptive anatomy of the viscera.

splanch′no·lith. Calculus of a viscus.

splanch″no·li·thi′a·sis. The condition of having a calculus of the intestine.

splanch·nol′o·gy. The branch of medical science pertaining to the viscera.

splanch″no·meg′a·ly. Enlargement of the viscera.

splanch″no·mi′cri·a (splank″no-migh′kree·uh, ·mick′ree·uh). Generalized reduction in the size of the visceral organs.

splanch·nop'a·thy. Disease of the viscera.

splanch'no·pleure. The wall of the gut, composed of endoderm and the splanchnic layer of lateral mesoderm. —**splanchnopleu'ral,** *adj.*

splanch"nop·to'sis (splank"nop-to'sis, splank"no-), **splanch"nop·to'si·a** (splank"nop·to'shuh, splank"-no-). A condition of relaxation of the abdominal viscera.

splanch"no·scle·ro'sis. Visceral induration.

splanch·nos'co·py. Visual examination of the viscera.

splanch'no·so·mat'ic. Pertaining to the viscera and the body.

splanch·not'o·my. Dissection of the viscera.

splanch'no·tribe. An instrument for crushing a segment of the intestine and so occluding its lumen, previous to resecting it.

spleen. One of the abdominal viscera, located immediately below the diaphragm on the left side; the largest lymphatic organ of the body. It is covered by a fibromuscular capsule continuous with trabeculae which radiate through the organ from the hilus, the portal of entry and exit of the splenic vessels. Between the trabeculae is white pulp, ensheathing branches of the splenic artery and composed of cords and nodules of lymphatic tissue, and red pulp, composed of atypical lymphatic tissue, the splenic cords, filling the spaces between venous sinuses. **accessory s.** Small mass of splenic tissue found either isolated or connected to the spleen by thin bands of splenic tissue. Also called *supernumerary s.* **floating s.** An abnormally movable and perhaps displaced spleen. Also called *movable s., wandering s.* **lardaceous s.** One affected with diffuse amyloid degeneration. Also called *waxy s.* **sago s.** One in which amyloid is present in the follicles showing on cut section numerous small glassy areas transmitting the red color of the spleen.

splen-. Same as *spleno-.*

sple·nal'gi·a. Pain originating in the spleen.

sple·nec'to·my. Excision of the spleen.

splen"ec·to'pi·a (splen"eck·to'pee-uh, splee"neck·), **sple·nec'to·py.** Displacement of the spleen.

sple·net'ic. 1. Pertaining to the spleen. 2. Having a diseased spleen.

splen'ic, sple'nic. Pertaining to the spleen.

splen'i·form, sple'ni·form. Resembling the spleen.

sple·ni'tis. Inflammation of the spleen.

sple'ni·us. One of two muscles of the back of the neck, splenius capitis and splenius cervicis. See Table of Muscles in the Appendix. —**splenial,** *adj.*

splen"i·za'tion. The stage of consolidation in the development of pneumonia during which lung tissue grossly, takes on an appearance resembling that of the normal spleen or liver, thus also called hepatization, *q.v.*

sple'no- (splee'no-, splen'o-), **sple'n'o-.** A combining form denoting *pertaining to the spleen.*

sple'no·cele. 1. Hernia of the spleen. 2. A tumor of the spleen.

sple'no·dyn'i·a (splee"no·din'ee·uh, splen"o·). Pain in the spleen.

sple'no·hep'a·to·meg'a·ly. Enlargement of the liver and spleen.

sple·nol'y·sis, splen"o·ly'sis. Destruction of splenic tissue.

sple'no·ma·la'ci·a (·ma·lay'shee·uh, ·see·uh). Softening of the spleen.

sple"no·meg'a·ly. Enlargement of the spleen; occurs in brucellosis, histoplasmosis, malaria, and other diseases

sple·nop'a·thy. Any disease of the spleen.

sple'no·pex'y. Fixation of the spleen to the abdominal wall by means of sutures.

sple"no·pneu·mo'ni·a. The stage of pneumonia producing splenization or hepatization of lung tissue.

sple"nop·to'sis. Downward displacement of the spleen, due to abnormal mobility.

sple·nor'rha·phy. Suture of the spleen.

sple·not'o·my. 1. The operation of incising the spleen. 2. Dissection of the spleen.

sple"no·tox'in (splee"no·tock'sin, splen"o·). A cytotoxin with specific action on the cells of the spleen.

splen'u·lus. Accessory spleen or rudimentary spleen.

splice. Join by suture, as to splice tendon.

splint. 1. A piece of wood, metal, plastic, wire, or other material for immobilizing the ends of a fractured bone or for restricting the movement of any movable part. 2. *In veterinary medicine* a form of periostitis in the foreleg of the horse. **acrylic s.** (a) *In dental surgery,* an apparatus or stent of plastic material used in fracture of the mandible and maxilla, or to give support in bone grafts of the jaws. (b) *In facial surgery,* one used to give support in fractures of the nasal bones and septum. **airplane s.** A special type which holds the arm in abduction with the forearm midway in flexion; generally of wire with an axillary strut and frequently incorporated in a plaster body support. **angular s.** One formed by two flat splints united at an angle, or a wire or other metal or plastic splint forming an angle appropriate to the condition to be treated. **banjo s.** A hand splint usually made of wire in the shape of a banjo or racket, attached to the forearm and sometimes incorporated in plaster. It is used generally for the attachment of rubber band traction devices for overriding and comminuted phalangeal fractures; the rubber bands are said to resemble the strings of a banjo, hence the name. **Böhler's s.** A wire extension splint used in the treatment of fractured fingers. **Bolles' s.** One used in the treatment of fracture of the coronoid process of the ulna. **caliper s.** One designed for the leg, consisting of two metal rods from a posterior thigh band or a padded ischial ring to a metal plate attached to the sole of the shoe at the instep. Also called *walking caliper.* **coaptation s.** A series of narrow splints of uniform size placed parallel to one another and held by adhesive plaster or leather, used to envelop a limb, such as the upper arm or thigh, where uniform and complete support is desired in the area covered. **cockup s.** A splint for immobilizing a hand in hyperextension during wound healing. **Fulton s.** One used in the treatment of dislocation of the radius. **Hodgen s.** A splint used in the treatment of fractures of the shaft of the femur. **pillow s.** A pillow support used as an emergency dressing for fractures of the lower leg. The pillow is compressed on either side and posteriorly with board splints held by several straps so as to exert firm pressure upon the leg. **Stader's s.** A metal bar with pins affixed at right angles. The pins are driven into the fragments of a fracture, and the bar maintains the alignment. **Thomas s.** One used to maintain traction in fractures of the humerus or femur, consisting of a ring which fits around the upper arm or thigh and two long metal rods extending from the ring on either side of the extremity. The rods are joined by a crosspiece below the hand or foot, and traction or fixation is applied to the crosspiece. Also used as an emergency splint for safe transportation in such injuries. **traction s.** One so devised that traction can be exerted on the distal fragment of a fracture to overcome muscle pull and maintain proper alignment of the fractured bone, such as the banjo, Thomas, or caliper splint. **T s.** One used to hold back the shoulders, and adapted by bandaging to hold the fragments in apposition in clavicular fractures.

splint'age. The application of splints.

splin'ter. 1. Colloquial term for a bit of wood or other material that pierces the skin. 2. *In veterinary medicine,* a vestigial second or fourth metacarpal or metatarsal of the horse; one of the splint bones extending, in the forelimb, from the "knee" and, in the hindlimb, from the hock, toward the fetlock.

splint'ing. Application of a splint, *q.v.*

split-prod'uct. A decomposition product as, for example, the aglycone produced by hydrolysis of a glycoside.

split'ting. A chemical change in which a compound is changed into two or more simpler bodies, as by hydrolysis.

spo"di·o·my"e·li'tis (spo"dee·o·migh"i·lye'tis, spod"ee·o·). Old term for acute anterior poliomyelitis, *q.v.*

spondylo-. See *spondylo-.*

spon"dy·lal'gi·a. Pain referred to a vertebra.

spon"dy·lar·throc'a·ce (spon"di·lahr·throck'uh·see). Caries of a vertebra.

spon"dy·li'tis. Inflammation of one or more vertebrae. —**spondylit'ic,** *adj.* **ankylosing s.** Arthritis of the spine affecting the vertebral and the sacroiliac joints leading to bony ankylosis with complete stiffness of the back. The costovertebral joints are included in the process when it involves the thoracic spine. Ossification of the anterior, lateral, and posterior, or yellow, ligaments produces the so-called bamboo spine. The intervertebral disks are not affected. It usually affects young men and is accompanied by severe debility. The peripheral joints, except for the hips, are usually spared. Also called *bamboo spine, rhizomelic spondylosis, spondylitis ankylopoietica, rheumatoid arthritis of the spine, poker back, poker spine, deforming spondylitis, Strümpell-Marie disease, Bekhterev's disease.* **deforming s.** (a) Ankylosing spondylitis. (b) Degenerative joint disease of the spine characterized by spur formation. It results, in part at least, from trauma with injury and deformity of the intervertebral disks. Limitation of motion is due to bony block, not to bony ankylosis. **tuberculous s.** Tuberculosis of the vertebral bodies leading to bone destruction, vertebral collapse, and kyphosis, healing by fusion of adjacent vertebrae. There may be accompanying psoas abscess and compression of the spinal cord. Also called *Pott's disease.*

spon'dy·lo-, spondyl-. A combining form signifying *pertaining to a vertebra.*

spon"dy·lo·di·dym'i·a. The condition of union of conjoined twins united by their vertebrae.

spon"dy·lo·dyn'i·a (spon"di·lo-din'ee-uh, ·dye'nee-uh). Pain in a vertebra.

spon"dy·lo·lis·the'sis. Deformity of the spinal column produced by the gliding forward of the lumbar vertebra in such a manner that they overhang the brim and obstruct the inlet of the pelvis; especially the forward displacement of the body of the last lumbar vertebra on the sacrum.

spon"dyl·ol'y·sis. Dissolution or destruction of a vertebra.

spon"dyl·op'a·thy. Any disease of the vertebrae.

spon"dy·lo·py·o'sis (spon"di·lo·pye·o'sis). Suppurative inflammation of one or more vertebrae.

spon"dy·lo'sis. Vertebral ankylosis. **rhizomelic s.** A variety of arthritis deformans with ankylosis of the vertebrae and arthritis of the hips and shoulders. See ankylosing *spondylitis*.

spon"dy·lo·syn·de'sis. Spinal fusion, *q.v.*

spon"dy·lot'o·my. Section of a vertebra in correcting a deformity.

spon'dy·lus. Old term for a vertebra. **—spondylous,** *adj.*

sponge. 1. An animal of the class Porifera. 2. The porous, horny skeleton of the animal, used as an absorbent. 3. Anything used like a sponge, as a rubber sponge. **—sponge,** *v.;* **spon'gi·form,** *adj.* **gauze s.** A flat folded piece of gauze of varying size, used by a surgical assistant to mop blood from the wound during the process of an operation. **gelatin s.** Sheet of gelatin, prepared to check bleeding when applied to a raw surface.

spon'gi·o·blast" (spon'jee·o·blast", spun'jee·o·). A nonnervous cell derived from the ectoderm of the embryonic neural tube, and later forming the neuroglia, the ependymal cells, the neurilemma sheath cells, the satellite cells of ganglions, and Müller's fibers of the retina.

spon"gi·o·blas·to'ma. A malignant, rapidly growing brain tumor, thought to be derived from embryonic spongioblasts, characterized by spindle cells and degenerative changes. Also called *spongiocytoma*.

spon'gi·ose. Full of pores, like a sponge.

spon'gy (spun'jee). Having the texture of sponge; very porous.

spontin. Trade-mark for ristocetin.

spoon. An instrument, usually made of metal, with a circular or oval bowl attached to a handle. A spoon is considered full when the contained liquid comes up to, but does not show a curve above, the upper edge or rim of the bowl. Household spoons are popularly used to measure the dose of medicines on the generally incorrect assumption that a teaspoon holds 4 cc. (1 drachm),

a tablespoon 15 cc. (half an ounce), and a dessertspoon 8 cc. (2 drachms). Medicine glasses are graduated on this basis. The actual spoons vary quite widely, teaspoons from 2 to 8 cc., averaging doses of 5 rather than of 4 cc. **cataract s.** A small spoon-shaped instrument used to remove the lens in cataract operations. **s. nail.** A fingernail with a concave outer surface. **surgical s.** A surgical instrument consisting of an oval or circular bowl fixed to a handle; it is used to scrape away dead tissue, granulations, etc.

spoon'er·ism. A psychic speech or writing defect characterized by the tendency to transpose letters or syllables of two or more words.

spo·rad'ic. Scattered; occurring in an isolated manner.

spore. A reproductive cell of a protozoan, bacterium, or higher plant. There is usually a thick cell wall enabling the cell to survive in adverse environments. **asexual s.** A spore formed without previous fusion of nuclear material. **resting s.** *In biology*, a spore, invested with a firm cell wall, which remains dormant during adverse environmental conditions before it germinates. **sexual s.** A spore formed subsequent to the union of two nuclei.

spo'ri·cide. Any agent which destroys spores. **—spori·ci'dal,** *adj.*

spo'ro-, spor-. A combining form signifying *relating to a spore or seed*.

spo'ro·cyst. A stage in the life cycle of the trematode worms. It occurs in the tissues of the first intermediate host. Two generations of sporocysts develop, the second generation giving rise to the redia larvae.

spo"ro·gen'e·sis. Production of spores.

spo·rog'o·ny. Reproduction by spores; especially applied to spore formation in Sporozoa which follows encystment of a zygote.

spo'ront. In Sporozoa, a cell which forms spores by encystment and subsequent division.

spo·rot'ri·chin (spo·rot'ri·kin). An antigenic filtrate of a culture of *Sporotrichum;* used for diagnostic complement fixation test.

spo"ro·tri·cho'sis (spor"o·tri·ko'sis, ·try·ko'sis). A subacute or chronic granulomatous disease caused by the fungus *Sporotrichum*. The lesions are usually cutaneous and spread along lymph channels; occasionally the internal organs and bones may be involved. The disease is reported among farmers, florists, and others working in soil.

Spo"ro·trich'um (spo"ro·trick'um). A genus of fungi which are the causative agents of sporotrichosis. The organisms are short, blunt, Gram-negative rods which occur singly or in groups, either in pus or in tissue. They may be free in the necrotic material or phagocytized by macrophages. **S. beurmanni** and **S. schencki** are the species most frequently isolated from cases of human infestation.

Spo″ro·zo′a. A class of parasitic Protozoa; the orders Coccidia, Sarcosporidia, and Haemosporidia are parasites of man.

spo″ro·zo′al. 1. Pertaining to Sporozoa. 2. A sporozoon.

spo″ro·zo′ite. 1. The organism resulting from sexual multiplication of the Sporozoa. 2. An animal spore.

spo″ro·zo′on. *In biology*, a member of the Sporozoa.

sport. An individual organism which differs from its parents to an unusual degree; a mutation.

spot. A small circumscribed area, differing in appearance or function from the surrounding area. **blind s. of Mariotte.** A scotoma in the visual field representing the entrance of the optic nerve, where the rods and cones are absent. Syn., *optic disk, optic papilla.* **blue s.** An integumentary spot, or spots, in the lumbar, sacral, or gluteal region; characteristic of the Mongolian race. Also called *Mongolian s.* **cherry-red s.** A bright red area seen in the retina in cases of amaurotic familial idiocy. **cold spots.** Areas on the surface of the skin overlying the nerve endings that are stimulated by cold. **germinal s.** The nucleolus of the egg nucleus. **hot spots.** Areas on the surface of the skin overlying the sense organs that are stimulated by heat. **Koplik's spots.** The characteristic exanthema of measles. See Koplik's *sign.* **milk s.** A patch of thickening and opacity of the epicardium, found post mortem, usually over the right ventricle; of common occurrence in persons who have passed middle life. **Mongolian s.** See blue s. **rose spots.** A red, papular eruption forming spots from 1 to 5 mm. in size which fade on pressure, occurring mostly on the abdomen and loins during the first seven days of typhoid fever. They are due to inflammation of the papillary layer of the skin from invasion of typhoid bacilli. Also called *typhoid roseola, typhoid spots.*

spot′ting. Small amounts of bloody vaginal discharge, usually intermenstrual, and of significance in certain obstetric and gynecologic conditions.

sprain. A wrenching of a joint, producing a stretching or laceration of the ligaments. **rider's s.** A sprain of the adductor longus muscle of the thigh, resulting from a sudden effort of the

horseman to maintain his seat owing to some unexpected movement of his horse. **s. fracture.** An injury in which a tendon or ligament, together with a shell of bone, is torn from its attachment.

spray. 1. A stream of air and finely divided liquid produced with an atomizer, nebulizer, or other device. 2. A liquid pharmaceutical preparation intended for applying medication to the nose, throat, or other cavities by spraying from an atomizer or nebulizer; may be aqueous or oily in character.

spread′ing. Growth of bacteria beyond the line of inoculation.

sprue. An afebrile, chronic disease characterized by the passage of voluminous, mushy, and often frothy stools, weakness, emaciation, changes in the tongue, and anemia. Common in white people in Southeastern Asia, East Indies, Ceylon, West Indies. Originally the disease was thought to be caused by the yeast *Monilia psilosis,* but recent work tends to show that the disease is basically a deficiency disease. Vedder stated that sprue may occur in individuals who have excellent diets. The question of defective absorption has been considered. Vedder also suggests that dysfunction of the anterior pituitary gland may be associated with the disturbed absorption from the intestine. Also called *psilosis, Ceylon sore mouth, diarrhea alba, Cochin-China diarrhea, tropical sprue.* **para-sprue.** A dietary disease characterized by chronic watery diarrhea, weight loss, a sore red tongue, and macrocytic anemia. It differs from true sprue in showing less emaciation, no swollen lower abdomen, dry skin, dysphagia, and pale, frothy stools with the fat content above 40%.

spud. 1. An instrument used in the detachment of the mucosa in flaps in operations necessitating the removal of bone. 2. A short, flattened blade used to dislodge a foreign substance.

spur. 1. A sharp projection. Also called *calcar.* 2. *In biology*, a pointed, spinelike outgrowth, either of the integument or of a projecting appendage. **calcaneal s.** A painful exostosis of the heel due to trauma, static conditions of the foot, improper shoes, or systemic infections. Also called *heel s.* **s. of the septum.** An outgrowth of the nasal septum.

spu′ri·ous. Counterfeit; false; not genuine, as spurious pregnancy.

spu′tum (pl. *sputums, sputa*). Material discharged from the surface of the air passages, throat, or mouth, and removed chiefly by spitting but in lesser degree by swallowing. It may consist of saliva, mucus, or pus, either alone or in any combination. It may also contain microörganisms, fibrin, blood or its decomposition products, or inhaled particulate foreign matter. **hailstone s.** That containing particles having the appearance of hailstones. **mucopurulent s.** That consisting of a mixture of mucus and pus. **mucous s.** Sputum consisting chiefly of mucus, often erroneously designated as mucoid sputum. **nummular s.** Sputum containing small, round, flattened masses of heavy material. **purulent s.** That consisting chiefly of pus. **rusty s.** That colored by various decomposition products of blood; seen chiefly in lobar pneumonia. Also called *prune-juice s., icteric s.*

squa'ma (pl. *squamae*). A scale or scalelike mass, as the squama of the temporal bone.

squa'mo-. A combining form denoting *relating to the squamous portion of the occipital or temporal bone.*

squa·mo'sa. The squamous portion of the temporal bone.

squa'mous. Of the shape of a scale, as the squamous portion of the temporal bone, or squamous epithelium, epithelium consisting of flat, scalelike cells.

squill. The cut and dried fleshy inner scale of the bulb of the white variety of *Urginea maritima,* or of *Urginea indica.* It contains scillipicrin, scillitoxin, scillin, scillenin, scillimarin, scillitin, and scillidiuretin. Work on the fresh drug has shown the existence of two glycosides, crystalline scillaren-A and an amorphous fraction, scillaren-B.

squint. See *strabismus.*

Sr. Chemical symbol for strontium.

Sr^{90}. Symbol for strontium-90.

ss, ss. *Semis,* one-half.

S.T. Surface tension.

stab. 1. A puncture wound. 2. Path formed by plunging an inoculation needle into nutrient media.

sta'bile (stay'bil, stab'll). Stationary; immobile; maintaining a fixed position.

sta'bi·li''zer. 1. A retarding agent, or a substance that counteracts the effect of a vigorous accelerator and preserves a chemical equilibrium. 2. A substance added to a solution to render it more stable, as acetanilid to hydrogen peroxide solution.

sta'ble. Unlikely to break down or dissolve; in the case of a compound, likely to retain its composition under the application of physical or chemical forces.

stac·ca'to (sta-kah'to). Denoting an abrupt, jerky manner of speech with a noticeable interval between words.

stach'y·drine. $C_7H_{13}NO_2$. N-Methylproline-methylbetaine, an alkaloid occurring in *Stachys tuberifera* and other plants.

stach'y·ose. A tetrasaccharide obtained from the tubers of *Stachys tuberifera* and some other plants. Also called *mannotetrose, lupeose.*

sta'di·um (pl. *stadia*). Stage. **s. acmes.** The height of a disease. **s. annihilationis.** The convalescent stage. **s. augmenti.** The period in which there is increase in the intensity of the disease. **s. caloris.** The period during which there is fever; the hot stage. **s. contagii.** The prodromal stage of an infectious disease. **s. convalescentiae.** The period of recovery from disease. **s. decrementi.** Defervescence of a febrile disease; the period in which there is a decrease in the severity of the disease. **s. decrustationis.** The stage of an exanthematous disease in which the lesions form crusts. **s. desquamationis.** The period of desquamation in an exanthematous fever. **s. eruptionis.** That period of an exanthematous fever in which the exanthem appears. **s. floritionis.** The stage of an eruptive disease during which the exanthema is at its height. **s. frigoris.** The cold stage of a fever. See *algid stage.* **s. incrementi.** The stage of increase of a fever or disease. **s. maniacale.** The last stage of excitement in mania, after which the nervous manifestations gradually subside. **s. nervosum.** The paroxysmal stage of a disease. **s. prodromorum.** The stage immediately prior to the appearance of the signs and symptoms of disease. **s. sudoris.** The sweating stage. **s. suppurationis.** The period in the course of smallpox in which suppuration occurs. **s. ultimum.** The final stage of a febrile affection.

staff. 1. An instrument for passing through the urethra to the bladder used as a guide in operations on the bladder or for stricture. It is usually grooved. 2. The personnel concerned with the care of patients in a hospital. **consulting s.** Specifically, a body of physicians, surgeons, or specialists attached to a hospital or medical unit who serve only in an advisory capacity. **house s.** The interns and residents living in the hospital. **visiting s.** The non-resident physicians and surgeons who supervise the care of patients in a hospital.

stage. 1. A definite period of a disease characterized by certain symptoms; a condition in the course of a disease. 2. The horizontal plate projecting from the pillar of a microscope for supporting the slide or object. **algid s.** A condition characterized by subnormal temperature, feeble, flickering pulse, and various nervous symptoms. It occurs in cholera and other diseases marked by exhausting intestinal discharges. **am-phibolic s.** The stage of a disease intervening between its height and its decline. **cold s.** The rigor or chill of an attack of a malarial paroxysm. **eruptive s.** That in which an exanthema makes its appearance. **expulsive s.** The stage of labor which begins when dilatation of the cervix uteri is complete and during which the child is expelled from the uterus. See stages of *labor*. **first s.** That stage of labor in which the molding of the fetal head and the dilatation of the cervix are effected. **hot s.** The febrile stage of a malarial paroxysm. **mechanical s.** A fixture on a microscope stage, with two horizontal screw adjustments at right angles to each other which permit the specimen to be moved as desired. Some have vernier scales for reading the amount of displacement to 0.1 mm. **microscope s.** The platform under the microscope tube which carries the specimen and is usually mounted permanently on the microscope pillar, although it may be mounted on a rack and pinion. **pre-eruptive s.** The period of an eruptive fever following infection and prior to the appearance of the eruption. **s. of invasion.** The period in the course of a disease in which the body comes under the influence of the infective agent. **s. of latency.** The incubation period of an infectious disease, or that period intervening between the entrance of the agent and the manifestations of the symptoms to which it gives rise. **sweating s.** The third or terminal stage of a malarial paroxysm, during which sweating occurs.

stag′gers. A term applied to various diseases which are manifested by lack of coördination in movement and a staggering gait, as gid of sheep, encephalomyelitis of horses, botulism, loco poisoning, and some cerebral affections of livestock.

stag′ing a′re·a. A military camp near a port of embarkation where troop units are assembled en route to overseas stations to await embarkation. Such areas include station hospitals and dispensary service, where immunizations against infectious disease are accomplished if necessary.

stag·na′tion. 1. A cessation of motion. 2. *In pathology*, a cessation of motion in any fluid; stasis. —**stag′nate**, *v*.

stain. (See Table of Special Stains and Staining Methods in next column.) 1. A discoloration produced by absorption of, or contact with, foreign matter. 2. *In microscopy*, a pigment or dye used (a) to render minute and transparent structures visible, (b) to differentiate

tissue elements, or (c) to produce specific microchemical reactions. **acid s.** A dye in which the anion is colored and does the staining. Acid stains are the common stains for cytoplasm and cytoplasmic inclusions. **basic s.** A dye in which the cation is colored and does the staining. Basic stains are the common stains for chromatin in nuclei, for nucleoproteins, for mucins, and for calcium-salt deposits in tissues. **Commission Certified s.** A stain which has been certified by the Biological Stain Commission. Abbreviated, C.C. **contrast s.** A double stain in which certain cell constituents take one stain and other constituents take the contrasting stain. **counterstain.** A second stain, usually a contrasting one, which is used after one which stains nuclei or desired constituents. **double s.** A mixture of two dyes of contrasting colors, usually an acid stain and a basic stain, or a method involving the successive use of contrasting stains. See contrast *s*. **fluorescent s. method.** A staining method using a fluorescent dye, such as the method for demonstrating *Mycobacterium tuberculosis* in smears using auramine O, and a fluorescence microscope. **intravital s.** A dye, introduced by injection into the body of man or animal, which stains certain tissues or cells selectively; the stain must be nontoxic so as not to kill any of the cells. **metachromatic s.** A stain which changes apparent color when absorbed by certain cell constituents, as mucin staining red instead of blue with toluidine blue. **neutral s.** A compound produced by the interaction of an acid and a basic dye, insoluble in pure water, and therefore employed in alcoholic solution when used as a stain. **nuclear s.** A stain, usually a basic dye, which stains nuclei selectively. **supravital s.** A stain applied to living cells removed from a living animal, or to still living cells within a recently killed animal; the stain may be perfused through the blood vessels of the animal. **vital s.** A nontoxic coloration of tissues produced by injection of a nontoxic dye into a living organism. Also called intravital *s*.

SPECIAL STAINS AND STAINING METHODS

Best's carmine (*for glycogen*). Prepare a stock solution by mixing 2 Gm. of carmine, 1 Gm. of potassium carbonate, 5 Gm. of potassium chloride, and 60 cc. of distilled water. Boil gently until color darkens, cool, and add 20 cc. of concentrated ammonia. A test for the selectivity of the glycogen staining is the pretreatment of the section with saliva, which digests the glycogen; Best's carmine should then stain nothing in the section. **Böhmer's hematoxylin.** An alum hematoxylin stain; used in histologic staining. Two solutions are required: *Solution I.* Hematoxylin crystals 1 Gm., absolute alcohol 12 cc. *Solution II.* Alum 20 Gm., warm distilled water 200 cc. Filter when cool. After 24 hours, mix both solutions. Place in a wide-mouth bottle and expose to air for 8 days. Filter through filter paper. Of historical interest only. **carbolfuchsin solution** *(for tubercle bacilli).* A staining fluid composed of basic fuchsin 0.3 Gm., alcohol 10 cc., liquefied phenol 5 cc., distilled water 95 cc. Used primarily for the staining of tubercle bacilli. Formerly called *Ziehl-Neelsen's carbolfuchsin.* **chromaffin reaction.** A brown coloration of a tissue, as adrenal medulla, when fixing fluids containing dichromate salts are used. **Delafield's hematoxylin.** An excellent nuclear stain. Dissolve 4 Gm. of hematoxylin in 25 cc. of absolute alcohol, and add 400 cc. of saturated aqueous solution of ammonium alum; expose to light and air for 3–4 days; filter; add to the filtrate 100 cc. each of glycerin and methyl alcohol; allow to ripen before use and dilute with water as desired. **Ehrlich's acid hematoxylin.** Used for staining sections and in the mass. Dissolve 1 Gm. of hematoxylin in 30 cc. of alcohol and add 50 cc. each of glycerin and water, alum in excess, and 4 cc. of glacial acetic acid. Allow the mixture to stand in the light until it acquires a deep red color. Stains nuclei, mucin, and calcium deposits deep blue. One of the most frequently used hematoxylin stains. **eosin.** Tetrabromofluorescein, an acid dye which occurs in red or yellowish crystals. Commercially, several rose-colored fluorescein dyes of the xanthine series are called eosins: eosin Y, ethyl eosin, eosin B, phloxine, and rose bengal. **eosin, bluish** (C.C.). Dinitro-dibromofluorescein, a useful counterstain for hematoxylin. Also called *eosin BN, B, BW,* or *DKV; saffrosin; eosin scarlet B* or *BB; scarlet J, JJ,* or *V; napolin G; imperial red.* **eosin Y.** Tetrabromofluorescein, a valuable stain; used most frequently as a counterstain for hematoxylin and the green or blue basic dyes. Dissolve 0.1–1.0 Gm. of eosin Y (85% dye content) in 100 cc. of distilled water. Also called *water-soluble yellowish eosin; eosin W* or *WS.* **Giemsa s.** (C.C.). A neutral stain used in staining blood, and as a general cytologic stain. It is the compound formed from eosin with one of the derivatives of methylene blue, known as azure II.

A stock solution may be prepared by dissolving 0.5 Gm. of Giemsa powder in 33 cc. of glycerin, C.P., and after several hours adding 33 cc. of absolute alcohol. Also called *azure II-eosin.* **Gram's s.** *(for staining bacteria).* Smear material to be examined on a glass slide, dry, and fix with heat. Stain with carbol-gentian violet for one-half minute. Wash with water. Stain with Gram's iodine for 1½ minutes. Wash with water. Destain with 95% ethyl alcohol for 2–3 minutes. Wash with water. Stain with 1% safranin for one-half to one minute. Wash with water, dry, and mount. Gram-positive organisms are dark violet or purple. Gram-negative organisms are faint pink. Numerous modifications are used. **Harris' hematoxylin.** Dissolve 1 Gm. of hematoxylin in 10 cc. of alcohol and add to 200 cc. of a saturated aqueous solution of alum; heat to boiling and add 0.5 Gm. of mercuric oxide. When the solution turns a dark purple, remove from the flame and cool quickly. For use dilute to the color of port wine with aqueous solution of alum. **Heidenhain's (azan) azocarmine.** A 2% aqueous solution of azocarmine G in distilled water. When used as a tissue stain it is acidified strongly with glacial acetic acid. Aniline blue and orange G are used as counterstains in Heidenhain's modification of the Mallory connective-tissue stain. **hematoxylin** (C.C.). $C_{16}H_{14}O_6$. A crystalline glycoside derived by extracting logwood with water in the presence of ether. It is oxidized to hematein which yields a deep blue coloration. An excellent nuclear stain. Various types are Harris' hematoxylin, iron hematoxylin, Mallory's ferric chloride hematoxylin, Mallory's phosphomolybdic acid hematoxylin, Mallory's phosphotungstic acid hematoxylin. **hematoxylin-eosin method.** Stain sections with hematoxylin (Harris'). Rinse with tap water, decolorize in 0.5% acid alcohol, washing thoroughly afterward with tap water, then with 0.5% ammonia water and again with tap water. Rinse in 70% alcohol, stain with alcoholic eosin, and rinse with 95% alcohol. Dehydrate in absolute alcohol, clear in carbolxylol and xylol, and mount. Many modifications are employed, such as the use of other hematoxylin solutions, or of water-soluble eosin. **India ink method.** A method of making spirochetes and other organisms visible under the microscope by means of India ink. Negative staining. The background is black with India ink, and the spirochetes, being unstained, show up clearly. **Leishman's s.** *(for blood)* A Romanovsky type of stain, the eosiate of polychrome methylene blue, available as a dry powder which is dissolved for use in pure methyl alcohol in the proportion of 0.15 Gm. to 100 cc. **Loeffler's s.** (for flagella). Treat air-dried film with freshly filtered mordant (100 cc. of 20% aqueous solution of tannic acid, 50 cc. of saturated aqueous solution of ferrous sulfate, 10 cc. of saturated basic fuchsin in 95% alcohol), heating gently for one-half to one minute; stain with carbolfuchsin. **MacNeal's tetrachrome s.** A blood stain containing eosin, methylene azure A, methylene blue, and methylene violet in methyl alcohol; it is used like Wright's stain. **May-Grünwald s.** (for blood). A saturated solution of methylene blue eosinate in methyl alcohol. Syn., Jenner's s. **medicinal methylene blue.** Methylthionine chloride. It is free of zinc, hence less toxic than commercial methylene blue. It is used as a urinary antiseptic, and for a kidney-function test. Also an antidote for carbon monoxide and cyanide poisoning. **Nocht-Romanovsky s.** This requires two solutions: a) Methylene blue 1.0 Gm., sodium carbonate 0.5 Gm., distilled water 100 cm. Heat at 60° C. for two days until solution shows a slight purplish color. b) Eosin soluble, yellowish, 1.0 Gm., distilled water 100 cc. Mix a few drops of each of these solutions with about 10 cc. of distilled water in an Esmarch dish; the smear, which has previously been fixed in absolute methyl alcohol, is then floated on this mixture for about 10 minutes. **Pappenheim's method** (for tubercle bacilli). Stain the fixed smear by steaming with carbolfuchsin (Ziehl-Neelsen). Pour off the dye, and, without washing, apply Pappenheim's solution 4–5 times. Wash, dry, and mount. **Romanovsky s.** Polychrome methylene blue eosinates used for staining blood. The modifications include the Leishman, Giemsa, Wright, MacNeal, and Jenner stains. **Shorr trichrome s.** (for vaginal epithelium). An alcoholic solution of Biebrich scarlet (water soluble), orange d, fast green FCF, aniline blue (water soluble), phosphomolybdic acid, phosphotungstic acid, and glacial acetic acid. It differentiates between cornified (brilliant orange-red) and noncornified (blue-green) cells. **tetrachrome s. (MacNeal's)** (C.C.) (for blood). A solution containing eosin, methylene blue, methylene violet, and methylene azure A in methyl alcohol; employed like Wright's stain. **tubercle bacilli, staining of.** The smear is stained with hot carbolfuchsin for 1–2 minutes, then rinsed with water, then decolorized with a 10% aqueous solution of sodium sulfite for 30–60 sec-

onds, then rinsed with water, then counterstained with malachite green (50 cc. of saturated aqueous solution of malachite green in 100 cc. of distilled water) for 15–30 seconds; the tubercle bacilli appear as dark red rods on a green background. Also see carbolfuchsin solution (for tubercle bacilli), under stain. **Wright's s.** (C.C.) (for blood). Wright's stain powder (methylene blue, polychromated with sodium bicarbonate and heat, to which eosin is added) 0.3 Gm., 100 cc. of absolute methyl alcohol (acetone free). Filter; let filtrate stand. Cover the dried film of blood for one minute. Add distilled water or buffered water (pH 6.4–7.0) for 4–10 minutes, the time for staining varying with different batches of stain. Wash with distilled water and dry. The nuclei of the leukocytes should stain a dark purple, the eosinophilic granules a bright red, and the erythrocytes an orange or buff.

stal″ag·mom′e·ter. An instrument for measuring the size of drops, or the number of drops in a given volume of liquid. It is used to measure the surface tension of liquids.

stalk. Any lengthened support to an organ. **body s.** The extraembryonic mesoderm connecting the chorion and the caudal region of the amnioembryonic vesicle. It forms a path for the allantoic blood vessels and the connective tissue of the future umbilical cord. **optic s.** The narrow medial part of the optic vesicle and cup which forms a pathway for the developing optic nerve.

sta′men. The male organ of the flower, consisting of stalk or filament and an anther containing pollen.

stam′i·na. Natural strength of constitution; vigor; inherent force.

stam′mer·ing. Interrupted or hesitating speech. Syn., anarthria, battarism, psellism. —stammer, v.

stand′ard. 1. An established form of quality or quantity. 2. A substance of known strength used for determining the strength of an unknown by comparison. **Harris and Benedict standards.** Multiple prediction equations and tables based on a statistical study of the available data for the basal metabolism of normal men and women. **reference standards.** Substances of defined purity used for comparison in conducting certain assays of the United States Pharmacopeia or National Formulary.

stand′ard con·di′tions. In gas analysis, an atmospheric pressure of 760 mm., and a temperature of 0° C., at latitude 45°. It is sometimes abbreviated S.T.P. (= standard temperature and pressure).

stand′ard de″vi·a′tion. Sigma (σ). The square root of the arithmetic average of the squares of the differences of each observation in a series from the mean of the series. The most commonly used measure of variation. Also called *the root-mean squared deviation from the mean.*

stand′ard er′ror. A measure of the variability which any statistical constant would be expected to show in taking repeated random samples of a given size from the same universe of observations.

stand′ard·i·za′tion. The procedure necessary to bring a preparation to an established or known quality, as the adjustment of a standard solution in volumetric analysis.

stand′ard·ized death rate. *In biometry,* the number of deaths per 1000 which would have occurred in some standard population with a known age-specific death rate. The rate may be standardized for race, sex, or other variables with known death rates.

stand′still. A state of quiescence dependent upon suspended action.

stan′nate. A salt of stannic acid.

stan′nic. 1. Pertaining to stannum, or tin. 2. Containing tin in the tetravalent state.

stan′nic ac′ids. A series of acids which vary in composition from H_2SnO_2 to H_2SnO_4.

stan′nous. Containing tin as a bivalent element.

stan′num. See *tin.*

sta″pe·dec′to·my. Resection of a stapes.

sta·pe′des (stay′pi·deez). Plural of stapes, *q.v.*

sta·pe′di·al. 1. Shaped like a stirrup. 2. Relating to the stapes.

sta·pe″di·o·te·not′o·my. Cutting of the tendon of the stapedius muscle.

sta·pe′di·us. A muscle in the middle ear, inserted on the stapes. See Table of Muscles in the Appendix.

sta′pes (stay′peez) (pl. *stapedes*). The stirrup-shaped bone of the middle ear, articulating with the incus and the fenestra ovalis. It is composed of the head, the crura or legs, and the foot plate. See Table of Bones in the Appendix.

staph″y·lec′to·my. Operation for removal of the uvula.

staph″yl·e·de′ma. Edema of the uvula; any enlargement of the uvula.

staph″y·he′ma·to′ma, staph″-yl·hae″ma·to′ma (staf″il-hee″-muh·to′muh, ·hem″uh·to′muh). An extravasation of blood into the uvula.

staph′y·line (staf′i·lyne, ·leen). Pertaining to the uvula or to the entire soft palate.

staph″y·li′tis. Inflammation of the uvula.

staph′y·lo-, staphyl-. A combining form denoting *relating to the uvula.*

staph″y·lo·coc′cal. Pertaining or caused by, staphylococci.

staph″y·lo·coc·ce′mi·a, staph″y·lo·coc·cae′mi·a (staf″i·lo-coc-see′mee·uh). A morbid condition due the presence of staphylococci in t blood.

staph″y·lo·coc′cic (staf″i·lo·cock sick). Pertaining to, or caused b staphylococci.

Staph″y·lo·coc′cus. A genus cocci of the family Micrococcace They are Gram-positive and often gr in groups resembling clusters of grap On nutrient agar the colonies are whi yellow, or orange; the pathogen strains are usually hemolytic and ela orate one or more staphylotoxins. T lesions are usually localized but m become widespread. **S. albus.** T colony is white, rarely hemolytic. T organism sometimes causes boils but usually considered of low pathogenicit Syn., *Micrococcus albus.* Also call *Micrococcus ascoformans, M. pyogen* var. *albus.* **S. aureus.** The colony golden or orange yellow; this spec has the highest pathogenicity. Sy *Micrococcus aureus.* Also called *Micr coccus ascoformans, M. pyogenes v aureus.*

staph″y·lo·coc′cus (pl. *staphyl cocci*). A member of the genera *Staph lococcus* and *Micrococcus.* **s. ant toxin.** An antitoxin prepared by im munizing horses with staphylococc toxoid and/or staphylococcus toxi **s. toxin.** See *staphylotoxin.* **s. tox oid.** Univalent or polyvalent, potent hemolytic and dermonecrotic toxins *Staphylococcus aureus* and *albus* a tered by the formaldehyde-detoxifyin process of Burnet (modified from R mon). Antigenicity is maintained b toxicity is greatly diminished.

staph″y·lo·der″ma·ti′tis. De matitis due to staphylococci.

staph″y·lo·di·al′y·sis (staf″i·l dye·al′i·sis). Relaxation of the uvul *Obs.*

staph″y·lol′y·sin (staf″i·lol′i·si staf″i·lo·lye′sin). A hemolysin pr duced by staphylococci.

staph″y·lo′ma. A bulging of th cornea or sclera of the eye. —**staph lomat′ic, staphylom′atous,** *ad* **equatorial s.** Staphyloma of th sclera in the equatorial region. **pos terior s.** A backward bulging of th sclerotic coat at the posterior pole the eye.

staph″y·lon′cus. Swelling of th uvula. *Obs.*

staph″y·lo·pha·ryn′ge·us (staf i·lo·fa·rin′jee·us, ·far″in·jee′us). Ol term for the palatopharyngeus muscl

staph'y·lo·phar"yn·gor'rha·phy. A plastic operation on the palate and pharynx, as for repair of a cleft palate.

staph'y·lo·plas"ty. A plastic operation on the soft palate or uvula.

staph'y·lop·to'sis. Abnormal elongation of the uvula.

staph'y·lor'rha·phy. Repair of a cleft palate by plastic operation and suture.

staph'y·los'chi·sis (staf"i·los'ki·sis). Cleft uvula, or cleft soft palate.

staph'y·lo·tome". A cutting instrument used in staphylotomy.

staph"y·lot'o·my. 1. The operation of incising the uvula. 2. *In ophthalmology,* the operation of incising a staphyloma.

staph"y·lo·tox'in. One of the toxins elaborated by staphylococci. Hemolysin, leukocidin, coagulase, fibrinolysin, necrotizing enterotoxin, and a lethal exotoxin are some of the toxins which have been identified.

star. *In biology,* any of various radiate structures, granules, cells, groups of cells, or organisms.

starch. 1. Any one of a group of carbohydrates or polysaccharides occurring as organized or structural granules of varying size and markings in many plant cells. It is insoluble in cold water and hydrolyzes to several forms of dextrin and glucose. The granules consist of at least two fractions: an inner portion called amylose or granulose, relatively soluble in water, and an outer portion called amylopectin, which is practically insoluble in water. 2. Corn starch. Consists of the granules separated from the grain of *Zea mays;* occurs as irregular, angular, white masses or as a fine powder; insoluble in cold water and alcohol. **animal s.** Glycogen. **soluble s.** Starch transformed into water-soluble dextrins by heating to about 200° C.

starch su'gar. See *dextrose.*

star grass. Aletris, the dried rhizomes of *Aletris farinosa.* Also called *star-wort, bitter grass, blazing star.*

star·va'tion. 1. Deprivation of food. 2. The state produced by deprivation of food.

stas"i·bas"i·pho'bi·a (stas"i·bas"i·fo'bee·uh, stay"si·bay"si··). A morbid fear of walking or of standing.

stas"i·pho'bi·a (stas"i·fo'bee·uh, tay"si··). A morbid fear of standing upright.

sta'sis. In blood vessels, complete cessation of the blood flow. The vessels are dilated and completely filled with a mass of red blood corpuscles. There is no transudation of fluid through the capillary walls and no diapedesis of red blood corpuscles. **intestinal s.** An undue delay in the passage of fecal matter along the intestines. **venous s.** Stasis due to venous congestion.

state. A condition. **anxiety s.** A psychoneurosis marked by more or less continuous diffuse anxiety and apprehension with acute episodes of fear and panic, manifested physically by palpitation, dyspnea, nausea, and diarrhea. **cataleptoid s.** A condition due to neuromuscular excitability and differing from true catalepsy in that the limbs must be held in fixed attitudes for a few seconds before they maintain themselves and then function causes them to become limp. **central excitatory s.** Degree of excitability of the synapses within the central nervous system. Abbreviated, c.e.s. **depressive state.** Certain mental disorders characterized by extreme depression. **hypnoidal s.** The state between sleeping and waking.

state'ment. A declaration. **antemortem s.** A declaration made immediately before death, which, if made with the consciousness of impending death, is legally held as binding as a statement sworn to.

stat'ic. At rest. In equilibrium. Pertaining to the laws of statics.

stat'ics. That science which deals with bodies at rest or at equilibrium relative to some given state of reference.

stat"i·den·sig'ra·phy. Measurement of the quantity of roentgen rays passing through a subject onto a radioscopic screen provided with a photoelectric cell; used to determine the local density of the lung.

stat'im, sta'tim. Immediately; at once.

sta'tion. 1. Standing position or attitude. 2. A place where first aid or treatment is given, as a dressing station, rest station.

sta'tion·ar"y. Standing still; not moving.

sta'tion hos'pi·tal. *In military medicine,* a hospital of from 25 to 2000 beds which functions as the general hospital of a post or station. Such a hospital may or may not have a complete professional staff of specialists.

sta·tis'ti·cal con'stant. A value such as the arithmetic mean, the standard error, or any other measure which characterizes a particular series of quantitative observations. Used as an estimate of the corresponding value for the universe from which the observations were chosen.

sta·tis'tics. A numerical collection of facts relating to any subject. **medical s.** That part of statistics relating to facts and data concerning human diseases. **vital s.** A term usually limited to data concerning births, marriages, and deaths; a branch of bio-statistics, *q.v.*

sta″to‑a‧cous′tic [NA]. The eighth cranial nerve.

stat″o‧ki‧net′ic (stat″o‧ki‧net′ick, ‧kigh‧net′ick). Pertaining to the position of the body or its parts during movement, as in locomotion.

sta‧tom′e‧ter. An instrument for measuring the degree of exophthalmos.

stat′ure. The height of any animal when standing. In quadrupeds, it is measured at a point over the shoulders. In man, it is the measured distance from the sole to the top of the head.

sta′tus. A state or condition; often, a severe or intractable condition. **s. an‧ginosus.** A severe or prolonged attack of angina pectoris, due to extreme coronary insufficiency with or without thrombosis of a coronary artery. **s. arthriticus.** The nervous manifestations preceding an attack of gout. **s. asthmaticus.** Intractable asthma characterized by extreme dyspnea, cyanosis, and exhaustion, lasting from a few days to a week or longer; sometimes fatal. **s. catarrhalis.** A condition characterized by a succession of inflammatory processes of a mucosa. **s. epilepticus.** A condition in which epileptic attacks occur in rapid succession, the patient not regaining consciousness during the interval. **s. praesens.** The state of a patient at the time of examination. **s. raptus.** Ecstasy.

S.T.D. Abbreviation for standard test dose of scarlet fever toxin. A skin test dose is the least amount of standard scarlet fever streptococcus toxin which, when injected intracutaneously into a person known to be susceptible to the toxin, will induce a red area in the skin measuring 1 cm. in diameter when observed 18 to 24 hours after the injection. The reaction is compared with that made by a control injection of the same amount of the material which has been heated to 100° C. for two hours. See Dick *test.*

steam. The vapor of water; water in a gaseous state.

ste‧ap′sin (ste‧ap′sin). A lipase present in pancreatic juice and capable of hydrolyzing fats to glycerin and fatty acids. Also called *pancreatic lipase.*

stear′ate (steer′ate). An ester or salt of stearic acid, as stearin (glyceryl stearate) or sodium stearate.

ste‧ar′ic ac′id (stee‧ar′ick, steer′-ick). A mixture of solid acids obtained from fats; consists chiefly of stearic acid, $CH_3(CH_2)_{16}COOH$, and palmitic acid, $CH_3(CH_2)_{14}COOH$; occurs as a hard, white, or faintly yellowish solid, or a white or yellowish powder; it is almost insoluble in water.

ste‧ar′i‧form. Having the appearance of, or resembling, fat.

stear′in (steer′in). $C_3H_5O_3(C_{17}F CO)_3$. Tristearin, glyceryl tristeara The glyceryl ester of stearic acid, occurring in many of the solid anim fats.

stear″o‧der′mi‧a. An affection the sebaceous glands of the skin.

stear‧op′tene. That portion of volatile oil, usually consisting of ox genated substances, which is solid ordinary temperatures.

stear′yl. The monovalent radic $C_{17}H_{35}CO—$, of stearic acid.

ste′a‧tin. 1. Stearin. 2. Any cer containing a considerable proporti of tallow.

ste″a‧ti′tis. Inflammation of adipo tissue.

ste′a‧to‑, steat‑. A combining fo meaning *fat.*

ste″a‧to‧cryp‧to′sis. Abnorm function of the sebaceous glands.

ste″a‧tol′y‧sis. The emulsify process by which fats are prepared absorption and assimilation. —**ste tolyt′ic,** *adj.*

ste″a‧to′ma. 1. A sebaceous cy *Obs.* 2. A lipoma. *Obs.*

ste″a‧to‧py′gi‧a (stee″uh‧to‧pye′ji uh, ‧pidj′ee‧uh). Excessive accumu tion of fat on the buttocks. —**ste top′ygous,** *adj.*

ste″a‧tor‧rhe′a. 1. An increased fl of the secretion of the sebaceous fol cles; see *seborrhea.* 2. Fatty stoo **s. simplex.** Excess of sebaceous e cretion of the face.

ste″a‧to′sis. An old term former used loosely for fatty degeneration, disease of sebaceous glands.

steel. Iron chemically combined wi a certain proportion of carbon, inte mediate between white cast iron a wrought iron.

Steenbock, Harry [*American ph iologist and biochemist,* 1886— Known for his investigations on vit mins. With Mariana Sell and Mary v Buell, separated vitamin D from vit min A (1921). Introduced a rachitogen diet, low in vitamin D and produci rickets when fed to rats. This was us for the biologic determination of vit min D (1925); known as *Steenbo. rachitogenic diet.* See also Steenbo *unit.*

steg‧no′sis. The closing of a passa —**stegnot′ic,** *adj.*

stel′late. Star-shaped, or with pa radiating from a center.

stem. 1. The pedicle or stalk of tumor. 2. A supporting stalk, as of leaf or plant. **brain s.** The porti of the brain remaining after the ce bral hemispheres and cerebellum ha been removed.

sten'o-. A combining form meaning *narrow* or *constricted.*

sten″o·ceph'a·ly, sten″o·ce·pha'li·a. Unusual narrowness of the head. —**stenocephalous,** *adj.*

sten″o·cho'ri·a (sten″o·kor'ee·uh). Narrowing; partial obstruction, particularly of a lacrimal duct.

sten″o·co·ri'a·sis. Narrowing of the pupil.

sten'o·dont. Provided with narrow teeth.

sten″o·pe'ic. 1. Pertaining to a narrow slit or minute hole. 2. A device of metal or other opaque substance with a very fine slit or minute hole or holes. Held before defective eyes, it facilitates vision. Duke-Elder's device enables a presbyope who has lost his glasses to read in an emergency. The slitted stenopeic (long used by Eskimos) protects from ultraviolet radiation from snow.

ste·nosed' (sti·nosed', sten″ozed). Constricted, narrowed.

ste·no'sis. A permanent narrowing, especially of a channel or aperture. —**stenosal, stenot'ic,** *adj.* **aortic s.** A narrowing of the aortic orifice at the base of the heart or a narrowing of the aorta itself. **cica·tricial s.** Stenosis due to a contracted cicatrix. **mitral s.** Disease of the mitral valve causing obstruction to the flow of blood through the left atrioventricular opening. It is a late (renote) effect of acute rheumatic fever. **post-tracheotomy s.** Stenosis after tracheotomy. **pyloric s.** Congenital obstruction of the pyloric orifice of the stomach caused by hypertrophy of the pyloric muscle.

sten″o·sto'mi·a. A reduction in the orifice of the mouth as a result of cicatrization. —**stenostom'atous,** *adj.*

ste·nos'to·my. Contracture of any mouth or aperture.

sten″o·ther'mal. Capable of resisting a small range of temperature.

sten″o·tho'rax. An unusually narrow chest.

stent. 1. A compound used for immobilizing some forms of skin graft. 2. A mold made of stent, used for immobilizing some forms of skin graft.

sten″to·roph'o·nous. Having a loud voice.

step'page gait. The peculiar highstepping gait seen in tabes dorsalis and certain forms of multiple neuritis, or neuropathy. It also occurs in toe drop.

ster″co·bi'lin. The chief constituent of the brown pigment found in feces. Derived from bilirubin by reduction due to bacteria in the intestine. Also called *hydrobilirubin, urobilin.*

ster″co·bi·lin'o·gen (stur″ko·buy'lin·o·jin, ·bi·lin'o·jin). A reduction product of stercobilin which occurs in the feces. Stercobilinogen is a colorless compound which becomes brown on oxidation. It is probably identical with urobilinogen.

ster'co·lith. A calcified, fecal concretion.

ster″co·ra'ceous. Fecal; having the nature of feces; containing feces, as stercoraceous vomiting.

ster″co·ro'ma. Fecalith; a hard fecal mass usually in the rectum.

Ster·cu'li·a. A large genus of tropical trees. **S. urens** of India and **S. tragacantha** of Africa afford karaya gum, which has been substituted for tragacanth. **S. acuminata** (*Cola nitida*) produces kola nut.

ster'cus. Feces.

stere (steer, stair). A measure of 1000 liters; a kiloliter.

ster'e·o- (sterr'ee·o-, steer'ee·o-), **ster'e-.** A combining form meaning *solid.*

ster″e·o·an″es·the'si·a (·an″essthee'zhuh, ·zee·uh). Inability to ascertain the form or size of objects by feeling them.

ster″e·o·ar·throl'y·sis. Loosening stiff joints by operation or manipulation in cases of ankylosis.

ster″e·o·blas'tu·la. A solid blastula; not having a blastocoele, but having all its cells bounding the external surface.

ster″e·o·chem'is·try. A branch of science that investigates the spatial arrangement of atoms in a molecule.

ster″e·o·cil'i·a. Nonmotile cilia.

ster″e·o·og·no'sis. The faculty of recognizing the form and size of objects by means of touch. —**stereognos'tic,** *adj.*

ster″e·o·i'so·mer. A compound containing the same number and kind of atoms as another compound, but with the atoms grouped differently in the molecule.

ster″e·o·i·som'er·ism (sterr″ee·oeye·som'ur·iz·um, steer″ee·o-). The condition in which two or more substances having the same molecular formulas have different properties; these differences are due to the different relative positions of the atoms in the molecule.

ster″e·o·phor'o·scope. A stereoscopic stroboscope, an instrument for producing a series of images apparently in motion; used in tests of visual perception.

ster″e·op'sis. Stereoscopic vision.

ster'e·op″ter. An instrument to provide a rapid quantitative test for depth perception.

ster″e·o·ra″di·og'ra·phy. Taking of two radiographs with the roentgenray tube in two positions, about six inches apart, and viewing of these two films in such a manner that the stereoscopic picture appears three-dimensional.

ster″e·o·roent″gen·og′ra·phy (sterr″ee·o·rent″ghin·og′ruh·fee, steer″ee·o·). A roentgenographic procedure for making stereoscopic roentgenograms.

ster″e·o·roent″gen·om′e·ter. Apparatus for determining the solid dimensions of a radiopaque object from its stereoscopic roentgenograms.

ster′e·o·scope. An instrument by which two similar pictures of the same object are so mounted that the images are seen as one, thereby giving a three-dimensional impression, as in binocular vision. —**stereoscop′ic,** *adj.*; **stereos′copy,** *n.*

ster′e·o·ty″py (sterr″ee·o·tye″pee). Morbid persistence of a volitional impulse when once started.

ster′id. A substance that is either a sterol or a steroid.

ster′ile. 1. Not fertile; not capable of reproducing. 2. Free from germs.

ste·ril′i·ty. The condition of being sterile, infertile, or incapable of reproducing.

ste·ril′i·ty clin′ic. Fertility clinic.

ster″i·li·za′tion. 1. The destruction of all forms of life. Substances may be sterilized by the use of physical or chemical agents, heat being the most important. Moist heat, at temperatures above the boiling point of water, will kill the most resistant spores formed by microörganisms within a relatively short period of time. Fractional or intermittent sterilization consists of the successive application of moist heat to destroy vegetative cells with intervening periods of sufficient duration to permit spores to germinate. 2. Any procedure which renders an individual incapable of reproduction.

ster′i·lize. 1. Render sterile or free from bacteria. 2. Render incapable of procreation.

ster′i·li″zer. An instrument for the destruction of all forms of life. The Arnold sterilizer utilizes steam at atmospheric pressure. The autoclave or pressure cooker uses steam under pressure at temperatures above the boiling point of water.

ster·nal′gi·a. Pain in the sternum.

ster′no-. A combining form denoting *breast* or *connection with the sternum.*

ster″no·clei″do·mas′toid (stur″-no·kly″do·mas′toyd). Pertaining to the sternum, the clavicle, and the mastoid process, as the sternocleidomastoid muscle. See Table of Muscles in the Appendix.

ster″no·dyn′i·a (stur″no·din′ee·uh, ·dye′nee·uh). Sternalgia; pain in the sternum.

ster″no·mas′toid. Unofficial term for sternocleidomastoid muscle.

ster·nos′chi·sis (stur·nos′ki·sis). Cleft or fissure of the sternum. A[l]so called *fissura sterni.*

ster·not′o·my. Cutting through t[he] sternum.

ster′num. The flat, narrow bone [in] the median line in the front of t[he] chest, composed of three portions—t[he] ma[n]ubri[um], the body, and the xipho[id] process. See Table of Bones in t[he] Appendix. —**ster′nal,** *adj.* **cleft —** Congenital fissure of the sternum.

ster′nu·ta″tor. A substance capab[le] of inducing sneezing, as certain w[ar] gases.

ster″o·chem′is·try (sterr″o·kem[·]is·tree, steer″o·). See *stereochemist[ry.]*

ster′oid, ste′roid. The gene[ric] name for the compounds comprisi[ng] the sterols, bile acids, heart poison[s], saponins, and sex hormones.

ster′ol, ste′rol. Any saturated [or] unsaturated alcohol derived from cycl[o-] pentanoperhydrophenanthrene; the s[te-] cohols occur both free and combined [as] esters or glycosides, and usually a[re] obtained as principal constituents [of] the nonsaponifiable fraction of fix[ed] oils and fats. Zoosterols are sterols [of] animal origin; *phytosterols* are ster[ols] from higher plants; *mycosterols* are t[he] sterols of fungi.

ster′one, ste′rone. A steroid po[s-] sessing one or more ketone groups.

sterosan. Trade-mark for chlo[r-] quinaldol.

ster′tor. Sonorous breathing or sno[r-] ing; the rasping, rattling sound pr[o-] duced when the larynx and the [air] passages are partially obstructed [by] mucus. —**stertorous,** *adj.*

steth′o-, steth-. A combining for[m] meaning *breast* or *chest.*

steth″o·pol′y·scope. A stethosco[pe] having several tubes for the simultan[e-] ous use of several listeners.

steth′o·scope. An instrument for t[he] detection and study of sounds arisi[ng] within the body. Invented by Laenne[c.] The early type was a slender wood[en] tube with a flange on each end. T[he] modern stethoscope has a bell or cu[p-] shaped end piece of metal or hard ru[b-] ber connected with rubber tubi[ng] which conducts the sound to both ea[rs] of the examiner. **binaural s.** O[ne] which connects to both ears of the us[er.]

steth″o·scop′ic. Pertaining to, [or] detected by means of, a stethoscope.

ste·thos′co·py. Examination w[ith] the aid of a stethoscope.

sthe′ni·a (sthee′nee·uh). Normal [or] excessive force or vigor; opposed [to] *asthenia.*

sthen′ic. Strong; active.

stib′a·mine glu′co·side. A nitr[o-] gen glucoside of sodium *p*-aminophe[n-] ylstibonate, a pentavalent antimo[ny] compound used in the treatment of kala-azar.

stib'i·al·ism. Antimonial poisoning.

stib'ine (stib'een, ·in). Antimonous hydride, SbH_3.

stib'i·um. Antimony.

sti·bo'ni·um. The monovalent radical, SbH_4^+, analogous to ammonium.

tib'o·phen. $(NaOS)_3C_6H_2O_2:SbOC_6$ $H_2(ONa)(SO_2Na)_3.7H_2O$. Sodium antimony-bispyrocatechol-3,5-sodium disulfonate; employed as a remedy in venereal lymphogranuloma and schistosomiasis. See *fuadin*.

tic·tac'ne (stick·tack'nee). Acne punctata; acne in which the pustules are tiny and surround a comedone.

tiff. Inflexible, unyielding, immovable in continuity; applied especially to normally movable parts.

ti'fle. Choke; kill by impeding respiration.

tig'ma (pl. **stigmas, stigmata**). 1. A small spot or mark, especially a spot of hemorrhage in the palm or sole, occurring in hysterical persons. 2. Any one of the marks or signs characteristic of a condition, as hysterical stigmas. 3. That part of a pistil which receives the pollen. 4. An opening between cells, especially one between the endothelial cells of a capillary, now considered an artifact. A stoma. —**stigmal, stigmat'ic,** adj. **hysterical stigmas.** The specific, peculiar phenomena or symptoms of hysteria, as anesthesia, hyperesthesia, hysterogenic zones, reversal of the color field, contraction of the visual field, the phenomena of transport amblyopia, impairment of the senses of hearing and of taste and of muscular sense, etc.

tig·mas'ter·ol. $C_{30}H_{49}O$. A sterol derived from the soybean.

tig'ma·tism. 1. A condition of the refractive media of the eye in which rays of light from a point are accurately brought to a focus on the retina. Also see *astigmatism*. 2. The condition of having stigmas.

tig"ma·ti·za'tion. The formation of stigmas.

tigmomene bromide. Trade-mark for benzpyrinium bromide.

til·bam'i·dine (stil·bam'i·deen, ·din). $NH:C(NH_2).C_6H_4.CH:CH.C_6H_4.$ $(NH_2)C:NH$; 4:4'-diamidinostilbene. One of a group of diamidines possessing trypanocidal activity.

til'bene. $C_6H_5CH=CH.C_6H_5$. The parent hydrocarbon from which the synthetic estrogen diethylstilbestrol may be considered to be derived.

til·bes'trol, stil·boes'trol (stil-bes'trole, ·trol, ·trawl). Diethylstilbestrol.

till'birth". The birth of a dead child.

till'born". Born dead.

stil·lin'gi·a. The dried root of *Stillingia sylvatica*. Syn., *queensroot*.

stim'u·lant. 1. Stimulating. 2. An agent that causes stimulation. **diffusible s.** One that has a prompt but transient effect. **local s.** One acting directly, as on the end organs of the sensory nerves of the skin.

stim'u·late. Quicken; stir up; excite; increase functional activity.

stim"u·la'tion. 1. The act of stimulating. 2. The effect of a stimulant.

stim'u·li (stim'yoo·lye). Plural of stimulus, *q.v.*

stim'u·lin. Metchnikoff's name for substances supposed to stimulate the phagocytes to destroy germs. *Obs.*

stim'u·lus (pl. **stimuli**). An excitant or irritant. **adequate s.** One effective in producing a response. **chemical s.** One due to, or produced by, chemical means. **conditioned s.** One to which a conditioned reflex response has been developed. **heterologous s.** One acting upon the nervous elements of the sensory apparatus along their entire course. **homologous s.** One acting only upon the end organ. **mechanical s.** One acting by mechanical means, as pinching or striking. **thermal s.** One acting through change in temperature. **threshold s.** One just adequate to wake a response.

sting. 1. The acute burning sensation caused by pricking, striking, or chemically stimulating the skin or a mucous membrane. 2. Cause such a sensation. 3. The wound caused. 4. The organ or part causing the wound, e.g. the sting of a bee or of a nettle.

stip'pling. 1. A change of a surface whereby the presence of tiny nodules produces an appearance like that of a stippled paper, as slight deposits of fibrin on a serous surface. 2. A change in erythrocytes whereby minute droplets with affinity for basic dyes occur, as in lead poisoning.

stir'pi·cul"ture. The improvement of animal stocks by scientific breeding. —**stirpicul'tural,** adj.

stitch. 1. A sudden, sharp, lancinating pain. 2. See *suture*, 2. **glover's s.** The continuous suture used especially in wounds of the intestines.

stock. A quantity of solution, or other material, kept on hand for use as occasion requires.

stock"i·net'. Cotton material or shirting, woven like a stocking, but of uniform caliber and used according to size to cover extremities or the body preparatory to the application of a fixed dressing, as plaster, splints.

stock'ing. A close-fitting covering for the leg and foot, sometimes designed and fitted for a special hygienic or therapeutic purpose; usually made of knitted or woven goods that sometimes contains an elastic thread. **elastic s.** One containing rubber so that it exerts a continuous pressure on the leg.

stoi″chi·om′e·try (stoy″kee·om′i-tree). The branch of chemistry that deals with the numerical relationship between elements or compounds (atomic weights), the determination of the proportions in which the elements combine (formulas), and the weight relations in reactions (equations). —**stoichiomet′ric,** adj.

sto′ma. A minute opening or pore in a surface; particularly, one of the stigmas, or minute openings, of a peritoneal surface, presumably for the drainage of fluid into lymphatics.

sto·mac′a·ce (sto-mack′uh·see). Ulcerative stomatitis.

stom′ach. The most dilatable part of the alimentary canal, situated below the diaphragm in the left hypochondriac, the epigastric, and part of the right hypochondriac regions. It is continuous at the cardiac end with the esophagus, at the pyloric end with the duodenum. Its wall consists of four coats: mucous, submucous, muscular, and serous. The mucous coat contains the gastric glands—cardiac, fundic, and pyloric—which secrete the gastric juice and mucus. **dumping s.** A condition following gastroenterostomy, marked by rapid emptying through the new opening with intestinal distention, discomfort, and colic. **hourglass s.** One divided more or less completely into two compartments by an equatorial constriction. **J s.** A long, vertically located stomach. **powdered s.** The dried and powdered, defatted wall of the stomach of the hog, Sus scrofa var. domesticus; it is a granular substance with a meaty odor, and is practically insoluble in water. It contains factors which cause an increase in the number of red blood cells in the blood of persons suffering from pernicious anemia. Also called dried stomach. **steerhorn s.** A high, transversely located stomach. Also called cow horn s.

sto·mach′ic (sto-mack′ick). 1. Pertaining to the stomach. 2. One of a class of substances which may stimulate the secretory activity of the stomach.

sto″ma·tal′gi·a. Pain in the mouth.

sto·mat′ic. Relating or belonging to the mouth.

sto″ma·ti′tis (sto″muh·tye′tis, stom″uh·). Inflammation of the soft tissues of the mouth. **aphthous s.** Herpetic stomatitis. **gangrenous s.** Stomatitis characterized by necrosis. See noma. **herpetic s.** Stomatitis believed to be caused by the herpes simplex virus, characterized by aphthous lesions. **membranous s.** Stomatitis

apparently caused by streptococcal infection, characterized by a grayish membranous covering on the oral mucous membranes. **ulcerative s.** Stomatitis characterized by the formation of ulcers and necrosis of oral tissue. **Vincent's s.** An infectious, painful inflammation of the gingival tissue with formation of a pseudomembrane. Vincent's spirillum and a fusiform bacillus are associated organisms. Syn. trench mouth, acute ulcerative gingivitis, Vincent's infection. Not to be confused with Vincent's angina.

sto′ma·to- (sto″muh·to-, stom″uh·to-. **stomat-.** A combining form meaning mouth.

sto″ma·toe′a·ce (sto″muh·tock′uh-see, stom″uh·). Ulcerative stomatitis.

sto″ma·to·ca·thar′sis. Salivation. q.v. Obs.

sto″ma·to·dyn′i·a. Pain in the mouth.

sto″ma·to·dy·so′di·a (sto″muh·to-di·so′dee·uh, stom″uh·to·). Ill-smelling breath.

sto″ma·tol′o·gy (sto″muh·tol′o·jee, stom″uh·). That branch of medical science which treats of the anatomy, physiology, pathology, therapeutics and hygiene of the oral cavity, of the tongue, teeth, and adjacent structures and tissues, and of the relationship of that field to the entire body. —**stomatolog′ic,** adj.

sto″ma·to·ma·la′ci·a (·ma·lay′shee-uh, ·see-uh). Sloughing or degeneration of the structures of the mouth.

sto″ma·to·me′ni·a. Vicarious bleeding in the mouth, associated with menstrual disorders.

sto″ma·to′mi·a (sto″muh·to′me-uh, stom″uh·). A general term for the incision of a mouth, as of the uterus.

sto·mat′o·my. Incision of the uteri.

sto″ma·to·my·co′sis (sto″muh·to-migh·ko′sis, stom″uh·to·). A disease of the mouth due to fungi, especially Monilia albicans. See thrush, 1.

sto″ma·to·no′ma. Gangrene of the mouth. Syn., stomatonecrosis.

sto″ma·top′a·thy (sto″muh·top′-uth·ee, stom″uh·). Any disease of the mouth.

sto″ma·to·plas″ty (sto″muh·to-plas″tee, stom″uh·to·, sto·mat′o·). plastic operation upon the mouth. —**stomatoplas′tic,** adj.

sto″ma·tor·rha′gi·a (·ray′ju-·radj′uh). Copious hemorrhage from the mouth.

sto″ma·to·scope′ (sto″muh·to-scope″, stom″uh·to·). An instrument used for inspecting the cavity of the mouth.

sto″ma·to′sis. Disease of the mouth.

sto″ma·tot′o·my. Incision of the uteri.

sto·men″or·rha′gi·a (sto·men″o-ray′juh, sto″men·o·). Vicarious bleeding in the mouth, associated with abnormal menstruation.

-sto′mi·a. A combining form denoting *a condition of the mouth*, as in *microstomia*.

sto″mo·de′um (sto″mo·dee′um, stom″o·). The primitive oral cavity of the embryo; an ectodermal fossa formed by the growth of the facial processes about the buccopharyngeal membrane. **—stomodeal,** *adj.*

sto·mos′chi·sis (sto·mos′ki·sis). Fissure of the mouth. There are the following special types: cheiloschisis, cleft lip; gnathoschisis, cleft jaw; uranoschisis or palatoschisis, cleft palate; staphyloschisis, cleft soft palate; uvula fissa, cleft uvula.

Sto·mox′ys. A genus of bloodsucking flies of the family Muscidae. It is similar to the common house fly. **S. calcitrans.** The common stable fly which aids in the transmission of trypanosomiasis and anthrax, and serves as an intermediate host of the nematode *Habronema*, parasitic in the stomach of the horse.

-stomy. 1. Same as *-stomia*. 2. A combining form denoting *an operation establishing a usually permanent artificial opening*, as in *gastrostomy*.

stone. 1. A hardened mass of mineral matter. See *calculus*. 2. An English unit of weight, 14 lb.

stone search′er. An instrument equipped with a porcelain tip, used for exploring the bladder, bile duct, etc., for concretions; now little used.

stool. Evacuation of the bowels. Also see *allochezia*. **acholic stools.** (a) Light gray or clay-colored stools having the consistency of putty, which follow obstruction of the flow of bile into the duodenum. The color is due to the presence of the normal urobilin. The stools show, under the microscope, an abnormal amount of fat. This form of acholic stool is accompanied by icterus and choluria. (b) Stools of the same color may occur in noninterference with the flow of bile, but then the stools do not contain an excessively large amount of fat and fatty acids. **fatty stools.** Stools in which fat is present; due to pancreatic disease. **lead-pencil stools.** Fecal discharges of very small caliber. Usually due to general nervousness causing local intestinal spasm, or to stricture or stenosis of the descending colon, sigmoid, or rectum. Also called *ribbon stools*. **mucous stools.** Stools containing mucus. They indicate the existence of intestinal inflammation. **pea soup stools.** The peculiar liquid evacuation of typhoid fever. **rice-water stools.** The stools of cholera, in which there is a copious

serous exudation containing detached epithelium. **tarry stools.** Stools having the color and consistency of tar, usually due to hemorrhage into the intestinal tract but also produced by iron, bismuth, barium, or other medication.

stop′cock. A turning cock, connected with a pipe, for regulating the flow of gases or liquids.

stop′page. Cessation of flow or action; closure or stenosis.

sto′rax. A balsam obtained from the trunk of *Liquidambar orientalis*, or of *L. styraciflua;* occurs as a semi-liquid, grayish to grayish brown, opaque mass, or a semi-solid or solid mass; insoluble in water. It consists largely of storesin, which is present in two forms—alpha and beta storesin—both free and in the form of a cinnamic ester. Cinnamic acid and its esters are also present. Also called *liquid s.*

sto·res′in (sto·rez′in). A hard resin from storax.

storm. Term sometimes used for sudden exacerbation of symptoms or crisis in a disease. **thyroid s.** Severe, acute thyrotoxicosis.

stovaine. Trade-mark for amylocaine hydrochloride.

stovarsol. Trade-mark for acetarsone.

S.T.P. Standard temperature and pressure. See *standard conditions*.

stra″bis·mom′e·try (stray″bizmom′i·tree, strab″iz·). The measurement of the degree of strabismus.

stra·bis′mus (stra·biz′mus). Squint; that abnormality of the eyes in which the visual axes do not meet at the desired objective point, in consequence of incoördinate action of the extrinsic ocular muscles. Syn., *heterotropia.* **—strabismal, strabismic,** *adj.* **concomitant s.** One in which the squinting eye has full range of movement. **convergent s.** Esotropia. **divergent s.** Exotropia. **paralytic s.** That due to paralysis of one or more muscles.

stra·bom′e·ter. An instrument for the measurement of the deviation of the eyes in strabismus.

stra·bom′e·try. The determination of the degree of ocular deviation in strabismus.

stra·bot′o·my. An operation for the correction of strabismus. *Obs.*

strain. 1. Excessive stretching; overuse of a part; overexertion. 2. The condition produced in a part by overuse or wrong use, as eyestrain. **—strain,** *v.* **ventricular s.** A term used in electrocardiography as either (a) **left ventricular strain,** designating the effect of increased left ventricular work as caused by hypertension or aortic valve disease, possibly reversible if the hypertension is removed; or (b)

right ventricular strain, designating the effect of increased right ventricular work as caused by pulmonary embolism (acute) or pulmonary disease or pulmonic stenosis (chronic).

strain. A group of organisms closely related to each other, characterized by a common peculiarity. **Flury s.** A rabies strain used in prophylactic vaccination of dogs; made from living virus modified by growth in chick embryos.

strain. In pharmacy, to separate insoluble substances from liquid; to filter.

strait. A narrow or constricted passage, as the inferior or superior strait of the pelvis.

strait′jack″et. A strong jacket placed on the insane or delirious to prevent injury to themselves or others.

stra·mo′ni·um. The dried leaf and flowering top of *Datura stramonium* (including *Datura Tatula*). It contains the alkaloid daturine, which is identical with hyoscyamine, and traces of scopolamine. The general physiologic and therapeutic action of stramonium is similar to that of belladonna. Syn., *Jamestown weed, Jimson weed.*

stran′gle. Choke or throttle by compression of the glottis or trachea.

stran″gu·la′tion. 1. The act of choking. 2. Constriction of a part producing arrest of the circulation, as strangulation of a hernia. —**stran′gulated,** adj.

stran′gu·ry. Painful urination, the urine being voided drop by drop.

strap. 1. A long band, as of adhesive plaster. 2. Compress a part by means of bands, especially bands of adhesive plaster.

stra′ta (strat′uh, stray′tuh). Plural of stratum, q.v.

strat″i·fi·ca′tion. Arrangement in layers.

strat′i·fied. Arranged in layers.

strat′o·sphere (strat′o·sfeer, stray′to·). The atmosphere above the troposphere, where temperature changes are small and winds essentially horizontal.

stra′tum (strat′um, stray′tum) (pl. *strata*). A layer. **s. cor′neum.** The layer of keratinized cells of the epidermis. **s. germinativum.** The deeper layer of the epidermis in which cell proliferation and growth take place. Syn., *Malpighian layer.* Formerly called **s. mucosum, rete mucosum. s. granulosum.** A layer of minute cells or one of cells containing many granules, especially the layer containing keratohyalin granules in volar epidermis. **s. spongiosum.** The deeper layer (about three-fourths) of the decidua parietalis. **s. submucosum.** The thin layer of the myometrium adjacent to the endometrium. **s. subserosum.** The thin layer of muscle of the myometrium adjacent to the serous coat. **s. supravasculare.** The layer of muscle of the myometrium between the stratum vasculare and the stratum subserosum. **s. vasculare.** The thickest layer of muscle in the myometrium next to the stratum submucosum.

straw′ber″ry mark. A vascular nevus which is visible at, or soon after, birth.

streak. 1. A furrow, line, or stripe. 2. In *bacteriology*, the process of distributing the inoculum over the surface of a solid culture medium. Cultures thus obtained are called streak cultures. **primitive s.** A dense, opaque band of ectoderm in the bilaminar blastoderm associated with the morphogenetic movements and proliferation of the mesoderm and notochord. It indicates the first trace of the embryo.

stream. Flow, especially in a definite direction; applied to movement in protoplasm.

streph″o·sym·bo′li·a (stref′o·simbo′lee·uh, ·sim·bol′ee·uh). Difficulty of children in learning to read; inability to distinguish between similar letters as *p* and *q* or *n* and *u*. It is the result of mixed motor dominance of right and left cerebral hemispheres.

strep′i·tus. A sound, a noise.

strep″ti·ce′mi·a. Streptococcal septicemia.

strep′ti·dine. $C_8H_{18}N_2O_4$. 1,3-Diguanidino-2,4,5,6-tetrahydroxycyclohexane, obtained when streptomycin undergoes acid hydrolysis; in the streptomycin molecule it is glycosidally linked to streptobiosamine.

strep′to-, strept-. A combining form meaning *twisted* or *curved*.

strep″to·an·gi′na (strep″to·anjye′nuh, ·an′ji·nuh). Streptococcal sore throat; septic sore throat; a pseudomembranous deposit in the throat due to streptococci.

strep″to·bi·o′sa·mine. $C_{13}H_{25}NO_7$. A nitrogen-containing disaccharide obtained when streptomycin undergoes acid hydrolysis; in the streptomycin molecule it is glycosidally linked to streptidine.

strep″to·coc′cal, strep″to·coc′cic (strep″to·cock′sick). Relating to or due to, streptococci.

strep″to·coc·ce′mi·a (·cock·see′mee·uh). The presence of streptococci in the blood.

Strep″to·coc′cus (pl. *Streptococci*). A genus of bacteria of the tribe Streptococcaceae, family Lactobacteriaceae; the bacterium is a Gram-positive coccus which forms chains. Colony reaction on blood agar plates is used to divide the genus into α hemolytic (*S. viridans*), β hemolytic (*S. pyogenes*) and γ hemolytic (*S. anhemolyticus*). Serologic studies have resulted in the

Lancefield groups A, B, C, D, and E. Organisms isolated from man usually are in groups A and C; those pathogenic for animals are in groups B and C. Disease-specific names have been abandoned. **s. hemolyticus.** Synonym for *S. pyogenes.* **s. mitis.** Synonym for *S. viridans.* **s. pyogenes.** Causative agent of scarlet fever, erysipelas, and frequently of sore throat, puerperal sepsis, pyogenic inflammations, and bronchopneumonia. **s. viridans.** A species which includes both pathogenic and saprophytic organisms. The pathogenic are recovered from cases of subacute bacterial endocarditis, bronchopneumonia, urinary-tract infection, and focal inflammations.

strep″to·der″ma·ti·tis. Inflammation of the skin due to streptococci.

strep″to·dor′nase. Deoxyribonuclease.

strep″to·du′o·cin. A mixture of equal parts of dihydrostreptomycin sulfate and streptomycin sulfate.

strep″to·ki′nase. A catalytic agent present in fibrinolysin, and possibly its active component, which activates the fibrin-lysing system present in the euglobulin fraction of human blood. Abbreviated, SK.

strep″to·ly′sin (strep″to·lye′sin, strep·tol′i·sin). The hemotoxins of hemolytic streptococci. They are filtrable. There are two types: **streptolysin S,** which is heat-sensitive and destroyed by acid, and **streptolysin O,** which is resistant to these factors but is destroyed by oxygen.

Strep″to·my′ces (strep″to·migh′-sees). A genus of aerobic fungi whose species are saprophytic soil forms. It includes several species that are sources of antibiotics.

strep″to·my′cin. $C_{21}H_{39}N_7O_{12}$. A water-soluble antibiotic obtained from *Streptomyces griseus.* It consists of a hydroxylated base, streptidine, glycosidally linked to the disaccharidelike molecule streptobiosamine. It is active almost exclusively against Gram-negative organisms.

strep″to·sep″ti·ce′mi·a. Septicemia due to streptococci.

strep″to·so′mus. A non-human form of celosoma in which the spine is twisted so that the legs are displaced laterally.

strep″to·thri′cin (strep″to·thry′sin, ·thriss′in). An antibiotic substance from *Streptomyces lavendulae.* It is an organic base, soluble in water.

strep″to·thri·co′sis. A disease resulting from infection with a streptothrix.

strep″to·thry′cin. Streptothricin, *q.v.*

stress. 1. Force exerted by load or other mechanical means. 2. The summation of stimuli which tends to up-

set the physiologic or psychologic equilibrium of an individual, thus making it difficult for him to fit his environment.

stretch. Draw out to full length.

stretch′er. See *litter.* **Neil Robertson s.** A canvas litter strengthened with slats of split bamboo. It is used to transport an injured man aboard a vessel.

stri′a (pl. *striae*). 1. Streak, stripe, narrow band. 2. Fibrinoid, *q.v.* **s. albicans gravidarum.** Stria strophica due to pregnancy. **s. atrophica.** One of the white, cicatricial lines seen in skin that has been stretched by adiposity, pregnancy, lactation, or repeated trauma.

stri′ae (stry′ee). Plural of stria, *q.v.*

stri′a·ted (stry′ay·tid). Striped, as striated muscle.

stric′ture. A narrowing of the lumen of a canal or hollow organ, as the esophagus, pylorus, ureter, or urethra, the result of inflammatory or other changes in its walls, and, occasionally, of external pressure. It may be temporary or permanent, depending upon the cause and the course of the disease producing it. **annular s.** A ringlike obstruction produced by a contracture which involves the entire circumference of the canal, bowel, etc. **bridle s.** A stricture caused by a delicate band stretched across the urethral lumen. **spasmodic s.** That involving the membranous urethra and caused by muscular spasm of the sphincter muscle, and usually associated with urethritis.

stri′dor. A peculiar, harsh, vibrating sound produced during respiration. **laryngeal s.** Stridor due to laryngeal spasm. **s. dentium.** Grinding of the teeth. **s. serratics.** A sound like sharpening a saw, sometimes produced by expiration through a tracheotomy tube.

strid′u·lous. Characterized by stridor; as stridulous laryngismus.

strin′gent. Binding.

string-gal″va·nom′e·ter. Instrument for measuring intensity and direction of minute currents. See *electrocardiograph.*

string′halt″ (string′hawlt″). An involuntary, convulsive movement of muscles in the hind leg of the horse; the leg is suddenly raised from the ground and lowered again with unnatural force. Also called *springhalt.*

strip. Press with a milking movement so as to force out the contents of a canal or duct.

stripe. A streak; a discolored mark.

strip′ping. 1. Uncovering; unsheathing. 2. In the plural, the last and richest milk given at any one milking; so called because it is slowly removed by the milker, who strips the teats between the fingers.

strob'ic. Resembling, or pertaining to, a top.

stro·bi'la. 1. The segmented body of the adult tapeworm. 2. The whole adult tapeworm including the scolex.

stro·bi'lus. The adult tapeworm.

stro'bo·scope, strob'o·scope. A device by which a moving object may appear to be at rest; a rapid motion may appear to be slowed, or motion can be depicted by a series of still pictures. The effect depends upon an accurately controlled, intermittent source of light or periodically interrupted vision. **—stroboscop'ic,** adj.

stroke. 1. A sudden and severe seizure or fit of disease. 2. A popular term for apoplexy. 3. Pass the hands gently over an object. **apoplectic s.** See apoplexy. **heat s.** See heat prostration. **paralytic s.** Sudden loss of muscular power from lesion of the brain or spinal cord.

stro'ma. 1. The supporting framework of an organ, including its connective tissue, vessels, and nerves, as contrasted with the epithelial or other tissues performing the special function of the organ, the parenchyma. 2. The substance of an erythrocyte less its hemoglobin. **—stromal,** adj.

stro'ma·tin, stro·ma'tin. The protein of the stroma of erythrocytes.

stro'muhr (stro'moor). Instrument for measuring velocity of blood flow.

Stron"gy·loi'de·a. A superfamily of roundworms, of the suborder Strongylinae, order Rhabditida. The genera *Ancylostoma* and *Necator* are included.

Stron"gy·loi'des (stron"ji·loy'deez). A genus of nematode worms. **S. stercoralis.** An intestinal parasite of man with the same distribution as hookworm. Other species are parasites of lower animals. Also called *S. intestinalis*.

stron"gy·loi·di·a·sis. Infestation with one of the roundworms of the genus *Strongyloides*. Formerly called *anguilluliasis*.

stron'ti·a (stron'shee·uh). Strontium oxide.

stron'ti·um (stron'shee·um, stron'-tee·um). Sr = 87.63. A silver-white to pale yellow, malleable, ductile metal; decomposes in water and alcohol. Strontium is used only as a carrier of therapeutically active acids. **s. bromide.** SrBr₂.6H₂O; occurs as colorless crystals; soluble in water. **s. salicylate.** (C₆H₄.OH.COO)₂Sr.2H₂O; occurs as a white, crystalline powder; soluble in water. Its use is identical with that of sodium salicylate.

stron'ti·um–90. A radioactive isotope of strontium, a product of uranium fission and dangerous because it concentrates in bone, but in the form of a strontium applicator used for the therapeutic effects of its beta radiation. Symbol, Sr^{90}.

stro·phan'thin. A glycoside or a mixture of glycosides obtained from *Strophanthus kombé*; occurs as a yellowish white powder; soluble in water. It can be separated into two portions, a crystalline and an amorphous fraction. The crystalline fraction can be separated into the glycosides *K-strophanthin-α*, and *K-strophanthin-β*. The amorphous fraction consists of glycosides, and the mixture is referred to as *amorphous K-strophanthin*. It is a cardiac stimulant.

stro·phan"tho·bi'ose. Disaccharide present in strophanthus, q.v.

stro·phan'thus. The dried ripe seed of *Strophanthus kombé*, or of *Strophanthus hispidus*, deprived of the awns. The activity of strophanthus is due to several glycosides. See *strophanthin*. Also called *s. seed*.

stroph'u·lus. A form of miliaria occurring in infants, and often unilateral. Also called *red gum*. **s. pruriginosus.** An eruption characterized by disseminated, intensely itching papules. Also called *prurigo*.

struc'ture. 1. The manner or method of the building up, arrangement, and formation of the different tissues and organs of the body or of a complete organism. 2. An organ, a part, or a complete organic body. **—structural,** adj.

stru'ma. Goiter. **s. aberranta.** A goiter of an accessory thyroid gland. **s. congenita.** Congenital goiter. **s. maligna.** Carcinoma of the thyroid gland.

stru"mi·priv'al (strōō"mi·priv'ul, stroo·mip'riv·ul), **stru"mi·pri'vous** (strōō"mi·pry'vus, stroo·mip'ri·vus). Deprived of the thyroid; due to removal of the thyroid gland.

stru·mi'tis. Inflammation of a goitrous thyroid gland.

strych'ni·a (strick'nee·uh). See *strychnine*.

strych'nine (strick'nin, ·neen, ·nyne). C₂₁H₂₂O₂N₂; an alkaloid obtained chiefly from nux vomica; occurs as a white, crystalline powder or as crystals; soluble in water. Strychnine is a powerful stimulant to the central nervous system, especially to the spinal cord and medullary centers. **s. sulfate.** (C₂₁H₂₂N₂O₂)₂.H₂SO₄.5H₂O, colorless or white crystals or powder that are soluble in water.

strych"nin·i·za'tion (strick"nin·i·zay'shun, ·eye·zay'shun). The condition produced by large doses of strychnine or nux vomica.

Strych'nos (strick'nos). A genus of

the Loganiaceae of which the most important is *S. nux-vomica.* See *nux vomica.*

stump. The extremity, pedicle, or base of the part left after surgical amputation, excision, or ablation.

stun. Render temporarily insensible, as by a blow.

stupe. A cloth used for applying heat or counterirritation; especially a cloth wrung out of hot water and sprinkled with a counterirritant, as turpentine-stupe.

stu″pe·fa′cient. Narcotic.

stu″pe·fac′tion. 1. Stupor. 2. The process of succumbing to stupor.

stu′por. 1. The condition of being but partly conscious; lethargy; insensibility. 2. Hysterical mutism. **—stuporous,** *adj.* **anergic s.** Stupor with immobility. Syn., *stuporous insanity.* **delusional s.** Melancholic dullness of mind, with delusions. **epileptic s.** The stupor following an epileptic convulsion. **s. melancholicus.** The stupor found in association with melancholia. **s. miliaris.** Paresthesia of the fingers and toes in connection with miliary fever. **s. vigilans.** Catalepsy.

stur′dy. 1. Vigorous; hardy. 2. See *staggers.*

stu′rine (stew′reen, ·rin). A protamine obtained from the spermatozoa of the sturgeon.

stut′ter. Hesitate or make repeated efforts to articulate a syllable. See *stammering.*

stut′ter·ing. A hesitation in speech due to an inability to enunciate the syllables without repeated efforts. **urinary s.** Hesitancy and involuntary interruptions in urination.

stye. See *hordeolum.*

sty′let (sty′lit, sty·let′). 1. A wire inserted into a soft catheter or cannula to secure rigidity. 2. A fine wire inserted into a hollow hypodermic needle or other hollow needle to maintain patency.

sty′lo-, styl-. A combining form meaning *pillar;* used to denote *connection with the styloid process of the temporal bone.*

sty″lo·glos′sus. A muscle arising from the styloid process of the temporal bone, and inserted into the tongue. See Table of Muscles in the Appendix. **—styloglossal,** *adj.*

sty″lo·hy′oid. Pertaining to the styloid process of the temporal bone and the hyoid bone, as the stylohyoid muscle. See Table of Muscles in the Appendix.

sty″lo·mas′toid. Relating to the styloid and mastoid processes, as stylo-mastoid foramen.

sty″lo·pha·ryn′ge·us (sty″lo·fa-rin′jee·us, ·far″in·jee′us). A muscle arising from the styloid process of the

temporal bone, and inserted into the pharynx. See Table of Muscles in the Appendix.

sty′lus. A pointed device in the form of a holder for applying medicines, as caustic potash. **—styloid,** *adj.*

styp′tic. An agent that checks hemorrhage by causing contraction of the blood vessels, as alum, tannic acid.

stypticin. Trade-mark for cotarnine chloride, *q.v.*

styr′ax. See *storax.*

sty′rene (sty′reen, stirr′een). Styrol.

sty′rol. $C_6H_5CH=CH_2$. Phenylethylene. A liquid hydrocarbon found in storax. It is also known as styrene, or cinnamene.

sty′ro·lene. Styrol, *q.v.*

suavitil. A trade-mark for benactyzine hydrochloride.

sub-. 1. A prefix denoting *under, beneath, deficient.* 2. *In chemistry,* a prefix denoting the *lower of two compounds of the same element* or *basic.*

sub·ac′e·tate (sub·ass′i·tayt). A basic acetate, as lead subacetate.

sub″a·cro′mi·al. Beneath the acromion, as the subacromial bursa.

sub″a·cute′. The stage of a disease when it is intermediate between an acute and a chronic form.

sub·al″i·men·ta′tion. Inadequate or deficient nourishment.

sub·a′que·ous. Living beneath the water.

sub″a·rach′noid (sub″a·rack′-noyd). Beneath the arachnoid membrane, as the subarachnoid space.

sub″a·tom′ic. Pertaining to the structure or components of atoms.

sub″au·di′tion (sub″aw·dish′un). The act or ability of comprehending what is not expressed.

sub·chron′ic. More nearly chronic than is indicated by the term subacute.

sub·cla′vi·an. Lying under the clavicle, as the subclavian artery. See Table of Arteries in the Appendix.

sub·clin′i·cal. Pertaining to a disease, in which manifestations are so slight as to be unnoticeable and even not demonstrable.

sub·con′scious. 1. *In psychiatry,* pertaining to material which, while being outside the range of clear consciousness, is capable of producing or determining conscious mental or physical reactions. 2. *In psychoanalysis,* that portion of the unconscious containing mental experiences which are not in the focus of immediate attention, but which may be recalled to consciousness.

sub·con′scious·ness. Imperfect consciousness; that state in which mental processes take place without the mind being distinctly conscious of its own activity.

sub·cos'tal. Lying beneath a rib or the ribs.

sub"cos·tal'gi·a. Pain beneath the ribs, or over a subcostal nerve.

sub"crep·i·ta'tion. An indistinctly crepitant sound.

sub·cul'ture. *In microbiology,* the procedure of transferring organisms from one culture to fresh culture medium; also, the resulting culture.

sub"cu·ta'ne·ous. Beneath the skin; hypodermic.

sub"de·lir'i·um. A slight or muttering delirium, with lucid intervals.

sub·del'toid. Beneath the deltoid muscle, as subdeltoid bursa.

sub"di·a·phrag·mat'ic (sub"dye-uh-frag·mat'ick). Under the diaphragm, as subdiaphragmatic abscess.

sub"di·vi'ded. Redivided; making secondary or smaller divisions.

sub·duct'. Draw downward.

su'ber·in. A waxy substance found in the cork cells of plants.

sub·gal'late. A basic salt of gallic acid. See *bismuth* subgallate.

sub"glos·si'tis. Inflammation of the tissues under the tongue. See *ranula.*

sub"grun·da'tion. The intrusion of one fragment of a cranial bone beneath another part in a fracture.

sub"in·fec'tion. A slight degree of infection.

sub"in·vo·lu'tion. Imperfect return to normal size after functional enlargement. **s. of the uterus.** The imperfect involution of the uterus after delivery.

sub·i'o·dide. That iodide of a series containing the least iodine.

sub·ja'cent. Lying beneath.

sub·jec'tive. 1. Pertaining to the individual himself. 2. Referring to symptoms, experienced by the patient himself, and not amenable to physical exploration.

sub·la'tion. Removal, ablation.

sub·le'thal. Less than fatal, as a sublethal dose of poison.

sub·li·mate. 1. A solid or condensed substance obtained by heating a material, which passes directly from the solid to the vapor phase and then back to the solid state. 2. *In psychiatry,* express or externalize instinctual impulses in a socially acceptable or conventional manner; purify instinctual modes of expression. **corrosive s.** Mercury bichloride.

sub"li·ma'tion. 1. The transformation of a solid to the gaseous state, followed by condensation to the solid state. 2. *In psychiatry,* a psychic device whereby undesirable primitive cravings and impulses gain outward expression

by converting their energies into socially acceptable activities.

sub·lime'. Successively volatilize and condense a solid.

sub·lim'i·nal. Below the threshold of consciousness or of sensation. See *threshold.*

sub·lin'gual. 1. Lying beneath the tongue. 2. Pertaining to the parts lying beneath the tongue.

sub"lin·gui'tis. Inflammation of a sublingual gland.

sub"lux·a'tion. Incomplete dislocation; sprain.

sub"mal·le'o·lar. Under the malleoli, as submalleolar amputation, removal of the foot at the ankle joint.

sub"man·dib'u·lar. Below or beneath the mandible, as the submandibular gland or ganglion.

sub"max"il·lar·i'tis. Inflammation of a submaxillary gland.

sub·max'il·lar"y (sub·mack'si-lerr"ee). Lying beneath the lower maxilla [O.T.], or mandible, as the submaxillary gland. *Syn., submandibular* [NA].

sub·men'tal. Situated under the chin.

sub"mi·cro·scop'ic (sub"migh-kro-skop'ick). Pertaining to a particle which is below the limit of resolution of the optical microscope.

sub·mor'phous. Having a structure intermediate between amorphous and true crystalline. Often applied to the indefinite, partially crystalline structure of calculi.

sub"mu·co'sa. The layer of fibrous connective tissue that attaches a mucous membrane to its subjacent parts. —**submu'cous,** *adj.*

sub"nar·cot'ic. Moderately narcotic.

sub·ni'trate. A basic nitrate.

sub·nor'mal. Below normal.

sub"nu·tri'tion (sub"new·trish'-un). Defective nutrition.

sub·or"di·na'tion. The condition of being under subjection or control; the condition of organs that depend upon or are controlled by other organs.

sub·par"a·lyt'ic. Slightly paralytic.

sub"per·i·os·te'al. Beneath the periosteum.

sub·phren'ic. See *subdiaphragmatic.*

sub·plan'ti·grade. Incompletely plantigrade; walking with the heel slightly elevated.

sub·scrip'tion. That part of a prescription containing the directions to the pharmacist, indicating how the ingredients are to be mixed and prepared.

sub·sib'i·lant. Having a sound like a muffled whistling.

sub·si'dence, sub'si·dence. The gradual cessation and disappearance of the manifestations of disease.

sub·sist'ence. That which nourishes or gives support; food.

sub′stage″. The parts beneath the stage of a microscope, including the diaphragm, condenser, mirror, and other accessories.

sub′stance. 1. The material of which anything is composed. 2. A tissue. **anterior pituitarylike s.** Chorionic gonadotropin; a hormone derived from the chorionic villi of the placenta, similar to the gonadotropic hormone of the pituitary gland; but active only in the presence of the pituitary gland and having a chiefly luteinizing effect on the ovaries. Also called *pregnancy urine hormone (P.U.).* See also *A.P.L.* **depressor s.** One whose pharmacodynamic action results in a lowering of arterial pressure. **desiccated ovarian s.** See *ovary.* 2. **ground s.** Homogeneous matrix or intercellular substance of a tissue in which the cellular elements and fibers are imbedded. **interprismatic s.** The cementing substance between enamel prisms. **Nissl s.** The chromophil substance of nerve cells. **posterior pituitary s.** An extract of the neurohypophysis containing oxytocic, pressor, and antidiuretic principles. The oxytocic principle stimulates the uterus, the pressor principle produces peripheral vasoconstriction, and the antidiuretic principle inhibits the renal tubules. **pressor s.** One whose pharmacodynamic action results in an elevation of arterial pressure. **vasodilator s.** A chemical compound capable of dilating blood vessels.

sub·stan′ti·a (sub-stan′shee-uh) (pl. *substantiae*). Substance, *q.v.*

sub·stan′ti·ae (sub-stan′shee-ee). Plural of substantia, *q.v.*

sub·stit′u·ent. *In chemistry,* an atom or a group that is substituted for another, or that enters a molecule in place of a part that is removed.

sub″sti·tu′tion. 1. The replacement of one thing by another. 2. *In chemistry,* the replacing of one or more elements or radicals in a compound by other elements or radicals.

sub′strate. 1. An under layer. 2. A substance upon which an enzyme acts.

sub·sul′to·ry. Leaping; twitching.

sub·sul′tus. A morbid jerking or twitching. **s. tendinum.** Involuntary twitching of the muscles, especially of the hands and feet, seen in low fevers.

sub″te·tan′ic. Pertaining to convulsions which are not distinctly clonic or tonic.

sub′ti·lin. An antibiotic substance obtained from *Bacillus subtilis.* It is active against Gram-positive bacteria.

sub·to′tal. Less than complete.

sub·trop′i·cal. Pertaining to regions almost tropical in climate.

sub·u′ber·es (sub-yoo′bur-eez). Children at the breast; suckling children.

sub·vir′ile (sub-virr′il, -vy′ril). Deficient in virility.

sub″vo·lu′tion. A method of operating for pterygium, in which a flap is turned over so that an outer or cutaneous surface comes in contact with a raw, dissected surface. Adhesions are thus prevented.

sub·wa′king. Pertaining to the condition between sleeping and complete wakefulness.

sucaryl. Trade-mark for cyclamate.

suc″ce·da′ne·ous (suck″si-day′nee-us). 1. Relating to, or acting as, a substitute. 2. Pertaining to that which follows after, as a permanent tooth that replaces a deciduous tooth.

suc′ci (suck′sigh). Plural of succus, *q.v.*

suc·cif′er·ous. Producing sap.

suc′ci·nate. A salt of succinic acid.

suc″cin·chlo′ri·mide. $C_4H_4O_2NCl.$ Occurs as white crystals or powder, soluble in water, with decomposition forming hypochlorous acid. Possesses powerful germicidal activity. Used as a water decontaminant.

suc·cin′ic ac′id. $COOH.CH_2.CH_2.COOH.$ A dibasic, crystalline acid occurring in amber and certain other resins; the sodium salt has been used as an analeptic in counteracting barbiturate poisoning. Succinates may possess protective action against depression of tissue metabolism.

suc·cin″o·de·hy′dro·gen·ase. The enzyme which catalyzes the oxidation of succinic acid to fumaric acid.

suc″cin·yl·sul″fa·thi′a·zole. $HOOC.(CH_2)_2CO.NH.C_6H_4.SO_2.NHC_6H_4NS.H_2O;$ 2-(p-succinylaminobenzenesulfonamide) thiazole monohydrate; occurs as a white or yellowish white, crystalline powder; soluble in water. Exerts a sulfonamide bacteriostatic action, chiefly on the intestinal contents, as it is poorly absorbed.

suc″cor·rhe′a, suc″cor·rhoe′a. An excessive flow of a secretion. **pancreatic s.** A pathologic increase of the pancreatic juice when the secretory activity of the gland is exaggerated.

suc′cu·lent. Juicy.

suc·cur′sal. Subsidiary.

suc′cus (pl. *succi*). 1. A vegetable juice. 2. An animal secretion. **s. entericus.** The intestinal juice, secreted by the glands of the intestinal mucous membrane. It is thin, opalescent, alkaline, and has a specific gravity of 1.011. It contains an amylolytic and a proteolytic ferment. **s. gastricus.** The gastric juice. **s. pancreaticus.** The pancreatic juice. **s. prostaticus.** The prostatic fluid, a constituent of the semen.

suc·cus′sion (suh-kush′un). A shaking, especially of the individual, from side to side, for the purpose of determining the presence of fluid in a cavity or hollow organ of the body. **s.-sound.** The splashing sound heard when the patient is shaken; occurs in hydropneumothorax, pyopneumothorax, or in cases of dilated stomach containing fluid.

suck. Take nourishment at the breast.

suck'er ap"pa·ra'tus. A contrivance for evacuating fluid from body cavities, operating by means of negative pressure. Syn., *suction apparatus.*

suck'le. Nurse at the breast.

suck'ling. 1. A nursling. 2. Nursing.

su'crase. See *saccharase.*

su'crate. A salt of saccharic acid.

su'crol. See *dulcin.*

su'crose. $C_{12}H_{22}O_{11}$. A sugar obtained from *Saccharum officinarum, Beta vulgaris,* and other sources; occurs as colorless or white crystals, crystalline masses, or powder; soluble in water. Used as a sweetening agent and preservative. Also called *saccharum, sugar.*

suc'tion. The act of sucking.

Suc·to'ri·a. 1. A synonym for *Siphonaptera,* the fleas. 2. A class of Protozoa, closely related to the Ciliata, without cilia in the mature stage, but possessing processes called tentacles, some of which are suctorial in function. A few species are parasitic on fish and other aquatic animals.

su·da'men (pl. *sudamina*). An eruption of translucent, whitish vesicles, due to a noninflammatory disturbance of the sweat glands, consisting in a collection of sweat in the ducts of the sweat glands. Is very transitory and occurs after excessive sweating. Syn., *miliaria crystallina.* **—sudam'inal,** *adj.*

Su·dan'. Any of a number of chemically related biological stains. **S. II.** $(CH_3)_2C_6H_3.N:N.C_{10}H_6OH.$ A fat stain. Also called *oil scarlet, fat ponceau.* **S. III** (C.C.). $C_6H_5N:N.C_6H_4N:N.C_{10}$-$H_6OH.$ A fat-soluble, diazo dye; used as a fat stain. Also called *fat ponceau G., oil red, Sudan G.* **S. IV** (C.C.). CH_3-$C_6H_4.N:N.C_6H_3(CH_3).N:N.C_{10}H_6OH.$ A dimethyl derivative of Sudan III; a fat stain, more intense than Sudan III. Also called *fat ponceau, oil red IV.* **S. R.** $CH_2O.C_6H_4N:N.C_{10}H_6OH.$ A stain suggested for use in the Kahn reaction for syphilis. Also called *oil vermilion.*

su·dan'o·phil. A leucocyte which, owing to fatty degeneration, is stained readily by Sudan III.

su·da'tion. The act of sweating.

su"da·to'ri·a. Hyperhidrosis, *q.v.*

su"da·to'ri·um. 1. A hot-air bath. 2. A room for the administration of a hot-air bath.

su'dor. Sweat. **—sudoral,** *adj.* **s. noc'turnus.** Night sweat. **s. san'guinosus.** See *hemathidrosis.*

su"do·re'sis. Excessive sweating.

su"dor·if'er·ous. Producing sweat.

su"dor·if'ic. 1. Inducing sweating. 2. An agent inducing sweating.

su"dor·i·ker'a·to'sis. Keratosis of the sweat glands.

su"dor·ip'a·rous. Secreting sweat.

su'et. Prepared suet, mutton suet; the internal fat of the abdomen of sheep or cattle. **mutton s.** See prepared *s.* **prepared s.** The purified internal fat of the abdomen of the sheep, *Ovis aries;* occurs as a white, solid fat. Used as an ointment base. Syn., *mutton s.*

suf'fo·cate. Asphyxiate.

suf"fo·ca'tion. Interference with the entrance of air into the lungs.

suf·fu'sion. 1. A spreading or flow of any fluid of the body into surrounding tissue; an extensive superficial extravasation of blood. 2. The pouring of water upon a patient as a remedial measure.

sug'ar. 1. Any carbohydrate, *q.v.,* having a sweet taste and the general formula $C_nH_{2n}O$ or $C_nH_{2n-2}O_{n-1}$. 2. Sucrose. **acid of s.** Oxalic acid. **acorn s.** Quercite. **beet s.** Sucrose. **blood s.** The carbohydrate of the blood, chiefly glucose. **brain s.** Cerebrose; galactose. **brown s.** Partially refined cane sugar. **cane s.** Sucrose. **corn s.** Glucose. **fruit s.** Levulose or fructose. **grape s.** Glucose. **gum s.** Arabinose. **honey s.** Glucose. **invert s.** A mixture of approximately equal parts of glucose and levulose obtained by hydrolysis of sucrose. **lead s.** See *lead* acetate. **liver s.** Glycogen. **malt s.** Maltose. **maple s.** The mixture of carbohydrates, chiefly sucrose, obtained from the sap of the sugar maple. **meat s.** Inositol. **milk s.** Lactose. **mucin s.** Levulose. **muscle s.** Inositol. **pectin s.** Arabinose. **refined s.** Purified cane sugar. **wood s.** Xylose.

sug·gest'i·bil'i·ty. The condition of being readily influenced by another; an abnormal state when the individual conforms with unusual readiness, as patients who too readily accept ideas of health or illness. **negative s.** Active negativism, *q.v.*

sug·gest'i·ble. Amenable to suggestion.

sug·ges'tion. 1. The artificial production of a certain psychic state in which the individual experiences such sensations as are suggested to him or ceases to experience those which he is instructed not to feel. 2. The thing suggested.

sug·ges'tion·ist. One who treats disease by means of suggestion. **—suggestionize,** *v.t.*

sug"gil·la'tion (sug"ji-lay'shun, sudj"i-). An ecchymosis or bruise.

su'i·cide. 1. Self murder; intention-

ally taking one's own life. 2. One who takes his own life. —**suicid'al**, *adj.*

su'int (sue'int, swint). A soapy substance rich in potassium salts of higher fatty acids and in cholesterol, derived from sheep's wool. Also called *wool-soap*.

sulamyd. Trade-mark for sulfacetimide.

sul'cus (pl. *sulci*). A furrow or groove; applied especially to the fissures of the brain. See also *fissure*. —**sulcal, sulcate,** *adj.* **anterolateral spinal s.** A broad, shallow groove on the anterolateral surface of the spinal cord, corresponding to the line of the origin of the ventral nerve roots. **central s.** A groove situated about the middle of the lateral surface of the cerebral hemisphere, separating the frontal from the parietal lobe. Formerly called *Rolandic sulcus, fissure of Rolando*. **posterior median s. of spinal cord.** A narrow groove extending the entire length of the spinal cord posteriorly in the midline.

sul"fa·cet'i·mide. NH₂.C₆H₄.SO₂.NH.CH₂CO. Para-aminobenzenesulfon-acetamide; a crystalline powder, soluble in water. A sulfonamide-type antibacterial agent. Also called *sulfacetamide.* See *sulamyd*.

sulf·ac'id. 1. A thioacid. 2. A sulfonic acid.

sul"fa·di'a·zine (sul"fuh-dye'uh-zeen, ·dye·az'een). NH₂.C₆H₄.SO₂.NH.C₄H₂N₃; p-amino-N-2-pyrimidylbenzene sulfonamide or 2-sulfanilylamidopyrimidine; occurs as a white or slightly yellow powder; soluble in water. An anti-infective agent of the sulfonamide group, effective against a variety of organisms. **s. sodium.** C₁₀H₉N₄O₂SNa. Occurs as a white powder; soluble in water.

sul"fa·di'me·tine. Sulfisomidine.

sul'fa drugs. A family of drugs of the sulfonamide type which have marked bacteriostatic properties.

sulf"a·eth'i·dole. N'-(5-Ethyl-1,3,4-thiadiazol-2-yl)sulfanilamide, an antibacterial sulfonamide. See *sulspansion, sul-spantab.*

sul"fa·guan'i·dine (sul"fuh-gwah'ni-deen). NH₂.C₆H₄.SO₂.NH.C(NH)NH₂.H₂O; p-aminobenzenesulfonyl-guanidine monohydrate; occurs as a white, needlelike, crystalline powder; soluble in water. Used primarily in the treatment of certain intestinal bacillary infections. Also called *sulfanilyl-guanidine monohydrate.*

sul"fa·mer'a·zine (sul"fuh-merr'uh-zeen, ·zin). 2-Sulfanilamido-4-methylpyrimidine; the 4-(mono)methyl derivative of sulfadiazine; it is more soluble in water than sulfadiazine. Its therapeutic uses are similar to those of sulfadiazine.

sul"fa·meth'a·zine (sul"fuh-meth'uh-zeen, ·zin). 2-Sulfanilamido-4,6-dimethylpyrimidine; the dimethyl derivative of sulfadiazine. Used like sulfadiazine.

sul"fa·meth'i·zole. N'-(5-Methyl-1,3,4-thiadiazol-2-yl)sulfanilamide, an antibacterial agent. See *thiosulfil.*

sul"fa·meth'ox·y·py·rid'a·zine. 3-Sulfanilamido-6-methoxypyridazine, a long-acting antibacterial sulfonamide. See *kynex.*

sul"fa·mex'a·thine (sul"fuh-mez'uh-theen, ·thin). Sulfamethazine, *q.v.*

sul·fam'ic ac'id. HO.SO₂.NH₂. A colorless, crystalline acid; has been used in the treatment of cholera.

sul"fa·min'ic ac'id. Sulfamic acid.

sulfamylon. Trade-mark for the hydrochloride of marfanil, *q.v.*

sul"fa·nil'a·mide. NH₂.C₆H₄.SO₂.NH₂; p-aminobenzenesulfonamide; occurs as white crystals, granules, or powder; soluble in water. It exerts a potent antibacterial effect against many organisms.

sul·fan'i·late. A salt of sulfanilic acid.

sul"fa·nil'ic ac'id. NH₂C₆H₄SO₂H. Para-aminobenzene sulfonic acid, occurring in colorless, water-soluble crystals. Used as a reagent.

sul"fa·pyr'a·zine (sul"fuh-pirr'uh-zeen, ·zin). NH₂.C₆H₄.SO₂.NH₄.C₄H₂N₃. p-Amino-N-2-pyrazinylbenzenesulfonamide, isomeric with sulfapyridine; soluble in water.

sul"fa·pyr'i·dine (sul"fuh-pirr'i-deen, ·din). NH₂.C₆H₄.SO₂.NH.C₅H₄N; 2-(p-aminobenzenesulfonamido)pyridine. Occurs as white or faintly yellowish white crystals, granules, or powder; soluble in water. A sulfonamide-type antibacterial agent.

sul"fa·quin·ox'a·line. 2-Sulfanilamidoquinoxaline, a drug used in veterinary medicine to control outbreaks of cecal and intestinal coccidiosis in poultry.

sulf·ars'phen·a·mine' (sulf·ars"fen-uh-meen', ·ars·fen'uh-meen). Consists chiefly of disodium 3,3'-diamino-4,4'-dihydroxyarsenobenzene-N-dimethylenesulfonate; it contains not less than 19% of arsenic; occurs as a yellow powder, very soluble in water. Used in treatment of syphilis.

sulfasuxidine. Trade-mark for a brand of succinylsulfathiazole.

sul'fa·tase. Any enzyme which hydrolyzes an ethereal sulfate (ester sulfate).

sul'fate. A salt of sulfuric acid of the type M₂SO₄.

sulfathalidine. Trade-mark for phthalylsulfathiazole.

sul″fa·thi′a·zole. $NH_2.C_6H_4.SO_2.-NH.C_3H_2NS$; 2-($p$-aminobenzenesulfonamido) thiazole; occurs as white or faintly yellowish white crystals, granules, or powder; soluble in water. A sulfonamide-type antibacterial agent. **s. sodium.** $C_9H_8N_3O_2S_2Na.1½H_2O$; the sodium salt of sulfathiazole; occurs as a white or faintly yellowish white powder; soluble in water. Also called *sulfathiazole sodium sesquihydrate*.

sulf″he·mo·glo′bin (sulf″hee·mo·glo′bin, ·hem·o·glo′bin). A greenish substance derived from hemoglobin by the action of hydrogen sulfide. Syn., *sulfmethemoglobin*.

sulf″he″mo·glo″bi·ne′mi·a (sulf″hee″mo·glo″bi·nee′mee·uh, ·hem″o·). A condition in which sulfhemoglobin is present in the blood; the symptoms are similar to those present in methemoglobinemia. Diagnosis is made by spectroscopic examination. Also see *methemoglobinemia*.

sulf·hy′drate. A compound of a base with the univalent radical sulfhydryl, SH.

sulf·hy′dryl. The univalent radical SH, usually attached to a carbon chain. The presence of active sulfhydryl groups is important for the activity of many enzymes. Often written *SH group*.

sul′fide. A compound of sulfur with an element or basic radical.

sul″fi·som′i·dine. N^1-(2,6-Dimethyl-4-pyrimidyl)-sulfonamide, a compound characterized by a very low degree of acetylation in the body and by maintenance of high blood and urine levels with moderate dosage. Formerly called *sulfadimetine*. See *elkosin*.

sul″fi·sox′a·zole. Nonproprietary title for the drug available under the trade-marked name gantrisin. *Obs.*

sul′fite. A salt of sulfurous acid of the type M_2SO_3.

sulf″met·he″mo·glo′bin (sulf″met·hee″mo·glo′bin, ·hem″o·glo′bin). Sulfhemoglobin.

sul′fo-. A combining form generally indicating *the presence of divalent sulfur or the sulfo- group*, $-SO_3H$.

sul″fo·ac′id (sul″fo·ass′id, sul″fo·ass″id). 1. A thioacid. 2. A sulfonic acid.

sul″fo·car′bo·late. A salt of phenolsulfonic acid.

sul″fo·car·bol′ic ac′id. Phenolsulfonic acid.

sul″fo·cy′a·nate. Thiocyanate, *q.v.*

sul′fo·nal. See *sulfonmethane*.

sul′fo·nal·ism (sul′fo·nul·iz·um, sulfon′ul·iz·um). A group of symptoms said to be occasioned by the prolonged administration of sulfonal. *Obs.*

sul·fon′a·mide (sul·fon′uh·mide, sul″fo·nam′ide). Any one of a group of compounds derived from sulfanilamide, $H_2N.C_6H_4.SO_2.NH_2$, and used in the treatment of various bacterial infections. The members of the group vary with respect to activity, degree and rate of absorption, metabolic alteration and excretion, and the toxic manifestations produced. The action of sulfonamides is blocked by p-aminobenzoic acid.

sul′fon·ate. 1. Treat an aromatic hydrocarbon with fuming sulfuric acid. 2. A sulfuric acid derivative. 3. The ester of a sulfonic acid.

sul″fo·na′tion. A chemical process resulting in the introduction in a compound of one or more sulfo groups.

sul′fone. An oxidation product of thio-compounds containing the group SO_2 attached to a hydrocarbon group.

sul″fone·phthal′e·in. Any one of a group of organic compounds made by the interaction of phenols with acid chlorides or anhydrides of ortho-sulfobenzoic acid and its derivatives; such as thymolsulfonephthalein and phenolsulfonephthalein.

sul″fon·eth″yl·meth′ane. $CH_3.C_2H_5.C.(SO_2C_2H_5)_2$. Diethylsulfonemethylethylmethane; occurs as colorless, crystalline scales; soluble in water. The sulfone group of hypnotics, which includes this drug and sulfonmethane, depress the cerebral centers. Syn., *methylsulfonal*.

sul·fon′ic ac′id. An organic acid containing the $-SO_3H$ or $-SO_2OH$ group.

sul″fon·meth′ane. $(CH_3)_2C.(SO_2-C_2H_5)_2$; diethylsulfonedimethylmethane; occurs as white crystals, or powder; soluble in water. A hypnotic. Also called *sulfonal*.

sul″fo·phe′nate, sul″fo·phen′yl·ate. 1. Phenolsulfonate, a salt or ester of phenolsulfonic acid, $C_6H_4(OH).SO_3H$. 2. Phenylsulfate, a salt of phenylsulfuric acid, $C_6H_5OSO_3H$.

sul″fo·phen′yl·ate. Sulfophenate, *q.v.*

sul″fo·sal″i·cyl′ic ac′id. $SO_2H.C_6H_3.OH.COOH.2H_2O$. A white or nearly white, crystalline powder, used as a reagent for albumin.

sul″fo·salt″ (sul″fo·sawlt″). A salt of sulfonic acid.

sul″fo·vi′nic ac′id (sul″fo·vy′nick, ·vin′ick). $C_2H_5HSO_4$, ethylsulfuric acid formed by the interaction of sulfuric acid and ethyl alcohol.

sul′fur. $S = 32.066$. A solid, nonmetallic element. Occurs as a yellow, brittle mass or in transparent monoclinic or rhombic crystals and exists in a number of modifications. It is insoluble in water. In contact with the skin, there forms either hydrogen sulfide or a polythionic acid which is poisonous to various pathogenic parasites. Precipitated sulfur, sublimed sulfur, and washed sulfur are official. **colloidal s.** A finely subdivided sulfur which may have some therapeutic action analogous, when injected intravenously, to that of foreign protein injections. **milk of s.** Precipitated sulfur. **precipitated s.** The form of sulfur obtained by adding hydrochloric acid to a solution prepared by boiling sublimed sulfur and lime with water. Because it is finely subdivided it is more readily suspended in liquids than are other forms of sulfur. **sublimed s.** The form of sulfur obtained by subliming native sulfur. **s. dioxide.** SO_2. A colorless, noninflammable gas with a strong suffocating odor; with water it forms sulfurous acid. It is a powerful reducing agent and disinfectant. **washed s.** Sublimed sulfur which has been washed with a dilute solution of ammonia to remove traces of acid. It is the preferred form for internal administration.

sul'fu·ra"ted. Combined with sulfur.

sul'fu·ra"tor. An apparatus for applying sulfur fumes for purposes of disinfection.

sul·fu'ric ac'id. An aqueous solution containing about 96% of H_2SO_4; occurs as a colorless, odorless liquid of oily consistency; it is miscible with water. It is widely employed in the arts and sciences. Also called *oil of vitriol.*

sul'fu·rous. 1. Of the nature of sulfur. 2. Combined with sulfur; derived from sulfur dioxide, SO_2.

sul·fu'rous ac'id. H_2SO_3. A solution of SO_2 in water. It has been used internally as a gastric antiseptic, and externally in the treatment of various skin diseases.

sul'phate. See *sulfate.*

sul·phe"mo·glo"bi·ne'mi·a. See *sulfhemoglobinemia.*

sulphetrone. A trade-mark for 4,4′-bis(γ-phenyl-n-propylamino)-diphenylsulfone-tetrasodium sulfonate, a crystalline, water-soluble compound which may be of value in the treatment of tuberculosis.

sul'phur. This spelling has been changed to *sulfur*, *q.v.*, which is now official in the U. S. Pharmacopeia and in the publications of the American Chemical Society.

sul·spansion. Trade-mark for a suspension dosage form of sulfaethidole.

sul·spantab. Trade-mark for a tablet dosage form of sulfaethidole.

sum. *Sume*, take; *sumendus*, to be taken; used as direction in prescriptions.

su'mac, su'mach (sue'mack, shōō'-mack). A name applied to various species of *Rhus* and *Toxicodendron.* Among the substances to which the irritant properties of the poison sumacs are ascribed are toxicodendrol, toxico-

dendrin, lobinol, urushiol. Also see *poison sumac.*

sum'bul. Consists of the dried rhizome and roots of *Ferula sumbul*, or of other closely related species of *Ferula* possessing a characteristic musklike odor. Also called *musk root.*

sum·ma'tion. The accumulation of effects, especially of those of muscular, sensory, or mental stimuli. **—summational**, *adj.* **s. of stimuli.** An aftereffect produced by several subthreshold stimuli on tissues causing succeeding equal stimuli to become effective.

sum'mer e·rup'tion. Miliaria.

sun'burn". 1. Discoloration of the skin due to exposure to the sun. 2. Inflammation of the skin, due to the action of the sun's rays, which may be of the first or second degree. 3. Affect, or be affected, with sunburn.

sun lamp. A lamp designed to give off radiations similar to those received from the sun. A mercury arc produces radiations ranging in wave length from infrared to visible and ultraviolet. A quartz bulb absorbs all ultraviolet radiations shorter than 2800 angstrom which are not present in sunlight.

sun'stroke". A form of heat stroke occurring on exposure to the sun. The body temperature rises because of faulty heat dissipation due to high environmental temperature and humidity as well as absorption of solar radiant energy. Rectal temperatures may go from 106° F. to 110° F. Syn., *insolation.*

su'per-. A prefix denoting *above, upon,* or *excessive.*

su"per·al"i·men·ta'tion. Overfeeding; feeding beyond ordinary metabolic requirements.

su"per·cil'i·um. The eyebrow. **—superciliary**, *adj.*

su"per·duct'. Elevate; lead upward.

su"per·e'go. *In psychoanalysis*, that subdivision of the psyche which acts as the conscience of the unconscious. Its components are derived from both the id and the ego.

su"per·fe"cun·da'tion. The fertilization of two or more ova, ovulated more or less simultaneously, by two or more successive coital acts not necessarily involving the same male.

su"per·fe·ta'tion, su"per·foe·ta'tion. The production or development of a second fetus after one is already present in the uterus.

su"per·fi'cial (sue"pur·fish'ul). Confined to or pertaining to the surface, as superficial fascia, a sheet of fatty areolar tissue under the skin.

su"per·fi'ci·es (sue"pur·fish'ee·eez, ·fish'eez). The outer surface.

su"per·in·duce'. Add a new factor or a complication of a condition already existing.

su″per·in·fec′tion. A second or subsequent infection by the same microorganism, as seen in tuberculosis.

su″per·in″vo·lu′tion. Hyperinvolution; excessive rolling up; return of the uterus after labor to less than normal size.

su·pe′ri·or. *In anatomy,* higher; denoting the upper of two parts; toward the vertex.

su·pe″ri·or′i·ty com′plex. A general attitude or character trait, often pathologic and usually arising out of an underlying feeling of inferiority, which is characterized by the occurrence of some form of real or assumed ascendancy and by feelings of conceit, vanity, envy, jealousy, or revenge.

su″per·mo′ron. A person whose mentality is slightly below normal, but who is of higher grade than a moron.

su·per·nate. The fluid which remains after the removal of suspended matter by centrifugation or other physical or chemical means. **—superna′tant,** *adj.*

su″per·nor′mal. 1. Pertaining to a faculty or phenomenon which is beyond the level of ordinary experience. 2. Superior to the average.

su″per·nu″mer·ar″y (sue″pur-new′mur-err″ee). Existing in more than the usual number, as supernumerary mammary gland.

su″per·nu·tri′tion. Excessive nourishment; hypernutrition. Nourishment in excess of ordinary metabolic requirements.

su″per·phos′phate. An acid phosphate.

su″per·sat′u·rate. Saturate to excess; add more of a substance than a liquid can normally and permanently dissolve.

su″per·scrip′tion. The sign ℞ (abbreviation of Latin *recipe,* take), at the beginning of a prescription.

su″per·sen″si·ti·za′tion. Excessive susceptibility to the action of a protein following its injection.

su″per·son′ic, su″pra·son′ic. Referring to waves of too high a frequency to produce sound that is audible to the human ear.

su″per·ve·nos′i·ty. The condition in which the blood has become venous to a high degree.

su″per·ven′tion. That which is added; a new, extraneous, or unexpected condition added to another, as the supervention of septicemia, or other complication in disease.

su′per·vi″sor. Term used to indicate a supervising or head nurse.

su′pi·nate. 1. Turn the arm so that the palm faces upward or to the front. 2. Turn the foot so that the sole is directed inward and downward. 3. Turn the body so that the chest and belly face upward while recumbent.

su″pi·na′tion. 1. The turning of the palm of the hand upward. 2. The condition of being supine; lying on the back.

su′pi·na″tor, su″pi·na′tor. A muscle of the forearm, which turns the radius outward. See Table of Muscles in the Appendix.

su·pine′. Lying on the back face upward, or the hand with the palm upward; the opposite of *prone.*

sup″pe·da′ne·ous. Pertaining to the sole of the foot.

sup″pe·da′ne·um. An application to the sole of the foot.

sup″ple·men′tal. Additional.

sup·port′. 1. The act of holding anything in its position. 2. Any appliance acting as a support, as an arch support.

sup·port′er. An apparatus intended to hold in place a low-hanging or prolapsed organ, as the uterus, the scrotum and its contents, the abdomen, etc., or to limit the use of certain joints, as the knee, ankle. See *pessary, jockey strap, binder, suspensory.*

sup·pos′i·to″ry (suh·poz′i·tor″ee). A medicated solid body of varying weight and shape, intended for introduction into different orifices of the body.

sup·pres′sion. 1. A sudden cessation of secretion, as of the urine, or of a normal process, as the menses. 2. *In psychiatry,* a mode of adjustment to urges and desires that are considered to be unacceptable, untenable or unworthy, through attempting, consciously and thoughtfully, to control or prevent their occurrence or expression in consciousness. Also see *repression.*

sup′pu·rant. 1. Promoting suppuration. 2. An agent promoting suppuration.

sup″pu·ra′tion. The formation of pus. **—sup′purate,** *v.*

sup″pu·ra′tive. 1. Producing pus. 2. An agent that favors suppuration.

su′pra-. A prefix signifying *upon* or *above.*

su″pra·cla·vic′u·lar. Above the clavicle, as supraclavicular nerves. See Table of Nerves in the Appendix.

su″pra·hy′oid. Above the hyoid bone, as a suprahyoid muscle.

su″pra·lim′i·nal. Lying above a threshold.

su″pra·oc·clu′sion. That condition created by the abnormal elongation of teeth in their sockets.

su″pra·or′bit·al. Above the orbit, as the supraorbital nerve. See Table of Nerves in the Appendix.

su″pra·pa·tel′lar. Above the patella.

su"pra·pu'bic. Above the pubes, as suprapubic prostatectomy.

su"pra·ren'-. For words beginning with *supraren-* not found here, see under *adren-*.

su"pra·re'nal. 1. The suprarenal gland. See adrenal *gland*. 2. The dried, partially defatted and powdered suprarenal gland of cattle, sheep, or swine; it is a light yellow to brown amorphous powder; it is only partially soluble in water. Over twenty crystalline steroid derivatives have been isolated from adrenal cortical extracts. Also called *desiccated suprarenal, dried adrenal substance.*

su"pra·re"nal·ec'to·my. Adrenalectomy; removal of an adrenal or suprarenal gland.

su"pra·ren'al·in (sue"pruh·ren'ul-in, -ree'nul-in). Epinephrine.

su"pra·re"nal·op'a·thy. A disordered condition resulting from disturbed function of the adrenal glands.

suprarenin. A trade-mark for epinephrine.

su"pra·son'ic. See *supersonic.*

su"pra·ster'ol, su"pra·ste'rol. A type of sterol produced by the irradiation of ergosterol. Suprasterols are toxic.

su"pra·verge'. Diverge from a vertical axis.

su"pra·vi'tal stain'ing. A method whereby stained cells may be studied in the living state. Janus green and neutral red are stains commonly employed. Of especial value in studying the immature leukocytes found in leukemia.

su'ra. The calf of the leg. **—sural,** *adj.*

sur"al·i·men·ta'tion. The method of forced feeding or overalimentation sometimes employed in pulmonary tuberculosis and other diseases.

sur·am'in, su"ram·in. $C_{51}H_{34}N_6O_{23}$-S_6Na_6. British Pharmacopoeia title for the symmetrical urea of the sodium salt of m-benzoyl-m-amino-p-methylbenzoyl-1-aminonaphthalene-4,6,8-trisulfonic acid. A white or faintly cream-colored powder used in various trypanosome infections, especially African sleeping sickness, and in pemphigus. Trade names are germanin, Fourneau 309, naganol, moranyl, and Bayer 205. **s. sodium.** The U. S. Pharmacopeia title for suramin. See *naphuride sodium.*

surd'i·ty. Deafness.

sur'face. 1. The exterior of a body. 2. The face or faces of a body; a term frequently used in anatomy in the description of various structures.

sur'face ten'sion. The contractile surface of a liquid by which it tends to assume a spherical form and to present the least possible surface (e.g., the formation of a meniscus). Abbreviated, S.T.

sur'face-ac'tive a'gent. Any substance, such as a wetting agent, that modifies the character of a surface, usually by lowering the interfacial tension. Syn. *surfactant.*

sur·fac'tant. A surface-active agent.

sur'geon. 1. One who practices surgery. The term implies the possession of a medical degree and license and is used irrespective of the field or limitation of practice. 2. In the United States Army, the ranking officer of the Medical Corps in a military command. **attending s.** One associated with the staff of a hospital, visiting the patients at specific times, performing major surgical operations, and supervising the postoperative care through directions to the house surgeon. **aural s.** An otologist. **dental s.** (a) One who limits his field to the surgery of the mouth and jaws. (b) In the United States Army, the ranking officer of the Dental Corps in a military command. **house s.** A chief resident surgeon in a hospital. **plastic s.** One who specializes in plastic surgery. **s. general.** In the United States armed forces and Public Health Service, the ranking officer and head of the Medical Service or Department. In foreign armies, in some cases, the title denotes the chief medical officer of a department or command. **veterinary s.** One whose practice is limited to the treatment of domestic, large and small animals, or to meat and food inspections on behalf of the national or state governments. **visiting s.** A surgeon whose duties require regular attendance at a hospital or dispensary as well as emergency visits to operate upon or care for patients himself or to supervise the care given by house surgeons.

sur'ger·y. The branch of medicine dealing with diseases requiring operative procedure, including manipulation. **—surgical,** *adj.* **antiseptic s.** The application of antiseptic methods in the treatment of wounds. **aseptic s.** Operative procedure in the absence of germs, everything coming in contact with the wound being sterile. **aural s.** That pertaining to the ear. **battle s.** Urgent surgery during active military operations in a forward area. **brain s.** That pertaining to any part within the cranium. **clinical s.** The practice of surgery in teaching. **conservative s.** Measures directed to the preservation rather than the removal of a part. **dental s.** That pertaining to the teeth and jaws. **general s.** Surgery as a whole and not confined to a particular specialty. **major s.** That in which the operations are important and involve risk to life. **military s.**

That pertaining to gunshot wounds and other injuries peculiar to military life. **minor s.** That part of surgery including procedures not involving serious hazard to life and usually not requiring general anesthesia; examples are bandaging, application of splints and casts, suturing of superficial lacerations, excision, incision, and drainage of superficial structures. **operative s.** That which refers to the performance of operations. **oral s.** That branch of dental science which is concerned with surgical procedures involving structures concerned with the oral cavity, particularly the teeth and jaws. **orthopedic s.** The remedy of deformities by manual and instrumental measures. **pelvic s.** That limited to the pelvic region. **plastic s.** Repair of absent or defective tissue by transference of tissue from another part or person. **reparative s.** Plastic surgery. **veterinary s.** The surgery of animals.

Su″ri·nam′ bark (soor″ĭ·nahm′, ·nam′). Cabbage tree bark; the bark of *Andira retusa*, which has been used as an anthelmintic in the West Indies.

Su″ri·nam′ quas′si·a. See under *quassia*.

surital sodium. Trade-mark for thiamylal sodium.

sur′ro·gate. Any medicine used as a substitute for a more expensive one, or for one to which there is a special objection in any particular case.

sur″sum·duc′tion. 1. The power of the two eyes of fusing two images when one eye has a prism placed vertically before it. 2. A movement of either eye alone upward. **right s.** The absolute power that the right eye has to rotate upward.

sur″sum·ver′sion. The upward movement of both eyes.

sur·vi′vor·ship. *In legal medicine,* the living of one of two or more persons after the death of the other or others.

sus·cep″ti·bil′i·ty. The opposite of immunity. A characteristic rendering an individual likely to acquire a disease if exposed to the causative agent. Susceptibility may be increased by certain traits, as racial, familial, etc.

sus·cep′ti·ble. 1. Sensitive to impression or influence. 2. *In immunology,* denoting one who has neither natural nor acquired immunity to a disease.

sus′ci·tate. Increase activity, stimulate.

sus·pend′ed. 1. Hung; applied to any structure attached to or hanging from another structure, and attached by a pedicle or cord. 2. Interrupted.

sus·pen′sion. 1. Hanging or fixation in a higher position; a method of treatment, as suspension of the uterus.

2. *In chemistry and pharmacy,* a dispersion of solid particles throughout the mass of a liquid. **tendon s.** Tenodesis, the surgical fixation of a tendon. Such an operation is suited to a variety of conditions, such as habitual dislocation of the shoulder, weakness in the extensor function of the thumb, disabilities of the extensor tendons of the foot, deformities of the feet, and certain disabilities of the knee.

sus·pen′soid. An apparent solution which actually consists of small particles of the solute in active Brownian movement.

sus·pen′so·ry. 1. Serving for suspension or support, as suspensory ligament, or suspensory bandage. 2. A device for suspending a part, as the scrotum. 3. A jockey strap.

sus″pi·ra′tion. 1. A sigh, *q.v.* 2. The act of sighing.

sus″ten·tac′u·lum. A support. **—sustentacular,** *adj.* **s. tali.** A process of the calcaneus supporting the talus.

su″sur·ra′tion. A murmur, or susurrus.

su·sur′rus. A soft murmur in aneurysm, cardiac diseases, contracting muscle, etc.

su·tu′ra (pl. *suturae*). A suture, *q.v.* **s. dentata.** One with toothlike interlocking processes, as the suture between the parietal bones. **s. harmonia.** One in which there is simple apposition of contiguous rough surfaces. **s. limbosa.** An interlocking suture, with beveling and overlapping of the articular surfaces, as in the coronal suture. **s. serrata.** One in which the edges of the bones are saw-toothed. **s. squamosa.** One formed by the overlapping of contiguous bones by broad, beveled margins. **s. vera.** A true suture, one in which the margins of the bones are connected by a series of processes and indentations interlocked together.

su′tur·al (sue′chur·ul). Pertaining to, or having the nature of, a suture.

su′ture. 1. *In osteology,* a line of junction or closure between bones, as a cranial suture. 2. *In surgery,* fine, cordlike structures used to close a wound. The term may mean either the material used, as gut, silk, etc., or the method of using the suture, as interrupted, mattress, etc. There are two main types of materials: absorbable, such as catgut, which are placed in deep tissue, and nonabsorbable, which usually are removed, as silk, linen, wire, etc., though some are used and left in deep tissue. 3. Close a wound by sewing. **approximating s.** One placed in deep tissue to pull together the edges of the wound. **button s.** A mattress suture which includes a button on either side of the wound to prevent cutting of the skin by the suture. **catgut s.** One in which the material employed is catgut. **coapting s.** One which brings the divided skin edges accurately together. **continuous s.** One in which the suture material is continued from one end of the wound to the other; may be of several types, the plain over-and-over sewing stitch being most common. **coronal s.** The union of the frontal with the parietal bones transversely across the vertex of the skull. **dermal s.** A fine linen suture impregnated with various chemicals used when a fine scar is desired. **harelip s.** One in which the edges of the wound are transfixed with pins and approximation secured by twisting or wrapping the ends of the pins with thread. **interrupted s.** A type in which each stitch is tied and cut individually. **lambdoid s.** The union between the two superior borders of the occipital bone and the parietal bones. **mattress s.** One in which the needle, after being drawn through both skin edges, is reinserted on the same side and drawn through the original side again. This may be continuous or interrupted. **relaxing s.** One placed deeply to and at a distance from the wound to relieve tension. **sagittal s.** The union between the superior borders of the parietal bones. **secondary s.** One done some time after the time of injury or operation. Also called *delayed s.* **shotted s.** One in which each end of the suture is passed through a perforated shot and then drawn tight. **subcuticular s.** A buried, continuous suture in which the needle is passed horizontally into the true skin back and forth until the wound is closed. **tension s.** One made at a distance from the wound edge and through the deeper tissues, to lessen the strain on the skin suture. **transfixion s.** A method of closing a wound by the use of a pin or needle which is placed through both wound edges and held by winding suture material over both ends in a figure-of-eight fashion. Also called *figure-of-eight s., harelip s.*

swab. A piece of cloth, sponge, or cotton upon the end of a stick, used in feeding the sick, making applications to the throat, cleansing the mouth and teeth, etc.

swab stick. A rod or shaft, one extremity of which is to be wound with cotton; a cotton stick.

swal′low·ing. Deglutition; the act of taking into the stomach through the esophagus. **tongue s.** A condition in which there is an abnormal flaccidity of the tongue, so that it falls backward, giving rise to danger of suffocation.

sway′-back″. Increased lumbar lordosis with a compensatory increased thoracic kyphosis.

sweat. The secretion of the sudoriferous glands, consisting of a transparent, colorless, aqueous fluid, holding in solution neutral fats, volatile fatty acids, traces of albumin and urea, free lactic acid, sodium lactate, sodium chloride, potassium chloride, and traces of alkaline phosphates, sugar, ascorbic acid, etc. Its excretion, largely by the cooling effect of evaporation, helps regulate the temperature of the body. **bloody s.** See *hemathidrosis.* **night s.** Drenching perspiration occurring at night or whenever the patient sleeps, in the course of pulmonary tuberculosis or other diseases.

sweat′ing. Perspiring.

Swe′dish move′ments. Gymnastics according to a system originated in Sweden and adapted to the health needs of individuals, especially for those having postural deformities.

sweet al′mond oil. Almond oil.

sweet oil. Olive oil.

swel′ling. 1. Any morbid enlargement, inflation, or abnormal protuberance. 2. A general embryologic term to denote a small eminence or ridge. **cloudy s.** Parenchymatous degeneration; a retrogressive change in cytoplasm of parenchymatous cells, as glandular epithelium, endothelial cells, and leukocytes, whereby the cell enlarges, the outline becomes irregular. In fresh tissue the nucleus is obscured, and the cytoplasm becomes coarsely granular. The basic change is imbibition of water, with agglomeration of protein particles and dispersal of lipid protein combinations. **white s.** *In orthopedics,* enlargement of a joint or part without increased local heat or redness; usually due to tuberculosis.

swiv′el stir′rup. An apparatus fashioned like a stirrup and used by attaching it to a Steinmann pin for traction in leg fractures.

sy·co′ma (sigh·ko′muh). A condyloma, or wart.

sy′cose. Saccharin.

sy·co′si·form (sigh·ko′si·form). Resembling sycosis.

sy·co′sis (sigh·ko′sis). An inflammatory disease affecting the hair follicles, particularly of the beard, and characterized by papules, pustules, and tubercles, perforated by hairs, together with infiltration of the skin and crusting. Also called *s. coccygenica, s. staphylogenes, folliculitis barbae, s. mentagra.*

syl·lab′ic ut′ter·ance. Scanning speech, as in multiple sclerosis; words are enunciated slowly and separately and there may be a staccato accentuation of some syllables.

syl′la·ble-stum′bling. A form of

dysphasia wherein each sound and syllable can be distinctly uttered, but the word as a whole is spoken with difficulty. Occurs in dementia paralytica.

syl′la·bus. 1. A compendium containing the heads of a discourse. 2. The main propositions of a course of lectures. 3. An abstract.

syl·lep″si·ol′o·gy. The physiology of conception and pregnancy. *Obs.*

syl·vat′ic plague. A name used in the U.S.A. for a bubonic plague transmitted by fleas from squirrels, chipmunks, and other rodents in California, Montana, and other Western states. The disease is gradually spreading eastward among wild rodents, according to reports of the United States Public Health Service.

sym-. See *syn-.*

sym·bal′lo·phone. A stethoscope equipped with two chest pieces for simultaneous use as a special aid in localizing or in comparing sounds.

sym′bi·on, sym′bi·ont. An organism living in symbiosis.

sym″bi·o′sis. A more or less intimate association or union between organisms of different species. In the restricted sense of the term, the organisms are mutually benefited and sometimes so dependent on each other that life apart is impossible. Symbiosis includes commensalism in which neither organism is injured and one may receive benefit, and parasitism in which the relation is detrimental to one organism, the host, and beneficial to the other, the parasite. Various gradations occur so that rigid classification cannot be maintained. —**symbiot′ic,** *adj.*

sym·bleph′a·ron. Adhesions of the eyelids to the eyeball. **anterior s.** Occurs when the edge of the lid is adherent. **posterior s.** Occurs when the adhesion is near the conjunctival fornix. **total s.** Occurs when the entire lid is adherent.

sym·bleph″a·ro′sis. Adhesion of the eyelids to the globe of the eye or to each other.

sym′bol. 1. A sign or character denoting an idea. The following are commonly employed in medicine: ℞, Recipe, take of; ℈, scruple; ℨ, dram; ℥, fluidrachm; ℥, troy ounce; f℥, fluidounce; ℳ, minim. See also Table of Signs and Symbols in the Appendix. 2. *In chemistry,* a conventional abbreviation of the name of an element, generally consisting of the initial letter or letters of the name in Latin or English. It denotes one atom of the element.

sym·bo′li·a. The ability to recognize an object by the sense of touch.

sym′bol·ism. The delusional or hallucinational interpretation of all events or objects as having a mystic significance, a habit not uncommon in certain forms of insanity.

sym″bol·i·za′tion. *In psychiatry,* the process by which mental disorder is expressed by substitute devices, as in dreams, the meaning of which is not clear to the conscious mind.

sy·me′li·a. A coalescence of the lower extremities. See *sympodia, sympus.*

sym′me·try. *In anatomy,* a harmonious correspondence of parts; also the relation of homologous parts at opposite sides or ends of the body. —**symmet′ric,** *adj.* **bilateral s.** Correspondence of both halves of an organism.

sym″pa·thec′to·my, sym·path″i·cec′to·my. Excision of a portion of the autonomic or sympathetic nervous system.

sym″pa·thet′ic. 1. Pertaining to or produced by sympathy. 2. Pertaining to the sympathetic nervous system. 3. The sympathetic nervous system.

sym·path″i·co·neu·ri′tis. Inflammation of the sympathetic system, particularly the sympathetic ganglionated chain.

sym·path″i·cop′a·thy. A disordered condition resulting from disturbance of the sympathetic nervous system.

sym·path″i·co·to′ni·a. Domination of bodily functions by the sympathetic nervous system, manifested by goose flesh, increased blood pressure, vascular spasm, etc.

sym·path″i·co·trop′ic. Possessing affinity for the sympathetic nervous system.

sym·path′i·cus. The sympathetic nervous system.

sym′pa·thin. A hormone similar to epinephrine, believed to be formed in the muscle cells by nerve impulses. Causes augmentation of blood pressure and heart rate. **s. E.** A postulated form of sympathin causing excitation and formed by combination of a chemical mediator released at sympathetic nerve endings with a hypothetical substance in excited effector cells. It is probably nor-epinephrine, also called arterenol. **s. I.** A postulated form of sympathin causing inhibition; formed by combination of a chemical mediator released at sympathetic nerve endings with a hypothetical substance in inhibited effector cells.

sym′pa·thism. Susceptibility to hypnotic suggestion. —**sympathist,** *n.*

sym′pa·thi″zer. An eye with sympathetic ophthalmia, *q.v.*

sym·path″o·blas·to′ma (sim-path″o·blas·to′muh, sim″puth·o·). A rare tumor of the sympathetic nervous system of the same order as the sympathogonioma, but less malignant and composed of the more mature sympathogonia, with processes and axons. A form of tumor intermediate between the sympathogonioma and the ganglioneuroma. Syn., *neuroblastoma.*

sym·path″o·go′ni·a. Primitive cells of the sympathetic nervous system derived from neuroblasts of the ganglionic crest of the neural tube. Differentiate to form along one line ganglion cells and along another line chromaffin cells. Also called *sympathogones.*

sym·path″o·go″ni·o′ma. A tumor of the sympathetic nervous system, usually of early life and situated in the adrenal gland, and highly malignant with early metastasis. Composed of small cells about the size of a lymphocyte, but actually sympathogonia, primitive neurocytes. Pseudorosettes and unidentified fibrils are often present.

sym·path″o·lyt′ic. Pertaining to an effect antagonistic to the activity produced by stimulation of the sympathetic system; the opposite of sympathomimetic.

sym·path″o·mi·met′ic (sim·path″o·mi·met/ick, sim″puth·o·). Having the power to cause physiologic changes similar to those produced by action of the sympathetic nervous system.

sym′pa·thy. The mutual relation between parts more or less distant, whereby a change in the one has an effect upon the other.

sym·pex′i·on. A concretion found in the seminal vesicles. Also called *sympexis.*

sym·phal′an·gism. Inherited condition of stiff fingers, or ankylosed finger joints.

sym·phy·ses (sim′fi·seez). Plural of symphysis.

sym″phy·si·ec′to·my (sim″fiz·ee·eck′to·mee). Excision of the symphysis pubis for the purpose of facilitating delivery. *Obs.*

sym·phys′i·on (sim·fiz′ee·on). The most anterior point of the alveolar process of the mandible, used as a craniometric point.

sym″phy·si·or′rha·phy (sim″fiz·ee·or′uh·fee). Suture of a divided symphysis.

sym·phys′i·o·tome″ (sim·fiz′ee·o·tome″). An instrument used in performing symphysiotomy.

sym″phy·si·ot′o·my (sim″fiz·ee·ot′o·mee). The dividing of the symphysis pubis for the purpose of increasing the diameters of the pelvic canal and facilitating labor. *Obs.*

sym′phy·sis (sim′fi·sis) (pl. *symphyses*). A synarthrosis, especially one in the sagittal plane. —**symphys′i·al,** *adj.* **s. mandibulae.** The midline osteochondral union of the halves of the mandible. **s. pubis.** The fibro-

cartilaginous union (synchondrosis) of the pubic bones.

sym″phy·so·ske′li·a. The condition in which the lower extremities are united. See *sympus.*

sym·po′di·a. The condition of united lower extremities. See *sympus.*

symp′tom. One of the phenomena of disease which lead to complaints on the part of the patient; a subjective sign in contrast to one which is objective. **concomitant symptoms.** Accessory phenomena occurring in connection with the essential phenomena of a disease. **constitutional s.** One produced by the effect of the disease on the whole body. Also called *general s.* **direct s.** One depending directly upon disease. **focal s.** One occurring at a given site. **local s.** One indicating the concentration of a disease in a certain part of the body. **negatively pathognomonic s.** One which never occurs in a certain disease and therefore by its presence shows the absence of that disease. **pathognomonic s.** A symptom which exhibits itself only in a certain disease and therefore undeniably proves its presence. **signal s.** The first disturbance of sensation preceding a more extensive convulsion, as the aura heralding an attack of epilepsy. **static s.** A symptom which indicates the condition in a single organ without reference to the rest of the body. **sympathetic symptoms.** Symptoms for which no adequate cause can be given other than so-called sympathy.

symp″to·mat′ic. 1. Pertaining to, or of the nature of, a symptom. 2. Affecting symptoms, as symptomatic treatment.

symp″tom·a·tog′ra·phy. A written or printed description of symptoms.

symp″tom·a·tol′o·gy. 1. The science of symptoms. 2. In common usage, the symptoms of disease taken together as a whole. —**symptomatolog′ic,** *adj.*

symp′tom com′plex. The ensemble of symptoms of a disease. Also see *syndrome.*

symp·to′sis. Wasting; emaciation; collapse.

sym′pus. A monster characterized by greater or less fusion of the legs, rotation of the legs, and marked deficiencies of the pelvic region and genitalia. Also called *cuspide fetus, sirenomelus, symelus, sirenoform fetus, mermaid fetus, uromelus, ankylomelus.*

syn-. A prefix signifying *with* or *together.*

syn″ac·to′sis. Malformations caused by the abnormal growing together of parts.

syn·al′gi·a. Pain felt in a distant

part from an injury or stimulation of another part. —**synalgic**, *adj*.

sy·nan'che (si-nang'kee, sigh-nang'-kee). Severe sore throat with choking, often caused by diphtheria organisms. Syn., *diphtheria*.

syn·an'the·ma (si-nan'thi-muh, sin"an-theem'uh). A group of elementary skin lesions of the same type.

syn'apse (sin'aps, si-naps'). The region of communication between neurons; the point at which an impulse passes from an axon of one neuron to a dendrite or to the cell body of another. The relation between the neurons is probably one of contiguity of plasma membranes, rather than one of continuity of protoplasm. A synapse is polarized, that is, nerve impulses are transmitted in only one direction, and is characterized by fatigability.

syn·ap'sis. The fusion of the male and female chromosome pair, either side to side or end to end without either univalent chromosome losing its identity, resulting in a bivalent chromosome which is responsible for transmitting mixed characteristics from the parents to the offspring.

syn·ap'tase (si-nap'tace, -taze). See *emulsin*.

syn·ap'tene. See *amphitene*.

syn·ap"to·lem'ma. The membrane at the synapse, separating the axonic ending from the body of the nerve cell.

syn"ar·thro·phy'sis. Progressive ankylosis of the joints.

syn"ar·thro'sis. A form of articulation in which the bones are immovably bound together without any intervening synovial cavity. The forms are suture, in which processes are interlocked; schindylesis, in which a thin plate of one bone is inserted into a cleft of another; and gomphosis, in which a conical process is held by a socket.

syn·can'thus. Adhesions between the orbital tissues and the eyeball.

syn·chi'li·a, syn·chei'li·a (sin-kigh'lee-uh). Fusion of the lips.

syn"chon·dro'sis (sing"kon-dro'-sis). A joint in which the surfaces are connected by a plate of cartilage. —**synchondrosial**, *adj*.

syn"chon·drot'o·my (sing"kon-drot'o-mee). A division of the cartilage uniting bones, especially of that of the symphysis pubis.

syn·chro'nism. Concurrence in time of two or more events. —**synchronous**, *adj*.

syn·chy·sis scin·til'lans (sing'-ki·sis sin'til·lanz, sin·til'anz). The presence of bright, shining particles in the vitreous body of the eye.

syn·cli'tism. A condition marked by parallelism or similarity of inclination; parallelism between the pelvic planes and those of the fetal head. —**syn·clit'ic**, *adj*.

syn·clo·nus. 1. Tremor, or cloni[c] spasm, of several muscles at the sam[e] time. 2. A disease thus characterized as chorea.

syn'co·pe (sing'ko·pee). Swooning o[r] fainting; temporary suspension of con[-] sciousness from cerebral anemi[a] —**syncopal, syncop'ic**, *adj*. **ca·rotid sinus s**. Spontaneous attack[s] of unconsciousness and convulsion[s] caused by a hyperactive carotid sinu[s]. **laryngeal s**. Spasm of the laryn[x] associated with vertigo and loss of con[-] sciousness. **local s**. Sudden pallor an[d] insensibility of a part. **s. anginosa** Synonym of angina pectoris. **vaso·vagal s**. That developing in person[s] with unstable vasomotor systems; emo[-] tional strain or pressure on the vagu[s] causes a lowering of blood pressure an[d] slowing of the pulse. Also see carot[id] sinus s.

syncurine. A trade-mark for th[e] bromide salt of decamethonium.

syn·cyt"i·o·ly'sin (sin-sit"ee-o·lye'-sin, sin·sish"ee·o·). A cytolysin pr[o] duced by injections of an emulsio[n] made from placental tissue.

syn·cyt"i·o·troph'o·blast (·tro'f[o] blast, ·trof'o·blast). Syncytial troph[o] blast. An irregular sheet or net o[f] deeply staining cytoplasm in whic[h] nuclei are irregularly scattered; it li[es] outside of the cytotrophoblast. Als[o] called *syncytium, plasmoditrophoblas[t]*.

syn·cyt'i·um (sin-sish'ee·um, si[n] sit'ee·um). A mass of cytoplasm wi[th] numerous nuclei. —**syncytial**, *adj*

syn·dac'tyl. Having the fingers o[r] toes joined together.

syn·dac'ty·lus. A person wit[h] webbed fingers or toes.

syn·dac'ty·ly, syn·dac'tyl·ism syn"dac·tyl'i·a. Adhesion of finger[s] or toes; webbed fingers; webbed toe[s]. —**syndactylous**, *adj*.

syn·de'sis, syn·de'sis. The state [of] being bound together.

syn·des"mec·to'pi·a (sin·dess[-] meck·to'pee·uh, sin·dez"·). Ligamen[-] tous displacement.

syn"des·mi'tis (sin"dess·my'ti[s] sin"dez·). 1. Inflammation of a lig[a] ment. 2. Conjunctivitis.

syn·des"mo·di·as'ta·sis (·dy[s] ass"tuh·sis). Separation of ligaments

syn"des·mol'o·gy. The study [of] ligaments.

syn·des'mo·pex"y. The attachmen[t] of a ligament in a new position.

syn"des·mor'rha·phy. Suture [or] repair of ligaments.

syn"des·mo'sis. A form of articula[-] tion in which the bones are connecte[d] by fibrous connective tissue.

syn"des·mot'o·my. The division [of] a ligament.

syn'drome (sin'drohm, sin'dr[o] mee"). A group of symptoms and sign[s] which, when considered together, cha[r] acterize a disease or lesion. **—syndrom'ic**, adj. **Adie's s.** Impairment of pupillary reaction to light and of accommodation associated with decrease or loss of the deep reflexes of the extremities. See Adie's *pupil.* **adiposogenital s.** See adiposogenital *dystrophy.* **adrenogenital s.** The clinical evidence of hypersecretion of the hormones of the adrenal cortex. This may lead in the fetus to pseudohermaphroditism, in the infant to pubertas praecox or pseudoprecocity in female children, virilism and hirsutism or the diabetes of bearded women in adults (Achard-Thiers syndrome), or Cushing's syndrome and rarely feminization in men. The term as usually employed refers to hirsutism, obesity, menstrual disorders, and other incomplete features similar to Cushing's syndrome in women. Also called *s. genitourrenale, hyperinterrenalism.* **Banti's s.** A symptom complex of enlarged spleen, hypochromic anemia, and leukopenia, often with cirrhosis and ascites. Also called *congestive splenomegaly.* **Budd-Chiari s.** Thrombosis of the hepatic veins associated with right upper quadrant abdominal pain, enlargement of the liver and spleen, ascites, edema of the lower extremities, and formation of collateral venous channels. **carotid sinus s.** Overirritability of the carotid sinus causing attacks of dizziness, fainting, and sometimes convulsions. During the attack there is a fall in arterial blood pressure and a marked slowing or standstill of the heart. Attacks may come on spontaneously, may follow an emotional upset, or may be caused by pressure over the carotid sinus. **compression s.** Crush syndrome. **crush s.** Nephrosis, involving chiefly distal convoluted renal tubules, consequent to crushing injuries of the extremities. **Cushing's s.** See pituitary *basophilism.* **dumping s.** A symptom complex sometimes occurring after complete or partial removal of the stomach, characterized by a feeling of warmth, weakness, vertigo, tightness or pain in the epigastrium, nausea, palpitation, and in some cases, collapse of the patient. **effort s.** A group of reactions evoked by moderate physical exercise and consisting principally of an abnormal degree of dyspnea, rapid heart action, palpitation, substernal oppression, and sometimes pain. It is usually described in connection with neurocirculatory asthenia, but is manifest also in other cardiac disorders. **Froelich's s.** Adiposogenital dystrophy. **Guillain-Barré s.** Benign, symmetrical paresthesia and paresis of the distal portions of the extremities, with increased albumin in the spinal fluid; occasionally

facial diplegia occurs; primary infectious polyneuritis. Also called *polyradiculoneuritis.* **hand-shoulder s.** Shoulder-hand syndrome. **Horner's s.** Unilateral ptosis of the eyelid, miosis, enophthalmos, flushing and diminished sweating of the face, caused by destruction of the cervical sympathetic nerves on the same side. **Korsakoff's s.** Polyneuritis with loss of memory, a retrograde amnesia associated with tendency to confabulation, caused by alcohol and severe deficiency of food intake. **Loeffler's s.** A disease of unknown origin, characterized by extensive pulmonary infiltration by eosinophils and by eosinophilia of peripheral blood. **low-salt s.** A clinical syndrome characterized by a low serum sodium concentration, occurring acutely in heat exhaustion or water intoxication, also in chronic cardiac or renal disease when sodium chloride intake has been long restricted. **Marfan's s.** A hereditary disorder of connective tissue, characterized by arachnodactyly, dislocation of the lenses of the eyes, bony abnormalities of the chest and palate, and a variety of congenital cardiovascular lesions, notably medial necrosis of the ascending aorta and defects of the interatrial septum of the heart. **Ménière's s.** A disease of the internal ear characterized by deafness, vertigo, and tinnitus. Frequently accompanied by nausea, vomiting, and nystagmus. The process may be an allergy because the mechanism is similar to angioneurotic edema. **Schüller-Christian s.** A disturbance of lipid metabolism characterized by abnormal deposits of cholesterol especially in the base of the skull. This primary xanthomatosis is seen mainly in children, is not hereditary, and is manifested principally by exophthalmos, diabetes insipidus, and often by xanthomatosis of the skin. **shoulder-hand s.** A disorder of the upper extremity, characterized by severe constant intractable pain in the shoulder and arm, limited motion, swelling of the hand, fibrosis and atrophy of muscles, and decalcification of underlying bones, thought to be similar to, or a form of, causalgia. **Stokes-Adams s.** A slowed pulse with syncopal attacks or convulsive seizures, usually epileptiform in character. The slowed cardiac action is a result of heart block; the cerebral symptoms are a direct result of the bradycardia. **thalamic s.** A symptom complex produced by thrombosis of the thalamogeniculate artery which supplies the posterior portion of the lateral nuclear mass of the thalamus. It includes contralateral partial hemianesthesia and hemiplegia, contralateral severe paroxysmal pain over the entire half of the body, contralateral increased response to stimuli, slight hemiataxia, and occasional hemichorea. Also called *Dejerine-Roussy* s. **Tietze's** s. A benign, self-limiting disease of unknown cause, characterized by nonsuppurative inflammation of the costal cartilages, frequently preceded or accompanied by upper respiratory tract infection.

syn·ech'i·a (si-neck'ee-uh, si-nee'kee-uh). A morbid union of parts; especially, adhesion of the iris to a neighboring part of the eye. **annular s.** Exclusion of the pupil. **anterior s.** Adhesion between the iris and transparent cornea. **posterior s.** Adhesion between the iris and crystalline lens. **total s.** Adhesion of the entire surface of the iris to the lens. See *iris bombé.*

syn·ech'o·tome (si-neck'o-tome). An instrument for the division of adhesions, particularly of the tympanic membrane.

syn"ech·ot'o·my (sin"i-kot'o-mee). The division of a synechia.

syn"en·ceph'a·lo·cele. An encephalocele with adhesions.

syn·er'e·sis. 1. Contraction of a clot (as blood, milk). 2. *In colloid chemistry,* the exudation of the liquid constituent of gels irrespective of the vapor pressure imposed upon the system. Lowered vapor pressure aids the process.

syn"er·get'ic. Exhibiting synergy; working together; synergic.

syn·er·gism (sin'ur-jiz-um, si-nur'jiz-um). 1. The harmonious and cooperative action of two or more agents or organs, as two muscles cooperating to produce a movement which neither alone could effect. 2. The joint action of two types of microörganisms on a carbohydrate medium, leading to the production of gas that is not formed by either organism when grown separately. **—synergis'tic,** *adj.*

syn·er·gist. An agent coöperating with another.

syn·er·gy. The coöperative action of two or more agents or organs. **—syner'gic,** *adj.*

syn"es·the'si·a, syn"aes·the'si·a (sin"ess-thee'zhuh, ·zee-uh). A secondary sensation or subjective impression accompanying an actual perception, as a sensation of color or sound aroused by a sensation of taste.

syn"es·the'si·al'gi·a, syn"aes·the'si·al'gi·a (sin"ess-thee"zee-al'juh, ·jee-uh). A painful sensation secondary to, and of a different quality from, that of a primary irritation.

Syn'ga·mus. A genus of nematode worms of the family Syngamidae which inhabits the upper respiratory tract of fowl and mammals. **S. laryngeus.**

A species which is usually a parasite ⸱ ruminants; incidental infestation ⸱ man has occurred.

syn·ga·my. Conjugation or union ⸱ gametes in fertilization. **—syng⸱ mous, syngam'ic,** *adj.*

syn·gig'no·sc:sm (sin-jig'no-siz-ur sin-ghig'·). Hypnotism.

syn·hex'yl. 1-Hydroxy-3-n-hexyl-⸱ 6,9-trimethyl-7,8,9,10-tetrahydro-6-d⸱ benzopyran, a synthetic analog of ⸱ tetrahydrocannabinol; a pale yello⸱ translucent, viscous and odorless resi⸱ insoluble in water. Employed as ⸱ euphoriant in the thalamic dysfunctio⸱ syndrome. Syn., *parahexyl, pyrahex*⸱

syn"hi·dro'sis. Concurrent swea⸱ ing; the association of perspiratio⸱ with another condition.

syn"i·ze·sis. Closure. **s. pupilla**⸱ Closure of the pupil.

synkamin. Trade-mark for 2-methy⸱ 4-amino-1-naphthol hydrochloride; r⸱ ferred to as vitamin K_5, a water-sol⸱ ble, active vitamin-K compound. S⸱ *menadione.*

synkayvite. Trade-mark for men⸱ diol sodium diphosphate.

syn"ki·ne'sis (sing"ki-nee'sis, ·kig⸱ nee'sis), **syn"ki·ne'si·a** (sing"⸱ nee'shuh, sing"kigh-nee'·). Involu⸱ tary movement taking place in one pa⸱ of the body synchronously with, or ⸱ consequence of, a voluntary or refl⸱ movement in another part, as swingi⸱ the arms while walking.

syn·oph'rys. Meeting of the ey⸱ brows.

syn"oph·thal'mi·a. A conditi⸱ characterized by fused orbits and va⸱ ous degrees of fusion of the eyes. Al⸱ called *cyclopia.*

syn·op'si·a. Congenital fusion of t⸱ eyes. See *cyclopia.*

syn·op'sis. A classified abbreviati⸱ of a treatise or article.

syn·or'chid·ism (sin-or'kid-iz-um⸱ **syn·or'chism** (sin-or'kiz-um). Pa⸱ tial or complete fusion of the two test⸱ within the abdomen.

syn·os'te·o·phyte". Congenit⸱ bony ankylosis. Syn., *synostosis co*⸱ *genita.*

syn"os·to'sis. A union of origina⸱ separate bones by osseous materi⸱ **—synostot'ic,** *adj.*

syn"o·vec'to·my (sin"o-veck'to-m⸱ sigh"no·). Excision of synovial me⸱ brane.

syn·o'vi·a (si-no'vee-uh, sigh-no've⸱ uh). The clear fluid which is norma⸱ present in joint cavities. See *synov⸱ fluid.* **—synovial,** *adj.*

syn·o·vi·o'ma (si-no"vee-o'mu⸱ sigh-no"·). A tumor of the synov⸱ membranes of joints, tendon sheat⸱ and bursas. Affects younger age grou⸱ especially in the knee, ankle, me⸱ tarsal joints, and elbow. It gro⸱ slowly but tends to recur after remov⸱

nd may metastasize. Accordingly it is
ften named *synovial sarcoma*. Micro-
copically it is composed of spindle,
uboidal, and round cells of fairly large
ize, arranged in sheets, papillary
tructures, and pseudoacini, sometimes
ccompanied by production of hya-
ronic acid. Syn., *synovioma*.

n″o·vi′tis (sin″o-vy′tis, sigh″no-).
nflammation of a synovial membrane.
cute suppurative s. An acute,
urulent form of infectious or trau-
atic origin. Syn., *pyarthrosis.*
hronic purulent s. Synonym of
ngous arthritis. **dry s.** Synovitis
ith little if any exudate. **gonor-
heal s.** Synonym of gonorrheal rheu-
atism. **lipomatous s.** Synovitis in
hich there is fatty degeneration.
etric s. A synovitis secondary to
terine infection. **puerperal s.** Syn-
vitis occurring after childbirth, due
ue to septic infection. **scarlati-
al s.** Synovitis occurring in an at-
ck of scarlet fever. **syphilitic s.**
novitis due to syphilitic inflammaon. **tendinous s.** Inflammation of
e synovial sheath surrounding a tenon. **tuberculous s.** Synovitis due
tuberculosis. **urethral s.** Gonor-
eal arthritis. **villous s.** A type of
novitis in which villous growths de-
lop within the articular cavity.

n′ta·sis. A stretching, or tension.

n′tha·lin. $NH_2.C:NH.NH(CH_2)_{12}$
H.C:NH.NH_2.2HCl. The dihydrochlo-
de of decamethylene bisguanidine,
aving hypoglycemic action through
imulation of secretion of insulin by
e pancreas. Its use has been aban-
ned because of harmful effects.

n′the·sis. 1. *In chemistry*, the proc-
ses and operations necessary to build
a compound. In general, a reaction,
series of reactions, in which a com-
ex compound is obtained from ele-
ents or simple compounds. 2. The
rmation of a complex concept by the
mbination of separate ideas. 3. *In
ychiatry*, the process in which the
o accepts unconscious ideas and feel-
gs and amalgamates them within it-
lf more or less consciously.

n·thet′ic. Produced by artificial
eans.

nthroid sodium. Trade-mark for
dium levothyroxine.

n·ton′ic. Pertaining to a type of
rsonality in which there is an ap-
opriate harmony of thinking, feeling,
d behavior.

n′to·nin. 1. A metaprotein obtained
the action of dilute acid on more
mplex proteins. 2. The specific meta-
otein thus obtained from the myosin
muscle.

ntropan. Trade-mark for the phos-
ate of the *dl*-tropic acid ester of
3-diethylamino-2,2-dimethyl-1-pro-
panol, an antispasmodic.

syph″il·el′cos. Syphilitic ulcer;
chancre.

syph″il·e′mi·a. The presence of the
Treponema pallidum in the blood
stream.

syph′i·lide, syph′i·lid. A skin
eruption due to syphilis. Nearly any
type of skin lesion can be produced by
the *Treponema pallidum.*

syph″il·i·on′thus. Any copper-
colored scaly eruption in syphilis.

syph′i·lis. A communicable venereal
disease, characterized by a variety of
lesions of which the chancre (primary
lesion), the mucous patch, and the
gumma are the most distinctive. A
spirochete, *Treponema pallidum*, is the
cause. The disease is usually acquired
in sexual congress, hence its earliest
manifestations appear on the genital
organs, but any abraded surface of the
body, if brought in contact with the
spirochete, may give entrance to the infection. The earliest lesion of acquired
syphilis is the chancre, initial sclerosis,
or primary sore, which appears after a
period of incubation varying from ten
days to three weeks. It is usually a
painless ulcer, and has a slight serous
or purulent discharge in which the
spirochetes may be seen on dark-field
examination. Microscopically it consists
of an accumulation of round cells, epithelioid cells, with, perhaps, a giant
cell here and there. The blood vessels
present a hyperplasia of the intima.
Very soon after the appearance of the
chancre the nearest lymph nodes become enlarged and indurated. The
mucous patch, condyloma latum, or
moist papule occurs on moist areas,
usually where two skin surfaces are in
contact. All these lesions harbor many
of the spirochetes. The gumma is a
rounded nodule, varying in size from
the dimensions of a pea to those of a
small apple. Its favorite seats are over
flat bones, the membranes of the brain,
the liver, spleen, and testis. It is usually
soft, and contains in its interior a
gelatinous gummy material. Spirochetes
are rarely found in these late lesions.
Another important though not distinctive lesion produced by syphilis is a
diffuse sclerosis of the blood vessels,
especially of the parenchymatous organs. The clinical course of syphilis is
generally divided into three stages: the
primary (primary syphilis), characterized by the presence of the chancre and
of the indolent bubo; the secondary
(secondary syphilis), by the mucous
patch, cutaneous eruptions, sore throat,
general enlargement of the lymph
nodes, and a systemic toxemia; the
tertiary (tertiary syphilis), by the
gumma and by severe skin lesions. Be-

tween the appearance of the chancre and the secondary manifestations a period of six weeks usually elapses. The tertiary phenomena follow the secondary after a stage of quiescence of variable length. Syphilis may involve any organ of the body. Typical late lesions are the aneurysm of the aorta, interstitial keratitis in congenital syphilis, and involvement of the central nervous system. Typical of the latter are syphilitic meningitis, tabes dorsalis, paresis, and other meningovascular lesions. Also called *lues*. **congenital s.** See prenatal *s.* **extragenital s.** Syphilis in which the first lesion is situated elsewhere than on the genital organs. **marital s.** Syphilis acquired in lawful wedlock. **meningovascular s.** Syphilis of the central nervous system involving the leptomeninges and the cerebral arteries causing the formation of large or small gummas and an endarteritis; parenchymatous changes in brain or spinal-cord tissue occur only secondary to vascular disease. **prenatal s.** Syphilis transmitted from mother to offspring. **s. technica.** Syphilis acquired in following one's occupation, as by physicians, midwives, nurses.

syph'i·lo-, syphil-. A combining form for *syphilis.*

syph'i·lo·derm, syph"i·lo·der'ma. Skin manifestations of syphilis. They are common, of many forms, and often diagnostic problems. While occurring in any stage of the disease, they are more common during the first two years of the infection. Early lesions are commonly a dull- to ham-red color and appear symmetrically over the body, palms, and soles. **—syphiloder'matous,** *adj.*

syph"i·lo·gen'e·sis. The origin or development of syphilis.

syph"i·log'ra·pher. One who writes about syphilis.

syph"i·log'ra·phy. A treatise on syphilis; any writing about the disease.

syph'i·loid. 1. Resembling syphilis. 2. A disease resembling syphilis.

syph"i·lol'o·gist. One who has made a study of syphilis; an expert in the diagnosis and treatment of the disease.

syph"i·lol'o·gy. The sum of knowledge regarding the origin, nature, and treatment of syphilis.

syph"i·lo'ma. 1. A syphilitic gumma. 2. Tumor due to syphilis. **—syphilom'atous,** *adj.*

syph"i·lo·ma'ni·a. A mental disorder resulting from syphilophobia.

syph"i·lo·nych'i·a (sif"i·lo·nick'-ee·uh). An onychia of syphilitic origin.

syph"i·lop'a·thy. Any syphilitic disease.

syph'i·lo·phobe". One affected wit[h] syphilophobia.

syph"i·lo·pho'bi·a. Morbid fear [of] syphilis.

syph"i·lo·phy'ma. 1. Syphiloma [of] the skin. 2. Any growth due to syphil[is].

syr. Syrup.

sy·rig'mo·pho'ni·a. 1. A piping [or] whistling state of the voice. 2. [A] sibilant rale.

sy·rig'mus. Any subjective hissin[g,] murmuring, or tinkling sound heard [in] the ear.

syr"ing·ad"e·no'ma. A swea[t] gland tumor.

syr"ing·ad"e·no'sus. Pertaining [to] the sweat glands.

syr'inge. An apparatus of meta[l,] glass, or plastic material, consisting [of] a nozzle, a barrel, and a plunger or rubber bulb; used to inject a liquid in[to] a cavity or under the skin. **aural s.** One used to wash out the external aud[i-] tory canal. **hypodermic s.** O[ne] used to administer drugs, as opiate[s,] under the skin. **penis s.** Urethral syringe. **rectal s.** A large syringe use[d] to administer an enen.a. **urethral s.** One adapted to force liquid into th[e] male urethra.

sy·rin"go·bul'bi·a. The presence [of] cavities in the medulla oblongata sim[i-] lar to syringomyelia.

sy·rin"go·cyst"ad·e·no'ma. Sy[r-] ingoma.

sy·rin'goid. Like a tube.

syr"in·go'ma. A multiple nevo[id] tumor of sweat glands, occurring mo[re] often in females and developing aft[er] puberty. Histologically the derma co[n-] tains numerous small cystic ducts wi[th] commalike tails of epithelium. Al[so] called *syringocystadenoma, syringocy[s-] toma.*

sy·rin"go·my·e'li·a (si·ring"g[o·] migh·ee'lee·uh). A chronic disea[se] characterized pathologically by th[e] presence of long cavities surrounded [by] gliosis, which are situated in relatio[n] to the central canal of the spinal co[rd] and frequently extend up into th[e] medulla (syringobulbia).

sy·rin"go·my'e·lo·cele". Spina b[i-] fida with protrusion of a meningeal s[ac] containing a portion of the spinal co[rd] whose central canal is greatly distende[d] with cerebrospinal fluid.

syr'inx. 1. Old term for a fistula [or] tube. 2. The organ of voice in birds, [at] bifurcation of the trachea.

syr'up. 1. A concentrated solution [of] sugar in aqueous fluids, with the a[d-] dition of medicating or flavoring i[n-] gredients. 2. The U.S.P. preparatio[n] containing sucrose, 850 Gm.; distille[d] water, a sufficient quantity to ma[ke] 1000 cc. Abbreviated, syr. Syn., *siru[p.]* Also called *simple s.* **—syrupy,** *adj.*

sys″sar·co′sis. The failure of union of bones after fracture by the interposition of muscular tissue. **—syssar·cot′ic,** *adj.*

rs·tal′tic. Pulsatory; contracting; having a systole.

sys′tem. 1. A methodical arrangement. 2. A combination of parts into a whole, as the digestive system, the nervous system. 3. The body as a whole. **—system′ic, systemat′ic,** *adj.* **alimentary s.** The alimentary canal with its accessory glands. **autonomic nervous s.** An aggregation of ganglia, nerves, and plexuses through which the viscera, heart, blood vessels, smooth muscles, and glands receive their motor innervation. It is divided into the craniosacral, or parasympathetic, and thoracicolumbar, or sympathetic, systems. **cardiovascular s.** The heart and blood vessels. **central nervous s.** The brain and spinal cord. Abbreviated, C.N.S. **cerebrospinal s.** The central nervous system. **digestive s.** The digestive tract from mouth to anus and usually considered as the alimentary canal. **endocrine s.** The ductless glands or glands of internal secretion considered as a whole. **exterofective s.** That part of the nervous system that is concerned with adapting the body to changes in its external environment. **fingerprint s.** A scientific system for the identification of persons in the military service, for the apprehension of criminals, and for the identification of the dead. A modern development of the Bertillon system. **Haversian s.** The concentric layers of bone about the blood vessels in the Haversian canals of compact bone. **hepatic duct s.** The biliary tract including the hepatic ducts, gallbladder, cystic duct, and common bile duct. **integumentary s.** That pertaining to the body covering, as the skin, hair, nails, etc. **locomotor s.** The extremities and their parts, as the bones, muscles, and joints concerned with locomotion, or the motor activities of the body. **lymphatic s.** A system of vessels and nodes accessory to the blood vascular system, conveying lymph. It begins as innumerable capillaries in interspaces of tissues. These form plexuses studded with lymph nodes that act as filters and finally all those below the diaphragm unite in the cisterna chyli in the second lumbar vertebra. From this the thoracic duct leads upward to empty into the junction of the left subclavian and internal jugular veins. The lymph from the upper left half of the body also empties here. The lymph from the upper right half of the body and head enters the right lymphatic duct, which empties into the junction of the right internal jugular and subclavian veins. **osseous s.** The bony skeleton of the body. **portal s.** A system of veins which drain a capillary bed at one end and supply a capillary bed at the other end. **redox s.** (*reductantoxidant*). A simple oxidation-reduction system in which two substances react reversibly with each other. The oxidized material is a reductant; the reduced material, an oxidant. **reproductive s.** The generative apparatus, as a whole, consisting in man of the penis, testes, deferential ducts, seminal vesicles, and prostate, and in woman of the vagina, uterus, uterine tubes (oviducts), and ovaries. **respiratory s.** All the passages by which air is conducted to, and including, the parts of the lungs where an exchange of oxygen and carbon dioxide takes place, such as the nasal cavities, pharynx, larynx, trachea, bronchi, bronchioles, and the pulmonary lobules with their alveoli. Other accessory structures, for example the diaphragm and muscles concerned with respiration, are included. **reticuloendothelial s.** The macrophage system, which includes all the phagocytic cells of the body, except the leukocytes. These cells, diverse morphologically, all have the capacity for the elective storage of certain colloidal dyes. They include: the histiocytes and macrophages of loose connective tissue, the reticular cells of lymphatic and myeloid tissues, the Kupffer cells of hepatic sinusoids, the cells lining the sinusoids of the adrenal and hypophysis, and the dust cells of the lungs. Abbreviated, RES. **urinary s.** The system made up of the kidneys, ureters, bladder, and urethra, whose function is the elaboration and excretion of urine. **urogenital s.** The combined urinary and genital systems which are intimately related embryologically and anatomically. **vasomotor s.** The nerve supply of the blood vessels.

sys′tem·oid. A term applied to tumors composed of a number of tissues resembling a system of organs.

sys′to·le (sis′to-lee). The contraction phase of the cardiac cycle.

sys·trem′ma (pl. *systremmata*). Cramp in the muscles of the leg.

Szymanowski, Julius von [*Russian surgeon,* 1829–68]. Developed a form of blepharoplasty called *Szymanowski's operation.* Developed operations for the restoration of the auricle, for ectropion, for restoration of the upper lip by lateral flaps brought together in the midline; also called *Szymanowski's operations.*

T. Tension, temperature.

T. A. Toxin-antitoxin.

Ta. Chemical symbol for tantalum.

tab″a·co′sis. A toxic state produced by the excessive use of tobacco, or by the inhalation of tobacco dust.

Ta·ban′i·dae (ta-ban′i-dee). A family of the Diptera, which includes the horseflies, deer flies, and gadflies. They are medium to large, robust flies, world-wide in distribution. The females of the well-known species are blood suckers which attack man and warm-blooded animals generally. Certain species distribute diseases such as anthrax among cattle and sheep; others transmit the trypanosomes of animals, especially the *Trypanosoma evansi*, the cause of surra in horses and cattle. The important genera are *Chrysops, Haematopota, Tabanus,* and *Pangonia*.

ta″ba‴tière′ an″a·to·mique′ (tah″baht″yair′ ahn″ah·to·meek′). The depression at the base of the thumb between the tendons of the abductor pollicis longus and the extensor pollicis longus. Also called *anatomist's snuffbox*.

ta·bel′la. A medicated troche or tablet, *q.v.*

ta′bes (tay′beez). A wasting or consumption. The word generally is used as a synonym for tabes dorsalis. **diabetic t.** A peripheral neuritis affecting diabetics. **spastic t.** Combined cord disease or posterolateral cord disease producing ataxia and spasticity of the lower extremities. **t. coxaria.** Wasting from hip disease. **t. dolorosa.** A form in which pain is the dominating feature. **t. dorsalis.** Locomotor ataxia, a disease dependent upon sclerosis of the posterior columns of the spinal cord. The symptoms are lightning pains; unsteadiness and incoördination of voluntary movements, extending to the upper extremities; disorders of the eye, such as the Argyll Robertson pupil; cutaneous anesthesia; pain crises in the gastric, laryngeal, and rectal zones; trophic disorders of the joints; girdle sense; abolition of the patellar reflex; diminution of sexual desire; and disturbance of the sphincters. **t. ergotica.** A toxemia resulting from the use of ergot; its symptomatology closely simulates that of tabes dorsalis. **t. mesenterica.** Tuberculous disease of mesenteric lymph nodes in children, with progressive wasting.

ta·bet′ic. 1. Affected with tabes; of, or pertaining to, tabes. 2. Pertaining to, or affected with, tabes dorsalis.

ta′ble. 1. A flat-topped piece of furniture, as an operating table, examining table. 2. A flat plate, especially one of bone, as the inner or outer table (of compact bone) of a flat bone of the cranium. 3. A presentation of data in the form of rows and columns.

ta′ble-spoon″. A large spoon, holding about 15 cc. or 4 fluidrachms. Abbreviated, tbsp.

tab′let. A friable solid dosage form. Hypodermic tablets must be readily soluble in water.

ta″bo·pa·ral′y·sis. A condition in which tabes is associated with general paralysis and with primary optic atrophy.

tab′u·lar. Having the form of a table, as a tabular bone.

tache (tahsh) (pl. *taches*). A spot. **t. bleuâtre.** A spot of a delicate bluish tint, sometimes observed in the skin of typhoid fever patients. **t. cérébrale.** The red line made when the fingernail is drawn over the skin, due to vasomotor reaction and occurring especially in connection with meningeal irritation. Also called *t. meningeale.*

ta·chet′ic (ta·ket′ick). Relating to the formation of reddish blue or purple patches (taches).

ta·chis′to·scope (ta·kis′to·scope). An instrument used in psychophysiology to observe the time rate and time conditions for apperception; also an instrument used in orthoptics for visual training, especially to overcome the suppression area in amblyopia from disuse. **—tachistoscop′ic,** *adj.*

tach′o·gram (tack′o·gram). The record made in tachography.

ta·chog′ra·phy (ta·kog′ruh·fee). The estimation of the rate of flow of arterial blood by means of a flowmeter, or tachygraph.

tach′y- (tack′i-). A combining form meaning *swift.*

tach″y·aux·e′sis. A condition in which the part grows more rapidly than the whole organism.

tach″y·car′di·a. Excessive rapidity of the heart's action. **atrial t.** Rapid and regular succession of P waves which are normal or abnormal in form. The QRS group may be normal or slightly or markedly aberrant. The rate is usually 160–200 per minute. **atrioventricular t.** Rapid and regular succession of systoles arising from the atrioventricular node at a rate of over 100 per minute; may be as fast as 270 per minute. In some records the P waves cannot be recognized. In other there is retrograde block and the basic atrial rhythm is undisturbed (His's bundle tachycardia or idioventricular tachycardia). **auricular t.** The rapid and regular succession of P waves which are normal or abnormal in form. The QRS group may be normal, or slightly or markedly aberrant. The rate is usually 160 to 200 per minute. **essential t.** That occurring in paroxysms, and due to functional disturbance of the cardiac nerves. **paroxysmal t.** Tachycardia occurring periodically in paroxysms. **reflex t.** Tachycardia due to causes other than those producing essential tachycardia. **t. strumosa exophthalmica.** The tachycardia occurring in exophthalmic goiter. **ventricular t.** A rapid succession of beats, each with the characteristics of a ventricular systole, occurring at rates from 150–250 per minute, regular or slightly irregular. The atrial rhythm, if recognized, is not disturbed.

tach′y·graph. An instrument for measuring the rate of blood flow.

ta·chyg′ra·phy (ta-kig′ruh-fee). The estimation of the rate of flow of arterial blood by means of the tachygraph.

tach″y·lo′gi·a. Morbid rapidity or volubility of speech; occurs in the manic phase of manic-depressive psychosis. Syn., *logorrhea, tachyphrasia, tachyphemia.*

ta·chym′e·ter (ta-kim′i-tur). An instrument for measuring the rate of speed of a moving object.

tach″y·pha′gi·a. Rapid eating.

tach″y·phre′ni·a. Morbidly accelerated mental activity.

tach″y·phy·lax′is (tack″i-fi-lack′-sis, -fligh-lack′sis). Rapid immunization.

tach″yp·ne′a, tach″yp·noe′a. Abnormal frequency of respiration. **nervous t.** Respiration of 40 or more to the minute accompanying neurotic disorders, particularly hysteria and neurasthenia.

tach″y·rhyth′mi·a. 1. Tachycardia. 2. *In electroencephalography,* an increase in the normal brain wave frequency to 12–50 per second.

ta·chys′ter·ol (ta-kis′tur-ole, tack″i-steer′·). The precursor of calciferol in the irradiation of ergosterol. It is an isomer of ergosterol.

tac′tile (tack′til). Pertaining to the sense of touch.

tae′di·um vi′tae (tee′dee-um vy′-tee). Weariness of life, a symptom occurring in many cases of depressive psychosis; it is sometimes a precursor of suicide.

Tae′ni·a (tee′nee-uh). A genus of parasitic worms of the class Cestoidea; they are ribbonlike segmental flatworms. The adult is an intestinal parasite of vertebrates; the larvae para-

sitize both vertebrate and invertebrate tissues. The adult consists of a scolex, an undifferentiated germinal neck, and two or more hermaphroditic segments or proglottids which contain fertile ova when mature. **T. echinococcus.** See *Echinococcus granulosus.* **T. saginata.** A tapeworm which passes its larval stages in cattle, its adult stage in the intestine of man. The human infestation is acquired by eating insufficiently cooked infested beef. Syn., *beef tapeworm.* **T. solium.** The larval stages occur in hogs; the adult is found in the intestine of man. Ingestion of ova may result in larval infestation in man; the larvae are then called *Cysticercus cellulosae.* Infestation is usually acquired by ingestion of viable larvae in pork. Syn., *pork tapeworm.*

tae′ni·a (pl. *taeniae*). 1. A band or bandlike structure. 2. See *tapeworm.* **t. coli.** One of the three tapelike bands of the longitudinal layer of the tunica muscularis of the colon.

tae′ni·a·cide″. 1. Destructive of tapeworms. 2. An agent that destroys tapeworms.

tae′ni·a·fuge″. 1. Expelling tapeworms. 2. An agent that expels tapeworms.

tae·ni·a′sis (tee-nigh′uh-sis, ti-nigh′·). The symptoms caused by infestation with any of the species of *Taenia, q.v.* Also see *tapeworm.*

tae″ni·o·pho′bi·a. Morbid dread of becoming the host of a tapeworm.

tag. A flap or appendage. **epithelial t.** A mass of epithelial cells projecting from the urethral groove on the glans of the embryonic phallus. Syn., *epithelial tubercle.*

tail. 1. The caudal extremity of an animal. 2. Anything resembling a tail.

tai′lor's spasm. An occupational neurosis occurring in tailors, characterized by spasm of the muscles of the arm and hand. Also called *tailor's cramp.*

taint. 1. Possessing a disposition or hereditary characters predisposing to disease, or affected by disease without outspoken manifestations. 2. Putrefaction or infestation, as tainted meat. 3. Local discoloration, as a blemish.

taka-diastase. Trade-mark for a powdered vegetable diastase.

take. Become infected, as by vaccine virus.

ta·lal′gi·a. Pain in the ankle.

talc, tal′cum. A native, hydrous magnesium silicate sometimes containing a little aluminum silicate. It occurs in various grades and degrees of purity, as potstone, soapstone, steatite, French chalk.

tal′cum. Talc, *q.v.*

tal′i·pes (tall′i-peez). Any one of a variety of deformities of the human foot, especially those of congenital origin, such as clubfoot or equinovarus. Also embraces paralytic deformities and the numerous simple varieties of foot distortion, according to whether the forefoot is inverted or everted and whether the Achilles tendon is shortened or lengthened. Combinations of the various types occur, called talipes equinovalgus, talipes equinovarus, talipes calcaneovalgus, talipes calcaneovarus, etc. **t. calcaneus.** Talipes in which the patient walks upon the heel alone. **t. cavus.** An increased curvature of the arch of the foot. **t. equinus.** Talipes in which the heel is elevated and the weight thrown upon the the anterior portion of the foot. **t. planus.** Flatfoot; splay foot. **t. spasmodica.** Noncongenital talipes due to muscular spasm. **t. valgus.** Talipes in which the outer border of the foot is everted, with inward rotation of the tarsus and flattening of the plantar arch. Also called *flatfoot, splay foot, pes planus, weak foot.* **t. varus.** A variety in which the foot is inverted, the weight falling on the outer border. If the inversion is extreme, with rotation of the forefoot, the condition is known as clubfoot.

tal″i·pom′a·nus (tal″i·pom′uh·nus, tal″i·po·may′nus). Clubhand, *q.v.*

tal′low. The fat extracted from suet, the solid fat of cattle, sheep, and other ruminants. It consists largely of stearin and palmitin.

ta′lo-. A combining form denoting *pertaining to the talus* or *astragalus.*

tal′ose. C₆H₁₂O₆. A monosaccharide isomeric with dextrose.

ta′lus. The bone of the ankle which articulates with the bones of the leg. The old term is *astragalus.* See Table of Bones in the Appendix.

ta′ma, tam′a. Swelling of the feet and legs.

tam′bour (tam′boor, tam-boor′). A drum; a drumlike instrument used in physiologic experiments for recording. It consists of a metal cylinder over which is stretched an elastic membrane, and to which passes a tube for transmitting changes in air pressure. Recording is done optically by means of a small mirror on the membrane, or mechanically by a stylus attached to the membrane.

tam′pon. 1. A plug of cotton, sponge, or other material inscrted into the vagina, nose, or other cavity. 2. Plug with a tampon.

tam″pon·ade′. The act of plugging with a tampon.

tam′pon·ing, tam′pon·ment (tam′pun·mint, tam·pon′mint). The act of inserting a pack or plug within a cavity for checking hemorrhage, etc.

tan. 1. Color the skin by exposure to sun or wind (or artificially, by use of a sun lamp). 2. The color so imparted.

tan′nase (tan′ace, ·aze). An enzyme found in cultures of *Penicillium* and *Aspergillus* which converts tannic acid to gallic acid.

tan′nic ac′id. A tannin usually obtained from nutgalls, the excrescences formed on the young twigs of *Quercus infectoria* and allied species. Yellow to light brown powder of astringent taste; very soluble in water. A styptic and astringent. Syn., *gallotannic acid, tannin, digallic acid.*

tan′nin. 1. Tannic acid. 2. Any one of a group of astringent plant principles characterized by their ability to precipitate collagen and to produce dark-colored compounds with ferric salts. The source is frequently identified by a prefix, as gallotannin, quercitannin, etc.

tan′sy (tan′zee). A perennial herb, *Tanacetum vulgare,* of the family Compositae.

tan′ta·lum. T₂ = 180.88. A rare metal element; silver white, very hard, malleable, and ductile. Unaffected by water, acids, or alkalies, and useful wherever resistance to corrosion is important. It is used in surgery. **Tantalum oxide** has been used as a dusting powder for wounds.

tan′trum. An expression of uncontrollable anger, sometimes accompanied by acts of violence, occurring in children and psychotics.

tap. A sudden slight blow.

tap. To withdraw fluid with a trocar or hollow needle.

tapazole. Trade-mark for methimazole.

ta·pe′tum (pl. *tapeta*). 1. The layer forming the roof of the posterior and middle horns of the lateral ventricles of the brain. It is composed of fibers from the corpus callosum. 2. The brilliant layer that makes the eyes of nocturnal animals visible by reflected light at night. **—tapet′al,** *adj.*

tape′worm′. Any of the species of the class Cestoidea; segmented, ribbon-like flatworms which are parasites of man and other animals. See *Bertiella Diphyllobothrium, Dipylidium, Echinococcus, Hymenolepis, Raillietina, Sparganum, Taenia.*

taph″e·pho′bi·a. Morbid fear of being buried alive.

tap″i·no·ceph′a·ly. Flatness of the top of the cranium; flat top. **—tapinocephal′ic,** *adj.*

tap″i·o′ca. A variety of starch obtained from the cassava or manioc plant, *Jatropha manihot.* Used as a food.

ta′pir mouth. A separation and thickening of the lips, with atrophy of the orbicularis oris muscle, causing the lips to resemble those of the tapir. It is sometimes seen in facial muscular atrophy of the Landouzy-Déjérine type.

ta'pir·oid (tay'pur·oyd, tap'ur·). Referring to an elongated cervix uteri, so called from its resemblance to a tapir's snout.

ta″pote″ment′ (tah″poht″mahng′). In massage, the operation of percussing or tapping.

tap'ping. Paracentesis of the abdomen, pleural cavity, hydrocele sac, etc.

tap'root. A main root which continues the axis of some plants downward.

tar. A thick brown to black liquid consisting of a mixture of hydrocarbons and their derivatives obtained by the destructive distillation of many kinds of carbonaceous matter.

ta·ran'tu·la. A large, hairy spider of the family Aviculariidae. The bite may be very painful, but is seldom dangerous to man, although small animals may be killed.

ta·rax'a·cum. Dandelion root. The dried rhizomes and roots of *Taraxacum officinale* or *T. laevigatum*, family Compositae.

ta·rax'is. A slight or mild conjunctivitis.

tar'dive. Tending to be late; tardy.

tare. 1. A counterweight. 2. A deduction made for the weight of a container. 3. Counterbalance.

tar'get. The point of metal in a roentgen-ray tube upon which the electrons are directed and from which the roentgen rays arise.

ta·rir'ic ac'id. $CH_3(CH_2)_{10}C\vdots C\cdot(CH_2)_4COOH$. An unsaturated acid occurring as a glyceride in the fat of tariri seeds.

ta'ro (tah'ro). The starchy root of *Colocasia antiquorum* or Indian kale. Used as a food in certain Pacific islands.

tars·al'gi·a. Pain, especially of neuralgic character, in the tarsus of the foot.

tars·ec'to·my. Excision of a tarsal bone or bones.

tar·si'tis. 1. Inflammation of the tarsus of the eyelid. 2. See *blepharitis.*

tar'so-, tars-. A combining form denoting *pertaining to a tarsus.*

tar″so·chei'lo·plas″ty (tahr″so·kigh'lo·plas″tee). Plastic surgery of the edge of the eyelid.

tar″so·ma·la'ci·a (tahr″so·ma·lay′shee·uh, ·see·uh). Softening of the tarsus of the eyelid.

tar″so·met'a·tar'sal. Relating to the tarsus and the metatarsus.

tar″so·phy'ma. Any morbid growth or tumor of the tarsus of the eye.

tar'so·plas″ty. Plastic surgery of the eyelid; blepharoplasty.

tar″sop·to'si·a (tahr″sop·to'shuh, ·zhuh). Flatfoot.

tar·sor'rha·phy. 1. The operation of sewing the eyelids together for a part or the whole of their extent. Also called *blepharorrhaphy.* 2. Suture of tarsal plate.

tar·sot'o·my. 1. Operation upon the tarsal plate. 2. Operation upon the tarsus of the foot.

tar'sus. 1. The instep, or ankle, consisting of the calcaneus, talus or astragalus, cuboid, navicular or scaphoid, first, second, and third cuneiform bones. See Table of Bones in the Appendix. 2. The dense connective tissue forming the support of an eyelid; the tarsal plate. **–tarsal,** *adj.*

tar'tar. 1. A hard deposit on the inside of wine casks, consisting mainly of acid potassium tartrate (cream of tartar). 2. That accretion, properly termed salivary calculus, which is deposited on the surface of the teeth. Its composition varies, but it consists of organic secretion and food particles into which are deposited various salts, as calcium carbonate, calcium phosphate, and ferric phosphate. **cream of t.** Potassium bitartrate. **soluble t.** Potassium tartrate. **t. emetic.** Antimony and potassium tartrate.

tar·tar'ic ac'id (tahr·tar'ick, tahr·tahr'ick). $HOOC.CHOH.CHOH.COOH$. White, crystalline powder; odorless, of acid taste, soluble in water. Also called *dextrotartaric acid.*

tar'tra·zine (tahr'truh·zeen, ·zin). $C_{16}H_9N_4O_9S_2Na_3$. Water-soluble yellow color suitable for use in foods, drugs, and cosmetics.

tar·tron'ic ac'id. $COOH.CHOH.COOH$. Hydroxymalonic acid, a product of oxidation of dextrose and several other substances.

taste. A sensation produced by stimulation of special sense organs in the tongue and pharynx by sweet, sour, bitter, or salty substances.

taste blind'ness. Inability to recognize the acid, bitter, salty, or sweet flavor of substances, readily detected by others; especially the inability to detect the bitter flavor of phenylthiocarbamide. Syn., *ageusia.*

tat·too'ing. The production of permanent colors in the skin by the introduction of foreign substances, vegetable or mineral, directly into the corium. **electrolytic t.** The treatment of skin diseases by introducing the negative pole of a galvanic current into the lesions. Drugs may be driven into the skin to treat certain diseases.

tau'rine (taw'reen, ·rin). Aminoethanesulfonic acid, $NH_2.CH_2.CH_2.SO_3.OH$. Occurs in bile combined with the cholic acids. White or yellowish crystals.

tau'ro-, taur-. A combining form meaning *bull.*

tau"ro·cho'lic ac'id (taw"ro·ko'-lick, ·kol'ick). $C_{26}H_{45}NSO_7$. An acid resulting from the conjugation of cholic acid with taurine and found in bile.

tau·tom'er·ism. The property of existing in a state of equilibrium between two isomeric forms and capable of reacting as either one.

tax'is. 1. A manipulation of an organ whereby it is brought into normal position; specifically, the reduction of a hernia by manual methods. 2. The involuntary response of an organism involving change of place toward (**positive taxis**) or away from (**negative taxis**) stimulus. Also see *tropism*.

-tax'is. A combining form denoting *involuntary movement in response to a stimulus*, as in chemo*taxis*, rheo*taxis*. See also *-tropic*. **__taxy**, *n*.

tax'on (pl. *taxa*). Taxonomic group.

tax·on'o·my. The science of the classification of organisms. **—taxonom'ic**, *adj*.

Tax'us. A genus of cone-bearing trees, the yews.

Tb. Chemical symbol for terbium.

t. b. Tubercle bacillus, tuberculosis.

tbsp. Tablespoon.

Tc. Chemical symbol for technetium.

Te. 1. Chemical symbol for tellurium. 2. Abbreviation for tetanic contraction.

tea. 1. The leaves of *Camellia sinensis* (*Thea sinensis*), family Theaceae. Tea contains 1–5% of caffeine, tannin, and a fragrant volatile oil. 2. An infusion or decoction prepared from the leaves of *C. sinensis*. 3. Any vegetable infusion or decoction used as a beverage.

TEAB. Tetraethylammonium bromide. See *tetraethylammonium*.

tea'ber"ry. See *gaultheria*.

teach'ers' nodes. Singer's nodes. White nodules appearing on the vocal folds of persons who use their voices excessively.

tears. 1. The secretion of the lacrimal gland. 2. Hardened lumps, or drops, of any resinous or gummy drug. **crocodile t.** A profuse, paroxysmal flow of tears observed in certain patients with facial paralysis, when they taste food. Also called *gustolacrimal reflex*.

tease. Tear or gently separate into its component parts, by the use of needles, a tissue which it is desired to examine microscopically.

tea'spoon". A spoon assumed to hold about 4 ml. or 1 fluidrachm but commonly holding about 5 ml. Abbreviated, tsp.

teat. A nipple.

tech·ne'ti·um (teck·nee'shee·um). Tc. Element number 43, prepared in 1937 by neutron or deuteron bombardment of molybdenum and later found among the fission products of uranium. Formerly called masurium, *q.v.*

tech·nic' (teck·neek'). The method of procedure in operations or manipulations of any kind.

tech·ni'cian. A person trained and expert in the technical details of certain medical fields, as bacteriology, pathology, roentgenology.

tech·nique' (tek·neek'). Same as *technic*.

tec"to·ceph'a·ly. The condition of having a roof-shaped skull.

te'di·ous. Unduly protracted, as tedious labor.

teel oil. Sesame oil.

teeth'ing. The eruption of the deciduous teeth; the process of dentition.

teg'men. A cover.

teg·men'tum (pl. *tegmenta*). A covering; specifically, the dorsal portion of the midbrain, exclusive of the corpora quadrigemina and the central gray substance. **—tegmental**, *adj*.

tegosept. Trade-mark for a brand of preservatives, consisting of esters of parahydroxybenzoic acid.

tei·chop'si·a (tye·kop'see·uh). Temporary amblyopia, with subjective visual images.

te'la (pl. *telae*). A web or tissue. **t. adiposa.** Adipose tissue. **t. choroidea.** The membranous roof of the third and fourth ventricles of the brain including the choroid plexuses. **t. subcutanea.** The subcutaneous connective tissue; the superficial fascia. **t. submucosa.** The layer of connective tissue which lies between a mucous membrane and subjacent tissues. Also called *tunica submucosa*.

tel·al'gi·a. Referred pain.

tel·an"gi·ec·ta'sis,　tel·an"gi·ec·ta'si·a (tel·an"jee·eck·tay'zhuh, ·shuh). Dilatation of groups of capillaries. They form elevated, dark red, wartlike spots, varying in size from 1 to 7 mm. **—telangiectat'ic**, *adj*. **hereditary hemorrhagic t.** A hereditary disease characterized by a tendency to hemorrhages of capillary origin.

tel·an"gi·i'tis. Inflammation of capillaries.

tel·an"gi·o'ma. A tumor composed of dilated capillaries.

tel·an"gi·o'sis. Disease of minute blood vessels.

tel"e·car'di·o·phone". An apparatus amplifying heart sounds.

tel"e·ki·ne'sis (tel"eh·ki·nee'sis, ·kigh·nee'sis). The power claimed by some people of causing inanimate objects to move without touching them.

tel"e·lec"tro·car'di·o·gram". An electrocardiogram taken in a laboratory, the galvanometer being connected by a wire with the patient who is elsewhere.

tel"e·lec"tro·ther"a·peu'tics (tel"eh·leck"tro·theer"uh·pew'ticks)

The treatment of hysterical paralysis by a series of electric discharges near the patient without actual contact.

tel″en·ceph'a·lon. The anterior subdivision of the primary forebrain that develops into olfactory lobes, cerebral cortex, and corpora striata. Syn., endbrain. **–telencephal'ic,** adj.

te″le·ol'o·gy (tee″lee·ol'o·jee). The doctrine that explanations of phenomena are to be sought in terms of final causes, purpose, or design in nature. **–teleolog'ic,** adj.

tel″e·op'si·a. A disorder in visual perception of space characterized by an excess of depth, or the illusion that close objects are far away.

tel″e·o·roent'gen·o·gram″ (tel″ee·o·rent'ghin·o·gram″, tee″lee·o·). A radiograph, usually of the heart, made at a distance of about 6 feet, to avoid distortion.

tel″e·o·ther″a·peu'tics (tel″ee·o·therr″uh·pew'ticks, tee″lee·o·). Suggestive therapeutics.

te·lep'a·thist. One who is versed in telepathy.

te·lep'a·thy. The action, real or supposed, of one mind upon another when the two persons are separated by a considerable distance and without the use of any sense perception; thought transference.

tel″e·ra″di·og'ra·phy. Radiography with the tube about 6 feet from the body to avoid distortion.

tel″e·re·cep'tors. Sense organs capable of receiving a stimulus from a distance, as the eyes, ears, and nose.

tel″e·ther'a·py. Absent treatment.

tel·lu'ri·um. Te = 127.61. A non-metallic element of bluish white color, obtained chiefly as a by-product in the refining of copper and lead.

tel'o·phase (tel'o·faze). 1. The final stage of mitosis in which the chromosomes reorganize to form an interstage nucleus. 2. The final phase of any process.

Tel″o·spo·rid'i·a. A subclass of Sporozoa, characterized by spore formation after the sporozoon has completed its growth. The orders included are Gregarinida, Coccidia, and Haemosporidia.

TEM (tee·ee·em). Abbreviation for triethylene melamine.

tem'per. Make metals hard and elastic by heating them and then suddenly cooling them.

tem'per·a·ment. In constitutional medicine, the mixture of motivational drives in a personality. The level of personality just above physiologic function and just below acquired attitudes and beliefs. The quantitative patterning of viscerotonia, somatotonia, and cerebrotonia in a personality.

tem'per·ate. Moderate; without excess.

tem'per·a·ture. The degree of intensity of heat of a body, especially as measured by the scale of a thermometer. Abbreviated, T. **absolute t.** That reckoned from the absolute zero, estimated at −273° C. **basal t.** That of the healthy body, usually obtained in the fasting stage and before arising after at least eight hours of relaxed sleep; used especially to detect ovulation. **body t.** The temperature of the body. Elevation above normal constitutes fever. **critical t.** The temperature at which a gas can, by pressure, be reduced to a liquid. **mean t.** The average temperature for a given period of time. **normal t.** The temperature of the body in health (37° C. or 98.6° F.). **optimum t.** That most favorable for cultivating microorganisms.

tem'ple. The portion of the head anterior to the ear and above the zygomatic arch.

tem'po·ral. 1. Pertaining to the temple, as the temporal bone, the temporal artery. See Tables of Arteries, of Bones, and of Muscles in the Appendix. 2. Pertaining to time.

tem'po·rar″y. Not permanent.

tem'po·ro-. A combining form denoting pertaining to the temple or to the temporal lobe of the cerebral hemisphere.

tem″po·ro·man·dib'u·lar. Pertaining to the temporal bone and the mandible, used specifically for a ligament of the mandibular joint.

te·na'cious. 1. Tough. 2. Cohesive.

te·nac'u·lum. A hook-shaped instrument for seizing and holding parts, approximating incised edges, etc., during surgical operations.

ten'der·ness. The condition of abnormal sensitiveness to touch; soreness.

ten'di·no·plas″ty. Plastic surgery of tendons. Also see tenoplasty. **–tendinoplas'tic,** adj.

ten'di·nous. Pertaining to, or having the nature of, tendon.

ten'do (pl. tendines). A tendon. **t. achillis.** The Achilles tendon or common tendon of the gastrocnemius and soleus muscles inserted into the heel. Also called tendo calcaneus.

ten·dol'y·sis, ten″do·ly'sis. The freeing of adhesions about a tendon.

ten″do·mn'oin, ten″do·mu'coid. A mucoid found in tendons.

ten'don. A band of dense fibrous tissue forming the termination of a muscle and attaching the latter to a bone. **–tendinous,** adj. **patellar t.** See patellar ligament.

ten″do·vag″i·ni'tis (·vadj″i·nigh'tis). Inflammation of a tendon and its sheath; tenosynovitis.

te·nec'to·my. 1. Excision of a lesion, as a ganglion or xanthoma, of a tendon or tendon sheath. 2. Tenoplasty.

te·nes'mus (tuh-nez'mus, tuh-ness'-mus). A straining, especially the painful straining to empty the bowels or bladder without the evacuation of feces or urine. **—tenesmic,** *adj.*

teni-. For words beginning with *teni-* not found here, see under *taeni-*.

ten'nis arm, ten'nis el'bow. An acute or chronic synovitis of the radiohumeral articulation common in tennis players. Radiohumeral bursitis.

ten'o-, ten-. A combining form meaning *pertaining to a tendon*.

ten''o·de'sis. Fixation of a tendon, as to a bone.

ten''o·dyn'i·a (ten''o·din'ee·uh, ·dye'nee·uh). Pain in a tendon.

ten''o·fi'bril. A small, delicate fibril connecting one epithelial cell with another; a tonofibril.

ten''o·my·ot'o·my (ten''o·migh·ot'-o·mee). *In ophthalmology,* a procedure for the treatment of squint, devised to enfeeble the action of one of the rectus muscles by incising portions of its tendon near the sclerotic insertion.

Tenon, Jacobus René [*French anatomist and surgeon,* 1724–1816]. Instrumental in bringing about hospital reform in eighteenth century Paris. See also Tenon's *capsule*.

ten''o·nec'to·my. Excision of a portion of a tendon.

ten''on·i'tis. Inflammation of a tendon sheath.

ten''o·nom'e·ter. An instrument for measuring the tension of the eyeball.

te·non''to·my'o·plas''ty. Reparative surgery involving both tendon and muscle; used particularly for hernia.

te·non''to·my·ot'o·my (ti·non''to·migh·ot'o·mee). Surgical division of tendons and muscles.

ten'o·phyte. A bony or cartilaginous growth on a tendon.

ten'o·plas''ty. Reparative or plastic surgery of a tendon. **—tenoplas'tic,** *adj.*

ten·or'rha·phy. The uniting of a divided tendon by sutures.

ten''os·to'sis. Ossification of a tendon.

ten''o·syn''o·vec'to·my (ten''o·sin''o·veck'to·mee, ·sigh''no·). Excision of a tendon sheath.

ten''o·syn''o·vi'tis (·sin''o·vy'tis, ·sigh''no·). Inflammation of a tendon and its sheath. **t. crepitans.** That form associated with cracking sounds during muscular activity.

ten'o·tome. A small, narrow-bladed knife mounted on a slender handle; a tenotomy knife.

te·not'o·my. The operation of cutting a tendon.

ten''o·vag''i·ni'tis (ten''o·vadj''i-nigh'tis). Inflammation of the sheath of a tendon.

ten''si·om'e·ter. An apparatus for measuring tension, as in the eyeball or blood vessels.

ten'sion. 1. The act of stretching; the state of being stretched or strained. 2. *In electricity,* the power of overcoming resistance. 3. Internal conflict of the psyche. Abbreviated, T. **arterial t.** The strain in the arterial walls at the height of the pulse wave. **interfacial t.** A measure of the work which must be done in increasing the interface between two phases by a given unit of surface. When one of the phases is gas, then the interfacial tension is commonly called the surface tension. **intraocular t.** The tension of the coats of the eyeball, produced by the pressure of the intraocular fluid. It may be estimated by means of an instrument called a tonometer, or by palpation with the fingers. **surface t.** The force operating at surfaces (commonly at the interface of a liquid and a gas) which is due to the unequal molecular attraction on either side of the molecules at the surface. The contractile force in the surface of a liquid by virtue of which the surface tends to shrink and assume the smallest area possible. Abbreviated, S.T.

ten'sor. A muscle that serves to make a part tense, as the tensor tympani. See Table of Muscles in the Appendix.

tent. 1. A plug or stuffing of soft material, such as gauze, sponge, or felt, that increases in volume by wetting; it is used for dilating an orifice or canal and for keeping a wound or sinus open. Except in gynecologic practice, the term in its strictest sense has almost disappeared from medical literature. 2. A portable shelter or covering. **laminaria t.** A cone-shaped plug made from *Laminaria digitata,* a seaweed. When wet, the plug dilates. **oxygen t.** An airtight chamber, enclosing the patient's head and shoulders, in which the oxygen content of the atmosphere can be maintained at a higher than normal level.

ten'ta·tive. Empirical; experimental.

tenth'me''ter. One ten-millionth of a millimeter, or one angstrom.

ten·tig'i·nous (ten·tidj'i·nus). Characterized by insane lust.

ten·to'ri·um (pl. *tentoria*). A partition of dura mater, roofing over the posterior cranial fossa, separating the cerebellum from the cerebral hemispheres. Also called *t. cerebelli.* **—tentorial,** *adj.*

ten'u·ate. Make thin.

ten'u·ous. Thin; minute.

teph''ro·my''e·li'tis. Inflammation of the gray matter of the spinal cord; poliomyelitis.

tep'id. About blood heat.

TEPP. Tetraethylpyrophosphate.

ter- (tur-). A combining form meaning *hree* or threefold.

er'a·tism. A congenital anomaly or monstrosity.

er"a·tol'o·gy. The science of malformations and monstrosities. —**teratolog'ic,** *adj.;* **teratologist,** *n.*

er"a·to'ma. A true tumor or neoplasm composed of multiple tissues, as teeth, hair, or other material not found in the part wherein it grows, and resulting from an embryonic misplacement of tissue or from the enclosure of parts of a rudimentary fetus. —**teratom'atous,** *adj.*

er"a·to·pho'bi·a. 1. Morbid fear of monsters or of deformed people. 2. Morbid dread, on the part of a pregnant woman, of giving birth to a monstrosity.

er"a·to'sis. 1. A congenital deformity. 2. Teratism.

er'bi·um. Tb = 158.93. A rare metallic element.

erchlorethylene. Tetrachloroethylene.

e're. Rub. Used in writing prescriptions.

er'e·bene. A mixture of hydrocarbons, chiefly dipentene and terpinene, prepared by the action of sulfuric acid on turpentine oil followed by steam distillation. A pale yellow liquid.

er"e·bin'thi·nate. Containing or resembling turpentine.

e"re·bra·che'sis (terr″i·bra·kee′-sis, teer″i·). The operation of shortening the round ligament of the uterus.

er'es (terr′eex) (pl. *teretes*). 1. Cylindrical, as the ligamentum teres. 2. A muscle having a cylindrical shape, as teres major, teres minor. See Table of Muscles in the Appendix.

eridax. Trade-mark for iophenoxic acid.

er in die. Three times a day; abbreviated, t.i.d.

erm. 1. A limit; the time during which anything lasts. 2. The time of expected delivery.

er'mi·nal. 1. Pertaining to the end; placed at or forming the end. 2. The pole of a battery or other electric source, or the end of the conductors or wires connected thereto.

er"mi·na'tion. Cessation; the end or ending.

er"mi·nol'o·gy. Nomenclature; a system of technical names or terms.

erms. The menses.

er'na·ry. Of chemical compounds, made up of three elements or radicals.

eropterin. A trade-mark for sodium pteroyltriglutamate, a derivative of folic (pteroylglutamic) acid.

erpane. Eucalyptol.

er'pene. Any one of the hydrocarbons of the general formula, $C_{10}H_{16}$ or $(C_5H_8)_2$, occurring in volatile oils and other plant sources. **Sesquiterpenes** are represented by the formula $C_{15}H_{24}$ or $(C_5H_8)_3$, while **polyterpenes** have the general formula $(C_5H_8)_n$, where n is greater than 3.

ter'pen·ism. Poisoning by terpene from internal use or inhalation.

ter'pi·lene di"hy·dro·chlo'ride (dye″high·dro·klor′ide). Eucalyptol, *q.v.*

ter·pin'e·ol. $C_{10}H_{17}OH$. A colorless, viscous liquid of lilac odor, occurring in many volatile oils and prepared from terpin hydrate; used in perfumes.

ter'pin hy'drate. $C_{10}H_{20}O_2.H_2O$. Colorless crystals prepared by the action of nitric acid on turpentine oil in the presence of alcohol. Soluble in water. An expectorant.

ter'pin·ol. An oily liquid, chiefly $C_{10}H_{16}$ and $C_{10}H_{18}O$, obtained by the action of dilute mineral acids on terpin hydrate.

ter'ra (pl. *terrae*). Earth. **t. alba.** Kaolin. **t. sigillata.** Sealed earth; kaolin. In medieval Europe, earth guaranteed to be genuine through the use of a seal.

terramycin. Trade-mark for oxytetracycline.

ter'tian. Recurring every other day, as tertian fever.

ter'ti·ar''y al'co·hol. An alcohol which contains the trivalent group COH.

ter·tip'a·ra. A woman who has borne three children.

ter·va'lence. See *trivalence.*

test. 1. A trial or examination. 2. A procedure to identify a constituent, to detect changes of a function, or to establish the true nature of a condition. 3. The reagent for producing a special reaction. **Abridged A. O. color vision t.** (Abridged version of American Optical Company's Charts.) A group of pseudo-isochromatic plates designed to detect color-vision deficiency. **acrolein t.** (for glycerol and fats). The suspected substance is heated with an equal quantity of potassium bisulfate. If glycerol or fats are present, acrolein is given off and is recognized by its characteristic irritating odor. **Addis and Shevky's t.** (for kidney function). A concentration test based upon the specific gravity of urine passed during the last 12 hours of a 24-hour period of fluid deprivation. **agglutination t.** (a) A test in which an agglomeration or clumping of particles produces masses which may be seen either with the unaided eye (**macroscopic agglutination test**) or with the aid of a microscope (**microscopic agglutination test**). The test also may be used for the identification of bacteria. (b) A test for the presence of specific antibodies (agglutinins) in the blood serum of infected individuals which will produce clumping of the specific bacteria causing the infection. **allergy t.** Any test used to demonstrate the presence of allergy, such as the conjunctival test, nasal test, patch test, or skin test. **alpha t.** A series of eight types of intelligence tests designed for group application and for rapid scoring; first used by the U. S. Army in World War I. **aptitude t.** A psychologic test given to determine a student's aptitude or ability for medicine or other pursuits. Also see Stanford scientific aptitude *t.* **Aschheim-Zondek t.** (*for pregnancy*). Urine from a woman is injected subcutaneously into immature white mice. If the woman is pregnant the ovaries of the mice will be enlarged, hyperemic, and hemorrhagic, and will show maturation of the ovarian follicles. **association t.** *In psychoanalysis,* the procedure used in the diagnosis of certain abnormal mental states; sometimes used in crime detection. The test is oral and consists of presenting the patient with a predetermined series of words and noting his word associations and his reaction time. **Babcock-Levy t.** An examination designed to measure intellectual deterioration by testing vocabulary, general information, symbol substitution, and the copying of designs with respect to correctness, speed, and accuracy; useful in organic cerebral deteriorative conditions. **Bárány's pointing t.** The patient points with finger or toe at a fixed object alternately with eyes open and closed. A constant error in pointing with the eyes closed in the presence of vertigo indicates peripheral labyrinthine disease or an intracranial lesion. **Benedict's t.** (*for glucose*). Eight drops of urine are added to 5 cc. of Benedict's qualitative sugar reagent (sodium citrate, copper sulfate, sodium carbonate, distilled water). Boil vigorously for 3 minutes. A green, yellow, or red precipitate indicates glucose. **benzidine t.** (*for blood*). To 3 cc. of a saturated solution of benzidine in glacial acetic acid add 1 cc. of 3% hydrogen peroxide and 1 cc. of the unknown. A blue or green color indicates blood. **Bernreuter personality inventory.** A test designed to measure neurotic tendency, self-sufficiency, introversion, dominance, sociability, and confidence. **beta t.** An intelligence test used, instead of the alpha test, for illiterates; carried out with signs and pictures. **Binet's t.** A method of estimating the intellectual capacity or measuring intelligence and expressing it as an intelligence quotient (I.Q.). **bitterling t.** (*for pregnancy*). A test made by placing the bitterling (a small carplike fish of Japan) in water to which some of the woman's urine has been added. If pregnancy is present, there is an outgrowth of the oviduct from the body of the fish. **blind t.** A comparison of two methods of treatment in which both the patient and the observer are ignorant of the identity until the results have been recorded. **bone conduction t.** The testing of hearing threshold by placing a tuning fork or audiometer oscillator directly against the mastoid process. The **absolute bone conduction test** is a similar test done when the external auditory meatus is blocked by any of several means. **Brown personality inventory.** A psychologic test designed for the detection of psychoneurotic problem children. **caloric t.** In the normal individual, nystagmus is produced by irrigating the external ear canal with hot (110° 120° F.) or cold (68° F.) water. When the vestibular nerve or labyrinth is destroyed, no nystagmus is produced upon testing the diseased side. **capillary resistance t.** A test of the tendency for blood capillaries to break down and produce petechial hemorrhages; usually performed by examining the skin of the forearm after the arm veins have been occluded for five minutes. **Cattell infant intelligence scale.** A modification of the revised Stanford-Binet test adapted for infants from 3–30 months of age. **Chi square t.** A test used to determine the probability that the difference between an actual and a theoretical distribution or between two or more distributions is the result of chance alone. **clearance t.** (*For kidney function*). A test of the excretory efficiency of the kidneys based upon the amount of blood cleared of a substance in 1 minute as determined by the ratio of the substance in the blood to the amount excreted in the urine during a fixed time. (*For liver function.*) A test based on the ability of the liver to remove a substance from the blood. **cold agglutination t.** (*for primary atypical pneumonia*). A test for the detection of the autohemagglutinins or so-called cold agglutinins which may occur in high titer in the serums of individuals with primary atypical pneumonia. **color vision t.** See Abridged A. O. color vision *t.* **complement-fixation t.** A test based on the complement-fixation reaction in which antigen uniting with its antibody combines with the complement and thus inactivates or fixes it. **concentration t.** (*for kidney function*). A test of kidney function based upon their normal ability concentrate or dilute urine. See Addis and Shevky's *t*. **conglutination t.** An antigen-antibody reaction in which a conglutinin is added. **Congo red t.** *(for amyloidosis)*. Congo red is injected intravenously. In normal persons, 30% of the dye disappears from the blood within an hour, but in amyloid disease from 40 to 100% disappears. **conjunctival t.** A test for allergy in which the antigen is instilled into the conjunctival sac. A positive test consists of injection of the conjunctival vessels with itching and lacrimation. **Dick t.** *(for susceptibility or immunity to scarlet fever)*. An immunologic skin test in which development of a local area of redness of the skin 18 to 24 hours after the intracutaneous injection of the filtrate of a culture of specific hemolytic streptococcus indicates susceptibility, and the absence of redness indicates immunity, to scarlet fever. **Eagle t.** (a) A complement-fixation test for syphilis. (b) A flocculation test for syphilis. **erythrocyte sedimentation t.** When citrated or oxalated blood is allowed to stand in a column, the erythrocytes settle to the bottom. The rate of this sedimentation varies in different pathologic conditions and may be determined by any of the different methods, such as Cutler's, Westergren's, Smith's, Wintrobe's, etc. **Exton's t.** *(for albumin)*. Equal volumes of clear urine and Exton's reagent (sodium sulfate, sulfosalicylic acid, bromphenol blue, water) are mixed in a test tube. Cloudiness appearing upon heating indicates albumin. **Fehling's t.** *(for glucose)*. Equal volumes of copper sulfate solution and alkaline tartrate solution are mixed. Equal volumes of this mixture (Fehling's solution) and urine are boiled. In the presence of glucose the solution turns green, yellow, or red depending on the amount present. **flicker fusion t.** A test of the minimal frequency of standard flashes of light which will be seen as a steady illumination; used as a test for fatigue and for tolerance to anoxia. Also used for diagnosing high blood pressure and some forms of heart disease, such as angina pectoris. **flocculation t.** A test in which the antibody reacts directly with the antigen to produce flocculi rather than to form a combination for the inactivation of complement as in a complement-fixation test. **Friedman t.** *(for pregnancy)*. The intravenous injection of urine from a pregnant woman into a female rabbit will bring about the formation of corpora hemorrhagica and corpora lutea in the ovaries of the rabbit. **galactose tolerance t.** *(for liver function)*. A test of the glycogenic function of the liver, performed by administering 40 Gm. of galactose to a fasting individual. The elimination of more than 3 Gm. of galactose over a 5-hour period indicates hepatic dysfunction. **Gesell developmental schedule.** A test of the mental growth of the preschool child which includes motor development, adaptive behavior, language development, and personal-social behavior. **glucose tolerance t.** *(for liver function)*. A test based on the ability of the liver to convert glucose to glycogen. It is useful in measuring the approximate severity of diabetes mellitus. **guaiac t.** *(for blood)*. An acetic acid or alcoholic solution of guaiac resin and hydrogen peroxide is mixed with the unknown. The development of a blue color is a positive test. **Haines's t.** A copper reduction test used for glucose in the urine. **hearing t.** See bone conduction *t.*, Rinne's *t.*, Weber's *t.* **heat and acid t.** *(for protein)*. Urine is boiled in a test tube for 1 or 2 minutes and then 3 to 5 drops of 5% acetic acid are added. A white precipitate indicates protein. **Heller's t.** *(for albumin)*. Stratify clear urine over concentrated nitric acid in a test tube. A white zone at the junction of the fluids indicates albumin. **hemolysin t.** One used for identification of streptococci performed by incubating the bacteria with blood agar and then noting the type of hemolysis produced. **hippuric acid t.** *(for liver function)*. A test based upon the ability of the liver to synthesize glycine and to conjugate it with benzoic acid to form hippuric acid. Given 6 Gm. of sodium benzoate, in 4 hours a normal person will eliminate 3 or more Gm. of hippuric acid in the urine, whereas a person with liver dysfunction will eliminate less than 3 Gm. **histamine t.** (a) The subcutaneous injection of histamine stimulates the gastric secretion of hydrochloric acid. (b) The precipitation of an attack of histaminic cephalalgia (vasomotor headache) by the injection of histamine done for purposes of diagnosis. **icterus index t.** A colorimetric test in which blood serum is compared with a standard solution of sodium dichromate. **insulin tolerance t.** *(for liver function)*. A test based upon the comparison of depression of blood sugar levels and rapidity of recovery from relative hypoglycemia following a standard intravenous dose of insulin as compared to the response of normal individuals. **intelligence t.** See alpha *t.*, Babcock-Levy *t.*, beta *t.*, Binet's *t.*, Cattell infant intelligence scale (under *test*), Gesell developmental schedule (under *test*), Kent mental *t.*, Minnesota preschool scale (under *test*), Stanford-Binet *t.*,

Wechsler-Bellevue intelligence scale (under *test*). **iodine t.** (*for bile pigments*). Tincture of iodine is slowly poured into urine. The development of a greenish blue color indicates bile pigments. **iodine t.** (*for starch*). A potassium iodide solution of iodine reacts with starch to produce a blue color. **Kent mental t.** An oral test for intelligence consisting of 25 questions for emergency use in clinics. **Kolmer's t.** (a) A complement-fixation test for syphilis. (b) A complement-fixation test for bacterial, spirochetal, viral, protozoan, or metazoan diseases. **levulose tolerance t.** (*for liver function*). A test based on the observation that the blood sugar level is normally unaffected by the oral administration of levulose, whereas it is increased in the presence of hepatic disease. **Marsh's t.** (*for arsenic or antimony*). Introduce the substance into a flask with dilute sulfuric acid and zinc. Light a jet, and permit it to impinge on cold porcelain, or heat the delivery tube, when a steel-white mirror of metallic arsenic is deposited. This may be distinguished from a similar deposit of antimony by the solubility of the arsenical mirror in potassium hypochlorite. **medicolegal tests for blood.** (a) Microscopical identification of the erythrocytes, (b) spectroscopic identification of blood solutions, (c) the guaiac or benzidine reaction, (d) preparation of hemin crystals, and (e) precipitin and other immunologic tests. **methylene blue t.** (*for renal permeability*). An injected solution of methylene blue normally appears in the urine in about 30 minutes. A longer interval indicates impaired renal permeability. Also called *Achard-Castaigne method*. **Minnesota multiphasic personality inventory.** A psychologic test designed to provide, in a single interview, scores on all the more important traits of personality, consisting of over 500 questions which the subject places into three categories as they apply to him. Abbreviated, MPI. **Minnesota preschool scale.** A test for measuring the learning ability of children from 18 months to 6 years of age. Being both verbal and nonverbal, it is particularly valuable in differentiating between the specific kinds of intellectual abilities. **patch t.** An allergy test in which material is applied to an intact skin surface in order to demonstrate tissue sensitivity. **paternity t.** The determination of the blood groups of an identified mother, an identified child, and a putative father in order to determine hereditary blood characters and to establish nonpaternity. **pregnancy t.** See Aschheim-Zondek *t.*,

bitterling *t.*, Friedman *t.*, prostigmine *t.* **prostigmine t.** (*for pregnancy*). The failure of injected prostigmine to bring about menstrual bleeding in the presence of amenorrhea is indicative of pregnancy. **psychologic t.** A planned situation in which an individual's behavior can be characterized by a numerical value or score. Also see aptitude *t.*, intelligence *t.* **psychomotor t.** An apparatus test, in contrast to a paper and pencil test, usually necessitating some form of muscular coördination and speed of reaction and often requiring certain perceptual abilities. **Purdy's t.** (*for albumin*). To a test tube two-thirds full of urine, add one-sixth of its volume of a saturated solution of sodium chloride and 5 to 10 drops of 50% acetic acid. Mix, boil the upper portion, and watch for white cloud. **Queckenstedt's t.** Pressure on the jugular veins causes a prompt rise in cerebrospinal fluid pressure. This is not seen in subarachnoid block or lateral sinus thrombosis. See also Queckenstedt's *sign*. **Rh testing.** Examination of blood for the Rh factor, using either anti-Rhesus serum or anti-Rh_0 serum alone. **Rinne's t.** A hearing test which compares the duration of bone conduction with that of air conduction. Normally air conduction is longer than bone conduction (Rinne positive; symbol, +R). Alteration in this relationship (Rinne negative; symbol, −R) indicates a lesion of the sound-conducting apparatus. **Roberts' t.** (*for albumin*). Overlay urine upon Roberts' reagent (saturated solution of magnesium sulfate and concentrated nitric acid). A white ring at the zone of contact indicates albumin. **Rorschach t.** A psychologic test in which the subject describes what he sees on a series of 10 standard ink blots. The subject's responses indicate personality patterns, special interests, general intelligence, deviations of affect, and neurotic or psychotic tendencies. **Rubin t.** (*for tubal patency*). One in which the patency or occlusion of the uterine tubes is demonstrated by insufflating them with air or gas. Also called *tubal insufflation*. **scarlet fever t.** See Dick *t.*, Schultz-Charlton blanching *t.* **Schick t.** (*for immunity to diphtheria*). An immunologic skin test performed by the intracutaneous injection of an amount of diluted diphtheria toxin equal to one-fiftieth of the minimal lethal dose. A positive reaction is interpreted on the fifth to seventh day. It consists of local erythema with edema, and indicates the lack of immunity. **Schultz-Charlton blanching t.** An immunologic skin test or aid in the diagnosis of scarlet fever performed by the intracutaneous injection of convalescent scarlet fever serum. A positive reaction which occurs in scarlet fever consists of blanching of the rash in a zone surrounding the point of injection. **scratch t.** An allergic skin test performed by scratching the epidermis and then applying the allergen to the scratch. **skin t.** Any test depending upon the production of an inflammatory or irritative reaction in the skin, usually performed for immunologic or allergic purposes. **Snellen t.** One testing central vision in which the subject stands a certain distance from a standard chart and reads the letters on the chart. It is based upon the fact that objects may be seen by the normal eye when they subtend an angle of one minute. **Stanford-Binet t.** A modification of the original Binet intelligence test; considered the standard individual test for pre-adult levels. **Stanford scientific aptitude t.** A test to detect the traits which comprise an aptitude for a science. **Teichmann's t.** (*for blood*). A crystal of sodium chloride and glacial acetic acid are added to the suspected liquid under a cover glass and the whole is heated without boiling and then cooled. The appearance of rhombic crystals of hemin indicates blood. **thematic apperception t.** A psychologic test consisting of 20 cards designed to reveal to the trained interpreter some of the dominant drives, emotions, sentiments, complexes, and conflicts of a personality. **therapeutic t.** A test in which the response to specific therapy is used to aid in the establishment of a diagnosis, such as liver extract in pernicious anemia and Lugol's solution in hyperthyroidism. **tuberculin t.** The introduction of measured quantities of tuberculin into superficial tissues of the body to establish the presence or absence of infection by the tubercle bacillus. A positive tuberculin reaction which may consist of erythema, edema, or necrosis indicates infection. Also see Vollmer patch *t.*, von Pirquet *t.* **two glass t.** A gross test for gonorrhea, in which urine is passed into two separate glasses. If that in the second glass is cloudy as well as that in the first, the posterior as well as the anterior urethra is involved. **urea clearance t.** (*for kidney function*). The excretory efficiency of the kidneys is tested by the amount of blood cleared of urea in 1 minute as determined by the ratio of the blood urea to the amount of urea excreted in urine during a fixed time. **van den Bergh's t.** (*The direct test.*) Diluted serum is added to diazo reagent. A bluish violet color becoming maximal in 10 to 30 seconds is an *immediate direct reaction*

supposedly indicating uncombined bilirubin and therefore the presence of obstructive jaundice. A red color beginning after 1 to 15 minutes and gradually turning to violet is a *delayed direct reaction*, indicating impaired liver function. A red color appearing at once and changing to violet is a biphasic direct reaction. (*The indirect test.*) Alcohol is added to serum which is then centrifuged. The diazo reagent is added to the supernatant fluid. An immediate violet-red color supposedly indicates bilirubin combined with protein and signifies a hemolytic jaundice. The tests are now used as a modification in which diazotized serum or plasma is compared with a standard solution of diazotized bilirubin. **Vollmer patch t.** A tuberculin test in which gauze saturated with tuberculin is applied to an intact skin surface under adhesive plaster. **von Pirquet t.** A tuberculin test in which the substance is applied to a superficial abrasion of the skin. **Wassermann's t.** A complement-fixation test for syphilis now used only as a modification of the original test. **Weber's t.** A hearing test in which the vibrations from a tuning fork placed on the forehead of a normal person are referred to the midline and heard equally in both ears. In unilateral middle-ear deafness, the sound is heard in the diseased ear. In deafness due to disease of the auditory nerve on one side, it is heard better in the normal ear. **Wechsler-Bellevue intelligence scale.** A verbal and performance test of information, comprehension, arithmetical reasoning, digit memory, similarities, configurational grasp, visual completion, object assembly, and vocabulary. **Widal t.** (*for typhoid fever*). An agglutination test for typhoid fever, using a living agglutinable culture of the typhoid bacillus as an antigen. The test is now performed by using H (formalized) and O (alcoholic) antigens.

tes′tis (pl. *testes*). One of the pair of male reproductive glands, after sexual maturity the source of the spermatozoa; a male gonad. **undescended t.** The condition in which a testis remains either in the pelvis or in the inguinal canal.

test meal. A specified quantity and type of food which, at a certain interval after ingestion, is removed from the stomach by means of a tube; the contents are studied chemically to ascertain the function of the stomach. **tes·tos′te·rone.** $C_{19}H_{28}O_2$. Δ⁴-Androstene-17(a)-ol-3-one. An androgenic hormone isolated first from the testis of the bull; also obtained by synthesis. **tet″a·nig′e·nous** (tet″uh·nidj′i-nus). Causing tetanus or tetanic spasms.

tet″a·nil′la. A mild form of tetanus.

tet′a·nism. A more or less continuous hypertonicity of muscle.

tet″a·ni·za′tion. Production of tetanus or of tetanic spasms by disease or by an electric current.

tet′a·no-. A combining form denoting *relating to tetanus.*

tet′a·node. The quiescent interval in tetanus, between the tonic spasms.

tet′a·noid. A spastic condition producing symptoms like tetanus.

tet″a·nom′e·ter. An instrument for measuring tetanic spasms.

tet″a·no·mo′tor. An instrument for stimulating a nerve mechanically and producing tetanus of the supplied muscle.

tet″a·no·pho′bi·a. A morbid fear of tetanus.

tet″a·no·spas′min (tet″uh-no-spaz′min). A toxin produced by the tetanus bacillus to which tetanic convulsions are due.

tet′a·nus. 1. An infectious disease, usually fatal, characterized by tonic spasm of the voluntary muscles, an intense exaggeration of reflex activity, and convulsions. It is due to the toxin produced by the tetanus bacillus, *Clostridium tetani,* which enters through a wound. Since the tetanus bacillus can grow only in the absence of oxygen, the character of the wound is important, the most dangerous being puncture, penetrating, and crushing injuries. Commonly called lockjaw. 2. A tense, contracted state of a muscle, especially when caused experimentally. **ascending t.** A type in which the muscular spasms are first noted at the site of injury, then spread to the rest of the body. **cephalic t.** A special form of tetanus occasionally observed following head injuries, especially those in the neighborhood of the eyebrow; trismus and facial paralysis occur at the site of the injury; there are dysphagia and epileptiform seizures, an early appearance of the disease, and usually a rapid fatal termination. Also called *cerebral t., kopf t.* **chronic t.** That occurring when a latent infection in a healed wound is reactivated by reopening the wound. Also called *delayed t.* **descending t.** A type in which the muscle spasms are first noted about the jaw and throat, later spreading to the rest of the body. **hydrophobic t.** Tetanus characterized by violent spasm of the muscles of the throat. **idiopathic t.** Tetanus in which there is no history of injury. **localized t.** Tetanic spasm of a part. **puerperal t.** That following labor. **surgical t.** That following operation, from contamination by infected catgut

or feces. **t. antitoxin.** Antitoxin produced in man or animals by the injection of tetanus toxin or tetanus toxoid. **t. neonatorum.** That due to infection of the umbilical stump. **t. toxoid.** Inactivated tetanus toxin used to produce active immunity against the disease.

tet′a·ny. A disease characterized by intermittent, bilateral, painful, tonic spasms of the muscles, in children and young adults. It is due to an abnormal calcium metabolism. Occurs in deficiency of parathyroid secretion, alkalosis, vitamin-D deficiency, and after extirpation of the parathyroid glands. **gutturotetany.** A stammering due to tetanoid spasm of the laryngeal muscles. **parathyreoprival t.** Tetany following removal of the parathyroid glands. **thyreoprival t.** A form following removal of the thyroid gland when the parathyroids have also been removed.

te·tar″to·co′nid (te-tahr″to-ko′nid, ·kon′id). Distolingual or fourth cusp of a lower molar tooth.

tet·i″o·thal′ein so′di·um (tet-eye″o-thal′in, ·thal′ee-in, tee″tee-o-). Iodophthalein sodium.

tet′ra-, tetr-. A combining form meaning *four.*

tet″ra·ba′sic. Having four atoms of replaceable hydrogen.

tet″ra·bo′ric ac′id. $H_2B_4O_7$. An acid obtained from boric acid by heating. Syn., *pyroboric acid.*

tet″ra·bra′chi·us (tet″ruh-bray′kee-us). Having four arms.

tet″ra·bro″mo·phthal′ein so′di·um (tet″ruh-bro″mo-thal′in, ·thal′ee-in). Sulfobromophthalein sodium.

tet′ra·caine hy″dro·chlo′ride. The hydrochloride of the *p*-n-butylaminobenzoic ester of β-dimethylaminoethanol; very soluble in water. A powerful local anesthetic. See also *pantocaine, pontocaine hydrochloride.*

tet″ra·chei′rus (tet″ruh-kigh′rus). Having four hands.

tet″ra·chlo″ro·eth′ane. $CHCl_2$·$CHCl_2$. A highly toxic solvent for fats, oils, waxes, resins, etc.

tet″ra·chlo″ro·eth′yl·ene. Cl_2C:CCl_2. Clear, colorless liquid, of characteristic ethereal odor, used as an anthelmintic. Also called *ethylene tetrachloride, perchloroethylene.*

tet″ra·chlo″ro·meth′ane. Carbon tetrachloride.

tet″ra·cy′cline (tet″ra-sigh′kleen). 1. The generic name for a group of antibiotics, including chlortetracycline and oxytetracycline. 2. The four-ring skeleton structure common to the tetracycline group. 3. A potent, broad-spectrum antibiotic, prepared from chlortetracycline and also obtained naturally, active against many Gram-positive and Gram-negative pathogens. See *achromycin, panmycin*.

tet′rad. 1. An element having a valence of four. 2. A group of four chromatids which arises during meiosis from the pairing and splitting of maternal and paternal homologous chromosomes.

tet″ra·dac′tyl. Having four digits in each limb.

tet″ra·eth″yl·am·mo′ni·um. The univalent cation $(C_2H_5)_4N^+$, used in the form of the bromide or chloride salt, which on intramuscular or intravenous injection produces reversible blockade of impulses of both sympathetic and parasympathetic divisions of the autonomic nervous system. See *etamon chloride, TEAB*.

tet″ra·eth′yl lead. A poisonous liquid, $Pb(C_2H_5)_4$, used in gasoline as an antiknock agent.

tet″ra·eth″yl·py″ro·phos′-phate. $(C_2H_5)_4P_2O_7$. A colorless liquid, having the power to inhibit cholinesterase. Syn., *TEPP*.

tet″ra·eth″yl·thi′u·ram·di·sul′-fide. $(C_2H_5)_2N.CS.S.S.CS.N(C_2H_5)_2$. A white or slightly yellow powder, insoluble in water; useful in treating alcoholism. Available under trademarked name *antabuse*.

tet″ra·hy′dric. Containing four replaceable atoms of hydrogen.

tet″ra·hy″dro·can·nab′in·ol. Any one of a group of substances obtained from cannabis possessing to a great degree the activity of that drug.

tet″ra·i·o′do·eth′yl·ene (tet″ruh-ye-o″do-eth′il-een, tet″ruh-eye″o-lo·). See *diiodoform*.

tet″ra·i·o″do·phe″nol·phthal′-in (·fee″nole·thal′in, ·thal′ee·in). Iodophthalein.

tet″ra·i·o″do·phthal′ein so′di-um. Iodophthalein sodium.

tet″ra·i·o″do·thy′ro·nine (·thigh′ro·neen, ·thigh·ro′nin). Thyroxin.

tetralogy of Fallot. A quadruple malformation of the heart, consisting of a high ventricular septal defect, dextroposition of the aorta so that it overrides and receives blood from both ventricles, stenosis of the pulmonary artery or atresia of the pulmonary valve and hypertrophy of the right ventricle.

tet″ra·mas′ti·a. The condition of having four breasts.

tet″ra·ma′zi·a. The presence of four breasts.

tet″ra·meth″yl·ene·di·am′ine (tet″ruh·meth″il·een·dye·am′een, ·dye′-ah·meen). $NH_2(CH_2)_4NH_2$. Putrescine.

tet″ra·meth″yl·pu·tres′cine (·pew·tress′een, ·in). $C_8H_{20}N_2$. A poisonous base from putrescine.

tet″ra·ni′trol. Erythrityl tetranitrate.

tet″ra·nu′cle·o·tide. The name sometimes given to nucleic acid from yeast from the fact that it contains four constituent nucleotides.

tet″ra·oph·thal′mus, tet″roph·thal′mus. Having four eyes. See *diprosopus*.

tet″ra·pep′tide. A polypeptide composed of four amino-acid groups.

tet″ra·ple′gi·a. Paralysis of all four extremities. Also called *quadriplegia*.

tet′ra·pus. Having four feet.

tet″ra·sac′cha·ride (tet″ruh·sack′-uh·ride, ·rid). A polysaccharide hydrolyzable into four molecules of monosaccharide.

te·tras′ce·lus (teh·trass′i·lus). Having four legs.

tet″ra·sti·chi′a·sis (tet″ruh·sti-kigh′uh·sis). Arrangement of the eyelashes in four rows.

tet″ra·thi′o·nate. The bivalent ion S_4O_6—.

tet″ra·thi′o·nate re·duc′tion. The reduction of a tetrathionate compound; used in bacteriologic isolations.

tet″ra·tom′ic. 1. Containing four atoms. 2. Having four hydroxyl radicals.

tet″ra·vac′cine (tet″ruh·vack′-seen, ·sin). A polyvalent vaccine containing four different cultures, as one containing typhoid, paratyphoid A and B, and cholera.

tet″ra·va′lent (tet″ruh·vay′lunt, teh·trav′uh·lunt). See *quadrivalent*.

tet·relle′. An appliance for enabling a weakly infant to obtain milk from its mother. It consists of a nipple shield and two tubes; the mother sucks one of the latter, and the milk flows to the infant's mouth through the other. *Obs.*

tet′rose. A monosaccharide whose molecule contains only four atoms of carbon, as erythrose, $C_4H_8O_4$.

te·tro′tus. Having four ears. See *diprosopus*.

te·trox′ide, te·trox′id. A binary compound containing four atoms of oxygen.

tet′ryl. 1. See *butyl*. 2. Tetranitro-methylaniline, picrylmethyl-nitramine, $C_7H_5N_5O_8$. Yellow powder used as explosive and as pH indicator. Also called *nitramine*.

tet′ter. A common term for various skin eruptions, particularly herpes, eczema, and psoriasis.

tex′is. Childbearing.

tex′ture. 1. Any organized substance or tissue of which the body is composed. 2. The arrangement of the elementary parts of tissue. *O.T.* **—textural,** *adj.*

Th. Chemical symbol for thorium.

thal'a·mo-. A combining form denoting *relating to the thalamus*.

thal'a·mus (pl. *thalami*). A mass of gray matter at the base of the brain, developed from the wall of the vesicle of the third ventricle, and forming part of the wall of the latter cavity. The posterior part is called the pulvinar. The thalamus sends projection fibers to the primary sensory areas of the cortex. The thalamus receives fibers from all parts of the cortex, and is also connected with the tegmentum and with fibers of the optic tract. **—thalam'ic,** *adj*.

tha·las″sa·ne'mi·a. A chronic hemolytic anemia with erythroblastosis, occurring in Mediterranean families and due to a specific gene influencing hemoglobin production. Also called *Cooley's anemia, thalassemia, Mediterranean anemia, familial erythroblastic anemia, target-cell anemia*.

thal″las·se'mi·a. See *thalassanemia*.

tha·las″so·pho'bi·a. A morbid fear of the sea.

tha·las″so·ther'a·py. Treatment of disease by sea voyages, sea bathing, sea air.

Tha·lic'trum. A genus of plants of the Ranunculaceae. Some species are cardiac poisons.

thal·lei'o·quin. The green substance produced when quinine or its salts is treated with a solution of chlorine or bromine followed by ammonia (called the *thalleioquin reaction*). Sometimes spelled *thalleoquin, thalleoquine*.

thal'li·um. Tl = 204.39. A bluish white metallic element; used in the manufacture of alloys, special glasses, and artificial gems. Salts of the metal have been used for epilation and for destruction of rodents; both uses are dangerous to humans since thallium is highly toxic.

tha·mu'ri·a. Frequent urination.

than'a·to-. A combining form meaning *death*.

than″a·to·bi'o·log'ic (than″uh-to-buy″o·lodj'ick). Pertaining to life and death.

than″a·to·gno·mon'ic (than″uh-to·no·mon'ick, than″uh·tog″no·). Indicative of death.

than″a·tog'ra·phy. 1. A dissertation on death. 2. A description of symptoms and feelings while dying.

than'a·toid. Resembling death.

than″a·tol'o·gy. The study of the phenomena of somatic death.

than″a·to·ma'ni·a. Death by autosuggestion, as in individuals who believe they are under the spell of a sorcerer.

than″a·to·pho'bi·a. A morbid fear of death.

than'a·tos. In *psychoanalysis*, all the instinctive tendencies which lead the organism toward death or senescence. Also called *death instinct*.

the·ba'ic. Pertaining to, or derived from, opium. *Obs.*

thi·ba'ine (theeb'uh·een, thi·bay'-een). $C_{19}H_{21}NO_3$. An alkaloid found in opium; it causes spasms like strychnine. Also called *paramorphine*.

the'ca (pl. *thecae*). A sheath, especially one of a tendon. **t. folliculi.** The capsule of a growing or mature ovarian (Graafian) follicle consisting of an inner vascular, cellular layer, the **theca interna,** and an outer fibrous layer, the **theca externa. —thecal,** *adj*.

the·ci'tis. Inflammation of the sheath of a tendon.

the·co'ma. A tumor of the ovary composed of cells derived from the ovarian stroma and sometimes resembling the thecal elements of the follicle.

the'e·lin (thee'uh·lin, thee'lin). See *estrone*.

the'e·lol (thee'uh·lohl, thee'lohl). See *estriol*.

the'ine (thee'een, tee'·). Caffeine.

the·lal'gi·a. Pain in a nipple.

the·las'is, the·las'mus (thi·laz'-mus). The act of sucking.

the'le·plas″ty. Plastic surgery of a nipple.

the·ler'e·thism. Erection of a nipple.

the·li'tis. Inflammation of a nipple.

the'li·um. 1. A papilla. 2. The nipple.

the·lon'cus. Tumor of a nipple.

the″lo·phleb″o·stem'ma. Venous circle around a nipple.

the″lor·rha'gi·a (theel″o·ray'juh·radj'uh). Hemorrhage from a nipple.

the·lo·thism. Projection of a nipple, caused by contraction of its smooth muscle.

thel'y·plas″ty. Plastic surgery of a nipple.

the'nar. 1. The palm of the hand. 2. The fleshy prominence of the palm corresponding to the base of the thumb. 3. Pertaining to the palm, as thenar muscles, the abductor and flexor muscles of the thumb.

thenfadil hydrochloride. Trade mark for thenyldiamine hydrochloride.

then″yl·di'a·mine hy″dro·chlo'ride. 2-[(2-Dimethylaminoethyl)-3-thenylamino]pyridine hydrochloride, used as an antihistaminic drug. See *thenfadil hydrochloride*.

thenylene hydrochloride. trade-mark for the antihistaminic substance methapyrilene hydrochloride *q.v.*

then″yl·pyr'a·mine (then″il·pirr'uh·meen, ·min). N,N-dimethyl-N'-(2-thenyl) -N' (2-pyridyl) -ethylenediamine or methapyrilene, used in the form of its hydrochloride salt as an antihistaminic agent.

the″o·bro′ma. A genus of trees of the Sterculiaceae. The seeds of **T. ca·cao** yield a fixed oil (theobroma oil) and contain the alkaloid theobromine. The seeds are used in the preparation of chocolate and cocoa.

he″o·bro′ma oil. A yellowish white solid consisting chiefly of the glycerides of fatty acids, obtained from the roasted seeds of *T. cacao*. Used in the preparation of suppositories, in ointments, and as an emollient. Also called *cocoa butter, cacao butter*.

he″o·bro′mine (thee″o·bro′meen, -min). An alkaloid, 3,7-dimethylxanthine, $C_7H_8N_4O_2$, isomeric with theophylline, found in cacao beans and kola nuts and obtained as a by-product in the manufacture of cocoa and chocolate. A diuretic and myocardial stimulant. **t. and sodium acetate.** An approximately equimolecular mixture of theobromine sodium and sodium acetate. It is a white, crystalline, hygroscopic powder which absorbs carbon dioxide from air with liberation of theobromine. Soluble in water. See *thesodate.* **t. and sodium salicylate.** An approximately equimolecular mixture of theobromine sodium and sodium salicylate. **t. calcium salicylate.** A mixture of theobromine calcium and calcium salicylate. See *theocalcin.*

heocalcin. Trade-mark for a brand of theobromine calcium salicylate.

he″o·ma′ni·a. 1. Religious mania. 2. Mental disorder in which the individual believes himself to be a divine being. **–theomaniac,** n.

he″o·pho′bi·a. Morbid fear of God.

he″o·phyl′line (thee″o·fil′een, -hee·off′il·een). An alkaloid, 1,3-dimethylxanthine, $C_7H_8N_4O_2.H_2O$, obtained from tea leaves and also prepared synthetically. It is isomeric with theobromine. It is a white, crystalline powder, soluble in water; diuretic and vasodilator. **t. and sodium acetate.** An approximately equimolecular mixture of theophylline sodium and sodium acetate. **t. calcium salicylate.** An approximately equimolecular mixture of theophylline calcium and calcium salicylate. **t. ethylenediamine.** Contains from 75–82% of anhydrous theophylline and 12.3–13.8% of ethylenediamine. It is a white or slightly yellow powder with a slight ammoniacal odor. It absorbs carbon dioxide from the air with the liberation of theophylline. Soluble in water. Also called *aminophylline.* **t. isopropanolamine.** Represents approximately 70% of theophylline. See *theopropanol.*

he″o·ple′gi·a. Apoplexy.

theopropanol. Trade-mark for theophylline isopropanolamine, *q.v.* under *theophylline.*

the″o·ret′i·cal. Based on theory; speculative.

the′o·ry. The abstract principles of a science. Also, a reasonable supposition or assumption, generally one that is better developed and more probable than a mere hypothesis. **cell t.** The theory that the cell is the unit of organic structure, and that cell formation is the essential process of life and its phenomena. Also called *cell doctrine.* **germ-layer t.** A young embryo establishes three superimposed cellular plates, the primary germ layers, which are called ectoderm, mesoderm, and entoderm. According to the germ-layer theory, the skin, nervous system and sense organs are derived from ectoderm, the inner lining of the primitive digestive canal from entoderm, and muscles, blood vessels, connective tissues and organs of excretion and reproduction from mesoderm. **monophyletic t. of hematopoiesis.** A conjecture or speculation that all blood cell types originate from a single primitive cell called a hemocytoblast. **quantum t.** According to Max Planck, radiant energy is given off from atoms or molecules in small discrete lots called quanta, and is absorbed in a like manner. The discharge of energy from an atom accompanies the passing of an electron from a high energy level to a lower level (from a larger to a smaller orbit), and the passage of an electron from a smaller to a greater orbit is accompanied by an absorption of energy. The energy discharged is equal to $h\nu$, where h is the Planck constant and ν is the frequency of the radiated energy. **recapitulation t.** The theory that the individual organism in its development from the ovum passes through a series of stages which resemble a series of ancestral types through which the species passed in its evolutionary history. This is also called the *biogenetic law.* Haeckel recognized a difference between those structures which are adaptive to the embryonic, larval, or fetal mode of life and those which may be regarded as inherited from the ancestral types. The former he included under cenogenesis and the latter under palingenesis. **side-chain t.** A chemical theory explaining the phenomena of immunity by the action of antibodies which, when circulating in an organism, unite with and render harmless the antigen and thereby prevent the antigen from attaching itself to the chemical system of the protoplasm. **unitarian t.** A theory of blood-cell formation which supposes that all blood cells come from a single parental blood cell, the hemocytoblast. Syn., *monophyletic t. of hematopoiesis.*

the″o·ther′a·py. The treatment of disease by prayer and religious exercises.

thephorin. A trade-mark for a brand of the antihistaminic substance phenindamine, *q.v.*

ther″a·peu′tics. The branch of medical science dealing with the treatment of disease. Also see *therapy, treatment.*

ther″a·peu′tist. One skilled in therapeutics.

ther′a·pist. One trained to administer treatment usually prescribed by a specialist, as in physical therapy, occupational therapy, or psychotherapy.

ther′a·py. Treatment. Also see *treatment.* **biologic t.** The use of biologic products such as serums, vaccines, antitoxins, and antibiotics. **cold t.** The use of cold in any form as a therapeutic agent. **collapse t.** The treatment of pulmonary tuberculosis by any surgical procedure designed to decrease lung volume, such as artificial pneumothorax, extrapleural thoracoplasty, or interruption of the phrenic nerve. **contact t.** Superficial x-ray therapy by means of a small, shockproof, low-voltage x-ray tube which may be placed in direct contact with the skin or introduced into body cavities. **electroshock t.** Treatment of mental patients, particularly those suffering with melancholia, mania, or catatonia, by passing a current through the brain (temple to temple), 85 to 110 volts and 500 milliamperes for $\frac{1}{10}$ to $\frac{1}{5}$ of a second. The patient does not recall the treatment. Better and safer than the metrazol shock therapy. **endocrine t.** The treatment of disease by the administration of extracts of the endocrine glands. **fever t.** Treatment of disease by artificially induced fever. **fluorine t.** The use of fluorine, as a fluoride, for the control of dental caries. The term is a general one and covers topical application of fluorine to the teeth, the addition of fluorine to water supplies, or the internal administration of fluorine. **glandular t.** The treatment of disease by glandular extracts, especially those obtained from organs which furnish internal secretions necessary to the bodily economy. **gold t.** The injection of various preparations of gold such as inorganic or organic salts or as a colloid for the treatment of lupus erythematosus, various dermatologic tuberculids, and rheumatoid arthritis. **heat t.** The treatment of disease with heat by means of hot baths, short-wave electric fields, heat lamps, hot-air cabinets. **hormone t.** The treatment of disease with hormones. **immuniza-**

tion t. Use of vaccines or antiserum to produce immunity against a specifi disease. **insulin shock t.** Treat ment of nervous disease by large dose of insulin. **interstitial irradia tion t.** Radium therapy with variou types of implants or seeds filled wit radium salts or radon. **intracavi tary irradiation t.** Radium ther apy by means of tubes, single or i strings of two or more, inserted into cavity of the body. **intravenous t** Introduction of therapeutic agents int the blood stream through a vein **maggot t.** The treatment of osteo myelitis by the introduction of liv larvae of the bluebottle fly into the open wound. The larvae clean the wound by eating the necrotic materia Also called *Baer's treatment.* **ma larial t.** The artificial induction o malaria for its therapeutic effect i central nervous system syphilis. **met razol shock t.** Treatment of per sons suffering with melancholia an with catatonic forms of schizophreni with an intravenous injection of met razol, which causes convulsions an produces temporary brain changes re sulting in elevation of the mood t normal levels and promotion of norma mental animation. Also see electro shock *t.* **musical t.** The use of musi for therapeutic effect, especially i treating mental disorders. **occupa tional t.** Giving to patients instruc tion in, and opportunity to pursue hobbies or trades for their sedative an psychologic effect. Used particularly i nervous and mental disease. **oxy gen t.** The administration of oxyge by means of nasal catheter, face mask or oxygen tent. It has also been give subcutaneously and intravenously **physical t.** The treatment of diseas by physical means such as light, heat cold, electricity, and massage. Als called *physical medicine.* **radian light t.** The use in physical therap of curative rays derived from the su or artificial sources as ultraviolet an infrared radiation. **radium t.** Ex posure of a part to high-voltage radiur emanations, usually for their destruc tive effect on malignant tissues. **re placement t.** The use of endocrin therapy to replace a function whicl has been destroyed surgically or ha ceased naturally. **shock t.** The treat ment of psychiatric patients by induc ing coma, with or without convulsions by means of drugs as insulin or metra zol or by passing an electric curren through the brain. Also see electro shock *t.,* insulin shock *t.,* metrazo shock *t.* **solar t.** Treatment of diseas by exposing the body to the direct ray of the sun or by the use of a su lamp; heliotherapy. **specific t.** On having a proved destructive effect against a specific etiologic factor or having a definite curative effect upon a particular disease. **suggestion t.** Treating disordered states by means of suggestion. **vaccine t.** Attempts to produce active immunity against disease by the use of specific antigens. See *vaccination*. **x-ray t.** Therapy with roentgen rays.

he·ri'a·ca. Treacle.

he"ri·od'ic. Malignant.

he"ri·o'ma. A malignant ulcer or tumor.

her'mal. Pertaining to heat.

her'mal·ge'si·a (thur"mal·jee'zee-uh, -see-uh). The condition in which heat causes pain.

her"ma·tol'o·gy. The scientific use or understanding of heat or of the waters of thermal springs in the cure of disease. **–thermatolog'ic,** *adj.*

herm"es·the'si·a (thurm"ess-thee'zhuh, -zee-uh). 1. Temperature sense for heat. 2. Sensitiveness to heat.

herm"es·the"si·om'e·ter (thurm"ess-thee"zee·om'i·tur, -see-om'i·tur). An instrument for measuring the sensibility to heat of different regions of the skin.

her'mite. Finely powdered aluminum mixed with iron oxide and capable of being ignited with a magnesium ribbon; the resulting reaction produces a temperature of about 3000° C.; used in welding.

her'mo-. A combining form meaning *heat*.

her"mo·an"al·ge'si·a (thur"mo-an"al·jee'zee-uh, -see-uh). Insensibility to heat or to contact with heated objects.

her"mo·an"es·the'si·a (thur"no-an"ess-thee'zhuh, -zee-uh). Loss of the perception of thermal impressions, a condition sometimes present in syringomyelia, severed nerve cases, and leprosy.

her"mo·cau'ter·y. A cautery which depends for its action upon heat delivered to the metal end of the instrument, either by a direct action of flame, aided by the passage of a current of hot air as in the Paquelin cautery, or by the passage of electric current. See *cautery*.

her"mo·chem'is·try. That branch of chemical science which treats of the mutual relations of heat and chemical changes.

her"mo·chro'ism. The property of transmitting some thermal radiations while absorbing or changing others.

her"mo·co·ag"u·la'tion. A method by which one or several layers of the cerebral cortex in a desired area can be destroyed by heat without alteration of the surrounding tissue.

ther'mo·cou'ple (thur'mo-cup"ul). A pair of metallic plates or wires forming a junction, in which a thermoelectromotive force is formed under the influence of heat. Thermocouple principle is also applied in the measurement of skin temperature.

ther"mo·dy·nam'ics (thur"mo-dye·nam'icks, -di·nam'icks). The science which treats of the relations of heat and other forms of energy.

ther"mo·gen'ics. The science of the production of heat.

ther"mo·hy"per·al·ge'si·a (-al-jee'zee-uh, -see-uh). The condition in which the application of heat causes excessive pain.

ther"mo·hy"per·es·the'si·a (-ess-thee'zhuh, -zee-uh). Abnormal sensitiveness to the application of heat.

ther"mo·hy"pes·the'si·a. Abnormal indifference or insensibility to heat or to contact with heated objects.

ther"mo·mas·sage' (thur"mo-ma-sahzh'). Massage with application of heat.

ther·mom'e·ter. An instrument for measuring temperatures or thermal states, generally consisting of a substance capable of expanding and contracting with different temperatures, and a graduated scale by means of which variations in the expansion of the substance can be determined. **centigrade t.** One in which the freezing point for water is at 0° and the boiling point at 100°. The interval is divided into 100 parts of 1° each. Also called *Celsius t.* **clinical t.** One used to ascertain the body temperature, so constructed that the maximum reading remains stationary after removal of thermometer from the patient. **Fahrenheit t.** One in which the interval between the freezing point and the boiling point for water is divided into 180 equal parts, each called a degree. 32° F. represents the freezing point and 212° F. the boiling point of water. **Réaumur t.** One in which the freezing point of water is 0° and the boiling point 80° with an interval of 80 points or degrees. **wet and dry bulb t.** A device for determining the relative humidity. It consists of two thermometers, the bulb of one of which is kept saturated with water vapor. The temperature difference between the two thermometers depends upon the relative humidity.

ther·moph'a·gy. The habit of swallowing very hot food.

ther'mo·phile (thur'mo-file, -fil). A microorganism for which the optimum temperature for growth is between 50°–55° C.; found in soil and water, especially hot springs.

ther"mo·pho'bi·a. Morbid dread of heat.

ther'mo·pile. An instrument for measuring temperatures; it consists of a series of thermocouples which permit measurement of minute temperature effects.

ther"mo·ple'gi·a. Sunstroke.

ther"mo·pol"yp·ne'a. Rapid respiration due to high temperature. **–thermopolypneic,** adj.

ther"mo·reg"u·la'tion. The regulation of heat production and heat loss to maintain normal temperature, as of the human body.

ther'mo·scope. An instrument for detecting changes or differences in temperature.

ther"mo·sta'ble. Resistant to temperatures above a certain critical temperature, 56° C. **–thermostabil'ity,** n.

ther'mo·stat. A device for automatically regulating and maintaining a constant temperature.

ther"mo·ste·re'sis. Deprivation of heat.

ther"mo·ther'a·py. Treatment of disease by heat of any kind.

ther"mo·tra"che·ot'o·my (thur"mo·tray"kee·ot'o·mee). Tracheotomy by means of the actual cautery.

thesodate. Trade-mark for a brand of theobromine and sodium acetate.

thev'e·tin. A poisonous glucoside with digitalislike action, from the seed of *Thevetia neriifolia.*

thi'a·mine hy"dro·chlo'ride (thigh'uh·meen, ·min). $C_{12}H_{17}ClN_4OS·HCl$. White crystals or powder, soluble in water. An essential vitamin occurring in many natural sources; frequently it occurs in the form of the pyrophosphoric acid ester known as cocarboxylase. Commercial thiamine hydrochloride is largely synthetic. A normal adult requires about 3 mg. daily. Syn., *thiamin chloride, vitamin B_1, aneurin, aneurine hydrochloride.* Also called *thiamin* and *thiamine,* although these names are sometimes given to the basic form of the vitamin.

thi·am'y·lal so'di·um. Sodium 5-allyl-5-(1-methylbutyl)-2-thiobarbiturate, an ultrashort-acting barbiturate. See *surital sodium.*

thi"a·zol·sul'fone. 2,4-Diamino-5-thiazolylphenyl sulfone, used in the treatment of leprosy. See *promizole.*

thigh. That part of the lower extremity from the pelvis to the knee.

thi'o-, thi-. A combining form denoting *the presence of sulfur.*

thi'o ac'id. An organic acid in which sulfur replaces oxygen.

thi'o al'co·hol. An alcohol in which sulfur replaces oxygen; a mercaptan.

thi"o·bar'bi·tal. 5,5-Diethylthiobarbituric acid. $C_8H_{12}N_2O_2S$.

thi"o·bar·bi·tu'rate (thigh"o·barbit·u'rate). A sulfur derivative of barbituric acid, which has analogous ac tivity.

thi'o·chrome. $C_{12}H_{14}N_4OS$. A fluorescent oxidation product of thiamine hydrochloride or other derivatives of the basic form of the vitamin. **t. assay.** A procedure for the analysis of thiamine hydrochloride or other derivatives of the basic form of the vitamin based on the intensity of the fluorescence produced by the thiochrome obtained by oxidation of the sample.

thi'o·cre'sol. D-Thiocresol. $C_6H_4SH·CH_3$. Crystalline leaflets of unpleasant odor, practically insoluble in water, soluble in alcohol. Used as cell proliferant in wounds, ulcers.

thi'o·cy'a·nate. Any compound containing the monovalent radical, $-SCN$

thi'o e'ther. An ether containing sulfur instead of oxygen.

thi"o·glyc'er·ol (thigh"o·gliss'uh·role, ·ol, ·awl). $CH_2OH.CHOH.CH_2SH$. Yellowish, viscous liquid, slightly soluble in water. Used as a cell proliferator.

thiomerin sodium. Trade-mark for mercaptomerin sodium.

thi'o·ne'ine. $C_9H_{15}N_3O_2S$. An amino acid derivative, the betaine of thiolhistidine, first isolated from ergot and later shown to be a normal constituent of blood. Also known as *ergothionein.*

thi·on'ic (thigh·on'ick). Pertaining sulfur.

thi'o·nin. See *thionine.*

thi'o·nine (thigh'o·neen, ·nin), **thi'o·nin.** $C_{12}H_{10}N_3S.HCl$. A dark green powder, solutions of which are purple, used as a stain in microscopy.

thi"o·pan'ic ac'id. Pantoyltaurin

thi"o·pen'tal so'di·um. The U. S. Pharmacopeia title for the barbiturate available under the trade-marked name pentothal sodium.

thi"o·pen'tone so'di·um. The British Pharmacopoeia title for the barbiturate available under the trade-marked name pentothal sodium.

thi'o·phene. A colorless liquid obtained from coal tar or produced synthetically. Insoluble in water.

thi"o·sin·am'ine (thigh"o·sin·am'een, ·sin'uh·meen). Allyl thiourea. $CH_2:CH.CH_2.NH.CS.NH_2$. White crystals, soluble in water. Syn., *rhodallin*

thi"o·sul'fate. Any salt containing the divalent radical, S_2O_3.

thiosulfil. Trade-mark for sulfamethizole.

thi"o·sul·fur'ic ac'id. $H_2S_2O_3$. An unstable acid, readily decomposing sulfurous acid and sulfur.

thi"o·u'ra·cil. $NH.CS.NH.CO.CH:C$ White, crystalline powder, soluble water. Used in the treatment of thyrotoxicosis. It interferes with the formation of thyroxin. See also *propy thiouracil.*

thi″o·u·re′a. $H_2N.CS.NH_2$. White crystals soluble in water. Has been used in the treatment of thyrotoxicosis. Syn., *thiocarbamide*. Also called *sulfocarbamide*.

thirst. A sensation associated with the need of the body for water. The sensory nerve endings for thirst are principally in the mucous membrane of the pharynx, and less than normal water content in this region supposedly produces thirst. Prolonged deprivation with dehydration of tissues produces severe unpleasant sensations probably of wide origin, which are more than thirst.

thix·ot′ro·py. The property of some gels, when mechanically agitated, to undergo a reversible isothermal solution and reconversion to a gel when allowed to stand. The tobacco mosaic virus has this property of thixotropy. —**thixotrop′ic,** *adj.*

tho″ra·cec·to′my. Resection of a rib.

tho″ra·cen·te′sis. Aspiration of the chest cavity for removal of fluid, usually for hydrothorax or empyema.

tho·rac′i·co-. A combining form denoting the *thorax.*

tho·ra·co-, thorac- (thor′uh·ko-, tho·ray′ko-). A combining form denoting the *thorax.*

tho″ra·co·cyl·lo′sis. Deformity of the thorax.

tho″ra·co·cyr·to′sis (·sur·to′sis). Excessive curvature of the thorax.

tho″ra·co·dyn′i·a. Pain in the chest.

tho″ra·co·lum′bar. Pertaining to the thoracic and lumbar portions of the spine, or to thoracic and lumbar ganglions and fibers of the sympathetic system.

tho″ra·cop′a·gus. Conjoined twins united by their thoraxes or epigastric regions. —**thoracopagous,** *adj.*

ho·ra′co·plas″ty. The mobilization of the chest wall by the resection of any number of ribs, wholly or in part, in order to produce collapse of the chest wall and obliteration of the pleural cavity. The operation is commonly extrapleural and may be partial or complete, the latter involving segments of the first to eleventh ribs. It is also referred to by location, as anterior, lateral, posterior, apical, etc.

tho·ra′co·scope, tho·rac′o·scope. An electrically lighted, tubular instrument designed for insertion between ribs into a pneumothorax space. Used for visual examination of the pleural surfaces and for the severance of pleural adhesion bands by electrocautery.

tho″ra·cos′co·py. Examination of the pleural cavity in the presence of a pneumothorax by means of a thoracoscope, *q.v.* Syn., *pleuroscopy.*

tho″ra·cos′to·my. Opening the chest; particularly, the removal of some ribs for drainage, or for access to the pleural cavity.

tho″ra·cot′o·my. Incision of the thoracic wall.

tho′rax (pl. *thoraxes, thoraces*). The chest; that portion of the trunk above the diaphragm and below the neck; the framework of bones and soft tissues bounded by the diaphragm below, the ribs and sternum in front, the ribs and thoracic portion of the vertebral column behind, and above by the structures in the lower part of the neck, and containing the heart enclosed in the pericardium, the lungs invested by the pleura, and the mediastinal structures. —**thorac′ic,** *adj.*

thorazine hydrochloride. Trademark for chlorpromazine hydrochloride.

tho′ri·um. Th = 232.05. A radioactive, grayish white, lustrous metal, the parent of a series of radioactive elements.

thorn′-ap″ple. See *stramonium.*

tho′ron. Tn = 220. A gaseous, radioactive element evolved from thorium X, one of the disintegration products of thorium. Also called *thorium emanation.*

thread′worm″. Commonly, any one of the long, thin worms, such as a pinworm or a filarial worm.

thre′o·nine (three′o·neen, ·nin). α-Amino-β-hydroxybutyric acid, CH_3·CHOH.CHNH_2.COOH. An amino acid essential to human nutrition.

thre′ose. $CHO.HOCH.HCOH.CH_2OH$. A monosaccharide having a spatial configuration similar to that of threonine.

threp·sol′o·gy. The science of nutrition.

thresh′old. 1. The lower limit of stimulus capable of producing an impression upon consciousness or of evoking a response in an irritable tissue. 2. The entrance to a canal. **flicker fusion t.** The minimal frequency of standard flashes of light which will be seen as steady illumination. Abbreviated, F.F.T. See flicker fusion *test.*

thrill. A fine vibration felt by the hand. A thrill may be felt on palpation over an aneurysm, over a heart which is the seat of valvular disease, and over hydatid cysts. **presystolic t.** A thrill which can sometimes be felt before the systole when the hand is placed over the apex beat (mitral stenosis).

thrix an″nu·la′ta. Hairs with alternating light and dark segments.

throat. The pharynx and the fauces. **sore t.** Pharyngitis and/or tonsillitis.

throb. A pulsation or beating.

throe. A violent pang, as in parturition.

throm·bec'to·my. Excision of a thrombus.

throm'bin. An enzyme elaborated in shed blood from an inactive precursor, prothrombin. It induces clotting by converting fibrinogen to fibrin and is used therapeutically as a topical hemostatic agent. Formerly called *fibrin ferment.*

throm·bin'o·gen. Prothrombin.

throm'bo-, thromb-. A combining form denoting *a thrombus* or *thrombosis.*

throm″bo·an″gi·i'tis. Thrombosis with inflammation of the intima of a vessel. **t. obliterans.** A disease characterized by minute, widespread, fugitive phlebitis with perivascular fibrosis involving the accompanying arteries and nerves. Seen chiefly in young or middle-aged males. Also called *Buerger's disease.*

throm″bo·ar″te·ri'tis. Inflammation of an artery associated with thrombosis. **t. obliterans.** See *thromboangiitis* obliterans.

throm·boc'la·sis. Breaking up or destruction of a thrombus; thrombolysis. **—thromboclas'tic,** *adj.*

throm'bo·cyte. Blood platelet; a small, colorless disk in the circulating blood of all mammals; it contains thromboplastin and is important in the clotting of blood. Normally, 1 cu. mm. of blood contains 250,000 to 500,000 platelets. Syn., *platelet, blood platelet.*

throm″bo·cy″to·pe'ni·a. Decrease in the number of blood platelets below normal. **—thrombocytopenic,** *adj.*

throm″bo·cy·to'sis (throm″bo-sigh·to'sis). A condition marked by the presence of a large number of thrombocytes in the blood.

throm″bo·em″bo·li·za'tion. The occlusion of a blood vessel by the lodgment of a portion of a thrombus.

throm″bo·en″do·car·di'tis. Bacterial or nonbacterial thrombotic vegetations on heart valves.

throm'bo·gen. Prothrombin.

throm″bo·kin'ase (throm″bo·kin'ace, ·kigh'nace). A substance considered capable of transforming prothrombin to thrombin. See also *thromboplastin.*

throm″bo·lym″phan·gi'tis. Lymphangitis with thrombosis.

throm·bol'y·sis. Destruction or dissolution of a thrombus; thromboclasis. **—thrombolyt'ic,** *adj.*

throm·bop'a·thy. Disease characterized by disturbance of platelet formation and consequent interference with the formation of blood clots.

throm″bo·pe'ni·a. A decrease in platelets. **—thrombopenic,** *adj.*

throm″bo·phil'i·a. A tendency t[o] form thrombi. **essential t.** Diffus[e] thrombosis of the arteries and vein[s] not accounted for by infection, stasi[s] or local inflammatory lesions. An in[-]crease of the coagulability of th[e] plasma seems to be the primary facto[r]

throm″bo·phle·bi'tis. Inflamma[-]tion of a vein associated with thromb[o]sis.

throm″bo·plas'tic. Causing or has[-]tening the coagulation of the blood.

throm″bo·plas'tin. A substanc[e] found in the platelets and tissues whic[h] is a factor in blood clotting. Thoug[ht] to be identical with thrombokinas[e] Also called *thrombozyme.*

throm″bo·plas″tin·o·pe'ni·a. [A] deficiency of thromboplastin in th[e] blood.

throm″bo·poi·e'sis. The produc[-]tion of blood platelets and other ele[-]ments necessary for thrombus forma[-]tion.

throm'bosed. 1. Affected with throm[-]bosis. 2. Clotted.

throm·bo'sis. The formation of [a] thrombus. **—thrombot'ic,** *ad[j.]* **atrophic t.** That due to gener[al] malnutrition. **cardiac t.** Thrombos[is] in the heart. **cavernous sinus t[.]** Inflammation of a cavernous sinu[s] with thrombus formation, usually sec[ondary] to staphylococcus infection [of] the nares and upper lip. **coagula[-] tion t.** That caused by fibrin coagula[-]tion. **compression t.** That due [to] compression of a vessel, as by a tumo[r] **coronary t.** Thrombosis of the coro[-]nary arteries of the heart. **dilata[-] tion t.** That which results from th[e] slowing of the blood current next to th[e] vessel walls as the result of dilatatio[n] of a vessel (as in aneurysms, varices[,] or of the heart. **lateral sinus t[.]** Thrombosis of a lateral sinus due t[o] extension of infection from mastoid a[ir] cells. The thrombus may be attached [to] the wall (mural thrombus) or it ma[y] completely obliterate the sinus. **pla[-] cental t.** That of the uterine veins [at] the site of a placenta. **puerpera[l] venous t.** Puerperal thrombosis [of] pelvic veins.

throm·bo·sta'sis. Stasis of bloo[d] leading to formation of a thrombus.

throm'bo·zyme. Thromboplastin.

throm'bus (pl. *thrombi*). A clot [of] blood formed within the heart or bloo[d] vessels, due usually to a slowing of th[e] circulation or to alteration of the bloo[d] or vessel walls. **—thromboid,** *ad[j.]* **annular t.** One that involves th[e] whole circumference of a vessel b[ut] does not entirely occlude it. **ball [t.]** A small or large, rounded, ante-morte[m] clot found in the heart, especially [in] an atrium. **coronary t.** One that a[f-]fects a branch of a coronary arter[y]

fibrolaminar t. One containing layers of connective-tissue fibers. Also called *stratified t.* **hyaline t.** One found in the smaller blood vessels, as a glossy fibrinous mass. Probably due to toxic injuries to the intima. **Laennec's t.** A globular thrombus formed in the heart, especially in cases where the latter is the seat of fatty degeneration. **lateral t.** A clot attached to a vessel wall, and not completely obstructing the lumen. **mural t.** One attached to the wall of a blood vessel. Also called *lateral t., parietal t.* **obstructing t.** One completely obstructing the lumen of a vessel. **parietal t.** One adherent to the wall of a vessel or the heart and not entirely occluding the lumen. **progressive t.** One that grows into the lumen of a vessel.

throt'tle. 1. The throat. 2. Choke, suffocate.

throw'back". A reversion to an ancestral type. See *atavism*.

thrush. 1. A form of moniliasis due to infection by *Candida albicans*. It occurs most often in children and is characterized by small, whitish spots on the tip and sides of the tongue and the buccal mucous membrane. Syn., *mycotic stomatitis, parasitic stomatitis*. 2. A diseased condition of the frog of the horse's foot, with a fetid discharge.

Thu'ja (thew'jah, thew'yah). A genus of trees of the Pinaceae.

thu'jone. A cyclic ketone, $C_{10}H_{16}O$, found in several volatile oils.

thu'li·um. Tm = 168.94. A rare earth metal.

thumb. The digit on the extreme radial side of the hand, differing from the other digits in having but two phalanges, and in that its metacarpal bone is freely movable.

thu'ya. See *Thuja*.

hy"la·ken'trin (thigh"luh·ken'-trin). Prolan-A, *q.v.*

thyme (time). The dried leaves and flowering tops of *Thymus vulgaris* of the Labiatae, yielding volatile oil. **t. camphor.** Thymol.

thy·mec'to·my (thigh·meck'to·mee). Excision of the thymus. —**thymectomize**, *v.*

thy'mene (thigh'meen, tigh'meen). $C_{10}H_{16}$. A terpene in thyme oil, identical with *l*-pinene.

hy"mer·ga'si·a (thigh"mur·gay'-zhuh, ·shuh). *In psychiatry*, Meyer's term for the affective-reaction psychoses such as manic-depressive psychosis and involutional melancholia. —**thymergasic**, *adj.*

thy'mi·a. A combining form denoting a *condition of mind*.

hy"mi·co·lym·phat'ic. Affecting the thymus and lymphatic structures such as spleen, lymph nodes, and lymphoid aggregates, as thymicolymphatic state.

thy'mine (thigh'meen, ·min). 2,4-Dihydroxy-5-methylpyrimidine; a substance isolated from thymus.

thy'mi·on. A wart; a condyloma.

thy·mi'tis (thigh·migh'tis). Inflammation of the thymus.

thy'mo-, thym-. A combining form denoting *thymol;* also referring to *thymus.*

thy"mo·cres'cin. A principle, claimed to be present in extracts of the thymus, that has growth-promoting properties.

thy"mo·ke'sis. Abnormal persistence or enlargement of the thymus.

thy'mol (thigh'mole, tigh'·). Methyl-propyl-phenol. A crystalline phenol, $C_{10}H_{14}O$, obtained from the volatile oils of many plants. It is also synthesized. A bactericide and fungicide. **t. blue.** Thymolsulfonphthalein. $C_{27}H_{30}O_5S$. Brownish green, crystalline powder soluble in alcohol. An indicator covering the pH ranges 1.2 to 2.8 and 8.0 to 9.6. **t. iodide.** A mixture of iodine derivatives of thymol, chiefly dithymoldiiodide. A reddish yellow powder, insoluble in water. Used as an antiseptic dusting powder. See *aristol*.

thy"mol·phthal'ein (·thal'in, ·thal'ee·in). A compound, analogous to phenolphthalein, used as an indicator; it is colorless below pH 9.3 and blue at pH 10.5.

thy"mol·sul'fon·phthal'e·in, thy"mol·sul'fone·phthal'e·in. Thymol blue.

thy·mo'ma (thigh·mo'muh). A primary tumor of the thymus. Frequently associated with myasthenia gravis, but no clear interrelationship is established. Also see thymic *carcinoma*.

thy"mo·no'ic. Pertaining to thoughts and ideas which are strongly influenced by deviations in mood.

thy"mo·nu·cle'ic ac'id. Deoxyribonucleic acid.

thy·mop'a·thy (thigh·mop'uth·ee). Any disease of the thymus.

thy'mo·pex"y. The fixation into a new position of thymus. *Obs.*

thy"mo·priv'ic. Related to, or caused by, removal of or premature involution of the thymus.

thy'mus. An organ situated in the anterior superior mediastinum. It continues to develop until the second year of life, afterward remains stationary until about the fourteenth, and then undergoes fatty metamorphosis and atrophy. It consists of lobules largely composed of lymphatic tissue in which are found minute concentric bodies, the remnants of epithelial structures, or thymic (Hassall's) corpuscles.

thy'mus nu·cle'ic ac'id. Deoxyribonucleic acid.

thy′re·o-. For words beginning with *thyreo-* not found here, see under *thyro-*.

thy′ro-. A combining form signifying *thyroid*.

thy″ro·ad″e·ni′tis. Inflammation of the thyroid gland.

thy″ro·ar″y·te′noid. Pertaining to the thyroid and arytenoid cartilages, as the thyroarytenoid ligaments, thyroarytenoid muscle. See Table of Muscles in the Appendix.

thy″ro·car′di·ac. Pertaining to thyroid disease with cardiac symptoms predominating.

thy′ro·cele. A tumor affecting the thyroid gland; goiter.

thy″ro·chon·drot′o·my (thigh″ro·kon·drot′o·mee). Incision of the thyroid cartilage; laryngotomy.

thy″ro·cri·cot′o·my (thigh″ro·cry·cot′o·mee, ·kri·cot′o·mee). Tracheotomy performed through the cricothyroid membrane.

thy″ro·ep″i·glot′tic. Pertaining to the thyroid cartilage and the epiglottis, as the thyroepiglottic muscle. See Table of Muscles in the Appendix.

thy″ro·glob′u·lin. The iodine-protein of the thyroid gland, secreted by it and lodged in the colloid substance.

thy″ro·glos′sal. Pertaining to the thyroid gland and the tongue.

thy″ro·hy′al. The greater cornu of the hyoid bone.

thy′roid. 1. Shield-shaped. 2. Pertaining to the thyroid gland. 3. Pertaining to the thyroid cartilage. 4. The thyroid gland. 5. The cleaned, dried, and powdered gland previously deprived of connective tissue and fat; it is obtained from domesticated animals that are used for food by man. Contains 0.17 to 0.23 per cent iodine in thyroid combination, especially as thyroxin. Administered in the treatment of thyroid deficiency states.

thy″roid·ec′to·my. Partial or complete excision of the thyroid gland.

thy′roid·ism. 1. Disturbances produced by hyperactivity of the thyroid gland. 2. A series of phenomena due to continued use of thyroid preparations.

thy″roid·i′tis. Inflammation of the thyroid gland.

thy″roid·i·za′tion. Treatment with thyroid gland preparations.

thy″roid·ot′o·my. Incision of the thyroid gland.

thy·roi′ge·nous (thigh·roy′ji·nus). Originating in disturbances of the thyroid gland.

thy″ro·pri′vus. 1. Deprived of the thyroid gland. 2. A disease due to loss of thyroid gland activity.

thy″ro·pro′te·in (thigh″ro·pro′tee·in, ·pro′teen). A protein from the thyroid gland.

thy″rop·to′sis. Displacement of goitrous thyroid so that it is partially or completely concealed in the thorax.

thy·ro′sis (thigh·ro′sis). Any disorder caused by abnormal function of the thyroid gland.

thy″ro·ther′a·py. Treatment of disease by thyroid gland preparations.

thy·rot′o·my (thigh·rot′o·mee). Incision or splitting of the thyroid cartilage.

thy″ro·tox′ic. Pertaining to disease caused by excessive activity of the thyroid gland or excessive thyroid hormone action.

thy″ro·tox″i·co′sis. Hyperthyroidism of any type.

thy·rot′ro·pin (thigh·rot′ro·pin). A thyroid-stimulating hormone produced by the adenohypophysis.

thy·rox′in (thigh·rock′sin), **thy·rox′ine** (thigh·rock′seen, ·sin). HO·C₆H₂I₂OC₆H₂I₂CH₂CH(NH₂)COOH. An active physiologic principle obtained from the thyroid gland or prepared synthetically; contains about 64 per cent iodine. Occurs as white crystals insoluble in water.

thy·rox″in·so′di·um. Thyroxin treated with sodium. Also spelled *thyroxine-sodium*.

Ti. Chemical symbol for titanium.

tib′i·a. The larger of the two bones of the leg, commonly called the shinbone; articulating with the femur, fibula, and talus. See Table of Bones in the Appendix. **—tibial,** *adj.* **saber t.** Anterior bowing and thickening of the tibia due to periostitis caused by congenital syphilis or yaws. Also called *saber shin; boomerang leg*.

tib″i·al′gi·a. Pain in a tibia; painful shin.

tib″i·a′lis (tib″ee·ah′lis, ·ay′lis). One of two muscles of the leg, **tibialis anterior** and **tibialis posterior**. See Table of Muscles in the Appendix.

tib′i·o-. A combining form signifying *tibia*.

tib″i·o·fib′u·lar. Pertaining to the tibia and the fibula.

tibione. Trade-mark for p-acetylaminobenzaldehyde-thiosemicarbazone, a tuberculostatic agent. See *conteben*.

tic. A twitching, especially of the facial muscles; a habit spasm. **convulsive t.** Spasm of the facial muscles. **painless t.** The occurrence, at intervals, of sudden rapid involuntary contraction in a muscle or group of muscles. **t. douloureux.** Paroxysmal neuralgia of the trigeminal nerve. **t. rotatoire.** Spasmodic torticollis; spinal accessory spasm; a spasm of certain muscles by which the head and neck are forcibly rotated to one side and from one side to the other.

tick. An arthropod of the order Acarrina infesting vertebrate animals. They are important vectors and reservoirs of rickettsial diseases. They also transmit many viral, bacterial, and protozoal diseases. Toxins produced by the female before oviposition produce tick paralysis. The important genera are *Amblyomma*, *Argas*, *Boöphilus*, *Dermacentor*, *Haemaphysalis*, *Hyalomma*, *Izodes*, *Ornithodorus*, and *Rhipicephalus*.

tick'ling. Stimulation of the skin or mucous membrane, either pleasant or annoying, which causes reflex responses.

tic·tol·o·gy. Obstetrics.

t. i. d. *Ter in die*, three times a day.

ti'dal drain'age. A method of draining a paralyzed urinary bladder with an automatic irrigation apparatus.

tide. A definite period of time. **acid t.** A period of increased excretion of acid radicals by the kidney after meals, while excessive alkali is secreted into the duodenum. **alkaline t.** The transient increase in the alkalinity of the urine during gastric digestion, presumably related to the secretion of hydrochloric acid into the stomach and the resulting relative excess of base in the blood. It is diminished or absent in achlorhydria.

ti'ger lil'y ap·pear'ance. The speckled appearance of the myocardium observed in pernicious anemia.

ti·gog'e·nin (ti-godj'i-nin). The aglycone of tigonin.

tig'o·nin. A saponin from *Digitalis purpurea*. On acid hydrolysis it yields the steroid aglycone tigogenin, glucose, galactose, and rhamnose.

ti'groid. A term applied to masses of chromophil substance in nerve cells.

tim'bre (tim'bur). The peculiar quality of a tone, other than pitch and intensity, that makes it distinctive. It depends upon the overtones of the vibrating body.

time. The duration of an event or phenomenon. **bleeding t.** The period elapsing between capillary puncture and the cessation of bleeding; in normal persons it usually is 1–3 minutes. **clot retraction t.** The period elapsing between the drawing of a blood specimen and the formation of contracted clot; usually is one hour. **clotting t.** The period elapsing between the drawing of a blood specimen and the formation of a normal clot; usually is 5–8 minutes. **inertia t.** In the stimulation of a muscle or sense organ the latent time required to overcome the inertia of the muscle or organ after the reception of the stimulus through the nerve. **prothrombin t.** The time required for oxalated plasma to clot after adding thromboplastin and recalcifying. The time is measured in seconds and is inversely proportional to the prothrombin content of the plasma.

reaction t. The interval between the application of a stimulus and the beginning of the response.

tim'o·thy. A common name for the most important meadow grass in America. It flowers during June and July, shedding quantities of pollen which is one of the more common causes of hay fever in the early summer.

tin. Sn = 118.70. An element and silver-white metal; used in alloys and the manufacture of tin salts. **t. chloride.** Stannous chloride, $SnCl_2.2H_2O$; used in chemical procedures as a reducing agent. **t. oxide.** Stannic oxide, SnO_2; used in combination with metallic tin for the treatment of furunculosis.

tin'cal. Crude or native borax.

tinc·to'ri·al. Pertaining to staining or dyeing.

tinc·tu'ra. Tincture. Abbreviated, tr.

tinc'ture. Alcoholic or hydroalcoholic solutions of medicinal substances, generally representing 10% or 20% (w/v) of drug and usually prepared by maceration or percolation of the drug with suitable menstruum. Abbreviated, tr. **mother t.** In *homeopathy*, a tincture, usually representing 10% of the drug, from which the standard dilutions are made.

tin'e·a. The lesions of dermatophytosis; ringworm. **t. barbae.** Ringworm of the bearded areas of the face and neck. Caused by various species of *Trichophyton* and *Microsporum*. Also called *barber's itch*, *t. sycosis*. **t. capitis.** Fungus infection of the scalp and hair. Caused by several species of *Trichophyton* and *Microsporum*. Also called *t. tonsurans*. **t. cruris.** A fungus infection involving the skin of the groin, perineum, and perianal regions. Caused by *Epidermophyton floccosum* and several species of *Trichophyton*. Also called *gym itch*, *jockey itch*. **t. favosa.** A chronic fungus infection which usually is limited to the scalp. Caused by *Trichophyton schoenleini* and *T. violaceum*. Also called *favus*, *honeycomb ringworm*. **t. imbricata.** A superficial fungus disease of the tropics characterized by the presence of concentric rings of papulosquamous patches scattered over the body. Caused by *Trichophyton concentricum*. Also called *gogo*, *scaly ringworm*, *Tokelau ringworm*, *tropical tinea circinata*. **t. pedis.** A fungus infection of the feet, especially the webs of the toes and the soles. Caused by *Epidermophyton floccosum*, various species of *Trichophyton*, and rarely by *Microsporum*. Also called *athlete's foot*. **t. unguium.** A chronic fungus infection involving the nails of the hands and feet. Caused by *Epidermophyton floccosum*, various species of *Trichophyton*, and *Candida albicans*. **t. versicolor.** A chronic superficial fungus infection of the skin, usually of the trunk. It is caused by *Malassezia furfur*. Also called *pityriasis versicolor, chromophytosis, t. flava, t. nigra.*

tin′gle. A pricking or stinging sensation; the feeling of a slight, sharp, and sudden thrill, as of pain; acanthesthesia.

tin·ni′tus, tin′ni·tus. A subjective ringing, roaring, or hissing sound in the ears or in one ear only.

tire. Weary; become exhausted; fag. The term is used extensively by the medical profession and laymen alike in reference to muscular and brain fatigue, general bodily and mental exhaustion, etc.

Tiselius, Arne [*Swedish biochemist,* 1902–]. Described a method for the separation of proteins from body fluids by means of electrophoresis. The apparatus used is called *Tiselius apparatus.* Nobel laureate (1948).

tis′sue. An aggregation of similar cells and their intercellular substance. **adipose t.** A form of connective tissue consisting of fat cells lodged in areolar tissue and arranged in lobules along the course of small blood vessels. **areolar t.** A form of loose connective tissue composed of cells and delicate collagenous and elastic fibers interlacing in all directions. **connective t.** A general term for all those tissues of the body that support the specialized elements or parenchyma. The most important varieties are adipose tissue, areolar tissue, osseous tissue, cartilaginous tissue, elastic tissue, fibrous connective tissue, and lymphatic tissue. **elastic t.** Connective tissue which is composed predominantly of yellow elastic fibers. **erectile t.** A spongelike system of vascular spaces in the penis and clitoris which becomes filled with blood causing enlargement and rigidity of the organ. **fibrous connective t.** The densest connective tissue of the body. Collagenous fibers form the main constituent and are arranged in parallel bundles between which are rows of connective-tissue cells. It includes tendons, ligaments, and fibrous membranes, as the dura mater. **glandular t.** A group of epithelial cells which elaborate secretions. **granulation t.** The mixture of newly formed capillaries and fibroblasts in inflammation, especially of exudative character, representing the early stages of healing. Followed by a growth into exudate or destroyed tissue, the process becomes one of organization. As it progresses to cicatrization by atrophy of blood vessels and maturation of connective tissue, inflammatory foci are cicatrized, or such foci or foreign bodies

are encapsulated; on surfaces, especially serous, fibrous adhesions are formed; wounds are healed. **hematopoietic t.** Blood-cell-forming tissue consisting of reticular fibers and primitive reticular cells which can be converted into all types of blood and connective-tissue cells. **keratinized t.** Tissue found in the nails, hair, or epidermis. **lymphatic t.** Tissue consisting of networks of reticular and collagenous fibers and lymphocytes. **lymphoid t.** (a) Lymphatic tissue, *q.v.* (b) Lymphatic tissue forming or occurring where it is not normally present. **muscular t.** The tissue of which muscles are composed. See *muscle,* 1. **myeloid t.** Red bone marrow consisting of reticular cells attached to argyrophile fibers which form wide meshes containing scattered fat cells, erythroblasts, myelocytes, and mature myeloid elements. **nervous t.** The nerve cells, their processes and accessory cells, such as the neuroglia. **osseous t.** Bone. **scar t.** Contracted dense connective tissue, the end result of healing. **subcutaneous t.** The layer of loose connective tissue under the derma. Also called *hypodermis.*

ti·ta′ni·um (tye-tay′nee-um, ti-tay′-nee-um). Ti = 47.90. A very hard, dark gray, lustrous, metallic element used in certain alloys to impart toughness. **t. dioxide.** TiO_2; extensively used as a white pigment in paints, plasters, etc.

ti′ter, ti′tre (ty′tur, tee′tur). 1. *In chemistry,* a titration figure. 2. An expression of the strength of a volumetric solution, usually grams of active constituent per cubic centimeter of solution. 3. The amount of one substance that corresponds to, reacts with, or is otherwise equivalent to a stated quantity of another substance.

tit″il·la′tion. The act of tickling; the sensation produced by tickling.

ti·tra′tion (tye-tray′shun, ti-tray′-shun). An operation in volumetric analysis involving the measurement of the volume of a standard solution required to react chemically with the sample being analyzed. —**ti′trate,** *v.*

ti′tre. See *titer.*

tit″u·ba′tion. A staggering gait seen especially in diseases of the cerebellum. **lingual t.** Stammering; stuttering.

Tl. Chemical symbol for thallium.

Tm. Chemical symbol for thulium.

Tn. Chemical symbol for thoron, *q.v.*

T.O. Original, or old, tuberculin. Also abbreviated O.T.

toad poi′sons. Toxic constituents of the skin glands of various toads, chiefly bufotoxins, bufagins, and bufotalins, all closely related to the digitalis principles in structure and action. Some contain the alkaloids bufotenin, bufotenidine, and bufothionine. Several tropical species yield epinephrine.

toad'skin". Abnormal dryness, scaling, and fissuring of the skin resulting from vasomotor disturbances. Seen in vitamin deficiencies and syringomyelia.

to·bac'co. A plant, *Nicotiana tabacum*, of the family Solanaceae, the dried leaves of which contain an alkaloid, nicotine. Its chief importance is as an enjoyment drug. It was formerly employed as an enema to overcome intestinal obstruction. **Indian t.** Lobelia.

toclase. Trade-mark for carbetapentane citrate.

toc"o·dy"na·mom'e·ter (tock"o-dye"nuh·mom'i·tur, to"ko·). An instrument for measuring the force of the expulsive efforts of the uterus in childbirth.

to·col'o·gy. The science of obstetrics.

toc"o·ma'ni·a (tock"o·may'nee·uh, to"ko·). Puerperal insanity.

tocopherex. Trade-mark for a distillate of vegetable oils containing mixed tocopherols.

to·coph'er·ol. Any one of several substances possessing vitamin-E activity, as α-, β-, or γ-tocopherol of which the α-variety is the most potent, found abundantly in wheat germ oil and also contained in cottonseed oil and in lettuce. See also *alphatocopherol*.

toc"o·pho'bi·a (tock"o·fo'bee·uh, to"ko·). Undue dread of childbirth.

toc'o·sine (tock'o·seen, ·sin). Tyramine hydrochloride.

to'cus. Childbirth.

toe. A digit of the foot. **t. drop.** The inability to raise or extend the toes, owing to paralysis of the peroneal nerve.

to'ko-. For words beginning with *toko-* not found here, see under *toco-*.

tol·az'o·line hy"dro·chlo'ride. 2-Benzyl-2-imidazoline hydrochloride, a sympatholytic, adrenolytic, and vasodilator drug. See *priscoline hydrochloride*.

tol·but'a·mide. 1-Butyl-3-*p*-tolylsulfonylurea, an orally active hypoglycemic agent. See *orinase*.

tol'er·ance, tol"er·a'tion. The ability of enduring the influence of a drug or poison, particularly when acquired by a continued use of the substance. **sugar t.** The tolerance of a diabetic patient for ingested sugar. It is measured by the maximum amount of sugar intake which does not produce glycosuria.

tol'er·ant. Withstanding the action of a drug without harm.

to·lo'ni·um chlo'ride. 3-Amino-7-dimethylamino - 2 - methylphenazothionium chloride, a dye having antihep-

arin activity. Syn., *toluidine blue O*. See *blutene chloride*.

tolserol. A trade-mark for mephenesin, *q.v.*

to·lu' bal'sam (to·loo' bawl'sum). Obtained from *Myroxylon balsamum*, a South American tree of the Leguminosae. It contains cinnamic and benzoic acids, esters of these acids and resins. A mild stimulant expectorant. Also called *tolu*.

tol'u·ene. Methylbenzene. $C_6H_5.CH_3$. A colorless liquid obtained chiefly from coal tar. Used as a solvent and reagent.

tol"u·ene·sul"fon·di"chlor·am'ide (para). Dichloramine-T. Also spelled *p-toluenesulfondichloroamide, p-toluenesulfonedichloramide, p-toluenesulfonedichloroamide.*

to·lu'i·dine (to·lew'i·deen, ·din). Aminotoluene. $H_2N.C_6H_4.CH_3$. The *o*- and *m*- varieties are liquids; the *p*- is a solid. **t. blue O.** Tolonium chloride.

tol'u·ol. Toluene.

tol·u·yl·ene, tol·u'yl·ene. Stilbene. **t. red.** Aminodimethylaminotoluphenazine hydrochloride. $C_{15}H_{16}N_4.HCl$. An indicator covering the pH range 6.8–8.0. Syn., *neutral red*.

tol'uyl. A univalent radical. $C_6H_4.CH_3$.

tolysin. Trade-mark for a brand of neocinchophen.

to·mat'i·dine. The aglycone portion, chemically a steroid secondary amine, resulting from hydrolysis of tomatine.

to·ma·tine. A glycosidal alkaloid, isolated from the tomato plant, having fungicidal activity.

-tome. 1. A combining form denoting *a part* or *a section*. 2. A combining form denoting *an instrument for cutting.*

to·mog'ra·phy. See *sectional radiography.*

to"mo·to'ci·a (to"mo·to'shee·uh, tom"o·). Cesarean section.

-tomy. A combining form denoting *a cutting operation.*

to'nal is'lands. Isolated areas in the range of human hearing in which some persons with practically no hearing have an appreciation of pure tones at maximum intensity.

to"na·pha'si·a (to"nuh·fay'zhuh, ton"uh·). Loss of the ability to sing (due to a cerebral lesion).

tone. 1. A distinct sound. 2. The normal state of tension of a part or of the body.

tongue. The movable muscular organ attached to the floor of the mouth, and concerned in tasting, masticating, swallowing, and speaking. It consists of a number of muscles, and is covered by mucous membrane from which project numerous papillae, and in which are placed the terminal organs of taste. **bifid t.** A tongue the anterior portion of which is cleft in the median line. **black, hairy t.** A tongue with a brown, furlike patch on the dorsum, due to hypertrophied filiform papillae and the presence of pigment. Also called *hyperkeratosis linguae*. **burning t.** Glossopyrosis. **fissured t.** A condition of the tongue in which there are deep furrows in the mucous membrane. Also called *furrowed t., lingua plicata*. **furred t.** A tongue the papillae of which are coated, giving the mucous membrane the appearance of a whitish fur. **geographic t.** Benign migratory glossitis. **strawberry t.** A hyperemic tongue, the fungiform papillae of which are very prominent; it is seen especially in scarlet fever.

tongue'-tie". A congenital abnormality of the frenulum of the tongue, interfering with its mobility. Syn., ankyloglossia.

ton'ic. 1. Pertaining to tone; producing normal tone or tension. 2. Characterized by continuous tension or contraction, as a tonic spasm, tonic convulsion. 3. An agent or drug given to improve the normal tone of an organ or of the patient generally.

to-nic'i-ty (to-niss'i-tee). The condition of normal tone or tension of organs.

ton"i-co-clon'ic (ton"i-ko-klon'ick, to"nick-o-). Both tonic and clonic, pertaining to muscular spasms.

ton'ka bean. The seed of *Dipteryx odorata*, a tree of South America; it contains coumarin, and is used as a flavoring agent.

to"no-a'brils (to"no-figh'brils, ton"o-). Delicate fibrils found particularly in epithelial cells, between which they run across intercellular bridges.

to-nom'e-ter. An instrument to measure tension, as that of the eyeball, or an instrument used to equilibrate samples of fluid, as blood, with gases at known tensions.

to'no-scope (to'no-scope, ton'o-). An instrument for examination of the interior of the cranium by means of sound.

ton'quin bean (tong'kin, ton-kwin'). Tonka bean, q.v.

ton'sil. 1. Aggregated lymph nodules and associated lymph vessels surrounding crypts or depressions of the pharyngeal mucosa. 2. A small lobe of the cerebellar hemisphere, on its inferior medial aspect. —tonsillar, adj. **lingual t.** Accumulations of lymphatic tissue more or less closely associated with crypts which serve also as ducts of the mucous glands of the base of the tongue. **palatine t.** One found on each side of the isthmus of the fauces and between the glossopalatine and pharyngopalatine arches, in the tonsillar sinus; almond-shaped and separated from the pharyngeal musculature by a well-defined thin capsule.

pharyngeal t. An unpaired tons found on the posterior wall of th nasopharynx, in folds of the mucos with grooves between, which simula crypts; more prominent during chil hood; when hypertrophied forms th "adenoids."

ton-sil'la (pl. *tonsillae*). 1. Tonsil. That lobe of the hemisphere of th cerebellum which is situated on the i ferior medial side of the hemispher by the vallecula.

ton"sil-lec'tome. An instrumen for the performance of tonsillectom

ton"sil-lec'to-my. Removal of th palatine tonsils.

ton"sil-li'tis. Inflammation of th tonsils. —tonsillit'ic, adj. **acute** Inflammation of the tonsils with su den onset, pyrexia, constitutional symp toms, and intense sore throat. **fo licular t.** A form in which the cryp are involved and their contents proje as whitish spots from the surface of th tonsil. **herpetic t.** A form chara terized by an eruption of herpetic ves cles, which soon rupture, leaving sma circular ulcers that coalesce and becon covered with a fibrinous exudation. Th disease has an acute onset, a continu ous fever, and a critical decline, affec those subject to herpes elsewhere, an tends to recur. **pustular t.** A for characterized by the formation of pu tules, as in smallpox.

ton-sil'lo-lith, ton'sil-lo-lith. concretion within a tonsil.

ton-sil'lo-tome, ton'sil-lo-tome. An instrument for removing a tonsil.

ton"sil-lot'o-my. The operation cutting away the whole or a part of tonsil.

ton"sil-sec'tor. A tonsillotome co sisting of a pair of circular or ov scissor blades moving inside a guardi ring.

ton'sure. The shaving or removal the hair from the crown of the head.

to'nus. The slight degree of contra tion usually present in muscles wh not undergoing active movement. skeletal muscles, it is a reflex respon to motor nerve impulses of low fr quency. In smooth muscle, it is an i herent property of the muscle cells.

tooth (pl. *teeth*). One of the calcifi organs supported by the alveolar pro esses and gums of both jaws, servi to masticate food, aid speech, and i fluence facial contour. Each tooth co sists of: (1) a main mass of denti surrounding a pulp cavity which co tains the dental pulp with its nerv and vessels, (2) a coronal porti (crown) covered by enamel, (3) radicular portion (root), which may single, bifid, or trifid, covered by bo called cementum, (4) a cervical porti (neck), the junction of crown a root. **bicuspid t.** See premolar *t.* **canine t.** A tooth with a conical crown, situated between the lateral incisor and the first premolar in each quadrant of the jaws. Also called *cuspid t.* **deciduous teeth.** The 20 temporary or milk teeth; those replaced by succedaneous permanent teeth. There are eight incisors, four canines, and eight molars. **eye t.** The upper canine tooth. **incisor t.** One of the two cutting teeth nearest the midline in each quadrant of the dentition. **molar t.** A multicuspidate tooth used for crushing, grinding, or triturating food. In the human deciduous dentition there are two in each quadrant immediately behind the canine; in the permanent dentition, three, behind the premolars. **permanent t.** One of the 32 teeth of the second dentition. There are eight incisors, four canines, eight premolars, and 12 molars. **premolar t.** One of the two teeth with two cusps situated between the canine and the first molar in each quadrant of the permanent dentition. Also called *bicuspid t.* **temporary teeth.** (a) The teeth of the first dentition; milk teeth; deciduous teeth. (b) A provisional set of artificial teeth. **wisdom t.** The third molar tooth in man.

tooth′ache. Any pain in or about a tooth; odontalgia.

tooth′ache″ tree. A tree whose bark, xanthoxylum, *q.v.*, has been used as a masticatory in toothache.

top″ag·no′sis. Loss of localization sensibility.

to·pal′gi·a. Localized pain, common in neurasthenia and hysteria; often appears suddenly after emotional disturbances.

to·pec′to·my. Excision of a portion of the cerebral cortex, usually in the frontal area, for the treatment of certain mental disorders or intractable pain.

top″es·the′si·a, top″aes·the′si·a (top″ess-thee′zhuh, to″pess·). Local tactile sensibility.

to′phus (pl. *tophi*). A mineral concretion in the body, especially about the joints. A sodium urate deposit in the skin about a joint, in the ear, or in bone, in gout.

top′ic, top′i·cal. Local.

top′o- (top′o-, to′po-), **top·.** A combining form meaning *place;* used to signify *localized.*

top″o·an″es·the′si·a (·an″ess-thee′zhuh, ·zee·uh). Inability to locate exactly a cutaneous sensation.

top″og·nos′tic. Pertaining to the recognition of changes, positions, or symptoms of parts of the body, as topognostic sensibility.

to·pog′ra·phy. A study of the regions of the body or its parts, as cerebral topography. **–topograph′ic,** *adj.*

top″o·nar·co′sis. Local insensibility or anesthesia.

top″o·neu·ro′sis. A localized neurosis.

top″o·pho′bi·a. Morbid dread of certain places.

tor′mi·na (sing., *tormen*). Griping pains in the bowel. **post-partum t.** The afterpains of parturition. **t. alvi.** Colic. **t.** Celsi. Dysentery. **t. intestinorum.** Dysentery.

Toronto unit. The anticoagulant activity of 0.01 mg. of a standard barium heparin employed at the University of Toronto.

tor′pid. Affected with torpor.

tor′por. Sluggishness; inactivity. **t. intestinorum.** Constipation. **t. retinae.** Dulled perceptive power of the retina.

tor′sion. 1. A twisting; also, the rotation of the eye about the visual axis. 2. The tilting of the vertical meridian of the eye. **t. of an artery.** Twisting of the free end of an artery to check hemorrhage. **t. of teeth.** The forcible turning of teeth in their alveoli for the purpose of correcting irregularity in position. **t. of the umbilical cord.** The spontaneous twisting of the umbilical cord. From eight to ten twists are normal; great torsion may occur after the death of the fetus.

tor′sive (tor′siv). Twisted; twisting.

tor′so. The trunk; the body without head or limbs.

tor″ti·col′lis. Wryneck, a contraction of the sternocleidomastoid muscle, usually of one side, resulting in an abnormal position of the head. **rheumatic t.** Old term for stiff neck, a form due to myositis of the sternocleidomastoid or other muscle of the neck. **spasmodic t.** Spasmodic contraction of the muscles of the neck of one side, especially the sternocleidomastoid, causing a drawing of the head toward the opposite side. Also called *torticollis spastica.*

tor′tu·ous. Twisted, sinuous.

tor′u·lus. An elevation.

to′rus (pl. *tori*). 1. A surface having a regular curvature with two principal meridians of dissimilar curvature at right angles to each other. 2. An elevation or prominence. **t. tubarius.** The arcuate elevation of the mucous membrane of the pharynx over the medial end of the cartilage of the auditory tube, above and behind the pharyngeal orifice of the tube. Also called *Eustachian cushion, tubal elevation.*

to′ta·quine (to′tuh·kween, ·kwin). A mixture of alkaloids from the bark of species of *Cinchona.* Yellowish white to gray powder affected by light. An anti-malarial.

touch. 1. Tactile sense. 2. Judging by the tactile sense; palpation. 3. *In obstetrics*, digital examination of the internal genitalia through the vagina. **abdominal t.** Application of the hands to the abdomen for the diagnosis of intraabdominal conditions. **double t.** Combined vaginal and abdominal or vaginal and rectal palpation. **rectal t.** An examination made by a finger in the rectum. **vaginal t.** Digital examination of the genital organs through the vagina.

tour de maî'tre (toor di may'truh). A method of passing a catheter into the male urinary bladder in which it is introduced into the urethra with the convexity upward. The shaft lies obliquely across the left thigh of the patient, and as the point enters the bulb, the handle is swept around toward the abdomen, when the beak passes into the membranous urethra. It is carried into the bladder by depressing the shaft between the patient's thighs.

tour'ne·sol' (toorn'sawl'). Litmus.

tour'ni·quet. Any apparatus for controlling hemorrhage from, or circulation in, a limb or part of the body, where direct pressure can be brought upon the blood vessels by means of straps, cords, rubber tubes, or pads. Tourniquets are made in a multiplicity of forms, from the simplest emergency adaptation of a handkerchief or piece of clothing wound about the limb and tightened with a stick, to elaborate instruments where pressure is made by means of screws acting upon metal pads or where a rubber hose encircling the limb is distended with air by means of a pump.

tous-les-mois' (too-lay-mwah'). A variety of arrowroot starch prepared from *Canna edulis*; canna starch.

tow. The coarse part of flax or hemp; used as an absorbent.

tox-. See *toxico-*.

tox''al·bu'min. A poisonous protein obtained from cultures of bacteria and from certain plants.

tox·e'mi·a. A condition in which the blood contains poisonous products, either those produced by the body cells or those due to the growth of microorganisms. It is a general involvement in which the blood contains toxins but not bacteria. **eclamptogenic t.** A condition associated with gestation. A disturbance of metabolism with fever, albuminuria, water retention, capillary injury, and acute hypertension. In severe cases, there are convulsions and coma. Also called *eclamptic t.*, *preeclamptic t. t.* **of pregnancy.** Eclamptogenic toxemia.

tox'ic. 1. Poisonous. 2. Of, pertaining to, or acting as a poison or a toxin.

toxic-. See *toxico-*.

tox'i·cant. 1. Poisonous or toxic. 2. A poisonous agent.

tox'i·cide. A remedy or principle that destroys toxic agents.

tox·ic'i·ty (tock·sis'i·tee). 1. The quality of being toxic. 2. The kind and amount of poison or toxin produced by a microorganism.

tox'i·co-, toxic-. A combining form meaning *poison*.

tox''i·co·den'drol. A toxic nonvolatile oil from poison ivy and poison oak, *Rhus toxicodendron* and *Rhus venenata*.

tox''i·co·der'ma. Disease of the skin due to poison.

tox''i·co·der''ma·ti'tis. Inflammation of the skin due to poison.

tox''i·co·der''ma·to'sis. Toxicoderma.

tox''i·co·gen'ic. Producing poisons.

tox'i·coid. Resembling a poison or a toxin.

tox'i·col'o·gist. One versed in toxicology; one who makes a special study of toxins.

tox'i·col'o·gy. The science of the nature and effects of poisons, their detection, and treatment of their effects. **–toxicolog'ic, toxicolog'ical,** *adj.*

tox''i·co·ma'ni·a. Morbid desire to consume poison. **–toxicomaniac,** *n.*

tox''i·co·mu'cin. A toxic substance from cultures of tubercle bacilli.

tox''i·co·path'ic. Pertaining to any morbid condition due to the action of a poison.

tox''i·co·pho'bi·a. Morbid dread of being poisoned.

tox''i·co'sis. A state of poisoning. **endogenic t.** That due to toxic substances produced within the body; autointoxication. **exogenic t.** One with clinical symptoms induced by the action of toxic bases taken into the system from without, as in botulism. **retention t.** One with clinical symptoms due to the retention of waste products, as in uremia.

tox·if'er·ous. Producing or conveying poison.

tox'in. A poisonous product of animal or vegetable cells which, on injection into animals or man, causes the formation of antibodies, called antitoxins The most important toxins are those produced by bacteria. See also *endotoxin, phytotoxin, zootoxin.*

tox'in-an''ti·tox'in. Abbreviated T. A. See *diphtheria toxin-antitoxin.*

tox''in·fec'tion. Infection by means of a toxin, the causative microorganism not being recognized.

tox·in'i·cide. Any substance that destroys a toxin.

tox·is'ter·ol. A product of the excessive irradiation of ergosterol. Although isomeric with calciferol, it has little antirachitic action and is highly toxic.

tox"i·ta·bel'la. A poison tablet, of an angular shape, and having the word poison and the skull and crossbones design distinctly stamped upon it.

tox"i·ther'a·py. The therapeutic use of antitoxins.

tox"i·tu·ber'cu·lide. A skin lesion due to the action of tuberculous toxin.

tox'o-, tox-. See *toxico-*.

tox'oid. A product formed by the treatment of toxin with physical or chemical agents. A toxoid is nontoxic but maintains the antigenic properties of the toxin. Toxoids are frequently used for immunization, particularly against diphtheria and tetanus.

tox"o·lec'i·thin (tock"so·less'i-thin). A mixture of a venom with a lecithin, the latter behaving as a complement for the former.

tox"on·o'sis. An affection resulting from a poison.

tox'o·phil, tox'o·phile (tock'so-file, -fil). Having an affinity for toxins or poisons.

Tox"o·plas'ma (tock"so·plaz'muh). A genus of parasitic protozoans. **T. gondii.** The causative agent of toxoplasmosis.

tox"o·plas·mo'sis (tock"so·plaz-mo'sis). The disease caused by infection with the protozoan, *Toxoplasma*. In infants and children the disease usually is characterized by an encephalomyelitis. In adults a form clinically resembling Rocky Mountain spotted fever has been reported.

TPN. Abbreviation for triphosphopyridine nucleotide.

tr. *Tinctura*; tincture.

tra·bec'u·la (pl. *trabeculae*). 1. Any one of the fibrous bands extending from the capsule into the interior of an organ. 2. One of the variously shaped spicules of bone in cancellous bone. **—trabec'ular,** *adj.*

trace el'e·ments. Substances or elements essential to plant or animal life, but present in extremely small amounts. Also called *trace substances*. Also see *tracer*.

tra'cer. An isotope which, because of its unique physical properties, can be detected in extremely minute quantity, and hence is used to trace the chemical behavior of the natural element. As isotopes of the same element differ in physical properties only, but have identical chemical properties (with a few exceptions), an isotope detectable by physical properties may be used to trace the pattern of biochemical reactions. Such use of isotopes is referred to as a

tracer study. The isotope itself is a tracer. Stable (by measurement of isotopic ratios) or unstable (by detection of their ionizing radiation) isotopes may be used. Also called *t. element*.

tra'che·a (tray'kee·uh, tra·kee'uh). The windpipe; the cartilaginous and membranous tube extending from the lower end of the larynx to its division into the two bronchi. **—tracheal,** *adj.*

tra"che·a·ec'ta·sy (tray"kee·uh-eck'tuh·see). Dilatation of the trachea.

tra"che·al'gi·a. 1. Pain in the trachea. 2. Croup.

tra"che·i'tis. Inflammation of the trachea.

trachel-. See *trachelo-*.

trach"e·lag'ra (track"i·lag'ruh). Rheumatic or gouty pain in the neck.

trach"e·lec'to·my (track"i·leck'to-mee). Excision of the neck of the uterus.

trach"e·le"ma·to'ma (track"i-lee"muh·to'muh, ·lem"uh·to'muh). A hematoma of the neck, or in a sternocleidomastoid muscle.

trach"e·lis'mus (track"i·liz'mus). Spasmodic contraction of the muscles of the neck.

trach"e·li'tis (track"i·lye'tis). Inflammation of the neck of the uterus. Also see *cervicitis*.

trach'e·lo- (track'i·lo-), **trachel-.** A combining form meaning *neck*.

trach"e·lo·cyl·lo'sis. Torticollis.

trach"e·lo·dyn'i·a. Pain in the neck.

trach"e·lo·ky·pho'sis (·kigh·fo'-sis). An abnormal anterior curvature of the cervical portion of the spinal column.

trach"e·lo·par"a·si'tus. Taruffi's term for any parasitic growth upon the neck or jaws.

trach"e·lo·pex'i·a. Surgical fixation of the neck of the uterus.

trach'e·lo·plas"ty. Plastic operation on the neck of the uterus.

trach"e·lor'rha·phy (track"i·lor'uh·fee). Repair of a laceration of the cervix uteri.

trach"e·lor·rhec'tes (·reck'teez). An instrument for crushing the cervical vertebrae; used in embryotomy.

trach"e·los'chi·sis (track"i·los'ki-sis). A congenital fissure of the neck.

trach"e·lo·syr"in·gor'rha·phy. An operation for vaginal fistula with stitching of the cervix uteri.

trach"e·lot'o·my (track"i·lot'o-mee). Incision into the cervix uteri.

tra'che·o- (tray'kee·o-, tra·kee'o-), **tra'che-.** A combining form denoting *connection with*, or *relation to*, the *trachea*.

tra"che·o·blen"nor·rhe'a. A profuse discharge of mucus from the trachea.

tra″che·o·bron·chi′tis (·brong-kigh′tis). Inflammation of the trachea and bronchi.

tra″che·o·bron·chos′co·py (tray″kee·o·brong·kos′ko·pee, tra-kee″o·). Inspection of the interior of the trachea and bronchi.

tra′che·o·cele. A hernia of the mucous membrane of the trachea.

tra″che·o·fis′sure. Congenital longitudinal cleft of the trachea.

tra″che·o·lar″yn·got′o·my. Incision into the larynx and trachea; combined tracheotomy and laryngotomy.

tra″che·o·path′i·a os″te·o·plas′ti·ca. A deposit of cartilage and bone in the mucosa of the trachea.

tra″che·oph′o·ny (tray″kee·off′o-nee). The sound heard over the trachea on auscultation.

tra″che·o·plas′ty. Plastic surgery of the trachea.

tra″che·o·py·o′sis (tray″kee·o·pye-o′sis, tra·kee″o·). Purulent tracheitis.

tra″che·or·rha′gi·a. Hemorrhage from the trachea.

tra″che·or′rha·phy. Suturing of the trachea.

tra″che·os′chi·sis (tray″kee·os′ki-sis). Congenital fissure of the trachea.

tra″che·os′co·py. Inspection of the interior of the trachea by means of a laryngoscopic mirror and reflected light, or through a bronchoscope. —**tracheoscop′ic,** adj.

tra″che·o·ste·no′sis. Abnormal constriction or narrowing of the trachea.

tra″che·os′to·my. The formation of an opening into the trachea, and suturing the edges of the opening to an opening in the skin of the neck, as in laryngectomy.

tra′che·o·tome. A cutting instrument used in tracheotomy; a tracheotomy knife.

tra″che·ot′o·mist. One skilled in tracheotomy.

tra″che·ot′o·mize. Perform tracheotomy upon a living subject.

tra″che·ot′o·my (tray″kee·ot′o-mee). The operation of cutting into the trachea. **inferior t.** One performed below the isthmus of the thyroid gland. **superior t.** One performed above the isthmus of the thyroid gland. The cut may be extended to include the cricoid cartilage. See laryngotomy.

tra″chi·el·co′sis (tray″kee·el·ko′-sis). Ulceration of the trachea.

tra″chi·el′cus. A tracheal ulcer.

tra·cho′ma (tra·ko′muh). An infectious disease of the conjunctiva and cornea producing photophobia, pain, and lacrimation; caused by *Chlamydozoon trachomatis*; characterized by pannus and redness, inflammation, and follicular and papillary hypertrophy of the conjunctiva. Syn., *Egyptian conjunctivitis, Egyptian ophthalmia, conjunctivitis granulosa, granular lids.* —**trachom′atous,** adj. **brawny t.** A late stage of trachoma, in which the conjunctiva is thickened due to lymphoid infiltration. **diffuse t.** A form in which large growths cover the tarsal conjunctiva. **t. deformans.** A form of kraurosis vulvae at the stage when it results in diffuse scar tissue. **t. of the vocal cords.** Nodular swellings on the vocal folds; singers' nodes.

tra″chy·pho′ni·a (tray″ki·fo′nee-uh, track″i·). Rough or hoarse voice.

tract. 1. A pathway or course. 2. A bundle or collection of nerve fibers. 3. Any one of the nervous pathways of the spinal cord or brain as an anatomic and functional entity. 4. A group of parts or organs serving some special purpose. **afferent t.** A nerve tract of the spinal cord conveying impulses toward the brain. Syn., *ascending t.* **alimentary t.** The alimentary canal, *q.v.* **biliary t.** The entire hepatic duct system, including hepatic ducts, gallbladder, cystic duct, and common bile duct. **comma t.** A tract, comma-shaped in cross section, in the dorsal funiculus of the spinal cord. Also called *fasciculus interfascicularis.* **corticospinal tracts.** Efferent tracts which descend from the frontal cortex through the internal capsule, cerebral peduncles, pons and medulla, where they undergo incomplete decussation to form the lateral and ventral corticospinal tracts. They are concerned in finely coördinated voluntary movements. Syn., *pyramidal tracts.* **digestive t.** The alimentary canal, *q.v.* **efferent t.** Nerve tract which conducts impulses toward the periphery. **lateral spinothalamic t.** A tract of nerve fibers which arise from cells of the posterior column, cross in the anterior white commissure, ascend in the lateral funiculus, and terminate in the thalamus; it conducts pain and temperature impulses. **motor t.** A nerve pathway for motor impulses from brain to muscle. **optic t.** A band of nerve fibers running around the lateral side of a cerebral peduncle from the optic chiasma to the lateral geniculate body and midbrain. **pyramidal tracts.** See *corticospinal tracts* under *tract.* **urinary t.** The passage for the urine, including the kidneys, renal pelves, ureters, bladder, and urethra. **ventral spinothalamic t.** A tract of nerve fibers which arise from cells in the posterior column, cross in the anterior white commissure, ascend in the ventral funiculus, and terminate in the thalamus; it conducts impulses from touch and pressure stimuli.

trac′tion. The act of drawing or pulling. **axis t.** Traction in the axis or direction of a channel, as of the pelvis, through which a body is to be drawn. **weight t.** That exerted by means of a weight, connected to the injured limb.

trac·tot'o·my. Section of a nerve fiber tract of the central nervous system, as of the spinothalamic tract, for the alleviation of intractable pain.

trag'a·canth. A gummy exudation from various Asiatic species of *Astragalus*, of the family Leguminosae. Almost white ribbons or powder; swells with water to make a mucilage.

Tra'gi·a. A genus of poisonous plants; some species have been used in folk medicine.

tra'gus. 1. The small prominence of skin-covered cartilage projecting over the meatus of the external ear. 2. One of the hairs at the external auditory meatus.

train'ing. Systematic exercise for physical development or for some special attainment.

trait. Any characteristic, quality, or property of an individual.

trance. 1. The hypnotic state; resembles sleep. See *hypnosis*. 2. A form of catalepsy, characterized by a prolonged condition of abnormal sleep, in which the vital functions are depressed and from which the patient ordinarily cannot be aroused. The breathing is almost imperceptible, and sensation abolished. The onset and awakening are both very sudden.

tran'quil·ize. To allay stress or tension; to calm; to pacify.

tran'quil·iz"er. A drug having a sedative or calming effect without inducing sleep; an ataraxic.

trans- (trans-, tranx-). A combining form denoting *through* or *across*.

trans·am'i·nase. The enzyme that catalyzes the transfer of the amino group of a dicarboxylic amino acid to a keto acid, to form another amino acid.

trans"am·i·na'tion. 1. The transfer of one or more amino groups from one compound to another. 2. The transposition of an amino group within a single compound.

trans·an"i·ma'tion. The performing of artificial respiration on a newborn infant.

tran·sec'tion. A section made across the long axis of a part, as transection of the spinal cord.

trans·fer'ence. *In psychoanalysis,* the revival of forgotten and repressed experiences of childhood which are relived not as they actually occurred but in a new relationship to the person of the analyst. An intense emotional attachment of the patient to the physician as a compensation for an inadequate adjustment to present reality.

trans·fix'ion. 1. The act of piercing

through and through. 2. A method of amputation in which the knife is passed directly through the soft parts, the cutting being done from within outward. **—transfix,** *v.*

trans"fo·ra'tion. The act of perforating the fetal skull. **—transfo·rate,** *v.*

trans·for·a"tor. An instrument for perforating the fetal head.

trans"for·ma'tion. A marked change in form, structure, or function.

trans·form'er. An apparatus for the transformation of lower potentials to higher potentials or vice versa. **step-down t.** A transformer to decrease voltage. **step-up t.** A transformer to increase voltage.

trans·fuse'. Perform transfusion.

trans·fu'sion. 1. A transfer of blood into a vein. 2. The introduction into a vessel of the body of blood, saline solution, or other liquid. 3. The pouring of liquid from one vessel to another. **arterial t.** Transfusion of blood into an artery. **blood t.** Transfer of blood from one individual to another. The blood of donor and recipient must be of the same type. **bone marrow t.** Transfusion into bone marrow cavities, especially those of the sternum, the femur, and the tibia. **citrate method of t.** An indirect method of blood transfusion; the donor's blood is collected in a bottle and mixed with sodium citrate to prevent clotting. **direct t.** The transfusion of blood from one person to another without exposure of the blood to the air. Also called *immediate t.* **indirect t.** The introduction of blood that was first drawn into a vessel. Also called *mediate t.* **peritoneal t.** Transfusion into the peritoneal cavity. **reciprocal t.** The exchange of equal volumes of blood between a patient suffering from a febrile disease and one who is convalescent from that disease. **replacement t.** A transfusion technic used in the newborn with erythroblastosis foetalis in which the greater part of the total blood volume is replaced in small amounts at a time with Rh negative donor blood, the theory being that the Rh positive antibodies remaining will be minimal. **sternal t.** That in which the donor's blood is introduced directly into the bone marrow of the recipient by puncture of the sternum. **venous t.** Transfusion into a vein.

trans·fu'sion·ist. One skilled in the transfusion of blood.

tran'sient or'ange. An unstable carotenoid pigment formed by the breakdown of visual purple exposed to light, which is rapidly transformed to indicator yellow and then to retinene.

trans"il·lu"mi·na'tion. 1. Illumination of an object by transmitted light. 2. Illumination of the paranasal sinuses by means of a light placed in the patient's mouth.

tran·sis'tor. A device, considerably smaller than a vacuum tube for similar use, that amplifies electric currents by means of the semiconductor property of germanium.

tran·si'tion·al (tran·zish'un·ul, tran·sish'·). 1. Denoting a change of form. 2. Ehrlich's name for a monocyte having a U-shaped nucleus, which he regarded as a transitional form in the development of a polymorphic granulocyte; now considered to be an older form of monocyte.

trans·lu'cent. Permitting a partial transmission of light; somewhat transparent.

trans·lu'cid. Semitransparent.

trans·meth'yl·a'tion. A type of metabolic chemical reaction in which a methyl group is transferred from a donor to a receptor compound. Methionine and choline are important sources of methyl groups.

trans"mi·gra'tion (trans"migh·gray'shun, tranz"·). A wandering across or through, as transmigration of an ovum, transmigration of white blood cells. See *diapedesis*. **external t.** The passage of an ovum from an ovary to the opposite oviduct without transversing the uterus. **internal t.** The passage of an ovum through its proper oviduct into the uterus and across to the opposite oviduct.

trans·mis"si·bil'i·ty. The capability of being transmitted or communicated from one person to another. **—transmis'sible,** *adj.*

trans·mis'sion. The communication or transfer of anything, especially disease, from one person or place to another. **duplex t.** The movement of impulses along a nerve in two directions. **placental t.** The conveyance of drug and disease products through the placental circulation from mother to offspring.

trans"mu·ta'tion. 1. The evolution of one species into another. *Obs.* 2. *In physics,* any process by which an atomic nucleus is converted into another of different atomic number.

trans·par'ent. Permitting the passage of light rays without material obstruction, so that objects beyond the transparent body can be seen.

tran·spi'ra·ble. Capable of passing in a gaseous state through the respiratory epithelium or the skin.

tran"spi·ra'tion (tran"spi·ray'shun, tran"spy·ray'shun). 1. The act of exhaling fluid through the skin. 2. The material exhaled. **pulmonary t.**

The exhalation of water vapor from the lungs.

trans'plant. Tissue removed from any portion of the body and placed in a different site. **—transplant',** *v.*

trans"plan·ta'tion. The operation of transplanting or of applying to a part of the body tissues taken from another body or from another part of the same body. Also see *graft*. **autoplastic t.** The exchange of different parts within the same individual. **heteroplastic t.** The exchange of parts between individuals belonging to different species. **heterotopic t.** That in which the graft is transplanted to a different location in the host than it had in the donor. **homotopic t.** That in which the graft is transplanted to the same location in the host that it had in the donor. **tendon t.** The removal of a tendon from its normal location and its reinsertion in another place, used to substitute a functioning muscle for a paralyzed one by transplanting its tendon.

trans·pose'. Displace; change about, as tissue from one location to another by operation.

trans"po·si'tion (trans"po·zish'un). Change or interchange of position or order of arrangement. **t. of the viscera.** A reversal of the normal position of the viscera.

trans"sub·stan"ti·a'tion. (trans"sub·stan"shee·ay'shun). The replacement of one tissue by another.

tran'su·date. A liquid or other substance produced by transudation.

tran"su·da'tion. The passing of fluid through a membrane, especially of blood serum through the vessel walls. **—transu'datory,** *adj.*

tran·sude'. Pass through a membrane.

trans"u·re'thral. Via the urethra, as transurethral operation.

trans·vag'i·nal (trans·vadj'i·nul, ·va·jy'nul). Across, or through, the vagina.

trans"ver·sa'lis (·vur·sah'lis, ·say'lis). Transverse, as transversalis fascia, the fascia on the inner surface of the transversus abdominis muscle between the latter and the peritoneum.

trans·verse'. Crosswise; at right angles to the longitudinal axis of the body.

trans"ver·sec'to·my. Excision of a transverse process of a vertebra; specifically, in orthopedic practice, the removal of the transverse process of the fifth lumbar vertebra for pain due to irritation of the lower spinal nerve roots.

trans·ves'ti·tism. The morbid desire to dress in the clothing of the opposite sex. See *eonism, sexo-esthetic inversion.*

tra·pe'zi·um. The multangulum majus, the first bone of the second row of the carpal bones. See Table of Bones in the Appendix.

tra·pe'zi·us. A muscle arising from the occipital bone, the nuchal ligament, and the spines of the thoracic vertebrae, and inserted on the clavicle, acromion, and spine of the scapula. See Table of Muscles in the Appendix.

trap'e·zoid. 1. A geometrical, four-sided figure having two parallel and two diverging sides. 2. The multangulum minus, the second bone of the second row of the carpus. See Table of Bones in the Appendix.

trasentine. Trade-mark for diphenylacetyldiethylaminoethanol hydrochloride, an antispasmodic.

trau'ma (trou'muh) (pl. *traumas, traumata*). 1. A wound or injury. 2. *In psychiatry,* an emotional shock leaving a deep psychologic impression.

trau·mat'ic (trou·mat'ick). Pertaining to, or caused by, a wound or injury.

trau·mat'ic ac'id. COOH.CH:CH(CH₂)₈COOH. A dibasic acid found in certain plants after they have been cut or bruised; stimulates resumption of division of mature cells.

trau'ma·tism (trou'muh·tiz·um). The general or local condition produced by a wound or injury. —**trau·natize,** *v.*

trau"ma·tol'o·gy. The science or description of wounds and injuries, especially as they occur in industry and transportation.

trau"ma·top'a·thy. Pathologic condition due to wounds or other injury.

trau"ma·top·ne'a. The passage of respiratory air through a wound in the chest wall.

trav'ail (trav'ail, trav'ul). Labor of childbirth.

tray. A flat, shallow vessel of glass, hard rubber, or metal, for holding instruments during a surgical operation. **impression t.** *In dentistry,* a metal receptacle used to hold wax or other plastic material used for making impressions of the teeth and gums.

treat. Combat disease by the application of remedies.

treat'ment. The means employed in effecting the cure of disease; the management of disease or of diseased patients. Also see *therapy.* **active t.** That which is vigorously applied to the disease. **after t.** The treatment of a convalescent patient, especially after a surgical operation or a crisis. **Carrel-Dakin t.** The frequent and regularly repeated irrigation of open wounds with a solution of chlorinated soda and sodium bicarbonate. **causal t.** That which is directed to the removal of the

cause of a disease. **closed plaster t.** A general descriptive term for a procedure in which plaster is used over a recent operative wound, the cast complementing the operation in the treatment. The encasement of the wound is carried out without suture. Except over the prominent bony points, plaster is applied directly to the skin over a petroleum jelly gauze. Joints proximal and distal to the wound are immobilized. Ordinarily, the dressing is not changed before a week or ten days. **conservative t.** Treatment which is entirely expectant and abstains from any interference until absolutely necessary; in surgical cases, it aims at preservation rather than mutilation. **dietetic t.** That depending entirely on the control of the type and amount of food. **drip t.** The continuous injection of fluid into the blood or a body cavity so slowly that the rate is measured in drops. **drug t.** That depending on the use of drugs. **electric light t.** The therapeutic application of electric light by means of cabinets in which the patient sits with the light directed upon the affected part. Its therapeutic effect depends on heat. Used in rheumatism, neuralgia, etc. **empiric t.** One based on practical observation rather than on scientific reasoning. **expectant t.** Watching the progress of a disease, and not interfering unless special symptoms arise. **holistic t.** Treatment of the patient as a whole. **palliative t.** That which is directed toward relief of symptoms rather than the cure of disease. **preseasonal t.** Prophylactic treatment by injection of pollen extract before the onset of hay fever. **specific t.** A treatment having a proved destructive effect against a specific etiologic factor or having a definite curative effect upon a particular disease. **Wagner-Jauregg t.** Treatment of central nervous system syphilis by fever of artificially induced malaria.

tre·ha'la (tri·hah'luh, tri·hay'luh). A sweet, gummy substance derived from the cocoons of *Larinus maculatus,* an insect that feeds upon a species of Asiatic thistle. Also called *Turkish manna.*

tre'ha·lose (tree'huh·loce, tri·hal'-oce). A disaccharide formed from trehala and certain fungi; it is hydrolyzed by acids to dextrose.

Trem"a·to'da (trem"uh·to'duh). A class of flatworms. The digenetic species are endoparasites of man. The life cycle is complex, involving sexual and asexual reproduction; two intermediate hosts are required. Some of the genera seen most often are *Clonorchis, Fasciola, Fasciolopsis, Opisthorchis, Paragonimus, Schistosoma,* and *Troglotrema.*

Also called *fluke*. **_trem'atode,** *n.,
adj.;* **trem'atoid,** *adj.*

trem"a·to·di'a·sis. Infestation with
a trematode.

trem'bles. A disease occurring in
humans who have ingested milk, butter,
or possibly beef of animals with the
disease. Animals are affected from eating white snakeroot, *Eupatorium ur-
ticaefolium*, or the rayless goldenrod,
Aplopappus heterophyllus. The disease
is afebrile, but there are weakness,
anorexia, vomiting, and sometimes
death. Also called *milk sickness*.

trem'bling. 1. A tremor; quivering.
2. Affected with involuntary muscular
agitation. **—tremble,** *v.*

trem'o·graph (trem'o·graf, tree'-
mo·). A device for recording tremor.

tre"mo·la'bile (tree"mo·lay'bil,
trem"o·). Easily inactivated or destroyed by agitation.

tre"mo·pho'bi·a (tree"mo·fo'bee-
uh, trem"o·). A morbid fear of trembling.

trem'or (trem'ur, tree'mur). A trembling of the voluntary muscles; involuntary rhythmic movements, involving
the entire muscle, or only a circumscribed group of muscle bundles.
coarse t. One with not more than six
or seven vibrations per second. **continuous t.** A form of tremor which
resembles that of paralysis agitans; it
is, however, likely to be remittent, and
may be diminished or arrested by voluntary effort. **essential t.** A familial tremor, associated with no other
stigmas, which is coarse and is exaggerated by action and emotional tension; it begins in adolescence and becomes progressive in old age. **fibrillary t.** Tremor caused by consecutive
contractions of separate muscle fibers.
fine t. One with ten or twelve vibrations per second. **forced t.** The convulsive movements persisting during
repose after voluntary motion, due to
an intermittent and rhythmic irritation of the nervous centers. **hysterical t.** The tremor observed in hysteria,
due to the irregularity of nervous impulses. **intention t.** A slow, coarse
tremor of the limbs which is intensified upon voluntary movement and
may cease on rest. It is present in certain diseases of the nervous system,
notably multiple sclerosis. **mercurial t.** A peculiar form of tremor
observed among smelters and others
exposed to the fumes of mercury. It is
sudden or gradual in onset, and usually
is unaccompanied by excessive salivation. The arms are first involved, and
then the entire muscular system. If
allowed to go on, paralysis and dementia may result. **passive t.** A resting
tremor, *q.v.* **physiologic t.** A tremor

in normal individuals, due to fatigu
apprehension, or overexposure to co
pill rolling t. The behavior of t
hand in Parkinsonism or shaking pals
the action is due to the static trem
and the exaggerated flexion of t
metacarpophalangeal joints. **res
ing t.** A tremor occurring during r
pose. **senile t.** Involuntary, rhyt
mic, oscillatory movements developi
with age; moderate movements are a
parently physiologic changes. **stri
cerebellar t.** That which is prese
while muscles are either at rest or
voluntary movement and which is a
sociated with ataxia and hypotoni
volitional t. A trembling of the e
tire body during voluntary effort,
observed in multiple sclerosis. See i
tention t.

trem"o·sta'ble. Not easily inact
vated or destroyed by agitation.

trem'u·lous. Trembling, quiverin
as tremulous iris.

trench foot. A condition of the fe
somewhat like frostbite; it occurs i
those exposed to cold and damp.

trench mouth. Vincent's stomatiti
q.v.

tre·pan'. See *trephine*.

tre·pan'ning. Boring; using the tre
phine.

tre·phine' (tre·fine', tre·feen'). A
instrument with circular, sawlike edge
for cutting out a disk of bone, usu
ally from the skull. **—trephine,** *v.*

tre·phin'ing (tre·figh'ning, tre·fee
ning). The operation of cutting bor
with a trephine; usually applied to re
moving a segment of cortical bone b
means of a special sawlike instrumen
also applied to removing a portion o
the sclera by means of a specially de
vised instrument, for the relief of ex
cessive intraocular pressure in chron
simple glaucoma.

treph'one. A growth-promoting ho
mone produced by leukocytes, said t
stimulate fibroblastic activity.

trep'i·dant. Trembling.

trep"i·da'tion. 1. Trembling.
Fear; trembling anxiety.

Trep"o·ne'ma. A genus of spiral or
ganisms of the family Treponemacea
T. pallidum. The organism whic
causes syphilis. **T. pertenue.** Th
organism which causes yaws.

trep"o·ne·mi'a·sis. Infection cause
by the *Treponema, q.v.*

trep"o·ne"mi·cid'al (trep"o·nee
mi·sigh'dul, ·nem"i·sigh'dul). 1. De
structive to any treponema. 2. Ant
syphilitic.

trep·op'ne·a. A respiratory distres
present in one recumbent posture an
absent in another.

trep'pe (trep'eh). A progressive, step
wise increase in contraction on re
peated stimulation of a muscle.

tri- (trye-). A combining form denoting *three*.

tri·ac″e·tyl·o″le·an·do·my′cin. The triacetyl ester of the antibiotic oleandomycin. See *cyclamycin*.

tri′ad. 1. A set of three related elements, objects, or symptoms. 2. *In chemistry*, a trivalent atom or radical. **Hutchinson's t.** The combination of notched teeth, interstitial keratitis, and eighth nerve deafness, found in subjects with prenatal syphilis.

tri″a·kai′de·ka·pho′bi·a (try″-ah·ky″di·kuh·fo′bee·uh). Superstitious fear of thirteen. Also called *triskaidekaphobia*.

tri′al. The act of trying or testing.

tri·al″kyl·a·mine′ (trye·al″kil·uh-meen′, trye·al″kil·am′in). See *alkylamine*.

tri′an″gle. 1. A geometrical figure having three sides and three angles. 2. A three-sided area or region having natural or arbitrary boundaries. —**tri·an′gular,** *adj.* **anal t.** One with the base between the two ischial tuberosities and the apex at the coccyx. Syn., *rectal t.* **bladder t.** The triangle formed by the openings of the ureters and the urethra. Syn., *trigone.* **femoral t.** One formed laterally by the medial margin of the sartorius, medially by the lateral margin of the adductor longus, and superiorly by the inguinal ligament. Also called *Scarpa's t.* **Hesselbach's t.** One bounded laterally by the inferior epigastric artery, medially by the rectus abdominis, and inferiorly by the medial half of the inguinal ligament. **t. of auscultation.** Area limited above by the trapezius, below by the latissimus dorsi, and laterally by the vertebral border of the scapula.

tri″a·tom′ic. 1. Consisting of three atoms. 2. Having three atoms of replaceable hydrogen.

tri′a·zol 156. Cyclohexyl-ethyl-triazole. A substance related chemically to metrazol; used as a convulsant in the treatment of schizophrenia.

tri·ba′sic (trye·bay′sick). Having three hydrogen atoms replaceable by bases.

tri″bo·lu″mi·nes′cence (try″bo-lew″mi·ness′uns, trib″o·). Luminosity induced by friction.

tri·bra′chi·us (trye·bray′kee·us). Having three arms.

tri·bro″mo·eth′a·nol (trye·bro″mo·eth′a·nole, ·nol). Tribromoethyl alcohol, Br₃CCH₂OH. White, crystalline powder, soluble in water. **t. solution.** Each cc. contains 1 Gm. of tribromoethanol in amylene hydrate. A clear, colorless liquid of camphoraceous odor. Used as a basal anesthetic. See *avertin with amylene hydrate*.

tri·bro″mo·eth′yl al′co·hol. Tribromoethanol, *q.v.*

tri·bro″mo·meth′ane. Bromoform.

tri·bu′ty·rin (trye·bew′ti·rin). A constituent of butterfat. See *butyrin*.

tri·cal′cic (trye·kal′sick). Containing three atoms of calcium. *Obs.*

tri·cal′ci·um phos′phate. See tribasic *calcium* phosphate.

tri′ceps. 1. Three-headed. 2. A muscle having three heads, as triceps brachii. See Table of Muscles in the Appendix.

trich- (trick-). See *tricho-*.

trich″an·gi·ec·ta′si·a (trick″an-jee·eck·tay′zhuh, ·shuh). Dilatation of the capillaries.

trich″a·tro′phi·a. A brittle state of the hair from atrophy of the hair bulbs.

trich″es·the′si·a, trich″aes·the′si·a (trick″ess·thee′zhuh, ·zee-uh). 1. A peculiar form of tactile sensibility in regions covered with hairs. 2. See *trichoesthesia*.

trich·i′a·sis (trick·eye′uh·sis). An abnormal position of the eyelashes which produces irritation by friction upon the globe. The acquired type usually follows an inflammatory condition that produces distortion.

Trich″i·nel′la (trick″i·nel′uh). A genus of nematode worms which are parasites of man, hogs, rats, dogs, cats, and many other mammals. **T. spiralis.** The species of *Trichinella* found in man.

trich″i·no·pho′bi·a. Morbid fear of trichinosis.

trich″i·no′sis. A disease produced by the ingestion of pork containing *Trichinella spiralis*. It it characterized by nausea, vertigo, fever, diarrhea, prostration, stiffness and painful swelling of muscles, and edema of the face. The intestinal symptoms are due to the development of the adult stage. The muscular and mental symptoms are due to the larval migration through the tissues.

trich·i′tis. Inflammation of the hair bulbs.

tri·chlo″ro·a·ce′tic ac′id (trye·klor″o·a·see′tick). CCl₃.COOH. Colorless, deliquescent crystals, soluble in water. A caustic and astringent.

tri·chlo″ro·bu′tyl al′co·hol. Chlorobutanol.

tri·chlo″ro·bu″tyl·al′de·hyde. Butyl-chloral hydrate.

tri″chlo·ro·bu·tyl′i·dene gly′col. Butyl-chloral hydrate.

tri·chlo″ro·eth′yl·ene. CHCl:CCl₂. A clear, colorless liquid of characteristic odor. An anesthetic administered by inhalation.

tri·chlo″ro·meth′ane. Chloroform.

tri·chlo″ro·phe′nol. C₆H₂Cl₃(OH). White crystals of pronounced germicidal power.

trich'o- (trick'o-), **trich-.** A combining form meaning *hair*.

trich"o·be'zoar. A hair ball or concretion in the stomach or intestine.

trich"o·car'di·a. Inflammation of the pericardium with pseudomembranous elevations.

trich"o·clas·ma'ni·a. An affection characterized by an abnormal desire to break off the hair, usually that of the scalp.

trich"o·ep"i·the"li·o'ma. A skin tumor originating from the hair follicles.

trich"o·es·the'si·a (trick"o-ess-thee'zhuh). The sensation received when a hair is touched.

trich"o·es·the"si·om'e·ter (·ess-thee"zee·om'i·tur, ·ess·thee"see·om'i-tur). An electric appliance for determining the amount of sensation when a hair is touched.

trich'o·gen (trick'o-jen). A substance that stimulates growth of hair.

trich"o·glos'si·a. Hairy tongue; a lengthening of the filiform papillae, producing an appearance as if the tongue were covered with hair.

trich'oid (trick'oyd). Resembling hair.

trich'o·lith. A calcified hair ball within the stomach or intestines.

trich"o·lo'gi·a. 1. Carphology. 2. The plucking out of one's hair.

trich·o'ma·tose (trick·o'muh·toce, ·toze). Matted together.

trich"o·ma·to'sis. An affection of the hair characterized by a matted condition, a result of neglect, filth, and the invasion of parasites.

Trich"o·mo'nas (trick"o·mo'nas, try"ko·). A genus of flagellate protozoa, belonging to the class Mastigophora. Three to five flagella, a thick rodlike axostyle extending throughout the pear-shaped body, and an undulating membrane characterize members of the genus. **T. hominis.** The intestinal form found in man; it is not pathogenic. **T. vaginalis.** The vaginal form which has been implicated in vaginitis.

trich"o·my·co'sis (trick"o·migh·ko'sis, try"ko·). A disease of the hair produced by fungi. **t. circinata.** Ringworm of the scalp. **t. nodosa.** A peculiar but common condition, generally nodose in character, affecting the hairs of the axilla and scrotum and due to the growth of masses of fungous and bacterial material along the hair. Also called *lepothrix*.

trich"o·no'sis (trick"o·no'sis, trikon'o·sis). Any disease of the hair.

trich"o·path"o·pho'bi·a. Undue anxiety and fear regarding the hair, its growth, color, or diseases.

trich·op'a·thy (trick·op'uth·ee). Any disease of the hair. **—trichopath'i** *adj.*

trich·oph'a·gy (trick·of'uh·jee). **trich"o·pha'gi·a.** The eating hair.

trich"o·pho'bi·a. 1. A morbid fe of hair. 2. Trichopathophobia.

trich"o·phy"to·be'zoar. A ball concretion in the stomach or intesti made of hair and fibers of vegetab matter and food detritus.

Trich"o·phy'ton, Trich·oph' ton. A genus of parasitic fungi whi attach to the hair, skin, and nails, a are common allergens. Species a identified by the size and position the spores and by the appearance the colonies on artificial mediums. T lesions of these fungi are included the dermatomycoses or ringworm fections. *In dermatology*, the genus grouped into three main division **Trichophyton ectothrix,** speci which invade the hair shaft but whi also form a persistent sheath of spor outside the shaft; **T. endothri** species which invade the hair she without forming a persistent sheath spores outside the shaft; **T. ne endothrix,** species intermediate character between ectothrix and e dothrix species.

trich"o·phy·to'sis (trick"o·fig to'sis). A contagious disease of sk and hair, occurring mostly in childre and due to skin invasion by the *Trich phyton* fungus. It is characterized circular scaly patches and partial lo of hair.

trich"or·rhe'a (trick"o·ree'uh Rapid loss of the hair.

trich"or·rhex'is. Brittleness of t hair. **t. nodosa.** An atrophic co dition of the hair, affecting more oft the male beard, and characterized irregular thickenings resembling nod on the hair shaft that are really part fractures of the hair. The hairs oft break, leaving a brushlike end; a ce tain amount of alopecia is thus pr duced.

trich"or·rhex"o·ma'ni·a. A con pulsion to break off hairs of the sca or beard with the fingernails.

tri·cho'sis. Any morbid affection the hair.

trich"o·til"lo·ma'ni·a. An u controllable impulse to pull out on hair.

tri·chot'o·my (try·cot'o·mee). vision into three parts.

tri'chro·ism. The property of hibiting three different colors wh viewed in three different aspects. **—t chro'ic,** *adj.*

tri'chro·mat. A person with norm color vision.

tri·chro'mic (try·kro'mick). Able

istinguish the three colors red, blue,
nd green.

·rich·u'ris. A genus of nematodes
f the superfamily Trichinelloidea.
C. trichiu'ra. The species infesting
nan. Transmission is from man to man
y ingestion of mature ova. Also called
*richocephalus dispar, Trichocephalus
richiurus, whipworm.*

·icoloid chloride. A trade-mark
or tricyclamol chloride.

·i·cre'sol (try·kree'sole, ·sol, ·sawl).
:resol. **t, phosphate.** Pale yellow
iquid, chiefly triorthocresyl phosphate,
$CH_3C_6H_4)_3PO_4$: used as plasticizer in
acquers and varnishes. Its ingestion
auses a degeneration of nerve cells.

·i·cus'pid (try·kus'pid). 1. Having
hree cusps, as a tricuspid tooth, or the
ricuspid valve. 2. Affecting, or pro-
lucing at, the tricuspid valve.

·i·cy'cla·mol chlo'ride. 1-Cyclo-
iexyl - 1 - phenyl - 3 - pyrrolidino - 1 - pro-
·anol methylchloride, an anticholiner-
ic agent. See *elorine chloride, tri-
·oloid chloride.*

·i·dac'tyl. Having three digits.

·idione. Trade-mark for trimetha-
lione.

·id'y·mus. Triplet.

·i·eth"a·nol'am·ine (try·eth"uh-
ioal'uh·meen, ·nol'uh·meen). $N(CH_2-$
:H_2.OH)_2. Colorless, viscid, hygroscopic
iquid miscible with water and alcohol.
he commercial article contains up to
5% of diethanolamine and up to 2.5%
f monoethanolamine. A solvent and
mulsifying agent.

·i·eth"yl·a·mine' (try·eth"il·uh-
ieen', ·am'een). $(C_2H_5)_3N$. A colorless
iquid of strong ammoniacal odor.

·i·eth'yl·ene gly'col. $HO.CH_2-$
:H_2.O.CH_2.CH_2.O.CH_2.CH_2.OH. Color-
ess, hygroscopic, practically odorless
iquid; miscible with water or alcohol.
.s an aerosol it is bactericidal in con-
entration of 0.005 mg. per liter of air.

·i·eth'yl·ene mel'a·mine. 2,4,6-
·ri(ethylenimino)-s-triazine, a com-
ound chemically related to one of
he nitrogen mustard analogs, used as
palliative in treating certain neo-
lastic diseases. Abbreviated, TEM.

·i·fa'cial nerve (try·fay'shul). Old
erm for the fifth cranial nerve, so
alled because it divides into three
nain branches that supply the face.

·i·for'mol. Paraformaldehyde.

·i·gem'i·nal. 1. Triple; dividing
nto three parts, as the trigeminal
erve. 2. Pertaining to the trigeminal
erve. See Table of Nerves in the Ap-
endix.

·i·gem'i·nus. The fifth cranial
erve.

·i'gone. 1. Triangle. 2. The smooth
riangular area on the inner surface of
he bladder between the orifices of the
wo ureters and the internal urethral

orifice. Also called *vesical t., t. of the
bladder.* Formerly called *t. of Lieu-
taud.* **—trig'onal,** *adj.*

Trig"o·nel'la (trig"o·nel'uh, try"-
go·). A genus of the Leguminosae.

tri'go·nid (try'go·nid, try·go'nid).
The first three cusps (viewed as one) of
a lower molar tooth.

tri"go·ni'tis (try"go·nigh'tis, trig"-
o·). Inflammation of the trigone of the
bladder.

tri"hex·y·phen'i·dyl. Nonproprietary name for 3-(1-piperidyl) -1-phenyl-
1-cyclohexyl-1-propanol hydrochloride,
an antispasmodic drug. See *artane.*

tri·hy'dric. Containing three atoms
of hydrogen replaceable by metals.

tri·hy'drol. An associated form of
water having the composition $(H_2O)_3$.

tri"hy·drox"y·ben·zo'ic ac'id.
Gallic acid, *q.v.*

tri"hy·drox"y·oes'trin (try"-
high·drock"see·es'trin). See *estriol.*

tri·i"o·do·meth'ane (try·eye"o·do-
meth'ane). Iodoform.

tri·i"o·do·thy'ro·nine. An amino
acid isolated from human blood and
prepared synthetically, chemically and
therapeutically similar to thyroxin,
but containing one less iodine atom
and exerting more rapid biological activity.

tri·ke"to·cho·lan'ic ac'id (try-
kee"to·ko·lan'ick). 3,7,12-Triketocho-
lanic acid. The compound resulting
from the oxidation of the three secondary alcohol groups of cholic acid to
ketone linkages.

tri·ke"to·pu'rine (try·kee"to·pew'-
reen, ·rin). Uric acid.

trilafon. Trade-mark for perphena-
zine.

tri·lam'i·nar (try·lam'i·nur). Three-
layered.

trilene. Trade-mark for a brand of
trichloroethylene.

tri"li·no'le·in. Glyceryl linoleate,
$(C_{18}H_{31}O_2)_3C_3H_5$, occurring in many
vegetable oils.

tri·lo'bate (try·lo'bayt). Three-lobed.

tri·man'u·al. Accomplished by the
aid of three hands.

tri·men'su·al. Occurring at periods
of three months.

tri·mes'ter (try·mes'tur). A stage or
period of three months.

tri"meth·a·di'one. Nonproprietary
title for the substance 3,5,5-trimethyl-
oxazolidine-2,4-dione, available under
the trade-marked name *tridione.*

**tri·meth'a·phan   cam"phor-
sul'fon·ate.** d-3,4-(1',3'-Dibenzyl-2'-
ketoimidazolido) -1,2-trimethylenethio-
phanium d-camphorsulfonate, a hypotensive agent. See *arfonad camphorsulfonate.*

tri·meth"yl·a·mine' (try·meth"il-
uh·meen', ·am'een). $(CH_3)_3N$. Colorless
gas of fishy ammoniacal odor, **very**

soluble in water. Produced by bacterial action on decayed animal matter or synthesized. Also called *secaline*.

tri·meth″yl·gly′cine (try-meth′-il-gly′seen, ·gly-seen′). See *betaine*.

tri·meth″yl·xan′thine (try-meth″il-zan′theen, ·thin). Caffeine.

trimeton. Trade-mark for a brand of the antihistaminic substance prophenpyridamine.

tri·ni″tro·phe′nol. $C_6H_2(NO_2)_3OH$. 2,4,6-Trinitrophenol, pale yellow crystals; soluble in water. It is germicidal and astringent. Syn., *carbazotic acid*, *picric acid*.

tri·o′le·in. See *olein*.

tri′ose. A monosaccharide containing three carbon atoms in the molecule.

tri″ose·phos·phor′ic ac′id. Triose phosphate. A phosphorylated three-carbon sugar. Several of these compounds are intermediaries in the breakdown of glycogen to pyruvic acid in carbohydrate metabolism.

tri·ox″y·meth′yl·ene. Paraformaldehyde.

tri·ox″y·pu′rine (try-ock″si-pew′reen, ·rin). Uric acid.

tri·pal′mi·tin. See *palmitin*.

trip′a·ra. A woman who has borne three children.

tri″pel·en′na·mine hy″dro·chlo′ride. Nonproprietary name for the antihistaminic substance N,N-dimethyl-N′-benzyl-N′-(α-pyridyl) ethylenediamine. See *pyribenzamine*.

tri·pep′tide, tri·pep′tid. A protein hydrolysis product representing condensation of three molecules of amino acids.

tri·phen″yl·eth′yl·ene. $(C_6H_5)_2$-C:CH(C_6H_5). A proestrogen potentiated as estrogen by passage through liver.

tri·phen″yl·meth′ane. Rosaniline dye.

tri·ple′gi·a. Hemiplegia with the additional paralysis of one limb on the opposite side.

trip′le point. The single temperature and pressure at which the solid, liquid, and vapor forms of a substance may coexist.

trip′le re·sponse′. See triple *response*.

trip′let. 1. One of three children born at one birth. 2. *In optics*, a system consisting of three lenses.

trip·lo′pi·a. A disturbance of vision in which three images of a single object are seen.

tris-. 1. A prefix meaning *thrice*. 2. *In chemistry*, a prefix denoting *the tripling of a complex expression*.

tri·sac′cha·ride (try-sack′uh·ride, ·rid). A carbohydrate which, on hydrolysis, yields three molecules of monosaccharides.

tris′mus (triz′mus). 1. Tonic spasm

of the muscles of mastication. 2. [ ] term for lockjaw. See *tetanus*, 1.

tris′tis. 1. Sad; gloomy. 2. Dull color.

tri·sul″fa·py·rim′i·dines. A m[ ] ture of equal parts of sulfadiaz[ ] sulfamerazine, and sulfamethazine[ ]

trit′i·cin. 1. A gumlike substa[ ] found in *Triticum repens*. 2. A p[ ] prietary food preparation.

Trit′i·cum. A genus of the G[ ] mineae. **T. sativum** is wheat.

trit′i·cum. The dried rhizome a[ ] roots of *Agropyron repens*, family G[ ] mineae. A diuretic. Syn., *couch gra[ ]* Also called *dog-grass*.

trit′i·um (trit′ee·um, trish′ee·un[ ] The hydrogen isotope with mass thr[ ] It is radioactive, displaying a be[ ] activity with a half-life of 12.3 yea[ ]

tri′ton. The nucleus of the trit[ ] atom, containing two neutrons and o[ ] proton thus bearing a positive cha[ ] of one.

trit′o·pine (trit′o·peen, ·pyne). alkaloid, $C_{20}H_{23}NO_4$, of opium. Sy[ ] *laudanine*.

tri″to·tox′in. One of the th[ ] group into which Ehrlich classi[ ] toxins, according to the avidity w[ ] which they combine with antitoxi[ ] tritotoxin combining least readily. S[ ] *prototoxin*.

trit·u·rate. 1. Reduce to a fine po[ ] der. 2. A finely divided powder. 3. [ ] powdered substances in a mortar w[ ] the aid of a pestle. **tablet t[ ]** molded tablet as distinguished from [ ] compressed tablet. Generally prepar[ ] in a base of sucrose and lactose.

trit′u·ra′tion. 1. The process of [ ] ducing a solid substance to a powder [ ] rubbing. 2. The product obtained [ ] triturating together 10 Gm. of a po[ ] dered medicinal substance and 90 G[ ] of powdered lactose.

tri·va′lence (try-vay′luns, triv′[ ] luns). The quality of having a valen[ ] of three.—**trivalent**, *adj*.

tri·valv′u·lar (try-valv′yoo·lu[ ] Having three valves.

tro′car. A surgical instrument [ ] puncturing cavities for the removal [ ] fluid contained therein. It consists [ ] hollow tube or cannula within which [ ] a snugly fitting bayonet-pointed sty[ ] or perforating core whose point p[ ] trudes beyond the beveled cann[ ] end. The entire instrument is used [ ] puncture a cavity, the perforator be[ ] removed when it is desired to be[ ] evacuation of the fluid.

troch. Trochiscus, troche.

tro·chan′ter (tro-can′tur). One [ ] two processes on the upper extrem[ ] of the femur below the neck. T[ ] **greater trochanter** is situated [ ] the outer, and the **lesser trocha[ ]**

ter on the inner, side of the bone. —**trochanter'ic**, adj.

tro'che (tro'kee). A lozenge. Abbreviated, troch.

tro·chis'cus (tro-kis'kus) (pl. *trochisci*). Troche. Abbreviated, troch.

troch'le·a (trock'lee-uh) (pl. *trochleae*). A part or process having the nature of a pulley.

troch'le·ar. 1. Of the nature of, or pertaining to, a pulley. 2 The trochlear nerve, the fourth cranial nerve. See Table of Nerves in the Appendix.

troch"o·car'di·a (trock"o-kahr'dee-uh, tro"ko-). Displacement of the heart by rotation on its long axis.

troch"or·i"zo·car'di·a (trock"or-eye"zo-kahr'dee-uh). Form of displacement of the heart characterized by rotation and change to horizontal position.

Trom·bic'u·la. A genus of mites; the larvae are blood suckers and cause a severe dermatitis. **T. akamushi.** A vector of *Rickettsia tsutsugamushi*, the cause of tsutsugamushi disease. **T. alfreddugesi.** The species which causes an annoying dermatitis; widely distributed in North America. Also called *chigger, red bug*, T. *irritans*. **T. irritans.** The chigger mite of eastern North America; attacks man and other mammals.

trom·bic"u·lo'sis. Infestation with *Trombicula*.

tromexan. A trade-mark for bis-3,3'-(4-oxycoumarinyl) ethyl acetate, an anticoagulant drug.

trom"o·ma'ni·a. Delirium tremens.

tro'na. A native compound of sodium carbonate and sodium bicarbonate. $Na_2.CO_2.NaHCO_3.2H_2O$.

tro"pa·co·caine' (tro"puh-ko-kayn', -ko'kayn). Benzoyl-pseudotropine. $C_{15}H_{19}NO_2$. An alkaloid in Java coca leaves; also prepared synthetically.

tro·pae'o·lin (tro-pee'o-lin). An indefinite name for several dyes used as pH indicators; so called because their colors resemble the flowers of *Tropaeolum*, the garden nasturtium. **t. D.** Methyl orange. **t. G.** Metanil yellow. **t. O.** Sodium azoresorcinol-sulfanilate. $NaSO_2.C_6H_4.N:N.C_6H_3(OH)_2$. Brown powder used as indicator. Yellow at pH 11; orange-brown at pH 12.7. Also called *resorcinol yellow*. **t. OO.** Sodium *p*-diphenylamine-azobenzenesulfonate. $NaSO_2.C_6H_4.N:N.C_6H_4.NH.C_6H_5$. Yellow powder used as indicator. Red at pH 1.4; yellow at pH 2.6. **t. OOO.** Sodium azo-α-naphtholsulfanilate. $NaSO_2.C_6H_4.N:N.C_{10}H_5.OH$. Reddish brown powder used as color for foods, drugs, and cosmetics, and as indicator. Brownish yellow at pH 7.6; purple at pH 8.9. Also called *orange I*. **t. R.** See t. O.

tro·pe·ine (tro'pee-een, -in). An ester

of tropine and an organic acid, as atropine and homatropine.

tro·pe'o·lin. See *tropaeolin*.

tro"phe·de'ma, tro"phoe·de'ma (tro"fi-dee'muh, trof"i-). Localized chronic edema due to damaged nourishment or nerve supply.

troph'e·sy. Defective nutrition of a part from disorder of the nerves regulating nutrition; trophoneurosis. —**trophe'sial, trophe'sic**, adj.

troph'ic. Pertaining to the functions concerned in nutrition, digestion, and assimilation.

-troph'ic. A combining form denoting *nourishing* or *of* or *pertaining to nutrition*. Also see -*tropic*. —**tro'phy**, n.

tro·phic'i·ty (tro-fiss'i-tee). Trophic influence or state.

troph'ism. 1. Nutrition. 2. Trophicity.

tro'pho-, troph'o-, troph-. A combining form denoting *relation to nutrition* or *to nourishment*.

tro'pho·blast (tro'fo-blast, trof'o-). The outer, ectodermal epithelium of the mammalian blastocyst or chorion and chorionic villi. See *cytotrophoblast, syncytiotrophoblast*. —**trophoblas'tic**, adj.

tro"pho·blas·to'ma. Chorionic carcinoma.

tro"pho·dy·nam'ics (tro"fo-dye-nam'icks, trof"o-). The laws governing nutrition.

tro·phol'o·gy. The science of nutrition.

tro"pho·neu·ro'sis. Any disease of a part due to disturbance of the nerves or nerve centers with which it is connected.

tro"pho·nu'cle·us. The nucleus which is concerned with the nutrition of a unicellular organism and not with its reproduction.

tro·phop'a·thy. A disorder of nutrition.

tro"pho·ther'a·py. Dietotherapy.

tro"pho·zo'ite. The final product of sexual multiplication of sporozoa of the genera *Coccidia* and *Plasmodium*. Found within the tissues of a host.

-trop'ic. A combining form denoting *a turning*. Also see -*trophic*. —**tro'py**, n.

trop'ic ac'id. $CH_2OH.CH(C_6H_5).$-$COOH$. α-Phenyl-β-hydroxypropionic acid. White crystals. Atropine is an ester of tropic acid and tropine.

trop'i·cal. Pertaining to the tropical zone of the earth, as the belt lying between the Tropic of Cancer and that of Capricorn.

tro'pin. Any one of the substances in the blood serum which make bacteria susceptible to phagocytosis. See *bacteriotropin*.

tro'pine (tro'peen, -pin). $C_8H_{15}NO$. A product of the hydrolysis of atropine.

White, hygroscopic crystals. See *tropic acid*.

tro'pi·none. $C_8H_{13}NO$. A substance formed by oxidation of tropine and used in the synthesis of atropine substitutes.

tro'pism. The involuntary bending, turning, or orientation of an organism toward **(positive tropism)**, or away from **(negative tropism)**, a stimulus. Also see *taxis*. 2. **chemotropism.** The response to chemical agents. **phototropism.** The response to light.

-tro·pism. A combining form meaning *a tendency to turn, an affinity for.*

tro·pom'e·ter. 1. An instrument for measuring the various rotations of the eyeball. 2. One for estimating the amount of torsion in long bones.

tro'po·sphere. The atmosphere which lies between the stratosphere and the earth's surface, a zone of marked changes in temperature, with ascending and descending air currents and cloud formation.

troy weight. See Tables of Weights and Measures in the Appendix.

true. Real; not false.

trun'cat·ed (trunk'ay·tid). 1. With the top cut off; shortened in height. 2. Deprived of limbs or accessory parts.

trun'cus (pl. *trunci*). Trunk, *q.v.*

trunk. 1. The torso; the body without head or limbs. 2. The main stem of a blood vessel, lymphatic, or nerve.

truss. Any mechanical apparatus for preventing the recurrence of a hernial protrusion which has been reduced. The term includes simple devices such as a yarn truss for the control of infantile inguinal hernia, as well as complicated pieces of apparatus with pressure pads designed to hold large inguinal or abdominal hernias.

trych"o·phy·to'sis. See *trichophytosis*.

trypaflavin. Trade-mark for acriflavine. **acid t.** Trade-mark for acriflavine hydrochloride.

tryp'an blue (trip'an, try'pan). A complex azo dye, occurring as a blue powder; used as a vital stain.

tryp'a·nide. Any eruption of the skin observed in trypanosomiasis.

try·pan'o·cide" (tri·pan'o·side", trip'uh·no·side"). An agent that destroys trypanosomes. **—trypanoci'dal,** *adj.*

Tryp"a·no·so'ma (trip"uh·no·so'muh, try"puh·no·). A genus of protozoa belonging to the class Mastigophora. They are slender, elongate organisms with a central nucleus, posterior blepharoplast, and an undulatory membrane, from which a free flagellum projects forward. Transmitted by insect vectors. **T. cruzi.** The cause of Chagas' disease in South America and of American trypanosomiasis. **T. gambiense.**

The cause of mid-African sleeping sickness. **T. rhodesiense.** An organism which causes East African sleeping sickness.

tryp"a·no·so·mi'a·sis (trip"uh·no·so·my'uh·sis, try"puh·no·, try·pan"o·). Any of the several diseases due to infection with the various species of *Trypanosoma*; characterized by irregular fever and palpable lymph nodes. **American t.** That in which the causative agent is *Trypanosoma cruzi*. Also called *barbiero fever, Brazilian t., Chagas' disease, South American t.* **Gambian t.** That in which the causative agent is *Trypanosoma gambiense*. Also called *mid-African sleeping sickness*. **Rhodesian t.** That in which the causative agent is *Trypanosoma rhodesiense*. Also called *East African sleeping sickness*.

tryp·pan'o·so·mide" (tri·pan'o·so·mide"). A skin lesion in any disease caused by a trypanosome.

tryp'an red (trip'an, try'pan). A complex azo dye, occurring as a reddish brown powder, recommended in the treatment of trypanosomiasis. Also used in vital staining.

tryp'an·roth. See *trypan red*.

tryp·ars'a·mide (tri·pahr'suh·mid) (HO) $OAs(ONa) C_6H_4.NH.CH_2.CO.NH_2$. Sodium N-phenylglycineamide-p-arsonate, a white, crystalline powder, soluble in water. Used in treatment of trypanosomiasis and syphilis.

tryp'sin. The proteolytic enzyme resulting from the action of the enterokinase of intestinal juice upon the trypsinogen secreted in the pancreatic juice. It catalyzes the hydrolysis of peptide linkages in proteins and partially hydrolyzed proteins. Syn., *tryptase. —tryptic, adj.*

tryp·sin'o·gen. The zymogen of trypsin, occurring in the pancreatic juice and converted to trypsin by enterokinase in the small intestine. Syn. *protrypsin.*

tryp'tase. See *trypsin*.

tryp"to·lyt'ic. Of, or pertaining to the hydrolysis of proteins caused by trypsin.

tryp'to·phan, tryp'to·phane. α-Amino-β-indole propionic acid, an essential amino acid widely distributed in animal and some plant proteins.

T. S. Test solution.

tset'se fly (tset'see, tet'see). Any dipterous insect of the genus *Glossina* almost wholly restricted to Africa. *Glossina* flies carry the flagellate trypanosomes, the causative agents of nagana in cattle, and of the African sleeping sickness in man.

tsp. Teaspoon.

tu'a·mine sul'fate (tew'uh·meen ·min). Trade-mark for 2-aminoheptane sulfate, $(C_7H_{15}NH_2)_2.H_2SO_4$, a local vasoconstrictor.

tu′ba (pl. *tubae*). A tube. **t. audi-tiva.** The auditory or Eustachian tube, *q.v.* **t. uterina.** The uterine or Fallopian tube.

tu′bage. The introduction of a tube or catheter. **t. of the glottis.** See *intubation.* Obs.

tube. A hollow, cylindrical structure, especially a uterine tube or an auditory tube. **auditory t.** The canal, lined by mucous membrane, with partly bony, partly cartilaginous support, connecting the pharynx with the tympanic cavity on each side. Also called *tuba auditiva* [BNA], *pharyngotympanic tube, Eustachian tube.* **cathode t.** An evacuated tube, frequently with a thin window opposite the cathode, to permit cathode rays to emerge from the tube. **Crookes t.** A highly exhausted vacuum tube used in producing x-rays. **drainage t.** A hollow tube of glass, rubber, or other material inserted into a wound or cavity to allow the escape of fluids. **Eustachian t.** See auditory *t.* **Fallopian t.** A uterine tube. See *oviduct.* **feeding t.** One for introducing food into the stomach. **Geiger-Müller t.** A tube which, when attached to a potential source, will produce an electric pulse each time an ionizing particle penetrates its walls. **hot cathode t.** A modern highly evacuated roentgen-ray tube with a hot filament cathode for the production of an abundant and controllable stream of cathode rays. **intubation t.** A tube for insertion into the larynx through the mouth in laryngeal diphtheria, etc. **Miller-Abbott t.** An intestinal catheter, approximately 2.5 meters in length, having a double lumen; the smaller lumen is for inflation of a small balloon near the end of the tube which acts as a bolus stimulating peristalsis to carry the tube to the desired location; the larger lumen is for aspiration of intestinal contents. The tube is used for relief of distention due to obstruction in the small intestine. **nasotracheal t.** A rubber tube or catheter inserted into the trachea by way of the nasal cavity and pharynx. **roentgen t.** An evacuated vessel containing a source of electrons and two electrodes, the positive anode and the negative cathode at a considerable potential difference; the cathode contains the source of electrons, as a hot filament, and the anode is of sturdy construction to withstand bombardment by the cathode rays. At the anode the energy of the cathode rays is converted into 98% of heat energy and 2% of roentgen rays. **stomach t.** A flexible tube used for irrigation or evacuation of the stomach. **test t.** A cylindrical

glass tube with one end open; used for growing cultures of bacteria, or for chemical analysis. **tracheotomy t.** A metal tube placed in the opening made in a tracheotomy, and through which breathing is carried on.

tu·bec′to·my. Salpingectomy; excision of a tube, specifically uterine tube.

tu′ber (pl. *tubera*). 1. A thickened portion of an underground stem. 2. Any rounded swelling or mass. Also see *tuberosity, eminence.*

tu′ber·cle. 1. A small nodule. 2. A rounded prominence on a bone. 3. The specific lesion produced by the tubercle bacillus, consisting of a collection of lymphocytes and epithelioid cells, at times with giant cells. **Darwin′s t.** A blunt tubercle projecting from the upper free margin of the helix toward the center of the auricle. **Ghon t.** The primary tubercle of air-borne tuberculosis formed in the periphery of a lung just beneath the pleura. **miliary t.** One of the many minute tubercles uniformly distributed throughout an organ or organs, caused by tubercle bacilli.

tu·ber′cu·lar. Characterized by the presence of small nodules or tubercles. Used erroneously for tuberculous, *q.v.*

tu·ber′cu·lid, tu·ber′cu·lide. A group of varied skin manifestations from tuberculosis of viscera. The skin changes often begin with necrosis in the derma; later there is involvement of the epidermis followed by ulceration. They are considered to be caused either by bacillary embolisms or by toxins from tubercle bacilli.

tu·ber′cu·lin. A material containing the proteins of the tubercle bacillus, or products derived from such proteins and capable of eliciting an inflammatory reaction in the tissues of a human or animal body which has been sensitized either by tuberculosis or by inoculation with living or dead tubercle bacilli. **old t.** A broth culture of tubercle bacilli, sterilized by heat, filtered, and concentrated by evaporation. Abbreviated, O.T., T.O.

tu·ber″cu·lo·der′ma. A cutaneous manifestation of the action of tubercle bacilli; a tuberculid.

tu·ber″cu·lo·fi′broid. Relating to a tubercle (3) that has undergone fibroid degeneration.

tu·ber′cu·loid. Resembling tuberculosis or a tubercle.

tu·ber″cu·lo′ma. A conglomerate caseous tubercle, usually solitary, which has attained such a size as to suggest the appearance of a tumor.

tu·ber″cu·lo·pho′bi·a. Morbid fear of tuberculosis.

tu·ber″cu·lo·sil″i·co′sis. Chronic inflammation of the lungs, caused by the combined action of tubercle bacilli and silicon dioxide. This term is preferred in South Africa to silicotuberculosis, which is in common use. See *silicotuberculosis*.

tu·ber″cu·lo'sis. An infectious disease caused by the *Mycobacterium tuberculosis*, commonly known as the tubercle bacillus. It may affect any organ or tissue of the body, but most deaths are due to tuberculosis of the lungs. The two characteristic types of tissue reaction are the exudative, consisting of acute inflammation, and the productive or proliferative, consisting of tubercle formation. Sometimes abbreviated, t. b. Formerly called *phthisis.* **active t.** That which is undergoing change, either progressive or retrogressive; causing, or threatening to cause, clinical symptoms or disability. Also called *acute disseminated t.* **acute generalized miliary t.** That in which miliary tubercles are widely distributed through the body by transmission of tubercle bacilli in large numbers through the blood stream. **avian t.** A form found in birds. **bovine t.** A form found in cattle, transmitted to man usually by raw milk from infected cows. Also see glandular *t.,* t. of bones and joints. **bronchogenic t.** That resulting from extension of infection within the lung by way of the air passages. Also called *bronchogenous t.* **bronchopneumonic t.** An exudative reaction in the lung caused by the tubercle bacillus, having the distribution of bronchopneumonia. Also see *pneumonia.* **caseous pneumonic t.** Exudative tuberculosis of the lung which has undergone a characteristic type of necrosis, simulating cheese in its gross appearance. **chronic fibroid t.** Slowly progressive pulmonary tuberculosis with extensive fibrosis and mild symptoms. **chronic miliary t.** A condition in which healing or healed miliary tubercles are distributed through one or more organs as a result of transmission of tubercle bacilli in small numbers through the blood stream. **chronic ulcerative t.** The most prevalent type of pulmonary tuberculosis in which necrosis has been followed by the formation of cavities surrounded by varying degrees of fibrosis. It represents a later stage in the evolution of either exudative or proliferative tuberculosis, and may coexist with lesions of either or both of these types. **closed t.** Pulmonary tuberculosis not discharging tubercle bacilli; it is therefore not capable of transmission to other persons. **cutis orificialis t.** Ulcerative tuberculosis of the skin. **endogenous t.** That arising from a source within the body; especially disease caused by bacilli transmitted through lymphatic

or blood vessels, or both, to anothe[r] organ, usually to the lungs. **exoge[-] nous t.** That arising from a sourc[e] outside the body. **extrapulmo[-] nary t.** That occurring in any par[t] of the body except in the lungs, as i[n] bones, joints, meninges, skin, or in[-] testines. **far advanced t.** (Ac[-] cording to the National Tuberculosi[s] Association classification). That i[n] which there are lesions more extensiv[e] than moderately advanced. **fibroid t[.]** Chronic tuberculosis, usually in th[e] upper lobe of the lung, associated wit[h] extensive fibrosis. **glandular t[.]** That affecting the lymph nodes, espe[-] cially the cervical, bronchial, and mes[-] enteric. Usually due to bovine tubercu[-] losis. **hematogenous t.** Any mani[-] festation resulting from the transmis[-] sion of tubercle bacilli through th[e] blood stream. **inactive t.** That whic[h] is in a state of partial or complete heal[-] ing, causing no clinical symptoms o[r] disability; it shows no change over [a] prolonged period of time. **incipient t[.]** The earliest stage of pulmonary tuber[-] culosis in point of time. Often confuse[d] with minimal tuberculosis which re[-] fers only to the extent of disease. **la[-] tent t.** That which shows no chang[e] over a prolonged period of time, but i[s] incompletely healed and potentiall[y] active. **lobar pneumonic t.** A[n] exudative reaction in the lung cause[d] by the tubercle bacillus, having th[e] characteristic distribution of loba[r] pneumonia. **lymphogenic t.** Me[-] tastasis from any focus to another b[y] way of the lymph channels. Also calle[d] *lymphogenous t.* **minimal t.** (Ac[-] cording to the National Tuberculosi[s] Association classification.) Tubercu[-] losis in which there are slight lesion[s] without demonstrable excavation con[-] fined to a small part of one or bot[h] lungs. The total extent of the lesion[s] regardless of distribution, shall no[t] exceed the equivalent of the volum[e] of lung tissue which lies above th[e] second chondrosternal junction an[d] the spine of the fourth or the body o[f] the fifth thoracic vertebra on one side[.] **moderately advanced t.** Tha[t] in which both lungs may be involve[d] but the total extent of the lesions sha[ll] not exceed the following limits: sligh[t] disseminated lesions which may exten[d] through not more than the volume o[f] one lung, or the equivalent of this i[n] both lungs; dense and confluent lesion[s] which may extend through not mor[e] than the equivalent of one-third th[e] volume of one lung. Any graduatio[n] within the above limits. Total diamete[r] of cavities, if present, is estimated no[t] to exceed 4 cm. **open t.** Pulmonar[y] tuberculosis in an infectious state; it i[s] capable of transmission to other per[-] sons. **pelvic t.** Tuberculosis of the uterine tubes which has spread to other pelvic structures or organs. **primary t.** The reaction which follows the first implantation of tubercle bacilli in the body. It consists of a caseous focal reaction in the parenchyma of the organ and a similar reaction in the regional lymph node or nodes. Both foci usually run a benign course and undergo healing with calcification. The most frequent site is the lung. Also called *primary phase, primary infection, primary focus, primary complex, childhood type t.* **pulmonary t.** Tuberculosis resulting from inhalation of tubercle bacilli. **reinfection t.** That which includes all manifestations of tuberculosis other than the primary phase. It exhibits in varying degree the influence of two factors not operative in primary tuberculosis; acquired resistance, and hypersensitivity of the tissues to tuberculin. It is characterized especially by an increased capacity for destruction of tissue, and by acceleration of both the early, exudative reaction and the subsequent, productive reaction. Also called *adult type t.* **t. cutis.** That affecting the skin. It occurs in many forms and is more frequent in Europe than in America. Also see *t. lichenoides, tuberculid.* **t. lichenoides.** A skin eruption consisting of groups of papules, usually on the trunk, seen in subjects suffering from tuberculosis, especially the glandular and bone types of the disease. Also called *lichen scrofulosus, chronic miliary t. of the skin.* **t. of bones and joints.** That affecting bones and joints, characterized by bone destruction and the formation of cold abscesses. Usually due to bovine tuberculosis. **t. verrucosa.** A type of warty skin eruption, usually on the hands and arms, due to inoculation with the tubercle bacillus from handling meat of infected cattle or infected human material.

tu·ber'cu·lous. Affected with, or caused by, tuberculosis.

tu·ber'cu·lum (pl. *tubercula*). Tubercle, *q.v.* **t. costae.** Tubercle of a rib.

tu"ber·os'i·ty. A protuberance on a bone. **deltoid t.** A rough elevation about the middle of the anterolateral surface of the humerus for the insertion of the deltoid muscle. **iliac t.** A rough, elevated area above the articular surface on the inner aspect of the ala of the ilium, which gives attachment to the posterior sacroiliac ligament, and from which the sacrospinalis and multifidus muscles take origin. **ischial t.** A protuberance on the posterior portion of the superior ramus of the ischium, upon which the body rests in sitting. **radial t.** The large emi-

nence on the medial side of the upper extremity of the radius, into which the tendon of the biceps brachii muscle is inserted. **t. of the tibia.** An oblong elevation on the anterior surface of the upper extremity of the tibia, to which the patellar tendon is attached. **t. of the ulna.** A rough eminence below coronoid process on anterior surface of ulna, which gives insertion to part of the brachialis muscle.

tu'bo-. A combining form denoting *pertaining to a tube.*

tu"bo·ad·nex'o·pex"y. Surgical fixation of the uterine adnexa.

tu"bo·cu·ra're (tew"bo-cue-rah'ree). Curare so named because of its tube shape, the result of being packed in hollow bamboo canes.

tu"bo·cu·ra'rine (·cue-rah'reen, ·rin). An alkaloid, $C_{19}H_{21}NO_4$, in tubocurare prepared from *Chondodendron tomentosum*. It is responsible for the typical action of curare. Also called *d-tubocurarine.* See *intocostrin.*

tu"bo·o·va"ri·ot'o·my. Excision of a uterine tube and ovary.

tu"bo·per"i·to·ne'al. Relating to the oviducts and the peritoneum.

tu'bu·lar. 1. Shaped like a tube. 2. Pertaining to or affecting tubules, as tubular nephritis. 3. Produced in a tube, as tubular breathing.

tu'bule. 1. A small tube. 2. *In anatomy,* any minute, tube-shaped structure. **collecting tubules.** The ducts conveying the urine from the renal tubules (nephrons) to the minor calyxes of the renal pelvis. **convoluted tubules.** (a) The contorted tubules of the testis. (b) The parts of the renal tubule which lie in the cortex, as the proximal and distal convoluted portions of the nephron. **seminiferous t.** Any one of the tubules of a testis. **uriniferous t.** One of the numerous winding tubules of the kidney; the tubule of a nephron.

tu"bu·li·za'tion. Protection of the ends of nerves, after neurorrhaphy, by an absorbable cylinder.

tu"bu·lo·al·ve'o·lar (·al-vee'o-lur, ·al'vee·o·lur). Consisting of a system of branching tubules which terminate in alveoli, as in the salivary glands. Also called *tubuloacinous.*

tu'bu·lo·cyst". A cystic dilatation occurring in an occluded canal or duct.

tu'bu·lus (pl. *tubuli*). A small, tube-like structure; a tubule.

tug, tug'ging. A jerking, pulling, or drawing.

tu"la·re'mi·a. An infectious disease due to the bacterium, *Pasteurella tularensis,* and transmitted to man by the handling of infected rabbits or other rodents or by the bite of a blood-sucking insect.

tu"me·fa'cient (tew"mi·fay'shunt).

Swelling; swollen, or tending to cause swelling.

tu″me·fac′tion. 1. A swelling. 2. The act of swelling.

tu′me·fy (tew′mi·figh). 1. Swell. 2. Cause to swell.

tu·men′ti·a (tew-men′shee-uh). Vasomotor disturbance characterized by irregular swellings in the legs and arms.

tu·mes′cence. 1. The condition of growing tumid. 2. A swelling.

tu·mid′i·ty. The state of being swollen. **_tumid_,** adj.

tu′mor. 1. A swelling. 2. Specifically, a new growth of cells or tissues characterized by autonomy, that is, independent of the laws of growth of the host. It is progressive, of unknown cause, and in malignant form limited only by the nutrition provided by the host. **—tumorous, tumoral,** adj. **adipose t.** Lipoma. **amyloid t.** A nonmalignant nodule situated usually on a vocal fold, a few millimeters in diameter, spherical and often pedunculated. Made up principally of a hyaline acidophilic substance which has staining reactions like primary amyloid. Less often found in the wall of the urinary bladder and rarely in other sites. **benign t.** One that grows by expansion, is usually encapsulated, and does not exhibit the features of malignant tumors. **Ewing's t.** Endothelial myeloma. A true bone tumor occurring usually in the shaft of a long bone, producing a fusiform swelling. It is invasive, does not metastasize, but is apt to recur. Presumed to be of endothelial origin. Syn., _angioendothelioma_. **fibroid t.** A fibroma; also often used to mean a fibromyoma of the uterus. **follicular t.** A sebaceous cyst. **giant-cell t.** (a) Epulis; a giant-cell tumor of the jaw. (b) One of bone occurring at the end of a long bone causing thinning of the compact bone and characterized by the presence of giant cells. **glomus t.** A tumor derived from a glomus body of the skin, especially of the digits, which is usually small, blue, painful, and benign. Also called _angioneuromyoma, pericytoma, glomangioma_. **granulosa-cell t.** A tumor of the ovary possessing endocrine activity. **histioid t.** One in which the tumor is made up almost entirely of a single type of cell. **homologous t.** A tumor consisting of tissue identical with that of the organ from which it springs. **hypophyseal-duct t.** An inclusive term applied to tumors derived from epithelial remnants of the involuted pouch of Rathke. Usually suprasellar, they include the adamantinoma and the so-called craniopharyngioma, which originate in the residual stalk, and cystic neoplasms,

which originate from the residual cleft. More frequent in children than in adults. **Krukenberg t.** See _fibrosarcoma mucocellulare carcinomatodes_. **malignant t.** One which grows peripherally, invades and destroys surrounding tissues, may extend directly, and may produce distant secondary tumors by metastasis. **metastatic t.** A secondary tumor produced by metastasis. **milk t.** A swelling of the breast due to the obstruction of milk ducts. **mixed t.** One composed of two or more tissue types or cell types. More specifically, a tumor originating from one or two of the primary germinal embryonal layers as contrasted with teratomas or teratoid tumors which contain elements of all three germinal layers. **phantom t.** A swelling simulating a tumor produced by the contraction of a muscle or by gaseous distention of the intestine. **recurrent t.** One recurring after surgical removal. **theca-cell t. of ovary.** A yellowish gray, firm tumor developing after the menopause. It has lipid-filled cells which are derived from the theca interna of the Graafian follicle. Also called _thecoma_. **tuberous t.** Any tumor, such as an angioma, which grossly resembles a tuber.

tu′mor·af″fin, tu″mor·af′fin. Substances (drugs, radiant energy, etc.) which are supposed to have some special affinity for tumor cells.

tu′mor·ous. Of the nature of a neoplasm or tumor.

tu·mul′tus. Tumult.

Tun′ga. A genus of fleas which burrow beneath the skin to lay their eggs, causing serious local inflammation. **T. penetrans.** A flea prevalent in the tropical regions of Africa and America. Also called _chigoe; jigger_.

tung′sten. W = 183.92. A heavy metallic element. Used in steel and other products where hardness and toughness are required. Recommended to be called _wolfram_.

tu′nic. A coat or membrane. See _tunica_.

tu′ni·ca (pl. _tunicae_). A tunic. **t. adventitia.** The outer connective-tissue coat of an organ where it is not covered by a serous membrane. **t. albuginea testis.** The dense fibrous capsule of the testis, deep to the tunica vaginalis propria. **t. dartos.** The layers of connective tissue containing smooth muscle in the corium and outer portion of the superficial fascia of the scrotum and penis. **t. externa.** The tunica adventitia of a blood or lymph vessel. **t. intima.** The inner coat of a blood or lymph vessel. **t. media.** The middle coat of a blood or lymph vessel. **t. muscularis.** The muscular coat of certain hollow organs; e.g., the digestive tube.

tu′ning fork. A two-tined metallic fork capable of vibrating at a rate which will produce a definite tone.

tu′ni·ver oil. Oil from the liver of the tuna fish.

tun′nel. A narrow, enclosed passageway.

tu·ran′ose (tew·ran′oce, tew′ran·oce). A disaccharide yielding on hydrolysis glucose and fructose.

tur′bid. Cloudy.

tur″bi·dim′e·ter. An instrument for measuring the degree of turbidity of a liquid. —**turbidimet′ric,** adj.; **turbidimetry,** n.

tur′bi·nate. A turbinate bone. See concha, 2. See Table of Bones in the Appendix.

tur′bi·na″ted. Top-shaped; scroll-shaped; as turbinated bone, one of the three bony projections (superior, middle, and inferior) upon the lateral wall of each nasal cavity. They are covered by an erectile vascular mucous membrane. See concha, 2.

tur″bi·nec′to·my. Excision of a nasal concha.

tur′bi·no·tome″. An instrument used in turbinotomy.

tur″bi·not′o·my. Incision into a nasal concha.

tur·ges′cence. Swelling.

tur·ges′cent. Swollen, tumid.

tur′gid. 1. Swollen. 2. Congested; hyperemic.

tur′gor. Active hyperemia; turgescence. **t. vitalis.** The normal fullness of the blood vessels.

Turlington′s balsam. See compound benzoin tincture.

tur′mer·ic. See curcuma.

turn. 1. Cause to revolve about an axis. 2. Change the position of the fetus so as to facilitate delivery.

tur′pen·tine. 1. A concrete or liquid oleoresin obtained from coniferous trees. 2. The concrete oleoresin from Pinus palustris and other species of Pinus. Yellow-orange, opaque masses, freely soluble in alcohol. Contains up to 32% of volatile oil. Occasionally used for local irritant effect. Also called gum thus, gum turpentine. **Canada t.** The liquid oleoresin from the American silver fir, Abies balsamea. Commonly used under the name Canada balsam as a mounting medium in microscopy. **larch t.** Venice turpentine. **t. oil.** The volatile oil distilled from turpentine. Colorless liquid soluble in alcohol. Consists essentially of terpenes, principally varieties of pinene. A local irritant and feeble antiseptic. Also called t. spirits. **Venice t.** From Larix decidua, yielding about 15% of volatile oil. Also called larch t. **wood t.** Pre-

pared from stumps, roots, sawdust, etc. Not equivalent to the official substance.

tur′peth. Ipomoea turpethum, a purgative plant resembling jalap, found in Asia. **t. mineral.** The yellow subsulfate of mercury, once used as an emetic.

turps. Turpentine oil.

tusk. A large, projecting, irregular tooth.

tus′sal. Pertaining to, or of the nature of, a cough.

Tus″si·la′go. A genus of plants of the Compositae. The leaves of T. farfara, coltsfoot, and also other parts of the plant have been used as a demulcent.

tus′sis. A cough. **t. convulsiva.** Whooping cough.

tus′sive. Pertaining to, or caused by, a cough.

twang. A nasal quality of the voice.

tweens. Trade-mark for a series of surface-active agents consisting of partial esters of long-chain fatty acids with polyoxyalkylene derivatives of hexitol anhydride. See spans.

tweez′ers. Delicate surgical forceps which are capable of seizing without crushing easily damaged structures, as nerves; they are also used for removing eyelashes or hairs.

twi′light sleep. In obstetrics, an injection of scopolamine and morphine to produce amnesia and analgesia.

twin. One of two born at the same birth. **conjoined twins.** Equal or unequal uniovular twins, united. Also called diplopagi. **fraternal twins.** Twins resulting from the simultaneous fertilization of two ova. They may be of the same or opposite sex, have a different genetic constitution, and each has a separate chorion. Also called biovular twins, dichorial twins, dissimilar twins, dizygotic twins. **identical twins.** Twins which are developed from a single ovum, always of the same sex, have the same genetic constitution, and have the same chorion. Also called monochorionic twins, uniovular twins, similar twins, enzygotic twins. **interlocking twins.** Those in which the neck of the first child becomes engaged with the head of the second above the superior strait. Such locking is possible when the first is a breech and the second a vertex presentation. The interlocking makes vaginal delivery virtually impossible.

twinge. A sudden short and sharp pain.

twin′ning. Production of like structures by division.

twitch. Give a short, sudden pull or jerk.

twitch′ing. An irregular spasm of a minor extent.

ty·lo′ma (tye·lo′muh). A callus.

ty·lo'sis (tye·lo'sis). 1. A localized patch of hyperkeratotic skin due to chronic pressure and friction. 2. A form of blepharitis with thickening and hardening of the edge of the lid. **—tylot'ic,** adj. **t. palmaris et plantaris.** An ectodermal anomaly of the palms and soles producing marked hyperkeratosis. Syn., *keratosis palmaris et plantaris.*

ty"lo·ste·re'sis. Removal of a callosity.

tym"pa·nec'to·my. Excision of the tympanic membrane.

tym"pa·ni'tes (tim"puh·nigh'teez). A distention of the abdominal wall from accumulation of gas in the intestine or peritoneal cavity.

tym"pa·ni'tis. Inflammation of the tympanum; otitis media.

tym"pa·no·mas'toid. Relating to the tympanum and the mastoid process or the mastoid cells.

tym"pa·no·mas"toid·i'tis. Inflammation of the tympanum and mastoid cells.

tym"pa·no·sym"pa·thec'to·my. The removal of the plexus on the medial wall of the middle ear for the relief of tinnitus.

tym"pa·not'o·my. Incision of a tympanic membrane. Syn., *myringotomy.*

tym'pa·nous. Distended with gas; relating to tympanism.

tym'pa·num. The middle ear. **—tym·pan'ic,** adj.

tym'pa·ny. 1. Tympanites. 2. A tympanitic percussion note. See tympanitic *resonance.*

Tyndall blue. The blue color produced when light is scattered by small particles suspended in a liquid or a gas. Also called the *Tyndall effect.*

Tyn"dall·i·za'tion. Fractional sterilization by the use of steam at atmospheric pressure. A sufficient period is permitted to elapse between treatments to allow spores of microorganisms to germinate.

type. 1. Imprint; emblem; symbol; character. 2. A normal average example. 3. *In pathology,* the distinguishing features of a fever, disease, etc., whereby it is referred to its proper class. **test t.** A chart of letters, most commonly the Snellen chart or its modifications, used to test the acuity of central vision.

typh·lat'o·ny, typh"la·to'ni·a. An atonic condition of the wall of the cecum.

typh"lec·ta'si·a (tif"leck·tay'zhuh, -shuh). Dilatation of the cecum.

typh·lec'to·my. Excision of the cecum.

typh·li'tis. Inflammation of the cecum.

typh·lo-, typhl-. A combining form meaning *cecum. Obs.*

typh"lo·di"cli·di'tis (tif"lo·dye"-kli·dye'tis, -dick"li·dye'tis). Inflammation of the ileocecal valve.

typh"lo·em"py·e'ma (tif"lo·em"-pye·ee'muh, -em"pee·ee'muh). Abscess attending typhlitis or appendicitis.

typh'loid. Having defective vision.

typh"lo·lex'i·a. Word blindness. See *aphasia.*

typh"lo·li·thi'a·sis. The formation of calculi in the cecum.

typh"lo·meg'a·ly. Enlarged cecum.

typh"lo·pto'sis (tif"lo·to'sis, tif"-lop·to'sis). Downward displacement or prolapse of the cecum.

typh·lo'sis. Blindness.

typh'lo·spasm. Spasm of the cecum.

typh"lo·ste·no'sis. Stenosis of the cecum.

typh·los'to·my. A cecal colostomy.

ty'pho-, typh-. A combining form denoting *typhus* or *typhoid.*

ty"pho·bac'te·rin. A vaccine prepared from the typhoid bacillus.

ty'phoid. 1. An old term for any condition resembling typhus. 2. Typhoid fever, an acute infectious disease caused by *Salmonella typhosa,* which enters the body with food and drinking water, and is found in the intestine, the spleen, and the fecal discharges, but may also occur in the various complicating lesions. The principal lesions of typhoid fever are an enlargement of the spleen and the mesenteric lymph nodes. The mucous membrane of the intestine is also the seat of a catarrhal inflammation. After a period of incubation of from two to three weeks, the disease sets in with weakness, headache, vague pains, the tendency to diarrhea, and nosebleed. The temperature gradually rises, being higher each evening than the previous evening, and reaches its maximum (104°–105° F.) in from one to two weeks. It then remains at this level for from one to two weeks, and finally sinks by lysis. The pulse is soft and dicrotic, but often not so rapid as would be expected from the high temperature. The tongue is at first coated on the dorsum and red at the tip and edges, but soon becomes dry, brown, and tremulous, and, like the teeth and lips, covered with sordes. There is usually complete anorexia, the bowels are loose, and the stools have a peculiar pea-soup color. At times constipation exists. Slight congestion of the lungs with cough is usually present. On the seventh, eighth, or ninth day the peculiar eruption appears; it consists of small, slightly elevated, rose-colored spots, disappearing on pressure, and coming out in successive crops. Nervous symptoms are prominent in typhoid, and consist of headache, slight deafness, stupor, muttering delirium, carphology, subsultus tendinum, and coma vigil. Complications are frequent, the most important being intestinal hemorrhage, perforation of the bowel, peritonitis, pneumonia, and phthisis. Relapses are fairly common, although second attacks are rare. **abortive t.** A form characterized by abrupt onset of symptoms, which subside quickly, convalescence following in a few days. **afebrile t.** Typhoid fever with the usual symptoms, positive diazo and Widal reaction, presence of rose spots, but no increased temperature. **ambulatory t.** Typhoid in which the patient does not take to his bed. **sudoral t.** Typhoid fever accompanied by profuse sweating and great prostration. **t. nodules.** Characteristic lesions in the liver after fatal typhoid. **t. vaccine.** A sterile suspension of killed typhoid bacilli (*Eberthella typhosa*) of a strain selected for high antigenic efficiency. The vaccine contains not less than 1,000,000,000 typhoid organisms in each cubic centimeter.

ty·phoi′dal (tye-foy′dul). Resembling typhoid.

ty″pho·ma′ni·a. The lethargic state, with delirium, sometimes observed in typhus, typhoid, and other fevers.

ty″pho·pneu·mo′ni·a. Pneumonia concurrent with typhoid fever.

ty′phus. An acute infectious disease; chiefly characterized by a petechial rash, marked nervous symptoms, and a high fever, ending by crisis in from 10 to 14 days. The only peculiar lesions noted post mortem are a dark fluid state of the blood and a staining of the endocardium and intima of the blood vessels. The disease is transmitted to man by the body louse and the rat flea infected with *Rickettsia prowazekii*. After a period of incubation of from a few days to two weeks, the disease sets in abruptly with pains in the head, back, and limbs, the fever rising rapidly to 104° or 105° F. The nervous symptoms resemble those of typhoid fever. The eruption appears on the fourth or fifth day as rose-colored spots scattered all over the body, and quickly becoming hemorrhagic. They do not disappear on pressure. The chief complications are hyperpyrexia, pneumonia, and nephritis. Also called *camp fever, Fleck typhus, jail fever, ship fever.* **epidemic t. vaccine.** A sterile suspension of the killed rickettsial organism of a strain or strains of epidemic typhus rickettsiae selected for antigenic efficiency. The rickettsial organisms are obtained by culturing in the yolk sac membrane of the developing embryo of the domestic fowl. Also called *typhus vaccine.*

typ′i·cal. 1. Constituting a type or form for comparison. 2. Illustrative. 3. Completely representative.

ty′ping. 1. The determination of a specific blood group or blood type. See under *blood.* See also *blood typing.* 2. The determination of the specific types into which certain bacteria (*e.g.*, *Diplococcus pneumoniae*) have been subdivided.

ty′po·scope. A small device to exclude extraneous light, for the use of cataract patients and amblyopes in reading.

ty″ra·mine′ (ty″ruh-meen′, tirr″-uh-). p-Hydroxyphenyl-ethylamine. $HO.C_6H_4.CH_2.CH_2NH_2$. An amine present in ergot and formed in putrefied animal tissue; also prepared synthetically. Syn., *tyrosamine.*

tyr′an·ism. Cruelty of morbid inception, of which sadism is an erotic variety.

ty·rem′e·sis (tye-rem′i-sis). The vomiting of caseous or curdy matter, often seen in infants.

ty′ro-, tyr-. A combining form meaning *cheese* or *cheeselike.*

ty″ro·ci′din, ty″ro·ci′dine. A component of tyrothricin, *q.v.*

Ty·rog′ly·phus (tye-rog′li-fus). A genus of sarcoptoid mites which usually infest dried vegetable products, cheese, and dead or living plants. Occasionally, they produce a temporary pruritus which is named by the occupation of the host. **T. farinor** causes grocer's itch, **T. siro** causes vanillism among handlers of vanilla pods, and **T. longior** causes copra itch and grocer's itch.

ty′roid. Cheeselike.

tyrosamine. Tyramine.

ty′ro·sin·ase (ty′ro-sin·ace, tye·ro′-sin·). A copper-containing enzyme found in plants, molds, crustacea, mollusks, and some bacteria. In the presence of oxygen, it causes the oxidation of mono- and poly-phenols with the introduction of —OH groups and/or formation of quinones. May be identical with monophenol oxidase and perhaps also with polyphenol oxidase.

ty′ro·sine (ty′ro·seen, tye·ro′sin). p-Hydroxyphenyl alanine. $p-HO.C_6H_4.CH_2.CH(NH_2)COOH$. An amino acid widely distributed in proteins, particularly in casein. It is closely related to, and a probable precursor of, epinephrine, thyroxin, and melanin.

ty″ro·si·nu′ri·a. The presence of tyrosine in the urine.

ty″ro·thri′cin. An alcohol-soluble, water-insoluble polypeptide mixture isolated from *Bacillus brevis* and consisting of the antibiotic substances gramicidin and tyrocidin; used topically as a bactericide in infections due to Gram-positive organisms.

ty″ro·tox′in. A curarelike poison claimed to be present in some specimens of cheese.

U

U. 1. Chemical symbol for uranium. 2. Abbreviation for unit.

u'ber·ty. Fertility; productiveness. **—uberous,** adj.

ud'der. The mammary gland of the cow and other animals.

u·lag″a·nac'te·sis (yōō-lag″uh-nack'ti·sis, ·nack·tee'sis). Irritation or uneasy sensations in the gums. Obs.

u″la·tro'phi·a. A shrinkage of the gums. Obs.

ul'cer. An interruption of continuity of a surface, with an inflamed base. **amputating u.** A penetrating ulcer encircling a part, such as a toe, leading ultimately to loss of the distal portion, as in yaws. **arterial u.** An ulcer of a part or surface due to arterial occlusion. **atonic u.** One which shows little or no disposition to heal. **creeping u.** One which slowly extends peripherally, sometimes with central healing. Syn., *serpiginous u.* **decubitus u.** A bedsore; that is, ulceration of skin and underlying tissue from prolonged pressure; seen especially in the aged or in paralysis. **diphtheritic u.** Specifically, an ulcer due to action of *Corynebacterium diphtheriae* or to detachment of a diphtheritic membrane. Also applied loosely to an ulcer, on or about which is a fibrinous exudate. One of the forms of tropical ulcer appears to be due to *C. diphtheriae*. **duodenal u.** A chronic ulcer, usually in the anterior wall of the duodenum, near the pylorus. Syn., *peptic u.* **endemic u.** One which is frequent in certain regions, as tropical ulcer. **follicular u.** An ulcer due to breakdown of a lymphatic aggregate, such as a solitary nodule of the ileum. **gastric u.** One affecting the mucosa of the stomach. May be a peptic ulcer or due to hemorrhagic erosion. **indolent u.** One with little tendency to heal, often accompanied by fibrosis of the base and margins with scanty granulation tissue. **inflamed u.** One accompanied by acute inflammation. **kissing u.** One which appears to be due to transmission from one apposing part to another, or due to pressure of apposing parts. **marginal u.** An ulcer of the jejunum along the stoma of a gastrojejunostomy; due to erosive action of acid gastric juice upon the jejunum. **penetrating u.** One which extends more deeply than the surface originally affected, as a peptic ulcer penetrating into muscular coats. **peptic u.** One due in part at least to digestive action of gastric juice, affecting the gastric or duodenal mucosa, or the mucosa of stomach and jejunum associated with gastrojejunal anastomosis. **perforating u.** One which extends through all coats of a viscus. **phagedenic u.** One accompanied by extensive necrosis or gangrene of neighboring tissues. **rodent u.** A basal-cell carcinoma with more or less deep penetration; microscopically of reticulated form, affecting especially the face, neck, and scalp and the mucocutaneous junctions of the eyes and nose. Metastasis is infrequent and late. **serpiginous u.** See creeping *u.* **trophic u.** One due to disturbances of nutrition of a part, such as varicose ulcer. **tropical u.** A cutaneous ulcer prevalent in tropical regions, not due to syphilis, yaws, leishmaniasis, or hookworm. May be acute, chronic, or phagedenic. Various microorganisms are associated with different ulcers in different regions, *Corynebacterium diphtheriae* being found most frequently. Syn., *Naga sore, Aden u., Annam u., Mozambique u., Yemen u.* **varicose u.** A chronic ulcer of skin due largely to malnutrition of the skin as a result of varicose veins, especially of the leg. Also called *leg u.*

ul'ce·ra. Plural of ulcus, q.v.

ul'cer·ate. Become converted into, or affected with, an ulcer.

ul″cer·a'tion. The process of formation of an ulcer.

ul″cer·o·mem'bra·nous. Pertaining to, or characterized by, ulceration, and accompanied by fibrinous inflammation with accompanying formation of a pseudomembrane.

ul'cus (pl. ulcera). An ulcer. **u. cancrosum.** (a) Cancer. (b) Rodent ulcer. **u. cruris.** Indolent ulcer of the leg. **u. exedens.** Old term for rodent ulcer. **u. induratum.** Chancre. **u. molle.** Chancroid. **u. phagedaenicum.** Phagedenic ulcer. **u. rodens.** Rodent ulcer. **u. tuberculosum.** Lupus vulgaris. **u. venereum.** (a) Chancre. (b) Chancroid.

–ule. A suffix designating a *diminutive,* as in tubule.

u·ler″y·the'ma. An erythematous disease marked by the formation of cicatrices.

u·let'ic. Pertaining to the gums.

u·li'tis. A general inflammation of the gums, as distinguished from simple gingivitis, which is confined to the free margins of the gums.

ul'mus. The inner bark of *Ulmus fulva* (slippery elm); mucilaginous and demulcent; has been used mainly in folk medicine.

ul'na. The bone on the inner side of the forearm, articulating with the humerus and the head of the radius above and with the radius below. See Table of Bones in the Appendix. **—ulnar,** adj.

u·loc'a·ce (yoo·lock'uh·see). Ulcerative inflammation of the gums.

u″lo·glos·si'tis. Inflammation of gums and tongue.

u'loid. Scarlike.

u″lor·rha'gi·a. Bleeding from the gums.

u·lo'sis. Cicatrization.

u·lot'ic. Pertaining to, or tending toward, cicatrization.

u·lot'o·my. Incision into the gum.

ul″ti·mo·gen'i·ture. The state of being the last born. **—ultimogenitary,** adj.

ul'tra-. A prefix denoting beyond, excess.

ul″tra·cen'tri·fuge. A high-speed centrifuge which will produce, according to type selected, centrifugal fields up to several hundred thousand times the force of gravity, used for the study of proteins, viruses, etc. **—ultracentrif'ugal,** adj.

ul″tra·fil'ter. A filter which will remove colloidal particles from their dispersion mediums and from crystalloids. Sometimes called jelly filter.

ul″tra·fil·tra'tion. 1. The removal of all but the smallest particles, such as viruses and chemical substances, by filtration. Either positive or negative pressure may be employed. 2. A method for the separation of colloids from their dispersion mediums and dissolved crystalloids by the use of ultrafilters.

ul″tra·mi'cro·scope. A microscope for examination, by powerful side illumination, of objects not visible with ordinary microscopes. Also called slit microscope. **—ultramicroscop'ic,** adj.; **ultramicros'copy,** n.

ul″tra·red'. Pertaining to radiations of shorter wave lengths than the red of the visible spectrum.

ul″tra·son'ic. Pertaining to sounds with frequencies above those ordinarily audible to the human ear.

ul″tra·son'ics. The science dealing with sound vibrations and waves having frequencies greater than 20 kilocycles, sometimes used in treating certain diseases.

ul″tra·vi'rus. A virus which is filtrable in an ultrafilter.

um'ber. A native ferric hydroxide containing manganese dioxide and silicate; occurs as a dark brown to brownish red powder. Used as a pigment. **burnt u.** A reddish brown pigment obtained by heating umber.

um″bi·lec'to·my. 1. Excision of the umbilicus. 2. An operation for the relief of umbilical hernia.

um·bil'i·cate, um·bil'i·ca″ted. Having a depression like that of the navel.

um·bil″i·ca'tion. 1. A depression like that of the navel. 2. The state of being umbilicated.

um·bil'i·cus, um″bi·li'cus. The navel; the round, depressed cicatrix in the median line of the abdomen, marking the site of the aperture which in fetal life gave passage to the umbilical vessels. **—umbil'ical,** adj.

um'bo (pl. umbos, umbones). A boss or bosselation; any central convex eminence, as the umbo of the tympanic membrane.

un'ci·a. Ounce.

un'ci·form. Hook-shaped.

Un″ci·na'ri·a. A generic name formerly applied to hookworms.

un'ci·nate. Hooked.

un'ci·nate fit. Episodic olfactory hallucinations associated with a peculiar dreamy state and smacking movements of the lips; due to irritative lesions of the uncus. Generally idiopathic; may be associated with gross lesions.

un·con'scious. 1. In psychiatry, pertaining to behavior or experiences not controlled by the conscious ego. 2. That part of the personality not in the immediate field of awareness. 3. Insensible; in a state lacking conscious awareness.

un·con'scious·ness. The state of being without sensibility and with reflexes abolished.

unc'tion. 1. The act of anointing. 2. An ointment.

unc'tu·ous. Greasy; oily.

un'cus. 1. A hook. 2. Hooklike anterior extremity of the hippocampal gyrus.

un·dec″y·len'ic ac'id (un·dess″i·len'ick, ·lee'nick). $CH_3CH:CH(CH_2)_7$·COOH. An unsaturated acid, melting at 24° C.; used therapeutically, generally in combination with one or more of its salts (copper, sodium, or zinc), as a fungicide.

un'der·weight'. A condition of the whole body which is characterized by a deficiency of body tissue, lack of fat being the most obvious. Usually the term is applied to persons whose body weight is at least 10% less than that of the average for persons of the same age, sex, and height.

un·dine' (un·deen', un'deen). A glass container for irrigating the eye.

un'du·lant fe'ver. Brucellosis, q.v.

un″du·la'tion. A wavelike motion; fluctuation. **jugular u.** The venous pulse. **respiratory u.** The variations in the blood pressure due to respiration.

un'du·la·to"ry. Moving like waves; vibratory.

ung. *Unguentum;* ointment.

un·guen'tum. Ointment. Abbreviated, ung.

un'guis (pl. *ungues*). A fingernail or toenail. **—ungual,** *adj.* **u. incar·natus.** Ingrowing nail.

un·gu·la. 1. An instrument for extracting a dead fetus. 2. A hoof; a claw. **—ungulate,** *adj.*

un·health'y. 1. Lacking health; sickly. 2. Injurious to health.

u'ni-. A combining form meaning *one.*

u"ni·ar·tic'u·lar. Pertaining to a single joint.

u"ni·cel'lu·lar. Composed of but one cell.

u"ni·cus'pid, u"ni·cus'pi·date. 1. Having but a single cusp, as a tooth. 2. A tooth with but a single cusp or point.

u"ni·fa·mil'i·al. Pertaining to a single family.

u"ni·grav'i·da. A woman who is pregnant for the first time. Also called *primigravida.*

u"ni·lat'er·al. Pertaining to, or affecting, but one side.

u"ni·loc'u·lar. Having but one loculus or cavity.

u"ni·oc'u·lar. 1. Pertaining to, or performed with, one eye. 2. Having only one eye.

un'ion. A joining; specifically, the consolidation of bone fractures. **immediate u.** That by first intention. **vicious u.** The healing of a fracture in improper position, with resulting deformity.

u"ni·ov'u·lar. Concerning, or derived from, one egg, as uniovular twins.

u·nip'a·ra. A woman who has borne but one child. **—uniparous,** *adj.*

u·nip'a·rous. Bearing one offspring, or producing one ovum, at a time.

u"ni·po'lar. 1. Having but one pole or process. 2. Pertaining to one pole.

u'nit. 1. A single thing or person or a group considered as a whole, as a hospital unit. 2. A standard of weight or measurement. Abbreviated, U. **angstrom u.** See *angstrom.* **antitoxic u.** The amount of antitoxin which neutralizes a definite number of minimum lethal doses, generally 100, of a given toxin. **Board of Trade u.** (*B.T.U.*). A unit of energy used in Britain equivalent to one kilowatt hour, 3,600,000 joules, or 3,415 American B.T.U. **British thermal u.** (B.Th.U. in British usage. American usage is B.T.U. In Britain, B.T.U. means Board of Trade unit.) The heat required to raise one pound of water 1° F. One B.T.U. is equivalent to 1,054 joules, 0.002928 kilowatt hours, 777.7 foot-pounds, 0.2520 large calories.

cat u. The amount of digitalis which will kill a cat when injected intravenously, calculated per kilogram of the animal. **C.G.S. u.** A unit in the centimeter-gram-second system. **clinical u.** That amount of a substance, e.g. liver extract, which will produce a desired response in a patient. Abbreviated, C.U. **electric u.** One for measuring the strength of an electric current. Three different systems of electric units are used: the electromagnetic, the electrostatic, and the ordinary or practical units. The commonly used practical units are the ampere or unit of current, the volt or unit of electromotive force, the ohm or unit of resistance, the coulomb or unit of quantity, the farad or unit of capacitance, and the watt or unit of power. **electromagnetic units.** Fundamental electric units expressed in the electromagnetic system; they are usually characterized by adding *ab-* to the unit, such as abampere, abvolt. Units measured in the electromagnetic system are 3×10^{10} times as large as electrostatic units. **electrostatic units.** Fundamental electric units expressed in the electrostatic system; they are usually characterized by adding *stat-* to the unit, such as statampere, statvolt. **e u.** See roentgen *u.* **Florey u.** See Oxford *u.* **gravitational u.** One gravitational unit equals one pound of force divided by one pound of mass. Abbreviated, G. **heat u.** The amount of heat required to raise the temperature of one kilogram of water from 0° to 1° C.; it is technically called a calorie. **immunizing u.** See antitoxic *u.* Abbreviated, I.U. **international u.** An arbitrarily defined weight of an international standard of reference adopted by the Permanent Commission on Biological Standardization of the League of Nations. Abbreviated, I.U. **International Units of vitamins.** See *vitamin* A, *vitamin* B₁, *vitamin* C, *vitamin* D. **M.K.S. units.** Meterkilogram-second system of fundamental units; mostly used by engineers. **mouse u.** That amount of estrusproducing substance which, when injected into a spayed mouse, will produce a characteristic change in the vaginal epithelium. **Oxford u.** The minimum quantity of penicillin which, when dissolved in 50 cc. of a meat broth, is sufficient to inhibit completely the growth of a test strain of *Micrococcus aureus.* Syn., *Florey u.* **previral u.** One related to early stages of intracellular virus multiplication; a number of such units surrounded by a matrix comprise a fully formed virus particle. **rat growth u.** The amount of vitamin A necessary to maintain a weekly gain of 3 Gm. in test rats previously depleted of vitamin A. Also called *Sherman-Munsell u.* **roentgen u.** Unit of x-ray dose in which the quantity of x- or gamma-radiation is such that the associated corpuscular emission per 0.001293 Gm. of air produces, in air, ions carrying one electrostatic unit of quantity of electricity of either sign. **Steenbock u.** The amount of vitamin D which will produce a line of calcification at the distal ulnar and radial epiphysis of rachitic rats within ten days. **thermal u.** The amount of heat required to raise the temperature of a pound of water one degree F. or C. **Toronto u.** The anticoagulant activity of 0.01 mg. of a standard barium heparin employed at the University of Toronto. **toxic u.** The smallest dose of a toxin which is capable of proving fatal to an experimental animal, usually a guinea pig, of definite weight, in a specified period of time. **u. character.** One of a pair of sharply contrasted traits which are inherited according to the Mendelian law of segregation. **u. of force.** The dyne; the force which, when acting for one second, will give to one gram a velocity of one centimeter per second. **u. of heat.** The calorie or B.T.U. **u. of length.** See Tables of Weights and Measures in the Appendix. **u. of light.** Foot-candle. The foot-candle is the illumination equal to one lumen per square foot or the illumination of a surface at a uniform distance of one foot from a point source of one candle. **u. of volume.** See Tables of Weights and Measures in the Appendix. **u. of weight.** See Tables of Weights and Measures in the Appendix. **u. of work.** The erg. Also called *u. of energy.* **U.S.P. u.** A certain amount of a substance as standardized by the United States Pharmacopeia.

unitensen. Trade-mark for cryptenamine.

u″ni·va′lent (yōo″ni-vay′lunt). 1. Having a valence of one. 2. An element that has only one valency and forms only one series of compounds.

u″ni·ver′sal do′nor. The blood donor of the group O type.

un″of·fi′cial. Describing a drug or remedy that is not included in the Pharmacopeia or National Formulary.

un·or′gan·ized. 1. Without organs. 2. Not arranged in the form of an organ or organs.

un·rest′. A condition characterized by vigorous and irregular movements of the gastrointestinal tract.

un·sat′u·ra″ted. 1. Not saturated. 2. Describing an organic compound having double or triple bonds.

un·sex′. Remove the testes in male, or the ovaries in female, animals.

un·sound′ness. The state of being not healthy, diseased, or not properly functioning. **—unsound,** *adj.* **u. of mind.** Incapacity to govern one's affairs.

un·stri′a·ted (un·stry′ay·tid). Not striated, as unstriated muscle.

un″u·ni′ted. Not joined, as an un-united fracture.

un·well′. 1. Ill; sick. 2. Lay term for menstruating.

up′take. That amount of a substance, as oxygen or radioactive iodine, that is accumulated or utilized by an organ or a system. Also see *intake,* 1.

u·ra·chus (yōo·ray′kus). An epithelial tube or cord connecting the apex of the bladder with the allantois, regarded as the stalk of the allantois or as the degenerate apex of the primitive bladder. Its connective tissue forms the median umbilical ligament. **—urachal,** *adj.* **patent u.** A condition in which the urachus of the embryo does not become obliterated, but persists as a tube from the apex of the bladder to the umbilicus.

u′ra·cil. A pyrimidine base; a constituent of nucleic acids.

u″ra·cra′si·a (yoor″uh·kray′zhuh, ·shuh), **u″ra·cra′ti·a** (yoor″uh·kray′shuh, ·shee·uh). Incontinence of urine; enuresis, *q.v.*

u′ra·gogue (yoor″uh·gog). Increasing urinary secretion; a diuretic.

u′ra·mine (yoor″uh·meen, yoo·ram′een). See *guanidine.*

u″ra·nal′y·sis. Same as *urinalysis.*

u′rane. 1. Uranium oxide. 2. A unit of radioactivity. See *kilurane.*

u′ra·nin. See *fluorescein* sodium.

u·ran′i·nite. Pitchblende. Native uranium oxide, a source of radium.

u″ra·nis′cus. The palate.

u·ra′ni·um. U = 238.07. A heavy metal of the radium group; occurs as silver-white, lustrous, radioactive crystals or powder. As concentrated from its ores uranium contains 99.3% of the isotope weighing 238, 0.7 per cent of the 235 isotope, and a negligible amount of the 234 isotope. Uranium 235 may be made to undergo fission with the release of a large amount of energy. Uranium 238 can absorb a neutron to produce uranium 239; this spontaneously loses a beta particle to form neptunium, which, in turn, loses another beta particle to form plutonium, the last also being fissionable.

u″ra·no·col′o·bo′ma. Cleft hard palate, not involving the alveolar process.

u″ra·no·plas′tic. Pertaining to repair of a cleft palate.

u″ra·no·ple′gi·a. Paralysis of the muscles of the soft palate.

u″ra·nor′rha·phy. Suture of a cleft palate; staphylorrhaphy.

u″ra·nos′chi·sis (yoor″uh·nos′ki·sis), **u·ran′o·schism** (yoo·ran′o·skiz·um, ·siz·um), **u″ra·no·schis′ma.** 1. Cleft hard palate. 2. Cleft hard palate and alveolar process. Also called *gnathopalatoschisis.*

u″ra·no·staph″y·lor′rha·phy. Repair of a cleft in both the hard and soft palates.

u′ra·nyl. The bivalent uranium radical UO_2, which forms salts with many acids, as, for example, uranyl acetate, $UO_2(C_2H_3O_2)_2.2H_2O$.

u″ra·ro′ma. Aromatic odor of urine.

u′rase (yoor′ace, ·aze). Urease, *q.v.*

u′ra·sin. A ferment derived from urea.

u′rate. A salt of uric acid. —**urat′ic,** *adj.*

u″ra·te′mi·a, u″ra·tae′mi·a. The presence of urates in the blood.

u″ra·tu′ri·a. The presence of urates in the urine.

ur″ban·i·za′tion. A term to express the tendency of modern society to develop cities at the expense of the country population, with a consequent influence upon disease, the death rate, etc.

u·re′a. $CO(NH_2)_2$. Carbonyldiamide, found in urine. Occurs as colorless to white crystals or powder; soluble in water. A diuretic, also employed externally in treating infected wounds. See Table of Normal Values of Blood Constituents in the Appendix. Syn., *carbamide.* —**ureal,** *adj.* **quinine and u. hydrochloride.** A salt employed as a local anesthetic and sclerosing agent. **u. nitrogen.** The nitrogen of urea. A term used to distinguish that nitrogen from the nitrogen in the form of protein. **u. peroxide.** A solid compound of urea and hydrogen peroxide; in contact with water it liberates urea and hydrogen peroxide. Also called *carbamide peroxide.*

u″re·am′e·ter. An apparatus for determining the amount of urea in a liquid by measuring the volume of nitrogen evolved.

u″re·am′e·try. The determination of the amount of urea in a liquid.

u′re·ase (yoor′ee·ace, ·aze). A urealytic enzyme obtained from the jack bean, the seed of *Canavalia;* occurs as a fine, white, or cream-colored powder; readily soluble in slightly alkaline water. Used in the estimation of urea.

u·rec′chy·sis (yoo·reck′i·sis). Extravasation of urine into the tissues.

urecholine chloride. Trade-mark for bethanechol chloride.

u″re·de′ma. Swelling of tissues from extravasation of urine.

u′re·ide. A compound of urea and an acid radical.

u·re′mi·a. The retention in the blood of urinary constituents, due to failure of the kidneys to excrete them, and the constitutional symptoms resulting. There may be headache, nausea, vomiting, and coma. —**uremic,** *adj.*

u·re″si·es·the′si·a (yoo·ree″see·ess·thee′zhuh, ·zee·uh). The impulse to urinate.

u·re′sis. Urination.

u·re′ter, u′re·ter. The long, narrow tube conveying the urine from the pelvis of a kidney to the bladder. —**ure′teral, ureter′ic,** *adj.* **aberrant ureters.** Ureters emptying at some point other than into the urinary bladder.

u·re″ter·ec′ta·sis. Dilatation of a ureter.

u·re″ter·ec′to·my. Excision of a ureter.

u·re″ter·i′tis. Inflammation of a ureter.

u·re′ter·o-, ureter-. A combining form denoting *the ureter.*

u·re″ter·o·cele. A cystlike dilatation at the termination of a ureter; of congenital origin or due to a narrowing of the terminal orifice. It is identified by cystoscopic examination.

u·re″ter·o·co·los′to·my. Implantation of a ureter, severed from the bladder, into the colon.

u·re″ter·o·cys·tos′to·my. The surgical formation of a communication between a ureter and the bladder.

u·re″ter·o·en″ter·os′to·my. Surgical formation of a passage from a ureter to some portion of the intestine.

u·re″ter·og′ra·phy. Radiography of the ureters after the injection of some opaque substance.

u·re″ter·o·hy″dro·ne·phro′sis. Distention of a ureter and the pelvis of its kidney, due to distal obstruction of outflow of urine.

u·re″ter·o·in·tes′ti·nal a·nas″·to·mo′sis. Surgical implantation of a ureter into the colon.

u·re′ter·o·lith. Calculus in a ureter.

u·re″ter·o·li·thi′a·sis. The presence or formation of a calculus in a ureter.

u·re″ter·o·li·thot′o·my. Incision of the ureter for removal of a calculus.

u·re″ter·ol′y·sis. Surgical repair of a tortuous or kinked ureter.

u·re″ter·o·ne″o·py″e·los′to·my. Suturing the distal end of a severed ureter into a new opening in the pelvis of its kidney.

u·re″ter·o·ne·phrec′to·my. Removal of a kidney and its ureter.

u·re′ter·o·plas″ty. A plastic operation on a ureter.

u·re″ter·o·py″e·li′tis. Inflammation of a ureter and the pelvis of a kidney.

u·re″ter·o·py″e·log′ra·phy. Roentgenographic visualization of the upper urinary tract by the injection of contrast mediums.

u·re″ter·o·py″e·lo·ne·os′to·my. Formation of a new passageway from the pelvis of a kidney to its ureter.

u·re″ter·o·py″e·lo·ne·phri′tis. Inflammation of a ureter and of a kidney and pelvis.

u·re″ter·o·py″e·lo·ne·phros′to·my. Surgical anastomosis of the ureter with the pelvis of the kidney.

u·re″ter·o·py′e·lo·plas″ty. Any plastic operation involving the upper portion of a ureter and the adjacent pelvis of the kidney.

u·re″ter·o·py″e·los′to·my. Excision of part of a ureter and implantation of the remaining part into a new aperture made into the pelvis of the kidney.

u·re″ter·or·rha′gi·a. Hemorrhage from a ureter.

u·re″ter·or′rha·phy. Suture of a ureter.

u·re″ter·o·sig″moid·os′to·my. Implantation of a ureter, severed from the bladder, into the sigmoid colon.

u·re″ter·os′to·my. Transplantation of a ureter to the skin; the formation of an external ureteral fistula.

u·re″ter·ot′o·my. Incision of a ureter.

u′re·than (yoor′i·thane, yōō·reth′-ane). 1. $C_2H_5O.CO.NH_2$. Ethyl carbamate, occurring as crystals or a white powder; soluble in water. Used as a somnifacient and, recently, in the treatment of myeloid and lymphatic leukemia. Also called *ethyl urethan.* 2. Any ester of carbamic acid.

u·re′thra. The canal through which the urine is discharged, extending from the neck of the bladder to the urethral meatus. It is divided in the male into the prostatic portion, the membranous portion, and the spongy or penile portion, and is from 8 to 9 inches long. In the female it is about 1½ inches in length. **—urethral,** *adj.* **membranous u.** The part of the urethra between the two layers of the urogenital diaphragm. **prostatic u.** That portion of the male urethra within the prostate gland. **spongy portion of u.** That contained in the corpus spongiosum of the penis; the penile urethra. Also called *cavernous u.*

u″re·three′to·my. Excision of the urethra or a portion of it.

u″re·thri′tis. Inflammation of the urethra. **anterior u.** Inflammation of the part situated anterior to the inferior layer of the urogenital diaphragm. **posterior u.** Inflammation of the prostatic and membranous portions.

u·re′thro-, urethr-. A combining form denoting *the urethra.*

u·re′thro·bulb′ar. Relating to the urethra and the bulb of the corpus spongiosum.

u·re′thro·cele. A urethral protrusion or diverticulum involving, usually, the female urethra.

u·re″thro·cys·ti′tis. Inflammation of the urethra and bladder.

u·re′thro·gram. A roentgenographic visualization of the urethra, obtained through the injection of a contrast medium.

u·re′thro·graph. A recording urethrometer.

u″re·throm′e·ter. An instrument for determining the caliber of the urethra or for measuring the lumen of a stricture.

u·re′thro·plas″ty. Plastic operation upon the urethra; surgical repair of the urethra.

u″re·thror′rha·phy. Surgical restoration of the continuity of the urethra.

u·re″thror·rhe′a. A morbid discharge from the urethra.

u·re′thro·scope. An instrument for inspecting the interior of the urethra. **—urethroscop′ic,** *adj.*

u″re·thros′co·py. Inspection of the urethra with the aid of a urethroscope.

u·re′thro·spasm. Spasmodic contraction of the urethral sphincters.

u·re″thro·ste·no′sis. Stricture of the urethra.

u″re·thros′to·my. Perineal section with permanent opening of the membranous urethra in the perineum.

u·re′thro·tome. An instrument used for performing urethrotomy. **dilating u.** A combined urethrotome and dilator.

u″re·throt′o·my. The operation of cutting a stricture of the urethra. **external u.** Division of a stricture by an incision from without. **internal u.** Division of a urethral stricture from within the urethra.

ur′gen·cy. Urgent desire to empty the urinary bladder.

Ur·gin′e·a. A genus of the Liliaceae. **U. maritima.** The plant that produces the official squill. See *squill.*

ur″hi·dro′sis (yoor″hi·dro′sis, ·high·dro′sis). A condition in which some of the constituents of the urine, chiefly urea, are excreted in excess of normal with the sweat.

-u′ri·a. A combining form meaning *a condition of the urine;* especially, *a diseased condition,* as in albumin*uria.*

u′ri·an. Urochrome, *q.v.*

u′ric. Pertaining to the urine, as uric acid.

u′ric ac′id. $C_5H_4N_4O_3$. Occurs in man as the end product of purine metabolism. It is a normal constituent of the blood and urine. Also called *triketo-purine*, 2,6,8-*trioxypurine*. See Table of Normal Values of Blood Constituents in the Appendix.

u″ric·ac″i·de′mi·a (yoor″ick·ass″i·dee′mee·uh). The presence of an abnormal amount of uric acid in the blood.

u″ric·ac″i·du′ri·a (·ass″i·dew′ree-uh). The presence of excessive amounts of uric acid in the urine.

u″ri·can′i·case. An enzyme in the liver which catalyzes conversion of urocanic acid to *l*-glutamic acid.

u′ri·case (yoor′i·kace, ·kaze). An enzyme present in the liver, spleen, and kidney of most mammals except man. In the presence of gaseous oxygen, it converts uric acid to allantoin.

u″ri·col′y·sis. The disintegration of uric acid.

u″ri·dyl′ic ac′id. A mononucleotide of yeast nucleic acid which yields uracil, ribose, and phosphoric acid upon complete hydrolysis.

u′ri·nal. A vessel for receiving urine.

u″ri·nal′y·sis. Analysis of the urine to determine specific gravity, presence or absence of albumin, sugar, pus, crystals, etc., and a microscopical examination of the sediment for abnormal constituents, such as casts and erythrocytes.

u′ri·nate. Discharge urine from the bladder. **—urina′tion**, *n*.

u′ri·na″tive. A drug which stimulates the flow of urine; a diuretic.

u′rine. The fluid excreted by the kidneys. In health, urine has an amber color, a slightly acid reaction, a faint odor, a saline taste, and a specific gravity 1.005 to 1.030. The quantity excreted in 24 hours varies with the amount of fluids consumed but averages between 1000 and 1500 cc. The amount of solids in the urine varies with the diet, more being excreted on a high protein, high salt diet. Normally between 40–75 Gm. of solids are present in the 24-hour urine, of which approximately 25% is urea, 25% chlorides, 25% sulfate and phosphates, and the remainder organic substances including organic acids, pigments, neutral sulfur, hormones, etc. The most important abnormal constituents present in disease are albumin, sugar, blood, pus, acetone, diacetic acid, fat, chyle, tube-casts, various cells, and bacteria. **—urinary**, *adj*. **incontinence of u.** Inability to retain the urine. See *enuresis*. **residual u.** Any considerable amount of urine remaining in the bladder after urination. The commonest causes are: in the male, prostatic hypertrophy and cystic disease; in the female, cystocele and pressure from uterine tumors. **retention of u.**

Inability to pass the urine. See *ischuria*. **suppression of u.** The sudden cessation of excretion of urine by the kidneys.

u″ri·nif′er·ous. Carrying or conveying urine, as uriniferous tubule.

u″ri·nif′ic. Excreting or producing urine.

u″ri·nip′a·rous. Producing urine.

u′ri·no-, urin-. A combining form denoting *urine*.

u″ri·no·gen′i·tal. Urogenital.

u″ri·no′ma. A cyst containing urine.

u″ri·nom′e·ter. A hydrometer for ascertaining the specific gravity of urine.

u″ri·nom′e·try. The determination of the specific gravity of urine.

u″ri·no·scop′ic. Pertaining to examination of urine. Syn., *uroscopic*.

u″ri·nose, u′ri·nous. Having the characters of urine, as a urinose or urinous odor.

u″ri·sol′vent. Dissolving uric acid.

u′ro-, ur-. A combining form denoting *urine*.

u″ro·ac″i·dim′e·ter (yoor″o·ass″i·dim′i·tur). An instrument for measuring the acidity of urine.

u″ro·am·mo′ni·ac. Relating to, or containing, uric acid and ammonia.

u″ro·an′thro·pos. An individual with a tail. Also called *Homo caudatus*.

u″ro·az″o·tom′e·ter. An apparatus for quantitative estimation of the nitrogenous substances in urine.

u″ro·bi′lin (yoor″o·buy′lin, ·bil′in). A bile pigment produced by the putrefaction of bilirubin in the gut and excreted by the kidneys or removed by the liver. Used as a reagent.

u″ro·bi″li·ne′mi·a (·buy″li·nee′mee·uh, ·bil″i·nee′mee·uh). The presence of urobilin in the blood.

u″ro·bi·lin′o·jen (·buy·lin′o·jen, ·bi·lin′o·jen). A chromogen from which urobilin is formed by oxidation when urine is allowed to stand.

u″ro·bi″li·noi′din (·buy″li·noy′din, ·bil″i·). A form of urinary pigment derived from hematin and resembling urobilin though not identical with it. It occurs in certain pathologic conditions.

u″ro·bi″li·nu′ri·a (·buy″li·new′ree·uh, ·bil″i·). The presence of an excess of urobilin in urine.

u·roch′e·ras (yoo·rock′ur·us). Gravel in urine.

u″ro·che′si·a (yoor″o·kee′zhuh, ·zee·uh). Discharge of urine through the anus.

u″ro·chlo·ral′ic ac′id. Trichlorethylglycuronic acid; a metabolic product of chloral hydrate.

u′ro·chrome. A yellow pigment in urine.

u″ro·chro′mo·gen. A substance occurring in tissues, which is oxidized to urochrome.

u″ro·clep′si·a. Involuntary or unconscious urination.

u″ro·cris′i·a (yoor″o·kriz′ee·uh, ·kriss′ee·uh). Diagnosis by means of urinary examination and analysis.

u″ro·cri′sis. 1. The critical stage of a disease distinguished by the excretion of a large volume of urine. 2. Severe pain in any part of the urinary tract occurring in tabes dorsalis.

u″ro·cy′a·nin. See *uroglaucin*.

u″ro·cy·an′o·gen (yoor″o·sigh·an′o·jen). A blue pigment found in urine.

u″ro·cy′a·nose. See *urocyanogen*.

u″ro·cy″a·no′sis. Blue discoloration of the urine, usually from the presence of excess amounts of indican oxidized to indigo blue; also from drugs such as methylene blue.

u″ro·er′yth·rin (yoor″o·err′ith·rin, ·i·rith′rin). A red pigment found in urine.

u″ro·fla′vin. A fluorescent compound of unknown structure, with properties similar to riboflavin, excreted in the urine along with the vitamin, following ingestion of riboflavin.

u″ro·fus′cin. A pigment found occasionally in urine in cases of porphyrinuria.

u″ro·fus″co·hem′a·tin (yoor″o·fus″ko·hem′uh·tin, ·hee′muh·tin). A red pigment derived from hematin, occurring in the urine.

u″ro·gas′trone. A substance extracted from urine which inhibits gastric secretion and motility; probably related to enterogastrone.

u″ro·gen′i·tal. Pertaining to the urinary and genital organs.

u·rog′e·nous (yoo·rodj′i·nus). Producing urine.

u″ro·glau′cin (yoor″o·glaw′sin). A blue pigment sometimes occurring in urine.

u′ro·gram. A radiograph or roentgenographic visualization of the urinary tract made after intravenous or retrograde injection of an opaque contrast substance.

u·rog′ra·phy. Roentgenographic visualization of the urinary tract by the use of contrast mediums.

u″ro·hem′a·tin (yoor″o·hem′uh·tin, ·hee′muh·tin). Altered hematin in the urine.

u″ro·hem″a·to·ne·phro′sis (·hem″uh·to·ni·fro′sis, ·hee″muh·to·). Distention of the pelvis of a kidney with blood and urine.

u″ro·hem″a·to·por′phy·rin. Urohematin; a urinary pigment occasionally occurring in urine in certain pathologic states.

u″ro·hy″per·ten′sin. A substance derived from urine which increases

blood pressure when it is injected intravenously.

u″ro·ki·net′ic (·ki·net′ick, ·kigh·net′ick). Due to a reflex from the urinary system; a term generally used to denote a form of indigestion secondary to irritation or disease of the urinary tract.

urokon sodium. Trade-mark for sodium acetrizoate.

u″ro·leu·kin′ic ac′id. An acid found in the urine in alkaptonuria.

u′ro·lith. A calculus occurring in urine. —**urolith′ic,** adj.

u″ro·li·thi′a·sis. 1. The presence of, or a condition associated with, urinary calculi. 2. The formation of urinary calculi.

u·rol′o·gist. One skilled in urology; a specialist in the diagnosis and treatment of diseases of the urogenital tract in the male and the urinary tract in the female.

u·rol′o·gy. The scientific study of the urine. That branch of medical science embracing the study and treatment of the diseases and the abnormalities of the urogenital tract in the male and the urinary tract in the female. —**urolog′ic,** adj.

u″ro·lu′te·in. A yellow pigment sometimes found in urine.

u″ro·mel′a·nin. A black pigment which sometimes appears in urine as a decomposition product of urochrome.

u·ron′ic ac′id. Any one of a group of acids of the formula $CHO.(CHOH)_x.-COOH$ derived from monosaccharides.

u″ron·on·com′e·try. Measurement of the quantity of urine passed or excreted in a definite period, as 24 hours.

u″ro·nos′co·py. Examination of urine by inspection and use of the microscope.

u·rop′a·thy. Old term for any disease involving the urinary tract, as indicated by urinary pathology.

u″ro·pla′ni·a. Urine elsewhere than in the urinary organs; discharge of urine from an orifice other than the urethra.

u″ro·por′phy·rin. A red pigment occurring in the urine and feces in porphyrinuria.

u″ro·ro′sein, u″ro·ro′se·in. A urinary pigment which does not occur preformed in the urine, but is present in the form of a chromogen, indoleacetic acid, which is transformed into the pigment upon treatment with a mineral acid. It is said to be identical with urorrhodin.

u″ror·rha′gi·a. Excessive discharge of urine.

u″ror·rho′din. A red pigment found in urine and derived from uroxanthin. Also see *urorosein*.

u″ror·rho·din′o·gen. The chromogen which by decomposition produces urorrhodin.

u″ro·ru′bin. A red pigment found in urine, seen only in disease.

u·ro·sa′cin. See *urorrhodin*.

u·ros′co·pist. One who makes a specialty of urinary examinations; a technician who examines urine for evidence of disease.

u·ros′co·py. Examination of urine.

u·ro′se·in. See *urorrhodin*.

u″ro·sep′sis. A systemic infection originating in the urinary tract. *Rare.* —**uroseptic,** *adj.*

u″ro·spec′trin. A pigment of normal urine.

u″ro·ste′a·lith. A fatlike substance occurring in some urinary calculi.

u″ro·tox′ic. 1. Pertaining to poisonous substances eliminated in urine. 2. Pertaining to poisoning by urine or some of its constituents. *Obs.*

urotropin. Trade-mark for a brand of methenamine.

u″ro·xan′thin (yoor″o·zan′thin). A yellow pigment in human urine which yields indigo blue on oxidation.

ur′rho·din (yoor′o·din, yoo·ro′din). See *urorrhodin*.

ur·sol′ic ac′id (ur·sol′ick). $C_{30}H_{48}O_3$. A triterpenic acid occurring in the waxlike coating of the skin or cuticle of fruits and in the leaves of certain plants. Used as an emulsifying agent.

ur″ti·ca′ri·a. Hives or nettle rash. A skin condition characterized by the appearance of intensely itching wheals or welts with elevated, usually white, centers and a surrounding area of erythema. They appear in crops, widely distributed over the body surface, tend to disappear in a day or two, and usually are unattended by constitutional symptoms. **allergic u.** That due usually to the ingestion, more rarely to inhalation of or contact with, a substance to which the individual is sensitive. Common food allergens are strawberries, citrus fruits, fish and shellfish, eggs, tomatoes, and chocolate. **factitious u.** Dermographia, *q.v.* **u. bullosa.** A type with the formation of fluid-filled vesicles or bullae on the surface of the wheals. **u. hemorrhagica.** A type of urticaria bullosa in which the vesicles contain bloody fluid. **u. medicamentosa.** That due to the ingestion of a drug to which the individual is allergic. **u. papulosa.** An intensely pruritic skin eruption seen in children, characterized by recurrent crops of erythematous patches and papules on the extensor surfaces of the extremities. Also called *lichen urticatus, prurigo simplex.* **u. pigmentosa.** A rare form of urticarial eruption, marked by more or less persistent, yellowish, brownish, or slate-colored lesions, which may be macules, papules, or nodules.

ur″ti·ca′tion. 1. A sensation as if one had been stung by nettles. 2. Production of wheals.

u·ru′shi·ol (yoo·roo′shee·ol). The irritant principle of poison ivy and poison oak.

U. S. P., U. S. Phar. United States Pharmacopeia.

U. S. P. H. S. United States Public Health Service.

us″ti·lag′i·nism (us″ti·ladj′i·nizum). Condition resembling ergot poisoning; caused by eating smutty corn.

Us″ti·la′go. A genus of parasitic fungi—the smuts. **U. maydis.** Corn smut, a fungus parasitic upon maize or Indian corn.

us′tion. *In surgery,* cauterization.

u″ter·al′gi·a. Pain in the uterus.

u′ter·ine (yoo′tur·in, yoo′tuh·ryne). Pertaining to the uterus.

u″ter·is′mus (yoo″tur·iz′mus). Uterine contraction of a spasmodic and painful character.

u″ter·i′tis. Inflammation of the uterus; metritis.

u′ter·o-, uter-. A combining form denoting *pertaining to the uterus.*

u″ter·o·cer′vi·cal. Relating to the uterus and the cervix of the uterus.

u″ter·o·ges·ta′tion. Gestation within the cavity of the uterus; normal pregnancy.

u″ter·og′ra·phy. Roentgenographic visualization of the uterine cavity by means of an iodized oil or other contrast medium injected therein through the cervical canal; metrography.

u″ter·om′e·ter. An instrument used to measure the uterus.

u″ter·o·pa·ri′e·tal. Pertaining to the uterus and the abdominal wall.

u″ter·o·plas′ty. A plastic operation on the uterus.

u″ter·o·rec′tal. Relating to the uterus and the rectum.

u″ter·o·sa′cral. Pertaining to the uterus and the sacrum.

u″ter·o·sal″pin·gog′ra·phy. Radiographic visualization of the cavities of the uterus and uterine tubes by means of an iodized oil contrast substance injected into the cervical canal under pressure. Also called *hysterosalpingography, metrosalpingography.*

u′ter·o·scope′. A uterine speculum.

u″ter·o·ton′ic. Increasing muscular tone of the uterus.

u′ter·o·trac′tor. 1. Old term for uterine tenaculum or volsella forceps. 2. A wide, heavy, sharp-toothed retractor used to make continuous traction on the anterior portion of the cervix of the uterus during surgery.

u″ter·o·tu′bal. Relating to the uterus and the uterine tubes.

ter·o·vag'i·nal (yoo"tur·o·vadj'-ul, ·va·jy'nul). Relating to the uterus d vagina.

ter·o·ven'tral. Relating to the rus and the abdomen.

ter·o·ves'i·cal. Relating to the rus and urinary bladder.

er·us (pl. *uteri*). The womb; the an of gestation which receives and ds the fertilized ovum, during the velopment of the fetus, and becomes principal agent in its expulsion ring parturition. It is a pear-shaped, scular organ, three inches long, two hes wide, and one inch thick, and is ided into three portions: the fundus, body, and the cervix. The fundus is upper and broad portion; the body dually narrows to the neck, which is contracted portion. The orifice, os ri, communicates with the vagina. e inner surface is covered with mu-is membrane continuous with that of vagina. The outer surface of the dus and body is covered with peri-eum. The whole organ is suspended the pelvis by means of the broad and nd ligaments and the uterosacral aments. The uterine tubes enter, one each side of the fundus, at the nua of the organ. **anteflexion u.** The normal position of the organ ne of anteflexion, that is, with the dus directed toward the symphysis is. Common usage of this term indi-es a greater degree of anteflexion n the accepted normal. **bipar-e u.** See *u. septus.* **fetal u.** One defective development, in which the gth of the cervical canal exceeds the gth of the cavity of the body. **avid u.** A pregnant uterus. **in-atile u.** A uterus normally formed, arrested in development. **pubes-at u.** An abnormality of the uterus which the characters of that organ uliar to the epoch preceding puberty sist in the adult. **retroflexion u.** Backward displacement of the dus of the uterus with the cervix in normal position. **retroversion u.** Backward displacement of the rus, with the cervix lying in the axis the vagina or pointing anteriorly. **acollis.** A uterus in which the inal part is absent. **u. bicornis.** terus divided into two horns or com-tments due to an arrest of develop-at. **u. bilocularis.** See *u. septus.* **didelphys.** Double uterus from ure of the paramesonephric ducts to

fuse. Syn., *u. duplex.* **u. duplex.** A uterus that is double from failure of the paramesonephric ducts to unite. **u. masculinus.** See *utricle,* 2. **u. septus.** A uterus in which a median septum more or less completely divides the lumen into halves. **u. uni-cornis.** A uterus having but a single lateral half with usually only one uterine tube; it is the result of faulty development.

u'tri·cle. 1. A delicate membranous sac communicating with the semicircu-lar canals of the ear. 2. The uterus masculinus, or prostatic utricle; a vestigial blind pouch in the colliculus seminalis opening into the prostatic urethra. The homolog of a part of the female vagina; derived from the fused distal ends of the paramesonephric ducts. Syn., *utriculus masculinus, sinus pocularis.* —**utric'ular,** *adj.*

u·tric"u·li'tis. Inflammation of the prostatic utricle.

u·tric"u·lo·sac'cu·lar. Pertaining to the utricle and saccule of the ear.

u'va ur'si (yoo'vuh ur'sigh). The dried leaf of *Arctostaphylos Uva-ursi* or its varieties *coactylis* and *adenotri-cha.*

u've·a. The pigmented, vascular layer of the eye, the iris, ciliary body, and choroid. —**uveal,** *adj.*

u"ve·i'tis. Inflammation of the uvea. —**uveit'ic,** *adj.*

u'vi·o·lize". Submit to the action of ultraviolet rays. *Rare.*

u"vi·o·re·sist'ant (yoo"vee·o·ri-zist'unt). Not responding to ultraviolet rays.

u'vu·la. The conical appendix hang-ing from the free edge of the soft palate, containing the uvular muscle covered by mucous membrane. —**uvu-lar,** *adj.* **u. cerebelli.** A small lobule of the inferior vermis of the cerebellum, forming the posterior boundary of the fourth ventricle. **u. fissa.** Cleft uvula.

u"vu·lec'to·my. Resection of the uvula.

u"vu·li'tis. Inflammation of the uvula.

u"vu·lop·to'sis. A relaxed and pen-dulous condition of the uvula.

u'vu·lo·tome, u"vu·la·tome. An instrument used in performing uvu-lotomy.

u"vu·lot'o·my, u"vu·lat'o·my. The operation of cutting off the uvula.

V

V. 1. Chemical symbol for vanadium. 2. Abbreviation for vision.

v. Volt.

vac'ci·na·ble. Susceptible of successful vaccination.

vac'ci·nate. Perform a vaccination.

vac''ci·na'tion. 1. Inoculation with the virus of vaccinia in order to protect against smallpox. 2. Inoculation with any organism to produce immunity against a given infectious disease. **compulsory** v. That legally required, as for admission to school or to a foreign country.

vac'cine (vack'seen, ·sin). 1. Smallpox vaccine. 2. Any organism used for preventive inoculation against a specific disease. **acne** v. One made from organisms cultured from the patient's lesions, or from a mixture of several strains of staphylococci, or from the acne bacillus, *Corynebacterium acnes.* **autogenous** v. A vaccine made from a culture obtained from the patient himself. **bacterial** v. An emulsion of bacteria, killed, living, or attenuated, in normal salt solution used hypodermically for the purpose of raising the immune response of a patient suffering from infection by the same organism. **BCG** v. (Bacillus Calmette-Guérin). One made from cultures of attenuated human tubercle bacilli, used orally to obtain immunity against tuberculosis. It has been suggested that the vaccine might also give some protection against leprosy. Also called *Calmette's v.* **brucella** v. One obtained from *Brucella melitensis, abortus* or *suis;* used in the treatment of undulant fever. **cholera** v. A sterile suspension of killed cholera vibrios (*Vibrio comma*), of strains selected for high antigenic efficiency, in isotonic sodium chloride solution or other suitable diluent. **Cox** v. A vaccine against typhus fever, prepared from *Rickettsia prowazekii* cultivated on the allantoic membrane of the developing chick embryo. **heterogenous** v. One prepared from organisms derived from some source other than the patient in whose treatment they are to be used; the source is usually a stock culture. **humanized** v. That obtained from vaccinal vesicles of man. **paratyphoid** v. A vaccine made from cultures of *Salmonella schottmuelleri* for immunization against paratyphoid. **pertussis** v. One made from cultures of *Hemophilus pertussis,* used in the prevention and treatment of whooping cough. **poliomyelitis** v. One prepared from strains of 3 types the poliomyelitis virus, usually in monkey kidney tissue culture mediu and deactivated with formaldehyd used to establish immunity again paralytic poliomyelitis in man. **polyvalent** v. A bacterial vaccine ma from cultures of two or more strai of the same species of bacteria. **rabies** v. An uncontaminated suspe sion of the attenuated, diluted, dri or dead, fixed virus of rabies. T virus is obtained from the tissue the central nervous system of an ar mal suffering from fixed virus rabi infection. Rabies vaccine is used e clusively as a prophylactic agent. treatment with rabies vaccine after t bite of a rabid animal, immunity often established before the incubati period of the disease is complete **Salk** v. Poliomyelitis vaccine. **sensitized** v. One prepared from kill microörganisms, to which has be added material containing homologo antibody material. **smallpox** v. glycerinated suspension of the ve cles of vaccinia or cowpox which ha been obtained from healthy vaccinat bovine animals. Smallpox vaccine used exclusively for the prevention this disease. Also called *virus vaccinu glycerinated v. virus, Jennerian antismallpox v.* Also see *vaccin* **staphylococcus** v. One made fro *Staphylococcus aureus* (*Micrococc aureus*), used in the treatment of f runculosis and other infections due the organism. **T.A.B.** v. Typho paratyphoid A and B vaccine. **triple v. for typhoid.** Typhoid-para phoid A and B vaccine. **typhoid paratyphoid A and B** v. O containing organisms of typhoid, a paratyphoid A and B strains, for sim taneous immunization against all thr diseases. **typhoid** v. A sterile suspe sion of killed typhoid bacilli used produce immunity against typhoid.

vac·cin'i·a (vack·sin'ee·uh). Cowpo a contagious disease of cows characte ized by vesicopustular lesions of t skin which are prone to appear on t teats and udder, and transmissible man by handling infected cows and vaccination; it confers immun against smallpox. In the human subje inoculated with cowpox, a small pap appears at the site of inoculation from one to three days, which becom a vesicle about the fifth day, and the end of the first week is pustul umbilicated, and surrounded by a r

772

reola. Desiccation begins in the second week and a crust forms, which soon falls off, leaving a white, pitted cicatrix.
vac·cin'i·fer (vack·sin'i·fur). 1. A person or animal from whom vaccine virus is taken. 2. A vaccine point.
vac·cin'i·o'la (vack·sin″ee·o'luh, vack″sin·eye'o·luh). A secondary eruption, sometimes following vaccinia, resembling the eruption of smallpox.
vac'ci·noid. Resembling vaccinia.
vac″ci·no·pho'bi·a. Morbid dread of vaccination.
vac″ci·no·ther'a·py. The therapeutic use of vaccines.
vac'u·o·lar (vack'yoo·o·lur, vack″oo·o'lur). Pertaining to, or of the nature of, a vacuole.
vac'u·o·late. Having, or pertaining to, vacuoles.
vac'u·o·la″ted. Containing one or more vacuoles; said of a cell or cytoplasm.
vac″u·o·la'tion. The formation of vacuoles; the state of being vacuolated.
vac'u·ole. A clear space in a cell.
contractile v. A vacuole in the cytoplasm of certain protozoa, which rhythmically gradually increases in size and then collapses.
vac″u·ol'i·za'tion. See vacuolation.
vac'u·ome. The internal reticular apparatus; consists of vacuoles found singly or forming a canalicular network near the centrosome and stainable with neutral red in living cells.
vac'u·um. A space from which most of the air has been exhausted.
va'gal. Pertaining to the vagus nerve.
va'gal at·tack'. A condition characterized by a feeling of impending death, dyspnea, cardiac discomfort, and a choking sensation; supposed to be due to vasomotor spasm.
va'gal es·cape'. One or more spontaneous beats of the heart, occurring in spite of the fact that the function of the sinus node that normally initiates heart beats has been arrested by stimulation of the vagus nerve.
va·gi'na (pl. *vaginas, vaginae*). 1. A sheath. 2. The musculomembranous canal from the vestibule to the cervix uteri, ensheathing the latter. It receives the penis during copulation. —**vag'i·nal** (vadj'i·nul, va·jy'nul), *adj.* **mucosa of v.** The mucous membrane lining the vagina.
vag″i·nec'to·my (vadj″i·neck'to·mee). 1. Excision of the vagina or a portion of it. 2. Excision of the tunica vaginalis.
vag″i·nic'o·line (vadj″i·nick'o·line, ·lin). Living in the vagina, as *Trichomonas vaginalis*.
vag″i·nis'mus (vadj″i·niz'mus, ·is'mus). Painful spasm of the vagina.
mental v. That due to extreme aver-

sion to the sexual act. **perineal v.** That due to spasm of the perineal muscles. **posterior v.** That due to spasm of the pubococcygeal portion of the levator ani muscle.
vag″i·ni'tis (vadj″i·nigh'tis). 1. Inflammation of the vagina. 2. Inflammation of a sheath. **atrophic v.** Inflammation of the vagina occurring after the menopause, surgical or otherwise. **senile v.** Inflammation of the vagina occurring after the menopause. It is more properly called *atrophic v.* **Trichomonas vaginalis v.** Vaginitis associated with, and thought to be caused by, *Trichomonas vaginalis*.
vag'i·no- (vadj'i·no-), **vagin-.** A combining form denoting *the vagina*.
vag″i·no·dyn'i·a. Neuralgic pain of the vagina.
vag″i·no·fix·a'tion. Fixation of the uterus to the vaginal peritoneum in the treatment of retroflexion.
vag″i·no·my·co'sis (vadj″i·no·migh·ko'sis, va·jy″no·). A fungus infection of the vagina, usually by *Candida albicans*.
vag'i·no·plas″ty (vadj'i·no·plas″tee, va·jy'no·). A plastic operation on the vagina.
vag'i·no·scope (vadj'i·no·scope, va·jy'no·). A vaginal speculum.
vag″i·nos'co·py. Inspection of the vagina.
vag″i·not'o·my. Incision of the vagina; colpotomy.
va·gi'tus. The cry of an infant. **v. uterinus.** The cry of a child while still in the uterus. **v. vaginalis.** The cry of a child while the head is still in the vagina.
va·got'o·mized. Pertaining to an individual or animal whose vagus nerves have been severed.
va·got'o·my. Surgical division of the vagus nerves.
va″go·to'ni·a. A condition due to overaction of the vagus nerves and modification of functions in organs innervated by them. —**vagoton'ic,** *adj.*
va·got'o·nin, vag″o·to'nin. A hormonal substance from the pancreas which stimulates the parasympathetic system.
va″go·trop'ic (vay″go·trop'ick, vag″o·). Having an effect upon, or influencing, the vagus nerve.
va'grant. Wandering, as a vagrant cell.
va'gus (pl. *vagi*). The tenth cranial nerve. Formerly called the *pneumogastric nerve*. See Table of Nerves in the Appendix.
va'lence, va'len·cy. 1. The capacity of an atom to combine with other atoms in definite proportions. 2. By analogy, also applied to radicals and atomic groups. Valence is measured with the

combining capacity of a hydrogen atom taken as unity. **-valent,** adj. **coör-dinate v.** Covalence in which one atom or ion contributes both electrons of the pair, and the other atom or ion supplies no electrons. **covalence.** The sharing of valence electrons between atoms. **residual v. forces.** The unsatisfied forces of ions or molecules which lead to formation of more complex substances from apparently saturated ions or molecules.

va'len·cy. See *valence.*

val'er·ate. A salt of valeric acid. Also called *valerianate.* **acid ammonium v.** NH₄C₅H₉O₂.2HC₅H₉O₂; occurs as colorless, quadrangular plates; soluble in water. Used as a nerve sedative and euphoric. Also called *ammonium valerianate.*

va·le'ri·an. The dried rhizome and roots of *Valeriana officinalis.* Contains a volatile oil. Used as a remedy for hysteria and other emotional states.

va·le'ri·a·nate. Valerate. **ammonium v.** Acid ammonium valerate.

va·le"ri·an'ic ac'id. Valeric acid, *q.v.*

va·ler'ic ac'id (va-lerr'ick, va-leer'-ick), **va·le"ri·an'ic ac'id.** C₅H₁₀O₂. Four isomeric modifications of this acid are known: 1. Normal valeric or propylacetic acid, CH₂(CH₂)₃COOH. 2. Isovaleric or isopropylacetic acid, (CH₃)₂CH.CH₂.COOH, the valeric acid of commerce. 3. Methylethylacetic acid, CH₃·(C₂H₅).CH.COOH. 4. Trimethylacetic acid, (CH₃)₃C.COOH.

val'er·o-, valer-. A combining form denoting *valeric.*

val"e·tu"di·na'ri·an·ism. Feeble or infirm state due to invalidism.

val'gus. A term denoting position; if of the foot it means eversion (talipes valgus); if of the knee it can mean either bowlegged, old term, or knockkneed, modern usage (genu valgum); if of the hip it refers to an increase in the angle between the neck and the shaft of the femur (coxa valga); if of the great toe it denotes a turning of that toe toward the other toes (hallux valgus). If the term is used alone it generally refers to the foot.

val'ine (val'een, vay'leen). (CH₃)₂·CHCH(NH₂)·COOH; α-aminoisovaleric acid, an amino-acid constituent of many proteins. It is essential to man, as well as to certain animals.

val'late. Surrounded by a walled depression; cupped.

val·lec'u·la (pl. *valleculae*). A shallow groove or depression. **v. cere·belli.** The depression between the cerebellar hemispheres. **v. epiglottica.** A depression between the lateral and median epiglottic folds on either side of the base of the tongue.

vallestril. Trade-mark for meth[...] lenestril.

valmid. Trade-mark for ethinama[...]

valve. A device in a vessel or passa[...] which prevents reflux of its conten[...] **anal valves.** Valvelike folds in a[...] mucous membrane which join togeth[...] the lower ends of the rectal colum[...] **aortic v.** One consisting of th[...] semilunar cusps situated at the ju[...] tion of the aorta and the left ventri[...] of the heart. **atrioventricul[...] valves.** The mitral and tricusp[...] valves of the heart. **bicuspid [...]** Mitral valve. **caval v.** The sem[...] lunar valve in the right atrium [...] the heart between the orifice of t[...] inferior vena cava and the right atr[...] ventricular orifice. Syn., *Eustachian [...] inferior vena caval v.* **coronary v.** [...] semicircular fold of the endocardi[...] of the right atrium at the orifice of t[...] coronary sinus. Syn., *Thebesian [...] Gerlach's v.* A mucosal fold som[...] times surrounding the orifice of t[...] appendix. **Houston's valves.** Th[...] transverse semilunar folds in the m[...] cous membrane of the rectum. **ile[...] cecal v.** The valve at the junction [...] the terminal ileum and the cec[...] which consists of a superior and [...] ferior lip and partially prevents ref[...] from the cecum into the ileum. Sy[...] *colic v.* Also called *ileocolic v.* Forme[...] called *Bauhin's v.* **mitral v.** A he[...] valve having two cusps, situated b[...] tween the left atrium and left vent[...] cle. Syn., *bicuspid valve.* **pulm[...] nary v.** One consisting of three sem[...] lunar cusps situated between the rig[...] ventricle and the pulmonary arter[...] **pyloric v.** The fold of mucous mem[...] brane at the pyloric end of the sto[...] ach together with the underlying [...] loric sphincter, a thickened ring [...] smooth muscle. **rectal valves.** S[...] *Houston's valves* under *valve.* **sem[...] lunar valves.** The valves situat[...] between the ventricles and aorta [...] pulmonary artery. **spiral v.** Col[...] mucomembranous folds in the neck [...] the gallbladder and cystic duct. Al[...] called *Heister's v.* **Thebesian v.** S[...] *coronary v.* **tricuspid v.** The thr[...] cusped valve situated between t[...] right atrium and right ventricle.

val·vot'o·my. Surgical incision i[...] a valve, especially the rectal folds. Sy[...] *diclidotomy.*

val'vu·la (pl. *valvulae*). A valve, q[...] **-valvular,** adj.

val"vu·li'tis. Inflammation of [...] valve, especially of a cardiac valve.

val'vu·lo·tome. An instrument d[...] signed especially for incising the val[...] of the heart.

val"vu·lot'o·my. The surgical in[...] sion of a valve of the heart, as [...] mitral stenosis.

al'zin. See *dulcin.*

an'a·date. A salt of vanadic acid.

a·nad'ic ac'id (va·nad'ick, va·ay'dick). H_3VO_4. An acid derived from anadium; forms salts called vanates.

a·na'di·um. V = 50.95. A rare metalc element.

a·na'di·um·ism. A chronic form of ntoxication due to the absorption of anadium; it occurs in workers using he metal or its compounds.

a·nil'la. The cured, full-grown, unipe fruit of *Vanilla planifolia*, or *V. ahitensis*. The fresh fruit possesses ione of the pleasant odor commonly ssociated with the fruit. Two enzymes, nder the influence of heat and moisure, produce vanillin from two of three lycosides, and perhaps another aroiatic substance from a third glycoside. anilla is used solely as a flavoring gent. Also called *vanilla bean*.

a·nil'lic ac'id. $CH_3O.C_6H_3(OH)-$ OOH. 3-Methoxy-4-hydroxybenzoic cid; the crystalline solid resulting rom the oxidation of vanillin.

an'il·lin, va·nil'lin. $CH_3.C_6H_3-$ OH) CHO. 3-Methoxy-4-hydroxybenzldehyde; occurs as fine, white to lightly yellow crystals; soluble in rater. Used as a flavoring agent.

a·nil'lism. A form of contact dernatitis characterized by marked itchng; occurring among vanilla workers.

anquin. Trade-mark for pyrvinium hloride.

a"po·cau"ter·i·za'tion. Cauteriation by live steam.

a'por. A gas, especially the gaseous orm of a substance which at ordinary emperatures is liquid or solid.

a"por·i·za'tion. The conversion of solid or liquid into a vapor. —**va'**orize, *v.*; **va'porizer**, *n.*

a"po·ther·a·py. The therapeutic mployment of medicated or nonmediated vapors, steam, or sprays.

a"ri·a·bil'i·ty. The property of rganisms which results in differences mong members of the same species, o that no two are alike in all their haracteristics.

a'ri·a·ble. *In biometry*, a quantity r magnitude which may vary in value inder differing conditions. Also see *urve*, 2.

a'ri·ance. The square of the standrd deviation. The second moment when deviations are taken from the nean.

a'ri·ant. *In bacteriology*, a colony vhich differs in appearance from the arent colony grown on the same meliums.

a'ri·a'tion. Deviation from a given ype as the result of environment, natural selection, or cultivation and domestication; diversity in characteristics among related organisms.

var"i·cec'to·my. Excision of a varix or varicose vein, as distinguished from avulsion of a vein.

var"i·cel'la. Chickenpox.

var"i·cel·la'tion. Preventive inoculation with the virus of varicella.

var'i·ces (valr'i·seez, var'i·seez). Plural of varix, *q.v.*

var"i·co·bleph'a·ron. A varicosity of an eyelid.

var"i·co·cele". Dilatation of the veins of the pampiniform plexus of the spermatic cord, forming a soft, elastic swelling that feels like a collection of worms.

var"i·co·ce·lec'to·my. Excision of dilated spermatic veins, with or without removal of a portion of the scrotum, for the radical cure of varicocele.

var"i·cog'ra·phy. Roentgenographic visualization of the course and extent of a collection of varicose veins.

var"ic·om'pha·lus. A varicosity at the navel.

var"i·co·phle·bi'tis. Inflammation of a varicose vein or veins.

var'i·cose. 1. Descriptive of blood vessels that are swollen, knotted, and tortuous. 2. Due to varicose veins, as varicose ulcer.

var"i·cos'i·ty. A varicose portion of a vein, usually of definite and limited extent.

var"i·cot'o·my. Excision of a varicose vein.

va·ric'u·la. A varix of the conjunctiva.

varidase. Trade-mark for a purified mixture of streptokinase and streptodornase, which causes liquefaction and the removal of necrotic tissue and thickened or clotted exudates from wounds or inflammatory processes, used to promote normal repair of tissue.

va·ri'e·ty. A subdivision of a species; a stock, strain, breed.

va'ri·form. Having diversity of form.

va·ri'o·la (va·rye'o·luh, va·ree'o·luh). Smallpox, *q.v.*

va·ri'o·lar. Pertaining to smallpox.

var"i·o·late (vair'ee·o·late, var'eeo·). 1. Having small pustules like those of variola. 2. Inoculate with smallpox virus.

var"i·o·la'tion (vair"ee·o·lay'shun, var"ee·o·). Inoculation of unmodified smallpox, usually from human to human; practice forbidden in most countries.

var"i·o'li·form (vair"ee·o'li·form, ·ol'i·form, var"ee·). Resembling variola.

var"i·o·loid (vair'ee·o·loyd, var'eeo·). A mild form of smallpox following the injection of smallpox virus in persons who previously had been successfully vaccinated or who previously had the disease.

va·ri″o·lo·vac′cine (va·rye″o·lo-vack′seen, va·ree″o·lo·). A vaccine obtained from the lymph in lesions produced in a heifer inoculated with smallpox virus. The virus may also be cultivated in a chick embryo by chorioallantoic inoculation.

va·ri″o·lo·vac·cin′i·a. A form of vaccinia or cowpox induced in a heifer by inoculating it with smallpox virus.

var′ix (vair′icks, var′icks) (pl. *varices*). A dilated and tortuous vein. See *cirsoid.*

va′rus. A term denoting position; if of the foot it means inversion (talipes varus); if of the knee it means bow-legged (genu varum); if of the hip it refers to a decrease in the angle between the neck and the shaft of the femur (coxa vara); if of the great toe it denotes a turning of that toe away from the other toes (hallux varus). If the term is used alone it generally refers to the foot.

vas (pl. *vasa*). A vessel. **v. afferens.** An afferent lymphatic vessel of a lymph node. **v. afferens glomeruli.** The arteriole supplying the capillary loops in a renal corpuscle. **vasa vasorum.** The blood vessels supplying the walls of arteries and veins having a caliber greater than 1 mm. **v. deferens.** The excretory duct of the testis; the ductus deferens (BNA). **v. efferens.** An efferent lymphatic vessel of a lymph node. **v. efferens glomeruli.** The precapillary draining the capillary loops in a renal corpuscle.

vas′cu·lar. Consisting of, pertaining to, or provided with, vessels.

vas′cu·lar bed. The total blood supply—arteries, capillaries, and veins—of an organ or region.

vas″cu·lar′i·ty. The quality of being vascular.

vas″cu·lar·i·za′tion. 1. The process of becoming vascular. 2. The formation and extension of vascular capillaries.

vas″cu·li′tis. See *angiitis.*

vas″cu·lo·gen′e·sis. The formation of the vascular system.

vas·ec′to·my. Resection of a ductus deferens.

vaseline. Trade-mark for a petroleum jelly and certain other products.

vas″i·fac′tion. The process of giving rise to new blood vessels.

vas·i′tis. Inflammation of the vas or ductus deferens.

vas′o- (vass′o-, vay′zo-), **vas-.** A combining form signifying *the blood vessels, ductus deferens,* or *vasomotor.*

vas″o·con·stric′tion. The constriction of blood vessels.

vas″o·con·stric′tor. 1. Causing constriction of blood vessels. 2. A nerve or a drug that causes constriction of blood vessels.

vas″o·de·pres′sor. Lowering blood pressure by relaxing blood vessels.

vas″o·dil″a·ta′tion (vay″zo·dil·uh·tay′shun, ·dye″luh·tay′shun). Dilatation of blood vessels.

vas″o·di·la′tin (·dye·lay′tin, ·dil·lay′tin). A widely distributed substance which lowers the blood pressure and stimulates gastric secretion. The substance is believed to be identical with histamine.

vas″o·di·la′tor (vay″zo·dye·lay′tur, ·di·lay′tur). 1. Pertaining to the relaxation of the smooth muscle of the vascular system. 2. Agent producing dilation of blood vessels.

vas″o·ep″i·did″y·mos′to·my (vaz″o·ep″i·did″i·mos′to·mee, vah″zo·). Anastomosis of a ductus deferens with its epididymal duct.

va·sog′ra·phy (vay·zog′ruh·fee, va·sog′·). Roentgenography of blood vessels.

vas″o·in·hib′i·tor. A drug or agent tending to inhibit the action of the vasomotor nerves. **—vasoinhibitory,** *adj.*

vas″o·li·ga′tion (vaz″o·lye·gay′shun, vah″zo·). Surgical ligation of a ductus deferens.

vas″o·mo′tion (vay″zo·mo′shun, vay″so·). Increase or decrease of the caliber of a blood vessel.

vas″o·mo′tor. Regulating the contraction (vasoconstriction) and expansion (vasodilatation) of blood vessels.

vas″o·or″chid·os′to·my (vaz″o-or″kid·os′to·mee, vah″zo-). Surgical anastomosis of a ductus deferens with any portion of its testis.

vas″o·pa·ral′y·sis. Paralysis of vasomotor mechanism.

vas″o·pa·re′sis (vay″zo·pa·ree′sis, ·par′i·sis). Paresis affecting the vasomotor nerves.

vas″o·pres′sin. The pressor principle of the neurohypophysis. Also called *beta-hypophamine.* See *pitressin.*

vas″o·punc′ture (vaz″o·punk′chur, vah″zo·). Surgical puncture of a ductus deferens.

vas″o·re″lax·a′tion (vay″zo·ree″lack·say′shun, vay″so·). Diminution of vascular tension.

vas·or′rha·phy (vaz·or′uh·fee, vahz·). End-to-end or end-to-side suture of a ductus deferens.

vas″o·sec′tion. Severing of a ductus deferens.

vas′o·spasm. Vasoconstriction, angiospasm.

as″o·stim′u·lant. Inducing or exiting vasomotor action.

as·os′to·my (va·zos′to·mee, va·sos′o·mee). The making of an artificial pening into a ductus deferens.

as·ot′o·my (va·zot′o·mee, va·sot′o-ee). Incision of a ductus deferens.

as″o·ton′ic (vay″zo·ton′ick, vay″o·). 1. Pertaining to the normal tone r tension of the blood vessels. 2. A asostimulant.

as″o·to′nin. A vasoconstrictor substance present in the blood.

as″o·troph′ic (vay″zo·trof′ick, ro′fick). Concerned in the nutrition f blood vessels.

as″o·va′gal. Pertaining to blood essels and vagus nerve, as paroxysmal asovagal attacks, or vasovagal synope.

as″o·va′gal at·tack′. Loss of conciousness, marked pallor, usually a rop in heart rate and rapid fall in ood pressure, occasionally profuse veating; due to exaggerated vagal ction through abnormal sensitivity of e carotid sinus. If it occurs in epiptiform diseases, it is called **paroxysmal vasovagal attack.** lso see carotid sinus *syncope.*

as″o·vas·os′to·my. Surgical anasmosis of one portion of a ductus deferens to another.

as″o·ve·sic″u·lec′to·my. Excion of a ductus deferens and seminal esicle.

soxyl hydrochloride. A tradeark for methoxamine hydrochloride. **s′tus.** 1. Large; extensive. 2. Any e of three muscles of the thigh. See able of Muscles in the Appendix.

ult. 1. An arched structure, as a me. 2. Specifically, the vault of the anium; calvaria.

cillin. A trade-mark for phenoxyethyl penicillin.

D. Venereal disease.

D. H. Valvular disease of the heart.

c′tion. The conveyance of disease rms from the sick to the well.

c′tis. An instrument similar to the ngle blade of a forceps, used in hasning the delivery of the fetal head in bor.

c′tor. 1. An arthropod which carries icroörganisms from a sick person to me other person. 2. A quantity inlving both magnitude and direction, velocity, force, momentum, which ay be represented by a straight line suitable length and direction. **—vec′rial,** *adj.*

g′e·tal (vedj′i·tul). Trophic.

g″e·ta′tion. An outgrowth resembing a plant in outline, as the projecns on the cardiac valves in endoditis, papillomas, polypoid growths, c.

ve′hi·cle. A liquid or solid substance, generally inactive therapeutically, employed as a medium or carrier for the active component of a medicine.

veil. A caul or portion of the amniotic sac covering the face of a newborn infant. **acquired v.** An obscuration or imperfection of voice from exposure to cold, catarrhal conditions, overuse, or bad training. **uterine v.** A cap fitted over the cervix uteri to prevent the entrance of semen.

vein. A blood vessel carrying blood from the tissues toward the heart. Veins, like arteries, have three coats, but the media is less developed; many possess valves. For veins unlisted here, see Table of Veins in the Appendix. **afferent veins.** Those conveying blood directly to an organ. **arcuate v.** A venous arch at the base of a renal pyramid, accompanying an arcuate artery. **central v.** (a) The vein in the center of a liver lobule into which the sinusoids empty. (b) That which receives blood from all vessels of the cortex and medulla of the adrenal gland. **collecting v.** A vein formed by the confluence of several intercalated veins of the liver. **common cardinal veins.** Paired primary veins located in the septum transversum, connecting the anterior and posterior cardinals with the sinus venosus. Syn., *ducts of Cuvier.* **diploic v.** One of the large, thin-walled veins occupying bony channels in the diploë of cranial bones, and communicating with each other, with meningeal veins and sinuses of the dura, and, through emissary veins, with the veins of the pericranium. **emissary v.** An emissary. **intercalated v.** Sublobular vein. **interlobar v.** In the kidney, one of the veins running in the renal columns and draining into the renal vein. **interlobular v.** In the kidney, a tributary of an arcuate vein, lying in the cortical substance between the medullary rays. **omphalomesenteric veins.** Embryonic veins uniting yolk sac and sinus venosus; their proximal fused ends form the portal vein. Syn., *vitelline veins.* **posterior cardinal veins.** Paired primary veins of the embryo draining body and mesonephros, located in the dorsolateral part of the urogenital fold; they unite with the anterior cardinal veins to form the common cardinal veins. **subcardinal veins.** Paired longitudinal veins of the embryo partly replacing the postcardinals; the prerenal part of the inferior vena cava develops largely from the right subcardinal. **sublobular v.** A vein formed by the joining of the central veins of several liver lobules. Syn., *intercalated v.* **supra-**

cardinal veins. Paired longitudinal venous channels of the embryo that replace the postcardinal and subcardinal veins and form the azygos-hemiazygos system of veins, and, on the right side, most of the postrenal part of the inferior vena cava. **systemic v.** One of those conveying venous blood from the systemic circuit to the right atrium of the heart. **Thebesian veins.** Small veins from the myocardium which open directly into the atria and ventricles. **umbilical veins.** Originally paired veins conveying blood from the placenta to the sinus venosus; the proximal right umbilical vein disappears early in development and the extraembryonic parts fuse to form a single vein in the cord. **varicose v.** Any vein that has become abnormally dilated and tortuous, due to interference with venous drainage or to weakening of its walls.

vein seek′er. A small pipet equipped with a teat-bulb, a glass sight filled with sodium citrate solution, and armed with an infusion needle. The teat is emptied by pressure of the fingers. The point of the needle is inserted under the skin where the vein is suspected, and the pressure released. The teat remains collapsed until a vein is entered, when blood appears in the tube. *Obs.*

ve·la′men. A veil or covering membrane.

veldt sore (velt, felt). A disease common in the African desert, but seen also in Australia and Burma; characterized by multiple, shallow, chronic, painful ulcers on exposed parts of the bodies of light-skinned individuals. It usually follows slight trauma, such as an insect bite. Exposure to sunlight is necessary, and there are usually secondary bacterial invaders. Also called *Barcoo disease, desert sore, septic sore.*

vel′li·cate. Twitch spasmodically.

vel·lo′sine (veh·lo′seen, vel′o·). $C_{22}H_{28}N_2O_4$. An alkaloid in Pao-Pereira bark, *Geissospermum vellosii laeve.*

ve′lum (pl. *vela*). A veil or veil-like structure. **—velar,** *adj.*

ve′na (pl. *venae*). A vein, *q.v.* **v. cava inferior.** A vein formed by the junction of the two common iliac veins and emptying into the right atrium of the heart. It receives the lumbar, right spermatic, renal, suprarenal, phrenic, and hepatic veins. **v. cava superior.** A vein formed by the union of the innominate veins, and conveying the blood from the head, chest wall, and upper extremities to the right atrium. **venae comitantes.** The veins accompanying an artery. **venae Thebesii.** Small veins from the myocardium which open directly into the atria and ventricles. **venae vorti-**

cosae. The stellate veins of th choroid coat of the eyeball.

ve·na′tion. Distribution of venou circulation to a part or organ.

ven·ec′to·my. Excision of a vein or portion of one.

ven″e·nif′er·ous (ven″i·nif′ur·u vee″ni·). Conveying poison.

ve·ne′re·al. Pertaining to, or pre duced by, sexual intercourse.

ve·ne″re·ol′o·gist. An expert i venereal diseases.

ve·ne″re·ol′o·gy. The study of vene real diseases.

ve·ne″re·o·pho′bi·a. Morbid fea of getting venereal disease.

ven′er·y. Copulation.

ven″e·sec′tion (ven″i·seck′shur vee″ni·). The abstraction of blood from the body by incising a vei popularly known as bleeding. In pra tice, blood is usually removed in mea ured quantity by the use of a needle o trochar passed into the lumen of vessel. Locally, a small amount of bloc may be removed by scarifying or leech ing.

ven″e·su′ture. The suturing of vein.

Ve·ne′tian red. A form of ferr oxide; used as a red pigment.

ven″i·punc′ture (ven″i·punk′chu ven′i·punk″chur). The surgical pun ture of a vein.

ve·noc′ly·sis. Injection of food drugs into a vein.

ve′no·gram. Roentgenogram of vein.

ven·og′ra·phy. Radiographic exam nation of veins following injectic of an opaque contrast medium.

ven′om. Poison, especially a poisc secreted by certain reptiles and insect

ve″no·mo′tor. Causing veins to co tract or dilate.

ven′om·ous. Poisonous.

ve″no·per″i·to·ne·os′to·m Surgical implantation of a divide greater saphenous vein into the per toneal cavity for drainage of ascite Also called *Ruotte's operation.*

ve″no·pres′sor. Pertaining to bloc pressure in the veins and right side the heart.

ve″no·scle·ro′sis. Induration veins; phlebosclerosis.

ve·nos′i·ty. A condition in which th arterial blood shows venous qualitie

ve″no·sta′sis, ve·nos′ta·sis. Pr vention of the return flow of the bloc by compression of veins or lowering venous pressure.

ve″no·throm·bot′ic. Having prop erty of producing venous thrombosis

ve·not′o·my. Phlebotomy; incision a vein.

ve′nous. Pertaining to the veins.

-no·ve·nos'to·my. The anastomosing of two veins.

-nt. Any aperture or outlet.

-nt'er. 1. The belly or abdomen. 2. he belly of a muscle. 3. The cavity of he abdomen.

-n'ti·late. 1. Renew the air in a lace. 2. Oxygenate the blood in the apillaries of the lungs.

-n'tral. 1. Pertaining to the belly. 2. *In human anatomy,* pertaining to he front portion of the body or of an rgan. _**ventrad, ventrally,** *adv.***

-n'tri·cle. A small cavity or pouch. _**ventric'ular,** *adj.* **fourth v.** he cavity of the metencephalon and yelencephalon. **laryngeal v.** The teral recess on either side between he ventricular and vocal folds. **lateral v.** The cavity of either cerebral emisphere communicating with the ird ventricle through the interventicular foramen, and consisting of a riangular central cavity or body and ree smaller cavities or cornua. **left v. of the heart.** That forcing the lood through the aorta and throughut the body. **right v. of the eart.** That forcing the blood rough the pulmonary artery into the ngs. **third v.** The cavity of the dincephalon, a narrow cleft between he two thalami. **ventricles of the rain.** Cavities in the interior of the rain, comprising the two lateral ventcles and the third and fourth ventcles.

-n·tric'u·lar es·cape'. Single or peated ventricular beats, arising from e A-V node, usually following a long iastole.

-n·tric'u·li'tis. Inflammation of e ependymal lining of the ventricles the brain. Syn., *ependymitis.*

-n·tric"u·lo·cor·dec'to·my. xcision of the wall of the laryngeal entricle and part of the vocal folds for e relief of bilateral abductor paralysis the vocal folds.

-n·tric'u·lo·gram". A roentgeno-am of the brain after the introducon of air or an opaque medium into e cerebral ventricles through trephine enings in the skull.

-n·tric"u·log'ra·phy. A method demonstrating the ventricles of the ain by roentgenography after the ntricular fluid has been replaced by r or by an opaque medium injected rough trephine openings in the skull.

-n·tric"u·lom'e·try. Measure-ent of the intraventricular pressure.

-n·tric"u·lo·punc'ture (ven-ick"yoo·lo·punk'chur, ven·trick'yoo-punk"chur). Puncture with a spinal uncture needle of a ventricle of the ain, particularly the lateral ventricle.

-n·tric"u·lo·scope". An instru-ent for inspecting the interior of the

cerebral ventricles and for electroco-agulation of the choroid plexus.

ven·tric"u·los'co·py. Examination of the ventricles of the brain by means of an endoscope.

ven·tric"u·los'to·my. The estab-lishment, by operative means, of drain-age of the cerebrospinal fluid from the ventricles of the brain.

ven·tric"u·lo·sub"a·rach'noid (·sub"a·rack'noyd). Pertaining to the subarachnoid space and the cerebral ventricles.

ven·tric'u·lus (pl. *ventriculi*). See *ventricle.* Old term for *stomach.*

ven"tri·cum'bent. Prone.

ven"tri·duc'tion. Drawing a part toward the abdomen.

ven·tril'o·quism. The art of speak-ing or singing without seeming to use the organs of speech. When the hearer's attention is properly directed, the voice seems to come from elsewhere, as from a dummy.

ven"tri·me'sal (ven"tri·mee'sul). In the middle in front.

ven·tro-. A combining form denoting *the abdomen* or *anterior aspect of the body.*

ven"tro·fix·a'tion. The stitching of a displaced viscus to the abdominal wall; specifically, the operative attach-ment of the uterus to the anterior ab-dominal wall for prolapse or displace-ment.

ven"tro·hys'ter·o·pex"y. Ventro-fixation of the uterus.

ven"tro·lat'er·al. Relating to the ventral and lateral aspects of a part.

ven"tro·me'di·an. At the middle of the ventral surface.

ven·tros'co·py. Direct examination of the abdominal and pelvic cavities by means of an apparatus resembling the cystoscope. Also called *peritoneoscopy.*

ven'trose. Having a belly, or a swell-ing like a belly (potbelly).

ven·tros'i·ty. Corpulence.

ven"tro·sus·pen'sion. The opera-tion of correcting a displacement of the uterus by shortening the round liga-ments or attaching them to the anterior abdominal wall.

ven"tro·ves"i·co·fix·a'tion. The suturing of the uterus to the urinary bladder and abdominal wall.

ven'ule (ven'yōōl, veen'yōōl). A small vein.

ve'nus. 1. Old term for sexual inter-course. 2. Alchemic name for copper.

ve·rat'ric ac'id. ($CH_3O)_2C_6H_3COOH$. Dimethoxybenzoic acid, found in sabadilla seeds.

ver·at'ri·dine (vuh·rat'ri·deen, ·din). $C_{26}H_{31}NO_{11}$. An alkaloid from veratrum viride and sabadilla seed. It slows the heart rate and has a vasodilator effect.

ve·ra'trum vi'ri·de (vi·ray'trum

virr'i·dee). Consists of the dried rhizome and roots of *Veratrum viride*. It contains a number of alkaloids, including germidine, germitrine, cevadine, veratridine, jervine, rubijervine, and pseudojervine. The outstanding physiologic actions of the drug are slowing of the respiration, slowing of the pulse, and fall of blood pressure. Also called *green hellebore*, *American hellebore*.

Ver·bas'cum. Mullein; a genus of plants of the family Scrophulariaceae.

ver·big'er·a'tion (vur·bidj″ur·ay′shun). The frequent and uncontrollable repetition of the same word, sentence, or sound without reference to its meaning.

ver'di·gris (vur′di·gree, ·griss). 1. A mixture of basic copper acetates. 2. A deposit upon copper, from the formation of cupric salts.

ver'do·fla·vin. A naturally occurring flavin of grass which is said to be identical with riboflavin.

ver″do·he'min. A green-colored bile pigment; a derivative of hemin in which the porphyrin ring has opened, rendering the iron labile.

ver″do·per·ox'i·dase. A green-colored peroxidase in leukocytes.

ver'gen·ces (vur′jin·seez). A term applied to associated disjunctive movements of the eyes, as convergence, divergence.

ver'gens (vur′jenz). Inclining. **v. deorsum.** Inclining downward, as of the axis of vision in one eye in strabismus. **v. sursum.** Upward inclination.

veriloid. Trade-mark for alkavervir.

ver'i·tol. OH.C₆H₄.CH₂.CH(CH₃) NH.CH₃. Para-hydroxyphenyl-isopropyl-methylamine; a base isomeric with ephedrine.

ver″mi·ci'dal. Destroying worms.

ver'mi·cide. An agent that destroys worms.

ver·mic'u·lar. Wormlike.

ver·mic'u·late. Resembling or shaped like a worm.

ver·mic'u·lose, ver·mic'u·lous. 1. Vermiform, vermicular. 2. Infested with worms or larvae.

ver'mi·form. Worm-shaped, as vermiform process.

ver'mi·fuge. Any agent that kills or expels intestinal worms. —**vermif'ugal,** *adj.*

ver″mi·lin'gual. Having a worm-shaped tongue.

ver'min. A term applied to animals which are obnoxious or harmful to man, especially those infesting his person, domesticated animals, or buildings, as flies, lice, rats, or mice.

ver'min·ous. Infested with, or pertaining to, vermin.

ver″mi·pho'bi·a. Morbid fear of worms or of worm infestation.

ver'mis. 1. A worm. 2. The media[l] lobe of the cerebellum, between th[e] hemispheres, or lateral lobes.

ver'nal. Pertaining to Spring.

ver'ni·er. A device attached to th[e] graduated scale of various instrumen[ts] which permits subdividing and measu[r]ing the smallest unit of this scale in[to] tenths or other fractions.

ver'nix ca″se·o'sa. A cheesy de[posit] posit on the surface of the fetus derive[d] from the stratum corneum, sebaceo[us] secretion, and remnants of the ep[i]trichium.

Ver·no'ni·a. A genus of plants of th[e] Carduaceae.

ver·o'di·gen. Gitalin, *q.v.*

veronal. Trade-mark for a brand [of] barbital. **v. sodium.** Trade-mark f[or] a brand of barbital sodium.

ver·ru'ca (pl. *verrucae*). Wart. **v[e]nereal v.** Condyloma acuminatu[m.] **v. acuminata.** A venereal wart oc[-]curring on the genitals. May occur i[n] the absence of venereal disease, b[ut] usually some discharge is present. Syn[.] *condyloma acuminatum*. **v. plan[a] juvenilis.** A smooth, flat, and sma[ll] type of wart seen most often in childre[n] on the back of the hands and fac[e.] Often arranged in lines. **v. plan[-] taris.** A wart on the sole of the foo[t.] It is often quite painful due to ingrowt[h] and pressure. Usually multiple b[ut] often grouped. Covered with a callu[s.] **v. senilis.** A brownish, pigmente[d,] hypertrophic lesion, usually seen on th[e] skin of the face, chest, and back [of] older people. It is usually scaly an[d] greasy. While listed with precancerou[s] lesions, it only occasionally become[s] malignant. There is no inflammatio[n] and the crust or scale is soft. Syn[.] *keratosis seborrheica.* **v. vulgari[s.]** The common wart, a disease caused b[y] a filtrable virus. It is usually seen o[n] the hands, about the nails, or on th[e] arms or legs, and is more common [in] children. Lesions are horny projection[s] of normal skin color but soon becom[e] dark with papillary projections. The[y] are of various sizes but usually a[re] round and from ¼ to 2 cm. in diamete[r.]

ver'ru·cose (verr′oo·kohss), **ver'r[u] cous** (verr′oo·kus, veh·roo′kus[.)] Warty; covered with, or having, wart[s.]

ver'ru·cous. See *verrucose.*

versenate. Trade-mark for edatham[ine] calcium-disodium.

ver′si·col″or, ver·sic'o·lor. De[-] noting change of color. See *tinea* vers[i]color.

ver'sion. Turning; manipulation du[r-] ing delivery to alter the presentation [of] the fetus. **abdominal v.** Manipul[a-] tions made exclusively through the ex[-] ternal abdominal wall. Also called *e[x-] ternal v.* **bimanual v.** Manipulatio[n] through the abdominal wall with one hand with the aid of one or more fingers of the other within the vagina. Also called combined v. **Braxton Hicks v.** Manipulation by the bimanual method to bring the fetal head into the pelvis. This has been advocated in treatment of placenta previa and prolapsed cord. **cephalic v.** Turning of the fetus to establish a vertex presentation. **combined v.** See bimanual v. **external v.** See abdominal v. **internal v.** Turning of the fetus by introducing the entire hand within the uterus. **pelvic v.** Turning the fetus to bring about a breech presentation. **podalic v.** One in which one or both feet are brought down to the outlet. **prophylactic v.** Converting a vertex into a breech presentation to avoid prolonged pressure on the head. Formerly employed in moderate dystocia. **spontaneous v.** Turning of the fetus without artificial assistance.

ver'te·bra (pl. vertebrae). One of the bones forming the spinal or vertebral column. There are 33 vertebrae, divided into seven cervical, 12 thoracic or dorsal, five lumbar, five sacral (the sacrum), four coccygeal (the coccyx). A typical vertebra consists of a body and an arch, the latter being formed by two pedicles and two laminas. The arch supports seven processes—four articular, two transverse, and one spinous. See Table of Bones in the Appendix. _vertebral, adj._

ver"te·brar·te'ri·al. Giving passage to the vertebral artery, as the vertebrarterial foramens in the transverse processes of the cervical vertebrae.

ver"te·bra'ta. One of the most important groups in the animal kingdom, comprising the fishes, amphibians, reptiles, birds, and mammals. They are characterized by a spinal column composed of bony, or, in the case of certain groups of fishes, cartilaginous, vertebrae. The spinal column also contains the spinal cord, which connects with a brain enclosed in a skull. The spinal column develops in embryonic life about a notochord; and the Vertebrata are commonly classified as a subphylum of the Chordata, q.v.

ver'te·brate, ver'te·bra"ted. 1. Having a vertebral column. 2. Resembling a vertebral column in flexibility, as a vertebrate catheter.

ver"te·brec'to·my. Excision of a portion of a vertebra.

ver'te·bro-, vertebr-. A combining form denoting vertebrae or vertebral.

ver'tex. 1. The highest point, in the sagittal plane, on the outer surface of a skull oriented on the Frankfort horizontal plane. 2. The crown. 3. The center of a lens surface; the point on either lens surface which lies on the principal axis.

ver'ti·cal. 1. Pertaining to the vertex. 2. Perpendicular; referring to the position of the long axis of the human body in the erect posture.

ver·tig'i·nous (vur·tidj'i·nus). Resembling or affected with vertigo.

ver'ti·go. The sensation that the outer world is revolving about the patient (objective vertigo) or that he himself is moving in space (subjective vertigo). The word frequently is used erroneously as a synonym for dizziness or giddiness to indicate an unpleasant sensation of disturbed relations to surrounding objects in space. **cerebral v.** That due to cerebral disorder. **epileptic v.** Vertigo associated with or preceding an attack of epilepsy. **gastric v.** That arising from dyspepsia. **intestinal v.** (a) That caused by intestinal disorder. (b) That caused by pressure on the terminal portions of the intestine by gas or feces, or even when the finger is introduced into the rectum and irritates the intestinal wall. It is thought to be due to pressure on the hemorrhoidal plexus of the sympathetic system. **labyrinthine v.** Vertigo, pallor, and aural, ocular, or gastric disturbances due to congestion or inflammation of the semicircular canals. See Ménière's syndrome. **neurasthenic v.** Psychologic vertigo found in neurasthenia. **ocular v.** That due to eye diseases. **organic v.** That due to brain lesion. **stomachal v.** Gastric vertigo caused by disorder of the stomach. **subjective v.** One in which the patient has a sensation as if he himself were moving. **toxemic v.** That due to some poison in the blood. **vertical v.** That caused by looking downward from or upward to a height.

ver"u·mon"ta·ni'tis (verr"oo-mon"tuh·nigh'tis, veer"oo·). Inflammation of the verumontanum.

ver"u·mon·ta'num (verr"oo·mon·tay'num, veer"oo·). An elevation on the posterior wall of the prostatic urethra; on it the prostatic utricle opens in the midline, and on its sides are the openings of the ejaculatory ducts. The colliculus seminalis. See also utricle, 2.

ves'i·ca. A bladder. **v. fellea.** The gallbladder. **v. urinaria.** The urinary bladder.

ves'i·cal. Pertaining to a bladder.

ves'i·cant. 1. Blistering. 2. A blistering agent. 3. A type of chemical used in warfare which is extremely irritating, causing blistering or even necrosis.

ves'i·cate. Blister.

ves″i·ca′tion. The formation of a blister; a blister.

ves′i·ca·to′ry. Vesicant.

ves′i·cle. 1. A small bladder; especially a small sac containing fluid. 2. A small blister, such as in herpes simplex or varicella. **auditory v.** The vesicular anlage of the inner ear. Also called *octocyst, otic v.* **brain vesicles.** The primary embryonic subdivisions of the brain. **cerebral vesicles.** The paired lateral outpouchings of the telencephalon which become the cerebral hemispheres; also called *telencephalic vesicles.* **chorionic v.** The gestation sac covered by chorionic villi and containing the embryo. **lens v.** The ectodermal vesicle that differentiates into the lens of the eye. **optic v.** The embryonic evagination of the diencephalon from which are derived the pigment and sensory layers of the retina. **primary brain v.** One of the first subdivisions of the embryonic brain; the prosencephalon, mesencephalon, or rhombencephalon. **seminal v.** The contorted, branched, saccular, glandular diverticulum of each ductus deferens with which its duct unites to form the ejaculatory duct.

ves′i·co-. A combining form denoting *bladder.*

ves″i·co·pro·stat′ic. Pertaining to the prostate gland and the urinary bladder.

ves′i·cot′o·my. Incision of the urinary bladder; cystotomy.

ve·sic′u·la (pl. *vesiculae*). A vesicle.

ve·sic′u·lar. 1. Pertaining to, or composed of, vesicles. 2. Produced in air vesicles, as vesicular breathing, vesicular murmur.

ve·sic″u·la′tion. The formation of vesicles; the state of becoming vesiculated.

ve·sic″u·lec′to·my. Resection, complete or partial, of the seminal vesicles.

ve·sic″u·li′tis. Inflammation of the seminal vesicles.

ve·sic″u·lo·gram″. A radiograph of the seminal vesicles, made by injecting a radiopaque substance by way of the ejaculatory ducts.

ve·sic″u·log′ra·phy. Radiography of the seminal vesicles. Also called *seminal vesiculography.*

ve·sic″u·lo·pap′u·lar. Consisting of vesicles and papules.

ve·sic″u·lo·pus′tu·lar. Consisting of vesicles and pustules.

ve·sic″u·lot′o·my. Division of a seminal vesicle.

ves′sel. A receptacle for fluids, especially a tube or canal for conveying blood or lymph.

ves·tib′u·lar ap″pa·ra′tus. The anatomical parts concerned with the vestibular portion of the acoustic nerve, including the saccule, utricle, semicircular canals, vestibular nerve, and vestibular nuclei.

ves·tib′u·lar nerve. That part of the acoustic nerve which transmits sensations from the vestibular apparatus.

ves·tib′u·lar nu′cle·us. A nucleus in the brain stem in which the fibers of the vestibular nerve end.

ves′ti·bule. An approach; an antechamber. **—vestib′ular,** *adj.* **aortic v.** The space formed by the left ventricle adjoining the root of the aorta. **pyloric v.** Antrum between the body of the stomach and the duodenal cap. **v. of the ear.** The cavity of the bony internal ear which communicates with the cochlea and the semicircular canals. **v. of the mouth.** The vestibular space; it is bounded internally by the teeth and gums, externally by the lips and cheeks. **v. of the nose.** The skin-lined portion of each nasal cavity, between the naris and the limen nasi. **v. of the vagina.** That portion of the vulva bounded by the minor lips.

ves·tib″u·lot′o·my. A surgical operation, making an opening into the vestibule of an ear.

ves′tige. A trace or remnant of something formerly present or more fully developed; a vestigium. **—vestig′ial,** *adj.*

ves·tig′i·um (ves·tidj′ee·um, ves·tig′ee·um). An anatomic relic of fetal or embryonic life; thus, the thymus becomes in adults a vestigium.

ve′ta (vay′tah, vee′tah). Mountain sickness.

vet″er·i·na′ri·an. One who practices veterinary medicine. **—veterinary,** *n.*

vet′er·i·nar″y (vet′ur·i·nerr″ee). 1. Pertaining to the practice of veterinary medicine. 2. Pertaining to a veterinarian.

Vi. Chemical symbol for virginium, now called francium, *q.v.*

vi′a·ble. Capable of living; likely to live; applied to a fetus capable of living outside of the uterus. **—viabil′ity,** *n.*

viadril. Trade-mark for hydroxydione sodium succinate.

vi′al. A small bottle.

vi′brate. To move to and fro. **—vi·bra′tion,** *n.*

vi′bra·tor. A device for conveying mechanical vibration to a part.

Vib′ri·o (vib′ree·o, vib′rye·o). A genus of the Spirillaceae. Short, bent, motile rods, single or united end-to-end spirals. Many species liquefy gelatin. **V. comma.** The causative organism of cholera.

vi·bris′sa (vye·briss′uh, vi·briss′uh). 1. One of the hairs in the vestibule the nose. 2. One of the long, coarse hairs on the face of certain animals; e.g., "cat-whiskers."

vi·bur'num o'pu·lus (vye·bur'num o'pew·lus, op'yoo·lus). The dried bark of *Viburnum Opulus*. Preparations containing it have been used empirically in various menstrual disorders. Also called *high-bush cranberry bark*, *true cramp bark*.

vi·bur'num pru"ni·fo'li·um. The dried bark of the root or stem of *Viburnum prunifolium* or *V. rufidulum*. It contains a crystalline glycoside, salicin, which has a relaxing action on uterine muscle. Also called *blackhaw*.

vi·car'i·ous (vye·kair'ee·us, vi·). Taking the place of something else; said of a habitual discharge occurring in an abnormal situation, as vicarious menstruation.

vice. 1. A physical defect. 2. Depravity. 3. Immorality. **—vicious**, *adj.*

Vi'chy wa"ter (vish'ee, vee'shee). A mildly laxative and antacid mineral water obtained from Vichy, France.

vi'ci·an·ose. A disaccharide which, on hydrolysis, yields L-arabinose and dextrose.

vid"e·og·no'sis. Television transmission of x-ray pictures; makes possible long distance consultation and diagnosis.

ig'il. Watchful wakefulness.

ig"il·am'bu·lism" (vidj"il·amb'yoo·liz"um). Ambulatory automatism in the waking state.

ig'i·lance. Insomnia, vigil.

vil'li (vil'eye). Plural of villus.

vil·lik'i·nine (vi·lick'i·neen, ·nin). The active principle of crude secretin extracts, which produces strong movements of the intestinal villi.

vil"lo·si'tis. Inflammation of the villous surface of the placenta.

vil'lous. Pertaining to a villus; covered with villi; characterized by the formation of villuslike projections.

vil'lus (pl. *villi*). A minute, elongated projection from the surface of a mucous membrane or other membrane. **anchoring v.** One of the placental villi with ends attached to the exposed surface of the decidua basalis by basal ectoderm. **arachnoid v.** See *arachnoidal granulations* under *granulation*. **chorionic v.** A villus of the chorion or the placenta. **intestinal villi.** The villi of the mucous membrane of the small intestine. Each consists of an epithelially covered, vascular core of connective tissue containing smooth muscle cells and an efferent lacteal endcapillary. **labial villi.** Minute, conical projections from the inner aspect (pars villosa) of the fetal lips, sometimes retained until birth. **synovial v.** One of the processes extending

from a synovial membrane into an articular cavity.

vil"lus·ec'to·my. Synovectomy; excision of a hypertrophied fold of the synovial membrane of a joint.

vin·bar'bi·tal. 5-Ethyl 5-(1-methyl-1-butenyl) barbituric acid. Delvinal sodium is a trade-mark for a brand of the sodium derivative.

Vincent's angina. See under *angina*.

vin'cu·lum (pl. *vincula*). A ligament, frenum. **v. tendinum.** One of the slender, tendinous filaments which connect the phalanges with the flexor tendons.

vin'e·gar. 1. A weak (approximately 6%) solution of acetic acid containing coloring matter and other substances (esters, mineral matter, etc.) formed by the fermentation of alcoholic liquids. 2. A pharmaceutical preparation obtained by macerating a drug with diluted acetic acid and filtering.

vinethene. A trade-mark for divinyl ether, $CH_2:CH.O.CH:CH_2$. The substance occurs as a clear, colorless liquid, with a slight purple fluorescence. An inhalation anesthetic used for short anesthesias.

vi'nyl, vin'yl. A univalent radical, $H_2C:CH$. **v. cyanide.** See *acrylonitrile*.

vioform. A trade-mark for iodochlorhydroxyquin.

vi"o·la·quer'cit·rin (vy"o·luh·kwur'sit·rin). Rutin.

vi"o·la'tion. Rape; the act of violating or ravishing. In a medicolegal sense, it is sometimes used to indicate the act of coitus without violence or force but by means of deception, by the influence of alcohol, or by intimidation.

vi'o·let. 1. A reddish blue color resembling the extreme blue end of the visible spectrum or the purple of violets; possesses the greatest refrangibility of the spectral colors. 2. A dyestuff imparting the above color. **gentian v.** Methylrosaniline chloride.

vi·o·my'cin. An antibiotic isolated from culture filtrates of the violet-colored soil microörganism *Streptomyces floridae* or *S. puniceus*, that is active against mycobacteria, including tubercle bacilli, and some Gram-negative organisms, but does not inhibit fungi, yeasts, protozoa, or viruses.

vi·os'ter·ol (vye·os'tur·ole, ·ol). Activated ergosterol. On activation (irradiation) with ultraviolet light, ergosterol undergoes a series of progressive molecular rearrangements forming several sterols of which calciferol possesses the greatest antirachitic activity. Viosterol, also known as vitamin D_2, is used to fortify fish liver oils, and, as a

vi′per. A poisonous snake of the genus *Vipera*.

Vi′per·a. A genus of the family Viperidae or true vipers.

Vi·per′i·dae (vye·perr′i·dee). True vipers, a family of venomous snakes possessing long, curved, movable front fangs which can be erected when striking. Some Viperidae are: *Bitis gabonica*, Gaboon viper; *B. lachesis*, puff adder; *B. nasicornis*, rhinoceros viper; *Echis carinatus*, saw-scaled viper; night adders of the genus *Causus*; *Aspis cornutus*, horned viper; and the pit viper. Outstanding representative in southern Asia is *Vipera russellii* (Russell's viper).

vi′per·ine (vy′puh·rin, ·reen). 1. Pertaining to a viper. 2. A toxalbumin extracted from the venom of vipers.

vir′gin. A chaste, unmarried woman; a woman who has never had sexual intercourse. **—virginal,** *adj.;* **vir·gin′i·ty,** *n.*

vir·gin′i·um. Element number 87, symbol Vi, reported in 1930 by Allison and Murphy but not isolated until 1939, by Perey, who named it francium, *q.v.*

vir′ile (virr′il, vy′ril). Pertaining to, or characteristic of, the male.

vir′i·lism. 1. Masculinity; the development of male traits or characteristics in the female. 2. A rare form of pseudohermaphroditism in which the subject is female, but has external genitals which appear in some degree like those of a male. Syn., *gynandry.*

vi·ril′i·ty (vi·ril′i·tee, vye·ril′i·tee). 1. The condition of being virile. 2. Procreative power.

vi·rip′o·tent (vi·rip′o·tunt, vye·rip′o·tunt). Sexually mature.

vi·rol′o·gist (vi·rol′o·jist, vye·). One who studies viruses and virus diseases.

vi·rol′o·gy (vi·rol′o·jee, vye·). The study of viruses and virus diseases.

vir″u·ci′din. An agent capable of destroying a virus.

vir′u·lence. Malignancy; noxiousness; infectiousness. The disease-producing power of a microörganism. **—virulent,** *adj.*

vir″u·lif′er·ous. Containing, or conveying, a virus.

vi′rus. 1. A general term for the poison of an infectious disease. 2. One of a group of pathogenic agents smaller than the accepted bacterial forms, some being visible by ordinary microscopical examination; others, also known as ultraviruses, are beyond this range. They are of particulate nature, and in each virus disease they are represented by particles of fairly constant size, ranging from 0.2μ ($200m\mu$) to 0.01μ ($10m\mu$). They multiply in the animal body much like pathogenic bacteria, but unlike bacteria, have never been cultivated on inanimate media. Virus cultures can be set up with surviving cells or proliferating embryonic cells. Cultivation is carried out in a number of cases on the chorioallantois of the developing chick. Among the well-known virus diseases of man are: rabies, poliomyelitis, encephalitis lethargica, St. Louis encephalitis, smallpox, chickenpox, herpes facialis, herpes zoster, molluscum contagiosum, common cold, influenza, measles, yellow fever, and mumps. The virus diseases of animals and plants are also numerous. See also *adenovirus, APC group,* Coxsackie *virus, ECHO virus.* **—viral,** *adj.* **attenuated v.** One whose disease-producing ability has been lessened by heat, chemicals, transfer through animals, or other means. **Coxsackie v.** Any one of a group of antigenically distinct enteric viruses, classified as group A and group B, resembling poliomyelitis viruses in size and in certain characteristics and capable of inducing destruction of striated muscle, paralysis, and death in infant mice; thought to be causative agents of herpangina and pleurodynia. **filtrable v.** One capable of passing through a fine filter, such as the porcelain or diatomaceous earth filters. Actually, all specific disease-producing viruses are filtrable. See *virus,* 2. **fixed rabies v.** Street rabies virus which is injected into rabbits and passed from one animal to another until it acquires a shorter and more constant incubation period than the naturally occurring virus. It is this fixed virus which is used for immunization. Also see rabies *vaccine.* **neurotropic v.** One that attacks and has its most serious effects upon nerve tissue. **smallpox v.** That which causes smallpox, one of three major types, all closely related, yet distinguishable by their effects in both man and animals. The viruses are smallpox or variola, alastrim, and vaccinia or cowpox. Smallpox and alastrim viruses, by animal passage, become transformed into vaccinia virus. Various strains of vaccinia virus are in use, the dermal strains, used for vaccine, being maintained by passage through calves, sheep, or rabbits. A strain widely used in experimental work is maintained by cerebral passage in rabbits, called neurovaccine, neurovaccinia, or neurovirus. Recently both the dermo- and neuro-viruses have been grown in tissue cultures and in the egg. **street rabies v.** The virus of rabies as found in dogs in nature or in the street as contrasted with the so-called fixed virus of rabbits. **tobacco mo**

saio v. A specific virus causing the mosaic disease of tobacco, frequently used in virus studies.

vis (pl. *vires*). Force; energy; power. **v. a fronte.** A force that attracts. **v. a tergo.** A force that pushes something before it. **v. formativa.** Energy manifesting itself in the formation of new tissue to replace that which has been destroyed. **v. inertiae.** That force by virtue of which a body at rest tends to remain at rest. **v. medicatrix naturae.** The healing power of nature apart from medicinal treatment.

vis·am/min. A more recent designation for khellin, *q.v.*

vis'ce·ra. Plural of viscus, *q.v.*

vis"cer·al'gi·a. Pain in a viscus.

vis'cer·o-. A combining form denoting the viscera.

vis"cer·o·in·hib'i·to"ry. Inhibiting the movements of viscera.

vis"cer·op·to'sis. The downward displacement of an abdominal organ.

vis"cer·o·sen'so·ry. Relating to sensation in the viscera.

vis"cer·ot'o·my. The process of cutting out a piece of liver or other viscus with the viscerotome.

vis"cer·o·to'ni·a. *In constitutional medicine,* the motivational drive in personality related to functions of the viscera and expressed in love of food and comfort, general relaxation, sociability, etc. The first component of temperament.

vis'cid. Adhesive; glutinous.

vis·cid'i·ty. See *viscosity*.

vis'co·li"zer. A machine used in reduction of size of fat particles, or in homogenization of a mixture or tissue. Also called *homogenizer*.

vis·com'e·ter (vis·kom'i·tur). See *viscosimeter*.

vis"co·sim'e·ter. An apparatus for determining the degree of viscosity of a fluid.

vis·cos'i·ty. The resistance which a liquid exhibits to the flow of one layer over another. The property of being glutinous or sticky; offering a resistance to a change of form, caused by the molecular attraction between the molecules of a liquid.

vis'cous. Glutinous; semifluid; sticky.

vis'cus (pl. *viscera*). Any one of the organs enclosed within one of the four great cavities, the cranial, thoracic, abdominal, or pelvic; especially an organ within the abdominal cavity. —**visceral,** *adj.*

vis'i·ble. Capable of being seen. —**visibil'ity,** *n.*

vi'sion. The act of seeing; sight. Abbreviated, V. —**vis'ual,** *adj.* **binocular v.** The faculty of using both eyes synchronously, without diplopia. **central v.** Vision with macula lutea.

chromatic v. That pertaining to the color sense. **double v.** See *diplopia.* **indirect v.** Vision with parts of the retina other than the macula. **qualitative v.** Vision in which there is ability to distinguish objects. **quantitative v.** Mere perception of light. **scotopic v.** Perception of shape and form without recognition of color, as occurs with very dim illumination. **solid v.** The perception of relief or depth of objects obtained by binocular vision. Also called *stereoscopic v.* **tubular v.** A hysterical phenomenon in which the constricted visual field defies the laws of physical projection and maintains a uniform small size, despite a change in distance of the patient from the tangent screen or the size of the test object. Also called *gunbarrel v., tunnel v.*

vis·na'gin, vis·nag'in. A crystalline constituent, chemically methoxymethyl-furanochrome, of *Ammi visnaga,* which yields also khellin (visammin) and khellinin. Visnagin relaxes smooth muscle.

vis"u·al·i·za'tion. The faculty of perceiving images in the mind with such distinctness that they seem to be seen by the eyes.

vis'u·al pur'ple. Erythropsin or rhodopsin. An organic pigment of the retina which is bleached to yellow by light. It is a conjugated protein closely related to vitamin A.

vis'u·al yel'low. A substance formed in the retina by visual purple in a photochemical reaction; it breaks up to yield colorless products and vitamin A.

vis"u·o·psy'chic (vizh"ōō·o·sigh'kick). Pertaining to the visual association areas of the occipital cortex, Brodmann's areas 18, 19.

vis"u·o·sen'so·ry. Pertaining to the visual projection area of the occipital cortex, Brodmann's area 17.

vi'sus. Vision.

vi'ta-. A combining form meaning *life.*

vi'ta·gen. A name suggested for one of the nutrients which meet a specific need for vital building material and a general need for fuel substance. These compounds are like vitamins in that a relatively small quantity is required, but are unlike vitamins in that they are utilized in animal metabolism as sources of energy.

vi'tal. Pertaining to life.

vi'tal·ism. The theory that the activities of a living organism are under the guidance of an agency which has none of the attributes of matter or energy. —**vitalist,** *n.*

vi·tal'i·ty. The power to grow, develop, perform living functions; vigor.

vi'tal·ize. Endow with the capacity to grow or develop as a living thing.

vitallium. Trade-mark for an alloy of cobalt, chromium, and molybdenum used in certain surgical appliances and procedures.

vi'tal red. A disazo dye, better known commercially as brilliant Congo R; used as a vital stain. Also called *brilliant vital red, acid Congo R, azidine scarlet R,* and *brilliant dianil red R.*

vi'tals. The organs essential to life.

vi'tal sen"si·bil'i·ties. The sensations which are of prime importance in self-preservation. Also called *paleo-s., affective s., autonomic s.*

vi'ta·mer. Any dietary factor or other substance which in a given species can produce a vitamin effect, as carotene in human subjects produces an effect of vitamin A.

vi'ta·min. One of a group of organic compounds present in variable, minute quantities in natural foodstuffs, required for the normal growth and maintenance of the life of animals, including man, who, as a rule, are unable to synthesize these compounds. They are effective in small amounts and do not furnish energy, but are essential for transformation of energy and for the regulation of the metabolism in the organism. **antiberi·beri v.** See *v.* B₁. **antidermatitis v.** See *v.* B₆. **antihemorrhagic v.** See *v.* K. **antiinfection v.** See *v.* A. **antineuritic v.** See *v.* B₁. **antipellagra v.** See *v.* B₂. **antirachitic v.** See *v.* D. **antiscorbutic v.** See *v.* C. **antisterility v.** See *v.* E. **antixerophthalmic v.** See *v.* A. **coagulation v.** See *v.* K. **fertility v.** Alphatocopherol. **neovitamin A.** See *v.* A. **sunshine v.** See *v.* D. **synthetic v. K.** See *menadione.* **v. A.** One necessary for maintenance of normal mucosal epithelium and visual acuity. Deficiency leads to atrophy of epithelial cells, and is conducive to susceptibility to local bacterial infections of mucous membranes, xerophthalmia, and night blindness. It is a highly complex alcohol derived from carotenoid precursors, plentiful in fish liver oil, milk fat, and many pigmented vegetables, and is now produced synthetically. The standard unit of vitamin A is the International unit which equals in activity 0.6 microgram of pure β-carotene. Also called *antixerophthalmic v., antiinfection v.* **v.-B complex.** Consists of an unknown number of different vitamins. So far eleven different vitamins have been identified: thiamine (vitamin B₁), riboflavin (vitamin B₂), niacin, pyridoxine (vitamin B₆), pantothenic acid, inositol, p-aminobenzoic acid, biotin, adenylic acid, folic acid,

and vitamin B₁₂. Occurs in high concentration in yeast and liver. **v. B_c.** See *folic acid.* **v. B_T.** A factor, not yet chemically characterized, required for growth and survival of the mealworm, *Tenebrio molitor.* **v. B_x.** Para-aminobenzoic acid. **v. B₁.** Thiamine hydrochloride or thiamine; necessary for normal carbohydrate metabolism, especially in nerves, for maintenance of normal appetite, muscular tissues, reproduction, and lactation. Deficiency leads to peripheral neuropathy and heart failure. Distributed in whole-grain cereals, meats (especially liver and pork), legumes, and yeast. Also called *aneurin, torulin, antineuritic v., antiberiberi factor.* See *thiamine hydrochloride.* **v. B₂.** Riboflavin; necessary for protection against pellagra. It is found in milk, lean meat, glandular organs, eggs, yeast, and certain leafy vegetables. Also called *antipellagra v., antipellagra factor, lactoflavin, ovoflavin, hepatoflavin, vitamin G.* Also see *riboflavin.* **v. B₆.** Pyridoxine; a vitamin essential to prevent edema and swelling of the skin in the rat. Found in rice bran, liver, yeast, and other sources rich in vitamin-B complex. Also called *antidermatitis v., anti-acrodynia factor, adermin.* See *pyridoxine.* **v. B₁₂.** An essential vitamin necessary for normal maturation of erythrocytes, and for normal neurologic function. It corrects both the hematologic and neurologic symptoms of pernicious anemia. Syn., *antianemia factor, extrinsic factor, maturation factor of liver, cyanocobalamin.* **v. C.** Ascorbic acid, cevitamic acid, cevitaminic acid; necessary for maintenance of intercellular substance of teeth, bones, and vascular walls. Deficiency leads to scurvy. Distributed in fruits, especially of the citrus variety, tomatoes, potatoes, and leafy vegetables. It is destroyed by heat. Also called *antiscorbutin, scorbutanin, antiscorbutic factor.* **v. D.** One of several vitamins having antirachitic activity, as calciferol (D₂), irradiated 7-dehydrocholesterol (D₃), irradiated 22-dihydroergosterol (D₄), and irradiated 7-dehydrositosterol (D₅). Vitamin D is necessary for normal deposition of calcium and phosphorus in bones and teeth. Deficiency leads to rickets in children, osteomalacia in adults. Found in fish liver oils (principally D₃), eggs, salmon, and produced after irradiation of ergosterol (to D₂) and other sterols or foods containing them. The action of sunshine on skin promotes the synthesis of vitamin D in the body. One United States Pharmacopeia or International unit is equal in activity, in standard rachitic rats, to 0.025 microgram of calciferol. Also called *antirachitic v., antiricketic v.* **v. E.** A topherol essential for maturation and differentiation of certain cells. Also called *antisterility vitamin*. See also *photocopherol*. **v. F.** A term formerly used for essential fatty acids, such as oleic acid ($C_{18}H_{32}O_2$), linolenic acid ($C_{18}H_{30}O_2$), and arachidonic acid ($C_{20}H_{32}O_2$). **v. G.** See *v. B₂*. **v. H.** A water-soluble component of the vitamin-B complex identical with biotin, *q.v.*, and enzyme R. **v. H′.** Para-aminobenzoic acid. **v. K.** Group of at least three phthoquinone derivatives, vitamin K₁, vitamin K₂, and vitamin K₃. Vitamin K is essential for formation of prothrombin. In vitamin-K deficiency, the blood clotting time is markedly prolonged and hemorrhages result. Principal dietary sources are spinach, cabbage, kale, cauliflower, tomatoes, and soybean oil. Also called *antihemorragic v.*, *prothrombin factor.* See *menadione*. **v. K₁.** Phylloquinone, *q.v.* **K₂.** See *menadione*. **v. L.** One of a group of lactation vitamins. Evidence indicates that these vitamins are distinct entities, but they have not been characterized chemically or extensively studied. **v. M.** A factor, which may be a member of the vitamin-B complex, believed to be necessary for the prevention of anemia and loss of weight in monkeys. Present in yeast and liver. **P-P.** Nicotinic acid. **v. U.** A supposed vitamin necessary for growth in the chick.

vi·ta·zyme. A substance having the properties of both a vitamin and an enzyme.

vi·tel′lin (vi·tel′in, vye·tel′in). A phosphoprotein found in egg yolk.

vi·tel′line (vi·tel′in, -een). Pertaining to the vitellus or yolk.

vi·tel″lo·ru′bin. A reddish pigment obtained from yolk of egg.

vi·tel′lus (vi·tel′us, vye·tel′us). A yolk; specifically, the yolk of the egg of the common fowl, *Gallus domesticus.*

vi·ti·a′tion (vish″e·ay′shun). A change which lessens utility or efficiency or neutralizes an action.

vit·i·li′go. A skin disease characterized by an acquired achromia in areas of various sizes and shapes. There is an almost complete lack of pigment with hyperpigmented borders. Lesions are more marked in areas exposed to sun. Also called *leukoderma*, *piebald skin*, *lichromia.*

vit″re·o·den′tin (vit″ree·o·den′tin). A variety of dentin with but few dentinal tubules.

vit′re·ous. 1. Glassy; hyaline. 2. The transparent, gelatinlike substance filling the greater part of the globe of the eye; the vitreous body; the vitreous humor.

vit·res′cence. The condition of be-

coming hard and transparent like glass.

vit′ri·ol. 1. Old term for any substance having a glassy fracture or appearance. 2. Sulfuric acid. Syn., *oil of v.* 3. Any crystalline salt of sulfuric acid. **—vitriolated,** *adj.* **blue v.** Copper sulfate. **green v.** Ferrous sulfate or copperas. **white v.** Zinc sulfate.

vit″ri·ol′ic ac′id. Sulfuric acid.

vit·ri′tis. Glaucoma.

vit′rum. Glass.

vi·vip′a·rous. (vye·vip′uh·rus, vi·vip′-). Bringing forth the young alive—distinguished from *oviparous.* **—vi·vipar′ity,** n.

viv″i·sec′tion. The surgical preparation of anesthetized animals for study of functions or their derangements. **—viv′isect,** v.

viv″i·sec′tion·ist. One who practices or defends experimental work on animals.

viv′i·sec″tor. One who uses surgical procedures on anesthetized animals to study functions or their derangements.

vo′cal. Pertaining to the voice; pertaining to the organs producing the voice.

voice. The sounds, especially articulate sounds, that are produced by the vibration of the vocal folds and modified by the resonance organs. **nasal v.** A peculiar, muffled timbre of the voice; it is especially marked in cases of perforated palate.

void. Evacuate.

vo′la. The palm of the hand or the sole of the foot. **—volar,** *adj.*

vol′a·tile. Readily vaporizing; evaporating. **—volatiliza′tion,** n.; **volatilize,** v.

vo·li′tion. The will or determination to act. **—volitional,** *adj.*

vol′ley. Approximately simultaneous discharges, as nerve impulses which travel simultaneously in different axons of a nerve or which are discharged simultaneously from groups of central neurons.

vol. %. Volume per cent.

vol·sel′la. A forceps having one or more hooks at the end of each blade. Also called *vulsella*, *vulsellum forceps.*

volt. The unit of electromotive force and of electric potential; the electromotive force that, steadily applied to a conductor whose resistance is 1 ohm, will produce a current of 1 ampere. Abbreviated, v. **electronvolt.** Unit of energy equivalent to the kinetic energy which an electron acquires in falling through a potential of one volt. **million electronvolts.** One million electronvolts; 1.59×10^{-6} erg. Abbreviated, *mev.*

volt′age. Electromotive force measured in volts. **effective v.** For alternating currents, 0.707 of the peak voltage.

vol·ta'ic (vol-tay'ick, voal-tay'ick). Described by, or named after, Volta.

vol·tam'e·ter (vol-tam'i·tur, voal-tam'i·tur). An instrument for ascertaining the electromotive force of a current in volts.

volt'am''me·ter. An instrument for measuring both voltage, or potential, and amperage, or amount of current.

volt'-am'pere. A watt; the rate of working in an electric circuit when the current is one ampere and the potential one volt.

volt'me''ter. An instrument for measuring voltage, or electromotive force. **electrostatic v.** One for measurement of high voltages; built on the principle that like electric charges repel and unlike charges attract each other.

vol'ume. In physics, the space which a substance fills. Cubic dimension. **atomic v.** The atomic weight of an element divided by the density; it represents the volume in cubic centimeters which would be occupied by the atomic weight of an element taken in grams. **molecular v.** The volume of one gram-molecule of substance; in the gaseous state under the same conditions of temperature and pressure, the molecular volumes of all substances are equal. **specific v.** The volume occupied by a definite weight of a substance, as the volume in cubic centimeters of 1 Gm. of substance. **v. per cent.** The number of cubic centimeters of a substance contained in 100 cc. of medium. Usually refers to gas (O_2 or CO_2) contained in blood. Symbol, vol. %.

vol''u·met'ric. Pertaining to measurement by volume.

vol'un·tar''y. Under control of the will; performed by an exercise of the will.

vol'vu·lus. A twisting of the bowel upon itself so as to occlude the lumen, occurring most frequently in the sigmoid flexure.

vo'mer. The thin plate of bone which is situated vertically between the nasal cavities, and which forms the posterior portion of the septum of the nose. See Table of Bones in the Appendix.

vom'it. 1. Expel from the stomach by vomiting. 2. Vomited matter. **bilious v.** Vomit stained with bile. **black v.** A dark fluid consisting of blood and the contents of the stomach. **coffee-ground v.** Vomit consisting of altered blood and the contents of the stomach.

vom'it·ing. The forcible ejection of the contents of the stomach through the mouth. **cyclic v.** Vomiting recurring at regular periods. **dry v.** Per-

sistent nausea with attempts at vomiting, but with ejection of nothing b gas. **pernicious v.** A variety vomiting occasionally occurring pregnancy and becoming at times excessive as to threaten life. **proje tile v.** A form observed in some d eases of the brain stem; the vomi is suddenly projected out of the mou to some distance, usually without na sea. **stercoraceous v.** Ejection fecal matter in vomit, usually due intestinal obstruction.

vom'i·tive. Emetic.

vom'i·to''ry. 1. Any agent that duces emesis. 2. A vessel used to rece ejecta.

vom''i·tu·ri'tion (vom''i·tew·ris un). Ineffectual attempt at vomiti retching.

vom'i·tus. 1. Vomited matter. 2. T act of vomiting. **v. cruentus.** Bloo vomit. **v. marinus.** Seasickne **v. matutinus.** Morning sickne

vonedrine. Trade-mark for phen propylmethylamine, a nasal vasoc strictor used by inhalation. See phen propylmethylamine.

von Graefe's knife. A small kn with a long, narrow blade, used ophthalmic surgery.

vo·ra'cious. Having an insatia appetite or desire for food.

vor'tex (pl. vortices). A struct having the appearance of being p duced by a rotary motion about an ax **v. coccygeus.** The point of c vergence of the lanugo hairs over coccyx. Also called vertex coccyge **v. of the heart.** The region at apex of the heart where the superfic layer of muscle of both ventricles (v tex fibers) passes into the deep layer the ventricles. **vortices pilorum** Hair whorls.

vor'ti·ces (vor'ti·seez). Plural of v tex, q.v.

vor'ti·cose. Whirling; having whorled appearance.

vox. The voice.

vo''yeur' (vwah''yur'). Peeping To One who obtains sexual gratificat from witnessing the sexual acts others or from viewing persons in nude. **—voyeurism,** n.

vn''e·rom'e·ter (view'i·rom'i·t view·rom'i·tur). An apparatus for termining the distance of the eyes fr each other.

vul'can·ize. Subject rubber to process wherein it is treated with sul at a high temperature, and ther rendered either flexible or very har **vul'ner·a·ble.** Susceptible to inju **vul'nus.** A wound. Obs.

vul·sel'lum (pl. vulsella). See sella.

vul'va. The external genital organs

a female. Syn., *pudendum muliebre.*
—vulvar, *adj.* **v. connivens.** A form of vulva in which the labia majora are in close apposition. **v. hians.** The form of vulva in which the labia majora are gaping.

vul·vec'to·my. Excision of the vulva.

vul·vi'tis. Inflammation of the vulva.
vul'vo-, vulv-. A combining form denoting *the vulva.*
vul"vo·vag"i·ni'tis (vul"vo-vadj"-i·nigh'tis). Inflammation of the vulva and of the vagina existing at the same time.

W

W. Chemical symbol for wolfram. In the U.S.A. usually called *tungsten.*

v. Watt or unit of electric energy.

wad'ding. 1. Carded cotton or wool, used for surgical dressings, generally not of the first quality. 2. Cotton batting, sometimes glazed to render it nonabsorbent.

wad'dle. A clumsy, swaying walk or gait.

Vade's urethral suppositories. Suppositories containing iodoform, bismuth subnitrate, chloral, and morphine.

va'fer. A thin sheet made by heating moistened flour and used to enclose powders that are taken internally. Also called *cachet.*

Vagner von Jauregg, Julius (*Austrian physician,* 1857–1940). Practiced fever therapy as treatment for neurosyphilis and dementia paralytica, using inoculation with malaria. Called *Wagner-Jauregg treatment.* Nobel laureate (1927).

va·hoo' bark (wah-hōō', wah'hōō). Euonymus.

vaist. The narrowest portion of the trunk above the hips.

vake'ful·ness. Insomnia; continued inability to sleep.

valk'ing i'ron. A metal support attached to a splint, shoe, or plaster cast designed to permit walking without the sole of the foot coming in contact with the ground.

vall. The bounding side or inside surface of a natural or artificial cavity or vessel. **cell w.** (a) The cellulose cell membrane of plant cells. (b) The outer boundary or membrane of some animal cells.

vall'eye". 1. Leukoma of the cornea. 2. Divergent strabismus. **—walleyed,** *adj.*

vall teeth. Molar teeth.

van'der·ing. 1. Moving about, as wandering cells. 2. Abnormally movable, as wandering spleen or kidney.

var'bles (wawr'bulz). The disease produced by infestation of domestic animals and man with the larva of the

warble fly or botfly, *Dermatobia hominis.*

ward. A division or room of a hospital.

war'far·in so'di·um. 3-(α-Acetonylbenzyl)-4-hydroxycoumarin sodium, an intravascular anticoagulant. See *coumadin sodium.*

warm'-blood'ed. Having a relatively high and constant body temperature, as in birds and mammals.

wart. A hyperplasia of the papillae of the skin, forming a small projection. See *verruca.* **—wart'y,** *adj.* **fig w.** A papillary growth of filiform or vegetating projections, often covered with an offensive-smelling secretion; usually found on the genitalia. Syn., *verruca acuminata, condyloma acuminatum, venereal w.* **moist w.** Condyloma acuminatum. **plantar w.** Verruca plantaris. **venereal w.** Condyloma acuminatum.

wash. A lotion. A class of pharmaceutical preparations (solutions or mixtures) intended for local application without friction or rubbing.

wash'ing so'da. Sodium carbonate, $Na_2CO_3.10H_2O$.

wasp's waist. Atrophy of trunk muscles in muscular dystrophy.

Wassermann, August von [*German bacteriologist,* 1866–1925]. Known internationally for his introduction, with Albert Neisser and Carl Bruck, of a specific blood test for the diagnosis of syphilis (1906). Called *Wassermann reaction* or *test, complement-fixation test.* See Wassermann's *test.*

waste. 1. Useless matter eliminated from the body. 2. Become thin; pine away. 3. Food no longer suitable for consumption.

wast'er (way'stur). 1. A child suffering from marasmus. 2. An animal affected with tuberculosis, usually bovine types.

watch'ma"ker's cramp. 1. An occupational neuritis, characterized by painful cramps of the muscles of the hands. 2. Spasm of the orbicularis oculi muscle, due to holding a jeweler's lens.

wa'ter. 1. The liquid consisting of

molecules of the composition H_2O, or aggregates thereof. 2. Pharmaceutically, any saturated aqueous solution of a volatile oil or other aromatic or volatile substance. Also called *aromatic w*. **deionized w.** Water purified by passage through substances which remove contaminating cations and anions and leave finally a water equivalent to distilled water in purity. **hard w.** Water containing soluble calcium or magnesium salts and not readily forming a lather with soap. **heavy w.** That which contains double-weight atoms of hydrogen (deuterium) instead of ordinary (lightweight) hydrogen atoms. Syn., *deuterium oxide*. **w. for injection.** Sterile distilled water for parenteral use, stored in suitable sterile containers to keep it free of pyrogens. **w. of crystallization.** Water entering into the crystalline structure of a compound in definite molecular proportions. **w. of hydration.** See *w. of crystallization*. **w. on the brain.** Hydrocephaly.

wa'ter brash. Watery acid fluid regurgitated from the stomach, accompanied by nausea.

wa'ter moc'ca·sin. The cottonmouth, *Ancistrodon piscivorus*.

wa'ters. Lay term for the liquor amnii; amniotic fluid. **bag of w.** The amnion and amniotic fluid.

watt. A unit of electric power, defined as the work done at the rate of one joule per second. Abbreviated, w. See *volt-ampere*.

watt'age. Consumption or output of an electric device in watts.

watt'me''ter. An instrument for measuring electric power or activity in watts.

wave. 1. A uniform movement in a body which is propagated with a continuous motion, each part of the body vibrating through a fixed path. 2. The course traced by a lever or a beam of light on a surface moving at right angles to the direction of lever or beam. **brain w.** Alpha wave. See *electroencephalography*, alpha *rhythm*. **coronary T w.** An inverted T wave with an upward convexity of the first limb, its apex peaked and its second limb rather straight. In some leads it may be upright. Frequently seen in electrocardiograms during various stages of myocardial infarction, but not confined to this exclusively. Also called *coveplane T w*. **electrocardiographic waves.** P, Q, R, S, T, U are signs arbitrarily chosen to signify various phases of the spread of depolarization and repolarization of cardiac muscle as seen in the electrocardiogram. **Hertzian waves.** Original term for radio waves; electromagnetic waves

resembling light waves, but having greater wave length. **pulse w.** The progressive expansion followed by contraction due to the flow of blood. It begins with each cardiac systole and is propagated along the aorta and other arteries, ending normally at the capillaries. **P w. of the electrocardiogram.** The first wave, due to depolarization of the atria. The average maximum height is 1.25 mm., and the average duration is 0.08 second. **QS w. of the electrocardiogram.** First and downward wave of the initial ventricular complex, not followed by an R wave. **Q w. of the electrocardiogram.** First and downward wave of the ventricular complex. It represents early ventricular depolarization. It is often absent normally. **R w. of the electrocardiogram.** The first upward deflection of the ventricular complex, usually of relatively large amplitude: it represents a major portion of ventricular depolarization. **R' w. of the electrocardiogram.** The second upward deflection of the normal electrocardiogram, if present. **S w. of the electrocardiogram.** The first downward deflection of the ventricular complex, following upon an R wave: it is often absent normally. **Ta w. of the electrocardiogram.** The deflection representing atrial repolarization. Normally it is opposite in direction to the P wave, which it follows. Usually it cannot be identified in a normal electrocardiogram. **T w. of the electrocardiogram.** The deflection which represents repolarization of the ventricles. In most leads it is normally upright, varying rather widely in amplitude and duration. **U w. of the electrocardiogram.** A deflection usually of low amplitude, following the T wave. It is often absent normally: its causation and significance are not certain. **w. length.** The distance from the crest of one wave to the crest of the succeeding wave. Abbreviated, w. l. **w. number.** The number of waves or cycles of light flux or radiant energy measured through a distance of 1 cm.

wax. Any substance, of plant, animal or mineral origin, consisting of a mixture of one or more of the following constituents: high molecular weight fatty acids, high molecular weight monohydric alcohols, esters of the fatty acids and alcohols, solid hydrocarbons. **white w.** Bleached yellow wax. For chemical composition and uses, see yellow *w*. Also called *bleached beeswax*. **yellow w.** The purified wax from the honeycomb of the bee, *Apis mellifera*. It consists chiefly of myricin (myricyl palmitate). It also contains cerotic acid (cerin), melissic acid, and hydrocarbons of the paraffin series. Also called *beeswax.*

weak. Not strong; feeble.

weak'ness. Loss or lack of strength.

wean. Cease to suckle or nurse offspring at a period when the latter is capable of taking substantial food from sources other than the breast.

weav'ers' bot'tom. Chronic ischial bursitis due to long-continued pressure in a sedentary occupation.

web. A membranelike structure; especially the skin and underlying tissue between the bases of fingers or toes.

wedge. An instrument or material used by dentists to separate adjoining teeth.

weep'ing. 1. Lacrimation. 2. Exudation or leakage of a fluid. 3. Exuding; applied to raw or excoriated surfaces bathed with a moist discharge.

weight. The force with which a body is attracted by the earth. For weights listed by name, see Tables of Weights and Measures in the Appendix. **atomic w.** A number representing the relative weight of an atom of an element compared with oxygen (= 16.000). It is the mean value of the isotopic weights of an element. **equivalent w.** The weight of an element which can replace or combine with a unit weight of hydrogen or is otherwise equivalent to the latter. **molecular w.** The weight of a molecule of any substance, representing the sum of the weights of its constituent atoms. Abbreviated, M. **specific w.** Specific gravity.

wen. A sebaceous cyst. The term is commonly used when the lesion occurs in the scalp.

wet. Not dry; moist.

wet'ting a'gent. A substance that causes a liquid to spread more readily upon a solid surface, chiefly through a reduction of surface tension.

W fac'tor. Biotin.

Wharton's duct. See submaxillary *duct.*

Wharton's jelly. See under *jelly.*

wheal. A primary lesion of the skin which is a circumscribed, edematous, usually transitory elevation that varies in size from that of a pinhead to that of the palm or larger. Lesions come and go quickly and are accompanied by tingling, burning, or intense itching. They occur classically in urticaria but also after insect bites, animal bites, trauma, or even physical agents as heat, cold, or sunlight. Syn., *pomphus, urtica.*

wheat germ oil. An oil derived from the embryo of wheat, *Triticum vulgare,* a rich source of tocopherols.

wheeze. A whistling or sighing noise

produced in the act of breathing. Often heard only by stethoscopic examination. It signifies partial obstruction of one or more of the air passages due to spasm, edema, inflammation, foreign body, tumor, or external pressure.

wheez'ing. The half-stertorous, sibilant sound occasionally heard in the breathing of persons affected with croup, asthma, or coryza.

whey. The liquid part of milk separating from the curd.

whiff. A puff of air. **oral w.** A peculiar sound heard during expiration from the open mouth, principally in cases of thoracic aneurysm.

whip'worm. An intestinal nematode, *Trichuris trichiura,* common to man and other mammals.

whis'per. A low, soft, sibilant sound produced by the passage of the breath through the glottis without vibrating the vocal folds.

white. 1. Having a color produced by reflection of all the rays of the spectrum; opposed to black. 2. Any white substance, as white of egg.

white pine. The dried inner bark of *Pinus strobus.* It contains a glycoside coniferin, tannin, mucilage, and oleoresin. Used as an ingredient in cough syrups. Also called *white pine bark.*

whites. A lay term for leukorrhea, *q.v.*

whi'ting. Prepared chalk or white clay; purified calcium carbonate.

whit'low. An old general term for any suppurative inflammation of the end of a finger or toe. See *felon, paronychia.*

whoop (hoŏp, whoŏp). The inspiratory crowing sound which precedes or occurs during a coughing paroxysm.

whoop'ing cough (hoŏp'ing, hoŏp'ing). An acute inflammation of the air passages caused by bacterial infection with *Hemophilus pertussis,* characterized by paroxysms of coughing that usually end in loud whooping inspirations. Also called *pertussis.*

wick'ing. Loosely twisted unspun cotton or gauze, employed in packing cavities; a gauze wick.

will. *In psychology,* the faculty by which the mind chooses its ends and directs action in carrying out its purpose.

wind'age (win'didj). Compression of air by the passage of a missile, shell, etc., near the body, causing blast injury, *q.v.*

wind' kes'sel. Compression-chamber-like action of the aorta and its immediate branches in buffering pressure and flow changes during the cardiac cycle, a function of the large capacity and elastic walls of the vessels.

wind'lass (wind'lus). Apparatus for exerting traction upon a limb by means of a winding device attached to the lower end of a splint, turned with a metal key. **Spanish w.** A temporary emergency expedient for accomplishing traction upon a limb supported by a splint; consists of cords which are tightened by twisting with a wooden skewer or similar object.

wind'lass trac'tion. A method for exerting traction on an extremity of the body. Extension straps are attached to the skin by means of adhesive tape or to a bone by means of a pin passed through it. The distal ends of the straps are attached to a fixed point, and traction is exerted by winding up the straps with a metal key or other device.

win'dow. 1. An opening in a wall usually enclosed by a movable frame of glass panes for the admission of light and air. 2. A small aperture in a bone or other unyielding tissue. See *fenestra*.

wind'pipe". See *trachea*.

wine'glass". A measure of nearly two fluidounces, or 60 cc.

wine spot. See port-wine *nevus*.

wing. See *ala*.

wink. Close and open the eyelids quickly.

win'tergreen". Gaultheria.

win'tergreen oil. Gaultheria oil.

win'ter itch. See *pruritus hiemalis*.

wir'ing. Securing in position, by means of wire, the fragments of a broken bone. **continuous loop w.** *In dentistry*, a procedure for reduction and immobilization of jaw fractures by the use of a long strand of wire wound around several selected teeth in each fragment. **eyelet w.** See single loop *w*. **single loop w.** *In dentistry*, a type of intermaxillary wiring used in fractures of the jaw.

Wirsung's duct. See pancreatic *duct*.

wir'y. Resembling wire; tough and flexible.

wis'dom teeth. The third permanent molars. Also called *dentes sapientes*.

witch ha'zel. *Hamamelis virginiana*.

witch's milk. Lay term for milk secreted in the breasts of a newborn infant.

wit'zel-sucht" (vit'sul-zōōkt"). A mental condition characterized by silly behavior, shallow facetiousness, and unstable mood; regarded as a symptom of frontal lobe disease such as brain tumor.

w. l. Wave length.

Wohl·fahr'ti·a (voal·fahr'tee·uh). A genus of flesh flies. See *Sarcophagidae*. **W. magnifica.** The Old World flesh fly; the larvae are deposited in cutaneous lesions or in one of the body openings. **W. meigeni.** A North American flesh fly. **W. vigil.** A North American flesh fly.

wolf'jaw. A bilateral cleft of the lip, jaw, and palate.

wolf'ram. Recommended name for tungsten, *q.v.*

wolfs'bane". 1. Aconite. 2. Any plant of the genus *Aconitum*, especially *A. lycoctonum*.

womb (wōōm). The uterus.

wood. The hard fibrous part of trees, the part within the bark.

wood al'co·hol. See *methyl alcohol*.

wood sor'rel. *Oxalis acetosella*, a low, tender pubescent herb of North America, Europe, Asia, and Northern Africa. Contains potassium binoxalate, which is sometimes obtained from it and sold as sorrel salt.

wood spir'it. See *methyl alcohol*.

wood sug'ar. Xylose.

wood vin'e·gar. Vinegar obtained by the dry distillation of wood.

wood wool. Prepared fibers of wood. Formerly used as a surgical dressing.

wool fat. The purified, anhydrous, fatlike substance from the wool of sheep, *Ovis aries*. Wool fat is chiefly composed of esters of high molecular weight alcohols, as cholesterol and lanosterol, with fatty acids. It is used as an ointment base. Also called *anhydrous lanolin, refined w. f.* **hydrous w. f.** Wool fat containing about 30% of water. Used as an ointment base. Syn., *lanolin*.

word blind'ness. See *alexia*.

word deaf'ness. See under *deafness*.

word-sal'ad. Meaningless words or neologisms emitted by psychotic patients, particularly those with schizophrenia. Syn., *schizophasia*.

work'ing dis'tance. *In microscopy*, the distance between the object and the objective.

work'up. A systematic examination or investigation; also, the compilation or elaboration of findings.

worm. A member of the phyla Annelida, Nemathelminthes, or Platyhelminthes. The medically important forms belong to the last two phyla. **dragon w.** The Guinea worm. **Guinea w.** A threadlike nematode, *Dracunculus medinensis*.

worm'seed. Santonica. **w. oil.** Chenopodium oil.

wound. A disruption of continuity of an external or internal surface of the body. **bullet splash w.** One caused by a fragmentation of steel armor from the impact of a bullet; this type of wound is small and frequently involves the neck; common in combat airmen. **contused w.** One produced by a blunt instrument or weapon. **gunshot w.** One made by a projectile from a gun or any small firearm. **in-**

cised w. One caused by a cutting instrument. **lacerated w.** One in which the tissues are torn. **open w.** One having a free external opening. **penetrating w.** One that pierces the walls of a cavity or enters into an organ. **punctured w.** One made by a pointed instrument. **shell w.** Usually a large lacerated one with accompanying devitalization of tissue and resulting from artillery fire or bombing. **spatter w.** One which is peppered superficially with a multitude of small splinters from an explosive. **tunnel w.** One having a small entrance and a small exit, the wound tract being the same diameter throughout.

wrin'kles. Minute crevices or furrows in the skin caused by habitual frowning, etc., but particularly by old age due to atrophy of the corium.

wrist. The part joining forearm and hand. See Table of Joints and Ligaments in the Appendix. **w. joint.** The articulation between the forearm and the carpus; the radiocarpal articulation.

wri'ting hand. A peculiar position assumed by the hand in paralysis agitans, with an exaggerated flexion of the metacarpophalangeal joints and an extension of the fingers.

wry'neck". Old term for torticollis, *q.v.*

w. s. Water soluble.

Wuch"er·er'i·a (wŏŏch″ur·err′ee·uh). A genus of filarial worms found in all the warm regions of the world. The larva or microfilaria must be ingested by a mosquito in order for metamorphosis to take place. **W. bancrofti.** A species of filaria of world wide distribution. Man is the only known definitive host. **W. malayi.** A species found in rural regions near ponds and rivers.

wuch″er·e·ri'a·sis (wŏŏch″ur·eh·rye′uh·sis). The disease caused by worms of the genus *Wuchereria*. The symptoms depend upon the location of the parasite within the body, but are due to obstruction of the lymph vessels by the adult worms. Also called *filariasis, Bancroft's filariasis, elephantiasis.*

wur'rus. A powder obtained in Arabia from the fruits of a leguminous plant, *Flemingia congesta;* used as an anthelmintic. Also called *waras, warras.*

w/v. Weight in volume; indicating that a weighed quantity of a solid substance is contained in solution in a measured quantity of liquid.

X

x. Symbol for the decimal scale of potency or dilution; used by the homeopaths.

xan"tha·line (zan″thuh·leen, ·lin). C₂₀H₁₉NO₅. An alkaloid from opium.

xan"the·las'ma (zan″thi·laz′muh, ·lass′muh). A type of xanthoma seen on the eyelids.

xan'thine (zan′theen, ·thin). C₅H₄N₄O₂. 2,6-Dioxopurine. An intermediate product in the transformation of adenine and guanine into uric acid. See *hypoxanthine.*

xan'thine ox'i·dase. A flavoprotein enzyme catalyzing the oxidation of certain purines.

xan"thi·nu'ri·a. The presence of xanthine in urine.

xan'tho-, xanth-. A combining form meaning *yellow.*

xan"tho·chroi'a. Yellow discoloration of the skin.

xan"tho·chro'mi·a. 1. A yellowish discoloration of the skin. 2. The yellow discoloration of the cerebrospinal fluid, diagnostic of hemorrhage in the spinal cord or brain. **—xanthochromic,** *adj.*

xan·thoch'ro·ous (zan·thock′ro·us). Yellow-skinned.

xan"tho·cy"a·no'pi·a, xan"tho·cy"a·nop'si·a. A defect of color vision in which yellow and blue are perceived, while red is imperceptible.

xan'tho·cyte. A cell containing a yellow pigment.

xan"tho·der'ma. A yellow discoloration of the skin.

xan'tho·dont, xan"tho·don'tous. Having yellow teeth.

xan"tho·gran"u·lo"ma·to'sis. A condition characterized by granulomalike deposits of cholesterol, chiefly in the flat bones, sometimes associated with hypercholesteremia. Exophthalmos and diabetes insipidus may occur, depending on the localization of the lipid deposits in the skull. Also see Schüller-Christian *disease.*

xan·tho'ma. A new growth of the skin occurring as flat or slightly raised patches or nodules from 2 to 12 mm. in size, and of a yellowish orange color. Several types are seen and often more than one type is seen in the same patient. They are all due to some disturbance of lipoid metabolism. Histologically, foam or xanthoma cells are seen with giant cells and some infiltrate. Various types of sterol crystals are seen with polariscopic examination. See *xanthelasma*. **juvenile x.** One occurring in children usually as xanthoma tuberosum, but often disseminated. May occur as an evidence of Schüller-Christian disease. **x. diabeticorum.** A rare disease of the skin associated with diabetes mellitus. The lesions are denser and firmer than those of true xanthoma, and are dull red, discrete, and solid, being more often seen on the palms and soles. **x. tuberosum.** One of the common types. Papules, nodules, plaques, or linear lesions are seen on the extensor surfaces. The yellow color is typical. Lesions are usually grouped together and are often found about the joints. Total blood lipids are usually elevated, as is cholesterol. Tendon sheaths or other internal structures may be involved, giving various and bizarre symptoms.

xan·tho″ma·to′sis. A condition marked by the deposit of a yellowish or orange lipoid material in the reticuloendothelial cells, the skin, and the internal organs. See *lipoidosis*, Schüller-Christian *disease*.

xan·thom′a·tous (zan·thom′uh·tus, zan·tho′muh·tus). Of the nature of, or affected with, xanthoma.

xan″tho·my′cin A. An antibiotic substance isolated from cultures of a strain of *Streptomyces*.

xan″tho·my′cin B. An antibiotic substance isolated from cultures of a strain of *Streptomyces*.

xan′tho·phane. A yellow pigment found in the retinal cones.

xan′tho·phyll. $C_{40}H_{56}O_2$. A yellow vegetable pigment similar to chlorophyll, found in plants.

xan″tho·pro·te′ic ac′id. The yellow compound resulting from the treatment of protein with nitric acid.

xan″tho·pro·te′in (zanth″o·pro′tee·in, ·pro′teen). A yellowish derivative formed by the action of concentrated nitric acid on proteins.

xan·thop′si·a. Yellow vision; the condition in which objects look yellow. It sometimes accompanies jaundice.

xan·thop′sin. Visual yellow, produced by the action of light on rhodopsin (visual purple).

xan·thop′ter·in. $C_6H_5N_5O_2$. A yellow pigment, widely distributed in animal organisms and representing an element of the structure of folic acid.

xan′tho·sine (zanth′o·seen, ·sin). A nucleoside made up of xanthine and ribose.

xan·tho′sis. A yellow discoloration of the skin due to a deposit of carotenoid pigment; occurs from eating

quantities of carrots, squash, sweet potatoes, etc. The reaction is readily reversible. A similar reaction is seen from another pigmentary deposit in the skin after taking atabrine over a period o. time. Also called *aurantiasis cutis* **—xan′thous,** *adj.*

xan·thox′y·lum (zan·thock′si·lum) The dried bark of *Zanthoxylum americanum*, or of *Z. clavaherculis*. Contain xanthoxylin-N, xanthyletin, volatile oil and resins. Also called *prickly ash bark* **x. fruit.** The dried, full-grown frui of *Z. americanum*, or of *Z. clavaherculis*. Contains a volatile oil and hesperidin. Also called *prickly ash berries.*

xan′thu·re′nic ac′id. A green pigment derived from quinoline found ir the urine of rats suffering from pyridoxine deficiency.

xan·thyl′ic. Pertaining to xanthine.

X chro′mo·some. See under *chromosome.*

Xe. Chemical symbol for xenon.

xen′o- (zen′o-), **xen-.** A combining form meaning *strange* or *foreign*.

xen″o·di′ag·no′sis. The procedure of using a suitable arthropod to transfer a disease from a patient to a susceptible laboratory animal.

xen″o·me′ni·a. Vicarious menstruation.

xe′non (zee′non, zen′on). Xe $= 131.3$. A chemically inert gaseous element found in the atmosphere.

xen″o·pho′bi·a. A morbid fear of strangers.

xen″oph·thal′mi·a. Conjunctivitis due to injury.

Xen″op·syl′la. A genus of fleas of the family Pulicidae. **X. cheopis** The Indian rat flea; found in tropica and subtropical regions. A vector for bubonic plague and *Hymenolepis diminuta*, a tapeworm. This flea attacks man and other mammals, ir addition to the rat, its natural host.

Xen′o·pus, Xen·o′pus. A genus of African toad belonging to the Pipidae used in laboratory tests for pregnancy **xe·ran′tic.** Having desiccative properties; drying. **—xeransis,** *n.*

xe·ra′si·a (zi·ray′zhuh, ·shuh). Old term for a disease of the hair marked by cessation of growth and excessive dryness.

xe′ro- (zeer′o-), **xer-.** A combining form meaning *dry*.

xe″ro·der′ma, xe″ro·der′mi·a, 1 An abnormal dryness of the skin. 2. A disease characterized by dryness and harshness of the skin, discoloration, and a fine scaly desquamation. Syn. *ichthyosis*. **x. pigmentosum.** A rare disease of the skin usually beginning in childhood, and characterized by disseminated pigment spots, telangiectasis, atrophy, and contraction of the skin. Occurs particularly in areas exposed to sunlight and is made worse by it. Patients have photophobia, and there is a definite familial tendency. Warty and keratolytic lesions occur that soon develop into malignant growths. The disease is eventually fatal. The skin develops many characteristics of the senile skin in early life. Also called *angioma pigmentosum atrophicum, atrophoderma pigmentosum, Kaposi's disease, melanosis lenticularis progressiva.*

xe·ro'ma. See *xerophthalmia.*

xe"ro·me'ni·a. The presence of the usual constitutional disturbances at the menstrual period but without the menstrual flow of blood.

xe"ro·myc·te'ri·a. Lack of moisture in the nasal passages.

xer·on'o·sus. A condition of dryness of the skin.

xe"ro·pha'gi·a. The eating of dry or desiccated food.

xe"roph·thal'mi·a. A dry and thickened condition of the conjunctiva, sometimes following chronic conjunctivitis, disease of the lacrimal apparatus, or vitamin-A deficiency. Also see *xerosis.*

xe·ro'sis. A state of dryness, especially of the skin (see *xeroderma*) or of the conjunctiva (see *xerophthalmia*). Syn., *asteatosis.* **x. conjuncti'vae.** A condition marked by silver-gray, shiny, triangular spots on both sides of the cornea, within the region of the palpebral aperture, consisting of dried epithelium, flaky masses, and microorganisms. The spots are observed in some cases of hemeralopia. See *xerophthalmia.* **x. infan'tilis.** Xerophthalmia marked by a lusterless, grayish white, foamy, greasy, very persistent deposit on the conjunctiva. Also called *keratitis sicca.*

xe"ro·sto'mi·a. Dry mouth, caused by insufficient secretion of saliva.

xe·rot'ic. Characterized by xerosis; dry.

xe"ro·to'ci·a (zeer"o·to'shee·uh, ·see·uh). Old term for dry labor.

xiph-. See *xipho-.*

xiph'i-. See *xipho-.*

xiph'o- (zif'o-, zy'fo-), **xiph-.** A combining form signifying *relation to the xiphoid cartilage.*

xiph"o·cos'tal. Pertaining to the xiphoid cartilage and to the ribs.

xiph·od'y·mus (zi·fod'i·mus, zye·fod'i·mus). A double monster with two heads, two thoraces, four arms, abdominal and pelvic regions in common, with two legs, or occasionally a rudimentary third leg. Also called *dicephalus tetrabrachius.*

xiph"o·dyn'i·a. Pain in the xiphoid cartilage.

xiph"oid·i'tis (zif"oy·dye'tis, zy"·foy·). Inflammation of the xiphoid process.

x'-ray pho·tog'ra·phy. See *radiography.*

x'-rays. See *roentgen rays* under *ray.*

x'-ray u'nit. 1. Any assemblage of equipment, primarily for diagnostic or therapeutic use of the roentgen ray. 2. A roentgen unit. See under *unit.*

xy'lem (zy'lem). The inner or woody portion of a vascular bundle of a plant, as opposed to the phloem.

xy'lene (zy'leen, zye·leen'). C_6H_4·$(CH_3)_2$. Dimethylbenzene; occurs as a colorless, mobile, inflammable liquid. The xylene of commerce is a mixture of the three isomerides—*o*-, *m*-, and *p*-xylenes. Syn., *xyloi.*

xy'lo-, xyl-. A combining form denoting *pertaining to* or *derived from wood.*

xylocaine hydrochloride. Trademark for lidocaine hydrochloride.

xy'lol. See *xylene.*

xy'lose. $C_5H_{10}O_5 = 150.1.$ Wood sugar. Obtained from vegetable fibers and used medicinally as a diabetic food.

Y

Y. Chemical symbol for yttrium.

yatren. Trade name for chiniofon.

yawn. To gape, to open the mouth widely. Also called *chasma.*

yawn'ing. A reflex stretching of the muscles accompanied by a deep inspiration, occurring during the drowsy state preceding the onset of sleep. Also called *hiant.*

yaws. An infectious, nonvenereal disease occurring in the hot, moist tropics; caused by *Treponema pertenue;* characterized by an initial cutaneous lesion, the mother *yaw,* followed by one or more crops of multiple, papillomatous raspberrylike lesions of the skin. Occasionally late destructive lesions occur involving especially skin and bones. This aspect of yaws, if the tissues about the nose and mouth are involved, is called *gangosa, q.v.* The spirochetes gain entrance through the skin. Flies, especially species of *Hippelates,* may be vectors. Serologic tests of the blood for syphilis are positive. Syn., *frambesia*, *pian*.

Yb. Chemical symbol for ytterbium.

Y chro′mo·some. See under *chromosome*.

yeast. The name applied to various species of *Saccharomyces*. Yeast is chiefly employed medicinally because of its richness in the water-soluble vitamins including thiamine, riboflavin, pyridoxine, nicotinic acid, and pantothenic acid. **autolyzed y.** Yeast digested by its own proteolytic enzymes; used for dietary deficiencies or to replace meat extracts. **brewer's y.** See dried *yeast*. **compressed y.** Consists of the moist, living cells of *Saccharomyces cerevisiae* or of other species of *Saccharomyces* combined with a starchy or absorbent base. It contains at least two enzymes: invertase which changes sucrose to monosaccharides, and zymase which converts monosaccharides to alcohol. **dried y.** Consists of the dry cells of any suitable strain of *Saccharomyces cerevisiae*. It may be obtained as a by-product from the brewing of beer when it is called brewer's dried yeast. Dried yeast may also be obtained by growing suitable strains of yeast, using mediums other than those required for the production of beer. This yeast is commonly known as primary dried yeast. Dried yeast is frequently fortified with vitamins of the B-complex group.

yel′low. Of a color like that of gold; producing such a color. **butter y.** See

butter yellow. **indicator y.** A hypothetical intermediary product in the breakdown of visual purple to retinene.

yel′low jack. See yellow *fever*.

yel′low-root′′. See *hydrastis*.

yodoxin. Trade-mark for 5,7-diiodo-8-hydroxyquinoline, an antiprotozoan agent.

yo·him′be′, yo·him′bi. The rubiaceous tree *Corynanthe Yohimbi* (*Pausinystalia Yohimbe*) growing in the southern Cameroons district in Africa. The bark contains several alkaloids of which the most important is yohimbine; both bark and yohimbine have been employed for reputed aphrodisiac effect.

yo·him′bine. The principal alkaloid of yohimbé, probably identical with quebrachine.

yolk. The nutritive part of an ovum. Also called *deuteroplasm*.

yolk sac. An extraembryonic membrane composed of endoderm and splanchnic mesoderm, enclosing the yolk when the latter is present; also the site of formation of the primitive blood cells.

youth. The period between childhood and maturity.

y′per·ite (ee″pur·ite, eye′pur·ite). Di(chloroethyl) sulfide; mustard gas (C₂H₄Cl)₂S. A vesicant liquid or vapor used in chemical warfare.

Yt. Chemical symbol for yttrium.

yt·ter′bi·um (i·tur′bee·um). Yb = 173.04. A rare metal.

yt′tri·um (it′ree·um). Y (or Yt) = 88.92. A rare metallic element.

Z

Z. 1. *Zuckung*, contraction; a term used in electrotherapeutics. 2. *Zwischenscheibe*, intermediate disk. See Z disk.

zanchol. Trade-mark for florantyrone.

xar·an′than. Scirrhous condition of the breast.

Z disk. See under *disk*. See also Z, 2.

ze′a. Consists of the fresh styles and stigmas of *Zea mays*. Contains maizenic acid, fixed oil, resin, and mucilage. Also called *corn silk*.

xe′′a·xan′thine (zee″uh·zan′theen, ·thin). A carotenoid from maize, egg yolk, and many plants.

xed′o·ar′′y (zed′o·err″ee). The dried rhizome of species of *Curcuma*; has actions similar to ginger.

xe′in (zee′in, tsee′in). A yellowish, soft, insipid prolamine of maize.

xe′o·lite. Any one of a group of hydrated aluminum and calcium or sodium silicates, of the type Na₂O.2Al₂O₃.5SiO₂ or CaO.2Al₂O₃.5SiO₂, certain of

which may be used for water softening by an ion exchange process.

xephiran chloride. Trade-mark for benzalkonium chloride.

ze′ro. 1. Any character denoting absence of quantity. 2. The point of thermometers from which temperatures are counted. **absolute z.** Approximately −273.2° C. or −459.8° F.

zinc. Zn = 65.38. Occurs as a bluish white, lustrous metal with a crystalline fracture. Most of the salts of zinc are astringent and antiseptic and employed as such in medicine. **medicinal z. peroxide.** A mixture consisting essentially of zinc peroxide with varying amounts of zinc oxide and zinc hydroxide; occurs as a fine, white, crystalline powder, insoluble in water. Used as an antiseptic deodorant and astringent application. **z. acetate.** Zn(C₂H₃O₂)₂.2H₂O. Occurs as white crystals or granules; soluble in water. Used as an astringent. **z. chloride.** $ZnCl_2$. Occurs as a white, or nearly white, crystalline powder; soluble in water; it is very deliquescent. It is an astringent. **z. iodide.** ZnI_2. Occurs as a white, or nearly white, granular powder, freely soluble in water; it is very deliquescent. Zinc iodide possesses astringent and caustic powers. **z. oxide.** ZnO. Occurs as a fine, amorphous, white or yellowish white powder; insoluble in water. Used as a mildly astringent and protective application. **z. phenolsulfonate.** $Zn(HOC_6H_4SO_3)_2.8H_2O$. Occurs as colorless, transparent crystals, or granules or powder; soluble in water. Used as an antiseptic and astringent. Also called **z. sulfocarbolate. z. stearate.** A compound of zinc with variable proportions of stearic and palmitic acids; occurs as a fine, white, bulky powder; insoluble in water. Used in eczema and other cutaneous diseases. **z. sulfanilate.** $Zn[C_6H_4(NH_2)SO_3]_2.4H_2O$. A salt used in 0.25-0.5% aqueous solution or in ointment as an astringent application. See *nizin*. **z. sulfate.** $ZnSO_4.7H_2O$. Occurs as colorless crystals, white granules, or powder; soluble in water. Internally, it is used for its emetic action in poisonings. Externally, it is actively astringent. **z. sulfocarbolate.** Zinc phenolsulfonate. **z. undecylenate.** A salt of zinc and undecylenic acid, used as a fungicide.

zinc'um. See *zinc*.

zin'ger·one (zin'jur·ohn). Gingerol. A pungent ketone, $C_{11}H_{14}O_3$, present in ginger.

zin'gi·ber. See *ginger*.

zir·co'ni·um. Zr = 91.22. A metallic element resembling titanium and silicon. **z. dioxide.** ZrO_2. Occurs as a heavy white powder. Used in x-ray photography as a substitute for bismuth salts.

Zn. Chemical symbol for zinc.

zo·an'thro·py. A form of mental disorder in which the person imagines himself transformed into or inhabited by an animal.

zo'na. 1. A belt or girdle. 2. See *herpes zoster*. **z. ciliaris.** The ciliary processes collectively. **z. columnaris recti.** The portion of the anal canal in which lie the rectal columns. **z. cutanea recti.** The portion of the anal canal lined by skin. **z. fasciculata.** The central portion of the cortex of the suprarenal gland in which the cellular cords are radially disposed. **z. glomerulosa.** The outer zone of the adrenal cortex in which the cells are grouped in rounded masses. **z. intermedia recti.** The portion of the anal canal which lies between the cutaneous and columnar zones. **z. pellucida.** The thick, solid, elastic envelope of the ovum, corresponding to the wall of a cell. **z. reticularis.** The inner zone of the adrenal cortex in which the cellular cords form a network.

zone. A delimited area or region. **–zo'nal,** *adj.* **androgenic z.** The hypertrophic, inner zone of the fetal adrenal cortex. It involutes rapidly after birth, has certain hormonal functions similar to the testes, and theoretically serves to protect the fetus against the excessive effect of maternal estrogens. Also called *z-zone, fetal cortex*. **ciliary z.** The ciliary processes collectively. **ependymal z.** The internal zone of the embryonic neural tube containing ependymal cells and undifferentiated, proliferative cells. **erotogenic z.** Any part of the body which, on being touched, causes sexual feelings. **trigger z.** Any area of hyperexcitability, stimulation of which will precipitate a specific response, such as an epileptic seizure or an attack of neuralgia.

zon"es·the'si·a, zon"aes·the'si·a (zo"ness·thee'zhuh, ·zee·uh). A sensation like that produced by a tight girdle encircling the waist. Syn., *girdle pain*.

zon'ule (zone'yool, zon'yool). A small band. **ciliary z.** The suspensory structure supporting the lens of the eye. Also called **z. of Zinn.**

zon"u·li'tis (zone"yoo·lye'tis, zon"·yoo·). Inflammation of the ciliary zonule.

zo'o-, zo-. A combining form denoting *animal* or pertaining to an animal.

zo"o·der'mic. Pertaining to, or taken from, the skin of some animal other than man; applied to a form of skin grafting.

zo"o·ge·og'ra·phy. The study of animals and animal life in various parts of the earth.

zo"o·glee'a (zo"o·glee'uh, zo·og'lee·uh). Microörganisms which are embedded in a jellylike matrix formed as the result of their metabolic activities. **–zooglecic,** *adj.*

zo·og'o·ny. The breeding of animals.

zo'o·graft. A graft of tissue taken from an animal.

zo·ol'o·gist. A scientist who studies animal life.

zo·ol'o·gy. The study of animals.

zo"o·par'a·site. An animal parasite.

zo·oph'a·gous. Subsisting on animal food.

zo·oph'i·lism. The love of animals; it is usually immoderate, and toward certain animals, illustrated in the fanaticism of antivivisection. **erotic z.** The desire or impulse to stroke or pet animals for sexual excitement.

zo"o·pho'bi·a. Morbid fear of animals.

zo′o·plas′ty. The surgical transfer of zoografts; the transplantation of tissue from any of the lower animals to man.

zo·op′si·a. The seeing of animals, as an illusion or as a hallucination or in a dream; occurs commonly in delirium tremens.

zo′o·tox′in. A poison or toxin produced by animals, as snake venom or spider poison.

zos′ter. An acute inflammatory disease, consisting of grouped vesicles corresponding in distribution to the course of a cutaneous nerve; accompanied by pain or burning, and usually unilateral. Syn., *herpes zoster.* **z. auricularis.** A form affecting the ear. **z. brachialis.** A form affecting the arm or forearm. **z. facialis.** That involving the sensory fibers of the trigeminal nerve distributed over the face. Any or all of the three branches may be involved. **z. femoralis.** That occurring over the sacrum and extending down the thighs. The perineal region may be involved. **z. ophthalmicus.** An eruption in the course of the ophthalmic division of the fifth nerve.

zos′ter·oid. Resembling zoster.

zox″a·zol′a·mine. 2-Amino-5-chlorobenzoxazole, a skeletal muscle relaxant. See *flexin.*

Zr. Chemical symbol for zirconium.

zuck′ung. Contraction; a term used in electrotherapeutics. Abbreviated, Z.

zwit′ter·i″on. Same as *zwitter ion.* See under *ion.*

Zy″ga·de′nus. A genus of herbs producing a crystalline alkaloid $C_{29}H_{63}NO_{10}$.

zy″ga·poph′y·sis (zy″guh·pof′i·sis). An articular process of a vertebra. —**zygapophys′eal,** *adj.*

zy·go′ma (zye·go′muh, zi·go′muh). 1. The arch formed by the union of the zygomatic processes of the temporal bone and maxilla, and the zygomatic bone. 2. The cheekbone. See Table of Bones in the Appendix. —**zygomat′ic,** *adj.*

zy″go·mat′ic (zy″go·mat′ik). One of several small subcutaneous muscles arising from, or in relation with, the zygoma. See Table of Muscles in the Appendix.

zy″go·mat′i·co- (zy″go·mat′i·ko-).

A combining form denoting *relating to the zygoma.*

zy″go·mat″i·co·fa′cial. Pertaining to the zygoma and the face, as zygomaticofacial foramen.

zy″go·mat″i·co·tem′po·ral. Pertaining to zygoma and temporal bone or fossa, as zygomaticotemporal foramen.

zy″go·my·ce′tes (zy″go·migh·see′teez). A group of fungi characterized by sexual reproduction through the union of two similar gametes.

zy′go·spore. The spore resulting from the fusion of two similar gametes, as in certain algae and fungi.

zy′gote (zy′goat). 1. An organism produced by the union of two gametes. 2. The fertilized ovum before cleavage.

zy′mase (zy′mace). 1. An enzyme. 2. An enzyme mixture of yeast causing alcoholic fermentation.

zy′mo-, zym-. A combining form denoting *pertaining to or produced by fermentation.*

zy″mo·gen. The inactive precursor of an enzyme which, on reaction with an appropriate kinase or other chemical agent, liberates the enzyme in active form.

zy″mo·hy·drol′y·sis (zy″mo·high·drol′i·sis). Hydrolysis produced by the action of an enzyme. Also called *enzymatic hydrolysis.*

zy·mol′o·gy (zye·mol′o·jee). The science of fermentation. —**zymolog′ic,** *adj.*

zy·mol′y·sis (zye·mol′i·sis). Fermentation. —**zymolyt′ic,** *adj.*

zy·mom′e·ter (zye·mom′i·tur). An instrument for measuring fermentation.

zy′mo·phore. The active part of an enzyme, that which bears the ferment That portion of the enzyme which possesses the characteristic activity. —**zymophor′ic,** *adj.*

zy″mo·pro′te·in (zy″mo·pro′tee·in·pro′teen). Any one of a class of proteins possessing catalytic powers.

zy·mo′sis (zye·mo′sis). 1. Fermentation. 2. An infectious disease due to a fungus. —**zymot′ic,** *adj.*

zy·mos′ter·ol (zye·mos′tur·ole, ·ol) $C_{27}H_{44}O$. A sterol from yeast; found in ergosterol residues.

zy′mur·gy. The branch of chemical technology dealing with the application of fermentation or enzymatic action to any industrial process.

APPENDIX

TABLES

APP.

TABLE OF ARTERIES

Name	Origin	Branches	Distribution
Aberrant	Brachial or axillary		Radial, radial recurrent, or, rarely, ulnar art.
Aberrant	Descending aorta		Anastomoses with an aberrant art. from the right subclavian, costocervical trunk, or superior intercostal art.
Acetabular or articular	Obturator		Round ligament of femur, synovial membrane, acetabular fat, head of femur
Acromial	Thoracoacromial		Deltoid m., acromial rete
Acromial	Transverse scapular		Trapezius m., acromial rete
Acromiothoracic	See *Thoracoacromial*		
Afferent	Interlobular of kidney		Glomeruli
Alveolar or gingival	Posterior superior alveolar		Gums of posterior portion of upper jaw
Alveolar, anterior superior (anterior su-	Infraorbital	Dental, antral	Upper incisor and canine teeth, mucous membrane of maxillary

Alveolar, inferior (inferior dental OT)	Internal maxillary	Mylohyoid, lingual, dental, mental, incisive	Mylohyoid m., buccal mucous membrane, lower teeth, mandible, gums
Alveolar, middle superior (inconstant)	Infraorbital		Upper premolar teeth
Alveolar, posterior superior (posterior superior dental OT)	Internal maxillary	Dental, antral, alveolar, muscular	Buccinator m., upper molar and premolar teeth, gums, mucous membrane of maxillary sinus
Anastomotic of inferior gluteal	Inferior gluteal		Anastomoses with first perforating and medial and lateral femoral circumflex art. in what is known as "crucial anastomosis"
Anastomotic of middle meningeal (also called perforating temporal)	Middle meningeal		Anastomoses with deep temporal
Anastomotica magna of brachial	See *Collateral, inferior ulnar*		
Angular	External maxillary	Muscular, lacrimal, terminal	Orbicularis oculi, nasalis, angular head of quadratus labii superioris and procerus mm.; lacrimal sac; anastomoses with dorsal nasal branch of ophthalmic
Antral	Anterior and posterior superior alveolar		Mucous membrane of maxillary sinus (antrum of Highmore OT)

TABLE OF ARTERIES—(Continued)

Name	Origin	Branches	Distribution
Aorta, abdominal	Continuation of descending (thoracic) aorta from level of inferior border of twelfth thoracic vertebra	(1) Visceral celiac superior mesenteric inferior mesenteric middle suprarenal renal internal spermatic (ovarian) (2) Parietal inferior phrenic lumbar (4 pairs) middle sacral (3) Terminal common iliac	Diaphragm, body wall, abdominal and pelvic viscera, lower extremities
Aorta, arch of	Continuation of ascending aorta outside pericardium	Innominate, left common carotid, left subclavian (occasionally thyreoidea ima and bronchial art.)	
Aorta, ascending	Base of left ventricle	Right and left coronary	
Aorta, descending (thoracic)	Continuation of arch of aorta at inferior border of left side of fourth thoracic vertebra	(1) Visceral pericardial bronchial esophageal mediastinal (2) Parietal intercostal superior phrenic subcostal (aber-	Body wall, thoracic viscera, diaphragm

Appendicular		Ileocolic	Cecal, appendicular	Apex of cecum, vermiform process
Arciform or arcuate of kidney		Interlobar	Interlobular	
Arcuate		Dorsalis pedis	Second, third, and fourth dorsal metatarsal	Dorsal metatarsal portion of foot
Auditory, Internal		Basilar or anterior inferior cerebellar		Internal ear
Auricular, deep		Internal maxillary	Meatal, tympanic, auricular	Skin of external acoustic meatus, external surface of tympanic membrane, temporomandibular articulation
Auricular, posterior		External carotid	Muscular, auricular, stylomastoid, occipital, parotid	Digastric, stylohyoid, sternocleidomastoid, auricularis posterior, occipitalis, and stapedius mm.; tympanic membrane and cavity, tympanic antrum, mastoid air cells, semicircular canals, auricle, scalp, parotid gland
Axillary		Continuation of subclavian	Highest thoracic, thoracoacromial, lateral thoracic, subscapular, posterior humeral circumflex, anterior humeral circumflex	Pectoralis major, pectoralis minor, biceps brachii, coracobrachialis, triceps (long head), subclavius, deltoid, serratus anterior, teres major, teres minor, latissimus dorsi, subscapularis, and infraspinatus mm.; mammary gland, shoulder joint, head of humerus, skin of pectoral region and shoulder, acromial rete

TABLE OF ARTERIES—(Continued)

NAME	ORIGIN	BRANCHES	DISTRIBUTION
Azygos of vagina	Uterine and vaginal		Vagina
Basilar	Formed by junction of the two vertebral	Anterior inferior cerebellar, internal auditory, pontine, superior cerebellar, posterior cerebral	Pons, internal ear, cerebellum, pineal body, anterior medullary velum, tela chorioidea of third ventricle, temporal and occipital lobes of cerebrum
Brachial	Axillary	Profunda brachii, nutrient, muscular, superior ulnar collateral, inferior ulnar collateral, radial, ulnar	Deltoid, triceps, brachioradialis, biceps brachii, brachialis, coracobrachialis, and anconeus mm.; shaft of humerus, elbow joint, forearm, and hand
Bronchial	(1) Descending (thoracic) aorta (upper and lower left) (2) First aortic intercostal (right) (3) Arch of aorta (occasionally)		Bronchial tubes, areolar tissue of lungs, bronchial lymph nodes, esophagus
Buccal	See *Buccinator*		
Buccinator	Internal maxillary		Buccinator m.; skin and mucous membrane of cheek, upper gums
Bulb of urethra, art. of	Internal pudendal	Muscular, glandular, spongiosal	Sphincter urethrae membranaceae m.; bulbourethral gland (Cowper's), bulb of urethra, corpus spongiosum urethrae
Bulb of vestibule, art.	Internal pudendal	Bulbar, glandular	Major vestibular glands (Bartho-

			Lining of tympanic cavity
Caroticotympanic	Internal carotid		Lining of tympanic cavity
Carotid, common	Right from innominate, left from arch of aorta	External and internal carotid, occasionally superior thyroid, ascending pharyngeal, and even vertebral	Region of neck and head
Carotid, external	Common carotid	Superior thyroid, ascending pharyngeal, lingual, external maxillary (facial), sternocleidomastoid (occasionally), occipital, posterior auricular, superficial temporal, internal maxillary	Anterior portion of neck, face, scalp, side of head, ear, dura mater
Carotid, internal	Common carotid	(1) Petrous portion: caroticotympanic, art. of pterygoid canal (Vidian) (inconstant) (2) Cavernous portion: cavernous, hypophyseal, semilunar, anterior meningeal, ophthalmic (3) Cerebral portion: anterior cerebral, middle cerebral, posterior communicating, choroid	Anterior portion of cerebrum, eye and its appendages, forehead, nose, internal ear, trigeminal nerve, dura mater, hypophysis

TABLE OF ARTERIES—(Continued)

Name	Origin	Branches	Distribution
Celiac	Abdominal aorta	Left gastric, hepatic, splenic	Esophagus, cardia and lesser curvature of stomach, liver, gall-bladder, pylorus, duodenum, pancreas, great omentum, spleen
Central art. of retina	Ophthalmic	Superior: nasal, temporal Inferior: nasal, temporal	Retina
Cerebellar, anterior inferior	Basilar		Anterior portion of inferior surface of cerebellum
Cerebellar, posterior inferior	Vertebral	Bulbar, choroid, nuclear, medial terminal, lateral terminal	Medulla oblongata, choroid plexus of third ventricle, dentate nucleus, nuclei of cranial nerves IX, X, XI
Cerebellar, superior	Basilar	Medial, lateral	Vermis cerebelli, superior surface of cerebellum, pineal body, anterior medullary velum, tela chorioides of third ventricle
Cerebral, anterior	Internal carotid	Anterior communicating, orbital, anterior medial frontal, recurrent, intermediate medial frontal, posterior medial frontal	Anterior perforated substance, lamina terminalis, rostrum of corpus callosum, septum pellucidum, head of caudate nucleus, frontal lobe of putamen, frontal lobe of globus pallidus, orbital surface of frontal lobe of cerebrum, gyrus rectus, medial orbital gyrus, olfactory lobe, superior frontal gyrus, middle frontal gyrus, corpus callosum, cinguli,

			sule, column of fornix, precuneus, upper part of ascending frontal gyrus, upper part of ascending parietal gyrus, superior parietal lobule
Cerebral, middle (art. fossae Sylvii OT)	Internal carotid	Medial striate, lateral striate, inferior lateral frontal, ascending frontal, ascending parietal, parietotemporal, temporal	Putamen, caudate nucleus, globus pallidus, internal capsule, inferior frontal gyrus (Broca's convolution), lateral part of orbital surface of frontal lobe, ascending frontal gyrus, ascending parietal gyrus, lower part of superior parietal lobule, supramarginal gyrus, angular gyrus, posterior parts of superior and middle temporal gyri, lateral surface of temporal lobe
Cerebral, posterior	Basilar	Anterior temporal, posterior temporal, posteromedial central, posterolateral central, posterior choroid, calcarine, parieto-occipital	Posterior perforated substance, cerebral peduncle, posterior part of thalamus, mammillary bodies, walls of third ventricle, corpora quadrigemina, medial and lateral geniculate bodies, uncus, hippocampal gyrus, fusiform gyrus, cuneus, precuneus, lingual gyrus, tela chorioidea of third ventricle, choroid plexus, fornix, posterior half of visual path, half of visual center of occipital lobe
Cervical, ascending	Inferior thyroid	Muscular, spinal, phrenic	Longus capitis, scalenus anterior and mm. of nape of neck, spinal medulla and its membranes, vertebrae, phrenic nerve

TABLE OF ARTERIES—(Continued)

NAME	ORIGIN	BRANCHES	DISTRIBUTION
Cervical, deep	Costocervical trunk	Muscular, spinal	Semispinalis cervicis, semispinalis capitis, and adjoining neck mm.; spinal, medulla and membranes via intervertebral foramen for eighth cervical nerve
Cervical, superficial	Transverse cervical	Muscular, glandular	Trapezius, levator scapulae, splenius cervicis, splenius capitis mm.; posterior chain of lymph nodes
Cervical, transverse	Thyrocervical trunk	Ascending or superficial cervical, descending	Trapezius, levator scapulae, splenii, rhomboids, latissimus dorsi mm.; posterior chain of lymph nodes
Choroid, anterior	Internal carotid	Optic, peduncular, ganglionic, choroid	Optic tract, cerebral peduncle, base of cerebrum, lateral geniculate body, tail of caudate nucleus, globus pallidus, internal capsule, choroid plexus of inferior horn of lateral ventricle
Choroid, posterior	Posterior cerebral		Tela chorioidea of third ventricle, choroid plexus
Ciliary, anterior	Muscular branches of ophthalmic and lacrimal	Episcleral, anterior conjunctival	Iris and conjunctiva
Ciliary, long posterior	Ophthalmic		Ciliary muscle and iris

Circumflex, anterior humeral	Axillary	Muscular, bicipital, pectoral	Coracobrachialis, biceps brachii, deltoid mm.; head of humerus, shoulder joint, tendons of pectoralis major and long head of biceps brachii mm.
Circumflex, deep iliac	External iliac	Muscular, cutaneous	Psoas, iliacus, sartorius, tensor fasciae latae, obliquus abdominis externus, obliquus abdominis internus, transversus abdominis mm.; skin over course of vessel
Circumflex, lateral femoral	Profunda femoris	Ascending, transverse, descending	Muscles of thigh
Circumflex, medial femoral	Profunda femoris	Muscular, superficial, deep, acetabular	Adductor, gracilis, obturator externus, quadratus femoris mm.; acetabular fat, round ligament of femur, head of femur
Circumflex, posterior humeral	Axillary	Muscular, articular, nutrient, acromial	Deltoid, teres minor, triceps brachii (long and lateral heads) mm.; greater tubercle of humerus, posterior portion of shoulder joint, acromial rete
Circumflex, scapular	Subscapular	Muscular, articular, nutrient	Subscapularis, infraspinatus, teres major, teres minor, deltoid, triceps brachii (long head) mm.; scapula, shoulder joint
Circumflex, superficial iliac	Femoral	Muscular, glandular, cutaneous	Sartorius, iliacus, tensor fasciae latae mm.; inguinal lymph nodes, skin over course of vessel

TABLE OF ARTERIES—(Continued)

NAME	ORIGIN	BRANCHES	DISTRIBUTION
Clitoris, deep art. of	Internal pudendal		Corpus cavernosum clitoridis
Clitoris, dorsal art. of	Internal pudendal		Dorsum, glans, corona and prepuce of clitoris
Colic, left	Inferior mesenteric	Ascending, descending	Left portion of transverse colon, upper portion of descending colon, splenic flexure
Colic, middle	Superior mesenteric	Right, left	Upper portion of ascending colon, hepatic flexure, right portion of transverse colon
Colic, right	Superior mesenteric	Ascending, descending	Ascending colon
Collateral, inferior ulnar (anastomotica magna OT)	Brachial	Posterior, anterior	Triceps brachii, brachialis, pronator teres mm.; articular rete of elbow joint
Collateral, middle	Profunda brachii	Muscular, anastomotic	Medial head of triceps brachii m.; articular rete of elbow joint
Collateral, radial	Profunda brachii	Muscular, anastomotic	Triceps brachii, brachioradialis mm.; articular rete of elbow joint
Collateral, superior ulnar (profunda inferior OT)	Brachial	Muscular, articular, anastomotic	Triceps brachii m.; skin, elbow joint, articular rete of elbow joint
Comes nervi mediani See Median			

Comes nervi phrenici, art.	See *Pericardiaco-phrenic*		
Comitans nervi ischiadici, art.	Inferior gluteal		Sciatic nerve
Communicating, anterior	Anterior cerebral	Anteromedial	Anterior perforated substance
Communicating, posterior	Internal carotid	Hippocampal, middle thalamic	Optic chiasm, optic tract, tuber cinereum, mammillary body, hippocampal gyrus, internal capsule, cerebral peduncle, interpeduncular region, thalamus
Conjunctival, anterior	Episcleral of anterior ciliary		Conjunctiva
Conjunctival, posterior	Medial and lateral palpebral arteries		Conjunctiva
Coronary, left	Left posterior aortic sinus	Anterior descending, circumflex, left marginal, left atrial, terminal	Left atrium, root of aorta and pulmonary art., myocardium of both ventricles, interventricular septum
Coronary, right	Anterior aortic sinus	Right atrial, posterior descending, right marginal, preventricular, transverse	Right atrium, root of pulmonary art. and aorta, anterior wall of right ventricle, septal myocardium, left ventricle adjoining posterior longitudinal cardiac sulcus

TABLE OF ARTERIES—(Continued)

Name	Origin	Branches	Distribution
Costocervical trunk	Subclavian	Superior intercostal, deep cervical, arteria aberrans on right	First and second intercostal spaces, mm. of neck, spinal cord and its membranes
Cremasteric	See *Spermatic, external*		
Cystic	Right hepatic	Superficial, deep	Free surface of gallbladder, attached surface of gallbladder, and liver substance
Deferential	Superior vesical, inferior vesical, or internal iliac	Ascending, descending	Seminal vesicle, ampulla of ductus deferens, ductus deferens, epididymis
Dental, anterior superior	See *Alveolar, anterior superior*		
Dental, inferior	See *Alveolar, inferior*		
Dental, posterior superior	See *Alveolar, posterior superior*		
Digital, common volar	Superficial volar arch	Proper volar digital	Contiguous sides of second to fifth fingers, flexor tendons and tendon sheaths, matrix of nails
Digital, dorsal, of	Radial		Dorsum and sides of thumb

Artery	Origin	Branches	Distribution
Digital, plantar	Plantar metatarsal arteries		Contiguous sides of toes, flexor tendons and sheaths, joints, skin
Digital, plantar, of lateral side of fifth toe	Lateral plantar		Lateral plantar part of fifth toe
Digital, proper volar, of medial side of little finger	Ulnar		Medial side of little finger, flexor tendon and sheath, matrix of nail
Digital, radial dorsal, of index finger	Radial		Radial dorsal surface of index finger
Dorsalis pedis	Anterior tibial	Cutaneous, lateral tarsal, medial tarsal, arcuate, first dorsal, metatarsal, deep plantar	Anastomoses with lateral plantar to form plantar arterial arch; plantar surface of first and second toes; tarsal, metatarsal, digital portions of dorsum of foot
Epigastric, deep	See *Epigastric, inferior*		
Epigastric, Inferior (deep epigastric OT)	External iliac	Cutaneous, muscular, external spermatic (cremasteric in male, art. of round ligament of uterus in female), pubic	Skin and muscles of anterior abdominal wall, cremaster m., spermatic cord (round ligament of uterus in female), peritoneum
Epigastric, superficial	Femoral		Skin of abdominal wall below umbilicus, superficial fascia (Camper's), inguinal lymph nodes
Epigastric, superior	Internal mammary	Cutaneous, muscular, hepatic, peritoneal, phrenic, xiphoid	Skin, fascia, muscles and peritoneum of upper abdominal wall, diaphragm, falciform ligament of liver

TABLE OF ARTERIES—(Continued)

Name	Origin	Branches	Distribution
Episcleral	Anterior ciliary	Anterior conjunctival	Iris, ciliary processes, conjunctiva
Esophageal (4 or 5)	Thoracic aorta		Esophagus
Ethmoidal, anterior	Ophthalmic	Ethmoidal, anterior meningeal, nasal, frontal, cutaneous	Anterior and middle ethmoidal air cells, dura mater of anterior cranial fossa, mucoperiosteum of middle meatus, lateral wall and septum of nose, frontal air sinus, skin of dorsum of nose
Ethmoidal, posterior	Ophthalmic	Ethmoidal, meningeal, nasal	Posterior ethmoidal air cells, dura mater around cribriform plate, superior meatus and superior nasal conchs
Facial	See *Maxillary, external*		
Facial, transverse	Superficial temporal	Glandular, muscular, cutaneous	Masseter m.; parotid gland, skin of face
Femoral	Continuation of external iliac	Superficial epigastric, superficial iliac circumflex, superficial external pudendal, deep external pudendal, muscular, profunda femoris, highest genicular (art. genus suprema)	Skin of lower part of abdomen and groin, external genitalia, inguinal lymph nodes; mm. of medial, lateral and anterior aspects of thigh; femur, knee joint

Femoral, deep	See *Profunda femoris*		
Fossae Sylvii, art. of	See *Cerebral, middle*		
Frenulum linguae, art. of	Sublingual		Frenulum of tongue
Frontal	Ophthalmic		Skin, mm. and pericranium of forehead
Gastric, left	Celiac	Esophageal, hepatic (occasionally)	Lesser curvature and cardia of stomach, lower end of esophagus, left lobe of liver (occasionally)
Gastric, right	Hepatic		Pyloric portion of stomach
Gastric, short (vasa brevia)	Splenic		Greater curvature of stomach
Gastroduodenal	Hepatic	Pylorus, right gastroepiploic, superior pancreaticoduodenal, omental	Pylorus, duodenum, pancreas, great omentum, common bile duct
Gastroepiploic, left	Splenic	Gastric, omental	Greater curvature of stomach, great omentum
Gastroepiploic, right	Hepatic	Gastric, omental	Greater curvature of stomach, great omentum
Genicular, highest (genus suprema OT)	Femoral	Saphenous, muscular, patellar, articular	Sartorius, gracilis, distal ends of vasti, adductor magnus mm., knee joint, skin of the medial-distal portion of thigh, arterial retia on medial and lateral sides of knee

TABLE OF ARTERIES—(Continued)

Name	Origin	Branches	Distribution
Genicular, lateral inferior	Popliteal		Knee joint, deep articular rete
Genicular, lateral superior	Popliteal	Superficial, deep	Vastus lateralis, vastus intermedius mm., knee joint, femur, patella, deep articular rete
Genicular, medial inferior	Popliteal		Popliteus m., proximal end of tibia, knee joint
Genicular, medial superior	Popliteal		Vastus medialis m., femur, patella, knee joint, deep articular rete
Genicular, middle (azygos articular OT)	Popliteal		Knee joint, cruciate ligaments, patellar synovial and alar folds
Genus suprema	See Genicular, highest		
Gluteal, inferior (sciatic OT)	Internal iliac, anterior trunk	Inside pelvis, muscular, vesical; outside pelvis, muscular, coccygeal, anastomotic, articular, comitans nervi ischiadici	Gluteus maximus, piriformis, coccygeus, levator ani, upper portion of hamstrings and mm. of buttocks; perirectal fat, fundus of bladder, seminal vesicle, prostate gland, hip joint, sciatic nerve, crucial anastomosis, skin over buttock, thigh, sacrum, and coccyx

Name	Origin	Branches	Distribution
Gluteal, superior	Internal iliac, posterior trunk	Muscular, iliac, superficial; deep	Iliacus, piriformis, obturator internus, gluteus medius, gluteus minimus, tensor fasciae latae mm., hip joint, ilium, skin over sacrum
Hallucis, art. dorsalis	See *Metatarsal, first dorsal*		
Hallucis, art. princeps	See *Metatarsal, first plantar*		
Helicine	Name applied by Müller to tortuous blood vessels in cavernous tissue such as corpora cavernosa penis (clitoridis), uterus, etc.		
Hemorrhoidal, inferior	Internal pudendal		Ischiorectal fat, anal canal, levator ani, sphincter ani externus mm., skin around anus and lower region of buttock
Hemorrhoidal, middle	Internal iliac		Rectum, ductus deferens, seminal vesicle, prostate gland
Hemorrhoidal, superior	Inferior mesenteric		Muscular and mucous coats of the pelvic colon and proximal portion of the rectum, mucous coat of distal portion of rectum
Hepatic	Celiac	Right gastric, gastroduodenal, cystic, right, left	Lesser and greater curvatures of stomach, pylorus, pancreas, great omentum, gallbladder, liver
Hepatic, accessory	Left gastric		Left lobe of liver

TABLE OF ARTERIES—(Continued)

Name	Origin	Branches	Distribution
Hypogastric	See *Iliac, internal*		
Ileocolic	Superior mesenteric	Ascending, descending, posterior cecal, anterior cecal, appendicular, ileal	Ascending colon, cecum, vermiform process, lower part of ileum
Iliac, common	Abdominal aorta	Internal iliac, external iliac (occasionally accessory renal, internal spermatic, middle sacral, lateral sacral, iliolumbar), small twigs to peritoneum, psoas major m., ureter	Psoas major m., peritoneum, fascia, pelvic viscera, external genitalia, gluteal region, lower extremity
Iliac, external	Common iliac	Inferior epigastric, deep iliac circumflex, muscular, glandular, continuing as femoral art.	Psoas major, iliacus, sartorius, tensor fasciae latae, cremaster, and mm. of abdominal wall; external iliac lymph nodes, peritoneum, skin of lower abdominal wall, spermatic cord (round ligament of uterus), lower extremity
Iliac, Internal (hypogastric OT)	Common iliac	Anterior trunk, superior vesical, middle vesical, middle hemorrhoidal, obturator, inferior pudendal, inferior gluteal; uterine and vaginal in female; posterior trunk, iliolumbar, lateral sacral, superior gluteal,	Pelvic wall and contents, gluteal region, medial portion of thigh, external genitalia, anal region

Name	Origin	Branches	Distribution
Illolumbar	Internal iliac, posterior trunk	Iliac, lumbar	Psoas major, quadratus lumborum, iliacus mm.; ilium, cauda equina
Infraorbital	Internal maxillary	Orbital, middle superior Alveolar, anterior superior Alveolar, terminal	Inferior rectus, inferior oblique of the eye, levator labii superioris, orbicularis oculi mm.; fat of the orbit, lacrimal gland and sac upper premolar, canine, and incisor teeth, mucosa of maxillary sinus
Innominate	Arch of aorta	Thyreoidea ima (occasionally), thymic, or bronchial (occasionally), right subclavian, right common carotid	Right side of neck and head, right shoulder girdle and arm, occasionally thymus gland, bronchus, Inferior portion of thyroid gland
Intercostal, aortic	Descending (thoracic) aorta	Anterior, collateral intercostal Muscular, lateral cutaneous, mammary Posterior, muscular, spinal	Intercostal, pectoral, serratus anterior, iliocostalis, longissimus dorsi, multifidus spinae, semispinalis dorsi mm.; abdominal wall, vertebrae, ribs, mammary gland, skin of body wall and back, contents of vertebral canal
Intercostal, highest	Costocervical trunk	Muscular, spinal	Posterior vertebral mm.; contents of first and second intercostal spaces, contents of vertebral canal
Interlober of kidney	Renal, primary branches	Arciform	
Interlobular of kidney	Arciform	Afferent glomerular (mostly)	Glomeruli of kidney

TABLE OF ARTERIES—(Continued)

Name	Origin	Branches	Distribution
Interosseous, common	Ulnar	Volar interosseous, dorsal interosseous	Deep mm. of forearm, radius, ulna, median nerve, volar carpal and dorsal carpal retia, rete olecrani
Interosseous, dorsal	Common interosseous	Muscular, interosseous recurrent	Mm. and skin on dorsal surface of forearm, dorsal carpal rete, rete olecrani
Interosseous, recurrent	Dorsal interosseous		Supinator, anconeus mm., rete olecrani
Interosseous, volar	Common interosseous	Muscular, nutrient, median, communicating, volar terminal, dorsal terminal	Flexor digitorum profundus, flexor pollicis longus, pronator quadratus mm.; radius, ulna, median nerve, volar carpal and dorsal carpal retia
Intestinal (vasa intestini tenuis OT) (10–16)	Superior mesenteric	Ileal, jejunal	Jejunum, ileum, mesentery, mesenteric lymph nodes
Labial, inferior	External maxillary		Mucous membrane, skin, mm. and glands of lower lip
Labial, posterior	Perineal		Labium majus
Labial, superior	External maxillary	Septal, alar	Mucous membrane, skin, mm. and glands of upper lip, nasal septum, ala of nose
Lacrimal	Dorsal nasal		Lacrimal sac

Lacrimal	Ophthalmic	Recurrent, muscular, zygomatic, lateral palpebral, anterior ciliary	Lacrimal gland, superior and lateral rectus mm.; eyelids, conjunctiva, region of cheek, dura mater, temporal fossa, sclera, iris, ciliary processes
Laryngeal, inferior	Inferior thyroid		Constrictor pharyngis inferior m. and mucous membrane of lower part of larynx
Laryngeal, superior	Superior thyroid		Muscles, mucous membrane, and glands of larynx
Lienal	See *Splenic*		
Ligamenti teretis uteri (equivalent to external spermatic in male)	Inferior epigastric		Round ligament of the uterus
Lingual	External carotid	Hyoid, dorsal lingual, sublingual, profunda linguae	Intrinsic and extrinsic mm. of tongue, mucous membrane of tongue and mouth, gums, sublingual gland, glossopalatine arch, tonsil, soft palate, epiglottis, frenulum linguae
Lumbalis ima (fifth lumbar)	Middle sacral	Dorsal	Iliacus, gluteus maximus mm.; vertebral canal
Lumbar (4 pairs)	Abdominal aorta	Vertebral, muscular, dorsal, renal, spinal	Psoas, quadratus lumborum, obliqui abdominis, sacrospinalis mm.; contents of vertebral canal, capsule of kidney, vertebrae, subperitoneal plexus of Turner
Malleolar, anterior lateral	Anterior tibial		Lateral side of ankle

TABLE OF ARTERIES—(Continued)

Name	Origin	Branches	Distribution
Malleolar, anterior medial	Anterior tibial		Medial side of ankle
Malleolar, posterior lateral	Peroneal		Lateral aspect of calcaneus, lateral malleolus
Malleolar, posterior medial	Posterior tibial		Medial side of ankle, medial malleolar rete
Mammary, external	See *Thoracic, lateral*		
Mammary, internal	Subclavian	Pericardiacophrenic, anterior mediastinal, thymic, pericardial, sternal, anterior intercostal, perforating, musculophrenic, superior epigastric	Phrenic nerve, pleura, pericardium, diaphragm, connective tissue of mediastinum, lymph nodes in mediastinum, thymus gland, sternum; transversus thoracis, intercostal, pectoral, rectus abdominis, obliqui abdominis mm.; skin over chest and upper abdomen, mammary gland, falciform ligament, subpleural mediastinal pleura
Masseteric	Internal maxillary		Masseter m.
Maxillary	See *Maxillary, internal*		
Maxillary, external (facial OT)	External carotid	Ascending palatine, tonsillar, glandular, submental, muscular, in-	Constrictor mm. of pharynx, stylopharyngeus, styloglossus, pterygoid internus, levator veli

		Branches	Distribution
		labial, lateral nasal. angular	buccinator, and mm. of facial expression; tonsil, auditory tube, root of tongue, submaxillary gland, lymph nodes of neck and face, skin of face, sis and dorsum of nose, lacrimal sac, nasal septum
Maxillary, Internal (maxillary OT)	External carotid	(1) Mandibular portion: anterior tympanic, deep auricular, middle meningeal, accessory meningeal, inferior alveolar	Tensor tympani, mylohyoid mm., lining of external acoustic meatus, temporomandibular joint, lining of tympanic cavity, dura mater, skull, facial nerve, semilunar ganglion, lower teeth, mandible, mucous membrane of mouth
		(2) Pterygoid portion: deep temporal, pterygoid, masseteric, buccinator	Temporalis, pterygoid internus, pterygoid externus, masseter, buccinator mm.; pericranium, mucous membrane of mouth
		(3) Pterygopalatine portion: posterior superior alveolar, infraorbital, descending palatine, artery of pterygoid canal, pharyngeal, sphenopalatine	Rectus inferior, obliquus inferior, quadratus labii superioris, caninus mm.; upper teeth, gums, mucous membrane of roof of mouth, soft palate, palatine tonsil, upper part of pharynx, auditory tube, conchae and meati of nose, nasal septum; mucous membrane of frontal, maxillary, sphenoidal, and ethmoidal air sinuses
Median (comes nervi mediani OT)	Volar interosseous		Median nerve
Median, anterior, of spinal cord	Anterior spinal		Pia mater of spinal cord, substance of spinal cord, cauda equina

TABLE OF ARTERIES—(Continued)

Name	Origin	Branches	Distribution
Mediastinal, anterior	Internal mammary		Connective tissue, fat, and lymph nodes of mediastinum, thymus gland
Meningeal, accessory	Internal maxillary		Semilunar ganglion, walls of cavernous sinus, dura mater of middle cranial fossa
Meningeal, anterior	(1) Internal carotid (2) Anterior ethmoidal		Dura mater of anterior cranial fossa
Meningeal, middle	Internal maxillary	Ganglionic, superficial petrosal, superior tympanic, perforating temporal, orbital, anterior terminal, posterior terminal, nutrient	Tensor tympani m.; semilunar ganglion, trigeminal nerve, dura mater of anterior and middle cranial fossae, skull, tympanic cavity, orbit, infratemporal fossa
Meningeal, posterior	Ascending pharyngeal		Dura mater of posterior and middle cranial fossae
Mental	Inferior alveolar		Lower lip and chin
Mesenteric, inferior	Abdominal aorta	Left colic, sigmoid, superior hemorrhoidal (occasionally hepatic, renal, middle colic)	Transverse colon, splenic flexure, descending colon, sigmoid flexure, proximal portion of rectum
Mesenteric, superior	Abdominal aorta	Inferior pancreaticoduodenal, intestinal, ileocolic, right colic, middle	Pancreas, duodenum, jejunum, ileum, mesentery, mesenteric lymph nodes, cecum, vermi-

		hepatic, splenic, pancreatic, gastric, gastroepiploic, or gastroduodenal)	flexure
Metacarpal, first dorsal	Radial		Adjacent sides of thumb and index finger
Metacarpal, second, third, and fourth dorsal	Dorsal radial carpal	Two dorsal digital, perforating	Adjacent sides of fingers
Metacarpal, volar (3)	Deep volar arch	Perforating	Interosseous and second, third, and fourth lumbrical mm.; common digital of superficial volar arch, metacarpal bones
Metatarsal, first dorsal (dorsalis hallucis OT)	Dorsalis pedis	Two dorsal digital	Adjacent sides of first and second toes
Metatarsal, first plantar (princeps hallucis OT)	Union of deep plantar with lateral plantar	Two plantar digital, medial digital to medial side of great toe	Great toe and medial side of second toe
Metatarsal, second, third, and fourth dorsal	Arcuate	Two dorsal digital, perforating	Adjacent sides of second, third, fourth, and fifth toes
Metatarsal, second, third, and fourth plantar	Plantar arch	Two plantar digital, perforating	Adjacent sides of second, third, fourth, and fifth toes
Musculophrenic	Internal mammary	Phrenic, anterior intercostal, muscular	Mm. of abdominal wall, diaphragm, lower six intercostal spaces
Nasal, dorsal	Ophthalmic	Lacrimal	Dorsum of nose, lacrimal sac

TABLE OF ARTERIES—(Continued)

Name	Origin	Branches	Distribution
Nasal, posterior lateral	Sphenopalatine		Nasal conchae and meati, mucosa of frontal, maxillary, sphenoidal, and ethmoidal air sinuses
Nasopalatine	See *Sphenopalatine*		
Neubauer's	See *Thyreoidea ima*		
Nutrient	Brachial		Shaft of humerus
Nutrient	Volar interosseous		Shaft of radius
Nutrient	Volar interosseous		Shaft of ulna
Nutrient	Second perforating art. of profunda femoris		Shaft of femur
Nutrient	Posterior tibial		Shaft of tibia
Nutrient	Peroneal		Shaft of fibula
Nutrient	Transverse scapular		Shaft of clavicle
Nutrient	Transverse scapular		Scapula
Nutrient	A general term used to designate a branch of any artery that supplies the substance of bone. Usage has lifted a certain number of this type of arterial branch to the status of "artery." This should not make us unmindful of the fact that		

Obturator	Internal iliac, anterior trunk	Iliac, vesical, pubic, anterior terminal, posterior terminal, muscular, acetabular	Iliacus, iliopsoas, obturator internus, obturator externus, adductors, pectineus, gracilis, semimembranosus, semitendinosus, biceps femoris (long head) mm.; pubis, hip joint, head of femur, bladder, ilium
Occipital	External carotid	Muscular, sternocleidomastoid, auricular, meningeal, descending, mastoid, medial terminal, lateral terminal	Digastric, occipitalis, stylohyoid, splenius capitis, longissimus capitis, sternocleidomastoid, trapezius, semispinalis capitis and cervicis mm.; posterior surface of auricle, mastoid cells, pericranium and scalp of posterolateral surface of the head
Ophthalmic	Internal carotid	Orbital lacrimal, supraorbital, posterior ethmoidal, anterior ethmoidal, medial palpebral, frontal, dorsal nasal / Ocular central artery of the retina, short posterior ciliary, long posterior ciliary, anterior ciliary, muscular	Contents of orbit, diploë of frontal bone, mucous membrane of frontal sinus and ethmoidal air cells, dura mater of anterior fossa of skull, superior nasal concha and meatus, lacrimal sac, skin of dorsum of nose
Ovarian (homolog of internal spermatic in male)	Abdominal aorta	Ureteric, ligamentous, uterine, tubal	Ovary, ureter, suspensory ligament of ovary, broad ligament of uterus, uterine tube, round ligament of uterus, skin of labium majus and groin

TABLE OF ARTERIES—(Continued)

Name	Origin	Branches	Distribution
Palatine, ascending	External maxillary	Palatine, tonsillar	Styloglossus, stylopharyngeus, superior constrictor of pharynx, levator veli palatini mm., auditory tube, lateral wall of upper part of pharynx, soft palate, palatine tonsil
Palatine, descending	Internal maxillary	Greater palatine, lesser palatine	Soft palate, palatine tonsil, mucous membrane of roof of mouth, gums, palatine glands, palatine bone, maxilla
Palatine, greater	Descending maxillary		Mucous membrane of hard palate, gums, palatine glands, palatine bone, maxilla
Palatine, lesser	Descending palatine		Soft palate, palatine tonsil
Palpebral, inferior medial	Ophthalmic		Conjunctiva, lacrimal caruncle, lacrimal sac, lower eyelid
Palpebral, lateral	Lacrimal		Upper and lower eyelids, conjunctiva
Palpebral, superior medial	Ophthalmic		Upper eyelid
Pancreatica magna	Splenic		Posterior surface of pancreas, following course of pancreatic duct

Pancreaticoduodenal, inferior	Superior mesenteric		Head of pancreas, descending and inferior parts of duodenum
Pancreaticoduodenal, superior	Gastroduodenal		Second part of duodenum, common bile duct, pancreas
Penis (clitoris), deep art. of	Internal pudendal		Corpus cavernosum penis (clitoridis)
Penis (clitoris), dorsal art. of	Internal pudendal		Dorsum of penis (clitoris), prepuce, glans, corpus cavernosum and its fibrous sheath
Perforating (3)	Profunda femoris	(1) Muscular	Pectineus, adductor brevis, adductor magnus, biceps femoris, gluteus maximus mm.; crucial anastomosis
		(2) Nutrient, ascending, descending	Posterior femoral mm., shaft of femur
		(3) Muscular, terminal	Adductor magnus m., posterior femoral mm.
Pericardiacophrenic (comes nervi phrenici OT)	Internal mammary		Phrenic nerve, pleura, pericardium, diaphragm
Perineal	Internal pudendal	Posterior scrotal (labial), transverse perineal	Transversus perinei superficialis, bulbocavernosus, ischiocavernosus mm.; posterior portion of scrotum (labium majus), subcutaneous structures in urogenital triangle
Perineal, transverse	Perineal		Transversus perinei superficialis m., structures between the anus and the bulb of the urethra, skin of perineum

TABLE OF ARTERIES—(Continued)

Name	Origin	Branches	Distribution
Peroneal	Posterior tibial	Muscular, nutrient to fibula, perforating communicating, lateral calcaneal, lateral posterior malleolar	Soleus, tibialis posterior, flexor hallucis longus, peroneus longus, peroneus brevis, extensor digitorum longus tius, extensor digitorum longus mm.; shaft of fibula, tibiofibular syndesmosis, dorsum of foot, ankle joint, lateral malleolar rete, rete calcaneum
Pharyngeal, ascending	External carotid	Pharyngeal, palatine, prevertebral, inferior tympanic, posterior meningeal	Longus colli, longus capitis, rectus capitis anterior, constrictors of pharynx (superior, medial, inferior), stylopharyngeus mm.; mucous membrane of pharynx, soft palate, palatine tonsil, auditory tube, cervical lymph nodes, tympanic cavity, dura mater of middle and posterior cranial fossae
Phrenic, inferior	Abdominal aorta	Right medial, lateral, superior suprarenal, caval, hepatic, pericardial Left medial, lateral superior suprarenal, hepatic, pericardial, esophageal, splenic	Inferior surface of diaphragm, suprarenal gland, vena cava inferior, liver, pericardium (from the right artery), esophagus, spleen (from the left)
Phrenic, superior	Descending (tho-		Posterior surface of diaphragm

Plantar arch	Lateral plantar	Perforating (3), plantar metatarsals (4)	Interosseous mm., toes
Plantar, deep	Dorsalis pedis	First plantar metatarsal	Plantar surface of first and second toes, unites with lateral plantar to form plantar arch
Plantar, lateral	Posterior tibial	Calcaneal, muscular, cutaneous, plantar metatarsal (4), perforating (3)	Flexor digitorum brevis, quadratus plantae, abductor digiti quinti, adductor hallucis, interossei mm.; toes, heel, skin on lateral side of foot
Plantar, medial	Posterior tibial	Deep, superficial	Abductor hallucis, flexor digitorum brevis mm., skin on medial surface of sole of foot
Pontine	Basilar		Pons
Popliteal	Continuation of femoral	Muscular, superior, medial, cutaneous, medial superior genicular, lateral superior genicular, middle genicular (azygos articular), medial inferior genicular, lateral inferior genicular	Adductor magnus, semimembranosus, semitendinosus, biceps femoris, gastrocnemius, soleus, vastus lateralis, vastus medialis, vastus intermedius, popliteus, plantaris mm.; femur, patella, tibia, knee joint, rete patellae, rete articulare genus
Preventricular	Right coronary		Anterior wall of right ventricle
Princeps cervicis (OT for descending branch)	Occipital	Superficial, deep	Splenius capitis, semispinalis capitis and cervicis, trapezius mm.
Princeps hallucis	See *Metatarsal, first plantar*		

TABLE OF ARTERIES—(Continued)

Name	Origin	Branches	Distribution
Princeps pollicis	Radial	Volar digital (2)	Dorsal interosseus, adductor pollicis obliquus, opponens pollicis, flexor pollicis brevis, lumbrical mm., sides of volar aspect of the thumb
Profunda brachii	Brachial	Deltoid, middle collateral, radial collateral, nutrient	Triceps (lateral and medial heads), brachioradialis, brachialis, deltoid, coracobrachialis, biceps brachii mm.; radial nerve, articular rete of elbow, shaft of humerus
Profunda femoris (deep femoral OT)	Femoral	Medial femoral circumflex, lateral femoral circumfler, perforating (3), muscular	Quadriceps femoris, iliopsoas, obturator externus, pectineus, tensor fasciae latae, quadratus femoris, adductors, semimembranosus, semitendinosus, biceps femoris, gracilis mm.; hip joint, head of femur, shaft of femur, crucial anastomosis
Profunda linguae (ranine OT)	Lingual		Genioglossus m., intrinsic mm. of the tongue, mucous membrane of inferior surface of tongue
Pterygoid canal, art. of (Vidian OT)	Internal maxillary	Pharyngeal, auditory, tympanic, muscular	Upper portion of pharynx; levator and tensor veli palatini mm.; auditory tube, tympanic cavity
Pudendal, deep external	Femoral	Anterior scrotal	Pectineus, adductor longus mm., scrotum (labium majus), skin of perineum

Pudendal, internal (cut off)	(cut off)	Muscular, inferior hemorrhoidal, perineal, art. of urethral bulb, urethral, deep art. of penis (clitoris), dorsal art. of penis (clitoris)	Levator ani, coccygeus, sphincter ani externus, bulbocavernosus, ischiocavernosus, transversus perinei superficialis, transversus perinei profundus, obturator externus, obturator internus, gemelli, quadratus femoris, gluteus maximus mm.; skin of anus and perineum, bulb of urethra, bulbourethral (vestibular gland), urethra, corpus cavernosum penis (clitoridis), dorsum of penis (clitoris), posterior surface of scrotum (labium majus)
Pudendal, superficial external	Femoral		Skin of lower part of abdomen, skin of penis (clitoris), scrotum (labium majus)
Pulmonary	Right ventricle of heart	Right, left	Lungs
Radial	Brachial	(1) In forearm radial recurrent muscular volar radial carpal superficial volar (2) At wrist dorsal radial carpal first dorsal metacarpal (3) In hand princeps pollicis volaris indicis radialis volar metacarpal (3) perforating (3) recurrent	Pronator teres, flexor pollicis longus, pronator quadratus, supinator, brachialis, brachioradialis, extensor carpi radialis longus, extensor carpi radialis brevis, flexor carpi radialis, flexor digitorum sublimis, interossei, lumbricales, and mm. of thenar eminence; metacarpals, elbow, wrist, and carpal joints; flexor tendon sheaths, volar carpal rete, dorsal carpal rete, superficial volar arch, deep volar arch, radius, skin of dorsum of hand and fingers, skin of volar surface of thumb and lateral side of index finger

TABLE OF ARTERIES—(Continued)

Name	Origin	Branches	Distribution
Radial recurrent	Radial		Supinator, brachialis, brachio-radialis, extensor carpi radialis longus, extensor carpi radialis brevis mm.; elbow joint, rete of elbow joint
Radialis, volaris indicis	Radial		Lateral volar aspect of index finger
Ranine	See *Profunda linguae*		
Renal	Abdominal aorta	Inferior suprarenal, capsular or perirenal, ureteric, terminal	Suprarenal gland, capsule of kidney, perirenal fat, upper end of ureter, aortic lymph nodes, kidney
Renales, arteriae propriae (4 or 5)	Renal		Kidney proper
Sacral, lateral inferior	Internal iliac	Spinal, rectal	Contents of sacral canal, sacral plexus, rectum; skin; piriformis and mm. on dorsal surface of sacrum; filum terminale
Sacral, lateral superior	Internal iliac		Piriformis and mm. on dorsal surface of sacrum, sacral dura mater, arachnoid, filum terminale, skin on dorsal surface of sacrum
Sacral, middle	Abdominal aorta	Lowest lumbar, lateral sacral, rectal	Iliacus, gluteus maximus mm.; contents of sacral canal, rectum, coccygeal body

Saphenous	Femoral or art. genus suprema	Cutaneous, muscular	Gracilis and sartorius mm.; skin on medial side of leg around knee, saphenous nerve, medial genicular rete
Scapular circumflex	See *Circumflex, scapular*		
Scapular, transverse (suprascapular OT)	Thyrocervical trunk	Nutrient, acromial, articular, subscapular, suprasternal, supraspinous, infraspinous	Sternocleidomastoid, subclavius, trapezius, subscapularis, supraspinatus, infraspinatus, omohyoid (inferior belly) mm.; clavicle, scapula, acromioclavicular and shoulder joints, acromial rete, periosteum, skin over upper part of chest and acromial area
Sciatic	See *Gluteal, inferior*		
Scrotal, anterior	Deep external pudendal		Anterior part of scrotum (labium majus), perineum
Scrotal, posterior	Perineal		Posterior part of scrotum (labium majus)
Septal, posterior	Sphenopalatine		Mucous membrane of posterior superior portion of nasal septum
Sigmoid (2 or 3)	Inferior mesenteric		Lower part of descending colon, iliac colon, and sigmoid or pelvic colon
Spermatic, external (cremasteric OT)	Inferior epigastric		Spermatic cord, cremaster m. (round ligament of uterus in female)

TABLE OF ARTERIES—(Continued)

NAME	ORIGIN	BRANCHES	DISTRIBUTION
Spermatic, Internal (ovarian in female)	Abdominal aorta	Ureteric, cremasteric, epididymal, testicular	Ureter, cremaster m., epididymis, body of testis
Sphenopalatine (naso-palatine OT)	Internal maxillary	Posterolateral nasal, posterior septal	Nasal conchae and meati, mucous membrane of frontal, maxillary, sphenoidal, and ethmoidal air sinuses, posterior portion of nasal septum
Spinal, anterior	Vertebral		Spinal cord and its coverings
Spinal, posterior	Vertebral		Fasciculi cuneatus and gracilis, spinal cord and its coverings
Splenic (lienal OT)	Celiac	Pancreatica magna, left gastroepiploic, short gastric, terminal splenic (or trabecular)	Pancreas, pancreatic duct, fundus of stomach, greater curvature of stomach, both surfaces of great omentum, body of spleen
Stapedial	Stylomastoid		Stapedius m. and tendon
Sternocleidomastoid	Occipital		Sternocleidomastoid m.
Stylomastoid	Posterior auricular	Mastoid, stapedial, posterior tympanic	Mastoid cells, stapes, stapedius m. and tendon, posterior portion of tympanic membrane
Subclavian	Right innominate, left arch of aorta	Vertebral, thyrocervical trunk, internal mam-	Mm. of neck and upper extremity, cervical vertebrae and canal

...mary, costocervical trunk			skin, brain and meninges, pericardium, pleura, mediastinum, bronchi, sternum, skin over shoulder and anterior body wall, mammary gland, peritoneum
Subcostal (twelfth thoracic OT)	Thoracic aorta	Posterior	Quadratus lumborum, transversus abdominis, obliquus abdominis internus mm.; lumbar vertebrae and contents of canal, skin of back
Sublingual	Lingual	Art. of the frenulum linguae	Mylohyoid, geniohyoid, genioglossus mm.; sublingual gland, frenulum linguae
Submental	External maxillary	Superficial, deep	Mylohyoid, digastric (anterior belly), platysma, triangularis, quadratus labii inferioris mm.; submaxillary and sublingual glands, skin over these parts
Subscapular	Axillary	Scapular circumflex, thoracodorsal	Subscapularis, teres minor, teres major, infraspinatus, triceps brachii (long head), latissimus dorsi, serratus anterior, deltoid mm.; scapula, shoulder joint, axillary lymph nodes
Supraduodenal art. of Wilkie	Gastroduodenal	Anterior, posterior	Anterior and posterior surfaces of first part of the duodenum
Supraorbital	Ophthalmic	Periosteal, muscular, diploic, trochlear, palpebral	Rectus superior, levator palpebrae superioris mm.; periosteum of roof of orbit, diploë of frontal bone, mucous membrane of frontal sinus, trochlea of obliquus superior m., upper eyelid

TABLE OF ARTERIES—(Continued)

Name	Origin	Branches	Distribution
Suprarenal, inferior	Renal		Suprarenal gland
Suprarenal, middle	Abdominal aorta		Suprarenal gland
Suprarenal, superior	Inferior phrenic		Suprarenal gland
Suprascapular	See *Scapular, transverse*		
Sural (2)	Popliteal		Gastrocnemius, soleus, plantaris mm., skin and fascia of calf of leg
Tarsal, lateral	Dorsalis pedis		Extensor digitorum brevis m., navicular and cuboid bones and joint between them
Tarsal, medial	Dorsalis pedis		Skin of medial surface of foot, tarsal joints
Temporal, deep Anterior Posterior	Internal maxillary		Temporal m., orbit, pericranium, skull
Temporal, middle	Superficial temporal		Temporal m., temporal fascia
Temporal, superficial	External carotid	Parotid, transverse facial, anterior auricular, middle temporal, zygomatico-orbital, frontal, parietal, articular	Temporal, masseter, frontalis, orbicularis oculi mm.; parotid gland and duct, skin of face, external ear, external acoustic meatus, scalp

Thalamic, middle	Posterior communicating		Thalamus
Thoracic, highest	Axillary		Pectoralis major, pectoralis minor, intercostal, serratus anterior mm., wall of thorax
Thoracic, lateral (external mammary OT)	Axillary	External mammary	Pectoralis major, pectoralis minor, serratus anterior, subscapularis mm.; axillary lymph nodes, mammary gland
Thoracic, twelfth	See *Subcostal*		
Thoracoacromial (acromiothoracic OT)	Axillary	Pectoral, acromial, clavicular, deltoid	Pectoralis major, pectoralis minor, deltoid, subclavius mm.; mammary gland, sternoclavicular joint, acromial rete
Thoracodorsal	Subscapular		Latissimus dorsi, teres major, serratus anterior mm.
Thymic	Internal mammary		Thymus gland
Thyreoidea ima (Neubauer's art. OT)	Innominate, arch of aorta, right common carotid, right subclavian, or internal mammary		Lower part of thyroid gland
Thyrocervical trunk	Subclavian	Inferior thyroid, transverse scapular (suprascapular), transverse cervical	Mm. of neck, scapular region and upper back; cervical spinal cord, cervical vertebrae, larynx and trachea, esophagus, thyroid gland, pharynx

TABLE OF ARTERIES—(Continued)

Name	Origin	Branches	Distribution
Thyroid, inferior	Thyrocervical trunk	Muscular, inferior laryngeal, tracheal, esophageal, pharyngeal, ascending cervical, terminal, glandular	Scalenus anterior, longus colli, sternohyoid, sternothyroid, omohyoid, inferior constrictor of pharynx, longus capitis mm.; esophagus, pharynx, larynx, trachea, posterior surface of thyroid gland, vertebrae, contents of vertebral canal
Thyroid, superior	External carotid	Hyoid, sternocleidomastoid, superior laryngeal, cricothyroid, muscular, glandular	Thyrohyoid, sternocleidomastoid, sternohyoid, cricothyroid, omohyoid, platysma, inferior constrictor of pharynx, and intrinsic mm. of larynx, mucous membrane of larynx, esophagus, thyroid gland
Tibial, anterior	Popliteal	Anterior tibial recurrent, fibular, posterior tibial recurrent, muscular, anterior lateral malleolar, anterior medial malleolar	Popliteus, tibialis anterior, extensor digitorum longus, peroneus tertius, soleus, peroneus longus, extensor hallucis longus mm.; knee joint, proximal tibiofibular joint, ankle joint, medial malleolar rete, lateral malleolar rete, fascia and skin over course of vessel on front of leg
Tibial, anterior recurrent	Anterior tibial		Tibialis anterior, extensor digitorum longus mm.; knee joint, overlying fascia and skin, rete

Tibial, posterior	Popliteal	Peroneal, nutrient to tibia, muscular; posterior medial malleolar, communicating, medial calcaneal, medial plantar, lateral plantar	Soleus, tibialis posterior, flexor hallucis longus, flexor digitorum longus, peroneus longus, peroneus brevis mm.; ankle joint, skin of medial and posterior part of leg and tarsus, lateral and medial malleolar retia, rete calcaneum, sole of foot, shaft of tibia, shaft of fibula
Tibial, posterior recurrent	Anterior tibial		Popliteus m., proximal tibio-fibular joint
Trabecular	Splenic	Lobular	Substance of spleen
Transverse facial	See *Facial, transverse*		
Transverse perineal	See *Perineal, transverse*		
Tympanic	Art. of pterygoid canal (Vidian OT)		Lining of wall of tympanic cavity
Tympanic, anterior	Internal maxillary		Mucous membrane of tympanic cavity
Tympanic, inferior	Ascending pharyngeal		Lining of medial wall of tympanic cavity
Tympanic, posterior	Stylomastoid		Tympanic membrane
Tympanic, superior	Middle meningeal		Tensor tympani m., lining of wall of tympanic cavity

TABLE OF ARTERIES—(Continued)

Name	Origin	Branches	Distribution
Ulnar	Brachial	(1) In forearm anterior ulnar recurrent posterior ulnar recurrent common, interosseous muscular (2) At wrist dorsal carpal volar carpal (3) In hand deep volar superficial volar arch	Flexor digitorum sublimis, flexor digitorum profundus, flexor carpi radialis, flexor carpi ulnaris, pronator teres, flexor pollicis longus, brachialis, pronator quadratus, anconeus, supinator, abductor pollicis longus, and superficial and deep extensor mm. of forearm; shafts of radius and ulna, median nerve, ulnar half of hand, dorsal carpal rete, volar carpal rete, carpal joints, skin over course of vessels
Ulnar, recurrent, anterior	Ulnar		Brachialis, pronator teres mm., skin over medial cubital region
Ulnar, recurrent, posterior	Ulnar		Flexor digitorum profundus, flexor digitorum sublimis, flexor carpi ulnaris mm.; cubital rete, elbow joint, ulnar nerve
Uterine (homolog of deferential art. in male)	Internal iliac, anterior trunk	Cervical, tubal, ovarian, vaginal, ligamentous	Uterus, broad ligament of uterus, round ligament of uterus, uterine tube, portion of vagina
Vaginal (corresponds to inferior vesical art. in male)	Internal iliac, anterior trunk	Rectal, vesical, vestibular	Vagina, fundus of bladder, rectum, vestibular bulb

Vertebral	Subclavian	(1) Cervical spinal		Semispinalis capitis, rectus capitis posterior major and minor, obliquus capitis superior, obliquus capitis inferior mm.; cervical vertebrae, cervical spinal cord and its membranes, intervertebral disks, bone and dura mater of posterior fossa of skull, falx cerebelli, cerebellum, medulla oblongata
		spinal muscular		
		(2) Cranial		
		meningeal		
		posterior spinal		
		anterior spinal		
		medullary		
		posterior inferior cerebellar		
Vesical, inferior (corresponds to vaginal art. in female)	Internal iliac	Vesical, prostatic, ureteric, deferential		Fundus of bladder, prostate gland, ductus deferens, seminal vesicle, lower part of ureter
Vesical, middle	Internal iliac, or superior vesical			Fundus of bladder, seminal vesicle
Vesical, superior	Internal iliac	Urachal, ureteric, vesical, deferential		Medial umbilical ligament (vestige of urachus), lower part of ureter, upper part of bladder, ductus deferens
Vidian	See *Pterygoid canal, art. of*			
Volar arch, deep	Radial and deep volar branch of ulnar	Volar metacarpal (3), recurrent, perforating		Interossei and second, third, and fourth lumbrical mm.; metacarpals, joints of fingers
Volar arch, superficial	Ulnar and superficial volar branch of radial	Common volar digital (3)		Flexor tendons and tendon sheaths, joints of fingers, bones of fingers, skin of palm and fingers
Volaris indicis radialis	Radial	Dorsal, communicating		First lumbrical, first dorsal interosseous, adductor pollicis mm., radial side of index finger
Zygomatico-orbital	Superficial temporal or middle temporal	Orbital		Orbicularis oculi m., fat between the two layers of temporal fascia, lateral portion of orbit

TABLE OF BONES

Name	Principal Features	Bones with Which Articulation Occurs and Type of Joint
Anvil	See *Incus*	
Astragalus [OT]	See *Talus*	
Atlas	First cervical vertebra; ringlike; lateral masses; anterior and posterior arches and tubercles; vertebral foramen; articular surfaces; transverse foramens; ossifies in cartilage	Occipital bone, *bilateral gliding* Epistropheus, 3 joints, *bilateral gliding* and *pivot* with dens
Axis [OT; BR]	See *Epistropheus*	
Calcaneus (calcaneum BR) (os calcis OT)	Heel bone; largest tarsal bone, irregularly cuboid; medial process (sustentaculum tali), lateral process (trochlear process), medial, lateral and anterior tubercles on inferior surface; articular surfaces; ossifies in cartilage	Talus (3 facets), } *gliding* Cuboid,
Calvaria or **calvarium**	Skull cap or upper part of skull	
Capitate (os magnum OT)	Usually largest carpal bone; in distal row of carpal bones; occupies center of wrist; head, neck, body; ossifies in cartilage	Navicular, Lunate, Lesser multangular, } *gliding* Hamate, Second Third } metacarpal, Fourth

Bone	Description	Articulations/Joints
Carpus (wrist)	Consists of 8 short bones: navicular, lunate, triquetrum, pisiform, greater multangular, lesser multangular, capitate, and hamate. See individual bones	
Clavicle	Collarbone; resembles the italic "f"; body, medial and lateral extremities; conoid tubercle, trapezoid ridge, coracoid tuberosity, costal tuberosity, subclavian groove; ossifies partly in cartilage and partly in membrane	Sternum, Scapula, Cartilage of first rib, } *gliding*
Coccyx	Last bone of vertebral column; usually composed of 4 small incomplete vertebrae fused together; base, apex, cornua, transverse processes; ossifies in cartilage	Sacrum, *amphiarthrosis*
Concha, Inferior nasal (inferior turbinate OT)	Irregular scroll-shaped bone situated on lateral wall of nasal cavity; lacrimal, ethmoidal, and maxillary processes; ossifies in cartilage	Ethmoid, Maxilla, Lacrimal, Palatine, } *synarthroses*
Costae	See *Ribs*	
Coxae (innominate OT)	Hipbone; large broad bone consisting of 3 parts; with its fellow, sacrum, and coccyx forms the bony pelvis or pelvic girdle; acetabulum; obturator foramen; pubic arch; greater and lesser sciatic notches; ossifies in cartilage. *Ilium*—broad, expanded upper portion; crest, spines, gluteal lines, fossa, iliopectineal eminence, tuberosity, auricular surface; ⅖ (about) of acetabulum	With its fellow of opposite side (symphysis pubis), *amphiarthrosis* Sacrum, *gliding* (very little movement) Femur, *ball-and-socket*

TABLE OF BONES—(Continued)

Name	Principal Features	Bones with Which Articulation Occurs and Type of Joint
Coxae—(Continued)	*Ischium*—heavy, posterior lower portion; body, tuberosity, ramus, spine, notches, lower boundary of obturator foramen; ⅖ (about) of acetabulum *Pubis*—anterior lower portion, body, superior and inferior rami, tubercle, crest, pectineal line, upper boundary of obturator foramen; ⅕ (about) of acetabulum	
Cranium	Brain case; composed of occipital, parietal (2), frontal, temporal (2), sphenoid, and ethmoid. See individual bones Sometimes cranium is used to designate entire skull without mandible	
Cuboid	Roughly cubical bone in lateral part of tarsus; tuberosity; ossifies in cartilage	Calcaneus, Third cuneiform, Fourth and fifth metatarsals, Navicular, } *gliding*
Cuneiform of carpus [OT]	See *Triquetrum*	
Cuneiform, first (inner cuneiform OT) (medial cuneiform BR)	Irregularly wedge-shaped; largest of the three; ossifies in cartilage	Navicular (of foot), Second cuneiform, First and second metatarsals, } *gliding*
Cuneiform, second (middle cuneiform OT) (intermediate cunei-	Wedge-shaped; smallest of the three; ossifies in cartilage	Navicular (of foot), First cuneiform, Third cuneiform, } *gliding*

Cuneiform, third (outer cuneiform OT) (lateral cuneiform BR)	Wedge-shaped; ossifies in cartilage	Navicular (of foot), Second cuneiform, Cuboid, Second Third Fourth metatarsal, } *gliding*
Epistropheus (axis OT; BR)	Second cervical vertebra; body, dens, thick spine, laminae, pedicles, transverse processes, articular surfaces, transverse foramens; vertebral foramen; ossifies in cartilage	Atlas, 3 joints, *bilateral gliding and pivot* with dens; Third cervical vertebra, *amphiarthrosis*
Ethmoid	Irregular shape; situated in anterior part of base of skull and forming medial wall of each orbit and a portion of roof and lateral walls of nasal cavities; horizontal or cribriform plates, nasal slit; perpendicular plate, crista galli, alar processes; labyrinth with air cells; superior and middle nasal conchae; ossifies in cartilage	Sphenoid, Frontal, Nasal (2), Maxilla (2), Lacrimal (2), Palatine (2), Inferior nasal concha (2), Vomer, } *synarthroses*
Face	Consists of nose and jaws; formed by maxilla, zygoma, nasal, lacrimal, palatine, inferior nasal conchs, vomer, mandible, and parts of ethmoid and sphenoid, q.v.	
Femur	Thigh bone; largest, longest, and heaviest bone in the body; shaft, head, neck, greater and lesser trochanters, quadrate tubercle, medial and lateral condyles, lines aspera, epicondylic lines, adductor tubercle; ossifies in cartilage	Coxae, *ball-and-socket*; Patella, *gliding*; Tibia, combined *hinge and gliding*

TABLE OF BONES—(Continued)

Name	Principal Features	Bones with Which Articulation Occurs and Type of Joint
Fibula	Splint bone; lateral bone of leg; head, body, interosseous crest, lateral malleolus; ossifies in cartilage	Tibia, *gliding* Talus with tibia and fibula, *hinge*
Foot	Composed of tarsus, metatarsus, and phalanges, *q.v.*	
Frontal	Forehead bone; flat bone; frontal part with tuberosities, zygomatic processes, temporal line, sagittal sulcus; orbital part, forming upper portion of each orbit, anterior and posterior ethmoidal canals; nasal part, frontal spine; ossifies in membrane	Parietal (2), Sphenoid, Ethmoid, Nasal (2), Maxilla (2), Lacrimal (2), Zygoma (2), } *synarthroses*
Greater multangular or multangulum majus (trapezium OT; BR)	In distal row of carpal bones; irregular bone with 6 surfaces, ridge; distal articular facet is saddle-shaped; ossifies in cartilage	Navicular, Lesser multangular, } *gliding* Second metacarpal, } First metacarpal, *saddle*
Hamate (unciform OT)	Wedge-shaped; in distal row of carpal bones; hooklike process (hamulus); ossifies in cartilage	Lunate, Fourth and fifth metacarpals, } *gliding* Triquetrum, Capitate,
Hammer	See *Malleus*	
Hand	Composed of carpus, metacarpus, and phalanges, *q.v.*	

Humerus	Largest bone of the arm; head, greater and lesser tubercles, intertubercular sulcus, surgical neck, deltoid tuberosity, capitulum, trochlea, coronoid and olecranon fossae; medial and lateral lines, condyles and epicondyles; ossifies in cartilage	Scapula (glenoid cavity), *ball-and-socket* Ulna, *hinge* Radius, *gliding*
Hyoid	U-shaped bone in front of neck; body, greater and lesser cornua; ossifies in cartilage	None
Ilium	See *Cozae*	
Incus (anvil)	Resembles a premolar tooth with two roots, body, long and short processes or crura, lenticular process; middle bone of chain of auditory ossicles; ossifies in cartilage	Malleus, *gliding* Stapes, *gliding*
Inferior maxilla [OT]	See *Mandible*	
Inferior turbinate [OT]	See *Concha, inferior nasal*	
Innominate [OT]	See *Cozae*	
Ischium	See *Cozae*	
Lacrimal	Small scale of bone resembling a finger nail; situated in anterior medial wall of orbit; crest, descending process, hamulus, groove; ossifies in membrane	Frontal, Ethmoid, Maxilla, Inferior nasal concha, } *synarthroses*
Lesser multangular or multangulum minus (trapezoid OT; BR)	Smallest bone of distal row of carpal bones; irregular bone with 6 surfaces; ossifies in cartilage	Navicular, Second metacarpal, Greater multangular, } *gliding* Capitate,

TABLE OF BONES—(Continued)

NAME	PRINCIPAL FEATURES	BONES WITH WHICH ARTICULATION OCCURS AND TYPE OF JOINT
Lunate (semilunar OT)	One of proximal row of carpal bones; named from lateral crescent-shaped articular facet; ossifies in cartilage	Radius, *biaxial* Capitate, Hamate, } *gliding* Triquetrum, Navicular,
Magnum [OT]	See *Capitate*	
Malar [OT]	See *Zygoma*	
Malleus (hammer)	Resembles a hammer; head, neck, spur, crista, handle, anterior and lateral processes; ossifies in cartilage	Incus, *gliding*
Mandible (inferior maxilla OT).	Lower jaw; body, 2 rami, coronoid and condyloid processes, symphysis, alveolus, mental protuberance and spine, mylohyoid line and groove, mandibular and mental foramens, notch; ossifies partly in membrane and partly in cartilage	Two temporal bones, combined *gliding* and *hinge*
Maxilla (superior maxilla OT)	Upper jaw; body with infraorbital foramen and canal, maxillary sinus, lacrimal groove, greater palatine foramen and canal; zygomatic process; frontal process, ethmoidal crest; alveolar process, maxillary tuberosity; palatine process, incisive crest, spine and canal, nasal crest; ossifies in membrane	Frontal, Ethmoid, Nasal, Zygoma, Lacrimal, Inferior nasal concha, } *synarthroses* Palatine, Vomer,

Metacarpus	Five bones of hand proper; each with head, shaft, and base; numbered from 1 to 5 beginning on thumb side; styloid process on base of third; each ossifies in cartilage	First metacarpal with greater multangular, *saddle* Four medial metacarpal bases with each other and with distal row of carpal bones, *gliding* Metacarpal heads with corresponding phalanges, *ball-and-socket*
Metatarsus	Five bones of foot proper; each with head, shaft, and base; numbered from 1 to 5 beginning on great toe side; tuberosity on lateral side of base of fifth; each ossifies in cartilage	Distal tarsal bones, Metatarsal bases with each other, } *gliding* Metatarsal heads with corresponding phalanges, *ball-and-socket*
Nasal	Rectangular plate; two form bridge of nose; ethmoidal sulcus, crest; ossifies in membrane	Frontal, Ethmoid, Maxilla, Nasal (opposite), } *synarthroses*
Navicular (of foot) (scaphoid of foot OT)	Boat-shaped; proximal articular surface markedly concave; plantar process, tuberosity; ossifies in cartilage	Talus, Three cuneiforms, } *gliding* Cuboid,
Navicular (of hand) (scaphoid of hand OT; BR)	Largest bone of proximal row of carpal bones; comma-shaped; tubercle; ossifies in cartilage	Greater multangular, Lesser multangular, } *gliding* Capitate, Lunate, Radius, *biaxial*

TABLE OF BONES—(Continued)

Name	Principal Features	Bones with Which Articulation Occurs and Type of Joint
Occipital	Posterior part and base of cranium; saucer-shaped; squamous part with internal and external protuberances, highest, superior and inferior nuchal lines, sagittal and transverse sulci; lateral part with condyles, canal for hypoglossal nerve, condyloid canal, jugular notch, process and tubercle; basal part with pharyngeal tubercle and foramen magnum; squamous part ossifies in membrane, the rest in cartilage	Parietal (2), ⎫ *synarthroses* Temporal (2), ⎭ Sphenoid, Atlas, *bilateral gliding*
Palatine	Forms portions of hard palate, orbits and nasal cavities; irregularly L-shaped; horizontal part, posterior nasal spine, greater palatine foramen, palatine crest, nasal crest; perpendicular part, conchal crest, ethmoidal crest, greater palatine canal, maxillary, pyramidal, orbital and sphenoidal processes, sphenopalatine foramen, lesser palatine canals and foramens; ossifies in membrane	Sphenoid, ⎫ Ethmoid, ⎪ Maxilla, ⎬ *synarthroses* Inferior nasal concha, ⎪ Vomer, ⎪ Palatine (opposite). ⎭
Parietal	Forms side and roof of cranium; quadrilateral plate of bone; eminence, superior and inferior temporal lines, parietal foramen; sagittal and transverse sulci; ossifies in membrane	Parietal (opposite), ⎫ Occipital, ⎪ Frontal, ⎬ *synarthroses* Temporal, ⎪ Sphenoid, ⎭
Patella	Knee cap; triangular; largest sesamoid; ossifies in cartilage	Condyles of femur, *gliding*

Pelvis	Pelvic girdle composed of 2 coxae, sacrum, and coccyx, *q.v.*	
Phalanges (of feet)	Two of great toe, three of each of others, 14 in all; usually fifth toe has only two; each phalanx is a miniature long bone with head, shaft, and base; each ossifies in cartilage	Proximal row with corresponding metatarsal bones, *ball-and-socket* Interphalangeal joints, *hinge*
Phalanges (of hand)	Two of the thumb, three of each of fingers, 14 in all; each phalanx is a miniature long bone with head, shaft, and base; each ossifies in cartilage	Proximal row with corresponding metacarpal bones, *ball-and-socket* Interphalangeal joints, *hinge*
Pisiform	Most medial of proximal row of carpus; smallest carpal; resembles half a pea; ossifies in cartilage	Triquetrum, *gliding*
Pubis	See *Coxae*	
Pyramidal [OT]	See *Triquetrum*	
Radius	Lateral bone of forearm; head, shaft, tuberosity, styloid process, interosseous crest, ulnar notch; ossifies in cartilage	Humerus, *gliding* Ulna, proximal, *pivot* Ulna, distal, *gliding* Lunate, Navicular, } *biaxial* Triquetrum,
Ribs	Twelve on each side; head, neck, body, tubercle, angle, costal groove; first is relatively broad and flattened; second, tubercle; 11 and 12 floating; each ossifies in cartilage	Head with vertebral bodies, Tubercle with transverse proc- } *gliding* ess, Sternum with first rib, *synchondroses* Sternum with others, *amphiarthroses*

TABLE OF BONES—(Continued)

Name	Principal Features	Bones with Which Articulation Occurs and Type of Joint
Sacrum	Large triangular bone composed of 5 fused vertebrae; base, apex, foramens, superior articular processes, promontory, auricular surface, sacral canal; ossifies in cartilage	Last lumbar vertebra, } *amphiarthroses* Coccyx, Coxae (2), *gliding* (very little movement)
Scaphoid of foot [OT]	See *Navicular (of foot)*	
Scaphoid of hand [OT; BR]	See *Navicular (of hand)*	
Scapula	Shoulder blade; flat, triangular bone of posterior portion of shoulder; head, neck, body, spine, acromion, coracoid, glenoid cavity, subscapular fossa, supraspinous fossa, infraspinous fossa, crest, greater and lesser scapular notches; ossifies in cartilage	Humerus, *ball-and-socket* Clavicle, *gliding*
Semilunar [OT]	See *Lunate*	
Sesamoid	Small seedlike nodules of bone which develop in muscular tendons where they play against a bone; patella, *q.v.*; one in each tendon of insertion of flexor hallucis brevis muscle and one in tendon of insertion of flexor pollicis brevis and of adductor pollicis are constant, others are variable; each develops in cartilage	

Skull	See *Cranium*. Sometimes used to include the mandible as well	
Sphenoid	Forms anterior part of base of skull and portions of cranial, orbital, and nasal cavities; in shape resembles a butterfly with extended wings; body, air sinuses, sella turcica, hypophyseal fossa, dorsum sellae, posterior clinoid processes, optic groove, spine, carotid groove, crest; optic groove, spine, carotid groove, crest; petrosal process, rostrum; small wings, optic foramen, anterior clinoid processes, superior orbital fissure; great wings, foramen rotundum, foramen ovale, foramen spinosum, pterygoid processes, medial and lateral pterygoid plates, hamulus, scaphoid fossa, pterygoid canal; ossifies partly in cartilage and partly in membrane	Frontal, Parietal (2), Occipital, Temporal (2), Ethmoid, Palatine (2), Zygoma (2), Vomer, $\Big\}$ *synarthroses*
Stapes (stirrup OT)	Resembles a stirrup; head, neck, base, anterior and posterior crura; smallest of auditory ossicles; ossifies in cartilage	Incus, *gliding* Fenestra ovalis, *gliding*
Sternum	Breastbone; dagger-shaped, manubrium, body, xiphoid process; ossifies in cartilage	Clavicle (2), *gliding* First rib (2), *synchondrosis* Costal cartilages of ribs 2 to 7, *amphiarthroses*
Stirrup [OT]	See *Stapes*	
Superior maxilla [OT]	See *Maxilla*	

TABLE OF BONES—(Continued)

Name	Principal Features	Bones with Which Articulation Occurs and Type of Joint
Sutural (Wormian OT)	Irregular variable bones occasionally found along cranial sutures; most frequent in lambdoid suture	
Talus (astragalus OT)	Second largest bone of tarsus; head, body, medial and posterior tubercles; ossifies in cartilage	Tibia, Fibula, } hinge Calcaneus (3 facets), } gliding Navicular (of foot), } gliding
Tarsus	Posterior portion of foot; consists of 7 bones; calcaneus, talus, cuboid, navicular, and 3 cuneiforms, q.v.	
Temporal	Forms a portion of lateral aspect of skull and part of base of cranium; squamous part, zygomatic process, mandibular fossa, petrotympanic fissure; tympanic part, auditory process, external acoustic meatus, styloid process and sheath, stylomastoid foramen, mastoid part, air cells, notch, foramen, sigmoid sulcus; petrous part, auditory tube, jugular fossa, carotid canal, internal acoustic meatus; ossifies partly in cartilage and partly in membrane	Occipital, Parietal, Sphenoid, Zygoma, } synarthroses Mandible, combined gliding and hinge
Tibia	Shinbone; large medial bone of leg; medial and lateral condyles, tuberosity, popliteal notch, intercondylar eminence, popliteal line, medial malleolus; ossifies in cartilage	Femur, combined hinge and gliding Fibula, superior, } gliding Fibula, inferior, } gliding Talus with fibula, hinge
Trapezium [OT; BR]	See Greater multangular	
Trapezoid [OT; BR]	See Lesser multangular	
Triquetrum (cuneiform of carpus OT) (pyramidal OT)	One of proximal row of carpal bones; wedge-shaped; ossifies in cartilage	Lunate, Pisiform, } gliding

Turbinate, middle [OT]	See *Ethmoid, middle nasal concha.* (Not a separate bone)	
Turbinate, superior [OT]	See *Ethmoid, superior nasal, concha.* (Not a separate bone)	
Tympanic	Includes 3 auditory ossicles: incus, malleus, and stapes, *q.v.*	
Ulna	Medial bone of forearm; olecranon, coronoid process, radial notch, semilunar notch, tuberosity, shaft, head, styloid process, interosseous crest; ossifies in cartilage	Humerus, *hinge* Radius, proximal, *pivot* Radius, distal, *gliding*
Unciform [OT]	See *Hamate*	
Vertebra	Backbone; composed of 33 in all, cervical 7, thoracic 12, lumbar 5, sacrum 5 (fused), coccyx 4 (fused); each has a body, arch, articular processes, transverse processes, spinous process, foramen; see *Atlas, Epistropheus, Coccyx, Sacrum*; each vertebra ossifies in cartilage	Between vertebral bodies, *amphiarthroses* Between articular processes, *gliding*
Vomer	Forms posterior part of nasal septum; alse; ossifies in membrane	Sphenoid, Ethmoid, Maxilla (2), Palatine (2), }*synarthroses*
Wormian [OT]	See *Sutural*	
Wrist	See *Carpus*	
Zygoma (malar OT)	Cheekbone; forms cheek and lateral aspect of orbit; tuberosity, zygomaticofacial foramen temporal process, frontosphenoidal process, marginal process, orbital process, zygomatic foramen, zygomaticotemporal foramen; ossifies in membrane	Frontal, Sphenoid, Temporal, Maxilla, }*synarthroses*

TABLE OF JOINTS AND LIGAMENTS

Name	Type	Named Ligaments

Acromioclavicular	Gliding	Articular disk (intraarticular fibrocartilage OT)
		Coracoclavicular
		  (1) Conoid
		  (2) Trapezoid
		Inferior acromioclavicular
		Superior acromioclavicular

Ankle	Hinge	Anterior
		Deltoid (internal lateral OT; medial BR)
		  (1) Anterior talotibial
		  (2) Calcaneotibial
		  (3) Deep talotibial
		  (4) Posterior talotibial
		  (5) Tibionavicular
		Interosseous membrane of leg
		Lateral (external lateral OT)
		  (1) Anterior talofibular
		  (2) Calcaneofibular
		  (3) Posterior talofibular
		Posterior

Atlantoepistrophic	See *Central* and *Lateral atlantoepistrophic*	
Atlanto-occipital	Gliding	Anterior atlanto-occipital membrane (anterior occipitoatlantal ligament OT) Membrana tectoria (occipitoaxial ligament OT)

Posterior atlanto-occipital membrane (posterior occipitoatlantal ligament OT)

Calcaneocuboid	Gliding	Dorsal calcaneocuboid Inferior calcaneocuboid (1) Long plantar (2) Plantar calcaneocuboid (short plantar OT; BR) Lateral calcaneocuboid Calcaneocuboid part of bifurcate (internal calcaneocuboid OT; medial calcaneocuboid BR)
Carpal	See *Intercarpal* and *Pisotriquetral*	
Carpometacarpal articulation of the thumb	Saddle	
Carpometacarpal articulations of fingers	Gliding	Dorsal carpometacarpal Interosseous carpometacarpal Volar carpometacarpal (palmar carpometacarpal BR)
Central atlantoepistrophic	Pivot	Alar (check or lateral odontoid OT; alar of odontoid process BR) Apical of dens (middle odontoid OT; apical of odontoid process BR) Cruciate atlantis (cruciform OT) (1) Inferior crus (2) Superior crus (3) Transverse crus (transverse of atlas BR)

1 This table does not include sutures, synostoses, synchondroses.
2 It is understood that every diarthrodial joint has a capsular ligament composed of two layers.

TABLE OF JOINTS AND LIGAMENTS—(Continued)

Name	Type	Named Ligaments
Costotransverse (upper 10 rib only)	Gliding	Anterior costotransverse (superior costotransverse OT; BR)
		Ligament of neck of rib (middle costotransverse OT; inferior costotransverse BR)
		Ligament of tubercle of rib (lateral costotransverse BR)
		Posterior costotransverse
Cuboideonavicular (cuboideoscaphoid OT) (inconstant)	Gliding	Dorsal cuboideonavicular (dorsal cuboideoscaphoid OT)
		Interosseous cuboideonavicular (interosseous cuboideoscaphoid OT)
		Plantar cuboideonavicular (plantar cuboideoscaphoid OT)
Cuneocuboid	Gliding	Dorsal cuneocuboid
		Interosseous cuneocuboid
		Plantar cuneocuboid
Cuneometatarsal	See *Intermediate* and *Medial tarsometatarsal*	
Cuneonavicular (cuneoscaphoid OT)	Gliding	Dorsal cuneonavicular (dorsal cuneoscaphoid OT)
		Plantar cuneonavicular (plantar cuneoscaphoid OT)

Distal radioulnar	Gliding	Anterior radioulnar Interosseous membrane of forearm Posterior radioulnar Triangular articular disk (triangular fibrocartilage OT)
Distal tibiofibular (variable)	When present, is an extension of ankle joint, q.v.	
Elbow (1) Humeroradial (2) Humeroulnar (3) Proximal radioulnar (sometimes described as a separate joint)	Gliding Hinge Pivot	Annular (orbicular OT) Anterior Interosseous membrane of forearm Posterior Quadrate [BR] Radial collateral (external lateral OT; lateral BR) Ulnar collateral (internal lateral OT; medial BR)
Heads of ribs	Combined hinge and gliding	Interarticular of head of rib (intervertebral OT; intraarticular BR) Radiate of head of rib (anterior costovertebral or stellate OT)
Hip	Ball-and-socket	Iliofemoral (Y-ligament of Bigelow OT) Ischiocapsular (ischiofemoral OT; BR) Labrum glenoidale (cotyloid OT; labrum acetabulare BR) Pubocapsular (pubofemoral OT; BR) Teres (round OT; ligament of head of femur BR) Transverse

[1] This table does not include sutures, synostoses, syndesmoses, synchondroses.

[2] It is understood that every diarthrodial joint has a capsular ligament composed of two layers.

TABLE OF JOINTS AND LIGAMENTS—(Continued)

Name	Type	Named[2] Ligaments
Humeroradial	See *Elbow*	
Humeroulnar	See *Elbow*	
Intercarpal (1) Distal (between 4 bones of distal row) (2) Proximal (between 3 bones of proximal row) (3) Transverse (between proximal and distal row)	Gliding	Dorsal carpal (extensor retinaculum BR) Dorsal intercarpal Interosseous intercarpal Radiate or volar carpal Radial collateral carpal (external lateral OT; lateral BR) Transverse carpal (flexor retinaculum BR) Ulnar collateral carpal (internal lateral OT; medial BR) Volar intercarpal (palmar intercarpal BR)
Intercuneiform	Gliding	Dorsal intercuneiform Interosseous intercuneiform Plantar intercuneiform
Intermediate tarsometatarsal	Gliding	Dorsal tarsometatarsal Interosseous cuneometatatarsal Interosseous intercuneiform Plantar tarsometatarsal
Intermetacarpal (4 medial metacarpal bases)	Gliding	Basal dorsal metacarpal (dorsal metacarpal BR) Basal interosseous metacarpal (interosseous metacarpal BR) Basal volar metacarpal (palmar metacarpal BR)

Intermetatarsal (4 lateral metatarsal bases)	Gliding	Basal dorsal metatarsal (dorsal metatarsal BR) Basal interosseous metatarsal (interosseous metatarsal BR) Basal plantar metatarsal (plantar metatarsal BR) Transverse metatarsal
Interphalangeal of fingers	Hinge	Collateral (lateral phalangeal OT)
Interphalangeal of toes	Hinge	Accessory plantar (plantar BR) Collateral (lateral phalangeal OT)
Intertarsal	See Cuboideonavicular, Cuneonavicular, Cuneocuboid, Intercuneiform, Talocalcaneal, Talocalcaneonavicular, Talonavicular, and Transverse tarsal	
Knee	Combined hinge and gliding	Alar folds (alar ligaments OT) Anterior cruciate Arcuate popliteal (arcuate BR) Coronary Fibular collateral (external lateral OT; lateral BR) Lateral meniscus (external semilunar cartilage OT; lateral semilunar cartilage BR)

[1] This table does not include sutures, synostoses, syndesmoses, synchondroses.

[2] It is understood that every diarthrodial joint has a capsular ligament composed of two layers.

TABLE OF JOINTS AND LIGAMENTS—(Continued)

Name	Type	Named[1] Ligaments
Knee—(Continued)		Lateral patellar retinaculum [BR]
		Medial meniscus (internal semilunar cartilage OT; medial semilunar cartilage BR]
		Medial patellar retinaculum [BR]
		Oblique popliteal (ligament of Winslow OT; oblique posterior BR)
		Patellar
		Patellar synovial fold (ligamentum mucosum OT)
		Posterior
		Posterior cruciate
		Superior patellar retinaculum [BR]
		Tibial collateral (internal lateral OT; medial BR)
		Transverse
Lateral atlantoepistrophic	Gliding	Accessory atlantoepistrophic (accessory atlantoaxial BR)
		Anterior atlantoepistrophic obturator (anterior atloaxoid OT; anterior atlantoaxial BR)
		Posterior atlantoepistrophic obturator (posterior atloaxoid OT; posterior atlantoaxial BR)
Lateral tarsometatarsal	Gliding	Dorsal tarsometatarsal
		Interosseous cuneocuboid

Mandibular (temporomandibular OT)	Combined gliding and hinge	Articular disk (intraarticular fibrocartilage OT); Sphenomandibular; Stylomandibular; Temporomandibular (external lateral OT)
Medial tarsometatarsal	Gliding	Dorsal tarsometatarsal; Interosseous cuneometatarsal; Plantar tarsometatarsal
Metacarpophalangeal	Ball-and-socket	Accessory volar (glenoid cartilage OT; palmar BR); Collateral (lateral phalangeal OT); Transverse of heads of metacarpals (deep transverse of palm BR)
Metatarsophalangeal	Ball-and-socket	Accessory plantar (glenoid OT; plantar of digits BR); Collateral (lateral phalangeal OT); Transverse of heads of metatarsals (transverse metatarsal OT; deep transverse of sole BR)
Midtarsal [OT]	See *Transverse tarsal*	
Pisotriquetral	Gliding	Pisohamate; Pisometacarpal
Proximal radioulnar	See *Elbow*	

[1] This table does not include sutures, synostoses, syndesmoses, synchondroses.
[2] It is understood that every diarthrodial joint has a capsular ligament composed of two layers.

TABLE OF JOINTS[1] AND LIGAMENTS—(Continued)

Name	Type	Named[1] Ligaments
Proximal tibiofibular	Gliding	Anterior of head of fibula (anterior superior tibiofibular OT) Interosseous membrane of leg Posterior of head of fibula (posterior superior tibiofibular OT)
Radioulnar	See *Elbow* and *Distal radioulnar*	
Sacroiliac	Gliding	Anterior sacroiliac Iliolumbar Interosseous sacroiliac Long posterior sacroiliac (oblique sacroiliac OT) Sacrotuberous (great or posterior sacrosciatic OT) Sacrospinous (lesser or anterior sacrosciatic OT) Short posterior sacroiliac

Shoulder	Ball-and-socket	Coracoacromial Coracohumeral Inferior glenohumeral Labrum glenoidale (glenoid ligament OT) Middle glenohumeral Superior glenohumeral Transverse humeral
Sternoclavicular	Gliding	Anterior sternoclavicular Articular disk (intraarticular fibrocartilage OT) Costoclavicular (rhomboid OT) Interclavicular Posterior sternoclavicular
Talocalcaneal (astragalocalcaneal OT)	Gliding	Anterior talocalcaneal (anterior calcaneo-astragaloid OT) Interosseous talocalcaneal (interosseous calcaneoastragaloid OT) Lateral talocalcaneal (external calcaneoastragaloid OT) Medial talocalcaneal (internal calcaneoastragaloid OT) Posterior talocalcaneal (posterior calcaneo-astragaloid OT)

[1] This table does not include sutures, synostoses, syndesmoses, synchondroses.

[2] It is understood that every diarthrodial joint has a capsular ligament composed of two layers.

TABLE OF JOINTS[1] AND LIGAMENTS—(Continued)

Name	Type	Named[2] Ligaments
Talocalcaneonavicular (anterior calcaneoastragaloid OT)	Gliding	Calcaneonavicular part of bifurcate (superior calcaneoscaphoid OT; lateral calcaneonavicular BR) Dorsal talonavicular (dorsal astragaloscaphoid OT) Interosseous talonavicular (interosseous astragaloscaphoid OT) Plantar calcaneonavicular or spring (inferior calcaneoscaphoid OT)
Talonavicular (taloscaphoid OT)	A portion of talocalcaneonavicular, q.v.	
Tarsal	See *Cuboideonavicular, Cuneonavicular, Cuneonavicular, Intercuneiform, Talocalcaneonavicular, Talonavicular,* and *Transverse tarsal*	

Tarsometatarsal	See *Intermediate*, *Lateral*, and *Medial tarsometatarsal*	
Temporomandibular [OT]	See *Mandibular*	
Tibiofibular	See *Distal* and *Proximal tibiofibular*	
Transverse tarsal (Chopart's) (midtarsal OT)	Combined calcaneocuboid and talocalcaneonavicular, *q.v.*	
Wrist	Biaxial	Dorsal radiocarpal (posterior radiocarpal OT; BR)
		Radial collateral carpal (external lateral OT; lateral BR)
		Triangular articular disk (triangular fibro-cartilage OT)
		Ulnar collateral carpal (internal lateral OT; medial BR)
		Volar radiocarpal (anterior radiocarpal BR)

[1] This table does not include sutures, synostoses, syndesmoses, synchondroses.

[2] It is understood that every diarthrodial joint has a capsular ligament composed of two layers.

TABLE OF MUSCLES

Name	Origin	Insertion	Innervation	Function
Abductor digiti quinti (of foot) (abductor digiti minimi BR)	Medial and lateral tubercles of calcaneus and plantar fascia	Lateral surface of base of proximal phalanx of little toe	Lateral plantar	Abducts little toe
Abductor digiti quinti (of hand) (abductor digiti minimi BR)	Pisiform and tendon of flexor carpi ulnaris	Medial surface of base of proximal phalanx of little finger	Ulnar	Abducts little finger
Abductor hallucis	Medial tubercle of calcaneus and plantar fascia	Medial surface of base of proximal phalanx of great toe	Medial plantar	Abducts and flexes great toe at metatarsophalangeal joint
Abductor ossis metatarsi quinti [BR]	Small variable portion of abductor digiti quinti of foot, q.v., inserting into fifth metatarsal			
Abductor pollicis brevis (abductor pollicis OT)	Navicular, ridge of greater multangular, and transverse carpal ligament	Lateral surface of base of proximal phalanx of thumb	Median	Abducts and flexes thumb
Abductor pollicis longus (extensor ossis metacarpi pollicis	Posterior aspect of ulna, radius, and interosseous membrane	Lateral aspect of base of first metacarpal and greater multangular	Dorsal interosseous branch of	Abducts and extends thumb

Accelerator urinae [OT]	See *Bulbocavernosus*		
Accesorius [OT]	See *Quadratus plantae*		
Accesorius [OT]	See *Iliocostalis dorsi*		
Adductor brevis	Pubis	Proximal part of linea aspera of femur and femur proximal to that line	Obturator	Adducts thigh
Adductor hallucis (1) Oblique head	Plantar fascia and bases of second, third, and fourth metatarsals	Lateral aspect of base of proximal phalanx of great toe	Lateral plantar	Adducts great toe
(2) Transverse head (adductor hallucis transversus OT) (transversus pedis OT)	Transverse metatarsal ligament and capsules of 4 lateral metatarsophalangeal joints			
Adductor hallucis, transversus [OT]	See *Adductor hallucis, transverse head*			
Adductor longus	Pubis	Linea aspera of femur	Obturator	Adducts thigh
Adductor magnus	(1) Inferior ramus of pubis and ramus of ischium	Linea aspera of femur	Obturator	Adducts thigh
	(2) Ischial tuberosity	Adductor tubercle of femur	Tibial	Extends hip joint
Adductor minimus (variable)	When present is a separate proximal portion of adductor magnus, *q.v.*			

TABLE OF MUSCLES—(Continued)

Name	Origin	Insertion	Innervation	Function
Adductor pollicis (1) Oblique head	Greater and lesser multangular, capitate, and bases of second, third, and fourth metacarpals	Medial aspect of base of proximal phalanx of thumb	Ulnar	Adducts and opposes thumb
(2) Transverse head (adductor pollicis transversus OT)	Third metacarpal			
Agitator caudae (variable)	Portion of gluteus maximus, q.v. Sometimes arises separately from coccyx			
Anconeus	Dorsal surface of lateral epicondyle of humerus	Olecranon of ulna	Radial	Extends elbow joint
Antitragicus (vestigial)	Lateral surface of antitragus	Antihelix and cauda helicis	Facial	
Arrectores pilorum (erector pili OT) (smooth muscle)	Found in corium	Hair follicles	Sympathetic	Elevate hairs of skin
Articularis genus (subcrureus OT)	Distal fourth of anterior surface of femur	Synovial membrane of knee joint	Femoral	Draws synovial membrane proximally during extension of knee
Aryepiglottic	Apex of arytenoid	Lateral margin of epi-	Recurrent	Closes inlet of

	Origin	Insertion	Nerve	Action
Arytenoepiglotticus [OT]	Continuation of oblique arytenoid, q.v.			Closes inlet of larynx
Arytenoid (1) Oblique portion	Dorsal aspect of muscular process of arytenoid cartilage	Apex of opposite arytenoid cartilage	Recurrent laryngeal	
(2) Transverse portion		Becomes continuous with thyroarytenoid, q.v.		Approximates arytenoid cartilages
Attollens aurem [OT] (vestigial)	See *Auricularis superior*			
Attrahens aurem [OT] (vestigial)	See *Auricularis anterior*			
Auricularis (vestigial) (1) Anterior (attrahens aurem OT)	Galea aponeurotica	Helix	Facial	Move external ear
(2) Oblique	Scattered fibers across transverse sulcus of antihelix			
(3) Posterior (retrahens aurem OT)	Mastoid	Auricle		
(4) Superior (attolens aurem OT)	Galea aponeurotica	Antihelix		
(5) Transverse	Scattered fibers from concha to scapha			
Axillary arches	Occasional slips of muscle in axillary fascia			

TABLE OF MUSCLES—(Continued)

Name	Origin	Insertion	Innervation	Function
Azygos uvulae [OT]	See *Uvulae*			
Biceps brachii (1) Short head (2) Long head	Tip of coracoid process of scapula Supraglenoid tuberosity of humerus	Tubercle of radius and deep fascia of forearm	Musculo-cutaneous	Flexes and supinates forearm
Biceps femoris (1) Short head	Linea aspera of femur	Head of fibula, lateral condyle of femur, and deep fascia on lateral aspect of knee	Peroneal	Flexes knee joint
(2) Long head	Ischial tuberosity		Tibial	Flexes knee joint and extends hip joint
Biventer cervicis [OT]	See *Semispinalis capitis*			
Brachialis (brachialis anticus OT)	Anterior aspect of humerus	Coronoid process of ulna	Musculo-cutaneous	Flexes elbow joint
Brachioradialis (supinator longus OT)	Lateral supracondylar ridge of humerus	Lower end of radius	Radial	Flexes elbow joint
Buccinator	Alveolar process of maxilla and of mandible and pterygomandibular raphe	Blends about mouth with orbicularis oris, q.v.	Facial	Compresses cheek and retracts angle of mouth

Buccopharyngeus	Portion of superior constrictor of pharynx, q.v.			
Bulbocavernosus (accelerator urinae OT) (compressor vaginae OT) (ejaculator urinae OT) (sphincter vaginae OT) (bulbospongiosus BR)	Central point of perineum and median raphe of bulb	Fascia of perineum and of penis (clitoris)	Perineal	In male, compresses urethra. In female, contracts vaginal orifice and compresses vestibular bulbs
Caninus (levator anguli oris BR; OT)	Maxilla	Skin of angle of mouth	Facial	Muscle of facial expression
Cephalopharyngeus [OT]	Portion of superior constrictor of pharynx, q.v.			
Ceratopharyngeus	Portion of middle constrictor of pharynx, q.v.			
Cervicalis ascendens [OT]	See *Iliocostalis cervicis*			
Chondroepitrochlearis (variable)	Occasional slip of muscle in axillary fascia			
Chondroglossus (variable portion of hyoglossus, q.v.)	Lesser cornu of hyoid	Side of tongue	Hypoglossal	Depresses tongue
Chondropharyngeus	Portion of middle constrictor of pharynx, q.v.			

TABLE OF MUSCLES—(Continued)

NAME	ORIGIN	INSERTION	INNERVATION	FUNCTION
Ciliary (smooth muscle)				
Meridional portion	Scleral spur	Ciliary processes	Oculomotor, parasympathetic	Visual accommodation
Circular portion	Sphincter of ciliary body			
Coccygeofemoralis (variable)	Occasional slip of gluteus maximus arising separately from coccyx			
Coccygeus (ischiococcygeus)	Ischial spine and sacrospinous ligament	Lateral border of lower sacrum and upper coccyx	Sacral	Helps to form pelvic diaphragm
Complexus [OT]	See *Semispinalis capitis*			
Compressor naris [BR] (compressor nasi OT)	See *Nasalis*			
Compressor urethrae [OT]	See *Sphincter urethrae membranaceae*			
Compressor vaginae [OT]	See *Bulbocavernosus*			
Constrictor of pharynx, Inferior	Oblique line of thyroid cartilage, side of cricoid cartilage	Median raphe of posterior wall of pharynx	Accessory via pharyngeal plexus, laryngeal branches of	Constricts pharynx

Constrictor of pharynx, middle	Stylohyoid ligament and both cornua of hyoid	Median raphe of pharynx	Accessory via pharyngeal plexus	Constricts pharynx
Constrictor of pharynx, superior	Medial pterygoid lamina, pterygomandibular raphe, and mylohyoid line of mandible	Pharyngeal tubercle of occiput and median raphe of pharynx	Accessory via pharyngeal plexus	Constricts pharynx
Coracobrachialis	Coracoid process of scapula	Medial aspect of shaft of humerus	Musculocutaneous	Flexes and adducts humerus
Coracobrachialis superior or brevis	Occasional proximal slip of coracobrachialis, q.v.			
Corrugator cutis ani (smooth muscle)	Found in skin about anus		Sympathetic	
Corrugator supercilii	Superciliary arch of frontal bone	Skin of forehead	Facial	Muscle of facial expression
Costalis [BR]	See *Iliocostalis dorsi*			
Costocervicalis [BR]	See *Iliocostalis cervicis*			
Costocoracoideus (variable)	Occasional slip of muscle in axillary fascia			
Cremaster	Inferior margin of internal oblique muscle of abdomen	Pubic tubercle	Genitofemoral	Elevates testis

TABLE OF MUSCLES—(Continued)

Name	Origin	Insertion	Innervation	Function
Cricoarytenoid, lateral	Lateral surface of cricoid cartilage	Muscular process of arytenoid cartilage	Recurrent laryngeal	Approximates vocal folds
Cricoarytenoid, posterior	Dorsal surface of cricoid cartilage	Muscular process of arytenoid cartilage	Recurrent laryngeal	Separates vocal folds
Cricopharyngeus	Portion of inferior constrictor of pharynx, q.v.			
Cricothyroid	Arch of cricoid cartilage	Lamina of thyroid cartilage	External branch of superior laryngeal	Tenses vocal cords
Crureus [OT]	See *Vastus intermedius*			
Dartos (smooth muscle)	Found in and beneath the skin of scrotum		Sympathetic	Corrugates skin of scrotum
Deltoid	Clavicle, acromion, and spine of scapula	Deltoid tuberosity of humerus	Axillary	Abducts humerus, anterior fibers flex and medially rotate humerus, posterior fibers extend and laterally rotate humerus
Depressor alae nasi	Incisor fossa of maxilla	Ala and septum of nose	Facial	Pulls ala and septum of nose downward. Muscle of facial expression

Name	Origin	Insertion	Nerve	Action
Depressor anguli oris [BR]	See *Triangularis*			
Depressor epiglottidis [OT]	Fibers of thyroepiglottic, q.v.			
Depressor labii inferioris [BR; OT]	See *Quadratus labii inferioris*			
Depressor septi [BR]	Portion of depressor alae nasi, q.v.			
Diaphragm	Xiphoid process of sternum, lower 6 costal cartilages, and lumbar vertebrae	Central tendon	Phrenic	Acts as main muscle of inhalation; aids in expulsive actions such as parturition
Digastric				
(1) Anterior belly	Inner surface of mandible near symphysis	Lesser cornu of hyoid via fascial sling	Nerve to mylohyoid	Elevates and fixes hyoid bone
(2) Posterior belly	Mastoid notch		Facial	
Dilator naris				
(1) Anterior portion	Alar cartilage	Ala	Facial	Muscle of facial expression
(2) Posterior portion	Nasal notch of maxilla			
Dilator naris [BR]	See *Nasalis*			
Dilator pupillae (smooth muscle)	Circumference of iris	Margin of pupil	Sympathetic	Dilates pupil
Dilator tubae [OT]	See *Tensor veli palatini*			

TABLE OF MUSCLES—(Continued)

Name	Origin	Insertion	Innervation	Function
Dorsoepitrochlearis (variable)	Occasional muscle slip in axillary fascia			
Ejaculator urinae [OT]	See *Bulbocavernosus*			
Epicranius (occipito-frontalis OT; BR)				
(1) Anterior belly (frontalis)	Galea aponeurotica	Skin of forehead	Facial	Elevates eyebrows and draws scalp forward
(2) Posterior belly (occipitalis)	Superior nuchal line of occiput	Galea aponeurotica	Facial	Draws scalp backward
Erector clitoridis [OT]	See *Ischiocavernosus*			
Erector penis [OT]	See *Ischiocavernosus*			
Erector pili [OT]	See *Arrectores pilorum*			
Extensor carpi radialis brevis (extensor carpi radialis brevior OT)	Lateral epicondyle of humerus	Base of second and third metacarpals	Radial	Extends wrist
Extensor carpi radialis longus (extensor carpi radialis longior OT)	Lateral epicondyle of humerus	Base of second metacarpal	Radial	Extends wrist

Extensor carpi ulnaris	Lateral epicondyle of humerus and dorsal margin of ulna	Base of fifth metacarpal	Radial	Extends wrist
Extensor digiti quinti proprius (extensor digiti minimi BR)	Lateral epicondyle of humerus	Dorsum of proximal phalanx of little finger	Radial	Extends metacarpophalangeal joint of little finger
Extensor digitorum brevis (of foot)	Dorsal surface of calcaneus	Extensor tendons of first, second, third, and fourth toes	Deep peroneal	Extends toes at metatarsophalangeal joints
Extensor digitorum communis (of hand) (extensor digitorum BR)	Lateral epicondyle of humerus	Common extensor tendon of each finger	Dorsal interosseous of forearm	Extends wrist and fingers at metacarpophalangeal joints
Extensor digitorum longus (of foot)	Anterior aspect of fibula, lateral aspect of lateral condyle of tibia, and interosseous membrane	Common extensor tendons of 4 lateral toes	Deep peroneal	Extends toes at metatarsophalangeal joints
Extensor hallucis brevis (most medial portion of extensor digitorum brevis, q.v.)	Dorsal surface of calcaneus	Base of proximal phalanx of great toe	Deep peroneal	Extends metatarsophalangeal joint of great toe
Extensor hallucis longus	Medial surface of fibula and interosseous membrane	Base of terminal phalanx of great toe	Deep peroneal	Dorsiflexes ankle joint and extends great toe
Extensor indicis proprius (extensor indicis BR; OT)	Dorsal surface of ulna	Common extensor tendon of index finger	Dorsal interosseous of forearm	Extends metacarpophalangeal joint of index finger

TABLE OF MUSCLES—(Continued)

Name	Origin	Insertion	Innervation	Function
Extensor ossis metacarpi pollicis [OT]	See *Abductor pollicis longus*			
Extensor ossis metatarsi hallucis [OT]	Occasional separate slip of insertion of extensor hallucis longus, *q.v.*, into first metatarsal			
Extensor pollicis brevis (*extensor primi internodii pollicis* OT)	Dorsal surface of radius and interosseous membrane	Dorsal surface of proximal phalanx of thumb	Dorsal interosseous of forearm	Extends metacarpophalangeal joint of thumb
Extensor pollicis longus (*extensor secundi internodii pollicis* OT)	Dorsal surface of ulna and interosseous membrane	Dorsal surface of distal phalanx of thumb	Dorsal interosseous of forearm	Extends and abducts thumb
Extensor primi internodii longus hallucis [OT]	Occasional separate slip of insertion of extensor hallucis longus, *q.v.*, into proximal phalanx of great toe			
Extensor primi internodii pollicis [OT]	See *Extensor pollicis brevis*			
Extensor secundi internodii pollicis [OT]	See *Extensor pollicis longus*			

Flexor carpi radialis	Medial epicondyle of humerus	Base of second metacarpal	Median	Flexes wrist joint
Flexor carpi ulnaris	Medial epicondyle of humerus and medial border of ulna	Pisiform, hamulus of hamate, and proximal end of fifth metacarpal	Ulnar	Flexes wrist joint
Flexor digiti quinti brevis (of foot) (flexor digiti minimi brevis BR)	Base of fifth metatarsal and plantar fascia	Lateral aspect of base of proximal phalanx of little toe	Lateral plantar	Flexes little toe at metatarsophalangeal joint
Flexor digiti quinti brevis (of hand) (flexor digiti minimi brevis BR) (variable)	Hamulus of hamate and transverse carpal ligament	Medial side of proximal phalanx of little finger	Ulnar	Flexes metacarpophalangeal joint of little finger
Flexor digitorum accessorius [BR]	See *Quadratus plantae*			
Flexor digitorum brevis	Medial tuberosity of calcaneus and plantar aponeurosis	Four tendons, one to middle phalanx of each of 4 lateral toes	Medial plantar	Flexes toes at metatarsophalangeal and proximal interphalangeal joints
Flexor digitorum longus	Posterior aspect of tibia	Four tendons, one to base of distal phalanx of each of 4 lateral toes	Tibial	Flexes toes at metatarsophalangeal and interphalangeal joints
Flexor digitorum profundus	Medial and anterior aspects of ulna and interosseous membrane	Four tendons, one to base of distal phalanx of each finger	Ulnar to medial portion, median to lateral portion	Flexes fingers primarily at distal interphalangeal joints, aids in flexing at wrist and other joints of the fingers

TABLE OF MUSCLES—(Continued)

Name	Origin	Insertion	Innervation	Function
Flexor digitorum sublimis	Medial epicondyle of humerus, coronoid process of ulna, and anterior margin of radius	Four tendons, one to base of middle phalanx of each finger	Median	Flexes fingers primarily at proximal interphalangeal joints. Aids in flexing wrist and metacarpophalangeal joints
Flexor hallucis brevis	Plantar aspect of cuboid and plantar fascia	Base of proximal phalanx of great toe	Medial plantar	Flexes metatarsophalangeal joint of great toe
Flexor hallucis longus	Posterior aspect of fibula	Base of distal phalanx of great toe	Tibial	Flexes great toe, plantar flexes foot, supports arches of foot
Flexor ossis metacarpi pollicis [OT]	See *Opponens pollicis*			
Flexor pollicis brevis	Transverse carpal ligament and ridge of greater multangular	Base of proximal phalanx of thumb	Median	Flexes metacarpophalangeal joint of thumb
Flexor pollicis longus	Anterior aspect of radius and interosseous membrane	Base of distal phalanx of thumb	Median	Flexes thumb
Frontalis	See *Epicranius*			

Muscle	Origin	Insertion	Nerve	Action
Gastrocnemius (1) Lateral head	Lateral condyle of femur	Posterior surface of calcaneus via tendo calcaneus (achillis)	Tibial	Plantar flexes ankle joint. Flexes knee joint
(2) Medial head	Medial condyle of femur			
Gemellus, inferior	Tuberosity of ischium	Greater trochanter of femur	Nerve to quadratus femoris	Rotates femur laterally
Gemellus, superior	Spine of ischium	Greater trochanter of femur	Nerve to obturator internus	Rotates femur laterally
Genioglossus (geniohyoglossus OT)	Superior genial tubercle of mandible	Hyoid and lateral portion of tongue	Hypoglossal	Protrudes and depresses tongue
Geniohyoid	Inferior genial tubercle of mandible	Body of hyoid	Descendens hypoglossi (first and second cervical)	Elevates and draws hyoid forward
Glossopalatine (palatoglossus OT; BR)	Inferior surface of soft palate	Side of tongue	Accessory	Elevates tongue and constricts anterior fauces
Glossopharyngeus	A portion of superior constrictor of pharynx, q.v.			
Gluteus maximus	Lateral surface of ilium, posterior surface of sacrum and coccyx, and sacro-tuberous ligament	Gluteal tuberosity and iliotibial tract	Inferior gluteal	Extends hip joint, extends trunk on legs when raising body from sitting position

TABLE OF MUSCLES—(Continued)

Name	Origin	Insertion	Innervation	Function
Gluteus medius	Lateral surface of ilium	Greater trochanter	Superior gluteal	Abducts femur
Gluteus minimus	Lateral surface of ilium	Greater trochanter	Superior gluteal	Abducts and medially rotates femur
Gracilis	Pubis	Medial surface of tibia	Obturator	Adducts femur, flexes knee joint
Hamstrings	Include semimembranosus, semitendinosus, and biceps femoris, q.v.			
Helicis major (vestigial)	Spina helicis	Ascending part of helix	Facial	
Helicis minor (vestigial)	Spina helicis	Crux of helix	Facial	
Hyoglossus	Body and greater cornu of hyoid	Side of tongue	Hypoglossal	Depresses tongue
Iliacus	Iliac fossa and sacrum	Lesser trochanter	Femoral	Flexes hip joint and trunk on lower extremity
Iliacus minor (iliocapsularis) (variable)	Iliac fossa and sacrum	Capsule of hip joint	Femoral	

Iliococcygeus	Portion of levator ani, q.v.			
Iliocostalis cervicis (costocervicalis BR) (cervicalis ascendens OT)	Upper 6 ribs	Posterior tubercles of transverse processes of fourth, fifth, and sixth cervical vertebrae	Posterior rami of cervical	The iliocostalis muscles form the lateral portion of the sacrospinalis, q.v. Extends vertebral column and assists in lateral movements of trunk
Iliocostalis dorsi (accessorius OT) (costalis BR)	Lower 6 ribs	Upper 6 ribs	Posterior rami of thoracic	Extends vertebral column and assists in lateral movements of trunk
Iliocostalis lumborum (sacrolumbalis OT) (iliocostalis BR)	Iliac crest, lumbar vertebrae, sacrum, and lumbodorsal fascia	Lower 6 ribs	Posterior rami of lumbar	Extends vertebral column and assists in lateral movements of trunk
Iliocostocervicalis [BR]	Composed of iliocostalis cervicis and iliocostalis dorsi, q.v.			
Iliopsoas	Combination of iliacus and psoas muscles, q.v.			
Infracostals [OT]	See *Subcostals*			
Infraspinatus	Infraspinous fossa of scapula	Greater tubercle of humerus	Suprascapular nerve	Rotates humerus laterally

TABLE OF MUSCLES—(Continued)

NAME	ORIGIN	INSERTION	INNERVATION	FUNCTION
Intercostal, external (11 pairs)	Lower border of rib above	Superior border of rib below	Anterior rami of thoracic	Accessory muscles of respiration (inhalation)
Intercostal, internal (11 pairs)	Lower border of costal cartilage and rib above	Superior border of costal cartilage and rib below	Anterior rami of thoracic	Accessory muscles of respiration (exhalation)
Interossei, dorsal (of foot) (4)	Each by two heads from sides of adjacent metatarsals	Extensor tendon of each of 4 lateral toes	Lateral plantar	Abduct toes. Plantar flex at metatarsophalangeal joints and extend at interphalangeal joints
Interossei, dorsal (of hand) (4)	Each by two heads from sides of adjacent metacarpals	Extensor tendons of second, third, and fourth fingers	Ulnar	Abduct fingers. Flex at metacarpophalangeal joints, and extend at interphalangeal joints
Interossei, plantar (3)	Medial side of third, fourth, and fifth metatarsals, respectively	Extensor tendons of third, fourth, and fifth toes	Lateral plantar	Adduct toes and assist the dorsal interossei, q.v.
Interossei, volar (interossei, palmar OT; BR) (3)	Sides of metacarpals	Extensor tendons of second, fourth, and fifth fingers	Ulnar	Adduct fingers and assist dorsal interossei, q.v.
Interspinales (variable may be absent	Spinous process of vertebra above	Spinous process of vertebra below	Posterior rami of	Extend vertebral column

	Origin	Insertion	Nerve	Action
Intertransversarii (intertransversales OT) (may be absent in thoracic region)	Transverse process of vertebra	Transverse process of vertebra	Anterior rami of spinal	Aid in lateral movements of vertebral column
Ischiobulbosus (variable)	Ischium	Perineal raphe	Perineal	Assists bulbocavernosus
Ischiocavernosus (erector penis OT) (erector clitoridis OT)	Ischium	Crus of penis (clitoris)	Perineal	Assists in erection of penis (clitoris)
Ischiofemoralis (variable)	Occasional slip of gluteus maximus, *q.v.*, arising from ischial tuberosity			
Ischiopubicus (variable)	Portion of sphincter urethrae membranaceae, *q.v.*			
Latissimus dorsi (latissimus thoracis BR)	Spines of lower 6 thoracic vertebrae, spines of lumbar vertebrae, lumbodorsal fascia, crest of ilium, lower ribs, and inferior angle of scapula	Intertubercular sulcus of humerus	Thoracodorsal	Adducts and extends humerus; used to pull body up in climbing; accessory muscle of respiration
Levator anguli oris [BR; OT]	See *Caninus*			
Levator anguli scapulae [OT]	See *Levator scapulae*			

TABLE OF MUSCLES—(Continued)

Name	Origin	Insertion	Innervation	Function
Levator ani (1) Iliococcygeal portion	Pelvic surface of ischial spine and pelvic fascia	Central point of perineum, anococcygeal raphe, and coccyx	Anterior rami of third and fourth sacral and perineal	Supports pelvic viscera
(2) Pubococcygeal portion	Pubic and pelvic fascia	Some fibers form a sling around the upper portion of anal canal		
Levator glandulae thyroideae (variable)	Hyoid	Isthmus of thyroid		
Levator labii superioris [OT; BR]	Portion of quadratus labii superioris, q.v.			
Levator labii superioris alaeque nasi [OT; BR]	See *Quadratus labii superioris*			
Levator menti [OT]	See *Mentalis*			
Levator palati [OT; BR]	See *Levator veli palatini*			
Levator palpebrae superioris	Roof of orbit	Skin of upper eyelid and superior tarsus	Oculomotor	Elevates upper lid
Levator prostatae	Medial fibers of pubococcygeal portion of levator ani, q.v.			

	Origin	Insertion	Nerve	Action
Levator scapulae (levator anguli scapulae OT)	Transverse processes of upper cervical vertebrae	Vertebral margin and medial angle of scapula	Dorsal scapular and anterior rami of third and fourth cervical	Elevates shoulder, rotates inferior angle of scapula medially
Levator veli palatini (levator palati OT; BR)	Apex of petrous part of temporal bone and cartilaginous part of auditory tube	Aponeurosis of soft palate	Accessory via pharyngeal plexus	Raises soft palate
Levatores costarum (12 pairs)	Transverse processes of seventh cervical and upper 11 thoracic vertebrae	Medial to angle of corresponding rib below	Anterior rami of thoracic	Aid in raising ribs in inspiration
Lingual, inferior [OT]	See *Longitudinalis, inferior, of tongue*			
Lingual, superior [OT]	See *Longitudinalis, superior, of tongue*			
Longissimus (portion of sacrospinalis) (1) **Capitis** (trachelomastoideus OT)	Transverse processes of upper sixth thoracic vertebrae and articular processes of lower 4 cervical vertebrae	Mastoid process of temporal bone	Posterior rami of spinal	Longissimus muscles form middle portion of sacrospinalis, q.v. Extends vertebral column and assists in rotation and lateral movements of trunk
(2) **Cervicis** (transversalis colli OT) (transversus colli OT)	Transverse processes of upper 6 thoracic vertebrae	Transverse processes of second to sixth cervical vertebrae		
(3) **Dorsi** (thoracis BR)	Iliac crest, sacroiliac ligament, spines of lumbar and sacral vertebrae	Ribs and transverse processes of thoracic and upper lumbar vertebrae		

TABLE OF MUSCLES—(Continued)

Name	Origin	Insertion	Innervation	Function
Longitudinalis, of tongue				
(1) Inferior (inferior lingual OT)	Base of tongue	Tip of tongue	Hypoglossal	Alters shape of tongue
(2) Superior (superior lingual OT)				
Longus capitis (rectus capitis anticus major OT)	Transverse processes of third to sixth cervical vertebrae	Basal portion of occipital bone	Anterior rami of upper 4 cervical	Flexes head
Longus colli (longus cervicis BR)				
(1) Inferior oblique portion	Bodies of first 3 thoracic vertebrae	Anterior tubercles of fifth and sixth cervical vertebrae	Anterior rami of cervical	Flexes vertebral column
(2) Superior oblique portion	Transverse processes of third to fifth cervical vertebrae	Anterior tubercle of atlas		
(3) Vertical portion	Bodies of last 3 cervical and first 3 thoracic vertebrae	Bodies of second to fourth cervical vertebrae		
Lumbricals (of fingers) (4)	Tendons of flexor digitorum profundus	One to extensor tendon of each finger	Two lateral by median and two medial by ulnar	Flex at metacarpophalangeal joints and extend at interphalangeal joints

	Origin	Insertion	Nerve	Action
Lumbricals (of toes) (4)	Tendons of flexor digitorum longus	One to extensor tendon of each of 4 lateral toes	Medial one by medial plantar, others by lateral plantar	Flex at metatarso-phalangeal joints and extend at interphalangeal joints
Masseter	Arch of zygoma	Ramus and angle of mandible	Mandibular	Muscle of mastication. Closes mouth and clenches teeth
Mentalis (levator menti OT)	Incisor fossa of mandible	Skin of chin	Facial	Muscle of facial expression
Multifidus (multifidus spinae OT)	Sacrum, sacroiliac ligament, mammillary processes of lumbar vertebrae, transverse processes of thoracic vertebrae, articular processes of lower 4 cervical vertebrae	Spines of vertebrae	Posterior rami of spinal	Extends and rotates vertebral column
Mylohyoid	Mylohyoid line of mandible	Hyoid	Nerve to mylohyoid	Elevates hyoid and supports floor of mouth
Mylopharyngeal	Portion of superior constrictor of pharynx, q.v.			
Nasalis (compressor nasi OT) (compressor naris BR) (dilator naris BR)	Maxilla	Skin over bridge of nose	Facial	Muscle of facial expression

TABLE OF MUSCLES—(Continued)

Name	Origin	Insertion	Innervation	Function
Obliquus abdominis externus	Lower 8 ribs	Xiphoid, linea alba, pubis, crest of ilium	Lower 6 thoracic	Supports abdominal viscera. Flexes vertebral column
Obliquus abdominis internus	Lumbodorsal fascia, iliac crest, inguinal ligament	Lower 3 ribs, linea alba, xiphoid, pubis	Lower 6 thoracic and iliohypogastric	Supports abdominal viscera. Flexes vertebral column
Obliquus auriculae (obliquus auris OT) (vestigial)	Helix	Antihelix	Facial	
Obliquus capitis inferior	Spine of epistropheus	Transverse process of atlas	Posterior ramus of first cervical	Aids in extension and lateral movements of head
Obliquus capitis superior	Transverse process of atlas	Occipital bone	Posterior ramus of first cervical	Aids in extension and lateral movements of head
Obliquus oculi inferior	Medial aspect of floor of orbit	Sclera	Oculomotor	Rotates eyeball upward and outward
Obliquus oculi superior (trochlearis OT)	Margin of optic foramen	Sclera	Trochlear	Rotates eyeball outward and downward
Obturator externus	Pubis, ischium, and superficial surface of obturator membrane	Trochanteric fossa of femur	Obturator	Rotates femur laterally

		Greater trochanter of femur	Nerve to obturator internus	Rotates femur laterally
Obturator internus	Pubis, ilium, ischium, and deep surface of obturator membrane	Greater trochanter of femur	Nerve to obturator internus	Rotates femur laterally
Occipitalis	See *Epicranius*			
Occipitofrontalis [OT; BR]	See *Epicranius*			
Omohyoid (1) Anterior belly. (2) Posterior belly	Intermediate tendon. Superior margin of scapula	Hyoid. Intermediate tendon	Descendens cervicis and hypoglossi	Depresses hyoid
Opponens digiti quinti (of foot) (opponens digiti minimi BR) (variable)	Occasional insertion of flexor digiti quinti brevis into fifth metatarsal			
Opponens digiti quinti (of hand) (opponens digiti minimi BR)	Transverse carpal ligament and hamulus of hamate	Medial aspect of fifth metacarpal	Ulnar	Deepens palm
Opponens hallucis (variable)	Occasional insertion of some fibers of flexor hallucis brevis, q.v., into shaft of first metatarsal			
Opponens pollicis (flexor ossis metacarpi pollicis OT)	Ridge of greater multangular and transverse carpal ligament	First metacarpal	Median	Opposes thumb

TABLE OF MUSCLES—(Continued)

Name	Origin	Insertion	Innervation	Function
Orbicularis oculi (orbicularis palpebrarum OT)	Medial aspect of orbit	Skin about eyelids	Facial	Closes lids
Orbicularis oris	Lies in skin about mouth		Facial	Muscle of facial expression; puckers mouth
Orbicularis palpebrarum [OT]	See Orbicularis oculi			
Orbitalis (smooth muscle)	Bridges inferior orbital fissure		Sympathetic	
Palatoglossus [OT; BR]	See Glossopalatine			
Palatopharyngeus [OT; BR]	See Pharyngopalatinus			
Palmaris brevis	Palmar aponeurosis	Skin of medial border of hand	Ulnar	Deepens hollow of hand
Palmaris longus (variable)	Medial epicondyle of humerus	Transverse carpal ligament and palmar aponeurosis	Median	Flexes wrist joint
Pectineus	Pubis	Femur distal to lesser trochanter	Femoral (occasionally obturator)	Adducts femur and flexes hip joint

Muscle	Origin	Insertion	Nerve	Action
Pectoralis major	Clavicle, sternum, first 6 ribs, aponeurosis of external oblique muscle of abdomen	Intertubercular sulcus of humerus	Medial and lateral anterior thoracic	Adducts and medially rotates humerus, flexes shoulder joint, depresses shoulder girdle
Pectoralis minor	Third to fifth ribs	Coracoid process of scapula	Medial and lateral anterior thoracic	Draws shoulder forward
Peroneocalcaneus (variable)	Occasional separate portion of tibialis posterior, q.v.			
Peroneocalcaneus externus (variable)	Occasional slip of insertion of peroneus longus or brevis, q.v., into calcaneus			
Peroneocuboideus (variable)	Occasional slip of insertion of peroneus longus or brevis, q.v., into cuboid			
Peroneus accessorius (variable)	Occasional extra portion of peroneus longus or brevis, q.v.			
Peroneus brevis	Lateral surface of fibula	Base of fifth metatarsal	Superficial peroneal	Everts and plantar flexes foot
Peroneus digiti quinti (variable)	Occasional extra slip of insertion of peroneus brevis, q.v., into fifth toe			

TABLE OF MUSCLES—(Continued)

Name	Origin	Insertion	Innervation	Function
Peroneus longus	Lateral condyle of tibia and lateral surface of fibula	First cuneiform and first metatarsal	Superficial peroneal	Everts and plantar flexes foot. Supports arches
Peroneus tertius	Medial surface of fibula	Fifth metatarsal	Deep peroneal	Everts and dorsiflexes foot
Pharyngopalatinus (palatopharyngeus OT; BR)	Soft palate and auditory tube	Aponeurosis of pharynx	Accessory via pharyngeal plexus	Aids in swallowing
Piriformis	Second to fourth sacral vertebrae, ilium, and sacrotuberous ligament	Greater trochanter of femur	Anterior rami of first and second sacral	Rotates femur laterally
Plantaris (variable)	Lateral condyle of femur	Calcaneus by tendo calcaneus (achillis)	Tibial	Flexes knee joint and plantar flexes ankle joint
Platysma (platysma myoides OT)	Deep fascia of cervical region	Mandible and skin around mouth	Facial	Muscle of facial expression
Popliteus	Lateral condyle of femur	Back of tibia	Tibial	Rotates tibia medially, flexes knee joint
Procerus (pyramidalis nasi OT)	Skin over nose	Skin of forehead	Facial	Muscle of facial expression
Pronator quadratus	Volar surface of ulna	Volar surface of radius	Volar interosseous	Pronates forearm

		Lateral surface of	Median	Pronates forearm
Pronator teres (pronator radii teres OT)	(1) Medial epicondyle of humerus (2) Coronoid of ulna	radius		
Psoas major (psoas magnus OT)	Lumbar vertebrae and fascia	Lesser trochanter of femur	Anterior rami of second and third lumbar	Flexes hip joint and trunk on lower extremities
Psoas minor (psoas parvus OT) (variable)	Last thoracic and first lumbar vertebrae	Iliopectineal eminence	Anterior ramus of first lumbar	Flexes trunk on pelvis
Pterygoideus externus (pterygoideus lateralis BR)	(1) Sphenoid (2) Lateral pterygoid plate	Neck of mandible and capsule of temporomandibular joint	Mandibular	Muscle of mastication, protrudes mandible
Pterygoideus internus (pterygoideus medialis BR)	(1) Lateral pterygoid plate (2) Tuberosity of maxilla	Medial surface of angle of mandible	Mandibular	Muscle of mastication, clenches teeth
Pterygopharyngeus	Portion of superior constrictor of pharynx, q.v.			
Pubecavernosus	Occasional slip of ischiocavernosus, q.v., arising from pubis			
Pubococcygeus	Portion of levator ani, q.v.			
Puborectalis	Middle fibers of pubococcygeal portion of levator ani, q.v.			

TABLE OF MUSCLES—(Continued)

NAME	ORIGIN	INSERTION	INNERVATION	FUNCTION
Pyramidalis abdominis (variable)	Pubis	Linea alba	Anterior ramus of lowest thoracic	Supports abdominal viscera
Pyramidalis auriculae (vestigial)	Portion of tragicus, q.v.			
Pyramidalis nasi [OT]	See *Procerus*			
Quadratus femoris	Ischial tuberosity	Quadrate tubercle of femur	Nerve to quadratus femoris	Adducts and laterally rotates femur
Quadratus labii inferioris (depressor labii inferioris BR; OT)	Mandible	Skin about mouth	Facial	Muscle of facial expression
Quadratus labii superioris (levator labii superioris alaeque nasi OT; BR)	Maxilla	Skin about mouth	Facial	Muscle of facial expression
Quadratus lumborum	Iliac crest, lumbodorsal fascia, and lumbar	Last rib	Anterior rami of first	Assists in lateral movements of ver-

...[flexor] digitorum accessorius BR) (accessorius OT)	*lesus*			
Quadriceps femoris (quadriceps extensor OT)	Includes rectus femoris and 3 vastus muscles, q.v.			
Rectus abdominis	Pubis	Xiphoid, fifth to seventh costal cartilages	Anterior rami of lower 6 thoracic	Supports abdominal viscera; flexes vertebral column
Rectus capitis anterior (rectus capitis anticus minor OT)	Lateral portion of atlas	Occipital bone	Anterior rami of first and second cervical	Flexes head
Rectus capitis anticus major [OT]	See *Longus capitis*			
Rectus capitis anticus minor [OT]	See *Rectus capitis anterior*			
Rectus capitis lateralis	Transverse process of atlas	Occipital bone	Anterior ramus of first cervical	Assists in lateral movements of head
Rectus capitis posterior major (rectus capitis posticus major OT)	Spine of epistropheus	Occipital bone	Posterior ramus of first cervical	Extends head
Rectus capitis posterior minor (rectus capitis posticus minor OT)	Posterior tubercle of atlas	Occipital bone	Posterior ramus of first cervical	Extends head

TABLE OF MUSCLES—(Continued)

NAME	ORIGIN	INSERTION	INNERVATION	FUNCTION
Rectus femoris (1) Straight head (2) Reflected head	Anterior inferior spine of ilium Dorsum ilii	Patella and ultimately into tubercle of tibia	Femoral	Extends knee joint Flexes hip joint
Rectus oculi inferior	Lower border of optic foramen	Sclera	Oculomotor	Rotates eyeball downward and somewhat inward
Rectus oculi lateralis (rectus oculi externus OT)	Lateral border of optic foramen	Sclera	Abducens	Rotates eyeball laterally
Rectus oculi medialis (rectus oculi internus OT)	Medial border of optic foramen	Sclera	Oculomotor	Rotates eyeball medially
Rectus oculi superior	Upper border of optic foramen	Sclera	Oculomotor	Rotates eyeball upward and somewhat inward
Retrahens aurem [OT] (vestigial)	See *Auricularis posterior*			
Rhomboideus major	Spines of second to fifth thoracic vertebrae	Vertebral margin of scapula	Dorsal scapular	Draws scapula backward and aids in rotating inferior angle of scapula medially

	vical and first thoracic vertebrae	scapula	ular	deus major
Risorius	Fascia over masseter	Skin at angle of mouth	Facial	Muscle of facial expression
Rotatores (11 pairs)	Transverse process of thoracic vertebra below	Lamina of thoracic vertebra above	Posterior rami of thoracic	Extend and rotate vertebral column
Sacrolumbalis [OT]	See *Iliocostalis lumborum*			
Sacrospinalis	Composed of longissimus, iliocostalis, and spinalis dorsi, q.v.			
Salpingopharyngeus	Portion of pharyngo-palatinus, q.v., arising from auditory tube			
Sartorius	Anterior superior spine of ilium	Tibia	Femoral	Flexes hip and knee joints, rotates femur laterally
Scalenus anterior (scalenus anticus OT)	Transverse processes of third to sixth cervical vertebrae	Tubercle of first rib	Anterior rami of third and fourth cervical	Flexes vertebral column laterally, accessory muscle of respiration (inhalation)
Scalenus medius	Transverse processes of second to sixth cervical vertebrae	First rib	Anterior rami of third and fourth cervical	Flexes vertebral column laterally, accessory muscle of respiration (inhalation)

TABLE OF MUSCLES—(Continued)

Name	Origin	Insertion	Innervation	Function
Scalenus posterior (scalenus posticus OT)	Tubercles of fourth to sixth cervical vertebrae	Second rib	Anterior rami of third and fourth cervical	Flexes vertebral column laterally, accessory muscle of respiration (inhalation)
Semimembranosus	Ischial tuberosity	Medial condyle of tibia	Tibial	Flexes knee joint and extends hip joint
Semispinalis capitis (complexus OT) (biventer cervicis OT)	Transverse processes of upper 6 thoracic and articular processes of lower 4 cervical vertebrae	Occipital bone	Posterior rami of spinal	Extends head
Semispinalis cervicis (semispinalis colli OT)	Transverse processes of upper 6 thoracic and lower 4 cervical vertebrae	Spines of second to fifth cervical vertebrae	Posterior rami of spinal	Extends and rotates vertebral column
Semispinalis dorsi (semispinalis thoracis BR)	Transverse processes of lower 6 thoracic vertebrae	Spines of last 2 cervical and first 4 thoracic vertebrae	Posterior rami of thoracic	Extends and rotates vertebral column
Semitendinosus	Ischial tuberosity	Medial aspect of proximal portion of tibia	Tibial	Flexes knee joint and extends hip joint
Serratus anterior (serratus anticus OT)	Upper 8 or 9 ribs	Vertebral border of scapula	Long thoracic	Draws scapula forward, draws inferior

Serratus posterior inferior (serratus posticus inferior OT)	Lumbodorsal fascia, spines of lowest thoracic and upper lumbar vertebrae	Last 4 ribs	Lower thoracic	Accessory muscle of respiration
Serratus posterior superior (serratus posticus superior OT)	Ligamentum nuchae, spines of seventh cervical and upper thoracic vertebrae	Second to fifth ribs	Second and third thoracic	Accessory muscle of respiration, elevates ribs
Soleus	Fibula, popliteal fascia, and tibia	Calcaneus by tendo calcaneus (achillis)	Tibial	Plantar flexes ankle joint
Sphincter ani externus (subdivided into subcutaneous, superficial, and deep portions)	Tip of coccyx	Surrounds anus	Pudendal	Closes anus
Sphincter pupillae	Circular fibers of iris		Oculomotor, parasympathetic portion	Constricts pupil
Sphincter urethrae membranaceae (sphincter urethrae BR) (compressor urethrae OT)	Ramus of pubis	Median raphe	Perineal	Compresses urethra
Sphincter vaginae [OT]	See *Bulbocavernosus*			

TABLE OF MUSCLES—(Continued)

NAME	ORIGIN	INSERTION	INNERVATION	FUNCTION
Spinalis capitis (variable)	Spines of upper thoracic and lowest cervical vertebrae	Occipital	Posterior rami of spinal	Extends head
Spinalis cervicis (spinalis colli OT) (variable)	Spines of lower cervical and upper thoracic vertebrae	Spines of second to fourth cervical vertebrae	Posterior rami of spinal	Extends vertebral column
Spinalis dorsi (spinalis thoracis BR)	Spines of lower 2 thoracic and upper 2 lumbar vertebrae	Spines of upper thoracic vertebrae	Posterior rami of spinal	Forms medial portion of sacrospinalis, q.v., extends vertebral column and assists in rotation and lateral movements of vertebral column
Splenius capitis	Ligamentum nuchae, spines of last cervical and upper thoracic vertebrae	Mastoid process	Posterior rami of spinal	Extends head
Splenius cervicis (splenius colli OT)	Ligamentum nuchae, spines of last cervical and upper thoracic vertebrae	Transverse processes of upper cervical vertebrae	Posterior rami of spinal	Extends vertebral column
Stapedius	Pyramidal eminence	Neck of stapes	Nerve to stapedius	Draws base of stapes toward tympanic

	Fascia of chest wall	Fascia of chest wall	Anterior thoracic	
Sternalis (variable)				
Sternoclavicularis (variable)	Small separate slip of subclavius, q.v., occasionally arising from sternum			
Sternocleidomastoid	Manubrium of sternum and clavicle	Mastoid process	Accessory and branch from second and third cervical	Flexes head
Sternocostalis [BR]	See *Transversus thoracis*			
Sternohyoid	Manubrium of sternum	Hyoid	Descendens cervicis and hypoglossi	Depresses hyoid
Sternothyreoid	Manubrium of sternum	Thyroid cartilage	Descendens cervicis and hypoglossi	Depresses larynx
Styloglossus	Styloid process	Side of tongue	Hypoglossal	Elevates tongue
Stylohyoid	Styloid process	Hyoid	Facial	Elevates hyoid
Stylopharyngeus	Styloid process	Lateral wall of pharynx	Glossopharyngeal	Pulls pharynx up
Subanconeus (variable)	Posterior distal surface of humerus	Posterior aspect of elbow joint	Radial	Pulls capsule back in extension of elbow joint

TABLE OF MUSCLES—(Continued)

Name	Origin	Insertion	Innervation	Function
Subclavius	First costal cartilage and first rib	Clavicle	Nerve to subclavius	Depresses lateral end of clavicle
Subcostals (infracostals OT) (variable)	Lower ribs	Lower ribs	Thoracic	Muscles of respiration
Subcrureus [OT]	See *Articularis genus*			
Subscapularis	Subscapular fossa of scapula	Lesser tubercle of humerus	Subscapular	Rotates humerus medially
Supinator (supinator radii brevis OT)	Lateral epicondyle of humerus, fascia about elbow joint, and shaft of ulna	Radius	Dorsal interosseous of forearm	Supinates forearm
Supinator longus [OT]	See *Brachioradialis*			
Supinator radii brevis [OT]	See *Supinator*			
Supraspinatus	Supraspinous fossa of scapula	Greater tubercle of humerus	Suprascapular	Abducts humerus
Temporal	Temporal fossa	Coronoid process of mandible	Mandibular	Closes mouth, clenches teeth, retracts lower jaw
Tensor fasciae latae (tensor vaginae femoris OT)	Iliac crest	Iliotibial tract and ultimately into tibia	Superior gluteal	Abducts leg, flexes hip joint, extends knee joint

Tensor fasciae suralis (variable)	Occasional insertion of long head of biceps femoris, *q.v.*, into tendo calcaneus (achillis)		
Tensor palati [OT; BR]	See *Tensor veli palatini*		
Tensor tarsi [OT]	Portion of orbicularis oculi, *q.v.*		
Tensor tympani	Cartilaginous portion of auditory tube	Manubrium of malleus	Mandibular	Tenses membrana tympani (ear drum)
Tensor vaginae femoris [OT]	See *Tensor fasciae latae*		
Tensor veli palatini (tensor palati OT; BR) (dilator tubae OT)	Scaphoid fossa of sphenoid and wall of auditory tube	Aponeurosis of soft palate	Mandibular	Tenses soft palate and opens auditory tube
Teres major	Axillary margin of scapula	Intertubercular sulcus of humerus	Subscapular	Adducts and medially rotates humerus
Teres minor	Axillary margin of scapula	Greater tubercle of humerus	Axillary	Laterally rotates humerus
Thyroarytenoid	Lamina of thyroid cartilage	Muscular process of arytenoid cartilage	Recurrent laryngeal	Relaxes vocal cords; closes vestibule of larynx

TABLE OF MUSCLES—(Continued)

NAME	ORIGIN	INSERTION	INNERVATION	FUNCTION
Thyroepiglottic (depressor epiglottidis OT)	Lamina of thyroid cartilage	Epiglottis	Recurrent laryngeal	Closes inlet of larynx
Thyrohyoid	Thyroid cartilage	Hyoid	Descendens hypoglossi (first and second cervical).	Draws thyroid and hyoid toward each other
Thyropharyngeus	Portion of inferior constrictor of pharynx, q.v.			
Tibialis anterior (tibialis anticus OT)	Tibia and interosseous membrane	First cuneiform and first metatarsal	Deep peroneal	Dorsiflexes and inverts foot
Tibialis posterior (tibialis posticus OT)	Fibula, tibia, and interosseous membrane	Bases of metatarsals and all tarsal bones except talus	Tibial	Plantar flexes and inverts foot, supports arches of foot
Tibiofascialis anterior (variable)	Occasional slip of insertion of tibialis anterior, q.v., into fascia of dorsum of foot			
Trachelomastoideus [OT]	See Longissimus capitis			
Tragicus (vestigial)	Crosses tragus		Facial	
Transversalis colli [OT]	See Longissimus cervicis			

Transversus abdominis (transversalis abdominis OT)	Costal cartilages of lower 6 ribs, lumbo-dorsal fascia, iliac crest, and inguinal ligament	Xiphoid, linea alba, inguinal ligament, and pubis	Anterior rami of lower 6 thoracic and iliohy-pogastric	Supports abdominal viscera and flexes vertebral column
Transversus auriculae (vestigial)	Crosses back of concha		Facial	
Transversus colli [OT]	See *Longissimus cervicis*			
Transversus linguae	Median raphe of tongue	Dorsum and sides of tongue	Hypoglossal	Alters shape of tongue
Transversus pedis [OT]	See *Adductor hallucis, transverse head*			
Transversus perinei profundus	Inferior ramus of ischium	Central point of perineum	Perineal	Supports perineum
Transversus perinei superficialis (variable)	Tuberosity of ischium	Central point of perineum	Perineal	Supports perineum
Transversus thoracis (sternocostalis BR) (triangularis sterni OT)	Mediastinal surface of xiphoid and body of sternum	Second to sixth costal cartilages	Thoracic	
Transversus urethrae (inconstant)	Occasional slip of sphincter urethrae membranaceae, q.v.			

TABLE OF MUSCLES—(Continued)

Name	Origin	Insertion	Innervation	Function
Transversus vaginae	Muscle in female which corresponds to sphincter urethrae membranaceae, q.v.			
Trapezius	Occipital bone, ligamentum nuchae, spines of seventh cervical and all thoracic vertebrae	Clavicle, acromion, and spine of scapula	Accessory and anterior rami of third and fourth cervical	Rotates inferior angle of scapula laterally, raises shoulder, draws scapula backward
Triangularis (depressor anguli oris BR)	Mandible	Skin at angle of mouth	Facial	Muscle of facial expression
Triangularis sterni [OT]	See *Transversus thoracis*			
Triceps brachii (1) Long head	Infraglenoid tuberosity	Olecranon of ulna	Radial	Extends elbow joint; long head also aids in adducting humerus
(2) Lateral head	Shaft of humerus			
(3) Medial head	Shaft of humerus			
Triceps surae [OT]	Combined gastrocnemius, soleus, and plantaris, q.v.			
Trochlearis [OT]	See *Obliquus oculi superior*			

Uvulae (azygos uvulae OT)	Posterior nasal spine	Aponeurosis of soft palate	Accessory (pharyngeal plexus)	
Vastus crureus [OT]	See *Vastus intermedius*			
Vastus externus [OT]	See *Vastus lateralis*			
Vastus intermedius (crureus OT) (vastus crureus OT)	Anterior and lateral aspects of femur	Patella and ultimately into tubercle of tibia	Femoral	Extends knee joint
Vastus internus [OT]	See *Vastus medialis*			
Vastus lateralis (vastus externus OT)	Capsule of hip joint and lateral aspect of femur	Patella and ultimately into tubercle of tibia	Femoral	Extends knee joint
Vastus medialis (vastus internus OT)	Medial aspect of femur	Patella and ultimately into tubercle of tibia	Femoral	Extends knee joint
Verticalis linguae	Dorsal aspect of tongue	Sides and base of tongue	Hypoglossal	Alters shape of tongue
Vocalis (medial fibers of thyroarytenoid)	Thyroid cartilage	Vocal process of arytenoid cartilage	Recurrent laryngeal	Adjusts vocal cords
Zygomatic (zygomaticus major OT; BR)	Zygoma	Skin about mouth	Facial	Muscle of facial expression
Zygomaticus major [OT; BR]	See *Zygomatic*			
Zygomaticus minor [OT; BR]	Portion of quadratus labii superioris, q.v.			

TABLE OF NERVES

NAME	CENTRAL ATTACHMENT	COMPONENTS	BRANCHES	DISTRIBUTION
Abducens (sixth cranial)	Brain stem at inferior border of pons	Motor	Muscular filaments	Lateral rectus muscle of eye
Accessory (eleventh cranial) (spinal accessory OT)				
(1) Bulbar part	Lateral aspect of medulla oblongata	Motor• Parasympathetic	Internal ramus to vagus	Striate muscles of larynx and pharynx Thoracic and abdominal viscera
(2) Spinal part	Upper 5 or 6 cervical segments of cord	Motor	External ramus to second, third, and fourth cervical (cervical plexus)	Trapezius and sternocleidomastoid muscles
Acoustic (eighth cranial) (auditory OT; BR)	See Cochlear and Vestibular			
Alveolar, anterior superior (anterior superior dental OT; BR)	Infraorbital	Somatic sensory	Filaments	Upper incisor and canine teeth, mucosa of nasal floor
Alveolar, inferior (inferior dental OT; BR)	Mandibular	Motor	N. to mylohyoid muscle	Mylohyoid and anterior belly of digastric muscles
		Somatic sensory	Mental and filaments	Lower teeth, skin of lower lip, and chin

		sory		teeth
rior (middle superior dental OT; BR)				
Alveolar, posterior superior (posterior superior dental OT; BR)	Maxillary	Somatic sensory	Filaments	Upper molar teeth and mucosa of maxillary sinus
Ampullary, inferior	Vestibular	Sensory (movement of head in space—dynamic)	Filaments	Ampulla of posterior semicircular duct
Ampullary, lateral	Vestibular	Sensory (movement of head in space—dynamic)	Filaments	Ampulla of lateral semicircular duct
Ampullary, superior	Vestibular	Sensory (movement of head in space—dynamic)	Filaments	Ampulla of superior semicircular duct
Anastomotic, peroneal	See *Peroneal, anastomotic*			
Anococcygeal	Fourth and fifth sacral and coccygeal segments of cord	Somatic sensory	Filaments	Skin in vicinity of coccyx
Arnold, N. of [OT]	See *Auricular*			
Auditory [OT; BR]	See *Acoustic*			
Auricular (N. of Arnold OT)	Vagus	Somatic sensory	Filaments	Skin of auricle and external acoustic meatus

* Nerves to muscles contain proprioceptive sensory fibers in addition to motor fibers; muscular branches of third, fourth, sixth, seventh, and twelfth cranial nerves may be exceptions.

TABLE OF NERVES—(Continued)

NAME	CENTRAL ATTACHMENT	COMPONENTS	BRANCHES	DISTRIBUTION
Auricular, great	Second and third cervical segments (cervical plexus)	Somatic sensory	Auricular, facial, and mastoid branches	Skin about ear
Auricular, posterior	Facial	Motor	Filaments	Occipitalis and intrinsic muscles of auricle
Auriculotemporal	Mandibular	Somatic sensory	Filaments	Skin of scalp and temple
Axillary (circumflex OT; BR)	Fifth and sixth cervical segments of cord (brachial plexus)	Motor	Muscular, articular, and cutaneous filaments	Deltoid and teres minor muscles
		Somatic sensory	Lateral cutaneous of arm	Shoulder joint, skin of lateral aspect of shoulder and arm
Bell, N. of [OT]	See *Thoracic, long*			
Bigeminus [OT]	Old term for third sacral nerve			
Buccinator (buccal BR)	Mandibular	Somatic sensory	Filaments	Skin and mucosa of cheek
Calcanean	Medial sural	Somatic sensory	Filaments	Skin of heel
Cardiac, inferior	Inferior cervical ganglion	Sympathetic. Visceral sensory	To cardiac plexuses	Heart

Cardiac, inferior or thoracic	Vagus and recurrent laryngeal	Parasympathetic. Visceral sensory	To cardiac plexuses	Heart
Cardiac, middle	Middle cervical ganglion	Sympathetic. Visceral sensory	To cardiac plexuses	Heart
Cardiac, superior	Superior cervical ganglion	Sympathetic. Visceral sensory	To cardiac plexuses	Heart
Cardiac, superior or cervical	Vagus	Parasympathetic. Visceral sensory	To cardiac plexuses	Heart
Caroticotympanic (small deep petrosal OT) (1) Inferior (2) Superior	Sympathetic plexus on internal carotid artery	Sympathetic	Tympanic plexus	Filaments
Carotid, external	Superior cervical ganglion	Sympathetic	Plexuses on external carotid artery and its branches	Filaments to smooth muscle and glands of head
Carotid, internal	Superior cervical ganglion	Sympathetic	Plexuses on internal carotid artery and its branches. See Petrosal, deep; Caroticotympanic	Filaments to smooth muscle and glands of head
Cervical, first (anterior division) (suboccipital OT)	First cervical segment of cord	Motor	Fibers to descendens hypoglossi, q.v.	Neck muscles

TABLE OF NERVES—(Continued)

NAME	CENTRAL ATTACHMENT	COMPONENTS	BRANCHES	DISTRIBUTION
Cervical, first (posterior division) (suboccipital OT)	First cervical segment of cord	Motor	Muscular	Deep muscles of back of neck
Cervical, second (anterior division)	Second cervical segment of cord	Motor. Somatic sensory	Fibers to descendens cervicis, q.v., and to third cervical	Neck muscles
Cervical, second (posterior division)	Second cervical segment of cord	Motor. Somatic sensory	Greater occipital and communicating to third cervical	Deep muscles of back of neck and skin of back of neck
Cervical, third (anterior division)	Third cervical segment of cord	Motor. Somatic sensory	Lesser occipital, great auricular, supraclavicular, phrenic, and cutaneus colli, q.v.	Levator scapulae, sternocleidomastoid, trapezius, scalenus medius, and scalenus posterior muscles; skin of neck
Cervical, third (posterior division)	Third cervical segment of cord	Motor. Somatic sensory	Third occipital, muscular	Deep muscles of neck; skin of back of neck
Cervical, fourth (anterior division)	Fourth cervical segment of cord	Motor. Somatic sensory	Phrenic, supraclavicular	Same as anterior division of third cervical
Cervical, fourth to eighth (posterior division)	Fourth to eighth cervical segments of	Motor. Somatic sensory	Muscular and cutaneous	Deep muscles of neck and upper por-

Cervical, fifth to eighth (anterior divisions)	Fifth to eighth cervical segments of cord	Motor. Somatic sensory	Nerves of brachial plexus	Muscles and skin of upper extremity
Cervical, superficial [OT]	See *Cutaneus colli*			
Chorda tympani	Intermedius	Parasympathetic Sensory (taste)	Filaments	Sublingual and submaxillary salivary glands Taste buds of anterior two-thirds of tongue
Ciliary, long	Nasociliary	Somatic sensory	Filaments	Eyeball
Ciliary, short	Ciliary ganglion Nasociliary	Parasympathetic Somatic sensory	Filaments	Ciliary muscle and constrictor fibers of iris Eyeball
Circumflex [OT; BR]	See *Axillary*			
Cluneal, inferior (gluteal BR)	Posterior cutaneous n. of thigh	Somatic sensory	Filaments	Skin of lower gluteal region
Cluneal, medial (gluteal BR)	First, second, and third sacral (posterior divisions)	Somatic sensory	Filaments	Skin of medial portion of gluteal region
Cluneal, superior (gluteal BR)	First, second, and third lumbar (posterior divisions)	Somatic sensory	Filaments	Skin of upper portion of gluteal region

TABLE OF NERVES—(Continued)

NAME	CENTRAL ATTACHMENT	COMPONENTS	BRANCHES	DISTRIBUTION
Coccygeal	Coccygeal segment of cord	Somatic sensory	Anococcygeal	Skin over coccyx
Cochlear	Brain stem at lower border of pons	Sensory (hearing)	Filaments	Spiral organ (of Corti) of cochlea
Crural, anterior [OT]	See Femoral			
Cutaneous, anterior, of abdomen	Iliohypogastric	Somatic sensory	Filaments	Skin of lower anterior abdomen
Cutaneous, dorsal, of forearm	Radial	Somatic sensory	Filaments	Skin of lower portion of posterior aspect of arm and dorsal aspect of forearm
Cutaneous, dorsal, of hand	Ulnar	Somatic sensory	Filaments	Skin of medial portion of dorsal aspect of hand
Cutaneous, dorsal intermediate, of foot	Superficial peroneal	Somatic sensory	Filaments	Skin of dorsum of foot
Cutaneous, dorsal medial, of foot	Superficial peroneal	Somatic sensory	Filaments	Skin of dorsum of foot
Cutaneous, intermediate, of thigh	Femoral	Somatic sensory	Filaments	Skin of anterior aspect of thigh
Cutaneous, lateral, of	Axillary	Somatic sensory	Filaments	Skin of lateral aspect of arm

Cutaneous, lateral, of forearm	Musculocutaneous	Somatic sensory	Filaments	Skin of lateral aspect of forearm
Cutaneous, lateral, of leg (lateral cutaneous of calf or lateral sural)	Common peroneal	Somatic sensory	Filaments	Skin of lateral aspect of leg
Cutaneous, lateral, of thigh	Second and third lumbar segments of cord (lumbar plexus)	Somatic sensory	Filaments	Skin of lateral aspect of thigh
Cutaneous, lateral palmar	Median	Somatic sensory	Digital branches	Skin of lateral portion of palm and fingers
Cutaneous, medial, of arm (lesser internal cutaneous OT)	First thoracic segment of cord (brachial plexus)	Somatic sensory	Filaments	Skin of medial aspect of arm
Cutaneous, medial, of forearm (internal cutaneous OT)	Eighth cervical and first thoracic segments of cord (brachial plexus)	Somatic sensory	Filaments	Skin of medial aspect of arm and forearm
Cutaneous, medial, of leg (medial sural) (tibial communicating OT) (sural BR)	Tibial	Somatic sensory	Filaments	Skin of medial aspect of leg
Cutaneous, medial, of thigh	Femoral	Somatic sensory	Filaments	Skin of posterior aspect of buttocks and medial aspect of thigh

TABLE OF NERVES—(Continued)

Name	Central Attachment	Components	Branches	Distribution
Cutaneous, medial palmar	Ulnar	Somatic sensory	Filaments. Digital	Skin of medial aspect of palm and fingers
Cutaneous, perforating (variable)	Second and third sacral segments of cord (pudendal plexus)	Somatic sensory	Filaments	Skin of posterior aspect of buttocks
Cutaneous, posterior, of arm	Radial	Somatic sensory	Filaments	Skin of posterior aspect of arm
Cutaneous, posterior, of thigh (small sciatic OT)	Second, third, and fourth sacral segments of cord (pudendal plexus)	Somatic sensory	Filaments	Skin of posterior aspect of buttocks, thigh, and perineum
Cutaneous colli (anterior cutaneous of neck BR) (superficial cervical OT)	Second and third cervical segments of cord (cervical plexus)	Somatic sensory	Filaments	Skin of anterior triangle of neck
Dental [OT; BR]	See Alveolar			
Descendens cervicis	Second and third cervical segments of cord (cervical plexus)	Motor	To ansa hypoglossi	Geniohyoid, thyrohyoid, sternothyroid, sternohyoid, and omohyoid mus-

Descendens hypoglossi	First and second cervical segments of cord (cervical plexus)	Motor	To ansa hypoglossi	Same as above
Digital (of fingers)	Median, ulnar, and superficial rami of radial, q.v.	Somatic sensory	Filaments	Skin of digits
Digital (of toes)	Superficial peroneal, deep peroneal, medial plantar, and lateral plantar, q.v.	Somatic sensory	Filaments	Skin of digits
Dorsal, of penis (clitoris)	Pudendal	Somatic sensory	Filaments	Skin of penis (clitoris)
Ethmoidal, anterior (internal nasal BR)	Nasociliary	Somatic sensory	External nasal, filaments	Mucosa of nasal cavity, mucosa of anterior ethmoidal air sinus
Ethmoidal, posterior	Nasociliary	Somatic sensory	Filaments	Mucosa of sphenoidal and posterior ethmoidal air sinuses
Facial (seventh cranial)	Brain stem at inferior border of pons	Motor	Stapedius, posterior auricular, temporal, zygomatic, buccal, mandibular, and cervical rami	Stapedius, stylohyoid, posterior belly of digastric, and muscles of facial expression
		Parasympathetic, Sensory (taste)	See *Intermedius*	

TABLE OF NERVES—(Continued)

Name	Central Attachment	Components	Branches	Distribution
Femoral (anterior crural OT)	Second, third, and fourth lumbar segments of cord (lumbar plexus)	Motor. Somatic sensory	Muscular, articular, saphenous, medial, and intermediate cutaneous of thigh	Pectineus, quadriceps femoris, articularis genus muscles; skin of anterior aspect of thigh and medial aspect of leg; hip and knee joints
Frontal	Ophthalmic	Somatic sensory	Supraorbital, supratrochlear, and nasociliary	Skin of upper eyelid, forehead, and scalp
Furcalis [OT]	Old term for fourth lumbar nerve			
Genitofemoral (genito-crural OT)	First and second lumbar segments of cord (lumbar plexus)	Somatic sensory	External spermatic and lumboinguinal	Skin of thigh and scrotum (labium majus)
Glossopalatine	See *Intermedius*			
Glossopharyngeal (ninth cranial)	Lateral aspect of medulla oblongata	Motor	Muscular, pharyngeal, tonsillar, lingual, tympanic	Stylopharyngeus and muscles of soft palate and pharynx via pharyngeal plexus;
		Visceral sensory		mucosa of posterior one-third of tongue.

			Sensory (taste) Parasympathetic	pharynx, middle ear and mastoid aircells; taste buds of posterior one-third of tongue; parotid gland via otic ganglion
Gluteal [BR] (cutaneous)	See *Cluneal*			
Gluteal, inferior	Fifth lumbar, first and second sacral segments of cord (sacral plexus)	Motor	Filaments	Gluteus maximus muscle
Gluteal, superior	Fourth and fifth lumbar and first sacral segments of cord (sacral plexus)	Motor	Filaments	Gluteus medius and minimus and tensor fasciae latae muscles
Hamstrings, N. to	Fourth and fifth lumbar, upper 3 sacral segments of cord (sacral plexus)	Motor	Filaments	Biceps femoris, semimembranosus, semitendinosus, and adductor magnus muscles
Hemorrhoidal, inferior	Pudendal	Motor. Somatic sensory	Filaments	External anal sphincter; skin about anus
Hypogastric	Aortic plexus	Sympathetic	To pelvic plexus	Pelvic viscera
Hypoglossal (twelfth cranial)	Medulla oblongata	Motor	Filaments	Intrinsic and extrinsic muscles of tongue

TABLE OF NERVES—(Continued)

Name	Central Attachment	Components	Branches	Distribution
Iliohypogastric	First lumbar segment of cord (lumbar plexus)	Motor. Somatic sensory	Filaments	Muscles of anterior abdominal wall; skin of buttocks and anterior abdominal wall
Ilioinguinal	First lumbar segment of cord (lumbar plexus)	Motor. Somatic sensory	Anterior scrotal (labial). Filaments	Muscles of anterior abdominal wall; skin of anterior abdominal wall and scrotum (labium majus)
Infraorbital	Maxillary	Somatic sensory	Anterior and middle superior alveolar, inferior palpebral, external nasal, and superior labial	Upper teeth, mucosa of nasal floor, and skin of face
Infratrochlear	Nasociliary	Somatic sensory	Filaments	Skin of eyelids and root of nose
Intercostobrachial (intercostohumeral OT)	Second thoracic segment of cord (brachial plexus)	Somatic sensory	Filaments	Skin of axilla and medial aspect of arm
Intermedius (glossopalatine) (Wrisberg's OT)	Brain stem at inferior border of pons	Parasympathetic. Sensory (taste)	Greater superficial petrosal, chorda tympani, anas-	Glands of palate and nose, taste buds of anterior two-

			tomotic ramus with tympanic plexus, external superficial petrosal (inconstant)	third of tongue, submaxillary and sublingual salivary glands
Interosseous, dorsal, of forearm (posterior interosseous OT; BR)	Radial	Motor. Somatic sensory	Muscular and articular filaments	Extensor carpi radialis brevis, supinator, extensor digitorum communis, extensor digiti quinti proprius, extensor carpi ulnaris; wrist joint
Interosseous, volar, of forearm (anterior interosseous OT; BR)	Median	Motor. Somatic sensory	Muscular and articular filaments	Flexor pollicis longus, flexor digitorum profundus, pronator quadratus; wrist joint
Jugular	Communicating branch of superior cervical ganglion to vagus			
Labial, inferior	Inferior alveolar	Somatic sensory	Filaments	Skin of lower lip
Labial, superior	Infraorbital	Somatic sensory	Filaments	Skin of upper lip and cheek
Lacrimal	Ophthalmic	Somatic sensory	Filaments	Skin of region of lateral commissure of eye

TABLE OF NERVES—(Continued)

Name	Central Attachment	Components	Branches	Distribution
Laryngeal, external [BR]	External branch of superior laryngeal nerve			
Laryngeal, inferior	Recurrent laryngeal	Motor	Filaments	Intrinsic muscles of larynx
Laryngeal, internal [BR]	Internal branch of superior laryngeal nerve			
Laryngeal, recurrent	Vagus	Motor. Parasympathetic	Inferior laryngeal, cardiac, and muscular	Intrinsic muscles of larynx, inferior constrictor of pharynx, trachea, and esophagus
Laryngeal, superior	Vagus	Motor. Visceral sensory	External and internal laryngeal branches	Cricothyroid and inferior constrictor of pharynx, mucosa of larynx, and base of tongue
Lingual	Mandibular	Somatic sensory	Filaments	Mucosa of floor of mouth and anterior two-thirds of tongue
Lumbar (5 pairs)	Lumbar segments of cord	Motor. Somatic sen-	Anterior and posterior divisions	Posterior divisions to muscles and skin

		sory. visceral sensory. Sympathetic (upper segments only)		of lower back, anterior divisions, lumbar plexus, to muscles and skin of lower abdomen and lower extremity, pelvic viscera, and genitalia
Lumboinguinal	Genitofemoral	Somatic sensory	Filaments	Skin of anterior aspect of thigh
Malar [OT]	See Zygomaticofacial			
Mandibular	Trigeminal	Motor (masticator n.). Somatic sensory	Spinosus, internal pterygoid, auriculotemporal, lingual, inferior alveolar, and branches to external pterygoid, temporal, and masseter muscles	Tensor tympani, tensor veli palatini, mylohyoid, anterior belly of digastric, and muscles of mastication; lower teeth, mucosa of anterior two-thirds of the tongue, floor of mouth, cheek and skin of lower portion of face, meninges
Masticator	Motor portion of trigeminal nerve			
Maxillary	Trigeminal	Somatic sensory	Middle meningeal, posterior superior alveolar, zygomatic, and infraorbital	Meninges, skin of upper portion of face, upper teeth, and mucosa of nose, palate, and cheeks

TABLE OF NERVES—(Continued)

Name	Central Attachment	Components	Branches	Distribution
Median	Fifth to eighth cervical and first thoracic segments of cord (brachial plexus)	Motor. Somatic sensory	Articular, muscular, and volar interosseous	Pronator teres, flexor carpi radialis, palmaris longus, flexor digitorum sublimis, flexor digitorum profundus, small muscles of thumb, two lateral lumbricals; skin of palm, hand, and fingers; elbow, wrist, and hand joints
Meningeal	Vagus	Somatic sensory	Filaments	Meninges
Meningeal, middle (recurrent OT)	Maxillary	Somatic sensory	Filaments	Meninges
Mental	Inferior alveolar	Somatic sensory	Filaments	Skin of lower lip and chin
Musculocutaneous (of lower extremity) [OT; BR]	See *Peroneal, superficial*			
Musculocutaneous (of upper extremity)	Fourth, fifth, and sixth cervical seg-	Motor. Somatic sen-	Lateral cutaneous of forearm, mus-	Coracobrachial, biceps brachii, and

	(brachial plexus)			skin of lateral aspect of forearm
Musculospiral [OT]	See *Radial*			
Mylohyoid, N. to	Inferior alveolar	Motor	Filaments	Mylohyoid and anterior belly of digastric muscles
Nasal, external	Infraorbital	Somatic sensory	Filaments	Skin of side of nose
Nasal, external (anterior nasal OT)	Nasociliary	Somatic sensory	Filaments	Skin of lower half and tip of nose
Nasal, lateral	Nasociliary	Somatic sensory	Filaments	Mucosa of lateral wall of nasal cavity
Nasal, medial	Nasociliary	Somatic sensory	Filaments	Mucosa of nasal septum
Nasal, posterior inferior lateral	Great palatine	Somatic sensory	Filaments	Mucosa of inferior nasal concha
Nasal, posterior superior lateral (short spheno-palatine BR)	Maxillary via sphenopalatine ganglion	Somatic sensory	Filaments	Mucosa of superior and middle nasal conchae
Nasociliary (nasal OT)	Ophthalmic	Somatic sensory	Anterior and posterior ethmoidal, infratrochlear, medial nasal, lateral nasal, external nasal, long and short ciliary	Eyeball, skin and mucosa of eyelids and nose, mucosa of ethmoidal and sphenoidal air cells

TABLE OF NERVES—(Continued)

Name	Central Attachment	Components	Branches	Distribution
Nasopalatine (long sphenopalatine BR)	Maxillary via sphenopalatine ganglion	Somatic sensory	Posterior superior medial nasal rami	Mucosa of nose and hard palate
Obturator	Second, third, and fourth lumbar segments of cord (lumbar plexus)	Motor. Somatic sensory	Muscular, cutaneous, and articular filaments	Obturator externus, gracilis, adductor brevis, adductor longus, adductor magnus muscles; skin of medial aspect of thigh; knee and hip joints
Obturator, accessory (variable)	Second, third, and fourth lumbar segments of cord (lumbar plexus)	Motor. Somatic sensory	Muscular and cutaneous filaments	Pectineus muscle, reinforces obturator n.
Obturator Internus, N. to	Fifth lumbar, first and second sacral segments of cord (sacral plexus)	Motor. Somatic sensory	Filaments	Obturator internus and superior gemellus muscles; sacro-iliac joint
Occipital, greater	Second cervical segment of cord	Somatic sensory	Filaments	Skin of posterior portion of scalp
Occipital, lesser	Second and third cervical segments of cord (cervical plexus)	Somatic sensory	Filaments	Skin of posterior portion of scalp and posterior aspect of auricle

Occipital, third (occipital minimus OT)	Third cervical segment of cord	Somatic sensory	Filaments	Skin of posterior aspect of neck and scalp
Oculomotor (third cranial)	Brain stem in region of posterior perforated substance	Motor. Parasympathetic	Muscular, root to ciliary ganglion	Levator palpebrae superioris, medial rectus, inferior rectus, superior rectus, inferior oblique muscles; ciliary and sphincter pupillae muscles
Olfactory (first cranial)	Olfactory bulb	Sensory (smell)	Filaments	Olfactory mucosa
Ophthalmic	Trigeminal	Somatic sensory	Tentorii, lacrimal, supratrochlear, frontal, nasociliary, communicating to oculomotor, trochlear, and abducens	Skin of forehead, upper eyelids, and anterior portion of scalp; orbit and eyeball; meninges; mucosa of nose, frontal, ethmoidal, and sphenoidal air sinuses
Optic (second cranial)	Optic tracts	Sensory (sight)	Filaments	Retina
Orbital	Maxillary via sphenopalatine ganglion	Somatic sensory	Filaments	Orbit
Orbital [OT]	See *Zygomatic*			
Palatine, anterior (great palatine BR) (large posterior palatine OT)	Maxillary via sphenopalatine ganglion	Somatic sensory	Filaments	Mucosa of hard and soft palates

TABLE OF NERVES—(Continued)

Name	Central Attachment	Components	Branches	Distribution
Palatine, middle (external) (lesser palatine BR) (accessory posterior palatine OT)	Maxillary via sphenopalatine ganglion	Somatic sensory	Filaments	Mucosa of soft palate, uvula, and palatine tonsil
Palatine, posterior (lesser palatine BR) (small posterior palatine OT)	Maxillary via sphenopalatine ganglion	Somatic sensory	Filaments	Mucosa of soft palate, uvula, and palatine tonsil
Palpebral, inferior	Infraorbital	Somatic sensory	Filaments	Lower eyelid
Palpebral, superior	Lacrimal, frontal, and nasociliary	Somatic sensory	Filaments	Upper eyelid
Pathetic [OT]	See *Trochlear*			
Perineal	Pudendal	Somatic sensory	Filaments	Skin of root of penis and scrotum (labium majus)
Peroneal, anastomotic (communicating fibular OT)	Common peroneal	Somatic sensory	Filaments; fibers may unite with fibers of medial cutaneous of leg	Skin of lateral aspect of leg, heel, and ankle
Peroneal, common (lateral popliteal BR) (external popliteal OT)	Fourth and fifth lumbar, first and second sacral seg-	Motor. Somatic sensory	Articular, muscular, lateral cutaneous of leg, peroneal anas-	Short head of biceps femoris, knee joint

	...ments of cord (sacral plexus)			tomotic, recurrent peroneal, deep peroneal, and superficial peroneal
Peroneal, deep (anterior tibial OT; BR)	Common peroneal	Motor. Somatic sensory	Muscular, articular, and cutaneous filaments	Tibialis anterior, extensor hallucis longus, extensor digitorum longus and brevis, and peroneus tertius muscles; skin of region between first and second toes; ankle joint and joints of feet
Peroneal, superficial (musculocutaneous OT; BR)	Common peroneal	Motor. Somatic sensory	Muscular and cutaneous filaments	Peroneus longus and peroneus brevis; skin of lower lateral aspect of leg and dorsum of foot
Petrosal, deep	Plexus on internal carotid artery	Sympathetic	N. of pterygoid canal	Along palatine branches of sphenopalatine ganglion
Petrosal, external superficial (inconstant)	Geniculate ganglion	Not known	Filaments	To plexus on middle meningeal artery
Petrosal, greater superficial	Geniculate ganglion	Visceral sensory. Parasympathetic	N. of pterygoid canal and on to sphenopalatine ganglion	Mucosa and glands of palate

TABLE OF NERVES—(Continued)

Name	Central Attachment	Components	Branches	Distribution
Petrosal, lesser superficial	Formed by union of anastomotic ramus from geniculate ganglion and tympanic branch of glossopharyngeal	Parasympathetic	To otic ganglion	Parotid gland
Petrosal, small deep [OT]	See *Caroticotympanic*			
Pharyngeal	Glossopharyngeal	Visceral sensory	Filaments	Mucosa of pharynx
Pharyngeal	Maxillary via sphenopalatine ganglion	Somatic sensory	Filaments	Mucosa of pharynx
Phrenic	Third, fourth, and fifth cervical (cervical plexus)	Motor	Filaments	Diaphragm
Piriformis, N. to	Fourth and fifth lumbar and first sacral segments of cord (sacral plexus)	Motor	Filaments	Piriformis
Plantar, lateral	Tibial	Motor. Somatic sensory	Muscular, cutaneous, and articular filaments	Quadratus plantae, adductor hallucis, small muscles of

				...ous soc, interossei, and lateral three lumbrical muscles of foot; skin of lateral aspect of sole; tarsal and metatarsal joints
Plantar, medial	Tibial	Motor. Somatic sensory	Muscular, cutaneous, and articular filaments	Abductor hallucis, flexor digitorum brevis, flexor hallucis brevis, and first lumbrical of foot; skin of medial aspect of sole; tarsal and metatarsal joints
Pneumogastric [OT]	See *Vagus*			
Popliteal, lateral [BR]	See *Peroneal, common*			
Popliteal, medial [BR]	See *Tibial*			
Pterygoid, external	Mandibular	Motor. Somatic sensory	Filaments	External pterygoid muscle; temporo-mandibular joint
Pterygoid, internal	Mandibular	Motor	Filaments	Internal pterygoid, tensor tympani, and tensor veli palatini muscles
Pterygoid canal, N. of (N. of Vidius OT)	Formed by union of greater superficial and deep petrosal nerves	Parasympathetic. Sympathetic	Filaments along branches of spheno-palatine ganglion	Glands of palate and nose

TABLE OF NERVES—(Continued)

Name	Central Attachment	Components	Branches	Distribution
Pudendal (pudic OT)	Second, third, and fourth sacral segments of cord (sacral plexus)	Motor. Somatic sensory	Inferior hemorrhoidal, perineal, and dorsal nn. of penis (clitoris)	Muscles and skin of perineal region
Quadratus femoris, N. to	Fourth and fifth lumbar and first sacral segments of cord (sacral plexus)	Motor. Somatic sensory	Filaments	Quadratus femoris and inferior gemellus; hip joint
Radial (musculospiral OT)	Fifth, sixth, seventh, and eighth cervical segments of cord (brachial plexus)	Motor. Somatic sensory	Muscular, superficial branch (radial OT), deep branch (posterior interosseous OT), dorsal interosseous, digital and articular	Triceps brachii, anconeus, extensor muscles of forearm, brachioradialis; skin of posterior aspect of arm and dorsal aspect of forearm and hand; elbow, carpal and hand joints
Recurrent	See *Laryngeal, recurrent*			
Recurrent [OT]	See *Spinosus*			
Recurrent [OT]	See *Tentorii*			
Rhomboids, N. to [OT; BR]	See *Scapular, dorsal*			

Saccular	Vestibular root of acoustic	Sensory (position of head in space—static)	Filaments	Macula acustica of saccule
Sacral (5 pairs)	Sacral segments of cord	Motor. Somatic sensory. Parasympathetic. Visceral sensory	Anterior and posterior divisions	Posterior divisions to muscles and skin of lower back and sacral region; anterior divisions to sacral plexus supplying muscles and skin of lower extremity and perineum; branches to hypogastric and pelvic plexuses supplying pelvic viscera and genitalia
Saphenous	Femoral	Somatic sensory	Filaments	Skin of medial aspect of leg and foot
Scapular, dorsal (N. to rhomboids OT; BR) (posterior scapular OT)	Fifth cervical segment of cord (brachial plexus)	Motor	Filaments	Levator scapulae, rhomboideus major, and rhomboideus minor
Sciatic	Fourth and fifth lumbar; first, second, and third sacral segments of cord (sacral plexus)	Composed of tibial, common peroneal, and n. to hamstrings, q.v.		
Sciatic, small [OT]	See *Cutaneous, posterior, of thigh*			

TABLE OF NERVES—(Continued)

Name	Central Attachment	Components	Branches	Distribution
Scrotal, anterior (labial)	Ilioinguinal	Somatic sensory	Filaments	Skin of pubic area and scrotum (labium majus)
Scrotal, posterior (labial)	Perineal	Somatic sensory	Filaments	Skin of posterior portion of scrotum (labium majus)
Spermatic, external	Genitofemoral	Somatic sensory	Filaments	Skin of scrotum (labium majus) and thigh near superficial inguinal ring
Sphenopalatine	Maxillary	Somatic sensory	Nasal and palatine branches of sphenopalatine ganglion	Via sphenopalatine ganglion and palatine nerves to nose and palate
Sphenopalatine, long [BR]	See *Nasopalatine*			
Sphenopalatine, short [BR]	See *Nasal, posterior superior lateral*			
Spinal (31 pairs)	See *Cervical, Thoracic, Lumbar, Sacral,* and *Coccygeal*			
Spinal accessory [OT]	See *Accessory*			

		Somatic sensory	Filaments	
Spinosus (recurrent OT)	Mandibular	Somatic sensory	Filaments	Meninges and mucosa of mastoid air cells
Splanchnic, greater	Fifth to ninth or tenth sympathetic ganglions	Sympathetic. Visceral sensory	Filaments	Cardiac, pulmonary, esophageal, and celiac plexuses
Splanchnic, lesser	Ninth and tenth sympathetic ganglions	Sympathetic. Visceral sensory	Filaments	Celiac plexus
Splanchnic, lowest	Last thoracic sympathetic ganglion	Sympathetic. Visceral sensory	Filaments	Renal plexus
Stapedius, N. to	Facial	Motor	Filaments	Stapedius muscle
Subclavius, N. to	Fourth, fifth, and sixth cervical (brachial plexus)	Motor	Filaments	Subclavius muscle
Subcostal [BR]	Anterior ramus of twelfth thoracic nerve			
Suboccipital [OT]	See *Cervical, first*			
Subscapular	Fifth and sixth cervical segments of cord (brachial plexus)	Motor	Filaments	Subscapularis and teres major muscles
Supraacromial [OT]	See *Supraclavicular, posterior*			

TABLE OF NERVES—(Continued)

NAME	CENTRAL ATTACHMENT	COMPONENTS	BRANCHES	DISTRIBUTION
Supraclavicular, anterior (medial supraclavicular BR) (suprasternal OT)	Third and fourth cervical segments of cord (cervical plexus)	Somatic sensory	Filaments	Skin of lower anterior aspect of neck and anterior chest wall; sternoclavicular joint
Supraclavicular, middle (intermediate supraclavicular BR) (supraclavicular OT)	Third and fourth cervical segments of cord (cervical plexus)	Somatic sensory	Filaments	Skin of lower anterior aspect of neck and anterior chest wall
Supraclavicular, posterior (lateral supraclavicular BR) (supraacromial OT)	Third and fourth cervical segments of cord (cervical plexus)	Somatic sensory	Filaments	Skin of lateral aspect of neck and shoulder
Supraorbital	Frontal	Somatic sensory	Filaments	Skin of upper eyelid and forehead, mucosa of frontal sinus
Suprascapular	Fourth, fifth, and sixth cervical segments of cord (brachial plexus)	Motor. Somatic sensory	Muscular and articular filaments	Supraspinatus and infraspinatus muscles; shoulder and acromioclavicular joints
Suprasternal [OT]	See *Supraclavicular, anterior*			
Supratrochlear	Frontal	Somatic sensory	Filaments	Skin of medial aspect of forehead,

				upper eyelid
Sural [BR]	Formed by union of medial sural and anastomotic ramus of common peroneal			
Sural, lateral (lateral cutaneous n. of calf or leg)	Common peroneal	Somatic sensory	Filaments	Skin of lateral aspect of leg
Sural, medial (tibial communicating OT)	Tibial	Somatic sensory	Cutaneous and articular filaments	Skin of back of leg; ankle and tarsal joints
Temporomalar [OT]	See Zygomatic			
Tentorii (recurrent OT)	Ophthalmic	Somatic sensory	Filaments	Meninges
Terminalis	Medial olfactory tract	Not known	Filaments associated with olfactory n.	Not known
Thoracic (12 pairs)	Thoracic segments of cord	Motor. Somatic sensory. Visceral sensory. Sympathetic	Anterior and posterior divisions	Posterior divisions to muscles and skin of back; anterior divisions to brachial plexus (muscles and skin of upper extremity) and muscles and skin of abdominal wall; sympathetic fibers and visceral sensory fibers for various viscera and blood vessels

TABLE OF NERVES—(Continued)

Name	Central Attachment	Components	Branches	Distribution
Thoracic, lateral anterior (lateral pectoral BR) (external anterior thoracic OT)	Fifth, sixth, and seventh cervical segments of cord (brachial plexus)	Motor	Filaments	Pectoralis major and minor muscles
Thoracic, long (N. to serratus anterior BR) (posterior thoracic OT) (N. of Bell OT)	Fifth, sixth, and seventh cervical segments of cord (brachial plexus)	Motor	Filaments	Serratus anterior muscle
Thoracic, medial anterior (medial pectoral BR) (internal anterior thoracic OT)	Eighth cervical and first thoracic segments of cord (brachial plexus)	Motor	Filaments	Pectoralis major and minor muscles
Thoracodorsal (long subscapular OT)	Sixth, seventh, and eighth cervical segments of cord (brachial plexus)	Motor	Filaments	Latissimus dorsi muscle
Tibial (internal popliteal OT) (medial popliteal BR)	Fourth and fifth lumbar and first, second, and third sacral segments of cord (sacral plexus)	Motor. Somatic sensory	Muscular, articular, medial sural, medial, and lateral plantar	Muscles of back of leg and sole of foot; skin of back of leg and foot; knee and ankle joints
Tibial, posterior [BR]	Posterior branch of tibial			

Tibial, recurrent	Common peroneal		Muscular and articular filaments	Tibialis anterior muscle; knee and proximal tibiofibular joints
Trigeminal (fifth cranial)	Brain stem at inferior surface of pons. See *Ophthalmic, Maxillary,* and *Mandibular*	Motor. Somatic sensory		
Trochlear (fourth cranial) (pathetic OT)	Dorsal surface of midbrain	Motor	Filaments	Superior oblique muscle of eyeball
Tympanic (N. of Jacobson OT)	Glossopharyngeal	Visceral sensory. Parasympathetic	Tympanic plexus	Mucosa of middle ear, mastoid air cells and auditory tube; filaments to otic ganglion and on to parotid gland
Ulnar	Eighth cervical and first thoracic segments of cord (brachial plexus)	Motor. Somatic sensory	Muscular, articular, and cutaneous filaments	Flexor carpi ulnaris, flexor digitorum profundus, adductor pollicis, muscles of hypothenar eminence, interossei and medial two lumbricals of hand; skin of medial portion of hand; elbow, wrist, carpal, and metacarpal joints
Ulnar, collateral (inconstant)	Radial	Proprioceptive	Filaments	Brachialis muscle

TABLE OF NERVES—(Continued)

Name	Central Attachment	Components	Branches	Distribution
Utricular	Vestibular	Sensory (position of head in space—static)	Filaments	Macula acustica of utricle
Vagus (tenth cranial) (pneumogastric OT)	Lateral aspect of medulla oblongata	Motor	Pharyngeal and laryngeal	Striate muscles of pharynx and larynx
		Parasympathetic	Cardiac, esophageal, and abdominal	Cardiac musculature, smooth muscle of thoracic and abdominal viscera
		Somatic sensory	Auricular (N. of Arnold OT), meningeal	Skin of external auditory meatus, meninges
		Visceral sensory	Pharyngeal, laryngeal, thoracic, and abdominal branches	Mucosa of pharynx, larynx, thoracic and abdominal viscera

Vestibular (part of eighth cranial)	Brain stem near restiform body	Sensory (movement and position of head in space—dynamic and static)	Utricular, ampullary, and saccular	Ampullae of semicircular canals and maculae acusticae of utricle and saccule
Vidius, N. of [OT]	See *Pterygoid canal, N. of*			
Wrisberg's [OT]	See *Intermedius*			
Zygomatic (temporomalar or orbital OT)	Maxillary	Somatic sensory	Zygomaticofacial and zygomaticotemporal	Skin in region of zygoma and temple
Zygomaticofacial (malar OT)	Zygomatic	Somatic sensory	Filaments	Skin over zygoma
Zygomaticotemporal (temporal OT)	Zygomatic	Somatic sensory	Filaments	Skin over anterior portion of temple

TABLE OF VEINS

The following list includes only those veins and venous sinuses and plexuses which have no accompanying artery of the same name, or which differ considerably from an accompanying artery. For all other veins—as, for example, the deep veins of the upper or lower extremity, or of the body wall—see the Table of Arteries for the accompanying artery of the same name; these veins have tributaries with the same distribution as the branches of the accompanying arteries.

NAME OF VEIN	REGION OR TRIBUTARY DRAINED	LOCATION	DRAINS INTO:
Accessory hemiazygos (v. hemiazygos accessoria BNA)	Three or four upper left intercostal spaces	Left side of vertebral column	Either azygos or hemiazygos
Anterior facial (v. facialis anterior BNA)	Continuation of angular vein	Anterior side of face	Joins with posterior facial to form common facial
Anterior jugular (v. jugularis anterior BNA)	Anterior part of neck	Near midline of neck	External jugular or subclavian
Azygos (v. azygos BNA)	Right chest wall; begins from ascending lumbar vein	Right side of vertebral column	Superior vena cava
Basilar plexus (plexus basilaris BNA)	Both inferior petrosal sinuses	Basilar part of occipital bone	Anterior part of vertebral plexus
Basilic (v. basilica BNA)	Ulnar side of hand and forearm	Medial side of biceps muscle	Joins the brachial to form the axillary
Basivertebral (vv. basivertebrales BNA)	Bodies of vertebrae	Bodies of vertebrae	External and internal vertebral plexuses
Cavernous sinus (sinus cavernosus BNA)	Superior ophthalmic	Lateral to sella turcica	Superior and inferior petrosal sinuses

Cephalic (v. cephalica BNA)	Radial side of hand and forearm	Lateral side of arm	Axillary
Common facial (v. facialis communis BNA)	Formed by junction of anterior and posterior facial veins	Below angle of mandible	Internal jugular
Coronary sinus (sinus coronarius BNA)	Most of the veins of the heart	Posterior part of coronary sulcus	Right atrium
Coronary v. of stomach (v. coronaria ventriculi BNA)	Both surfaces of stomach	Lesser curvature of stomach	Portal
Diploic veins (vv. diploicae BNA)	Diploë of cranium	Inside cranial bones	Either internally into the sinuses or externally into veins like the occipital or supraorbital
Emissary veins	Venous sinuses inside cranial cavity, such as the transverse sinus	Apertures in skull, named as follows according to location: condyloid, mastoid, occipital, parietal, and postcondyloid	Veins external to the skull, as the posterior auricular or occipital
External Jugular (v. jugularis externa BNA)	Posterior auricular and posterior division of posterior facial	Side of neck	Subclavian
External vertebral plexus (plexus venosi vertebrales externi BNA)	Vertebrae and surrounding muscles	Anterior and posterior to vertebral column	Basivertebral and intervertebral veins
Great cardiac (v. cordis magna BNA)	Anterior side of ventricles	Anterior longitudinal sulcus of heart	Coronary sinus

TABLE OF VEINS—(Continued)

Name of Vein	Region or Tributary Drained	Location.	Drains into:
Great cerebral (great v. of Galen) (v. cerebri magna [Galeni] BNA)	Internal cerebral veins	Below and behind splenium of. corpus callosum	Straight sinus
Great saphenous (v. saphena magna BNA)	Medial side of leg and thigh	Medial side of leg and thigh	Femoral
Hemiazygos (v. hemiazygos BNA)	Left ascending lumbar	Left side of vertebral column	Azygos
Hemorrhoidal plexus (plexus haemorrhoidalis BNA)	Rectum	Rectum, submucosa, and external to muscular coat	Superior, middle, and inferior hemorrhoidal veins
Hepatic	Substance of the liver	Converge at posterior surface of liver	Inferior vena cava
Inferior ophthalmic (v. ophthalmica inferior BNA)	Lower part of orbit	Floor of orbit	Pterygoid plexus and cavernous sinus
Inferior petrosal sinus (sinus petrosus inferior BNA)	Cavernous sinus	Inferior petrosal sulcus	Internal jugular
Inferior sagittal sinus (sinus sagittalis inferior BNA)	Falx cerebri	Lower edge of falx cerebri	Straight sinus
Inferior vena cava (vena cava inferior BNA)	Common iliac veins, blood from lower extremities and abdomen	Front of vertebral column, right of aorta	Right atrium

Innominate (vv. anonymae dextra et sinistra BNA)	Internal jugular and subclavian	Root of neck	Superior vena cava
Intercavernous sinuses (anterior and posterior) (sinus intercavernosus anterior et posterior BNA)	Connect the two cavernous sinuses		
Internal cerebral (vv. cerebri internae BNA)	Terminal and choroid veins	Beneath splenium of corpus callosum	Great cerebral
Internal jugular (v. jugularis interna BNA)	Brain, face, and neck; transverse sinus	Side of neck	Innominate
Internal vertebral plexus (plexus venosi vertebrales interni BNA)	Vertebrae and meninges	Within the vertebral canal anterior and posterior to the spinal cord	Intervertebral veins
Middle cardiac (v. cordis media BNA)	Posterior side of heart	Posterior longitudinal sulcus of heart	Coronary sinus
Oblique v. of left atrium (oblique v. of Marshall OT) (v. obliqua atrii sinistri BNA)	Left atrium	Back of left atrium	Coronary sinus
Occipital sinus (sinus occipitalis BNA)	Region around foramen magnum	Attached margin of falx cerebelli	Confluence of the sinuses
Parumbilical (vv. parumbilicales [Sappeyi] BNA)	Commences at umbilicus	Round ligament of liver	Portal
Portal (v. portae BNA)	Superior mesenteric and lienal veins	Lesser omentum	Sinusoids of liver
Posterior facial (v. facialis posterior BNA)	Superficial temporal and internal maxillary veins	In parotid gland	Common facial and external jugular veins

TABLE OF VEINS—(Continued)

Name of Vein	Region or Tributary Drained	Location	Drains into:
Posterior v. of left ventricle (v. posterior ventriculi sinistri BNA)	Left ventricle	Diaphragmatic surface of left ventricle of heart	Coronary sinus
Prostatic plexus (plexus prostaticus BNA)	Prostatic veins	Fascial sheath of prostate gland	Pudendal and vesical plexuses
Pterygoid plexus (plexus pterygoideus BNA)	Veins corresponding to branches of internal maxillary artery	Between pterygoid muscles	Internal maxillary
Pudendal plexus (plexus pudendalis BNA)	Deep dorsal vein of penis	Behind symphysis pubis, in front of bladder	Vesical and hypogastric veins
Pyloric (v. coronaria ventriculi BNA)	Stomach	Lesser curvature of stomach	Portal
Sigmoid sinus (sinus transversus BNA)	Transverse sinus	Groove on posterior surface of temporal bone	Internal jugular
Small cardiac (v. cordis parva BNA)	Back of right atrium and ventricle	Coronary sulcus	Coronary sinus
Small saphenous (v. saphena parva BNA)	Leg and foot	Back of leg	Popliteal
Straight sinus (sinus rectus BNA)	Inferior sagittal sinus and great cerebral vein	Junction of falx cerebri with tentorium cerebelli	Transverse sinus

Superior ophthalmic (v. ophthalmica superior BNA)	Tributaries corresponding to branches of ophthalmic artery	Orbit	Cavernous sinus
Superior petrosal sinus (sinus petrosus superior BNA)	Cavernous sinus	Superior petrosal sulcus of temporal	Transverse sinus
Superior sagittal sinus (sinus sagittalis superior BNA)	Superior cerebral veins, diploic veins, and dura mater	Attached margin of falx cerebri	Confluence of the sinuses or transverse sinus
Superior vena cava (vena cava superior BNA)	Head, chest wall, and upper extremities; is formed by junction of two innominate veins	Behind first and second intercostal spaces and right margin of sternum	Right atrium
Transverse sinus (sinus transversus BNA)	The right one is usually continuation of the superior sagittal sinus, the left of the straight sinus	Attached margin of tentorium cerebelli	Internal jugular; the terminal portion is often called the sigmoid sinus
Vesical plexus (plexus vesicalis BNA)	Pudendal and prostatic plexuses	Lower part of bladder and base of prostate gland	Hypogastric
Vorticose (venae vorticosae BNA)	Veins of eyeball	Eyeball	Ciliary and superior ophthalmic veins

TABLE OF NORMAL VALUES OF BLOOD CONSTITUENTS

All Values Expressed in mg. per 100 cc. of Whole Blood Unless Otherwise Stated. Figures Represent Weighted Averages of the Observations of Several Investigators

Acetone bodies, total (as acetone)	0.5–1.0
Albumin (serum)	4–5 Gm. %
Amino acids (as amino acid N)	5.0–8.0
Amylase (serum or plasma)	70–200 Somogyi units
Ascorbic acid (reduced)	0.6–2.5
Base, total (serum)	150–160 mEq./l.
Bilirubin (serum)	0.1–0.5
Bromides (as sodium bromide)	0.2–1.5
Calcium, total (serum)	9–11
Carbon dioxide combining power (plasma)	4.5–5.5 mEq./l.
	55–75 vol. %
Carbon dioxide content (arterial)	45–55 vol. %
Carbon dioxide content (venous)	50–60 vol. %
	22–27 mEq./l.
Carotene (plasma or serum)	0.1
Chlorides (as chloride ion) (plasma or serum)	350–380
	97–106 mEq./l.
Chlorides (as sodium chloride) (plasma or serum)	570–620
Cholesterol, total (plasma or serum)	150–250
Cholesterol esters	60–75% of total cholesterol
Creatine	3–7
Creatinine	1–2
Fat, neutral (serum)	0–370
Fatty acids	190–450
Fibrinogen (plasma)	0.2–0.4 Gm. %
Globulin (serum)	1.5–3 Gm. %
Glucose	70–120
Guanidine	0.1–0.4
Hemoglobin	
For children	13 ± 1 Gm. %
For men	16 ± 2 Gm. %
For women	14 ± 2 Gm. %

Hydrogen-ion concentration	pH 7.3–7.5
Icterus index (serum)	4–6 units
Iodine (total)	3–13 micrograms %
Iron, inorganic (serum)	0.05–0.18
Lactic acid	5–20
Lipase (serum) in terms of N/20 NaOH used per cc. of serum	0.2–1 cc.
Lipids, total (serum)	400–800
Magnesium (serum)	1–3
Nitrogen, nonprotein	25–35
Nitrogen, undetermined	4–18
Oxygen capacity	16–24 vol. %
Oxygen content (arterial)	15–23 vol. %
Oxygen content (venous)	10–18 vol. %
Phenols (free)	1–2
Phosphatase (acid)	0.1–1.1 Bodansky units
Phosphatase (alkaline)	
For adults	1–5.4 Bodansky units
For children	5–12 Bodansky units
Phospholipid (serum) (as lecithin)	150–300
Phosphorus (serum), inorganic	
For adults	2.5–4.0
For children	3.5–6.0
Potassium (serum)	16–22
	4–6 mEq./l.
Proteins (serum)	6–8 Gm. %
Sodium (serum)	310–335
	135–145 mEq./l.
Solids, total	19–23%
Specific gravity	1.055
Specific gravity (plasma)	1.052–1.063
Sugar (see *Glucose*)	
Sulfates, inorganic as S (serum)	0.9–1.5
Urea	17–32
Urea nitrogen	8–15
Uric acid	2–4
Water content	77–81%

DIET TABLES

Guide for a Calorie-restricted Diet*†

100-Calorie Portions of Food	
Apple	1 large
Asparagus	20 medium tips
Bacon	3 strips, lean
Beans, string	2½ cups (1-in. pieces)
Beef, lean	2⅓ oz., uncooked
Berries	1⅛ cups
Bread, white	1⅓ oz.
Bread, whole-wheat	1⅓ oz.
Butter	1 tbsp.
Cabbage	¾ lb. (5 cups, shredded)
Cantaloupe	1 medium-sized
Carrots	3–4 medium-sized
Cauliflower	Half a medium-sized head
Celery	4 cups ¼-in. pieces (about 1 lb.)
Chicken, lean	2½ oz., cooked
Cocoa	2 tbsp.
Codfish	5 oz., uncooked
Cottage cheese	5–6 tbsp.
Crackers, soda	5–6
Cucumbers	3 small (1¼ lb.)
Eggs	1⅓ small or 1 large
Figs	2 medium-sized
Grapes	1 bunch (about 4 oz.)
Halibut	3 by 2 by 2 in. (small serving)
Lettuce	2 large heads (1¼ lb.)
Milk, skim	1¼ cups
Milk, whole	⅝ cup (1 qt. contains about 700 cal.)
Oatmeal, uncooked	4 tbsp.

Onions	3–4 medium-sized
Orange	1 large juicy
Oysters	12–14
Peaches, canned	2 large halves plus 3 tbsp. of juice
Peaches, fresh	3 medium-sized
Pears	$1\frac{1}{2}$
Pineapple, canned	1 slice plus 3 tbsp. of juice
Pineapple, fresh	2 slices 1 in. thick
Potatoes	4 oz, raw
Raisins	37
Rhubarb	4 cups (1-in. pieces)
Spinach	$2\frac{1}{2}$ cups, cooked
Steak, round	$1\frac{1}{2}$ oz. (2.5 by 1 by 1 in.)
Sugar	2 tbsp.
Tomatoes	$1\frac{3}{4}$ cups, cooked (2 medium-sized)
Turnips	$\frac{1}{2}$ lb., raw (2 cups $\frac{1}{2}$-in. cubes)

STANDARD PORTIONS

1 serving of bacon	2 strips (20 Gm.)
1 serving of bread	1 slice, $\frac{1}{2}$ in. thick (30 Gm.)
1 serving of butter	1 "square" (10 Gm.)
1 serving of cereal	$\frac{2}{3}$ cup (20 Gm., dry; 140 Gm., cooked)
1 serving of fruit	2 heaping tbsp. (100 Gm.)
1 serving of meat	1 piece, 3 by 2 by $\frac{1}{2}$ in. (50 Gm.)
1 serving of milk	1 glass $\frac{4}{5}$ full (200 Gm.)
1 serving of soup	1 cup (200 Gm.)
1 serving of vegetables	2 heaping tbsp. (100 Gm.)

* From W. M. Yater's "Fundamentals of Internal Medicine," 3d ed., New York, Appleton-Century-Crofts, Inc.

† This table makes it easy to measure the comparative caloric values of various foods in various amounts.

DIET TABLES—(Continued)
Composition of Various Foods

	Average Composition of 100 Gm.		
	Carbohydrate Gm.	Protein Gm.	Fat Gm.
Vegetables and fruits:			
3 % vegetables	3	1	0
6 % vegetables	6	1	0
15 % vegetables	15	2	0
20 % vegetables:			
Green corn	20	3	1
Potato	20	2	0
Shelled beans	20	7	0
5 % fruits	5	1	0
10 % fruits	10	1	0
15 % fruits	15	1	0
20 % fruits	20	2	0
Green olives	2	1	10
Ripe olives	4	1	20
Cereals and breadstuffs:			
Breakfast cereals, dry	80	10	5
Breakfast cereals, cooked	11	1	0
White bread	53	9	2
Whole wheat bread	49	10	1
Rye bread	53	9	1
Wheat flour	76	8	1
Soda crackers	73	10	9
Soybeans	8	38	15
Dairy products:			
Whole milk	5	3	4
Skimmed milk	5	3	1
Cream, 20 % fat	5	3	20
Cream, 30 % fat	3	2	30
Cream, 40 % fat	3	2	40
Buttermilk	5	3	1
Cheese	0	29	38
Cottage cheese	4	21	1
Eggs, each	0	6	6
Dairy products—(Continued):			
Egg white (one)	0	3	0
Egg yolk (one)	0	3	6
Meats and fish:			
Meat, cooked	0	25	15
Fat meat, cooked	0	25	30
Liver	2	20	3
Fat bacon	0	10	67
Lean bacon	0	16	43
Cooked bacon	0	25	50
Fish (halibut, lake trout, perch, white fish)	0	18	5
Fish (salmon, fresh or canned)	0	22	13
Oysters	4	6	1
Fats:			
Butter	0	0	85
Lard, tallow, oleomargarine, crisco, bacon fat	0	0	85–100
Mayonnaise	0	0	85
Olive oil and other oils	0	0	100
Peanut butter	6	29	46
Nuts:			
Almonds	3	21	55
Beechnuts	13	22	57
Black walnuts	12	28	56
Brazil nuts	7	17	67
Butternuts	3	28	61
Chestnuts	42	6	5
English walnuts	16	17	63
Filberts	13	16	65
Hickory nuts	11	15	65
Peanuts	6	30	50
Pecans	13	11	71

Classification of Vegetables and Fruits According to Percentage of Carbohydrate Content*

VEGETABLES

5% Carbohydrate Av.
Asparagus
Beans, green or wax
Broccoli
Brussels sprouts
Cabbage
Cabbage, Chinese
Cauliflower
Celery
Chard or Swiss chard
Collards
Cucumbers
Eggplant
Endive
Escarole
Greens: beet, dandelion, mustard, or turnip greens
Kale or sea kale
Leeks
Lettuce
Okra
Olives, ripe or green
Onions, cooked
Peppers, green or red
Pickles, unsweetened, dill or sour
Radishes
Rhubarb
Sauerkraut
Spinach
Summer squash or cymlings
Tomatoes or tomato juice
Water cress

6% Carbohydrate Av.
Artichokes, globe or French
Beets
Carrots
Kohlrabi
Onions, raw
Oyster plant or salsify
Pumpkin
Rutabagas
Squash, winter or Hubbard
Turnips, white or yellow

15% Carbohydrate Av.
Artichokes, Jerusalem
Green peas
Parsnips

20% Carbohydrate Av.
Corn
Hominy, cooked
Lima beans, canned
Macaroni, boiled
Noodles, cooked
Potatoes
Rice, boiled
Shelled beans, cooked
Spaghetti, cooked

FRUITS

5% Carbohydrate Av. (canned without sugar)
Apricots
Blackberries
Cherries, red or white
Loganberries
Peaches
Raspberries
Rhubarb, fresh
Strawberries

10% Carbohydrate Av.
Blackberries, fresh
Cantaloupe, muskmelon, honeydew, Spanish melon
Cranberries
Gooseberries
Grapefruit or grapefruit juice
Lemons
Oranges or orange juice
Peaches, fresh
Pears, alligator or avocado
Pineapple, fresh
Strawberries, fresh
Tangerines or tangelos
Watermelon

* From W. M. Yater's "Fundamentals of Internal Medicine," 3d ed., New York, Appleton-Century-Crofts, Inc.

DIET TABLES—(Continued)

Classification of Vegetables and Fruits According to Percentage of Carbohydrate Content* (Cont.)

15% Carbohydrate Av.		20% Carbohydrate Av.
Apples	Currants	Bananas
Apricots, fresh	Loganberries, fresh	Grapes or grape juice
Blueberries or huckleberries	Nectarines	Plums
Cherries, sour	Pears	Prunes
	Raspberries, red or black, fresh	

High-vitamin Acid-ash Diet*

In cases of *renal calculi* and *infections* a high-vitamin, acid-ash diet is sometimes used in an attempt to dissolve the stones, prevent their secretion, and reduce infection by acidifying the urine.

Include in the daily diet the following foods:

Soups: Broths and cream soups of meats or allowed vegetables

Meats: All meats, poultry, fish, cheese—twice daily

Eggs: 1 or 2 daily

Fruits: Prunes, cranberries, and plums as desired

Watermelon, grapes, fresh pears, apples, and orange juice—not more than 2 servings daily

Vegetables: Corn (fresh or canned) as desired

Asparagus, green peas, onions, pumpkin, squash, turnips, and radishes—1 or 2 servings daily

If only 1 of the above group of vegetables is chosen, 1 of the following may be included: mushrooms, cauliflower, string beans, tomatoes, cabbage, tomato juice

Salads: Of the allowed fruits and vegetables

Bread: Soda crackers, whole wheat bread, white bread—at least 3 slices daily, and as many more as desired

Cereals: Wheat germ, oatmeal, corn meal, shredded wheat, macaroni, rice, noodles, spaghetti—at least 2 servings daily

Milk: 1 pint

Cream: 1/2 pint

Nuts: Walnuts, peanuts—as desired

Yeast: 2 cakes daily

Cod liver oil: 2 tsp. daily

Miscellaneous: Butter, sugar, cornstarch, tapioca, tea, coffee—as desired

Foods to be omitted:

Vegetables of all kinds except those listed.

Fruits of all kinds except those listed.

Evaporated or condensed milk.

Dried or fresh chestnuts, coconuts, almonds.

Olives, olive oil, and molasses.

For *oxalate calculi* foods containing oxalic acid should be avoided. These are mainly tea, coffee, cocoa, pepper, rhubarb, spinach, beetroot, beans, tomatoes, strawberries, cranberries, radishes, grapes, currants, and figs.

Standard Diabetic Diets for Adults*

	Diets for Women				Diets for Men				
	I	II	III	IV	I	II	III	IV	V
Vegetable, 3%	400	400	400	400	400	400	400	400	400
Fruit, 10%	300	300	300	300	300	300	300	300	300
Vegetable or fruit, 20%	100	100	100	100	100	100	100	100	150
Cereal		14		20		20	20	20	20
Bread	60	100	120	120	60	80	120	120	120
Cream, 20%	15	100	100	230	15	50	100	230	300
Milk	400	200	400	400	400	400	100	400	400
Bacon									
Eggs	1	1	1	1	2	2	2	2	2
Meat	100	100	100	100	100	100	125	125	125
Composition:				*Grams*					
Carbohydrate	115	141	162	174	115	143	167	174	187
Protein	57	59	67	72	63	69	80	84	90
Fat	41	52	60	86	47	56	70	96	116
Calories	1057	1268	1456	1758	1135	1352	1618	1896	2143
				Calories					
For calories required, add butter or equivalents (*Grams Butter*)									
30	1290								
40	1360	1570	1760	2060	1370	1660	1920	2200	2450
50	1440	1660	1840	2150	1440	1740	2010	2280	2530
60	1520	1730	1920	2220	1520	1810	2080	2360	2600
70		1810	2000	2300	1590	1890	2160	2440	2680
80									2760

* From W. M. Yater's "Fundamentals of Internal Medicine," 3d ed., New York, Appleton-Century-Crofts, Inc.

DIET TABLES—(Continued)

Low-calorie (1200 Calories) Reducing Diet**†

BREAKFAST

Food	Household Measure	Grams
Fruit, 10%........................	Large serving, 5 oz........	150
or Fruit, 15%.....................	Medium serving, 3 oz......	100
Egg.............................	1 medium-sized...........	50
or crisp bacon....................	2 thin strips.............	15
Milk, partially skimmed...........	1 glass.................	200
Bread, toasted if desired..........	1 thin slice.............	20
Coffee, if desired................	1 or 2 cups.............	..
Cream...........................	2 tbsp.................	30
or butter........................	½ square or 1 level tsp...	5
No sugar, saccharin, if desired.		

LUNCH

Clear broth, if desired............	1 cup (no food value)......	..
Cottage cheese...................	1 heaping tbsp..........	50
Vegetable, 3%....................	Generous serving, as ⅓ to ⅔ cup or 2 heaping tbsp..........................	100
	Or half this amount 6% vegetable.	
Vegetable, 3%....................	Generous serving, preferably as a salad........	100

Mayonnaise or French dressing made with mineral oil	As desired (no food value)	..
Lister's Golden Spread	As desired (no food value)	..
Butter	1 square or 2 level tsp	10
Bread	½ thin slice	10
Milk, partially skimmed, or buttermilk	1 glass	200
Fruit	Same choice as at breakfast	..
Coffee or tea, if desired.		

DINNER

Lean meat or fish	Generous serving (2½ oz.)	75
Vegetable, 6%	Generous serving, as ½ to ⅔ cup, or 2 heaping tbsp	100
Vegetable, 3%	Generous serving	100
Vegetable, 3%	Generous serving, preferably as a salad	100
Salad dressing made with mineral oil	As desired (no food value)	..
Lister's Golden Spread	As desired (no food value)	..
Butter	1 square or 2 level tsp	10
Bread	1 thin slice	20
Milk, partially skimmed	1 glass	200
Fruit, 10%	Same choice as at breakfast	..
Coffee or tea, if desired.		

*From W. M. Yater's "Fundamentals of Internal Medicine," 3d ed., New York, Appleton-Century-Crofts, Inc.

†Approximate food value of this diet: Carbohydrates, 121; protein, 68; fats, 50.

DIET TABLES—(Continued)

High-calorie (3000 Calories) Diet*†

BREAKFAST

Food	Household Measure	Grams
Fruit..	1 serving.............	100
Cereal (cooked).............................	⅔ cup...............	140
Bacon..	2 slices.............	10
Egg...	1...................	50
Bread (toast)................................	1 slice..............	30
Butter...	2 squares............	20
Sugar..	1 tbsp..............	15
Jam or jelly.................................	2 tbsp..............	30
Cream, 20%.................................	½ glass.............	100
Milk..	½ glass.............	100
Beverage—coffee, tea, or coffee substitute.		
10 A.M. Fruit juice........................	1 glass.............	200

LUNCH

Egg or substitute...........................	1 serving.............	50
Potato or substitute.......................	1 small serving......	75
Vegetable.....................................	1 serving.............	100

Salad:

Vegetable	1 serving	100
Salad dressing with oil	1 tbsp.	15
Bread	1 slice	30
Butter	2 squares	20
Cream, 20%	¼ glass	50
Milk	¾ glass	150
3 P.M. Fruit juice	1 glass	200

DINNER

Meat	1 serving	60
Potato	1 small serving	75
Vegetable	1 serving	100
Salad:		
Fruit	1 serving	100
Salad dressing with oil	1 tbsp.	15
Bread	1 slice	30
Butter	2 squares	20
Dessert	1 serving	100
Cream, 20%	¼ glass	50
Milk	¾ glass	150

*From W. M. Yater's "Fundamentals of Internal Medicine," 3d ed, New York, Appleton-Century-Crofts, Inc.

†This table represents a suggested distribution of the total food allowance for one day.

TABLE OF ELEMENTS

Name	Symbol	Atomic Weight *,†	Atomic Number
Actinium	Ac	[227]	89
Alabamine (now *astatine*)			
Aluminum	Al	26.98	13
Americium	Am	[243]	95
Antimony (*stibium*)	Sb	121.76	51
Argentum. See *Silver*.			
Argon	Ar	39.944	18
Arsenic	As	74.91	33
Astatine (formerly *alabamine*)	At	[210]	85
Aurum. See *Gold*.			
Barium	Ba	137.36	56
Berkelium	Bk	[249]	97
Beryllium (formerly *glucinum*)	Be	9.013	4
Bismuth	Bi	209.00	83
Boron	B	10.82	5
Bromine	Br	79.916	35
Cadmium	Cd	112.41	48
Calcium	Ca	40.08	20
Californium	Cf	[251]	98
Carbon	C	12.011	6
Cerium	Ce	140.13	58
Cesium	Cs	132.91	55
Chlorine	Cl	35.457	17
Chromium	Cr	52.01	24
Cobalt	Co	58.94	27
Columbium (now *niobium*)			
Copper (*cuprum*)	Cu	63.54	29
Cuprum. See *Copper*.			
Curium	Cm	[247]	96
Cyclonium (now *promethium*)			
Dysprosium	Dy	162.51	66
Einsteinium	Es	[254]	99
Erbium	Er	167.27	68
Europium	Eu	152.0	63
Fermium	Fm	[253]	100
Ferrum. See *Iron*.			
Florentium (now *promethium*)			
Fluorine	F	19.00	9
Francium (formerly *virginium*)	Fr	[223]	87
Gadolinium	Gd	157.26	64
Gallium	Ga	69.72	31

* Adopted by International Union of Pure and Applied Chemistry, 1957.
† A value in brackets denotes the mass number of the isotope of either the one of longest known half-life or of a better known one.

TABLE OF ELEMENTS—(Continued)

Name	Symbol	Atomic Weight *,†	Atomic Number
Germanium	Ge	72.60	32
Glucinum. See *Beryllium.*			
Gold (*aurum*)	Au	197.0	79
Hafnium	Hf	178.50	72
Helium	He	4.003	2
Holmium	Ho	164.94	67
Hydrargyrum. See *Mercury.*			
Hydrogen	H	1.0080	1
Illinium (now *promethium*)			
Indium	In	114.82	49
Iodine	I	126.91	53
Iridium	Ir	192.2	77
Iron (*ferrum*)	Fe	55.85	26
Kalium. See *Potassium.*			
Krypton	Kr	83.80	36
Lanthanum	La	138.92	57
Lead (*plumbum*)	Pb	207.21	82
Lithium	Li	6.940	3
Lutetium	Lu	174.99	71
Magnesium	Mg	24.32	12
Manganese	Mn	54.94	25
Masurium (now *technetium*)			
Mendelevium	Md	[256]	101
Mercury (*hydrargyrum*)	Hg	200.61	80
Molybdenum	Mo	95.95	42
Natrium. See *Sodium.*			
Neodymium	Nd	144.27	60
Neon	Ne	20.183	10
Neptunium	Np	[237]	93
Nickel	Ni	58.71	28
Niobium (formerly *columbium*)	Nb	92.91	41
Niton. See *Radon.*			
Nitrogen	N	14.008	7
Nobelium	No		102
Osmium	Os	190.2	76
Oxygen	O	16	8
Palladium	Pd	106.4	46
Phosphorus	P	30.975	15
Platinum	Pt	195.09	78
Plumbum. See *Lead.*			
Plutonium	Pu	[242]	94
Polonium	Po	[210]	84

TABLE OF ELEMENTS—(Continued)

Name	Symbol	Atomic Weight *,†	Atomic Number
Potassium (*kalium*)	K	39.100	19
Praseodymium	Pr	140.92	59
Promethium (formerly also *cyclonium, florentium, illinium*)	Pm	[147]	61
Protactinium	Pa	[231]	91
Radium	Ra	[226]	88
Radon	Rn	[222]	86
Rhenium	Re	186.22	75
Rhodium	Rh	102.91	45
Rubidium	Rb	85.48	37
Ruthenium	Ru	101.1	44
Samarium	Sm	150.35	62
Scandium	Sc	44.96	21
Selenium	Se	78.96	34
Silicon	Si	28.09	14
Silver (*argentum*)	Ag	107.880	47
Sodium (*natrium*)	Na	22.991	11
Stannum. See *Tin.*			
Stibium. See *Antimony.*			
Strontium	Sr	87.63	38
Sulfur	S	32.066 ‡	16
Tantalum	Ta	180.95	73
Technetium (formerly *masurium*)	Tc	[99]	43
Tellurium	Te	127.61	52
Terbium	Tb	158.93	65
Thallium	Tl	204.39	81
Thorium	Th	232.05	90
Thulium	Tm	168.94	69
Tin (*stannum*)	Sn	118.70	50
Titanium	Ti	47.90	22
Tungsten (*wolfram*)	W	183.86	74
Uranium	U	238.07	92
Vanadium	V	50.95	23
Virginium (now *francium*)			
Wolfram. See *Tungsten.*			
Xenon	Xe	131.30	54
Ytterbium	Yb	173.04	70
Yttrium	Y	88.92	39
Zinc (*zincum*)	Zn	65.38	30
Zincum. See *Zinc.*			
Zirconium	Zr	91.22	40

‡ Because of natural variations in the relative abundances of the isotopes of sulfur, the atomic weight of sulfur has a range of ±0.003.

ELY'S TABLE OF THE DURATION OF PREGNANCY

Explanation.—In the upper horizontal row of numbers, find the date of last menstruation; the number beneath, set in *italics*, will show the expiration of 280 days or ten months of 28 days each.

Last menstruation	1	2	3	4	5	6	7	8	9	10	11	12	13	14	15	16	17	18	19	20	21	22	23	24	25	26	27	28	29	30	31	Expiration
January / *October*	*8*	*9*	*10*	*11*	*12*	*13*	*14*	*15*	*16*	*17*	*18*	*19*	*20*	*21*	*22*	*23*	*24*	*25*	*26*	*27*	*28*	*29*	*30*	*31*	*1*	*2*	*3*	*4*	*5*	*6*	*7*	*November*
February / *November*	*8*	*9*	*10*	*11*	*12*	*13*	*14*	*15*	*16*	*17*	*18*	*19*	*20*	*21*	*22*	*23*	*24*	*25*	*26*	*27*	*28*	*29*	*30*	*1*	*2*	*3*	*4*	*5*				*December*
March / *December*	*6*	*7*	*8*	*9*	*10*	*11*	*12*	*13*	*14*	*15*	*16*	*17*	*18*	*19*	*20*	*21*	*22*	*23*	*24*	*25*	*26*	*27*	*28*	*29*	*30*	*31*	*1*	*2*	*3*	*4*	*5*	*January*
April / *January*	*6*	*7*	*8*	*9*	*10*	*11*	*12*	*13*	*14*	*15*	*16*	*17*	*18*	*19*	*20*	*21*	*22*	*23*	*24*	*25*	*26*	*27*	*28*	*29*	*30*	*31*	*1*	*2*	*3*	*4*		*February*
May / *February*	*5*	*6*	*7*	*8*	*9*	*10*	*11*	*12*	*13*	*14*	*15*	*16*	*17*	*18*	*19*	*20*	*21*	*22*	*23*	*24*	*25*	*26*	*27*	*28*	*1*	*2*	*3*	*4*	*5*	*6*	*7*	*March*
June / *March*	*8*	*9*	*10*	*11*	*12*	*13*	*14*	*15*	*16*	*17*	*18*	*19*	*20*	*21*	*22*	*23*	*24*	*25*	*26*	*27*	*28*	*29*	*30*	*31*	*1*	*2*	*3*	*4*	*5*	*6*		*April*
July / *April*	*7*	*8*	*9*	*10*	*11*	*12*	*13*	*14*	*15*	*16*	*17*	*18*	*19*	*20*	*21*	*22*	*23*	*24*	*25*	*26*	*27*	*28*	*29*	*30*	*1*	*2*	*3*	*4*	*5*	*6*	*7*	*May*
August / *May*	*8*	*9*	*10*	*11*	*12*	*13*	*14*	*15*	*16*	*17*	*18*	*19*	*20*	*21*	*22*	*23*	*24*	*25*	*26*	*27*	*28*	*29*	*30*	*31*	*1*	*2*	*3*	*4*	*5*	*6*	*7*	*June*
September / *June*	*8*	*9*	*10*	*11*	*12*	*13*	*14*	*15*	*16*	*17*	*18*	*19*	*20*	*21*	*22*	*23*	*24*	*25*	*26*	*27*	*28*	*29*	*30*	*1*	*2*	*3*	*4*	*5*	*6*	*7*		*July*
October / *July*	*8*	*9*	*10*	*11*	*12*	*13*	*14*	*15*	*16*	*17*	*18*	*19*	*20*	*21*	*22*	*23*	*24*	*25*	*26*	*27*	*28*	*29*	*30*	*31*	*1*	*2*	*3*	*4*	*5*	*6*	*7*	*August*
November / *August*	*8*	*9*	*10*	*11*	*12*	*13*	*14*	*15*	*16*	*17*	*18*	*19*	*20*	*21*	*22*	*23*	*24*	*25*	*26*	*27*	*28*	*29*	*30*	*31*	*1*	*2*	*3*	*4*	*5*	*6*		*September*
December / *September*	*7*	*8*	*9*	*10*	*11*	*12*	*13*	*14*	*15*	*16*	*17*	*18*	*19*	*20*	*21*	*22*	*23*	*24*	*25*	*26*	*27*	*28*	*29*	*30*	*1*	*2*	*3*	*4*	*5*	*6*	*7*	*October*

TABLE OF THE MORE COMMON LATIN OR GREEK TERMS AND ABBREVIATIONS USED IN PRESCRIPTION WRITING

TERM OR ABBREVIATION	LATIN OR GREEK	TRANSLATION
āā, aa	ana	of each
a.c.	ante cibum	before meals
ad	ad	to, up to
ad lib.	ad libitum	at pleasure
alternis horis	alternis horis	every other hour
ante	ante	before
aq.	aqua	water
aq. dest.	aqua destillata	distilled water
b.i.d.	bis in die, bis in dies	twice daily
bis	bis	twice
c̄, c	cum	with
caps.	capsula	a capsule
chart.	charta	a paper
collyr.	collyrium	an eyewash
divid.	divide	divide (thou)
d.t.d. No. iv	dentur tales doses No. iv	let 4 such doses be given
elix.	elixir	an elixir
enem.	enema	an enema
et	et	and
fldxt.	fluidextractum	fluidextract
ft.	fac; fiat; fiant	make (thou); let it be made; let them be made
ft. chart. vi	fiant chartulae vi	let 6 powders be made
ft. pulv. et div. in char. xii	fiat pulvis et divide in chartulas xii; *or*, fiat pulvis in chartulas xii dividenda	let 12 powders be made
gtt.	gutta(e)	drop(s)
H.	hora	an hour
hor. som., H.S.	hora somni	at bedtime
in d.	in dies	from day to day, daily
inf.	infusum	an infusion
Inject.	injectio	an injection
inter	inter	between
lin.	linimentum	a liniment
liq.	liquor	a solution
lot.	lotio	a lotion
M.	misce	mix (thou)
m.	minimum	a minim
min.	minimum	a minim
mist.	mistura	a mixture
no.	numero, numerus	number
noctis	noctis	of the night
non	non	not
non rep.	non repetatur	do not repeat
O.D.	oculus dexter	the right eye

TABLE OF THE MORE COMMON LATIN OR GREEK TERMS AND ABBREVIATIONS USED IN PRESCRIPTION WRITING—(Continued)

TERM OR ABBREVIATION	LATIN OR GREEK	TRANSLATION
O.L.	oculus laevus	the left eye
omn. hor.	omni hora	every hour
omni nocte	omni nocte	every night
p.c.	post cibos; post cibum	after eating; after food
pil.	pilula(e)	pill(s)
p.r.n.	pro re nata	as occasion arises, occasionally
pulv.	pulvis; pulveres; pulveratus	powder; powders; powdered
q.h.	quaque hora	each hour, every hour
q. 2 h.	quaque secunda hora	every 2 hours
q.i.d.	quater in die	4 times a day
q.s.	quantum sufficit; quantum sufficiat; quantum satis	a sufficient quantity; as much as is sufficient
S.	signa; signetur	write (thou); let it be written; label (thou)
S.A.	secundum artem	according to art
sig.	signa; signetur	write (thou); let it be written; label (thou)
sine	sine	without
sol.	solutio	a solution
sp.	spiritus	spirit
ss, s̄s̄	semis	a half
suppos.	suppositorium	a suppository
syr.	syrupus	syrup
tabel.	tabella (dim. of *tabula*, a table)	a lozenge
talis	talis	such; like this
t.d.	ter die	3 times a day
t.i.d.	ter in die	3 times a day
tinct.	tinctura	a tincture
tr.	tinctura	a tincture
ung.	unguentum	an ointment
ut dict.	ut dictum	as directed

Symbols made up of letters in the English alphabet are in their proper alphabetic places in the vocabulary section and defined there; those which form specific categories, as chemical elements and radioactive isotopes, are also listed in tables in the Appendix. (See also Table of Signs and Symbols.)

Abbreviations with medical significance appear in their proper alphabetic places in the vocabulary section. For lexical abbreviations used in definitions, see table on page ix.

TABLE OF RADIOACTIVE AND OTHER ISOTOPES COMMONLY USED IN MEDICINE AND BIOLOGY *

Name and Symbol †	Radiation: Type and Energy ‡	Radioactive Half-life	Medical Uses
Deuterium (hydrogen, heavy) $_1H^2$	None; naturally occurring		*Investigative:* tracer studies
Tritium $_1H^3$	Beta (0.02)	12.3 years	*Investigative:* tracer studies
Carbon 13 $_6C^{13}$	None; naturally occurring		*Investigative:* tracer studies
Carbon 14 $_6C^{14}$	Beta (0.154)	5,700 years	*Investigative:* tracer studies
Nitrogen 15 $_7N^{15}$	None; naturally occurring		*Investigative:* tracer studies
Oxygen 18 $_8O^{18}$	None; naturally occurring		*Investigative:* tracer studies

Element	Radiation (MeV)	Half-life	Use
Sodium 24 $_{11}Na^{24}$	Beta (1.39) Gamma (1.38, 2.76)	14.9 hours	*Diagnostic:* study of peripheral vascular disease, extracellular fluid volume, formation of cerebrospinal fluid, and sodium metabolism
Phosphorus 32 $_{15}P^{32}$	Beta (1.71)	14.3 days	*Therapeutic:* chronic myeloid leukemia, polycythemia vera, lymphomas, and widespread carcinomatosis *Diagnostic:* determination of blood volume; study of peripheral vascular disease; localization of brain tumors
Sulfur 35 $_{16}S^{35}$	Beta (0.167)	87.1 days	*Investigative:* tracer studies
Potassium 42 $_{19}K^{42}$	Beta (3.56, 2.04) Gamma (1.51)	12.5 hours	*Diagnostic:* localization of brain tumors; determination of intracellular fluid volume; study of potassium metabolism
Chromium 51 $_{24}Cr^{51}$	Gamma (0.32)	26 days	*Diagnostic:* study of blood volume with radioactively labeled erythrocytes
Iron 59 $_{26}Fe^{59}$	Beta (0.26, 0.46) Gamma (1.1, 1.3)	46 days	*Diagnostic:* study of blood volume, iron metabolism, and blood transfusion
Cobalt 60 $_{27}Co^{60}$	Beta (0.31) Gamma (1.17, 1.33)	5.2 years	*Therapeutic:* source of teleoroentgen therapy and interstitial radiation for malignancies sensitive to gamma radiation

TABLE OF RADIOACTIVE AND OTHER ISOTOPES COMMONLY USED IN MEDICINE AND BIOLOGY *—(Continued)

Name and Symbol †	Radiation: Type and Energy ‡	Radioactive Half-Life	Medical Uses
Strontium 90 $_{38}Sr^{90}$	Beta (0.65)	25 years	*Therapeutic:* benign conditions of the eye such as pterygia, traumatic corneal ulceration, corneal scars, vernal conjunctivitis, and hemangioma of the eyelid and in preparation for corneal transplant
Ruthenium 106 $_{44}Ru^{106}$	Beta (0.04)	330 days	*Therapeutic:* same as *strontium 90*
Iodine 131 $_{53}I^{131}$	Beta (0.60, 0.3) Gamma (0.364, 0.636, 0.284, 0.080)	8 days	*Therapeutic:* cancer of the thyroid, hyperthyroidism, and severe heart disease *Diagnostic:* study of thyroid and antithyroid drugs; determination of thyroid activity When incorporated in diiodofluorescein, used to localize brain tumors With iodinated serum globulin, studies of blood volume, cardiac output
Gold 198 $_{79}Au^{198}$	Beta (0.965) Gamma (0.411)	2.69 days	*Therapeutic:* widespread abdominal carcinomatosis with ascites; carcinomatosis of the pleural cavity; lymphomas; and lymphatic metastases from other malignant tumors

Lead 210 (radium D) $_{82}Pb^{210}$	Beta (0.028) Gamma (0.046, 0.0078, 0.0258) Naturally occurring	22 years	*Therapeutic:* same as *strontium 90*
Radon $_{86}Rn^{222}$	Alpha (5.486) Average gamma energy of decay products (1.8) Naturally occurring	3.825 days	*Therapeutic:* treatment of malignancies by interstitial radiation; used in cancer of uterine cervix and fundus, oral pharynx, urinary bladder, skin, and in metastatic cancer of the lymph nodes
Radium $_{88}Ra^{226}$	Alpha (4.79, 4.61) Gamma (0.19) Average gamma energy of decay products (1.8) Naturally occurring	1590–1690 years	*Therapeutic:* same as *radon*

* This table is organized on the basis of atomic number. See Table of Elements (pages 966 to 968) for the atomic number of any element in question.

† The subscript preceding the normal abbreviation is the atomic number of the isotope. The superscript following the nominal abbreviation is the atomic weight; in common practice, it is this number which characterizes the isotope, thus $_6C^{14}$ is often called carbon 14.

‡ Alpha (α) radiation refers to emission of helium nuclei consisting of two protons and two neutrons; beta (β) radiation refers to emission of electrons; gamma (γ) radiation refers to emission of gamma rays. The energy of the characteristic radiation is given in million electron volts (mev); two or more values indicate two or more components of the radiation

TABLE OF SIGNS AND SYMBOLS *

A, Å	angstrom unit	μrfd	microrutherford
C'	complement	mμ	millimicron, micromillimeter
E$_0$	electroaffinity	σ	$\frac{1}{1000}$ of a second
F$_1$	first filial generation	π	3.1416—ratio of circumfer-
F$_2$	second filial generation		ence of a circle to its diameter
L$_+$	limes death	℔.	pound (usually apothe-
L$_0$	limes zero		caries')
℞	[*L. recipe*]. Take	®	registered trade-mark status
c̄, c	[*L. cum*]. With	□, ♂	male
s̄s̄, ss	[*L. semis*]. One-half	○, ♀	female
m, M	[*L. misce*]. Mix	*	birth
°	degree	†	death
♏	minim	−	negative; levorotatory (*l*−)
℈	scruple	+	positive; dextrorotatory
ℨ	drachm (apothecaries')		(*d*−)
f℥	fluidrachm	±	either positive or negative,
℥	ounce (troy)		not definite; racemic (*dl*−)
f℥	fluidounce	⇌	denotes a reversible reaction
α	alpha	<	less than
β	beta	>	more than
γ	gamma	#	number
μ	micron	%	per cent
$\mu\mu$	micromicron	∧	value considered as a vector
μc	microcurie		in electrocardiography
μg.	microgram		

* Symbols made up of letters in the English alphabet are in their proper alphabetic places in the vocabulary section and are defined there; those which form specific categories, as chemical elements or radioactive isotopes, are also listed in separate tables in the Appendix.

All abbreviations are entered alphabetically in the vocabulary section, and the more common abbreviations of Latin or Greek terms used in prescription writing are also listed in a table in the Appendix.

TABLE OF THERMOMETRIC EQUIVALENTS

Centigrade to Fahrenheit Scales

$$\tfrac{9}{5}\,C.^\circ + 32 = F.^\circ$$

C.°	F.°	C.°	F.°	C.°	F.°	C.°	F.°	C.°	F.°
−20	−4.0	21	69.8	61	141.8	101	213.8	141	285.8
−19	−2.2	22	71.6	62	143.6	102	215.6	142	287.6
−18	−0.4	23	73.4	63	145.4	103	217.4	143	289.4
−17	1.4	24	75.2	64	147.2	104	219.2	144	291.2
−16	3.2	25	77.	65	149.	105	221.	145	293.
−15	5.	26	78.8	66	150.8	106	222.8	146	294.8
−14	6.8	27	80.6	67	152.6	107	224.6	147	296.6
−13	8.6	28	82.4	68	154.4	108	226.4	148	298.4
−12	10.4	29	84.2	69	156.2	109	228.2	149	300.2
−11	12.2	30	86.	70	158.	110	230.	150	302.
−10	14.	31	87.8	71	159.8	111	231.8	151	303.8
−9	15.8	32	89.6	72	161.6	112	233.6	152	305.6
−8	17.6	33	91.4	73	163.4	113	235.4	153	307.4
−7	19.4	34	93.2	74	165.2	114	237.2	154	309.2
−6	21.2	35	95.	75	167.	115	239.	155	311.
−5	23.	36	96.8	76	168.8	116	240.8	156	312.8
−4	24.8	37	98.6	77	170.6	117	242.6	157	314.6
−3	26.6	38	100.4	78	172.4	118	244.4	158	316.4
−2	28.4	39	102.2	79	174.2	119	246.2	159	318.2
−1	30.2	40	104.	80	176.	120	248.	160	320.
0	32.	41	105.8	81	177.8	121	249.8	161	321.8
1	33.8	42	107.6	82	179.6	122	251.6	162	323.6
2	35.6	43	109.4	83	181.4	123	253.4	163	325.4
3	37.4	44	111.2	84	183.2	124	255.2	164	327.2
4	39.2	45	113.	85	185.	125	257.	165	329.
5	41.	46	114.8	86	186.8	126	258.8	166	330.8
6	42.8	47	116.6	87	188.6	127	260.6	167	332.6
7	44.6	48	118.4	88	190.4	128	262.4	168	334.4
8	46.4	49	120.2	89	192.2	129	264.2	169	336.2
9	48.2	50	122.	90	194.	130	266.	170	338.
10	50.	51	123.8	91	195.8	131	267.8	171	339.8
11	51.8	52	125.6	92	197.6	132	269.6	172	341.6
12	53.6	53	127.4	93	199.4	133	271.4	173	343.4
13	55.4	54	129.2	94	201.2	134	273.2	174	345.2
14	57.2	55	131.	95	203.	135	275.	175	347.
15	59.	56	132.8	96	204.8	136	276.8	176	348.8
16	60.8	57	134.6	97	206.6	137	278.6	177	350.6
17	62.6	58	136.4	98	208.4	138	280.4	178	352.4
18	64.4	59	138.2	99	210.2	139	282.2	179	354.2
19	66.2	60	140.	100	212.	140	284.	180	356.
20	68.								

TABLE OF THERMOMETRIC EQUIVALENTS—(Continued)

Fahrenheit to Centigrade Scales

$$(F.° - 32) \times \tfrac{5}{9} = C.°$$

F. °	C. °	F. °	C. °	F. °	C. °	F. °	C. °	F. °	C. °
0	−17.78	51	10.56	101	38.33	151	66.11	201	93.8
1	−17.22	52	11.11	102	38.89	152	66.67	202	94.4
2	−16.67	53	11.67	103	39.44	153	67.22	203	95.
3	−16.11	54	12.22	104	40.	154	67.78	204	95.5
4	−15.56	55	12.78	105	40.56	155	68.33	205	96.1
5	−15.	56	13.33	106	41.11	156	68.89	206	96.6
6	−14.44	57	13.89	107	41.67	157	69.44	207	97.2
7	−13.89	58	14.44	108	42.22	158	70.	208	97.7
8	−13.33	59	15.	109	42.78	159	70.56	209	98.3
9	−12.78	60	15.56	110	43.33	160	71.11	210	98.8
10	−12.22	61	16.11	111	43.89	161	71.67	211	99.4
11	−11.67	62	16.67	112	44.44	162	72.22	212	100.
12	−11.11	63	17.22	113	45.	163	72.78	213	100.5
13	−10.56	64	17.78	114	45.56	164	73.33	214	101.1
14	−10.	65	18.33	115	46.11	165	73.89	215	101.6
15	−9.44	66	18.89	116	46.67	166	74.44	216	102.2
16	−8.89	67	19.44	117	47.22	167	75.	217	102.7
17	−8.33	68	20.	118	47.78	168	75.56	218	103.3
18	−7.78	69	20.56	119	48.33	169	76.11	219	103.8
19	−7.22	70	21.11	120	48.89	170	76.67	220	104.4
20	−6.67	71	21.67	121	49.44	171	77.22	221	105.
21	−6.11	72	22.22	122	50.	172	77.78	222	105.5
22	−5.56	73	22.78	123	50.56	173	78.33	223	106.1
23	−5.	74½	23.33	124	51.11	174	78.89	224	106.6
24	−4.44	75	23.89	125	51.67	175	79.44	225	107.2
25	−3.89	76	24.44	126	52.22	176	80.	226	107.7
26	−3.33	77	25.	127	52.78	177	80.56	227	108.3
27	−2.78	78	25.56	128	53.33	178	81.11	228	108.8
28	−2.22	79	26.11	129	53.89	179	81.67	229	109.4
29	−1.67	80	26.67	130	54.44	180	82.22	230	110.
30	−1.11	81	27.22	131	55.	181	82.78	231	110.5
31	−0.56	82	27.78	132	55.56	182	83.33	232	111.1
32	0.	83	28.33	133	56.11	183	83.89	233	111.6
33	0.56	84	28.89	134	56.67	184	84.44	234	112.2
34	1.11	85	29.44	135	57.22	185	85.	235	112.7
35	1.67	86	30.	136	57.78	186	85.56	236	113.3
36	2.22	87	30.56	137	58.33	187	86.11	237	113.8
37	2.78	88	31.11	138	58.89	188	86.67	238	114.4
38	3.33	89	31.67	139	59.44	189	87.22	239	115.
39	3.89	90	32.22	140	60.	190	87.78	240	115.5
40	4.44	91	32.78	141	60.56	191	88.33	241	116.1
41	5.	92	33.33	142	61.11	192	88.89	242	116.6
42	5.56	93	33.89	143	61.67	193	89.44	243	117.2
43	6.11	94	34.44	144	62.22	194	90.	244	117.7
44	6.67	95	35.	145	62.78	195	90.56	245	118.3
45	7.22	96	35.56	146	63.33	196	91.11	246	118.8
46	7.78	97	36.11	147	63.89	197	91.67	247	119.4
47	8.33	98	36.67	148	64.44	198	92.22	248	120.
48	8.89	99	37.22	149	65.	199	92.78	249	120.5
49	9.44	100	37.78	150	65.56	200	93.33	250	121.1
50	10.								

TABLES OF WEIGHTS AND MEASURES

Metric Doses with Approximate Apothecary Equivalents*

The *approximate* dose equivalents in the following table represent the quantities which would be prescribed, under identical conditions, by physicians trained, respectively, in the metric or in the apothecary system of weights and measures.

When prepared dosage forms such as tablets, capsules, pills, etc., are prescribed in the metric system, the pharmacist may dispense the corresponding *approximate* equivalent in the apothecary system, and vice versa. This does not, however, authorize the alternative use of the approximate dose equivalents given below for specific quantities on a prescription which requires compounding, nor in converting a pharmaceutical formula from one system of weights or measures to the other system; for such purposes exact equivalents must be used.

LIQUID MEASURES		LIQUID MEASURES	
Metric	Approximate Apothecary Equivalents	Metric	Approximate Apothecary Equivalents
1000 cc.	1 quart	0.75 cc.	12 minims
750 cc.	1½ pints	0.6 cc.	10 minims
500 cc.	1 pint	0.5 cc.	8 minims
250 cc.	8 fluidounces	0.3 cc.	5 minims
200 cc.	7 fluidounces	0.25 cc.	4 minims
100 cc.	3½ fluidounces		
		0.2 cc.	3 minims
50 cc.	1¾ fluidounces	0.1 cc.	1½ minims
30 cc.	1 fluidounce	0.06 cc.	1 minim
15 cc.	½ fluidounce (4 fluidrachms)	0.05 cc.	¾ minim
10 cc.	2½ fluidrachms	0.03 cc.	½ minim
8 cc.	2 fluidrachms		
5 cc.	75 minims (1¼ fluidrachms)		
4 cc.	1 fluidrachm		
3 cc.	45 minims	1 Troy or Apothecary ounce	31.1 Gm.
2 cc.	30 minims	1 Avoirdupois ounce	28.35 Gm.
1 cc.	15 minims	1 Avoirdupois pound	453.6 Gm.

TABLES OF WEIGHTS AND MEASURES—(Continued)

| WEIGHTS | | WEIGHTS | |
Metric	Approximate Apothecary Equivalents	Metric	Approximate Apothecary Equivalents
30 Gm.	1 ounce	30 mg.	½ grain
15 Gm.	4 drachms		
10 Gm.	2½ drachms	25 mg.	⅜ grain
7.5 Gm.	2 drachms	20 mg.	⅓ grain
6 Gm.	90 grains	15 mg.	¼ grain
		12 mg.	⅕ grain
5 Gm.	75 grains	10 mg.	⅙ grain
4 Gm.	60 grains (1 drachm)		
3 Gm.	45 grains	8 mg.	⅛ grain
2 Gm.	30 grains (½ drachm)	6 mg.	⅒ grain
1.5 Gm.	22 grains	5 mg.	½₂ grain
1 Gm.	15 grains	4 mg.	⅟₁₅ grain
0.4 Gm.	6 grains		
		3 mg.	½₀ grain
0.75 Gm.	12 grains	2 mg.	⅟₃₀ grain
0.6 Gm.	10 grains	1.5 mg.	⅟₄₀ grain
0.5 Gm.	7½ grains	1.2 mg.	⅟₅₀ grain
0.45 Gm.	7 grains	1 mg.	⅟₆₀ grain
0.3 Gm.	5 grains	0.8 mg.	⅟₈₀ grain
		0.6 mg.	⅟₁₀₀ grain
0.25 Gm.	4 grains	0.5 mg.	⅟₁₂₀ grain
0.2 Gm.	3 grains		
0.15 Gm.	2½ grains	0.4 mg.	⅟₁₅₀ grain
0.12 Gm.	2 grains	0.3 mg.	⅟₂₀₀ grain
0.1 Gm.	1½ grains	0.25 mg.	⅟₂₅₀ grain
		0.2 mg.	⅟₃₀₀ grain
75 mg.	1¼ grains	0.15 mg.	⅟₄₀₀ grain
60 mg.	1 grain	0.1 mg.	⅟₆₀₀ grain
50 mg.	¾ grain		
40 mg.	⅔ grain		

NOTE—A cubic centimeter (cc.) is the approximate equivalent of a milliliter (ml.).
 • Reprinted through the courtesy of "New and Nonofficial Remedies, 1951," published in Philadelphia by J. B. Lippincott Co.

TABLES OF WEIGHTS AND MEASURES—(Continued)

Comparative Values of Metric Liquid and Apothecaries' Measures

Cubic Centimeters	Fluid-ounces	Cubic Centimeters	Flui-drachms	Cubic Centimeters	Minims
30	1.01	5	1.35	0.05	0.81
50	1.69	6	1.62	0.07	1.14
75	2.54	7	1.89	0.09	1.46
100	3.38	8	2.17	1	16.23
200	6.76	9	2.43	2	32.5
300	10.15	10	2.71	3	48.7
400	13.53	25	6.76	4	64.9
473	16.00				
500	16.91				
600	20.29				
700	23.67				
800	27.05				
900	30.43				
1000	33.82				

Comparative Values of Avoirdupois and Metric Weights

Avoir. Ounces	Grams	Avoir. Pounds	Grams
1/16	1.772	1	453.59
1/8	3.544	2	907.18
1/4	7.088	2.2	1000.00
1/2	14.175	3	1360.78
1	28.350	4	1814.37
2	56.699	5	2267.96
3	85.049	6	2721.55
4	113.398	7	3175.15
5	141.748	8	3628.74
6	170.097	9	4082.33
7	198.447	10	4535.92
8	226.796		
9	255.146		
10	283.495		
11	311.845		
12	340.194		
13	368.544		
14	396.893		
15	425.243		

Comparative Values of Apothecaries' and Metric Liquid Measures

Minims	Cubic Centimeters	Flui-drachms	Cubic Centimeters	Fluid-ounces	Cubic Centimeters
1	0.06	1	3.70	1	29.57
2	0.12	2	7.39	2	59.15
3	0.19	3	11.09	3	88.72
4	0.25	4	14.79	4	118.29
5	0.31	5	18.48	5	147.87
6	0.37	6	22.18	6	177.44
7	0.43	7	25.88	7	207.01
8	0.49			8	236.58
9	0.55			9	266.16
10	0.62			10	295.73
11	0.68			11	325.30
12	0.74			12	354.88
13	0.80			13	384.45
14	0.86			14	414.02
15	0.92			15	443.59
16	0.99			16	473.17
17	1.05			17	502.74
18	1.11			18	532.31
19	1.17			19	561.89
20	1.23			20	591.46
25	1.54			21	621.03
30	1.85			22	650.60
35	2.16			23	680.18
40	2.46			24	709.75
45	2.77			25	739.32
50	3.08			26	768.90
55	3.39			27	798.47
				28	828.04
				29	857.61
				30	887.19
				31	916.76
				32	946.33
				48	1419.49
				56	1656.08
				64	1892.66
				72	2129.25
				80	2365.83
				96	2839.00
				112	3312.16
				128	3785.32

TABLES OF WEIGHTS AND MEASURES—(Continued)

Table for Converting Metric Weights into Apothecaries' Weights

Grams	Exact Equivalents in Grains	Grams	Exact Equivalents in Grains
0.01	0.1543	12.0	185.189
0.02	0.3086	13.0	200.621
0.03	0.4630	14.0	216.054
0.04	0.6173	15.0	231.486
0.05	0.7716	16.0	246.918
0.06	0.9259	17.0	262.351
0.07	1.0803	18.0	277.783
0.08	1.2346	19.0	293.216
0.09	1.3889	20.0	308.648
0.1	1.543	21.0	324.080
0.2	3.086	22.0	339.513
0.3	4.630	23.0	354.945
0.4	6.173	24.0	370.378
0.5	7.716	25.0	385.810
0.6	9.259	26.0	401.242
0.7	10.803	27.0	416.674
0.8	12.346	28.0	432.107
0.9	13.889	29.0	447.538
1.0	15.432	30.0	462.971
2.0	30.865	31.0	478.403
3.0	46.297	32.0	493.835
4.0	61.730	40.0	617.294
5.0	77.162	45.0	694.456
6.0	92.594	50.0	771.618
7.0	108.027	60.0	925.942
8.0	123.459	70.0	1080.265
9.0	138.892	80.0	1234.589
10.0	154.324	90.0	1388.912
11.0	169.756	100.0	1543.236

Table for Converting Apothecaries' Weights into Metric Weights

Grains	Grams	Grains	Grams
1/50	0.00130	50	3.240
1/32	0.00202	51	3.305
1/20	0.00324	52	3.370
1/18	0.00360	53	3.434
1/16	0.00405	54	3.499
1/15	0.00432	55	3.564
1/12	0.00540	56	3.629
1/10	0.00648	57	3.694
1/8	0.00810	58	3.758
1/6	0.01080	59	3.823
1/5	0.01296	60	3.888
1/4	0.01620	61	3.953
1/3	0.02160	62	4.018

Table for Converting Apothecaries' Weight into Metric Weights —(Continued)

Grains	Grams	Grains	Grams
1/2	0.03240	63	4.082
3/4	0.04860	64	4.147
1	0.0648	65	4.212
2	0.1296	66	4.277
3	0.1944	67	4.342
4	0.2592	68	4.406
5	0.3240	69	4.471
6	0.3888	70	4.536
7	0.4536	71	4.601
8	0.5184	72	4.666
9	0.5832	73	4.730
10	0.6480	74	4.795
11	0.7128	75	4.860
12	0.7776	76	4.925
13	0.8424	77	4.990
14	0.9072	78	5.054
15	0.9720	79	5.119
16	1.037	80	5.184
17	1.102	81	5.249
18	1.166	82	5.314
19	1.231	83	5.378
20	1.296	84	5.443
21	1.361	85	5.508
22	1.426	86	5.573
23	1.490	87	5.638
24	1.555	88	5.702
25	1.620	89	5.767
26	1.685	90	5.832
27	1.749	91	5.897
28	1.814	92	5.962
29	1.879	93	6.026
30	1.944	94	6.091
31	2.009	95	6.156
32	2.074	96	6.221
33	2.138	97	6.286
34	2.203	98	6.350
35	2.268	99	6.415
36	2.333	100	6.480
37	2.398	120	7.776
38	2.462	150	9.720
39	2.527	180	11.664
40	2.592	200	12.958
41	2.657	480	31.103
42	2.722	500	32.396
43	2.786	600	38.875
44	2.851	700	45.354
45	2.916	800	51.833
46	2.981	900	58.313
47	3.046	960	62.207
48	3.110	1000	64.799
49	3.175		

Troy Weight

1 pound = 22.816 cubic inches of distilled water at 62° F.

| Grains | Pennyweights | Ounces | Pound |
gr.	dwt.	oz.	lb.
24 =	1		
480 =	20 =	1	
5760 =	240 =	12 =	1

Apothecaries' Weight

| Grains | Scruples | Drachms | Ounces | Pound |
gr.	Ə	Ʒ	℥	lb.
20 =	1			
60 =	3 =	1		
480 =	24 =	8 =	1	
5760 =	288 =	96 =	12 =	1

Metric Weights

1 cubic centimeter of distilled water at 4° C.

	Grams		Avoir. Ounces
Milligram =	0.001 =	0.01543	
Centigram =	0.01 =	0.15432	
Decigram =	0.1 =	1.54324	
Gram =	1. =	15.43248 =	.03528
Decagram =	10. =		.3528
Hectogram =	100. =		3.52758
Kilogram =	1,000. =		35.2758

Avoirdupois Weight

1 pound = 1.2153 pounds troy

| Grains | Drachms | Ounces | Pound |
gr.	dr.	oz.	lb.
27.34375 =	1		
437.5 =	16 =	1	
7000 =	256 =	16 =	1

Apothecaries' Measure

| Minims | Fluidrachms | Fluidounces | Pints | Gallon |
♏	fƷ	f℥	O.	C.
60 =	1			
480 =	8 =	1		
7,680 =	128 =	16 =	1	
61,440 =	1024 =	128 =	8 =	1

Comparative Values of Standard and Metric Measures of Length

Inches	Centimeters	Inches	Millimeters
1	2.54	1/25	1.00
2	5.08	1/12	2.12
3	7.62	1/8	3.18
4	10.16	1/4	6.35
5	12.70	1/3	8.47
6	15.24	1/2	12.70
7	17.78	5/8	15.88
8	20.32	2/3	16.93
9	22.86	3/4	19.05
10	25.40	5/6	21.16
11	27.94	7/8	22.22
12	30.48	11 1/12	23.28